Practical Strategies
in Pediatric Diagnosis
and Therapy

Practical Strategies in Pediatric Diagnosis and Therapy Second Edition

Edited by

Robert M. Kliegman, MD
Professor and Chair
Department of Pediatrics
Medical College of Wisconsin
Pediatrician-in-Chief
Pam and Les Muma Chair in Pediatrics
Children's Hospital of Wisconsin
Milwaukee, Wisconsin

Larry A. Greenbaum, MD, PhD
Associate Professor
Department of Pediatrics
Medical College of Wisconsin
Children's Hospital of Wisconsin
Milwaukee, Wisconsin

Patricia S. Lye, MD
Associate Professor
Department of Pediatrics
Medical College of Wisconsin
Children's Hospital of Wisconsin
Milwaukee, Wisconsin

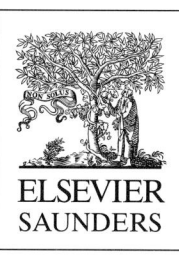

ELSEVIER
SAUNDERS

ELSEVIER
SAUNDERS

The Curtis Center
170 S Independence Mall W 300E
Philadelphia, Pennsylvania 19106

PRACTICAL STRATEGIES IN PEDIATRIC DIAGNOSIS AND THERAPY   ISBN: 0–7216–9131–5
Second Edition

NOTICE

Medicine is an ever-changing field. Standard safety precautions must be followed, but as new research and clinical experience broaden our knowledge, changes in treatment and drug therapy may become necessary or appropriate. Readers are advised to check the most current product information provided by the manufacturer of each drug to be administered to verify the recommended dose, the method and duration of administration, and contraindications. It is the responsibility of the licensed prescriber, relying on experience and knowledge of the patient, to determine dosages and the best treatment for each individual patient. Neither the publisher nor the authors assumes any liability for any injury and/or damage to persons or property arising from this publication.

First Edition copyrighted 1996.

Library of Congress Cataloging-in-Publication Data
Practical strategies in pediatric diagnosis and therapy / [edited by] Robert M. Kliegman,
    Larry A. Greenbaum, Patricia S. Lye.—2nd ed.
       p. ; cm.
    Includes bibliographical references and index.
    ISBN 0–7216–9131–5
      1. Pediatrics—Decision making. 2. Pediatrics. I. Kliegman, Robert. II. Greenbaum,
    Larry A. III. Lye, Patricia S.
      [DNLM: 1. Pediatrics. WS 200 P895 2004]
RJ47.P724 2004
618.92—dc22   2003069724

Executive Publisher: Judith Fletcher
Developmental Editors: Wendy Buckwalter Coffman/Dana Lamparello
Senior Project Manager: Robin E. Davis
Book Designer: Gene Harris

Printed in the United States of America.

Last digit is the print number: 9   8   7   6   5   4   3   2   1

This book is dedicated to those master clinician-educators who have inspired us with their clinical wisdom, enthusiasm, empathy, and insight. At no time in the history of pediatrics have these adaptable master clinician-educators been needed more to inspire young students and residents and to provide encouragement and clinical guidance to the practicing pediatrician.

In this light, we dedicate this edition to the memory of **Dr. David A. Lewis**, Associate Professor of Pediatrics, Director of Residency Training, Pediatric Cardiologist, and master clinician at the Children's Hospital of Wisconsin. His teaching will be missed by us all.

Contributors

Uri S. Alon, MD
Professor of Pediatrics, University of Missouri at Kansas City School of Medicine; Pediatric Nephrologist and Director, Bone and Mineral Disorders Clinic, Children's Mercy Hospital, Kansas City, Missouri
Acid-Base and Electrolyte Disturbances

R. Stephen S. Amato, MD, PhD
Clinical Professor of Pediatrics, Tufts University School of Medicine, Boston, Massachusetts; Chief, Pediatrics Service and Director, Medical Genetics, Eastern Maine Medical Center, Bangor, Maine
Dysmorphology

Stephen C. Aronoff, MD
Professor and Chair, Department of Pediatrics, Temple University School of Medicine; Temple University Children's Medical Center, Philadelphia, Pennsylvania
Fever of Unknown Origin

Jane P. Balint, MD
Clinical Associate Professor, Ohio State University; Pediatric Gastroenterologist, Columbus Children's Hospital, Columbus, Ohio
Jaundice

Sharon Bartosh, MD
Associate Professor of Pediatrics, University of Wisconsin School of Medicine; Chief, Division of Pediatric Nephrology, University of Wisconsin Children's Hospital, Madison, Wisconsin
Hypertension

Stuart Berger, MD
Professor of Pediatrics, Medical College of Wisconsin; Medical Director, Herma Heart Center, Children's Hospital of Wisconsin, Milwaukee, Wisconsin
Heart Failure

Brian W. Berman, MD
Professor of Pediatrics, Case Western Reserve University School of Medicine; Vice Chair for Community–Physician Affairs and Chief, Division of General Academic Pediatrics, Rainbow Babies and Children's Hospital, Cleveland, Ohio
Lymphadenopathy; Pallor and Anemia

David J. Beste, MD
Medical Director, Speech and Audiology, Children's Hospital of Wisconsin, Milwaukee, Wisconsin
Neck Masses in Childhood

R. Alexander Blackwood, MD, PhD
Associate Professor of Pediatrics and Pediatric Infectious Diseases, University of Michigan Medical School, Ann Arbor, Michigan
Recurrent Infection

Andrew Bleasel, MBBS, PhD
Staff Specialist, Neurology and Neurophysiology, Westmead Hospital and Children's Hospital at Westmead, Sydney, Australia
Paroxysmal Disorders

Laurence A. Boxer, MD
Henry and Mala Dorfman Family Professor in Pediatric Hematology/Oncology, University of Michigan Medical School; Director, Pediatric Hematology/Oncology, C. S. Mott Children's Hospital, Ann Arbor, Michigan
Recurrent Infection

Ben H. Brouhard, MD
Professor of Pediatrics and Associate Dean, Case Western Reserve University School of Medicine; Executive Vice President of Medical Affairs and Chief of Staff, MetroHealth System, Cleveland, Ohio
Hematuria

Gale R. Burstein, MD, MPH
Medical Officer, Division of HIV/AIDS Prevention, Centers for Disease Control and Prevention, Atlanta, Georgia
Sexually Transmitted Diseases

Vimal Chadha, MD
Assistant Professor of Pediatrics, Virginia Commonwealth University School of Medicine; Chair, Section of Pediatric Nephrology, Virginia Commonwealth University Medical Center, Richmond, Virginia
Acid-Base and Electrolyte Disturbances

John C. Chandler, MD
Pediatric Surgeon, Children's Hospital of the Greenville Hospital System, Greenville, South Carolina
Abdominal Masses

Bruce H. Cohen, MD
Staff, Section of Pediatric Neurology, Department of Neurology, Cleveland Clinic Foundation, Cleveland, Ohio
Headaches in Childhood

Robert J. Cunningham III, MD
Chair, Medical Subspecialty Pediatrics and Head, Section of Pediatric Nephrology, Cleveland Clinic Foundation, Cleveland, Ohio
Proteinuria

Leona Cuttler, MD
Professor of Pediatrics, Case Western Reserve University School of Medicine; Chief, Division of Endocrinology, Diabetes, and Metabolism, Rainbow Babies and Children's Hospital, Cleveland, Ohio
Short Stature

Jack S. Elder, MD
Professor of Pediatrics and Carter Kissell Professor of Urology, Case Western Reserve University School of Medicine; Director, Pediatric Urology, Rainbow Babies and Children's Hospital, Cleveland, Ohio
Acute and Chronic Scrotal Swelling; Ambiguous Genitalia

Susan Feigelman, MD
Associate Professor of Pediatrics, University of Maryland School of Medicine, Baltimore, Maryland
Failure to Thrive and Malnutrition

Thomas Ferkol, MD
Associate Professor of Pediatrics, Washington University School of Medicine; Director, Cystic Fibrosis Center, St. Louis Children's Hospital, St. Louis, Missouri
Respiratory Distress

Michele A. Frommelt, MD
Associate Professor of Pediatrics, Medical College of Wisconsin; Children's Hospital of Wisconsin, Milwaukee, Wisconsin
Cyanosis

Peter C. Frommelt, MD
Associate Professor of Pediatrics, Medical College of Wisconsin; Director of Pediatric Echocardiography, Children's Hospital of Wisconsin, Milwaukee, Wisconsin
Cyanosis

Michael W. L. Gauderer, MD
Professor of Surgery, University of South Carolina School of Medicine; Adjunct Professor of Bioengineering, Clemson University; Chief, Pediatric Surgery, Children's Hospital of the Greenville Hospital System, Greenville, South Carolina
Abdominal Masses

Mitchell E. Geffner, MD
Professor, University of Southern California Keck School of Medicine; Physician and Director of Fellowship Training, Division of Endocrinology, Diabetes, and Metabolism, Childrens Hospital Los Angeles, Los Angeles, California
Disorders of Puberty

Manju E. George, MD
Resident in Dermatology, University of Kansas Medical Center, Kansas City, Kansas
Rashes and Skin Lesions

William M. Gershan, MD
Associate Professor of Pediatrics, Medical College of Wisconsin; Pediatric Pulmonologist, Children's Hospital of Wisconsin, Milwaukee, Wisconsin
Cough

Larry A. Greenbaum, MD, PhD
Associate Professor, Department of Pediatrics, Medical College of Wisconsin; Children's Hospital of Wisconsin, Milwaukee, Wisconsin
Delirium and Coma

Marjorie Greenfield, MD
Associate Professor of Reproductive Biology, Case Western Reserve University School of Medicine; Associate Professor of Obstetrics and Gynecology and Pediatrics, University Hospitals of Cleveland, Cleveland, Ohio
Menstrual Problems and Vaginal Bleeding

Ajay Gupta, MD
Staff, Section of Pediatric Neurology and Epilepsy, Department of Neurology, Cleveland Clinic Foundation, Cleveland, Ohio
Headaches in Childhood

Peter L. Havens, MD
Professor of Pediatrics and Epidemiology, Medical College of Wisconsin; Consultant in Infectious Diseases, Children's Hospital of Wisconsin, Milwaukee, Wisconsin
Meningismus and Meningitis

Jeffrey S. Hyams, MD
Professor of Pediatrics, University of Connecticut School of Medicine, Farmington, Connecticut; Head, Division of Digestive Diseases, Connecticut Children's Medical Center, Hartford, Connecticut
Gastrointestinal Bleeding

David M. Jaffe, MD
Dana Brown Professor of Pediatrics, Washington University School of Medicine; Director, Division of Emergency Services, St. Louis Children's Hospital, St. Louis, Missouri
Fever without Focus

Candice E. Johnson, MD, PhD
Professor of Pediatrics, University of Colorado School of Medicine; Attending Physician, Children's Hospital, Denver, Colorado
Dysuria

Hugh F. Johnston, MD
Professor, Departments of Psychiatry and Educational Psychology, University of Wisconsin Medical School; University of Wisconsin Hospital and Clinics, Madison, Wisconsin
Unusual Behaviors

Virginia Keane, MD
Associate Professor of Pediatrics, University of Maryland School of Medicine, Baltimore, Maryland
Failure to Thrive and Malnutrition

Carolyn M. Kercsmar, MD
Professor of Pediatrics, Case Western Reserve University School of Medicine; Director, Children's Asthma Center, Rainbow Babies and Children's Hospital, Cleveland, Ohio
Respiratory Distress

Robert M. Kliegman, MD
Professor and Chair, Department of Pediatrics, Medical College of Wisconsin; Pediatrician-in-Chief and Pam and Les Muma Chair in Pediatrics, Children's Hospital of Wisconsin, Milwaukee, Wisconsin
Airway Obstruction in Children; Acute and Chronic Abdominal Pain

Subra Kugathasan, MD
Associate Professor of Pediatrics, Medical College of Wisconsin; Children's Hospital of Wisconsin, Milwaukee, Wisconsin
Diarrhea

Robert M. Lembo, MD
Associate Professor of Clinical Pediatrics and Director, Medical Education, Department of Pediatrics, New York University School of Medicine; Attending Physician, Bellevue Hospital Center, New York, New York
Fever and Rash

David A. Lewis, MD
Associate Professor of Pediatrics, Division of Pediatric Cardiology; Director, Graduate Medical Education Program, Medical College of Wisconsin, Milwaukee, Wisconsin *(Deceased)*
Syncope and Dizziness

Gregory S. Liptak, MD, MPH
Professor of Pediatrics, University of Rochester Medical Center; Attending Physician, Strong Memorial Hospital, Rochester, New York
Mental Retardation and Developmental Disability

Patricia S. Lye, MD
Associate Professor, Department of Pediatrics, Medical College of Wisconsin; Children's Hospital of Wisconsin, Milwaukee, Wisconsin
Earache

Saleem I. Malik, MD
Associate Director, Comprehensive Epilepsy Center, Cook Children's Hospital, Fort Worth, Texas
Hypotonia and Weakness

Kelly W. Maloney, MD
Assistant Professor of Pediatrics, Medical College of Wisconsin, Milwaukee, Wisconsin
Splenomegaly

Andrea C. S. McCoy, MD
Associate Professor of Pediatrics, Temple University School of Medicine and Temple University Children's Medical Center, Philadelphia, Pennsylvania
Fever of Unknown Origin

Daniel W. McKenney, MD
Associate Professor of Pediatrics, Nephrology and Hypertension Division, University of Louisville, Louisville, Kentucky
Renal Failure

James J. Nocton, MD
Associate Professor of Pediatrics, Medical College of Wisconsin; Director, Pediatric Residency Training Program, Children's Hospital of Wisconsin, Milwaukee, Wisconsin
Arthritis

Amy Jo Nopper, MD
Associate Professor of Pediatric Dermatology, University of Missouri–Kansas City School of Medicine; Chief, Section of Pediatric Dermatology, Children's Mercy Hospital, Kansas City, Missouri
Rashes and Skin Lesions

Susan R. Orenstein, MD
Professor of Pediatrics, Division of Pediatric Gastroenterology, University of Pittsburgh School of Medicine; Children's Hospital of Pittsburgh, Pittsburgh, Pennsylvania
Vomiting and Regurgitation

Michael J. Painter, MD
Professor of Neurology and Pediatrics, Division of Child Neurology, University of Pittsburgh School of Medicine; Children's Hospital of Pittsburgh, Pittsburgh, Pennsylvania
Hypotonia and Weakness

Cynthia G. Pan, MD
Associate Professor of Pediatrics, Medical College of Wisconsin; Medical Director, Dialysis Unit and Nephrology, Children's Hospital of Wisconsin, Milwaukee, Wisconsin
Polyuria and Urinary Incontinence

Andrew N. Pelech, MD
Associate Professor of Pediatrics, Division of Cardiology, Medical College of Wisconsin; Children's Hospital of Wisconsin, Milwaukee, Wisconsin
Heart Sounds and Murmurs

John M. Peters, DO
Assistant Professor of Pediatrics, Division of Pediatric Gastroenterology, University of Pittsburgh School of Medicine; Children's Hospital of Pittsburgh, Pittsburgh, Pennsylvania
Vomiting and Regurgitation

Emory M. Petrack, MD
Associate Clinical Professor, Department of Pediatrics, Case Western Reserve University School of Medicine; President, Petrack Consulting, Inc., Cleveland, Ohio
The Irritable Infant

Philip A. Pizzo, MD
Professor of Pediatrics and of Microbiology and Immunology; Dean, Stanford University School of Medicine, Stanford, California
Fever and Neutropenia

Robert M. Reece, MD
Clinical Professor of Pediatrics, Tufts University School of Medicine; Visiting Professor of Pediatrics, Dartmouth Medical School; Director of Child Protection Program, The Floating Hospital for Children at New England Medical Center, Boston, Massachusetts
Child Abuse

Michael J. Rivkin, MD
Associate Professor of Neurology, Harvard Medical School; Attending Physician, Department of Neurology; Director, Developmental Neuroimaging Laboratory, Children's Hospital, Boston, Massachusetts
Stroke in Childhood

Mark S. Ruttum, MD
Professor of Ophthalmology, Medical College of Wisconsin; Chief of Pediatric Ophthalmology, Children's Hospital of Wisconsin, Milwaukee, Wisconsin
Eye Disorders

John R. Schreiber, MD, MPH
Professor of Pediatrics and Pathology, Case Western Reserve University School of Medicine; Chief, Division of Infectious Diseases, Allergy, Immunology, and Rheumatology, Rainbow Babies and Children's Hospital, Cleveland, Ohio
Lymphadenopathy

J. Paul Scott, MD
Professor, Medical College of Wisconsin; Attending Physician, Children's Hospital of Wisconsin, Milwaukee, Wisconsin
Bleeding and Thrombosis

Stanford T. Shulman, MD
Professor of Pediatrics, Northwestern University Feinberg School of Medicine; Chief, Division of Infectious Diseases, Children's Memorial Hospital, Chicago, Illinois
Sore Throat

Garry S. Sigman, MD
Professor, Northwestern University Feinberg School of Medicine; Director, Adolescent Medicine, Evanston Northwestern Healthcare, Evanston, Illinois
Chest Pain

Mark L. Splaingard, MD
Professor of Pediatrics, Medical College of Wisconsin; Director of Pediatric Pulmonary Care, Children's Hospital of Wisconsin, Milwaukee, Wisconsin
Apnea and Sudden Infant Death Syndrome

Charles A. Stanley, MD
Professor of Pediatrics, University of Pennsylvania School of Medicine; Chief, Division of Endocrinology, Children's Hospital of Philadelphia, Philadelphia, Pennsylvania
Hypoglycemia

Rita Steffen, MD
Staff, Department of Pediatric Gastroenterology, Cleveland Clinic Foundation, Cleveland, Ohio
Constipation

Frederick J. Suchy, MD
Professor and Chair, Department of Pediatrics, Mount Sinai School of Medicine; Pediatrician-in-Chief, Mount Sinai Hospital, New York, New York
Hepatomegaly

William J. Swift, MD
Professor Emeritus of Child and Adolescent Psychiatry, University of Wisconsin Medical School and Wisconsin Psychiatric Institute and Clinic, Madison, Wisconsin; Regional Medical Officer and Psychiatrist, U.S. Department of State, Pretoria, South Africa
Unusual Behaviors

Francisco A. Sylvester, MD
Associate Professor of Pediatrics, University of Connecticut School of Medicine; Pediatric Gastroenterologist, Connecticut Children's Medical Center, Hartford, Connecticut
Gastrointestinal Bleeding

Robert R. Tanz, MD
Professor and Director of Medical Education, Department of Pediatrics, Northwestern University Feinberg School of Medicine; Attending Physician, Division of General Academic Pediatrics, Children's Memorial Hospital, Chicago, Illinois
Sore Throat

John G. Thometz, MD
Professor of Orthopaedic Surgery, Medical College of Wisconsin; Chief, Pediatric Orthopaedic Surgery and Medical Director, Orthopaedic Surgery, Children's Hospital of Wisconsin, Milwaukee, Wisconsin
Back Pain in Children and Adolescents

George H. Thompson, MD
Professor of Orthopaedic Surgery and Pediatrics, Case Western Reserve University School of Medicine; Director, Pediatric Orthopaedics, Rainbow Babies and Children's Hospital, Cleveland, Ohio
Gait Disturbances

George F. Van Hare, MD
Associate Professor of Pediatrics, Stanford University School of Medicine; Director, Pediatric Arrhythmia Center, Lucile Packard Children's Hospital at Stanford University Medical Center; Director, Pediatric Arrhythmia Center, University of California, San Francisco, Children's Hospital, San Francisco, California
Palpitations and Arrhythmias

Kristine G. Williams, MD, MPH
Instructor of Pediatrics, Division of Pediatric Emergency Medicine, Washington University School of Medicine, St. Louis, Missouri
Fever without Focus

Martha S. Wright, MD
Associate Professor of Pediatrics, Case Western Reserve University School of Medicine; Associate Director, Pediatric Emergency Medicine, Rainbow Babies and Children's Hospital/University Hospitals of Cleveland, Cleveland, Ohio
Bites

Elaine Wyllie, MD
Head, Section of Pediatric Neurology and Pediatric Epilepsy, Cleveland Clinic Foundation, Cleveland, Ohio
Paroxysmal Disorders

Robert Wyllie, MD
Chair, Department of Pediatric Gastroenterology, Cleveland Clinic Foundation, Cleveland, Ohio
Constipation

Preface

Most children's hospitals and pediatric residency training programs have multiple educational conferences, such as professor rounds, patient management conference, clinicopathologic conference, and senior resident intake rounds. In these high-quality learning activities, experienced master clinician-educators lead a discussion of a particular patient-based issue, permitting the trainees to see how a master clinician thinks through diagnostic or therapeutic challenges. The advice given is derived from the knowledge accumulated over many years of clinical experience and careful analysis of the medical literature. The synthesis of the facts of the case with the clinician's practical experience and knowledge of the literature often results in the diagnosis and the appropriate treatment strategy. These master clinician-educators provide wisdom that gives clarity to confusing clinical cases and helps to reconcile discrepancies between practice and theory.

In addition, master clinician-educators focus on the importance of a detailed history and a complete physical examination. The chief complaint directs the questioning during the history, whereas the physical examination focuses on clues obtained by the history. Laboratory and other studies are then employed to support the diagnosis, not to make the diagnosis.

The goal of this book is to put into a written text the oral teaching rounds–based approaches toward clinical problem solving of the many expert clinician-educators who present at teaching conferences. The combination of clinical experience and evidenced-based strategies will provide guidance in developing a differential diagnosis, then a specific diagnosis, and finally the appropriate therapy of common pediatric problems. This book is arranged in chapters that cover specific chief complaints, mirroring clinical practice. Patients do not usually present with a chief complaint of cystic fibrosis; rather, they may present with a cough, respiratory distress, or chronic diarrhea.

This text is intended to help the reader begin with a specific chief complaint that may encompass many disease entities. In a user-friendly, well-tabulated, and illustrated approach, the text will help the reader differentiate between the many disease states causing a common chief complaint. The inclusion of many original tables and figures should help the reader identify distinguishing features of diseases and work through a diagnostic and/or therapeutic approach to the problem using decision trees. Modified, adapted, and borrowed artwork and tables from other outstanding sources have been added as well. The combination of all of these illustrations and tables will help provide a quick visual guide to the differential diagnosis or treatment of the various diseases under discussion.

We greatly appreciate the hard work of our contributing authors. Writing a chapter in this type of format is quite different from writing in the format of a disease-based book. In addition, we greatly appreciate the efforts of Judy Fletcher of Elsevier, whose patience and expertise contributed to the publication of this book. We are all also greatly appreciative of Carolyn Redman of the Department of Pediatrics at the Medical College of Wisconsin, whose editorial assistance and organization has made this edition a reality. The authors also wish to make a special acknowledgment to Dr. Brendan M. Reilly, for his courtesy and assistance. Finally, we acknowledge the support and, at times, sacrifice of our families: Sharon, Jonathan, Rachel, Alison, and Matthew Kliegman; Jordan, Harry, and Irene Greenbaum; and Dale, Erin, John, and Therese Lye, whose understanding helped make the time and effort put into this book meaningful.

ROBERT M. KLIEGMAN

LARRY A. GREENBAUM

PATRICIA S. LYE

Contents

RESPIRATORY DISORDERS

1 Sore Throat

Robert R. Tanz   Stanford T. Shulman

Sore throat is a common chief complaint. Each year approximately 20 million patients in the United States visit physicians because of throat complaints. The majority of these illnesses are nonbacterial and neither necessitate nor are alleviated by antibiotic therapy (Tables 1-1 to 1-3). Acute streptococcal pharyngitis, however, warrants accurate diagnosis and therapy to prevent serious suppurative and nonsuppurative complications. Furthermore, life-threatening infectious complications of streptococcal and nonstreptococcal oropharyngeal infections may manifest with mouth pain, pharyngitis, parapharyngeal space infectious extension, and airway obstruction (Tables 1-4 and 1-5).

VIRAL PHARYNGITIS

Most episodes of pharyngitis are caused by viruses (see Tables 1-2 and 1-3). It is difficult to clinically distinguish between viral and bacterial pharyngitis with a very high degree of precision, but certain clues may help the physician. Accompanying symptoms of conjunctivitis, rhinitis, croup, or laryngitis are common with viral infection but rare in bacterial pharyngitis.

Many viral agents can produce pharyngitis (see Tables 1-2 and 1-3). Some cause distinct clinical syndromes that are readily diagnosed without laboratory testing (see Tables 1-1, 1-4, and 1-6). In pharyngitis caused by parainfluenza and influenza viruses, rhinoviruses, coronaviruses, and respiratory syncytial virus (RSV), the symptoms of coryza and cough often overshadow sore throat, which is generally mild. Influenza virus may cause high fever, cough, headache, malaise, myalgias, and cervical adenopathy in addition to pharyngitis. In young children, croup or bronchiolitis may develop. RSV is associated with bronchiolitis, pneumonia, and croup in young children. RSV infection in older children is usually indistinguishable from a simple upper respiratory tract infection. Pharyngitis is not a prominent finding of RSV infection in either age group. Parainfluenza viruses are associated with croup and bronchiolitis; minor sore throat and signs of pharyngitis are common at the outset but rapidly resolve. Infections caused by parainfluenza, influenza, and RSV are often seen in seasonal (winter) epidemics.

Adenoviruses can cause upper and lower respiratory tract disease, ranging from ordinary colds to severe pneumonia. The incubation period of adenovirus infection is 2 to 4 days. Upper respiratory tract infection typically produces fever, erythema of the pharynx, and follicular hyperplasia of the tonsils, together with exudate. Enlargement of the cervical lymph nodes occurs frequently. When conjunctivitis occurs in association with adenoviral pharyngitis, the resulting syndrome is called *pharyngoconjunctival fever*. Pharyngitis may last as long as 7 days and does not respond to antibiotics. There are many adenovirus serotypes; adenovirus infections may therefore develop in children more than once. Laboratory studies may reveal a leukocytosis and an elevated erythrocyte sedimentation rate. Outbreaks have been associated with swimming pools and contamination in health care workers.

The *enteroviruses* (coxsackievirus and echovirus) can cause sore throat, especially in the summer. High fever is common, and the throat is slightly red; tonsillar exudate and cervical adenopathy are unusual. Symptoms resolve within a few days. Enteroviruses can

Table 1-1. Etiology of Sore Throat

Infection
Bacterial (see Tables 1-2, 1-3)
Viral (see Tables 1-2, 1-3)
Fungal (see Table 1-3)
Neutropenic mucositis (invasive anaerobic mouth flora)
Tonsillitis
Epiglottitis
Uvulitis
Peritonsillar abscess (quinsy sore throat)
Retropharyngeal abscess (prevertebral space)
Ludwig angina (submandibular space)
Lateral pharyngeal space cellulitis-abscess
Buccal space cellulitis
Suppurative thyroiditis
Lemierre disease (septic jugular thrombophlebitis)
Vincent angina (mixed anaerobic
   bacteria–gingivitis–pharyngitis)

Irritation
Cigarette smoking
Inhaled irritants
Reflux esophagitis
Chemical toxins (caustic agents)
Paraquat ingestion
Smog
Dry hot air
Hot foods, liquids

Other
Tumor, including Kaposi sarcoma, leukemia
Wegener granulomatosis
Sarcoidosis
Glossopharyngeal neuralgia
Foreign body
Stylohyoid syndrome
Behçet disease
Kawasaki syndrome
Posterior pharyngeal trauma—pseudodiverticulum
Pneumomediastinum
Hematoma
Systemic lupus erythematosus
Bullous pemphigoid
Syndrome of periodic fever, aphthous stomatitis,
   pharyngitis, cervical adenitis (PFAPA)

Table 1-2. Infectious Etiology of Pharyngitis
Definite Causes
Streptococcus pyogenes (Group A streptococci)
Corynebacterium diphtheriae
Arcanobacterium haemolyticum
Neisseria gonorrhoeae
Epstein-Barr virus
Parainfluenza viruses (types 1–4)
Influenza viruses
Rhinoviruses
Coronavirus
Adenovirus (types 3, 4, 7, 14, 21, others)
Respiratory syncytial virus
Herpes simplex virus (types 1, 2)
Probable Causes
Group C streptococci
Group G streptococci
Chlamydia pneumoniae
Chlamydia trachomatis
Mycoplasma pneumoniae

cause meningitis, rash, and two specific syndromes that involve the oropharynx:

Herpangina is characterized by distinctive discrete, painful, gray-white papulovesicular lesions distributed over the posterior oropharynx (Table 1-6). The vesicles are 1 to 2 mm in diameter and are initially surrounded by a halo of erythema before they ulcerate. Fever may reach 39.5°C. The illness generally

Table 1-3. Additional Potential Pathogens Associated with Sore Throat
Bacteria
Fusobacterium necrophorum (Lemierre disease)
Neisseria meningitidis
Yersinia enterocolitica
Tularemia (orpharyngeal)
Yersinia pestis
Bacillus anthracis
Chlamydia psittaci
Secondary syphilis
Mycobacterium tuberculosis
Lyme disease
Corynebacterium ulcerans
Leptospira species
Mycoplasma hominis
Virus
Coxsackievirus A, B
Cytomegalovirus
Viral hemorrhagic fevers
Human immunodeficiency virus (HIV) (primary infection)
Human herpesvirus 6
Measles
Varicella
Rubella
Fungus
Candida species
Histoplasmosis
Cryptococcosis

lasts less than 7 days, but severe pain may impair fluid intake and necessitate medical support.

Coxsackievirus A16 causes *hand-foot-mouth disease*. Vesicles can occur throughout the oropharynx; they are painful, and they ulcerate. Vesicles also develop on the palms, soles, and, less often, on the trunk or extremities. Fever is present in most cases, but many children do not appear seriously ill. This disease lasts less than 7 days.

Primary infection caused by herpes simplex virus (HSV) usually produces high fever with acute *gingivostomatitis,* involving vesicles (which become ulcers) throughout the anterior portion of the mouth, including the lips. There is sparing of the posterior pharynx in herpes gingivostomatitis; the infection usually occurs in young children. High fever is common, pain is intense, and intake of oral fluids is often impaired, which may lead to dehydration. In addition, HSV may manifest in adolescents with pharyngitis. Approximately 35% of new-onset HSV-positive adolescent patients have herpetic lesions; most patients with HSV pharyngitis cannot be distinguished from patients with other causes of pharyngitis. The classic syndrome of herpetic gingivostomatitis in infants and toddlers lasts up to 2 weeks; data on the course of more benign HSV pharyngitis are lacking. The differential diagnosis of vesicular-ulcerating oral lesions is noted in Table 1-6. A common cause of a local and large lesion of unknown etiology is aphthous stomatitis (Fig. 1-1). Some children have a combination of periodic fever (recurrent at predictable fixed times), aphthous stomatitis, pharyngitis, and cervical adenitis (PFAPA); this syndrome is idiopathic and may respond to oral prednisone or cimetidine. PFAPA usually begins before the age of 5 years and is characterized by high fever lasting 4 to 6 days, occurring every 2 to 8 weeks, and resolving spontaneously.

Infants and toddlers with measles often have prominent oral findings early in the course of the disease. In addition to high fever, cough, coryza, and conjunctivitis, the pharynx may be intensely and diffusely erythematous, without tonsillar enlargement or exudate. The presence of *Koplik spots,* the pathognomonic white or blue-white enanthem of measles, on the buccal mucosa near the mandibular molars provides evidence of the correct diagnosis before the rash develops.

INFECTIOUS MONONUCLEOSIS

PATHOGENESIS

Acute exudative pharyngitis commonly occurs with infectious mononucleosis caused by primary infection with Epstein-Barr virus (EBV) (Table 1-7). Mononucleosis is a febrile, systemic, self-limited lymphoproliferative disorder that is usually associated with hepatosplenomegaly and generalized lymphadenopathy. The pharyngitis may be mild or severe, with significant tonsillar hypertrophy (possibly producing airway obstruction), erythema, and impressive tonsillar exudates. Regional lymph nodes may be particularly enlarged and slightly tender.

Infectious mononucleosis usually occurs in adolescents and young adults; EBV infection is generally milder or subclinical in preadolescent children. In United States high school and college students, attack rates are 200 to 800 per 100,000 population per year. EBV is transmitted primarily by saliva.

CLINICAL FEATURES

After a 2- to 4-week incubation period, patients with infectious mononucleosis usually experience an abrupt onset of malaise, fatigue, fever, and headache, followed closely by pharyngitis. The tonsils are enlarged with exudates and cervical adenopathy. More generalized adenopathy with hepatosplenomegaly often follows. Fever and pharyngitis typically last 1 to 3 weeks, while lymphadenopathy and

Table 1-4. Distinguishing Features of Parapharyngeal–Upper Respiratory Tract Infections

	Peritonsillar Abscess	Retropharyngeal Abscess (Cellulitis)	Submandibular Space (Ludwig Angina)*	Lateral Pharyngeal Space*	Masticator Space*	Epiglottitis	Laryngotracheobronchitis (Croup)	Bacterial Tracheitis	Postanginal Sepsis* (Lemierre Disease)
Etiology	Group A streptococci, oral anaerobes[†]	*Staphylococcus aureus,* oral anaerobes,[†] group A streptococci, "suppurative adenitis"	Oral anaerobes[†]	Oral anaerobes[†]	Oral anaerobes[†]	*Haemophilus influenzae* type b	Parainfluenza virus; influenza adeno-virus and respiratory syncytial virus less common	*Moraxella catarrhalis, S. aureus, H. influenzae* type b or nontypable	*Fusobacterium necrophorum*
Age	Teens	Infancy, preteens, occasionally teens	Teens	Teens	Teens	2–5 yr	3 mo–3 yr	3–10 yr	Teens
Manifestations	Initial episode of pharyngitis, followed by sudden worsening of unilateral odynophagia, trismus, hot potato (muffled) voice, drooling, displacement of uvula	Fever, dyspnea, stridor, dysphagia, drooling, stiff neck, pain, cervical adenopathy, swelling of posterior pharyngeal space; Descending mediastinitis (rare); Lateral neck radiograph reveals swollen retropharyngeal prevertebral space: infants, >1 × width of adjacent vertebral body (>2–7 mm); teens, > ⅓ × width of vertebral body (>1–7 mm); CT distinguishes cellulitis from abscess	Fever, dysphagia, odynophagia, stiff neck, dyspnea; airway obstruction, swollen tongue and floor of mouth (tender); Muffled voice	Severe pain, fever, trismus, dysphagia, edematous appearing; painful lateral facial (jaw) or neck swelling (induration); May lead to Lemierre disease	Pain, prominent trismus, fever; Swelling not always evident	Sudden-onset high fever, "toxic" appearance, muffled voice, anxiety, pain, retractions, dysphagia, drooling, stridor, sitting up, leaning forward tripod position, cherry-red swollen epiglottis; Usually not hoarse or coughing; Lateral neck radiograph shows "thumb sign" of swollen epiglottis	Low-grade fever, barking cough, hoarseness–aphonia, stridor; mild retractions; radiograph shows "steeple sign" of subglottic narrowing on anteroposterior neck view	Prior history of croup with sudden onset of respiratory distress, high fever, "toxic" appearance, hoarseness, stridor, barking cough, tripod sitting position; radiograph as per croup plus ragged tracheal air column	Prior pharyngitis with sudden-onset fever, chills, odynophagia, neck pain, septic thrombo-phlebitis of internal jugular vein with septic emboli (e.g., lungs, joints), bacteremia
Treatment	Penicillin for abscess and cellulitis; Aspiration for abscess (needle or I and D); Needle is preferred	Airway management, nafcillin, ceftriaxone, ampicillin-sulbactam; Surgical drainage if an abscess	Airway management; Penicillin, clindamycin, ampicillin-sulbactam; Rarely surgical drainage	Penicillin, clindamycin, ampicillin-sulbactam; Surgical drainage usually required	Penicillin, clindamycin, ampicillin-sulbactam	Airway management (intubation), ceftriaxone	Airway management (rare); Cool mist, racemic epinephrine, dexamethasone	Airway management (frequent intubation); Ceftriaxone with or without nafcillin	Clindamycin, penicillin, or cefoxitin

[†]*Peptostreptococcus, Fusobacterium, Bacteroides* (usually *melaninogenicus*).

*Often odontogenic; check for tooth abscess, caries, tender teeth.

CT, computed tomography.

Table 1-5. "Red Flags" Associated with Sore Throat
Fever > 2 weeks
Duration of sore throat > 2 weeks
Trismus
Drooling
Cyanosis
Hemorrhage
Asymmetric tonsillar swelling or asymmetric cervical adenopathy
Respiratory distress (airway obstruction or pneumonia)
Suspicion of parapharyngeal space infection
Suspicion of diphtheria (bull neck, uvula paralysis, thick membrane)
Apnea
Severe, unremitting pain
"Hot potato" voice
Chest or neck pain
Weight loss

hepatosplenomegaly subside over 3 to 6 weeks. Malaise and lethargy can persist for several months, possibly leading to impaired school or work performance.

DIAGNOSIS

Laboratory studies of diagnostic value include atypical lymphocytosis; these lymphocytes are primarily EBV-specific, cytotoxic T lymphocytes that represent a reactive response to EBV-infected B lymphocytes. A modest elevation of serum transaminase levels, reflecting EBV hepatitis, is common. Tests useful for diagnosis include detection of heterophile antibodies that react with bovine erythrocytes (most often detected by the monospot test) and specific antibody against EBV viral capsid antigen (VCA), early antigen (EA), and nuclear antigen (EBNA). Acute infectious mononucleosis is usually associated with a positive heterophile test result and antibody to VCA and EA (Fig. 1-2).

The findings of acute exudative pharyngitis together with hepatomegaly, splenomegaly, and generalized lymphadenopathy suggest infectious mononucleosis. Early in the disease and in cases without liver or spleen enlargement, differentiation from other causes of pharyngitis, including streptococcal pharyngitis, is difficult. Indeed, a small number of patients with infectious mononucleosis have a throat culture positive for group A streptococci. Serologic evidence of mononucleosis should be sought when splenomegaly or other features are present or if symptoms persist beyond 7 days.

TREATMENT

Patients with infectious mononucleosis require supportive treatment. Corticosteroids may be indicated for acute life-threatening conditions, such as airway obstruction caused by enlarged tonsils.

GROUP A STREPTOCOCCAL INFECTION

In the evaluation of a patient with sore throat, the primary concern is usually accurate diagnosis and treatment of pharyngitis caused by group A streptococci, which accounts for about 15% of all episodes of pharyngitis. The sequelae of group A streptococcal pharyngitis, especially acute rheumatic fever and acute glomerulonephritis, at one time resulted in considerable morbidity and mortality in the United States and continue to do so in other parts of the world. Prevention of acute rheumatic fever in particular depends on timely diagnosis of streptococcal pharyngitis and prompt antibiotic treatment.

Group A streptococci are characterized by the presence of group A carbohydrate in the cell wall, and they are further distinguished by several kinds of cell wall protein antigens (M, R, T). These protein antigens are useful for studies of epidemiology and pathogenesis.

EPIDEMIOLOGY

Group A streptococcal pharyngitis has been endemic in the United States; epidemics occur sporadically. Episodes peak in the late winter and early spring; rates of group A streptococcal pharyngitis are highest among children aged 5 to 11 years old.

Spread of group A streptococci in classrooms and among family members, especially in crowded living conditions, is common. Transmission occurs primarily by inhalation of organisms in large droplets or by direct contact with respiratory secretions. Pets do not appear to be a frequent reservoir. Untreated streptococcal pharyngitis is particularly contagious early in the acute illness and for the first 2 weeks after the organism has been acquired. Antibiotic therapy effectively prevents disease transmission. Within 24 hours of institution of therapy with penicillin, it is difficult to isolate group A streptococci from patients with acute streptococcal pharyngitis, and infected children can return to school.

Molecular epidemiology studies of streptococcal pharyngitis have shown that numerous distinct strains of group A streptococci circulate simultaneously in the community during the peak season. "DNA-fingerprinting" techniques further demonstrate that children with streptococcal pharyngitis serve as a community reservoir for strains that cause invasive disease (e.g., sepsis, streptococcal toxic shock syndrome, cellulitis, necrotizing fasciitis) in the same geographic area and season.

CLINICAL FEATURES

The classic patient with acute streptococcal pharyngitis has a sudden onset of fever and sore throat. Headache, malaise, abdominal pain, nausea, and vomiting occur frequently. Cough, rhinorrhea, conjunctivitis, stridor, diarrhea, and hoarseness are distinctly unusual and suggest a viral etiology.

Examination of the patient reveals marked pharyngeal erythema. Petechiae may be noted on the palate, but they can also occur in viral pharyngitis (see Table 1-7). Tonsils are enlarged, symmetric, and red, with patchy exudates on their surfaces. The papillae of the tongue may be red and swollen; hence the designation "strawberry tongue." Anterior cervical lymph nodes are often tender and enlarged.

Combinations of these signs can be used to assist in diagnosis; in particular, tonsillar exudates in association with fever, palatal petechiae, and tender anterior cervical adenitis strongly suggest infection with group A streptococci. However, other diseases can produce this constellation of findings. Some or all of these classic characteristics may be absent in patients with streptococcal pharyngitis. Younger children often have coryza with crusting below the nares, more generalized adenopathy, and a more chronic course, a syndrome called *streptococcosis*.

When rash accompanies the illness, accurate clinical diagnosis is easier. *Scarlet fever,* so-called because of the characteristic fine, diffuse red rash, is essentially pathognomonic for infection with group A streptococci. Scarlet fever is rarely seen in children younger than 3 years old or in adults.

SCARLET FEVER

The rash of scarlet fever is caused by infection with a strain of group A streptococci that contains a bacteriophage encoding for production of an erythrogenic (redness-producing) toxin, usually erythrogenic (or pyrogenic) exotoxin A. Scarlet fever is simply group A streptococcal pharyngitis with a rash and should be explained as such to patients and their families. Although patients with the *streptococcal*

Table 1-6. Vesicular-Ulcerating Eruptions of the Mouth and Pharynx

	Gingivostomatitis	Herpangina	Hand-Foot-Mouth Disease	Chickenpox	Systemic Lupus Erythematosus (SLE)	Inflammatory Bowel Disease (IBD)	Aphthous Stomatitis	Behçet Disease	Vincent Stomatitis	Recurrent Scarifying Ulcerative Stomatitis (Sutton Disease)
Etiology	Herpes simplex virus (HSV) I	Coxsackievirus A, B; echovirus or HSV (rarely)	Coxsackievirus A, coxsackievirus B (rarely)	Varicella-zoster virus	Unknown; autoimmune	Unknown; autoimmune	Unknown	Unknown; vasculitis	Unknown; or anaerobic bacteria	Unknown
Location	Ulcerative vesicles of pharynx, tongue, and palate plus lesions of mucocutaneous (perioral) margin	Anterior fauces (tonsils), soft palate (uvula), less often pharynx	Tongue, buccal mucosa, palate, palms, soles, anterior oral cavity	Tongue, gingiva, buccal mucosa, marked cutaneous lesions; trunk > face	Oral, nasal mucosa; palate, pharynx, buccal mucosa	Lips, tongue, buccal mucosa, oropharynx	As in IBD	Oral (similar to IBD); genital ulcers	Gingiva; ulceration at base of teeth	Tongue; buccal mucosa
Age	Less than 5 yr	3–10 yr	1 yr–teens	Any age	Any age	Any age	Teens and adulthood	Teens, adulthood, occasionally <10 yr	Teens; if younger, consider immunodeficiency and blood dyscrasia	Teens
Manifestations	Fever, mouth pain, toxic, fetid breath, drooling, anorexia, cervical lymphadenopathy; cracked, swollen hemorrhagic gums; secondary inoculation possible (fingers, eye, skin); reactivation with long latency (any age)	Fever, sore throat, odynophagia; summer outbreaks; 6–12 lesions (2 to 4 mm papule → vesicle → ulceration; headache, myalgias	Painful bilateral vesicles, fever	Fever, pruritic cutaneous vesicles, painful oral lesions	Renal, central nervous system, arthritis, cutaneous, hematologic, other organ involvement; ulcers minimally to moderately painful; may be painless	Multiple recurrences; painful ulcerations 1–2 mm, but may be 5–15 mm	Similar to IBD	Painful ulcerations (heal without scarring); uveitis, arthralgia, arthritis, lower gastrointestinal ulceration (similar to IBD); recurrences; spontaneous remissions	Fever, bleeding gums; gray membrane	Deep, large, painful ulcerations; relapsing; scarring with distortion of mucosa
Treatment	Avoid dehydration; acyclovir if immunocompromised	Avoid dehydration; rarely, secondary aseptic meningitis or myocarditis	Avoid dehydration;	Avoid dehydration, secondary infection; acyclovir if immunocompromised	Specific therapy for SLE	Specific therapy for IBD	Topical corticosteroids; must exclude SLE, IBD, human immunodeficiency virus (HIV), Behçet disease	Topical corticosteroids; oral (viscous) lidocaine	Oral hygiene; tetracycline wash	Topical corticosteroids, analgesics; must rule out malignancy by biopsy

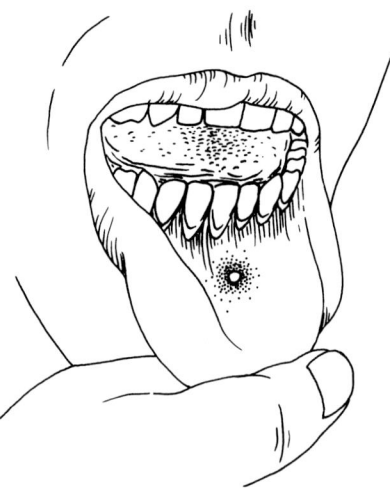

Figure 1-1. Aphthous stomatitis ("canker sore"). (From Reilly BM: Sore throat. In Practical Strategies in Outpatient Medicine, 2nd ed. Philadelphia, WB Saunders, 1991.)

toxic shock syndrome are infected with group A streptococci that produce erythrogenic toxin A, most infections with group A streptococci are not associated with unusual severity (Table 1-8). Streptococcal toxic shock syndrome is usually associated with a primary cutaneous rather than a pharyngeal focus of infection.

The rash of scarlet fever has a texture like sandpaper and blanches with pressure. It usually begins on the face, but after 24 hours it becomes generalized. The face, especially the cheeks, is red, and the area around the mouth often appears pale in comparison (circumoral pallor). Accentuation of erythema occurs in flexor skin creases, especially in the antecubital fossae (Pastia's lines). The erythema begins to fade within a few days. Desquamation begins within a week of

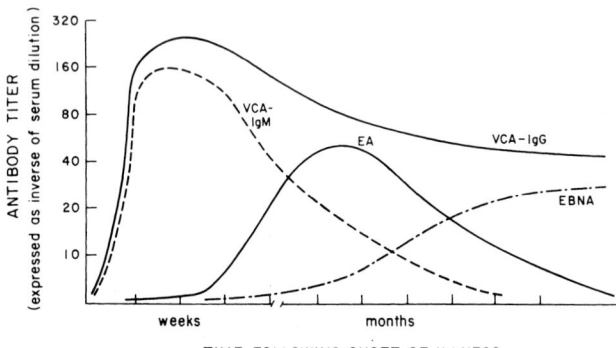

Figure 1-2. Typical human serologic response to Epstein-Barr virus infection. At time of clinical presentation (usually 2 to 7 weeks after exposure), anti–viral capsid antigen (VCA) response may consist of IgM and IgG antibodies; anti–early antigen (EA) response is often present; and anti–nuclear antigen (EBNA) is usually negative. The IgM anti-VCA response usually subsides within 2 to 4 months, and the anti-EA response usually disappears within 2 to 6 months. (Data from Andiman WA, McCarthy P, Markowitz RI, et al: Clinical, virologic, and serologic evidence of Epstein-Barr virus infection in association with childhood pneumonia. J Pediatr 1981;99:880-886; Fleisher G, Henle W, Henle G, et al: Primary infection with Ebstein-Barr virus in infants in the United States: Clinical and serological observations. J Infect Dis 1979;139:553-558; Brown NA: The Epstein-Barr virus (infectious mononucleosis, B-lymphoproliferative disorders). In Feigin RD, Cherry JD [eds]: Textbook of Pediatric Infectious Diseases, 2nd ed. Philadelphia, WB Saunders, 1987.)

Table 1-7. Manifestations of Infectious Mononucleosis (Epstein-Barr Virus)

Common

Fever (1–2 weeks)
Lymphadenopathy (bilateral, minimally tender, primarily cervical nodes with axillary, inguinal, epitrochlear, supraclavicular nodes)
Tonsillopharyngitis (exudative)
Splenomegaly
Hepatomegaly
Elevated liver enzymes (transaminases)
Malaise
Fatigue

Less Common

Rash (spontaneous or associated with ampicillin or allopurinol)
Oropharyngeal petechiae
Jaundice
Eyelid edema
Abdominal pain
Thrombocytopenia—purpura
Hemolytic or aplastic anemia—pallor
Severe upper airway obstruction
Meningoencephalitis
Guillain-Barré syndrome
Bell palsy (seventh cranial nerve)
Hemophagocytic syndrome
X-linked lymphoproliferative disorder (Duncan syndrome)
Lymphoproliferative disorder in immunocompromised hosts
Splenic rupture
Glomerulonephritis
Orchitis

---

onset on the face and progresses downward, often resembling that seen after a mild sunburn. On occasion, sheetlike desquamation occurs around the free margins of the fingernails and is usually more coarse than the desquamation seen with Kawasaki disease. The differential diagnosis of scarlet fever includes Kawasaki disease, measles, and staphylococcal toxic shock syndrome (Table 1-9).

DIAGNOSIS

Although signs and symptoms may strongly suggest acute streptococcal pharyngitis, laboratory diagnosis is highly recommended, even for patients with scarlet fever (Fig. 1-3). Scoring systems for diagnosing acute group A streptococcal pharyngitis on clinical grounds have not proved very useful. Using clinical criteria alone, physicians overestimate the likelihood that patients have streptococcal infection. The throat culture has traditionally been used to diagnose streptococcal pharyngitis. Plating a swab of the posterior pharynx and tonsils on sheep blood agar, identifying β–hemolytic colonies, and testing them for the presence of sensitivity to a bacitracin-impregnated disk is the "gold standard" diagnostic test, but it takes 24 to 48 hours to obtain results. There are a number of rapid diagnostic tests that take less than 15 minutes. These "rapid strep" tests detect the presence of the cell wall group A carbohydrate antigen after acid extraction of organisms obtained by throat swab. Rapid strep tests are highly *specific* (generally >95%), with the throat culture used as the standard. Unfortunately, the *sensitivity* of most of these rapid tests can be considerably lower. In comparison to hospital or reference laboratory throat culture results, the sensitivities of these tests are generally 80% to 85% and can be lower. However, when both throat cultures and rapid tests performed in physicians' offices are compared with cultures performed in reference laboratories,

Table 1-8. Characteristics of Severe Invasive and/or Toxigenic Group A Streptococcal Infection

Positive Culture Sites
Blood
Soft tissue abscess
Synovial fluid
Throat
Peritoneal fluid
Surgical wound
Cellulitis aspirate

Clinical Manifestations	**Laboratory Manifestations**
Fever	Leukocytosis
Toxic Shock*	Lymphopenia
Confusion	Thrombocytopenia
Headache	Hyponatremia
Abdominal pain	Hypoalbuminemia
Vomiting	Hyperbilirubinemia (direct)
Local extremity pain and	Elevated AST, ALT, BUN
swelling	Renal sediment abnormalities
Hypesthesia	Coagulopathy
Cellulitis	Hypoxia
Scarlatiniform rash (40%)	
Erythroderma (25%)	
Conjunctival injection	
Red pharynx	
Pneumonia with or	
without empyema	
Osteomyelitis	
Vaginitis	
Proctitis	
Desquamation	
Necrotizing fasciitis	
Diarrhea	

*Case definition of streptococcal toxic shock syndrome requires (I) isolation of group A streptococci from (a) a normally sterile site (blood, synovial or peritoneal fluid) or (b) a nonsterile site (throat, wound). (II) Severity is defined by (a) hypotension and (b) two or more of renal impairment, coagulopathy, liver involvement, adult respiratory distress syndrome, a generalized erythematous macular rash (with or without later desquamation), and soft tissue necrosis (necrotizing fasciitis, myositis, gangrene). The definitive diagnosis requires criteria IA and IIA plus B. Criteria IB and IIA plus B are considered probable if no other identifiable cause is present.

ALT, alanine aminotransferase; AST, aspartate aminotransferase; BUN, blood urea nitrogen.

the sensitivities, specificities, and overall accuracy of the office culture and the office rapid test are quite similar; the latter often performs better than the culture.

The low sensitivity of these tests, coupled with their excellent specificity, has led to the recommendation that two swabs be obtained from patients with suspected streptococcal pharyngitis. One swab is used for a rapid test. When the rapid antigen detection test result is positive, it is highly likely that the patient has group A streptococcal infection, and the extra swab can be discarded. When the rapid test result is negative, group A streptococci may nonetheless be present; thus, the extra swab should be processed for culture. Physician offices that have demonstrated that their rapid test and throat culture results are comparable may be able to rely on the rapid test result even when it is negative, without performing a backup culture.

In general, patients with a negative result of the rapid test do not require treatment before culture verification unless there is a particularly high suspicion group A streptococcal infection (e.g., scarlet fever, peritonsillar abscess, or tonsillar exudates in addition to tender cervical adenopathy, palatal petechiae, fever, and recent exposure to a person with group A streptococcal pharyngitis).

Testing patients for serologic evidence of an antibody response to extracellular products of group A streptococci is not useful for diagnosing acute pharyngitis. Because it generally takes several weeks for antibody levels to rise, streptococcal antibody tests are valid only for determining past infection. Specific antibodies include antistreptolysin O (ASO), anti-DNase B, and antihyaluronidase (AHT). When antibody testing is desired in order to evaluate a possible post-streptococcal illness, more than one of these tests should be performed to improve sensitivity.

TREATMENT

Treatment begun within 9 days of the onset of group A streptococcal pharyngitis is effective in preventing acute rheumatic fever. Therapy does not appear to affect the risk of the other nonsuppurative sequela, acute post-streptococcal glomerulonephritis. Antibiotic therapy also reduces the incidence of suppurative sequelae of group A streptococcal pharyngitis, such as peritonsillar abscess and cervical adenitis. In addition, treatment produces a more rapid resolution of signs and symptoms and terminates contagiousness within 24 hours. For these reasons, antibiotics should be instituted as soon as the diagnosis is supported by laboratory studies.

There are numerous antibiotics available for treating streptococcal pharyngitis (Table 1-10). The drug of choice is penicillin. Despite the widespread use of penicillin to treat streptococcal and other infections, penicillin resistance among group A streptococci has not developed. Penicillin can be given by mouth for 10 days or intramuscularly as a single injection of benzathine penicillin. Intramuscular benzathine penicillin alleviates concern with patient compliance. A less painful alternative is benzathine penicillin in combination with procaine penicillin. Intramuscular procaine penicillin alone is inadequate for prevention of acute rheumatic fever because adequate levels of penicillin are not present in blood and tissues for a sufficient time. Other β-lactams, including semisynthetic derivatives of penicillin and the cephalosporins, are at least as effective as penicillin for treating group A streptococcal pharyngitis. Their broader spectrum, their higher cost, and the lack of formal data concerning prevention of acute rheumatic fever relegate them to second-line status. The decreased frequency of dose administration of some of these agents may improve patient compliance and makes their use attractive in selected circumstances.

Patients who are allergic to penicillin should receive erythromycin or another non–β-lactam antibiotic, such as clarithromycin, azithromycin, or clindamycin. Resistance of group A streptococci to erythromycin has increased dramatically in areas such as Japan, France, Spain, Taiwan, and Finland, where erythromycin has been widely used. This has not yet emerged as a major problem in the United States, where the rate of macrolide resistance is about 5%. Sulfa drugs (including sulfamethoxazole combined with trimethoprim), tetracyclines, and chloramphenicol should not be used for treatment of acute streptococcal pharyngitis because they do not eradicate group A streptococci.

COMPLICATIONS

Suppurative Complications

Antibiotic therapy has greatly reduced the likelihood of developing suppurative complications caused by spread of group A streptococci from the pharynx or middle ear to adjacent structures. *Peritonsillar abscess* ("quinsy") manifests with fever, severe throat pain, dysphagia, "hot potato voice," pain referred to the ear, and bulging of the peritonsillar area with asymmetry of the tonsils and sometimes displacement of the uvula (Fig. 1-4; see Table 1-4). On occasion, there is peritonsillar cellulitis without a well-defined abscess cavity. Trismus may be present. When an abscess is found clinically or by an imaging study such as a computed tomographic scan, surgical drainage is indicated. Peritonsillar abscess occurs most commonly in older children and adolescents.

Table 1-9. Differential Diagnosis of Scarlet Fever

	Scarlet Fever	Kawasaki Disease	Measles	Staphylococcal Toxic Shock Syndrome	Staphylococcal Scalded Skin Syndrome
Agent	Group A streptococci	Unknown	Measles virus	*Staphylococcus aureus*	*S. aureus*
Age range	All (peak, 5–15 yr)	Usually <5 yr	<2 yr, 10–20 yr	All (especially > 10 yr)	Usually <5yr
Prodrome	No	No	Fever, coryza cough, conjunctivitis	Usually no	No
Enanthem	No	Occasionally	Koplik spots	No	Limited
Mouth	Strawberry tongue, exudative pharyngitis, palatal petechiae	Erythema; red, cracked lips, strawberry tongue	Diffusely red, no cracked lips	Usually normal	Erythema
Rash	Fine, red, "sandpaper," membranous desquamation, circumoral pallor, Pastia lines	Variable polymorphic erythematous face, trunk, and diaper area; tips of fingers and toes desquamate 10–28 days after onset	Maculopapular; progressing from forehead to feet; may desquamate	Diffuse erythroderma; desquamates	Erythema, painful bullous lesions; positive Nikolsky sign; desquamates
Other	Cervical adenitis, gallbladder hydrops, fever	Coronary artery disease; fever >5 days; conjunctival (nonpurulent) injection; tender, swollen hands and feet; cervical adenopathy (size >1.5 cm); thrombocytosis; pyuria (sterile); gallbladder hydrops	"Toxic" appearance; dehydration; encephalitis, pneumonia; fever	Shock (hypo-tension, including orthostatic); encephalopathy; diarrhea; headache	Fever, cracked lips; conjunctivitis

Retropharyngeal abscess represents extension of infection from the pharynx or peritonsillar region into the retropharyngeal (prevertebral) space, which is rich in lymphoid structures (Figs. 1-5 and 1-6; see Table 1-4). Children younger than 4 years old are most often affected. Fever, dysphagia, drooling, stridor, extension of the neck, and a mass in the posterior pharyngeal wall may be noted. Surgical drainage is often required if frank suppuration has occurred. Spread of group A streptococci via pharyngeal lymphatic vessels to regional nodes can cause *cervical lymphadenitis.* The markedly swollen and tender anterior cervical nodes that result can suppurate.

Otitis media, mastoiditis, and sinusitis also may occur as complications of group A streptococcal pharyngitis. Additional parapharyngeal suppurative infections that may mimic streptococcal disease are noted in Table 1-4. Furthermore, any pharyngeal infectious process may produce torticollis if there is inflammation that extends to the paraspinal muscles and ligaments, producing pain, spasm, and, on occasion, rotary subluxation of the cervical spine.

The differential diagnosis of torticollis is presented in Table 1-11. Oropharyngeal torticollis lasts less than 2 weeks and is not associated with abnormal neurologic signs or pain over the spinous process.

Nonsuppurative Sequelae

Nonsuppurative complications include acute rheumatic fever (see Chapters 11 and 44), acute post-streptococcal glomerulonephritis (see Chapter 25), and possibly reactive arthritis/synovitis. In addition, an association between streptococcal infection and neuro-psychiatric disorders such as obsessive-compulsive disorder and Tourette syndrome has been postulated. This possible association has been called PANDAS (pediatric autoimmune neuropsychiatric disorders associated with streptococci). Therapy with an appropriate antibiotic within 9 days of onset of symptoms is highly effective in preventing rheumatic fever, but acute glomerulonephritis is not prevented by treatment of the antecedent streptococcal infection. Pharyngitis caused by one of the nephritogenic strains of group A streptococci precedes the glomerulonephritis by about 10 days. Unlike acute rheumatic fever, which occurs only after group A streptococcal pharyngitis, acute glomerulonephritis also can follow group A streptococcal skin infection.

TREATMENT FAILURE AND CHRONIC CARRIAGE

Treatment with penicillin cures group A streptococcal pharyngitis but is unable to eradicate group A streptococci from the pharynx in approximately 25% of patients (Fig. 1-7). This causes considerable consternation among such patients and their families. Penicillin resistance is not the cause of treatment failure. A small proportion of these patients are symptomatic and are thus characterized as having *clinical treatment failure.* Reinfection with the same strain or a different strain is possible, as is intercurrent viral pharyngitis. Some of these patients may be chronic pharyngeal carriers of group A streptococci who are suffering from a new superimposed viral infection; others may be noncompliant with regard to therapy.

Many patients who do not respond to antimicrobial treatment are asymptomatic and are identified when follow-up culture specimens are obtained, a practice that is usually unnecessary. Patients who are compliant with regard to therapy are at minimal risk for acute rheumatic fever. One explanation for asymptomatic persistence of group A streptococci after treatment is that these patients were chronic carriers of group A streptococci who were initially symptomatic because of a concurrent viral pharyngitis and who did not truly have acute streptococcal pharyngitis.

Patients who are chronically colonized with group A streptococci are called *chronic carriers.* Carriers do not appear to be at risk for acute

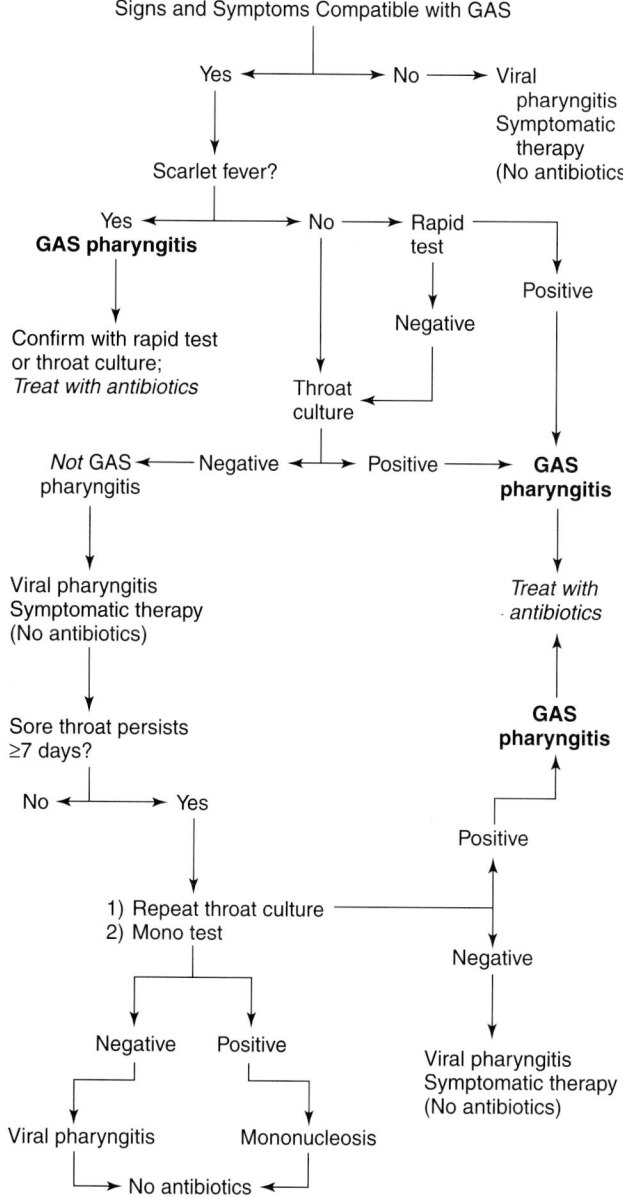

Figure 1-3. Management of patients with sore throat. GAS, group A streptococci.

rheumatic fever or for development of suppurative complications, and they are rarely sources of spread of group A streptococci in the community. There is no reason to exclude these carriers from school.

There is no easy way to identify chronic carriers prospectively among patients with symptoms of acute pharyngitis. The clinician should consider the possibility of chronic group A streptococcal carriage when a patient or a family member has multiple culture-positive episodes of pharyngitis, especially when symptoms are mild or atypical. A culture specimen is usually positive for group A streptococci when the suspected carrier is symptom-free or is receiving treatment with penicillin (intramuscular benzathine penicillin is recommended in order to eliminate concern about compliance).

Carriers often receive multiple unsuccessful courses of antibiotic therapy in attempts to eliminate group A streptococci. Physician and patient anxiety is common and can develop into "streptophobia." Unproven and ineffective therapies include tonsillectomy, prolonged administration of antibiotics, use of β-lactamase–resistant antibiotics, and culture or treatment of pets.

Available treatment options for the physician faced with a chronic streptococcal carrier include the following:

1. Obtaining a rapid test, throat culture, or both each time the patient has pharyngitis with features that suggest streptococcal pharyngitis, and treating with penicillin each time a test is positive.
2. Treating with one of the regimens effective for terminating chronic carriage.

The first option is simple, as safe as penicillin, and appropriate for many patients. The second option should be reserved for particularly anxious patients; those with a history of acute rheumatic fever or living with someone who had it; or those living or working in nursing homes, chronic care facilities, hospitals, and perhaps schools.

The two antibiotic treatment regimens that have been effective for eradication of the carrier state are:

- Intramuscular benzathine penicillin plus oral rifampin (10 mg/kg/dose up to 300 mg, given twice daily for 4 days beginning on the day of the penicillin injection)
- Oral clindamycin, given for 10 days (20 mg/kg/day up to 450 mg, divided into three equal doses)

Clindamycin may be preferred because it is easier to use than intramuscular penicillin plus oral rifampin and may be somewhat more effective. In controlled, comparative trials, no other antibiotic regimens have been demonstrated to reliably terminate the chronic streptococcal carrier state. Successful eradication of the carrier state makes evaluation of subsequent episodes of pharyngitis much easier, although chronic carriage can recur upon reexposure to group A streptococci.

RECURRENT ACUTE PHARYNGITIS

Some patients seem remarkably susceptible to group A streptococci. The reasons for frequent bona fide acute group A streptococcal pharyngitis are obscure, but appropriate antibiotic treatment results in resolution of symptoms and eradication of group A streptococci.

The role of tonsillectomy in the management of patients with multiple episodes of streptococcal pharyngitis is controversial. Fewer episodes of sore throat have been reported among patients treated with tonsillectomy (in contrast to patients treated without surgery) during the first 2 years after operation. The patients enrolled in that study had experienced numerous episodes of pharyngitis, but it appears that not all episodes were caused by group A streptococci. Of particular concern is the reported tonsillectomy complication rate of 14% and the improvement over time noted among the nontonsillectomy patients.

In addition, the presence of tonsils is not necessary for group A streptococci to infect the throat. Tonsillectomy cannot be recommended except in unusual circumstances. It seems preferable to treat most patients with penicillin whenever symptomatic group A streptococcal pharyngitis occurs. Obtaining follow-up throat specimens for culture helps distinguish recurrent pharyngitis from chronic carriage.

NON–GROUP A STREPTOCOCCAL INFECTION

Certain β–hemolytic streptococci of serogroups other than group A cause acute pharyngitis. Well-documented epidemics of food-borne group C and group G streptococcal pharyngitis have been reported in young adults. In these situations, a high percentage of individuals who have ingested the contaminated food promptly developed acute pharyngitis, and throat cultures yielded virtually pure growth of the epidemiologically linked organism. There have been outbreaks of group G streptococcal pharyngitis among children. However, the role of these non–group A streptococcal organisms as etiologic agents of acute pharyngitis in endemic circumstances has been difficult to establish. Group C and group G β streptococci may be responsible for acute pharyngitis, particularly in adolescents.

Table 1-10. Treatment Regimens for Acute Streptococcal Pharyngitis

	Children	Adolescents/Adults	Frequency	Route	Duration
Standard					
Penicillin V	250 mg	500 mg	bid-tid	Oral	10 days
Benzathine penicillin G	600,000 U (weight < 27 kg)	1.2 million U (weight ≥ 27 kg)	Once	IM	Once
Amoxicillin	125 mg (weight < 15 kg)	250 mg (weight ≥ 15 kg)	tid	Oral	10 days

Penicillin-Allergic Patients	Oral Dose	Frequency	Duration
Erythromycin			
Ethylsuccinate	40 mg/kg/day up to 1000 mg/day	bid	10 days
Estolate	20-40 mg/kg/day up to 1000 mg/day	bid	10 days
Clarithromycin	15 mg/kg/day up to 500 mg/day	bid	10 days
Azithromycin*	12 mg/kg/day	Once daily	5 days
Clindamycin	10-25 mg/kg/day up to 450 mg/day	tid	10 days
Cephalosporins†	Varies with agent chosen		10 days

Once Daily and Short Duration Treatment Schedules	Oral Dose	Frequency	Duration
Azithromycin*	12 mg/kg	Once daily	5 days
Amoxicillin‡	50 mg/kg up to 750 mg	Once daily	10 days
Cefadroxil	30 mg/kg up to 1000 mg	Once daily	10 days
Cefixime	8 mg/kg up to 400 mg	Once daily	10 days
Cefdinir	14 mg/kg up to 600 mg	Once daily	10 days
Ceftibuten	9 mg/kg up to 400 mg	Once daily	10 days
Cefpodoxime	10 mg/kg/day up to 200 mg/day	bid	5 days
Cefdinir	14 mg/kg/day up to 600 mg/day	bid	5 days
Cefuroxime‡	20 mg/kg/day up to 500 mg/day	bid	4 or 5 days

*Maximum dose for children is 500 mg/day. Adult dosage: 500 mg the first day, 250 mg the subsequent 4 days.

†First-generation cephalosporins (e.g., cephalexin, cefadroxil) are preferred; dosage and frequency vary among agents. Avoid use in patients with history of immediate (anaphylactic) hypersensitivity to penicillin or other beta-lactam antibiotics.

‡Not approved by the U.S. Food and Drug Administration for use in this manner.

From Tanz RR, Shulman ST: Pharyngitis. In Long SS, Pickering LK, Prober CG (eds): Principles and Practice of Pediatric Infectious Diseases. New York, Churchill Livingstone, 1997, p 204.

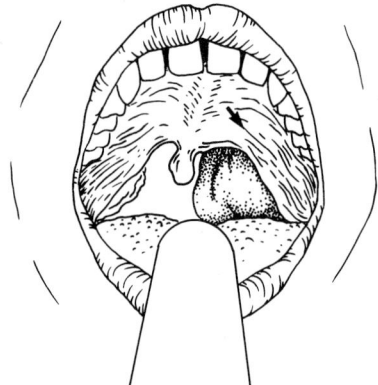

Figure 1-4. Peritonsillar abscess (quinsy, sore throat). The left tonsil is asymmetrically inflamed and swollen; there is displacement of the uvula to the opposite side. The supratonsillar space (*arrow*) is also swollen; this is the usual site of the surgical incision for drainage. Prominent unilateral cervical adenopathy typically coexists. (From Reilly BM: Sore throat. In Practical Strategies in Outpatient Medicine, 2nd ed. Philadelphia: WB Saunders, 1991.)

However, the exact role of these agents, most of which are carried asymptomatically in the pharynx of some children and young adults, remains to be fully characterized.

When they are implicated as agents of acute pharyngitis, groups C and G organisms do not appear to necessitate treatment, inasmuch as they cause self-limited infections. Acute rheumatic fever is not a sequela to these infections, although post-streptococcal acute glomerulonephritis has been documented in rare cases after epidemic group C and group G streptococcal pharyngitis.

ARCANOBACTERIUM INFECTION

Arcanobacterium (formerly *Corynebacterium*) *haemolyticum* is a gram-positive rod that has been reported to cause a scarlet fever–like illness with acute pharyngitis and scarlatinal rash, particularly in teenagers and young adults. Detecting this agent requires special methods for culture, and it has not routinely been sought in patients with scarlet fever or pharyngitis.

The clinical features of *A. haemolyticum* pharyngitis are indistinguishable from group A streptococcal pharyngitis; pharyngeal erythema is present in almost all patients, patchy white to gray exudates in about 70%, cervical adenitis in about 50%, and moderate fever in 40%. Palatal petechiae and strawberry tongue may also occur. The scarlatiniform rash usually spares the face, palms, or soles. It is erythematous and blanches; it may be pruritic and demonstrate minimal desquamation.

Erythromycin appears to be the treatment of choice.

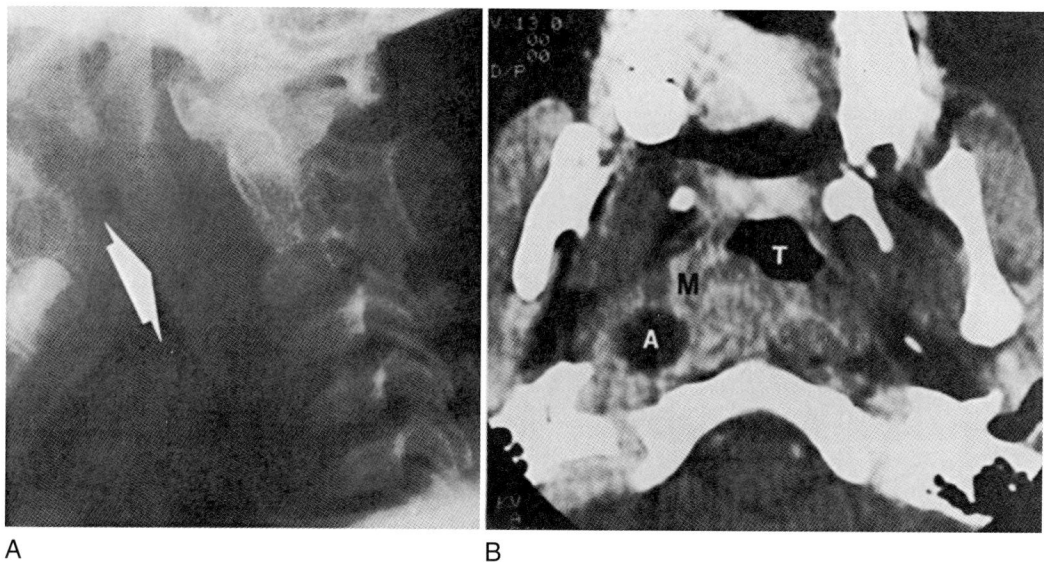

Figure 1-5. Retropharyngeal abscess. **A,** Lateral neck radiograph shows marked increased soft tissue (*arrow*) between the upper airway and cervical spine. **B,** Axial computed tomographic scan shows the lower attenuation center of the abscess (A), the anterior and leftward shift of the trachea (T), and the soft tissue mass (M) of abscess and surrounding edema. (Courtesy of A. Oestreich, M.D., Cincinnati, Ohio.)

DIPHTHERIA

Diphtheria is a very serious disease that is caused by pharyngeal infection by toxigenic strains of *Corynebacterium diphtheriae*. It has become very rare in the United States and other developed countries as a result of immunization. The handful of diphtheria cases recognized annually in the United States usually occur in unimmunized individuals, and the fatality rate is about 5%. A relatively large outbreak of diphtheria in the former Soviet Union has been recorded (1990 to 1995), and infection has been documented in several travelers from Western Europe.

PATHOGENESIS

The pathogenesis of diphtheria involves nasopharyngeal mucosal colonization by *C. diphtheriae* and toxin elaboration after an incubation period of 1 to 5 days. Toxin leads to local tissue inflammation and necrosis (producing an adherent grayish membrane made up of fibrin, blood, inflammatory cells, and epithelial cells) and it is absorbed into the blood stream. Fragment B of the polypeptide toxin binds particularly well to cardiac, neural, and renal cells, and the smaller fragment A enters cells and interferes with protein synthesis. Toxin fixation by tissues may lead to fatal myocarditis (with arrhythmias) within 10 to 14 days and to peripheral neuritis within 3 to 7 weeks.

CLINICAL FEATURES

Acute tonsillar and pharyngeal diphtheria is characterized by anorexia, malaise, low-grade fever, and sore throat. The grayish membrane forms within 1 to 2 days over the tonsils and pharyngeal walls and occasionally extends into the larynx and trachea. Cervical adenopathy varies but may be associated with development of a "bull neck." In mild cases, the membrane sloughs after 7 to 10 days and the patient recovers. In severe cases, an increasingly toxic appearance can lead to prostration, stupor, coma, and death within 6 to 10 days. Distinctive features include palatal paralysis, laryngeal paralysis, ocular palsies, diaphragmatic palsy, and myocarditis. Airway obstruction (from membrane formation) may complicate the toxigenic manifestations.

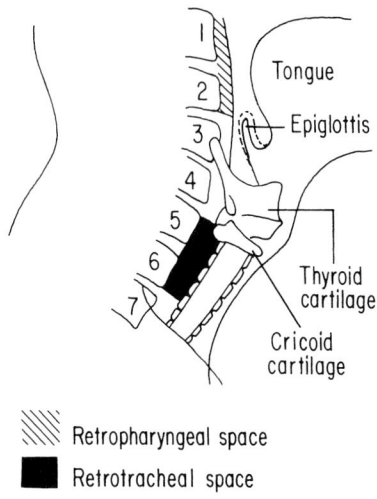

Figure 1-6. In a teenager, the retropharyngeal space normally does not exceed 7 mm when measured from the anterior aspect of the C2 vertebral body to the posterior pharynx. In infants, the retropharyngeal space is usually less than one width of the adjacent vertebral body. However, during crying, this distance may be three widths of the vertebral body. Also, under normal circumstances, the retrotracheal space does not exceed 22 mm in teenagers when measured from the anterior aspect of C-6 to the trachea. *Dotted lines* depict the "thumbprint" sign, noted on a lateral neck radiograph, made by a swollen epiglottis. (From Reilly BM: Sore throat. In *Practical Strategies in Outpatient Medicine*, 2nd ed. Philadelphia: WB Saunders, 1991.)

DIAGNOSIS AND TREATMENT

Accurate diagnosis requires isolation of *C. diphtheriae* on culture of material from beneath the membrane, with confirmation of toxin production by the organism isolated. Laboratories must be forewarned that diphtheria is suspected. Other tests are of little value.

Treatment includes equine antitoxin to neutralize circulating toxin, as well as systemic penicillin or erythromycin.

Table 1-11. Differential Diagnosis of Torticollis (Wryneck)

Congenital

Muscular torticollis
Positional deformation
Hemivertebra (cervicosuperior dorsal spine)
Unilateral atlanto-occipital fusion
Klippel-Feil syndrome
Unilateral absence of sternocleidomastoid
Pterygium colli

Trauma

Muscular injury (cervical muscles)
Atlanto-occipital subluxation
Atlantoaxial subluxation
C2–C3 subluxation
Rotary subluxation
Fractures

Inflammation

Cervical lymphadenitis
Retropharyngeal abscess
Cervical vertebral osteomyelitis
Rheumatoid arthritis
Spontaneous (hyperemia, edema) subluxation with adjacent head and neck infection (rotary subluxation syndrome)
Upper lobe pneumonia

Neurologic

Visual disturbances (nystagmus, superior oblique paresis)
Dystonic drug reactions (phenothiazines, haloperidol, metoclopramide)
Cervical cord tumor
Posterior fossa brain tumor
Syringomyelia
Wilson disease
Dystonia musculorum deformans
Spasmus nutans

Other

Acute cervical disk calcification
Sandifer syndrome (gastroesophageal reflux, hiatal hernia)
Benign paroxysmal torticollis
Bone tumors (eosinophilic granuloma)
Soft-tissue tumor
Hysteria

From Behrman RE (ed): Nelson Textbook of Pediatrics; 14th ed. Philadelphia: WB Saunders, 1992, p 1718.

GONOCOCCAL PHARYNGITIS

Acute symptomatic pharyngitis caused by *Neisseria gonorrhoeae* occurs occasionally in sexually active individuals as a consequence of oral-genital contact. In cases involving young children, sexual abuse must be suspected. The infection usually manifests as an ulcerative, exudative tonsillopharyngitis but may be asymptomatic and resolve spontaneously. Gonococcal pharyngitis occurs in homosexual men and heterosexual women after fellatio and is less readily acquired after cunnilingus. Gonorrhea rarely is transmitted from the pharynx to a sex partner, but pharyngitis can serve as a source for gonococcemia.

Diagnosis requires culture on appropriate selective media (e.g., Thayer-Martin medium). Recommended therapeutic regimens include a single intramuscular dose of 125 mg of ceftriaxone or a single oral 500-mg dose of ciprofloxacin. Spectinomycin is ineffective

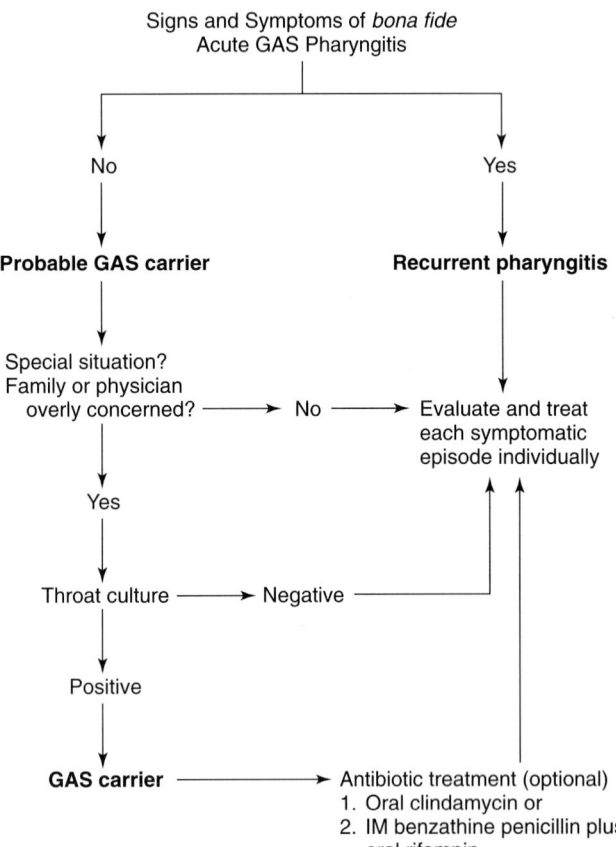

Figure 1-7. Management of patients with repeated or frequent positive rapid tests or throat cultures. GAS, group A streptococci; IM, intramuscular.

Table 1-12. Spectrum of *Mycoplasma Pneumoniae* Infection

Common

Primary atypical pneumonia* (with or without pleural effusion)
Pharyngitis
Tracheobronchitis

Less Common

Wheezing
Rhinitis
Bullous myringitis
Otitis media
Myocarditis
Pericarditis
Meningoencephalitis—aseptic meningitis
Polyneuritis—Guillain-Barré syndrome
Transverse myelitis
Sinusitis
Erythema multiforme—Stevens Johnson syndrome
Erythema nodosum
Urticaria
Intravascular hemolysis (high-titer cold agglutinins)
Arthralgia

*Manifestations during pneumonia include sore throat, hoarseness, malaise, headache, cough, earache, chills, and fever >102°F (38.9°C). Less often there may be coryza, rash, pleuritis, diarrhea, or leukocytosis > 10,000/mm³.

in gonococcal pharyngitis. Examination and testing for other sexually transmitted diseases and pregnancy are recommended.

CHLAMYDIAL AND MYCOPLASMAL INFECTIONS

Chlamydia species and *Mycoplasma pneumoniae* may cause pharyngitis, although the frequency of these infections is disputed. *Chlamydia trachomatis* has been implicated serologically as a cause of pharyngitis in as many as 20% of adults with pharyngitis, but isolation of the organism from the pharynx has proved more difficult. *Chlamydia pneumoniae* has also been identified as a cause of pharyngitis. Because antibodies to this organism show some cross-reaction with *C. trachomatis*, it is possible that infections formerly attributed to *C. trachomatis* were really caused by *C. pneumoniae*.

Diagnosis of chlamydial pharyngitis is difficult, whether by culture or serologically, and neither method is readily available to the clinician.

M. pneumoniae most likely causes pharyngitis. Serologic (positive mycoplasma immunoglobulin M [IgM]) or, less often, culture methods can be used to identify this agent, which was found in 33% of college students with pharyngitis in one study. Polymerase chain reaction (PCR) is diagnostic.

There is no need to seek evidence of these organisms routinely in pharyngitis patients in the absence of ongoing research studies of nonstreptococcal pharyngitis. The efficacy of antibiotic treatment for *M. pneumoniae* and chlamydial pharyngitis is not known, but these illnesses appear to be self-limited. Treatment of more complicated *M. pneumoniae* infections, such as pneumonia (Table 1-12), is indicated with erythromycin, azithromycin, or clarithromycin; doxycycline may be used if the patient is older than 10 years.

REFERENCES

Group A Streptococci

Attia MW, Zaoutis T, Klein JD, et al: Performance of a predictive model for streptococcal pharyngitis in children. Arch Pediatr Adolesc Med 2001; 155:687-691.

Bisno AL: Group A streptococcal infections and acute rheumatic fever. N Engl J Med 1991;325:783-793.

Bisno AL: Acute pharyngitis. N Engl J Med 2001;344:205-211.

Gerber MA, Tanz RR, Kabat W, et al: Optical immunoassay test for Group A ß-hemolytic streptococcal pharyngitis: An office-based, multicenter investigation. JAMA 1997;277:899-903.

Gerber MA, Tanz RR, Kabat W, et al: Potential mechanisms for failure to eradicate group A streptococci from the pharynx. Pediatrics 1999;104:911-917.

Hoge CW, Schwartz B, Talkington DF, et al.: The changing epidemiology of invasive group A streptococcal infections and the emergence of streptococcal toxic shock-like syndrome: A retrospective population-based study. JAMA 1993;269:384-389.

Podbielski A, Kreikemeyer B: Persistence of group A streptococci in eukaryotic cells—A safe place? Lancet 2001;358:3.

Tanz RR, Gerber MA, Shulman ST: What is a throat culture? Adv Exp Med Biol 1997;418:29-33.

Tanz RR, Shulman ST: Streptococcal pharyngitis: The carrier state, definition and management. Pediatric Annals 1998;27:281-285.

Torres-Martinez C, Mehta D, Butt A, et al: Streptococcus associated toxic shock. Arch Dis Child 1992;67:126-130.

Veasy LG, Tani LY, Hill HR: Persistence of acute rheumatic fever in the intermountain area of the United States. J Pediatr 1994;124:9-16.

Wheeler MC, Roe MH, Kaplan EL, et al: Outbreak of group A streptococcus septicemia in children: Clinical, epidemiologic, and microbiological correlates. JAMA 1991;266:533-537.

Working Group on Severe Streptococcal Infections: Defining the group A streptococcal toxic shock syndrome: Rationale and consensus definition. JAMA 1993;269:390-391.

Other Pathogens

Gerber MA, Randolph MF, Martin NJ, et al: Community-wide outbreak of group G streptococcal pharyngitis. Pediatrics 1991;87:598-603.

Feder HM Jr: Periodic fever, aphthous stomatitis, pharyngitis, adenitis: a clinical review of a new syndrome. Curr Opin Pediatr 2000;12:253-256.

Karpathios T, Drakonaki S, Zervoudaki A, et al: *Arcanobacterium haemolyticum* in children with presumed streptococcal pharyngotonsillitis or scarlet fever. J Pediatr 1992;121:735-737.

Komaroff AL, Branch WT, Aronson MD, et al: Chlamydial pharyngitis. Ann Intern Med 1989;111:537-538.

Lajo A, Borque C, Del Castillo F, et al: Mononucleosis caused by Epstein-Barr virus and cytomegalovirus in children: A comparative study of 124 cases. Pediatr Infect Dis J 1994;13:56-60.

McMillan JA, Weiner LB, Higgins AM, et al: Pharyngitis associated with herpes simplex virus in college students. Pediatr Infect Dis J 1993; 12:280-284.

Nakayama M, Miyazaki C, Ueda K, et al: Pharyngoconjunctival fever caused by adenovirus type 11. Pediatr Infect Dis J 1992;11:6-9.

Straus SE, Cohen JI, Tosato G, et al: Epstein-Barr virus infections: Biology, pathogenesis, and management. Ann Intern Med 1993;118:45-58.

Sumaya CV, Ench Y: Epstein-Barr virus infectious mononucleosis in children: I. Clinical and general laboratory findings. Pediatrics 1985;75 1003-1010.

Sumaya CV, Ench Y: Epstein-Barr virus infectious mononucleosis in children: II. Heterophil antibody and viral-specific responses. Pediatrics 1985;75:1011-1019.

Waagner DC: *Arcanobacterium haemolyticum*: Biology of the organism and diseases in man. Pediatr Infect Dis J 1991;10:933-939.

Complications

Chow AW: Life-threatening infections of the head and neck. Clin Infect Dis 1992;14:991-1004.

de Marie S, Tham RT, van der Mey AGL, et al: Clinical infections and nonsurgical treatment of parapharyngeal space infections complicating throat infection. Rev Infect Dis 1989;11:975-982.

Fiesseler FW, Riggs RL: Pharyngitis followed by hypoxia and sepsis: Lemierre syndrome. Am J Emerg Med 2001;19:320-322.

Savolainen S, Jousimies-Somer HR, Makitie AA, et al: Peritonsillar abscess: Clinical and microbiologic aspects and treatment regimens. Arch Otolaryngol Head Neck Surg 1993;119:521-524.

Wald ER, Guerra N, Byers C: Upper respiratory tract infections in young children: Duration of and frequency of complications. Pediatrics 1991; 87:129-133.

White B: Deep neck infections and respiratory distress in children. Ear Nose Throat J 1985;64:30-38.

Treatment

Gerber MA, Tanz RR: New approaches to the treatment of group A streptococcal pharyngitis. Curr Opin Pediatr 2001;13:51-55.

Markowitz M, Gerber MA, Kaplan EL: Treatment of streptococcal pharyngotonsillitis: Reports of penicillin's demise are premature. J Pediatr 1993;123:679-685.

Massel BF, Chute CG, Walker AM, et al: Penicillin and the marked decrease in morbidity and mortality from rheumatic fever in the United States. N Engl J Med 1988;318:280-286.

Paradise JL, Bluestone CD, Bachman RZ, et al: Efficacy of tonsillectomy for recurrent throat infection in severely affected children: Results of parallel randomized and nonrandomized clinical trials. N Engl J Med 1984; 310:674-683.

Randolph MF, Gerber MA, DeMeo KK, et al: Effect of antibiotic therapy on the clinical course of streptococcal pharyngitis. J Pediatr 1985;106: 870-875.

Seppala H, Nissinen A, Jarvinen H, et al: Resistance to erythromycin in group A streptococci. N Engl J Med 1992;326:292-297.

Shulman ST, Gerber MA, Tanz RR, et al: Streptococcal pharyngitis: The case for penicillin therapy. Pediatr Infect Dis J 1994;13:1-7.

Snellman LW, Stang HJ, Stang JM, et al: Duration of positive throat cultures for group A streptococci after initiation of antibiotic therapy. Pediatrics 1993;91:116-117.

Tanz RR, Poncher JR, Corydon KE, et al: Clindamycin treatment of chronic pharyngeal carriers of group A streptococci. J Pediatr 1991;119:123-128.

2 Cough

William M. Gershan*

Cough is an important defense mechanism of the lungs and is a common symptom, particularly during winter months. In most patients, it is self-limited. However, cough can be ominous, indicating serious underlying disease, because of accompanying problems (hemoptysis) or because of serious consequences of the cough itself (e.g., syncope and hemorrhage).

PATHOPHYSIOLOGY OF COUGH

The cough reflex serves to prevent the entry of harmful substances into the tracheobronchial tree and to expel excess secretions and retained material from the tracheobronchial tree. Cough begins with stimulation of cough receptors, located in the upper and lower airways, and in many other sites such as the ear canal, tympanic membrane, sinuses, nose, pericardium, pleura, and diaphragm. Receptors send messages via vagal, phrenic, glossopharyngeal, or trigeminal nerves to the "cough center," which is in the medulla. Because cough is not only an involuntary reflex activity but also one that can be initiated or suppressed voluntarily, "higher centers" must also be involved in the afferent limb of the responsible pathway. The neural impulses go from the medulla to the appropriate efferent pathways to the larynx, tracheobronchial tree, and expiratory muscles.

The act of coughing (Fig. 2-1) begins with an inspiration, followed by expiration against a closed glottis (compressive phase), resulting in the buildup of impressive intrathoracic pressures (50 to 300 cm H_2O). These pressures may be transmitted to vascular, cerebrospinal, and intraocular spaces. Finally, the glottis opens, allowing for explosive expiratory air flow (300 m/second) and expulsion of mucus, particularly from the larger, central airways. The inability to seal the upper airway (tracheostomy) impairs, but does not abolish, the effectiveness of cough. Weak ventilatory muscles (muscular dystrophy) impair both the inspiratory and the compressive phase.

HISTORY

The history often provides the most important body of information about a child's cough. A diagnosis can often be discerned with relative certainty from the family history, the environmental and exposure history, and the acuteness and characterization of the cough.

DEMOGRAPHICS

The patient's age (Table 2-1) helps to focus the diagnostic possibilities. Congenital anatomic abnormalities may be symptomatic from birth, whereas toddlers, who may have incomplete neurologic control over swallowing and often put small objects in their mouths, are at risk for foreign body aspiration; adolescents may experiment with smoking

or inhaled drugs. Socioeconomic factors must be considered; a family that cannot afford central heating may use a smoky wood-burning stove; spending time at a day care center may expose an infant to respiratory viruses; and several adult smokers in a small home expose children to a high concentration of respiratory irritants.

CHARACTERISTICS OF THE COUGH

The various cough characteristics can help determine the cause of cough. The causes of acute, recurrent, and chronic coughs may be quite different from each other (Fig. 2-2; see Table 2-1). A cough can be paroxysmal, brassy, productive, weak, volitional, and "throat-clearing," and it may occur at different times of the day (Tables 2-2 and 2-3).

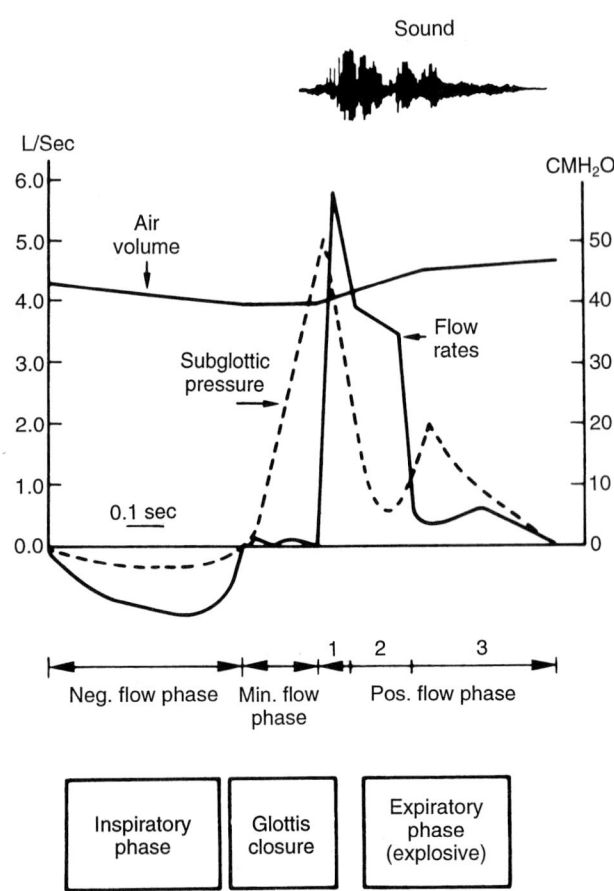

Figure 2-1. Cough mechanics, showing changes in expiratory flow rate, air volume, subglottic pressure, and sound recording during cough. (Adapted from Yanagihara N, et al: The physical parameters of cough: The larynx in a normal single cough. Acta Otolaryngol 1996;61:495-510.)

---

*This chapter is an updated and edited version of the chapter by David M. Orenstein that appeared in the first edition.

Table 2-1. Causes of Cough

Age Group	Acute	Recurrent	Chronic (>3 weeks)
Infants	Infection[1]* Aspiration[2] Foreign body[3]	Reactive airways[1] CF[1] GER[1] Aspiration[2] Anatomic abnormality[3†] Passive smoking[3]	Reactive airways[1] CF[1] GER[1] Aspiration[2] Pertussis[2] Anatomic abnormality[3†] Passive smoking[3] Miscellaneous[3] (see Table 2-26)
Toddlers	Infection[1] Foreign body[2] Aspiration[3]	Reactive airways[1] CF[1] GER[1] Aspiration[2] Anatomic abnormality[3] Passive smoking[3]	Reactive airways[1] CF[1] GER[1] Aspiration[2] Pertussis[2] Anatomic abnormality[3] Passive smoking[3] Miscellaneous[3]
Children	Infection[1] Foreign body[3]	Reactive airways[1] CF[1] GER[1] Passive smoking[3]	Reactive airways[1] CF[1] GER[2] Pertussis[2] *Mycoplasma*[3] Psychogenic[3] Anatomic abnormality[3] Passive smoking[3] Miscellaneous[3]
Adolescents	Infection[1]	Reactive airways[1] CF[1] GER[1] Aspiration[2] Anatomic abnormality[3]	Reactive airways[1] CF[1] GER[2] Smoking[2] *Mycoplasma*[2] Psychogenic[2] Pertussis[3] Aspiration[3] Anatomic abnormality[3] Miscellaneous[3]

*Infections include upper (pharyngitis, sinusitis, tracheitis, rhinitis, otitis) and lower (pneumonia, abscess, empyema) respiratory tract disease.

†Anatomic abnormality includes tracheobronchomalacia, tracheoesophageal fistula, vascular ring, abnormal position, or take-off of large bronchi.

[1]common; [2]less common; [3]much less common.

CF, cystic fibrosis; GER, gastroesophageal reflux.

RESPONSES TO PREVIOUS TREATMENT: DRUG HISTORY

The previous response or lack of response to some therapies for recurrent and chronic cough can provide important information (see Table 2-3). Furthermore, some coughs may be caused or worsened by medications (Table 2-4).

ASSOCIATED SYMPTOMS

A history of accompanying signs or symptoms, whether localized to the respiratory tract (wheeze, stridor) or elsewhere (failure to thrive, frequent malodorous stools) can give important clues (Table 2-5; see Tables 2-2 and 2-3). It is essential to remember that the daily language of the physician is full of jargon that may be adopted by parents but with a different meaning from that understood by physicians. If a parent says that a child "wheezes" or "croups" or is "short of breath," it is important to find out what the parent means by that term.

FAMILY AND PATIENT'S MEDICAL HISTORY

Because many disorders of childhood have genetic or nongenetic familial components, the family history can provide helpful information:

Are there older siblings with cystic fibrosis (CF) or asthma?
Is there a coughing sibling whose kindergarten class has been closed because of pertussis?

Similarly, the key to today's problems may be found in the past:

Was the child premature and, if so, did he or she spend a month on the ventilator, and does he or she now have chronic lung disease (bronchopulmonary dysplasia)?
Did the toddler choke on a carrot or other food 3 months ago?
Did the child receive a bone marrow transplant a year ago?
Is the child immunized?
Did the infant have a tracheoesophageal fistula repaired in the neonatal period?

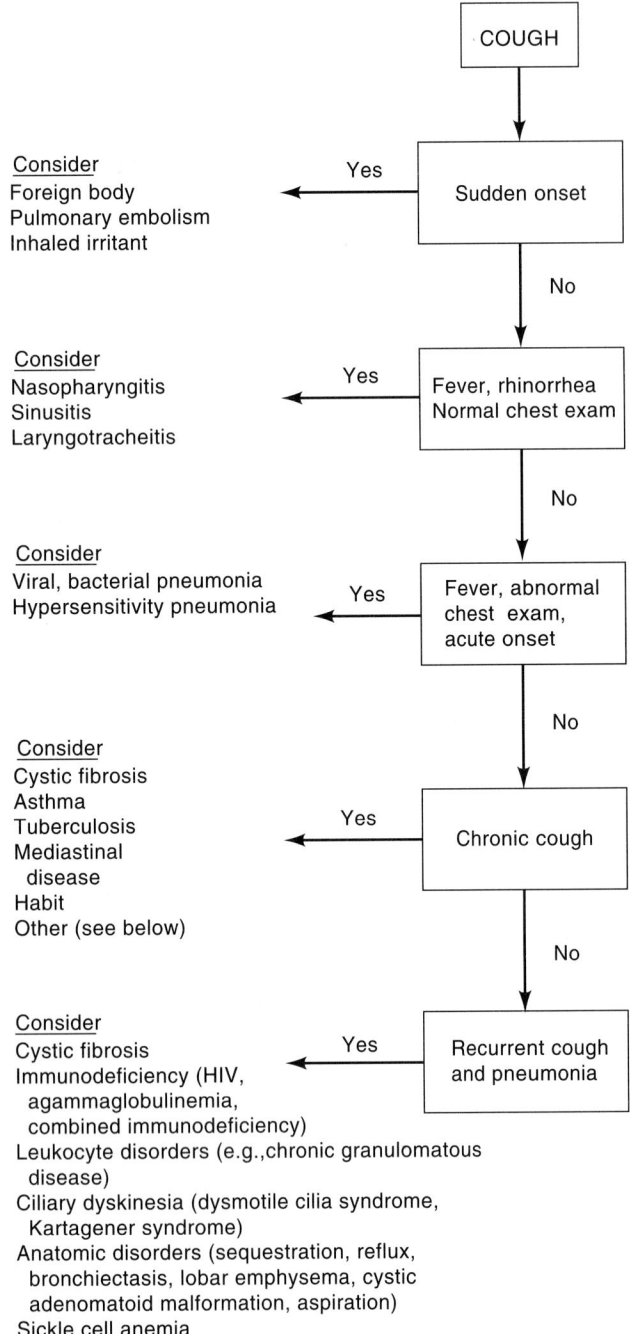

Figure 2-2. Algorithm for differential diagnosis of cough. HIV, human immunodeficiency virus.

PHYSICAL EXAMINATION

INSPECTION

Initial inspection often reveals the seriousness of an illness:

Is the child struggling to breathe (dyspnea)?
Does the child have an anxious look?
Can the child be calmed or engaged in play?
Is the child's skin blue (representing cyanosis) or ashen?
Does the child appear wasted, with poor growth that may indicate a chronic illness?

The respiratory rate is often elevated with parenchymal lung disease or extrathoracic obstruction. Respiratory rates vary with the age of the child (Fig. 2-3) and with pulmonary infection, airway obstruction, activity, wakefulness and sleep, fever, metabolic acidosis, and anxiety.

Odors may also give helpful clues. Does the examining room or the clothing smell of stale cigarette smoke? Is there a foul odor from a diaper with a fatty stool, which may suggest pancreatic insufficiency and CF? Is the child's breath malodorous, as can be noticed in sinusitis, nasal foreign body, lung abscess, or bronchiectasis?

Fingers

It has been said that the examination of the lungs begins at the fingertips. Cyanotic nail beds suggest hypoxemia, poor peripheral circulation, or both. The examiner looks for the presence of digital clubbing (Fig. 2-4), which makes asthma or acute pneumonia extremely unlikely. The absence of digital clubbing but a history of severe chronic cough in an older child makes CF unlikely.

Chest and Abdomen

The shape of the chest gives information. Is the anteroposterior (AP) diameter increased, which indicates hyperinflation of the lungs from obstruction of small airways (asthma, bronchiolitis, CF)? Is this diameter small, as can be seen with some restrictive lung diseases with small lung volumes (muscular dystrophy, spinal muscular atrophy)? The normal infant has a "round" chest configuration, with the AP diameter of the chest about 84% of the transverse (lateral) diameter. With growth, the chest becomes more flattened in the AP dimension, and the AP-to-transverse ratio is closer to 70% to 75%. Although obstetric calipers can be used to give an objective assessment of the AP diameter of the chest, most clinicians rely on their subjective assessment of whether the diameter is increased: Does the patient look "barrel-chested"?

Intercostal, subcostal, suprasternal, and supraclavicular *retractions* (inspiratory sinking in of the soft tissues) indicate increased effort of breathing and reflect both the contraction of the accessory muscles of respiration and the resulting difference between intrapleural and extrathoracic pressure. Retractions occur most commonly with obstructed airways (upper or lower), but they may occur with any condition leading to the use of the accessory muscles. Any retractions other than the mild normal depressions seen between an infant's lower ribs indicate a greater-than-normal work of breathing.

Less easy to notice than intercostal retractions is their bulging out with expiration in a child with expiratory obstruction (asthma). Contraction of the abdominal muscles with expiration is easier to notice and is another indication that a child is working harder than normal to push air out through obstructed airways.

Spine

Inspection of the spine may reveal kyphosis or scoliosis. There is a risk of restrictive lung disease or static pneumonia if the curvature is severe.

PALPATION

Palpating the trachea, particularly in infants, may reveal a shift to one side, which suggests loss of volume of the lung on that side or extrapulmonary gas (pneumothorax) on the other side. Placing one hand on each side of the chest while the patient breathes may enable the examiner to detect asymmetry of chest wall movement, either in timing or in degree of expansion. The former indicates a partial bronchial obstruction, and the latter suggests a smaller lung volume, voluntary guarding, or diminished muscle function on one side. Palpating the abdomen gently during expiration may allow the examiner to feel the contraction of the abdominal muscles in cases of expiratory obstruction.

Table 2-2. **Clinical Clues about Cough**

Characteristic	Think of
Staccato, paroxysmal	Pertussis, cystic fibrosis, foreign body, *Chlamydia* species, *Mycoplasma* species
Followed by "whoop"	Pertussis
All day, never during sleep	Psychogenic, habit
Barking, brassy	Croup, psychogenic, tracheomalacia, tracheitis, epiglottitis
Hoarseness	Laryngeal involvement (croup, recurrent laryngeal nerve involvement)
Abrupt onset	Foreign body, pulmonary embolism
Follows exercise	Reactive airways disease
Accompanies eating, drinking	Aspiration, gastroesophageal reflux, tracheoesophageal fistula
Throat clearing	Postnasal drip
Productive (sputum)	Infection
Night cough	Sinusitis, reactive airways disease
Seasonal	Allergic rhinitis, reactive airways disease
Immunosuppressed patient	Bacterial pneumonia, *Pneumocystis carinii*, *Mycobacterium tuberculosis*, *Mycobacterium avium–intracellulare*, cytomegalovirus
Dyspnea	Hypoxia, hypercarbia
Animal exposure	*Chlamydia psittaci* (birds), *Yersinia pestis* (rodents), *Francisella tularensis* (rabbits), Q fever (sheep, cattle), hantavirus (rodents), histoplasmosis (pigeons)
Geographic	Histoplasmosis (Mississippi, Missouri, Ohio River Valley), coccidioidomycosis (southwest), blastomycosis (north and midwest)
Workdays with clearing on days off	Occupational exposure

Palpation for *tactile fremitus,* the transmitted vibrations of the spoken word ("ninety-nine" is the word often used to accentuate these vibrations), helps determine areas of increased parenchymal density and hence increased fremitus (as in pneumonic consolidation) or decreased fremitus (as in pneumothorax or pleural effusion).

PERCUSSION

The percussion note determined by the examiner's tapping of one middle finger on the middle finger of the other hand, which is firmly placed over the patient's thorax, may be dull over an area of consolidation or effusion and hyperresonant with air trapping. Percussion can also be used to determine diaphragmatic excursion. The lowest level of resonance at inspiration and expiration determines diaphragmatic motion.

AUSCULTATION

Because lung sounds tend to be higher-pitched than heart sounds, the diaphragm of the stethoscope is better suited to pulmonary auscultation than is the bell, whose target is primarily the lower-pitched heart sounds (Table 2-6). The adult-sized stethoscope generally is far superior to the smaller pediatric or neonatal diaphragms, even for listening to small chests, because its acoustics are better. The two-headed stethoscope enables the user to hear homologous segments of both lungs simultaneously (Fig. 2-5) in order to identify instances in which there is a delay in air entry or exit. The traditional single-headed stethoscope is adequate in most children with cough. The ability to recognize normal breath sounds comes with practice (Fig. 2-6).

Adventitious Sounds

Adventitious sounds come in a few varieties, namely, stridor, crackles, rhonchi, and wheezes. Other sounds should be described in clear, everyday language.

Stridor is a continuous musical sound usually heard on inspiration and is caused by narrowing in the extrathoracic airway, as with croup or laryngomalacia.

Crackles are discontinuous, representing the popping open of air-fluid menisci as the airways dilate with inspiration. Fluid in

Table 2-3. **Cough: Some Aspects of Differential Diagnosis**

Cause	Only Abrupt Onset	When Awake	Responds to Inhaled Yellow Sputum	Responds to Bronchodilator (by History)	Responds Antibiotics (by History)	to Steroids (by History)	Failure to Thrive	Wheeze	Digital Clubbing
Reactive airways disease/asthma	+	++	++	+++	+	+++	+	+++	−
Cystic fibrosis	+	++	++	+	+++	+	++	++	+++
Infection	+	+	++	−	++	−	+	+	−
Aspiration	+	+	+	+	+	+	++	++	+
Gastroesophageal reflux	+	++	−	−	−	+	++	++	−
Foreign body	+++	+	++	+	++	+	+	++	+
Habit	−	+++	−	−	−	−	−	−	−

+++, Very common and suggests the diagnosis; ++, common; +, uncommon; −, almost never and makes examiner question the diagnosis.

Table 2-4. Drugs Causing Cough

Drug	Mechanism
Tobacco, marijuana	Direct irritants
β-Adrenergic blockers	Potentiate reactive airways disease
ACE inhibitors	(?) Possibly potentiate reactive airways disease
Bethanechol	Potentiates reactive airways disease
Nitrofurantoin	(?) Via oxygen radicals versus via autoimmunity
Antineoplastic agents	Various (including pneumonitis/fibrosis, hypersensitivity, noncardiogenic pulmonary edema)
Sulfasalazine	(?) Causes bronchiolitis obliterans
Penicillamine	(?) Causes bronchiolitis obliterans
Diphenylhydantoin	Hypersensitivity pneumonitis
Gold	(?) Causes interstitial fibrosis
Aspirin, NSAIDs	Potentiate reactive airways disease
Nebulized cromolyn	Potentiates reactive airways disease via hypotonicity
Nebulized antibiotics	(?) Direct irritant
Inhaled/nebulized bronchodilators	Increases tracheal/bronchial wall instability in airway malacia; or via reaction to vehicle
Theophylline, caffeine	Indirect, via worsened gastroesophageal reflux (relaxation of lower esophageal sphincter)
Metabisulfite	Induces allergic reactive airways disease
Cholinesterase inhibitors	Induce mucus production (bronchorrhea)

ACE, angiotensin-converting enzyme; NSAIDs, nonsteroidal anti-inflammatory drugs.

larger airways causes crackles early in inspiration (congestive heart failure); crackles that tend to be a bit lower in pitch ("coarse" crackles) than the early, higher-pitched ("fine") crackles are associated with fluid in small airways (pneumonia). Although crackles usually signal the presence of excess airway fluid (pneumonia, pulmonary edema), they may also be produced by the popping open of noninfected fibrotic or atelectatic airways. Fine crackles are not audible at the mouth, whereas coarse crackles may be. *Crackles* is the preferred term, rather than the previously popular "rales."

Rhonchi, or "large airway sounds," are continuous gurgling or bubbling sounds typically heard during both inhalation and exhalation. These sounds are caused by movement of fluid and secretions in larger airways (asthma, viral URI). Rhonchi, unlike other sounds, may clear with coughing.

Wheezes are continuous musical sounds (lasting longer than 200 milliseconds), caused by vibration of narrowed airway walls, as with asthma, and perhaps vibration of material within airway lumens. These sounds are much more commonly heard during expiration than inspiration.

LABORATORY FINDINGS

RADIOGRAPHY

The chest radiograph is often the most useful diagnostic test in the evaluation of the child with cough. Table 2-7 highlights some of the

Table 2-5. Nonpulmonary History Suggesting Cystic Fibrosis

Maldigestion, malabsorption, steatorrhea (in 80%-90%)
Poor weight gain
Family history of cystic fibrosis
Salty taste to skin
Rectal prolapse (up to 20% of patients)
Digital clubbing
Meconium ileus (in 10%-15%)
Intestinal atresia
Neonatal cholestatic jaundice

radiographic features of the most common causes of cough in pediatric patients. Radiographic findings are often similar for a number of disorders, and thus these studies may not indicate a definitive diagnosis. Chest films are normal in children with psychogenic (habit) cough and in children with sinusitis or gastroesophageal reflux (GER) as the *primary* cause of cough. A normal chest radiograph indicates the unlikelihood of pneumonia caused by respiratory syncytial virus (RSV), influenza, parainfluenza, adenovirus, *Chlamydia* species, or bacteria. Although children with cough resulting from CF, *Mycoplasma* species, tuberculosis, aspiration, a bronchial foreign body, or an anatomic abnormality usually have abnormal chest radiographs, a normal radiograph does not exclude these diagnoses. Hyperinflation of the lungs is commonly seen on chest films of infants with RSV bronchiolitis or *Chlamydia* pneumonia, and a lobar or round (coin lesion) infiltrate is the radiographic hallmark of

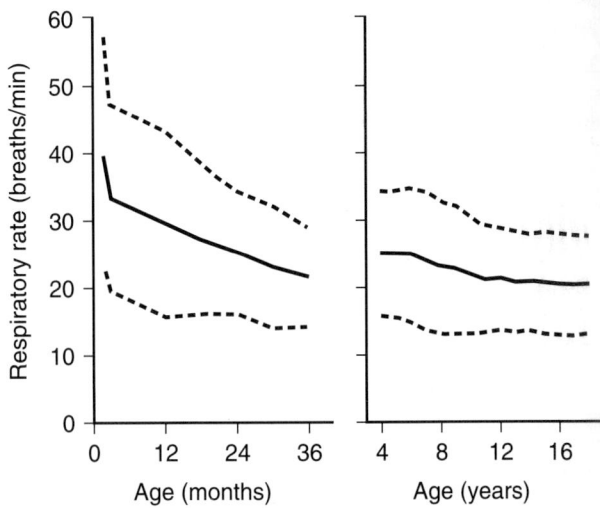

Figure 2-3. Mean values (*solid line*) ±2 standard deviations (*dotted lines*) of the normal respiratory rate at rest (during sleep in children younger than 3 years). There is no significant difference between the sexes. (Data from Pasterkamp H: The history and physical examination. In Chernick V [ed]: Kendig's Disorders of the Respiratory Tract in Children, 6th ed. Philadelphia, WB Saunders, 1998, p 88.)

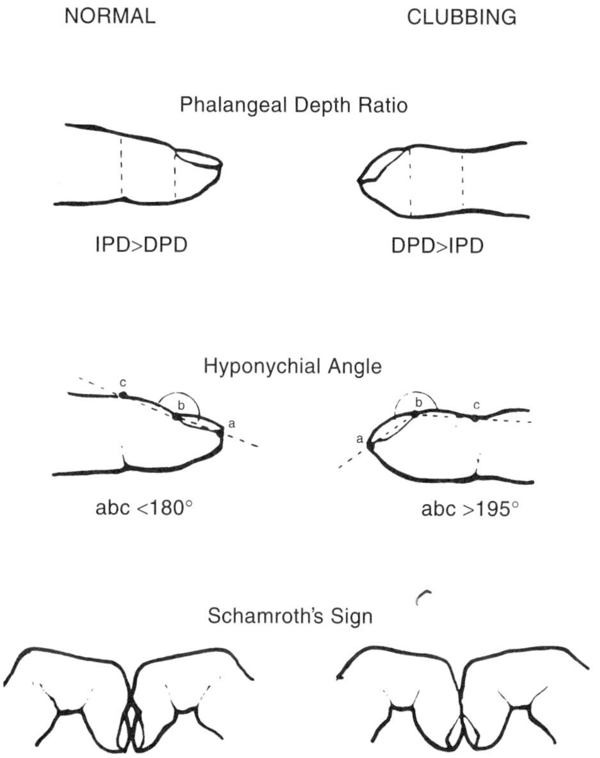

NORMAL   CLUBBING

Phalangeal Depth Ratio

IPD>DPD   DPD>IPD

Hyponychial Angle

abc <180°   abc >195°

Schamroth's Sign

Figure 2-4. Measurement of digital clubbing. The ratio of the distal phalangeal depth (DPD) to the interphalangeal depth (IPD), or the *phalangeal depth ratio,* is normally less than 1 but increases to more than 1 with finger clubbing. The DPD/IPD ratio can be measured with calipers or, more accurately, with finger casts. The *hyponychial angle* is measured from lateral projections of the finger contour on a magnifying screen and is normally less than 180 degrees but greater than 195 degrees with finger clubbing. *Schamroth's sign* is useful for bedside assessment. The dorsal surfaces of the terminal phalanges of similar fingers are placed together. With clubbing, the normal diamond-shaped aperture or "window" at the bases of the nail beds disappears, and a prominent distal angle forms between the end of the nails. In normal subjects, this angle is minimal or nonexistent. (From Pasterkamp H: The history and physical examination. In Chernick V [ed]: Kendig's Disorders of the Respiratory Tract in Children, 6th ed. Philadelphia, WB Saunders, 1998.)

bacterial pneumonia. The diagnosis of sinusitis cannot be sustained with normal sinuses on radiograph or computed tomography (CT) scan.

HEMATOLOGY/IMMUNOLOGY

The white blood cell (WBC) count may help exclude or include certain entities for a differential diagnosis, but, with the possible exception of pertussis, can seldom establish a diagnosis with certainty. A WBC count of 35,000 with 85% lymphocytes strongly suggests pertussis, but not every child with pertussis presents such a clear hematologic picture. The presence of a high number or large proportions of immature forms of WBCs suggests an acute process, such as a bacterial infection. Immunoglobulins provide supportive evidence for a few diagnoses, such as chlamydial infection, which rarely occurs without elevated serum concentrations of immunoglobulins G and M.

BACTERIOLOGY/VIROLOGY

Specific bacteriologic or virologic diagnoses can be made in a number of disorders causing cough, including RSV, influenza, parainfluenza, adenovirus, and *Chlamydia* pneumonia. In most cases, these diagnoses

are based on culturing the organism from nasopharyngeal washings. In some cases, the viruses can be rapidly identified with immunofluorescence or amplification of viral genome through polymerase chain reaction (PCR). In bacterial pneumonia, the offending organism can be cultured from the blood in a small proportion (10%) of patients. A positive culture provides definitive diagnosis, but a negative culture specimen is not helpful. Throat cultures are seldom helpful (except in CF) in identifying lower respiratory tract organisms. Sputum cultures and Gram stains may help guide initial empirical therapy in older patients with pneumonia or purulent bronchitis, but their ability to identify specific causative organisms with certainty (again with the exception of CF) has not been shown clearly.

Infants and young children usually do not expectorate but, rather, swallow their sputum. Specimens obtained via bronchoscopy may be contaminated by mouth flora, but heavy growth of a single organism in the presence of polymorphonuclear neutrophils certainly supports the organism's role in disease. If pleural fluid or fluid obtained directly from the lung via needle aspiration is cultured, the same rules apply: Positive cultures are definitive, but negative cultures are not. Bacterial antigen detection in serum or urine by various techniques (latex agglutination) can help identify pneumococcus and *Haemophilus influenzae* type b.

OTHER TESTS

A number of specific tests can help to establish diagnoses in a child with cough (see Table 2-7). These include a positive response to bronchodilators in a child with asthma; visualizing the red, swollen epiglottis in epiglottitis (to be done only under very controlled conditions, as described later); the bronchoscopic visualization of the peanut, plastic toy, or other offender in foreign body aspiration; a positive purified protein derivative in tuberculosis; and several studies of the esophagus in GER. Several imaging techniques, such as CT or magnetic resonance imaging (MRI), can help to delineate various intrathoracic anatomic abnormalities. Finally, multiple tests can be employed to confirm the diagnosis of CF (Table 2-8).

DIFFERENTIAL DIAGNOSIS AND TREATMENT

INFECTION

Infections are the most common cause of acute cough in all age groups and are responsible for some chronic coughs. The age of the patient has a large impact on the type of infection.

Infants

Viral upper respiratory infections (common cold); croup (laryngotracheobronchitis); viral bronchiolitis, particularly with RSV; and viral pneumonia are the most frequently encountered respiratory tract infections and hence the most common causes of cough in infancy. Viral illness may predispose to bacterial superinfection (croup and *Staphylococcus aureus* tracheitis or influenza and *H. influenzae* pneumonia).

Common Cold

Cold symptoms and signs usually include stuffy nose, with nasal discharge (rhinorrhea); sore throat and sneezing frequently occur. There may be fever, constitutional signs (irritability, myalgias, headache), or both. Cough is common and may persist for 5 to 7 days. The mechanism by which upper respiratory infections cause cough in children is undetermined. In adults, it is generally thought that "postnasal drip"—that is, nasal or sinus secretions draining into the posterior nasopharynx—causes cough and, in fact, may be one of the most frequent causes of cough. Indeed, sinus CT in older patients

Table 2-6. Physical Signs of Pulmonary Disease

Disease Process	Mediastinal Deviation	Chest Motion	Fremitus	Percussion	Breath Sounds	Adventitious Sounds	Voice Signs
Consolidation (pneumonia)	No	Reduced over area, splinting	Increased	Dull	Bronchial or reduced	Crackles	Egophony,* whispering pectoriloquy increased†
Bronchospasm	No	Hyperexpansion with limited motion	Normal or decreased	Hyperresonant	Normal to decreased	Wheezes, crackles	Normal to decreased
Atelectasis	Shift toward lesion	Reduced over area	Decreased	Dull	Reduced or absent	None or crackles	None
Pneumothorax	Tension deviates trachea and PMI to opposite side	Reduced over area	None	Resonant, tympanitic	None	None	None
Pleural effusion	Deviation to opposite side	Reduced over area	None	Dull	None	Friction rub; splash, if hemopneumothorax	None
Interstitial process	No	Reduced	Normal to increased	Normal	Normal	Crackles	None

Adapted from Dantzker D, Tobin M, Whatley R: Respiratory diseases. In Andreoli TE, Carpenter CJ, Plum F, Smith LH (eds): Cecil Essentials of Medicine. Philadelphia, WB Saunders, 1986, p 126-180.

*Egophony is present when e sounds like a.

†Whispering pectoriloquy produces clearer sounding whispered words (e.g., "ninety-nine").

PMI, point of maximal impulse.

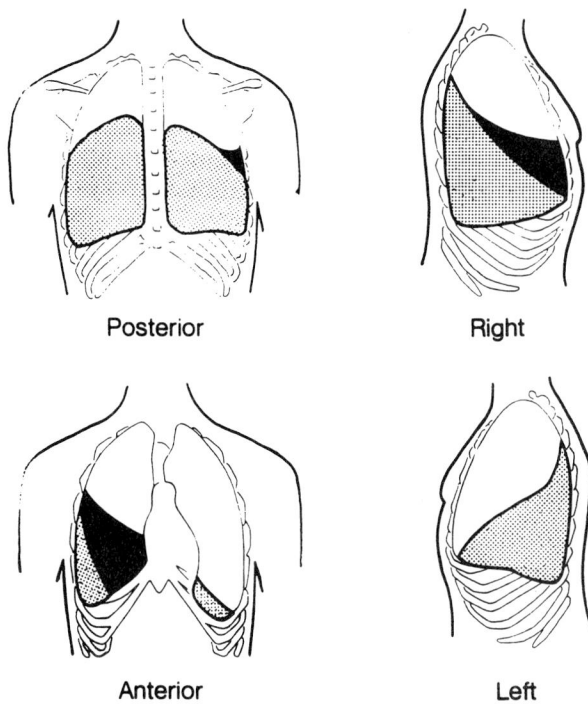

Figure 2-5. Projections of the pulmonary lobes on the chest surface. The upper lobes are white, the right-middle lobe is black, and the lower lobes are dotted. (From Pasterkamp H: The history and physical examination. In Chernick V [ed]: Kendig's Disorders of the Respiratory Tract in Children, 6th ed. Philadelphia, WB Saunders, 1998.)

Posterior

Right

Anterior

Left

with colds often reveals involvement of the sinus mucosa. Whether this is true in children remains undetermined. Other authorities believe that cough in a child with a cold indicates involvement (inflammation or bronchospasm) of the lower respiratory tract. The physician's bias on this matter will probably influence how to treat the child with cough accompanying a cold. In adults, the cough of the common cold may respond to a combination antihistamine-decongestant preparation, presumably from the decreased postnasal drip. It is uncertain whether such treatment is effective or indicated in children, particularly young infants, in whom toxicity of the drugs may be a greater concern than in adults.

Common viral pathogens include rhinovirus, RSV, and parainfluenza virus. The differential diagnosis includes allergic rhinitis, which often demonstrates clear nasal secretions with eosinophils and pale nasal mucosa, in contrast to mucopurulent nasal secretions with neutrophils and erythematous mucosa.

Croup (Laryngotracheobronchitis)

Infectious croup (see Chapter 5) is most common in the first 2 years of life. Its most dramatic components are the barking ("croupy") cough and inspiratory stridor, which appear a few days after the onset of a cold. In most cases, the patient has a low-grade fever, and the disease resolves within a day or two. In severe cases, the child can be extremely ill and is at risk for complete laryngeal obstruction. There may be marked intercostal and suprasternal retractions and cyanosis. Stridor at rest signifies significant obstruction. Diminishing stridor in a child who is becoming more comfortable is a good sign, but diminishing stridor in and of itself is not necessarily good: If the child becomes fatigued because of the tremendous work of breathing through an obstructed airway and can no longer breathe effectively, smaller-than-needed tidal volumes make less noise.

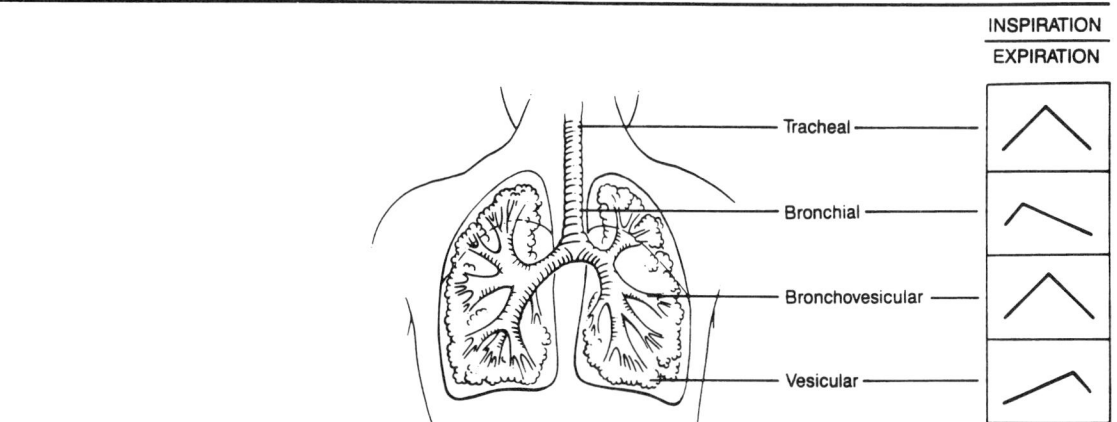

Characteristic	Tracheal	Bronchial	Bronchovesicular	Vesicular
Intensity	Very loud	Loud	Moderate	Soft
Pitch	Very high	High	Moderate	Low
I:E Ratio*	1:1	1:3	1:1	3:1
Description	Harsh	Tubular	Rustling, but tubular	Gentle rustling
Normal locations	Extrathoracic trachea	Manubrium	Over mainstem bronchi	Most of peripheral lung

* Ratio of duration of inspiration to expiration.

Figure 2-6. Characteristics of breath sounds. *Tracheal* breath sounds are very harsh, loud, and high-pitched; they are heard over the extrathoracic portion of the trachea. *Bronchial* breath sounds are loud and high-pitched; normally, they are heard over the lower sternum and sound like air rushing through a tube. The expiratory component is louder and longer than the inspiratory component; a definite pause is heard between the two phases. *Bronchovesicular* breath sounds are a mixture of bronchial and vesicular sounds. The inspiratory (I) and expiratory (E) components are equal in length. They are usually heard only in the first and second interspaces anteriorly and between the scapulae posteriorly, near the carina and mainstem bronchi. *Vesicular* breath sounds are soft and low-pitched; they are heard over most of the lung fields. The inspiratory component is much longer than the expiratory component; the latter is softer and often inaudible. (From Swartz MH: The chest. In Textbook of Physical Diagnosis: History and Examination. Philadelphia: WB Saunders, 1989.)

Table 2-7. Cough: Laboratory Evaluation

	Chest Radiograph						Complete Blood Count								
	Normal	Hyper	Lobar Infil	Diff Infil	Other	Abnormal Sinus Radiograph	↑WBC	↑LY	↑EOS	↑PMN	↑IgG	↑IgM	↑IgE	+NP Cult	Other
RAD/asthma	+	++	-	-	-	+	+	+	++	-	+	+	++		+bdilator[1]
Cystic fibrosis	+	++	+	+	++	++	++	+	+	++	++	++	+		See Table 2-8
Other infection															
Croup	++	+	+	+	++[2]	-	-	+	+	-				Paraflu +++	+PCR
Epiglottitis	++	+	+	+	++[3]	-	+++	+	+	+++					Direct look
Sinusitis	+++	-	+	-	-	++	++	-	+	+++	++		+		
Bronchiolitis	-	+++	+	++	+	-	+	+	+	+				RSV	+PCR
Pneumonia															
Influenza	-	++	+	++	+	-	++	-	+	+				+++	+PCR
Paraflu	-	+	+	++	+	-	++	+	+	+				+++	+PCR
Adenovirus	-	+	-	++	+	-	++	+	+	+	++	+	-	+[4]	
Pertussis	++	+	+	+++	++[5]	-	+	+++	++	+	+++	+++	-	+++	
Chlamydia	-	+		+		-	+	++	+	+	-	++			
Mycoplasma	+	+	+	+	++[5]	+	+	+	+	+					+Cold agglutinin, PCR
TB	+	-	++	+	++[5]	-	+	+	+	+++					+PPD
Bacterial	-	-	+++	+	++[5]	-	+++	-	-	++	++	+	+	+	+Bld cult[6]
Foreign body	-	+[7]	++	-	++[7]	-	-	-	+	-					Bronch
GE reflux	+++	+	-	-	-	+	-	-	+	-	-	-	+	-	Esoph pH[8]
Aspiration	+	+	+	-	++[9]	+	+	-	-	+	-	-	+	-	[10]
Anatomic	+	+	+	-	++[11]	-	-	-	-	+	-	-	-	-	[12]
Habit	+++	-	-	-	-	-	-	-	-	-				-	

[1] Positive response to bronchodilators, either as a home therapeutic trial or in a pulmonary function test in the laboratory.

[2] "Steeple" sign: narrowing of upper tracheal air column.

[3] "Swollen thumb": sign of thickened epiglottis.

[4] Low yield on culture in paroxysmal stage.

[5] Pleural effusion relatively common.

[6] Blood culture positive in 10%; needle aspiration of pleural fluid or lung fluid may yield organism; bacterial antigen in urine. In older infants and children, common pathogens include pneumococci and group A streptococci; *Staphylococcus aureus* is rare and may be associated with pneumatoceles or empyema.

[7] Localized hyperinflation is common; localized atelectasis in common; inspiratory-expiratory films may show ball-valve obstruction.

[8] Esophageal biopsy specimen shows esophagitis.

[9] Multilobular or multisegmental, dependent lobes.

[10] (?) Lipid-laden macrophages from bronchoscopy or gastric washings; barium swallow or radionuclide study showing aspiration.

[11] Right-sided arch, mass effect on airways, mass identified; magnetic resonance imaging (MRI).

[12] Bronchoscopy; computed tomography; MRI.

+++, almost always—if not present, must question diagnosis; ++, common; +, less common; -, seldom—if present, must question diagnosis; +Bld Cult, blood culture may be positive; Bronch, bronchoscopy can reveal the foreign body; Diff, diffuse or scattered; ↑EOS, increased eosinophil count; Esoph pH, prolonged esophageal pH probe monitoring; GE, gastroesophageal; Hyper, hyperinflated; Ig, immunoglobulin; Infil, infiltrates; ↑LY, increased lymphocyte count; +NP Cult, nasopharyngeal culture positive for specific organism; Paraflu, parainfluenza virus; PCR, polymerase chain reaction; ↑PMN, increased polymorphonuclear neutrophil count; PPD, purified protein derivative (TB); RAD, reactive airways disease; RSV, respiratory syncytial virus; TB, tuberculosis; ↑WBC, increased white blood cell count.

Table 2-8. Laboratory Tests for Cystic Fibrosis

Usefulness	Test	Sensitivity	Specificity	Cost
Definitive	"Sweat test"	.99+	.95+	$175
	DNA analysis	.85-.90	.99	$35
Suggestive	Throat or sputum culture* positive for mucoid			$140
	Pseudomonas aeruginosa	.70-.80	.85	
	Sinus radiographs			$179
	Pansinusitis	.95	.90	
	Positive IRT newborn screen	.98	.25	$1
	Typical histologic appearance of appendix	.95	.98	—
Supportive	Absent stool trypsin	.40-.75	.75(?)	$103
	Abnormal Chymex test result for pancreatic insufficiency	.70-.90	.90+	$98
	Pulmonary function tests:			$100-$800
	Obstructive pattern, especially small airways and especially if patient is poorly responsive to bronchodilator	.70+	?	
	Chest film:			$160
	Hyperinflation, ± other findings; especially with right upper lobe infiltrate/atelectasis	.70+	?	
	Throat or sputum culture*:			$140
	Positive for *Staphylococcus aureus*	.20	.20	
	Positive for *Haemophilus influenzae*	.05-.20	.15	

*Throat is usually deep pharyngeal culture.

IRT, immunoreactive trypsinogen.

It is important to distinguish croup from epiglottitis in the child with harsh, barking cough and inspiratory stridor because the natural histories of the two diseases are quite different (see Table 2-7). Epiglottitis occurs more commonly in toddlers than in infants (see Chapter 5).

Treatment of mild croup is usually not needed. For decades, pediatricians have recommended putting a child with croup in a steamy bathroom or driving to the office or emergency room with the car windows rolled down. (It is likely that these remedies are effective because of the heat exchange properties of the upper airway; air that is cooler or more humid than the airway mucosa will serve to cool the mucosa, thus causing local vasoconstriction and probably decreasing local edema.)

In a child who has stridor at rest, hospitalization is indicated. Symptomatic, often dramatic relief through decreased laryngeal edema can usually be achieved with aerosolized racemic epinephrine (2.25% solution, 0.25 to 0.5 mL/dose). It is essential to remember that the effects of the epinephrine are transient, lasting only a few hours, although the course of the illness is often longer. The result is that when the racemic epinephrine's effect has worn off, the child's cough and stridor will probably be as bad or even worse than before the aerosol was administered. This is *not* a "rebound" effect: The symptoms are not worse because of the treatment but, rather, because of the natural progression of the viral illness. Repeating the aerosol will probably again have a beneficial effect and reduce the likelihood of requiring a tracheotomy or endotracheal intubation. A child who responds favorably to such an aerosol needs to be observed for several hours because further treatment may be needed. A single dose of dexamethasone (0.6 mg/kg orally, intramuscularly, or intravenously) reduces the severity and hastens recovery. Aerosolized steroids (budesonide) may also be effective in patients with mild to moderately severe croup.

Bronchiolitis

Bronchiolitis is a common and potentially serious lower respiratory tract disorder in infants (see Chapters 3 and 5). It is caused usually by RSV but on occasion by parainfluenza, influenza, or adenovirus. It occurs in the winter months, often in epidemics. RSV bronchiolitis is seen uncommonly in children older than 4 years. Typically, "cold-like" symptoms of rhinorrhea precede the harsh cough, increased respiratory rate, and retractions. Respiratory distress and cyanosis can be severe. The child's temperature is seldom elevated above 38°C.

The chest is hyperinflated, widespread crackles are audible on inspiration, and wheezing marks expiration. The most striking laboratory abnormalities are in the chest radiograph, which invariably reveals hyperinflation, as depicted by a depressed diaphragm, with an enlarged retrosternal air space in as many as 60% of patients, peribronchial thickening in approximately 50%, and consolidation and/or atelectasis in 10% to 25%.

The diagnosis is confirmed with demonstration of RSV by immunofluorescent stain or PCR of nasopharyngeal washings. In most cases, no treatment is needed because the disease does not interfere with the infant's eating or breathing. Apnea is a common complication of RSV bronchiolitis in young infants and may necessitate close monitoring. In severe cases, often those in which there is underlying chronic heart, lung, or immunodeficiency disease, RSV can be life-threatening. In these cases, hospital care with supplemental oxygen and intravenous fluids is indicated. The effect of aerosolized bronchodilators is not clear but is probably beneficial in some infants. The aerosolized antiviral agent ribavirin may be beneficial for the sickest infants. It is expensive and difficult to administer; it needs to be given 12 to 18 hours per day (some studies advocate 2 hours three times a day) and may block ventilator tubing and valves. Ribavirin may improve oxygenation but should not be used in lieu of mechanical ventilation in patients with hypoxia and hypercarbia (respiratory failure).

Viral Pneumonia

Viral pneumonia can be similar to RSV bronchiolitis in its manifestation, with cough and tachypnea, after a few days of apparent upper respiratory infection. There can be variable degrees of fever and of overall illness. Infants and children with viral pneumonia may appear relatively well or, particularly with adenovirus, may have a rapidly progressive course, which ends in death within a few days after the onset of illness. Frequent symptoms include poor feeding, cough, cyanosis, fever (some patients may be afebrile), apnea, and rhinorrhea. Frequent signs include tachypnea, retractions, crackles, and cough. Cyanosis is less common.

The most common agents causing viral pneumonia in infancy and childhood are RSV, influenza, and parainfluenza. Adenovirus is less common, but it is important because it can be severe and leave residua, including bronchiectasis and bronchiolitis obliterans. Adenovirus pneumonia is often accompanied by conjunctivitis and pharyngitis, in addition to leukocytosis and an elevated erythrocyte sedimentation rate (ESR); the ESR and leukocyte count are usually not elevated in other types of viral pneumonia. Additional viral agents include enteroviruses and rhinovirus. Radiographs most often reveal diffuse, bilateral peribronchial infiltrates, with a predilection for the perihilar regions, but occasionally lobar infiltrates are present. Pleural effusions are not common. On occasion, if an infant is extremely ill, bronchoscopy with bronchoalveolar lavage may be indicated to isolate the virus responsible for the pneumonia.

Treatment is largely supportive, with oxygen and intravenous fluids. Mechanical ventilation may be necessary in a small minority of infants. In young infants, the *afebrile pneumonia syndrome* may be caused by *Chlamydia, Ureaplasma,* or *Mycoplasma* species; cytomegalovirus; or *Pneumocystis carinii.* In this syndrome, cough and tachypnea are common. Severe pneumonia may develop in neonates as a result of herpes simplex.

Pertussis (Whooping Cough)

Pertussis is an extremely important cause of lower respiratory tract infection in infants and children. The causative organism, *Bordetella pertussis,* has a tropism for tracheal and bronchial ciliated epithelial cells; thus, the disease is primarily bronchitis, but spread of the organism to alveoli, or secondary invasion by other bacteria, can cause pneumonia. The disease can occur at any age, from early infancy onward, although its manifestations in young infants and in those who have been partially immunized may be atypical.

Most commonly, pertussis has three stages:

- catarrhal, in which symptoms are indistinguishable from the common cold
- paroxysmal, dominated by repeated forceful, paroxysmal coughing spells; many spells may be punctuated by an inspiratory "whoop," post-tussive emesis, or both
- convalescent, in which the intensity and frequency of coughing spells gradually diminish

Each stage typically lasts 1 to 2 weeks, except the paroxysmal stage, which lasts many weeks. The Chinese term for pertussis translates to "100 days of cough." Most children are entirely well between coughing spells, when physical findings are remarkably benign. Infants younger than 3 months of age may have the most severe illness, and in this age group, the rate of mortality from pertussis is as high as 40%.

Diagnosis can be difficult because the definitive result—namely, culturing the organism from nasopharyngeal secretions—requires special culture medium (Bordet-Gengou, which must be prepared fresh for each collection). Culture specimens are much less likely to be positive during the paroxysmal stage than during the catarrhal stage, when the diagnosis is not being considered. Fluorescent antibody stains (for the antigen) of secretions are also helpful if they are positive, but, similarly, they are more likely to be positive before the paroxysmal stage. Serum antibodies against *B. pertussis* may occasionally be helpful, although they are often difficult to interpret in immunized individuals. Perhaps the laboratory test that is most helpful is the WBC count, which is typically elevated; values are as high as 20,000 to 50,000, with lymphocytes predominating. PCR is also useful. Chest radiographic findings are nonspecific. Infants with severe disease may require hospitalization.

Treatment is largely supportive, with oxygen, fluids, and small frequent feedings for patients who do not tolerate their normal feedings. Treatment with erythromycin estolate (50 mg/kg/day for 14 days, every 6 hours, orally) decreases infectivity and may ameliorate the course of the disease if given during the catarrhal stage. Studies suggest that azithromycin or clarithromycin may also be effective. In some patients, aerosolized bronchodilators (albuterol) or systemic steroids may help, although such treatment is controversial. Cough suppressants are not helpful, but good hydration, oxygenation, and nutrition, in addition to not disturbing the infant, are important.

Complications include those related to severe coughing (Table 2-9) and those specific to pertussis, such as seizures and encephalopathy. Pertussis is prevented by three primary immunizations (at 2, 4, and 6 months of age) and regular booster immunizations at 15 to 18 months and 4 to 6 years of age. Pertussis infection produces lifelong immunity.

Chlamydial Infection

Chlamydia trachomatis can cause pneumonia in young infants, particularly those aged 3 to 12 weeks. Cough, nasal congestion, low-grade or no fever, and tachypnea are common. Conjunctivitis is an important clue to chlamydial disease but is present in only 50% of infants with chlamydial pneumonia at the time of presentation. Affected infants may have a paroxysmal cough similar to that of pertussis, but post-tussive emesis is less common. Crackles are commonly heard on auscultation, but wheezing is much less common than the overinflated appearance of the lungs on radiographs would suggest. The organism may be recovered from the nasopharynx by culture or antigen testing. The complete blood cell count may reveal eosinophilia. Chlamydial infection responds to oral erythromycin therapy (40 to 50 mg/kg/day, every 6 hours for 10 to 14 days).

Table 2-9. Potential Complications of Cough

Musculoskeletal	Rib fractures
	Vertebral fractures
	Rupture of rectus abdominis muscle
	Asymptomatic elevation of serum creatine phosphokinase
Pulmonary	Chest wall pain*
	Bronchoconstriction
	Pneumomediastinum
	Pneumothorax
	Mild hemoptysis
	Subcutaneous emphysema
	Irritation of larynx and trachea
Cardiovascular	Rupture of subconjunctival,* nasal,* and anal veins
	Bradycardia, heart block
	Transient hypertension
Central nervous system	Cough syncope
	Headache
	Subarachnoid hemorrhage
Gastrointestinal	Hernias (ventral, inguinal)
	Emesis
	Rectal prolapse
	Pneumoperitoneum
Miscellaneous	Anorexia*
	Malnutrition
	Sleep loss*
	Urinary incontinence
	Disruption of surgical wounds
	Vaginal prolapse
	Displacement of intravenous catheters

*Common.

Ureaplasmal Infection

Ureaplasma urealyticum pneumonia is difficult to diagnose but causes cough in some infants. There are no particularly outstanding features to distinguish this relatively uncommon infection from viral pneumonias.

Bacterial Pneumonia

Bacterial pneumonia is relatively less common in infants than is viral pneumonia but can cause severe illness, with cough, respiratory distress, and fever. Chest films are strikingly abnormal; the WBC count is elevated.

Treatment is with broad-spectrum intravenous antibiotics effective against pneumococci, group A (possibly B) streptococci, and, if illness is severe, *S. aureus.* Cefotaxime with or without nafcillin may be effective.

Toddlers and Children

Colds

In early childhood, as children attend day care and nursery schools, they are constantly exposed to respiratory viruses to which they have little or no immunity (e.g., rhinoviruses, adenoviruses, parainfluenza, and coxsackievirus). Such children may have as many as 6 to 8 or even more colds in a year. The remarks concerning colds and cough in infants (see previous discussion) apply to this older age group. The differential diagnosis of rhinorrhea is noted in Table 2-10.

Sinusitis

The sinuses may become the site for viral and subsequent secondary bacterial infection spreading from the nasopharynx (Fig. 2-7). The signs and symptoms are usually localized, including nasal congestion, a feeling of "fullness" or pain in the face (Fig. 2-8), headache, sinus tenderness, day or night cough, and fever. Maxillary toothache, purulent nasal discharge for more than 10 days, a positive transillumination (opacification), and a poor response to oral antihistamines or nasal decongestants are important clues. Sinus radiographs or (more accurate) CT scan may facilitate the diagnosis of sinusitis by demonstrating opacification of the sinus with mucosal thickening. Sinusitis is thought to be a cause of cough in adults and can probably be listed, with lower certainty, as a cause of cough in children.

Sinusitis is frequently seen in other conditions known to cause cough, especially CF, asthma, and ciliary dyskinesia. It may be difficult to ascertain whether the cough is a direct result of the sinus infection or the underlying problem (purulent bronchitis in the child with CF or ciliary dyskinesia, exacerbation of asthma). In the first two situations, it may not matter because treatment is the same. In the case of the child with asthma, it is important to treat the asthma with bronchodilating and antiinflammatory agents, as well as to treat the infected sinuses with antibiotics.

The treatment of sinusitis involves the use of oral antibiotics active against the common pathogens (*Streptococcus pneumoniae,* nontypable *H. influenzae, Moraxella catarrhalis,* and, in rare cases, anaerobic bacteria or *Streptococcus pyogenes*). Treatment regimens include the use of amoxicillin, amoxicillin-clavulanate, cefuroxime, cefpodoxime, or cefdinir. Amoxicillin is considered the initial agent of choice. Oral (pseudoephedrine, phenylephrine) or topical (phenylephrine, oxymetazoline) decongestants may be of benefit by increasing the patency of the sinus ostia, which permits drainage of the infected and obstructed sinuses. Oral antihistamines may benefit patients with an allergic history. Treatment with antimicrobial agents should continue for at least 7 days after the patient has responded. This may require 14 to 21 days of therapy. Many patients with presumed sinusitis recover without antibiotic therapy.

Table 2-10. Differential Diagnosis of Rhinorrhea				
Etiology	**Frequency**	**Duration***	**Discharge**	**Comment**
Viral	Common	Acute	Purulent	Polymorphonuclear neutrophils in smear
Allergic	Common	Acute/chronic	Clear	Eosinophils in smear, seasonal
Vasomotor	Common	Chronic	Variable	? Environmental triggers
Sinusitis	Common	Chronic	Purulent	Sinus tenderness
Rhinitis medicamentosus	Common	Chronic	Variable	Medication use
Response to stimuli	Common	Acute	Clear	Odors, exercise, cold air, pollution
Nasal polyps	Uncommon	Chronic	Variable	Consider cystic fibrosis
Granulomatous disease	Uncommon	Chronic	Bloody	Sarcoid, Wegener granulomatosis, midline granuloma
Cerebrospinal fluid fistula	Uncommon	Chronic	Watery	Trauma, encephalocele
Foreign body	Uncommon	Chronic	Purulent	Often malodorous
Tumor	Uncommon	Chronic	Clear to bloody	Angiofibroma, hemangioma, rhabdomyosarcoma, lymphoma, nasopharyngeal carcinoma, neuroblastoma
Choanal atresia, stenosis	Uncommon	Chronic	Clear to purulent	Congenital
Nonallergic eosinophilic rhinitis syndrome	Uncommon	Chronic	Clear	Eosinophils in smear
Septal deviation	Unknown	Chronic	Clear	Congenital, trauma
Drugs	Uncommon	Chronic	Variable	Cocaine, glue and organic solvents, angiotensin-converting enzyme inhibitors, β blockers
Hypothyroidism	Uncommon	Chronic	Clear	
Cluster headache	Uncommon	Intermittent	Clear	Associated tearing, headache
Horner syndrome	Uncommon	Chronic	Clear	Ptosis, miosis, anhidrosis

*Less than 1 week is considered acute.

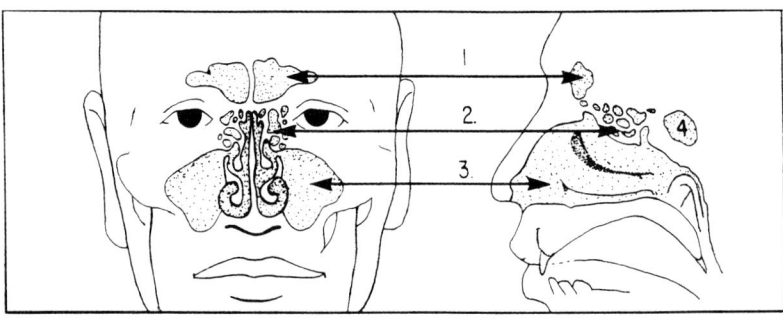

Figure 2-7. The paranasal sinuses. 1, Frontal. 2, Ethmoid. 3, Maxillary. 4, Sphenoid. (From Smith RP: Common upper respiratory tract infections. In Reilly B [ed]: Practical Strategies in Outpatient Medicine, 2nd ed. Philadelphia, WB Saunders, 1991.)

Complications of acute sinusitis include orbital cellulitis, abscesses (orbital, cerebral), cranial (frontal) osteomyelitis (Pott puffy tumor), empyema (subdural, epidural), and thrombosis (sagittal or cavernous sinus).

Croup and Epiglottitis

See previous text and Chapter 5.

Pneumonia

Viral Pneumonia. The features discussed for viral pneumonia in infants are relevant for viral pneumonia in older children. The differentiation of viral or atypical pneumonia from classical bacterial pneumonia is noted in Table 2-11.

Bacterial Pneumonia. Bacterial pneumonia is more common in toddlers and older children than in infants. The most common pathogen is *S. pneumoniae;* other bacterial causes vary with age (Table 2-12). Cough may not be as prominent a presenting symptom or sign as tachypnea and grunting, sometimes (especially in infants) with vomiting (see Table 2-11). Raised respiratory rates (≥50 in infants 2 to 12 months old, ≥40 in children 1 to 5 years old) plus retractions and grunting with or without hypoxia (oxygen saturation <90%) have a high specificity and sensitivity for pneumonia. Chest pain, abdominal pain, headache, or any combination of these symptoms may occur. Upper lobe pneumonia may produce meningeal signs, and lower lobe involvement may cause abdominal pain and an ileus.

Examination of the chest shows tachypnea but may be otherwise surprisingly normal. In older children, there may be localized dullness to percussion, with crackles or amphoric (bronchial) breath sounds over a consolidated lobe. The chest film may be normal in the first hours of the illness, inasmuch as the radiographic findings often lag behind the clinical manifestations. Nonetheless, both posteroanterior and lateral views are the main diagnostic tools; lobar consolidation is usual, with or without pleural effusion. In infants, the pattern may be more diffuse and extensive.

Some clinical and radiographic features may be suggestive of the bacterial cause of pneumonia. Children (especially infants) with staphylococcal pneumonia are more likely to have a rapid overwhelming course. Staphylococcal pneumonia may be accompanied by more extensive radiographic abnormalities, including multilobar consolidation, pneumatocele formation, and extensive pleural (empyema) fluid. The presence of a pleural effusion is not helpful in indicating the specific bacterial diagnosis because other bacterial pneumonias may be accompanied by pleural effusion. Pleural effusions may represent a reactive parapneumonic effusion or an empyema. Pleural fluid may be characterized as transudate, exudate, or complicated empyema, the latter necessitating closed chest drainage with a chest tube (Table 2-13). If the effusion is of sufficient size, as demonstrated by a lateral decubitus film or ultrasonography, a thoracentesis is indicated to differentiate the nature of the effusion and to identify possible pathogens.

Differentiating among the causes of bacterial pneumonia can be done with certainty only with positive cultures from blood, pleural fluid, fluid obtained by direct lung tap, or, in rare cases, sputum. Current or previous antibiotic treatment diminishes the yield of such cultures. The presence of bacterial antigens in the urine for *S. pneumoniae* or *H. influenzae* provides strong evidence of the causative agent. Bronchoscopy with or without lavage may yield helpful specimens from the progressively ill child or the child who has not responded promptly to empirical antibiotics.

Treatment is with antibiotics. Cefotaxime or ceftriaxone is the drug of choice for the previously healthy child who requires hospitalization with lobar pneumonia. For the critically ill child, vancomycin may be considered for possible resistant *S. pneumoniae*. Many children with pneumonia do well with oral antibiotics (amoxicillin, amoxicillin-clavulanate, oral cephalosporins) and respond within hours to the first dose. A smaller number may require hospitalization and intravenous antibiotics along with supportive measures (e.g., oxygen and intravenous fluids). Repeated or follow-up chest films may remain abnormal for 4 to 6 weeks after pneumonia and are not indicated for a single episode of uncomplicated pneumonia (i.e., no effusion, no abscess, and good response to treatment). Children with suspected pneumococcal pneumonia must be monitored carefully because of the possibility of resistance to penicillin and cephalosporin.

Mycoplasma pneumoniae is a common cause of pneumonia among school-aged children. The disease often occurs in community outbreaks in the fall months. The illness typically begins with

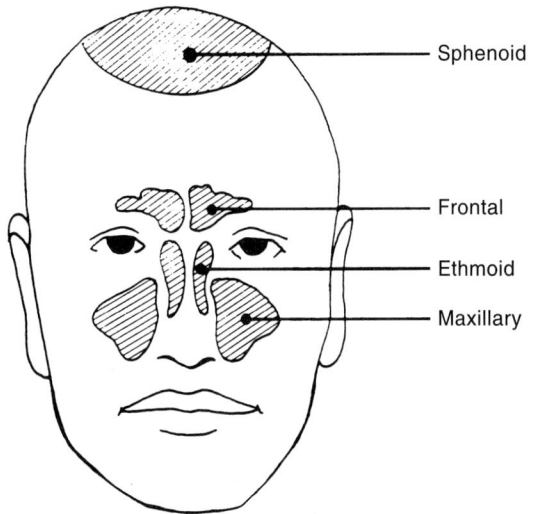

Sphenoid

Frontal

Ethmoid

Maxillary

Figure 2-8. Typical pain locations in patients with various anatomic sites of acute sinusitis. (From Smith RP: Common upper respiratory tract infections. In Reilly B [ed]: Practical Strategies in Outpatient Medicine, 2nd ed. Philadelphia, WB Saunders, 1991.)

Table 2-11. Differentiation of Classical Bacterial Pneumonia from Viral and Atypical Pneumonias*

	Bacterial	Viral/Atypical
History	Precedent URI	Headache, malaise, URI, myalgias
Course	Often biphasic illness	Often monophasic
Onset	Sudden	Gradual
Temperature	High fever	Low-grade fever
Rigors	Common	Uncommon
Vital signs	Tachypnea, tachycardia	Less toxic
Pain	Pleuritic	Unusual
Chest examination	Crackles, signs of consolidation	Consolidation unusual
Sign of pleural effusion	Common	Uncommon
Sputum	Productive, purulent, many PMNs, one dominant organism on Gram stain	Scant, no organisms; PMNs or mononuclear cells
ESR	Elevated	Usually normal
WBC count	15,000–25,000; left shift	Often normal; predominant lymphocytes
Chest radiography	Lobar consolidation, round infiltrate, parapneumonic effusion; may be "bronchopneumonia"	Diffuse, bilateral, patchy, interstitial or bronchopneumonia; lower lobe involvement common; chest film may look worse than patient's condition
Progression	May be rapid	Rapid if *Legionella* species, hantavirus, SARS, herpesvirus, adenovirus
Diagnosis	Blood, sputum, and pleural fluid specimens for culture; antigen detection possible; BAL if progressive	Viral, chlamydial culture or antigen detection; acute and convalescent titers; BAL if progressive

*Atypical pneumonias include *Chlamydia pneumoniae, Mycoplasma pneumoniae, Legionella* species (*L. pneumophila, L. micdadei*), Q fever, psittacosis.

BAL, bronchoalveolar lavage; ESR, erythrocyte sedimentation rate; PMNs, polymorphonuclear neutrophils; SARS, severe acute respiratory syndrome; URI, upper respiratory tract infection; WBC, white blood cell.

Table 2-12. Causes of Infectious Pneumonia

Bacterial

Common

Streptococcus pneumoniae	See Table 2-11
Group B streptococci	Neonates
Group A streptococci	See Table 2-11
*Mycoplasma pneumoniae**	Adolescents; summer-fall epidemics
*Chlamydia pneumoniae**	Adolescents (see Table 2-11)
Chlamydia trachomatis	Infants
Mixed anaerobes	Aspiration pneumonia
Gram-negative enteric	Nosocomial pneumonia

Uncommon

Haemophilus influenzae type B	See Table 2-11
Staphylococcus aureus	Pneumatoceles; infants
Moraxella catarrhalis	
Neisseria meningitides	
Francisella tularensis	Animal, tick, fly contact
Nocardia species	Immunosuppressed persons
*Chlamydia psittaci**	Bird contact
Yersinia pestis	Plague
Legionella species*	Exposure to contaminated water; nosocomial

Viral

Common

Respiratory syncytial virus	See Table 2-11
Parainfluenza types 1-3	Croup
Influenza A, B	High fever; winter months
Adenovirus	Can be severe; often occurs between January and April

Viral *(continued)*

Uncommon

Rhinovirus	Rhinorrhea
Enterovirus	Neonates
Herpes simplex	Neonates
Cytomegalovirus	Infants, immunosuppressed persons
Measles	Rash, coryza, conjunctivitis
Varicella	Adolescents
Hantavirus	Southwestern United States
SARS agent	Asia

Fungal

Histoplasma capsulatum	Geographic region; bird, bat contact
Cryptococcus neoformans	Bird contact
Aspergillus species	Immunosuppressed
Mucormycosis	Immunosuppressed
Coccidioides immitis	Geographic region
Blastomyces dermatitides	Geographic region

Rickettsial

*Coxiella burnetii**	Q fever, animal (goat, sheep, cattle) exposure
Rickettsia rickettsiae	Tick bite

Mycobacterial

Mycobacterium tuberculosis	See Table 2-14
Mycobacterim avium–intracellulare	Immunosuppressed persons

Parasitic

Pneumocystis carinii	Immunosuppressed, steroids
Eosinophilic	Various parasites (e.g., Ascaris *Strongyloides* species)

*Atypical pneumonia syndrome (see Table 2–11); atypical in terms of extrapulmonary manifestations, low-grade fever, patchy diffuse infiltrates, poor response to penicillin-type antibiotics, and negative sputum Gram stain.

SARS, severe acute respiratory syndrome.

Table 2-13. Differentiation of Pleural Fluid

	Transudate	Exudate	Complicated Empyema
Appearance	Clear	Cloudy	Purulent
Cell count	<1000	>1000	>5000
Cell type	Lymphocytes, monocytes	PMNs	PMNs
LDH	<200 U/L	>200 U/L	>1000 U/L
Pleural/serum LDH ratio	<0.6	>0.6	>0.6
Protein >3 g	Unusual	Common	Common
Pleural/serum protein ratio	<0.5	>0.5	>0.5
Glucose*	Normal	Low	Very low* (<40 mg/dL)
pH*	Normal (7.40–7.60)	7.20-7.40	<7.20, chest tube placement required
Gram stain	Negative	Usually positive	>85% positive unless patient received prior antibiotics

*Low glucose or pH may be seen in malignant effusion, tuberculosis, esophageal rupture, pancreatitis (positive pleural amylase), and rheumatologic diseases (e.g., systemic lupus erythematosus).

LDH, lactate dehydrogenase; PMNs, polymorphonuclear neutrophils.

extrapulmonary symptoms (i.e., sore throat, myalgias, headache, fever), which then progress to include worsening cough, paroxysmal at times. Patients do not often appear acutely ill, but cough may persist for weeks. There may be no specific abnormalities on the chest examination, although a few crackles may be heard, and about one third of younger patients wheeze.

The radiographic findings in mycoplasmal pneumonia can mimic almost any intrathoracic disease; scattered infiltrates with non-specific "dirty" lung fields, predominantly perihilar or lower lobes, are common, and lobar infiltrates and pleural effusion are occasionally seen. Laboratory data (complete blood cell count, ESR, sputum culture) may not be helpful. A rise in antimycoplasmal immunoglobulin G over 1 to 2 weeks may be demonstrated but is seldom helpful in guiding therapy. A positive immunoglobulin M response may be useful, although it can persist in serum for several months and, consequently, may not indicate current infection. PCR may be helpful. The cold agglutinin test yields positive results in about 70% of patients with mycoplasmal pneumonia, but they are also positive in other conditions, including adenovirus infection. The more severe the illness is, the greater is the frequency of positive cold agglutinins. The diagnosis is often made from the history of an older child who has a lingering coughing illness in the setting of a community outbreak, unresponsive to most (non-erythromycin) antibiotic regimens.

Treatment is with erythromycin (azithromycin or clarithromycin are alternatives in children younger than 8 years, whereas tetracycline or doxycycline can be administered to older children), which usually shortens the course of the illness. Extrapulmonary complications of mycoplasmal infection include aseptic meningitis, transverse myelitis, peripheral neuropathy, erythema multiforme, myocarditis, pericarditis, hemolytic anemia, and bullous otitis media (myringitis). In patients with sickle cell anemia, severe respiratory failure and acute chest syndrome may develop. Infection with *Chlamydia pneumoniae* mimics respiratory disease resulting from *M. pneumoniae*, inasmuch as it occurs in epidemics, is seen in older children, and produces an atypical pneumonia syndrome and pharyngitis.

Tuberculosis

The incidence of tuberculosis is increasing as a result of acquired immunodeficiency syndrome, homelessness, urban poverty, and immigration from endemic countries. Tuberculosis must be considered in the child with chest disease that is not easily explained by other diagnoses, especially if the child has been exposed to an adult with active tuberculosis. Nonetheless, tuberculosis is an infrequent cause of cough in children, even in those with active disease.

The diagnosis is made primarily by skin testing (purified protein derivative [PPD]); a history of contact with a person who has tuberculosis; and recovery of the organism from sputum, bronchoalveolar lavage, pleural fluid or biopsy, or morning gastric aspirates (Table 2-14). The yield from these procedures is relatively low, even from children with active pulmonary tuberculosis.

The patterns of disease in normal hosts include primary pulmonary tuberculosis, with subsequent inactivation usually noted in young children and reactivation pulmonary disease among adolescents. Primary pulmonary disease is often noted as a lower or middle lobe infiltrate during the period of T lymphocyte reaction to the initial infection. Before resolution, the *Mycobacterium tuberculosis* infection may disseminate to the better oxygenated upper lobes and extrathoracic sites, such as bone, or the central nervous system. If the immune response contains the initial infection, the radiographic

Table 2-14. Definitions of Positive Tuberculosis (TB) by Mantoux Skin Test (5 TU)*

Cutaneous Induration ≥ 5 mm

Close exposure to known or suspected active TB
Chest radiograph consistent with TB (old or active)
Clinical evidence of TB
Immunosuppressed children (with HIV, taking corticosteroids, with lymphoma, with Hodgkin disease)

Cutaneous Induration ≥ 10 mm

Age < 4 yr of age
Medical *high risks* (chronic renal failure, malnutrition, diabetes mellitus)
High-risk social environment (incarcerated youth, homeless persons, intravenous drug users, medically indigent, migrant workers, nursing home residents, immigrants from regions with TB)

Cutaneous Induration ≥ 15 mm

All children ≥ 4 yr of age without any identifiable risk

Data from American Academy of Pediatrics: Tuberculosis. In Pickering LK, (ed): 2003 *Red Book: Report of the Committee on Infectious Diseases,* 26th ed. Elk Grove Village, Ill, American Academy of Pediatrics, 2003, p 643.

*BCG vaccination status not relevant.

BCG, bacille Calmette-Guérin; HIV, human immunodeficiency virus; TU, tuberculin units.

findings may be indistinguishable from those of any other pneumonic process. With altered immune function, however, there may be progressive local disease, dissemination to miliary pulmonary disease, or early reactivation (months to 5 years) at distal sites, which produces tuberculous meningitis or osteomyelitis. Reactivation of upper lobe pulmonary disease may produce cavities that are similar to the disease among adults. Cavitary and endobronchial lymph node involvement are highly infectious, in contrast to the much less contagious nature of the hypersensitivity reaction noted in primary pulmonary disease.

Treatment of active disease, especially in regions of multidrug-resistant tuberculosis, consists of three or four drug regimens, including isoniazid, rifampin, pyrazinamide with or without streptomycin, and ethambutol. Risk of infection based on history and PPD induration size are presented in Table 2-14.

ASPIRATION

Inhaling food, mouth or gastric secretions, or foreign bodies into the tracheobronchial tree causes acute, recurrent, or chronic cough. Interference with normal swallowing disrupts the coordination of swallowing and breathing that prevents aspiration. Structural causes of disordered swallowing include esophageal atresia (in neonates), strictures, webs, or congenital stenoses. Mediastinal lesions (tumors, lymph nodes), including vascular rings, may compromise the esophageal lumen and esophageal peristalsis, increasing the likelihood of aspiration. Functional disorders include central nervous system dysfunction (e.g., coma, myopathy, neuropathy) or immaturity, dysautonomia, achalasia, and diffuse esophageal spasm. Prior neck surgery, including tracheostomy, may alter normal swallowing. Tracheoesophageal fistula and laryngeal clefts are congenital malformations with direct physical connections between the tracheobronchial tree and the upper gastrointestinal tract; oral contents enter the lungs directly.

Making the diagnosis of aspiration as the cause of cough may be difficult. Barium contrast studies during swallowing may help characterize these disorders if barium enters the trachea. Because most patients aspirate sporadically, a normal barium swallow does not rule out aspiration. Radionuclide studies can be helpful if ingested radiolabeled milk or formula is demonstrated over the lung fields at several-hour intervals after the meal. Bronchoscopy and bronchoalveolar lavage that recover large numbers of lipid-laden macrophages suggest that milk aspiration has taken place; however, the finding is neither sensitive nor specific for aspiration.

Treatment depends largely on the cause of aspiration. Because many patients who aspirate do so because of lack of neurologic control of swallowing and breathing, it is often difficult to prevent. Even gastrostomy feedings cannot prevent aspiration of oral secretions. In extreme cases, tracheostomy with ligation of the proximal trachea has been employed. This prevents aspiration but also prevents phonation, and it must be considered only in unusual situations. Aspiration pneumonia is often treated with intravenous penicillin or, preferably, clindamycin to cover mouth flora of predominant anaerobes. Additional coverage against gram-negative organisms (an aminoglycoside or cefepime) may be indicated if the aspiration is nosocomial.

FOREIGN BODY

Any child with cough of abrupt onset should be suspected of having inhaled a foreign body into the airway. Toddlers, who by nature put all types of things into their mouths and who have incompletely matured swallowing and airway protective mechanisms, are at high risk. Infants with toddlers or young children in the household who may "feed" the baby are also at risk. In older children, it is usually possible to obtain an accurate history of the aspiration event. These events are described as choking, gagging, and coughing while

something (e.g., peanuts, popcorn, small toys, sunflower seeds) is in the mouth. The child may come to the physician with cough and wheeze immediately after the event, with a clear history and a straightforward diagnosis. In many children with a tracheobronchial foreign body, however, the initial episode is not recognized; these children may not come to medical attention for days, weeks, or even months (Fig. 2-9). The initial episode may be followed by a relatively symptomless period lasting days or even weeks, until infection develops behind an obstructed segmental or lobar bronchus. At this point, cough, perhaps with hemoptysis, with or without wheeze, recurs.

On physical examination early after an aspiration episode, there is cough, wheeze, or both, often with asymmetry of auscultatory findings. There may be locally diminished breath sounds. Later, localized wheeze or crackles may be detected. In some cases, the two-headed stethoscope may enable the examiner to recognize that a lobe or lung has delayed air entry or exit in comparison with the other side. The triad of wheezing, coughing, and decreased breath sounds is present in fewer than 50% of patients. The presence of laryngotracheal foreign bodies often manifests with stridor, retractions, aphonia, cough, and normal radiographs.

Chest radiographs may be normal in 15% of patients with intrathoracic foreign bodies but should be obtained in both inspiration and expiration, because in some cases the only abnormality is unilateral or unilobar air trapping, which is occasionally more clearly identified with a view in expiration. In this view, an overdistended lung that had appeared normal on the inspiratory view does not empty, but the normal, unobstructed lung empties normally. This phenomenon causes a shift of the mediastinum toward the emptying lung (away from the side with the obstructing foreign body). In other patients, localized infiltrate or atelectasis may be present behind the obstructing object. In a few patients, it may be possible to identify the foreign body itself; nonetheless, most inhaled food particles are not radiopaque and cannot be seen on radiographs. Aspiration is usually unilateral (80%); 50% to 60% of the objects are in the right lung (the lobe depends on body position-supine versus standing-but is often the right middle lobe). The definitive diagnostic and therapeutic maneuver is bronchoscopy; either the flexible or rigid open-tube bronchoscope enables direct visualization of the object; the rigid instrument also enables its removal.

GASTROESOPHAGEAL REFLUX

GER is a common cause of cough in all age groups (see Chapter 16). The typical patient is an infant in the first 6 months of life who spits up small amounts of milk frequently after feedings. This "regurgitant reflux" most commonly resolves by 1 year of age. However, many toddlers and children continue to have reflux, although it may be "silent" or nonregurgitant (without spitting up).

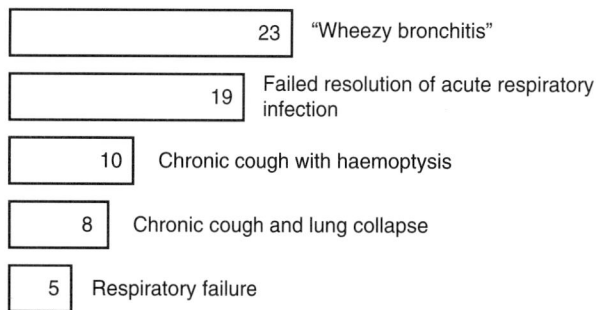

23	"Wheezy bronchitis"
19	Failed resolution of acute respiratory infection
10	Chronic cough with haemoptysis
8	Chronic cough and lung collapse
5	Respiratory failure

Figure 2-9. *Presenting problems in children who aspirated foreign bodies in whom diagnosis was delayed over 1 month and the number of children with each problem. (From Phelan PD, Olinsky A: Respiratory Illness in Children. Oxford, United Kingdom, Blackwell, 1994.)*

In most people with GER, it is merely a nuisance or not noticed. In some there are sequelae, and this condition is designated *gastroesophageal reflux disease* (GERD). One manifestation is cough; the mechanisms for the cough are not fully understood. Aspiration of refluxed material is one mechanism for cough but is probably not very common in neurologically intact children. A major mechanism for GERD with cough is mediated by vagal esophagobronchial reflexes (bronchoconstriction), stimulated by acid in the esophagus. Whether acid in the esophagus is sufficient stimulus to cause bronchoconstriction by itself or whether it merely heightens bronchial reactivity to other stimuli is not yet clear (see Chapter 3). Many children with reactive airways disease have cough or wheeze that is difficult to control until their concurrent GER is also treated. Many episodes of cough caused by GERD occur in children with asthma that is difficult to control.

The diagnosis of GERD must also be considered in the child with chronic or recurrent cough with no other obvious explanation. The child who coughs after meals or at night, when the supine position may provoke GER, should be evaluated for GER. If GER is confirmed, the next step is a therapeutic trial of antireflux therapy (see Chapter 16). If the results of the therapeutic trial are negative or equivocal, it may make sense to establish a causal relationship between the GER and the cough, by using the modified Bernstein test. During this test, hydrochloric acid and saline are alternately infused into the esophagus through a nasoesophageal tube while the child is observed for cough or wheeze or while the older child undergoes serial pulmonary function tests. If the symptoms occur or if pulmonary function deteriorates during acid but not saline infusion, it is likely that esophageal acidification through GER is the cause of the child's cough or wheeze.

Treatment in a child whose cough is related to GER may be accomplished by treating the reflux (see Chapter 16) or by a combination of antireflux and antiasthma treatment (see Chapter 3). Theophylline may worsen GER by lowering the tone of the lower esophageal sphincter, and some drugs that increase lower esophageal sphincter tone may cause bronchoconstriction. On occasion, the cough may be abolished by stopping all antiasthma medications. In such cases, the cough was a manifestation of reactive airways with esophageal acidification as the trigger for bronchospasm; the esophageal acidification was caused by the bronchodilator effects on the lower esophageal sphincter. Inhaled bronchodilators are less likely than oral or intravenous drugs to cause GER.

REACTIVE AIRWAYS DISEASE (ASTHMA)

Cough is frequently the sole or most prominent manifestation of asthma; wheezing may be entirely absent. In fact, reactive airway disease or asthma (see Chapter 3) is almost certainly the most common cause of recurrent and chronic cough in childhood. Some of the features that characterize the cough of a child with asthma are listed in Table 2-15. Treatment for asthma manifesting as cough is the same as the treatment for asthma (see Chapter 3).

CYSTIC FIBROSIS

CF is a common cause of recurrent or chronic cough in infancy and childhood. CF occurs in 1 in 2500 live births among white persons, is far less common among African Americans (1 in 17,000), and is rare among Native Americans and Asians. Early diagnosis improves the poor prognosis for untreated CF; if untreated, many patients die in infancy or early childhood. With current state-of-the-art care, median length of survival is to age 31.

CF is a genetic disorder, inherited as an autosomal recessive trait. The CF gene is on the long arm of chromosome 7; more than 1000 mutations have been identified at the CF locus. Of these mutations, one (ΔF508, indicating a deletion, Δ, of a single phenylalanine, F, at position 508 of the protein product) is the most common, responsible

Table 2-15. Reactive Airways Disease (Asthma) as a Cause of Cough: History
Any age (even infants)
Coexistence of allergy increases likelihood, but absence of allergy does not decrease likelihood
Wheeze need not be present
↑Cough with upper respiratory infections
↑Cough with (and especially after) exercise
↑Cough with hard laughing or crying
↑Cough with exposure to cold
↑Cough with exposure to cigarette smoke
Usually a history of dramatic response to inhaled β agonists
May not have responded to oral β agonists

for 70% to 75% of all CF chromosomes. The currently recognized mutations account for approximately 90% of cases. The mutation affects the gene's protein product, termed *cystic fibrosis transmembrane regulator*, which acts as a chloride channel and affects other aspects of membrane transport of ions and water. Not all the consequences of the defective gene and protein have been determined. Most explain the long-observed clinical manifestations of the disease, including thick, viscid mucus in the tracheobronchial tree, leading to purulent bronchiolitis and bronchitis with subsequent bronchiectasis, pulmonary fibrosis, and respiratory failure; pancreatic duct obstruction, leading to pancreatic insufficiency with steatorrhea and failure to thrive; and abnormally high sweat chloride and sodium concentrations. The airway disease in CF is characterized by infection, inflammation, and endobronchial obstruction. The infection begins with *S. aureus, H. influenzae, Escherichia coli, Klebsiella* species, or combinations of these organisms but eventually is dominated by nonmucoid or mucoid *Pseudomonas aeruginosa*. Other organisms, such as *Burkholderia cepacia, Xanthomonas maltophilia, Alcaligenes xylosoxidans, Aspergillus fumigatus*, or nontuberculous mycobacteria may also appear; their significance remains undetermined. In some patients, *B. cepacia* has been associated with rapid deterioration and death, and in others, *Aspergillus* species has caused allergic bronchopulmonary aspergillosis. The airway inflammation in all patients with CF appears to be the result of toxic substances, including elastase, released by neutrophils as they respond to the endobronchial infection and by similar enzymes released by the invading organisms.

CF may manifest at birth with meconium ileus (10% to 15% of patients) or later, with steatorrhea and failure to thrive despite a voracious appetite, in an apparent effort to make up for the calories that are lost in the stool (see Chapter 15). The most common presenting symptom is cough, which may appear within the first weeks of life or may be delayed for decades. The cough can be dry, productive, or paroxysmal. Cough may respond to antibiotics or perhaps steroids, but it is less likely to improve with bronchodilators (see Tables 2-3 and 2-5). Although CF is a genetic disease, there is often no family history. Furthermore, in atypical cases, patients may not have pancreatic insufficiency (usually present in 85% to 90%) and thus may not demonstrate steatorrhea and failure to thrive. In addition, malabsorption may not be evident in the neonatal period.

There is no such thing as a child who looks "too good" to have CF; common abnormalities found on physical examination are noted in Table 2-16. One of the most important physical findings is digital clubbing. In most patients with CF, clubbing develops within the first few years of life. Although the list of conditions associated with digital clubbing (Table 2-17) is long, they are less common than CF, or the incidence of digital clubbing with these conditions is low. There is some relationship between the degree of pulmonary disease severity and the degree of digital clubbing. A child who has had years of severe respiratory symptoms without digital clubbing is not likely to have CF.

Table 2-16. Physical Examination Features of Cystic Fibrosis

General
  Low weight for height (>50% of patients)
Head, eyes, ears, nose, and throat
  Nasal polyps (20%)
Chest
  Cough
  Barrel chest (↑ anteroposterior diameter)
  Intercostal, suprasternal retractions
  Crackles, especially upper lobes
  Wheeze
Abdomen
  Hepatomegaly (10%)
  Right lower quadrant fecal mass (5%-10%)
Extremities
  Digital clubbing (80%)
Reproductive tract
  Bilateral atresia or absence of vas deferens (>95% of males)

The diagnosis is confirmed by a positive sweat test or confirming the presence of two CF mutations on chromosome 7. The sweat test, if not performed correctly in a laboratory with extensive experience with the technique (as, for example, in an accredited CF center), yields many false-positive and false-negative results. The proper technique is to use the Gibson-Cooke method, with quantitative analysis of the concentration of sodium, chloride, or both, in the sweat produced after pilocarpine iontophoretic stimulation. Chloride (and sodium) concentrations higher than 60 mEq/L are considered positive indications, and those lower than 40 mEq/L are negative (normal). Healthy adults have slightly higher sweat chloride concentrations than do children, but the same guidelines hold for positive tests in adults. The non-CF conditions yielding elevated sweat chloride concentrations are listed in Table 2-18. False-negative results of sweat tests can be seen in CF children presenting with edema or hypoproteinemia and in samples from children with an inadequate sweat rate. Sweat testing can be performed at any age; newborns within the first few weeks of life may not produce a large enough volume of sweat to analyze (75 mg minimum), but in those who do (the majority), the results are accurate. Indications for sweat testing are noted in Table 2-19.

In patients for whom sweat testing is difficult (e.g., because of distance from an experienced laboratory, small infants who have not produced enough sweat, patients with extreme dermatitis, or patients with intermediate-range sweat chloride concentrations), DNA testing can be useful. Demonstration of two known CF mutations confirms the diagnosis. Finding one or no known mutation makes the diagnosis less likely but is not exclusive, inasmuch as there are patients with not-yet-characterized mutations. Furthermore, commercial laboratories do not identify all of the 1000-plus mutations.

Recovery of mucoid *P. aeruginosa* from respiratory tract secretions is strongly suggestive of CF. Similarly, pansinusitis is nearly universal among CF patients but is quite uncommon in other children. Some states are using a neonatal screen for CF. The CF screen is for immunoreactive trypsinogen (IRT) levels, which are elevated in most infants with CF for the first several weeks of life. (Some states do genetic testing on DNA.) Because of the very high sensitivity of this test (almost no one with CF has normal IRT levels) and because early institution of treatment is beneficial, this test may come into wider use. Its main drawback is that it has relatively poor specificity; as many as 90% of the positive results on the initial screen are false-positive results. If an infant's IRT screen is positive, the test should be repeated; at 2 to 3 weeks of age, which is when the test is repeated, the false-positive rate has fallen dramatically but is

---

Table 2-17. Causes of Digital Clubbing in Children

Pulmonary
Cystic fibrosis ++
Non–cystic fibrosis bronchiectasis +
Ciliary dyskinesia
Bronchiolitis obliterans
Empyema
Lung abscess
Malignancy
Tuberculosis
Mesothelioma
Pulmonary arteriovenous fistula

Cardiac
Cyanotic congenital heart disease ++
Subacute bacterial endocarditis +
Chronic congestive heart disease

Gastrointestinal
Crohn disease
Ulcerative colitis
Celiac disease +
Severe gastrointestinal hemorrhage
Small bowel lymphoma
Multiple polyposis

Hepatic
Biliary cirrhosis
Chronic active hepatitis

Hematologic
Thalassemia
Congenital methemoglobinemia

Miscellaneous
Familial
Thyroid deficiency
Thyrotoxicosis
Chronic pyelonephritis
Heavy metal poisoning
Scleroderma
Lymphoid granulomatosis
Hodgkin disease
Human immunodeficiency virus

++, very common cause of digital clubbing; +, common cause of digital clubbing.

Table 2-18. Conditions Other than Cystic Fibrosis with Elevated Sweat Electrolytes

Adrenal insufficiency (untreated)
Ectodermal dysplasia
Autonomic dysfunction
Hypothyroidism
Malnutrition, including psychosocial dwarfism
Mucopolysaccharidosis
Glycogen storage disease (type I)
Fucosidosis
Hereditary nephrogenic diabetes insipidus
Mauriac syndrome
Pseudohypoaldosteronism
Familial cholestasis
Nephrosis with edema

Table 2-19. Indications for Sweat Testing

Pulmonary Indications

Chronic or recurrent cough
Chronic or recurrent pneumonia (especially RUL)
Recurrent bronchiolitis
Atelectasis
Hemoptysis
Staphylococcal pneumonia
Pseudomonas aeruginosa in the respiratory tract (in the absence of such circumstances as tracheostomy or prolonged intubation)
Mucoid *P. aeruginosa* in the respiratory tract

Gastrointestinal Indications

Meconium ileus
Neonatal intestinal obstruction (meconium plug, atresia)
Steatorrhea, malabsorption
Hepatic cirrhosis in childhood (including any manifestations such as esophageal varices or portal hypertension)
Pancreatitis
Rectal prolapse
Vitamin K deficiency states (hypoprothrombinemia)

Miscellaneous Indications

Digital clubbing
Failure to thrive
Family history of cystic fibrosis (sibling or cousin)
Salty taste when kissed; salt crystals on skin after evaporation of sweat
Heat prostration, especially under seemingly inappropriate circumstances
Hyponatremic hypochloremic alkalosis in infants
Nasal polyps
Pansinusitis
Aspermia

From Kercsmar CM: The respiratory system. In Behrman RE, Kliegman RM (eds): Nelson Essentials of Pediatrics, 2nd ed. Philadelphia, WB Saunders, 1994, p 451.

RUL, right upper lobe.

Table 2-20. Complications of Cystic Fibrosis

Pulmonary Complications

Bronchiectasis, bronchitis, bronchiolitis, pneumonia
Atelectasis
Hemoptysis
Pneumothorax
Nasal polyps
Sinusitis
Reactive airways disease
Cor pulmonale
Respiratory failure
Mucoid impaction of the bronchi
Allergic bronchopulmonary aspergillosis

Gastrointestinal Complications

Meconium ileus
Meconium peritonitis
Distal intestinal obstruction syndrome (meconium ileus equivalent) (nonneonatal obstruction)
Rectal prolapse
Intussusception
Volvulus
Appendicitis
Intestinal atresia
Pancreatitis
Biliary cirrhosis (portal hypertension: esophageal varices, hypersplenism)
Neonatal obstructive jaundice
Hepatic steatosis
Gastroesophageal reflux
Cholelithiasis
Inguinal hernia
Growth failure
Vitamin deficiency states (vitamins A, D, E, K)
Insulin deficiency, symptomatic hyperglycemia, diabetes

Other Complications

Infertility
Edema/hypoproteinemia
Dehydration/heat exhaustion
Hypertrophic osteoarthropathy/arthritis
Delayed puberty
Amyloidosis

From Kercsmar CM: The respiratory system. In Behrman RE, Kliegman RM (eds): Nelson Essentials of Pediatrics, 2nd ed. Philadelphia: WB Saunders, 1994, p 451.

still quite high (25%). Definitive testing needs to be carried out on infants with two elevated IRT levels. In the unusual older child whose appendix is removed and examined carefully by a knowledgeable pathologist, the diagnosis may be suggested by the typical histologic appearance of the appendix (the mucus-secreting glands are overdistended with eosinophilic material).

Laboratory data that may support the diagnosis of CF include absence of stool trypsin or chymotrypsin. This suggests pancreatic insufficiency, which occurs most commonly in CF but can be seen in other diseases. The test is not perfect even for confirming pancreatic insufficiency, because intestinal flora may produce or destroy trypsin. Pulmonary function test findings with an obstructive pattern, incompletely responsive to bronchodilators, are consistent with CF but, of course, can be seen in other conditions. Conversely, some patients with CF also have asthma and may show a marked response to a bronchodilator. Complications of CF that should suggest the diagnosis are noted in Table 2-20.

The treatment of patients with CF requires a comprehensive approach, best performed in, or in conjunction with, an approved CF center. Several studies have shown survival to be significantly better in center-based care than in non–center-based care.

The treatment of the pulmonary aspects of CF involves approaching the obstruction, infection, and inflammation that cause the cough. Cough should be monitored closely, and any increase in frequency or in the intensity should be taken as an indication that there is worsening endobronchial infection, inflammation, or both. Because active

infection and inflammation lead to irreversible lung damage, such changes need to be taken seriously and treated aggressively. This is just as true for the appearance of a mild morning cough in the child who was previously cough free as it is for severe coughing spells that keep a child awake through the night.

Obstruction is treated with physical means (chest physical therapy, with percussion, vibration, and postural drainage) to dislodge the mucus into the large central airways, where cough can then effectively clear it. Studies have shown this rather crude and time-consuming procedure to be effective in helping to maintain lung function acutely and over a period of years. Variations on the physical maneuvers to help with mucus clearance include forced expiratory technique, positive airway pressure face masks, and masks with expiratory flutter valves. The frequency with which any of these physical means of expelling mucus should be used varies but should be increased with signs of active infection and obstruction.

Other approaches to relieving obstruction in the bronchial tree include the use of inhaled bronchodilators (despite a paucity of studies showing their long-term efficacy) and mucolytic agents.

N-acetylcysteine (Mucomyst) has been available for years, but it may cause tracheobronchial irritation, with bronchorrhea, bronchospasm, or both, in an unacceptably high proportion of patients. An inhaled drug, dornase alfa, or recombinant human DNase (Pulmozyme), is clearly effective in the test tube for liquefying the thick mucus associated with CF. This occurs because 40% of the mucus viscosity in CF is attributed to DNA released from dying polymorphonuclear cells. Another drug that appears promising is amiloride. Long available as a diuretic, amiloride can bring about a partial correction of the membrane transport defects in CF. Amiloride aerosols seem to decrease sputum viscosity and increase cough clearance. In a small 6-month study, aerosolized amiloride appeared to slow the decline in lung function.

The approach to endobronchial infection in children with CF includes prevention and treatment. Prevention involves immunizing patients with CF against preventable respiratory pathogens, particularly influenza, measles, and pertussis. Prevention also means avoiding unnecessary exposure to respiratory viruses (e.g., at day care centers). It should not mean avoiding school or other social functions and settings, because this approach is invariably futile and can cause severe emotional damage. However, spread of bacteria, especially resistant organisms such as *B. cepacia*, between patients is a concern.

Treatment of infection usually proceeds in a stepwise manner. If colonies of *H. influenzae* or *S. aureus* are present, appropriate antibiotics should be initiated. If no recent throat or sputum specimens for culture are available, and if the patient is young with very mild lung disease, empirical therapy can also be directed at those organisms. In the older or sicker patient who has any sign of chronic pulmonary involvement, such as pulmonary overinflation, infiltrates on a chest film, digital clubbing, or severe coughing spells, it makes sense to include antibiotics effective against *P. aeruginosa* (Fig. 2-10; Table 2-21).

Treatment of the inflammation associated with CF is evolving. Some patients benefit from short-term oral prednisone. A 4-year study of alternate-day prednisone showed improved pulmonary function but unacceptable side effects (e.g., glucose intolerance, growth failure) in those taking 2 mg/kg/day and similar side effects (although less severe) in those taking 1 mg/kg/day. The beneficial role of oral nonsteroidal antiinflammatory agents has been demonstrated; the role of inhaled topical steroids and α1-antitrypsin is being investigated.

ANATOMIC ABNORMALITIES

Table 2-22 lists the main anatomic abnormalities (most of them congenital) that cause cough.

Vascular Rings and Slings

Vascular rings and slings are often associated with inspiratory stridor because the abnormal vessels compress central airways, most commonly the trachea (see Chapter 5). The patient may also have difficulty swallowing if the esophagus is compressed.

The diagnosis may be suspected from plain films of the chest, especially those showing tracheal deviation and a right-sided aortic arch. Further support for the diagnosis can be found at bronchoscopy (which shows extrinsic compression of the trachea or a mainstem bronchus), barium swallow study (which shows esophageal compression), or both. The definitive diagnosis is made with magnetic resonance imaging, angiography, or magnetic resonance angiography. Treatment is surgical.

Pulmonary Sequestration

Pulmonary sequestration is relatively unusual, occurring in 1 in 60,000 children. It occurs most commonly in the left lower lobe and

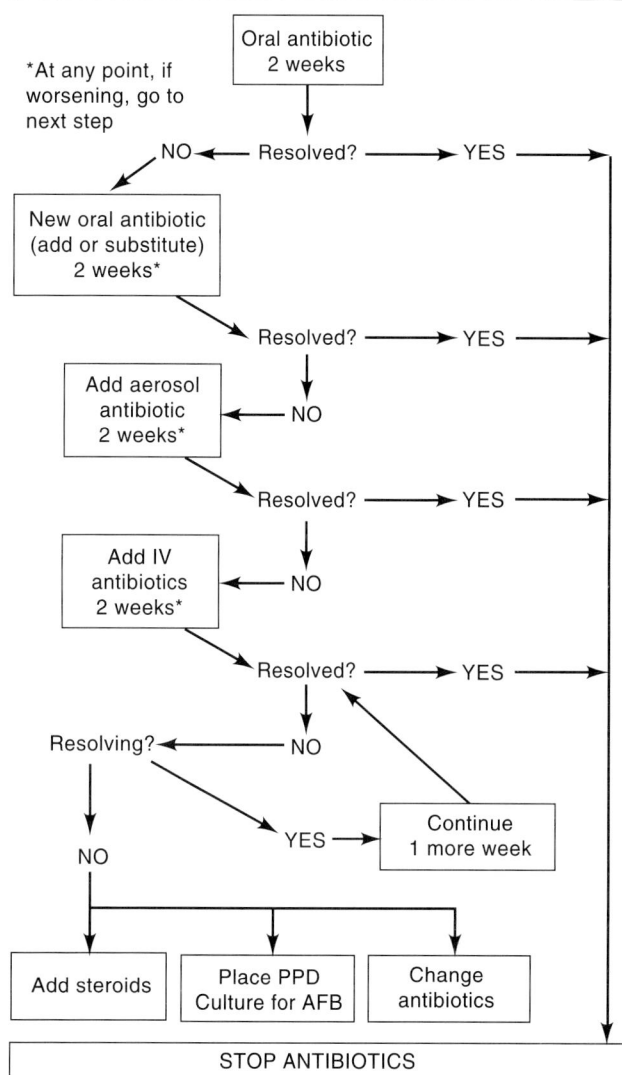

Figure 2-10. Stepwise therapeutic approach to increased cough in patients with cystic fibrosis and airway colonization with *Pseudomonas aeruginosa*. AFB, acid-fast bacillus; IV, intravenous; PPD, purified protein derivative.

can manifest in several ways (Fig. 2-11; see Table 2-22). The chest radiograph usually shows a density in the left lower lobe; this density often appears to contain cysts. The feature distinguishing a sequestered lobe from a complicated pneumonia is that the blood supply arises from the aorta and not the pulmonary circulation. Doppler ultrasonography and angiography provide the definitive diagnosis. The treatment is surgical removal.

Cystic Adenomatoid Malformation

Cystic adenomatoid malformation is a rare condition. It manifests in infancy with respiratory distress in nearly 50% of cases; the other half may manifest as cough with recurrent infection later in childhood or even adulthood. The chest film reveals multiple cysts, separated by dense areas. Chest CT scans can help make the diagnosis with near certainty. Surgical removal is the treatment.

Table 2-21. Antibiotic Treatment of Cough in Cystic Fibrosis

Route	Organism	Agent	Dosage (mg/kg/24 hr)	Doses Per 24 Hours	Cost* ($) for 2 Weeks	Comments
Oral	*Staphylococcus aureus*	Cloxacillin	50–100	3–4	22	
		Clindamycin	20	3–4	93	
		Clarithromycin	15	2	77	Less gastrointestinal upset than erythromycin
		Erythromycin	50–100	2–4	12	Gastrointestinal upset common
		Amoxicillin/ clavulanate	40	3	105	
	Haemophilus influenzae	Amoxicillin	50–100	3	19	
		Trimethoprim- sulfamethoxazole	10–20	2–3	29	Dose based on trimethoprim
		Chloramphenicol	50–100	3–4	64	Bone marrow suppression
	Pseudomonas aeruginosa	Ciprofloxacin	15–30	2	141	Not for young children
		Ofloxacin	20	2	98	Also active against *Staphylococcus* species
	Empirical	Tetracycline	50–100	3–4	5	Not for children <12 yr
		Doxycycline	2.5–5.0	1–2	88	Total dose, 50–100 mg b.i.d.
		Chloramphenicol	50–100	3–4	64	Also active against *Staphylococcus* species
Intravenous	*S. aureus* *P. aeruginosa*	Oxacillin	150–200	4	665	
		Gentamicin or tobramycin	8–20	1–3	78	Nephrotoxicity, ototoxicity; doses based on serum levels
		Amikacin	15–30	2–3	1380	Nephrotoxicity, ototoxicity; doses based on serum levels
		Netilmicin	6–12	2–3	392	Nephrotoxicity, ototoxicity; doses based on serum levels
		Carbenicillin	250–450	4–6	495	Large sodium load
		Ticarcillin	250–450	4–6	653	Large sodium load
		Piperacillin	250–450	4–6	1171	Sodium < carbohydrate, ticarcillin
		Mezlocillin	250–450	4–6	883	
		Azlocillin	250–450	4–6	—	
		Ticarcillin/ clavulanate	250–450	4–6	730	Also active against *Staphylococcus* species
		Imipenem/ cilistatin	45–90	3–4	1881	Nausea with infusion
		Ceftazidime	150	3	1195	
		Aztreonam	200	4	1544	
Aerosol	*P. aeruginosa*	Gentamicin or tobramycin (TOBI)	—	2–4	43–186	80–600 mg/dose
		Colistin	—	2–4	960	75–150 mg/dose in saline
		Carbenicillin	—	2–4	77	500 mg–1 g; strong odor
		Ceftazidime	—	2–4	597	May foam

Modified from Boat TF: Cystic fibrosis. In Behrman RE, Kliegman RM, Nelson WE, Vaughn VC (eds): Nelson Textbook of Pediatrics, 14th ed. Philadelphia, WB Saunders, 1992, p 1113.

*Costs are for an intermediate dose and for drug alone (no delivery devices).

Congenital Lobar Emphysema

Congenital lobar emphysema occurs in one of 50,000 live births. It can manifest dramatically with respiratory distress in the neonatal period or later (Fig. 2-12), with cough or wheeze, or as an incidental finding on a chest radiograph. Radiography shows localized overinflation, often dramatic, with compression of adjacent lung tissue and occasionally atelectasis of the contralateral lung because of mediastinal shift away from the involved side. The appearance on chest CT scan is typical, with widely spaced blood vessels (as opposed to congenital cysts, for example, which have no blood vessels within the overinflated area). Bronchoscopy can document patent bronchi and should probably be performed in older children, in whom congenital lobar emphysema can be confused with acquired overinflation of a lobe as the result of bronchial obstruction, as with a foreign body. If the disease is symptomatic, treatment is surgical.

Tracheoesophageal Fistula

Tracheoesophageal fistula is common, with an incidence of about one in 5000 live births. Of these fistulas, the large majority (85%) are associated with esophageal atresia; only 3% are the isolated, H-type fistula (a patent esophagus with fistulous tract connecting the esophagus and trachea). A neonate with esophageal atresia experiences respiratory distress, excessive drooling, and choking and gagging with feeding. The H-type fistula causes more subtle signs and may be undiagnosed for months or even years. The child may have only

Table 2-22. Anatomic Abnormalities Causing Cough

Condition	Other Symptoms	Diagnostic Evidence	Treatment
Vascular ring/sling	Stridor; dysphagia, emesis	Radiographic: deviated trachea, right-sided arch Barium swallow: esophageal indentation Bronchoscopy: extrinsic compression MRI/angiography: definitive	Surgical
Pulmonary sequestration	Fever, dyspnea; may be asymptomatic	Radiographic: left lower lobe density, usually with cysts Angiography: blood supply from aorta	Surgical
Cystic adenomatoid malformation	Respiratory distress; recurrent infection	Radiographic: multiple cysts alternating with solid areas CT: typical appearance	Surgical
Congenital lobar emphysema	Respiratory distress; wheeze; may be asymptomatic	Radiographic: localized overinflation, other lobes (even other lung) collapsed CT: typical pattern Bronchoscopy in older patients to rule out foreign body	Surgical (if symptomatic)
Tracheoesophageal fistula, cleft	Gagging, choking with feeds; respiratory distress (especially with esophageal atresia)	Barium swallow: barium in tracheobronchial tree Bronchoscopy: direct visualization	Surgical
Airway hemangioma	Stridor; wheeze; dysphagia; hemoptysis	Bronchoscopy	Steroids; laser; interferon-α; occasionally tracheostomy required
Mediastinal lymph nodes	Stridor	Radiographic: hilar nodes; compressed tracheal air column	Treat cause
Bronchial stenosis	Wheeze; recurrent pneumonia	Bronchoscopy	Balloon dilatation; surgery
Bronchogenic cysts	Wheeze, stridor	Radiographic: hyperinflation of one lung; visible mass (carina, posterior mediastinum) Bronchoscopy: extrinsic compression CT: often definitive	Surgical

CT, computed tomography; MRI, magnetic resonance imaging.

intermittent feeding trouble, especially with liquids. There may be recurrent lower respiratory tract infections.

The diagnosis is not challenging in the infant with esophageal atresia; a nasogastric tube cannot be passed, and swallowed barium outlines the trachea. In the older child with H-type fistula, a barium esophagogram may or may not reveal the fistula. Bronchoscopy and esophagoscopy should permit direct visualization of the fistula; however, the opening may be hidden in mucosal folds.

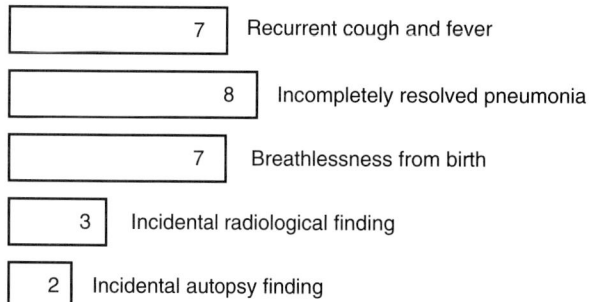

7	Recurrent cough and fever
8	Incompletely resolved pneumonia
7	Breathlessness from birth
3	Incidental radiological finding
2	Incidental autopsy finding

Figure 2-11. Different modes of presentation of sequestered lobe and number of children with each problem. (From Phelan PD, Olinsky A: *Respiratory Illness in Children.* Oxford, United Kingdom, Blackwell, 1994.)

Treatment is surgical. Many children born with tracheoesophageal fistula have recurrent cough and lower respiratory tract infection for many years, even after successful surgical correction. The cough is characteristically the harsh cough of tracheomalacia, which is present at the site of the fistula. The infections result from several causes, including GER, with or without aspiration, and altered mucociliary transport. Treatment involves regular chest physical therapy and early and aggressive use of antibiotics whenever there is evidence of increased pulmonary symptoms.

Hemangiomas

Hemangiomas may be present within the airway and can cause cough, rarely with hemoptysis; stridor (if the hemangioma is high in the airway) and respiratory distress (if the hemangioma is large) may also occur. In rare cases, with very large airway hemangiomas, there may even be dysphagia from extrinsic compression. About 50% of children with airway hemangiomas have cutaneous hemangiomas as well.

The diagnosis is made with bronchoscopy. As with cutaneous hemangiomas, these lesions may resolve spontaneously over the first year or so. However, if they cause symptoms, it may not be advisable or possible to wait for them to resolve.

Many airway hemangiomas regress with steroid treatment, although others have been shown to respond to interferon-α. Laser ablation may be indicated in some refractory cases. In the case of a

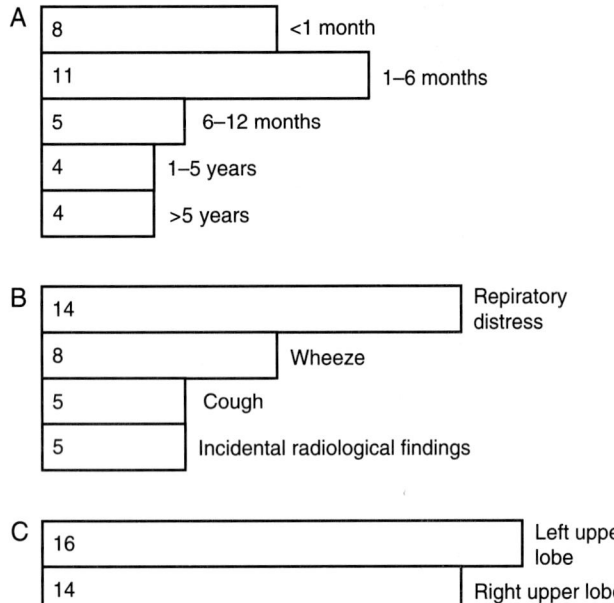

Figure 2-12. Different modes of presentation of congenital lobar emphysema. **A,** Age at presentation. **B,** Symptoms at presentation. **C,** Involved lobe. Numbers refer to the number of children in each category. (From Phelan PD, Olinsky A: Respiratory Illness in Children. Oxford, United Kingdom, Blackwell, 1994.)

Table 2-23. Intrathoracic Mass Lesions
Anterior Mediastinum
Thymus tumor
T cell lymphoma
Teratoma
Thyroid lesions
Pericardial cyst
Hemangioma
Lymphangioma
Hilar–Middle Mediastinum
Tuberculosis
Histoplasmosis
Coccidioidomycosis
Acute lymphocytic leukemia/lymphoma
Hodgkin disease
Sarcoidosis
Hiatal hernia
Pericardial cyst
Bronchogenic or enteric cyst
Posterior Mediastinum
Neuroblastoma/ganglioneuroma
Other neural tumors
Neuroenteric lesions
Esophageal lesions (duplication)
Vertebral osteomyelitis
Diaphragmatic hernia
Meningocele
Aortic aneurysm

---

large subglottic hemangioma, a tracheostomy is frequently performed and maintained until the mass regresses.

Enlarged Lymph Nodes

Enlarged mediastinal lymph nodes, such as those resulting from tuberculosis, leukemia, other hematologic malignancies, or other infections, are occasionally a cause of cough in children (Tables 2-22 and 2-23). These nodes are usually seen on plain films of the chest. The x-ray study or bronchoscopy may show extrinsic compression of the trachea. Treatment is directed at the underlying cause.

Bronchial Stenosis

Occasionally bronchial stenosis, either congenital or acquired, may cause cough. The diagnosis is made with bronchoscopy, after suspicion has been raised by the child's having recurrent infiltrates in the same lobe, especially with localized wheeze.

Treatment may be difficult. In some cases, endoscopic balloon dilatation or airway stent placement is successful; in others, surgical resection of stenotic areas may be necessary.

Bronchogenic Cysts

Bronchogenic cysts are uncommon, but they can cause cough, wheeze, stridor, or any combination of these. They may also cause recurrent or persistent pneumonia if they block a bronchus sufficiently to interfere with normal drainage of the segment or lobe. Radiography may show localized overinflation if the cyst causes a ball-valve–type obstruction. The cyst itself may or may not be seen on plain films. Bronchoscopy reveals extrinsic compression of the airway. CT studies often definitively show the lesion. Surgical removal is indicated.

HABIT (PSYCHOGENIC) COUGH

On occasion, a school-aged child may develop a cough that lasts for weeks, often after a fairly typical cold. This cough occurs only during wakefulness, never during sleep. In many cases, the cough is harsh and foghorn-like. It often disrupts the classroom, and the child is asked to leave. The child is otherwise well and may seem rather unbothered by the spectacle created. There has been no response to medications. It seems that this type of cough, often termed "psychogenic," or "psychogenic cough tic," but perhaps more accurately and humanely thought of as habit cough, has given the child valuable attention. This attention then serves as the sustaining force, and the cough persists beyond the original airway inflammation. In the small minority of cases, there may be deep-seated emotional problems, of which the cough is the physical expression.

During the history or physical examination, the child appears completely well and may cough when attention is drawn to the child or when the word "cough" is uttered. The physical examination findings are otherwise completely normal, as are laboratory values. Because this may occur in any child, evidence of mild reactive airways disease (history or pulmonary function testing) does not rule out the diagnosis. Once a physician has seen a child with this problem, it is usually possible to make the diagnosis with certainty on entering the examining room or, indeed, from the hallway outside the room.

Treatment can prove more difficult. There are several treatment schools, summarized in Tables 2-24 and 2-25. One approach is "the bed sheet," in which the child is told that he or she coughs because of weak chest muscles. A bed sheet is wrapped tightly and uncomfortably around the chest "to serve as added support for the muscles … [and] with this support, the muscles would then be able to suppress [the] cough." The child is to go to school wearing the bulky bed sheet under his or her clothes and may not remove the sheet until he or she is certain that the cough will not return. The authors who describe this method call it a "reinforcement suggestion technique." Some

Table 2-24. Therapeutic Approaches to Habit Cough

Approach	Advantages	Disadvantages
Perform all possible tests	Can tell patient and family: "We've ruled out all physical problems." In one study, resolution followed bronchoscopy ("aversive stimulus"?)	Reinforces the idea of a physical cause
Apply an aversive stimulus (e.g., an electric shock to forearm)	Has worked in some patients	By definition, this treatment is unpleasant
Try the "bed sheet" (see text)	Seems to work in most patients	Demeans the patient
Try placebo drugs	Probably works in some patients	Is a dishonest technique
Provide psychotherapy	May work in some patients	Is unnecessary in most patients; labels the patient as having a psychological problem
Gently explain that there is no physical cause and this is a habit that the body has sustained	Works in some patients	Is resented by some families focused on an organic cause or treatment
Prevent mouth breathing by holding a button between the patient's lips	Has worked in some patients	Not known
Apply speech therapy techniques (see Table 2–25)	Works in many patients: can be presented as specific therapy; nonthreatening	Is resented by some families focused on organic cause or treatment

view this approach as demeaning to the child. Whatever its mechanism of action, this method was reported to have been successful in 31 of 33 patients.

OTHER CAUSES OF COUGH

Table 2-26 lists several miscellaneous causes of cough in children.

Postnasal Drip

Postnasal drip is thought to be a major cause of cough in adults. The mechanism by which this occurs is unclear, and most pulmonologists believe that this must remain a diagnosis of exclusion for explaining cough in children.

Bronchiectasis

Bronchiectasis is defined as an abnormal dilation of the subsegmental bronchi and is usually associated with chronic cough and purulent sputum production. It occasionally occurs after severe pneumonias (bacterial or viral); it eventually develops in nearly all patients with CF. Diagnosis may, on occasion, be made with plain chest radiographs, but high-resolution CT scanning is the diagnostic procedure of choice, replacing bronchography. Treatment of bronchiectasis consists of chest physiotherapy and postural drainage, occasionally bronchodilators and mucolytic agents, and antibiotic therapy during exacerbations. Surgical resection may be indicated in cases that are progressive and localized when medical therapy has failed. The

prognosis of bronchiectasis depends on the underlying cause. Bronchiectasis associated with CF is fatal, although many cases of bronchiectasis remain stable or may even regress with therapy.

Ciliary Dyskinesia

Conditions in which the cilia do not function properly (dysmotile cilia or ciliary dyskinesia) lead to cough, usually because infection (and bronchiectasis) occurs in the absence of normal mucociliary transport. Treatment is similar to that for CF, with regular chest physical therapy and frequent and aggressive use of antibiotics at the first sign of airways infection, most commonly increased cough.

Interstitial Lung Disease

There are several varieties of interstitial lung disease: desquamative, lymphoid, and "usual" (see Chapter 3). All are very uncommon in childhood, and little is known about their causes, courses, or treatment. One type of pediatric interstitial lung disease, the lymphoid type, is becoming much more common, inasmuch as it is seen in human immunodeficiency virus (HIV) infection. Interstitial lung disease manifests with cough, dyspnea, and crackles on examination. Because the diagnosis is based on histologic findings, lung biopsy is required. The only exception to this may be in the child with documented acquired immunodeficiency syndrome who has new pulmonary infiltrates and symptoms, in whom bronchoscopy and bronchoalveolar lavage are initially used to diagnose infection (*P. carinii*, cytomegalovirus).

Interstitial lung disease in a patient with a chronic seborrhea-like dermatitis should suggest the diagnosis of histiocytosis X.

Heart Failure

Heart failure can cause cough but seldom as its sole clinical manifestation.

Pulmonary Hemosiderosis

Pulmonary hemosiderosis is a rare, and often fatal, condition of bleeding into the lung that can manifest with cough. If sputum is produced, it is often frothy and blood-tinged. There may be frank hemoptysis. However, the cough may be nonproductive, or the sputum may be swallowed. Some cases are associated with milk

Table 2-25. Speech Therapy Techniques for Treating Habit Cough

Increase abdominal breathing
Reduce muscle tension in neck, chest, and shoulders
Interrupt early cough sensation by swallowing
Substitute gentle cough for racking cough
Interrupt cough sequence with diaphragm breathing and tightly pursed lips
Increase the patient's awareness of initial sensations that would trigger cough

Table 2-26. Miscellaneous Causes of Cough in Children

Postnasal drip (?)	Cerumen impaction
Bronchiectasis	Irritation of external auditory canal
Ciliary dyskinesia	Obliterative bronchiolitis
Interstitial lung disease	Follicular bronchiolitis
Heart failure/pulmonary edema	Mediastinal disease (nodes, pneumomediastinum)
Pulmonary hemosiderosis	Nasal polyps
Drug-induced (see Table 2-4)	Hypersensitivity pneumonitis (extrinsic allergic alveolitis)
α_1-antitrypsin deficiency	Thyroid lesions
Graft-versus-host disease	Subphrenic abscess
Bronchopulmonary dysplasia	Sarcoidosis
Tumor (bronchial adenoma, carcinoid; mediastinal)	Anaphylaxis
Alveolar proteinosis	Pulmonary embolism
Tracheomalacia, bronchomalacia	Lung contusion
Spasmodic croup	

hypersensitivity (Heiner syndrome), and affected children may have upper airway obstruction. Some cases are associated with collagen vascular disorders. Radiographs usually show diffuse fluffy infiltrates, and there is invariably iron deficiency anemia. The diagnosis is based on lung biopsy findings.

Treatment is often unsatisfactory; the mortality rate is as high as 50%. Milk products should be eliminated from the patient's diet, and underlying collagen vascular disease should be treated. Some affected children seem to respond to corticosteroids or cytotoxic drugs (e.g., azathioprine, cyclophosphamide, and chlorambucil), but the episodic nature of the disease, with some clear cases of spontaneous resolution, makes it difficult to evaluate therapies.

Bronchopulmonary Dysplasia

See Chapter 3.

Tumors

Tumors, which fortunately are rare in childhood, can cause cough, usually because of bronchial blockage, either extrinsic or endobronchial (see Table 2-23). The diagnosis is usually made from bronchoscopy, chest CT, or both. Treatment depends on the cell type, but it usually involves at least some surgical removal. Chemotherapy or radiation may be used in some cases.

Tracheomalacia and Bronchomalacia

Isolated tracheomalacia or bronchomalacia is uncommon but can cause cough in some children. The cough of tracheomalacia is typically harsh and brassy. Treatment is difficult but, fortunately, is seldom needed.

Spasmodic Croup

Some children, usually preschoolers, may episodically awaken at night with stridor and a harsh, barking cough indistinguishable from that of viral croup. This entity is termed *spasmodic croup* and is of unclear origin. Viral and allergic causes have been postulated. GER may be the cause in some patients.

Treatment with cool mist or racemic epinephrine is effective in most patients. If GER is the underlying cause, antireflux treatment is beneficial.

Obliterative Bronchiolitis

Obliterative bronchiolitis is very rare except in lung transplant recipients. In other instances, it may arise after adenovirus, measles, or influenza pneumonia; after exposure to certain toxins; or in other rare circumstances. Children may exhibit cough, respiratory distress, and exercise intolerance.

The diagnosis is suggested by the pulmonary function or radiographic evidence of small airways obstruction; however, these findings are not always present. Not all chest films show overinflated lungs, and not all pulmonary function tests show decreased small airways function.

The definitive diagnosis is histologic via open or transbronchial biopsy. No specific treatment is available. Most children with obliterative bronchiolitis recover, but many progress to chronic disability or death.

HEMOPTYSIS

The child who coughs out blood or bloody mucus presents special diagnostic and therapeutic challenges. Although hemoptysis is relatively uncommon in children, particularly among those without CF, many conditions can cause it (Table 2-27). It is important (and not always easy) to distinguish cases in which blood has originated in the tracheobronchial tree (true hemoptysis), the nose (*epistaxis*), and the gastrointestinal tract (*hematemesis*). Table 2-28 gives some guidelines to help localize sites of origin of blood that has been reported or suspected as hemoptysis. None of these is foolproof, partly because blood that has originated in one of these sites might well end in another before being expelled from the body; for instance, blood from the nose can be swallowed and vomited or aspirated and coughed out.

Infection is among the most common causes of hemoptysis. Lung abscess and tuberculosis need to be considered. Bronchiectasis can readily cause erosion into bronchial vessels, often made tortuous by years of local inflammation, and produce hemoptysis. Other infectious settings are less common and include necrotizing pneumonias and fungal and parasitic lung invasion.

Foreign bodies in the airway can cause hemoptysis by direct irritation, by erosion of airway mucosa, or by secondary infection.

Pulmonary embolus is uncommon in children and adolescents, but it needs to be considered in the differential diagnosis of an adolescent with hemoptysis of unclear origin. Clues to the diagnosis of pulmonary embolus include a positive family history, severe dyspnea, chest pain, hypoxia, a normal chest film, an accentuated second heart sound, an abnormal compression ultrasonographic study of the leg veins, a positive Homans sign, a positive helical CT scan, and a high-probability lung ventilation-perfusion scan.

The diagnosis of several causes of hemoptysis is straightforward. For example, hemoptysis that occurs immediately after a surgical or invasive diagnostic procedure in the chest should suggest an iatrogenic problem. The chest film can help suggest lung abscess, pulmonary

Table 2-27. Hemoptysis: Differential Diagnosis

Infection	Lung abscess	Pulmonary	Idiopathic or with milk allergy (Heiner
	Pneumonia*	hemosiderosis	syndrome)
	Tuberculosis	Trauma	Contusion*
	Bronchiectasis* (cystic fibrosis, ciliary dyskinesia)		Fractured trachea, bronchus
	Necrotizing pneumonia	Iatrogenic	After surgery
	Fungus (especially allergic bronchopulmonary aspergillosis or mucormycosis)		After transbronchial lung biopsy*
			After diagnostic lung puncture*
		Tumors	Benign (neurogenic, hamartoma, hemangioma, carcinoid)
	Parasite		
	Herpes simplex		Malignant (adenoma, bronchogenic carcinoma)
Foreign body	Retained		
Congenital defect	Heart (various)		Metastatic (Wilms tumor, osteosarcoma, sarcoma)
	Primary pulmonary hypertension		
	Eisenmenger syndrome	Pulmonary	Cardiogenic
	Abnormal arteriovenous connections	embolus	Deep venous thrombosis
	Arteriovenous malformation	Other	Factitious
	Telangiectasia (Osler-Weber-Rendu)		Endometriosis
	Pulmonary sequestration		Coagulopathy*
	Bronchogenic cyst		Congestive heart failure
Autoimmune-	Henoch-Schönlein purpura		After surfactant therapy in neonates
inflammatory	Goodpasture syndrome		Kernicterus
	Wegener granulomatosis		Hyperammonemia
	Systemic lupus erythematosus		Intracranial hemorrhage
	Sarcoidosis		Epistaxis*
			Idiopathic

*A common cause of hemoptysis.

sequestration, bronchogenic cyst, or tumor. Chest CT can help with cases of arteriovenous malformations, and additional laboratory values can support the diagnosis of collagen-vascular disease. Bronchoscopy can sometimes localize a bleeding site, identify a cause (e.g., a foreign body or endobronchial tumor), or recover an offending bacterial, fungal, or parasitic pathogen. In many instances, bronchoscopy does not help except by excluding some possibilities, because either no blood or blood throughout the tracheobronchial tree is found. Bronchial artery angiography may help to identify the involved vessel or vessels.

Treatment of hemoptysis depends on the underlying cause. It can be a terrifying symptom to children and their parents, and a calm, reassuring approach is essential. Because hemoptysis is seldom fatal in children, reassurance is usually warranted. Furthermore, hemoptysis most often resolves, and treatment of the bleeding itself is not often needed. What is required is treatment of the underlying cause of the hemoptysis, such as therapy for infection, removal of a foreign body, or control of collagen-vascular disease. When death occurs from hemoptysis, it is more likely to be from suffocation than from exsanguination. In cases of massive bleeding, the rigid open-tube bronchoscope may help suction large amounts of blood while ventilating and keeping unaffected portions of lung clear of blood. Interventional radiologists treat as well as localize a bleeding site by injecting the offending vessel with occlusive substances, such as Gelfoam or silicone coils. In extremely rare instances, emergency lobectomy may be indicated.

WHEN COUGH ITSELF IS A PROBLEM

Cough itself seldom necessitates specific treatment. Nonetheless, cough is not always completely benign (see Table 2-9). Most complications are uncommon, and most accompany only very severe cough, but some are serious enough to justify treatment of the cough itself.

Cough suppressants include codeine and hydrocodone (two narcotics) and dextromethorphan (a nonnarcotic D-isomer of the codeine analogue of levorphanol). Such agents should be used only for severe cough that may produce significant complications (see Table 2-9). For most diseases, suppressing the cough offers no advantage. Disadvantages include narcotic addiction and loss of the protective cough reflex with subsequent mucus retention and possible superinfection. Demulcent preparations (sugar-containing, bland soothing agents) temporarily suppress the cough response from pharyngeal sources, and decongestant-antihistamine combinations may reduce postnasal drip and thus cough in adults.

Table 2-28. Hemoptysis: Differentiating Sites of Origin of Blood

	Pulmonary	Gastrointestinal Tract	Nose
Hisory	Cough, with or without gurgling in lung before episode	Nausea, vomiting, pain	With or without nosebleed dripping in back of throat
Physical	Cough; localized crackles or decreased breath sounds; digital clubbing	↑ Liver, spleen, epigastric tenderness	Blood in nose

Table 2-29. Cough: Red Flags and When to Refer

If associated with severe, acute
  Hemoptysis
  Dyspnea
  Hypoxemia
If associated with chronic
  Failure to thrive
  Steatorrhea
  Decreased exercise tolerance
  Digital clubbing
Persistence of
  Cough for 6 weeks or more
  Radiographic abnormality, especially if asymmetric
Failure to respond to empirical therapy
  Antibiotics for presumed infection
  Bronchodilators for presumed reactive airways

SUMMARY: RED FLAGS AND WHEN TO REFER

Cough is important because it is a symptom and sign of underlying disease that frequently merits treatment. In the acute setting, severe disease, including massive hemoptysis or profound dyspnea or hypoxemia, warrants immediate attention, rapid diagnosis, and rapid management. Certain chronic conditions, including those that suggest CF and those in which symptoms have persisted and interfere with a child's daily activities and quality of life, warrant further evaluation and treatment. Finally, a child whose cough fails to respond to what should have been reasonable treatment should be referred to a pulmonary specialist (Table 2-29).

REFERENCES

Cough

Black P: Evaluation of chronic or recurrent cough. In Hilman BC (ed): Pediatric Respiratory Disease: Diagnosis and Treatment. Philadelphia, WB Saunders, 1993, pp 143-154.
Cohlan S, Stone E: The cough and the bedsheet. Pediatrics 1984;74:11-15.
Irwin RS, Boulet LP, Cloutier MM, et al: Managing cough as a defense mechanism and as a symptom. A consensus panel report of the American College of Chest Physicians. Chest 1998;114(2, Suppl):133S-181S.

Upper Respiratory Infection

Donnelly BW, McMillan JA, Weiner LB: Bacterial tracheitis: Report of eight new cases and review. Rev Infect Dis 1990;12:729-735.
Gwaltney JM, Phillips CD, Miller RD, et al: Computed tomographic study of the common cold. N Engl J Med 1994;330:25-30.
Turner RB: Epidemiology, pathogenesis, and treatment of the common cold. Ann Allergy Asthma Immunol 1997;78:531-539.
Williams JW, Simel DL: Does this patient have sinusitis? Diagnosing acute sinusitis by history and physical examination. JAMA 1993;270:1242-1246.

Pneumonia

American Academy of Pediatrics: [Tuberculosis]. In Pickering LK (ed): 2003 Red Book: Report of the Committee on Infectious Diseases, 26th ed. Elk Grove Village, Ill, American Academy of Pediatrics, 2003, pp 642-660.
Bourke SJ: Chlamydial respiratory infections. BMJ 1993;306:1219-1220.
Brasfield DM, Stagno S, Whitley RJ, et al: Infant pneumonitis associated with cytomegalovirus, *Chlamydia, Pneumocystis,* and *Ureaplasma:* Follow-up. Pediatrics 1987;79:76-83.
Gibson NA, Hollman AS, Paton JY: Value of radiological follow-up of childhood pneumonia. BMJ 1993;307:117.
McCracken GH Jr: Etiology and treatment of pneumonia. Pediatr Infect Dis J 2000;19:373-377.

McIntosh K, Halonen P, Ruuskanen O: Report of a workshop on respiratory viral infections: Epidemiology, diagnosis, treatment, and prevention. Clin Infect Dis 1993;16:151-164.
Meduri GU, Stein DS: Pulmonary manifestations of acquired immunodeficiency syndrome. Clin Infect Dis 1992;14:98-113.
Mulholland EK, Simoes EAF, Costales MOD, et al: Standardized diagnosis of pneumonia in developing countries. Pediatr Infect Dis 1992;11:77-81.
Nohynek H, Eskola J, Laine E, et al: The causes of hospital-treated acute lower respiratory tract infection in children. Am J Dis Child 1991;145:618-622.
Onyango FE, Steinhoff MC, Wafula EM, et al: Hypoxaemia in young Kenyan children with acute lower respiratory infection. BMJ 1993;306:612-614.
Rubin BK: The evaluation of the child with recurrent chest infections. Pediatr Infect Dis 1985;4:88-98.
Smith KC: Tuberculosis in children. Curr Probl Pediatr 2001;31:1-30.

Foreign Bodies

Black RE, Choi K-J, Syme WC: Bronchoscopic removal of aspirated foreign bodies in children. Am J Surg 1984;148:778-781.
Friedman EM: Tracheobronchial foreign bodies. Otolaryngol Clin North Am 2000;33:179-185.
Gay BB, Atkinson GO, Vanderzalm T, et al: Subglottic foreign bodies in pediatric patients. Am J Dis Child 1986;140:165-168.
Puhakka H, Svedstrom E, Kero P, et al: Tracheobronchial foreign bodies. Am J Dis Child 1989;143:543-545.

Cystic Fibrosis

Hamos A, Corey M: The cystic fibrosis genotype-phenotype consortium. Correlation between genotype and phenotype in patients with cystic fibrosis. N Engl J Med 1993;329:1308-1316.
Jaffe A, Bush A, Geddes DM, et al: Prospects for gene therapy in cystic fibrosis. Arch Dis Child 1999;80:286-289.
Kerem E, Reisman J, Corey M, et al: Prediction of mortality in patients with cystic fibrosis. N Engl J Med 1992;326:1187-1191.
Kerem E, Reisman J, Corey M, et al: Wheezing in infants with cystic fibrosis: Clinical course, pulmonary function, and survival analysis. Pediatrics 1992;90:703-706.
Prasad SA, Tannenbaum EL, Mikelsons C: Physiotherapy in cystic fibrosis. J R Soc Med 2000;93(Suppl):27-36.
Ranasinha C, Assoufi B, Shak S, et al: Efficacy and safety of short-term administration of aerosolised recombinant human DNase I in adults with stable stage cystic fibrosis. Lancet 1993;342:199-202.
Rosenstein BJ, Cutting GR: The diagnosis of cystic fibrosis: A consensus statement. Cystic Fibrosis Foundation Consensus Panel. J Pediatr 1998;132:589-595.
Rubin BK: Emerging therapies for cystic fibrosis. Chest 1999;115:1120-1126.
Taylor RFH, Gaya H, Hodson ME: *Pseudomonas cepacia:* Pulmonary infection in patients with cystic fibrosis. Respir Med 1993;87:187-192.

Asthma

Agertoft L, Pederson S: Effect of long-term treatment with inhaled budesonide on adult height in children with asthma. N Engl J Med 2000;343:1064-1069.
Castro-Rodriguez JA, Holberg CJ, Wright AL, et al: A clinical index to define risk of asthma in young children with recurrent wheezing. Am J Respir Crit Care Med 2000;162:1403-1406.
Palmer LJ, Rye PJ, Gibson NA, et al: Airway responsiveness in early infancy predicts asthma, lung function, and respiratory symptoms by school age. Am J Respir Crit Care Med 2001;163:37-42.
Suissa S, Ernst T, Benayoun S, et al: Low-dose inhaled corticosteroids and the prevention of death from asthma. N Engl J Med 2000;343:332-336.
Warner JO, Naspitz CK: Third International Pediatric Consensus Statement on the Management of Childhood Asthma. International Pediatric Asthma Consensus Group. Pediatr Pulm 1998;25:1-17.

Hemoptysis

David M, Andrew M: Venous thromboembolic complications in children. J Pediatr 1993;123:337-346.
Jean-Baptiste E: Clinical assessment and management of massive hemoptysis. Crit Care Med 2000;28:1642-1647.
Jones DK, Davies RJ: Massive haemoptysis: Medical management will usually arrest the bleeding. BMJ 1990;300:889-890.
Panitch HB, Schidlow DV: Pathogenesis and management of hemoptysis in children. Int Pediatr 1989;4:241-244.

3 Respiratory Distress

Carolyn M. Kercsmar   Thomas Ferkol

Respiratory distress occurs for a variety of reasons and with many levels of severity. *Dyspnea,* the sensation of difficult, labored, or uncomfortable breathing, may arise from an increase in work of breathing caused by a change in respiratory drive, impaired neuromuscular reserve, or increased ventilatory demand, which in turn may be caused by an altered metabolic state. True respiratory distress arises when there is impaired air exchange that leads to decreased ventilation and oxygenation. Physical findings typically associated with respiratory distress include dyspnea, tachypnea, stridor, cough, and wheezing. Respiratory failure ensues if the respiratory efforts and ventilation/perfusion ratios are inadequate for maintaining arterial oxygen saturation and carbon dioxide (CO_2) clearance necessary to provide appropriate tissue oxygenation and maintenance of blood pH. In general, an arterial oxygen pressure (PaO_2) of less than 50 mm Hg (hypoxemia) while a person is breathing room air and an arterial carbon dioxide pressure ($PaCO_2$) level greater than 50 mm Hg (hypercapnia) suggest respiratory failure. The causes of acute respiratory distress are legion, but they often can be identified by considering the associated clinical findings, the history and setting of symptoms, and the age of the patient (Table 3-1).

THE PULMONARY EXAMINATION

HISTORY

An appropriate medical history is important in the child with acute respiratory distress (see also Chapter 2). The chief complaint provides insight into the nature of the distress (i.e., cough, wheezing, stridor, dyspnea, or chest pain); some indication of the onset and duration of symptoms should be obtained. Data regarding prodrome, exacerbating or ameliorating factors, history of trauma, previous occurrence of similar symptoms, and response to any therapy should be sought. Past medical history of neonatal events (prematurity), previous endotracheal intubation, recurrent infections, hospitalizations, and gagging or choking episodes may provide valuable information. A family history of asthma and allergies, travel, and environmental exposure (e.g., smoking, pets, or irritants) may uncover etiologic clues. Finally, a review of systems with regard to systemic signs and symptoms associated with respiratory disease, such as fever, weight loss, night sweats, or dysphagia, is useful.

PHYSICAL EXAMINATION

The physical examination begins with measurement of vital signs, with attention paid to respiratory rate, heart rate, and blood pressure. Tachypnea is often the most prominent manifestation of respiratory distress caused by airway obstruction or parenchymal lung disease. Age-dependent normal values for resting respiratory rates are listed in Table 2-7. A resting respiratory rate higher than 40 breaths per minute in an infant younger than 1 year or higher than 30 breaths per minute in an older child is abnormal.

Inspection

Inspection of the patient should focus on skin color, level of consciousness, presence of nasal flaring, grunting, use of accessory muscles of respiration, chest wall symmetry, and respiratory excursion. Altered mental status (either agitation or somnolence) may be indicative of severe respiratory distress, hypoxemia, and/or hypercapnia. The presence of grunting, nasal flaring, chest wall retractions, and the use of accessory muscles of respiration, particularly the strap muscles of the neck, all suggest airway obstruction. Cyanosis suggests severe hypoxemia.

Palpation

Palpation of the chest wall and cervical region may enable the examiner to detect the presence of subcutaneous emphysema indicative of pulmonary air leak. A hyperresonant note during percussion of the chest wall indicates hyperinflation, whereas dullness to percussion suggests atelectasis, pulmonary consolidation, or pleural effusion.

Auscultation

Auscultation of the chest should focus on identifying the degree of air exchange and the presence, timing, and symmetry of adventitious breath sounds. Air entry should be evaluated over all discrete anatomic locations bilaterally. Homologous segments of each lung should be examined sequentially to compare similar areas. The presence of adventitious sounds should be determined next (Table 3-2). The most commonly encountered sounds are wheezing, stridor (a subclass of wheezing), crackles, and rhonchi.

- Crackles (previously called "rales") are intermittent, low- or higher pitched, largely inspiratory noises that are produced by the opening of airways closed during the previous expiration.
- Wheezing is a continuous, high-pitched musical noise, similar to a hiss or whistle.
- Rhonchi are also continuous sounds that are lower pitched and more rumbling or sonorous.
- Stridor, a type of wheezing, is harsher, often localized over the central intrathoracic airways or trachea, and predominates in inspiration.

Determination of the timing (inspiration, expiration, or biphasic) and distribution of the adventitious sounds offers clues as to the site of airway involvement. For example, wheezing that is continuous and heard equally over both lung fields is likely to arise from above the tracheal bifurcation, whereas late inspiratory crackles may emanate from the smaller airways. Unilateral or very localized wheezing or decreased breath sounds suggest segmental airway obstruction, such as that found with retained foreign body aspiration, mucus plugging, or atelectasis (Fig. 3-1).

Table 3-1. Age-Related Causes of Respiratory Distress

Cause	Preterm Neonate	Full-Term Neonate	Infant-Toddler	Child	Adolescent
Common	RDS	Meconium aspiration pneumonia	Afebrile pneumonia[4]	Pneumonia[7]	Pneumonia[9]
	Congenital pneumonia[1]	Congenital heart disease	Pneumonia[5]	Asthma	Asthma
	Nosocomial pneumonia[2]	Transient tachypnea	Aspiration[6]	Cystic fibrosis	Sickle cell acute chest crisis
	BPD	Persistent fetal circulation	Croup (infectious, spasmodic)	Sickle cell acute chest crisis	Tonsillitis
	Congenital heart disease (cyanotic, heart failure, or both)	Congenital pneumonia	Bronchiolitis (RSV)	Aspiration[6]	Peritonsillar abscess
	Pneumothorax		Cystic fibrosis	Tonsillitis	Cystic fibrosis
	Transient tachypnea		Laryngotracheomalacia		Panic attack
			Asthma		
Uncommon	Congenital anomalies[3]	Pneumothorax	Congenital anomalies	ARDS	ARDS
	Pulmonary hemorrhage	Congenital anomalies[3]	Epiglottitis	Anaphylaxis	Spontaneous pneumothorax
	Pneumopericardium	Pneumopericardium	Near drowning	Interstitial lung disease[8]	Pulmonary embolism
	Vocal cord paralysis	Polycythemia	Pulmonary hemosiderosis	Hemoptysis	Drug-induced[10]
	Pulmonary hypoplasia	Vocal cord paralysis	Pulmonary hemorrhage	Retropharyngeal abscess	Interstitial lung disease[8]
		Pleural effusions	Retropharyngeal abscess	Near drowning	Collagen vascular disease[11]
		Severe anemia	Trauma	Hydrocarbon aspiration	Hypersensitivity pneumonitis[12]
		Pulmonary hypoplasia	Hydrocarbon aspiration	Trauma	Allergic bronchopulmonary aspergillosis
		Surfactant protein deficiency	Smoke inhalation (burn)	Pulmonary fibrosis	Alveolar proteinosis
		Pulmonary lymphangiectasia	Airway hemangioma	Desquamating interstitial pneumonia	Trauma
			Papilloma of vocal cords	Pulmonary alveolar proteinosis	Anaphylaxis
			Bacterial tracheitis	Smoke inhalation (burn)	Smoke inhalation (burn)
			Heart failure	HIV associated[14]	Scoliosis
			HIV associated[14]		Bronchiectasis
					Mediastinal mass[13]
					Hemoptysis
					HIV associated[14]

[1]Congenital pneumonia = group B streptococcus, *Escherichia coli, Listeria monocytogenes,* herpes simplex; possible *Ureaplasma urealyticum* and *Mycoplasma hominis.*

[2]Nosocomial pneumonia = *Staphylococcus epidermidis, Staphylococcus aureus, Candida albicans, Klebsiella, Pseudomonas aeruginosa,* adenovirus, RSV.

[3]Congenital anomalies = tracheoesophageal fistula; choanal atresia; tracheal web-stenosis-atresia-cleft; diaphragmatic hernia; eventration of the diaphragm; cystic adenomatoid malformation; lobar emphysema; cleft palate–macroglossia (Pierre Robin syndrome); thyroid goiter; pulmonary hypoplasia, including Potter syndrome (renal agenesis, oligohydramnios, pulmonary hypoplasia); lung cysts; chylothorax; pulmonary lymphangiectasia; asphyxiating thoracic dystrophy; vascular rings and slings; arteriovenous malformation; subglottic stenosis.

[4]Afebrile pneumonia = *Chlamydia trachomatis,* cytomegalovirus, RSV, *Pneumocystis carinii, U. urealyticum, M. hominis.*

[5]Pneumonia (infant–toddler): see Chapter 2.

[6]Aspiration = gastric fluid or formula aspiration in gastroesophageal reflux (see Chapter 16); foreign body aspiration (see Chapter 2).

[7]Pneumonia (child): see Chapter 2.

[8]Interstitial lung disease = (see Tables 3-10 to 3-13) idiopathic, rheumatoid, infection (*P. carinii*), histiocytosis X, hypereosinophilia syndromes, Goodpasture syndrome, LIP, alveolar proteinosis, familial fibrosis, chronic active hepatitis, inflammatory bowel disease, vasculitis (Wegener granulomatosis, Churg-Strauss syndrome, hypersensitivity), graft-versus-host disease, pulmonary venooclusive disease, sarcoidosis, leukemia, lymphoma, neurofibromatosis, tuberous sclerosis, Gaucher disease, Niemann-Pick disease, Weber Christian disease, organic dusts (e.g., farmer's lung, humidifier/air-conditioner lung, bird feeder, pancreatic extract, rodent handler, cheese worker), inorganic dusts (pneumoconiosis), irradiation.

[9]Pneumonia (adolescent): see Chapter 2.

[10]Drugs = azathioprine, bleomycin, cyclophosphamide, methotrexate, nitrosoureas, busulfan, nitrofurantoin, penicillin, sulfonamides, erythromycin, isoniazid, hydralazine, phenytoin, carbamazepine, imipramine, naproxen, penicillamine, cromolyn sodium, mineral oil, paraquat, inhaled drugs (cocaine, hydrocarbons), talc, shoe spray.

[11]Collagen vascular disease = rheumatoid arthritis, progressive systemic sclerosis, systemic lupus erythematosus, dermatomyositis, mixed connective tissue disease.

[12]Hypersensitivity pneumonia (also called *extrinsic allergic alveolitis*): see No. 8 above for some specific organic dusts (antigens).

[13]Mediastinal masses = *anterior* (teratoma, T-cell lymphoma, thymus, thyroid); *middle* (lymph nodes–infection–tumor–sarcoidosis, cysts); *posterior* (neuroenteric cysts–duplication, meningocele, neural tumors–neuroblastoma, ganglioneuroblastoma, neurofibroma, pheochromocytoma), and parenchymal tumors (hamartoma, arteriovenous malformation, carcinoid, adenoma, metastatic–osteogenic sarcoma, Wilms tumor).

[14]HIV associated = *P. carinii,* LIP, CMV, *Mycobacterium tuberculosis,* atypical mycobacteria, measles, common bacterial pathogens (see Chapter 2).

ARDS, acute respiratory distress syndrome; BPD, bronchopulmonary dysplasia; CMV, cytomegalovirus; HIV, human immunodeficiency virus; LIP, lymphocytic interstitial pneumonia; RDS, respiratory distress syndrome; RSV, respiratory syncytial virus.

Table 3-2. Description of Adventitious Lung Sounds

Acoustic Qualities	American Thoracic Society Nomenclature	Common Synonyms
Discontinuous, explosive, loud, low-pitched	Coarse crackle	Coarse rale
Softer, higher-pitched than above; shorter duration than coarse crackles	Fine crackle	Fine or crepitant rale
Continuous, high-pitched, hissing or whistling, musical sound*	Wheezing	Sibilant rhonchus or fine wheezing
Longer-duration, lower-pitched than wheezing, continuous, sonorous	Rhonchus	Sonorous rhonchus

Modified from Loudon R, Murphy RLH: Lung sounds. Am Rev Respir Dis 1984;130:663-673.

*Also describes stridor, when heard over central extrathoracic airways.

Cardiac Examination

Other elements of the physical examination that may have direct bearing on the respiratory system include the cardiac examination and inspection of the distal extremities. Congenital heart disease that results in a large left-to-right shunt, pulmonary hypertension, congestive heart failure, and increased pulmonic blood flow may result in respiratory distress (see Chapter 8). The presence of digital clubbing in the absence of cardiac or gastrointestinal disease usually indicates a significant pulmonary abnormality (see Chapter 2).

DIAGNOSIS

Signs and symptoms of respiratory distress can vary, depending on the severity and cause. Not all causes of respiratory distress arise within the respiratory tract. Heart failure, pulmonary edema, neuromuscular disorders, toxic ingestion, and central nervous system disorders may all manifest with respiratory signs and symptoms (Table 3-3). The manifestations of respiratory distress include dyspnea, shortness of breath, cough, wheezing, stridor, and chest wall retractions; however, anxiety, pallor, and cyanosis may also herald respiratory embarrassment.

LABORATORY TESTS

A number of laboratory tests and diagnostic aids can be useful in determining the causes and degree of severity of respiratory distress. The arterial blood gas analysis, obtained while the patient is breathing a known fraction of inspired oxygen (FiO_2), is the "gold standard" for assessing oxygenation, ventilation, and acid-base status. In lieu of an arterial blood gas determination, noninvasive measure of oxygenation by pulse oximetry may provide valuable information. Oximetry measures the degree of hemoglobin saturation with oxygen and should not be confused with partial pressure of oxygen in blood, as measured by blood gas analysis or estimated by transcutaneous measures. A hemoglobin oxygen saturation lower than 93% indicates that significant hypoxemia may be present, and saturations of 90% or lower are clearly abnormal. An arterial blood gas analysis may be necessary to confirm the presence and degree of hypoxemia, as well as information on acid-base status (pH) and ventilation ($PaCO_2$). Hemoglobin oxygen saturation, measured by pulse oximetry, *cannot* detect significant hyperoxia; it is relatively accurate (±3%) at oxygen saturations of 70% or more. Various conditions, such as poor circulation, presence of carboxyhemoglobin or methemoglobin, nail polish, and improper sensor alignment and motion, can result in inaccurate oximetry measures.

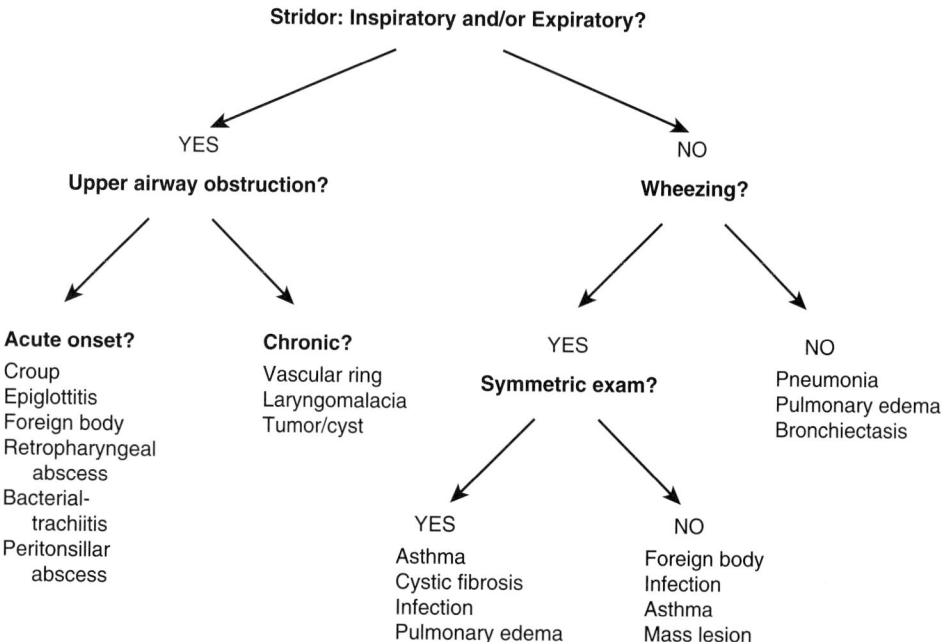

Figure 3-1. Algorithm for a child with respiratory distress.

Table 3-3. Causes of Respiratory Distress

Extrathoracic	Intrathoracic
Nervous System–Metabolic	**Pulmonary**
Intracranial hemorrhage	Airway obstruction
Acidosis	Parenchymal lesions:
Ingestion (aspirin)	pneumonia, hemorrhage,
Ketoacidosis (diabetes)	malformation
Meningitis	Air leaks:
Shock/sepsis	pneumomediastinum,
Neuromuscular disease	pneumothorax
Diaphragmatic paralysis,	Pleural effusion, empyema
paresis	Acute respiratory distress
Psychologic (anxiety), vocal	syndrome
cord dysfunction	Chest wall trauma
Panic attack	Pulmonary embolus
	Foreign body (airway or
	esophagus)
	Tumor (cyst, adenoma)
	Cystic fibrosis
Anatomic Lesions of Upper	**Cardiac**
Airway	Myocarditis,
Malacia	cardiomyopathy
Web	Shunt (left to right)
Cyst	Congestive heart failure
Hemangioma	Pulmonary edema
Stenosis (glottic or choanal)	Pericardial effusion
Papillomatosis	
Miscellaneous	
Abdominal masses, distention	
Ascites	
Anemia	

IMAGING

Radiography

Radiographic imaging of the respiratory tract may be obtained with a variety of techniques and can yield a great deal of insight into the causes of respiratory distress. A plain film of the chest, taken in the posterior-anterior and lateral projections, should be obtained in any patient with respiratory distress. Important information regarding the presence of parenchymal infiltrates, effusion, airway obstruction, cardiac size, pulmonary vascular markings, extrapulmonary air leaks, and the presence of radiopaque foreign bodies may be obtained from this test. Plain films of the chest taken during inspiration and expiration may be helpful in identifying the presence of intraluminal bronchial obstruction, such as that seen with a retained endobronchial foreign body. Demonstration of unilateral hyperinflation or a mediastinal shift during expiration suggests localized bronchial obstruction. A lateral decubitus positioning of the patient during the radiographic procedure can reveal a pleural effusion in the lower dependent lung. Ultrasonography of the chest is also useful in detecting pleural fluid and loculations within pleural effusions. For patients with stridor, radiographs of the neck and upper airway should be obtained.

Computed Tomography

Computed tomography (CT) of the upper airway and chest can help detect the relationship of the vasculature to the airways (trachea and large central airways), pulmonary parenchymal lesions (infiltrates, abscesses, cysts) or masses in the airway, and central airway caliber. Rapid, fine-cut CT is a technique of high resolution and short duration, which increases its acceptability for pediatric patients.

It is the method of choice for noninvasive detection and evaluation of bronchiectasis and interstitial lung disease. Helical CT is a valuable method of detecting pulmonary embolism.

Magnetic Resonance Imaging

Magnetic resonance imaging (MRI) of the pulmonary system may also be useful in elucidating the relationship of the great vessels to the airways and may be superior to CT for this purpose. MRI is less useful for imaging the lung parenchyma. The need for long imaging times often means sedation for young children, and this limits the utility of MRI imaging of the chest for some pediatric patients.

Fluorography

Fluoroscopic examination of the chest may be useful in determining the cause of respiratory distress. Real-time visualization of the diaphragm can determine whether paralysis or paresis of this major muscle of respiration is contributing to respiratory embarrassment. Asymmetric chest wall motion or unilateral hyperinflation during the respiratory cycle suggests bronchial obstruction, such as that seen with a retained foreign body in the airways. Likewise, a barium swallow study can help detect an esophageal foreign body, as well as most types of closed vascular rings.

CLINICAL OBSERVATION

Assessing the severity of respiratory distress can be aided by clinical observations. The presence of chest wall retractions signifies airway obstruction. In infants, the particularly compliant chest wall predisposes to intercostal and sternal retractions; in older children, these features may be less prominent. Flaring of the alae nasi also signifies airway obstruction and significant distress in both infants and older children. Infants may grunt during expiration; as fatigue and increased respiratory efforts commence, a head bob may appear. Use of neck strap (accessory) muscles to aid in respiratory efforts is also a harbinger of severe respiratory distress and airway obstruction. Alteration in the child's mental status signifies impending respiratory failure; hypoxemia typically results in agitation and anxiety, whereas hypercapnia can usually produce somnolence and mental confusion.

Pulsus paradoxus, the difference between the systolic blood pressure obtained during inspiration and that during exhalation, is exaggerated by airway obstruction and pulmonary hyperinflation. As pulmonary overinflation worsens, pulsus paradoxus values increase and correlate well with the degree of airway obstruction. It is difficult to measure pulsus paradoxus in young children with rapid heart rates. A method that allows a reasonable approximation of the pulsus paradoxus can be obtained by using a sphygmomanometer and noting the difference between the pressures at which the first sporadic faint pulse sounds and the pressure at which all sounds are heard. Values greater than 10 mm Hg are abnormal, and values greater than 20 mm Hg are consistent with severe airway obstruction.

Although digital clubbing is occasionally seen as a normal and familial variant, its presence in a child with respiratory distress suggests an acute illness superimposed on an underlying chronic condition. The most common pulmonary causes of digital clubbing in pediatric patients are cystic fibrosis, bronchiectasis, and other destructive pulmonary diseases (see Chapter 2). Digital clubbing is rarely seen in children with asthma.

CAUSES OF RESPIRATORY DISTRESS

WHEEZING

Wheezing is best characterized as a continuous, "musical" sound most often heard on expiration, but it may occur in both phases of respiration. The sound is a result of flow limitation in large or medium-sized airways; obstruction of the airways may result from intraluminal or extraluminal causes.

Intraluminal obstruction is most typically caused by smooth muscle constriction, mucosal edema, hypersecretion of mucus, or cellular infiltrate, all of which are commonly associated with airway inflammation or infection. Other less common sources of intraluminal obstruction include aspirated foreign body and tumors.

Extraluminal obstruction is typically caused by external compression from enlarged lymph nodes, vascular structures, pulmonary cysts, tumors, or intrinsic defects of the airway wall. Because extraluminal obstruction usually involves a fairly localized segment of airway, the wheezing is often restricted to the portion of the chest containing the affected airways. In small infants, it may be difficult to define the site of obstruction because breath sounds are transmitted throughout the thorax.

ASTHMA

The most common cause of intraluminal obstruction is asthma. Asthma is a common disorder that affects nearly 5 million children in the United States; 5% to 10% of children experience symptoms of asthma at some time. The prevalence of asthma is higher among African American children than among white children; the morbidity and mortality are likewise increased among African American children. Asthma is defined as airway obstruction that is reversible either spontaneously or with the use of medication. Chronic airway inflammation and bronchial hyperresponsiveness are the proposed causes of the airway obstruction. The airways of patients with even mild asthma demonstrate inflammation, manifested as mucosal edema, hypersecretion of mucus, smooth muscle constriction, and inflammatory cell infiltrate. Even when asthma symptoms are not present, airway inflammation may be demonstrated. Furthermore, bronchial hyperresponsiveness, the tendency of airway smooth muscle to constrict in response to a variety of environmental stimuli, is present in virtually all children with asthma and may be exacerbated by airway inflammation. Airway remodeling, the deposition of collagen in the subepithelial basement membrane area, occurs in some but not all asthmatic patients. Fixed airway obstruction can occur as a result of airway remodeling.

Diagnosis

The diagnosis of asthma is made by a combination of clinical observations and laboratory tests (Fig. 3-2). For the child with acute wheezing and respiratory distress, a therapeutic trial of an inhaled or, less often, a subcutaneous adrenergic agonist is also the best "diagnostic test" for reversible airway obstruction. Once the acute symptoms have improved, other diagnostic studies can be undertaken. Spirometry, particularly measurement of the forced expiratory volume in 1 second (FEV_1) and mid-maximal forced expiratory flow rates ($FEF_{25-75\%}$), provides a good indication of airflow obstruction in the larger and smaller airways, respectively. If airway obstruction is detected in the resting state, a bronchodilating aerosol (albuterol) is administered, and spirometry (pulmonary function tests) is repeated. An improvement of 12% and 200 mL in FEV_1 above baseline is considered significant and indicative of reversible airway obstruction. If the baseline spirometry is normal, an inhalation challenge test, with either increasing doses of methacholine or hyperventilation of cold, dry air can provoke a statistically (but usually not clinically) significant decrease in FEV_1; a fall in FEV_1 of 10% or greater is considered diagnostic of airway hyperresponsiveness and asthma. In children too young to perform spirometry, the repeated nature of wheezing episodes and the improvement in symptoms after treatment with antiinflammatory agents and bronchodilators, peripheral blood eosinophilia (>4%), a family history of asthma or allergy, and a personal history of eczema or food allergy

are strongly suggestive of the diagnosis of asthma. Other studies include measurement of total serum immunoglobulin E (IgE) levels; this immunoglobulin is often elevated in individuals with asthma and/or allergy, as well as in those predisposed to asthma.

Radiographic findings are nonspecific, but the films usually show symmetric hyperinflation and increased peribronchial thickening. A chest radiograph may also help to rule out other causes of wheezing, such as foreign body, pneumonia, or atelectasis (Table 3-4). The peripheral white blood cell count may reveal eosinophilia; if sputum is available, it may also demonstrate eosinophils.

Patients with acute asthma typically present with shortness of breath, wheezing, cough, and increased work of breathing. Persistent cough may be the most prominent or even sole feature of acute asthma. Many asthma episodes are misdiagnosed as bronchitis (see Chapter 2). Chest wall and suprasternal notch retractions and nasal flaring may be present. Chest wall retractions and the use of neck strap (accessory) muscles indicate significant airway obstruction. Acute asthma exacerbations that are unresponsive to aggressive bronchodilator administration are termed *status asthmaticus*. The severity of asthma may be assessed with the parameters presented in Tables 3-5 and 3-6. Common triggers of acute episodes include upper respiratory tract infections, exposure to cold air, exercise, allergens, pollutants, strong odors, and tobacco smoke.

A brief but pertinent history should be obtained for every child with acute asthma to determine the duration of symptoms, the character of previous episodes (severity, need for hospitalization, and need for intensive care, including mechanical ventilation), antecedent illness, symptoms, exposures, and both chronic and acute use of medications, including dose and time of last administration.

It is critical to rule out other causes of wheezing that are not asthma and that necessitate different therapy (see Table 3-4). Anatomic abnormalities of the airway, such as vascular ring, tracheobronchomalacia, ciliary dyskinesia, and foreign body aspiration, may cause airway obstruction and wheezing, especially in infants and young children. Viral infections, notably those of respiratory syncytial virus (RSV), metapneumovirus, adenovirus, parainfluenza, and influenza, are also common causes of wheezing in infants and young children. Infection with *Mycoplasma* species may produce airway hyperactivity in older children. Other entities to consider are cystic fibrosis, interstitial lung disease, or a behavioral disorder, such as vocal cord dysfunction. In comparison with asthma, the key distinguishing feature of these diagnoses is that the wheezing does not respond to treatment with bronchodilators.

The *physical examination* should focus on respiratory rate, air exchange, degree and localization of wheezing, other adventitious lung sounds, mental status, presence of cyanosis, and degree of fatigue (see Tables 3-5 and 3-6). An arterial blood gas analysis should be obtained if the clinical evaluation reveals moderate to severe airway obstruction. The presence and degree of hypoxemia and hypoventilation can be determined. Pulse oximetry is a noninvasive means of rapidly assessing oxygenation; when used in conjunction with measurement of the venous CO_2 pressure or pH, it is an acceptable alternative to an arterial blood gas determination in mildly to moderately ill patients.

Chest roentgenograms should be obtained for all patients with a first episode of wheezing. Patients with recurrent asthma should have a chest radiograph if there is fever, localized crackles or wheezing, decreased breath sounds, a poor response to therapy, or significant tachypnea.

Spirometry has limited efficacy in the emergency management of status asthmaticus. Although peak expiratory flow meters are often available in the emergency department, the test with this device is a measure of large airway function only, is effort dependent, and may be most unreliable in an anxious, untrained patient. The major value of peak flow measurements in acute asthma is to provide an objective trend indicative of improvement (or lack thereof) in airway caliber.

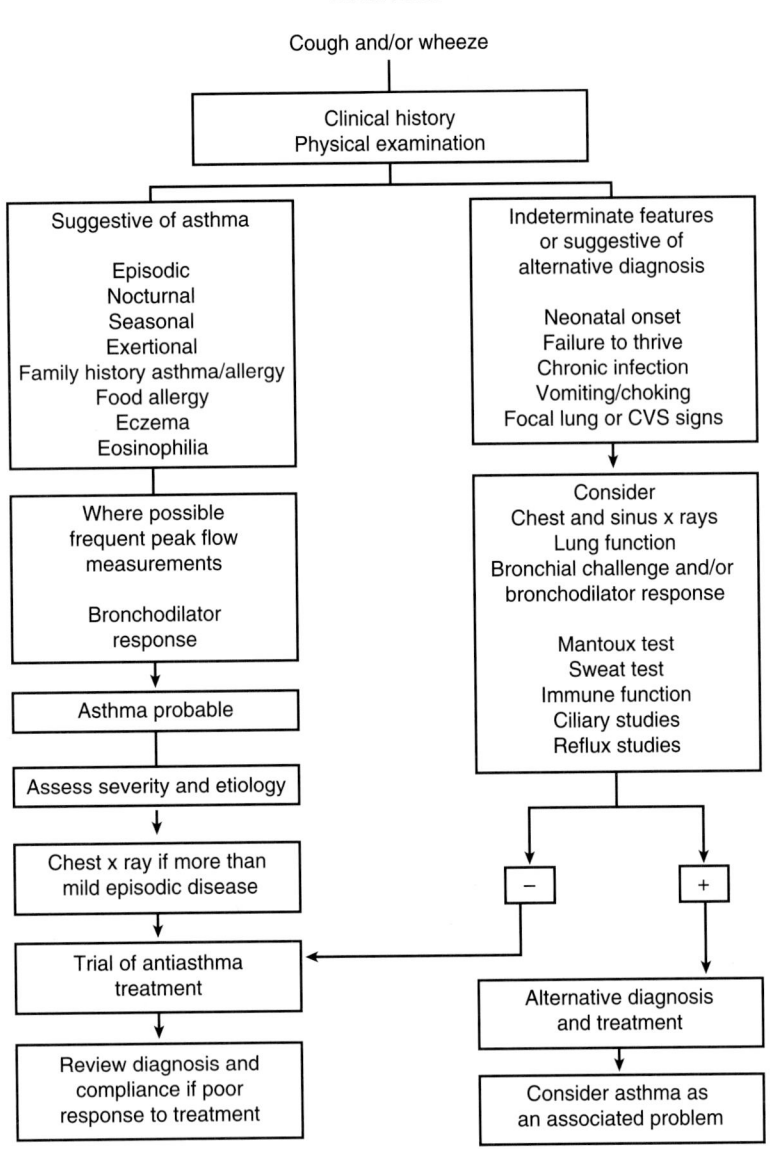

Figure 3-2. Diagnostic algorithm for asthma. CVS, cardiovascular system; −, negative; +, positive. (From Special Report of the Steering Committee: Asthma: A follow-up statement from an international paediatric asthma consensus group. Arch Dis Child 1992;67:240-248.)

A complete blood cell count is not of use unless other complicating conditions (e.g., infection, anemia, hemoglobinopathy) are suspected. Serum electrolyte measurements are of little value unless dehydration is suspected. Hypokalemia is associated with the frequent administration of β-adrenergic agonists. Most children cannot produce sputum, but if sputum is available, it should be examined for the presence of bacteria and inflammatory cells.

Treatment

Acute Asthma

Treatment of acute asthma should be instituted in any child with wheezing, dyspnea, cough, and no other immediately discernible cause of the symptoms.

Patients with moderate to severe airway obstruction have significant hypoxemia as a result of ventilation-perfusion mismatch. Consequently, supplemental humidified oxygen, usually 30% by face mask, is of benefit. Oxygen should be administered to any child who has significant wheezing, accessory muscle use, or an oxygen saturation of less than 93%.

The mainstay of treatment for status asthmaticus is the administration of an inhaled (or, less often, subcutaneous) β-adrenergic agonist. Inhalation of nebulized medication is the route of choice because the onset of action is rapid, sustained, and relatively free of significant side effects even in the most severely affected patients (Table 3-7). Patients who do not respond to initial therapy with aerosolized medication or cannot comply with the regimen should be given a subcutaneous injection. Although subcutaneous injection of epinephrine or a β agonist are equally effective, the procedure causes some discomfort and anxiety and may yield a higher incidence of side effects. Administration of β agonists from metered-dose inhalers with a valved holding chamber is also effective treatment of acute asthma in most children.

Anticholinergic agents (ipratropium bromide), when combined with β agonists as inhaled treatment, can provide additional bronchodilation. The effect is most marked in children who present to the emergency department with significant airway obstruction. Corticosteroids are potent antiinflammatory agents that are extremely useful in treating acute asthma exacerbations. With few exceptions, any patient who presents with other than mild wheezing responsive to minimal bronchodilator therapy or any patient requiring hospital

Table 3-4. Causes of Wheezing in Childhood

Acute

Reactive Airways Disease

Asthma*
Exercise-induced asthma*
Hypersensitivity reactions

Bronchial Edema

Infection* (bronchiolitis, ILD, pneumonia)
Inhalation of irritant gases or particulates
Increased pulmonary venous pressure

Bronchial Hypersecretion

Infection
Inhalation of irritant gases or particulates
Cholinergic drugs

Aspiration

Foreign body*
Aspiration of gastric contents (reflux, H-type TEF)

Chronic or Recurrent

Reactive Airways Disease (same as in Acute)
Hypersensitivity Reactions, Allergic Bronchopulmonary
Aspergillosis

Dynamic Airways Collapse

Bronchomalacia
Tracheomalacia*
Vocal cord adduction*

Airway Compression by Mass or Blood Vessel

Vascular ring/sling
Anomalous innominate artery
Pulmonary artery dilation (absent pulmonary valve)
Bronchial or pulmonary cysts
Lymph nodes or tumors

Chronic or Recurrent *Continued*

Aspiration

Foreign body
Gastroesophageal reflux*
Tracheoesophageal fistula (repaired of unrepaired)

Bronchial Hypersecretion or Failure to Clear
Secretions

Bronchitis, bronchiectasis
Cystic fibrosis*
Dyskinetic (immotile) cilia syndrome
Immunodeficiency disorder
Vasculitis
Lymphangiectasia
α_1-antitrypsin deficiency

Intrinsic Airway Lesions

Endobronchial tumors
Endobronchial granulation tissue
Plastic bronchitis syndrome
Bronchial or tracheal stenosis
Bronchiolitis obliterans
Sequelae of bronchopulmonary dysplasia
Sarcoidosis

Congestive Heart Failure

Modified from Kercsmar CM: The respiratory system. In Behrman RE, Kliegman RM (eds): Nelson Essentials of Pediatrics, 2nd ed. Philadelphia, WB Saunders, 1994, p 445.
*Common.

ILD, interstitial lung disease; TEF, tracheoesophageal fistula.

admission should receive corticosteroids (Table 3-8; see Table 3-7). Although theophylline (or the intravenous formulation amino-phylline) is an effective bronchodilator in chronic use, when optimal amounts of inhaled or parenteral β-adrenergic agonists are administered, the addition of theophylline does not consistently provide further significant improvement. Some severely affected patients respond to intravenous magnesium therapy. Intravenous fluids should be administered to any patient who has clinical or laboratory signs of dehydration. Fluids other than those required for normal homeostasis should not be routinely given. Chest physiotherapy may be useful for the patient who has significant atelectasis or sputum production.

A small percentage of children with acute asthma progress to severe status asthmaticus and respiratory failure. A number of clinical signs and symptoms define respiratory failure in such severely affected patients: a PaO_2 less than 60 mm in room air or cyanosis in 40% FiO_2, a $PaCO_2$ of 40 mm or higher or rising and accompanied by respiratory distress, deterioration in clinical status in spite of aggressive treatment, a change in mental status, and fatigue (see Tables 3-5 and 3-6). Patients meeting any of these criteria should be observed in an intensive care unit, and they should receive maximal medical therapy. Algorithmic approaches to the treatment of asthma are presented in Figure 3-3 and Tables 3-8, 3-9, and 3-10.

Chronic Asthma

Treatment of chronic asthma requires careful assessment of the severity of the disease, according to frequency and intensity of symptoms, and subsequent grading into mild, moderate, and severe categories (see Table 3-9 and 3-10). In general, all patients except those with mild intermittent disease are best managed with chronic administration of an inhaled antiinflammatory agent (corticosteroids) and the intermittent use of an inhaled β-adrenergic agonist for treatment of acute wheezing episodes. Leukotriene receptor antagonists may be considered as an alternative preventive therapy for mild asthma. Oral corticosteroids are administered for short intervals to control more severe exacerbations. Avoidance of environmental triggers (allergens, tobacco smoke) is also paramount to successful management.

RESPIRATORY DISTRESS IN INFANTS AND TODDLERS

VIRAL BRONCHIOLITIS

Bronchiolitis is a frequent manifestation of acute viral infections of the distal lower respiratory tract and a cause of wheezing and

Table 3-5. Classifying Severity of Asthma Exacerbations*

	Mild	Moderate	Severe	Respiratory Arrest Imminent
Symptoms				
Breathlessness	While walking	While talking (infant—softer, shorter cry; difficulty feeding)	While at rest (infant—stops feeding)	—
Posture	Can lie down	Prefers sitting	Sits upright	—
Talks in	Sentences	Phrases	Words	—
Alertness	May be agitated	Usually agitated	Usually agitated	Drowsy or confused
Signs				
Respiratory rate	Increased	Increased	Often >30/min	—

Guide to rates of breathing in awake children:

Age	Normal Rate
<2 months	<60/minute
2-12 months	<50/minute
1-5 years	<40/minute
6-8 years	<30/minute

	Mild	Moderate	Severe	Respiratory Arrest Imminent
Use of accessory muscles; suprasternal retractions	Usually not	Commonly	Usually	Paradoxical thoracoabdominal movement
Wheeze	Moderate, often only end expiratory	Loud; throughout exhalation	Usually loud; throughout inhalation and exhalation	Absence of wheeze
Pulse/minute	<100	100-120	>120	Bradycardia

Guide to normal pulse rates in children:

Age	Normal Rate
2-12 months	<160/minute
1-2 years	<120/minute
2-8 years	<110/minute

	Mild	Moderate	Severe	Respiratory Arrest Imminent
Pulsus paradoxus	Absent at <10 mm Hg	May be present at 10-25 mm Hg	Often present at >25 mm Hg (adult) 20-40 mm Hg (child)	Absence suggests respiratory muscle fatigue
Functional Assessment				
PEF % predicted or % personal best	80%	Approx. 50%-80%	<50% predicted or personal best or response lasts <2 hrs	—
PaO_2 (on air)	Normal (test not usually necessary)	>60 mm Hg (test not usually necessary)	<60 mm Hg: possible cyanosis	—
and/or PCO_2	<42 mm Hg (test not usually necessary)	<42 mm Hg (test not usually necessary)	≥42 mm Hg: possible respiratory failure (see text)	—
SaO_2% (on air) at sea level	>95% (test not usually necessary)	91%-95%	<91%	—

Hypercapnia (hypoventilation) develops more readily in young children than in adults and adolescents.

*The presence of several parameters, but not necessarily all, indicates the general classification of the exacerbation. Many of these parameters have not been systematically studied, so they serve only as general guides.

PaO_2, arterial oxygen pressure; PCO_2, carbon dioxide pressure; PEF, peak expiratory flow; SaO_2, arterial oxygen saturation.

respiratory distress. RSV is the most important respiratory pathogen in infants and young children. It has been identified as the etiologic agent in 5% to 40% of pneumonias in young children. Although infections with other viruses, such as adenovirus, metapneumovirus, and parainfluenza, can produce inflammation of the bronchioles, RSV causes most cases of bronchiolitis in the first 2 years of life. The most severe disease occurs in infants younger than 6 months, although the occurrence of lower respiratory tract disease during the first month of life is uncommon. When RSV infection does occur in neonates, it is often characterized by nonspecific signs such as poor feeding, lethargy, and apnea. By 5 years of age, 95% of all children have serologic evidence of RSV infection. Reinfections are common in older children and adults, because immunity to RSV is short-lived and incomplete. In older children and adolescents, infections with RSV are often limited to the upper respiratory tract.

In temperate climates, RSV epidemics occur yearly, beginning in midwinter and persisting through early spring. Intervals between epidemics often alternate between long (13 to 16 months) and short (7 to 12 months) duration; outbreaks may last 1 to 5 months.

Table 3-6. Factors Associated with Risk of Severe Status Asthmaticus or Death From Asthma

History

Chronic steroid-dependent asthma
Prior intensive care admission
Prior mechanical ventilation for asthma
Recurrent visits to emergency unit in past 48 hr
Sudden onset of severe respiratory distress
Poor compliance with therapy
Poor recognition by patient, family, or physician of severity of attack
Family dysfunction, crisis
Respiratory arrest
Hypoxic seizures, encephalopathy
Low socioeconomic status
Central urban residence
Black race
Other chronic obstructive pulmonary disease or cardiovascular disease
Sensitivity to *Alternaria* species

Physical Examination

Pulsus paradoxus >20 mm Hg
Hypotension, tachycardia, tachypnea
Cyanosis
One- to two-word dyspnea
Lethargy
Agitation
Sternocleidomastoid, intercostal, suprasternal retractions
Poor air exchange (e.g., quiet chest with severe distress)

Laboratory Tests

Hypercapnia
Hypoxia with supplemental oxygen
FEV_1 <30% expected; no improvement 1 hr after aerosol therapy
Chest radiograph (pneumothorax, pneumomediastinum)

Therapy

Overreliance on aerosol, inhaler therapy (>2 cannisters per month)
Delayed use of systemic corticosteroids
Sedation
Delayed admission to hospital or intensive care unit

From National Asthma Education and Prevention Program Expert Panel Report 2: Guidelines for the diagnosis and management of asthma (NIH Publication No. 97-4051). Rockville, MD, National Institutes of Health/National Heart, Lung, and Blood Institute, 1997.

Nosocomial acquisition of RSV poses a major and severe threat to hospitalized infants and children. As many as 35% of hospitalized infants may acquire RSV infection, and 40% of the hospital staff caring for infected infants also may become ill. Control of nosocomial spread is particularly difficult. RSV infection is readily spread by contact with contaminated secretions; subsequent self-inoculation via the ocular or nasal routes is common. The virus can survive for hours in secretions contaminating surfaces, such as countertops or hands. Masks and gowns are of minimal benefit, but groupings of patients and staff in cohorts and good hand washing are the most efficacious control mechanisms.

Infants with congenital heart disease and pulmonary hypertension have a much increased rate of morbidity and a somewhat increased rate of mortality from RSV. The course of illness is usually prolonged, and intensive care and mechanical ventilation are frequently needed. Among about 4% of infants with RSV and congenital heart disease, the outcome is fatal, in contrast to 1.5% of infected infants who were otherwise normal. Chronic obstructive pulmonary disease, immunosuppression from transplantation or chemotherapy, and primary immunodeficiency also increase the risk of severe morbidity or death from RSV infection.

In infected infants, upper respiratory tract symptoms usually precede the lower respiratory tract involvement by 3 to 7 days. Low-grade fever, rhinitis, and pharyngitis are common signs. Cough and wheezing are consistent and prominent features of RSV infection. Chest wall retractions and dyspnea are frequently observed, and adventitious sounds (wheezing, crackles) are appreciated on auscultation of the chest. Most children with bronchiolitis or pneumonia demonstrate clinical improvement after 3 to 4 days, but the duration of illness can be as long as 21 days. Bacterial superinfection of the lower respiratory tract is rare. Approximately 30% of infants with bronchiolitis caused by RSV have recurrent episodes of wheezing caused by bronchial hyperactivity, in part because of persistent inflammation of the distal respiratory tract produced by the viral infection.

Impaired gas exchange can occur as a result of airway obstruction and ventilation-perfusion inequalities. The clinical determination of the severity of the lower respiratory tract involvement in infants infected with RSV can be difficult. Physical findings often associated with respiratory distress, such as tachypnea, intercostal retractions, and wheezing, are not necessarily correlated with the level of hypoxemia. Cyanosis is an insensitive sign of mild arterial hypoxemia. Carbon dioxide retention secondary to alveolar hypoventilation is not a common finding in otherwise normal children, but hypercapnia and acute respiratory acidosis can be serious problems in infants with chronic pulmonary disease (e.g., bronchopulmonary dysplasia) or heart disease. Roentgenographic findings include a diffuse interstitial pneumonitis and bilateral lung overinflation; alveolar infiltrates or consolidation is present in approximately 20%

Table 3-7. Drugs for Treatment of Acute Asthma

Drug	Form	Dosage
Albuterol	Nebulizer solution, 0.5% (5 mg/mL)	0.15-0.3 mg/kg/dose every 20 min for 1-2 hours; minimum dose, 1.25 mg; maximum dose, 5 mg
OR Levalbuterol	1.25 mg/3 mL	0.63-1.25 mg every 20 min for 1-2 hours; minimum dose, 0.63 mg; maximum dose, 1.25 mg
Epinephrine HCl	1:1000 (1 mg/mL)	0.01 mg/kg subcutaneous injection every 20 min up to 3 injections; maximum dose, 0.3 mg
Terbutaline	0.1% (1 mg/mL)	0.01 mg/kg subcutaneous injection every 2 hr; maximum dose, 0.5 mg
Systemic corticosteroid	Oral prednisone or prednisolone Intravenous methylprednisolone	Prednisone, 1-2 mg/kg/day as single dose; maximum dose, 60 mg
		Prednisolone, 1-2 mg/kg/day; maximum dose, 125 mg

Table 3-8. Management of Acute Exacerbations of Asthma in a Child Who Is Capable of Using a Peak Flow Meter

Assessment	Recommended Actions
Initial Assessment and Emergency Treatment	
Does the patient have Altered level of consciousness Marked dyspnea, speaks only in single words or short phrases Severe intercostal or sternocleidomastoid retractions Cyanosis, pallor, or diaphoresis Inaudible breath sounds Subcutaneous or other extrapulmonary air Oxygen saturation <90% PEFR <50% of predicted norm or baseline PCO$_2$ >40 mm Hg if arterial blood gases are available	If any of these conditions exist: Give oxygen by Ventimask or nasal cannula. If unable to generate PEFR, give epinephrine subcutaneously (SC), 0.01 mL/kg/dose of 1:1000 epinephrine with a maximum dose of 0.3 mL or SC terbutaline, 0.005–0.010 mg/kg/dose with a maximum dose of 0.25 mg. If able to generate PEFR, give nebulized albuterol, 0.15 mg/kg/dose or 0.03 mL/kg/dose up to a maximum of 10 mg with 6 L/min of O$_2$ flow or levalbuterol, 1.25 mg. Give systemic steroids at a prednisone equivalent of 2 mg/kg. Consider transfer to an appropriate emergency setting at an FiO$_2$ of 0.40 or greater and intermittent albuterol treatments every 20 min or continuous albuterol treatments at 0.5 mg/kg/hr if initial response is inadequate. If patient responds well to initial albuterol treatment, repeat twice every 20 min and go to **Follow-up Treatment.**
Does the patient have a history of Steroid-dependent asthma Panic attacks with acute exacerbations Duration of asthma >12 hr History of respiratory failure Premonitions of death ≥2 visits to office or ED in 24 hr >3 visits in 48 hr Paroxysmal attacks, especially at night	*This is a high-risk patient!* Begin therapy immediately as outlined in **Initial Treatment:** Assess the severity of the current episode. These are high-risk factors that should be considered in the decision to urgently transfer the patient to an appropriate emergency setting. If there is not a prompt clinical response to therapy, consider transfer and give systemic steroids (oral or parenteral) at a prednisone equivalent of 2 mg/kg before transfer.
Initial Treatment	
If the exacerbation is in the mild category	Give albuterol by nebulizer at 0.1 mg/kg/dose or 0.02 mL/kg/dose with a minimum dose of 1.25 mg or 2–4 puffs by metered-dose inhaler (with spacer). This may be repeated every 20 min for up to 1 hr as needed.
If the exacerbation is in the moderate or severe category	Give oxygen. If an oximeter is available, keep O$_2$ saturation ≥93%–95%. Give nebulized albuterol at 0.15 mg/kg/dose or 0.03 mL/kg/dose up to a maximum of 5 mg or 1 mL at 6 L/min of O$_2$ flow. This may be repeated every 20 min for up to 1 hr.

Follow-up Treatment

For patients who were in the mild category, if the PEFR is >80% of predicted norm or baseline with no more than one sign in the moderate category after initial treatment

Discharge home *and* have patient continue albuterol every 4 hr while awake at the same dose previously given. If the patient is receiving inhaled steroids, theophylline or oral β agonists, continue medications and consider monitoring theophylline levels. Give systemic steroids (oral or parenteral) at a prednisone equivalent of 2 mg/kg. Give patient education and follow up with patient in 24 hr by phone call, and schedule visit in 3 days to reevaluate need for continuing corticosteroids.

For patients who were in the moderate or severe category, if the PEFR >80% of predicted norm or baseline with no more than one sign in the moderate category after initial treatment

Give systemic steroids (oral or parenteral) at a prednisone equivalent of 2 mg/kg and monitor the patient every 20 min for 1 hr. If stable after this time, discharge home as described above, and if patient is not stable, go to **Additional Treatment or Transfer to ED.**

Additional Treatment or Transfer to ED or Direct Admission to Appropriate Hospital Unit

If the patient is in the severe category *or* if the clinician is uncomfortable with additional treatment *or* if facilities to monitor the patient with pulse oximetry are unavailable

Transfer to ED with O_2, albuterol, and steroids, or order direct admission to a hospital unit.

If the patient is in the mild or moderate category with a PEFR <80% of predicted norm or baseline *and* the clinician is comfortable with further treatment *and* facilities are available to monitor the patient with pulse oximetry

Give systemic steroids (oral or parenteral) at a prednisone equivalent of 2 mg/kg. Repeat nebulized albuterol at 0.15 mg/kg/dose or 0.03 mL/kg/dose up to a maximum of 10 mg or 2 mL at 6 L/min of O_2 flow. This may be repeated every 20 min for up to 1 hr *and* give oxygen (mandatory) by Ventimask or nasal cannula; monitor with pulse oximeter to keep O_2 saturation ≥93%–95%.

Additional Treatment and/or Hospitalize

If after additional treatment the patient has a PEFR >80% of predicted norm or baseline and no more than one clinical sign in the moderate category and if after monitoring every 20 min for 1 hr the patient remains stable

Discharge home as described above and have patient continue corticosteroids (oral or parenteral) at a prednisone equivalent of 2 mg/kg/d.

If after additional treatment the PEFR is <80% of predicted norm or baseline

Transfer to an appropriate emergency setting or hospitalize in appropriate unit.

Modified from Provisional Committee on Quality Improvement. Practice parameter: The office management of acute exacerbations of asthma in children. Reproduced by permission of Pediatrics 1994;93:119-126. ED, emergency department; FiO_2, fraction of inspired oxygen; PEFR, peak expiratory flow rate.

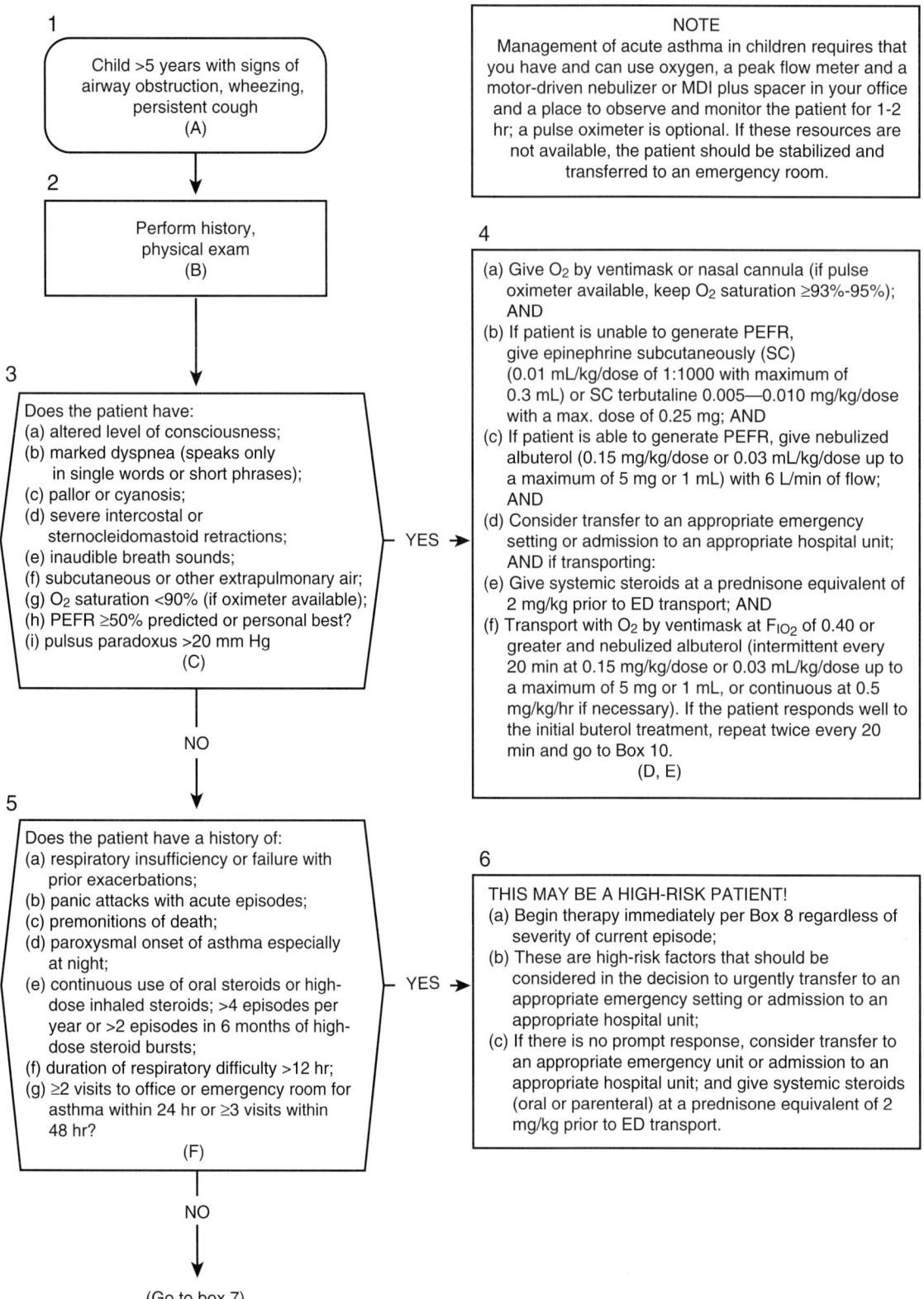

1

Child >5 years with signs of
airway obstruction, wheezing,
persistent cough
(A)

2

Perform history,
physical exam
(B)

NOTE
Management of acute asthma in children requires that
you have and can use oxygen, a peak flow meter and a
motor-driven nebulizer or MDI plus spacer in your office
and a place to observe and monitor the patient for 1-2
hr; a pulse oximeter is optional. If these resources are
not available, the patient should be stabilized and
transferred to an emergency room.

3

Does the patient have:
(a) altered level of consciousness;
(b) marked dyspnea (speaks only
    in single words or short phrases);
(c) pallor or cyanosis;
(d) severe intercostal or
    sternocleidomastoid retractions;
(e) inaudible breath sounds;
(f) subcutaneous or other extrapulmonary air;
(g) O_2 saturation <90% (if oximeter available);
(h) PEFR ≥50% predicted or personal best?
(i) pulsus paradoxus >20 mm Hg
(C)

— YES →

4

(a) Give O_2 by ventimask or nasal cannula (if pulse
    oximeter available, keep O_2 saturation ≥93%-95%);
    AND
(b) If patient is unable to generate PEFR,
    give epinephrine subcutaneously (SC)
    (0.01 mL/kg/dose of 1:1000 with maximum of
    0.3 mL) or SC terbutaline 0.005—0.010 mg/kg/dose
    with a max. dose of 0.25 mg; AND
(c) If patient is able to generate PEFR, give nebulized
    albuterol (0.15 mg/kg/dose or 0.03 mL/kg/dose up to
    a maximum of 5 mg or 1 mL) with 6 L/min of flow;
    AND
(d) Consider transfer to an appropriate emergency
    setting or admission to an appropriate hospital unit;
    AND if transporting:
(e) Give systemic steroids at a prednisone equivalent of
    2 mg/kg prior to ED transport; AND
(f) Transport with O_2 by ventimask at F_{IO_2} of 0.40 or
    greater and nebulized albuterol (intermittent every
    20 min at 0.15 mg/kg/dose or 0.03 mL/kg/dose up to
    a maximum of 5 mg or 1 mL, or continuous at 0.5
    mg/kg/hr if necessary). If the patient responds well to
    the initial buterol treatment, repeat twice every 20
    min and go to Box 10.
(D, E)

NO

5

Does the patient have a history of:
(a) respiratory insufficiency or failure with
    prior exacerbations;
(b) panic attacks with acute episodes;
(c) premonitions of death;
(d) paroxysmal onset of asthma especially
    at night;
(e) continuous use of oral steroids or high-
    dose inhaled steroids; >4 episodes per
    year or >2 episodes in 6 months of high-
    dose steroid bursts;
(f) duration of respiratory difficulty >12 hr;
(g) ≥2 visits to office or emergency room for
    asthma within 24 hr or ≥3 visits within
    48 hr?
(F)

— YES →

6

THIS MAY BE A HIGH-RISK PATIENT!
(a) Begin therapy immediately per Box 8 regardless of
    severity of current episode;
(b) These are high-risk factors that should be
    considered in the decision to urgently transfer to an
    appropriate emergency setting or admission to an
    appropriate hospital unit;
(c) If there is no prompt response, consider transfer to
    an appropriate emergency unit or admission to an
    appropriate hospital unit; and give systemic steroids
    (oral or parenteral) at a prednisone equivalent of 2
    mg/kg prior to ED transport.

NO

(Go to box 7)

Figure 3-3. Algorithm presenting the management of asthma by pediatricians in an office setting; this version is for a child using a peak expiratory flow meter. ED, emergency department; FIO_2, fraction of inspired oxygen; MDI, metered-dose inhaler; PEFR, peak expiratory flow rate. (From Provisional Committee on Quality Improvement: Practice parameter: The office management of acute exacerbations of asthma in children. Reproduced by permission of Pediatrics 1994;93:119-126.)

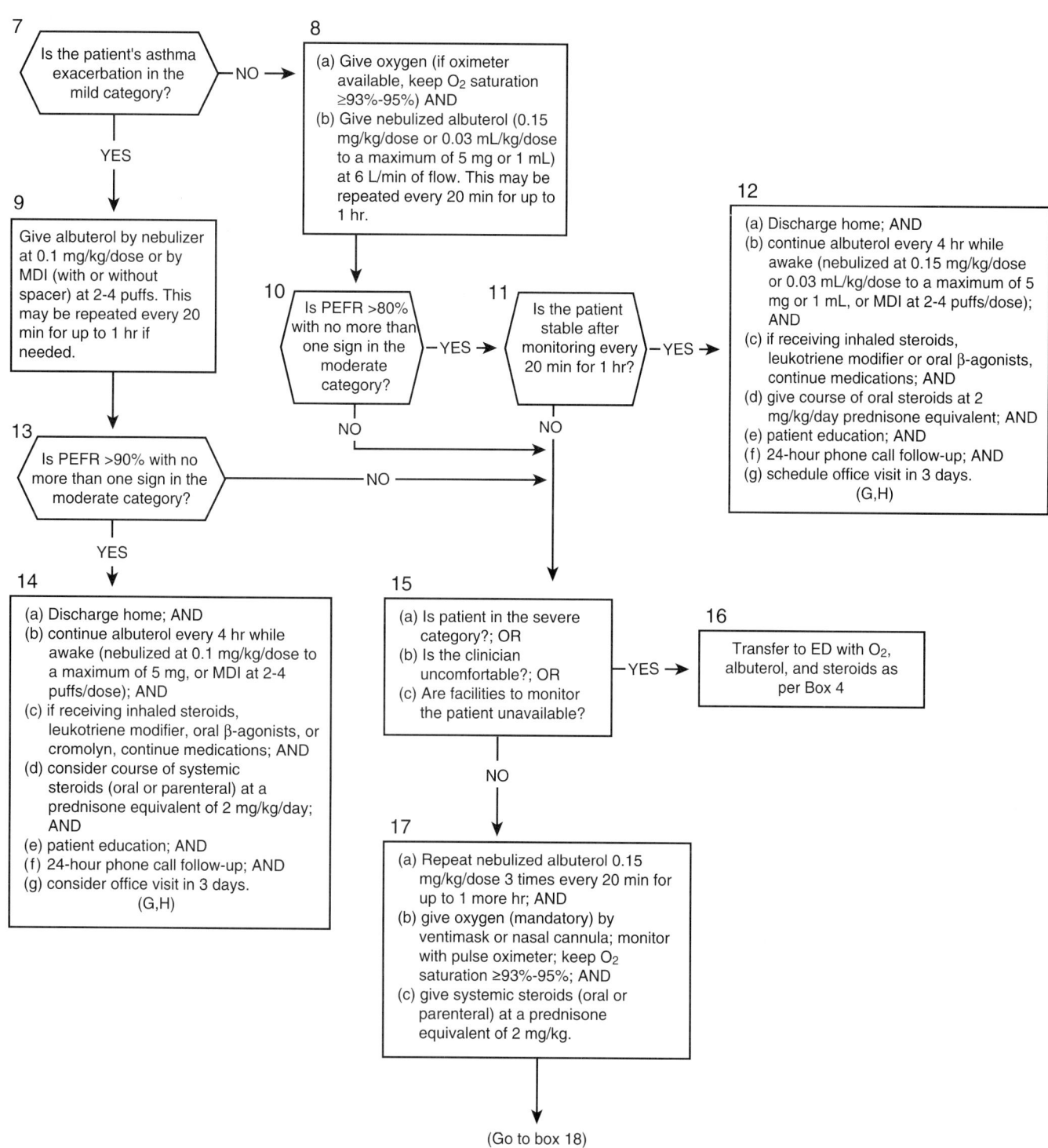

Figure 3-3, cont'd.

of children with lower respiratory disease. Roentgenographic abnormalities frequently persist longer than the clinical symptoms, and areas of lung consolidation are often the last abnormalities to resolve.

The diagnosis of viral bronchiolitis is usually made on clinical grounds. Bronchiolitis is most common in children under 2 years of age and should be suspected in the wheezing child who has current or antecedent upper respiratory tract infection symptoms in the late fall or winter months. The definitive diagnosis of RSV infection is based on the presence of virus or viral antigens or genome in respiratory secretions. Nasopharyngeal washings readily yield the virus when placed into cell culture. Alternatively, fluorescent antibody staining of epithelial cells obtained from washing or swabbing the nasopharynx can reveal viral infection. When properly performed, the technique is highly sensitive and specific. Moreover, in comparison with cell culture, fluorescent antibody staining is rapid and readily available. Enzyme-linked immunosorbent assay can also be used to detect RSV in nasopharyngeal secretions. Polymerase chain reaction is often specific and diagnostic.

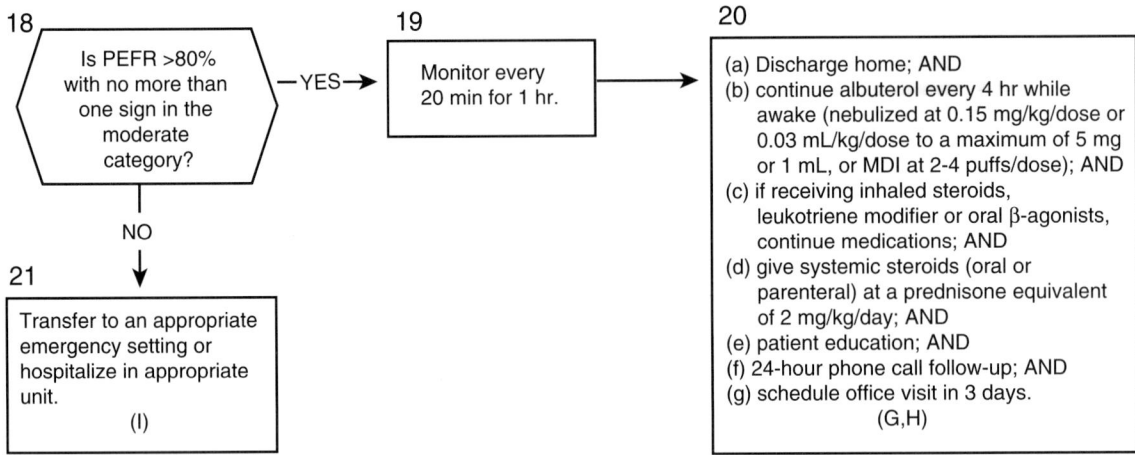

Figure 3-3, cont'd.

Unlike asthma, the wheezing accompanying bronchiolitis is often less responsive to bronchodilators. Nonetheless, patients with significant hypoxia and hypercapnia may receive a trial treatment with aerosol bronchodilators. Infants with bronchiolitis do not usually respond to treatment with antiinflammatory agents, such as corticosteroids and cromolyn sodium. Treatment with exogenous surfactant or helium-oxygen mixtures for severely ill infants requiring intubation and mechanical ventilation has yielded mixed results and remains experimental. Although a successful vaccine for RSV remains to be developed, several candidate vaccines are under investigation.

Ribavirin is a synthetic triazole nucleoside that exhibits in vitro antiviral activity against a number of RNA and DNA viruses, notably influenza A and B and RSV. Infants treated with ribavirin experience slightly more rapid resolution of lower respiratory tract signs and improvement in oxygenation than do untreated infants; however, the effect is modest at best. Several limitations (difficulty in administration, duration of therapy, expense, teratogenicity) prevent its widespread use. Moreover, the small degree of improvement provided by ribavirin does not warrant its use in all patients. Because bronchiolitis is typically a self-limited disease, only infants with underlying cardiopulmonary disorders and those with life-threatening infection should be considered for therapy.

Monthly administration (intramuscularly) of a humanized monoclonal antibody (palivizumab) against RSV can reduce morbidity from bronchiolitis but does not completely prevent infection. Infants at high risk (infants who had been premature, those with bronchopulmonary dysplasia or other forms of chronic obstructive pulmonary disease, those with complex congenital heart disease) who are younger than 2 years are most likely to benefit.

CYSTIC FIBROSIS

Cystic fibrosis is a multisystem disorder that involves the eccrine and mucous secretory glands (see Chapter 2). Inherited as an autosomal recessive trait, cystic fibrosis is the most common lethal genetic disease in white children and is an important cause of chronic suppurative lung disease. The earliest pulmonary defect exists in the peripheral airways, where viscous, mucopurulent material accumulates in the lumen of the bronchi and bronchioles and obstructs the airways. The involved bronchi become infiltrated with inflammatory cells and infected with *Pseudomonas aeruginosa* and *Staphylococcus aureus*, secondary to impaired mucociliary clearance. Chronic infection and inflammation lead to the weakening and destruction of the airway wall, which results in *bronchiectasis*, the abnormal dilatation of the subsegmental airways, and in pulmonary abscesses.

In general, the pulmonary deterioration characteristic of cystic fibrosis is rather insidious and is characterized by increasing airway obstruction over a period of years. Respiratory failure is typically seen late in the disease. However, some infants and children with cystic fibrosis can present in acute respiratory distress because of pneumonia, empyema (usually caused by *S. aureus* infection), or pneumothorax. Wheezing and eosinophilia should suggest allergic bronchopulmonary aspergillosis.

DYSKINETIC CILIA SYNDROME

Dyskinetic (immotile) cilia syndrome, another progressive lung disease, occurs in approximately 1 in 16,000 children and is the result of ultrastructural abnormalities of the cilia. The absence of dynein arms (inner and outer) is the most common form of the syndrome, but other structural abnormalities can result in decreased or absent ciliary movement. Acquired ciliary dyskinesia may be caused by a number of different environmental and infectious agents and is usually a temporary condition. The abnormal mucociliary clearance of endobronchial secretions causes a chronic bronchitis; wheezing is a common clinical manifestation resulting from the obstruction of the airways by mucus. Repeated or persistent severe upper respiratory tract infections, usually in the form of chronic pansinusitis or recurrent suppurative otitis media, are typical. Male sterility resulting from the impaired movement of spermatozoa is also present. Although Kartagener initially described several patients with situs inversus totalis, chronic sinusitis, and bronchiectasis, dextrocardia is present in only 50% of patients with this syndrome.

Arriving at a diagnosis necessitates a high index of suspicion and warrants pursuit in the child with recurrent wheezing, bronchitis, sinusitis, and otitis media. Findings on chest roentgenograms are generally nonspecific, but these films frequently demonstrate areas of pulmonary consolidation. Extensive atelectasis with significant respiratory distress has been described in neonates with this condition. Bronchiectasis is a late sequela of dyskinetic cilia syndrome. Functional assays for mucociliary clearance or examination of respiratory epithelial cells for ultrastructural ciliary defects with electron microscopy is necessary to establish a diagnosis.

GASTROESOPHAGEAL REFLUX

Gastroesophageal reflux can be a primary cause of or an exacerbating factor in wheezing in infants and young children (see Chapters 2 and 16). Direct inhalation of stomach contents into the lungs can produce bronchospasm and a chemical pneumonitis. Gastroesophageal reflux with aspiration has also been implicated in cases of bacterial pneumonia, bronchiectasis, obliterative bronchiolitis, and lung abscesses. Tachypnea, wheezing, and cough are the usual clinical findings, typically occurring within 1 hour of the aspiration event. The signs and symptoms of the pneumonitis, however, can be delayed.

Although pulmonary aspiration of gastric contents was once assumed to be the basis of reflux-induced wheezing, reflex bronchoconstriction in response to esophageal acidification can also produce bronchospasm in some patients. Other respiratory symptoms associated with gastroesophageal reflux, such as stridor and obstructive apnea, can manifest as the result of reflex laryngospasm. Gastroesophageal reflux can also complicate and worsen underlying lung diseases, such as asthma or subglottic stenosis, by provoking bronchospasm and potentiating airway or laryngeal inflammation and possibly bronchial hyperactivity.

PULMONARY ASPIRATION OF OROPHARYNGEAL CONTENTS

Central nervous system or neuromuscular disease in infants and children can result in dysfunction of the swallowing mechanism, leading to repeated episodes of pulmonary aspiration. This is the most common cause of respiratory distress in such children and typically manifests with intractable wheezing, chronic airway inflammation, and recurrent pneumonias.

Barium esophagograms, in which barium-laced foods of a variety of textures and consistencies are fed to a child under direct visualization and fluoroscopy, can be useful in making the diagnosis and establishing that the child has an abnormal swallowing mechanism. In addition, modified barium esophagography can be helpful with regard to therapy and may determine the appropriate feeding techniques, food consistencies, and feeding volumes that are less likely to cause aspiration in a vulnerable child.

Nasogastric tube or gastrostomy tube feedings may be necessary in children who do not respond to conservative management and who continue to have repeated episodes of pulmonary aspiration. Nevertheless, the affected child can continue to have periodic inhalation of oropharyngeal secretions (saliva) despite these interventions. A Nissan fundoplication may be needed to reduce the incidence of gastric aspiration.

ANATOMIC AIRWAY MALFORMATIONS

Anatomic or structural anomalies of the intrathoracic airways (see Chapters 2 and 5) can cause recurrent or persistent wheezing in infants and children (see Table 3-1). Conversely, malformations that obstruct the extrathoracic airway produce stridor predominantly. The lumina of the large proximal airways (trachea and bronchi) are maintained by cartilaginous rings. However, if these support structures are absent, malformed, or excessively pliant, the airways collapse during expiration, thus producing symptoms of airway obstruction (see Chapter 5).

Tracheobronchomalacia, in which excessively collapsible central airways produce wheezing, cough, and tachypnea, is usually generalized throughout the airways and is a congenital anomaly. Acquired bronchomalacia or tracheomegaly has also been described in premature infants after prolonged mechanical ventilatory support, presumably because of barotrauma. Tracheobronchomalacia can be focal, particularly if the malformation is associated with extrinsic compression of the involved airway. Extrinsic compression of the intrathoracic airway by enlarged hilar lymph nodes, mediastinal tumors, and bronchogenic cysts, or vascular rings can produce progressively worsening airway obstruction. Congenital bronchial stenosis and absence of bronchial cartilage are rare conditions that produce fixed obstruction of the involved airway, resulting in persistent, localized wheezing refractory to treatment with bronchodilators. All these conditions are associated with persistent wheezing

(which may be localized over the affected segment), recurrent lower respiratory infections, and a chronic, productive cough.

Abnormalities of the lung parenchyma usually lead, in infants, to tachypnea and respiratory distress. In addition, congenital lobar hyperinflation, pulmonary sequestrations, and cystic adenomatoid malformations can cause wheezing secondary to compression of the intrathoracic airways.

Tracheoesophageal fistula, an unusual malformation of the respiratory tract, is a congenital communication between the airways and gastrointestinal tract. The most frequent form of this anomaly, distal tracheoesophageal fistula with esophageal atresia, typically becomes symptomatic early in life (see Chapter 2). Wheezing often persists despite appropriate surgical repair, inasmuch as gastroesophageal reflux or bronchomalacia may be present.

VASCULAR RINGS

Several types of vascular malformations caused by irregularities in the development of the primitive aortic arches can produce extrinsic compression and narrowing of the intrathoracic trachea (see Chapter 5). The three most common types of complete vascular rings that affect the airway are

- double aortic arch
- right aortic arch with left ligamentum arteriosum
- anomalous left carotid artery

In the case of the double aortic arch, the right dorsal aorta persists, courses posterior to the esophagus, and joins the left dorsal aorta, which lies anterior to the trachea. This type of malformation produces a complete vascular ring that surrounds both the trachea and esophagus and compresses both structures.

Similarly, a persistent right aortic arch associated with ductus or ligamentum arteriosum completely entraps the trachea and esophagus, thus frequently leading to difficulties in breathing and swallowing. The anomalous left carotid artery anteriorly compresses the trachea and does not represent a complete vascular ring unless it is accompanied by an associated malformation.

An anomalous innominate artery, probably the most common form of this vascular malformation, also is not a complete ring; instead, it produces an anterior compression of the trachea. Consequently, the symptoms associated with this abnormality (i.e., harsh cough, stridor, and wheezing) are usually not as severe.

The clinical presentation of these vascular rings depends on the type of vascular malformation, its relative location in the airway, and the extent of airway compression. The pulmonary signs and symptoms of vascular defects are usually manifested during the first year of life as progressively worsening and ultimately persistent stridor, tachypnea, dyspnea, dysphagia, and respiratory distress. Cough is prominent and is typically harsh and stridulous. A prolonged expiratory phase and wheezing may also be appreciated on auscultation. Most of these conditions in children are mistakenly diagnosed as bronchiolitis or asthma.

Chest roentgenograms usually do not demonstrate parenchymal lesions of the lung, and the airways may appear normal. However, leftward deviation of the trachea by a right aortic arch should alert the examiner to the possibility of a vascular ring, particularly in a patient who has chronic respiratory symptoms. In patients with "complete" vascular rings, posterior compression of the esophagus is evident on contrast esophagram. Chest CT scan (with intravenous contrast media) or MRI can also identify the vascular anomaly. Bronchoscopy usually reveals a pulsatile (anterior) compression of the trachea.

FOREIGN BODY ASPIRATION

Aspiration of a foreign body into the intrathoracic airways must be considered in the differential diagnosis of a child with the *sudden onset* of respiratory distress or wheezing (see Chapter 2). Aspiration

Table 3-9. Stepwise Approach for Managing Infants and Young Children (5 Years of Age and Younger) with Acute or Chronic Asthma (Updates EPR-2)

Classify Severity: Clinical Features Before Treatment or Adequate Control		Medications Required to Maintain Long-Term Control
Symptoms/Day		
Symptoms/Night		*Daily Medications*
Step 4: Severe Persistent	Continual Frequent	**Preferred treatment:** High-dose inhaled corticosteroids AND Long-acting inhaled beta$_2$-agonists AND, if needed, Corticosteroid tablets or syrup long term (2 mg/kg/day, generally do not exceed 60 mg per day). (Make repeat attempts to reduce systemic corticosteroids and maintain control with high-dose inhaled corticosteroids.)
Step 3: Moderate Persistent	Daily >1 night/week	**Preferred treatment:** Low-dose inhaled corticosteroids and long-acting inhaled beta$_2$-agonists OR Medium-dose inhaled corticosteroids. Alternative treatment: Low-dose inhaled corticosteroids and either leukotriene receptor antagonist or theophylline. If needed (particularly in patients with recurring severe exacerbations): **Preferred treatment:** Medium-dose inhaled corticosteroids and long-acting beta$_2$-agonists. Alternative treatment: Medium-dose inhaled corticosteroids and either leukotriene receptor antagonist or theophylline.
Step 2: Mild Persistent	>2/week but <1x/day >2 nights/month	**Preferred treatment:** Low-dose inhaled corticosteroids (with nebulizer or MDI with holding chamber with or without face mask or DPI). Alternative treatment (listed alphabetically): Cromolyn (nebulizer is preferred or MDI with holding chamber) OR leukotriene receptor antagonist.
Step 1: Mild Intermittent	≤2 days/week ≤2 nights/month	No daily medication needed.

Quick Relief: All Patients	Bronchodilator as needed for symptoms. Intensity of treatment will depend upon severity of exacerbation. **Preferred treatment:** Short-acting inhaled beta$_2$-agonists by nebulizer or face mask and space/holding chamber Alternative treatment: Oral beta$_2$-agonists With viral respiratory infection Bronchodilator q 4–6 hours up to 24 hours (longer with physician consult): in general, repeat no more than once every 6 weeks Consider systemic corticosteroid if exacerbation is severe or patient has history of previous severe exacerbations Use of short-acting beta$_2$-agonists >2 times a week in intermittent asthma (daily, or increasing use in persistent asthma) may indicate the need to initiate (increase) long-term-control therapy.
Step down: *Step up:*	Review treatment every 1 to 6 months; a gradual stepwise reduction in treatment may be possible. If control is not maintained, consider step up. First, review patient medication technique, adherence, and environmental control.
Goals of Therapy: *Asthma Control*	Minimal or no chronic symptoms day or night Minimal or no exacerbations No limitations on activities; no school/parent's work missed Minimal use of short-acting inhaled beta$_2$-agonist Minimal or no adverse effects from medications

Notes:
- The stepwise approach is intended to assist, not replace, the clinical decisionmaking required to meet individual patient needs.
- Classify severity: assign patient to most severe step in which any feature occurs.
- There are very few studies on asthma therapy for infants.
- Gain control as quickly as possible (a course of short systemic corticosteroids may be required): then step down to the least medication necessary to maintain control.
- Minimize use of short-acting inhaled beta$_2$-agonists. Over-reliance on short-acting inhaled beta$_2$-agonists (e.g., use of short-acting inhaled beta$_2$-agonist every day, increasing use or lack of expected effect, or use of approximately one canister a month even if not using it every day) indicates inadequate control of asthma and the need to initiate or intensify long-term-control therapy.
- Provide parent education on asthma management and controlling environmental factors that make asthma worse (e.g., allergies and irritants).
- Consultation with an asthma specialist is recommended for patients with moderate or severe persistent asthma. Consider consultation for patients with mild persistent asthma.

From National Institutes of Health, National Heart, Lung, and Blood Institute: Guidelines for the Diagnosis and Management of Asthma—Update on Selected Topics 2002. NIH Publication No. 02-5075, July 2002.

Table 3-10. Stepwise Approach for Managing Asthma in Adults and Children Older Than 5 Years of Age: Treatment (Updates EPR-2)

Classify Severity: Clinical Features Before Treatment or Adequate Control			Medications Required to Maintain Long-Term Control
Symptoms/Day / Symptoms/Night	PEF or FEV$_1$ / PEF Variability		Daily Medications
Step 4: Severe Persistent	Continual / Frequent	≤60% / >30%	**Preferred treatment:** High-dose inhaled corticosteroids AND Long-acting inhaled beta$_2$-agonists AND, if needed, Corticosteroid tablets or syrup long term (2 mg/kg/day, generally do not exceed 60 mg per day). (Make repeat attempts to reduce systemic corticosteroids and maintain control with high-dose inhaled corticosteroids.)
Step 3: Moderate Persistent	Daily / >1 night/week	>60%–<80% / >30%	**Preferred treatment:** Low-to-medium dose inhaled corticosteroids and long-acting inhaled beta$_2$-agonists. Alternative treatment (listed alphabetically): Increase inhaled corticosteroids within medium-dose range OR Low-to-medium dose inhaled corticosteroids and either leukotriene modifier or theophylline. If needed (particularly in patients with recurring severe exacerbations): **Preferred treatment:** Increase inhaled corticosteroids within medium-dose range and add long-acting inhaled beta$_2$-agonists. Alternative treatment: Increase inhaled corticosteroids within medium-dose range and add either leukotriene modifier or theophylline.
Step 2: Mild Persistent	>2/week but <1x/day / >2 nights/month	≥80% / 20–30%	**Preferred treatment:** Low-dose inhaled corticosteroids Alternative treatment (listed alphabetically): cromolyn, leukotriene modifier, nedocromil, OR sustained release theophylline to serum concentration of 5–15 mcg/mL.
Step 1: Mild Intermittent	≤2 days/week / ≤2 nights/month	≥80% / <20%	No daily medication needed. Severe exacerbations may occur, separated by long periods of normal lung function and no symptoms. A course of systemic corticosteroids is recommended.

Quick Relief: All Patients	Short-acting bronchodilator: 2–4 puffs short-acting inhaled beta$_2$-agonists as needed for symptoms. Intensity of treatment will depend on severity of exacerbation up to 3 treatments at 20-minute intervals or a single nebulizer treatment as needed. Course of systemic corticosteroids may be needed. Use of short-acting beta$_2$-agonists >2 times a week in intermittent asthma (daily, or increasing use in persistent asthma) may indicate the need to initiate (increase) long-term-control therapy.
Step down:	Review treatment every 1 to 6 months; a gradual stepwise reduction in treatment may be possible.
Step up:	If control is not maintained, consider step up. First, review patient medication technique, adherence, and environmental control.
Goals of Therapy: Asthma Control	Minimal or no chronic symptoms day or night Minimal or no exacerbations No limitations on activities: no school/work missed Maintain (near) normal pulmonary function Minimal use of short-acting inhaled beta$_2$-agonist Minimal or no adverse effects from medications

Notes:

- The stepwise approach is meant to assist, not replace, the clinical decisionmaking required to meet individual patient needs.
- Classify severity: assign patient to most severe step in which any feature occurs. (PEF is % of personal best: FEV$_1$ is % predicted).
- Gain control as quickly as possible (consider a short course of systemic corticosteroids): then step down to the least medication necessary to maintain control.
- Minimize use of short-acting inhaled beta$_2$-agonists. Over-reliance on short-acting inhaled beta$_2$-agonists (e.g., use of short-acting inhaled beta$_2$-agonist every day, increasing use or lack of expected effect, or use of approximately one canister a month even if not using it every day) indicates inadequate control of asthma and the need to initiate or intensify long-term-control therapy.
- Provide education on self-management and controlling environmental factors that make asthma worse (e.g., allergens and irritants).
- Refer to an asthma specialist if there are difficulties controlling asthma or if step 4 care is required. Referral may be considered if step 3 care is required.

From National Institutes of Health, National Heart, Lung, and Blood Institute: Guidelines for the Diagnosis and Management of Asthma—Update on Selected Topics 2002. NIH Publication No. 02-5075, July 2002.

of foreign bodies is most common in children between 1 and 4 years of age, particularly in boys. It is rare in children younger than 6 months. The most common objects aspirated by children are food products. Endobronchial aspiration of peanuts, raisins, popcorn kernels, or seeds tends to produce more difficulties than other kinds of foreign bodies (metallic or plastic objects), because, in addition to causing physical obstruction of the airway, vegetable matter tends to produce an intense, local inflammatory response secondary to chemical and allergic bronchitis. Larger objects, such as coins, are also frequently aspirated but usually lodge in the esophagus. Esophageal foreign bodies can produce significant respiratory symptoms as a result of extrinsic compression of the posterior trachea.

The typical clinical manifestation after the acute event is abrupt respiratory distress, characterized by choking, gagging, cyanosis, and a harsh, paroxysmal cough. However, because many aspiration events occur while children are unsupervised, the history of foreign body ingestion or aspiration is frequently not elicited. Chronic cough, dyspnea, hemoptysis, and wheezing may develop. Because the object is most frequently aspirated into mainstem or segmental bronchi, the wheezing is typically unilateral. Physical examination may also reveal a decrease in breath sounds on the obstructed side, prolongation of the expiratory phase, and a tracheal shift.

In some instances, retained foreign bodies in the airways can produce a persistent pneumonitis, and the chronic inflammatory response can result in bronchiectasis or lung abscess. If both mainstem bronchi and the trachea are obstructed, the patient may have asphyxia; inhalation of foreign bodies is a leading cause of accidental death in children younger than 6 years. Large foreign bodies in the proximal esophagus can also produce respiratory distress, stridor, and wheezing by the extrinsic compression of the posterior wall of the trachea, especially in infants and young children. Dysphagia and vomiting can be late symptoms associated with an esophageal foreign body.

The diagnosis of foreign body aspiration can be difficult to establish and necessitates a combination of clinical examination, radiographic studies, and ultimately endoscopic visualization. Because most inhaled objects are not radiopaque, chest roentgenograms frequently do not demonstrate the foreign body. In a clinical series, chest roentgenograms were interpreted as normal in 25% of patients with foreign bodies and did not contribute to the diagnosis. However, the abrupt interruption of a bronchus (air bronchograms), persistent pulmonary infiltrates, and lobar or segmental atelectasis may be evidence of the presence of a retained, radiolucent foreign body. Unilateral hyperaeration on expiratory plain films, lateral decubitus films, or fluoroscopy indicates a check-valve obstruction of the airway. Nevertheless, the fluoroscopic evaluation is negative in approximately 10% of patients with a retained endobronchial foreign body.

The definitive diagnostic procedure for foreign body aspiration is bronchoscopy. Obviously, an unambiguous history of foreign body aspiration is a clear indication for bronchoscopy. However, bronchoscopic evaluation of the airways should also be considered in a child who has a history of recurrent or persistent atelectasis or pneumonia in a single lobe, particularly if the pneumonia is refractory to treatment.

BRONCHOPULMONARY DYSPLASIA

Bronchopulmonary dysplasia (BPD), also called chronic lung disease, is a chronic pulmonary disorder that is a sequela of mechanical ventilation and supplemental oxygen therapy for neonatal respiratory distress syndrome. It is probably the response of an immature lung to oxygen toxicity, barotrauma, and the resultant inflammation. The histologic features of the pulmonary disease include squamous metaplasia of the airways, peribronchial smooth muscle hypertrophy, alveolar septal fibrosis, and hyperinflation. The risk for development of BPD increases with decreasing gestational age and birth weight and with the duration of oxygen and ventilator therapy.

BPD is clinically characterized by prolonged oxygen requirements (either more than 1 month or after 36 weeks of gestational age), tachypnea, wheezing, scattered rhonchi, and increased respiratory effort. Chest roentgenograms typically show alternating areas of subsegmental atelectasis and hyperinflation. Persistent hypoxemia, secondary to abnormal lung mechanics and ventilation-perfusion inequalities, is common, especially in patients with severe lung injury. Patients with BPD have an increased susceptibility to viral infections of the lower respiratory tract, and exacerbations caused by infections with RSV can be life-threatening. Airway hyperactivity resulting in episodes of acute bronchospasm is common in infants with BPD and often persists into adolescence. However, clinical symptoms abate in most children after 3 years of age. Pulmonary function studies in older children may show improvement, but elevated residual lung volumes, decreased lung compliance, decreased expiratory air flows, and bronchial hyperresponsiveness can persist into adulthood.

The diagnosis of BPD is based on clinical history and typical radiographic findings. The best treatment is prevention. Acute exacerbations are generally treated in much the same manner as asthma, with inhaled bronchodilators and corticosteroids. Theophylline and inhaled antiinflammatory and anticholinergic agents may be of benefit.

RESPIRATORY DISTRESS IN CHILDREN AND ADOLESCENTS

Asthma is the most common cause of respiratory distress in children and adolescents, although infectious agents (e.g., viruses) may produce wheezing in children. Furthermore, persistent bronchial hyperactivity after acute lower respiratory tract infections can also result in recurrent episodes of wheezing. Nevertheless, other less common causes of persistent wheezing or respiratory distress should be sought, particularly if therapeutic interventions do not affect the patient's clinical condition.

HYPERSENSITIVITY PNEUMONITIS

Hypersensitivity pneumonitis, or extrinsic allergic alveolitis, results from the inhalation of organic dust particles. Although numerous causes have been identified, the clinical features of the various types of hypersensitivity pneumonitis are similar and depend on the intensity and frequency of exposure to the allergen; both acute and chronic forms have been described.

In the acute form of the disease, the patient typically has fever, rigors, cough, and dyspnea several hours after exposure. The symptoms usually resolve within 24 hours of the onset once the offending material is removed. In the chronic or subacute forms of hypersensitivity pneumonitis, the affected individual may have exercise intolerance, anorexia, weight loss, and a productive cough. Diffuse crackles (rales) are the prominent finding on physical examination, although the patient may be cyanotic if gas exchange is significantly impaired. Digital clubbing is an unusual finding. In acute cases, inflammation of the alveoli and pulmonary interstitium are common reactions, whereas the chronic form can result in interstitial fibrosis and noncaseating granulomas. Chronic hypersensitivity pneumonitis can insidiously lead to respiratory failure and cor pulmonale.

A number of laboratory studies may be helpful in confirming the diagnosis of hypersensitivity pneumonitis. Chest roentgenograms demonstrate diffuse reticulonodular infiltrates; lung hyperinflation is atypical. Pulmonary function studies characteristically show a restrictive defect, and the carbon monoxide diffusion capacity is reduced. During the acute phase of the disease, the patient may have a peripheral leukocytosis and eosinophilia. Serologic studies for precipitating immunoglobulin G antibodies to specific antigens are useful in identifying the offending agent. However, these antibodies may be found in asymptomatic individuals exposed to the allergen, and thus their presence is not necessarily correlated with severity of pulmonary disease. Percutaneous or intradermal tests may also be useful, particularly if an avian hypersensitivity pneumonitis is suspected.

Removal of the specific organic dust from the patient's environment is critical. Mild episodes of hypersensitivity pneumonitis may resolve spontaneously once the offending allergen is eliminated. Severe exacerbations often necessitate treatment with systemic corticosteroids; bronchodilators may be beneficial if the patient is experiencing symptoms of bronchospasm.

Hypersensitivity pneumonitis must be differentiated from other causes of interstitial lung disease (Tables 3-11 to 3-13). A diagnostic approach to interstitial lung disease is presented in Table 3-14.

ALLERGIC BRONCHOPULMONARY ASPERGILLOSIS

Allergic bronchopulmonary aspergillosis (ABPA) is an immunologic disorder identified in patients with chronic lung disease, in which airway colonization (but not invasive infection) with *Aspergillus fumigatus* causes chronic antigen exposure and increased bronchial hyperactivity. This condition can lead to pulmonary fibrosis,

---

Table 3-11. Known Causes of Interstitial Lung Disease in Children

Infectious or Postinfectious

Viral

Cytomegalovirus
Human immunodeficiency virus (HIV)
Respiratory syncytial virus
Adenovirus
Influenza virus
Parainfluenza viruses
Mycoplasma species
Measles

Mycobacterial
Fungal
*Pneumocystis carinii**
Aspergillus species

Bacterial
Legionella pneumophila
Bordetella pertussis

Environmental Inhalants, Toxic Substances, Foreign Materials, or Antigenic Dusts

Inorganic Dusts

Silica
Asbestos
Talcum powder
Zinc stearate

Organic Dusts

Hypersensitivity pneumonitis
Bird-fancier's lung
Farmer's lung

Fumes

Sulfuric acid
Hydrochloric acid

Gases

Chlorine
Nitrogen dioxide
Ammonia

Drug-Induced Disorders

Antineoplastic Drugs

Cyclophosphamide
Nitrosoureas (carmustine, lomustine)
Azathioprine
Cytosine arabinoside
6-Mercaptopurine
Vinblastine

Antineoplastic Drugs Continued

Bleomycin
Methotrexate

Miscellaneous Drugs

Nitrofurantoin
Penicillamine
Gold salts

Neoplastic Diseases

Leukemia
Hodgkin disease
Non-Hodgkin lymphoma
Letterer-Siwe disease
Hand-Schüller-Christian disease
Eosinophilic granuloma
Histiocytosis X

Lymphoproliferative Disorders

Familial erythrophagocytic lymphohistiocytosis
Angioimmunoblastic lymphadenopathy
Lymphoid interstitial pneumonitis
Pseudolymphomas of the lung

Metabolic Disorders

Storage Disorders

Hermansky-Pudlak syndrome

Pulmonary Lipidosis

Gaucher disease
Niemann-Pick disease

Disorders of Ion Transport

Cystic fibrosis

Other

Cardiac failure
Renal disease
Surfactant protein deficiency

Degenerative Disorders

Idiopathic pulmonary alveolar microlithiasis

Neurocutaneous Syndromes with Interstitial Lung Disease

Tuberous sclerosis
Neurofibromatosis
Ataxia-telangiectasia

Adapted from Hilman BC: Interstitial lung disease in children. In Hilman BC (ed): Pediatric Respiratory Disease: Diagnosis and Treatment. Philadelphia, WB Saunders, 1993, p 362.
**P. carinii*, previously considered a protozoan, is now classified as a fungus.

Table 3-12. Interstitial Lung Disease in Children with Unknown Causes

Usual interstitial pneumonitis	Pulmonary alveolar
Idiopathic pulmonary fibrosis	proteinosis
and familial idiopathic	Pulmonary infiltrates with
pulmonary fibrosis	eosinophilia
Sarcoidosis	Chronic eosinophilic
Pulmonary hemosiderosis	pneumonia
Idiopathic pulmonary	
hemosiderosis	

From Hilman BC: Interstitial lung disease in children. In Hilman BC (ed): Pediatric Respiratory Disease: Diagnosis and Treatment. Philadelphia, WB Saunders, 1993, p 363.

Table 3-13. Interstitial Lung Disease in Children Associated with Other Conditions

Interstitial Lung Disease Associated with Collagen Vascular Disease

Juvenile rheumatoid arthritis
Dermatomyositis/polymyositis
Scleroderma
Progressive systemic sclerosis
Ankylosing spondylitis
Sjögren syndrome
Behçet syndrome

Interstitial Lung Disease Associated with Pulmonary Vasculitides

Polyarteritis
Wegener granulomatosis
Churg-Strauss syndrome
Lymphomatoid granulomatosis
Hypersensitivity vasculitis
Systemic necrotizing vasculitides
"Overlap" vasculitis

Interstitial Lung Disease Associated with Liver Disease

Chronic active hepatitis
Primary biliary cirrhosis

Interstitial Lung Disease Associated with Bowel Disease

Ulcerative colitis
Crohn disease

Interstitial Lung Disease Caused by Failure of Other Organs

Chronic left ventricular failure
Chronic left-to-right intracardiac shunt
Chronic renal disease with uremia

Amyloidosis
Graft-Versus-Host Disease
Post-transplantation Lymphoproliferative Disorder
Recovering Phase of Adult Respiratory Distress Syndrome
Goodpasture Syndrome
Hypereosinophilic Syndrome
Pulmonary Veno-occlusive Disease

From Hilman BC: Interstitial lung disease in children. In Hilman BC (ed): Pediatric Respiratory Disease: Diagnosis and Treatment. Philadelphia, WB Saunders, 1993, p 362.

Table 3-14. Investigations for Interstitial Lung Disease in Children

Pediatric Acquired Immunodeficiency Syndrome (AIDS)

Testing for HIV antibodies or antigen or viral load
ELISA or Western blot for HIV antibodies
Polymerase chain reaction (PCR) for HIV

Cystic Fibrosis

Quantitative analysis of sweat electrolytes
Genetic (DNA) testing

Gastroesophageal Reflux/Chronic Aspiration

Barium swallow
pH probe
BAL for lipid-laden macrophages

Immunodeficiency

Quantitative immunoglobulins
Immunoglobulin G subclasses
Assay of antibody response to tetanus, diphtheria,
    Pneumovax, *Haemophilus influenzae* type b
T and B lymphocyte subset quantitation
Anergy panel

Ciliary Disorders

Electron microscopy of nasal scrapings or tracheal biopsy
    for ciliary morphology study

Collagen-Vascular Disorders

Antinuclear antibody (ANA)
Rheumatoid factor (RF)
Antineutrophil cytoplasmic antibodies (ANCA)

Infectious Disease

Viral cultures/serology/viral probe studies, ELISA for
    respiratory syncytial virus
Cultures/serology tests for *Mycoplasma*
Culture for bacterial pathogens/Gram stain
Fungal cultures/smears, lung biopsy
Mycobacterial cultures/smear for acid-fast bacilli; PPD
Silver stains (*Pneumocystis carinii*)
Fluorescent antibodies for *Chlamydia, Legionella* species
Immunofluorescence for *Pneumocystis carinii*

Hypersensitivity Pneumonitis

Serum precipitins

Pulmonary Hemosiderosis

Cytology (gastric lavage, BAL fluid, lung biopsy) for
    hemosiderin-laden macrophages

Adapted from Hilman BC: Interstitial lung disease in children. In Hilman BC (ed): Pediatric Respiratory Disease: Diagnosis and Treatment. Philadelphia, WB Saunders, 1993, p 361.

BAL, bronchoalveolar lavage; ELISA, enzyme-linked immunosorbent assay; HIV, human immunodeficiency virus; PPD, purified protein derivative of *Mycobacterium tuberculosis*.

bronchiectasis, and progressive respiratory insufficiency. Hypersensitivity to other fungal species that produces a clinical picture similar to that of ABPA has been reported.

It is important that the diagnosis of ABPA be made and that appropriate therapy with systemic corticosteroids be instituted, because this condition can result in irreversible lung damage. ABPA is characterized by fever, weight loss, wheezing, and productive cough yielding purulent or rust-colored sputum. This condition should be considered in patients with chronic or atypical and progressive or frequently relapsing lung diseases (e.g., asthma) who have undergone clinical deterioration. ABPA is associated with peripheral eosinophilia and markedly elevated serum IgE levels. Although these laboratory findings are not pathognomonic for this condition, the presence of a normal serum IgE makes the diagnosis of active disease unlikely. Affected individuals have evidence of hypersensitivity to *A. fumigatus,* and sputum evaluation may demonstrate *Aspergillus* hyphal elements. Elevated levels of specific IgE and immunoglobulin G antibodies to *A. fumigatus* can be useful in establishing the diagnosis.

The typical radiographic findings include increased bronchopulmonary markings, opacification of the affected area, and localized pulmonary consolidation. Linear radiolucencies and parallel markings radiating from the hilum ("tram lines") caused by dilated, thickened bronchi may also be present. Chest CT may demonstrate a localized (central) saccular bronchiectasis.

The treatment of choice is systemic corticosteroids, administered for weeks to months. Antifungal agents, such as itraconazole, may be effective in this disorder in some cases or may be a useful adjunct to corticosteroid therapy.

MYCOPLASMAL INFECTIONS

One of the basic tenets regarding respiratory infections in children is that "bacteria do not make you wheeze." *Mycoplasma pneumoniae* is an exception to that rule and should be considered in an older child who presents with new-onset wheezing (see Chapter 2). In addition, infections with *M. pneumoniae* can precipitate exacerbations in patients with asthma. The incidence of *M. pneumoniae* infection peaks between the ages of 5 and 19 years; the organism usually does not produce disease in children younger than age 2. Infections with *M. pneumoniae* tend to be seasonal, occurring most frequently during autumn and early winter.

The findings during *M. pneumoniae* infection on chest roentgenograms are variable. A diffuse, bilateral, reticular infiltrate is the classic roentgenographic appearance of mycoplasmal pneumonia. However, lobar, alveolar, and interstitial infiltrates have also been described. Enlargement of hilar or peritracheal lymph nodes may also be evident. Pleural effusions (usually small) are found in 14% of patients with *M. pneumoniae* pneumonia. Atypical pneumonia (diffuse infiltrates with nonlobar pattern; fever, malaise, myalgias) is often caused by *M. pneumoniae* but may also be caused by *Chlamydia pneumoniae, Legionella* species, and other related pathogens. *M. pneumoniae* tracheobronchitis may produce only subtle roentgenographic changes. PCR or antibody titers (IgM) help to confirm a diagnosis.

VOCAL CORD DYSFUNCTION

A functional disorder that mimics asthma, vocal cord dysfunction is typically manifested as wheezing, dyspnea, and shortness of breath refractory to treatment with inhaled bronchodilators. The wheezing is produced by the adduction of the vocal cords during inspiration and expiration, and the resultant high-pitched inspiratory and expiratory noises are transmitted to the chest, although the sounds are best appreciated over the larynx. Despite the patient's apparent dyspnea, gas exchange is usually unaffected. Pulmonary function studies may demonstrate variable extrathoracic airway obstruction but only during an "attack." The diagnosis is established by direct laryngoscopy, which demonstrates paradoxical motion of the vocal cords. Speech therapy is effective, whereas medications are not.

PNEUMOTHORAX

A pneumothorax occurs when air leaks from the alveoli or airways into the pleural space. The most common cause of pneumothorax in children is chest wall trauma. However, spontaneous pneumothorax can occur in otherwise healthy children with no antecedent illness or injury. This probably affects adolescent boys or young adult men who are typically tall, thin, and athletic; the presence of Marfan syndrome should be considered. Children with asthma may develop a pneumothorax. Clinical presentation usually includes acute onset of dyspnea and chest or shoulder pain.

The physical examination reveals hyperresonance to percussion over the ipsilateral chest, with decreased breath sounds auscultated on the affected side. If the air dissects up through the mediastinum, it may escape into the subcutaneous tissues, producing subcutaneous emphysema. Progressive air leak without air escape can lead to a tension pneumothorax. With increasing pressure, there is mediastinal shift, airway compression, and a decrease in cardiac output. Tension pneumothorax can be life-threatening if it is not recognized and treated rapidly.

The treatment of choice for a pneumothorax of greater than 20% volume is drainage with needle aspiration or with an indwelling chest tube.

NONPULMONARY CAUSES OF RESPIRATORY DISTRESS

Cardiac disease is probably the most important and common nonpulmonary cause of respiratory distress. Increased work of breathing and respiratory distress most commonly occur in cardiac diseases caused by large left-to-right shunts, dysfunction of the systemic ventricle, and vascular lesions that obstruct the airway (see previous discussion). Cardiac failure from any cause is often manifested as respiratory distress. Infants with congenital heart defects that produce a large left-to-right shunt that results in pulmonary vascular engorgement, edema formation, and reduced lung compliance demonstrate tachypnea, dyspnea, and grunting. Wheezing or "cardiac asthma" can occur when there is compression of intrathoracic airways by vascular engorgement and edema. With most congenital heart defects with left-to-right shunts, an abnormal heart murmur and cardiomegaly are prominent clues to diagnosis (see Chapters 8 and 11). Acute myocarditis, usually of viral etiology, can manifest with tachypnea, dyspnea, grunting, and diaphoresis.

The physical examination reveals tachycardia and decreased heart sounds, and chest radiography shows a massively enlarged heart. Cardiomyopathy may be congenital, may have a metabolic or toxic cause, may be familial, or may be idiopathic. Other causes of cardiac failure, such as severe hypertension, renal failure, and severe anemia, should also be sought. Systemic ventricular failure caused by obstructing lesions, such as aortic stenosis, coarctation of the aorta, or mitral stenosis, also causes increased pulmonary vascular engorgement and edema, which results in the same symptoms as those for a large left-to-right shunt. Depending on the severity of the left ventricular outflow obstruction, systemic blood flow may be decreased, resulting in poor perfusion and metabolic acidosis. If blood flow into the systemic ventricle from the pulmonary veins or left atrium is decreased or obstructed, as in total anomalous pulmonary venous return or mitral stenosis, then severe pulmonary edema, hypoxemia, and respiratory distress ensues. Many of these lesions manifest early in infancy. Tachypnea, wheezing, cyanosis, and metabolic acidosis are typical presenting signs. Accurate diagnosis depends on echocardiography; cardiac catheterization may be needed in complex cases.

Children with certain primary neurologic disorders (e.g., increased intracranial pressure or neuromyopathic weakness) may present in respiratory distress. Common symptoms include irregular respirations, hypoventilation, or hyperventilation. These symptoms, accompanied by an altered mental status, should prompt an evaluation of the central nervous system for problems such as meningitis, cerebritis or encephalitis, intracranial hemorrhage, mass lesion, or toxic ingestion. Metabolic derangement that results in acidosis produces tachypnea and possible dyspnea. Common causes of acidosis include diabetic ketoacidosis, sepsis, and ingestions (e.g., aspirin). The presence of multisystem involvement in addition to respiratory distress should lead to arterial blood gas determination, urinalysis, and possibly a toxicologic screen.

Table 3-15. Differentiation of Respiratory Distress in the Neonatal Period

	Respiratory Distress Syndrome	Transient Tachypnea of Newborn	Congenital Pneumonia	Persistent Fetal Circulation	MAS	Congenital Heart Disease*
Gestational age	Preterm	Preterm, full term	Preterm, full term	Full term	Full term; postdates (>40 wk)	Preterm, full term
Perinatal history	Preterm labor, no antenatal corticosteroids; Vaginal bleeding; Fetal distress; Second twin; IDM	Cesarean section; No labor; CNS depressant drugs; IDM	PROM; Maternal fever and leukocytosis; Group B streptococcal cervical colonization; Uterine tenderness; Fetal tachycardia; Amnionitis; May be negative	Fetal distress; MSAF; Low Apgar score; Amnionitis; Oligohydramnios (if pulmonary hypoplasia)	MSAF; Fetal distress	Family history; Abnormal fetal echocardiography; Fetal nonimmune hydrops; Fetal arrhythmia; IDM syndrome–malformation complex
Onset	Birth–12 hr	Birth–12 hr	Birth–1 wk	Birth–6 hr	Birth–6 hr	Birth–1 wk
Neonatal history	Grunting, flaring, retractions, cyanosis, tachypnea, borderline hypotension, edema, oliguria	Tachypnea, flaring, minimal cyanosis or retractions; Hypotonia; Lasts 2–3 days	As per RDS plus hypotension, mottling, cold extremities, apnea, bradycardia; Multiorgan system dysfunction secondary to sepsis–shock†	Tachypnea, cyanosis; Minimal retraction; Multiorgan system dysfunction from perinatal asphyxia†	Meconium below vocal cords; Meconium-stained umbilical cord and fingernails; Failure to suction trachea at birth	Heart murmur; Cyanosis; Minimal flaring, grunting, retraction unless pulmonary edema–heart failure; Poor pulses, active precordium
Arterial blood gas analysis	Progressive but varying hypoxia; Hypercapnia as the disease progresses; Acidosis is mixed respiratory and metabolic	Mild hypoxia (requires ≤50% FiO_2)	Profound, often fixed hypoxia, poorly responsive to therapy; Severe metabolic acidosis secondary to sepsis syndrome–shock	Profound but fluctuating: labile hypoxia; at times therapy-responsive hyperoxia; patient may have minimal or no hypercapnia or therapy-induced hypocapnia; Arterial oxygen gradient between right radial and umbilical arteries secondary to intracardiac shunts (RRA >UA)	As per PFC	Fixed, profound hypoxia, especially if ductus arteriosus is closed; Minimal or no hypercapnia; Profound metabolic acidosis secondary to hypoxia or left-sided heart failure
Chest radiograph	Air bronchogram; Ground glass–bilateral white-out; Atelectasis	Normal, hyperinflated; Perihilar edema	As per RDS; Often bilateral white-out; Focal infiltrates	Normal	Normal or meconium-induced pneumothorax–pneumomediastinum, atelectasis, marked hyperinflation	Unusual heart shape or location; Right-sided aortic arch; Decreased or increased pulmonary vascular markings

	Immature amniotic fluid (RDS)	(TTN)	Pneumonia/Sepsis (GBS)	PPHN/PFC	Meconium Aspiration (MAS)	CHD
Laboratory findings	Immature amniotic fluid, tracheal or gastric aspirate L/S ratio Hypoalbuminemia	None	Neutropenia, leukocytosis, or high band count Positive Gram stain of tracheal aspirate or buffy coat Positive blood culture Positive latex agglutination for GBS Elevated CRP	Occasionally polycythemia (Hct >65%)	None	Abnormal ECG Echocardiogram is definitive test Cardiac catheterization for complex lesions
Treatment	Oxygen, CPAP mechanical ventilation, exogenous intratracheal surfactant Because congenital pneumonia–sepsis can be indistinguishable, add IV ampicillin and gentamicin	Oxygen	Oxygen, mechanical ventilation,‡ broad-spectrum antibiotics (ampicillin and gentamicin) Blood pressure support (IV fluids, dopamine, epinephrine) Possibly hyperimmune globulin for GBS ECMO	Oxygen, mechanical ventilation,‡ surfactant, INO, ECMO	As per PFC	Initial palliation with prostaglandins, then surgery Digoxin, inotropic agents (dopamine, dobutamine)
Prevention	Antenatal dexamethasone or betamethasone Exogenous surfactant Prevent preterm birth	Avoid unnecessary cesarean section	Intrapartum ampicillin for GBS	Prevent and treat fetal distress and neonatal hypoxia	Suction (DeLee) oropharynx after delivery of head Suction trachea after birth if born through thick meconium, if signs of fetal or neonatal distress, or if no DeLee suctioning of oropharynx on perineum	Avoid teratogenic drugs or chromosomal syndromes

*See Chapters 10 and 11.

†Multisystem organ dysfunction includes myocardial depression (shock, heart failure, tricuspid regurgitation), pulmonary hypertension (hypoxia), acute tubular necrosis (oliguria–anuria, renal failure), hepatic abnormalities (direct reacting jaundice, elevated liver enzymes, prolonged prothrombin time), hematologic abnormalities (disseminated intravascular coagulation, neutropenia, anemia, thrombocytopenia), and CNS dysfunction (coma, seizures).

‡Mechanical ventilation includes conventional rate, flow or pressure-regulated ventilators, or high-frequency jet or oscillator ventilators.

CHD, congenital heart disease; CNS, central nervous system; CPAP, continuous positive airway pressure; CRP, C reactive protein–acute phase reactant; ECG, electrocardiogram; ECMO, extracorporeal membrane oxygenation (heart-lung or lung bypass); FiO_2, fraction of inspired oxygen; GBS, group B streptococci; Hct, hematocrit; IDM, infant of diabetic mother; INO, inhaled nitric oxide; IV, intravenous; L/S, lecithin-sphingomyelin ratio: determines active surfactant maturity and reduced risk for RDS; MAS, meconium aspiration syndrome (pneumonia); MSAF, meconium-stained amniotic fluid; PFC, persistent fetal circulation—also known as persistent pulmonary hypertension of the newborn; PROM, premature, prolonged rupture of the fetal membranes (>18–24 hr); RDS, respiratory distress syndrome; RRA, right radial artery (preductal blood); UA, umbilical artery (postductal blood).

RESPIRATORY DISTRESS IN THE NEONATAL PERIOD

Preterm and full-term infants can have respiratory distress for several reasons (Table 3-15; see also Table 3-1), many of which do not directly involve the respiratory system (e.g., hypoglycemia, sepsis, anemia, intracranial hemorrhage, and necrotizing enterocolitis). Respiratory distress in the neonate is usually characterized by cyanosis, tachypnea, grunting, chest wall retractions, and nasal flaring. Cyanosis is common and may be caused by congenital heart disease with right-to-left shunt, severe pulmonary disease, methemoglobinemia, central nervous system depression, shock, or sepsis.

In the preterm infant, *respiratory distress syndrome,* caused by surfactant deficiency, alveolar collapse, and hyaline membrane formation, is the most common cause of respiratory distress. Although it can be recognized on the basis of diffuse bilateral atelectasis (ground-glass appearance with air bronchograms) on chest radiographs, hypoxemia, and late-onset hypercapnia, bacterial pneumonia and sepsis can present in an almost identical manner (see Tables 3-1 and 3-15).

Meconium aspiration at the time of delivery can cause severe respiratory distress and pneumonia in full-term infants. *Persistent fetal circulation,* also called persistent pulmonary hypertension of the newborn, can also accompany meconium aspiration, pneumonia, and sepsis. Profound but fluctuating hypoxemia refractory to treatment with supplemental oxygen and occurring in the absence of cyanotic congenital heart disease helps confirm the diagnosis of persistent fetal circulation.

Other pulmonary causes of respiratory distress in the newborn include *spontaneous pneumothorax,* which can occur in up to 2% of all live births (see Table 3-1). Most pneumothoraces are small (<20%) and resolve spontaneously or with only the administration of supplemental oxygen.

Pulmonary hypoplasia is a rare condition that generally occurs in infants with oligohydramnios with or without renal dysgenesis or agenesis and abnormal facies (*Potter syndrome*). In these infants, bilateral pneumothoraces may develop, particularly after resuscitative efforts in the delivery room.

Transient tachypnea of the newborn is a relatively benign condition most often seen in more mature preterm and some full-term infants delivered by cesarean section after an uneventful pregnancy. The disorder is characterized by tachypnea without significant distress and usually normal arterial blood gas values (an FiO_2 of 30% to 40% may be needed to treat mild hypoxemia). Although grunting may occur, other signs of dyspnea are not present, and the infant is otherwise well. Chest radiography may demonstrate central perihilar streaking. The condition is self-limited and usually resolves within 2 to 3 days.

Hematologic abnormalities that cause profound anemia (erythroblastosis, nonimmune hydrops) or polycythemia can also result in respiratory distress. These conditions are often recognized prenatally or in the immediate neonatal period because of the significant pallor or plethora exhibited, respectively.

A newborn with severe respiratory distress, absence of left-sided breath sounds, bowel sounds in the chest, and a scaphoid abdomen should be suspected of having a *congenital diaphragmatic hernia* (CDH). This lesion occurs five times more frequently on the left than on the right side and is identified when loops of bowel are seen within the thoracic cavity on a chest radiograph. In many cases, the lung on the affected side is hypoplastic, and this accounts for the residual pulmonary symptoms seen after surgical repair of the defect. Diaphragmatic hernias are often detected on prenatal ultrasound examination and are surgically repaired after stabilization on mechanical ventilation, inhaled nitric oxide, or extracorporeal membrane oxygenation. The survival rate of affected infants remains approximately 60%. Extracorporeal membrane oxygenation is beneficial to patients with CDH, both preoperatively and in the immediate postoperative period. Although infants affected with CDH are usually profoundly ill in the immediate neonatal period, an occasional patient may present later in infancy or even childhood and with milder symptoms. These patients tend to do quite well and have few, if any, long-term sequelae.

The diagnostic, therapeutic, and preventive approaches to common disorders associated with neonatal respiratory distress are noted in Table 3-15. The hyperoxia test is another diagnostic test used to attempt to differentiate cyanotic congenital heart disease from pulmonary diseases such as respiratory distress syndrome. If the response to breathing 100% oxygen, often with continuous positive airway pressure (+ 4 to 6 cm H_2O), does not improve the umbilical arterial oxygenation to greater than 150 mm Hg, cyanotic heart disease may be considered. However, this test may not produce a hyperoxic response if the patient has persistent fetal circulation, or it may produce a hyperoxic response if the umbilical arterial catheter is misplaced. Therefore, immediate evaluation with echocardiography is indicated if the differential diagnosis includes cyanotic heart disease or persistent fetal circulation (see Chapter 11).

RED FLAGS AND THINGS NOT TO MISS

Respiratory distress may be a result of disorders of the extrathoracic or intrathoracic airways (intrinsic or extrinsic compression-obstruction), alveoli, pulmonary vasculature (pulmonary emboli), pleural spaces, or thorax. The distress may be secondary to respiratory, cardiovascular, hematologic, or central nervous system diseases. Red flags include sudden onset of distress (pulmonary embolism, foreign body aspiration), chronicity (asthma, mass, immune deficiency, congenital anomaly, cystic fibrosis), digital clubbing (see Chapter 2), weight loss, fever, hemoptysis (see Chapter 2), focal physical findings, pleural effusions, positive family history, dyspnea, and cyanosis. Hypoxia in the presence of a normal chest film suggests a pulmonary embolism.

In the neonatal period, respiratory distress syndrome must be differentiated from infections, meconium aspiration, persistent fetal circulation, and congenital respiratory, hematologic, or cardiovascular anomalies.

REFERENCES

Asthma

Bahrainwala AH, Simon MR: Wheezing and vocal cord dysfunction mimicking asthma. Curr Opin Pulm Med 2001;7:8-13.

Chang AB: Cough, cough receptors, and asthma in children. Pediatr Pulmonol 1999;28:59-70.

Ciarallo L, Brousseau D, Reinert S: Higher-dose intravenous magnesium therapy for children with moderate to severe asthma. Arch Pediatr Adolesc Med 2000;154:979-83.

Gibson PG, Henry RL, Coughlan JL: Gastro-oesophageal reflux treatment for asthma in adults and children. Cochrane Database Syst Rev 2000;(2): CD001496.

Gries DM, Moffett DR, Pulos E, Carter ER. A single dose of IM administered dexamethasone acetate is as effective as oral prednisone to treat asthma exacerbations in young children. J Pediatr 2000;136:298-303.

National Asthma Education and Prevention Program Expert Panel Report 2: Guidelines for the diagnosis and management of asthma (NIH Publication No. 97-4051). Rockville, MD, National Institutes of Health/National Heart, Lung, and Blood Institute, 1997.

Payne DN, Balfour-Lynn IM. Children with difficult asthma: A practical approach. J Asthma 2001;38:189-203.

Sontag SJ: Why do the published data fail to clarify the relationship between gastroesophageal reflux and asthma? Am J Med 2000;108:159S-169S.

Theodoropoulos DS, Lockey RF, Boyce HW Jr, Bukantz SC: Gastroesophageal reflux and asthma: a review of pathogenesis, diagnosis, and therapy. Allergy 1999;54:651-661.

Werner HA: Status asthmaticus in children: A review. Chest 2001;119: 1913-1929.

Anatomic Anomalies

Bakker DA, Berger RM, Witsenburg M, Bogers AJ: Vascular rings: A rare cause of common respiratory symptoms. Acta Pediatr 1999;88:947-952.

Schwartz DS, Reyes-Mugica M, Keller MS: Imaging of surgical diseases of the newborn chest. Intrapleural mass lesions. Radiol Clin North Am 1999; 37:1067-1078.

Sebening C, Jakob H, Tochtermann U, et al: Vascular tracheobronchial compression syndromes—Experience in surgical treatment and literature review. Thorac Cardiovasc Surg 2000;48:164-174.

Infections

Bauer TT, Torres A: Acute respiratory distress syndrome and nosocomial pneumonia. Thorax 1999;54:1036-1040.

Bochud PY, Moser F, Erard P, et al: Community-acquired pneumonia. A prospective outpatient study. Medicine 2001;80:75-87.

Esposito S, Blasi F, Arosio C, et al: Importance of acute *Mycoplasma pneumoniae* and *Chlamydia pneumoniae* infections in children with wheezing. Eur Respir J 2000;16:1142-1146.

Hall CB: Respiratory syncytial virus and parainfluenza virus. N Engl J Med 2001;344:1917-1928.

Lerou PH: Lower respiratory tract infections in children. Curr Opin Pediatr 2001;13:200-206.

Panitch HB: Bronchiolitis in infants. Curr Opin Pediatr 2001;12:256-260.

Principi N, Esposito S, Blasi F, et al: Role of *Mycoplasma pneumoniae* and *Chlamydia pneumoniae* in children with community-acquired lower respiratory tract infections. Clin Infect Dis 2001;32:1281-1289.

Tan TQ, Mason EO, Barson WJ, et al: Clinical characteristics and outcome of children with pneumonia attributable to penicillin-susceptible and penicillin-nonsusceptible *Streptococcus pneumoniae.* Pediatr 1998;102: 1369-1375.

Wark PA, Gibson PG: Allergic bronchopulmonary aspergillosis: new concepts of pathogenesis and treatment. Respirology 2001;6:1-7.

Zambon M: Active and passive immunisation against respiratory syncytial virus. Rev Med Virol 1999;9:227-236.

Neonatal Disorders

Ballard PL, Nogee LM, Beers MF, et al: Partial deficiency of surfactant protein B in an infant with chronic lung disease. Pediatrics 1995;96: 1046-1052.

Bancalari E: Changes in the pathogenesis and prevention of chronic lung disease of prematurity. Am J Perinatol 2001;18:1-9.

Barrington KJ, Finer NN: Inhaled nitric oxide for respiratory failure in preterm infants. Cochrane Database Syst Rev 2000;(2):CD000509.

Bhuta T, Henderson-Smart DJ: Rescue high frequency oscillatory ventilation versus conventional ventilation for pulmonary dysfunction in preterm infants. Cochrane Database Syst Rev 2000;(2):CD000438.

Christou H, Van Marter LJ, Wessel DL, et al: Inhaled nitric oxide reduces the need for extracorporeal membrane oxygenation in infants with persistent pulmonary hypertension of the newborn. Crit Care Med 2000;28: 3722-3727.

Jobe AH, Ikegami M: Prevention of bronchopulmonary dysplasia. Curr Opin Pediatr 2001;13:124-129.

Soll RF: Synthetic surfactant for respiratory distress syndrome in preterm infants. Cochrane Database Syst Rev 2000;(2):CD001149.

Management

Arnold JH, Anas NG, Luckett P, et al: High-frequency oscillatory ventilation in pediatric respiratory failure: a multicenter experience. Crit Care Med 2000;28:3913-3919.

Baumann MH: Treatment of spontaneous pneumothorax. Curr Opin Pulm Med 2000;6:275-280.

Chou KJ, Fisher JL, Silver EJ: Characteristics and outcome of children with carbon monoxide poisoning with and without smoke exposure referred for hyperbaric oxygen therapy. Pediatr Emerg Care 2000;16: 151-155.

Curley AE, Halliday HL: The present status of exogenous surfactant for the newborn. Early Hum Dev 2001;61:67-83.

Lewandowski K: Extracorporeal membrane oxygenation for severe acute respiratory failure. Crit Care 2000;4:156-168.

Moriette G, Brunhes A, Jarreau PH: High-frequency oscillatory ventilation in the management of respiratory distress syndrome. Biol Neonate 2000;77(Suppl. 1):14-16.

Moyle JTB: Uses and abuses of pulse oximetry. Arch Dis Child 1996;74:77.

Shapiro MB, Anderson HL 3rd, Bartlett RH: Respiratory failure. Conventional and high-tech support. Surg Clin North Am 2000;80: 871-883.

Cystic Fibrosis

Davis PB Drumm ML, Konstan MW: Cystic fibrosis—State of the art. Am J Respir Crit Care Med 1996;154:1229-1256.

Koch C, Hoiby N: Diagnosis and treatment of cystic fibrosis. Respiration 2000;67:239-247.

Nixon GM, Armstrong DS, Carzino R, et al: Clinical outcome after early *Pseudomonas aeruginosa* infection in cystic fibrosis. J Pediatr 2001; 138:699-704.

Rosenstein BJ, Cutting GR: The diagnosis of cystic fibrosis: A consensus statement. J Pediatr 1998;132:589-595.

Zeitlin PL: Future pharmacological treatment of cystic fibrosis. Respiration 2000;67:351-357.

Other Disorders

Goldberg BJ, Kaplan MS: Non-asthmatic respiratory symptomatology. Curr Opin Pulm Med 2000;6:26-30.

Homnick DN, Pratt HD: Respiratory diseases with a psychosomatic component in adolescents. Adolesc Med 2000;11:547-565.

Howenstine MS, Eigen H: Current concepts on interstitial lung disease in children. Curr Opin Pediatr 1999;11:200-204.

Irwin RS, Bochet LP, Cloutier, MM, et al: Managing cough as a defense mechanism and as a symptom. A consensus panel report of the American College of Chest Physicians. Chest 1998;114:133s-181s.

Meeks , Bush A: Primary ciliary dyskinesia (PCD). Pediatr Pulmonol 2000; 29:307-316.

Sahn SA, Heffner JE: Spontaneous pneumothorax. N Engl J Med 2000; 342:868-874.

Skoulakis CE, Doxas PG, Papadakis CE, et al: Bronchoscopy for foreign body removal in children. A review and analysis of 210 cases. Int J Pediatr Otorhinolaryngol 2000;53:143-148.

Ware LB, Matthay MA: The acute respiratory distress syndrome. N Eng J Med 2000;342:1334-1349.

4 Earache

Patricia S. Lye*

Earache (otalgia) is pain that arises from a pathologic process in the external, middle, or inner ear or that is referred to the ear from another structure. The most common cause of ear pain in children is otitis media (Tables 4-1 and 4-2). Otitis media accounts for approximately 25% of all physician office visits for children, and the number of visits for this illness has increased nearly twofold since 1980. The second most common cause of ear pain is otitis externa, followed by dermatitis and infections of the pinna. All other causes are rare (Table 4-3). A careful examination of the pinna, external auditory canal, and tympanic membrane can help the clinician identify most causes of ear pain. When the findings are normal, the clinician should consider referred pain (Table 4-4).

DIAGNOSTIC APPROACH

HISTORY

Verbal children with ear pain are usually able to localize and accurately describe their symptoms. Younger children often cannot localize their pain and may present with a variety of nonspecific symptoms, including fever, irritability, rhinorrhea (from an associated upper respiratory tract infection), and ear pulling. Even though ear pulling is associated with ear pain, it is neither specific nor sensitive in the

diagnosis of ear disease. In addition, infants with acute otitis media may be afebrile and present with various degrees of irritability, such as sleep disturbances and/or eating or drinking inadequately. The clinician should be highly suspicious of ear disease in infants during the first year of life or in any preschool child with fever, irritability, or an upper respiratory tract infection.

The clinician must be careful in taking a history from a child who presents with ear pain, to distinguish between true ear pain and the fullness that children experience when they have an effusion or discomfort from a retracted tympanic membrane secondary to a dysfunctional eustachian tube. With an older child, the clinician can ask about a sensation of pressure or if their ears need to "pop," such as when they are flying in an airplane. Children with a middle ear effusion also may have decreased hearing acuity.

Risk factors for acute otitis media include a sibling's or personal history of recurrent acute otitis media, trisomy 21, household cigarette smoke exposure, formula-feeding, Native American or Eskimo heritage, lower socioeconomic status, male gender, cleft palate, immunodeficiency, and group day care attendance or siblings in the household.

Children with otitis externa ("swimmer's ear") present with ear pain and/or purulent otorrhea. When the pinna and tragus are manipulated, there is extreme pain. The canal is red, and there is drainage from the external ear canal. Relapsing polychondritis also involves

Table 4-1. Differential Diagnoses of Painful External Ear and Auditory Canal Disorders

Disorder	Clinical Features
Acute otitis externa	Diffuse redness, swelling, and pain of the canal with greenish to whitish exudate; often very tender pinna
Malignant otitis externa	In immunocompromised hosts and poorly controlled diabetics; rapidly progressive, severe swelling and redness of pinna; pinna may be laterally displaced
Dermatitis	
Eczema	History of atopy, presence of lesions elsewhere; lesions are scaly, red, pruritic, and weeping
Contact	History of cosmetic use or irritant exposure; lesions are scaly, red, pruritic, and weeping
Seborrhea	Scaly, red, papular dermatitis; scalp may have thick, yellow scales
Psoriasis	History or presence of psoriasis elsewhere; erythematous papules that coalesce into thick, white plaques
Cellulitis	Diffuse redness, tenderness, and swelling of the pinna
Furuncles	Red, tender papules in areas with hair follicles (distal third of the ear canal)
Infected periauricular cyst	Discrete, palpable lesions; history of previous swelling at same site; cellulitis may develop, obscuring cystic structure
Insect bites	History of exposure; lesions are red, tender papules
Herpes zoster	Painful, vesicular lesions in the ear canal and tympanic membrane in the distribution of cranial nerves V and VII
Perichondritis	Inflammation of the cartilage, usually secondary to cellulitis
Tumors	Very rare, palpable mass, destruction of surrounding structures
Foreign body	Almost any type of foreign body is possible; the foreign body may cause secondary trauma to the ear canal or become a nidus for an infection of the ear canal
Trauma	Bruising and swelling of external ear; there may be signs of basilar skull fracture (cerebrospinal fluid otorrhea, hemotympanum)

*This chapter is an updated and edited version of the chapter by Colin Marchant that appeared in the first edition.

Table 4-2. Differential Diagnosis of Painful Middle Ear Disorders

Disorder	Clinical Features
Acute otitis media	Immobile tympanic membrane that may appear bulging, red, and/or opaque
Myringitis bullosa	Presumably viral vesicles and bullae, often with hemorrhage on the tympanic membrane; illness may also be caused by the same bacterial pathogens of acute otitis media
Acute mastoiditis with periostitis	Tenderness and erythema over mastoid process; no destruction of bone trabeculae
Acute mastoid osteitis	Destruction of bone trabeculae; tenderness and erythema over mastoid process coupled with outward displacement of pinna
Wegener granulomatosis	Severe necrotizing vasculitis; ulcerative and destructive granulomatous lesions of upper and lower respiratory tract
Histiocytosis	Pituitary dysfunction, exophthalmos, seborrheic dermatitis, and bone lesions; if bone lesions involve the ear, patient presents with mastoid tenderness and otorrhea

Table 4-3. Causes of Otalgia and Sources for Referred Pain

Intrinsic

I. External Ear

A. External otitis
B. Cerumen impaction
C. Foreign body
D. Perichondritis
E. Preauricular cyst or sinus
F. Insects
G. Myringitis
H. Trauma
I. Tumor

II. Middle Ear, Eustachian Tube, and Mastoid

A. Barotrauma
B. Middle ear effusion
C. Negative intratympanic pressure (eustachian tube dysfunction)
D. Acute otitis media
E. Mastoiditis
F. Aditus block
G. Complication of otitis media
H. Tumor
I. Eosinophilic granuloma
J. Wegener granulomatosis

Extrinsic

I. Trigeminal Nerve

A. Dental
B. Jaw
C. Temporomandibular joint
D. Oral cavity (tongue)
E. Infratemporal fossa tumors

II. Facial Nerve

A. Bell palsy
B. Tumors
C. Herpes zoster

III. Glossopharyngeal Nerve

A. Tonsil
B. Oropharynx
C. Nasopharynx

IV. Vagus Nerve

A. Laryngopharynx
B. Esophagus
C. Gastroesophageal reflux
D. Thyroid

V. Cervical Nerves

A. Lymph nodes
B. Cysts
C. Cervical spine
D. Neck infections

VI. Miscellaneous

A. Migraine
B. Neuralgias
C. Paranasal sinuses
D. Central nervous system
E. Drug induced (mesalazine, sulfasalazine)
F. Munchausen syndrome

From Bluestone CD, Stool SE, Alper CM, et al: Pediatric Otolaryngology, vol 1, 4th ed. Philadelphia, WB Saunders, 2003, p 288.

swelling and redness of the pinna; however, this condition is usually bilateral and recurrent, and other cartilaginous structures are affected.

With referred ear pain, such as from tooth decay or teething, there are often additional symptoms associated with the respective head and neck structures (see Table 4-4). For example, patients with ear pain secondary to maxillary sinusitis may also complain of headaches and purulent rhinorrhea.

PHYSICAL EXAMINATION

In a child presenting with a chief complaint of ear pain, the general examination includes the temperature, the respiratory rate, and a determination of whether the infant or child has a toxic appearance. Then the clinician proceeds with the complete head, eyes, ears, nose, and throat examination and with an appropriately focused physical examination of other pertinent systems.

The examination of the ear begins with inspection of the pinna and adjacent tissues for dermatitis, redness, and edema. In mastoiditis, the redness is over the mastoid process; in otitis externa, it is localized to the external auditory canal and the pinna. In both conditions, the swelling may be so severe that the pinna is laterally displaced. The opening of the external ear canal is also examined for the presence of discharge or exudate. The pinna, including the cartilaginous portions, and the mastoid process are palpated for any tenderness. Most disorders of the external ear can be detected through this examination (see Tables 4-1 and 4-3).

Otoscopy provides an opportunity to indirectly view the middle ear through the tympanic membrane. The middle ear is normally an air-filled cavity that transmits sound from the eardrum to the ossicle and then into the internal ear (Fig. 4-1). Otoscopy begins by properly positioning and, if necessary, restraining the patient. Both shoulders and hips need to be stabilized so that the patient cannot roll during the examination. Infants are best examined on an examining table in the prone position, with a parent or an attendant firmly holding the patient's shoulders, thus preventing the patient from moving. Toddlers should sit on a parent's lap, with the examiner sitting in a chair opposite them. The child is held against the parent's chest, with

Table 4-4. Causes of Referred Ear Pain

Neck

Cervical lymphadenitis
Infected cervical cysts
Subluxation of the atlantoaxial joint (torticollis and otalgia)

Salivary Glands

Parotitis

Thyroid

Thyroiditis

Teeth and Gums

Dental abscess
Impacted teeth
Gingivitis

Temporomandibular Joint

Arthritis, juvenile rheumatoid arthritis
Spasm from bruxism or dental malocclusion

Tonsils

Tonsillitis
Peritonsillar abscess
Post-tonsillectomy neuralgia

Pharynx

Pharyngitis

Paranasal Sinuses

Maxillary sinusitis

Other

Herpes zoster (Ramsey-Hunt syndrome: postherpetic
  neuralgia, migraine, Bell palsy)
Tumors (e.g., of facial nerve)

one of the parent's hands and arms holding the child's arms and the other around the child's head so that one ear is exposed.

The eardrum is often obscured by cerumen (ear wax). Failure to remove the debris is the major reason for diagnostic errors. To view the eardrum properly, the examiner first removes the wax by irrigating the ear canal gently with lukewarm water, by lifting the wax out with a blunt curette, or by dissolving the wax by placing 1 to 2 drops of docusate sodium liquid in the canal for 10 to 15 minutes. Contraindications for irrigation or use of a ceruminolytic solution are the presence of a tympanostomy tube, a perforated tympanic membrane, or an organic foreign body (e.g., legumes swell in contact with fluids).

During the insertion of the speculum, the clinician should note any redness, edema, tenderness, exudate, furuncles, or vesicles that may be present in the external auditory canal. In some illnesses (otitis externa), the ear canal may be so edematous that the speculum cannot be inserted and the eardrum cannot be seen. In addition, in neonates and in some children with craniofacial anomalies such as trisomy 21, the external canal may be so tiny as to preclude an accurate assessment of the tympanic membrane.

Because pneumatic otoscopy is more accurate than otoscopy in detecting middle ear effusion, it should be part of every ear examination. In performing pneumatic otoscopy, the examiner first selects a speculum that will fit snugly in the external auditory canal. The examiner partially depresses the rubber bulb of the pneumatic otoscope and inserts the otoscope into the ear canal (Fig. 4-2). Once the eardrum is seen, the examiner should observe the color, appearance, position, bone landmarks, and mobility of the tympanic membrane (Table 4-5, Fig. 4-3). If the eardrum is not perforated, the clinician observes its mobility by alternating positive and negative pressure by gently depressing and releasing the bulb of the pneumatic otoscope. Poor mobility of the eardrum may be secondary to middle ear effusion, a perforated tympanic membrane, or lack of an airtight seal (Fig. 4-4).

In neonates and young infants, the eardrum is less perpendicular to the observer, the bony landmarks are less distinct, and the eardrum

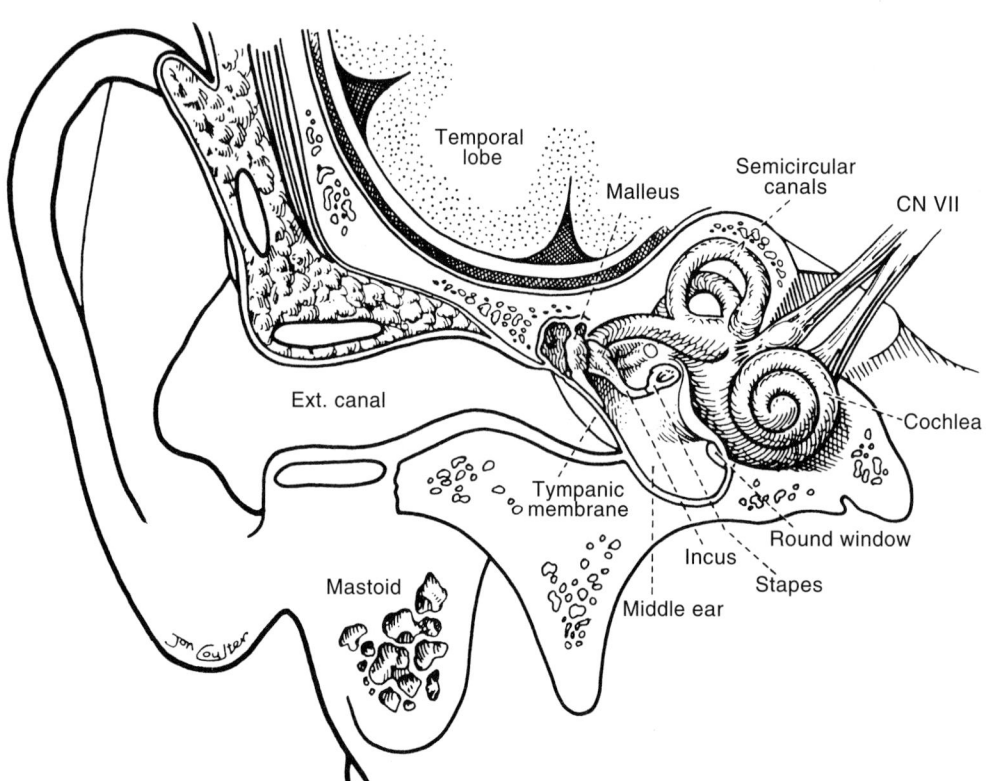

Figure 4-1. Anatomy of the ear. CN, cranial nerve; ext, exterior. (From Bluestone CD, Klein JO: Otitis Media in Infants and Children, 2nd ed. Philadelphia, WB Saunders, 1995, p 11.)

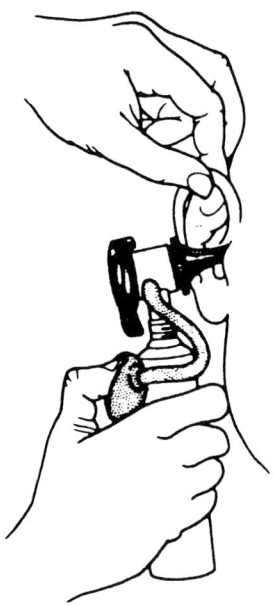

Figure 4-2. Technique for pneumatic otoscopy. (From Bluestone CD, Klein JO: Otitis Media in Infants and Children, 2nd ed. Philadelphia, WB Saunders, 1995, p 92.)

is less mobile than in older infants and children. Failure to appreciate these normal otoscopic findings may lead to the overdiagnosis of middle ear effusion.

In the first few hours of acute otitis media, the middle ear cavity may not yet be filled with fluid, and the mobility may be normal. By the time the patient is examined, however, the middle ear cavity is usually filled with fluid, and the eardrum is opaque, is bulging, and has decreased mobility (see Fig. 4-4). A reddened eardrum may indicate inflammation of the tympanic membrane, but the specificity of this physical finding is reduced because crying alone induces diffuse redness of the eardrum. In addition, differentiation of color is highly variable among observers, which may in part result from the intensity and type of light source used in otoscopy.

Otitis media with effusion (OME) is also called *serous otitis media*. The cardinal sign is decreased mobility of the eardrum.

The eardrum may also be opaque, but it should not be bulging or grossly inflamed. A challenge for the clinician is the child with symptoms consistent with acute otitis media (ear pain) but with the physical findings of OME. In such cases, it is difficult to decide whether there is an acute infection of the middle ear or whether it is OME with an illness at another site causing the symptoms.

When the external ear and tympanic membrane are normal in a child with an earache, the clinician must consider the possibility of referred pain (see Table 4-4). Innervation of the external and middle ear includes pain fibers of the trigeminal, glossopharyngeal, and vagus nerves and, to a lesser extent, the facial nerve and upper cervical nerves. The clinician should examine the neck, parotid gland, thyroid, mouth, tongue, teeth, temporomandibular joint, tonsils, and throat. In children, the cause of referred pain is usually infectious rather than noninfectious (e.g., a tumor).

DIAGNOSTIC TESTS

Bacterial Cultures

Routine cultures of middle or external ear fluid are not required because most infections are self-limited and respond to empirical antimicrobial therapy. In selected instances (e.g., persistent treatment failure or severe pain, an immunocompromised host, a neonate), culture of otorrhea from the external auditory canal or cultures of middle ear fluid by tympanocentesis may guide therapy (Fig. 4-5). In a child with acute otitis media, the offending pathogen is usually present in the nasopharynx. Unfortunately, nasopharyngeal cultures are not helpful in directing therapy because it is not known which organism is actually causing the middle ear infection. With the emergence of strains of *Streptococcus pneumoniae* that are resistant to commonly used antibiotics, the incidence of treatment failures may increase. This may necessitate a greater reliance on tympanocentesis for culture of middle ear fluid to determine the appropriate antimicrobial agent.

Tympanometry

Tympanometry is an objective method for detecting the presence of middle ear effusion. A soft plastic probe is inserted into the opening of the external auditory canal in order to obtain an airtight seal. The tympanometer measures the flow of sound energy into the middle ear under conditions of changing air pressure. When the air pressure

Table 4-5. The Tympanic Membrane in Acute Otitis Media and Otitis Media with Effusion

Characteristic	Normal Findings	Acute Otitis Media	Otitis Media with Effusion	Comments
Color	Gray to pink	Often red from inflammation; yellow to white from purulent fluid behind eardrum	Usually gray to pink, but may still be yellow or white; not red (inflamed)	Interobserver variation of color is high; redness occurs from crying alone
Appearance	Translucent	Opaque	Translucent or opaque	Opacity is caused by opaque fluid or by scarring of eardrum
Position	Neutral	Fluid under pressure produces bulging of eardrum; bony landmarks may be distorted and the light reflux lost	Not bulging; may be retracted by negative middle pressure (caused by eustachian tube obstruction)	
Mobility (to positive and negative pressure)	Tympanic membrane moves freely	Mobility to positive and negative pressure reduced	Mobility to positive and negative pressure reduced	
Other findings		Perforation with otorrhea		

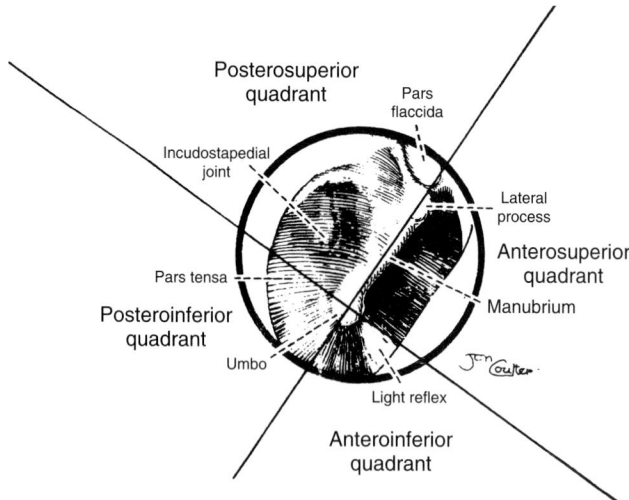

Figure 4-3. The four quadrants of a right tympanic membrane. (From Bluestone CD, Stool SE, Alper CM, et al: Pediatric Otolaryngology, vol 1, 4th ed. Philadelphia, WB Saunders, 2003, p 179.)

is equal on both sides of an intact eardrum, with the drum in neutral position, the transmission of sound energy through the tympanic membrane is at its maximum. The peak on the tympanogram represents the pressure at which the flow of sound energy is maximal. For example, in a normal air-filled middle ear cavity, the peak occurs at ambient atmospheric pressure (Fig. 4-6A). With eustachian tube dysfunction (a retracted eardrum but no middle ear effusion), the peak occurs in the negative pressure range on the recording (see Fig. 4-6C). With middle ear effusion, the sound energy flow into the middle ear is reduced, which produces a flat tympanogram (see Fig. 4-6B). A flat tympanogram may also result from cerumen or from occlusion of the opening of the probe by the wall of the external auditory canal. In a perforated eardrum, the sound energy is readily transmitted through the hole in the drum throughout the entire pressure range, which results in a flat tympanogram with a markedly elevated baseline.

The sensitivity and specificity of tympanometry depend on the patient population, the instrument, and the criteria for interpretation. When performed by experts, tympanometry and pneumatic otoscopy have equivalent sensitivity (approximately 90%) and specificity (70% to 80%). Tympanometry is neither more accurate nor more convenient than is properly performed pneumatic otoscopy. Some tympanometers do not perform well in infants younger than 6 months of age. Tympanometry is advantageous if the clinician is unsure of the otoscopic findings, and it provides an objective and printed record documenting the status of the middle ear effusion.

Acoustic Reflectometry

The acoustic reflectometer detects middle ear effusion by directing a sound of varying frequency toward the tympanic membrane and measuring the intensity of reflected sound. This hand-held instrument is similar in size to that of an otoscope. The tip of the reflectometer is inserted in the external opening of the ear canal. In contrast to tympanometry, an airtight seal is not required. The frequency of maximal reflected sound depends on the arbitrary distance of the probe from the eardrum. Middle ear effusion is detected not by the frequency but by the magnitude of maximal reflected sound. When middle ear effusion is present, reflectance is increased in comparison with that in the air-filled ear.

Reflectometry is easily learned, quick, convenient, and useful in a crying child. With a sensitivity of 80% to 87% and a specificity of 54% to 70%, reflectometry is less accurate than properly performed pneumatic otoscopy in detecting middle ear effusion. Because the accuracy of current models decreases in infants younger than 1 year, this technique should not be used in infants younger than 6 months of age. Like tympanometry, reflectometry can reveal only whether middle ear effusion is present and cannot reveal whether the effusion is secondary to acute otitis media or otitis media with effusion. Reflectometry is useful if otoscopic findings are indefinite.

Diagnostic Imaging

Radiologic techniques are rarely required in the evaluation of external or middle ear disease, but they may be useful in the assessment of intratemporal and intracranial complications of otitis media. Roentgenograms of the mastoid are helpful in the diagnosis of acute and chronic mastoiditis. Opacification of the normally aerated mastoid air cells is usually seen in acute otitis media because the mastoid air cells communicate with the middle ear space. By definition, this is acute *mastoiditis;* however, this opacification resolves concomitantly with the successful treatment of acute otitis media. In contrast, in *acute mastoid osteitis,* also called *acute coalescent mastoiditis,* there is destruction of bone trabeculations in the mastoid air cells.

Computed tomographic scans of the mastoid yield clearer images of the destructive process in the bone trabeculations. Other imaging studies that may be useful in evaluating a patient for complications of acute otitis media include computed tomographic scans of the head for suspected cholesteatomas and intracranial mass lesions (brain abscess) and magnetic resonance venography for sinus thrombosis.

DIFFERENTIAL DIAGNOSIS

Most disorders of the external and middle ear are readily apparent after the examination of the ear (see Tables 4-1 to 4-3). If examination findings are unremarkable, the clinician should consider referred pain (see Table 4-4). Most cases of otitis media are uncomplicated; however, the clinician should be alert to the complications and sequelae of acute otitis media (Tables 4-6 and 4-7).

SPECIFIC ILLNESSES

OTITIS EXTERNA

Otitis externa, an infection of the external ear canal, is linked to warm humid weather, moisture in the canal, and swimming. The moisture may cause small abrasions in the protective lipid layer of skin in the ear canal. These abrasions become infected on exposure to pathogenic bacteria. *Pseudomonas aeruginosa* is the predominant organism causing otitis externa, followed by *Staphylococcus aureus, S. pneumoniae,* and *Proteus mirabilis.* Less commonly, otorrhea draining from a perforated tympanic membrane secondary to otitis media may cause otitis externa. The patient may complain of intense pain (especially with manipulation of the pinna), redness, and otorrhea. On physical examination, the ear canal is red, edematous, and tender.

Treatment consists of a topical suspension containing ofloxacin or ciprofloxacin or a preparation combining polymyxin and neomycin with hydrocortisone. Most patients respond quickly in a few days. If there is marked edema of the canal, antibiotics may not reach the site of infection. In this case, the canal should be cleaned with gentle suction, and a cotton wick should be inserted into the auditory canal. Antibiotic suspension is then dripped into the wick, which allows the medication to diffuse further into the ear canal. In some cases, daily cleaning and replacement of the wick are necessary. If the infection progresses, the patient may need parenteral antibiotics and a consultation with an otolaryngologist.

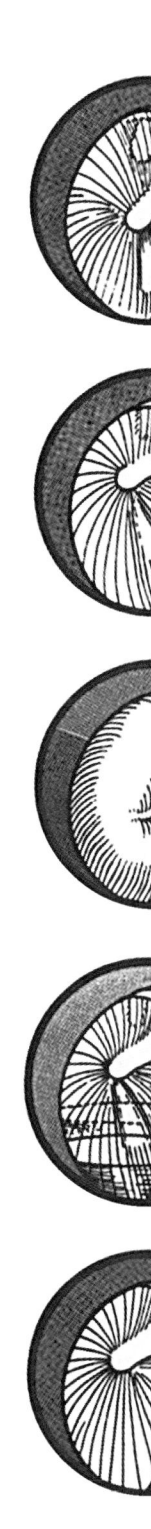
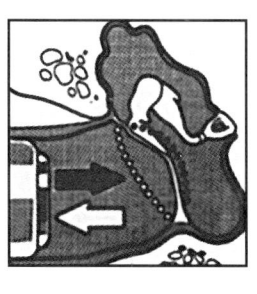

NORMAL
Position—neutral
Color—normal
Translucency—translucent
Mobility—moves briskly with slight
  positive and negative pressure

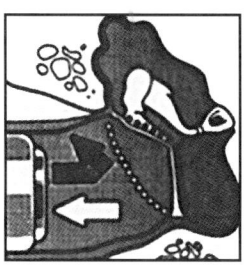

NEGATIVE MIDDLE EAR
  PRESSURE
Position—retracted
Color—normal
Translucency—translucent
Mobility—moves only with applied
  negative pressure

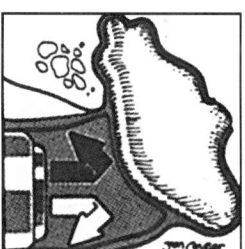

ACUTE OTITIS MEDIA
Position—full to bulging
Color—red (can be pink, white, or
  yellow)
Translucency—opaque
Mobility—poor when both positive
  and negative pressures are
  applied

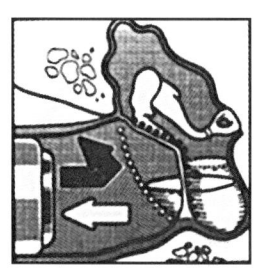

FLUID LEVEL
Position—retracted
Color—yellow or amber
Translucency—translucent
Mobility—same as with high
  negative pressure, but fluid level
  and bubbles change with applied
  pressure

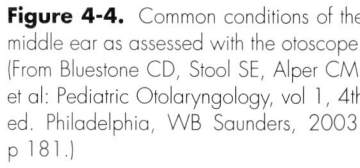

Figure 4-4. Common conditions of the middle ear as assessed with the otoscope. (From Bluestone CD, Stool SE, Alper CM, et al: Pediatric Otolaryngology, vol 1, 4th ed. Philadelphia, WB Saunders, 2003, p 181.)

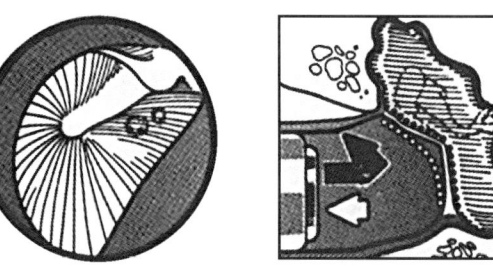

OTITIS MEDIA WITH EFFUSION
Position—usually retracted
Color—white (or yellow or blue)
Translucency—opaque (may be
  translucent)
Mobility—poor when both positive
  and negative pressures are
  applied

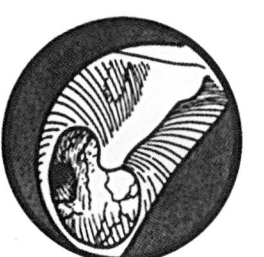
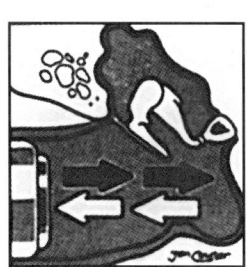

PERFORATION (OR PATENT
  TYMPANOSTOMY TUBE)
Position—neutral or retracted
Color—white, pink, red, or normal
Translucency—translucent or
  opaque
Mobility—none

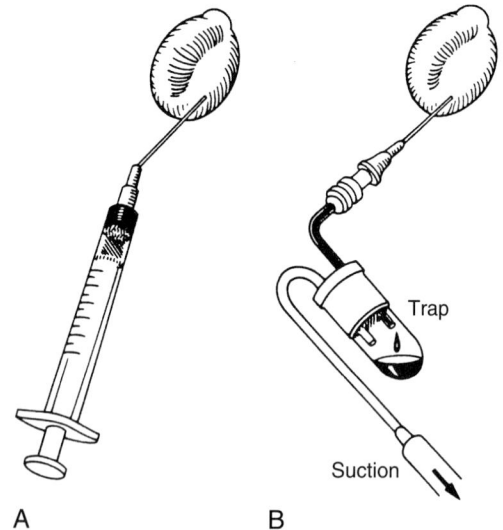

Figure 4-5. Tympanocentesis using a sterile spinal needle attached to a tuberculin syringe (**A**) or an Alden-Senturia suction trap (**B**). (From Bluestone CD, Klein JO: Otitis Media in Infants and Children, 2nd ed. Philadelphia, WB Saunders, 1995, p 127.)

Chondritis is a potential complication of severe otitis externa. It occurs when the infection progresses into the cartilaginous structures of the ear. This complication is rare without a history of previous trauma or surgery.

MALIGNANT OTITIS EXTERNA

Malignant otitis externa is a fulminant condition that causes extensive tissue destruction. The illness may result in chondritis and osteitis of both the middle and inner ears. This condition occurs primarily in patients with poorly controlled diabetes mellitus and in those who are immunocompromised. The pinna is markedly swollen and laterally displaced. Aggressive treatment with broad-spectrum parenteral antibiotics, including antibiotics directed against *P. aeruginosa* and *S. aureus*, is indicated.

ACUTE OTITIS MEDIA

Acute otitis media is usually a bacterial complication of a preceding or concurrent viral upper respiratory tract illness. It usually occurs several days after the onset of a viral upper respiratory tract infection. The viral infection enables pathogenic bacteria in the nasopharynx to ascend through the eustachian tube into the middle ear either by impairing local host defenses or by eustachian tube dysfunction. The bacterial pathogens then cause a secondary infection. The diagnosis is suspected when fever, irritability, and/or ear pain is coupled with otoscopic findings of decreased mobility, opacity, and bulging of the tympanic membrane (see Table 4-5).

Bacteriology/Virology

The leading bacterial pathogens isolated from middle ear fluid in children with acute otitis media are *S. pneumoniae* (25% to 30%), nontypable *Haemophilus influenzae* (20% to 30%), and *Moraxella catarrhalis* (15% to 20%); group A streptococci and staphylococci are uncommon pathogens. In the first month of life (especially the first 2 weeks), gram-negative enteric bacteria (e.g., *Escherichia coli*, *Klebsiella pneumoniae*) or group B streptococcus may also be isolated. Otitis media with ipsilateral conjunctivitis is often caused by nontypable *H. influenzae*.

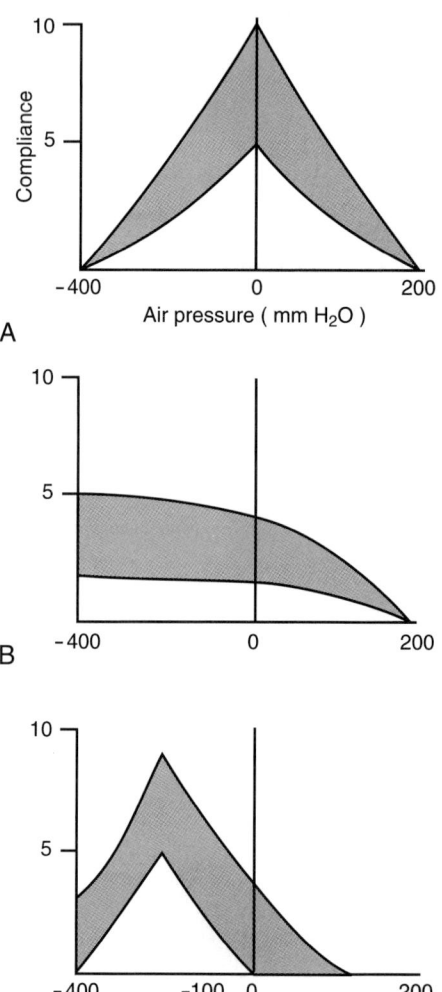

Figure 4-6. **A,** A normal tympanogram with a peak at atmospheric pressure, indicating an air-filled middle ear with normal (atmospheric) pressure. **B,** A "flat" tympanogram, indicating middle ear effusion. **C,** A tympanogram with a negative peak pressure, indicating eustachian tube obstruction.

The three most common organisms may not be equally virulent. There is some evidence that nontypable *H. influenzae* is more likely to clear spontaneously than is *S. pneumoniae*. The spectrum of disease associated with *M. catarrhalis* and *H. influenzae* is not as severe as that seen with *S. pneumoniae*.

Viruses also have an important etiologic role. It is not clear whether the virus alone or a combination of virus and bacteria are involved in the pathogenesis. Several studies have documented the presence of viruses (10% to 44% with or without bacteria) in the middle ear fluid of children with otitis media. Respiratory syncytial virus and rhinovirus are the most commonly recovered agents, but many others (influenza, parainfluenza) have also been found. Viruses appear to enhance or prolong inflammation in the middle ear and thus worsen the clinical outcome.

Strains of *S. pneumoniae* have emerged with altered penicillin-binding proteins on the bacterial cell wall, which makes them less susceptible to β-lactam drugs (penicillins and cephalosporins). Strains of *S. pneumoniae* may be classified as susceptible, intermediate, or resistant. *Susceptible* strains are inhibited by less than 0.1 μg/mL of penicillin (minimal inhibitory concentration ≤ 0.1). The minimal inhibitory concentrations of intermediate and resistant strains are 0.1 to 1.0 μg/mL and greater than 1.0 μg/mL, respectively. The proportion of invasive disease caused by penicillin-nonsusceptible strains (intermediate and

Table 4-6. **Classification of Otitis Media and Its Complications and Sequelae**

Acute otitis media
Otitis media with effusion
  Acute (short duration)
  Subacute
  Chronic
Eustachian tube dysfunction
Intratemporal (extracranial) complications and sequelae
  Hearing loss
    Conductive
    Sensorineural
  Vestibular, balance, and motor dysfunctions
  Perforation of tympanic membrane
    Acute perforation
      Without otitis media
      With otitis media (acute otitis media with perforation)
        Without otorrhea
        With otorrhea
    Chronic perforation
      Without otitis media
      With otitis media
        Acute otitis media
          Without otorrhea
          With otorrhea
        Chronic otitis media (and mastoiditis) (chronic
          suppurative otitis media)
          Without otorrhea
          With otorrhea
  Mastoiditis
    Acute
      Acute mastoiditis without periosteitis or osteitis
      Acute mastoiditis with periosteitis
      Acute mastoiditis with osteitis
        Without subperiosteal abscess
        With subperiosteal abscess
    Subacute
    Chronic
      Without chronic suppurative otitis media
      With chronic suppurative otitis media
  Petrositis
    Acute
    Chronic

Intratemporal (extracranial) complications and sequelae *continued*
  Labyrinthitis
    Acute
      Serous
        Localized (circumscribed)
        Generalized
      Suppurative
        Localized
        Generalized
    Chronic
    Labyrinthine sclerosis
  Facial paralysis
    Acute
    Chronic
  External otitis
    Acute external otitis
    Chronic external otitis
  Atelectasis of the middle ear
    Localized
      Without retraction pocket
      With retraction pocket
    Generalized
  Adhesive otitis media
  Cholesteatoma
    Without infection
    With infection
      Acute
        Without otorrhea
        With otorrhea
      Chronic (cholesteatoma with chronic suppurative otitis media)
        Without otorrhea
        With otorrhea
  Cholesterol granuloma
  Tympanosclerosis
  Ossicular discontinuity
  Ossicular fixation
Intracranial complications
  Meningitis
  Extradural abscess
  Subdural empyema
  Focal otitic encephalitis
  Brain abscess
  Dural sinus thrombosis
  Otitic hydrocephalus

From Bluestone CD, Klein JO: Otitis Media in Infants and Children, 3rd ed. Philadelphia, WB Saunders, 2001.

resistant) ranges from 8% to 34% in the United States. In addition, because resistance genes are frequently linked, organisms with resistance to β-lactam drugs are more likely to be resistant to sulfa antibiotics and to the macrolide class. Nonetheless, high-dose amoxicillin is the best oral antibiotic available for drug-resistant *S. pneumoniae.* Also, several antibiotics formerly used commonly for the treatment of otitis media (cefaclor, ceftibuten, and loracarbef) are used less frequently now because they have significantly less activity against the pneumococci. Currently, 30% to 40% of *H. influenzae* strains and 90% of *M. catarrhalis* strains produce β-lactamase enzymes, which hydrolyze penicillins and some cephalosporins.

Treatment

The goals of treatment in acute otitis media are to relieve discomfort and to prevent infectious complications (Fig. 4-7). Evaluating the treatment of otitis media is complicated by the high rate of spontaneous

resolution of the infection. Approximately 87% of children not treated with antibiotics have resolution of pain and fever within 2 to 3 days. Spontaneous resolution is least likely for otitis media caused by *S. pneumoniae.* The emergence of drug-resistant *S. pneumoniae* strains and concerns about treating a disease with a high rate of spontaneous resolution has led to change in the recommended treatment for otitis media (Tables 4-8 and 4-9).

Some authorities suggest not administering antibiotics to a child with a low risk for complications. In the Netherlands, antibiotic therapy is commonly delayed until 48 to 72 hours after the diagnosis, to determine whether there is spontaneous resolution of the infection. The benefits of antibiotic treatment are most clearly seen in children younger than 2 years.

When an antibiotic is used, efficacy against *S. pneumoniae* is the most important consideration. In addition, the clinician must consider the drug's safety, convenience, palatability, and the costs of therapy. In view of all these factors, high-dose amoxicillin (80 to

Table 4-7. Manifestations of the Sequelae and Complications of Otitis Media

Complications	Clinical Features
Acute	
Perforation with otorrhea	Immobile tympanic membrane secondary to visible perforation, exudate in ear canal
Acute mastoiditis with periostitis	Tenderness and erythema over mastoid process, no destruction of bony trabeculae
Acute mastoid osteitis	Destruction of bony trabeculae; tenderness and erythema over mastoid process coupled with outward displacement of pinna
Petrositis	Infection of perilabyrinthine cells; may present with otitis, paralysis of lateral rectus, and headache (Gradenigo syndrome)
Facial nerve palsy	Peripheral cranial nerve VII paralysis
Labyrinthitis	Vertigo, fever, ear pain, nystagmus, hearing loss, tinnitus, nausea and vomiting
Lateral sinus thrombophlebitis	Headache, fever, seizures, altered states of consciousness, septic emboli
Meningitis	Fever, headache, nuchal rigidity, seizures, altered states of consciousness
Extradural abscess	Fever, headache, seizures, altered states of consciousness
Subdural abscess	Fever, headache, seizures, altered states of consciousness
Brain abscess	Fever, headache, seizures, altered states of consciousness, focal neurologic examination
Nonacute	
Chronic perforation	Immobile tympanic membrane secondary to perforation
Otitis media with effusion (OME)	Immobile, opaque tympanic membrane
Adhesive otitis	Irreversible conductive hearing loss secondary to chronic OME
Tympanosclerosis	Thickened white plaques, may cause conductive hearing loss
Chronic suppurative otitis media	Following acute otitis media with perforation, secondary infection with *Staphylococcus aureus, Pseudomonas aeruginosa,* or anaerobes develops, causing chronic otorrhea
Cholesteatoma	White, pearl-like destructive tumor with otorrhea arising near or within tympanic membrane; may be secondary to chronic negative middle ear pressure
Otitic hydrocephalus	Increased intracranial pressure secondary to AOM; signs and symptoms include severe headaches, blurred vision, nausea, vomiting, papilledema, diplopia (abducens paralysis)

90 mg/kg/day given b.i.d. or t.i.d.) is the appropriate initial therapy for most cases. Because otitis media is usually a self-limited illness, some authorities believe that the use of broad-spectrum antibiotics for the initial treatment should be discouraged because of their high cost, the increased risk of adverse reactions, and the increased likelihood of the development of resistant strains.

The dose of amoxicillin depends on the risk for the presence of drug-resistant pneumococci. Risk factors for drug resistance include age younger than 2 years, day care attendance, recent antibiotic exposure, and cigarette smoke exposure. In addition, clinicians should consider resistance patterns within their own community. In the setting of multiple risk factors, high-dose amoxicillin should be considered for initial therapy.

The effect of widespread use of heptavalent pneumococcal conjugate vaccine on the incidence of acute otitis media caused by *S. pneumoniae* is unclear; preliminary studies suggest that the incidence appears to decrease by approximately 6% to 8%.

Patients with Persistent Symptoms

After 72 hours of antibiotic therapy, most patients are either asymptomatic or experiencing improvement. If tympanocentesis is performed and a specimen from the middle ear is analyzed, bacterial cultures are sterile in more than 50% of cases. Many patients may have an active viral infection, whereas others may have a persistent inflammatory reaction despite elimination of viable bacteria. Other cases involve bacterial species that are sensitive to the prescribed antibiotic, which suggests noncompliance or failure of the prescribed drug to achieve adequate concentrations in middle ear fluid. Some patients have resistant bacteria, primarily *S. pneumoniae*. To address the causes of persistent symptoms, the clinician should

1. prescribe analgesic-antipyretic medications for relief of symptoms
2. discuss the issues of drug compliance, including palatability and dosing interval

3. prescribe an alternative antibiotic effective against possible resistant *S. pneumoniae* and β-lactamase–producing *H. influenzae* and *M. catarrhalis,* such as amoxicillin-clavulanic acid (80 to 90 mg/kg/day of the amoxicillin component), cefuroxime axetil, or 3 days of intramuscular ceftriaxone.

With the emergence of *S. pneumoniae* resistance, it may become necessary to perform tympanocentesis more frequently to guide antibiotic therapy.

Early Recurrences of Acute Otitis Media

Up to 30% of patients who respond to initial antibiotic treatment of acute otitis media have a recurrent infection within a few weeks after discontinuing therapy. In only 20% of these cases is the organism the same. Thus, most recurrences are not a result of failure of the previous antibiotic regimen. With recurrent otitis media, the clinician must consider drug-resistant pneumococci and β-lactamase–producing *H. influenzae.*

Recurrent Acute Otitis Media

Recurrent otitis media does not have as favorable a natural history as uncomplicated otitis media. Risk factors for recurrent acute otitis media include

- onset of acute otitis media in the first year of life, especially if the first episode is before the patient is 6 months of age
- Native American or Eskimo heritage
- male gender
- a sibling's history of recurrent acute otitis media
- cleft palate
- craniofacial anomalies
- trisomy 21
- day care attendance
- household cigarette smoke

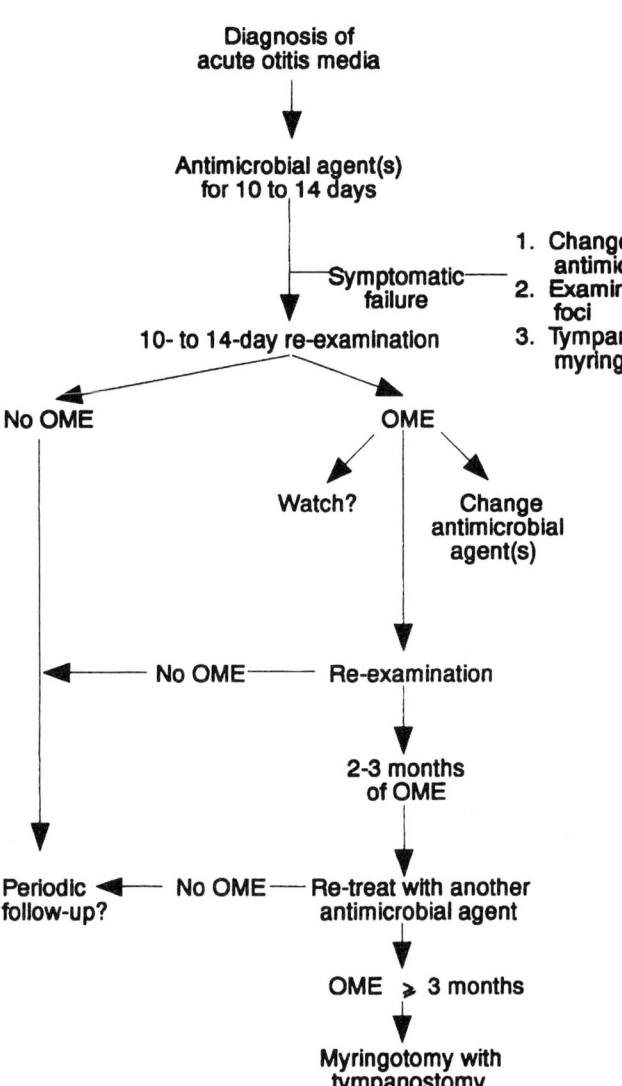

Figure 4-7. Recommended algorithm for management of acute otitis media. OME, otitis media with effusion. (From Bluestone CD, Klein JO: Otitis Media in Infants and Children, 3rd ed. Philadelphia, WB Saunders, 2001.)

Table 4-8. Antimicrobial Agents approved for Therapy for Acute Otitis Media: United States, 2000

Drug	Trade Name
Amoxicillin	Amoxil
Amoxicillin-clavulanate	Augmentin
Cephalexin	Keflex
Cefaclor	Ceclor
Loracarbef	Lorabid
Ceftibuten	Cedax
Cefprozil	Cefzil
Cefpodoxime	Vantin
Cefuroxime axetil	Ceftin
Cefdinir	Omnicef
Ceftriaxone	Rocephin
Erythromycin + sulfisoxazole	Pediazole
Azithromycin	Zithromax
Clarithromycin	Biaxin
Trimethoprim-sulfamethoxazole	Bactrim, Septra
Ofloxacin otic	Floxin Otic

From Bluestone CD, Klein JO: Otitis Media in Infants and Children, 3rd ed. Philadelphia, WB Saunders, 2001.

- human immunodeficiency virus infection
- the absence of breast milk in the diet

Children with frequent episodes of otitis media (three or more episodes in the past 6 months or four or more episodes during the past year) present a particular challenge. Previously, antimicrobial chemoprophylaxis was recommended to prevent subsequent infections and reduce the time spent with middle ear effusion. A meta-analysis of antibiotic prophylaxis (with sulfisoxazole, trimethoprim-sulfamethoxazole, or amoxicillin) decreased the number of episodes by approximately 0.11 episodes per patient per month. In view of the risks of promoting antibiotic resistance, this is not commonly recommended.

Myringotomy and tympanostomy tube placement may have some benefit. One study demonstrated decreased number of episodes of acute otitis media with bulging eardrums. Tympanostomy tubes are eventually extruded from the eardrum by the normal process of epithelial growth. Recurrent episodes of otitis media may then resume.

Otitis Media with Effusion

OME may occur after an acute episode of otitis media or because of eustachian tube obstruction resulting from another cause (most commonly, an upper respiratory tract infection). After acute

Table 4-9. **Antimicrobial Agents for Otitis Media: Dosage Schedules**

Drug (Trade Name)	Number of Doses × Days	Dosage (per kg/day)
Amoxicillin (Amoxil)	2-3/day × 10	40-80 mg
Amoxicillin-clavulanate (Augmentin)	2/day × 10	40-80 mg
Azithromycin (Zithromax)	1/day × 5	10 mg day 1; 5 mg days 2-5
Clarithromycin (Biaxin)	2/day × 10	15 mg
Erythromycin + sulfisoxazole (Pediazole)	4/day × 10	40 mg
Ceftriaxone (Rocephin)	1/day × 1	50 mg
Ceftibuten (Cedax)	1/day × 10	9 mg
Loracarbef (Lorabid)	2/day × 10	30 mg
Cefprozil (Cefzil)	2/day × 10	30 mg
Cefpodoxime (Vantin)	2/day × 10	10 mg
Cefuroxime axetil (Ceftin)	2/day × 10	30 mg
Cefaclor (Ceclor)	2-3/day × 10	40 mg
Cefdinir (Omnicef)	1-2/day × 10	14 mg
Trimethoprim-sulfamethoxazole (Bactrim, Septra)	2/day × 10	10 mg/40 mg

From Bluestone CD, Klein JO: Otitis Media in Infants and Children, 3rd ed. Philadelphia, WB Saunders, 2001.

otitis media, middle ear fluid can persist for weeks. Three weeks after an acute otitis media, an effusion is still present in 10% to 15% of patients. Because most cases of OME resolve without treatment, a period of observation is the most appropriate initial strategy.

Medical therapy of otitis media with effusion has not been consistently successful. Antihistamines, decongestants, and nonsteroidal antiinflammatory agents do not promote the resolution of middle ear effusion. With systemic corticosteroids (prednisone), the effusion may resolve in up to 50% of the cases, but it recurs within a few weeks of stopping the steroids. Although bacteria may be present in up to 30% of cases, antibiotic therapy has only a minimal effect on the resolution of effusion. A period of observation for 4 to 6 months is recommended before surgical intervention is considered.

To assist the clinician in the management of persistent middle ear effusion, the Otitis Media Guideline Panel from the Agency for Health Care Policy and Research (AHCPR) has developed a set of practice guidelines for affected children between 1 and 3 years. The panel recommends documentation of effusion with pneumatic otoscopy, confirmation of effusion by tympanometry when pneumatic otoscopy is inconclusive, reduction of risk factors for otitis media, and myringotomy with tympanostomy tube placement in children with bilateral effusion lasting longer than 3 months and coupled with bilateral hearing loss. In addition, a course of antibiotics may be tried before the clinician decides to place tympanostomy tubes. The panel does not recommend decongestants, steroids, antihistamines, tonsillectomy, or adenoidectomy in the management of persistent OME. The panel also recommends against tympanostomy tube placement with unilateral hearing loss secondary to OME unless the patient has an underlying sensorineural hearing loss or has only one functional ear. As with any set of guidelines, the clinician needs to individualize these recommendations.

When these guidelines were developed, the panel considered the then available evidence that persistent middle ear effusion, which usually produces a 20- to 30-db conductive hearing loss, might affect language development and cognitive abilities. The report stated that there was insufficient evidence available to support a causal relationship. Since then, several studies have shown that the presence of asymptomatic middle ear effusions in otherwise normal children is unlikely to cause harm. If a child has persistent OME *and* other risks for or documented language or behavior problems, the clinician may elect to follow the previously recommended guidelines. Without these additional risk factors, however, most effusions can be monitored without intervention.

Mastoiditis

Mastoiditis is a potentially serious acute or chronic suppurative complication of otitis media. Life-threatening complications of mastoiditis are related to intracranial extension of the suppurative process.

Mastoiditis begins with the development of hyperemia and edema, which then progresses to a suppurative process that may produce demineralization and necrosis of bone, abscess formations, and contiguous spread to intracranial or other head and neck areas.

Mastoiditis with periosteitis manifests most commonly in children younger than 3 years, although children of any age may be affected. Otalgia, posterior ear pain, fever, and otorrhea are frequent symptoms. Posterior auricular tenderness and erythrema, anterior-inferior pinna protrusion, loss of the posterior auricular crease, middle ear effusion, a bulging or perforated tympanic membrane, and sagging of the posterior auditory canal wall are observable signs.

Common pathogens include pneumococci, *P. aeruginosa,* and group A streptococci. The computed tomographic scan is usually diagnostic and reveals various stages of mastoiditis:

- mastoiditis with periosteitis
- mastoiditis with osteitis with or without subperiosteal abscess

Treatment is based on the stage of the process (periosteitis, osteitis, abscess). High-dose intravenous antibiotics plus tympanostomy and myringotomy with or without a tympanostomy tube are important therapeutic (for drainage) and diagnostic (for culture) procedures. Mastoidectomy is usually indicated for severe osteitis, mastoid abscess formation, and all intracranial suppurative complications.

SUMMARY AND RED FLAGS

A careful examination of the pinna, external auditory canal, and tympanic membrane can identify most causes of ear pain. If findings are normal, the clinician should consider pain referred from another source (see Table 4-3). Because young children may have trouble localizing their pain, clinicians should be highly suspicious of ear disease in any examination conducted during a patient's first year of life or in any preschool child with fever, irritability, or upper respiratory tract infection.

Even though most conditions causing ear pain respond readily to therapy, the clinician must be aware of the following red flags associated with these conditions:

laterally displaced pinna (malignant otitis externa, mastoid osteitis)
mastoid tenderness (mastoid osteitis)

perforated tympanic membrane

a pearl-like tumor in the tympanic membrane (cholesteatoma)

subacute headache, meningismus, altered mental status (brain abscess, subdural-epidural empyema)

REFERENCES

Black S, Shinefield H, Fireman B, et al: Efficacy, safety and immunogenicity of heptavalent pneumococcal conjugate vaccine in children. Pediatr Infect Dis J 2000;19:187-195.

Dowell SF, Butler JC, Giebink GS, et al: Acute otitis media: Management and surveillance in an era of pneumococcal resistance—A report from the Drug-resistant *Streptococcus pneumoniae* Therapeutic Working Group. Pediatr Infect Dis J 1999;18:1-9.

Eskola J, Kilpi T, Palmu A, et al: Efficacy of pneumococcal conjugate vaccine against otitis media. N Engl J Med 2001;344:403-409.

Faden H, Duffy L, Boeve M: Otitis media: Back to basics. Pediatr Infect Dis J 1998;17:1105-1113.

Feldman HM, Dollaghan CA, Campbell TF, et al: Parent-reported language and communication skills at one and two years of age in relation to otitis media in the first two years of life. Pediatrics 1999;104(4):e52. Available at http://www.pediatrics.org/cgi/content/full/104/4/e52.

Heikkinen T, Ruuskanen O: Signs and symptoms predicting acute otitis media. Arch Pediatr Adolesc Med 1995;149:26-29.

Heikkinen T, Thint M, Chonmaitree T: Prevalence of various respiratory viruses in the middle ear during acute otitis media. N Engl J Med 1999;340:260-264.

Hendley JO: Otitis media. N Engl J Med 2002;347:1169-1174.

Kilpi T, Herva E, Kaijalainen T, et al: Bacteriology of acute otitis media in a cohort of Finnish children followed for the first two years of life. Pediatr Infect Dis J 2001;20:654-662.

Minter KR, Roberts JE, Hooper SR, et al: Early childhood otitis media in relation to children's attention-related behavior in the first six years of life. Pediatrics 2001;107:1037-1042.

Olson L, Jackson MA: Only the pneumococcus…. Pediatr Infect Dis J 1999;18:849-850.

Otitis Media Guideline Panel: Clinical Practice Guideline Number 12: Otitis media with effusion in young children (AHCPR Publication No. 94-0622). Rockville, Md: U.S. Department of Health and Human Services, Agency for Health Care Policy and Research, July 1994. [Summary published in Pediatrics 1994;94:766-773.]

Paradise JL, Rockette HE, Colborn DK, et al: Otitis media in 2253 Pittsburgh-area infants: Prevalence and risk factors during the first two years of life. Pediatrics 1997;99:318-333.

Pichichero ME: Evaluating the need, timing and best choice of antibiotic therapy for acute otitis media and tonsillopharyngitis infections in children. Pediatr Infect Dis J 2000;19:S131-S140.

Piglansky L, Leibovitz E, Raiz S, et al: Bacteriologic and clinical efficacy of high dose amoxicillin for therapy of acute otitis media in children. Pediatr Infect Dis J 2003;22:405-412.

Ruben RJ: Efficacy of ofloxacin and other otic preparations for otitis externa. Pediatr Infect Dis J 2001;20:108-110.

U.S. Department of Health and Human Services, Agency for Healthcare Research and Quality: Management of acute otitis media. Evidence Report/Technology Assessment No. 15 (AHRQ Publication No. 00-E008). Washington, DC: U.S. Department of Health and Human Services, June 2000.

5 Airway Obstruction in Children

Robert M. Kliegman*

A child with an upper airway obstruction may require immediate life-saving medical or surgical intervention or simply extended observation with various diagnostic studies to determine the site and cause of obstruction before medical treatment is begun. In the absence of imminent respiratory failure or respiratory arrest, a brief directed history should be obtained. The pattern (acute versus chronic versus recurrent), time of onset, and rapidity of progression of the obstruction should be noted along with possible previous episodes of airway compromise, their therapy, and outcome. A review of the birth and neonatal history is important in determining a prior need for airway intervention, such as aggressive suctioning or endotracheal intubation. Questions should be directed toward any change in voice or cry and toward feeding problems. Although a foreign body is not always observed, its possibility should be raised and, of course, a short review of any underlying medical problems and their therapy should be briefly determined. Most cases (~80%) of upper airway obstruction (with or without stridor) are acute infections (Table 5-1). An age-related differential diagnosis is noted in Table 5-2.

PHYSICAL EXAMINATION

The physical examination is most important and should be performed in a warm, well-lit room, preferably with the child in the parent's lap and the child's chest exposed. An examination of the oropharynx or auscultation of the lungs is not as important as taking a few seconds to note the child's general appearance, sense of well-being, degree of dyspnea, and respiratory pattern. The respiratory rate (see Chapter 3) and the presence of cyanosis, degree of anxiety, and any posture assumed in an effort to minimize the airway difficulties should be determined (see Table 5-1).

Stridor is a high-pitched musical noise generated by turbulent flow of air through the large upper airways and should be categorized as inspiratory, expiratory, or biphasic. Nasal flaring, the use of accessory muscles of respiration (neck), and the degree of retractions, which may vary from a slight sternal tug to intercostal, and significant deep sternal, should be observed. The patient's cry or voice (pitch, aphonia, muffled, hoarse), and difficulty in a child's ability to handle oral secretions should be noted. A feeding trial should not be attempted, because some children may require control of their airway (endotracheal intubation) or other diagnostic or therapeutic procedures in the operating room with anesthesia; feeding may increase the risk of aspiration or further airway compromise. Other physical findings include mouth breathing and morphologic features suggestive of craniofacial anomalies, such as maxillary hypoplasia, nasal septal deflection, micrognathia, retrognathia, absent nasal air flow (choanal obstructions), platybasia, or macroglossia.

Radiologic evaluations are needed only if the diagnosis is not clear on the basis of history and physical examination; if there is

concern for the degree of the acute respiratory distress, that patient should be accompanied to the radiology suite by a person able to evaluate and control any airway problems. Physical restraints are sometimes needed to limit a child's motion, but in general, these should be avoided because they often are more upsetting and may precipitate airway problems. Anteroposterior and lateral soft tissue radiographic studies of the neck and chest are frequently needed. Neck films should be obtained during inspiration, because the soft tissues of the pharynx may bulge with expiration, causing a false-positive finding of a soft tissue mass that may mimic a retropharyngeal infection. Radiopaque foreign bodies are generally seen easily on a radiograph. If there is a possibility of a radiolucent foreign body, inspiratory and expiratory chest radiographic studies are performed. These identify air trapping distal to a foreign body, which acts as a ball valve with airway obstruction on expiration as the bronchial diameter decreases. Hyperinflation causes a mediastinal shift away from the obstructed side.

A barium swallow study, directed to assess either any associated abnormalities in swallowing or tracheoesophageal problems, such as a vascular ring, may also be obtained. The use of computed tomographic (CT) or magnetic resonance image (MRI) scanning provides excellent soft tissue and, particularly with MRI, vascular definition. These studies usually require that the patient be very cooperative or sedated. Sedatives must be used very carefully and only in monitored situations with the availability of personnel and equipment to provide possible resuscitation. The developmental relative anatomy of the upper airway is shown in Figure 5-1.

Once the clinical and radiologic examinations have been completed, the examiner determines the site of the airway obstruction, its likely cause, and type of treatment needed (see Tables 5-1 and 5-2). The key physical findings (see Table 5-1) in determining the site of obstruction involve the character of the stridor, retractions, the voice, and the ability to handle secretions.

Inspiratory stridor is characteristic of airway obstruction at or above the vocal cords and is caused by collapse of the soft tissues with the normal negative pressure generated by inspiration; it is usually soft and muffled.

Biphasic (inspiratory and expiratory) stridor indicates little change in airway size with respiration caused by a fixed obstruction. In one phase, a stethoscope may be necessary to hear the sound, whereas in the other, no assistance is necessary for it to be heard. The cricoid cartilage immediately below the vocal cords is the only rigid circumferential structure in the upper airway; narrowing in this site (as in subglottic stenosis or croup) is a common cause of biphasic stridor.

Obstruction within the larger portions of the intrathoracic tracheobronchial tree causes *expiratory stridor* because there is a decrease in airway diameter with expiration. This mechanism is similar to that of the generation of the typical expiratory wheeze heard from the smaller airways in a patient with reactive airways disease (see Chapter 3).

The degree of retractions varies greatly and depends on the site of obstruction. Pharyngeal or supraglottic (above the vocal cords) laryngeal obstructions often produce minimal retractions, inasmuch as the patients may sense that increased respiratory effort actually

*This chapter is an updated and edited version of the chapter by James E. Arnold that appeared in the first edition.

increases the amount of soft tissue obstruction and collapse. These patients may have very shallow respirations with no retractions until the airway obstruction is severe. At the level of the vocal cords or subglottic larynx, the degree of retractions is generally correlated with the degree of obstruction. If the obstruction is in the trachea, retractions are not present unless the obstruction is severe, because the tracheobronchial diameter increases with inspiration. A muffled "hot potato" voice is typical of pharyngeal obstruction caused by inflammation or mass effect. *Hoarseness* is present with involvement of the vocal cords, usually by an inflammatory process. Tracheal obstructions generally do not affect the voice.

Neonates are predominantly nasal breathers, and nasal obstruction usually interferes greatly with their ability to feed. Neonates may be able to switch to oral respirations either spontaneously or with crying, but while feeding, they may be unable to swallow before stopping to breathe. Obstruction in the pharynx and larynx above the vocal cords often makes feeding and swallowing difficult; these children often present with drooling. If the site of obstruction is at or below the vocal cords or in the trachea, feedings are usually normal, except as determined by the degree of respiratory obstruction, unless an esophageal foreign body or vascular ring is narrowing the trachea by compressing the soft posterior tracheal wall.

Endoscopy can provide direct visualization of the cause of the airway obstruction; however, its use involves manipulation of the airway, which should not be undertaken unless the personnel and equipment are present to manage possible worsening airway compromise. Short, flexible fiberoptic nasopharyngolaryngoscopes are widely used to visualize the upper airway. Flexible pediatric bronchoscopy provides visualization of both the upper and lower airways, and cardiopulmonary monitoring and intravenous access for sedative administration are required. In cases of significant upper airway obstruction necessitating intervention, or if there is any likelihood of a foreign body, direct laryngoscopy and rigid bronchoscopy in the operating room are the safest procedures that can secure the airway, provide a diagnosis, and accomplish treatment, such as extraction of the foreign body.

ANATOMIC CAUSES OF AIRWAY OBSTRUCTION

NASAL OBSTRUCTION

Nasal obstruction is often an uncomfortable nuisance for the older child. It may sometimes contribute to sinusitis (by obstructing the sinus ostia) and may be exacerbated by allergic inflammation. Obstruction in the neonate who is a predominant nasal breather is very significant; it can cause respiratory distress and, by interfering with feeding, can cause a delay in growth and development. The differential diagnosis of nasal obstruction is noted in Table 5-3.

Choanal atresia (Fig. 5-2) is a lack of the opening of the posterior nasal airway. In approximately 66% of the cases, it is unilateral. In 90%, there is a bony obstruction between the posterolateral wall of the nose and the nasal septum; in the remaining 10%, the obstruction is membranous. The incidence is 1 to 1.5 in 5000 births. In *unilateral* cases, there is usually no respiratory distress but a constant, persistent unilateral nasal drainage. This is usually diagnosed in an older child; it is important to be sure that a foreign body does not cause obstruction. *Bilateral* choanal atresia may cause severe neonatal respiratory distress that is often relieved by crying; a pattern of cyclic cyanosis may develop in which infants become cyanotic while trying to breathe through the nose and then recover as they begin to cry.

The diagnosis is suspected on the basis of the clinical presentation and is confirmed by the inability to pass a small catheter or feeding tube through the nose into the pharynx. Care must be taken to ensure that a small catheter has not curled in the nose and seemingly passed further than choanal atresia would allow; this is best done by being able to visualize the catheter in the oropharynx. CT scanning

is needed to define the anatomy (bony versus membranous, complete versus incomplete).

At least 50% of children with choanal atresia have other congenital anomalies (such as the CHARGE* association); initial management is directed toward maintaining the airway, often with a McGovern nipple (a modified baby bottle nipple used as an oral airway) and tube feedings, while an evaluation for other congenital anomalies is being performed.

Surgical correction of choanal atresia is usually performed through either a transnasal or a transpalatal route. The operative timing depends on the severity and in unilateral cases can be delayed until the child is several years of age. Because the repaired choanae often scar, form contractures, and re-stenose, long-term follow-up is needed. Patients with the CHARGE association often have associated feeding problems over and above that caused by their nasal obstruction; management often entails a tracheotomy and gastrostomy tube with delayed repair of the choanal atresia when the child's nasal structures are larger and less likely to have postoperative problems.

DEVIATED SEPTUM

Passage through the birth canal may cause a neonatal septal deviation, which can often be corrected with minor manipulation immediately after delivery. This problem manifests with asymmetric nares, is often asymptomatic, and is less common in Asian American and African American children, who have a lower nasal profile than do white children. Other causes of nasal obstruction include intranasal cysts, bony narrowing of the anterior portion of the nose, and a reactive nasal mucosa secondary to vigorous suctioning or other manipulation. Evaluation with flexible nasal endoscopy and the use of CT scanning give the best analysis of any abnormal anatomy.

NASAL FOREIGN BODY

Nasal aspiration of foreign bodies usually occurs in toddlers and young children. The foreign bodies include small toy parts, buttons, button batteries, sponges, insects, beads, and food (nuts, seeds, pits, beans). Food is not inert; it may absorb water and swell or cause chemical irritation (batteries are also caustic). A spontaneous rhinolith also acts as a foreign body. A foreign body should be suspected when there is a chronic mucopurulent or bloody unilateral nasal discharge. The discharge may improve temporarily with the use of decongestants or antibiotics. Treatment includes topical nasal decongestants and removal of the foreign body with a simple forceps, a cerumen curette, a wire loop, Hartmann forceps, or a nasopharyngoscope.

LARYNGOMALACIA

Laryngomalacia is the most common cause of inspiratory stridor and noisy respiration in neonates and infants. It is caused by the inspiratory collapse of the laryngeal cartilages, with prolapse of the epiglottis or arytenoid cartilages into the airway during inspiration. This may occur at birth, but the onset is often delayed, occurring at 2 to 4 weeks of age. The condition is usually self-limited and resolves with time, often by 8 to 12 months of age but occasionally not until 18 to 24 months of age.

The diagnosis is made on the basis of the clinical presentation (stridor is worse when the patient is supine or during activity, and exacerbations occur with upper respiratory tract infections) and

---

*Coloboma (iris, retina), *h*eart disease (tetralogy of Fallot, patent ductus arteriosus, ventricular septal defect, atrial septal defect), *a*tresia choanae, *r*etarded growth and mental deficiency, *g*enital hypoplasia (males), and *e*ar anomalies (external ear plus deafness). Four of six categories must be present in order to diagnose CHARGE syndrome.

Table 5-1. Differential Diagnosis of Upper Airway Obstruction

	Laryngotracheo-bronchitis (Croup)	Laryngitis	Spasmodic Croup	Epiglottitis	Membranous Croup (Bacterial Tracheitis)
Age	3 mo–3 yr	5 yr–teens	3 mo–3 yr	2–6 yr	Any age (3–10 yr)
Location	Subglottic	Subglottic	Subglottic	Supraglottic	Trachea
Etiology	Parainfluenza influenza virus, RSV; rarely *Mycoplasma,* measles, adenovirus	As per croup	Unknown	*Haemophilus influenzae* b	Prior croup or influenza virus with secondary bacterial infection by *Staphylococcus aureus, Moraxella catarrhalis, H. influenzae*
Prodrome onset	Insidious, URI	As per croup	Sudden onset at night; prior episodes	Rapid, short prodrome	Bisphasic illness with sudden deterioration
Stridor	Yes—biphasic	No	Yes	Yes—soft inspiratory	Yes
Retractions	Yes	No	Rare	Yes	Yes
Voice	Hoarse	Hoarse; whispered	Hoarse	Muffled	Normal or hoarse
Position and appearance	Normal	Normal	Normal	Tripod sitting, leaning forward; agitation	Normal
Swallowing (dysphagia)	Normal	Normal	Normal	Drooling	Normal
Barking cough	Yes	Rare	Yes	No	Yes
Toxicity	Rare	No	No	Severe	Severe
Fever	<101°F	<101°F	None	>102°F	>102°F
Radiographic findings	Subglottic narrowing; steeple sign	Normal	Subglottic narrowing	Thumb sign of thickened epiglottis	Ragged irregular tracheal border; as per croup
WBC count	Normal	Normal	Normal	Leukocytosis with left shift	Leukocytosis with left shift
Therapy	Racemic epinephrine: aerosol, systemic steroids, aerosolized steroids, cool mist	None	Cool mist; occasionally as for croup	Endotracheal intubation, ceftriaxone	Ceftriaxone; intubation if needed
Prevention	None	None	None	*H. influenzae* b conjugated vaccine	None

FFP, fresh-frozen plasma; HPV, human papillomavirus; IV, intravenous; RSV, respiratory syncytial virus; URI, upper respiratory tract infection, coryza, sneezing; WBC, white blood cell.

findings of outpatient flexible laryngoscopy, which can generally be performed safely with topical anesthesia. Complete airway evaluation has been recommended in children with laryngomalacia, because 15% to 25% have other airway lesions. This approach has been used on selected referral patient populations and should be considered if the stridor of laryngomalacia does not follow the typical course of being mild and resolving spontaneously. Unusually severe cases of laryngomalacia may necessitate operative intervention, such as an epiglottoplasty to trim redundant soft tissue or even a temporary tracheotomy. Laryngomalacia may be accompanied by *tracheomalacia,* a partial collapse of the tracheal cartilages with respiration. Tracheomalacia may be congenital or secondary to extrinsic compression by vascular rings or tumors. Patients with tracheomalacia manifest wheezing, cough, stridor, dyspnea, tachypnea, or cyanosis. Some have opisthotonic posturing, and some have absence of the ear cartilage.

Retropharyngeal Abscess	Foreign Body	Angioedema	Peritonsillar Abscess	Laryngeal Papillomatosis
<6 yr	6 mo–5 yr	All ages	>10 yr	3 mo–3 yr
Posterior pharynx	Supraglottic, subglottic, variable	Variable	Oropharynx	Larynx, vocal cords, trachea
S. aureus, anaerobes	Small objects, vegetable, toys, coins	Congenital C-1 esterase deficiency; acquired anaphylaxis	Group A streptococci, anaerobes	HPV
Insidious to sudden	Sudden	Sudden	Biphasic with sudden worsening	Chronic
No	Yes	Yes	No	Possible
Yes	Yes—variable	Yes	No	No
Muffled	Complete obstruction—aphonic; other variable	Hoarse, may be normal	"Hot potato," muffled	Hoarse
Arching of neck or normal	Normal	Normal; may have facial edema	Normal	Normal
Drooling	Variable, usually normal	Normal	Drooling, trismus	Normal
No	Variable; brassy if tracheal	Possible	None	Variable
Severe	No, but dyspnea	No, unless anaphylactic shock or severe anoxia	Dyspnea	None
>101°F	None	None	>101°F	None
Thickened retropharyngeal space	Radiopaque object may be seen	As per croup	None needed	May be normal
Leukocytosis with left shift	Normal	Normal	Leukocytosis with left shift	Normal
Nafcillin; ampicillin-sulbactam; ceftriaxone; surgical drainage if abscess	Endoscopic removal	Anaphylaxis; epinephrine, IV fluids, steroids; C-1 esterase deficiency; replacement infusion therapy	Penicillin; aspiration	Laser therapy, repeated excision, interferon
None	Avoid small objects; supervision	Avoid allergens; FFP for congenital angioedema	Treat group A streptococci early	Treat maternal genitourinary lesions; possible cesarean section?

VOCAL CORD PARALYSIS

Vocal cord paralysis is a common cause of congenital neonatal laryngeal obstruction. It can also occur in older children. It is usually bilateral and associated with neurologic syndromes, such as the Arnold-Chiari malformation. Traction on the brain stem or increased intracranial pressure and herniation puts pressure on the vagus nerve. Tracheotomy may be necessary to maintain the airway, and neurologic and MRI evaluation should be performed to identify any central causes. Children with Arnold-Chiari malformation in whom a ventriculoperitoneal shunt has been placed may present with airway obstruction secondary to increased intracranial pressure if the ventriculoperitoneal shunt is obstructed. Vocal cord paralysis may also be a result of traction on the recurrent laryngeal nerve secondary to a difficult delivery; it is usually unilateral, resolves with time, and causes few airway problems. Vocal cord paralysis also occurs in older children and may be caused by a polyneuropathy (Guillain-Barré syndrome), brain stem encephalitis, neck or thoracic surgery, or compression by local masses.

Table 5-2. **Age-Related Differential Diagnosis of Airway Obstruction**

Newborn

Foreign material (meconium, amniotic fluid)
Congenital subglottic stenosis (uncommon)
Choanal atresia
Congenital cysts
Micrognathia (Pierre Robin syndrome, Treacher Collins syndrome, DiGeorge syndrome)
Macroglossia (Beckwith-Wiedemann syndrome, hypothyroidism, Pompe disease, trisomy 21, hemangioma)
Laryngeal web, clefts, atresia
Laryngospasm (intubation, aspiration, hypocalcemia, transient)
Lingual thyroid
Vocal cord paralysis (weak cry; unilateral or bilateral, with or without increased intracranial pressure from Arnold-Chiari malformation or other CNS pathology; birth trauma)
Tracheal web, stenosis, malacia, atresia
Pharyngeal collapse (cause of apnea in preterm infant)
Tumors*

Infant

Laryngomalacia (most common cause)
Subglottic stenosis (congenital; acquired after intubation)
Tumors*
Tongue tumor (dermoid, teratoma, ectopic thyroid)
Laryngeal papillomatosis
Vascular rings

Toddler

Viral croup (most common etiology in children 3 mo–4 yr of age)
Bacterial tracheitis (toxic, high fever)
Foreign body (sudden cough; airway or esophageal)
Spasmodic (recurrent) croup
Laryngeal papillomatosis
Retropharyngeal abscess
Diphtheria (uncommon)

Older than 2-3 Yr

Epiglottitis (epiglottis, aryepiglottic folds)
Inhalation injury (burns, toxic gas, hydrocarbons)
Foreign bodies
Angioedema (familial history, cutaneous angioedema)
Anaphylaxis (allergic history, wheezing, hypotension)
Trauma (tracheal or larynx fracture)
Peritonsillar abscess (adolescents)
Ludwig angina
Diphtheria
Parapharyngeal abscess
Tumors*
Trauma

Modified from Kercsmar C: The respiratory system. In Behrman RE, Kliegman RM (eds): Nelson Essentials of Pediatrics, 2nd ed. Philadelphia, WB Saunders, 1994, p 444.

*Tumors include lymphangiomas, hemangiomas, papillomas, neuroblastoma, lymphoma, rhabdomyosarcoma, and chondrosarcomas.

CNS, central nervous system.

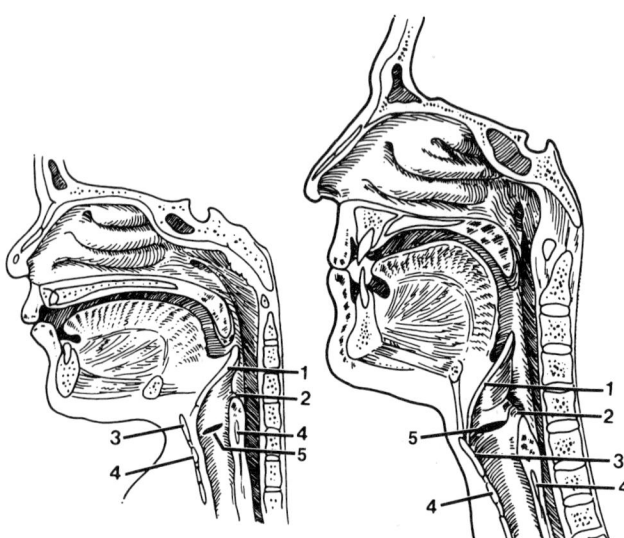

Figure 5-1. Relative comparative anatomy of the larynx in an infant (*left*) and an adult (*right*). Specific landmarks: 1, epiglottis; 2, arytenoid cartilages; 3, thyroid cartilage; 4, cricoid cartilage; 5, laryngeal ventricle, the air space below the false vocal cords and above the true vocal cords. Its radiolucency is an excellent landmark on lateral radiograph. The infant larynx is situated relatively high in the cervical region. In addition, the base of the infant's tongue is close to the larynx, and the epiglottis is located near the palate. These anatomic differences partially explain the predominantly obligate nose breathing of the young infant, as well as the relative ease with which upper airway obstructions develop in infants. (From Grad R, Taussig LM: Acute infections producing upper airway obstruction. In Chernick V, Kendig EL [eds]: Kendig's Disorders of the Respiratory Tract in Children, 5th ed. Philadelphia, WB Saunders, 1990.)

VASCULAR RINGS

Vascular rings are common and can produce symptoms related to compression of the trachea and/or the esophagus (Table 5-4). Feeding often exacerbates manifestations when the obstructed esophagus acts as an additional extrinsic force on the trachea. Patients present with cough, dysphagia, odynophagia, tachypnea, emesis, noisy breathing, stridor, wheezing, and opisthotonos. Because they handle oral secretions poorly, they may develop pulmonary aspiration pneumonia. They also do not tolerate neck flexion well. The two most common symptomatic lesions are the right aortic arch with a left ligamentum arteriosus (or patent ductus arteriosus) and the double aortic arch.

The diagnosis may be suspected on a chest radiograph by a demonstrated right-sided aortic arch or a narrow displaced trachea. Barium esophagograms demonstrate the indentation of the anterior and or posterior esophagus, whereas endoscopy demonstrates the pulsatile extrinsic compressing vessels. MRI or echocardiography is usually diagnostic; angiography is not needed to find most of these lesions (see Table 5-4).

OTHER LESIONS

The cricoid cartilage immediately below the vocal cords and above the trachea is the only circumferential rigid structure of the upper airway. On occasion, a child is born with a smaller than normal cricoid cartilage that may have an elliptic shape. These children may present at birth with airway obstruction or within the first year of life with recurrent atypical crouplike episodes that may not completely clear. In children, the subglottic space is the narrowest part of the upper airway. Laryngoscopy and bronchoscopy can help assess the airway size, and if the stenosis is only minimal, the child may be observed with nighttime cardiorespiratory monitors, with the expectation of improvement as growth occurs. Most often, surgical correction is required. *Acquired subglottic stenosis* may develop secondary to endotracheal intubation, particularly if the intubation

Table 5-3. Nasal Obstruction and Rhinorrhea

Congenital

Total nasal agenesis
Proboscis lateralis
Congenital occlusion of anterior nares
Posterior choanal atresia
Choanal stenosis
Mandibulofacial dysostoses
  Treacher Collins syndrome
  Crouzon syndrome
Coronal craniosynostosis
Cleft palate
Congenital cysts of nasal cavity
  Dermoid cysts
  Nasoalveolar cysts
  Dentigerous cysts
  Mucous cysts of floor of nose
  Jacobson organ cysts
Meningoencephalocele
Encephalocele
Pharyngeal bursa (Tornwaldt)
Hamartomas
Craniopharyngiomas
Chordomas
Teratoid tumors
Epignathus
Possible third branchial cleft cyst (presenting in
  Rosenmüller fossa)
Congenital squamous cell carcinoma of nasopharynx

Inflammatory
Infectious

Bacterial
  Secondary invaders
    Haemophilus influenzae
    Streptococcus pneumoniae
    Other streptococci
    Staphylococcus species
    Branhamella catarrhalis
  Primary agent
    Diphtheria
    Pertussis
    Tuberculosis
    Rhinoscleroma
    Leprosy
    Chlamydia species
Viral
  Primary agent
    Acute viral rhinonasopharyngitis
    Rhinovirus
    Adenovirus
    Coxsackieviruses A and B
    Myxoviruses
      Influenza
      Parainfluenza
      Respiratory syncytial virus
  Prodromal stage of virus disease
    Mumps
    Poliomyelitis
    Measles (rubella, rubeola)
    Roseola infantum
    Erythema infectiosum
    Infectious mononucleosis
    Hepatitis
  Acquired immunodeficiency syndrome
Spirochetal
  Congenital "snuffles"
  Acquired "snuffles"
Protozoan
  Leishmaniasis

Fungal
  Moniliasis
  Mucormycosis (immunocompromised children)
  Aspergillosis (immunocompromised children)
Parasitic

Allergic

Acute: type I (anaphylactic, reagin dependent)
Chronic: nasal polyposis

Toxic

External stimuli
  Inhalants (e.g., urban pollutants)
  Ingested (hormones, iodides, bromides, aspirin)
  Topically applied (nose drops, cocaine) (rhinitis medicamentosa)

Nasopharyngeal

Adenoid hyperplasia
Nasopharyngeal or gastroesophageal reflux

Traumatic
External Deformity

In utero
Neonatal
Acquired in childhood

Internal Deformity

Neonatal
Septal hematoma acquired in childhood
Septal abscess acquired in childhood

Foreign Bodies

Rhinolith

Cerebrospinal Fluid Rhinorrhea

Traumatic
Spontaneous

Neoplastic

Ectodermal origin
Mesodermal origin
Neurogenic origin
  Olfactory neuroblastoma
Odontogenic origin
Idiopathic origin
  Juvenile angiofibroma
  Nasopharyngeal carcinoma

Metabolic

Cystic fibrosis
Calcium abnormalities
Thyroid disease
  Hypothyroidism
  Hyperthyroidism
Diabetes mellitus
Immunodeficiency disease

Idiopathic

Ciliary dyskinesia (Kartagener syndrome, congenital and acquired
  immotile cilia syndrome)
Atrophic rhinitis
Chronic catarrhal rhinitis
Granulomatosis and vasculitis diseases
  Lupus erythematosus
  Rheumatoid arthritis
  Psoriatic arthritis
  Scleroderma
  Sarcoidosis
  Wegener granulomatosis
  Midline lethal granuloma
  Churg-Strauss syndrome
  Pemphigoid: cicatricial or benign mucoid

From Bluestone CD, Stool SE, Alper CM, et al (eds): Pediatric Otolaryngology, vol 2, 4th ed. Philadelphia, WB Saunders, 2003, p 912.

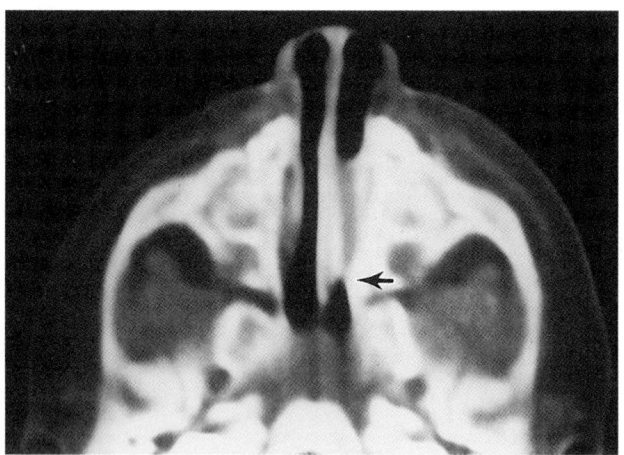

Figure 5-2. Computed tomography scan of unilateral bony choanal atresia (*arrow*) with mucus collected within left nasal cavity.

has been prolonged for several months, if an oversized tube was used, or if multiple intubations were required. Subglottic stenosis should be suspected in any child with these risk factors who does not respond to extubation because of upper airway obstruction. Laryngoscopy and bronchoscopy are required for evaluation. Acquired subglottic stenosis is often more severe than the congenital type. In both types of subglottic stenosis, infection and gastroesophageal reflux may exacerbate symptoms and contribute to narrowing of the airway. A cricoid split operation, tracheotomy, or laryngotracheal reconstruction may be needed. Serial dilatations are no longer commonly used because they may continue to injure the cartilage and its overlying mucosa. Apparently successful dilatations have probably been used for mild stenotic areas and have allowed time for growth of the airway.

A variety of other lesions may cause laryngotracheal obstruction in children. *Laryngeal cysts* may occur as mucoceles from minor salivary glands that are present within the laryngeal mucosa whose secretions do not drain externally. Similar *subglottic cysts* have been reported in children who have undergone prolonged endotracheal intubation; it is thought that a soft tissue reaction secondary to the intubation has obstructed the drainage of these glands into the airway, causing the cyst fluid to accumulate. Cysts may occur deeper within the laryngeal

---

Table 5-4. Vascular Rings

Lesion	Symptoms	Plain Film	Barium Swallow	Bronchoscopy	MRI/Echo-cardiography	Treatment
Double arch	Stridor Respiratory distress Swallowing dysfunction Reflex apnea	AP—wider base of heart Lat.—narrowed trachea displaced forward at C3-C4	Bilateral indentation of esophagus	Bilateral tracheal compression—both pulsatile	Diagnostic	Ligate and divide smaller arch (usually left)
Right arch and ligamentum/ductus	Respiratory distress Swallowing dysfunction	AP—tracheal deviation to left (right arch)	Bilateral indentation of esophagus R > L	Bilateral tracheal compression—r. pulsatile	Diagnostic	Ligate ligamentum or ductus
Anomalous innominate	Cough Stridor Reflex apnea	AP—normal Lat.—anterior tracheal compression	Normal	Pulsatile anterior tracheal compression	Unnecessary	Conservative Apnea, then suspend
Aberrant right subclavian	Occasional swallowing dysfunction	Normal	AP—oblique defect upward to right Lat.—small defect on right posterior wall	Usually normal	Diagnostic	Ligate artery
Pulmonary sling	Expiratory stridor Respiratory distress	AP—low l. hilum, r. emphysema/atelectasis Lat.—anterior bowing of right bronchus and trachea	±Anterior indentation above carina between esophagus and trachea	Tracheal displacement to left Compression of right main bronchus	Diagnostic	Detach and reanastomose to main pulmonary artery in front of trachea

Modified from Keith HH: Vascular rings and tracheobronchial compression in infants. Pediatr Ann 1977;6:540–549.

AP, anteroposterior; L and l., left; Lat., lateral; MRI, magnetic resonance imaging; R and r., right.

Table 5-5. Anomalies of the Pharynx

Supraglottic	Glottic	Subglottic
Congenital flaccid larynx	Vocal cord paralysis	Subglottic hemangioma
Supraglottic atresia	Laryngeal web	Subglottic web
Supraglottic hemangioma	Cri du chat syndrome	Subglottic atresia
Laryngocele	Laryngeal atresia	Subglottic stenosis
Bifid epiglottis	Anterior laryngeal cleft	Posterior laryngeal cleft
Anomalous cuneiform cartilage	Duplication of vocal folds	G syndrome
Absent epiglottis	Neurofibroma of larynx	
Supraglottic web	Plott syndrome	
Lymphangioma of vallecula	Arthrogryposis multiplex	
	Laryngoptosis	

From Cotton RT, Reilly JS: Congenital malformations of the larynx. In Bluestone CD, Stool SE, Scheetz MD (eds): Pediatric Otolaryngology, 2nd ed. Philadelphia, WB Saunders, 1990, p 1122.

tissue when the saccule, an air-containing appendage of the laryngeal ventricle, becomes blocked and fills with mucus. Excision, either endoscopically or with an external neck incision, is necessary.

Laryngeal webs may form as a result of the incomplete canalization of the laryngeal airway. These usually manifest soon after birth with absence of or a very weak cry. Webs may be thick, and complex surgical reconstruction with a tracheotomy to maintain the airway is often required.

Complete tracheal rings, which may not increase in size with growth, are another source of airway obstruction. In rare cases, the esophagus may fail to separate from the larynx and trachea, which results in a posterior *laryngeal cleft,* causing both feeding and airway difficulties. The cleft may involve only part of the larynx, or it may extend to the carina.

A *subglottic hemangioma* is a vascular tumor occurring just below the vocal cords. It usually manifests a few weeks to a few months after birth. As with all hemangiomas, there is a postnatal proliferative phase with increase in size and, therefore, an increase in obstruction, followed by a plateau phase and then a spontaneous resolution phase (at 1 to 5 years of age). Airway obstruction is usually severe, and treatment with carbon dioxide (CO_2) laser vaporization of the tumor, often supplemented by intermittent use of steroids and interferon (α_{2a}), may help avoid a tracheotomy. Care must be used to avoid aggressive intervention, because increased scarring may occur, causing long-term subglottic stenosis.

The differential diagnosis of congenital anomalies of the pharynx and tracheobronchial tree that may produce airway obstruction is noted in Tables 5-5 and 5-6.

INFLAMMATORY DISORDERS OF THE UPPER AIRWAY

MONONUCLEOSIS AND RETROPHARYNGEAL ABSCESS

Infections that cause significant airway obstruction in children are considered according to their site of involvement (see Table 5-1). Oropharyngeal obstruction may occur in severe cases of mononucleosis (tonsil, adenoid hypertrophy) or with a retropharyngeal abscess. Children with mononucleosis (see Chapter 47) and upper airway obstruction usually respond to steroid therapy, although intubation is sometimes needed. Tonsillar and adenoid hypertrophy from mononucleosis or other causes may obstruct the airway and produce acute pulmonary edema or cor pulmonale (see Chapters 6 and 8). With resolution of the infection, the tonsil size usually returns to normal and causes no further problems.

Table 5-6. Classification of Congenital Anomalies of the Tracheobronchial Tree

I. Anomalies of the Trachea
  A. Agenesis or atresia
  B. Constriction
    1. Fibrous strictures
      a. Webs
      b. Fibrous stenosis of tracheal segments
    2. Absence or deformity of tracheal cartilages
      a. Tracheomalacia
      b. Deformity caused by vascular anomalies
      c. Individual cartilage deformity
  C. Tracheal enlargement (congenital trachiectasis)
  D. Tracheal evaginations or outgrowths
    1. Tracheoceles, cysts
    2. Fistulas
  E. Abnormal bifurcation
    1. Tracheal bronchus
    2. Other gross morphologic anomalies

II. Anomalies of Bronchi and Lungs
  A. Agenesis or atresia
  B. Constriction
    1. Fibrous strictures
      a. Webs
      b. Fibrous stenosis of bronchial segments
    2. Absence or deformity of bronchial cartilages
      a. Bronchomalacia
      b. Bronchial hypoplasia
  C. Bronchial enlargements
    1. Congenital bronchiectasis
    2. Kartagener syndrome
  D. Bronchial evaginations
    1. Bronchoceles, cysts
    2. Fistulas
  E. Abnormal bifurcation
  F. Anomalous attachments
    1. Sequestered lung
    2. Lung tissue attached to the gastrointestinal tract

Adapted from Holliner PH, Zimmerman AA, Schild JA: Tracheobronchial tree malformations. In Ferguson CF, Kendig EL Jr (eds): Pediatric Otolaryngology, vol 2, 2nd ed. Philadelphia, WB Saunders, 1972, p 1286. Reprinted from Bluestone CD, Stool SE, Scheetz MD (eds): Pediatric Otolaryngology, 2nd ed. Philadelphia: WB Saunders, 1990, p 1129.

A retropharyngeal abscess causes a child to have difficulty swallowing, and because of inflammation of the prevertebral muscle, there is usually limitation of neck motion and sometimes a slight torticollis.

The diagnosis of either enlarged tonsils or a retropharyngeal abscess can be made by direct inspection or with a lateral soft tissue radiograph of the neck . Cases that are difficult to visualize are best evaluated with a contrast-enhanced CT scan, which shows the exact location of the infection and helps distinguish it from other deep neck infections (see Chapter 1). A retropharyngeal abscess may not always cause severe respiratory compromise.

Treatment of retropharyngeal abscesses consists of intravenous antibiotics directed at anaerobes and gram-positive bacteria, plus incision and drainage. After surgical drainage, the patient needs continued observation because of the rare possibility of edema formation. Rare causes of oropharyngeal airway obstruction include tonsillitis, not associated with mononucleosis; this usually responds to antibiotics. A peritonsillar abscess, which usually manifests with trismus, uvular deviation, and fullness to the superior pole of the tonsil, is usually not associated with airway obstruction unless the abscess is particularly large. It responds to intravenous antibiotics, to incision and drainage, or, less often, to an immediate tonsillectomy (see Table 5-1).

EPIGLOTTITIS

Epiglottitis, sometimes called *supraglottitis* because it involves the larynx above the vocal cords, is the most serious life-threatening infection in this area. Croup involves the subglottic larynx and trachea; bacterial tracheitis is usually a secondary bacterial infection after a viral prodrome (see Table 5-1).

Epiglottitis is an acute, rapidly progressive, potentially lethal infection of the epiglottis, aryepiglottic folds, and false vocal cord area. It is a surgical emergency because of the potential for rapid airway obstruction; evaluation and treatment are directed toward establishing an airway while the physician is confirming the diagnosis and treating the infection. In the past, pediatric epiglottitis was caused by *Haemophilus influenzae* type b in nearly 100% of cases. Blood cultures are positive in 90% of the cases and are used to confirm the diagnosis. Epiglottic or throat cultures are unreliable, with only approximately 50% producing positive results.

Since the introduction of the polysaccharide conjugated *H. influenzae* type b vaccine, there has been a dramatic fall in the incidence of acute epiglottitis in the United States. However, in an internationally mobile world, patients who have not been vaccinated may acquire epiglottitis in any country. In addition, other, less common pathogens may produce epiglottitis. Because the new generation of pediatricians and otolaryngologists is not familiar with epiglottitis, it may actually become a more dangerous disease on a case-by-case basis. Unusual presentations will also become more common, with children presenting at a younger age range and immunosuppressive diseases being caused by atypical organisms.

Typically, there is an abrupt onset, usually without an obvious prodrome, with rapid progression toward airway compromise. Initially, complaints of sore throat and odynophagia are common. Patients are usually febrile, and drooling is present. The typical presentation is an ill-appearing child sitting forward with her or his head hyperextended who does not want to lie down (Fig. 5-3). There is a "hot potato" voice and drooling, the mouth is open, and the tongue is protruding. Mild inspiratory stridor and retractions may be present, but these are usually not obvious, because the patient generally takes short, shallow breaths. An intraoral examination is contraindicated because it may predispose to laryngospasm and airway obstruction.

If there is any question as to the diagnosis, a lateral soft tissue radiograph of the neck can be confirmatory (Fig. 5-4). Someone who has the expertise and equipment to handle sudden airway decompensation should accompany the patient to the radiology suite.

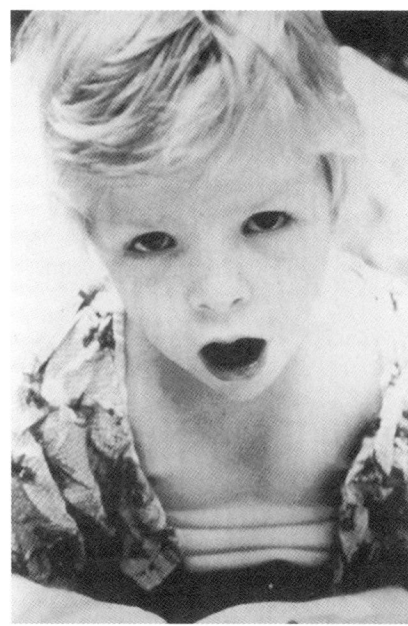

Figure 5-3. Characteristic posture in a patient with epiglottitis. The child is leaning forward and drooling, and the neck is hyperextended. (From Grad R, Taussig LM: Acute infections producing upper airway obstruction. In Chernick V, Kendig EL [eds]: Kendig's Disorders of the Respiratory Tract in Children, 5th ed. Philadelphia, WB Saunders, 1990.)

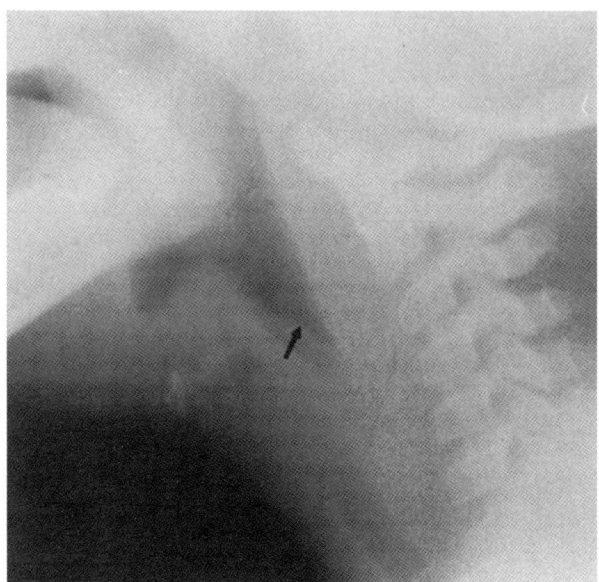

Figure 5-4. Epiglottitis. The patient is a 3½-year-old child with fever and sudden onset of stridor. Lateral radiograph shows an enlarged epiglottis ("thumb-print" sign) and aryepiglottic folds (*arrow*) and distention of the pharynx. Such films are unnecessary if the clinical manifestations are classic for epiglottitis. The patient should be taken immediately to the operating room for intubation. If the diagnosis is uncertain, a physician accompanies the patient to the radiology department. (From Effmann EL: Pediatric chest diseases. In Putman CE, Ravin CE [eds]: Textbook of Diagnostic Imaging. Philadelphia, WB Saunders, 1988.)

When a clinical diagnosis of epiglottitis is at all likely, the patient should be taken immediately to the operating room and cared for by experienced pediatric anesthesiology and otolaryngology personnel.

Once the airway is secured and the diagnosis confirmed, blood specimens are obtained for culture and treatment is begun with ceftriaxone or cefotaxime. Patients usually require 36 to 48 hours of endotracheal intubation, with observation in the pediatric intensive care unit (PICU). A nasotracheal tube is easier to secure and is more comfortable for the patient. Development of an air leak and the patient's clinical improvement can be used as indicators for extubation, which is generally done in the PICU. If a patient self-extubates prematurely, there is not an immediate loss of airway because the previously placed endotracheal tube has acted as a stent. It takes a few minutes for the inflammatory edema to reaccumulate. Depending on the time of self-extubation and the presence of airway obstruction, some patients may be managed with observation in the PICU to avoid reintubation. If there is a question of safety of extubation, a second laryngoscopy, in either the PICU or the operating room, is indicated.

CROUP

Laryngotracheal bronchitis (croup) is generally a slowly progressive, mild, self-limited viral inflammation of the subglottic larynx occurring in infants and young children (see Table 5-1). The most common causes are parainfluenza virus types 1 and 3, influenza A, respiratory syncytial virus, and adenovirus. The circumferential cricoid cartilage, which comprises the subglottic airway just below the vocal cords, is the narrowest part of the upper airway in a child. The inflammation associated with a viral infection in this location causes airway obstruction as edema develops within the confines of the cricoid cartilage (Fig. 5-5). The cry or voice is usually normal, although occasionally hoarse. There is biphasic stridor with retractions. Unless the airway obstruction is severe, the child generally has no trouble handling saliva; the typical barking cough of croup is present.

Management varies from outpatient observation with parent education to endotracheal intubation. For mild cases, the patient must be well hydrated; the use of extra humidity is soothing to the airways and helps to keep secretions from being tenacious, so that they are less likely to become obstructive. In more severe cases (stridor at rest, retractions), nebulized epinephrine used as a mucosal vasoconstrictor may provide relief. Usually, patients being treated in this manner are observed in the hospital for a possible rebound effect that may occur 2 to 6 hours after treatment. Parenteral or oral dexamethasone is a safe and effective additional therapy for moderate to severe croup. Aerosolized steroids may be beneficial in patients with mild to moderate croup. Patients with severe croup are usually admitted to the hospital for observation; steroid use has decreased the requirement for endotracheal intubation. If intubation is needed, an endotracheal tube one-half to one size smaller than that used for a child with a normal airway of the same age and size is chosen. A nasotracheal tube is more comfortable, and guidelines for extubation are similar to those for patients who have epiglottitis. In atypical cases of recurrent croup or in patients in whom extubation is difficult, an endoscopic evaluation of the airway with laryngoscopy and bronchoscopy is necessary to exclude an anatomic abnormality (see Tables 5-2 and 5-5).

Spasmatic croup is a poorly defined process that is generally self-limited with a very short course. It may be related to allergic tendencies (see Table 5-1).

BACTERIAL TRACHEITIS

Bacterial tracheitis is a bacterial superinfection of a previous tracheal (croup, influenza virus) viral process and is usually caused by *Staphylococcus aureus*. A variety of other organisms, including *Moraxella catarrhalis*, *Streptococcus pneumoniae*, and *H. influenzae* (nontypable) have also been identified as being occasionally involved. There is generally a virus-like mild phase, followed by a rapid deterioration of the airway, during which the patient clinically appears more ill with an elevated temperature and white blood cell count. Neck and chest films often show irregular scalloping of the trachea. Radiopaque densities from inspissated mucus may be seen. Close monitoring and intensive intravenous antibiotic treatment (ceftriaxone, nafcillin), directed toward the likely causative organisms are required. Endotracheal intubation for control of the airway is usually necessary, particularly in younger patients.

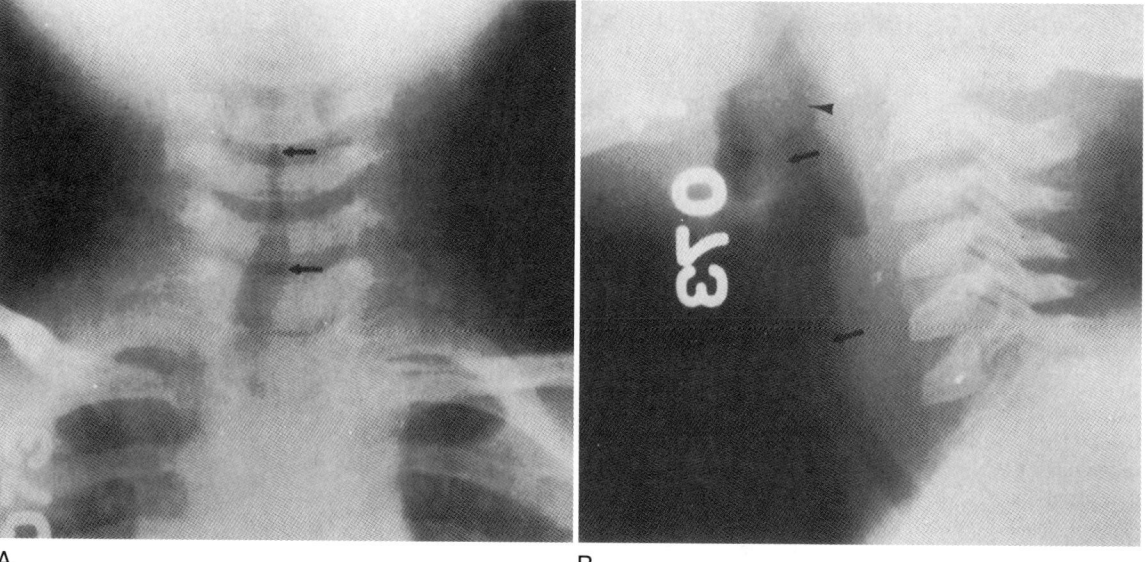

A   B

Figure 5-5. Croup in a 1-year-old infant with stridor. **A,** Frontal radiograph of the neck shows a tapered reduction of the subglottic tracheal caliber from the level of the vocal cords (*upper arrow*) to the normal caliber trachea below (*lower arrow*). The right mild tracheal deviation is a normal sign resulting from the left aortic arch. **B,** Lateral view shows a normal epiglottis (*upper arrow*), distention of the pharynx, normal palatine tonsils (*arrowhead*), and increased density in the subglottic trachea (*lower arrow*). (From Effman EL: Pediatric chest diseases. In Putman CE, Ravin CE [eds]: Textbook of Diagnostic Imaging. Philadelphia, WB Saunders, 1988.)

Extubation is performed on the basis of clinical improvement and a resolution of excessive amounts of purulent secretions. Sometimes the exudate secondary to the tracheitis is thick and can cause airway obstruction similar to that from a foreign body; bronchoscopy is needed. Extubation is performed on the basis of clinical improvement and a resolution of purulent secretions.

OTHER CAUSES OF PEDIATRIC AIRWAY OBSTRUCTION

FOREIGN BODY

Whenever a child presents with airway obstruction, the possibility of a foreign body should be considered (see Chapters 2 and 3). Not all foreign body ingestions or aspirations are witnessed; it is important to question the adult who accompanies a child with airway obstruction. Common foreign bodies include small toy parts, coins, marbles, balloons, and foods (hot dog, seeds, nuts, grapes, carrots, beans). Foreign body aspiration is seen most often in boys younger than 3 years or children with neurologic disorders or delayed development. Radiopaque foreign bodies are generally easily visualized by radiographic studies. Radiolucent foreign bodies may become apparent on inspiratory or expiratory chest radiographs, lateral decubitus films, fluoroscopy, or barium swallow studies when an esophageal foreign body could be compressing the posterior tracheal wall. Because an occasional foreign body may not lodge in a bronchus, typical radiologic findings may not be seen. If a foreign body is likely to be present, rigid bronchoscopy for examination of the lower airway and foreign body removal is indicated. Flexible bronchoscopy provides an excellent look at the airway and should be reserved for when other diagnoses appear to be much more likely. A typical clinical course for an aspirated foreign body is for there to be an *immediate* onset of coughing, gagging, drooling, and voice changes with dyspnea, often followed by a day or two of minimal symptoms, then recurrence of paroxysms of coughing and sometimes localized physical diagnostic (wheezing) and radiographic findings. Laryngeal foreign bodies carry high rates of morbidity and mortality because of the possibility of complete airway obstruction. This is often manifested by sudden inability to speak or cry or cough, cyanosis, severe dyspnea, and, in older children, clutching at the neck (the universal sign of distress). This must be treated immediately as described in Table 5-7.

Foreign bodies remain a cause of significant morbidity and mortality and must be sought in an atypical presentation of airway obstruction. With significant improvements in pediatric anesthesia techniques as well as instrumentation for removal of foreign bodies, rigid bronchoscopy is indicated in their management, and maneuvers such as bronchodilators and percussion and postural drainage, used in the hope that the patient will cough out a foreign body, have no place in the management of this problem.

RECURRENT RESPIRATORY PAPILLOMA

Recurrent respiratory papillomas are exophytic wartlike growths caused by human papillomaviruses 6 and 11 and may occur

---

Table 5-7. First Aid for the Choking Child: Recommendations of the American Heart Association and the International Liaison Committee on Resuscitation

Relief of foreign body airway obstruction in the *responsive infant*:

1. Infant is held prone with the head slightly lower than the chest, resting on the forearm of the rescuer. Rescuer's forearm is rested on the thigh with the hand supporting infant's jaw.
2. Five back blows are administered forcefully with the heel of the rescuer's hand between infant's shoulder blades.
3. If obstruction is not relieved, infant is turned supine as a unit onto rescuer's free forearm with rescuer's hand supporting the occiput of infant's head. Rescuer's forearm is again rested on the thigh with infant's head lower than the trunk.
4. Five rapid chest thrusts are administered over the lower third of the infant's sternum, one fingerbreadth below the intermammary line. Chest thrusts are delivered at a rate of 1 per second.
5. If the airway remains obstructed, the sequence is repeated until the object is removed or victim becomes unresponsive.

Relief of foreign body airway obstruction in the *responsive child*:

1. Rescuer stands or kneels behind victim, arms under the victim's axillae, encircling the torso.
2. Rescuer places flat, thumb side of one fist against victim's abdomen in the midline slightly above the navel and well below the tip of the xiphoid process.
3. Rescuer grabs own fist with other hand and exerts a series of five quick inward and upward thrusts. The xiphoid process and lower portions of the victim's rib cage are avoided, because force applied to these structures may damage internal organs. Each thrust should be a separate, distinct movement, delivered with the intent to relieve the obstruction.

4. If the airway remains obstructed, the series may be repeated, or back blows and chest thrusts may be substituted as described for the unresponsive infant. The rescue attempt continues until the foreign body is expelled or the victim becomes unresponsive.

Relief of foreign body airway obstuction in the *unresponsive infant or child*:

1. Rescuer opens victim's airway with tongue-jaw lift and looks for an object in the pharynx. It the object is visible, it is removed with a finger sweep. *Blind finger sweep should not be performed.*
2. Rescuer opens victim's airway with a head tilt–chin lift and attempts to provide rescue breaths. If the breaths are not effective, victim's head is repositioned and ventilation reattempted.
3. If breaths are still not effective:
   • For infant:
     a. Rescuer performs sequence of five back blows and five chest thrusts.
     b. Steps 1 through 3a are repeated until the object is dislodged and the airway is patent, or for approximately 1 minute. If infant remains unresponsive after approximately 1 minute, rescuer activates EMS system.
   • For child:
     a. Rescuer performs sequence of five abdominal thrusts.
     b. Steps 1 through 3a are repeated until the object is retrieved or rescuer breaths are effective.
4. Once effective breaths are delivered, rescuer assesses for signs of circulation and provides additional cardiopulmonary resuscitation as needed or places victim in a recover position if victim demonstrates adequate breathing and signs of circulation.

From Bluestone CD, Stool SE, Alper CM, et al (eds): Pediatric Otolaryngology, vol 2, 4th ed. Philadelphia, WB Saunders, 2003, p 1545.

EMS, emergency medical services.

anywhere in a child's airway (see Table 5-1). The most common location for their involvement is the larynx, followed by the uvula, tonsillar area, nose, and nasopharynx. The virus is acquired by passage through a birth canal infected with condyloma acuminata (also human papillomaviruses 6 and 11). The papilloma may appear shortly after birth, but it more commonly occurs when the child is several years of age. Lesions have previously been called "laryngeal papillomas," but because they can occur anywhere in the respiratory tract and have a high likelihood of recurrence, the name has been changed. Although the natural history has not been well studied, there is a tendency toward spontaneous regression. As the child's airway enlarges with growth, the papillomas also become less obstructive.

Treatment is directed toward conservative removal of the papillomatous lesions to allow maintenance of an airway that will allow full activities and normal function of the voice. CO_2 laser vaporization is most commonly used. It is not unusual for some children to require dozens of procedures, inasmuch as the viral genome has been found to persist in the airway epithelium and total removal is impossible. Tracheotomies are avoided, unless upper airway obstruction is severe, because the placement of a tracheotomy predisposes to distal pulmonary parenchymal involvement. Interferon has been used for refractory cases with mixed results. Radiation therapy is avoided, to lower the risk of malignant degeneration or secondary (thyroid) malignancies.

OBSTRUCTIVE SLEEP APNEA

The epidemiologic and etiologic features of obstructive sleep apnea (OSA) in children are different from those in adults. Although the causes in children (Table 5-8) are diverse, the most common is adenotonsillar hypertrophy. Additional causes include syndromes with craniofacial anomalies: Pierre Robin, Crouzon, Apert, Treacher Collins, and Cornelia de Lange syndromes; trisomy 21; the mucopolysaccharidoses; and neuromuscular disorders (myopathies, anterior horn cell diseases, neuropathies, cerebral palsy). OSA occurs in 3% of all children.

The manifestations occur in children between 2 and 8 years of age, with no gender predilection. Young patients may have failure to thrive (adolescents may be obese), hyperactivity, developmental delay, morning headaches, cor pulmonale (with pulmonary hypertension), and systemic hypertension, but usually no daytime sleepiness. Additional features include snoring (Table 5-9), mouth breathing, respiratory pauses and enuresis during sleep, and nighttime diaphoresis. Not all patients who snore have OSA.

The patients may be evaluated with radiology of the neck, but polysomnography is the most helpful diagnostic procedure, demonstrating obstructive apnea and poor arousal.

Treatment in patients with hypertrophied tonsils and adenoidal tissue usually consists of adenoidectomy and tonsillectomy, which are quite effective in most patients. Complications of surgery include bleeding, postoperative respiratory compromise, and a delayed onset of velopharyngeal incompetence or nasopharyngeal stenosis.

Alternative therapies include nasal or mask continuous positive airway pressure, topical nasal steroids, and, in neurologically impaired children, uvulopharyngopalatoplasty. Oxygen should be used cautiously because it may depress respirations and produce hypercapnia.

RED FLAGS AND THINGS NOT TO MISS

The most important aspect of the evaluation of a child with airway obstruction is the observation of the child's breathing pattern and a brief, directed history. Supplemental radiologic studies may be needed, and once the site of the obstruction and likely cause are

---

Table 5-8. Causes of Upper Airway Obstuction Associated with Obstructive Sleep Apnea and Related Disorders

I. Anatomic
- A. Nasal
  1. Anterior nares (fetal warfarin syndrome)
  2. Nasal septal hematoma
  3. Trauma: septal deviation
- B. Nasopharyngeal
  1. Choanal atresia, stenosis
  2. Choanal polyp
  3. Nasopharyngeal cyst
  4. Adenoid hypertrophy
  5. Cleft palate repair
  6. Velopharyngeal repair
- C. Oropharyngeal
  1. Tonsillar hypertrophy
  2. Macroglossia (Down syndrome)
  3. Retrognathia, micrognathia
     a. Pierre Robin, Cornelia de Lange syndromes
     b. Achondroplasia
- D. Supraglottic
  1. Laryngotracheomalacia
  2. Vallecular cyst
- E. Craniofacial
  1. Crouzon syndrome
  2. Apert syndrome
  3. Treacher Collins syndrome
  4. Down syndrome

II. Neuromuscular
- A. Cerebral palsy
- B. Down syndrome
- C. Myotrophic dystrophy
- D. Arnold-Chiari malformation
  1. Type I with Klippel-Feil syndrome
  2. Type II with spina bifida
- E. Syringomyelobulbia

III. Miscellaneous
- A. Congenital myxedema
- B. Prader-Willi syndrome (mental retardation, short stature, obesity, hypogonadic hypogonadism)
- C. Obesity
  1. Endogenous
  2. Exogenous
- D. Sickle cell disease

From Bluestone CD, Stool SE, Alper CM, et al (eds): Pediatric Otolaryngology, vol 2, 4th ed. Philadelphia, WB Saunders, 2003, p 1226.

---

identified, treatment is instituted. Because patients with airway obstruction may require operative intervention, these patients should not receive feedings during the evaluation period.

Red flags include sudden onset (as with epiglottitis, foreign body), lack of resolution with normal therapy (as with foreign body, anatomic narrowing), chronic noisy respiration from birth (as in anatomic narrowing, laryngomalacia), positional worsening (acute with epiglottitis, chronic with laryngomalacia), and exacerbations by upper respiratory tract infections. Feeding difficulties (emesis, dysphagia) combined with respiratory manifestations (cough, stridor, noisy respiration) should suggest the presence of an esophageal foreign body, a vascular ring, or other connecting congenital anomalies (e.g., clefts). Additional danger signs include cyanosis, sitting up–leaning forward posture, dysphagia and drooling, aphonia, severe retractions, dyspnea, and lethargy (possibly

Table 5-9. Classification of Obstructive Sleep Disorders and Related Disorders, Based on Clinical Features and Symptoms

I. Primary snoring (alone)

Excessive oropharyngeal noise associated with sleep; more prominent with inspiration

Respirations orderly and regular

II. Snoring with

Respiratory pattern changes

Irregular breathing cycle

Irregular breathing with short pauses (up to 5 seconds)

III. Snoring with

Breathing pauses up to 6 seconds

Periodic breathing (three or more pauses of 3 seconds in a 20-second period)

Hypopnea (limitation of airflow)

IV. Obstructive sleep apnea syndrome

A. Obstructive apnea (cessation of airflow for >6 seconds)
   Airway obstruction
   Apnea, 20-30 episodes of obstructive type per evening (obstructive sleep apnea syndrome)

B. Snoring with behavioral changes
   Hyperactivity, excessive daytime somnolence, aggression, depression
   Deteriorating school performance caused by poor attentiveness, behavior changes, or hypersomnolence

C. Obstructive apnea with major clinical features
   Poor growth and development
   Heart failure
   Cor pulmonale
   Hypertension (other primary causes of hypertension ruled out)
   Hypoxemia with sleep

From Bluestone CD, Stool SE, Alper CM, et al (eds): Pediatric Otolaryngology, vol 2, 4th ed. Philadelphia, WB Saunders, 2003, p 1227.

CO_2 narcosis). It is imperative not to miss epiglottitis or delay endotracheal intubation with unnecessary clinical or radiologic studies. It is also important not to miss a foreign body, which with time may produce chronic respiratory disease that is often confused with pneumonia or asthma.

REFERENCES

Anatomic Abnormalities

Burch M, Balaji S, Deanfield JE, et al: Investigation of vascular compression of the trachea: The complementary roles of barium swallow and echocardiography. Arch Dis Child 1993;68:171-176.

Cozzi F, Steiner M, Rosati D, et al: Clinical manifestations of choanal atresia in infancy. J Pediatr Surg 1988;23:203-206.

Donnelly LF, Strife JL, Myer CM III: Glossoptosis (posterior displacement of the tongue) during sleep: A frequent cause of sleep apnea in pediatric patients referred for dynamic sleep fluoroscopy. AJR Am J Roentgenol 2000;175:1557-1559.

Drazen JM: Sleep apnea syndrome. N Engl J Med 2002;346:390.

Ezekowitz RAB, Mulliken JG, Folkman J: Interferon alfa-2a therapy for life-threatening hemangiomas of infancy. N Engl J Med 1992;326:1456-1463.

Flemons WW: Obstructive sleep apnea. N Engl J Med 2002;347:498-504.

Holinger PH, Brown WT: Congenital webs, cysts, laryngoceles and other anomalies of the larynx. Ann Otol Rhinol Laryngol 1967;76:744-752.

Kaplan LC: The CHARGE association: Choanal atresia and multiple congenital anomalies. Otolaryngol Clin North Am 1989;22:661-672.

Marcus CL: Nasal steroids as treatment for obstructive sleep apnea: Don't throw away the scalpel yet. J Pediatr 2001;138:795-797.

Marcus CL: Sleep-disordered breathing in children. Am J Respir Crit Care Med 2001;164:15-30.

McNamara F, Sullivan CE: Obstructive sleep apnea in infants: Relation to family history of sudden infant death syndrome, apparent life-threatening events, and obstructive sleep apnea. J Pediatr 2000;136:318-323.

Nieminen P, Tolonen U, Lopponen H: Snoring and obstructive sleep apnea in children. Arch Otolaryngol Head Neck Surg 2000;126:481-486.

Shvero J, Koren R, Hadar T, et al: Clinicopathologic study and classification of vocal cord cysts. Pathol Res Pract 2000;196:95-98.

Steward DL, Welge JA, Myer CM: Do steroids reduce morbidity of tonsillectomy? Meta-analysis of randomized trials. Laryngoscope 2001;111:1712-1718.

Thomson AH, Beardsmore CS, Firmin R, et al: Airway function in infants with vascular rings: Preoperative and postoperative assessment. Arch Dis Child 1990;65:171-174.

Zalzal GH: Stridor and airway compromise. Pulm Clin North Am 1989;36:1389-1402.

Infectious Etiologies

Aaltonen LM, Rihkanen H, Vaheri A: Human papillomavirus in larynx. Laryngoscope 2002;112:700-707.

Bisno AL: Acute pharyngitis. N Engl J Med 2001;344:205-211.

Brook I: Microbiology of retropharyngeal abscesses in children. Am J Dis Child 1987;141:202-204.

Chipps BE, McClurg D Jr, Friedman FM, et al: Respiratory papillomas: Presentation before six months. Pediatr Pulmonol 1990;9:125-130.

Chirinos JA, Lichtstein DM, Garcia J, et al: The evolution of Lemierre Syndrome. Report of 2 cases and review of the literature. Medicine 2002;81:458-465.

Coulthard M, Isaacs D: Retropharyngeal abscess. Arch Dis Child 1991;66:1227-1230.

Cressman WR, Myer CM: Diagnosis and management of croup and epiglottitis. Pediatr Clin North Am 1994;41:265-276.

Donnelly BW, McMillan JA, Weiner LB: Bacterial tracheitis: Report of eight new cases and review. Rev Infect Dis 1990;12:729-735.

Gorelick MH, Baker MD: Epiglottitis in children, 1979 through 1992: Effects of *Haemophilus influenzae* type b immunization. Arch Pediatr Adolesc Med 1994;148:47-50.

Klassen TP, Feldman ME, Watters LK, et al: Nebulized budesonide for children with mild-to-moderate croup. N Engl J Med 1994;331:285-289.

Leventhal BG, Kashima HK, Mounts P, et al: Long-term response of recurrent respiratory papillomatosis to treatment with lymphoblastoid interferon alfa-N1. N Engl J Med 1991;325:613-617.

Mauro RD, Poole SR, Lockhart CH: Differentiation of epiglottitis from laryngotracheitis in the child with stridor. Am J Dis Child 1988;142:679-682.

Saipe C: Respiratory emergencies in children. Pediatr Ann 1990;19:637-646.

Super DM, Cartelli NA, Brooks LJ, et al: A prospective randomized double-blind study to evaluate the effect of dexamethasone in acute laryngotracheitis. J Pediatr 1989;115:323-329.

6 Apnea and Sudden Infant Death Syndrome

Mark L. Splaingard*

Apnea is the cessation of airflow for longer than 20 seconds or for a shorter duration in the presence of pallor, cyanosis, or bradycardia. Apneic episodes may be classified as central, obstructive, or mixed (combined central/obstructive). *Periodic breathing* includes three or more consecutive respiratory pauses of longer than 3 seconds; respirations interrupting the apneas are less than 20 seconds. *Cheyne-Stokes respiration,* a form of periodic breathing, is characterized by cycles of increasing rate and amplitude of respirations, followed by progressive diminution until the cycle ends in apnea. Cheyne-Stokes respiration occurs in heart failure, increased intracranial pressure, narcotic use, and high altitude.

Central apneas may be primary (resulting from central nervous system mechanisms) or secondary (resulting from systemic disorders). The causes of apnea vary with the age of the patient and the presence of other identifiable demographic, biologic, or environmental risk factors (Tables 6-1 through 6-4). The most common causes of primary central apnea include apnea of prematurity, sudden infant death syndrome (SIDS), and breath-holding spells. Infections, central nervous system diseases, trauma, and poisonings are common secondary causes of central apnea.

APNEA OF PREMATURITY

Apnea of prematurity (AOP) is caused by a maturational delay in brainstem function. The frequency and severity of AOP are inversely related to gestational age. AOP is defined by central apnea (no ventilatory effort, no respiratory muscle activity) of longer than 15 to 20 seconds or obstructive apnea associated with bradycardia (<100 beats per minute) with or without cyanosis. AOP is a diagnosis of exclusion after other potential common causes of apnea have been eliminated (see Table 6-2). Preterm infants with AOP have partial deficits in respiratory center output, as manifested by decreased ventilatory responsiveness to hypercarbia, in comparison with matched preterm infants without AOP. In affected infants, resting carbon dioxide pressure (PCO_2) levels are higher, and resting minute ventilation is decreased.

Apnea spells in the preterm infant can be central (10% to 25% of spells), obstructive (12% to 20%), or mixed (53% to 71%). Obstruction is usually in the pharynx. Because many electronic surveillance monitors detect only central apnea (respiratory pauses), obstructive apnea is recognized only if it is associated with a significant central component (mixed apnea), bradycardia, or cyanosis. Color changes (erythema, plethora) other than cyanosis are uncommon. AOP with or without bradycardia and cyanosis is usually sleep related.

HISTORY

The initial manifestation of AOP includes episodes of apnea with bradycardia (heart rate < 100) and cyanosis. If the apneic spells are predominantly obstructive, the initial clinical manifestation may be limited to the bradycardia, cyanosis, or both. The onset of symptoms is unusual in the first day after birth or after a postconceptional age of 34 weeks, and by definition the condition does not begin after 37 weeks. AOP can become evident any time after spontaneous respirations have been established, even as early as 1 to 2 days of age. AOP does not manifest in the delivery room (see Table 6-3).

PHYSICAL EXAMINATION

Important aspects of the physical examination are assessment of gestational age and physical findings associated with a specific cause of apnea other than AOP (see Table 6-2). Particular attention must be directed at signs of intraventricular hemorrhage, cardiovascular compromise from sepsis, necrotizing enterocolitis, heart failure, or other acute life-threatening disorders.

DIAGNOSTIC EVALUATION

The diagnosis of AOP is one of exclusion, based on the clinical symptoms and the absence of specific medical causes (see Table 6-2). Laboratory evaluation includes measurements of arterial blood gases (or capillary blood gas plus pulse oximetry) to determine hypoxia or acidosis, serum electrolyte levels (Na^+, K^+, Cl^-, HCO_3^-), and serum glucose and calcium levels; a complete blood cell count (to detect anemia, leukocytosis or leukopenia for infection); a head ultrasonographic study (to detect intracranial hemorrhage); and other diagnostic studies according to the history or physical examination (abdominal radiograph for necrotizing enterocolitis, chest radiograph for pneumonia or postextubation atelectasis). Multichannel cardiorespiratory recordings may document the extent of periodic breathing, hypercarbia, oxygen desaturation, and relative distribution of central, obstructive, and mixed apneas. Such recordings are usually unnecessary for clinical care. *Severity* is defined by the frequency of spells and the extent of any necessary intervention. Resolution is best determined by clinical observation.

DIFFERENTIAL DIAGNOSIS

In preterm infants weighing less than 1500 g at birth, symptomatic apnea occurs at least once in approximately 70% of appropriate weight-for-gestational-age infants, of whom approximately 80% (57% of all such infants) have AOP (see Table 6-2). Severe hypoxemia from any cause can cause apnea. Apnea may be the first clinical indication of hypoglycemia, hypocalcemia, sepsis, and/or meningitis. Patients with seizures may have apnea-related symptoms. Although patients with AOP are generally not anemic, hematocrit levels are lower in preterm infants with AOP than in matched infants without AOP; symptoms often improve after transfusion or erythropoietin therapy. Thermal stress (fever or overheating) can cause apnea. In premature infants, especially those weighing less than 1000 g, apnea-bradycardia-cyanosis spells may be related to feeding and not necessarily to AOP. Gastroesophageal reflux is common in preterm infants and is sometimes associated with significant wakefulness-related apnea-bradycardia-cyanosis symptoms; although infants with AOP with sleep-related symptoms may also have evidence of gastroesophageal

---

*This chapter is an updated and edited version of the chapter by Carl E. Hunt that appeared in the first edition.

Table 6-1. Categories of Apnea

Disease	Example	Mechanism	Signs	Treatment
Apnea of prematurity	Premature baby (<36 wk gestation)	Central control, airway obstruction	Apnea, bradycardia	Theophylline, caffeine, transfusion, nasal CPAP, intubation
Congenital central hypoventilation	Previously called Ondine curse	Central control	Apnea, hypoventilation	Mechanical ventilation
SIDS	Previously normal child; increased incidence with prematurity, SIDS in sibling, maternal drug abuse, cigarette smoking, males; may have preceding minor URI	Central respiratory control?	Child (2–3 mo) found cyanotic, apneic, and pulseless in bed	No treatment; prevention with home apnea monitor unproved, but supine sleep position decreases risk
Cyanotic "breath-holding spells"	Breath holder <3 yr old	Prolonged expiratory apnea, cerebral anoxia	Cyanosis, syncope, brief tonic-clonic movements	Reassurance that the condition is self-limiting; must exclude seizure disorder
Pallid "breath-holding spells"	Breath holder	Asystole, reflex anoxic seizures	Rapid onset, with or without crying; pallor; bradycardia; opisthotonos; seizures; follows painful stimuli	Atropine (?); must exclude seizure disorder; less benign than cyanotic breath holding
Obstructive sleep apnea (OSA)	Obesity, chronic tonsil hypertrophy, Pierre Robin syndrome, Down syndrome, cerebral palsy, myotonic dystrophy, myopathy	Airway obstruction by enlarged tonsils and/or adenoids, choanal stenosis and/or atresia, large tongue, temporomandibular joint dysfunction, micrognathia, velopharyngeal incompetence. Also may be central	Daytime sleepiness, loud snoring, nighttime insomnia and enuresis, hyperactivity, poor school performance, behavior problems, mouth breathing inspiratory stridor, hypertension	Tonsillectomy, adenoidectomy, nasal trumpets, nasal CPAP, uvulopalatoplasty; tracheostomy
Obesity (subcategory of OSA) (pickwickian syndrome)	Obesity, Prader-Willi syndrome	Airway obstruction, central control	Obesity, nocturnal wakefulness, daytime somnolence, hypoxia, hypercarbia, polycythemia, cor pulmonale (see obstructive sleep apnea)	Theophylline, weight loss, nasal CPAP or BiPAP, tracheostomy

BiPAP, bilevel positive airway pressure; CPAP, continuous positive airway pressure; SIDS, sudden infant death syndrome; URI, upper respiratory infection.

? = unproven questionable effects.

reflux, the AOP and gastroesophageal reflux episodes are not temporally related. A sudden increase or new onset of apnea in a preterm infant older than 2 to 3 weeks is not AOP and warrants an evaluation to exclude more serious diseases (see Table 6-2). Similarly, apnea at birth is always caused by a more serious disorder (see Table 6-3).

TREATMENT

Mild infrequent episodes of apnea that resolve spontaneously and are not associated with cyanosis do not necessitate treatment. Contributing acid-base imbalance, hypoxemia, or anemia should be corrected. Tactile stimuli that nonspecifically increase central adrenergic input, including mild shaking, stroking (massage), or the use of an air mattress with low-frequency intermittent inflation or a water mattress, may be helpful. If multiple episodes occur daily and

necessitate vigorous stimulation, or if any episodes require bag-and-mask ventilation with supplemental oxygen, more aggressive treatment is indicated. Although no consensus exists as to when a methylxanthine should be used, both theophylline (loading dose, 5 to 6 mg/kg; maintenance dose, 1 to 2 mg/kg every 8 hours; therapeutic serum maintenance level, 5 to 10 μg/mL) and caffeine (loading dose, 10 mg/kg; maintenance dose, 2.5 mg/kg every day; serum level, 8 to 20 μg/mL) are effective treatments. For the same extent of central respiratory stimulation, caffeine appears to be associated with fewer systemic side effects (tachycardia), and fewer doses per day are necessary. Both agents are central respiratory stimulants and increase diaphragmatic contraction, decrease muscle fatigue, and increase metabolic rate and catecholamine activity. Treatment with methylxanthines results in rapid and significant clinical improvement and eliminates symptoms in 50% or more of preterm patients.

Table 6-2. Etiology of Apnea-Related Spells in Preterm Infants

Cause	Comment
Idiopathic*	Apnea of prematurity with immaturity of respiratory center; modified by sleep state, position, upper airway collapse
CNS	IVH,[†] seizure,[†] depressant drugs, hypoxic injury
Respiratory	Pneumonia, obstructive airway lesions, atelectasis,[†] severe RDS, laryngeal reflex, phrenic or vocal cord paralysis, pneumothorax, hypoxia, hypercarbia, nasal occlusion caused by phototherapy eye patches, tracheal occlusion caused by neck position
Cardiovascular	Heart failure, hypotension, hypertension, hypovolemia, increased vagal tone
Gastrointestinal	Gastroesophageal reflux, nasogastric tube feeding,[†] esophagitis, necrotizing enterocolitis, intestinal perforation, bowel movement
Infection	Sepsis; meningitis: bacterial, viral, fungal
Metabolic	Hypoglycemia, hypocalcemia, hyponatremia, hypernatremia, hyperammonemia, elevated organic acid levels, fluctuations of ambient temperature, hypothermia, hyperthermia
Hematologic	Anemia[†]

*Most common cause, with onset in first week of life (not on first day) and generally resolution by 40 weeks' postconceptional age.

[†]Common.

CNS, central nervous system; IVH, intraventricular hemorrhage; RDS, respiratory distress syndrome.

Whether administered parenterally or orally, methylxanthines appear to be effective for mixed, obstructive, and central apnea. If the patient requires intubation, endotracheal tube placement and mechanical ventilation should not be delayed while the physician waits for a drug to start working.

Nasal continuous positive airway pressure (NCPAP) is usually started after methylxanthine administration or simultaneously with these agents in severe AOP. NCPAP is generally effective in improving and often eliminating clinical symptoms of AOP. In addition to reducing hypoxia and splinting the upper airway, thus reducing upper airway resistance, this therapy may also have some effect related to increased sensory input and secondary changes in sleep state. Since the advent of NCPAP, assisted ventilation has seldom been required for uncomplicated AOP.

OUTCOME

Most symptoms of AOP resolve by a postconceptional age of 35 to 37 weeks. Symptoms occasionally persist until 40 weeks or, in rare cases, longer. Infants should be symptom free for at least 3 days before they are discharged from the hospital. If a methylxanthine is used, the drug should be discontinued in symptom-free infants at least 3 days and preferably 4 to 5 days before discharge.

There is no increased risk of a subsequent cardiorespiratory control deficit, such as SIDS, as a consequence of AOP. The incidence of SIDS is increased in preterm infants; this risk is related to gestational age and is unrelated to presence or severity of AOP. Neurodevelopmental sequelae in preterm infants are correlated with young gestational age and low birth weight and are unaffected by the presence of appropriately treated AOP.

Table 6-3. Etiology of Apnea at Birth

Cause	Comment
Intrauterine asphyxia*	Antenatal, perinatal, postnatal
Placental transfer of CNS-depressant drugs*	Narcotics, magnesium sulfate
Airway obstruction	Choanal atresia, macroglossia–mandibular hypoplasia (Pierre Robin syndrome), tracheal web or stenosis, airway mass lesions
Neuromuscular disorders	Congenital myotonic dystrophy, congenital myopathies or neuropathies
Trauma*	Intracranial hemorrhage, spinal cord transection, phrenic nerve palsy
Infection*	Consolidated congenital pneumonia
Severe immaturity*	Weight <1000 g
CNS lesions	Infantile thalamic degeneration, familial multisystem atrophy, infantile neuroaxonal dystrophy, Pena-Shokeir syndrome, CNS brainstem tumor, Arnold-Chiari malformation, Dandy-Walker malformation, Joubert syndrome, lissencephaly, Miller-Dieker syndrome, medullary hypoplasia, Möbius syndrome, congenital central hypoventilation
Skeletal lesions	Osteogenesis imperfecta, camptomelic dysplasia, achondroplasia, asphyxiating thoracic dystrophies, short-rib polydactyly syndromes, chondroectodermal dysplasia (Ellis–van Creveld syndrome)

Data from Brazy JE, Kinny HC, Oakes WJ: Central nervous system structural lesions causing apnea at birth. J Pediatr 1987;111:163-175.

*Common.

CNS, central nervous system.

PREVENTION

The only definitive way to prevent AOP is to prevent prematurity. If this goal cannot be achieved, the risk for symptoms can be minimized by maintaining optimal acid-base balance, oxygenation, hemoglobin level, and thus oxygen-carrying capacity and oxygen delivery. Because frequent blood transfusions to treat anemia of prematurity have other potential risks, the use of recombinant erythropoietin may be a useful adjunctive treatment.

APPARENT LIFE-THREATENING EVENT

Apparent life-threatening event (ALTE) is a clinical label for any acute episode of apnea that was thought to be potentially life-threatening. An ALTE has some combination of apnea, bradycardia, cyanosis, and loss of tone or consciousness. An ALTE may necessitate cardiopulmonary resuscitation. Apnea of infancy (AOI), the major subcategory of ALTE, can be diagnosed only after the exclusion of all other diagnoses that could explain the acute episode (Fig. 6-1; see Table 6-4). AOI is an idiopathic sleep state–dependent episode associated with bradycardia, cyanosis, and

Table 6-4. Condition that May Cause Apparent Life-Threatening Events or Sudden Death

Cause	Comment
CNS	Arteriovenous malformation, seizures, congenital central hypoventilation (see also Table 6-1), neuromuscular disorders (Werdnig-Hoffmann disease), Arnold-Chiari crisis, Leigh syndrome
Cardiac	Subendocardial fibroelastosis, aortic stenosis, anomalous coronary artery, myocarditis, cardiomyopathy, arrhythmias (prolonged QT syndrome, Wolff-Parkinson-White syndrome, congenital heart block)
Pulmonary	Pulmonary hypertension, vocal cord paralysis, aspiration, laryngotracheal disease
Gastrointestinal	Pancreatitis, diarrhea and/or dehydration, gastroesophageal reflux, volvulus
Endocrine-metabolic	Congenital adrenal hyperplasia, malignant hyperpyrexia, long- or medium-chain acyl coenzyme A deficiency, hyperammonemias (urea cycle enzyme deficiencies), glutaricaciduria, carnitine deficiency (systemic or secondary), glycogen storage disease type I, maple syrup urine disease, congenital lactic acidosis, biotinidase deficiency
Infection	Sepsis, meningitis, encephalitis, brain abscess, hepatitis, pyelonephritis, bronchiolitis (RSV), infant botulism, pertussis
Trauma	Child abuse (see Chapter 36), suffocation, physical trauma, Munchausen syndrome by proxy
Poisoning	Boric acid, carbon monoxide, salicylates, barbiturates, ipecac, cocaine, insulin

CNS, central nervous system; RSV, respiratory syncytial virus.

hypotonia; AOI and ALTE were formerly called "aborted" or "near-miss" SIDS.

HISTORY

The typical history is that a previously normal full-term infant has an acute sleep-related episode of color change, hypotonia, and apnea at home. The history needs to include a number of specific questions to focus the differential diagnosis and diagnostic evaluation (Table 6-5) and to determine the severity of the episode. Risk factors may be similar to those of SIDS (Table 6-6). Conditions that may cause sudden death or an ALTE are noted in Table 6-4.

PHYSICAL EXAMINATION

The role of the physical examination is to identify any specific abnormality that is sufficient to explain the ALTE (see Fig. 6-1, Table 6-4). Abnormal results of a neurologic examination might suggest the presence of a central nervous system lesion, neurode-generative disease, trauma, or a seizure-related cause, especially if multiple episodes have occurred. If the infant is lethargic or unresponsive, intoxication, inborn errors of metabolism, hypo-glycemia, and meningitis are prominent considerations. Severe hypoxia caused by an ALTE also produces a hypoxic-ischemic encephalopathy. The presence of midfacial hypoplasia, micro-gnathia, or both suggests obstructive sleep apnea. A cardiac cause for the episode is not common, but its presence is usually evident from the examination. Evidence of neglect or unexplained bruising necessitates consideration of child abuse. Delay in seeking care, a physical finding unexplained by the history, and inconsistent historical information from the same or multiple family members should raise suspicions for abuse (see Chapter 36). Depending on parental behavior and consistency of the history and clinical findings, Munchausen syndrome by proxy with intentional suffocation may also need to be considered.

DIAGNOSTIC EVALUATION

If the examination findings are normal and the history is consistent with an idiopathic ALTE (AOI), the laboratory evaluation can be limited. If the patient is seen within 2 to 4 hours of the episode, a serum bicarbonate level might show evidence of hypoxia-induced metabolic acidosis if the episode was of significant severity and duration. A urine toxicology screen should be obtained; 10% to 15% of screens demonstrate a drug that can explain the ALTE, related to either well-intentioned but overzealous parents or to intentional poisoning. Tests such as electroencephalography, chest roentgenography, electrocardiography, complete blood cell count, evaluation for gastroesophageal

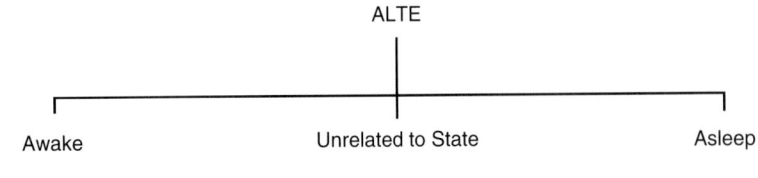

ALTE

Awake	Unrelated to State	Asleep
Gastroesophageal reflux	Airway obstruction (severe)	Obstructive sleep apnea
Breath-holding spells	Neurologic dysfunction	Suffocation
Airway obstruction	Infection	Idiopathic (apnea of infancy)
	Cardiac disturbance	Alveolar hypoventilation
	Metabolic error	
	Toxic–poisoning	
	Autonomic dysfunction	
	Child abuse, including Munchausen syndrome by proxy	

Figure 6-1. Possible causes of an apparent life-threatening event (ALTE) in infancy and their relationship to sleep state. Causes classified as "unrelated to state" can occur while the child is awake or asleep.

Table 6-5. Questions that Guide the Evaluation of Apparent Life-Threatening Events*

1. Who discovered the infant?
2. Was the infant awake or asleep?
3. Where was the infant sleeping (cosleeping)? What were the circumstances related to sleeping surface, bedding, and covering (swaddling)?
4. In what sleep position was the infant found? If the position was prone, what was the position of the face?
5. What were the specific observations in regard to color, muscle tone, pulse, and respiratory effort?
6. What was the timing and the sequence of intervention, and what was required for a response?
7. When was the last feeding?
8. Has there been a recent febrile illness?
9. Have any other spells occurred?
10. How long did it take the infant to fully recover after the episode?
11. If available, what were the objective findings of the Emergency Medical Service or ambulance personnel?
12. Is there a family history of such events?

*Responses to all of these questions are necessary as part of the assessment of an apparent life-threatening event.

reflux, or lumbar puncture should be performed if they are indicated by the history (including family history) and physical examination.

No specific diagnostic evaluation can provide positive confirmation that the ALTE is idiopathic and is thus appropriately labeled as AOI. A partial deficit in central inspiratory drive, as indicated by blunted ventilatory or arousal responsiveness to hypercarbia or hypoxemia and perhaps mild alveolar hypoventilation, occurs in approximately 30% to 40% of infants with AOI. Pneumography has often been performed, but results are abnormal in no more than 50% of infants with AOI. The respiratory pattern abnormalities that can be

Table 6-6. Epidemiologic Risk Factors for Sudden Infant Death Syndrome (SIDS)

Low birth weight (<2500 g)
Very low birth weight (<1500 g)
Male sex
Black race
Winter months
Formula (versus breast) feeding
Prone sleeping position*
Prior ALTE
Cosleeping
Natural fiber mattress use*†
Swaddling*†
Recent respiratory illness*†
Thermal stress*†
Poor or no prenatal care
Previous sibling with SIDS
Maternal urinary tract infection
Maternal cigarette smoking
Maternal illicit drug use
Low socioeconomic status
Maternal age <19 yr

*The combination of these factors may impose the greatest and most significant risk.

†If sleeping prone.

ALTE, apparent life-threatening event.

observed include prolonged apnea, excessive respiratory pauses, and excess periodic breathing. Furthermore, the pneumographic results do not predict risk for recurrence and are not correlated with the potential future risk for SIDS. Polysomnograms may be obtained in patients with AOI, but results may be normal in 90%; a normal result does not contradict the diagnosis of AOI. An interval of documented monitoring can be a useful diagnostic test to better characterize the diagnosis by recording any alterations in cardiorespiratory pattern that occur during a clinical event that are sufficient to exceed the alarm thresholds.

DIFFERENTIAL DIAGNOSIS

In a large series of infants with ALTE, 62% had a known cause; among these, the diagnoses included 47% digestive, 29% neurologic, 15% respiratory, 3.5% cardiovascular, 2.5% endocrine-metabolic, and 3% miscellaneous (see Table 6-4). The other 38% had AOI: 61% of these infants had mild AOI, and 39% had severe AOI, requiring vigorous stimulation or cardiopulmonary resuscitation.

The ALTE should first be classified as awake-related, sleep-related, or unrelated to state (see Fig. 6-1). If the ALTE is exclusively wakefulness-related, the possible diagnoses are limited; if it is postprandial and especially if it is associated with regurgitation or vomiting, gastroesophageal reflux is a likely consideration. If the ALTE is associated with behavioral or vagally induced antecedents, a breath-holding spell is the likely diagnosis. There is a continuum between breath-holding spells and autonomic spells, the latter generally not being associated with any behavioral antecedents; autonomic spells (familial dysautonomia, autoimmune neuropathy) are not common but need to be considered when spells predominately or exclusively during wakefulness are severe and recurrent, and especially if the severity seems to be increasing after the initial manifestation. Acute upper airway obstruction can also cause an ALTE (see Chapter 5).

If the cause of the ALTE is a respiratory control abnormality, such as obstructive sleep apnea or central hypoventilation syndrome, then the symptoms are sleep related and extend into wakeful periods only in the most severe instances. If the cause for the ALTE is related to infectious, metabolic, neurologic, cardiac, or toxic causes, there is generally no clear relationship to sleep state. Child abuse by suffocation has to be considered. In some instances, the child abuse is related to Munchausen syndrome by proxy, in which the infant is a victim of illness imposed for the psychological benefit of a parent, generally the mother. Although this syndrome is an uncommon cause of an ALTE, presentation as an ALTE may account for 40% to 50% of cases of Munchausen syndrome by proxy in infancy. If the suspicion for Munchausen syndrome by proxy seems warranted, covert video surveillance may be necessary (see Chapter 36).

TREATMENT

If the ALTE is attributed to a specific cause, the appropriate treatment should then be apparent. If the final diagnosis by exclusion is AOI, then the predominant treatment strategy has been the use of a home monitor until the infant is free of recurrent symptoms for at least 2 to 3 months, often until the child is 5 or 6 months of age. Although there are no data to indicate that home monitoring for AOI reduces the risk for SIDS, home monitors are indicated to alert the family to any potentially life-threatening recurrences and thus permit timely intervention and prevention of serious morbidity. The availability of documented monitoring with stored events and respiratory patterns in computerized memory permits a more objective use of the home monitor. These event recordings permit characterization of any clinically significant events that recur and establish whether any of the alarms occurring at home are of clinical or physiologic significance.

In patients with AOI with an abnormal respiratory pattern, a methylxanthine has also been recommended. As with AOP (see earlier discussion), the respiratory pattern abnormalities generally resolve with such treatment, and the clinical symptoms also tend to resolve. Although methylxanthines have been used as an adjunct or even as an alternative to home monitoring in patients with AOI, only anecdotal data regarding their efficacy are available. All families of infants with AOI should be taught basic cardiopulmonary life support.

OUTCOME

The outcome of an ALTE depends on the cause. If the cause is idiopathic (AOI), 40% to 50% of affected infants are likely to have no further life-threatening episodes, and those having recurrences generally show progressive improvement over the ensuing months. Of patients with AOI, 90% or more have at least one episode of apnea (≥20 seconds) at home as determined by monitor alarms. Most infants triggering alarms receive stimulation, divided approximately equally among gentle stimulation, vigorous stimulation, and resuscitation. Although not necessary for routine clinical care, hypoxic arousal responses do help identify patients with AOI who are at highest risk for severe recurrent ALTE; patients with deficient hypoxic arousal responsiveness have a higher incidence of subsequent apnea episodes than do those with normal arousal responsiveness. Although most true alarm signals occurring at home are caused by apnea, about 15% are associated with bradycardia and about 15% are isolated bradycardia. These outcome data are based on undocumented home monitoring. More detailed studies have demonstrated that parental observations and home monitor logs significantly overstate the occurrence of events; that is, approximately 90% of home alarms are not caused by a clinically significant event. Loose monitor leads and movement artifact alarms account for 65% to 70%, and false alarms account for the remaining 20% to 25% of nonphysiologic alarms.

Follow-up studies have not been performed with sufficient frequency to clarify the extent to which immature or abnormal brainstem respiratory output later improves. Infants with AOI may have a small but increased risk for respiratory control disorders in later years, such as alveolar hypoventilation or obstructive sleep apnea. Previous reports in patients with AOI indicate a risk of SIDS as low as zero and as high as 5% to 6%. The natural risk is probably closer to 5%, and the extent to which home monitoring may reduce this risk is unknown.

Follow-up studies of patients with AOI to 7 to 10 years of age reveal no neurodevelopmental differences between affected and normal children. Nevertheless, a small number of children in whom the ALTE was of sufficient severity to cause a hypoxic-ischemic event have significant neurobehavioral sequelae. Children with AOI do have a higher frequency of breath-holding spells and of minimal behavioral problems.

PREVENTION

It is not possible to prevent the first episode of AOI, because there is no way to predict which infants will develop the condition. There may be an increased incidence of AOI in families with a history of SIDS or AOI, but 95% or more of subsequent siblings are normal, and there is no accurate means of prospectively identifying the few who might be at an increased risk for developing AOI.

SUDDEN INFANT DEATH SYNDROME

SIDS is the most common cause of sudden and unexpected death in infants after the neonatal period (Fig. 6-2); 40% to 50% of post-neonatal infant mortality is caused by SIDS. The peak incidence is at 2 to 4 months of postconceptional age; 95% of all cases of SIDS occur by age 6 months. SIDS is the sudden death of an infant that remains unexplained despite a complete autopsy, examination of the death scene, and review of the history. An autopsy is thus required in all instances of sudden infant death because the history and death scene investigation are not sufficient to exclude most congenital or acquired causes (Table 6-7; see Table 6-4).

HISTORY

The location, time, and circumstances of the death need to be ascertained as soon as possible. If the infant was asleep, which is usually the case, the position in which he or she was found and the nature of the sleeping surface (hard or soft mattress, pillow, blanket) also need to be documented (see Table 6-5). Approximately 50% of SIDS victims have a history of a recent or intercurrent minor upper respiratory or other febrile illness, such as gastroenteritis. Decreased activity or listless appearance on the last day is also common, but an autopsy is needed to exclude severe infection. Many epidemiologic risk factors are associated with SIDS (see Table 6-6); absence of risk factors does not eliminate the risk for SIDS. Because most SIDS victims have not been identified in advance, most of the assessments of biologic risk factors have been evaluated in surviving infants who presented with AOI.

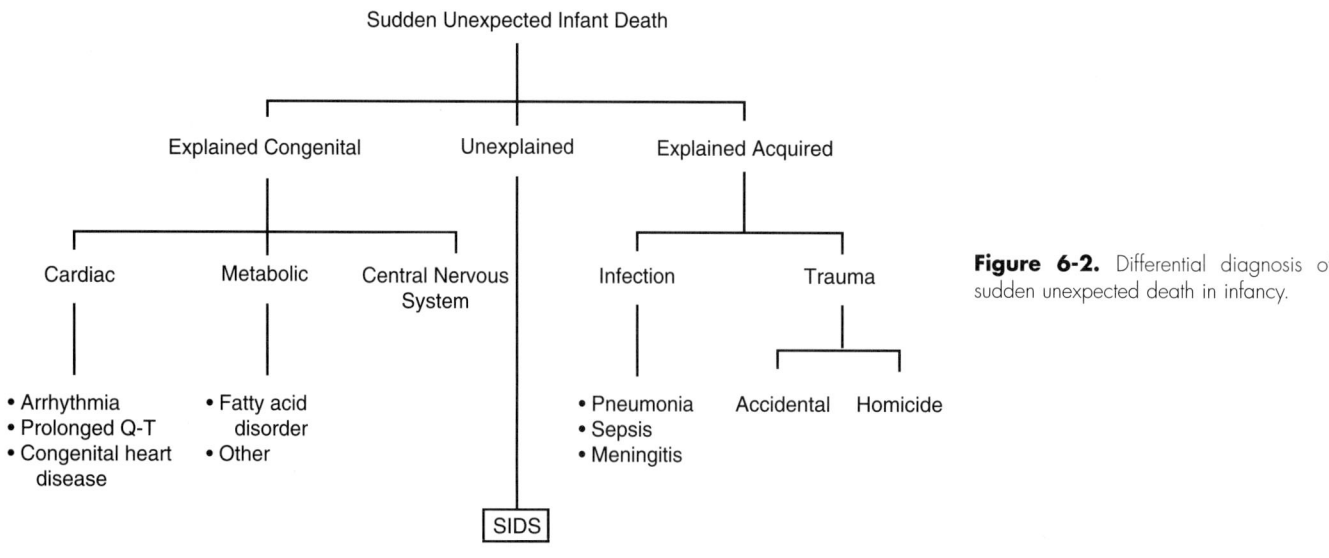

Figure 6-2. Differential diagnosis of sudden unexpected death in infancy.

Table 6-7. Differential Diagnosis of Recurrent Sudden Infant Death in a Sibship

Idiopathic	Recurrent true sudden infant death syndrome
CNS	Congenital central hypoventilation, neuromuscular disorders, Leigh syndrome
Cardiac	Endocardial fibroelastosis, Wolff-Parkinson-White syndrome, prolonged QT syndrome, congenital heart block
Pulmonary	Pulmonary hypertension
Endocrine-metabolic	See Table 6-4
Infection	Disorders of immune host defense (see Chapter 51)
Child abuse	Filicide, infanticide, Munchausen syndrome by proxy

CNS, central nervous system.

PHYSICAL EXAMINATION

The examination begins with the death scene investigation and ends with the autopsy. The body needs to be examined for any evidence of trauma. Even in the absence of any external evidence, the presence of internal hemorrhage or fracture needs to be ascertained. It is necessary to rule out unsuspected congenital defects, such as cardiac defects (e.g., critical aortic stenosis), or central nervous system anomalies. Blood and urine need to be examined for toxic substances and for medium-chain fatty acid metabolism defects. The presence of a significant infection, such as meningitis, sepsis, or overwhelming pneumonia, needs to be determined.

Minimal pulmonary edema and diffuse intrathoracic petechiae are commonly observed in SIDS; they are associated and not diagnostic findings, because neither has been of sufficient specificity and sensitivity to prove or explain SIDS. Numerous other findings suggestive of chronic prenatal or postnatal asphyxia have been reported. Detailed examination of the brain has also revealed other subtle findings that suggest delayed maturational changes that may contribute to the causation of SIDS.

DIFFERENTIAL DIAGNOSIS

The diagnosis of SIDS is based on exclusion of all known causes of sudden infant death (see Fig. 6-2 and Tables 6-4 and 6-7) by the history, death scene, and pathologic investigations. Episodes of recurrent ALTE in a patient or of SIDS in a sibship may be clues to other identifiable disorders (see Table 6-7). Perhaps as many as 10% of deaths consistent with SIDS are in fact explained by child abuse (filicide).

Inborn errors of metabolism may manifest as an ALTE or SIDS. Hepatomegaly (glycogen storage disease), hypoglycemia (glycogen storage disease, disorders of fat metabolism such as carnitine deficiency, medium acyl coenzyme A dehydrogenase deficiency), absence of fasting ketosis (disorders of fat metabolism), hypotonia (carnitine deficiency), cardiomyopathy (glycogen storage disease, carnitine deficiency), and recurrences of SIDS in a family increase the possibility of an inborn error of metabolism.

TREATMENT

The only available "treatment" strategy pertains to the surviving family. Local SIDS support groups are available to provide information and support to the family. The increased focus on filicide is

justified, but a negative consequence of this has been the delayed implementation of the support process, even when SIDS is the correct final diagnosis. A primary forensic approach to all sudden and unexpected deaths can thus unduly delay the support process for the 90% or more of such deaths that are indeed SIDS.

PREVENTION

It is not possible to prospectively identify infants who, in the absence of effective intervention, will die of SIDS. Therefore, preventive measures have been suggested for all infants.

Public education campaigns in numerous countries have advocated large-scale efforts to reduce SIDS rates by interventions such as supine position for sleep, breast-feeding, parental smoking cessation, solitary sleeping, avoidance of overheating, and early evaluation of any febrile illness. Although the epidemiology of SIDS is complex, the mechanism is unknown, and the determination of position at death is imprecise and generally retrospective, epidemiologic studies now support the "Back to Sleep" campaign for infants (see Table 6-6). The American Academy of Pediatrics recommends placing all infants in the supine position before sleep, to reduce the risk of SIDS. In addition, soft pillows and soft mattresses should be avoided.

OBSTRUCTIVE SLEEP APNEA

Obstructive sleep apnea (OSA), a common disorder in adults, is also a significant clinical entity in children (see Table 6-1). OSA is a sleep-related phenomenon associated with severe, prolonged, partial airway obstruction; intermittent episodes of reversible complete obstruction; or both. In children, this condition is usually a result of adenoidal-tonsillar hypertrophy or obesity. The incidence in childhood peaks at 2 to 5 years of age, but the specific age at presentation depends on the underlying mechanism (see Table 6-1). Brainstem respiratory center output is generally normal to increased in response to obstruction in patients with OSA. In obese children, however, OSA may indeed be associated with diminished central respiratory drive and resultant alveolar hypoventilation that may remain even if the obstruction is treated. Additional causes include micrognathia, midfacial hypoplasia, extrinsic or intrinsic anatomic lesions obstructing the airway, and functional obstruction from pharyngeal muscle dysfunction (see Table 6-1).

HISTORY

A careful delineation of symptoms during wakefulness (hyperactivity, irritability, daytime sleepiness) and during sleep (snoring, arousals, nocturnal enuresis, nonrestorative sleep) is essential. Snoring is loud and can persist through most or all of sleep. Brief episodes of respiratory silence indicate episodic complete obstruction. Sleep disturbances are related to both the severity of obstruction-related sleep asphyxia and repetitive arousals that lead to sleep fragmentation.

The occurrence of daytime symptoms is a direct consequence of chronic sleep deprivation. Depending on the patient's age and the severity of the sleep disturbance, the history may reveal hypersomnolence, behavioral disturbances, morning headache, or decreased school performance. A history of inability to sleep lying flat—that is, preferring sitting up, knee-chest position, or neck hyperextension—suggests possible OSA.

PHYSICAL EXAMINATION

Craniofacial abnormalities, low muscle tone, cerebral palsy, or Down syndrome all predispose children to OSA. Mouth breathing suggests significant nasal obstruction (adenoids), and the presence of midfacial underdevelopment indicates an anatomic predisposition. Although marked adenoidal or tonsillar hypertrophy confirms the most likely cause for OSA, the absence of significant adenotonsillar hypertrophy does not exclude OSA, inasmuch as the nasopharyngeal airway narrowing may be present only during sleep.

Heavy or persistent snoring strongly suggests significant partial upper airway obstruction, especially if the snoring is associated with color change or bradycardia or with cor pulmonale. The occurrence of episodes of complete obstruction is indicated by intervals of silent breathing despite severe retractions.

DIAGNOSTIC EVALUATION

To determine the severity and to clarify the underlying mechanism, polysomnography is necessary. This assessment requires referral to a sleep laboratory experienced in the evaluation of infants and young children. The diagnosis of OSA in children is confirmed by (1) episodes of partial or complete airway obstruction during sleep that result in an oxygen saturation of less than 90%, frequent electrocortical arousals fragmenting sleep continuity, or an end-tidal PCO_2 of greater than 45 mm Hg or by (2) sleep-related asphyxia and sleep deprivation that result in failure to thrive, cor pulmonale, or neurobehavioral disturbance.

The presence of polycythemia or elevated serum bicarbonate levels is consistent with a greater severity of chronic sleep-disordered breathing or chronic hypoxia and hypercarbia, respectively. Radiographic examination of the sinuses and nasopharynx may be helpful in some children, but lateral neck radiography performed during wakefulness may significantly underrepresent the degree of sleep-related nasopharyngeal collapse that would be evident on airway fluoroscopy performed while the patient is asleep. The presence and severity of cor pulmonale (cardiomegaly, hepatomegaly, hypoxia, right ventricular hypertrophy on electrocardiography, accentuated P_2 sound on cardiac auscultation, and narrow splitting of the second heart sound) also need to be evaluated.

DIFFERENTIAL DIAGNOSIS

Other airway conditions can potentially be confused with OSA. Any condition causing stenosis or collapse of the airway can secondarily be associated with snoring and partial airway obstruction asleep; the absence of significant symptoms during wakefulness, however, indicates OSA (see Chapter 5). Reactive airway disease should be distinguished by the history and the results of the physical examination. Gastroesophageal reflux can cause stridor and coughing and can certainly be present as an additional finding, but the history and polysomnographic results distinguish between

OSA and gastroesophageal reflux as the primary diagnosis (see Chapter 16). Excessive daytime sleepiness or neurobehavioral problems such as attention-deficit/hyperactivity disorder may be caused by OSA but can also be a symptom of primary sleep disorders such as narcolepsy, periodic limb movement disorder, or idiopathic hypersomnia.

Narcolepsy is manifested by daytime sleepiness and cataplexy, sleep paralysis, or hypnagogic hallucinations. Narcolepsy is a severely disabling sleep disorder that may or may not be associated with apnea.

TREATMENT

In otherwise normal children, OSA can be cured by both tonsillectomy and adenoidectomy. Children younger than 2 years who have craniofacial abnormalities or neurologic disorders are at high risk of postoperative complications after tonsillectomy and adenoidectomy. They should have careful postoperative monitoring in a setting capable of managing pediatric airway obstruction. Children with OSA that is unresponsive to surgery or for which no surgery is possible may benefit from NCPAP. Acting as a splint to maintain higher end-expiratory nasopharyngeal cross-sectional area, NCPAP has been a very successful treatment strategy in children. Tracheostomy may be necessary in some children with severe craniofacial or neurologic disorders. Children with significant obesity or pickwickian syndrome who fail to achieve significant weight reduction and in whom therapy with CPAP fails may require tracheostomy (see Table 6-1).

OUTCOME

The outcome for children with OSA is generally excellent. Because most cases are related to adenotonsillar hypertrophy, tonsillectomy and adenoidectomy should be curative. Chronic problems generally occur only if permanent consequences of severe sleep-related asphyxia occurred before diagnosis and treatment (Fig. 6-3). Hypoxic-ischemic encephalopathy is rare, but it is a consideration. In children with midfacial hypoplasia or other discrete causes of airway obstruction, the outcome depends on the specific problem.

PREVENTION

The occurrence of severe long-term sequelae can be prevented by an awareness of the presenting symptoms in children and by timely interventions.

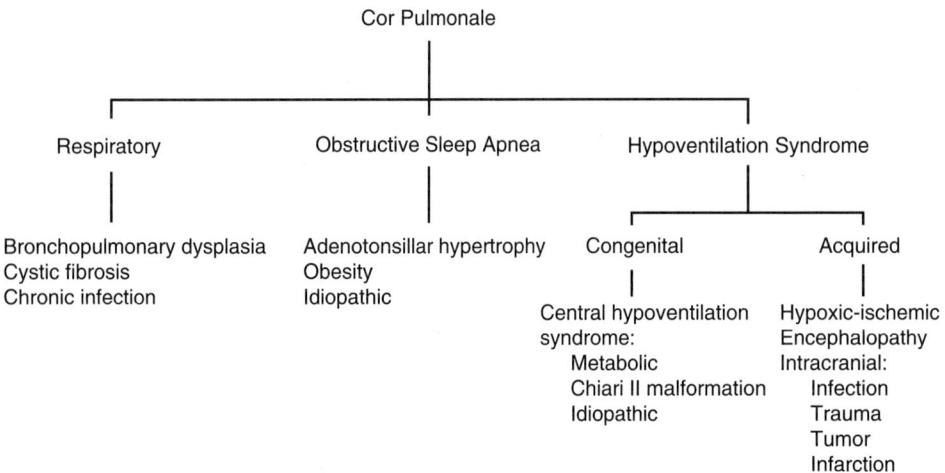

Figure 6-3. Causes of cor pulmonale in infants and children.

HYPOVENTILATION SYNDROMES

HISTORY

Alveolar hypoventilation encompasses all respiratory control deficits associated with decreased central respiratory drive and resultant deficiency of autonomic control of ventilation. *Alveolar hypoventilation* is also a descriptive label for the milder form of hypoventilation syndromes. *Central hypoventilation syndrome* (CHS) represents the severe end of the respiratory control spectrum, in which output of the brainstem respiratory centers is not sufficient to sustain spontaneous ventilation (Table 6-8). The range of severity encompasses milder forms that are evident only during quiet sleep; ventilation may be sufficient for avoiding acute symptoms but insufficient for preventing progressive cor pulmonale. In severe cases, spontaneous sleep ventilation is inadequate for survival. In the most severe cases, the deficient respiratory center output extends to variable degrees into wakefulness. Patients with CHS typically have normal respiratory rates associated with shallow breathing (hypopnea). These rates do not increase in response to progressive asphyxia, because of the underlying deficiency in automatic control of respiration. Voluntary ventilation is normal but cannot be adequately regulated. Overt apnea is uncommon.

Infants with a severe congenital CHS have persistent hypopnea that necessitates ventilatory support. If the extent of hypoventilation is not severe, the diagnosis may not be clinically evident until cor pulmonale develops or an acute respiratory infection occurs. In children with alveolar hypoventilation, the extent of sleep-related asphyxia may thus be minimal, so that diagnosis does not occur until adolescence. As with any respiratory control deficit, the history is not complete until sleep-related symptoms have been evaluated by polysomnography.

PHYSICAL EXAMINATION

The findings with mild alveolar hypoventilation are unremarkable while the patient is awake unless the presentation was precipitated by acute respiratory infection or cor pulmonale. Examination during the patient's sleep reveals hypopnea, a normal respiratory rate, mild cyanosis or pallor, and perhaps sweating. Obesity may be an associated finding.

The manifestations depend on the severity of the hypoventilation and the patient's age. Infants with severe congenital CHS are likely to be symptomatic in the delivery room or within the first 12 to 24 hours, with marked hypopnea, secondary bradycardia, and cyanosis that necessitate assisted ventilation.

The examination must include a search for associated congenital or acquired abnormalities. In the newborn, hypoventilation may be associated with a myelomeningocele and Chiari II malformation. Patients with CHS generally have mild hypotonia, but more substantial degrees of hypotonia might indicate a specific metabolic or neuromuscular disorder (see Chapter 38). If the deficit is acquired, the physical examination should reveal the underlying cause, such as severe central nervous system infection, trauma, or tumor.

DIFFERENTIAL DIAGNOSIS

Regardless of the patient's age at presentation, the differential diagnosis of CHS includes acute cardiac and respiratory conditions capable of causing cardiorespiratory failure. If the severity of hypopnea is not sufficient to cause acute cardiorespiratory failure, the sleep-related hypopnea and secondary asphyxia result in right-sided heart failure or cor pulmonale. The differential diagnosis for cor pulmonale (see Fig. 6-3) then needs to be considered.

TREATMENT

Drug therapy is effective in the milder degrees of alveolar hypoventilation. Theophylline or caffeine may be sufficient to normalize sleep ventilation; progesterone has sometimes been effective. Intravenous doxapram improves ventilation in most CHS patients but seldom to the extent that ventilatory support can be withdrawn. Long-term treatment with doxapram is not realistic because of its generalized adrenergic side effects.

Mechanical ventilatory support is an essential component of the treatment for CHS. The options include positive- and negative-pressure ventilation and diaphragm pacing. In infants and young children, negative-pressure methods are generally not practical, and chronic tracheostomy is usually necessary. Positive-pressure ventilation has been the most commonly used long-term treatment for CHS. Home ventilators are most practical and least intrusive when children require support only during sleep. As an alternative to chronic tracheostomy, limited success with positive-pressure ventilation or bilevel positive airway pressure delivered by nasal mask has been achieved in a few older children. Negative-pressure ventilation has been successful in some older children who require mechanical assistance only during sleep. Both a chest shell (cuirass) and a jump suit (wrap ventilator) have been advocated. The primary advantage of negative-pressure or nasal mask ventilation is that the ventilation may be successful without a tracheostomy.

There has been substantial clinical experience with diaphragm pacing in infants and children. The pacer system includes an external transmitter, a loop antenna, and three internal components: a receiver, unipolar phrenic nerve electrodes, and an indifferent electrode (anode). A radiofrequency signal is emitted from the antenna, converted by the receiver to an electrical impulse, and transmitted to the phrenic nerve. To be eligible for diaphragm pacing, the child must have intact phrenic motoneurons and must not have any significant reduction in lung compliance. If wakefulness pacing is being contemplated, age-appropriate activities are fully achievable if supplemental oxygen is not required. Diaphragmatic pacing requires a tracheostomy. The primary complication of pacing is periodic failure of an implanted pacemaker component, generally a receiver or, less commonly, an electrode wire. Chronic phrenic nerve or diaphragm damage ("burnout") has not occurred in children enrolled in a recommended clinical pacing regimen.

OUTCOME

Except for patients with CHS caused by associated congenital abnormalities, optimal long-term outcome appears to be related primarily

---

Table 6-8. Respiratory Control Abnormalities Characteristic of Central Hypoventilation Syndrome

1. Hypoventilation (hypopnea) during quiet sleep, all sleep, or all states, depending on severity of the condition, leading to progressive hypercarbia and hypoxemia
2. Absent or negligible ventilatory and arousal sensitivity to hypercarbia during sleep
3. Absent or negligible hypercarbic ventilatory responsiveness during wakefulness, regardless of the adequacy of awake ventilation
4. Variable deficiency in hypoxic ventilatory responsiveness in all states, being absent in the most severe cases
5. Absent or negligible hypoxic arousal responsiveness during sleep
6. General unresponsiveness to respiratory stimulants, especially during sleep
7. Absence of autoresuscitation or gasping (during sleep) and inability to perceive asphyxia or to experience dyspnea during wakefulness

to the avoidance of cor pulmonale. Timely diagnosis, establishment of an effective home ventilation program, and effective long-term surveillance combining noninvasive blood gas monitoring with periodic sleep laboratory evaluations should be sufficient for preventing cor pulmonale.

The neurodevelopmental outcome is generally good for infants with congenital CHS. Although neurodevelopmental data are limited and variable in CHS patients, full-scale intelligence quotient scores are typically above 70. Extensive neuropsychological assessments

suggest that CHS may actually be a more generalized central nervous system process. In individual cases, severe pretreatment asphyxia or subsequent chronic or recurrent asphyxia may be a cause of sequelae.

There is no evidence that children with congenital CHS later outgrow the central respiratory control deficiency. There is a tendency for such children to later demonstrate some stabilization and amelioration of symptoms but not to the extent that ventilatory support becomes unnecessary. In acquired deficiencies, later normalization

Table 6-9. Etiology of Sudden Unexpected Death in Children, Adolescents, and Young Adults*

Cause	Comment
Respiratory	
Foreign body aspiration	Sudden-onset cough, gagging
Severe asthma[†]	Sudden onset, often at night
Spontaneous pneumothorax	Tension pneumothorax
Pulmonary embolism	Chest pain, hypoxia, normal chest radiograph
Cardiac	
Pericardial tamponade	Pericardial effusion, trauma
Myocarditis[†]	Kawasaki disease, viral infection, rheumatic fever
Cardiomyopathy	Hypertrophic, familial, dilated, metabolic
Right ventricular cardiomyopathy[†]	Also known as right ventricular dysplasia (arrhythmogenic right ventricle)
Mitral valve prolapse	Arrhythmia, embolism, indefinite as a cause of sudden death
Marfan syndrome	Aortic dissection, mitral valve prolapse
Blunt chest trauma	Commotio cordis, cardiac contusion, concussion
Coronary arteritis	Kawasaki disease, Takayasu disease, periarteritis nodosa
Anomalous position of coronary artery[†]	Anomalous origin of ostia (right artery from left sinus or vice versa or from pulmonary artery), anomalous deep intramyocardial course
Idiopathic coronary artery dissection	More common in females
Coronary ostia obstruction	Congenital webs
Atherosclerotic coronary artery disease	Idiopathic or familial hyperlipidemia, s/p heart transplant
Aortic valve stenosis	Congenital
Shone syndrome	Parachute mitral valve and subaortic stenosis
Conduction system pathway	Fibrosis, congenital heart block, tumor
Sinus node disturbance	Idiopathic, after atrial surgery, sick sinus syndrome
Preexcitation-induced arrhythmia	Wolff-Parkinson-White or other accessory pathways
Prolonged QT syndrome	Familial; risk of ventricular arrhythmia
Recent cardiac surgery	Sinus node, atrioventricular node (heart block) or ventricular arrhythmia, obstructed baffle
Neurological	
Ruptured berry aneurysm	Severe headache, meningismus, coma
Cerebrovascular accident	Paradoxical embolism through patent foramen ovale; carotid or left-sided cardiac source; spontaneous thrombosis (hypercoagulable state secondary to hereditary [protein C, protein S, antithrombin III deficiency] or acquired [antiphospholipid antibodies]), homocystinuria
Miscellaneous	
Drug abuse[†]	Cocaine, amphetamines, and inhalants (Freon, cleaning fluid [trichloroethylene], gasoline, glue, typewriter correction fluid, nitrites [amyl, butyryl]), emetine
Suicide[†]	Poisoning (carbon monoxide), firearms
Sickle cell anemia	Risk is also increased in persons with sickle cell trait with intense exercise and/or high altitude (hypoxia)
Anaphylaxis[†]	Drug or food induced
Anorexia nervosa, severe starvation	Electrolyte disturbance, emetine abuse, arrhythmia
Heat stroke	Risk increased with exercise and high humidity

*For cardiac pathology, the cause may be myocardial infarction or fatal ventricular arrhythmia (ventricular fibrillation or tachycardia; rarely asystole or bradyarrhythmia). In many cardiac-related deaths, there is often a history of chest pain (see Chapter 9), palpitations (see Chapter 7), or syncope (see Chapter 42). Exertion is often a preceding event for cardiac-based sudden death. Sudden cardiac death occurs within 1 hour of the onset of acute symptoms and is unexpected even in the presence of existing disease.

[†]Common cause of unexplained death.

Data from McCaffrey FM, Braden DS, Strong WB: Sudden cardiac death in young athletes. Am J Dis Child 1991;145:177-183; Corrado D, Thiene G, Cocco P, Frescura C: Non-atherosclerotic coronary artery disease and sudden death in the young. Br Heart J 1992;68:601-606; Corrado D, Thiene G, Nava A, et al: Sudden death in young competitive athletes: Clinicopathologic correlations in 22 cases. Am J Med 1990;89:588-596.

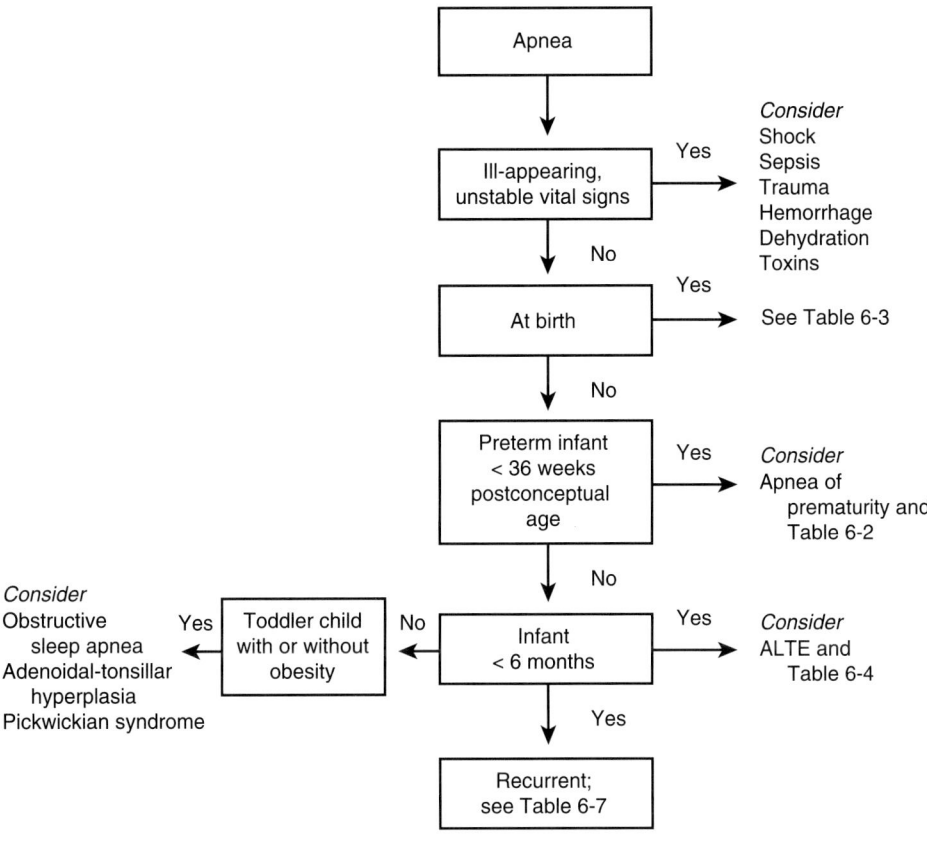

Figure 6-4. Algorithm for evaluation and differential diagnosis of apnea. ALTE, apparent life-threatening event.

Table 6-10. Red Flags for Apnea and Sudden Unexpected Death

Problem	Suspect
Repeated episodes in patient or family	Child abuse or neglect, inborn errors of metabolism, carbon monoxide or other poisoning (see Table 6-7)
Retinal hemorrhages	Child abuse
Hypotension, fever, poor capillary perfusion, persistent tachycardia	Sepsis, shock hemorrhage, dehydration, myocarditis
Onset at birth	Asphyxia, birth trauma (see Table 6-3)
Onset at ≥6 mo of age	Primary CNS pathology (seizure, increased intracranial pressure, drug overdose, trauma), primary cardiovascular disorder, obstructive apnea, systemic infection, shock (see Table 6-4)
Obesity	Obstructive sleep apnea
Daytime drowsiness, nighttime restlessness	Obstructive sleep apnea, narcolepsy
Syncope	See Chapter 42
Chest pain	See Chapter 9
Palpitations	See Chapter 7

CNS, central nervous system.

should not be anticipated if the ventilatory control deficit has been stable for 6 months.

PREVENTION

There is no way to prevent congenital hypoventilation syndromes. The ultrastructural or biochemical abnormality is unknown, as is the molecular genetics. Periconceptional folic acid supplementation does reduce the occurrence of myelomeningocele, however, and thus there is a potential for prevention of congenital CHS associated with Chiari II malformation.

SUDDEN UNEXPECTED DEATH

Sudden unexpected death is much less common in older children and adolescents than in adults. Respiratory, cardiac, vascular, or neurologic disorders may be identified at postmortem examination or by history. The causes of sudden unexpected death in children are listed in Table 6-9.

SUMMARY AND RED FLAGS

An algorithm for the differential diagnosis of apnea is noted in Figure 6-4. Red flags for apnea and SIDS are noted in Table 6-10.

REFERENCES

Apnea

Brazy JE, Kinney HC, Oakes WJ: Central nervous system structural lesions causing apnea at birth. J Pediatr 1987;111:163-175.

Erenberg A, Leff RD, Haack DG, et al: Caffeine citrate for the treatment of apnea of prematurity: A double-blind, placebo-controlled study. Pharmacotherapy 2000;20:644-652.

Huon C, Rey E, Mussat P, et al: Low-dose doxapram for treatment of apnoea following early weaning in very low birthweight infants: A randomized, double-blind study. Acta Paediatr 1998;87:1180-1184.

Larsen, PB, Brendstrup L, Skov L, et al: Aminophylline versus caffeine citrate for apnea and bradycardia prophylaxis in premature neonates. Acta Paediatr 1995;84:360-364.

Poets CF, Pauls U, Bohnhorst B: Effect of blood transfusion on apnoea, bradycardia and hypoxaemia in preterm infants. Eur J Pediatr 1997;156:311-316.

Ruggins NR: Pathophysiology of apnea in preterm infants. Arch Dis Child 1991;66:70-73.

Apparent Life-Threatening Event

Arens R, Gozal D, Williams JC, et al: Recurrent apparent life-threatening events during infancy: A manifestation of inborn errors of metabolism. J Pediatr 1993;123:415-418.

Cote A, Hum C, Broouillette R, et al: Frequency and timing of recurrent events in infants using home cardiorespiratory monitors. J Pediatr 1998;132:783-789.

Hunt CE: Familial small upper airways and sleep-disordered breathing: Relationship to idiopathic apparent-life-threatening events. Pediatr Res 2001;50:3-5.

McMurray JS, Holinger LD: Otolaryngic manifestations in children presenting with apparent life-threatening events. Otolaryngol Head Neck 1997;116:575-579.

Ramanathan R, Corwin M, Hunt C, et al: Cardiorespiratory events recorded on home monitors. JAMA 2001;285:2199-2207.

Samuels MP, Poets CF, Noyes JP, et al: Diagnosis and management after life threatening events in infants and young children who received cardiopulmonary resuscitation. BMJ 1993;306:489-492.

Steinschneider A, Santos V: Parental reports of apnea and bradycardia: Temporal characteristics and accuracy. Pediatrics 1991;88:1100-1105.

Sudden Infant Death Syndrome

American Academy of Pediatrics Task Force on Infant Positioning and SIDS: Changing concepts of sudden infant death syndrome: Implications for infant sleeping environment and sleep position. Pediatrics 2000;105:650-656.

Blair PS, Fleming PJ, Smith IJ, et al: Babies sleeping with parents: Case-control study of factors influencing the risk of the sudden infant death syndrome. CESDI SUDI research group. BMJ 1999;319:1457-1462.

Committee on Child Abuse and Neglect, 1993-1994: Distinguishing sudden infant death syndrome from child abuse fatalities. Pediatrics 1994;94:124-126.

Cote A, Russo P, Michaud J: Sudden unexpected deaths in infancy: What are the causes? J Pediatr 1999;135:437-443.

Emery JL: Child abuse, sudden infant death syndrome, and unexpected infant death. Am J Dis Child 1993;147:1097-1100.

Guntheroth WG, Spiers PS: Thermal stress in sudden infant death: Is there an ambiguity with the rebreathing hypothesis? Pediatrics 2001;107:693-698.

Harper RM, Kinney HC, Fleming PJ, Thach BT: Sleep influences on homeostatic functions: Implications for sudden infant death syndrome. Respir Physiol 2000;119:123-132.

Hauck FR, Hunt C: Sudden infant death syndrome in 2000. Curr Probl Pediatr 2000;30:239-261.

Holton JB, Allen JT, Green CA, et al: Inherited metabolic diseases in the sudden infant death syndrome. Arch Dis Child 1991;66:1315-1317.

Kemp JS, Livne M, White DK, et al: Softness and potential to cause rebreathing: Differences in bedding used by infants at high and low risk for sudden infant death syndrome. J Pediatr 1998;132:234-239.

Ponsonby AL, Dwyer T, Gibbons LE, et al: Factors potentiating the risk of sudden infant death syndrome associated with the prone position. N Engl J Med 1993;329:377-382.

Schwartz PJ, Stramba-Badiale M, Segantini A, et al: Prolongation of the QT interval and the sudden infant death syndrome. N Engl J Med 1998;338:1709-1714.

Southall DP, Plunkett MCB, Banks MW, et al: Covert video recordings of life-threatening child abuse: Lesson for child protection. Pediatrics 1997;100:735-760.

Thogmartin JR, Siebert CE, Pellan WA: Sleep position and bed-sharing in sudden infant deaths: An examination of autopsy findings. J Pediatr 2001;138:212-217.

Willinger M, Hoffman HJ, Wu KT, et al: Factors associated with the transition to nonprone sleep positions of infants in the United States: The National Infant Sleep Position Study. JAMA 1998;280:329-335.

Willinger M, Ko CW, Hoffman HJ, et al: Factors associated with caregivers' choice of infant sleep position, 1994-1998: The National Infant Sleep Position Study. JAMA 2000;283:2135-2142.

Obstructive Sleep Apnea

Carroll JL, McColley SA, Marcus CL, et al: Inability of clinical history to distinguish primary snoring from obstructive sleep apnea syndrome in children. Chest 1995;108:610-618.

Guilleminault C, Pelayo R, Clerk A, et al: Home nasal continuous positive airway pressure in infants with sleep-disordered breathing. J Pediatr 1995;127:905-912.

Guilleminault C, Pelayo R, Leger D, et al: Recognition of sleep-disordered breathing in children. Pediatrics 1996;98:871-882.

Marcus CL. Sleep-disordered breathing in children. Am J Respir Crit Care Med 2001;164:16-30.

Marcus CL, Ward SL, Mallory GB, et al: Use of nasal continuous positive airway pressure as treatment of childhood obstructive sleep apnea. J Pediatr 1995;127:88-94.

Nieminen P, Tolonen U, Lopponen H: Snoring and obstructive sleep apnea in children. Arch Otolaryngol Head Neck Surg 2000;126:481-486.

Rosen GM, Muckle RP, Mahowald MW, et al: Postoperative respiratory compromise in children with obstructive sleep apnea syndrome: Can it be anticipated? Pediatrics 1994;93:784-788.

Suen JS, Arnold JE, Brooks LJ: Adenotonsillectomy for treatment of obstructive sleep apnea in children. Arch Otolaryngol Head Neck Surg 1995;121:525-530.

Hypoventilation Syndromes

Frates RC, Splaingard ML, Smith EO, Harrison GM: Outcome of home mechanical ventilation in children. J Pediatr 1985;106:850-856.

Hunt CE, Silvestri JM: Pediatric hypoventilation syndromes. Curr Opin Pulm Med 1997;3:445-448.

Weese-Mayer DE, Hunt CE, Brouillette RT, et al: Diaphragm pacing in infants and children. J Pediatr 1992;120:1-8.

Weese-Mayer DE, Shannon DC, Keens TG, Silvestri JM: Idiopathic congenital central hypoventilation syndrome—Diagnosis and management. Am J Respir Crit Care Med 1999;160:368-373.

Weese-Mayer DE, Silvestri JM, Menzies LJ, et al: Congenital central hypoventilation syndrome: Diagnosis, management, and long-term outcome in thirty-two children. J Pediatr 1992;120:381-387.

SECTION TWO

CARDIAC DISORDERS

7 Palpitations and Arrhythmias

George F. Van Hare

Palpitation refers to a patient's conscious and often uncomfortable or frightening awareness of the heart's actions. Palpitations may be slow or fast, regular or irregular. The sensation is described as pounding, fluttering, flopping, skipping or missing of beats, stopping, or jumping. Some patients report feeling as if the heart has turned over. Palpitations are often caused by a change in the rate, rhythm, or contractibility of the heart. Although arrhythmias may cause palpitations, many arrhythmias are imperceptible by the patient. A broad overview of factors associated with palpitations is presented in Table 7-1. Common arrhythmias according to patients' ages are noted in Table 7-2, and arrhythmias associated with congenital heart disease are noted in Table 7-3.

Because palpitations raise the possibility of cardiac disease, their occurrence is frequently associated with anxiety. However, most patients with palpitations do not have a serious cardiac condition. Although evaluation and, on occasion, invasive testing are required for some patients, most patients can be safely reassured. One goal is to identify patients in whom the symptom of palpitations is a manifestation of a life-threatening or otherwise clinically significant arrhythmia and to evaluate them appropriately. Another is to identify the cause to aid in further therapy if appropriate.

DIAGNOSTIC METHODS

HISTORY

The only definitive way to diagnose the cause of the palpitations is to record an electrocardiogram during the symptom. Nonetheless, information from the patient's history may be helpful in diagnosing the problem and in assessing the urgency of reaching a diagnosis. The patient's description of the sensation is important. Sustained tachycardia is usually described as a "racing" heartbeat, whereas premature beats are usually described as skipping of a beat. For the latter symptom, the sensation of the heart stopping is probably caused by the pause that follows a premature beat. Abrupt onset of palpitations, with equally abrupt spontaneous termination, especially if paroxysmal, suggests supraventricular tachycardia and not sinus tachycardia. The duration and rate of the symptoms should be noted; for sustained fast rhythms, some assessment of the likely rate may be obtained by asking the patient or parent to imitate the rhythm by tapping it out. Parents or patients may be taught to measure the pulse during such episodes. Patients can usually tell whether the fast rhythm is regular or irregular. Some fast rhythms, such as atrial fibrillation and often atrial flutter (with block), are irregular, whereas supraventricular tachycardia and ventricular tachycardia are usually regular.

Symptoms associated with palpitations give clues to the severity of the problem. The most ominous sign is *syncope,* defined as a sudden loss of consciousness with inability to maintain posture (see Chapter 42). Syncope occurs as a result of central nervous system hemodynamic compromise caused by the arrhythmia (rapid supraventricular tachycardia, ventricular tachycardia, atrioventricular [AV] block). Patients with syncope associated with possible arrhythmia require full cardiac evaluation because of the possibility that future episodes may result in sudden death, depending on the underlying cardiac problem. Patients may complain of transient dizziness or lightheadedness, which also suggests hemodynamic compromise of a lesser degree. Chest pain is occasionally reported, but it is often caused by the strong rapid heartbeat rather than any coronary artery abnormality. Sensation of the palpitation in the neck may signify AV nodal reentrant tachycardia or ventricular tachycardia and is caused by contraction of the atria against closed AV valves, resulting in jugular venous regurgitation (cannon a waves).

Factors that elicit the symptom are important to note; certain forms of ventricular tachycardia are elicited only by exercise. These causes of arrhythmia may depend on sympathetic activity, and "stress" is frequently reported as an eliciting factor. Such patients may respond best to β-adrenergic receptor blocking agents.

Factors that terminate the episodes help in the diagnosis, as does the manner of termination. Sustained fast heart rhythms that terminate suddenly are more likely to have reentrant causes, whereas those that slow gradually are more likely to have an automatic focus. Termination of the episode by the Valsalva maneuver, gagging, coughing, straining, or facial immersion in cold water suggests reentrant supraventricular tachycardia, although atrial flutter may also terminate with these maneuvers.

The medical history and review of systems are important, primarily for identifying structural cardiac disease (see Table 7-3), which may affect the prognosis and therefore the urgency of evaluation. However, the history may provide other clues. The most important example is hyperthyroidism, which may manifest as sinus tachycardia or as atrial fibrillation (see Table 7-1). Deafness is present in some cases of *prolonged QT syndrome.* In *Kearns-Sayre syndrome,* a mitochondrial disorder, patients have progressive ophthalmoplegia and pigmentary retinal degeneration; many develop right bundle branch block or complete AV block. Distal muscle weakness and myotonia are present in the autosomal dominant disorder *myotonic dystrophy,* which is also associated with AV block.

PHYSICAL EXAMINATION

Few specific physical findings aid in the diagnosis. However, any signs of structural cardiac disease (see Chapter 11) are important because patients with serious structural cardiac disease are likely to tolerate arrhythmias poorly and to have more complex and dangerous cardiac rhythms than are those without heart disease. Several specific cardiac abnormalities are strongly associated with arrhythmias. Patients with *dilated cardiomyopathy* may have ventricular arrhythmias, including ventricular fibrillation, and often have a gallop rhythm on cardiac auscultation or signs of heart failure (see Chapter 8). Those with *hypertrophic cardiomyopathy* may have nonspecific ejection murmurs and may also have an increased apical impulse; these patients are at risk for ventricular arrhythmias. Arrhythmias are often noted in patients with congenital heart disease, both before and after corrective or palliative surgery (see Table 7-3).

Table 7-1. Possible Etiologic Factors in Palpitations*

Sinus Tachycardia

Arrhythmias

Paroxysmal atrial or ventricular tachycardia
Paroxysmal atrial flutter or fibrillation
Sinus bradycardia
Junctional rhythm
Complete heart block
Premature atrial or ventricular beats
Prolonged QT interval
Wolff-Parkinson-White syndrome

Drugs

Tobacco
Tea
Coffee
Colas
Cocaine
Amphetamines
Atropine
Tricyclic antidepressant agents
Amyl nitrate
Epinephrine
Ephedrine, *Ephedra* (mahuang)
Aminophylline
Albuterol
Terbutaline
Carbon monoxide
Digitalis

Proarrhythmia Agents†

Erythromycin lactobionate
Terfenadine (ketoconazole)
Astemizole
Quinidine (and other class Ia agents)
Cisapride
Flecainide
Encainide

Endocrine

Hyperthyroidism
Pheochromocytoma
Insulin excess (hypoglycemia)

Others

Anemia
Panic-anxiety syndrome (panic attacks)
Epilepsy
Arteriovenous malformation
Fever
Porphyria
Guillain-Barré syndrome (autonomic neuropathy)
Myocarditis
Rheumatic fever
Endocarditis
Lyme disease
Mitral valve prolapse
Cardiomyopathies, including mitochondrial disorders
Arrhythmogenic right ventricular dysplasia
Kawasaki disease

*Many of these etiologic factors are interrelated; for example, anemia produces sinus tachycardia, as do various drugs (e.g., caffeine, cocaine).

†Proarrhythmia agents induce arrhythmias by prolonging the QT interval, resulting in ventricular tachycardia, often of the torsades de pointes type.

During an episode, the rate, rhythm, blood pressure, and arterial and venous (jugular cannon a wave) pulsations should be determined.

ELECTROCARDIOGRAPHIC MONITORING

Resting

The resting 15-lead electrocardiogram (ECG), which is obtained when the patient is asymptomatic, may provide a diagnosis, but a normal result does not rule out a transient arrhythmia. Complete electrocardiography should always be performed in any patient with such symptoms.

A standard cardiac cycle as noted on the ECG is shown in Figure 7-1; the corresponding conduction system is noted in Figure 7-2. The *P wave* represents atrial depolarization, and the *PR interval* represents the time for the signal to travel from the sinus node to the ventricles, with most time spent in the AV node. The PR interval increases with age. Conduction time is shortened when an accessory pathway bypasses the AV node, as is seen in Wolff-Parkinson-White syndrome. A prolonged PR interval indicates prolonged conduction anywhere between the sinus node and the myocardium but usually indicates AV node block.

The *QRS complex* represents ventricular depolarization, and the *QT interval* represents ventricular repolarization. Examples of diagnoses that may be evident on the ECG include the Wolff-Parkinson-White syndrome (Fig. 7-3), the long QT syndrome, and conduction abnormalities, such as second-degree and third-degree AV block. In addition, patients who are symptomatic as a result of premature beats—atrial (Fig. 7-4) or ventricular (Fig. 7-5)—may have these on the resting ECG. Nonspecific changes, such as T-wave abnormalities, suggest the presence of a myocardial problem. Left ventricular hypertrophy is a more specific finding that may indicate the presence of hypertrophic cardiomyopathy.

If the ECG captures the arrhythmia, it may reveal supraventricular tachycardia (Fig. 7-6), atrial flutter (Fig. 7-7), ventricular tachycardia (Figs. 7-8 and 7-9), polymorphous ventricular tachycardia, torsades de pointes (Fig. 7-10), or, in rare cases, ventricular fibrillation (Fig. 7-11).

Ambulatory Electrocardiographic Monitoring

Twenty-four-hour ambulatory monitoring (*Holter monitoring*) is used to attempt to capture the abnormality on the ECG when symptoms occur. With Holter monitoring, the ECG is continuously recorded digitally or on magnetic tape for 24 hours, capturing as many as three separate leads simultaneously, for later playback and analysis. The patient keeps a diary of events and symptoms, and the Holter recording is examined at these times to determine the heart rhythm during the symptom. If symptoms are a daily occurrence, Holter monitoring is probably the most efficient method of diagnosis. It is particularly valuable in patients with very frequent symptoms (many times per day) that are not clearly the result of an arrhythmia. In such patients, the recording of many episodes that turn out to be normal electrocardiographically provides strong and reassuring evidence against a dangerous cardiac arrhythmia. In addition, information about cardiac conduction, average heart rates, response of sinus rates to normal daily exertion, and the prominence of atrial ectopy, ventricular ectopy (premature beats), or both is also available and may be useful if an episode of palpitations is not captured.

ECHOCARDIOGRAPHY

Echocardiography is usually helpful in diagnosing structural cardiac disease. Because many of the structural abnormalities (congenital heart disease, hypertrophic cardiomyopathy, rhabdomyoma, mitral valve prolapse, aberrant coronary artery) associated with arrhythmias

Table 7-2. Common Arrhythmias by Patient Age

Age	Arrhythmia	Comment
Fetus	Sinus bradycardia (<100 bpm)	Fetal hypoxic stress
	Complete heart block (<60 bpm)	Isolated, or associated with maternal
		SLE or fetal congenital heart disease; may cause hydrops fetalis
	Sinus tachycardia (>180 bpm)	Maternal fever, drugs, fetal stress, anemia
	Supraventricular tachycardia (>200 bpm)	Causes hydrops if sustained
	Atrial flutter (280-450 bpm; conduction delay, 2:1)	Causes hydrops if sustained
	Ventricular tachycardia (>120 bpm)	Rare; causes hydrops if sustained
Neonate	Continuation of fetal arrhythmias	
	Sinus bradycardia	Associated with apnea of prematurity as primary event
Infant	Sinus tachycardia (<250 bpm)	Fever, anxiety, shock, dehydration, heart failure, pain
	Supraventricular tachycardia	Primary or sympathomimetic drug administration, fever, myocarditis, trauma
Older child and adolescent	Premature atrial beats, premature ventricular beats, paroxysmal atrial tachycardia	Thyrotoxicosis, idiopathic, atrial enlargement, mitral stenosis, sympathomimetic drugs
	Sinus bradycardia	Trained athlete, vasodepressor syncope
	Sinus tachycardia	As for infant (see earlier comment), plus drug abuse (cocaine, amphetamine)
	Various post–cardiac surgery arrhythmias	See Table 7-3

bpm, beats per minute; SLE, systemic lupus erythematosus.

are difficult to rule out on the basis of the physical examination and electrocardiographic results, certain patients require echocardiography. Patients whose symptoms are very worrisome (syncope, chest pain, dyspnea, prolonged duration) and who may have life-threatening episodes of tachycardia should undergo echocardiography. In most cases, the echocardiogram is normal.

TRANSTELEPHONIC INCIDENT MONITORING

When symptoms are not a daily occurrence, Holter monitoring is inefficient, because several consecutive Holter recordings are often needed to capture a single episode. Such an approach frequently fails altogether. Transtelephonic incident recorders are small, battery-powered devices that the patient carries for 1 month or more. When the symptom occurs, the patient makes a recording by placing the device on the chest or connecting it to wrist electrodes. A single ECG lead is recorded into the device's memory for 60 to 90 seconds. The patient then plays the recording back over the telephone to the clinician's office or monitoring center. The unit generates a series of signals that are decoded by the monitoring center into the ECG. For very transient symptoms, there are devices that are connected to the patient like a Holter monitor and continuously record the heart rhythm in a memory loop. When the patient experiences a symptom, he or she presses a button, which causes the device to store the ECG for the 30 to 45 seconds before as well as for a short period after the button was pushed.

For patients with very severe but very infrequent symptoms that have not been captured on a standard memory loop recorder, implantable loop recorders (Reveal, Medtronic) are now available. These devices are implanted in a prepectoral location, like a pacemaker, and are activated by the patient or family member by using a hand-held device. Stored ECGs are available for electronic downloading later.

EXERCISE TESTING

In some patients, an exercise test elicits an episode of tachycardia or irregular heart rhythm and is a reasonable approach when symptoms are primarily exercise related. The patient's ECG and blood pressure are monitored while the patient runs on a treadmill or rides a stationary bicycle. During the test, the workload is increased in discrete steps. The ECG is monitored both during exercise and in the recovery phase. Formal exercise testing, however, is limited in its ability to reproduce the exercise stress actually experienced by athletes, particularly the competitive stress, and so lack of an arrhythmia at exercise testing does not rule out exercise-related arrhythmias.

ELECTROPHYSIOLOGIC STUDY

For carefully selected patients, the definitive method of diagnosing the mechanism of an arrhythmia is the invasive electrophysiologic study, which is done through cardiac catheterization. Two to four electrode catheters are inserted into the cardiac chambers via the veins or arteries and are positioned in various sites for pacing and for recording of intracardiac conduction signals. AV conduction may be carefully studied, and sustained tachycardias may be induced and diagnosed by programmed stimulation of the heart. Such testing is also useful in determining appropriate drug treatment of the arrhythmia, and catheter ablation is also available as a curative option for most sustained tachyarrhythmias.

MECHANISMS OF TACHYCARDIAS

REENTRANT VERSUS AUTOMATIC TACHYCARDIAS

Two common mechanisms for the tachyarrhythmias are seen in clinical practice: those caused by *reentry* and those caused by *increased automaticity*. Reentry is the circular movement of impulses within the myocardium or conduction system. Increased automaticity is present when there is automatic repetitive depolarization of localized cardiac cells at a faster rate than normal.

For a tachycardia to be termed reentrant, three conditions must be met. First, an anatomically distinct reentrant circuit must be present, allowing for the circular movement of excitation conduction. Second, an area of this potential reentrant circuit must be subject to delay in conduction, or the circuit must be large enough to allow for recovery by the time the next reentrant wave arrives. Third, unidirectional conduction block must occur in one segment, but with subsequent reversed conduction in that segment (Fig. 7-12).

Table 7-3. Arrhythmias Associated with Congenital Heart Disease

Anomaly	Arrhythmia		
	Preoperative	*Postoperative*	*Delayed–Late Onset*
Ostium secundum ASD	Mild prolonged PR interval Occasional atrial tachyarrhythmias	Atrial tachycardia Junctional tachycardia Atrial fibrillation Atrial flutter Sinus bradycardia	Atrial tachycardia Sinus bradycardia
Ostium primum ASD	Prolonged PR interval	As in ostium secundum ASD plus AV block	As in ostium secundum ASD
Complete AV canal	Prolonged PR interval	Atrial tachycardia Junctional tachycardia Transient complete AV block	Complete AV block
Total anomalous venous return	As in ASD	As in ASD	As in ASD
Transposition of great arteries: Mustard or Senning repair	—	Sinus bradycardia Atrial flutter Accelerated junctional tachycardia AV block	Sinus bradycardia Atrial tachycardia
Arterial switch repair	—	Premature atrial contractions	—
Tricuspid atresia	Atrial fibrillation	Junctional tachycardia	Supraventricular tachycardia
Fontan repair	Preexcitation	Atrial fibrillation Atrial flutter Complete AV block Sinus bradycardia	—
VSD	—	Right bundle branch block Bifascicular block Transient complete AV block	Complete AV block Right bundle branch block
Tetralogy of Fallot	Ventricular tachycardia (rare) Supraventricular tachycardia (rare)	As in VSD, plus ventricular premature contractions	As in VSD, plus sustained ventricular tachycardia
Ebstein anomaly	Wolff-Parkinson-White preexcitation Atrial flutter or fibrillation Supraventricular tachycardia	Transient AV block Atrial flutter or fibrillation Premature ventricular contractions	Complete AV block
Corrected transposition (L-transposition) of the great arteries	Complete AV block	As in VSD if present AV block	As in VSD if present AV block

ASD, atrial septal defect; AV, atrioventricular; VSD, ventricular septal defect.

An example of a reentrant supraventricular tachyarrhythmia is the reciprocating AV reentrant tachycardia seen in patients with the Wolff-Parkinson-White syndrome (Fig. 7-13; see Fig. 7-3). A premature atrial contraction may be blocked in the accessory pathway but is conducted down the AV node, where the impulse is slowed, and then travels to the ventricle via the rapid His-Purkinje system. Impulses arriving in the ventricle are then conducted in a retrograde direction via the accessory pathway back to the atrium. The conduction delay in the AV node allows the accessory pathway and atrium sufficient time to recover and thus allows establishment of sustained tachycardia.

The reentrant tachycardias include sinoatrial and intraatrial reentry, AV node reentry, AV reciprocating tachycardia involving an accessory pathway, atrial flutter, the permanent form of junctional reciprocating tachycardia, and the reentrant form of ventricular tachycardia. Tachycardias caused by increased automaticity include sinus tachycardia, atrial ectopic tachycardia, junctional ectopic tachycardia, and (automatic focus) ventricular tachycardia. Atrial fibrillation has been shown to exhibit characteristics both of abnormal automaticity and of complex reentrant patterns in the atrium.

A major characteristic of the reentrant tachycardias that allows differentiation from the automatic tachycardias is their tendency to start and stop suddenly. Premature atrial and ventricular contractions may initiate or terminate these rhythms, or they start during normal episodes of sinus bradycardia with junctional escape rhythm. Direct current cardioversion is usually successful in terminating reentrant tachycardias but not automatic focus tachycardias.

SINUS TACHYCARDIA

Sinus tachycardia may masquerade as paroxysmal supraventricular tachycardia in children and is usually secondary to some other problem (see Table 7-2). The gradual slowing of a narrow QRS tachycardia after an intravenous fluid bolus in a patient thought to have intravascular depletion provides strong evidence for sinus tachycardia and against other forms of paroxysmal supraventricular tachycardia. Other causes of sinus tachycardia include high fever, pain, hypoxia, hyperthyroidism, seizures, chronotropic agents (isoproterenol or dobutamine), and sedation in paralyzed patients undergoing ventilation.

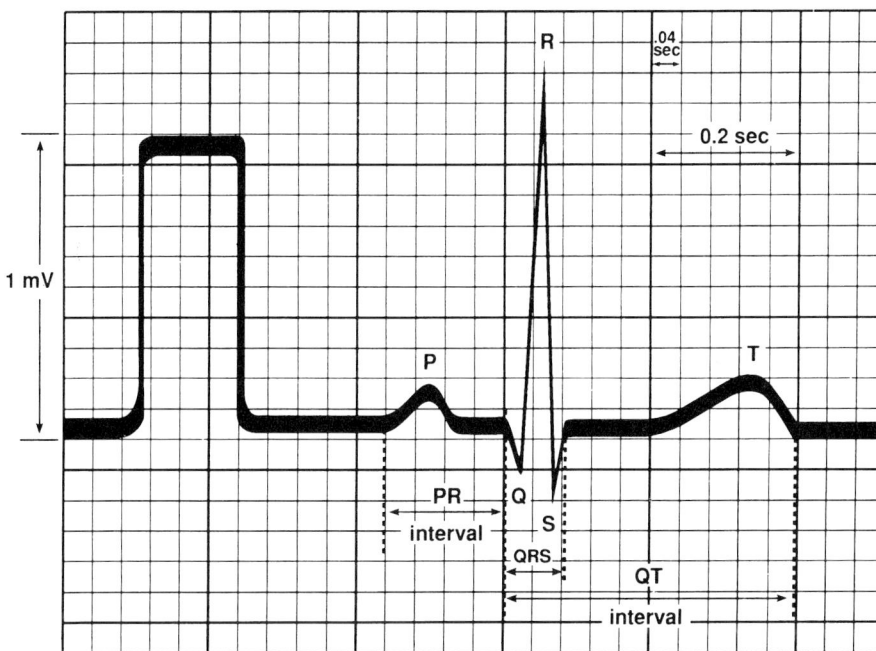

Figure 7-1. Waves and intervals in a P-QRS-T complex. Standard calibration is 1 mV = 10 mm; paper speed is 25 mm/second. (From Victorica BE: Electrocardiogram interpretation and diagnostic value. In Gessner IH, Victorica BE [eds]: Pediatric Cardiology: A Problem Oriented Approach. Philadelphia, WB Saunders, 1993.)

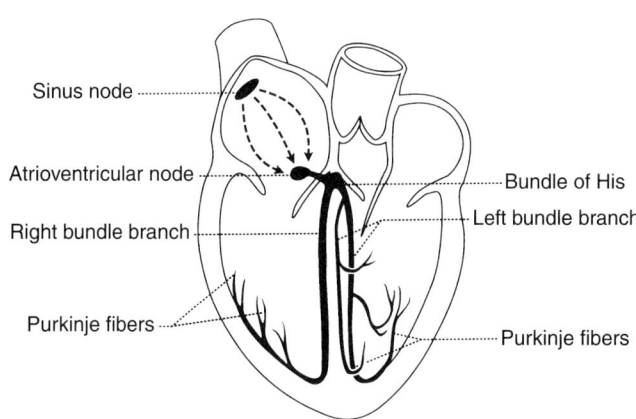

Figure 7-2. Cardiac conduction system. (From Epstein ML: Disturbances of cardiac rhythm. In Gessner IH, Victorica BE [eds]: Pediatric Cardiology: A Problem Oriented Approach. Philadelphia: WB Saunders, 1993.)

The criteria for sinus tachycardia are

- normal P-wave axis
- normal (not prolonged) PR interval
- gradual onset and termination
- heart rates of less than 250 beats per minute (bpm)

Rates exceeding 250 bpm rule out sinus tachycardia, whereas narrow complex tachycardias of less than 250 bpm often represent sinus tachycardias.

Sinus tachycardia must be ruled out, if possible, before antiarrhythmic therapy is instituted. The diagnosis may be quite difficult in children because the P wave may be hidden on the preceding T wave. Several leads should be carefully analyzed for deformation of the T wave by a P wave. Vagal maneuvers and other methods for converting supraventricular tachycardia do not terminate sinus tachycardia. Vagal maneuvers may briefly slow the rhythm, but because the underlying cause of sinus tachycardia is unaffected by such maneuvers, the rhythm resumes immediately. Therapy should be directed to the likely underlying causes of the sinus tachycardia. The response to such measures may well be diagnostic.

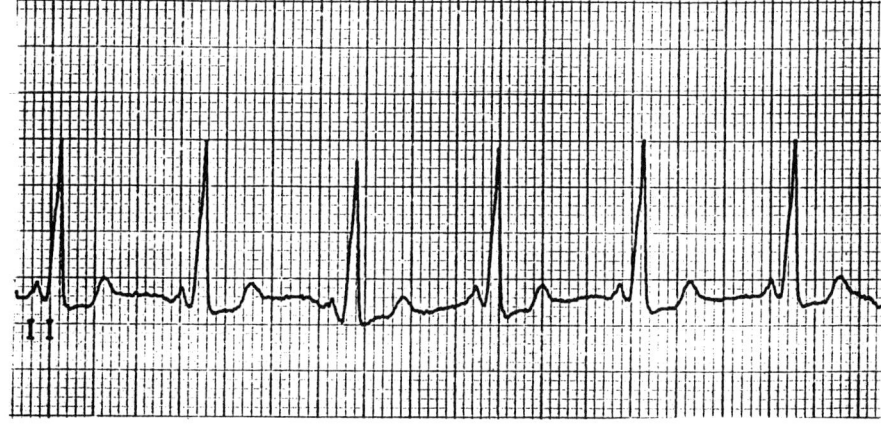

Figure 7-3. Rhythm strip, lead II, in a patient with Wolff-Parkinson-White syndrome. Note the lack of an isoelectric interval between the end of the P wave and the start of the QRS complex, as well as the slurred QRS upstroke.

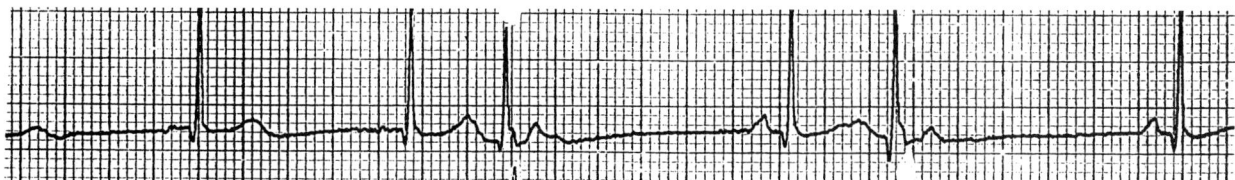

Figure 7-4. Rhythm strip, lead AVF, in a patient with premature atrial contractions. The clear deformation of the T wave before the premature beat indicates the presence of a premature P wave.

MECHANISMS OF BRADYCARDIA

SINUS BRADYCARDIA

Sinus bradycardia is recognized as a regular, slow atrial rate with normal P waves and 1:1 conduction. Causes include hypoxia, acidosis, increased intracranial pressure, abdominal distention, and hypoglycemia. Agents such as digoxin, organophosphate pesticides, and β-blocking agents (propranolol) may cause sinus bradycardia. Mild heart rate slowing may also be caused by increased vagal tone or cardiac conditioning in a trained athlete.

ATRIOVENTRICULAR BLOCK

AV block is classified as follows:

- *First degree:* prolonged PR interval; no missed ventricular beats. This may be idiopathic or associated with myocarditis, congenital heart disease, hypoxia, hyperkalemia, or drug toxicity (e.g., from digoxin).
- *Second degree:* some impulses are not conducted to the ventricles. This is classified as either *Mobitz type I (Wenckebach)* or *Mobitz type II.* Wenckebach conduction is characterized by progressive PR interval prolongation followed by a blocked beat, followed by recovery of conduction. Mobitz type II block lacks this characteristic PR prolongation with shortening after the blocked beat. Mobitz type I block generally carries a better prognosis than does Mobitz type II block and responds readily to medication. Mobitz type II block may progress to complete heart block.
- *Third degree (complete):* there is no conduction between the atria and the ventricles. Complete AV block may be congenital, may be surgically induced, or may occur suddenly as a result of myocarditis. It is recognized as AV dissociation and regular RR intervals, regular PP intervals, an atrial rate greater than the ventricular rate, and the absence of capture beats. Congenital AV block, in the absence of structural heart disease, is caused by maternal systemic lupus erythematosus (diagnosed or asymptomatic; associated with anti-Ro autoantibody) in about 80% of cases. In other cases, congenital heart block may be seen with congenital heart anomalies. Causes of acquired heart block include Lyme disease, Kearns-Sayre syndrome (weakness, progressive external ophthalmoplegia, pigmentary retinal degeneration), and myotonic dystrophy (myotonia, weakness).

Other causes of bradycardia are (1) sinus exit block, in which sinus P waves intermittently disappear as a result of block of impulses leaving the region of the sinus node, and (2) frequent premature atrial contractions, which occur too early to be conducted to the ventricles and therefore slow the resulting ventricular rate.

MECHANISMS OF PREMATURE BEATS

PREMATURE SUPRAVENTRICULAR CONTRACTIONS

Supraventricular premature contractions are narrow and early QRS beats. They occasionally also have wide QRS complexes as a result of an associated bundle branch aberration. Those that originate in the atrium *(premature atrial contractions)* may be recognizable by the finding of a premature P wave superimposed on the previous T wave, deforming it (see Fig. 7-4). This sign may be subtle, necessitating the examination of multiple leads.

PREMATURE VENTRICULAR COMPLEXES

Premature ventricular complexes (PVCs) are recognizable as wide, often bizarre early beats, generally without preceding P waves. The differentiation between ventricular contractions and aberrantly conducted supraventricular contractions is sometimes difficult or impossible from the surface ECG. Although premature ventricular beats are traditionally differentiated from supraventricular beats by the presence of a full compensatory pause (see Fig. 7-5), this sign is unreliable in children. The identification of fusion beats, in which a sinus beat occurs simultaneously with a premature beat, thus creating an intermediate morphologic pattern, is helpful and establishes the premature beat as ventricular in origin.

DIAGNOSTIC EVALUATION OF PALPITATIONS

The starting point in the diagnostic evaluation of palpitations is a thorough history and careful physical examination and the recording of a baseline ECG (i.e., while the patient is not having the symptom).

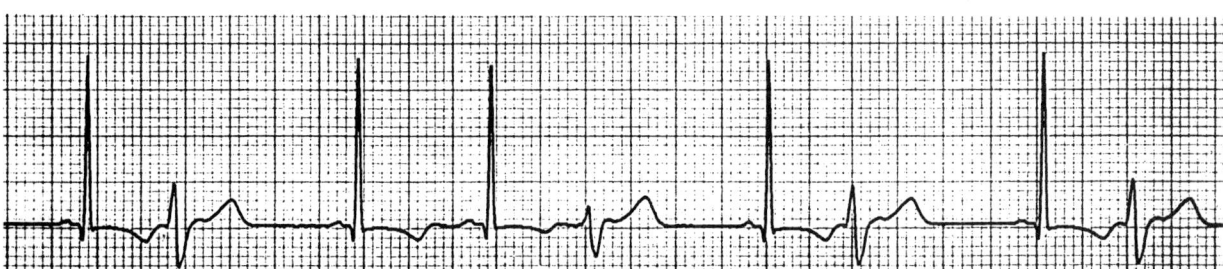

Figure 7-5. Rhythm strip, lead V₅, in a patient with frequent premature ventricular contractions. Note the lack of clear deformation of the T wave preceding the premature beat, the prolonged QRS duration of the premature beat, and the full compensatory pause.

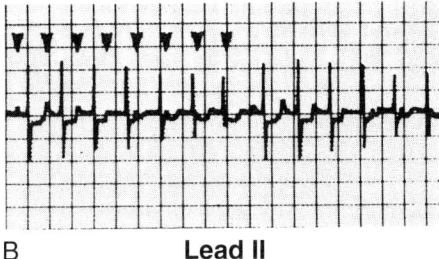

A   **Lead II**

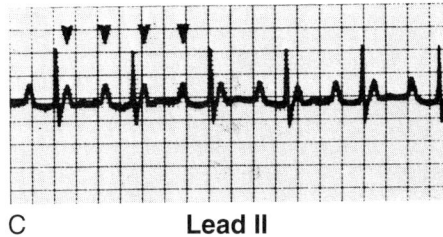

B   **Lead II**

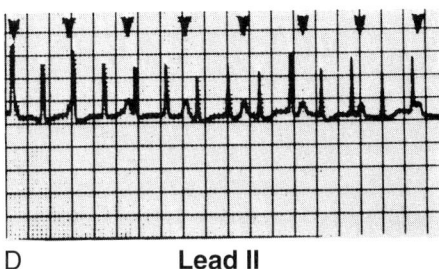

C   **Lead II**

Figure 7-6. P-QRS relationship in supraventricular tachycardia. P waves are marked by *arrowheads*. **A**, There is a 1:1 relationship between P waves and QRS complexes. **B**, Supraventricular tachycardia with type II second-degree atrioventricular (AV) block. **C**, Supraventricular tachycardia with 2:1 AV block. **D**, Rare supraventricular tachycardia with AV dissociation. (From Garson A: Arrhythmias in pediatric patients. Med Clin North Am 1984;68:1171-1208.)

The approach is summarized in the flow diagram in Figure 7-14. In obtaining the patient's history, the examiner is attempting to determine (1) whether the rhythm abnormality might be caused by a life-threatening problem; (2) whether it is likely that the patient is experiencing episodes of tachycardia, premature beats, or bradycardia; (3) whether the symptoms are exercise related; and (4) whether there is structural cardiac disease.

During the physical examination, the examiner is looking for evidence of structural heart disease. On the ECG, the examiner is looking for obvious evidence of a problem, such as a prolonged QT interval or the Wolff-Parkinson-White syndrome. The QT interval varies with the heart rate. A corrected QT (QTc) interval is determined

by dividing the QT interval by the square root of the RR interval. A normal QTc interval is less than 0.44 second.

A life-threatening problem may be suspected if the episodes of palpitations are associated with near-syncope, syncope, severe chest pain, or aborted sudden death or if there is a family history of the long QT syndrome or unexplained sudden death. Patients with a long QT interval are treated with β-adrenergic receptor blocking agents and avoidance of proarrhythmia drugs that prolong the QT interval (see Table 7-1). Patients with a potentially life-threatening problem but a normal QT interval are referred for invasive electrophysiologic evaluation to avoid delay in capturing an episode and to initiate appropriate treatment of a dangerous arrhythmia.

Patients who do not have obvious evidence of a life-threatening arrhythmia are then differentiated by whether they are likely to be experiencing episodes of tachycardia versus premature beats or bradycardia. Those with tachycardia proceed to a noninvasive evaluation (discussed later), with the goal of capturing an episode electrocardiographically for the purpose of diagnosis. If there is evidence of structural cardiac disease, an echocardiogram is obtained. Likewise, if there is electrocardiographic evidence of Wolff-Parkinson-White syndrome, an echocardiogram is obtained, primarily to rule out the possibility of an associated Ebstein anomaly of the tricuspid valve or, in rare cases, hypertrophic cardiomyopathy. In patients who are likely to have premature beats or bradycardia with no evidence of structural cardiac disease or an abnormal ECG, noninvasive evaluation is considered optional and is performed according to the severity of the symptoms. If there is structural cardiac disease or an abnormal ECG (e.g., complete AV block), an echocardiogram is obtained, followed by a noninvasive evaluation. An invasive electrophysiologic study may be recommended, depending on the results of the noninvasive evaluation and the severity of the symptoms.

Noninvasive evaluation involves the use of any of the modalities for diagnosis that do not involve intracardiac electrophysiologic study. The goal is to capture an episode of the patient's symptom electrocardiographically. The approach is summarized in the flow diagram shown in Figure 7-15. Patients whose symptoms are brought on by exercise may be referred for exercise testing in hopes that the test will reproduce the abnormal rhythm. If the results of the exercise test are negative or if the symptoms are unrelated to exercise, consideration of the frequency of symptoms leads to use of either a Holter monitor, for those with daily symptoms, or transtelephonic incident recording, for those with less frequent symptoms. If incident recording is used, it is important to choose the correct mode for recording. In general, if the episodes last less than 30 seconds, it is difficult for the patient or parent to produce the monitor, connect it, and make a recording before the symptom resolves. In such patients, the use of a continuous memory loop recorder is recommended.

When a symptomatic episode is recorded, it is important to determine, by discussion with the patient, whether the symptom was in fact typical, because benign arrhythmias and sinus tachycardia may coexist with more serious conditions. Recording of multiple episodes may increase the reliability of the diagnosis, particularly in patients who do not have a cardiac arrhythmia when they are symptomatic.

ELECTROCARDIOGRAPHIC DIAGNOSIS

The electrocardiographic diagnosis of the arrhythmia's mechanism is vital for determining the best treatment, particularly when antiarrhythmic medications are contemplated. Failure to document the tachycardia can often lead to inappropriate treatment of patients experiencing sinus tachycardia or benign premature contractions.

An initial determination is made as to whether the QRS duration and morphologic pattern during tachycardia are normal or increased. The "narrow" QRS tachycardias are usually caused by supraventricular tachycardia (Table 7-4). The "wide" QRS tachycardias may be caused by either ventricular tachycardia or supraventricular tachycardia

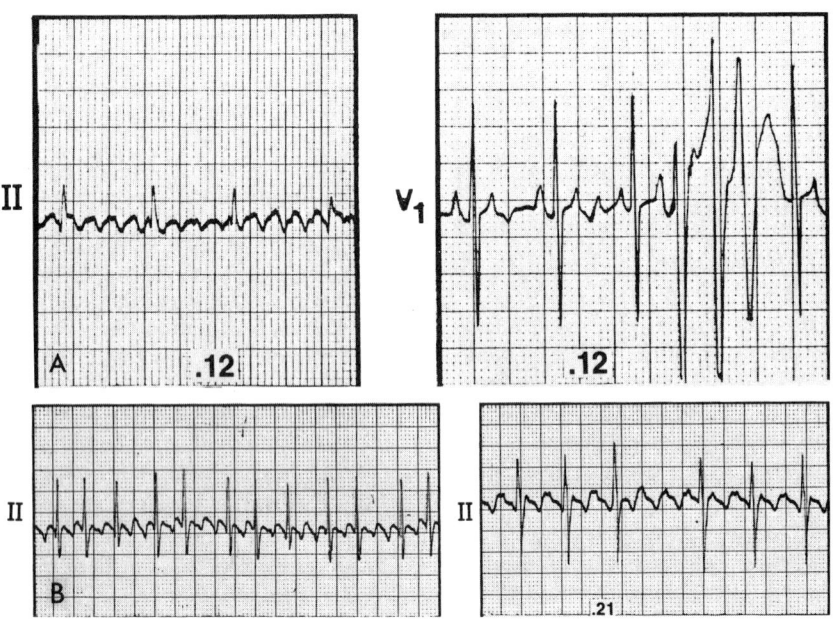

Figure 7-7. A, Atrial flutter in infants. In the left tracing, classic flutter waves (sawtooth waves) are seen at an atrial rate of 500 per minute with 4:1 and 5:1 atrioventricular (AV) conduction. In the right tracing, blocked premature atrial contractions follow the first two QRS complexes. Then there are two beats of atrial flutter. The rapid wide QRS rhythm on the right results from 1:1 AV conduction of atrial flutter at a ventricular rate of 460 per minute. B, The tracing on the left is taken from a 3-month-old. The atrial rate is 375 per minute with 2:1 and 3:1 conduction. The tracing on the right is taken from a 16-year-old. The atrial rate is 285 per minute with varying 4:1 and 2:1 AV conduction. (From Garson A: Arrhythmias in pediatric patients. Med Clin North Am 1984;68:1171-1208.)

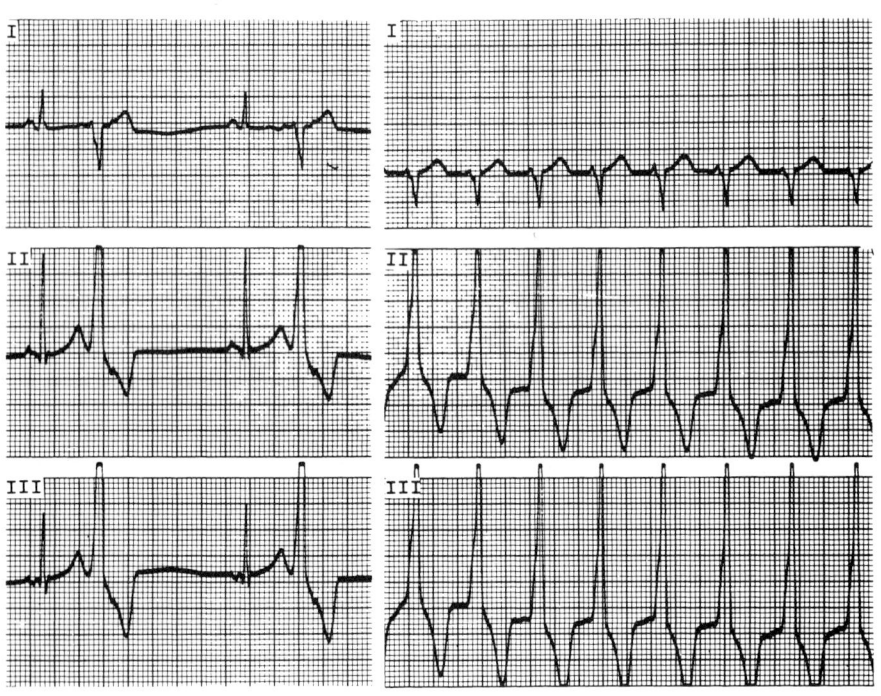

Figure 7-8. Paroxysmal ventricular tachycardia in a 14-year-old boy with no other evidence of organic heart disease. The ectopic ventricular beats are probably left ventricular in origin. Retrograde atrial capture is present. (From Chou T-C: Sinus rhythms. In Chou T-C [ed]: Electrocardiography in Clinical Practice, 3rd ed. Philadelphia, WB Saunders, 1991, p 395.)

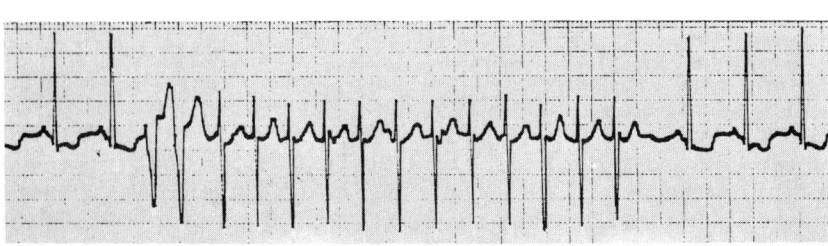

Figure 7-9. Tracing from a newborn with ventricular tachycardia and a "narrow" QRS complex. After two sinus beats, there are two obviously wide premature ventricular contractions. This initiates ventricular tachycardia. There is atrioventricular dissociation. The QRS complexes are narrow but have a completely different morphologic pattern from that of the sinus QRS. (From Garson A: Arrhythmias in pediatric patients. Med Clin North Am 1984;68:1171-1208.)

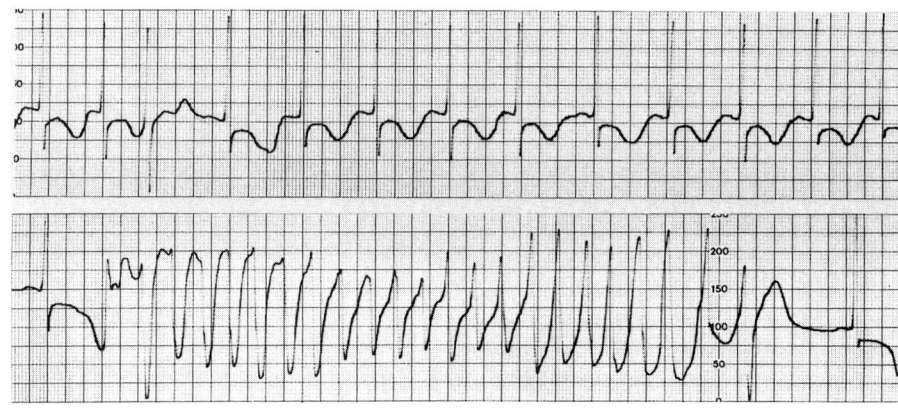

Figure 7-10. Torsades de pointes resulting from quinidine administration. The tracings show a basic sinus rhythm. There is a marked prolongation of the QT interval, measuring 0.56 second. In the bottom strip, there is an ectopic ventricular beat falling on the T wave of the preceding sinus beat. The ectopic beat initiates an episode of ventricular tachyarrhythmia. The tachycardia has a rate of about 200 beats per minute. The RR interval is irregular. The QRS complexes have a negative polarity in the first part of the episode and an upright polarity in the second part. (From Chou T-C: Sinus rhythms. In Chou T-C [ed]: Electrocardiography in Clinical Practice, 3rd ed. Philadelphia, WB Saunders, 1991, p 399.)

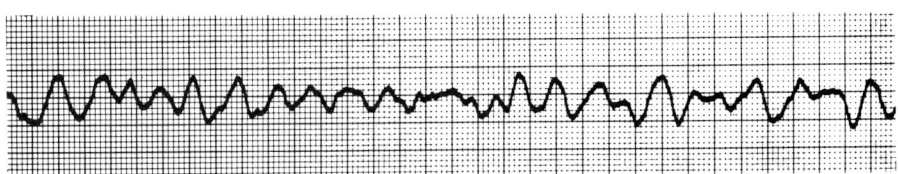

Figure 7-11. This tracing of ventricular fibrillation with no distinct QRS complex or T waves demonstrates irregular undulations with varied amplitude and contour and shows no palpable pulse. (From Chou T-C: Sinus rhythms. In Chou T-C [ed]: Electrocardiography in Clinical Practice, 3rd ed. Philadelphia, WB Saunders, 1991, p 403.)

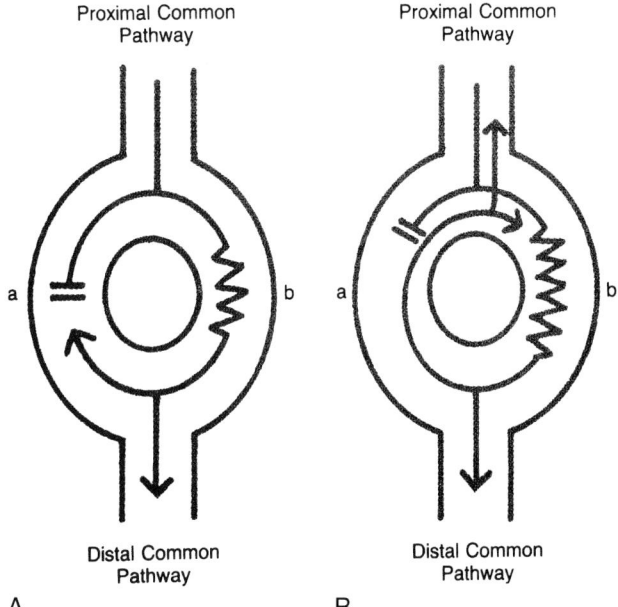

Figure 7-12. Mechanism of reentry. Reentry requires the presence of two separate pathways that join proximally and distally. **A,** A premature impulse blocks in an antegrade manner in pathway "a" (*double bars*) but conducts down pathway "b," albeit with a moderate conduction delay (*serpentine arrow*). The impulse attempts to return up pathway "a" but meets refractory tissue. **B,** A more premature impulse blocks earlier in pathway "a" and experiences more conduction delay in pathway "b." This impulse finds pathway "a" recovered from its previous activation and returns in a retrograde manner to the proximal common pathway. If able to again travel in an antegrade manner over pathway "b," it would activate the distal common pathway prematurely. If this cycle were to continue, a circus movement or reentrant tachycardia would result. For example, in atrioventricular (AV) nodal reentrant tachycardia, the atrium represents the proximal common pathway and the His bundle represents the distal common pathway, with the reentrant circuit located within the AV node. (From Andreoli TE, Bennett JC, Carpenter CCJ, et al [eds]: Cecil Essentials of Medicine, 2nd ed. Philadelphia: WB Saunders, 1990, p 82.)

with sustained aberrant conduction or bundle branch block; in children, most wide-complex tachycardias are ventricular tachycardias (Table 7-5).

Next, the relationship between P waves and QRS complexes is determined, if possible; this relationship is often diagnostic (see Table 7-4). For example, a narrow QRS tachycardia with AV dissociation and an atrial rate lower than the ventricular rate may be diagnosed as junctional ectopic tachycardia. For rhythms with a 1:1 relationship between P waves and QRS complexes, the relative timing of the respective waves is often helpful (i.e., P waves close to preceding QRS, close to following QRS, or on top of QRS). These characteristics help to differentiate among accessory pathway tachycardia, atrial tachycardia, and AV node reentry. These observations are not completely reliable, but an exact electrophysiologic diagnosis may not be necessary for initial decisions concerning treatment.

GENETIC DISEASES

PROLONGED QT SYNDROME

Children with prolonged QT syndrome come to medical attention because of syncope, cardiac arrest, palpitations, seizures, or a positive family history. Clinical episodes are usually associated with either physical or emotional stress (i.e., fright, surprise). The patient develops ventricular tachycardia with torsades de pointes, which may degenerate into ventricular fibrillation. The resting ECG is usually associated with a prolonged QTc interval, although not all patients with a prolonged QTc interval have the syndrome and affected patients may not have a prolonged QTc interval by classic definition (QTc interval > 440 milliseconds or age-appropriate standards). Other ECG findings may include T-wave alternans and relative bradycardia. Diagnosis is based on the degree of QTc prolongation, the clinical history, and on the family history.

Familial disease is due to two syndromes. *Romano-Ward syndrome* (RWS), the much more common entity, is an autosomal dominant disorder (a few families show autosomal recessive inheritance) due to mutations in either sodium or potassium channel

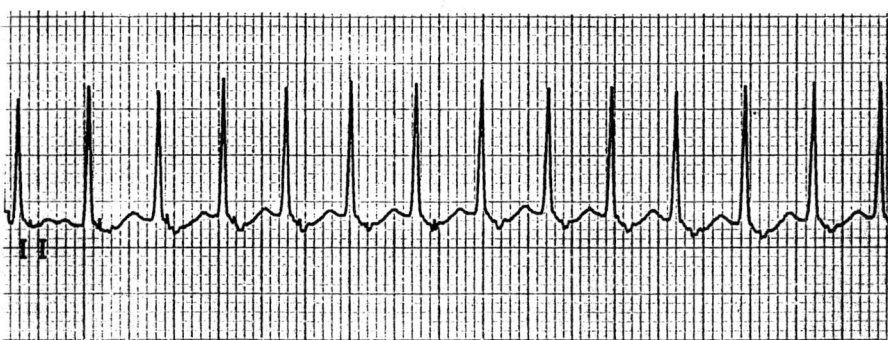

Figure 7-13. Rhythm strip, lead II, in a patient with supraventricular tachycardia caused by an accessory pathway (same patient as in Fig. 7-3). Note the normalization of QRS duration in tachycardia versus the prolonged QRS duration in sinus rhythm (Fig. 7-3) as a result of the loss of antegrade accessory pathway conduction in favor of retrograde accessory pathway conduction during tachycardia, as well as the clear P wave seen on the upstroke of the T wave, closest to the previous QRS complex.

subunits. In *Jervell and Lange-Nielsen syndrome,* an autosomal recessive disorder, there is the combination of prolonged QT syndrome (usually longer than in RWS) and sensorineural deafness. The course is more malignant than RWS. Jervell and Lange-Nielsen syndrome is caused by homozygous mutations in one subunit of a potassium channel; heterozygous mutations of this channel cause Romano-Ward syndrome.

BRUGADA SYNDROME

Brugada syndrome is the combination of ST-segment elevation in leads V_1 to V_3 (which mimics right bundle branch block) and sudden cardiac death from ventricular arrhythmias. Most cases of Brugada syndrome are diagnosed in 30- to 40-year-old men, although it can

manifest in childhood; cases in infants are described. This autosomal dominant disorder arises from a mutation in a sodium channel. Interestingly, mutations in this channel are seen in RWS, conduction system disease, and sudden infant death syndrome.

TREATMENT

TACHYCARDIA

Immediate treatment of patients with sustained symptomatic tachycardia starts with an assessment of the patient's hemodynamic status. Patients with signs of shock require immediate cardioversion, whatever the mechanism of tachycardia. Other modalities may be tried

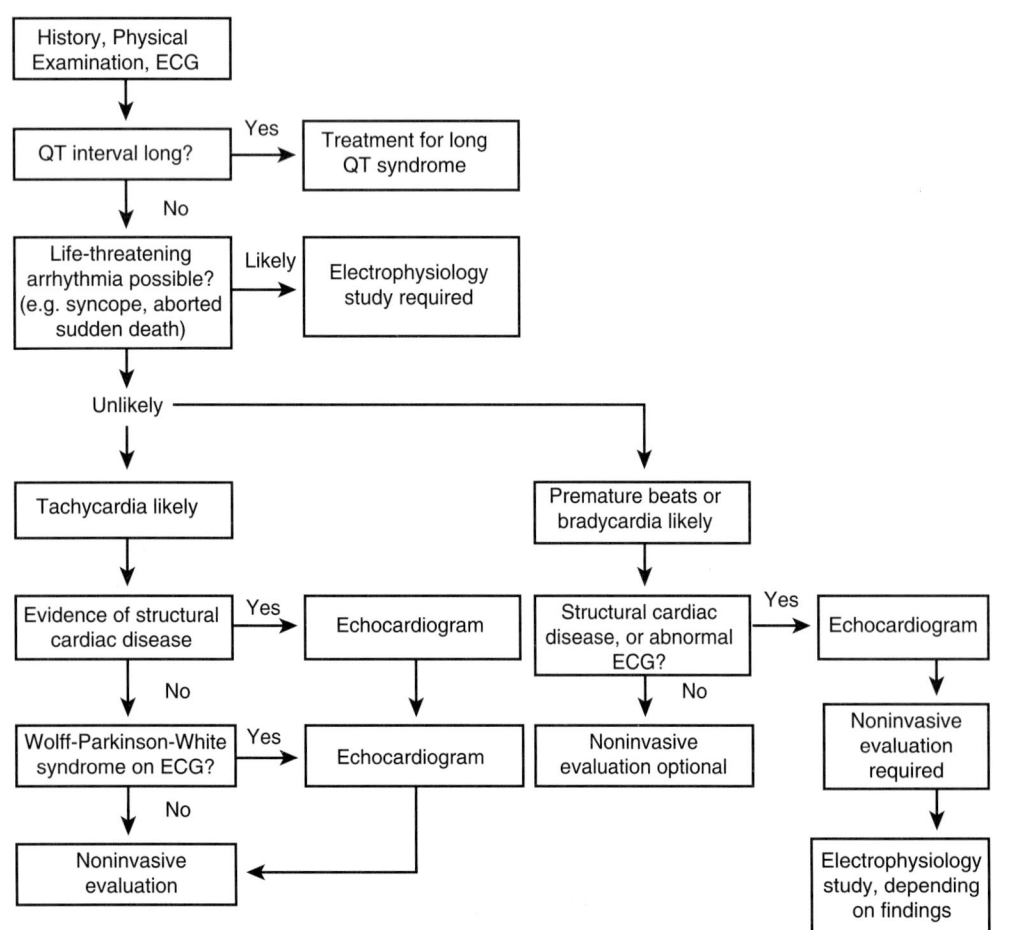

Figure 7-14. Flow diagram for evaluation of palpitations. ECG, electrocardiogram.

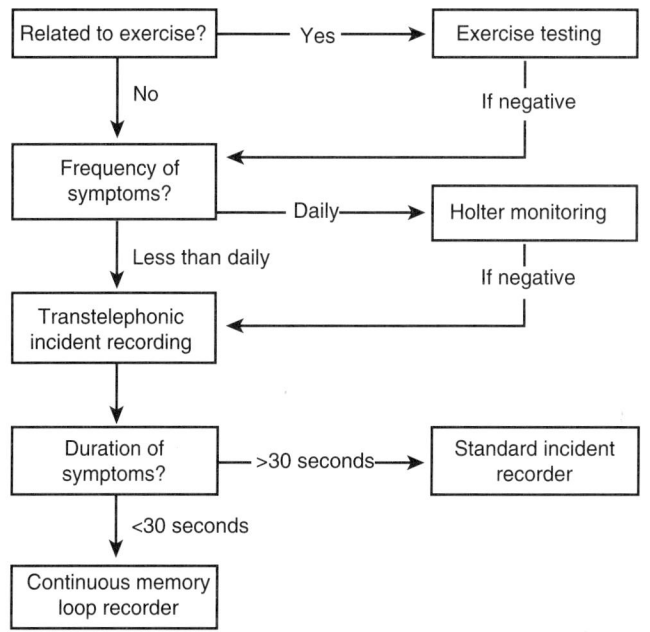

Figure 7-15. Flow diagram for noninvasive evaluation of palpitations.

first in patients who are less symptomatic. Patients with prolonged QRS durations during tachycardia should probably undergo electrical cardioversion because of the high likelihood that the prolonged durations are caused by ventricular tachycardia. Intravenous lidocaine is an alternative treatment, provided that the diagnosis of ventricular tachycardia is certain and the hemodynamic status is stable. In uncertain cases, intravenous procainamide may be used because it is effective in ventricular tachycardia as well as in most forms of supraventricular tachycardia.

Patients with normal QRS durations should initially be approached with several maneuvers designed to increase vagal tone. Older children may be coached through a Valsalva maneuver or facial immersion in ice water, whereas younger children may have gagging induced, have rectal stimulation, or, more often, have an ice bag applied to the face. Although these measures often work, a time limit should be placed on them, so that the patient's hemodynamic status does not deteriorate during prolonged unsuccessful attempts. If maneuvers fail, the administration of adenosine intravenously is the preferred approach (Table 7-6), with continuous electrocardiographic monitoring in a room with a cardioverter-defibrillator available. Adenosine is given by very rapid intravenous injection at an initial dose of 0.05 mg/kg, and the ECG is observed for 10 to 15 seconds. If there is no effect, the dose is doubled repeatedly until a maximum dose of 0.40 mg/kg is reached (24 mg in adolescents and adults). In patients with tachycardia involving the AV node (accessory pathway

Table 7-4. Mechanisms of Tachycardia with Normal QRS Duration

Diagnosis	Electrocardiographic Findings
Reentrant Tachycardias	
Atrial and sinoatrial reentry	P waves present, precede next QRS complex
	Terminates with QRS rather than P wave
	Variable AV conduction possible: AV block does not terminate atrial rhythm
	P-wave axis may be superior or inferior, depending on origin
Atrial flutter	Sawtooth flutter waves
	AV block does not terminate atrial rhythm
	Atrial rate 300 in older children, up to 500 in newborns
Accessory pathway–mediated tachycardia (Wolff-Parkinson-White syndrome and concealed accessory pathway)	P waves follow QRS, typically on upstroke of T wave
	Superior or rightward P-wave axis
	AV block always terminates tachycardia
	Typically terminates with P wave
	After termination, those wih Wolff-Parkinson-White syndrome have preexcitation
Permanent form of junctional reciprocating tachycardia	Incessant
	P waves precede QRS
	Inverted P waves in II, III, AVF leads
	AV block always terminates tachycardia
	May terminate with QRS or with P wave
	No preexcitation after termination
AV node reentry	AV block usually terminates tachycardia
Atrial fibrillation	"Irregularly irregular"—no two RR intervals exactly the same
	P waves difficult to see or bizarre and chaotic
Increased Automaticity	
Sinus tachycardia	Normal P-wave axis
	P waves precede QRS
	Caused by extrinsic factor, such as heart failure, fever, anemia, or catecholamine or theophylline infusion
	Continues in presence of AV block
Atrial ectopic tachycardia	Incessant
	Abnormal P-wave axis, which predicts location of focus
	P waves precede QRS
	Continues in presence of AV block
Junctional ectopic tachycardia	Capture beats with no fusion

AV, atrioventricular.

Table 7-5. Mechanisms of Tachycardia with Prolonged QRS Duration

Diagnosis	Findings on Electrocardiogram
Ventricular tachycardia	Often with AV dissociation
	Capture beats with narrower QRS interval than on other beats
	Fusion beats
Supraventricular tachycardia with preexisting bundle branch block	QRS morphology similar to that in sinus rhythm
	QRS morphology is that of right or left bundle branch block
Supraventricular tachycardia with rate-dependent bundle branch block	QRS morphology usually similar to that of right or left bundle branch block
	Rare in small children
	Difficult to distinguish from ventricular tachycardia in children
Antidromic supraventricular tachycardia in Wolff-Parkinson-White syndrome	QRS morphology similar to preexcited sinus rhythm but wider
	Never occurs with AV dissociation
Atrial fibrillation with Wolff-Parkinson-White syndrome	"Irregularly irregular" wide QRS tachycardia

AV, atrioventricular.

tachycardia, AV node reentry), adenosine terminates the arrhythmia by stopping AV conduction for 1 to 2 seconds. In patients with sinus or atrial tachycardia or atrial flutter, adenosine causes a short episode of AV block, and the underlying atrial rhythm is revealed on the continuous electrocardiographic recording. If the diagnosis is shown to be atrial tachycardia or flutter, patients older than 6 months may receive intravenous verapamil. Those younger than 6 months should never receive verapamil; instead, they may undergo pace conversion with esophageal pacing or cardioversion, or they may receive intravenous procainamide.

Many patients do not require long-term treatment if the episodes are not severely symptomatic and are either self-limited or easily converted with vagal maneuvers. If suppressive drug therapy is indicated, various medications may be used, including digoxin, β blockers, verapamil, flecainide, sotalol, and amiodarone. The last three antiarrhythmic agents are more potent but are associated with increased risk of side effects. The choice of medication is determined by the likely diagnosis; the less benign agents are usually reserved for children who do not respond to the initial choice.

Intracardiac catheter ablation techniques during cardiac catheterization with radiofrequency energy are available for pediatric patients with nearly all forms of abnormal tachycardia and may be offered for life-threatening tachycardia. In older children, this treatment may be used as an alternative to long-term medication therapy; in younger children, it may be used when medication fails to control the tachycardia.

In selected patients who are found to have life-threatening ventricular arrhythmias not amenable to ablation and not reliably prevented or controlled by medication, the use of implantable cardioverter-defibrillators may be appropriate. These devices are implanted in a procedure similar to that used for pacemaker placement; they detect and terminate dangerous ventricular arrhythmias

Table 7-6. Intravenous Antiarrhythmic Agents

Agent	Dosage	Comments
Verapamil	0.1-0.2 mg/kg IV, 5-10 mg maximum	Beware of hypotension
		Definitely contraindicated in children <6 months of age, probably <12 months of age
		Do *not* give with β blockers
Propranolol (β blocker)	0.02 mg/kg IV every 5 minutes, to 0.1 mg/kg	Monitor pulse, blood pressure
		Contraindicated in patients with asthma and those with congestive heart failure
		Do *not* give with verapamil
Procainamide	10-15 mg/kg IV over 30 minutes	May cause hypotension; continuous monitoring is essential
		Cardiologic guidance is recommended
Digoxin	10 µg/kg IV as initial load	Do not use in patients with hypokalemia or if digoxin toxicity is suspected
	Second dose in 6 hr, third at 24 hr	
Lidocaine	1-2 mg/kg IV over 15 minutes	May cause hypotension, respiratory depression, or central nervous system symptoms
	Continuous infusion: 30-50 µg/kg/min	
Phenylephrine	0.02 mg/kg IV slowly	Used for raising blood pressure and eliciting a baroreceptor vagal reflex
Adenosine	Starting IV dose: 0.05 mg/kg; double dose repeatedly until effect is seen, to maximum of 0.4 mg/kg	Contraindicated in preexisting second- or third-degree AV block without pacemaker
		Use with caution in patients with severe asthma; half-life is 10 sec in serum

AV, atrioventricular; IV, intravenously.

Table 7-7. Red Flags: Palpitations

Family history of sudden death
Syncope
Heart failure
Chest pain
Stroke
Prior cardiac surgery
Heart surgery for structural congenital defects
Drug overdose
Hypotension
Exercise-induced
Prolonged duration
Exercise intolerance
Suicide attempt (drug overdose)
Prolonged QT intervals

either by rapid pacing or by the delivery of a high-voltage shock to the heart.

BRADYCARDIA

The hemodynamic effect of a slow heart rate depends on how different it is from the patient's usual heart rate. Sudden decreases in rate may be poorly compensated by increases in stroke volume, particularly in patients with preexisting poor cardiac function. Moderate sinus bradycardia in normal children rarely necessitates treatment. Underlying causes, such as hypothyroidism, should be corrected. Patients with third-degree AV block and those with severe sinus node dysfunction may require permanent artificial cardiac pacing. In all cases, the occurrence of symptoms (over and above the symptom of palpitations), such as syncope, exercise intolerance, or dizziness, is an indication for pacing. With severe sinus node dysfunction, pacing may be required if the patient is to be given antiarrhythmic agents to suppress episodes of tachycardia because of the danger that such medications will worsen sinus node dysfunction. Patients with persisting complete AV block as a result of cardiac surgery generally require permanent pacing, even in the absence of symptoms. Prophylactic cardiac pacing may be recommended in completely asymptomatic patients with complete congenital AV block if daytime average heart rates fall below 50 bpm, if nighttime rates are below 30 bpm, or if long pauses (>3 seconds) are recorded on Holter monitoring. This is because patients with these findings are at greater risk for progressing to syncope or sudden death.

PREMATURE BEATS

In the absence of tachycardia, patients rarely need to be treated for premature beats of any kind. Patients with premature supraventricular contractions virtually never require treatment; those with premature ventricular contractions may require treatment in a few situations:

1. when the contractions are multiform
2. when the contractions occur in couplets or in short runs of ventricular tachycardia
3. when the contractions are seen in association with a recently converted ventricular tachycardia
4. when the contractions exhibit the "R-on-T" phenomenon (i.e., they fall repeatedly on the early part of the T wave of the preceding beat)

Decisions concerning treatment of premature beats are difficult and should be made in consultation with a cardiologist. Possible inciting factors, such as drugs, hypoxia, and acidosis, should be corrected. If premature ventricular contractions necessitate emergency treatment, the agent of choice is lidocaine, given by a continuous intravenous infusion. Some cardiologists have used bretylium to terminate ventricular tachycardia.

RED FLAGS

Table 7-7 lists the red flags associated with palpitations that warrant immediate attention and evaluation.

REFERENCES

Etiology and Pathogenesis

Ackerman MJ: The long QT syndrome: Ion channel diseases of the heart. Mayo Clin Proc 1998;73:250-269.
Berger S, Dhala A, Friedberg DZ: Sudden cardiac death in infants, children, and adolescents. Pediatr Clin North Am 1999;46:221-234.
Boutjdir M: Molecular and ionic basis of congenital complete heart block. Trends Cardiovasc Med 2000;10:114-122.
Narchi H: The child who passes out. Pediatr Rev 2000;21:384-388.
Priori SG, Napolitano C, Giordano U, et al: Brugada syndrome and sudden cardiac death in children. Lancet 2000;355:808-809.
Roberts R, Brugada R: Genetic aspects of arrhythmias. Am J Med Genet 2000;97:310-318.
Schwartz PJ, Stramba-Badiale M, Segantini A, et al: Prolongation of the QT interval and the sudden infant death syndrome. N Engl J Med 1998; 338:1709-1714.
Towbin JA, Vatta M: Molecular biology and the prolonged QT syndromes. Am J Med 2001;110:385-398.
Towbin JA, Wang Z, Li H: Genotype and severity of long QT syndrome. Arch Pathol Lab Med 2001;125:116-121.

Diagnosis and Treatment

Bevilacqua L, Hordof A: Cardiac pacing in children. Curr Opin Cardiol 1998;13:48-55.
Bink-Boelkens MT: Pharmacologic management of arrhythmias. Pediatr Cardiol 2000;21:508-515.
Case CL: Diagnosis and treatment of pediatric arrhythmias. Pediatr Clin North Am 1999;46:347-354.
Cecchin F, Jorgenson DB, Berul CI, et al: Is arrhythmia detection by automatic external defibrillator accurate for children? Circulation 2001;103:2483-2488.
Dubin AM, Van Hare GF: Radiofrequency catheter ablation: Indications and complications. Pediatr Cardiol 2000;21:551-556.
Eronen M, Siren MK, Ekblad H, et al: Short- and long-term outcome of children with congenital complete heart block diagnosed in utero or as a newborn. Pediatrics 2000;106:86-91.
Kugler JD, Danford DA: Management of infants, children, and adolescents with paroxysmal supraventricular tachycardia. J Pediatr 1996;129: 324-338.
Moss AJ, Zareba W, Hall WJ, et al: Effectiveness and limitations of beta-blocker therapy in congenital long-QT syndrome. Circulation 2000; 101:616-623.
Paul T, Pfammatter JP: Adenosine: An effective and safe antiarrhythmic drug in pediatrics. Pediatr Cardiol 1997;18:118-126.
Pfammatter JP, Paul T: New antiarrhythmic drug in pediatric use: Sotalol. Pediatr Cardiol 1997;18:28-34.
Sliz NB Jr, Johns JA: Cardiac pacing in infants and children. Cardiol Rev 2000;8:223-239.
Tanel RE, Rhodes LA: Fetal and neonatal arrhythmias. Clin Perinatol 2001;28:187-207, vii.
Tipple MA: Usefulness of the electrocardiogram in diagnosing mechanisms of tachycardia. Pediatr Cardiol 2000;21:516-521.

8 Heart Failure

Stuart Berger*

The chief complaint and presenting symptoms of heart failure are variable and nonspecific (Table 8-1). None are pathognomonic. The presenting symptoms depend on the age of the patient, the severity of the heart failure, the acuity (chronicity) of the presentation, and the efficiency of the physiologic compensatory mechanisms (Fig. 8-1).

DEFINITION

Heart failure is defined as inadequate oxygen delivery by the circulatory system so that the needs of the body are not met. This process depends on adequate cardiac performance. Symptoms during periods of increased oxygen needs, such as exercise in the older child or feeding in the infant, are often the first manifestation of heart failure.

Oxygen delivery is calculated by multiplying the systemic oxygen content by the cardiac output. Oxygen content is the oxygen saturation multiplied by the hemoglobin concentration plus the small amount of dissolved oxygen. Cardiac output is equal to the product of stroke volume and heart rate. The preload, the afterload, and the contractility determine stroke volume. Alterations in any of these parameters can alter oxygen delivery to the tissues; optimization of these parameters, which is the basis for the treatment of heart failure, can improve oxygen delivery and ameliorate the symptoms of heart failure.

MECHANISMS, PHYSIOLOGY, COMPENSATION/OVERCOMPENSATION

Manifestations of heart failure may be the result of exhausted compensatory mechanisms. In addition, many features of heart failure are caused by the physiologic compensation or overcompensation that the body invokes in order to combat inadequate oxygen delivery (Fig. 8-2; see Fig. 8-1). The renal system (activation of renin-angiotensin system) is a very important compensation mechanism in heart failure. Renal hypoperfusion stimulates renal salt and water retention to increase the circulating blood volume (preload). By the Frank-Starling mechanism, an increase in preload causes an increase in stroke volume within a wide physiologic range. Salt retention occurs by activation of the renin-angiotensin system. The secretion of renin by the kidney leads to the release of angiotensin I. Angiotensin I is then converted to angiotensin II, a very potent vasoconstrictor. This effect increases the blood pressure and the systemic vascular resistance (afterload). Angiotensin stimulates the synthesis and secretion of aldosterone, causing further sodium and fluid retention (preload).

Organ hypoperfusion causes an increase in levels of circulating catecholamines, including epinephrine and norepinephrine. Stretching of mechanoreceptors in the heart potentiates catecholamine activity. Circulating catecholamines and their direct stimulation of β-adrenergic receptors on the heart increase the heart rate (chronotropic) and contractility (inotropic). As a result of these mechanisms, there may be a redistribution of cardiac output to the vital organs such as the heart, the brain, and the kidneys with a decrease in perfusion of the skin and skeletal muscle system. Nonetheless, chronic sympathetic nervous system stimulation of the heart may produce an increase in myocardial oxygen demand, poor relationships between muscle contraction and relaxation, increased intracellular calcium concentrations, and a risk for arrhythmias and uncoupling of mitochondrial oxidation, thus increasing energy needs.

The very delicate balance of hormonal and mechanical compensation can improve tissue perfusion by increasing circulating blood volume, cardiac output, and blood pressure. The compensatory mechanisms may also contribute to the signs and symptoms of heart failure if the underlying problem persists and/or intensifies. Salt and water retention may cause peripheral and/or pulmonary edema. Adrenergic stimulation is associated with tachycardia, diaphoresis, and cool, clammy skin because of decreased cutaneous perfusion. Vasoconstriction may adversely affect afterload, which can cause a further demand on myocardial oxygen consumption, producing hypertrophy, further decreasing cardiac output, and thereby resulting in a vicious cycle (see Fig. 8-2). Chronic heart failure may produce ventricular hypertrophy and a reversion to fetal cardiac gene expression. Hypertrophy may compensate for volume overload by decreasing wall tension and afterload. However, cardiac muscle remodeling with myocyte death, fibrosis, and poor capillary penetration may produce uncompensated chamber dilatation.

Increased blood volume, initially a beneficial compensation, is ultimately associated with increased left ventricular volume and left atrial volume. Left ventricular end-diastolic pressure can then increase in proportion to the ventricular volume overload. Eventually, the systemic vascular resistance increases. The elevation in left ventricular end-diastolic pressure is transmitted to the left atrium, to the pulmonary veins, and to the lung parenchyma, thereby contributing to the pulmonary edema seen in congestive heart failure. This potentiates the tachypnea and dyspnea noted in patients with heart failure.

The compensatory mechanisms may lead to tachycardia, chamber dilatation, and arrhythmias. Chamber dilatation occurs as a result of increased volume but can also be increased by dilatation of the atrioventricular (AV) valve rings or the failing chamber itself. AV valve dilatation can produce AV valve regurgitation, which further potentiates volume overloading of the atria and ventricles. Arrhythmias that can occur in association with heart failure are potentiated by atrial or ventricular chamber dilatation, as well as by the direct effect of circulating catecholamines.

Systolic dysfunction results from impaired contractility and is noted when the ventricle is less able to respond to an increased preload with an enhanced stroke volume. The impaired ventricle is less able to increase cardiac output in response to a small increase in afterload, whereas a small decrease of afterload may dramatically improve cardiac output. When systolic dysfunction improves, the end-systolic volume increases, and if this improvement is associated with an increase in preload (venous return), there is improvement in cardiac output.

*This chapter is an updated and edited version of the chapter by Dennis P. Ruggerie that appeared in the first edition.

Table 8-1. Signs and Symptoms of Congestive Heart Failure and Their Mechanisms and Treatment

Signs and Symptoms	Mechanisms	Treatment
Pulmonary venous congestion	↑Left-sided filling pressures	Diuretics
Tachypnea	Interstitial pulmonary edema	Oxygen
Wheezing	Bronchiolar edema	Surgery
Rales	Alveolar edema	
Feeding difficulties	↑Work of breathing	
Irritability	↓Oxygen transport	
Systemic venous congestion	↑Right-sided filling pressure	Diuretics
Hepatomegaly	Hepatic venous congestion	Spironolactone
Peripheral edema	↑Fluid transudation,	
	↑aldosterone	
Impaired cardiac output	Decreased inotropic state	Digoxin
↓Precordial activity	↓Inotropic function	Dopamine
↓Arterial pulsations	↓Systemic perfusion	Dobutamine
↓Capillary refill	↓Systemic perfusion	Afterload reduction
Volume loading	Chamber dilatation	Digoxin
↑Precordial activity	Preserved inotropic state	Diuretics
Gallop sounds	↑Ventricle filling	Surgery
Pressure loading	↑Afterload	Catheterization or surgical
Gallop sounds	↓Compliance	stenosis relief
Murmurs	Poststenotic turbulence	
Adaptive changes	↑Neurohumoral responses	Digoxin
Tachycardia	↑β_1-adrenergic activity	β_1 Blockers
Pallor	↑α_1 and angiotensin response (vasoconstriction)	Afterload reduction
Low urine output	↓Renal perfusion	Dopamine
Growth failure	↑Metabolic demands	
Sweating	↑Sympathetic and cholinergic	

From O'Laughlin MP: Congestive heart failure in children. Pediatr Clin North Am 1999;46:264.

↑, increased; ↓, decreased.

Diastolic dysfunction results when the ventricular compliance requires a higher than normal venous pressure to permit adequate filling and cardiac output. Diastolic dysfunction with poor cardiac output may be present in the absence of systolic dysfunction. Lesions associated with diastolic dysfunction include obstructive lesions to ventricular filling (AV valve stenosis, obstructed anomalous pulmonary venous return, cor triatriatum), poorly functioning Fontan procedures, pericardial tamponade, and poorly compliant ventricles (hypertrophy, cardiac transplant rejection, cardiomyopathy, hypertension). The medical management of systolic and diastolic dysfunction must be based on the underlying pathophysiology, and at times it is different for the two types of dysfunction.

CLASSIFICATION/CAUSES OF CONGESTIVE HEART FAILURE

Classification can be based on age at presentation, whether it is congenital or acquired, whether it is acute or chronic, the presence of

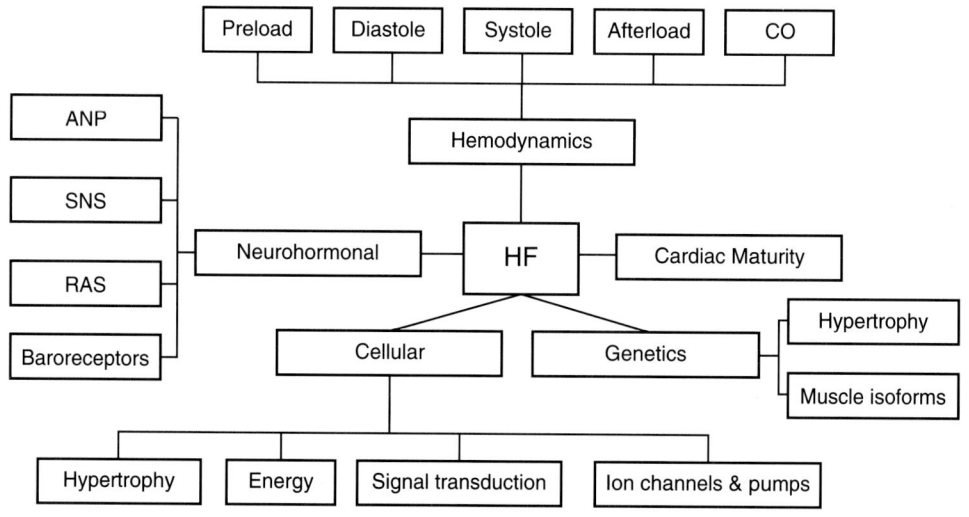

Figure 8-1. The heart failure pathophysiology paradigm. Current pathophysiologic paradigm that unifies the understanding of mechanisms that are active in the syndrome of heart failure. ANP, atrial natriuretic peptide; CO, cardiac output; HF, heart failure; RAS, renin-angiotensin system; SNS, sympathetic nervous system. (From Balaguru B, Artman M, Auslender M: Management of heart failure in children. Curr Probl Pediatr 2000;30:6.)

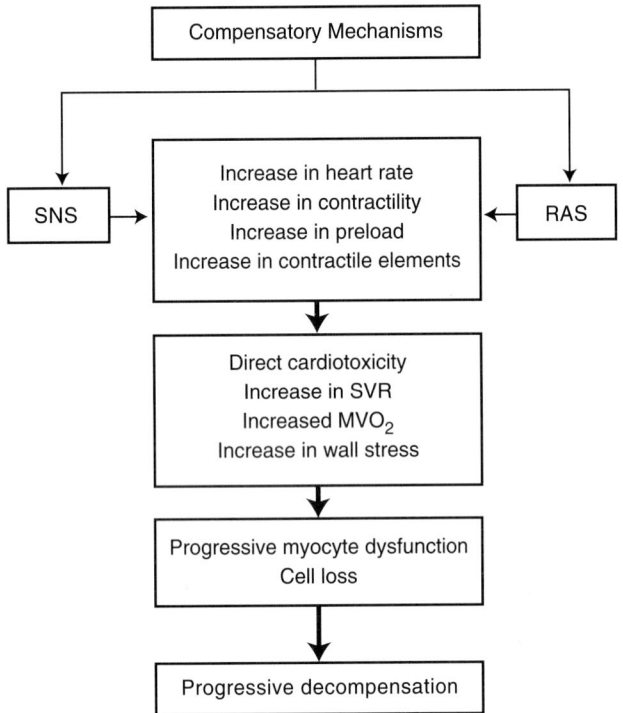

Figure 8-2. Path to decompensation in heart failure. During the decompensated phase of heart failure, the sympathetic nervous system (SNS) and the renin-angiotensin system (RAS) are activated as compensatory mechanisms. A progression of cardiac and vascular remodeling can be observed. Continued activation of these compensatory mechanisms is initially adaptive, but eventually they become maladaptive mechanisms that lead to decompensation. MVO_2, myocardial oxygen consumption; SVR, systemic vascular resistance. (From Balaguru B, Artman M, Auslender M: Management of heart failure in children. Curr Probl Pediatr 2000;30:9.)

right- or left-sided heart failure, and whether there is low- or high-output failure (Tables 8-2 and 8-3; Figs. 8-3 to 8-5).

Heart failure in the fetus and/or during the first few hours of life is generally uncommon. At this time, it is relatively unusual for structural heart disease to be the cause, because most forms of congenital heart disease are well tolerated in utero (Table 8-4; see Table 8-3). Fetal heart failure is manifested by cardiomegaly and hydrops with pleural effusions and ascites (see Table 8-3). This is often detected by fetal ultrasonography. The most common causes include fetal arrhythmias, most often supraventricular tachycardia. Ventricular tachycardia or heart block can also be associated with fetal hydrops. Less common causes include fetal myocarditis, severe anemia, and hemolysis from immune hydrops. In rare cases, congenital cardiac abnormalities with severe AV valve regurgitation can manifest with in utero heart failure.

Symptoms of heart failure within the first several days after birth indicate the presence of a congenital heart anomaly for which survival requires a patent ductus arteriosus. Left-sided obstructive heart lesions in particular, such as hypoplastic left heart syndrome or coarctation of the aorta, are examples. Critical aortic stenosis is another lesion manifesting early with heart failure.

Lesions that manifest several weeks to months after birth usually have left-to-right shunts, such as a ventricular septal defect or a patent ductus arteriosus (PDA). Symptoms of heart failure in this group are related to pulmonary overcirculation and left-sided heart volume overload that can occur when the normal postnatal decline in pulmonary vascular resistance occurs. It is typical for these pulmonary vascular changes to occur at several weeks of age, and this is thus the most likely time for symptoms of heart failure to manifest in this group.

CLINICAL PRESENTATION AND PHYSICAL EXAMINATION

The clinical presentation is somewhat variable, depending on the cause of heart failure and the age at presentation (see Tables 8-1 and 8-4).

NEWBORNS

Common symptoms in newborns include poor feeding and growth failure with tachypnea and/or respiratory distress. In the later stages or in severe heart failure, cyanosis, poor perfusion, and poor capillary refill may be present. Feeding difficulties may be caused by labored breathing. It may take the neonate up to 60 minutes to finish a feed that normally would take 10 to 15 minutes.

The approach to the newborn with structural heart disease is discussed in Chapters 10 and 11; Figure 8-6 offers a critical pathway approach to the newborn and infant with structural heart disease that is based on whether the presenting symptom is cyanosis, cyanosis with respiratory distress, or low cardiac output.

Physical examination should include careful attention to vital signs, including heart rate and respiratory rate (Table 8-5). Four limb blood pressure measurements are essential for assessing the possibility of aortic obstruction. It is critical to compare the carotid pulse to limb pulses because, in rare cases, an interrupted aortic arch with an anomalous right subclavian artery can manifest with equal extremity pulses. Differential cyanosis may also be noted in newborns with left-sided obstructive heart lesions because of right arm and upper body perfusion from the left ventricle and descending aortic perfusion from the ductus arteriosus, which has poorly oxygenated blood.

In some forms of heart failure, the pulses may actually be increased or bounding (high-output failure); in the neonate, this may be caused by a PDA or an arteriovenous malformation of the brain or liver. In rare cases, large coronary arteriovenous fistulae can manifest in this manner. Careful auscultation of the skull and abdomen for bruits or continuous murmurs that get louder farther away from the precordium should accompany the cardiac examination of any neonate or infant with signs of congestive heart failure.

Chest palpation is an important part of the physical examination. A hyperactive precordium may be an important indicator of cardiac disease. Auscultation may show a systolic murmur in many forms of neonatal congenital heart disease, although the absence of a murmur certainly does not rule out serious heart disease in any age group (Table 8-6).

INFANTS

Symptoms in infants are not significantly different from those in neonates and often include poor feeding, lethargy, tachypnea, respiratory distress, tachycardia, and diaphoresis.

There are two important congenital heart lesions that can manifest later in infancy and that should not be missed. These include certain forms of total anomalous pulmonary venous return (TAPVR) and anomalous left coronary artery arising from the pulmonary artery (ALCAPA).

Total Anomalous Pulmonary Venous Return

Patients who are not initially symptomatic have no obstruction to pulmonary venous return and have a nonrestrictive atrium level communication. However, the atrium level communication may become restrictive over the first several months of life. Affected infants then become progressively symptomatic as the pulmonary venous return becomes progressively obstructed. The symptoms usually encountered are tachypnea, wheezing, and respiratory distress.

Table 8-2. Age-Based Approach to the Etiology of Heart Failure*

Fetus

Severe anemia
Supraventricular tachycardia
Congenital heart block
Ventricular tachycardia
Complex congenital anomalies
Myocarditis-cardiomyopathy
Nonimmune hydrops fetalis (see Table 8-3)

Premature Infant

Fluid overload
Patent ductus arteriosus
Ventricular septal defect
Bronchopulmonary dysplasia (cor pulmonale)
Hypertension (aortic–renal artery thrombosis)

First Week of Life

Left-sided heart obstructive defects
  Hypoplastic left heart syndrome
  Coarctation of aorta
  Interrupted aortic arch
  Critical aortic stenosis
  Mitral valve stenosis, atresia
  Total anomalous pulmonary venous return (obstructed)
Left-to-right shunt
  Patent ductus arteriosus
  Arteriovenous malformations
  Aortopulmonary window
  Total anomalous venous return (unobstructed)
Other lesions
  Truncus arteriosus
  Single ventricle
  Transposition of great arteries with intact ventricular septum
  Transposition of great arteries with ventricular septal defect
  Severe Ebstein anomaly
  Tetralogy of Fallot with absent pulmonary valve
Other
  Hypoxic-ischemic cardiomyopathy (asphyxia)
  Anemia
  Arrhythmias
  Sepsis
  Myocarditis
  Hypoglycemia
  Hypocalcemia

Older Neonate, Infant, or Toddler

Left-to-right shunts
  Ventricular septal defect
  Patent ductus arteriosus
  Atrial septal defect (rare)
  Endocardial cushion defect
  Tricuspid atresia
Other congenital heart defects
  Coarctation of the aorta
  Aortic stenosis
  Anomalous left coronary artery from the pulmonary artery
  Ebstein anomaly
  Absent pulmonary valve
  Critical pulmonary stenosis
Acquired
  Arrhythmia (tachyarrhythmia, bradyarrhythmia)
  Anemia
  Myocarditis
  Cardiomyopathy
  Hypertension
  Endocarditis
  Airway obstruction
  Arteriovenous malformation
  Kawasaki disease

School-Aged Child or Adolescent

Myocarditis
Cardiomyopathy
Rheumatic fever
Endocarditis
Hypertension
Thyrotoxicosis
Hemochromatosis
Cancer therapy (radiation, adriamycin)
Cor pulmonale (cystic fibrosis, chronic airway obstruction–sleep apnea syndrome)

*After corrective or palliative heart surgery, ventricular failure may occur acutely in the postoperative period or may develop 1 to 20 years later. It may be caused by prosthetic valve malfunction, progressive valve insufficiencies, endocarditis, ischemia, intrinsic myocardial failure resulting from cardiopulmonary bypass, surgical shunts, or natural progression of disease (i.e., single-ventricle, right pump failure after a Mustard operation, long-term cyanosis).

It is common for these infants to be mistakenly treated for pneumonia, bronchiolitis, or asthma.

Anomalous Origin of the Left Coronary Artery from the Pulmonary Artery (ALCAPA)

Manifestation of this condition in the neonatal period is uncommon because of the high fetal pulmonary artery pressure and pulmonary vascular resistance, which allows for coronary artery perfusion albeit with desaturated blood. When the pulmonary artery pressure and pulmonary vascular resistance normally decrease after birth, coronary blood flow decreases and the ventricular muscle becomes ischemic with resultant myocardial infarction and mitral valve regurgitation. Profound congestive heart failure and dilated cardiomyopathy (DCM) occurs. Any infant with DCM should undergo thorough investigation of the coronary artery anatomy to rule out ALCAPA.

Early discovery and surgical reimplantation of the anomalous coronary artery into the aorta may lead to complete recovery of the left ventricular function.

CHILDREN AND YOUNG ADULTS

Older children, adolescents, and young adults are able to report more specific symptoms such as exercise intolerance or tiredness that accompanies fairly routine activities. Tachypnea, shortness of breath, or dyspnea on exertion may be present. Examination may reveal some of the features described for neonates or infants but may also reveal ascites or peripheral edema, which are less common in infants and younger children. A new onset of symptoms of heart failure in this age group should prompt the examiner to consider myocarditis or DCM, as well as less common forms of acquired cardiac disease such as endocarditis and rheumatic fever.

Table 8-3. Selected Causes of Heart Failure in the Fetus

I. Nonimmune Hydrops Fetalis*

A. Cardiovascular
1. Congenital heart disease
2. Dysrhythmias (supraventricular tachycardia, congenital heart block)
3. Myocarditis
4. Complicated congenital heart disease
5. Rhabdomyoma

B. Hematologic
1. Twin-twin transfusion, fetomaternal hemorrhage
2. Arteriovenous malformation
3. α-Thalassemia

C. Chromosomal
1. Turner syndrome
2. Trisomies 13, 18, 21

D. Metabolic diseases
1. Maternal diabetes (poor control)
2. Gaucher and other storage diseases

E. Infection
1. Syphilis
2. Cytomegalovirus
3. Parvovirus (anemia)
4. Chagas disease
5. Toxoplasmosis

F. Pulmonary
1. Cystic adenomatoid malformation
2. Diaphragmatic hernia
3. Lymphangiectasia

G. Hepatic-gastrointestinal
1. Hepatitis
2. Hepatic fibrosis
3. Atresia
4. Volvulus
5. Chylous ascites
6. Cystic fibrosis

H. Renal
1. Nephrosis
2. Prune-belly syndrome

I. Tumor
1. Neuroblastoma
2. Placental chorioangioma

J. Malformation complex
1. Arthrogryposis
2. Thanatophoric dysplasia
3. Noonan syndrome

II. Erythroblastosis Fetalis (Immune Hydrops Fetalis)

*Represents the most common etiologic factors.

GENERAL EXAMINATION

The history and physical examination remain essential both for the detection of heart disease and for the evaluation of its severity at any age. Achieving calmness in a patient in a quiet room helps the undisturbed observation of appearance and respiration. Spending a few minutes talking with the family may allow the patient to become familiarized with the physician. A good stethoscope is essential because auscultation is the primary means of assessing the heart (see Chapter 11). Because inflation of the blood pressure cuff may induce anxiety in the infant or child, it may be best to leave this until the end of the examination.

A systemic head-to-toe inspection should be performed. Most major congenital anomalies recognizable at birth have an increased incidence of associated structural heart disease. Some syndromes may not become apparent until later infancy or childhood (Noonan and Williams syndromes) or adolescence (Marfan syndrome).

In the newborn, complete history taking often follows stabilization efforts, because the manifestation of heart failure is often acute, severe, and life-threatening. Initially, a brief birth history is obtained, including gestational age, Apgar scores, and any difficulties with pregnancy, labor, and delivery. Details of the prenatal course, delivery, maternal history (i.e., maternal diabetes, systemic lupus erythematosus, and drug usage), and further information about difficulties should be obtained after the newborn has been stabilized.

Children and adolescents in whom heart failure develops may have a personal or family history of known congenital or acquired heart disease or surgical interventions for congenital heart disease. Midline sternotomy and lateral thoracotomy incision scars provide evidence of previous cardiac surgery. Patients may have a history of general malaise; weight loss over several weeks; increasing respiratory effort with activity; difficulty with everyday activities, such as walking up a flight of stairs; breathlessness; palpitations; or possible delayed sexual maturation. A history of recurrent lower respiratory tract infections should prompt an investigation of possible underlying heart disease. In some children, the onset of febrile illness may "unmask" symptoms of heart failure that have previously been compensated, or the illness may be the cause of heart failure (endocarditis, rheumatic fever).

THE 3-MINUTE EXAMINATION

A brief, age-independent, focused examination to rapidly assess for the symptoms of congestive heart failure begins with the counting of the sleeping or resting respiratory rate for 30 to 60 seconds. The patient's general status, including distress, color, and perfusion, should then be evaluated. Capillary refill is checked, as are signs of edema in the pretibial area. The precordium can be palpated for hyperactivity; the abdomen is examined for hepatomegaly; and the pulses, including simultaneous arm and leg pulses as well as carotid pulses, are palpated. Auscultation of the head, abdomen, and chest for bruits, murmurs, and gallops should follow. Finally, the lungs are auscultated for rales or rhonchi.

PATTERN RECOGNITION

The key to the diagnosis of heart failure is the recognition of patterns of signs and symptoms as manifestations of physiologic events. The clinical manifestations of heart failure may differ in the fetus, infant, child, and adolescent (see Table 8-4).

The hallmarks (pattern recognition) of heart failure are

- tachypnea
- tachycardia
- cardiomegaly
- hepatomegaly

Tachycardia and cardiomegaly are early signs of heart failure, followed by tachypnea. Hepatomegaly is a late sign. Splenomegaly is rarely associated with heart failure; its presence suggests inferior vena cava obstruction, portal hypertension, anemia, infectious processes, or a myeloproliferative disorder (see Chapter 19).

Heart failure leads to alterations in respiratory function. Ventilation is assessed by auscultation of breath sounds and observation of respiratory effort; the adequacy of oxygenation is assessed by the absence of cyanosis. Respiratory distress is a clinical state of increased respiratory rate and work of breathing (intercostal-supraclavicular-subcostal retractions, nasal flaring, grunting) developed in an effort to maintain minute ventilation. Respiratory failure is characterized by inadequate ventilation and/or inadequate oxygenation, manifested by pallor or central cyanosis, labored respiratory effort, irregular or apneic respiratory pattern, air hunger (anxiety), and altered mental status (see Chapters 3 and 10).

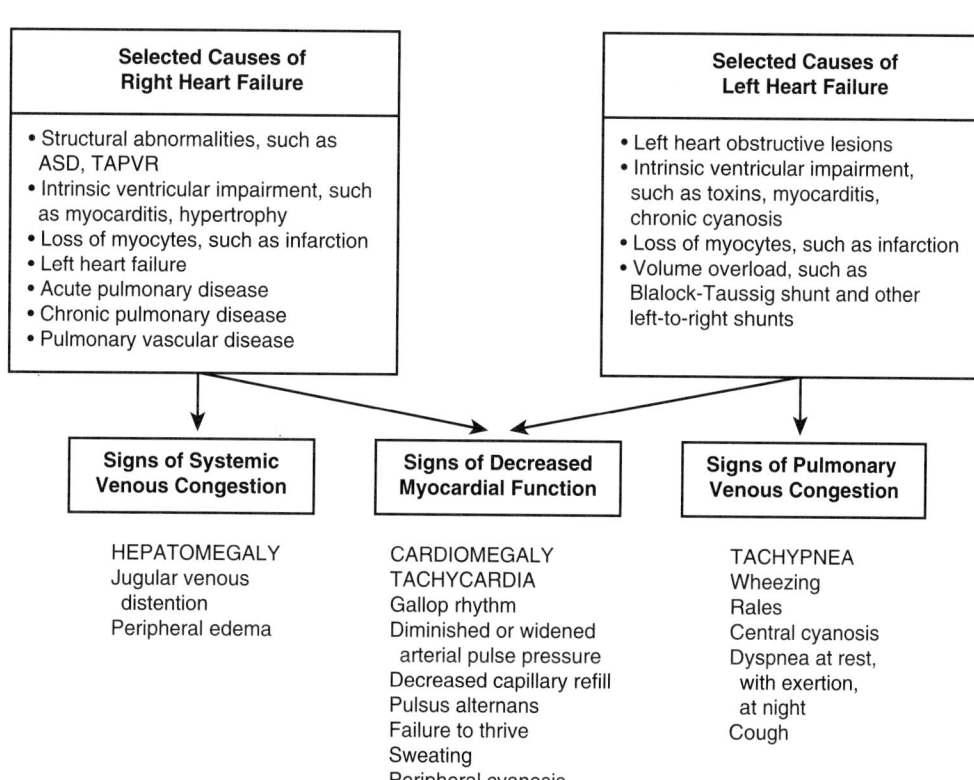

┌─────────────────────────────┐   ┌─────────────────────────────┐
│ **Selected Causes of**   │   │ **Selected Causes of**   │
│ **Right Heart Failure**   │   │ **Left Heart Failure**   │
├─────────────────────────────┤   ├─────────────────────────────┤
│ • Structural abnormalities, such as   │ • Left heart obstructive lesions   │
│   ASD, TAPVR   │ • Intrinsic ventricular impairment,   │
│ • Intrinsic ventricular impairment, such │ such as toxins, myocarditis,   │
│   as myocarditis, hypertrophy   │   chronic cyanosis   │
│ • Loss of myocytes, such as infarction │ • Loss of myocytes, such as infarction │
│ • Left heart failure   │ • Volume overload, such as   │
│ • Acute pulmonary disease   │   Blalock-Taussig shunt and other   │
│ • Chronic pulmonary disease   │   left-to-right shunts   │
│ • Pulmonary vascular disease   │   │

Figure 8-3. Physiologic paradigm of heart failure, emphasizing which ventricle is predominantly dysfunctional, and associated clinical signs and symptoms. ASD, atrial septal defect; TAPVR, total anomalous pulmonary venous return. (From Ruggerie DP: Congestive heart failure. In Blumer J [ed]: Practical Guide to Pediatric Intensive Care, 3rd ed. St. Louis, Mosby–Year Book, 1990.)

Signs of Systemic Venous Congestion

HEPATOMEGALY
Jugular venous distention
Peripheral edema

Signs of Decreased Myocardial Function

CARDIOMEGALY
TACHYCARDIA
Gallop rhythm
Diminished or widened arterial pulse pressure
Decreased capillary refill
Pulsus alternans
Failure to thrive
Sweating
Peripheral cyanosis

Signs of Pulmonary Venous Congestion

TACHYPNEA
Wheezing
Rales
Central cyanosis
Dyspnea at rest, with exertion, at night
Cough

Tachycardia, a sensitive but nonspecific sign of heart failure, is caused by increased circulating endogenous catecholamines that augment cardiac output by increasing myocardial contractility and heart rate. The heart rate is increased and often fixed without respiratory variation. Sustained resting tachycardia faster than 160 beats per minute (bpm) in infants and faster than 100 bpm in children is common. Sustained heart rates faster than 220 bpm in infants and 150 bpm in children should prompt investigation into the possibility of supraventricular tachycardia, which may be the etiology of the heart failure (see Chapter 7).

Tachypnea is caused by increased pulmonary artery flow (left-to-right shunt), obstruction to pulmonary venous return (left-sided obstructive heart defects or ventricular failure), or pulmonary edema and, on occasion, the respiratory compensation for the metabolic acidosis resulting from poor perfusion. Mild to moderate degrees of hypoxemia or decreased cardiac output usually do not cause tachypnea; respiratory distress develops when either severe hypoxemia is present or cardiac output is severely diminished. When heart failure progresses and tachypnea alone cannot maintain minute ventilation, further signs of increased work of breathing develop. Crackles, uncommon in infancy, are common in children and adolescents with heart failure and represent pulmonary edema from advanced myocardial failure. Wheezing is more likely to be a result of intercurrent bronchiolitis, pneumonitis, or asthma, but it may result from large airway compression by enlarged pulmonary arteries or a dilated left atrium and bronchial edema associated with interstitial pulmonary edema.

In addition to hepatomegaly, evidence of systemic venous congestion can be seen in older children and adolescents in the presence of distention of the neck veins. In children 6 years of age or older who are sitting upright, jugular venous distention should not be visible above the clavicle unless central venous pressure is elevated. If the patient is supine at 45 degrees, jugular venous pulsations should not rise above an imaginary straight line from the clavicle across to the manubrium of the sternum. In the supine position, venous pulsations are always present unless the superior vena cava is

not connected to the right atrium, as with Glenn or Fontan palliative cardiac operations.

Cardiac examination does not always reveal *cardiomegaly.* Inspection of the precordium may reveal a prominent precordium caused by an enlarged heart. Nearly all shunt lesions are associated with increased palpable precordial activity, whereas heart failure from cardiomyopathy may have a relatively quiet precordium. The asymmetrical precordium noted in infants and children with prolonged cardiomegaly is uncommon in affected neonates. When present, a precordial prominence in the neonate is associated with lesions with altered prenatal hemodynamics, including arteriovenous malformations, tetralogy of Fallot with absence of the pulmonary valve, Ebstein anomaly with severe tricuspid insufficiency, fetal dysrhythmias, and myocarditis. A visible precordial impulse is a normal finding frequently present in full-term newborns and may result from transient patency of a ductus arteriosus. In the absence of cardiopulmonary disease, this sign frequently disappears by 12 hours after birth. A visible precordial impulse in the absence of ventricular overload is common in premature infants, in whom there is less development of anterior thoracic and abdominal musculature. Premature infants who subsequently develop left-to-right shunts through a PDA may have visible and marked precordial activity.

A third heart sound may be a common and normal auscultatory finding in children, but a fourth heart sound is never normal, and its presence is limited to advanced cardiomyopathy. A gallop rhythm may be heard in many infants with heart failure. Additional auscultatory findings, such as first and second heart sounds, clicks, rubs, and murmurs, vary, depending on the underlying reason for the heart failure (see Chapter 11).

The physical examination also defines the adequacy of the cardiac output. This is best accomplished by measuring heart rate and blood pressure and evaluating the adequacy of end-organ perfusion. Perfusion is assessed by cutaneous blood flow, central nervous system function, and urine output. A rule for minimally acceptable systolic blood pressure in patients older than 2 years has been approximated

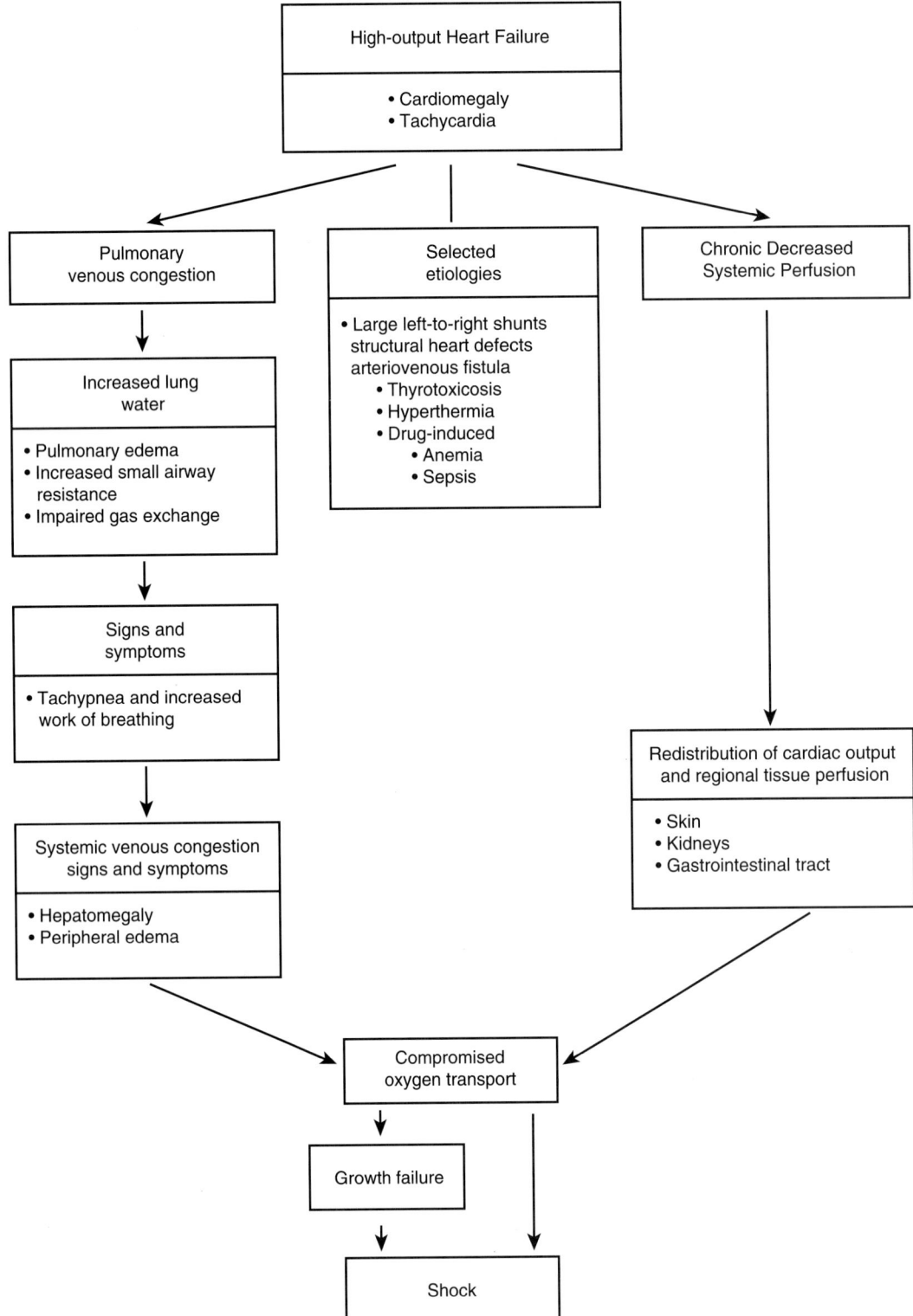

Figure 8-4. Hemodynamic classification of heart failure based on increased cardiac output. Physiologic emphasis is on abnormalities of pulmonary function that result from increased pulmonary blood flow. The majority of signs and symptoms are pulmonary. Symptoms of heart failure ensue when oxygen delivery can no longer meet metabolic demands. (From Ruggerie DP: Congestive heart failure. In Blumer J [ed]: Practical Guide to Pediatric Intensive Care, 3rd ed. St. Louis, Mosby–Year Book, 1990.)

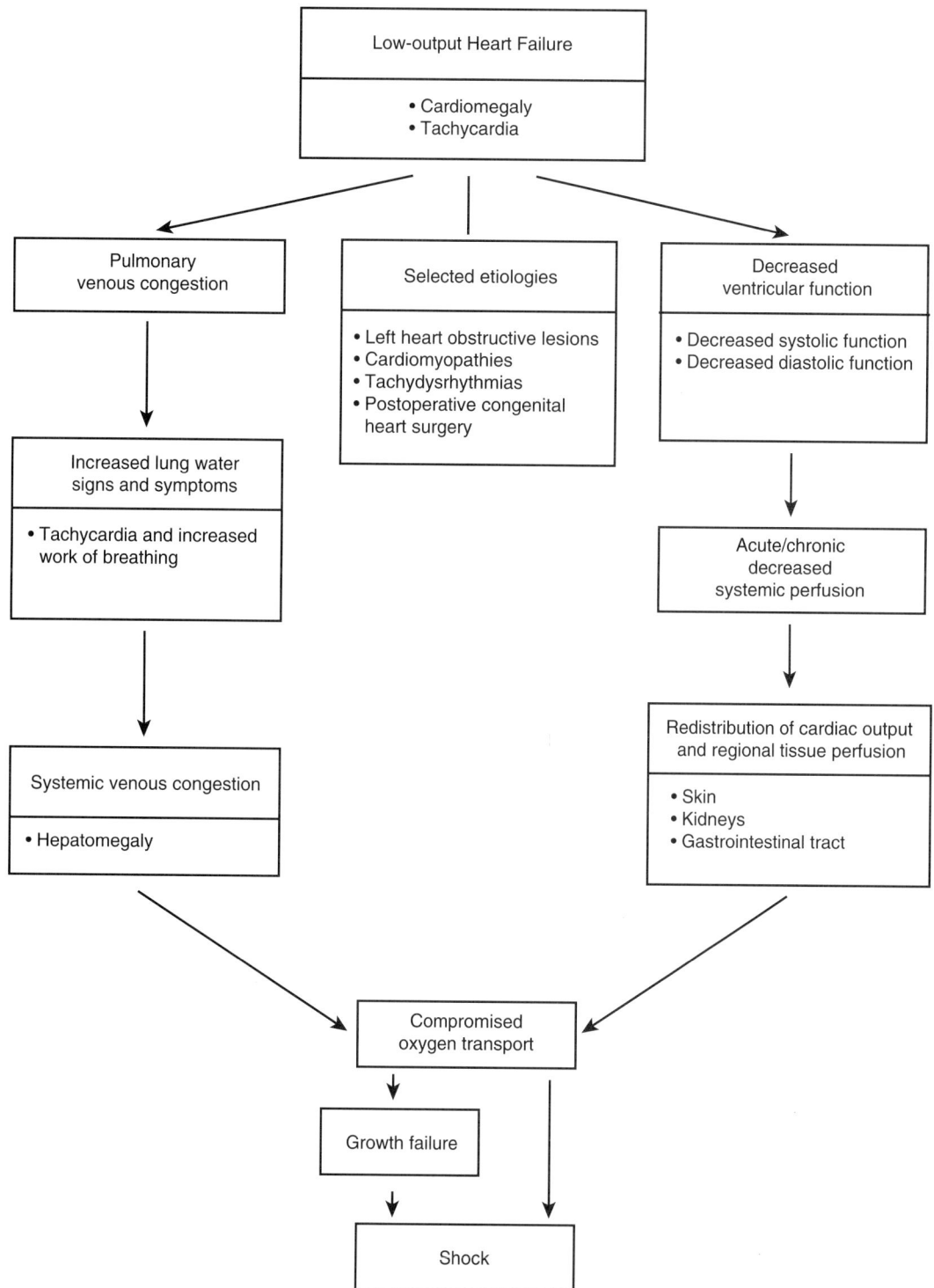

Figure 8-5. Hemodynamic classification of heart failure, based on decreased cardiac output. Physiologic emphasis is on decreased tissue perfusion and redistribution of blood flow. Once oxygen delivery can no longer meet the metabolic needs, symptoms develop.

by the formula 70 + (2 × age in years). Decreases in cardiac output are balanced by increases in heart rate and systemic vascular resistance aimed at maintaining blood pressure. Initial increases in systemic vascular resistance are clinically manifested in the extremities as prolonged capillary refill (normal < 2 to 3 seconds), cool temperature to touch, mottling or paleness of the skin, and peripheral pulses that are weaker than central pulses. Altered brain perfusion may be characterized by irritability, inconsolability, lethargy, unresponsiveness to voice or pain, and decreased muscle tone from decreased oxygen delivery. Urine output is normally 1 to 3 mL/kg/hour; oliguria indicates poor renal perfusion, hypovolemia, or acute tubular necrosis. Signs and symptoms of altered perfusion with normal blood pressure define compensated heart failure; the same manifestations with hypotension define decompensated shock.

Table 8-4. Signs and Symptoms of Heart Failure by Age

Fetus	Premature Infant	Full-Term Neonate-Infant	Child	Adolescent
Hydrops fetalis*	Tachycardia*	Tachycardia*	Breathlessness*	Same as child*
Polyhydramnios	Cardiomegaly*	Tachypnea*	Tachycardia*	Delayed sexual maturity*
Tachycardia*	Pallor*	Feeding difficulties*	Tachypnea*	Orthopnea
	Peripheral vasoconstriction*	Excessive perspiration*	Cardiomegaly*	Syncope
	Respiratory distress*	Cardiomegaly*		
	Wide pulse pressure*	Gallop rhythm*	Hepatomegaly*	Peripheral edema
	Increased oxygen requirement (cyanosis)		Peripheral edema	Rales
	Hepatomegaly	Hepatomegaly*	Eyelid puffiness	Gallop rhythm
		Failure to thrive*	Rales, wheezes cough	
		Shock*	Neck vein distention	
		Hepatic dysfunction	Fatigue, weakness	
		Wheezing	Ascites, effusion	
		Rales		
		Cough		

Adapted from Ruggerie DP: Congestive heart failure. In Blumer J (ed): Practical Guide to Pediatric Intensive Care, 3rd ed. St. Louis, Mosby–Year Book, 1990.

*Common findings.

Figure 8-7 presents a critical pathway for using pattern recognition of the symptoms of heart failure, a rapid cardiopulmonary assessment based on simple physiologic relationships of cardiac output and minute ventilation, that leads the examiner to subsequent physiologic diagnoses, etiologic diagnosis, and therapies.

ASSESSMENT AND DIAGNOSIS

LABORATORY DATA

Laboratory tests (glucose, serum electrolytes, complete blood count, blood gas analysis) help assess the severity of heart failure but rarely provide a diagnosis. Exceptions include heart failure caused by hypoglycemia, endocrine disorders, poisoning, anemia, or electrolyte disturbances. Markers of inflammation (leukocytosis, C-reactive protein, elevated sedimentation rate, and other acute-phase reactants) are helpful indicators of systemic illness but lack diagnostic specificity. The value of laboratory data includes the abilities to

- serve as a marker of specific physiologic disturbances (i.e., anemia, acidosis, hypoglycemia, hypoxemia, renal and liver dysfunction)
- guide therapeutic decisions and interventions (airway management, drug administration, transfusion therapies)
- provide a baseline against which therapies and interventions are monitored (improved acidosis, oxygenation, blood glucose, and hypokalemia, as well as hypomagnesemia that results from diuretic therapy and resolving inflammation)
- allow ongoing monitoring of anticipated alterations caused by the disease process (oxygen delivery, vital organ function, and nutritional support)

CARDIOPULMONARY MONITORING

Cardiopulmonary monitoring provides continuous heart rate, respiratory rate, and rhythm surveillance. Continuous pulse oximetry identifies oxygen needs and helps direct oxygen therapy. Blood pressure should be assessed at the initial examination and frequently thereafter in acutely ill hospitalized patients. Certain clinical conditions may demand more frequent and invasive monitoring. Cardiac output may be clinically assessed at the bedside or may be directly measured by echocardiographic techniques. Placement of a central venous catheter at the level of the right atrium and an arterial catheter permits cardiac output determination by the Fick principle or indicator dye technique. Pulmonary artery catheterization allows for thermodilution cardiac output determination.

CHEST RADIOGRAPHY

If heart failure is present, chest radiography shows an enlarged cardiac silhouette; if not, the diagnosis of heart failure should be questioned. Cardiomegaly on a chest radiograph more reliably reflects volume overload than pressure overload. Pressure overload is more reliably represented by electrocardiographic evidence of ventricular hypertrophy and by echocardiography. Pulmonary venous congestion on chest radiography suggests left-sided obstructive lesions or left ventricular failure; increased pulmonary arterial markings suggest left-to-right shunt. Cardiomegaly ("boggy water bottle heart") with normal vascular patterns suggests pericardial effusion. Pleural effusions should prompt the possibility of superior vena cava obstruction, right-sided or left-sided heart failure, or noncardiac disease.

ELECTROCARDIOGRAPHY

The electrocardiogram (ECG) is helpful in identifying ventricular hypertrophy, atrial enlargement, and changes in ST-T wave segments. Although lacking diagnostic specificity, the ECG is helpful in the diagnosis of heart failure caused by myocarditis (ST-T wave changes, decreased QRS voltage), dysrhythmia (supraventricular tachycardia, complete heart block, sick sinus syndrome), or myocardial infarction (Q-wave pattern). When ischemic ECG findings are present, the examiner must consider the diagnoses of anomalous origin of the left coronary artery, Kawasaki disease (acute or long-term sequelae), myopericarditis, cocaine ingestion, and, in the premature infant, a PDA.

Rare causes of ECG ischemia include coronary obstruction caused by metabolic heart disease, familial hypercholesterolemia, and coronary stenosis in Williams syndrome. Long-term survivors of Kawasaki disease, cardiac transplantation, and the Jantene arterial switch operation for transposition of the great vessels are populations potentially at risk for myocardial ischemia.

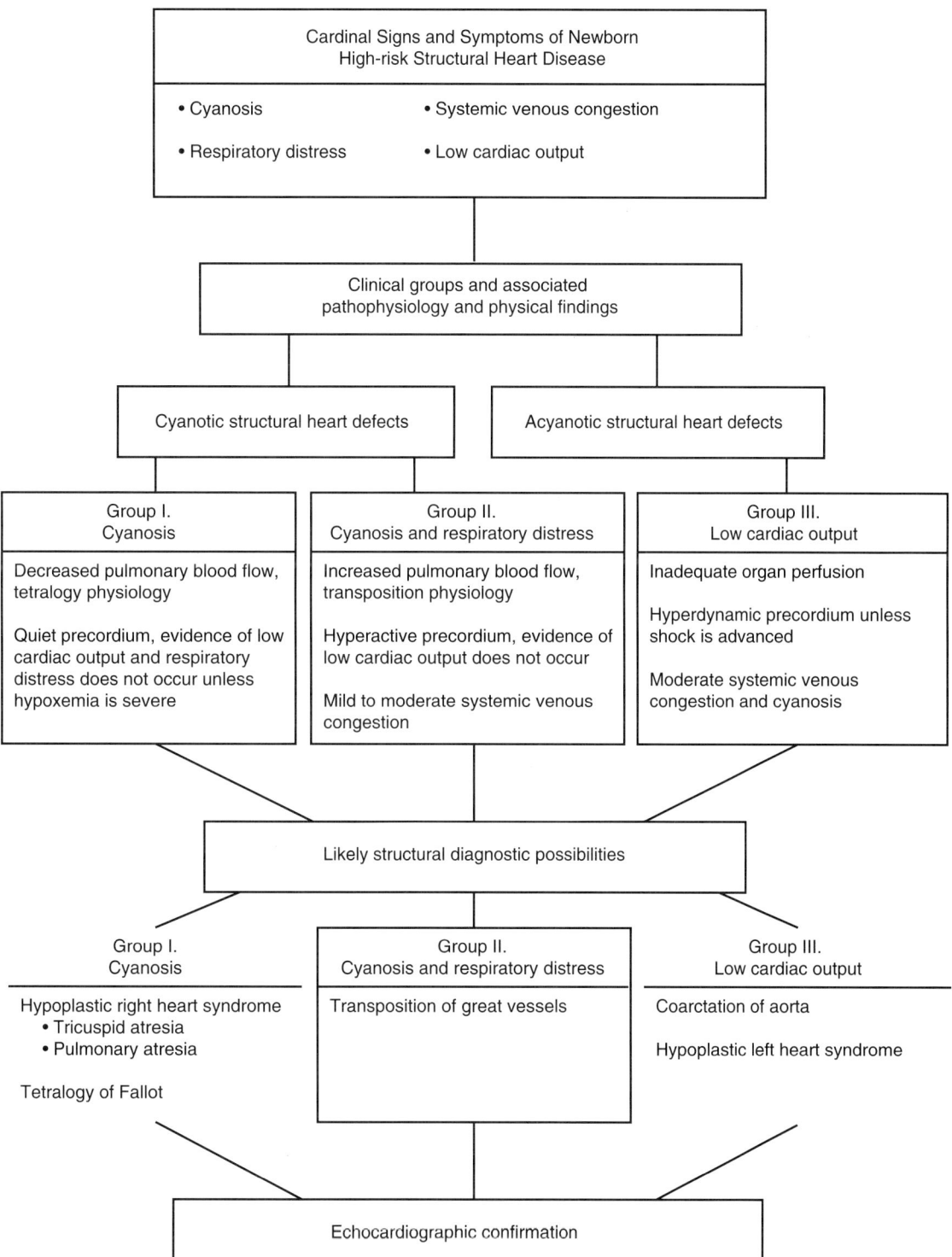

Figure 8-6. Critical pathway approach to the neonate and infant with high-risk structural heart disease.

ECHOCARDIOGRAPHY

Echocardiography is the most applicable, cost-effective imaging modality for identifying the cause of heart failure and for monitoring therapeutic interventions as well as long-term sequelae. All patients suspected of having heart failure must undergo echocardiography. Echocardiography significantly narrows the field of potential causes and usually identifies a specific diagnosis. Images may be obtained with the conventional transthoracic approach or by the transesophageal technique. Complete echocardiographic evaluation permits rapid, simultaneous acquisition of anatomic detail, blood flow analysis (Doppler color echocardiography), and hemodynamic data. Echocardiographic indices of left ventricular function include shortening fraction (normal, 30% to 40%), ejection fraction (normal, 67% ± 8%), cardiac output, and velocity of circumferential shortening (contractility index).

Table 8-5. Age-Related Normal Respiratory and Heart Rates

Age	Respiratory Rate	Heart Rate (Mean)
Premature	<60	110-180 (150)
Newborn	40-60	85-205 (140)
Infant to 2 years old	24-40	100-190 (130)
2 to 10 years old	20-24	60-140 (80)
Older than 10 years	18-20	60-100 (75)

CARDIAC CATHETERIZATION

Diagnostic catheterization is rarely needed but is beneficial when questions regarding anatomy or hemodynamics (i.e., shunt quantification, magnitude of pulmonary hypertension, degree of ventricular dysfunction) remain unanswered after echocardiographic imaging or when a discrepancy exists between clinical presentation and noninvasive diagnostic findings. Certain circumstances may require diagnostic or therapeutic catheterization. Examples include complex heart defects requiring surgical repair, balloon valvuloplasty, blade or balloon atrial septostomy to decompress the left atrium, endomyocardial biopsy in a patient with cardiomyopathy or suspected cardiac transplant rejection, and electrophysiologic catheterization with or without ablation therapy in a patient with heart failure caused by a dysrhythmia (see Chapter 7).

RADIONUCLIDE IMAGING

Radionuclide angiography and myocardial perfusion imaging are useful in assessing myocardial blood flow and function in response to exercise. As a part of long-term management, nuclear cardiac imaging may help to assess the sequelae and the efficacy of therapeutic interventions when combined with exercise (bicycle or treadmill) or pharmacologic stress exercise protocols (dipyridamole, dobutamine, or adenosine). For myocardial inflammation, gallium citrate Ga 67 has shown adequate specificity but lacks sensitivity to be clinically useful. Indium In 111–labeled antimyosin antibody has shown high sensitivity (80% to 100%) but low specificity (<60%). Therefore, myocardial biopsy remains the diagnostic procedure of choice for cardiac inflammation.

PHYSIOLOGIC BASIS FOR THERAPY OF HEART FAILURE

It is clinically useful to distinguish left-sided from right-sided heart failure and from biventricular failure. Failure of one ventricle may produce hemodynamic abnormalities of the other ventricle. Physical findings are dominated by signs and symptoms of right-sided or left-sided heart failure or both.

Another concept recognizes two hemodynamic states underlying heart failure. High-output failure often results from volume overloading conditions caused primarily by left-to-right shunts (see Fig. 8-4). Low-output failure results primarily from left-sided obstructive lesions, cardiomyopathies, and tachydysrhythmias (see Fig. 8-5). Myocardial contractility is usually, although not always, preserved in high-output failure, and the principal signs and symptoms of heart failure result from pulmonary vascular congestion and the increased work of breathing. Myocardial contractility is diminished in patients with low-output states in which principal signs and symptoms are those of markedly decreased systemic perfusion with altered vital organ function.

A third concept describes the relationship among ventricular pressure and volume, stroke volume, and the Frank-Starling law of the heart. This approach is the most useful therapeutically (Fig. 8-8). Pressure-volume diagrams relate cardiac output (stroke volume), preload, afterload, and contractility with the two phases of the cardiac cycle: systole and diastole (Fig. 8-9; see Fig. 8-8). The end-systolic pressure-volume curve represents an index of contractility. Pressure-volume loops can then be used to conceptualize a family of loops representing various contractility states (Fig. 8-10).

In a normal heart, the stroke volume increases with increasing left ventricular volume (or pressure), as noted in Figure 8-8, curve C. Heart failure, represented by the lowest curve, is caused by decreased contractility and myocardial dysfunction. Digitalis or arterial vasodilating agents move the curve upward (e.g., to A). Venodilation and diuretic agents move function to a safer position (e.g., from A to B) on the same curve, thus reducing the risk of pulmonary edema.

In addition to optimizing pressure-volume relationships, interventions may be titrated against known physiologic signs of improvement. Oxygen may be given in sufficient amounts to improve oxygen saturation; diuretics may be given to reduce edema, reduce pulmonary venous congestion, and improve urine output.

Another possible means to optimize treatment is to titrate multidrug regimens against a biochemical marker of heart failure. Brain natriuretic peptide (BNP) is produced in the cardiac ventricles in

Table 8-6. Heart Failure Without a Significant Murmur

I. **Myocarditis***

II. **Cardiomyopathy***

III. **Arrhythmias***

IV. **Severe Anemia***
   A. Sickle cell anemia
   B. Hemorrhage
   C. Fetal maternal hemorrhage
   D. Hemolytic anemias
   E. Nonproductive anemia (bone marrow hypoplasia-aplasia)

V. **Coronary Artery Lesions**
   A. Kawasaki disease: aneurysms*
   B. Anomalous origin
   C. Anomalous intramyocardial course
   D. Periarteritis nodosa
   E. Spontaneous dissection
   F. Medial necrosis
   G. Idiopathic calcification
   H. Premature arteriosclerosis (familial hyperlipidemia, after heart transplantation): ischemic cardiomyopathy
   I. Embolization-thrombosis

VI. **Congenital Heart Disease**
   A. Coarctation of aorta
   B. Critical aortic stenosis (neonate)
   C. Ebstein anomaly

VII. **Cor Pulmonale**

VIII. **Catecholamine Excess**
   A. Pheochromocytoma
   B. Drug of abuse (e.g., cocaine, amphetamine)
   C. Hyperthyroidism

IX. **Hypertension**

X. **Arteriovenous Malformation**
   A. Intracranial
   B. Hepatic
   C. Extremity
   D. Pulmonary

*Potentially common causes of heart failure without a significant heart murmur.

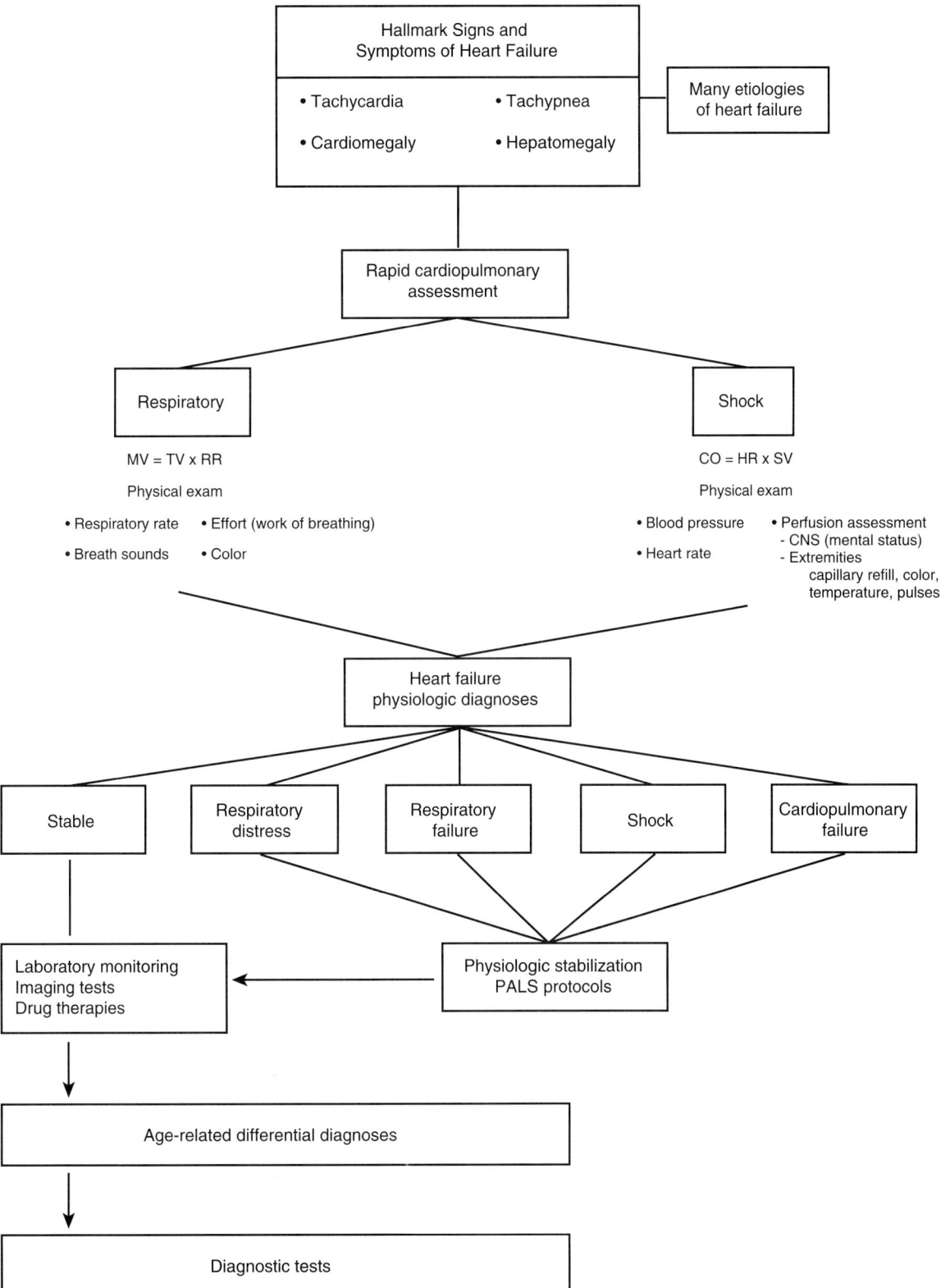

Figure 8-7. Critical pathway for heart failure diagnosis and treatment. Initial recognition and therapy rely on the "3-minute examination" and on pattern recognition of signs and symptoms. This approach allows the examiner to make the diagnosis of heart failure, institute stabilizing interventions, and even make an etiologic diagnosis. CNS, central nervous system; CO, cardiac output; HR, heart rate; MV, minute ventilation; PALS, pediatric advanced life support; RR, respiratory rate; SV, stroke volume; TV, tidal volume.

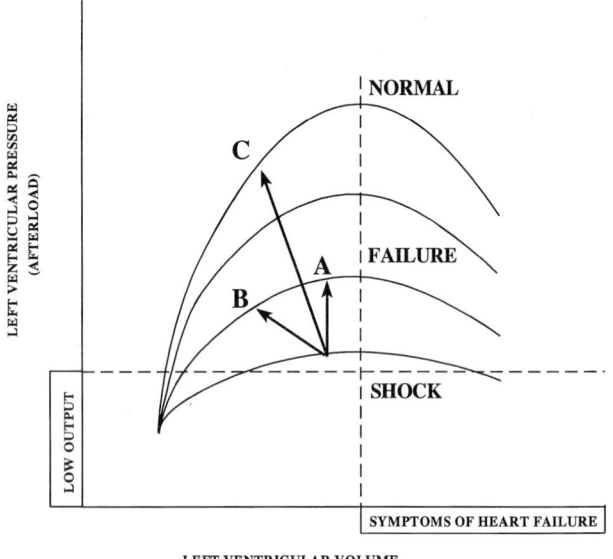

Figure 8-8. Effects of inotropic and afterload-reducing agents on ventricular function curve. Beginning on the shock curve, positive inotropic stimulation improves cardiac performance to point A and afterload reduction to point B. Combination therapy (point C) enhances cardiac performance to a greater degree than does therapy focused on a single determinant of cardiac output. (Adapted from Friedman WF, George BL: Treatment of congestive heart failure by altering loading conditions of the heart. J Pediatr 1985;106:704.)

response to increased transmural wall stress. BNP (like atrial natriuretic peptide) increases the glomerular filtration rate and sodium excretion. It also produces peripheral vasodilation and decreases neurohumoral responses to heart failure; plasma levels predict left ventricular function. Using improvements in plasma levels of BNP as a surrogate end point helps guide therapy in adults with heart failure.

TREATMENT

Treatment includes supportive, symptomatic, pharmacologic, mechanical, and surgical approaches (Table 8-7). The goals of therapy are to restore the balance between sodium and free water, to optimize vascular tone (preload and afterload), to improve myocardial performance (heart rate and contractility), and to accomplish these goals in a cost-effective manner.

SYMPTOMATIC TREATMENT

Symptomatic measures address oxygen needs and correction of metabolic, hematologic, and endocrine abnormalities adversely affecting cardiac performance. These may involve positioning the patient to maintain minute ventilation, maintaining normothermia, and administering supplemental oxygen, glucose, calcium, or magnesium. Oxygen should be given, but it should be administered cautiously in patients with a left-to-right shunt because oxygen-induced pulmonary vasodilation may potentially worsen the shunting. Patients with anemia may require a transfusion, and those with polycythemia may require partial exchange transfusion or phlebotomy, which thereby reduces viscosity and enhances oxygen delivery. Specific management of systemic illness, such as sepsis, Kawasaki disease, collagen vascular disease, trauma, and envenomation, is indicated with antibiotics, aspirin and gamma globulin, steroids, neurocardiopulmonary resuscitation, and antivenin, respectively.

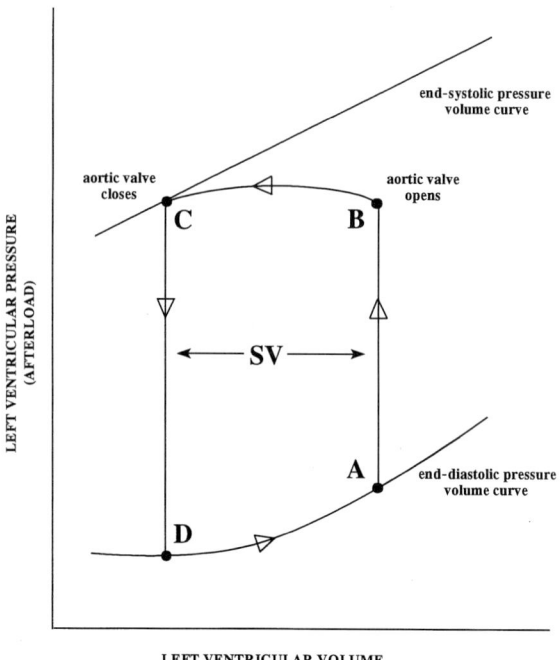

Figure 8-9. Pressure-volume loop. Contraction begins at point A, representing end-diastolic volume preload. Isovolumetric contraction occurs along line A to B. At point B, the aortic valve opens and ejection begins. Ejection ends at point C, at which the aortic valve closes. Isovolumetric relaxation occurs along line C to D, with a fall in ventricular pressure. At point D, the mitral valve opens to fill the left ventricle, generating the preload for the next cardiac cycle. Stroke volume (SV) is represented by the distance from line CD to AB. A similar curve can be drawn for the right ventricle. The end-systolic pressure-volume curve is a measure of contractility. The end-diastolic pressure-volume curve represents the Frank-Starling relationship.

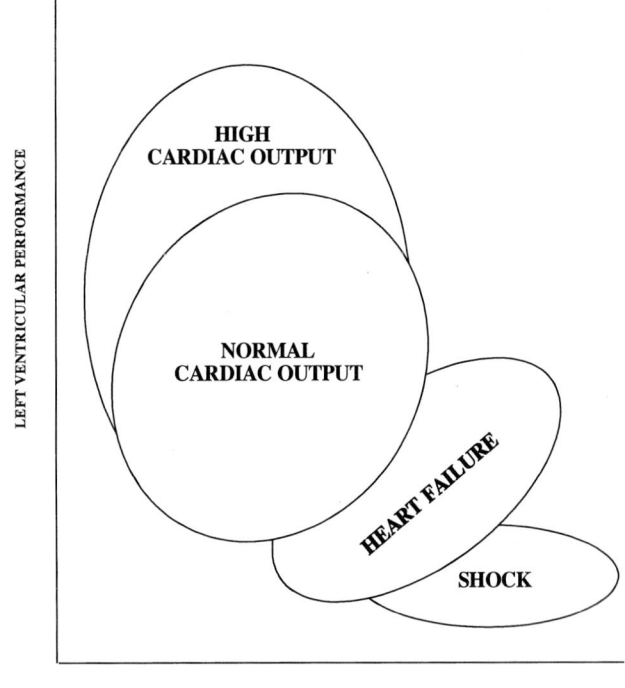

Figure 8-10. A family of pressure-volume loops representing various contractility states.

Table 8-7. Treatment of Heart Failure	
Therapy	**Mechanism**
General Care	
Rest	Reduces cardiac output
Oxygen	Improves oxygenation in presence of pulmonary edema
Sodium, fluid restrictions	Decreases vascular congestion; decreases preload
Diuretics	
Furosemide	Increases salt excretion by ascending loop of Henle; reduces preload; afterload reduced if hypertension improves; also may cause venodilation
Combination of distal tubule and loop diuretics	Increases sodium excretion
Spironolactone	Inhibits angiotensin II action
Inotropic Agents	
Digitalis	Inhibits membrane Na^+,K^+-ATPase and increases intracellular Ca^{2+}; improves cardiac contractility; increases myocardial oxygen consumption
Dopamine	Releases myocardial norepinephrine plus direct effect on β receptor; may increase systemic blood pressure; at low infusion rates, dilates renal artery, facilitating diuresis
Dobutamine	β ($β_1$)-receptor agent; often combined with dopamine
Amrinone	Nonsympathomimetic, noncardiac glycosides with inotropic effects; also may produce vasodilation
Afterload Reduction	
Hydralazine	Arteriolar vasodilation
Nitroprusside	Arterial and venous relaxation; venodilation reduces preload
Prazosin	Oral α-adrenergic blocking agent; arterial and venous dilator; venodilation reduces preload
Captopril/enalapril	Inhibition of angiotensin-converting enzyme; reduces angiotensin II production
β-Adrenergic Blocking Agents	
Carvedilol	Nonselective β blocker with α-adrenergic blocking properties; also an antioxidant; controls excessive-persistent neurohumoral cardiac stimulation
Propranolol	Classic β blocker; reduces rate and inotropy; useful in hypertrophic cardiomyopathy and cardiomyopathy of IDMs

Modified from Behrman RE, Kliegman RM (eds): Nelson Essentials of Pediatrics, 2nd ed. Philadelphia, WB Saunders, 1994.

IDMs, infants of diabetic mothers.

DRUG THERAPY

Drug therapy is the cornerstone of management (Table 8-8; see Table 8-7). The initial pharmacologic approach is directed by physiologic assessment and stabilization. Drug therapy targets the determinants of cardiac output, as well as alterations in salt and water balance.

MULTIPLE THERAPIES

Multiple drug therapies improve ventricular function to a greater extent than does therapy focused on a single determinant of cardiac output. This is because the failing circulation typically has multiple hemodynamic abnormalities. Multimodal pharmacodynamic effects may be obtained by combining agents such as digoxin and a diuretic, digoxin and captopril, or, in more severe life-threatening disease, epinephrine and nitroprusside, or by using single agents with multiple effects, such as dobutamine and amrinone. Unless there is heart block or a tachyarrhythmia, treatment is not directed at the heart rate component of cardiac output. With successful therapy, sinus tachycardia may resolve.

Diuretics are most useful if circulatory congestion (pulmonary overcirculation edema, peripheral edema) is present. In addition to producing diuresis, furosemide also reduces venous return by rapid vasodilation, thus reducing fluid overload even before the actual diuresis. Preload is the most commonly manipulated determinant of stroke volume. The right ventricle appears to be more readily responsive to afterload reduction than to inotropic stimulation, whereas the left ventricle appears equally responsive to modulation of either determinant. If there is biventricular failure, positive inotropic agents may improve right ventricular performance by reducing the portion of right-sided heart dysfunction that is attributable to impaired left-sided heart function.

Patients with chronic heart failure may be given oral furosemide (2 mg/kg/24 hours divided b.i.d.). The hypokalemia and metabolic alkalosis associated with chronic diuretic therapy can be minimized with the addition of spironolactone. Hyperkalemia can potentially occur, especially with the use of spironolactone in combination with oral potassium replacement therapy or angiotensin-converting enzyme inhibitors. Renal calculi can be minimized with the use of alternative diuretics such as hydrochlorothiazide.

INOTROPIC AGENTS

There are three classes of inotropic agents: cardiac glycosides, catecholamines, and phosphodiesterase inhibitors. Figure 8-11 outlines a rational use of inotropic agents in heart failure.

Cardiac Glycosides

Digoxin is an important agent for the long-term therapy of chronic heart failure. Digoxin has a low toxic-therapeutic index, a long half-life, and a slow onset of action and is arrhythmogenic. In addition, altered renal function and hence altered renal elimination make its administration challenging. Electrolyte abnormalities (hypokalemia) may further potentiate the toxicity of digoxin.

The mechanism of action of digoxin involves blockage of the myocardial cellular sodium-potassium pump with resultant uptake of calcium into the cells by means of a sodium-calcium exchange mechanism. The increased intracellular concentration of calcium allows for more actin and myosin cross bridges to form during the activation of cardiac muscle, thereby increasing the efficiency of contraction (inotropic). The typical maintenance dose of digoxin is 8 to 10 μg/kg/24 hours divided b.i.d. The maximum dose in children should be 100 to 150 μg/24 hours. A small adult should receive 125 μg/24 hours, whereas the typical adult dose is 250 μg/24 hours.

Table 8-8. Dosage of Drugs Commonly Used for the Treatment of Congestive Heart Failure

Drug	Dosage
Digoxin	
Digitalization (PO) (3 doses q8h)	Premature: 0.02-0.025 mg/kg
	Neonate (≤1 mo): 0.03-0.04 mg/kg
	Infant or child: 0.04-0.06 mg/kg
	Adolescent or adult: 1.0-1.5 mg in divided doses
Digitalization (IV) (timing of dosage variable, depending on clinical indications)	75% of PO dose
Maintenance	¼-⅓ of digitalizing dose, divided q12h
Furosemide	
IV	1-2 mg/kg/dose, prn
PO	1-4 mg/kg/24 hr, q.d., b.i.d., or q.i.d.
Bumetanide	
IV	0.01-0.2 mg/kg/dose
PO	0.04-0.8 mg/kg/24 hr, q6-8h
Chlorothiazide (PO)	20-50 mg/kg/24 hr, b.i.d., or q.i.d.
Spironolactone (PO)	2-3 mg/kg/24 hr, b.i.d.
β Agonists (IV)	
Isoproterenol	0.01-0.5 µg/kg/min
Dopamine	2-20 µg/kg/min
Dobutamine	2-20 µg/kg/min
Amrinone (IV)	0.75 mg/kg bolus 5-10 µg/kg
Afterload-reducing agents	
Nitroprusside (IV)	0.5-8 µg/kg/min
Hydralazine	
IV	0.5 mg/kg
PO	0.5-7.5 mg/kg/24 hr, t.i.d.
Captopril (PO)	0.5-6 mg/kg/24 hr, q.i.d.
β-Blocking agents	
Carvedilol	0.08 mg/kg/24 hr, b.i.d. initial dose, titrated doubling every 2 wk
	0.46 mg/kg/24 hr, b.i.d. maintenance dose
Propranolol	0.01-0.10 mg/kg dose IV, repeat q6-8h prn
	0.5-4 mg/kg/24 hr, PO q6-8h

Modified from Behrman RE (ed): Nelson Textbook of Pediatrics, 14th ed. Philadelphia, WB Saunders, 1992, p 1214.

IV, intravenous; PO, orally; prn, as needed.

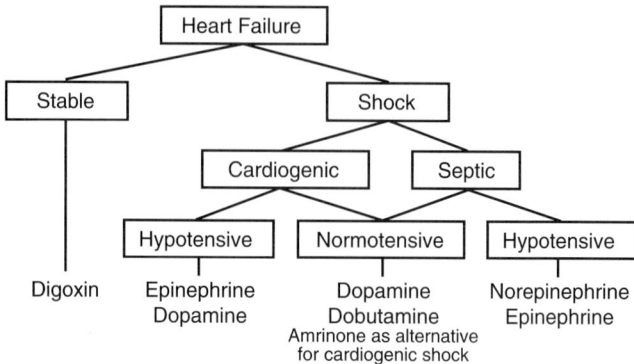

Figure 8-11. Suggested initial selection of inotropic agents.

increased myocardial oxygen consumption, and, in rare cases, a catecholamine-induced hypertrophic cardiomyopathy (HCM).

Dopamine can improve contractility and at lower doses may improve renal perfusion by renal arterial vasodilation. Dobutamine has a greater effect on heart rate and contractility and may also have an afterload-reducing effect at lower doses. Epinephrine tends to have an inotropic effect at lower doses but causes potent vasoconstriction at higher doses. Catecholamines with both inotropic and chronotropic effects can increase left ventricular outflow obstruction in patients with HCM and in infants of diabetic mothers. Catecholamines can increase right ventricular obstruction in patients with tetralogy of Fallot, especially during a cyanotic spell.

Phosphodiesterase Inhibitors

These inotropic agents (amrinone and milrinone) have the added benefit of being peripheral vasodilators and, therefore, afterload-reducing agents. Advantages include a nonadrenergic mechanism and the combined effects of inotropic and afterload reduction unaffected by β-adrenergic downregulation. Disadvantages include hypotension and thrombocytopenia; the latter is less common with milrinone.

AFTERLOAD-REDUCING AGENTS

There is a physiologic rationale for the use of afterload-reducing agents in the therapy of heart failure when afterload is abnormally elevated. According to Laplace's law, any condition that results in excessive dilatation of the left ventricle will also result in an increase in wall tension. This can occur in DCM or with severe AV valve regurgitation and ventricular dilatation. Therefore, vasodilator or afterload reduction therapy along with other therapies has the potential to increase the cardiac output.

There are three classes of vasodilators. Venous dilators such as nitroglycerin reduce preload. They have relatively little effect on afterload. Sodium nitroprusside has dilator effects on both preload and afterload and therefore is a mixed vasodilator. It has potent effects as an arterial vasodilator and has the ability to increase cardiac output in situations of elevated afterload. It is administered as continuous intravenous drip, and it can be titrated to a desired effect.

Chronic afterload reduction is an important part of the therapy for heart failure and typically employs the use of angiotensin-converting enzyme inhibition with agents such as captopril, enalapril, or lisinopril. These medications can be given orally, and with the blockade of angiotensin II production (a potent vasoconstrictor), systemic afterload is reduced and hence cardiac output can be improved. These medications are not given to patients with right-to-left shunts because they can worsen the cyanosis by increasing systemic output at the expense of pulmonary blood flow. Angiotensin-converting enzyme inhibitors are relatively contraindicated in patients with

Catecholamines

Catecholamines by continuous intravenous drip are an important class of drugs for the critically ill patient in the intensive care unit with low cardiac output. They work rapidly and continuously, and the dosage can be titrated to the desired effect. Side effects include tachycardia, arrhythmias, excessive vasoconstriction, renal compromise. These agents are also contraindicated in patients with bilateral renovascular hypertension or unilateral vascular disease in a solitary kidney. This class of drugs tends to be most effective in patients with congestive heart failure secondary to myocardial dysfunction, as well as in most patients with systemic hypertension. In addition, it has been administered successfully to patients with intracardiac left-to-right shunts. Side effects include hypotension, rash, cough, and throat pain. Angiotensin receptor blocking agents are also effective; there is little clinical experience in children.

β-ADRENERGIC RECEPTOR BLOCKADE

Low-dose β blockade is a promising therapy for patients with chronic, severe heart failure, usually in the setting of DCM. Studies have shown that β blockade seems to upregulate β receptors and may actually allow more receptors to become available on the cell surface, increasing overall contractility. It has also been suggested that the chronically elevated levels of circulating catecholamines in patients with heart failure produce β-receptor downregulation as well as direct myocardial damage. These observations support the use of β blockade in the situation of chronic DCM. Clinical studies performed in adults with DCM have suggested that carvedilol, a β blocker that also has free radical scavenger effects, may be superior to other β blockers. This may support the theory that ongoing myocardial damage in chronic DCM may be a result of both circulating catecholamines as well as free radicals.

The efficacy of β-blocker therapy for children with heart failure has not been clearly established, although some studies advocate their use. The dose should be progressively increased every few weeks, and the drug should not be abruptly discontinued (see Table 8-8). β-Blocking agents have also been effective in conditions in which dynamic contraction of the left ventricle increases a preexisting left ventricle obstruction, as noted in HCM and in the cardiomyopathy of the infant of a diabetic mother.

SURGICAL MANAGEMENT/MECHANICAL PALLIATION

Specific surgical management depends on the underlying cause of heart failure. If heart failure is secondary to a congenital heart defect, surgical repair of the heart defect is often the treatment of choice. An excellent prognosis should be expected for the surgical repair of most congenital heart defects. It is appropriate to stabilize the patient with medical therapy initially, before early surgical intervention (see Chapters 10 and 11). Examples include transposition of the great arteries, ventricular septal defect, TAPVR, atrial septal defect, PDA, interrupted aortic arch, ALCAPA, coarctation of the aorta, hypoplastic left heart syndrome, and truncus arteriosus.

Cardiac transplantation may be the only effective therapy for patients with end-stage cardiomyopathy, complex congenital heart anomalies, or other forms of heart disease causing severe heart failure when symptoms are unresponsive to aggressive medical therapy. Currently in affected children, the 1-year survival rate is 80% to 85%, the 5-year survival rate is 70%, and the 10-year survival rate is 50% to 60%. Donor shortage and potential long-term complications such as rejection, infection, post-transplantation lymphoproliferative disease, and graft coronary artery atherosclerosis limit the long-term success of transplantation.

Alternative surgical therapies have been reported in adults with DCM. Both left ventricular volume reduction surgery (the Batista operation) and the latissimus dorsi wrap have been reported to yield success; there is little experience in children. The rationale for the former approach is based on Laplace's law. Surgical resection of the free wall of the extremely dilated left ventricle along with mitral valve repair would theoretically improve wall tension and might allow for remodeling of the left ventricle. Although the mortality rate with this approach is high, there have been several reports in adults that suggest that in a select group of patients with DCM, improvement

in left ventricular function can occur, symptoms can improve, and cardiac transplantation can be avoided.

Mechanical support of the heart is an important palliative or bridging procedure in the pediatric population. It is appropriate to use support such as extracorporeal membrane oxygenation (ECMO) in the critically ill patient with severe heart failure that is unresponsive to medical therapy. This intervention can be coupled with corrective surgical intervention for patients with congenital heart disease or can be used as a short-term bridge to transplantation in patients with end-stage heart failure. In patients with acute, severe myocarditis, ECMO or other mechanical support devices, coupled with left-sided heart decompression either surgically or through a transcatheter approach, can be used to "rest" the heart and allow for recovery.

Longer term support with mechanical devices other than ECMO also exists for children. Most devices are limited by patient size. The youngest patient supported with such a long-term device was 7 years of age. ECMO support can be used for 1 to 3 weeks before a complication such as bleeding or infection limits the length of therapy. Implantable mechanical devices are designed for use for several months.

DIFFERENTIAL DIAGNOSIS: SPECIFIC DISEASE PROCESS

Age at heart failure presentation is an initial guide to identifying common causes. Table 8-2 provides expanded etiologic features, including common and uncommon causes; Table 8-6 and Table 8-9 present more in-depth comparisons.

CONGENITAL HEART DISEASE

Congenital heart defects are the most common cause of heart failure in infancy and childhood. Of infants with significant structural heart disease, 80% manifest heart failure. Approximately 50% of critically ill infants have one of the following high-risk cardiac defects, which manifest as heart failure with or without cyanosis:

- hypoplastic left heart syndrome
- coarctation of the aorta
- transposition of the great vessels
- truncus arteriosus
- single ventricle

Low-risk lesions are simple left-to-right shunt lesions. Ventricular septal defect and PDA are the two most common defects (left-to-right shunts) manifesting with heart failure in infancy. Although atrial septal defects are frequently diagnosed in young children or adolescents, 10% of symptomatic atrial septal defects manifest in infants younger than 1 year of age.

The signs and symptoms of neonatal heart disease are

- central cyanosis
- respiratory distress
- systemic venous congestion
- low cardiac output

Heart murmurs are not consistently the presenting sign; murmurs may be soft even in the sickest neonates (see Chapter 11).

Central cyanosis caused by cardiac disease is the result of right-to-left shunting in which systemic venous (blue) blood does not enter the lungs but is shunted to the left side of the heart and into the systemic circulation (see Chapter 10). As a result of right-to-left shunting, cyanosis occurs in structural defects associated with right-sided heart obstruction, resulting in decreased total pulmonary blood flow, sometimes referred to as *tetralogy physiology*. Heart failure is unusual with tetralogy physiology. Central cyanosis may also occur in complex cardiac defects in which fully oxygenated (red) blood

Table 8-9. Etiology of Myocardial Disease

Familial-Hereditary

Carnitine deficiency syndromes*
Mitochondrial myopathy syndromes*
Hypertrophic cardiomyopathy*
Dilated cardiomyopathy*
Arrhythmogenic right ventricular dysplasia
Barth syndrome
Duchenne muscular dystrophy*
Other muscular dystrophies (Becker, limb girdle)
Myotonic dystrophy
Kearns-Sayre syndrome (progressive external
  ophthalmoplegia)
Friedreich ataxia
Mucopolysaccharidosis
Hemochromatosis
Fabry disease
Pompe disease (glycogen storage disease)
Primary endocardial fibroelastosis
Mucopolysaccharidosis (Hurler, Hunter, others)

Infection

Viruses: coxsackievirus A and B,* human immunodeficiency
  virus (AIDS), echovirus, rubella, varicella, influenza, mumps,
  Epstein-Barr virus, measles, poliomyelitis
Rickettsiae: Coxiella, Rocky Mountain spotted fever, typhus
Bacteria: diphtheria, *Mycoplasma,* meningococcus,
  leptospirosis, Lyme disease, typhoid fever, tuberculosis,
  streptococcus, listeriosis, psittacosis
Parasites: Chagas disease, toxoplasmosis, *Loa loa, Toxocara
  canis,* schistosomiasis, cysticercosis, *Echinococcus,* trichinosis
Fungi: histoplasmosis, coccidioidomycosis, actinomycosis

Metabolic, Nutritional, Endocrine

Beriberi (thiamine deficiency)
Keshan disease (selenium deficiency)
Kwashiorkor
Hypothyroidism
Hyperthyroidism
Carcinoid
Pheochromocytoma
Hypercholesterolemia
Infant of diabetic mother*
Hypoglycemia
Hypocalcemia
Type II X-linked 3-methylglutaconic aciduria

Connective Tissue–Granulomatous Disease

Systemic lupus erythematosus
Scleroderma
Churg-Strauss vasculitis
Rheumatoid arthritis
Rheumatic fever*
Sarcoidosis
Amyloidosis
Dermatomyositis
Periarteritis nodosa

Drugs-Toxins

Doxorubicin*
Cyclophosphamide
Chloroquine
Ipecac (emetine)
Iron overload (hemosiderosis)
Sulfonamides
Mesalazine
Chloramphenicol
Hypersensitivity reaction (penicillin)
Alcohol
Irradiation
Envenomations (snake, scorpion)

Coronary Arteries

Kawasaki disease*
Medial necrosis
Anomalous left coronary artery

Other

Anemia*
Sickle cell anemia (sickling)*
Hypertension*
Cor pulmonale*
Hypereosinophilic syndrome (Loeffler syndrome)
Tachyarrhythmias*
Endomyocardial fibrosis
Ischemia-hypoxia
Peripartum cardiomyopathy
Idiopathic dilated cardiomyopathy
Arrhythmogenic right ventricular dysplasia (nonfamilial)
Uhl right ventricular anomaly
Histiocytoid (oncocytic, lipidosis) cardiomyopathy
Acute eosinophilic necrotizing myocarditis
Rhabdomyoma
Left ventricular noncompaction

Adapted from Behrman RE (ed): Nelson Textbook of Pediatrics, 14th ed. Philadelphia, WB Saunders, 1992.
*Relatively common causes of myocarditis-cardiomyopathy.

mixes at the ventricular level with systemic venous (blue) blood via a large ventricular septal defect, which results in recirculation of a mixture of oxygenated and unoxygenated blood into the pulmonary and systemic circulations (see Table 8-2). Therefore, fully oxygenated blood recirculates to the lungs and does not reach the systemic circulation, which instead receives mainly unoxygenated blood returning from the body, and this results in central cyanosis. This type of cardiac shunting is known as *transposition physiology.* In these lesions, as pulmonary vascular resistance falls, and in the absence of pulmonary obstruction, total pulmonary blood flow increases, which results in heart failure with cyanosis.

An approach to differentiating causes of heart failure in the high-risk neonate is noted in Figure 8-6.

MYOCARDITIS

Myocarditis is an enigmatic disease. Manifestation is variable, ranging from an acute presentation with fever, malaise, heart failure, and dysrhythmia to a chronic end-stage DCM.

Diagnosis relies on clinical suspicion. The "gold standard" for diagnosis is evidence of myocardial inflammation by endomyocardial biopsy and, less persuasive, by nuclear scintigraphy. Newer molecular techniques (polymerase chain reaction amplification of viral genomes in myocardial biopsy specimens) help increase the sensitivity and specificity of diagnostic criteria and help target new therapy.

Treatment involves supportive efforts (diuretics, digoxin, captopril), rest, anticoagulation if indicated, and evaluation for cardiac transplantation for some patients. Immunosuppression (with prednisone and/or cyclosporine) is controversial but may be useful as a short-term measure for the sickest patients. If enteroviruses are identified, the patient should be treated with the effective antiviral agent pleconaril. Considerable evidence suggests a link between acute viral myocarditis and the later onset of idiopathic DCM (see later section on DCM).

CARDIOMYOPATHY

Cardiomyopathy is a primary disease of the myocardium and is classified as hypertrophic (HCM), dilated (DCM), arrhythmogenic right ventricular (ARVC), and restrictive (RCM) (Table 8-10). Overall DCM is more comon than HCM; together they make up 80% to 90% of all pediatric cardiomyopathies. Other categories with some overlap with this classification include familial, metabolic storage (Pompe disease, carnitine deficiency), postpartum, hypersensitivity (eosinophilic), toxic (daunorubicin), and unclassified cardiomyopathies. Cardiomyopathies may be caused by abnormalities in the cardiac myocyte cytoskeleton (sarcomeres, desmoglobin), or in the ability to generate (mitochondria DNA mutations) or utilize

energy (actin, myosin mutations). Risks associated with all cardiomyopathies include heart failure, arrhythmias, sudden death, syncope, and end-stage heart disease. Possible causes and an approach to diagnosis are noted in Tables 8-9 and 8-10 and Figure 8-12.

HYPERTROPHIC CARDIOMYOPATHY

HCM is linked to specific genetic defects in myosin, dystrophin, or other cardiac muscle components (see Table 8-10). HCM is familial in 50% of patients; other cases may represent new sporadic mutations. There are more than 10 genes associated with HCM and multiple (>130) allelic mutations for these genes, and thus there is a wide spectrum of severity. The typical echocardiographic findings include asymmetrical hypertrophy of the intraventricular septum of varying degrees; systolic anterior motion of the mitral valve, which can contribute to obstruction of the left ventricular outflow tract; and mitral insufficiency. HCM can be progressive and at its later stages may evolve into a DCM.

The majority of patients with HCM are asymptomatic and are identified either because of a known symptomatic family member, which prompts screening, or because of referral for a heart murmur. The majority of children do not have left ventricular outflow tract obstruction; its presence results in a loud systolic murmur. A minority of children are symptomatic, usually with symptoms of tiredness and

Table 8-10. Cardiomyopathies

Features	Dilated Cardiomyopathy	Hypertrophic Cardiomyopathy	Arrhythmogenic Right Ventricular Cardiomyopathy	Restrictive Cardiomyopathy
Prevalence	50:100,000	1:500	Unknown	Unknown
Familial	30%: AD, AR, X-L, Mt	50%: AD	30%: AD, rare AR (Naxos disease)	Unknown
Genes	Dystrophin Tafazzin Troponin T Sarcoglycan Actin Lamin A/C Desmin tRNA-Lys	β myosin heavy chain Troponin T or I α-Tropomysin Myosin binding protein C Actin Myosin light chain 1 or 2	Plakoglobin Desmoplakin Ryanodine receptor	None identified
Sudden death	Yes	Depends on gene 0.7%-11% per year ↑ with exercise	Yes	1.5% per year
Arrhythmias	Atrial and ventricular and conduction disturbances	Atrial and ventricular	Ventricular and conduction disturbances	Atrial fibrillation
Ventricle function	Systolic and diastolic dysfunction	Diastolic dysfunction Dynamic systolic outflow obstruction	Normal to reduced systolic Reduced diastolic	Severely reduced diastolic
Diagnosis	Dilated left ventricular cavity with normal to thin wall thickness	Asymmetrical left ventricular hypertrophy	Right ventricular fibrofatty replacement on biopsy, right ventricular dilation	Normal or reduced ventricles cavity size and thickness Biatrial enlargement
Management	ACE inhibitors, spironolactone, β-blocking agents ICD Transplantation	Propranolol Pacemaker ICD Surgery Transplantation	β-Blocking agents, class III antiarrhythmic agents Catheter ablation ICD Transplantation	Antiarrhythmic agents support diastolic dysfunction ICD Transplantation

ACE, angiotensin-converting enzyme; AD, autosomal dominant inheritance; AR, autosomal recessive inheritance; ICD, implantable cardiac defibrillator; Mt, mitochondrial inheritance; X-L, X-linked inheritance.

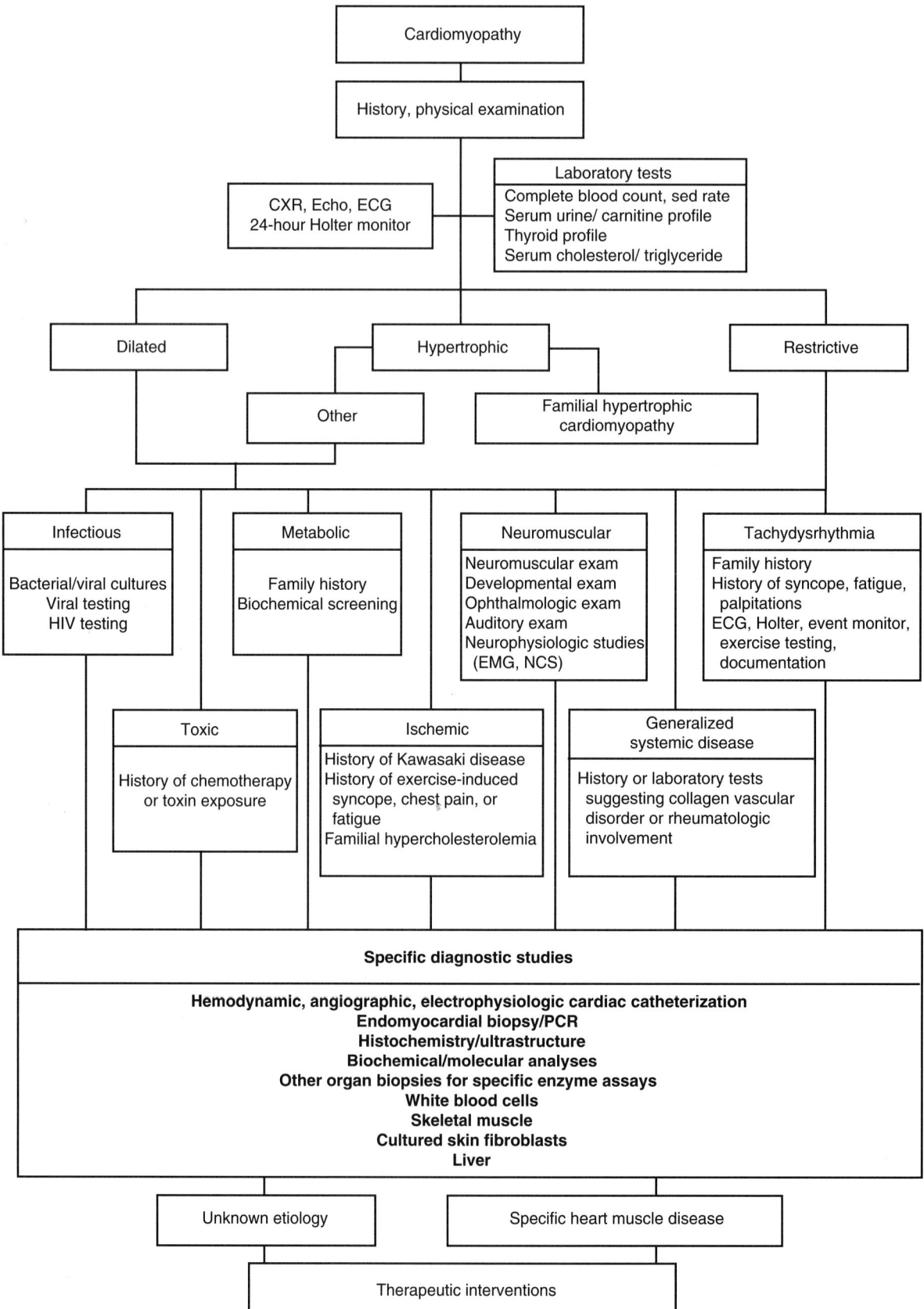

Figure 8-12. Cardiomyopathy critical pathway; unknown versus specific heart muscle disorders. The metabolic category includes endocrine causes. CXR, chest roentgenogram; ECG, electrocardiogram; Echo, echocardiogram; EMG, electromyography; HIV, human immunodeficiency virus; NCS, nerve conduction studies; PCR, polymerase chain reaction; sed, sedimentation.

activity intolerance. Chest pain, dizziness, or syncope are serious symptoms and may be indicative of ischemia and/or arrhythmias. Sudden cardiac death is a well-known risk. Risk factors for sudden cardiac death include a positive family history of HCM or of sudden cardiac death, previous episodes of syncope, a high degree of left ventricular wall thickness, a fall in blood pressure with exercise, specific genes (β-myosin heavy chain, troponin T or I, α-tropomysin carry the highest risks), and documented ventricular arrhythmias.

Patients with HCM should avoid competitive sports and strenuous exercise. β-blocker therapy and/or implantable cardoverter-defibrillator (ICD) placement may be appropriate for patients with symptoms or in the higher risk category. Significant left ventricular outflow tract obstruction from septal hypertrophy and/or systolic anterior motion may necessitate intervention either because of symptoms or because of progressive severe obstruction. Calcium channel blockers such as verapamil may be used. β-blockers and calcium channel blockers do not eliminate the risk of sudden death. Myomectomy surgery may be performed if the obstruction is related primarily to outflow obstruction from muscle hypertrophy. If systolic anterior motion appears to be the major mechanism of severe obstruction, mitral valve replacement may be necessary. In situations in which HCM progresses to a severe, symptomatic DCM or in which life-threatening arrhythmias persist, cardiac transplantation may be recommended.

DILATED CARDIOMYOPATHY

DCM is an abnormality of the heart muscle characterized by systolic ventricular dysfunction. It manifests with heart failure or cardiomegaly without a significant murmur. The majority of pediatric cases of DCM are idiopathic. However, many of the cases of chronic idiopathic DCM may be linked to an earlier presentation of acute viral myocarditis. There is also increasing evidence that some cases may be genetically linked and familial. It is critical to consider the different origins of DCM so that a treatable cause is not overlooked. For example, a careful analysis of the coronary artery anatomy is essential in every patient with a diagnosis of DCM so that ALCAPA is ruled out. Other rare treatable causes of DCM include chronic atrial tachycardias and carnitine deficiency. In the former, it may be difficult to determine whether the tachyarrhythmia is secondary to the cardiomyopathy or the cause of the cardiomyopathy. Aggressive treatment of the tachycardia may improve symptoms and may reverse the cardiomyopathic process.

Myocarditis may be the most common precursor to DCM in children. Its manifestation can be quite variable, ranging from early presentation with fever and lethargy and progressing to heart failure and arrhythmias. Manifestation can also be very mild or can involve symptoms of severe low cardiac output, shock, and death. Myocarditis is most commonly viral in origin; coxsackievirus B and adenovirus are the most frequent etiologic agents (see Table 8-9).

The outcomes associated with myocarditis are also variable; one third of patients with myocarditis die, one third survive and require either several medications or cardiac transplantation for treatment of chronic heart failure, and one third survive with either full recovery of cardiac function or minimal to no symptoms with medical management. Because even the most critically ill patient with myocarditis has the capacity for full recovery, aggressive therapy, including mechanical support with ECMO and antiviral therapy with pleconaril during the acute enteroviral infection, is warranted.

The diagnosis of myocarditis is based on clinical suspicion. Although the "gold standard" for diagnosis is endomyocardial biopsy, the need to perform this procedure is not universally accepted. Because the current therapy for myocarditis is primarily supportive (diuretics, inotropic agents, afterload reduction, and anticoagulation),

the results of the biopsy may not change the treatment. In addition, although endomyocardial biopsy can be performed relatively safely, there is a potential for significant complications, especially in neonates and infants. Immunosuppression with prednisone and/or cyclosporine is not efficacious in the treatment of myocarditis, even though there is pathophysiologic evidence to suggest that myocarditis may be an autoimmune disease process rather than directed viral injury to the myocardium.

Evaluation for transplantation is appropriate if the patient's symptoms are progressive and severe. The physician should be very cautious in this regard, especially with the patient with acute heart failure, because full recovery may ultimately occur. Aggressive medical therapy should be instituted in the hope of recovery. The usual time for such recovery is over a 1- to 2-week period. In the patient in whom the disease has reached the chronic phase, with little or no recovery of cardiac function *and* with significant symptoms despite maximal medical therapy, cardiac transplantation evaluation is appropriate.

Metabolic causes of cardiomyopathy should always be considered and should not be missed. Two such examples include carnitine deficiency and Pompe disease.

Carnitine Deficiency

Carnitine is an essential cofactor for the transport of long-chain fatty acids into the mitochondria, where oxidation takes place. Because long-chain fatty acids are the primary and preferred cardiac substrate, carnitine deficiency can result in depressed mitochondrial oxidation of fatty acids and accumulation of lipids within the cytoplasm. The result can be significant organ dysfunction. Both HCM and DCM have been reported in primary and secondary carnitine deficiency. A child with DCM may recover complete cardiac function with L-carnitine replacement therapy.

Because inherited primary or secondary disorders of carnitine metabolism can be one of the treatable causes of familial cardiomyopathy, it is important to screen all patients with idiopathic DCM for plasma carnitine levels and to begin therapy with carnitine (100 mg/kg/24 hours) immediately.

Pompe Disease

Pompe disease, a glycogen storage disease, is an inheritable (autosomal recessive) disorder of glycogen metabolism resulting from a defect of a specific enzyme, lysosomal 1,4-α-glucosidase. The result of this defect is an accumulation of glycogen within the myocardium and within other organs such as the skeletal muscle (causing hypotonia), nervous system, diaphragm, and tongue (causing macroglossia). Accumulation within the myocardium leads to extreme thickening of the heart, which ultimately compromises function. In the classic infantile form of Pompe disease, death generally occurs by 2 years of age. The heart can become very globular and be 3 to 10 times the normal weight. Pompe disease is often accompanied by an enlarged tongue and generalized hypotonia. The ECG shows the typical pattern of very high voltage in all QRS segments, representing severe combined left and right ventricular hypertrophy. It also shows a classic short PR interval. Death generally occurs as a result of progressive respiratory compromise from a combination of congestive heart failure, primary respiratory failure, and/or aspiration pneumonia related to poor muscle tone and an enlarged tongue that may contribute to abnormal deglutition. Because of the involvement of multiple organ systems, cardiac transplantation has not been an option for infants with Pompe disease. The diagnosis should be suspected in an infant with poor muscle tone and failure to thrive, who has cardiomegaly with severe left ventricular hypertrophy, and who has a short PR interval on ECG. A skeletal muscle biopsy confirms the diagnosis. Therapy with the recombinant enzyme is currently being evaluated.

Additional genetic causes of DCM include mutations in the genes for dystrophin and tafazzin. The dystrophin mutation is not the same mutation seen in classic Becker or Duchenne muscular dystrophy; skeletal muscle involvement is minimal, but the disorder progresses rapidly to end-stage heart failure. The mutation of tafazzin is associated with Barth syndrome, a lethal metabolic disease that is usually fatal in infancy; however, a few spontaneous recoveries have been noted. In addition to the disorders, fatty acid oxidation defects resulting from multiple steps in the oxidative pathway (including carnitine) have been reported to cause DCM, especially in children younger than 10 years. Skeletal muscle weakness is a potential clue to fatty acid oxidation defects; consanguinity may be present in autosomal recessive disorders, whereas a matrilineal pattern suggests mutations in mitochondrial DNA.

ARRHYTHMOGENIC RIGHT VENTRICULAR CARDIOMYOPATHY

ARVC is characterized by progressive loss of right ventricular myocytes by fibrofatty tissue (see Table 8-10). Most causes are inherited through autosomal dominance except for those associated with Naxos disease (palmoplantar keratoderma and woolly hair). There is a high risk of arrhythmias, syncope, sudden cardiac death, and heart failure. A high percentage of sudden cardiac death in young adults in one community in Italy was associated with under-diagnosed ARVC. Management is noted in Table 8-10.

RESTRICTIVE CARDIOMYOPATHY

This is the least common form of cardiomyopathy. The cause of RCM is not known, although there exists speculation that either a viral infection or a primary muscle abnormality, or both, may be involved. Physiologically, it is noted that there is diastolic dysfunction of the left ventricle, producing an abnormality of ventricular filling (see Table 8-10). Although the systolic function tends to be preserved, the diastolic dysfunction can impair cardiac output and result in symptoms of a moderate degree, including syncope and ischemia. Sudden cardiac death is also a risk.

Patients with moderate symptoms should avoid competitive sports. There does not seem to be adequate medical therapy for this condition, inasmuch as both diuretics and calcium channel blockers have not been associated with either symptomatic or echocardiographic improvement. An ICD may be appropriate for minimizing the risk of sudden cardiac death. Because of the lack of medical therapy and the risk of sudden cardiac death, some authorities have advocated that children with RCM and moderate symptoms should be placed on the cardiac transplantation list at the time of diagnosis.

SYSTEMIC HYPERTENSION

Severe acute or chronic hypertension may manifest with heart failure by causing a significant increase in afterload with or without expansion of the blood volume. It can occur at any age, including the neonatal and infancy periods, and is often overlooked because it is relatively uncommon. In many cases, hypertension is asymptomatic until significant organ damage occurs. Because of this, all children older than 3 years should have their blood pressure checked at all physician visits. The causes of hypertension are variable and are age dependent. Tables 8-11 and 8-12 list the causes of acute and chronic hypertension, respectively. In a neonate or an infant, it is important to rule out coarctation of the aorta or aortic thrombi; the latter is probably related to a previous umbilical arterial line or clotting abnormality. Older children and adolescents with hypertension may have post-streptococcal glomerulonephritis, structural

renal disease, renovascular stenosis, or essential hypertension. Potential clues to other causes include the family history and findings suggestive of other diseases such as rash (systemic lupus erythematosus, Henoch-Schönlein purpura), neurofibromas, café-au-lait spots, hirsutism, buffalo hump, moon facies, abdominal bruits, abdominal masses, edema, poor femoral pulses, and thyromegaly; pregnancy; or diseases such as tuberous sclerosis, von Hippel-Lindau disease, Turner or Williams syndrome, and signs of hypertensive crisis (retinopathy, encephalopathy, Bell palsy). Treatment requires the careful use of antihypertensive agents as well as the specific approach aimed at the underlying disorder. Commonly used antihypertensive agents and their dosages are listed in Tables 8-13 and 8-14. Normal blood pressure levels are noted in Tables 8-15 and 8-16.

BACTERIAL ENDOCARDITIS

Endocarditis is uncommon but can cause heart failure by causing valve dysfunction, associated myocarditis, and/or arrhythmias. Endocarditis typically occurs on a congenitally abnormal valve or cardiac structure or is associated with previous endocarditis or a prosthetic valve. It may also affect a previously normal valve. The more common pathogens associated with endocarditis include the streptococcus viridans group *(Streptococcus sanguis, S. mutans, S. mitis), Staphylococcus aureus,* and coagulase-negative staphylococcus. In addition to heart failure, complications include stroke, arrhythmias, systemic emboli, arthritis, nephritis, and pericarditis (see Chapter 11).

RHEUMATIC FEVER

Heart failure can result from rheumatic carditis. It is usually associated with the murmur of mitral insufficiency and may also be associated aortic valve insufficiency. Diagnostic Jones criteria for the diagnosis of rheumatic fever continue to be useful in confirming the diagnosis (see Chapter 11).

SUMMARY AND RED FLAGS

Heart failure manifests with variable, nonspecific symptoms that may be dependent on the age of the patient, the cause of the heart failure, and its severity. The typical constellation of symptoms that should raise a "red flag" includes tachypnea, tachycardia, hepatomegaly, and cardiomegaly. Neonates and infants also present with poor feeding, irritability, lethargy, and poor growth. Because of the frequent involvement of the pulmonary system in patients with heart failure, additional signs and symptoms such as respiratory distress, wheezing, crackles, and rhonchi must not always be assumed to be caused by a primary pulmonary process.

The degree of heart failure and hence the severity of illness are very easily assessed by physical examination and evaluation of end-organ perfusion. It is critical to emphasize that the blood pressure is a poor indicator of cardiac output; because of the compensatory mechanisms in heart failure, the changes in blood pressure occur very late in the evolution of the symptoms associated with heart failure. Rather, the examination of the skin, including warmth, color, capillary refill and pulses, the examination of the central nervous system (including assessment for irritability and lethargy), and the examination of renal perfusion as manifested by urine output are the best clinical indicators of systemic cardiac output. Nonetheless, hypotension signifies cardiogenic shock and is a life-threatening emergency. Signs of severe respiratory distress with inadequate or worsening cardiac output in the setting of heart failure are danger

Table 8-11. Conditions Associated with Acute Transient or Intermittent Hypertension in Children

Renal

Acute postinfectious glomerulonephritis
Henoch-Schönlein purpura and other vasculitides
Hemolytic-uremic syndrome
Thrombotic thrombocytopenic purpura
Acute tubular necrosis
After renal transplantation (immediately and during
  episodes of rejection)
After blood transfusion in patients with azotemia
Hypervolemia
After surgical procedures on genitourinary tract
Pyelonephritis
Renal trauma
Leukemic infiltration of kidney
Obstructive uropathy

Drugs and Poisons

Cocaine
Oral contraceptives
Sympathomimetic agents
Amphetamines
Phencyclidine
Corticosteroids and adrenocorticotropic hormone
  (ACTH)
Cyclosporine
Licorice (glycyrrhizic acid)
Lead, mercury, cadmium, thallium
Antihypertensive withdrawal (clonidine, methyldopa,
  propranolol)
Vitamin D intoxication
Monoamine oxidase inhibitor plus sympathomimetic
  agents

Central and Autonomic Nervous System

Increased intracranial pressure
Guillain-Barré syndrome
Burns
Familial dysautonomia
Stevens-Johnson syndrome
Posterior fossa lesions
Porphyria
Poliomyelitis
Encephalitis

Miscellaneous

Preeclampsia-eclampsia
Pheochromocytoma
Fractures of long bones
Hypercalcemia
Postcoarctation repair
White cell transfusion
Extracorporeal membrane oxygenation
  (ECMO)
Chronic upper airway obstruction

Modified from Behrman RE (ed): Nelson Textbook of Pediatrics, 14th ed. Philadelphia, WB Saunders, 1992, p 1223.

Table 8-12. Conditions Associated with Chronic Hypertension in Children

Renal

Chronic pyelonephritis
Chronic glomerulonephritis
Hydronephrosis
Congenital dysplastic kidney
Multicystic kidney
Solitary renal cyst
Vesicoureteral reflux nephropathy
Segmental hypoplasia (Ask-Upmark kidney)
Ureteral obstruction
Renal tumors (Wilms tumor)
Renal trauma
Rejection damage after transplantation
Postirradiation damage
Systemic lupus erythematosus (and other connective
  tissue diseases)

Vascular

Coarctation of thoracic or abdominal aorta
  (preoperative or postoperative)
Renal artery lesions (stenosis, fibromuscular dysplasia,
  thrombosis, aneurysm)
Umbilical artery catheterization with thrombus
  formation
Neurofibromatosis (intrinsic or extrinsic narrowing of
  vascular lumen)
Renal vein thrombosis
Vasculitis
Arteriovenous shunt
Williams-Beuren syndrome

Endocrine

Hyperthyroidism
Hyperparathyroidism
Congenital adrenal hyperplasia (11β-hydroxylase
  and 17-hydroxylase defect)
Cushing syndrome
Primary aldosteronism
Dexamethasone-suppressible hyperaldosteronism
Pheochromocytoma
Other neural crest tumors (neuroblastoma,
  ganglioneuroblastoma, ganglioneuroma)
Diabetic nephropathy

Central Nervous System

Intracranial mass
Hemorrhage
Residual damage after brain injury
Quadriplegia

Essential Hypertension

Low renin
Normal renin
High renin

From Behrman RE (ed): Nelson Textbook of Pediatrics, 14th ed. Philadelphia, WB Saunders, 1992.

Table 8-13. Treatment of Chronic Hypertension in Children

Drug	Dosage	Comments
Diuretics		
Hydrochlorothiazide	20-30 mg/kg/day PO divided q12h	Monitor for ↓ K, ↑ glu, ↑ uric acid
Chlorothiazide	2-3 mg/kg/day PO divided q12h	Monitor for ↓ K, ↑ glu, ↑ uric acid
Chlorthalidone	Dose not established in pediatrics	Longer acting than thiazides
Furosemide	2-3 mg/kg/day PO divided q6-12h	Monitor for ↓ K, ↑ glu, ↑ uric acid, loop diuretic, hypercalciuria
Ethacrynic acid	2-3 mg/kg/day PO divided q6-12h	Monitor for ↓ K, ↑ glu, ↑ uric acid, loop diuretic
Bumetanide	0.02-0.3 mg/kg/day PO divided q6-12h	Monitor for ↓ K, ↑ glu, ↑ uric acid, loop diuretic
Spironolactone	1-3 mg/kg/day PO divided q6-12h	Aldosterone antagonist; ↑ K
Triamterene	2-3 mg/kg/day PO divided q6-12h	Distal tubule blocker of Na:K exchange
Acetazolamide	5 mg/kg/day PO	Carbonic anhydrase inhibitor not useful in patients with hypertension
Vasodilators		
Hydralazine	0.75-3.0 mg/kg/day PO divided q6-8h	↑ Heart rate, headache, lupus-like syndrome (rare in pediatrics)
Minoxidil	0.05-1.0 mg/kg/day PO divided q12h	Salt and water retention, hirsutism
Prazosin	0.05-0.5 mg/kg/day PO divided q8-12h	Give first dose with patient supine
Nifedipine (extended release)	0.25-3 mg/kg/day PO divided q12-24h	↑ Heart rate, flushing, headache, dizziness
β-Adrenergic Antagonist		
Propranolol	0.5-6.0 mg/kg/day PO divided q6-12h	Avoid in patients with asthma or CHF, ↓ glu
Atenolol	1-2 mg/kg/day PO divided q12-24h	↓ Bronchospasm and bradycardia
Labetalol	1-3 mg/kg/day PO divided q6-12h	α- and β-blockade
α-Adrenergic Antagonist		
Clonidine	0.05-0.6 mg/kg/day PO divided q6-12h	Initial drowsiness, rebound HTN with abrupt discontinuation
Angiotensin-Converting Enzyme Inhibitors		
Captopril	0.02-2.0 mg/kg/day PO divided q12h (infants) 0.5-6.0 mg/kg/day PO divided q8h (children)	↑ K, ↓ platelets, neutropenia, cough, caution in renal artery stenosis, ↓ GFR
Enalapril	0.15-? mg/kg/day PO divided q12-24h	↓ GFR, ↑ K, ↓ platelets, ↓ WBC

From Bartosh SM, Aronsen AJ: Childhood hypertension: An update on etiology, diagnosis and treatment. Pediatr Clin North Am 1999;46:248.

CHF, congestive heart failure; GFR, glomerular filtration rate; glu, glucose level; HTN, hypertension; K, potassium level; Na, sodium; WBC, white blood cell count.

Table 8-14. Pharmacologic Therapy for Hypertensive Emergencies in Children

Drug	Dose	Onset of Action
Nifedipine	0.25-0.5 mg/kg/dose SL/PO	Minutes
Sodium nitroprusside*	0.5-1.0 μg/kg/min IV (max, 8 μg/kg/min)	Seconds
Labetalol	0.2-1.0 mg/kg/dose IV, 0.25-2.0 mg/kg/hr mtn (bolus or continuous)	Minutes
Esmolol[†]	500 μg/kg IV, load over 1-2 min, then 50-250 μg/kg/min	Minutes
Diazoxide[‡]	1-3 mg/kg IV (max, 150 mg/dose)	Minutes
Hydralazine	0.2-0.4 mg/kg IV	Minutes
Minoxidil	0.1-0.2 mg/kg PO	Minutes
Captopril	0.01-0.25 mg/kg/dose PO (infants)	Minutes
	0.1-0.2 mg/kg/dose PO (children)	Minutes
Phentolamine mesylate[§]	0.1-0.2 mg/kg IV	Seconds

From Bartosh SM, Aronsen AJ: Childhood hypertension: An update on etiology, diagnosis and treatment. Pediatr Clin North Am 1999;46:247.

*Check thiocyanate blood levels every 48 hours.

[†]Limited pediatric data available.

[‡]No longer recommended because of potential abrupt decrease in blood pressure.

[§]α-Adrenergic blocking agent for treatment of pheochromocytoma.

IV, intravenously; max, maximum; mtn, maintenance; PO, by mouth; SL, sublingual.

Table 8-15. Blood Pressure Levels for the 90th and 95th Percentiles of Blood Pressure for Boys Aged 1 to 17 Years by Percentiles of Height

Age (yr)	Blood Pressure Percentile*	Systolic Blood Pressure by Percentile of Height (mm Hg)†							Diastolic Blood Pressure by Percentile of Height (mm Hg)†						
		5%	*10%*	*25%*	*50%*	*75%*	*90%*	*95%*	*5%*	*10%*	*25%*	*50%*	*75%*	*90%*	*95%*
1	90th	94	95	97	98	100	102	102	50	51	52	53	54	54	55
	95th	98	99	101	102	104	106	106	55	55	56	57	58	59	59
2	90th	98	99	100	102	104	105	106	55	55	56	57	58	59	59
	95th	101	102	104	106	108	109	110	59	59	60	61	62	63	63
3	90th	100	101	103	105	107	108	109	59	59	60	61	62	63	63
	95th	104	105	107	109	111	112	113	63	63	64	65	66	67	67
4	90th	102	103	105	107	109	110	111	62	62	63	64	65	66	66
	95th	106	107	109	111	113	114	115	66	67	67	68	69	70	71
5	90th	104	105	106	108	110	112	112	65	65	66	67	68	69	69
	95th	108	109	110	112	114	115	116	69	70	70	71	72	73	74
6	90th	105	106	108	110	111	113	114	67	68	69	70	70	71	72
	95th	109	110	112	114	115	117	117	72	72	73	74	75	76	76
7	90th	106	107	109	111	113	114	115	69	70	71	72	72	73	74
	95th	110	111	113	115	116	118	119	74	74	75	76	77	78	78
8	90th	107	108	110	112	114	115	116	71	71	72	73	74	75	75
	95th	111	112	114	116	118	119	120	75	76	76	77	78	79	80
9	90th	109	110	112	113	115	117	117	72	73	73	74	75	76	77
	95th	113	114	116	117	119	121	121	76	77	78	79	80	80	81
10	90th	110	112	113	115	117	118	119	73	74	74	75	76	77	78
	95th	114	115	117	119	121	122	123	77	78	79	80	80	81	82
11	90th	112	113	115	117	119	120	121	74	74	75	76	77	78	78
	95th	116	117	119	121	123	124	125	78	79	79	80	81	82	83
12	90th	115	116	117	119	121	123	123	75	75	76	77	78	78	79
	95th	119	120	121	123	125	126	127	79	79	80	81	82	83	83
13	90th	117	118	120	122	124	125	126	75	76	76	77	78	79	80
	95th	121	122	124	126	128	129	130	79	80	81	82	83	83	84
14	90th	120	121	123	125	126	128	128	76	76	77	78	79	80	80
	95th	124	125	127	128	130	132	132	80	81	81	82	83	84	85
15	90th	123	124	125	127	129	131	131	77	77	78	79	80	81	81
	95th	127	128	129	131	133	134	135	81	82	83	83	84	85	86
16	90th	125	126	128	130	132	133	134	79	79	80	81	82	82	83
	95th	129	130	132	134	136	137	138	83	83	84	85	86	87	87
17	90th	128	129	131	133	134	136	136	81	81	82	83	84	85	85
	95th	132	133	135	136	138	140	140	85	85	86	87	88	89	89

From Update on the 1987 Task Force Report on High Blood Pressure in Children and Adolescents: A working group report from the National High Blood Pressure Education Program. Pediatrics 1996;98:653.

*Blood pressure percentile was determined by a single measurement.

†Height percentile was determined by standard growth curves.

signs that mandate immediate attention and treatment in an intensive care setting.

There are several conditions that can manifest with heart failure and that should not be missed. These include coarctation of the aorta, TAPVR, cor triatriatum, anomalous origin of the left coronary artery from the pulmonary artery, systemic hypertension, bacterial endocarditis, rheumatic fever, and Kawasaki syndrome. Early diagnosis of and intervention for these lesions can be lifesaving as well as curative. In the neonate, it is important to identify ductal dependent lesions that must be initially managed with prostaglandins (hypoplastic left heart syndrome, coarctation of the aorta, interrupted aortic arch).

The category of heart failure without a significant murmur represents a more frequently diagnosed entity, DCM. Many of these cases are initially caused by acute viral myocarditis, especially in very young children. It is critical that this diagnosis not be delayed or missed. Early and aggressive supportive therapy, even in the most severe cases of heart failure associated with acute viral myocarditis, can stabilize the patient and optimize the possibility for eventual complete recovery.

Table 8-16. Blood Pressure Levels for the 90th and 95th Percentiles of Blood Pressure for Girls Aged 1 to 17 Years by Percentiles of Height

Age (yr)	Blood Pressure Percentile*	Systolic Blood Pressure by Percentile of Height (mm Hg)[†]							Diastolic Blood Pressure by Percentile of Height (mm Hg)[†]						
		5%	10%	25%	50%	75%	90%	95%	5%	10%	25%	50%	75%	90%	95%
1	90th	97	98	99	100	102	103	104	53	53	53	54	55	56	56
	95th	101	102	103	104	105	107	107	57	57	57	58	59	60	60
2	90th	99	99	100	102	103	104	105	57	57	58	58	59	60	61
	95th	102	103	104	105	107	108	109	61	61	62	62	63	64	65
3	90th	100	100	102	103	104	105	106	61	61	61	62	63	63	64
	95th	104	104	105	107	108	109	110	65	65	65	66	67	67	68
4	90th	101	102	103	104	106	107	108	63	63	64	65	65	66	67
	95th	105	106	107	108	109	111	111	67	67	68	69	69	70	71
5	90th	103	103	104	106	107	108	109	65	66	66	67	68	68	69
	95th	107	107	108	110	111	112	113	69	70	70	71	72	72	73
6	90th	104	105	106	107	109	110	111	67	67	68	69	69	70	71
	95th	108	109	110	111	112	114	114	71	71	72	73	73	74	75
7	90th	106	107	108	109	110	112	112	69	69	69	70	71	72	72
	95th	110	110	112	113	114	115	116	73	73	73	74	75	76	76
8	90th	108	109	110	111	112	113	114	70	70	71	71	72	73	74
	95th	112	112	113	115	116	117	118	74	74	75	75	76	77	78
9	90th	110	110	112	113	114	115	116	71	72	72	73	74	74	75
	95th	114	114	115	117	118	119	120	75	76	76	77	78	78	79
10	90th	112	112	114	115	116	117	118	73	73	73	74	75	76	76
	95th	116	116	117	119	120	121	122	77	77	77	78	79	80	80
11	90th	114	114	116	117	118	119	120	74	74	75	75	76	77	77
	95th	118	118	119	121	122	123	124	78	78	79	79	80	81	81
12	90th	116	116	118	119	120	121	122	75	75	76	76	77	78	78
	95th	120	120	121	123	124	125	126	79	79	80	80	81	82	82
13	90th	118	118	119	121	122	123	124	76	76	77	78	78	79	80
	95th	121	122	123	125	126	127	128	80	80	81	82	82	83	84
14	90th	119	120	121	122	124	125	126	77	77	78	79	79	80	81
	95th	123	124	125	126	128	129	130	81	81	82	83	83	84	85
15	90th	121	121	122	124	125	126	127	78	78	79	79	80	81	82
	95th	124	125	126	128	129	130	131	82	82	83	83	84	85	86
16	90th	122	122	123	125	126	127	128	79	79	79	80	81	82	82
	95th	125	126	127	128	130	131	132	83	83	83	84	85	86	86
17	90th	122	123	124	125	126	128	128	79	79	79	80	81	82	82
	95th	126	126	127	129	130	131	132	83	83	83	84	85	86	86

From Update on the 1987 Task Force Report on High Blood Pressure in Children and Adolescents: A working group report from the National High Blood Pressure Education Program. Pediatrics 1996;98:654.

*Blood pressure percentile was determined by a single reading.

[†]Height percentile was determined by standard growth curves.

REFERENCES

Heart Failure

Davies MK, Gibbs CR, Lip GYH: ABC of heart failure. Investigation. BMJ 2000;320:297-300.

Dreyer WJ, Fisher DJ: Clinical recognition and management of chronic congestive-cardiac failure. In Garson A Jr, Bricker JT, Fisher DJ, et al (eds): The Science and Practice of Pediatric Cardiology, 2nd ed. Baltimore, Williams & Wilkins, 1998, pp 2309-2325.

O'Laughlin MP: Congestive heart failure in children. Pediatr Clin North Am 1999;46:263-273.

Perloff JK: The jugular venous pulse and third heart sound in patients with heart failure. N Engl J Med 2001;345:612-614.

Towbin JA: Pediatric myocardial disease. Pediatr Clin North Am 1999; 46:289-312.

Tripp ME, Shug AI: Plasma carnitine concentrations in cardiomyopathy patients. Biochem Med 1984;32:199-206.

Etiology

Baltimore RS: Infective endocarditis in children. Pediatr Infec Dis J 1992; 11:907-913.

Bartosh SM, Aronson AJ: Childhood hypertension. Pediatr Clin North Am 1999;46:235-252.

Beevers G, Lip GYH, O'Brien E: ABC of hypertension. The pathophysiology of hypertension. BMJ 2001;322:912-916.

Bousa E, Menasalvas A, Munoz P, et al: Infective endocarditis—A prospective study at the end of the twentieth century. Medicine 2001;80: 298-307.

Brook MM: Pediatric bacterial endocarditis. Pediatr Clin North Am 1999; 46:275-287.

Clark AL, Coats AJS: Screening for hypertrophic cardiomyopathy. BMJ 1993;306:409-410.

Dalakas MC, Park KY, Semino-Mora C, et al: Desmin myopathy, a skeletal myopathy with cardiomyopathy caused by mutations in the desmin gene. N Engl J Med 2000;342:770-780.

Dluby RG, Anderson B, Harlin B, et al: Glucocorticoid-remediable aldosteronism is associated with severe hypertension in early childhood. 2001;138:715-720.

Drugs for hypertension. Med Lett 2001;43:17-22.

Elliott PM, Gimeno Blanes JR, Mahon NG, et al: Relation between severity of left-ventricular hypertrophy and prognosis in patients with hypertrophic cardiomyopathy. Lancet 2001;357:420-424.

Felker GM, Thompson RE, Hare JM, et al: Underlying causes and long-term survival in patients with initially unexplained cardiomyopathy. N Engl J Med 2000;342:1077-1084.

Figueroa FE, Fernandez MS, Valdes P, et al: Prospective comparison of clinical and echocardiographic diagnosis of rheumatic carditis: Long term follow up of patients with subclinical disease. Heart 2001;85: 407-410.

Franz WM, Müller OJ, Katus HA: Cardiomyopathies: From genetics to the prospect of treatment. Lancet 2001;358:1627-1637.

Franz WM, Müller M, Müller OJ, et al: Association of nonsense mutation of dystrophin gene with disruption of sarcoglycan in X-linked dilated cardiomyopathy. Lancet 2000;355:1781-1785.

Kamisago M, Sharma SD, DePalma SR, et al: Mutations in sarcomere protein genes as a cause of dilated cardiomyopathy. N Engl J Med 2000;343:1688-1696.

Khogali SS, Mayosi BM, Beattie JM, et al: A common mitochondrial DNA variant associated with susceptibility to dilated cardiomyopathy in two different populations. Lancet 2001; 357:1265-1268.

Lipshultz SE, Sleeper LA, Towbin JA, et al: The incidence of pediatric cardiomyopathy in two regions of the United States. N Engl J Med 2003;348:1647-1655.

McCoy G, Protonotarios N, Crosby A, et al: Identification of a deletion in plakoglobin in arrhythmogenic right ventricular cardiomyopathy with palmoplantar keratoderma and woolly hair (Naxos disease). Lancet 2000; 355:2119-2124.

Michels VV: Progress in defining the causes of idiopathic dilated cardiomyopathy. N Engl J Med 1993;329:960-961.

Michels VV, Moll PP, Miller FA, et al: The frequency of familial dilated cardiomyopathy in a series of patients with idiopathic dilated cardiomyopathy. N Engl J Med 1992;326:77-82.

Mylonakis E, Calderwood SB: Infective endocarditis in adults. N Engl J Med 2001;345:1318-1330.

Nugent AW, Daubeney PEF, Chondros P, et al: The epidemiology of childhood cardiomyopathy in Australia. N Engl J Med 2003;348: 1639-1646.

Pearson GD, Veille JC, Rahimtoola S, et al: Peripartum cardiomyopathy. JAMA 2000;283:1183-1188.

Saiman L, Prince A, Gersony WM: Pediatric infective endocarditis in the modern era. J Pediatr 1993;122:847-853.

Seliem MA, Mansara KB, Palileo M, et al: Evidence for autosomal recessive inheritance of infantile dilated cardiomyopathy: Studies from the eastern province of Saudi Arabia. Pediatr Res 2000;48:770-775.

Veasy LG: Time to take soundings in acute rheumatic fever. Lancet 2001; 357:1994-1995.

Management

Balaguru D, Artman M, Auslender M: Management of heart failure in children. Curr Probl Pediatr 2000;30:5-30.

Bruns LA, Kichuk Chrisant M, Lamour JM, et al: Carvedilol as therapy in pediatric heart failure: An initial multicenter experience. J Pediatr 2001; 138:505-511.

Chan KY, Iwahara M, Benson LN, et al: Immunosuppressive therapy in the management of acute myocarditis in children: A clinical trial. J Am Coll Cardiol 1991;17:458-460.

Davies MK, Gibbs CR, Lip GY: ABC of heart failure. Management: diuretics, ACE inhibitors, and nitrates. BMJ 2000;320:428-431.

Fisher DJ, Feltes TF, Moore JW, et al: Management of acute congestive cardiac failure. In Garson A Jr, Bricker JT, Fisher DJ, et al (eds): The Science and Practice of Pediatric Cardiology, 2nd ed. Baltimore, Williams & Wilkins, 1998, pp 2329-2343.

Gibbs CR, Davies MK, Lip GY: ABC of heart failure. Management: Digoxin and other inotropes, β blockers, and antiarrhythmic and antithrombotic treatment. BMJ 2000;320:495-498.

Gilbert EM, Anderson JL, Deitchman D, et al: Long-term β-blocker vasodilator therapy improves cardiac function in idiopathic dilated cardiomyopathy: A double-blind, randomized study of bucindolol versus placebo. Am J Med 1990;88:223-229.

Helton E, Darragh R, Francis P, et al: Metabolic aspects of myocardial disease and a role for L-carnitine in the treatment of childhood cardiomyopathy. Pediatrics 2000;105:1260-1270.

Kulick DL, Rahimtoola SH: Current role of digitalis therapy in patients with congestive heart failure. JAMA 1991;265:2995-2997.

Lewis AB, Chabot M: The effect of treatment with angiotensin-converting enzyme inhibitors on survival of pediatric patients with dilated cardiomyopathy. Pediatr Cardiol 1993;14:9-12.

Millane T, Jackson G, Gibbs CR, et al: ABC of heart failure. Acute and chronic management strategies. BMJ 2000;320:559-562.

O'Connell JB: Immunosuppression for dilated cardiomyopathy. N Engl J Med 1989;321:1119-1121.

Packer M, Bristow MR, Cohn JN, et al: The effect of carvedilol on morbidity and mortality in patients with chronic heart failure. N Engl J Med 1996; 334:1349-1355.

Parrillo JE, Cunnion RE, Epstein SE, et al: A prospective, randomized, controlled trial of prednisone for dilated cardiomyopathy. N Engl J Med 1989;321:1061-1068.

Raithel SC, Pennington DG, Boegner E, et al: Extracorporeal membrane oxygenation in children after heart surgery. Circulation 1992;86(Suppl 5): 305-310.

Troughton RW, Frampton CM, Yandle TG, et al: Treatment of heart failure guided by plasma aminoterminal brain natriuretic peptide (N-BNP) concentrations. Lancet 2000;355:1126-1130.

Vaughan CJ, Delanty N: Hypertensive emergencies. Lancet 2000;356:411-417.

Waagstein F, Bristow MR, Swedberg K, et al: Beneficial effects of metoprolol in idiopathic dilated cardiomyopathy. Lancet 1993;342: 1441-1446.

9 Chest Pain

Garry S. Sigman

Chest pain in children and adolescents is common and is responsible for 650,000 physician visits annually in patients between the ages of 10 and 21 years. Chest pain is one of the most common reasons for referral to pediatric cardiology clinics, second only to heart murmur.

Because chest pain is sometimes indicative of significant cardiovascular disease in the adult population, this symptom commonly invokes fear in the patient and family. In the pediatric population, chest pain is less likely to be caused by cardiac disease. Nevertheless, it is a challenge because life-threatening disease must be ruled out, and specific noncardiac causes are not always easy to diagnose.

Chest pain affects preadolescents and adolescents of both sexes with equal frequency. The mean age at presentation is about 12 years.

Some basic facts have emerged:

- Chest pain in children and adolescents is associated with serious illness in the minority of cases.
- The majority of cases can be attributed to noncardiac causes.
- Chest pain can be chronic and an ongoing source of concern and morbidity.
- The precise diagnosis is not made in a high percentage of cases (Table 9-1).
- The complaint of chest pain is of significant concern to children and their parents.

The possible causes of the pain are extensive (Tables 9-1 to 9-3) because most patients do not have serious disease (see Table 9-2); an awareness of indicators (red flags) that might suggest serious disease is required (Table 9-4). The first priority is to identify causes of pain that necessitate immediate treatment. Most patients have a more benign cause that may become chronic. Because precise diagnosis is not always possible, the physician must deal with uncertainty, must not overtest or overrefer, and must provide ongoing care that minimizes disability. Finally, because the complaint is one that engenders fear in patients and in parents, the physician must reassure patients and help those who have psychosocial contributions to their chest pain receive the care that is needed.

COMMON CAUSES OF CHEST PAIN

The diagnoses that are responsible for the highest percentage of cases that present in a primary care setting include

- pain from chest wall–musculoskeletal causes (Table 9-5)
- respiratory causes (cough, asthma, pneumonia, pleural effusion, pneumothorax)
- psychological causes (anxiety, somatoform disorder, hyperventilation)

Chest pain in younger children is more likely to have respiratory causes. Adolescents are more likely to have chest wall pain or psychogenic causes. Most of the common causes of chest pain can be diagnosed by a careful history and physical examination. One common diagnostic category is "idiopathic," signifying that (1) many cases of chest pain are not referable to a specific organ system and

that (2) they are clinically undiagnosable. In these cases, the history and physical examination indicate the absence of serious organic disease and, therefore, no further need for extensive testing.

CHEST WALL AND MUSCULOSKELETAL PAIN

Discomfort emanating from the chest wall is the most common identifiable cause of chest pain. Pain can involve the ribs, costochondral junctions, costal cartilages, intercostal muscles, sternum, clavicle, and spine. Figure 9-1 illustrates the chest wall structures important in the etiology of chest pain. Musculoskeletal causes are characterized by an insidious onset (except for acute trauma) and the demonstration of localized tenderness over specific areas of the chest wall or of pain elicited by specific manipulation of the thorax (Fig. 9-2). The pain is nagging and localized to the affected area but might radiate; on occasion there is pain on deep breathing. General features of musculoskeletal chest wall pain are listed in Tables 9-3 and 9-5. Most causes are benign conditions but can be slow to resolve.

Exertion (Strain)

Various forms of physical exertion, especially some athletic pursuits and repetitive lifting, can readily strain chest wall muscles. New activities tend to stress chest muscles that have not been used; it is important to determine whether the patient has recently started training for a sport or a new job. Weight lifting has a particular predilection for causing postexercise chest wall pain. Coughing for a prolonged duration may strain chest muscles and cause pain (see Chapter 2).

Trauma

Direct trauma to the thoracic cavity may also cause chest wall pain. Contusion or rib fracture causes a particularly painful syndrome with pain on inspiration and exquisite tenderness on palpation. Palpable crepitus may be present along the rib. Trauma to the intercostal muscles and the chondrosternal areas is common.

Trauma or strain to specific muscles on the chest wall may be recognized as pain in a certain distribution:

In *pectoral syndrome*, the pain is in a band across the anterior parasternal chest wall on the right or left. On the left, this ache may be mistaken for angina or cardiac disease.

The *coracoid syndrome* is characterized by a strain of the pectoralis minor muscle and tenderness at its insertion into the coracoid process.

The *xiphoid process syndrome* results in pain in the anterior chest and epigastrium and tenderness over the xiphoid process. Pain in the lateral upper back is caused by strain of the *trapezius muscle*. Pain in the anterior lateral chest wall can be caused by strain of the *serratus anterior muscle*.

Strain of the *deltoid* and other muscles of the shoulder girdle may cause chest pain.

The diagnosis of specific injured muscle groups can be aided by the chest wall maneuvers described in Figure 9-2.

Table 9-1. Differential Diagnosis of Pediatric Chest Pain

Musculoskeletal	**Cardiac**
Trauma (accidental, abuse)	Structural cardiac abnormalities
Exercise, overuse injury (strain, bursitis)	Congenital aortic stenosis
Tietze syndrome	Congenital coronary artery abnormalities
Costochondritis	Mitral valve prolapse
Precordial catch syndrome	Acquired cardiac abnormalities
Herpes zoster (cutaneous)	Hypertrophic cardiomyopathy
Pleurodynia	Dilated cardiomyopathy
Fibromyalgia	Myocarditis
Slipping rib	Ischemic heart disease
Sickle cell anemia vasoocclusive crisis (rib infarction)	Idiopathic atherosclerotic heart disease
Osteomyelitis (rare)	Familial hypercholesterolemia
Primary or metastatic tumor	Kawasaki disease
	Diabetes mellitus
Pulmonary	Systemic lupus erythematosus
Pneumonia	Cocaine, sympathomimetic drugs
Pleurisy	Acute pericarditis
Asthma	Endocarditis
Cough	Primary cardiac arrhythmias
Pneumothorax, pneumomediastinum	Idiopathic ventricular tachycardia
Pulmonary eosinophilic granuloma	Exercise-induced ventricular tachycardia
Sickle cell anemia vasoocclusive crisis	Wolff-Parkinson-White syndrome
Infarction (sickle cell anemia, embolism)	Other cardiac abnormalities
Foreign body	Postpericardiotomy syndrome
Tumor	Marfan syndrome (dissecting aortic aneurysm)
	Pulmonary hypertension: any cause
Gastrointestinal	
Achalasia	**Psychiatric**
Constipation	Anxiety, hyperventilation
Esophagitis (gastroesophageal reflux)	Panic disorder
Esophageal foreign body	
Esophageal spasm	**Drug-Related**
Esophageal rupture (related to bulimia nervosa)	Cigarette smoking
Cholecystitis	Cocaine use
Subdiaphragmatic abscess	Sympathomimetic use
Perihepatitis (Fitz-Hugh–Curtis syndrome)	Tetracycline ingestion (esophagitis, esophageal ulceration)
Peptic ulcer disease	
Pancreatitis	**Other**
Splenic rupture	Anorexia nervosa
	Spinal cord or nerve root compression
	Breast-related disease
	Castleman disease (lymph node neoplasm)

Precordial Catch Syndrome

Episodes of very brief (30 seconds to 3 minutes), nonradiating, sharp pains in the left parasternal area or near the cardiac apex related to deep inspiration may be caused by the precordial catch syndrome. It is unrelated to trauma and to exertion. This syndrome occurs more commonly in the slouched or bent-over posture, is completely benign, and responds to reassurance, stretching the painful area, and attention to posture.

Table 9-2. Causes of Chest Pain in Children and Adolescents by Frequency of Causes

Idiopathic	(12%-85%)
Musculoskeletal	(15%-31%)
Pulmonary	(12%-21%)
Psychiatric	(5%-17%)
Gastrointestinal	(4%-7%)
Cardiac	(4%-6%)
Other	(4%-21%)

Costochondritis

Pain emanating from the costal cartilages, *costochondritis,* is a common cause of chest pain. Tietze syndrome, a rare condition, causes visible swelling in that location with pain. In contrast, costochondritis is more common, and pain and tenderness in the costal cartilage are demonstrated without visible swelling. The pain is often unilateral (left-sided more than right-sided) and affects girls more than boys. The fourth left sternocostal cartilage is most frequently involved.

Slipping Rib Syndrome

The slipping rib syndrome causes pain at the lower costal margin and is associated with increased mobility of the 8th, 9th, or 10th rib, resulting in one rib rubbing against another and irritating the intercostal nerve. The pain is sharp and intense, lasts several minutes, and is often brought on by exertion. It is occasionally associated with abdominal pain. The pain can be duplicated by hooking the fingers under the anterior costal margins and pulling the ribs anteriorly (see Fig. 9-2).

Table 9-3. **Differentiation of Chest Pain**

Cause	Example	Clinical Pleuritic*	Laboratory Characteristic	Data	Comments
Angina	Anomalous left coronary artery from pulmonary artery	No	Infant with poor feeding, diaphoresis, tachycardia, irritability	Q-wave infarction pattern or ST-segment changes; echo demonstrates anomalous vessels	Difficult diagnosis, may demonstrate heart failure, cyanosis
	Anomalous origin (ostia) or course of coronary artery Hyperlipidemia	No	Adolescent with exercise-induced, oppressive, constricting, retrosternal anterior pain; episodic, brief duration, radiation to neck, shoulder interscapular area	ST-segment depression	Infarction demonstrates Q-wave pattern; more prolonged pain (>30 min); elevated CPK (MB); history of prior angina, sudden death
Reactive airway disease	Asthma	No	Exercise-induced dyspnea, dull or sharp pain lasting 1-5 min, may occur at rest	Pulmonary function (exercise or metha-choline) tests with response to β-agonist aerosols	Very common; cough or wheeze may be absent.
Chest wall syndrome (see Table 9-5)	Tietze syndrome, pleurodynia, overuse exercise	Yes	Pain and palpable local tenderness or swelling; pain with chest movement	CXR may demonstrate rib fracture or, rarely, other pathology	Exclude trauma, pneumonia, pleural effusion
Pericarditis (see Table 9-9)	Viral, SLE	Possibly	Sharp pain worse while recumbent, better while sitting up leaning forward; three-component pericardial friction rub: atrial systole, ventricular systole, diastolic filling Tachycardia	ECG: ST-segment elevation, T-wave flattening, electrical alternans Echo: pericardial fluid CXR: large heart, normal pulmonary vasculature	If severe dyspnea and fever, suspect purulent bacterial pericarditis and tamponade
Pulmonary embolism	Hypercoagulable state, deep venous thrombosis, central catheter related	Possibly	Sudden pain, dyspnea, hypoxia, apprehension, palpitation; pain is pressure-like or pleuritic Hemoptysis rare	CXR: normal or small pleural effusion or atelectasis ECG: RV strain; positive (high probability) ventilation-perfusion scan	CT is standard
Pneumonia	Viral, bacterial	Usually	Cough, fever, dyspnea, crackles	CXR: infiltrate CBC: leukocytosis Positive sputum or blood culture	See Chapter 2
Pleural effusion	Viral, bacterial, parapneumonia; SLE	Yes	Sudden onset, dullness to chest percussion, diminished breath sounds	CXR: effusion	See Chapter 2
Pneumothorax	Secondary to asthma, trauma, cystic fibrosis, severe cough, idiopathic, Valsalva maneuver	Possibly	Sudden onset dyspnea, pain, cough, cyanosis (if tension pneumothorax), hyperresonant to chest percussion	CXR: pneumothorax	Treat with chest tube if patient is symptomatic
Trauma (nonpenetrating)	Pneumothorax, rib fracture, hemothorax, pulmonary contusion	Yes	As per specific diagnosis	As per specific diagnosis	Chest tube if needed
Esophagitis	Reflux, hiatal hernia, chalasia	No	Heartburn, worse if bending over	Endoscopy, upper GI study, pH probe study	See Chapter 16
Peptic ulcer disease	Gastric, duodenal ulcer	No	Epigastric, preprandial, nighttime sharp pain; relief with food, antacids	Endoscopy	See Chapters 14 and 17

*Pleuritic chest pain results from stimulation of pain receptors of the parietal pleura (inner chest wall, diaphragm, mediastinum, hilum), the inferior pericardium, and the bone and soft tissue of the chest wall.

CBC, complete blood count; CPK, creatine phosphokinase; CT, computed tomography; CXR, chest x-ray study; ECG, electrocardiogram; Echo, echocardiogram; GI, gastrointestinal; RV, right ventricular; SLE, systemic lupus erythematosus.

Table 9-4. Red Flags Associated with Chest Pain

Sudden onset of severe pain with exercise
Syncope
Palpitations and/or dysrhythmias
Family history of sudden death
High fever
Severe dyspnea
Cyanosis
Tachycardia
Hypotension
Congenital heart disease (unoperated or repaired)
Family history of DVT or PTE
Significant other disease (SLE, Kawasaki disease, sickle cell anemia, Marfan syndrome, cystic fibrosis, pneumonia)
Previous esophageal surgery (esophageal rupture)
History of bulemia (esophageal rupture)
Night pain that awakens the patient

DVT, deep venous thrombosis; PTE, pulmonary thromboembolism; SLE, systemic lupus erythematosus.

Puberty

On occasion, adolescents and their parents are not aware of normal early pubertal development. The small breast nodule that normally develops in girls and some boys can produce discomfort, especially if it is palpated by the patient repeatedly. Other breast abnormalities in girls may manifest with pain; these include fibroadenoma, cystosarcoma phyllodes, breast infections, and other breast tumors.

Herpes Zoster

Herpes zoster occurs occasionally in childhood. Chest area pain may precede a typical rash. Neurologic symptoms ranging from hypoesthesia to hyperesthesia may occur.

Fibromyalgia Syndrome

Primary fibromyalgia is a benign syndrome characterized by chronic musculoskeletal aching and stiffness associated with fatigue and sleep disturbance. Its onset peaks between adolescence and middle adulthood, and so it is a common cause of chest discomfort in adolescents. The pain syndrome, in addition to other systemic symptoms, causes areas of point tenderness of muscle. The diagnosis is based on multiple tender points (predetermined sites that evoke pain with minimal pressure). The most common areas of chest wall tenderness are on the trapezius muscle and at the second costochondral junction areas.

Diseases of the Spine

Diseases of the lower cervical or upper thoracic spine can cause chest pain. *Cervical spinal root compression* causes referred pain in the region of the serratus anterior and pectoral muscles. Thoracic root disease causes pain in the skin of the chest wall and intercostal muscles. Spinal root pain, when sharp, may radiate widely and lead to spasm in the muscles innervated by the nerve root. Pain and tenderness over the anterior chest wall therefore may indicate spinal disease. Clues to the correct diagnosis include history of back pain in addition to anterior pain; a history of vertigo, headache, or pain after prolonged recumbency or straining; tenderness over the spine; and elicitation of pain with maneuvers that stress the cervical and thoracic spine (see Fig. 9-2).

Ankylosing spondylitis causes disease of the sacroiliac joints and variable involvement in the thoracic and cervical spine. Although typically a disease of young adults, it may occur in boys as young as 9 years. Chest pain may be present before the onset of lower spinal symptoms. Other disease processes of the spine may cause back and radiating chest pain in children; these include trauma, transverse myelitis, kyphosis, spondylolysis, spondylolisthesis, disk herniation, Scheuermann disease, neoplasms, diskitis, epidural abscess, and osteomyelitis (see Chapter 44). Cervical ribs may, in rare cases, cause chest pain. These ribs arise from C7 (or, less commonly, C5 or C6). Pain involves the shoulder girdle, extremities, and upper chest; pain may radiate down the arms and cause paresthesia of the fingers. The cervical ribs may impinge on the brachial plexus or subclavian artery. The symptoms and signs of nerve or vascular compression at the thoracic outlet may be caused by supernumerary scalene muscles in addition to cervical ribs. The costoclavicular angle between the first rib and the clavicle may compress the brachial plexus or the subclavian artery. Patients may have chest pain in addition to paresthesia; muscle weakness; or vascular signs of blanching, cyanosis, or edema of the upper extremity.

Table 9-5. Chest Wall Syndromes

Syndrome	Manifestation
Female breast	Fibroadenoma, hypertrophy, cystic disease, menstrual swelling, pregnancy, panniculitis, malignancy (rare)
Male breast	Gynecomastia
Pleurodynia	Intercostal muscle infection with coxsackievirus (group B), rarely other enteroviruses; epidemics; sudden onset of spasmodic, paroxysmal, stitchlike chest and abdominal pain; lasts 4-6 days
Rib fractures	Traumatic, pathologic (tumor, rickets), cough induced; localized tenderness with local crepitus
Xiphoidalgia	Idiopathic or traumatic; sternal tenderness rarely caused by hematologic malignancy
Costochondritis	Idiopathic, traumatic, or rheumatologic; tenderness over costochondral junction
Myodynia	Idiopathic, sickle cell anemia; tenderness of intercostal or pectoralis muscles
Fibrositis	Fibromyalgia; point tenderness in parasternal-intercostal area
Herpes zoster	Vesicular rash over unilateral dermatome
Tietze syndrome	Idiopathic: must consider osteomyelitis, tumor, rheumatoid arthritis, and fracture in differential diagnosis; characterized by painful, tender bulbous or fusiform swelling of costal cartilages with or without warmth, erythema
Slipping rib syndrome	Recurrent subluxation of usually the eighth, ninth, or tenth costal cartilage
Pectoralis major syndrome	Exertional overuse; pain in parasternal area or with contraction of the muscle
Thoracic outlet syndrome	Multiple causes; suspect if pain and dysesthesia are predominantly in arm, forearm, or hand

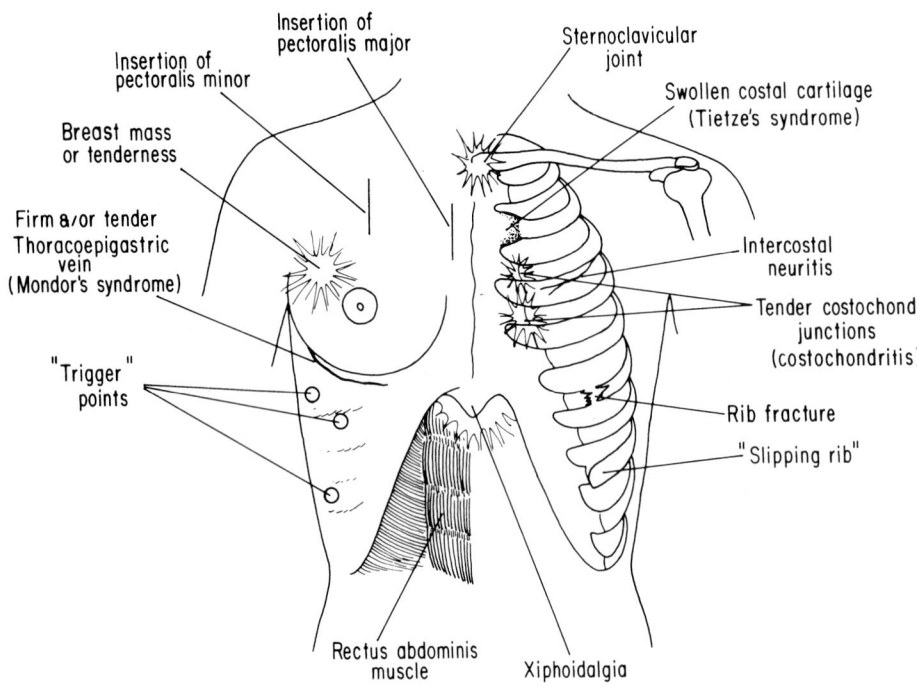

Insertion of pectoralis minor

Insertion of pectoralis major

Sternoclavicular joint

Swollen costal cartilage (Tietze's syndrome)

Breast mass or tenderness

Firm a/or tender Thoracoepigastric vein (Mondor's syndrome)

Intercostal neuritis

Tender costochondral junctions (costochondritis)

"Trigger" points

Rib fracture

"Slipping rib"

Rectus abdominis muscle

Xiphoidalgia

Figure 9-1. Palpable and/or visible abnormalities of the chest wall that may be found in different chest wall syndromes. In addition, various proximal abdominal causes of chest pain, such as disease of the gallbladder, liver, stomach, pancreas, or subdiaphragmatic space, must be considered. (From Reilly BM: Chest pain. In Practical Strategies in Outpatient Medicine, 2nd ed. Philadelphia, WB Saunders, 1991.)

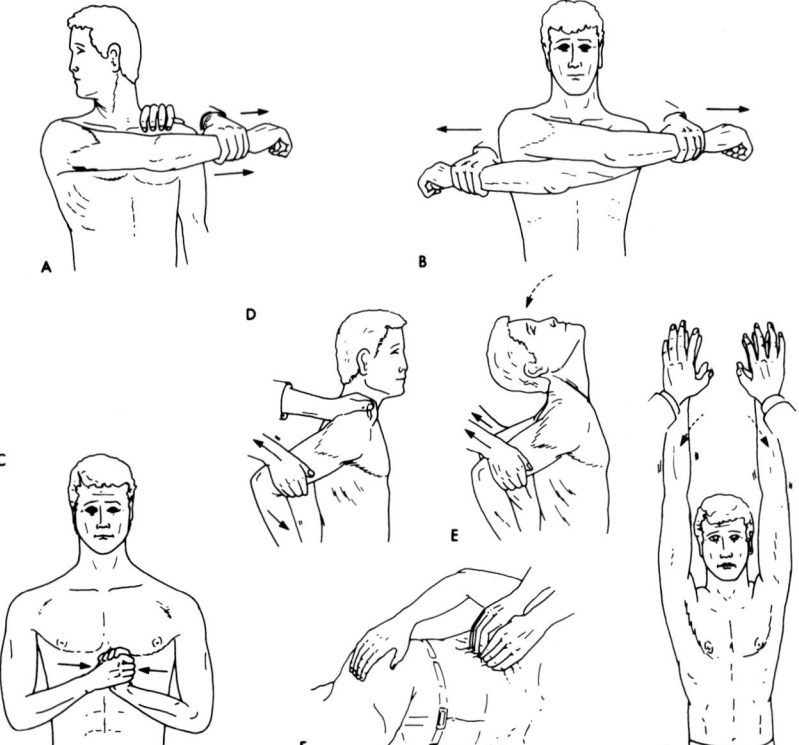

Figure 9-2. Chest wall maneuvers. A, B, The "scissors" maneuver. The patient's arm is adducted across the anterior chest, and the examiner pulls the patient's hand beyond the contralateral shoulder (**A**). When both arms are tested together, traction is applied to both (**B**), the patient turns the head to either side, and the arms form a "scissors." Pain originating in the scapula, thoracic spine, pectoral muscles, or ribs and intercostal structures is often precipitated by the scissors maneuver. **C,** The "hedge clipper" maneuver. The pectoralis major muscles are stressed by the patient's pressing the palms forcefully together with the elbows flexed anterior to the chest. The pectoral muscles are thus more clearly defined, and pain is often appreciated within the muscles or at their insertion in the upper parasternal area (see Fig. 9-1). **D,** The "racing dive" maneuver. The pectoralis minor muscles are stressed by forcefully resisting the patient's attempt to throw forward the shoulder and upper arm from an initial position behind (dorsal to) the chest wall. The attempted arm motion is that of flinging the arm and hand forward, as a swim racer would when beginning a racing dive. The examiner resists this forward arm and shoulder motion. **E,** The "crowing rooster" maneuver. The patient hyperextends the neck while the examiner lifts both of the patient's arms backward and superiorly. Pain originating in the cervical spine or anterior chest wall or both is often thus reproduced. **F,** The "hooking" maneuver. With the patient supine, the examiner stands at the patient's side, facing the patient's feet. The examiner then "hooks" his or her fingers around the lower costal margin of the patient's rib cage and pulls anteriorly (ventrally) and superiorly (cephalad). This maneuver may elicit pain when costochondritis or traumatic rib injuries involve the lower rib cage, when the upper rectus abdominis muscle is torn, or when a "slipping rib" is the problem. **G,** The "high ten" maneuver. The patient raises both hands overhead, elbows extended, and then presses forward with the hands against resistance offered by the examiner. Pain originating in the anterior rib cage, thoracic spine, or pectoral muscles may be elicited here. (**A, B,** and **G,** From Reilly BM: Chest pain. In Practical Strategies in Outpatient Medicine, 2nd ed. Philadelphia, WB Saunders, 1991.)

PSYCHOLOGICAL CAUSES OF PAIN

Psychological symptoms contributing to chest pain are more common in adolescents than in younger children (Table 9-6).

There are two basic precepts for recognizing these disorders:

1. Patients do not usually have only a psychological problem. Most have biomedical or physiologic causes of pain, usually of a benign nature, in addition to psychological factors that exacerbate (or amplify) the clinical presentation.
2. Patients with chest pain may have more than one psychological phenomenon (see Table 9-6). Anxiety, depression, and psychosomatic features often coexist.

Patients who have psychological problem–related chest pain may also have other somatic symptoms, including breathlessness, fatigue, nervousness, faintness, near-syncope, and palpitation. Adolescents with chronic chest pain, in comparison with a pain-free control group, may demonstrate more bodily worries, more limitation of general activity, and more school absences. Many have a family history of chest pain, sleep disturbance, and recurrent somatic complaints. The symptom of acute or chronic chest pain causes concern in children and their parents because most adolescents associate such pain with heart disease. This concern is so pervasive that reassurance by physicians is not always simple. The effectiveness of physicians in reassuring a patient and family has significant implications for the chronicity of the pain and the functional outcome. Effectiveness depends on awareness of anxiety levels, awareness of cognitive developmental factors, and proper use of tests and consultants (see treatment section).

Hyperventilation

Hyperventilation is the cause in about 20% of patients with chest pain. Hyperventilation is also commonly associated with other causes of chest pain, such as costochondritis or asthma. Dyspnea, chest discomfort (tightness), and cough during exercise may indicate hyperventilation rather than asthma, but this is difficult to distinguish without exercise testing.

The syndrome of hyperventilation is defined as overbreathing accompanied by dyspnea and anxiety to a degree that results in systemic symptoms, including paresthesia and lightheadedness. It may also be accompanied by palpitation and confusion. Symptoms of hyperventilation syndrome are physiologic phenomena caused by hypocapnia, respiratory alkalosis, and chest muscle strain (Table 9-7, Fig. 9-3). It may be caused by stomach distention from aerophagia or spasm of the left hemidiaphragm. Typically, adolescents complain of sharp, nonradiating pain that is located over the left precordium.

Hyperventilation is often a symptom of underlying acute or chronic psychologic problems. On occasion, hyperventilation might manifest as an acute, nonrecurrent event; however, it often indicates a long-term disorder that necessitates psychological management. When chronic and recurrent, hyperventilation most commonly represents a panic disorder. Forty percent of children who hyperventilate continue to do so as adults.

Table 9-6. Psychological Causes of Chest Pain in Children and Adolescents

Functional effects of nonspecific chest pain
Hyperventilation syndrome
Anxiety and panic disorder
Depression
Somatization disorder

Table 9-7. Type and Incidence of System Involvement during Hyperventilation in Children

System	Percentage of Cases
Cardiovascular	
Chest pain	86
Palpitation	74
Pallor	72
Cold extremities	42
Respiratory	
Deep, sighing respirations	100
Dyspnea, breathlessness	68
Neurologic	
Numbness	66
Dizziness	58
Tingling	34
Loss of consciousness	22
Musculoskeletal	
Aches and pains	38
Limping	20
Tetany	10
Gastrointestinal	
Dry mouth	52
Abdominal bloating and pain	40
Belching	26

Anxiety

Anxiety disorders are common in children of all ages. Many children with anxiety disorder or panic disorder have episodic chest pain either with or without hyperventilation. Children with anxiety conditions manifest the same spectrum of symptoms as do adults (see Chapter 35). Many of the acute symptoms are related temporally to stressful situations, such as death, divorce, separation from friends, school failure, pregnancy, or physical illness. Stressors also include a family member with chest pain; psychogenic pain is four times as likely to occur with a family history of chest pain. Children with anxiety disorders also manage everyday common stresses with difficulty, and so their history does not always indicate a significant identifiable life event. School or athletic activities might be initiating events. Athletes with chest pain and psychological causes are challenging to treat because of the necessary concerns about the cardiovascular system.

Depression

Depression is demonstrated in approximately 10% of children with chest pain. Multiple studies have reported the common association of depression in children with somatic complaints that include chest pain. Depression may be a primary etiologic factor in chest pain, or it might be related to a reaction to an underlying physical illness.

Somatoform Disorders (Conversion Disorder, Somatization Disorder)

Another common psychological cause of chest pain in children is somatoform disorder, formerly known as psychosomatic illness. These disorders occur more commonly in adolescents than in children and are two to three times more common in girls. Somatoform disorders fall along a spectrum that includes severe problems, such as conversion hysteria, to more mild forms of bodily concerns. Anxiety and depressive symptoms may be present. Chest symptoms are included in the many bodily concerns of these patients, along

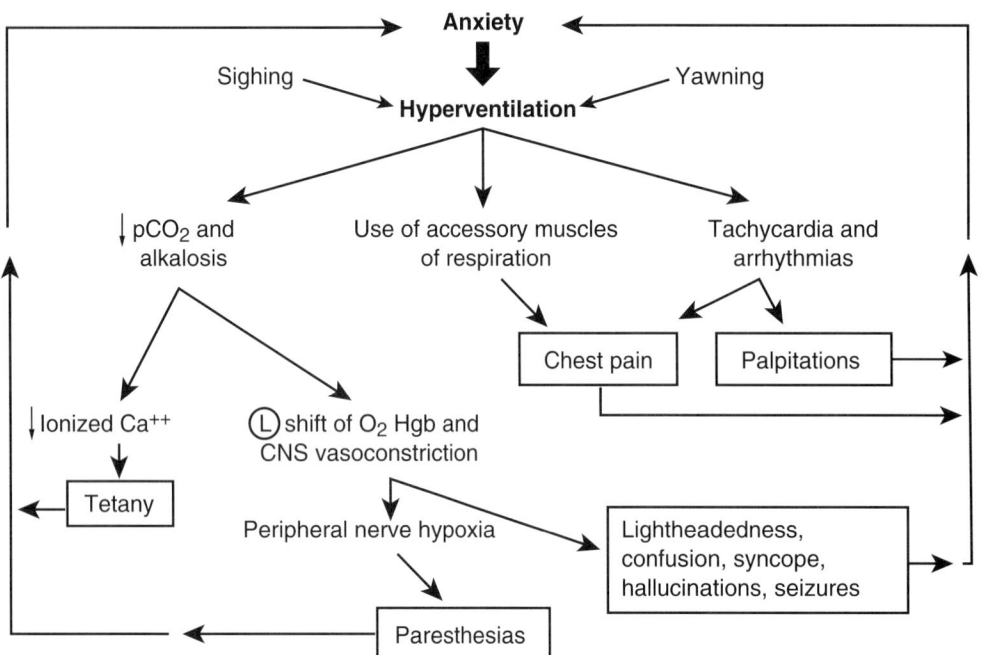

Figure 9-3. Pathophysiologic mechanisms of hyperventilation. CNS, central nervous system; Hgb, hemoglobin; pCO₂, carbon dioxide pressure; O₂ Hgb, oxyhemoglobin dissociation curve. (From Herman SP, Stickler GB, Lucas AR: Hyperventilation syndrome in children and adolescents: Long-term follow-up. Pediatrics 1981;67:183-187.)

with headaches, abdominal symptoms, dizziness, and other sensory-related symptoms (see Chapter 35).

RESPIRATORY CAUSES OF PAIN

Asthma and Respiratory Infection

Asthma and acute respiratory infections are common entities that cause cough and respiratory distress (see Chapters 2 and 3). Prolonged symptoms are likely to stress chest wall muscles, causing pain. Pain from prolonged cough or respiratory distress might be a constant ache or pain with respiratory excursions; the pain might be localized to a specific area of the chest wall, or it may be a diffuse discomfort. Pain recedes with the cessation of cough and with amelioration of tachypnea and labored respirations.

Asthma may cause chest pain with or without significant respiratory distress. Some patients with asthma may have chest pain as a primary symptom. Patients with chest pain associated with exercise often have bronchospasm provoked by exercise and no cardiac abnormalities. The location of the pain is mostly midsternal but can also be parasternal, left- or right-sided, or diffuse. The character of the pain is mostly sharp but can also be tight, stabbing, or dull. Patients with chest pain from undiagnosed causes have a greater likelihood than do normal control subjects to have abnormal results on methacholine challenges and exercise testing, which provides further support for the association of bronchial hyperactivity with chest pain. For some patients with asthma, the chest pain may result from esophageal disease (reflux esophagitis). In such patients, chest pain resolves with treatment for esophagitis.

Pneumonia and Pleurisy

Chest pain can be caused by pneumonia and pleurisy (see Chapters 2 and 3). Patients with chest pain secondary to these respiratory diseases have symptoms of lung infection at the time of the pain. These illnesses are the most common identifiable causes of acute chest pain *with fever*. Inflammation of the pleural surface of the lung causes chest discomfort during inspiration as the pleural surfaces rub together. Bacterial pneumonia is the most common cause of pleuritis in children. Pain is exaggerated by deep breathing, coughing, or straining. The sensation might be sharp, stabbing, or dull. Localization may be over the anterior chest wall but may radiate to the back or shoulder. Characteristic physical and radiographic findings are usually present (see Table 9-3).

Pneumothorax

Pneumothorax may cause acute chest pain with or without dyspnea. The severity of the pain is not correlated with the degree of the pneumothorax. A known predisposing pulmonary disease may be evident, such as acute asthma, pneumonia with empyema, trauma, or cystic fibrosis, but it most commonly occurs spontaneously in previously healthy adolescent boys. A tympanitic percussion note over decreased breath sounds is the characteristic physical finding. Chest x-ray study confirms the diagnosis.

CARDIOVASCULAR CAUSES

Heart Disease

Although a rare cause of chest pain, heart disease is more commonly found in adolescents than in children who complain of chest pain. Adolescents represent the largest group of patients between ages 1 and 21 years who die suddenly from cardiac causes (see Chapters 7 and 42). Therefore, despite the fact that heart disease is uncommon, the importance of accurate diagnosis derives from the potential for dangerous morbidity and mortality.

The possibility of heart disease must be carefully evaluated to detect a causative lesion or to reassure the patient and family that such a lesion does not exist. This is necessary because of the general belief that chest pain indicates heart disease.

Evidence is limited for the prevalence of the various cardiac causes of chest pain (see Table 9-2). Structural abnormalities of the heart that produce ischemic chest pain might also produce altered cardiac output, leading to syncope or sudden death (see Chapter 42). *Hypertrophic cardiomyopathy* (HCM), *aortic valve*, and *subvalvular stenosis* are common causes of cardiac chest pain. If these structural disorders are severe, increased systolic wall stress and shortening of the diastolic period of perfusion can compromise blood flow to the myocardium. Exercise would be expected to provide the hemodynamic stress that worsens chest discomfort in these patients; a history of chest pain with exercise is a significant finding. A family history of recurrent syncope or premature sudden death is significant because HCM is inherited in an autosomal dominant pattern. The most common presenting symptoms of HCM are heart murmur, shortness of breath with exercise, chest pain, syncope, and presyncope.

Children with pulmonic stenosis or pulmonary vascular obstructive disease (Eisenmenger complex) are at risk for ischemia, arrhythmia, and sudden death. Pulmonary hypertension, whether primary or secondary, may manifest with chest pain.

Ischemic chest pain is not common in children and adolescents. If present, it should prompt investigation of the possibility of the obstructive lesions mentioned earlier or various anomalies of the coronary arteries (see Chapter 42). The characteristic pain gradually increases during physical exertion or other stress. It usually persists for a short time (1 to 5 minutes) and is relieved by rest. The pain is typically diffuse, not easily localized but characteristically retrosternal, and occasionally epigastric, with radiation to the neck, jaw, arms, or interscapular area. The sensation is a constricting, choking, tight feeling. If the history indicates previous episodes of chest discomfort similar to this description that is now persistent and associated with syncope, diaphoresis, tachycardia, tachypnea, and hypotension, myocardial infarction must be considered (see Table 9-3). It is important to recognize that this classic presentation may be absent, especially in children who cannot verbalize the experience of pain.

Physical findings might allow recognition of left ventricular outflow tract obstruction (Table 9-8; see Chapter 11). The fixed obstruction of aortic stenosis results in a harsh ejection murmur heard best at the upper right sternal border, radiating to the carotid arteries, and sometimes associated with a thrill. Many children with high-output states (fever, anemia, hyperthyroidism, pregnancy) have basilar ejection murmurs, but the relative harshness of the murmur and the presence of a thrill would be important clues of an anatomic valve abnormality. Diagnostic studies in this group of patients are necessary to determine the anatomic diagnosis and severity. The sensitivity of the chest film and electrocardiogram (ECG) is low; these studies do not always demonstrate left ventricular hypertrophy.

The presence of a prominent septal Q wave strongly suggests HCM. Echocardiography is the most important test because it determines the nature and the degree of outflow obstruction, as well as the degree of ventricular hypertrophy. Exercise electrocardiography may also be useful.

Mitral Valve Prolapse

Mitral valve prolapse (MVP) is much less common in children than in adults. It is a phenomenon in which the mitral valve leaflets protrude during ventricular systole beyond the boundary of the mitral ring, toward the left atrium (see Chapter 11). Varying degrees of mitral insufficiency can occur. MVP may be seen in conjunction with an atrial septal defect (secundum type) and with generalized connective disease disorders, such as Marfan syndrome, osteogenesis imperfecta, pseudoxanthoma elasticum, and Ehlers-Danlos syndrome. Isolated MVP has a familial incidence, with a probable dominant inheritance pattern. The syndrome is more common in girls than in boys.

Most pediatric patients with MVP are asymptomatic; chest pain does not occur in most patients, even in those with thickened and furled mitral valve leaflets. In older adolescents, it can be associated with postural hypotension, palpitations, or syncope. In adults, 40% to 50% complain of chest pain. Some children with prolapsing mitral valves may have vague, nonexertional chest discomfort. Possible pain mechanisms include papillary muscle and endocardial ischemia, as well as discomfort from supraventricular and ventricular dysrhythmia. It is not known why some patients with MVP have chest discomfort.

Cardiac examination should be performed with the patient supine, sitting, standing, squatting, and standing after squatting. Findings are accentuated when the patient stands after squatting, which leads to less ventricular filling. Any maneuver that decreases left ventricular volume (e.g., standing, Valsalva maneuver) accentuates the posterior protrusion of the leaflets and makes the auscultatory findings more prominent. The ECG may be normal or may demonstrate T-wave abnormalities or prominent U waves. Echocardiography is highly specific and permits exclusion of other cardiac defects. Patients with thoracoskeletal deformity (scoliosis, straight back) should be carefully examined to rule out MVP.

Table 9-8. **Systolic Murmurs Important in the Diagnosis of Chest Pain***

Cardiac Diagnosis	Physical Findings	Maneuvers
Innocent ejection murmur	Loudest left sternal border at base, 1 to 3 intensity, peaks early in systole; no click, gallop, heave, or diastolic murmur	Diminishes with standing and Valsalva maneuver

Valvular aortic stenosis	Mild:
	    Similar to innocent murmur but ejection click is possible
	Severe:
	    Loudest over right second intercostal space, peaks late in systole; delayed carotid upstroke, thrill present; left ventricular heave; audible S_4 gallop; aortic insufficiency murmur may also be present	

Hypertrophic cardiomyopathy	Loudest over left second intercostal space, peaks in midsystole; carotid upstroke brisk or bisferiens; no diastolic murmur	Increases with standing or Valsalva maneuver; decreases on squatting

Pulmonic stenosis	Mild:
	    Similar to innocent murmur but ejection click is possible
	Severe:
	    Loudest over left second intercostal space; loud, widely split S_2; thrill present; right ventricular heave; ejection click at left second intercostal space	

Mitral valve prolapse	Loudest at left sternal border and apex; mid- to late-systolic murmur; click precedes murmur	Increases with standing after squatting and during expiration

Modifed from Reilly BM: Practical Strategies in Outpatient Medicine, 2nd ed. Philadelphia, WB Saunders, 1991, p 458.

*See Chapter 11, Heart Sounds and Murmurs.

Ventricular arrhythmias are present in 4% of children with MVP on exercise testing and in 8% on Holter monitoring. Sudden death is unusual in affected children younger than 16 years. There is however, a subgroup of adolescents who are at risk from sudden death from arrhythmia. Nonetheless, the prognosis of MVP in children is usually excellent.

Recognition of MVP provides a challenge because it may not necessarily be the cause of the chest pain. Chest pain has no prognostic significance in a patient with no family history and with an isolated midsystolic click. Noncardiac causes of chest pain might be present in children with benign forms of MVP. Anxiety is a common noncardiac cause of chest pain in young people with MVP that bears closer investigation. There may be an association of panic disorder and MVP.

Acute Pericarditis

Acute pericarditis must be considered when a child presents with chest pain (Table 9-9). Patients with idiopathic or viral pericarditis often have a preceding or accompanying flulike illness with myalgias, arthralgias, and fever. Most commonly, the pain is sharp and stabbing and is aggravated by deep inspiration, coughing, or straining. The patient with a large pericardial effusion may feel less pain while leaning forward in the sitting position. Dysphagia, dyspnea, or hiccup may accompany the pain. Pain is typically in the substernal area, but it may refer elsewhere. Pain may be intermittent or constant. A pericardial rub with three components (one systolic and two diastolic) may be present; if so, it greatly aids in the diagnosis (see Table 9-3). ECGs might reveal a diffuse ST elevation and a low QRS voltage (Fig. 9-4). The chest x-ray study, if positive, may show a globe-shaped, enlarged cardiac shadow. Echocardiography is the definitive test for diagnosis to quantify the amount of pericardial fluid and the degree of ventricular dysfunction.

Myocarditis and Acquired Cardiomyopathy

Most cases of acute myocarditis are caused by viral infection, but some are caused by toxic reactions or autoimmune processes. Typically the patient presents with lethargy, pallor, low-grade fever, anorexia, chest or abdominal pain, and signs of congestive heart failure (see Chapter 8).

Dilated cardiomyopathy is another possible cause of chest pain. While many cases are considered idiopathic, previous myocarditis is thought to be a common cause. Chest radiographs usually demonstrate an enlarged heart and pulmonary edema. Echocardiograms reveal a dilated and poorly contractile left ventricle.

Rhythm Disturbances

Chest pain may be caused by various rhythm disturbances (see Chapter 7). This pain may be caused by an imbalance of myocardial

---

Table 9-9. Etiology of Pericarditis and Pericardial Effusion

Idiopathic (Presumed Viral)

Infectious Agents

Bacterial: Group A streptococci, *Staphylococcus aureus*, pneumococci, meningococci,* *Haemophilus influenzae*,* *Salmonella* species, *Mycoplasma pneumoniae, Borrelia burgdorferi, Mycobacterium tuberculosis*, rickettsiae, tularemia

Viral†: Coxsackievirus (group A, B), echovirus, mumps, influenza, Epstein-Barr virus, cytomegalovirus, herpes simplex, herpes zoster, hepatitis B virus

Fungal: *Histoplasma capsulatum, Coccidioides immitis, Blastomyces dermatitidis, Cryptococcus neoforms, Candida* species, *Aspergillus* species

Parasitic: *Toxoplasma gondii, Entamoeba histolytica*, schistosomes

Collagen Vascular-Inflammatory and Granulomatous Diseases

Rheumatic fever
Systemic lupus erythematosus (idiopathic and drug induced)
Rheumatoid arthritis
Kawasaki disease
Scleroderma
Mixed connective tissue disease
Reiter syndrome
Inflammatory bowel disease
Wegener granulomatosus
Dermatomyositis
Behçet syndrome
Sarcoidosis
Vasculitis
Familial Mediterranean fever
Serum sickness
Stevens-Johnson syndrome

Traumatic

Cardiac contusion (blunt trauma)
Penetrating trauma
Postpericardiotomy syndrome
Radiation

Contiguous Spread

Pleural disease
Pneumonia
Aortic aneurysm (dissecting)

Metabolic

Hypothyroidism
Uremia
Gaucher disease
Fabry disease
Chylopericardium

Neoplastic

Primary
Contiguous (lymphoma)
Metastatic
Infiltrative (leukemia)

Others

Drug reaction
Pancreatitis
After myocardial infarction
Thalassemia
Central venous catheter perforation
Heart failure
Hemorrhage (coagulopathy)
Biliary-pericardial fistula

*Infectious or immune complex.

†Common (viral pericarditis or myopericarditis is probably the most common cause of acute pericarditis in a previously normal host).

A

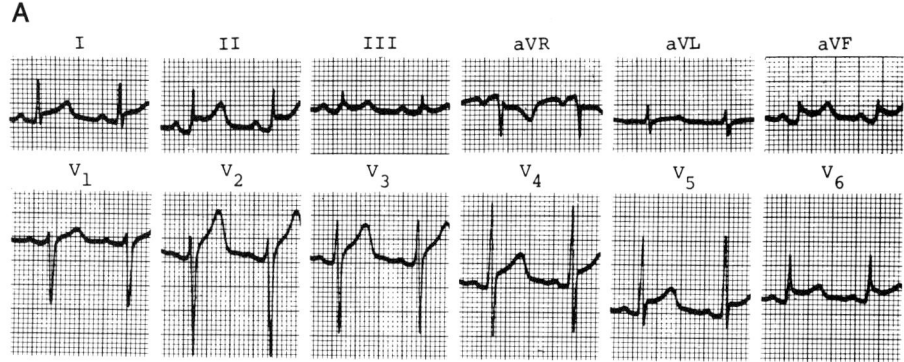

B

2-16-71

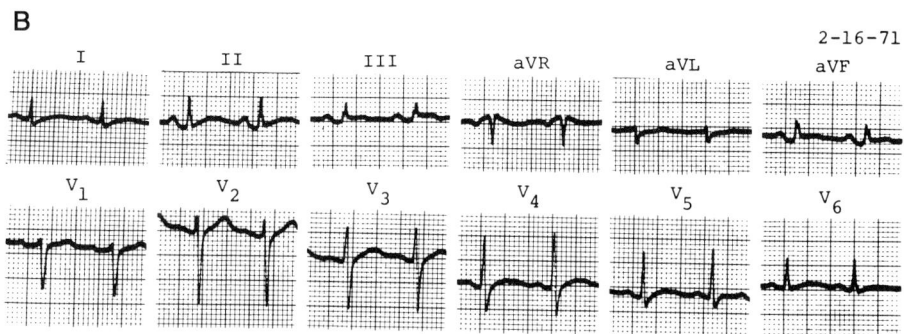

Figure 9-4. Serial changes of acute idiopathic pericarditis. **A,** Diffuse ST-segment elevation involving all the leads except aV_R and aV_L. In lead aV_R, the ST segment is depressed. The QRS complex is normal. **B,** The ST segment is almost isoelectric, and the T waves are flattened or notched. (From Chou T-C: Pericarditis. In Electrocardiography in Clinical Practice, 3rd ed. Philadelphia, WB Saunders, 1991.)

oxygen supply and demand, subendocardial wall stress, and diminished diastolic coronary perfusion. Any of the tachyarrhythmias, ventricular or supraventricular, may bring about these events. Many of these abnormalities have a paroxysmal nature, so that intermittent symptoms are expected. The pain is not classically related to exercise. Chest pain associated with dizziness, palpitations, or syncope may be the presenting complaint and should prompt the physician to perform electrocardiography.

Acute Aortic Dissection and Acute Pulmonary Embolism

Two acute, potentially catastrophic cardiovascular events, acute aortic dissection and acute pulmonary embolism, deserve mention in the consideration of acute chest pain. In patients with Marfan syndrome, Ehlers-Danlos syndrome, and Erdheim familial cystic necrosis, acute aortic dissection may occur. In addition, there have been case reports of aortic dissection in otherwise healthy, recreational weight-lifting athletes. Dissection causes acute, tearing chest pain in the anterior or posterior areas of the chest that migrates to the arms, abdomen, and legs. Clinical clues include pulse deficits, an aortic insufficiency murmur, and a normal ECG.

Pulmonary embolism may occur in adolescents (see Chapter 3). This condition manifests with acute, pleuritic-type pain, dyspnea, cough, and, occasionally, hemoptysis. Usually, factors that might predispose to venous thrombosis are present. These include oral contraceptive use; recent elective abortion; the early postoperative period; protein C, protein S, or antithrombin III deficiency; the antiphospholipid antibody syndrome (anticardiolipin, lupus anticoagulant); and immobilization (see Chapter 50).

GASTROINTESTINAL CAUSES

Esophagitis (acid reflux, infectious) and esophageal motility disorders (diffuse esophageal spasm, achalasia) can cause chest pain in adults and children (see Chapter 16).

If esophageal manometry or esophagoscopy is performed in children with chest pain, abnormal findings are occasionally discovered.

It is possible that some of the patients in the large idiopathic group in empirical studies have esophageal disease. Furthermore, esophageal disease may be associated with asthma and MVP. A gastrointestinal cause might be suggested by symptoms with some association with meals or body position, hematemesis, or melena. Trials of antacids are often helpful diagnostically.

Peptic Esophagitis

Peptic esophagitis occurs in children when gastric contents enter the esophagus. Typical "heartburn," a substernal burning sensation, occurs in children but less commonly than in adults. Indwelling esophageal pH probe studies, barium swallows, scintigraphy, or esophagoscopy are used to diagnose the condition. Unfortunately, the percentage of patients with reflux esophagitis who present primarily with chest pain is not known because most patients have not been evaluated with these investigations.

Esophageal Motility Disorders

Motility disorders of the esophagus are probably less common than reflux esophagitis. Chest pain from a motility disorder may last only for a few seconds, or it may continue for several hours. The pain is nonexertional but may be exacerbated by bending forward. This type of pain is typically substernal but may radiate to the infrascapular area and into the neck. It may therefore resemble the pain of coronary obstruction.

Achalasia is a condition that classically causes dysphagia, nocturnal regurgitation, and chest pain. The symptoms may not be dramatic, and the diagnosis may be elusive. Achalasia may occur at any age. Chest pain occurs in 19% to 95% of patients with achalasia.

Esophageal Rupture

Acute rupture of the esophagus occurs rarely. It has been described in patients with bulimia nervosa, a condition that is prevalent in the adolescent age range, or after surgery for a tracheoesophageal fistula.

Other Gastrointestinal Problems

Any of the gastrointestinal disorders that affect organs in the upper aspect of the abdominal cavity may cause pain that is sensed in the chest. Disorders such as esophageal foreign body, gastric and duodenal ulcers, cholecystitis, pancreatitis, hepatitis, and infections of the subdiaphragmatic space can cause chest discomfort.

Other Causes of Chest Pain

Substance Abuse

Adolescent substance use or abuse can cause chest pain. Cigarette smokers complain more often of chest pain than do nonsmokers. Cocaine has also been implicated as a cause of chest pain in adolescents. Chest pain in acute cocaine intoxication frequently resembles myocardial infarction. Abnormal ST-segment and T-wave changes and the quality of the pain contribute to the diagnostic difficulty. Nonetheless, the incidence of myocardial infarction in young patients presenting with acute chest pain after cocaine use is low. The incidence may be increased in cocaine-using patients who smoke cigarettes. The use of sympathomimetic substances has also been recognized as a cause of chest pain.

Foreign Bodies

Foreign bodies in the airways and esophagus might be unusual causes of chest discomfort in younger children. Usually, there are other symptoms that suggest the diagnosis, including dysphagia, drooling, choking, wheezing, stridor, and dyspnea. Both solid bodies, such as coins, and caustic substances, such as acid or alkaline liquid cleaners, which damage the esophagus, can cause chest pain.

Neoplastic Diseases

Neoplastic diseases may be characterized by chest pain. A mediastinal tumor may cause a constant boring pain that may be associated with cough or dysphagia. Hodgkin disease, non-Hodgkin lymphoma, neural-derived neoplasms, and other tumors may manifest in this manner.

THE APPROACH TO THE PATIENT WITH CHEST PAIN

The practical approach to chest pain requires a detailed history and physical examination. The process not only is necessary to make a diagnosis but also can serve as a therapeutic intervention. A deliberate, orderly, and complete approach to the clinical evaluation can do much to calm an anxious child and parent. Physicians must not forget that chest pain is, in the minds of many, an ominous symptom that needs immediate attention.

Because the most common causes of chest pain are discernible by history and physical examination, it is highly likely that the diagnosis can be made solely on the merits of this clinical evaluation (Table 9-10, Fig. 9-5; see Tables 9-2 to 9-6). Identifying one cause does not eliminate others. Many adolescents present with a benign or more serious organic problem made worse by anxiety or depression.

A primary goal in evaluating a patient with chest discomfort is to prioritize on the basis of the history and physical examination (Table 9-11). The examination allows the physician to attribute the pain to one of these categories:

- Life-threatening emergency
- Chronic condition with possible serious complications
- Specific acute cause
- Specific chronic cause

> **Table 9-10. Historical Features of Chest Pain that are Essential to its Assessment**
>
> Duration of pain (how long present but also duration of each episode)
> Acuteness of onset
> Severity of pain (use scale of 1 to 10)
> Associated symptoms
> Precipitating and ameliorating factors
> Quality of pain (pleuritic, sharp, dull)
> Location of pain
> Limitation of activities by pain
> Radiation of pain
> Time of day that pain occurs
> Recent activity, injury, and stresses
> Full psychosocial review, including behaviors
> Medical history
> Family medical history

HISTORY

Much can be learned by the way the symptoms are reported by patient and parent, together and separately. The parental response to the child's symptoms and the intensity of the parents' concern are important to observe. It is always helpful to elicit beliefs about the symptom from the parent and child. Asking, "What are you concerned that this pain is caused by?" can give much information about previous communications between parent and child and about overriding fears. In assessing the severity of pain, it is useful to ask a parent about how the symptom is being expressed by the child. Asking, "Would you know that she has pain if she didn't tell you?" is a good way of obtaining this information.

For older children and adolescents, it is necessary to interview the patient alone. This measure allows the practitioner to assess the child's level of concern, to clarify the nature of the symptoms in the words of the patient, and to explore areas that might be easier to talk about in private. It is hard for children to discuss areas of difficulty in their family life or school or concern about physical changes (like breast development) unless they are given some degree of confidentiality.

Table 9-10 reviews the appropriate historical features to explore. Duration of pain is first. Sudden, significant pain in a patient who appears ill suggests acute pneumothorax, pericarditis, pulmonary embolism, or dissecting aneurysm (see Table 9-11). Acute pain of a less severe nature might suggest chest wall injury or strain or the onset of a pulmonary infection. Longer term pain or recurrent pain suggests a chronic cause such as a psychological problem, a dysrhythmia, or a gastrointestinal problem. Pain that has persisted for months rarely has a serious organic cause. However, if long-term pain persists and increases in severity and is associated with night sweats, fever, or weight loss, a malignancy should be considered.

The character of pain is not always useful in sorting out its cause. Children are often vague in their descriptions. Pain that is "sharp" or "achy" suggests a chest wall pain or pleural irritation, whereas pain that is "burning" or "gnawing" suggests a thoracic or abdominal visceral origin. Pain that is associated with respiration suggests chest wall discomfort or pleural irritation.

It is helpful to determine factors that exacerbate or reduce pain. Pain that is worse when the patient is lying down or after a large meal or after the consumption of particular foods is consistent with reflux esophagitis. This pain is often relieved by antacids. Pain that is relieved by sitting up and leaning forward might be caused by pericarditis. Pain that is worsened by any movement or sneezing might be related to pleuritic irritation. Pain that is present only during intense exercise may be consistent with myocardial ischemia and must be actively explored. Pain that is temporally related to perceived

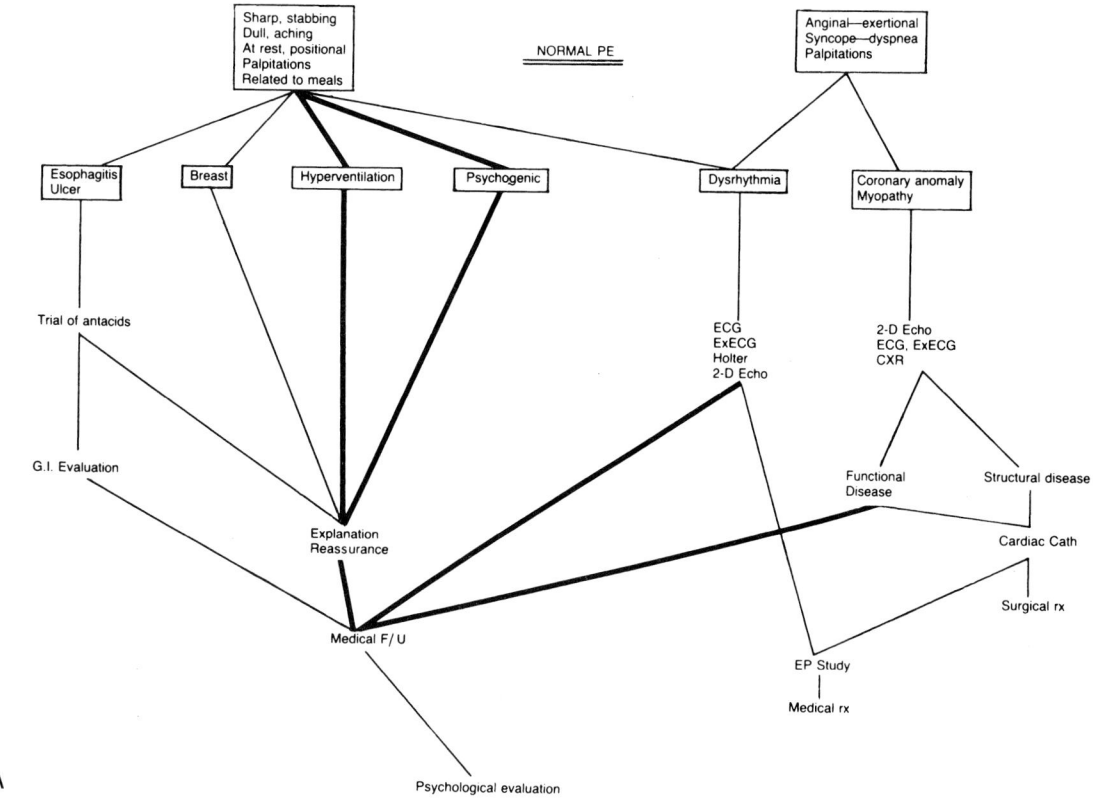

Figure 9-5. These flow diagrams are designed to differentiate the types of chest pain likely to be encountered, with management options based on whether the physical examination (PE) is normal or abnormal. The *heavy lines* indicate the pathway that would be most commonly encountered. Diagnostic possibilities are listed across the page; pertinent laboratory evaluation and further therapy (rx) are suggested. **A,** In patients with normal physical findings, unless the pain is anginal or associated with syncope, progressive dyspnea, or suspected rhythm disturbance, laboratory evaluation is rarely necessary. Cardiac disease is divided into structural abnormalities (coronary lesions), functional disease (myopathy), or dysrhythmia. CXR, chest x-ray; ECG, electrocardiogram; 2-D Echo, two-dimensional echocardiogram or color Doppler echocardiogram; EP study, intracardiac electrophysiologic study; ExECG, exercise electrocardiogram; F/U, follow-up; G.I., gastrointestinal; Holter, 24-hour ambulatory ECG monitor. *Continued*

stress and is relieved by relaxation is an important historical feature for anxiety-related chest pain. Pain that awakens a patient at night is more likely to have an organic cause.

Localization of the pain is useful. Noncardiac pain is often diffuse and radiates to the abdomen. However, in children, pain may also be noncardiac when it is substernal. When pain radiates to the left shoulder, a cardiac origin is more common. Chest wall syndromes have specific locations (see Table 9-5 and Figs. 9-1 and 9-2).

Determination of associated symptoms is helpful. Fever suggests an acute infectious process; cough, dyspnea, or wheezing suggests a bronchospastic condition or acute infection. Vomiting, postprandial discomfort, or abdominal pain suggests a gastrointestinal cause. Tachypnea is consistent with pneumonia, asthma, and hyperventilation. Tingling sensation in the extremities suggests hyperventilation. Multisystemic complaints are evocative of psychogenic causes, unless they include weight loss, intermittent chronic fevers, or syncope.

Information about the recent past can be helpful. Paroxysmal, chronic coughing causes chest wall pain. If the child or adolescent has recently begun to participate in a new sporting activity, especially weight lifting or football, the chest wall may be strained. Recent trauma to the chest is sometimes remembered only with direct questioning.

A full psychosocial review should be performed for each patient. This action ensures that details regarding personal stressors and behaviors will emerge. Asking about school attendance, family relationships, and recent personal and family stressors is necessary. Children with somatoform disorders might have a history of school absences out of proportion to their degree of illness. It is helpful to

ask older children whether anyone close to them has had a recent illness. This question may yield information that there is an adult with chest pain and an anxious reaction in the young person.

Review of symptoms and of medical history is sought for specific features. A history of unexplained syncope might suggest a psychogenic condition, a left-sided cardiac obstruction, or a recurrent arrhythmia (see Chapter 42). The examiner should always seek the history of recognized or unrecognized Kawasaki disease. The history of sickle cell anemia is usually known. Previous history of vague, recurrent symptoms for which no specific diagnosis has been made might indicate that the child has a psychosomatic disorder.

A family medical history should be sought. Not only does the history of chest disease or heart disease in adults put families at risk for anxiety but it is also possible that some diseases are genetically transmitted. Idiopathic hypertrophic subaortic stenosis (hypertrophic cardiomyopathy) and familial hypercholesterolemia might have caused premature death in a relative. Other inherited conditions that may cause chest pain include asthma, sickle cell disease, Marfan syndrome, other forms of myocardiopathy, peptic ulcer disease, and reflux esophagitis.

PHYSICAL EXAMINATION

The examiner should start by observing the child for general states of distress, respirations, splinting, and interaction with parents. Does the child look distressed or ill? Who looks worse, the child or the parent? Vital signs should be checked next. Catastrophic causes of

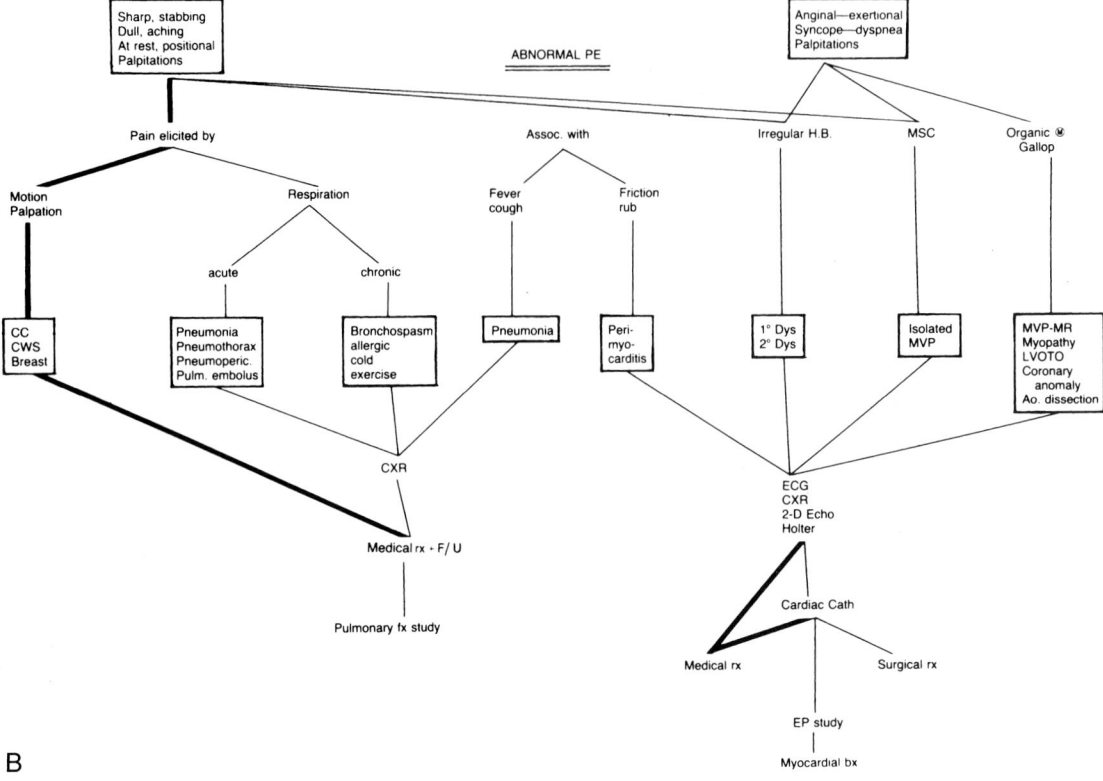

Figure 9-5, cont'd. B, In patients with chest pain and abnormal physical findings, the diagnostic pathway is determined by the physical examination. If pain is produced by palpation or trunk motion or is associated with gynecomastia or breast nodule, a chest x-ray study is only occasionally needed. Acute or chronic respiratory disorders generally necessitate radiographic assessment. An irregular rhythm may be a primary problem or may be secondary to myocardial inflammation or mitral valve prolapse (MVP). Chest pain associated with fever and cough may be caused by bronchopneumonitis. The addition of pericardial friction rub with a history of fever and cough raises concern about perimyocarditis and should prompt specific cardiac studies. Isolated MVP may be confirmed by two-dimensional echo (2-D Echo) or color Doppler echocardiography, but when it is associated with mitral regurgitation or if other structural cardiac disease is suspected, a more detailed evaluation is suggested. 1°, primary; 2°, secondary; Ao, aortic; bx, myocardial biopsy; CC, costochondritis; CWS, chest wall syndrome (rib, vertebral, muscle abnormalities); CXR, chest radiograph; Dys, dysrhythmia; ECG, electrocardiogram; EP study, intracardiac electrophysiologic study; F/U, follow-up; fx, function; H.B., heartbeat; LVOTO, left ventricular outflow obstruction; MR, mitral regurgitation; MSC, mid-systolic click; Pneumoperic., pneumopericardium; Pulm., pulmonary. (From Brenner JI, Ringel RE, Berman MA: Cardiologic perspectives of chest pain in childhood: A referral problem? To whom? Pediatr Clin North Am 1984;31:1241-1258.)

chest pain increase the resting heart rate and increase or decrease the blood pressure. Fever suggests an acute infectious or inflammatory cause.

The examiner should observe the chest wall for signs of trauma, for abnormal breathing patterns, and for deformity. Dilated jugular venous pulsations consistent with heart failure should be sought. The most helpful physical finding is the elicitation of chest wall tenderness. This is the most common physical finding in patients who have no cardiac diseases. Palpation and percussion over the chest, including the ribs, intercostal areas, sternum, xiphoid, manubrium, axilla, clavicles, epigastric area, spinous processes, and paraspinal areas, should be performed. Tenderness is pathognomonic for chest wall pain. Pain over the breasts helps diagnose chest pain caused by gynecomastia. Dullness over the thorax suggests consolidation, effusion, or atelectasis (see Chapter 2). Hyperresonance suggests pneumothorax or asthma. Palpation should also detect evidence of a cardiac heave or cardiac thrill, as well as determine the point of maximal intensity and peripheral pulses (see Chapter 11).

Auscultation of the lungs and heart is next. Presence of a friction rub or gallop rhythm helps make an immediate cardiac diagnosis. Systolic heart murmurs provide the clinical evidence of a cardiac cause of the chest pain (see Table 9-8).

Palpation of the abdomen should be performed for tenderness and the presence of organomegaly.

LABORATORY TESTING

Testing is of little use if the history is unrevealing and the physical examination results are normal. Testing might be helpful in confirming a positive physical finding. Laboratory tests that may be helpful include the chest radiograph, ECG, and echocardiogram. None of these should be ordered routinely.

Radiographic studies are indicated if there is a history of trauma, if there is pleuritic chest pain or fever, and if history and physical findings give positive evidence of heart disease. The likelihood of finding unexpected bone or intrathoracic abnormalities in the absence of other features is low.

Electrocardiography should not be thought of as routine, but it is useful if the history and physical examination indicate the possibility of arrhythmia, pericarditis, myocardial ischemia, or MVP.

Echocardiography is helpful if MVP, valvular heart disease, HCM, or pericarditis is suspected. Exercise testing with the ECG is useful if the history suggests angina-type pain and the rest of the

Table 9-11. Categorization and Prioritization of Chest Discomfort

Category 1: Does complaint indicate life-threatening emergency, such as...

Acute ischemic heart disease?
Aortic dissection?
Pulmonary embolism?
Spontaneous pneumothorax/pneumomediastinum?
Acute arrhythmia?

Indicators:

Acute onset
Severe pain
High or low blood pressure
Significant tachycardia
Cyanosis
Loss of consciousness
Pleuritic-type pain

Category 2: Does the complaint indicate a chronic condition that might result in serious complications, such as...

Aortic stenosis?
Pulmonary hypertension?
Coronary disease?
Hypertrophic cardiomyopathy?
Marfan syndrome?
Nonbenign cardiac arrhythmias, such as Wolf-Parkinson-White syndrome, long QT syndrome, ventricular arrhythmias?

Indicators:

Recurrent intermittent discomfort, especially with exercise
History of syncope
Family history heart disease
Heart murmur

Category 3: Does the complaint indicate specific acute causes, such as...

Asthma?
Pericarditis?
Pneumonia?
Pleural effusion?
Herpes zoster?
Chest wall injury?
Hyperventilation?

Indicators:

Acute onset
Fever
Associated signs and symptoms of lung disease, such as cough or dyspnea

Category 4: Does the complaint indicate specific chronic causes, such as...

Gastroesophageal reflux disease?
Fibromyalgia?
Panic disorder?

Indicators:

Chronic intermittent symptoms
Other gastrointestinal symptoms
Psychosocial indicators such as school absences, mood symptoms, family problems

---

tests are normal. A 24-hour recording by Holter monitor is indicated if arrhythmia is suspected but the resting ECG is normal.

Testing might be indicated to determine whether bronchospasm is present. Exercise testing and methacholine challenge testing with concurrent monitoring of pulmonary function are the most sensitive methods. If exercise-induced asthma is suspected, the testing protocol should include an exercise stimulus.

Overtesting and overreferring to subspecialists can cause harm to the patient. Because the prevalence of chest pain caused by heart disease is low, the physician should avoid reinforcing this association. Patients may experience increased anxiety after their medical encounter.

The patient and family need the physician to make a resolute, clear, and confident diagnosis. If heart disease is strongly suspected from a carefully taken history and carefully performed physical examination, it is unreasonable to cquate negative results on chest film and ECG with the absence of heart disease. It is best to refer the patient to a qualified pediatric cardiologist for further evaluation.

TREATMENT

For patients who have pain at rest and no abnormal physical finding or unusual historical clues, reassurance is the most important treatment. As simple as it sounds, physicians are not uniformly successful at implementing it, especially in just one visit. Successful reassurance demands trust, a symptomatic treatment approach, and a follow-up plan. Successful reassurance occasionally helps the patient recognize that the acute chest pain is benign and does not

merit concern. Performing this step successfully can help the patient avoid a chronic course with possible disability. It is not normal to have pain; therefore, the persistence of chest pain indicates that the diagnosis has not yet been adequately made or that the treatment is either ineffective or has not had sufficient time to help the patient.

All patients with chest pain should be given follow-up appointments. Because chest pain has a predilection to chronicity and can cause disability in young people, the physician's role is to see the complaint to its resolution, rather than dismissing the patient once it is known to be a benign process.

A symptomatic treatment plan is needed so that patients go home with specific directions as to how they can help themselves. If musculoskeletal pain is thought to be present, application of heat, administration of antiinflammatory medication, or specific exercises may be helpful.

Psychogenic pain calls for an active treatment plan developed and implemented by the primary care physician. Making the diagnosis of hyperventilation syndrome does not help the patient deal with the causative psychological illness. Similarly, prescribing rebreathing into a paper bag is not an adequate treatment without more specific treatment for the psychological disorder.

Specific treatments have been shown to be successful for chest pain that is primarily of psychogenic origin. Treatments for hyperventilation have been developed, including breathing retraining, behavioral treatment, and group treatment. Specific treatments for anxiety disorders, depression, and somatoform disorders are warranted if they cause chest pain. These treatments include behavioral techniques for relaxation, guided imagery, individual or group psychotherapy, and/or the use of psychotropic medications.

A *pain diary,* which charts frequency, severity, and circumstances by the patient, is a useful device for follow-up discussion of how the patient can learn to reduce the symptoms. If the physician is not equipped to work with patients in this way, or if the patient is not responding to treatment, a referral should be made to a behavioral pediatrician, an adolescent medicine specialist, a pain specialist, or a mental health professional with experience in somatoform disorders in children. Referral to mental health professionals may be warranted but requires that the physician stay actively involved and instrumental in the treatment plan. This involvement is important to provide ongoing treatment of symptoms of pain and to verify that the patient and family are following through with the mental health treatment plan.

If gastroesophageal reflux is thought to be present, a trial of antacids, H_2-blocking agents, or proton pump inhibitors seems reasonable, as is education regarding limiting foods that seem to worsen the condition, not eating at a time close to bedtime, and raising the head of the bed at night. If the patient does not respond to this approach, or if other gastrointestinal disease is suspected, referral to a pediatric gastroenterologist is indicated.

Because many patients have more than one interacting influence that results in chest pain, the primary care physician must stay involved even if referrals are made. Patients and families are not always sure who is "in charge" of the plan. A complaint such as chest pain, which, if chronic, can have a complex variety of causes, requires a primary physician to coordinate consultations and to interpret the specialist's recommendations to the patient.

REFERENCES

General

Knapp JE, Padalik S, Conner J, et al: Recurrent stabbing chest pain. Pediatr Emerg Care 2002;18:460-465.
Kocis KC: Chest Pain in Pediatrics. Pediatr Clin North Am 1999;46:189-203.
Leung A, Robson W, Cho H: Chest pain in children. Can Fam Physician 1996;42:1156-1164.
Owens TR: Chest pain in the adolescent. Adolesc Med 2001;12:95-104.
Rowe BH, Dulberg CS, Peterson RG, et al: Characteristics of children presenting with chest pain to a pediatric emergency department. Can Med Assoc J 1990;143:388-394.
Selbst SM: Adolescent chest pain and cardiac emergencies. Adolesc Med 1993;4:23-33.
Selbst SM: Chest pain in children. Pediatr Rev 1997;18:169-173.
Swenson JM, Fischer DR, Miller SA, et al: Are chest radiographs and electrocardiograms still valuable in evaluating new pediatric patients with heart murmurs or chest pain? Pediatrics 1997; 99:1-3.

Cardiac Disorders

Alpert MA, Mukerji V, Sabeti M, et al: Mitral valve prolapse, panic disorder, and chest pain. Med Clin North Am 1991;75:1119-1133.
Bor I: Myocardial infarction and ischemic heart disease in infants and children. Arch Dis Child 1969;44:268-281.
Duvernoy CS, Bates ER, Fay WP, et al: Acute myocardial infarction in two adolescent males. Clin Cardiol 1998;21:687-690.
Gitter MJ, Goldsmith SR, Dunbar DN, et al: Cocaine and chest pain: Clinical features and outcome of patients hospitalized to rule out myocardial infarction. Ann Intern Med 1991;115:277-282.
Lam JC, Tobias SC: Follow-up survey of children and adolescents with chest pain. South Med J 2001;94:921-924.
Owens TR: Sudden cardiac death: Is your patient at risk? (Part 1). J Respir Dis 1998;19:152-165.
Owens TR: Sudden cardiac death: Is your patient at risk? (Part 2). J Respir Dis 1998;19:384-396.
Perry RF, Garlisi AP, Allison EJ, et al: Acute myocardial infarction in a 16-year-old boy with no predisposing risk factors. Pediatr Emerg Care 1997;13:413-416.

Roodpeyma S, Sadeghian N: Acute pericarditis in childhood. A 10-year experience. Pediatr Cardiol 2000;21:363-367.
Schor JS, Horowitz MD, Livingstone AS: Recreational weight lifting and aortic dissection: Case report. J Vasc Surg 1993;17:774-776.

Noncardiac Causes

Archer TP, Qualman SJ, Mazzaferri EL: Chest pain and dyspnea in a 17-year-old smoker. Hosp Pract (Off Ed) 1998;33(5):97-98.
Berezin S, Medow MS, Glassman MS, Newman LJ: Esophageal chest pain in children with asthma. J Pediatr Gastroenterol Nutr 1991;12:52-55.
Birmingham CL, Stigant C, Goldner EM: Chest pain in anorexia nervosa. Int J Eating Disord 1999;25:219-222.
Buskila D, Press J, Gedalia A, et al: Assessment of nonarticular tenderness and prevalence of fibromyalgia in children. J Rheumatol 1993;20:368-370.
Corrado G, Bastianon V, Frandina G, et al: Exertional chest pain in a child due to gastroesophageal reflux with a family history of rumination. Panminerva Med 1997;39:312-314.
Dammen T, Ekeberg O, Arnesen H, Friis S: Personality profiles in patients referred for chest pain. Investigation with emphasis on panic disorder patients. Psychosomatics 2000;41:269-276.
Gelfand MJ, Daya SA, Rucknagel DL, et al: Simultaneous occurrence of rib infarction and pulmonary infiltrates in sickle cell disease patients with acute chest syndrome. J Nucl Med 1993;4:614-618.
Greydanus DE, Parks DS, Farrell EG: Breast disorders in children and adolescents. Pediatr Clin North Am 1989;36:601-638.
Hammo AH, Weinberger MM: Exercise-induced hyperventilation: A pseudoasthma syndrome. Ann Allergy Asthma Immunol 1999;82:574-578.
Hotopf M, Mayou R, Wadsworth M, Wessely S: Psychosocial and developmental antecedents of chest pain in young adults. Psychosom Med 1999;61:861-867.
James LP, Farrar HC, Komoroski EM, et al: Sympathomimetic drug use in adolescents presenting to a pediatric emergency department with chest pain. J Toxicol 1998;36:321-328.
Langevin S, Castell DO: Esophageal motility disorders and chest pain. Med Clin North Am 1991;75:1045-1063.
Leffert RD: Thoracic outlet syndromes. Hand Clin 1992;8:285-297.
Luder AS, Segal D, Saba N: Hypoxia and chest pain due to acute constipation: An underdiagnosed condition? Pediatr Pulmonol 1998;26:222-223.
Makhoul RG, Machleder HI: Developmental anomalies at the thoracic outlet: An analysis of 200 consecutive cases. J Vasc Surg 1992;10:534-542.
Malleson PN, al-Mater M, Petty RE: Idiopathic musculoskeletal pain syndromes in children. J Rheumatol 1992;19:1786-1789.
Medow S, Glassman MS, Newman LJ: Esophageal chest pain in children with asthma. J Pediatr Gastroenterol Nutr 1991;12:52-55.
Nakshabendi IM, Maldonado ME, Brady PG: Chest pain: Overlooked manifestation of unsuspected esophageal foreign body. South Med J 2001;94:333-335.
Palmer KM, Selbst SM, Shaffer S, Proujansky R: Pediatric chest pain induced by tetracycline ingestion. Pediatr Emerg Care 1999;15:200-201.
Papo M, Mearin F, Castro A, et al: Chest pain and reappearance of esophageal peristalsis in treated achalasia. Scand J Gastroenterol 1997;32:1190-1194.
Pittman JA, Pounsford JC: Spontaneous pneumomediastinum and ecstasy abuse. J Accid Emerg Med 1997;14:335-336.
Schikler KN: Is it rheumatoid arthritis or fibromyalgia? Med Clin North Am 2000;84:967-982.
Vichinsky EP, Styles LA, Colangelo LH, et al: Acute chest syndrome in sickle cell disease: Clinical presentation and course. Cooperative Study of Sickle Cell Disease. Blood 1997;89:1787-1792.
Voskuil J, Cramer MJ, Breumelhof R, et al: Prevalence of esophageal disorders in patients with chest pain newly referred to the cardiologist. Chest 1996;109:1210-1214.
Wiens L, Sabath R, Ewing L, et al: Chest pain in otherwise healthy children and adolescents is frequently caused by exercise-induced asthma. Pediatrics 1992;90:350-353.

10 Cyanosis

Michele A. Frommelt   Peter C. Frommelt*

Cyanosis is one of the most dramatic and challenging emergencies in pediatric practice. Detection of cyanosis, understanding the physiology of oxygenation, and differentiating the causes of cyanosis are important for successful treatment of the affected child.

DEFINITION

True or *central cyanosis* is a bluish discoloration of the skin, mucous membranes, lips, and conjunctiva, and it indicates significant arterial oxygen desaturation. Central cyanosis should be distinguished from *acrocyanosis,* a bluish discoloration of the hands and feet only. Acrocyanosis indicates the presence of peripheral vasoconstriction rather than arterial oxygen desaturation. Vasoconstriction causes decreased peripheral perfusion and increased oxygen extraction from peripheral capillary blood. This results in decreased oxygen content of venous return, which produces the peripheral bluish discoloration. Acrocyanosis can be associated with fever, hypovolemia, exposure to cold temperatures, sympathomimetic agents, sepsis, congestive heart failure, or shock. Acrocyanosis in an otherwise healthy 1- to 2-day-old infant is relatively common and probably physiologic.

Differential cyanosis and *reverse differential cyanosis* are special variants of central cyanosis that may occur in the newborn. Differential cyanosis is defined as relative cyanosis in the postductal circulation: the circulation supplied by the aorta distal to the origin of the patent ductus. In this case, the lower abdomen, legs, and feet are diffusely cyanotic but the right arm, face, and often the left arm appear less cyanotic or even normal in color. Reverse differential cyanosis indicates relative cyanosis in the preductal circulation. Either condition may be clinically inapparent and may need to be confirmed by comparing pulse oximetry or arterial blood gas partial pressure of oxygen (PO_2) from sites representing preductal circulation (usually the right arm or hand) and postductal circulation (usually the umbilical artery or feet). The detection of differential or reverse differential cyanosis streamlines the differential diagnosis of cyanosis.

DETECTION AND CONFIRMATION OF CYANOSIS

Pulse oximetry has improved the detection of cyanosis, and a low "pulse-ox" reading may often be the "chief complaint." The detection of cyanosis by physical examination requires an absolute amount of at least 3 to 5 g/dL of deoxygenated or desaturated hemoglobin. Clinical cyanosis is therefore directly related to the degree of oxygen saturation and to the total hemoglobin. Cyanosis is usually evident at arterial oxygen saturation levels below 78% to 80%.

Oxygen saturation is the percentage of circulating hemoglobin that binds oxygen. This percentage is determined by the arterial PO_2 and the hemoglobin-oxygen dissociation curve (Fig. 10-1). This curve represents a sigmoidal rather than a linear relationship. When the arterial PO_2 is 60 mm Hg or higher, the arterial oxygen saturation is usually above 90%. As the PO_2 falls below 60 mm Hg, there is a precipitous decrease in oxygen saturation to a level of 50% at a PO_2 of 27 (the oxygen half-saturation pressure [P_{50}] for adult hemoglobin).

The dissociation curve shifts rightward or leftward under various conditions. The fetal hemoglobin curve is shifted to the left because this hemoglobin has a higher affinity for oxygen (oxygen is released less easily to the tissues). Thus, a given PO_2 produces a higher oxygen saturation of fetal hemoglobin than of adult hemoglobin. Acidosis, carbon dioxide (CO_2) retention, hyperthermia, or elevated levels of erythrocyte 2,3-diphosphoglycerate (DPG) shifts the curve to the right (oxygen is released more easily to the tissues). Under these conditions, the oxygen saturation is lower than normal for any given PO_2. Some abnormal hemoglobins have altered affinity for oxygen and functionally shift the curve to the right.

Methemoglobinemia occurs when ferric (Fe^{+3}) rather than ferrous (Fe^{+2}) ion is bound to the hemoglobin molecule. The Fe^{+3} ion has a poor affinity for oxygen at any given PO_2. In this case, the hemoglobin oxygen saturation can be severely depressed, even though arterial PO_2 is normal. Thus, with the exception of methemoglobinemia, arterial oxygen desaturation implies arterial hypoxemia (a depression of arterial PO_2).

The detection of cyanosis requires the presence of an absolute amount of 3 to 5 g/dL desaturated hemoglobin. Therefore, the total hemoglobin also affects the examiner's ability to detect cyanosis. For example, in a newborn with a normal hemoglobin count of 18 g/dL, cyanosis can be detected more easily. If 3 g/dL hemoglobin must be desaturated to detect cyanosis, 15 g/dL (18 − 3 g/dL) is the amount of hemoglobin that is saturated with oxygen. The amount of hemoglobin that is saturated is 15 g/dL (amount saturated) divided by 18 g/dL (total hemoglobin), or 83% (oxygen saturation is 83%). Thus, oxygen saturation of 83% or less produces detectable cyanosis in a neonate with normal hemoglobin. If the child is anemic (hemoglobin of 9 g/dL), detection of cyanosis may be more challenging. Because 3 g/dL hemoglobin must be desaturated before cyanosis can be detected, only 6 g/dL is saturated. Dividing saturated hemoglobin (6 g/dL) by total hemoglobin (9 g/dL) reveals that the child must have 67% or less oxygen saturation for cyanosis to be detected.

The arterial blood gas provides the clinician with information about the patient's acid-base status as well as the arterial PO_2. *Hypoxemia* is defined as a PO_2 less than 60 mm Hg during the first day of life and less than 80 mm Hg thereafter. Normal arterial partial pressure of oxygen (PaO_2) is higher than 90% after the first week of life in infants born at term. Because the arterial saturation reported on an arterial blood gas measurement is not measured directly with a cooximeter (it is calculated from the measured PO_2 and the hemoglobin-oxygen dissociation curve for adult hemoglobin), the report may be inaccurate. This value may not be correlated with pulse oximetry in neonates, who have high levels of fetal rather than of adult hemoglobin, or in patients with methemoglobinemia.

*This chapter is an updated and edited version of the chapter by Frank Smith that appeared in the first edition.

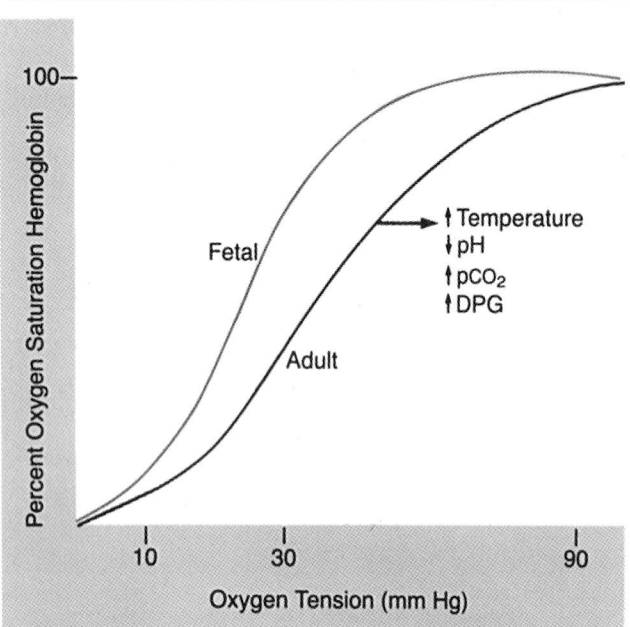

Figure 10-1. Hemoglobin-oxygen dissociation curves. The position of the adult curve depends on the binding of adult hemoglobin to 2,3-diphosphoglycerate (DPG), temperature, carbon dioxide tension (pCO$_2$), and hydrogen ion concentration (pH). (From Behrman RE, Kliegman RM [eds]: Nelson's Essentials of Pediatrics, 2nd ed. Philadelphia, WB Saunders, 1994, p 166.)

A capillary blood gas sample cannot be used to measure arterial oxygenation.

PHYSIOLOGY OF OXYGENATION

Oxygenation requires adequate ambient oxygen, an intact central nervous system, normal hemoglobin, and normal respiratory and cardiac systems. Mechanisms of cyanosis (hypoxemia) include alveolar hypoventilation, abnormalities of hemoglobin oxygen affinity, ventilation-perfusion imbalance, oxygen diffusion defects (rare), and shunts (intrapulmonary or cardiac right-to-left shunts), respectively.

The normal circulation of the fetus and newborn is noted in Figure 10-2. Differential and reverse differential cyanosis is based on this physiologic change (Fig. 10-3). *Differential cyanosis* (relatively more cyanosis in the postductal circulation) occurs when pulmonary vascular resistance remains abnormally high after birth. Flow into the pulmonary artery does not reach the pulmonary vascular bed; it passes across the patent ductus into the descending aorta, in a manner similar to that of the fetal circulation. This condition is known as *persistent pulmonary hypertension of the newborn* (PPHN). A right-to-left ductal shunt may also occur when descending aortic flow is dependent on the patent ductus because of obstruction of flow upstream, as in critical coarctation of the aorta.

Reverse differential cyanosis (relatively more cyanosis in the preductal circulation) occurs when pulmonary vascular resistance remains abnormally high after birth *and* there is transposition of the great arteries. In this case, the pulmonary artery arises from the oxygenated left ventricle. If pulmonary vascular resistance is abnormally high, this oxygenated blood passes from the pulmonary artery into the descending aorta via the patent ductus arteriosus. The ascending aorta, however, arises from the deoxygenated right ventricle, and thus the preductal aortic circulation receives desaturated blood. Reverse differential cyanosis occurs with transposition of the great arteries and patent ductus arteriosus with PPHN or with transposition and either critical coarctation of the aorta or interrupted aortic arch (Fig. 10-4).

THE NEWBORN

Determining the underlying cause of cyanosis requires different approaches for the neonate, infant, and older child.

HISTORY

An accurate history is critical for evaluating a newborn with cyanosis (Table 10-1). A history of fetal distress, difficult delivery, low Apgar scores, intracranial hemorrhage, seizures, or neuromuscular disease in the newborn, or excessive maternal sedation may implicate central nervous system depression or disease resulting in *central hypoventilation*. *Respiratory disease* can be suspected when there is a history of prematurity (respiratory distress syndrome), prolonged rupture of

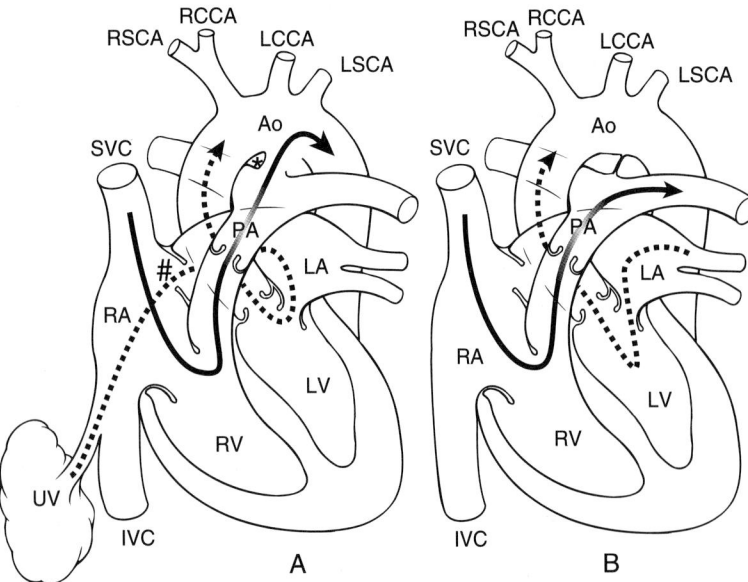

Figure 10-2. Prenatal (**A**) and postnatal (**B**) circulation. **A,** Prenatal circulation: Relatively oxygenated blood (*dashed line with arrow*) from the placenta returns to the umbilical vein, coursing through the foramen ovale to the left side of the heart and ascending aorta. Deoxygenated blood (*unbroken line with arrow*) returns to the right side of the heart, pulmonary artery, and then mainly to the descending aorta through the patent ductus arteriosus, because pulmonary vascular resistance is very high in utero. **B,** Postnatal circulation: Oxygenated blood (*dashed line with arrow*) from the lungs returns to the left side of the heart and aorta. Deoxygenated blood (*unbroken line with arrow*) returns to the right side of the heart, pulmonary artery, and lungs. *Asterisk* (*) represents patent ductus arteriosus; *pound sign* (#) represents patent foramen ovale. Ao, aorta; IVC, inferior vena cava; LA, left atrium; LCCA, left common carotid artery; LSCA, left subclavian artery; LV, left ventricle; PA, pulmonary artery; RA, right atrium; RCCA, right common carotid artery; RSCA, right subclavian artery; RV, right ventricle; SVC, superior vena cava; UV, umbilical vein.

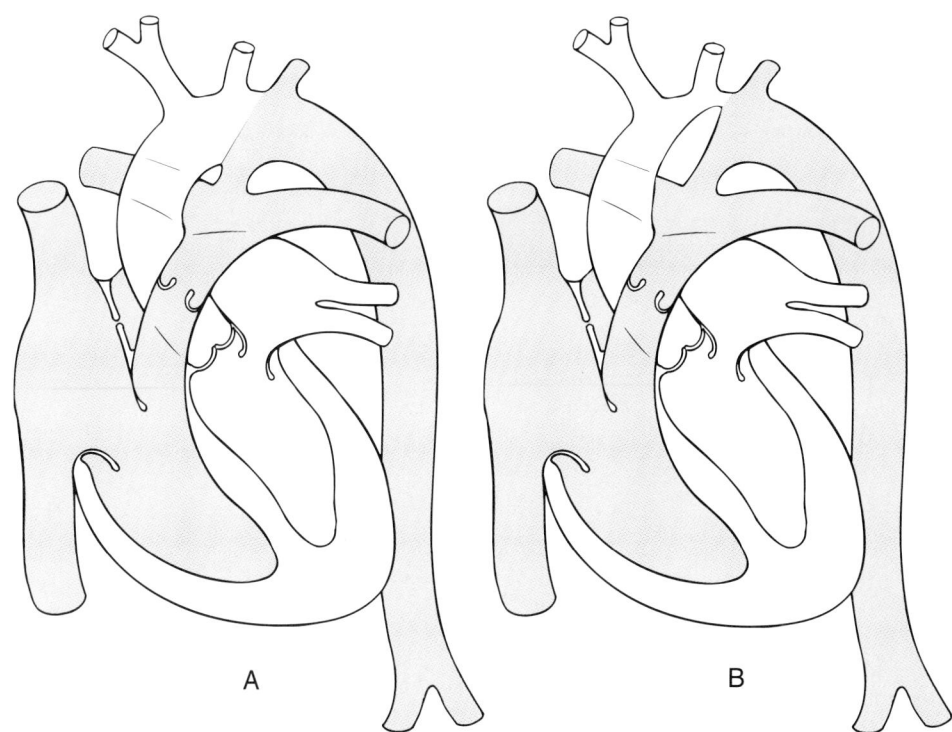

Figure 10-3. Differential cyanosis. **A,** Differential cyanosis occurs when pulmonary vascular resistance remains abnormally high after birth. Flow into the pulmonary artery avoids the pulmonary vascular bed and passes across the patent ductus into the descending aorta. **B,** Critical coarctation of the aorta with dependence on a patent ductus arteriosus. *Shading* represents deoxygenated blood.

membranes or maternal fever (neonatal sepsis or pneumonia), meconium-stained amniotic fluid (meconium aspiration, PPHN), respiratory distress in the delivery room (pneumothorax, diaphragmatic hernia), or cyanosis, particularly with feedings (choanal stenosis or atresia, Pierre Robin syndrome).

Methemoglobinemia is rarely a cause of cyanosis in a newborn, but a family history of abnormal hemoglobin should be elicited when the baby is cyanotic for seemingly unexplained reasons. A history of exposure to oxidizing agents, including drugs or nitrate-rich well water may be obtained for infants or children.

Cardiac disease is an important cause of cyanosis in the neonate. The newborn with cyanotic heart disease is usually full term with a history of normal labor and delivery. The Apgar scores are often 8 and 8 at 1 and 5 minutes, respectively, because of the central cyanosis. Often this initial cyanosis improves enough so that many infants are transferred to the normal nursery. However, they are soon found to be cyanotic with the gradual closure of the foramen ovale and ductus arteriosus. Even if cyanosis is observed within hours after delivery, a history of severe respiratory distress (retractions, flaring) is usually absent.

PHYSICAL EXAMINATION

Patients with central nervous system depression or disease that results in hypoventilation can have a low respiratory rate or diminished lung air entry. The physician should also focus on possible hypotonia; flaccid posture; weak cry; poor response to stimuli; obvious abnormalities in size, shape, or transillumination of the head; brachial plexus palsy; or signs of phrenic palsy associated with shoulder dystocia.

Signs of neonatal pulmonary disease include tachypnea, dyspnea with retractions, nasal flaring, stridor, grunting, wheezes, or rales. Severe respiratory distress with cyanosis and a scaphoid abdomen shortly after birth are signs of a diaphragmatic hernia. Unilateral breath sounds suggest this diagnosis but may also be consistent with a pleural effusion, pneumothorax, or hemidiaphragm palsy. Transillumination of the thorax may confirm the presence of a

pneumothorax. Inability to pass a feeding tube through each nostril indicates airway obstruction from choanal stenosis or atresia.

A neonate with a slate-gray appearance who has brown-red "chocolate" discoloration of the blood that fails to become bright red when exposed to room air may have congenital methemoglobinemia.

The infant with cardiac cyanosis is remarkably alert and comfortable for the degree of cyanosis. Usually, the child has normal tone and no abnormal respiratory signs other than mild tachypnea. Exceptions to this scenario include infants with cyanotic heart lesions associated with either pulmonary edema or severe congestive heart failure. Pulmonary edema may occur early with lesions that cause severe pulmonary venous obstruction (total anomalous pulmonary venous return [TAPVR] with obstruction). Congestive heart failure can occur precipitously with the *hypoplastic left heart syndrome,* in which ductal closure leads to circulatory collapse as well as commitment of all the cardiac output to the pulmonary artery.

Although the cardiac examination findings may be deceptively normal in newborns with cyanotic heart disease, the presence of abnormalities increases the likelihood of a cardiac cause. Specific signs include abnormal parasternal activity (present in right ventricular enlargement/hypertrophy or left ventricular hypoplasia), abnormal apical activity (present in right ventricular hypoplasia), single second heart sound (present in pulmonary hypertension, transposition of the great arteries, atretic pulmonic or aortic valve, truncus arteriosus), murmurs, a systolic ejection click (present in pulmonic stenosis, truncus arteriosus), and diminished or unequal pulses (present in coarctation of the aorta or interrupted aortic arch) (see Chapter 11). Signs of congestive heart failure such as gallop rhythm, tachypnea, tachycardia, or hepatomegaly (hypoplastic left heart syndrome) are seen in certain cyanotic infants (see Chapter 8). Stigmata of certain genetic syndromes suggest particular heart defects (Table 10-2).

DIFFERENTIAL DIAGNOSIS

The general causes of cyanosis in the neonate can often be identified or excluded by a complete history and physical examination in combination with a chest radiograph, an electrocardiogram (ECG), and

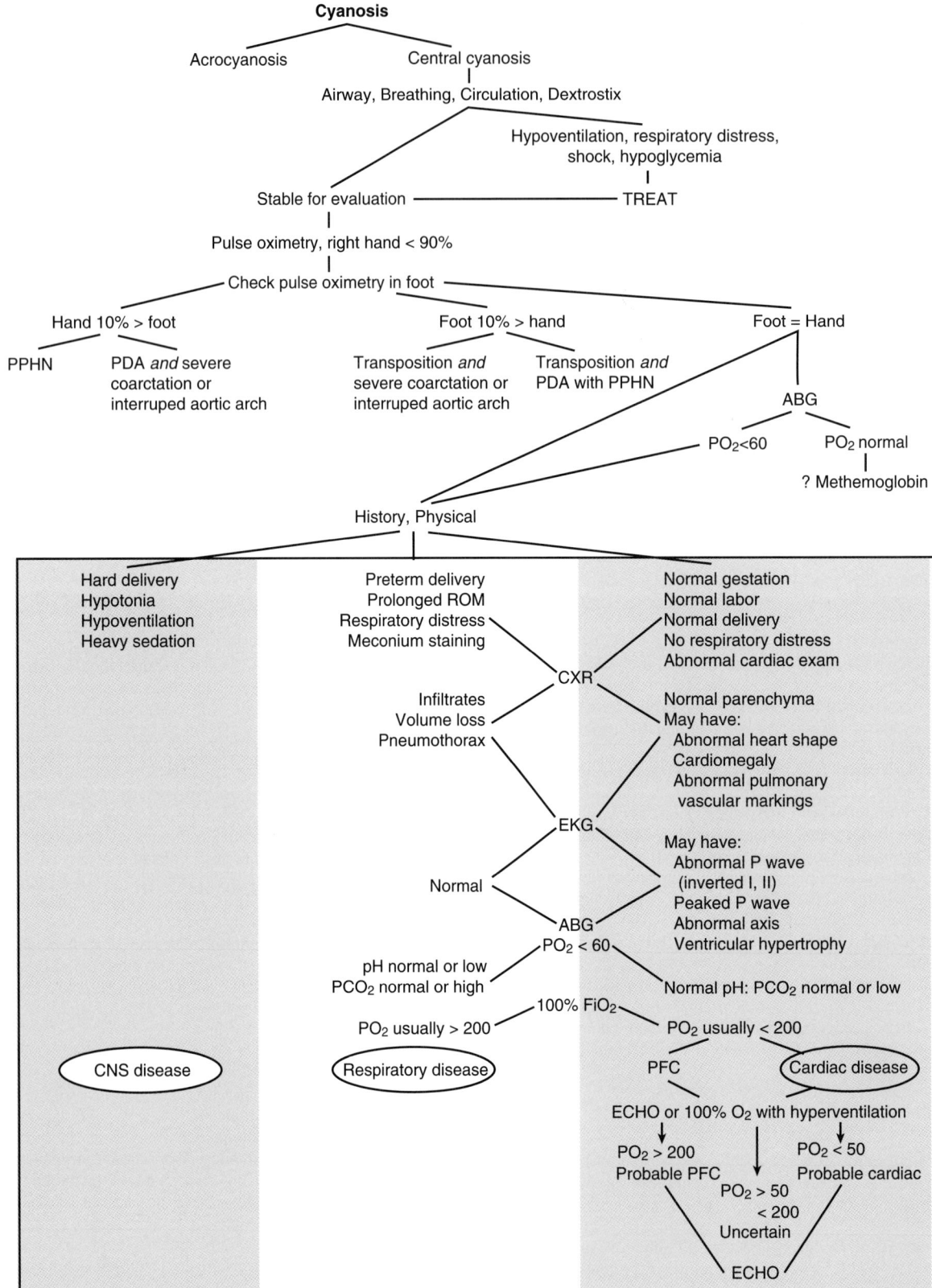

Figure 10-4. Approach to neonatal cyanosis. ABG, arterial blood gas; CNS, central nervous system; CXR, chest radiograph; ECHO, echocardiogram; EKG, electrocardiogram; FiO$_2$, fraction of inspired oxygen; nl = normal; PCO$_2$, partial pressure of carbon dioxide; PDA, patent ductus arteriosus; PFC, persistent fetal circulation; PO$_2$, partial pressure of oxygen; PPHN, persistent pulmonary hypertension of the newborn; ROM, rupture of membranes.

Table 10-1. Differential Diagnosis of Cyanosis in the Newborn

Inadequate Ambient O₂ or Less O₂ Delivered Than Expected (rare)
Incubator malfunction
Disconnection of oxygen supply to nasal cannula, head hood
Connection of air, rather than oxygen, to a mechanical ventilator
Central or Peripheral Nervous System Hypoventilation
Birth asphyxia
Intracranial hypertension, hemorrhage
Oversedation (direct or through maternal route)
Diaphragm palsy
Neuromuscular diseases
Seizures
Respiratory Disease
Upper airway
  Choanal atresia/stenosis
  Pierre Robin syndrome
  Intrinsic airway obstruction (laryngeal/bronchial/tracheal stenosis)
  Extrinsic airway obstruction (bronchogenic cyst, duplication cyst, vascular compression)
Lower airway
  Respiratory distress syndrome
  Transient tachypnea
  Meconium aspiration
  Pneumonia/pneumonitis
  Pneumothorax
  Congenital diaphragmatic hernia
  Pulmonary hypoplasia
  Persistent fetal circulation (persistent pulmonary hypertension of newborn)
Cardiac Right-to-Left Shunt
Abnormal connections (pulmonary blood flow normal or increased)
  Transposition of the great vessels
  Total anomalous pulmonary venous return
  Truncus arteriosus
  Hypoplastic left heart syndrome
  Single ventricle or tricuspid atresia with large ventricular septal defect without pulmonic stenosis
Obstructed pulmonary blood flow (pulmonary blood flow decreased)
  Pulmonic atresia with intact ventricular septum
  Tetralogy of Fallot
  Critical pulmonic stenosis with patent foramen ovale or atrial septal defect
  Tricuspid atresia
  Single ventricle with pulmonic stenosis
  Ebstein malformation of the tricuspid valve
  Persistent fetal circulation (persistent pulmonary hypertension of newborn)
Methemoglobinemia
Congenital (hemoglobin M, methemoglobin reductase deficiency)
Acquired (e.g., nitrates, nitrites)
Spurious/artifactual
Oximeter artifact (poor contact between probe and skin, poor pulse searching)
Arterial blood gas artifact (contamination with venous blood)
Other
Hypoglycemia
Adrenogenital syndrome
Polycythemia
Blood loss

Table 10-2. Syndromes Associated with Cyanotic Heart Disease

Down syndrome	Endocardial cushion defects (including complete atrioventricular septal defect with or without pulmonic stenosis)
DiGeorge syndrome	Interrupted aortic arch, conotruncal defects (tetralogy of Fallot, truncus arteriosus)
CHARGE syndrome	Conotruncal defects
Turner syndrome	Hypoplastic left heart syndrome, coarctation of the aorta
Asplenia and polysplenia syndromes (see Chapter 11)	Complex cyanotic heart disease with multiple lesions: endocardial cushion defect, pulmonic stenosis or atresia, transposition of the great arteries, anomalous pulmonary venous return

CHARGE, coloboma, heart disease, atresia choanae, retarded growth, ears (deafness). (The Shprintzen syndrome [velocardiofacial] is also related.)

an arterial blood gas analysis on room air and maximum (~100%) fraction of inspired oxygen (FiO_2) (hyperoxia test) (see Table 10-1).

Chest Radiography

The chest radiograph in the newborn with apparent respiratory disease may show abnormalities of the upper airway or tracheal air column or tracheal bifurcation. There may be a reticulogranular appearance consistent with respiratory distress syndrome or sepsis, infiltrates or interstitial densities (pneumonia, hemorrhage), pneumothorax, pleural effusion, or air-filled densities consistent with a diaphragmatic hernia or cystic adenomatoid malformation. With partial airway obstruction, there may be air trapping with hyperaeration of one or both lungs and flattening of the hemidiaphragms.

The chest radiograph in the newborn with cyanotic heart disease usually lacks findings of parenchymal lung disease and may also not show abnormalities of the cardiac silhouette and pulmonary vascular markings. Evidence of abnormal cardiac size and shape, and especially abnormal pulmonary vascular markings, may help identify whether a cardiac defect is present (Table 10-3). A large right atrial shadow suggests the presence of tricuspid incompetence. The "wooden shoe"–shaped cardiac silhouette resulting from an upturned apex (right ventricular dominance) and absence of the main pulmonary segment may be seen with tetralogy of Fallot. Other shapes ("egg on a string," "snowman," "globular heart") may be seen with transposition of the great arteries, TAPVR, and tricuspid atresia, respectively, but they are inconsistent findings, and their absence does not exclude these diagnoses. Aneurysmal dilatation of the proximal pulmonary artery branches, which may cause air trapping by compression of mainstem bronchi, is seen with tetralogy of Fallot with absence of the pulmonary valve.

The location of the stomach may provide an important clue. Both the cardiac apex and stomach are normally left-sided (*situs solitus*). When both structures are right-sided, *situs inversus totalis* is present. In this case, there is a slightly higher risk of congenital heart disease. When the cardiac apex and the stomach bubble are on opposite sides, *situs ambiguus* is likely. This often occurs with asplenia and polysplenia syndromes, both of which are associated with complex heart disease (see Chapter 11). The presence of a right aortic arch is suggested by a round density at the upper right border of the cardiac silhouette, displacing the distal trachea to the left. This is frequently

Table 10-3. Differentiating Cardiac Cyanosis by Radiograph

Normal or Increased Pulmonary Vascular Markings
Transposition of the great arteries
Total anomalous pulmonary venous return
Truncus arteriosus
Single ventricle without pulmonic stenosis
Tricuspid atresia with ventricular septal defect and mild or
  no pulmonic stenosis

Decreased Pulmonary Vascular Markings
Pulmonary atresia with intact ventricular septum
Tetralogy of Fallot
Tricuspid atresia with small ventricular septal
  defect/pulmonic stenosis
Ebstein malformation of the tricuspid valve
Single ventricle with pulmonic stenosis

Right Aortic Arch
Truncus arteriosus
Tetralogy of Fallot/pulmonic atresia
Transposition complex

Discordant Situs of Heart and Stomach
Complex cardiac disease (polysplenia and asplenia
  syndrome)

Cardiomegaly
Total anomalous pulmonary venous return
Truncus arteriosus
Single ventricle with mild or no pulmonic stenosis
Ebstein malformation of the tricuspid valve

Abnormal Cardiac Shape
Transposition of the great arteries ("egg on a string")
Total anomalous pulmonary venous return ("snowman")
Tetralogy of Fallot ("wooden shoe," "boot-shaped")

Table 10-4. Differential Cardiac Cyanosis by Electrocardiographic Abnormalities

Peaked P wave lead II (right atrial enlargement)	Pulmonary atresia with intact ventricular septum, tricuspid atresia
Inverted P waves lead I, II (atrial situs inversus)	Situs inversus, complex cyanotic heart disease, lead malposition
Wolff-Parkinson-White syndrome	Ebstein malformation of the tricuspid valve, complex transposition of the great arteries
Prolonged PR interval, heart block	Complex transposition of the great arteries, asplenia and polysplenia syndromes
Severe left axis deviation (superior axis)	Endocardial cushion defects with or without pulmonic stenosis
Mild left axis deviation	Tricuspid or pulmonic atresia
Absent right ventricular forces	Tricuspid or pulmonary atresia
Absent left ventricular forces	Hypoplastic left heart syndrome

seen with truncus arteriosus and tetralogy of Fallot with or without pulmonary atresia.

Detection of increased or decreased (decreased pulmonary blood flow with cyanosis) pulmonary vascular markings not only suggests congenital heart disease but also helps determine which particular defects are present (see Table 10-3).

Electrocardiography

Although the ECG may be normal in newborns with cyanotic congenital heart disease, certain ECG abnormalities suggest particular cardiac defects (Table 10-4). Abnormally peaked P waves may be seen with lesions associated with right atrial enlargement (tricuspid atresia, pulmonic stenosis or atresia with intact ventricular septum, Ebstein malformation of the tricuspid valve). Preexcitation, a short PR interval with wide QRS complex consisting of an initial slurred "delta wave" (otherwise known as *Wolff-Parkinson-White syndrome* when associated with supraventricular tachycardia) is seen with Ebstein malformation of the tricuspid valve and less commonly with complex transposition of the great arteries. An abnormal left axis deviation is associated with diminished right ventricular forces (tricuspid atresia). Severe left axis deviation is seen with an endocardial cushion defect, such as atrioventricular septal defect or "atrioventricular canal."

Arterial Blood Gas Analysis and Pulse Oximetry

Pulse oximetry is a sensitive noninvasive instrument to confirm the visual suspicion of cyanosis. The pulse oximeter can estimate the oxygen saturation with reasonable accuracy for an oxygen saturation of 60% or greater. Pulse oximetry may not estimate the true oxygen saturation when methemoglobinemia is present. In this case, the estimated oxygen saturation is usually low (~85%). If an abnormally low oxygen saturation is detected when cyanosis appears unlikely, another sensor should be used and different extremities sampled. Finally, pulse oximetry cannot detect hyperoxemia. A pulse oximetry saturation of 95% or higher could correspond to an arterial PO_2 of 80 or 380.

Transcutaneous monitors require placement of a heated probe on the infant's skin. These monitors can estimate arterial partial pressure of carbon dioxide (PCO_2) as well as PO_2 and are particularly useful for management of the premature infant, inasmuch as PO_2 can be monitored and hyperoxemia can be avoided. The pulse oximeter is currently preferred for most other noninvasive oxygen monitoring.

When significant desaturation (<80%) is detected by pulse oximetry, an arterial blood gas analysis should be performed to confirm hypoxemia. The arterial PO_2 may be artifactually depressed if the arterial specimen is contaminated with venous blood or if the child is sufficiently agitated to produce a transient right-to-left shunt across the patent foramen ovale. The arterial blood gas measurement confirms arterial hypoxemia, and the pH and PCO_2 help differentiate respiratory (hypercarbia may be present) from cardiac causes of hypoxemia. An arterial blood gas analysis that is repeated while the infant breathes the maximum (~100%) FiO_2 (the *hyperoxia test*) may further differentiate respiratory from cardiac cyanosis (see later discussion).

With respiratory disease, the elimination of CO_2 is often impaired. With compensated cyanotic heart disease, the PCO_2 is either normal or slightly lower than normal as a result of mild hyperventilation. Carbon dioxide retention occurs with cyanotic heart disease only when pulmonary blood flow is extremely limited or if there is concomitant pulmonary disease. If arterial hypoxemia is significant enough to depress oxygen delivery to the tissues (in spite of a relatively high hemoglobin and the presence of fetal hemoglobin), a metabolic (lactic) acidosis develops with respiratory compensation.

If a low arterial PO_2 is originally obtained from the postductal circulation (usually the umbilical artery), differential cyanosis should be considered and excluded. Pulse oximetry or an arterial blood gas measurement performed in the right radial artery should be obtained. If the preductal PO_2 is 20 mm Hg higher than the postductal value, differential cyanosis is present.

For the *hyperoxia test,* an arterial blood gas analysis is performed after the child inhales maximum (~100%) FiO_2 for at least 10 to 15 minutes. If the hypoxemia is caused by respiratory disease, the arterial PO_2 often rises significantly unless respiratory disease is severe or unless there is concomitant PPHN. If the PO_2 is less than 50 mm Hg, respiratory disease is still possible, but cyanotic heart disease should be seriously considered. The two most common cyanotic heart defects in the newborn (transposition of the great arteries, pulmonic atresia) are characteristically associated with an arterial PO_2 less than 50 mm Hg both on room air and with hyperoxia in the absence of respiratory acidosis or clinical respiratory distress.

When the PO_2 is higher than 200 mm Hg with hyperoxia, primary respiratory disease is much more likely. Only cyanotic heart defects with torrential pulmonary blood flow (present in truncus arteriosus, unobstructed anomalous venous return, or variants of single ventricle with minimal pulmonic stenosis) may be associated with an arterial PO_2 higher than 200 mm Hg. In these cases, cyanosis in room air is usually mild, but abnormal cardiac or chest findings often suggest a cardiac cause.

When the arterial PO_2 remains low during the hyperoxia test and the differential diagnosis is limited to cyanotic heart disease or PPHN, intubation and mechanical hyperventilation can be performed. If PPHN is present, hyperventilation may cause pulmonary vasodilation, a reduction in right-to-left shunting at the atrial or ductal levels, and a dramatic increase in arterial PO_2. If cyanotic heart disease is present, the arterial PO_2 remains low. A response to inhaled nitric oxide occurs in patients with PPHN but not in most cases of cyanotic congenital heart disease.

INITIAL APPROACH TO THE CYANOTIC NEWBORN

A stepwise approach to the newborn with cyanosis is presented in Figure 10-4. First, the airway, breathing, and circulation must be assessed and stabilized. Hypoglycemia should be excluded. Pulse oximetry of the right hand and foot can be performed while an arterial blood gas value is obtained from the right radial artery. A history and physical examination should focus on the predisposing factors and manifestations of neurologic, pulmonary, or cardiac disease. A chest radiograph, the ECG, detection of differential cyanosis, and the hyperoxia test help establish the diagnosis.

ESTABLISHING THE CAUSE OF CARDIAC CYANOSIS IN THE NEWBORN

Certain cyanotic heart defects manifest earlier than others. Those defects that depend on ductal patency usually produce significant cyanosis within the first 3 days of life. Age at presentation may help focus the differential diagnosis (Table 10-5).

Once the diagnosis of cyanotic congenital heart disease is suspected, the infant should be stabilized with plans made for transfer to a tertiary care facility with pediatric cardiology and pediatric cardiothoracic surgery availability. Prostaglandin E_1 (PGE_1) therapy may be indicated in the severely cyanotic newborn with acidosis before transfer. The physician must be aware that significant apnea can develop with prostaglandin infusion, and prophylactic intubation before transfer might be considered. It is also important to create a stable metabolic milieu for these newborns; acidosis, anemia, hypothermia, and hypoglycemia may contribute to a poorer outcome.

The pediatric cardiologist is able to confirm the suspicion of cyanotic congenital heart disease, using two-dimensional and Doppler echocardiography, and can perform palliative procedures and refer the patient to the pediatric cardiothoracic surgeon.

Table 10-5. Presentation of Cyanotic Heart Disease by Age

Newborn–1 day
Transposition of the great arteries with intact ventricular septum
Pulmonic atresia
Tricuspid atresia with small ventricular septal defect or intact ventricular septum and pulmonic stenosis
Hypoplastic left heart syndrome
Ebstein malformation
Total anomalous venous return (obstructed)

1–7 days
Transposition of the great arteries with or without ventricular septal defect
Tetralogy of Fallot
Hypoplastic left heart syndrome
Tricuspid atresia with or without ventricular septal defect
Truncus arteriosus
Ebstein malformation of the tricuspid valve
Total anomalous venous return (obstructed)

>7 days
Tetralogy of Fallot
Transposition of the great arteries with ventricular septal defect
Tricuspid atresia with ventricular septal defect
Single ventricle with or without pulmonary stenosis
Total anomalous pulmonary venous return (unobstructed)

CYANOTIC LESIONS WITH NORMAL OR INCREASED PULMONARY BLOOD FLOW

Transposition of the Great Arteries

Complete transposition or dextrotransposition of the great arteries (d-TGA) is defined as the aorta arising from the right ventricle and the pulmonary artery arising from the left ventricle (Fig. 10-5). This leads to parallel circulations, in which the deoxygenated blood returns to the aorta without passing through the lungs. If there is no site of mixing between the systemic and pulmonary circulations, survival is not possible. It is the second most common cyanotic defect but the most common to manifest in the neonatal period.

Newborns with d-TGA usually do not have extracardiac or chromosomal abnormalities; there is a slight male predominance. Most infants have severe cyanosis; the cardiac physical findings are subtle. The second heart sound is single and loud secondary to the anteriorly positioned aorta; a murmur may be present if there is any degree of pulmonary stenosis (in about one third of patients). Chest radiographs may reveal an increased heart size with increased pulmonary vascular markings but a narrow mediastinum ("egg on a string") (Fig. 10-6); the chest radiograph may also be normal. The ECG is often normal but may show right ventricular hypertrophy. Echocardiography rapidly identifies the presence of d-TGA and should also identify any associated abnormalities as well as the adequacy of the atrial level communication.

Although infusion of PGE_1 can maintain patency of the ductus and improve mixing, many affected babies also require an adequate interatrial communication. With echocardiographic guidance, creation of an atrial communication can be performed at the infant's bedside with a balloon atrial septostomy (Rashkind procedure). This procedure is life-saving in infants with severe cyanosis and allows stabilization of the infant before complete surgical repair.

The surgical procedure of choice for these infants is the Jatene or arterial switch procedure, in which the great arteries are transected

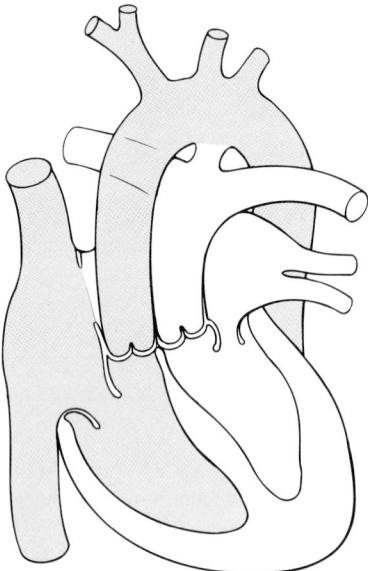

Figure 10-5. *Illustration of the anatomic features and blood flow patterns in d-transposition of the great arteries. Deoxygenated blood (shaded) returns to the right side of the heart and recirculates to the body through the transposed aorta. Oxygenated blood (not shaded) returns to the left side of the heart and recirculates to the lungs through the transposed pulmonary artery. Mixing of blood occurs at the patent ductus arteriosus as well as at the patent foramen ovale.*

above the valves and then repositioned and reanastomosed above the appropriate ventricles. The arterial switch procedure is generally performed in the first 2 weeks of life because, with time, the pulmonary artery pressures fall and the left ventricle becomes unprepared to handle the systemic circulation. Results of the arterial switch operation are excellent, with a perioperative mortality rate of less than 5%; the long-term outcome also appears good, as the heart is anatomically corrected.

Total Anomalous Pulmonary Venous Return

TAPVR is present when all pulmonary veins connect anomalously to the systemic venous circulation. Total mixing of systemic and pulmonary blood occurs at the level of the right atrium, and an interatrial communication is necessary for survival. The anatomic classification is based on the location of pulmonary venous drainage (supracardiac, cardiac, or infracardiac). TAPVR is rare, representing only 1% of all congenital heart disease. When TAPVR is associated with complex heart disease, the diagnosis of asplenia should be considered.

Infants with isolated TAPVR are generally otherwise normal, without extracardiac abnormalities. The clinical presentation of these patients is variable and dependent on the presence of pulmonary venous obstruction. The newborn with infracardiac TAPVR has severe cyanosis and respiratory distress shortly after birth, because the pulmonary veins are obstructed as they course through the diaphragm into the portal system. Cardiac findings can be minimal, although the second heart sound is usually single and loud. Hepatomegaly is also common. The ECG demonstrates right ventricular hypertrophy (RVH); the chest radiograph demonstrates a small heart size with interstitial pulmonary edema, and this can be incorrectly interpreted as "diffuse interstitial pneumonia" (Fig. 10-7). Echocardiography is diagnostic but technically challenging, because the pulmonary veins drain away from the heart via an anomalous venous channel. Other echocardiographic features include a dilated dysfunctional right ventricle, a relatively small left atrium and left ventricle, and Doppler evidence of severe pulmonary artery hypertension.

Many infants with supracardiac or cardiac TAPVR present later, because pulmonary venous obstruction is less common, and cyanosis

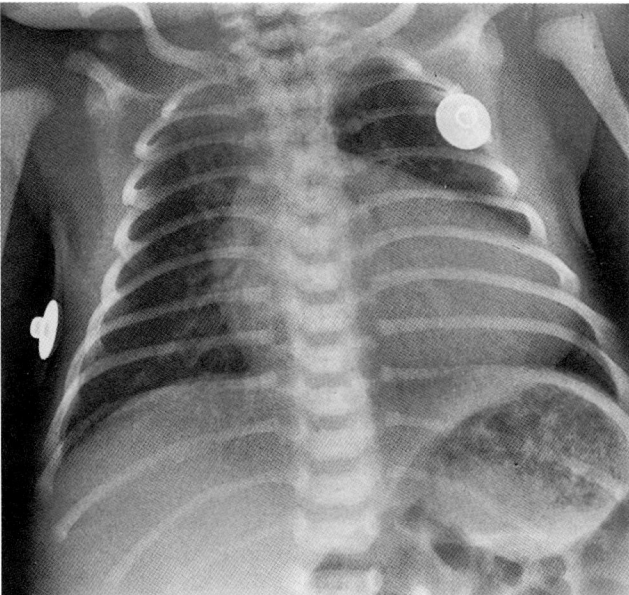

Figure 10-6. *Chest radiograph of a patient with transposition of the great arteries, demonstrating narrow superior mediastinum and enlarged heart ("egg on a string").*

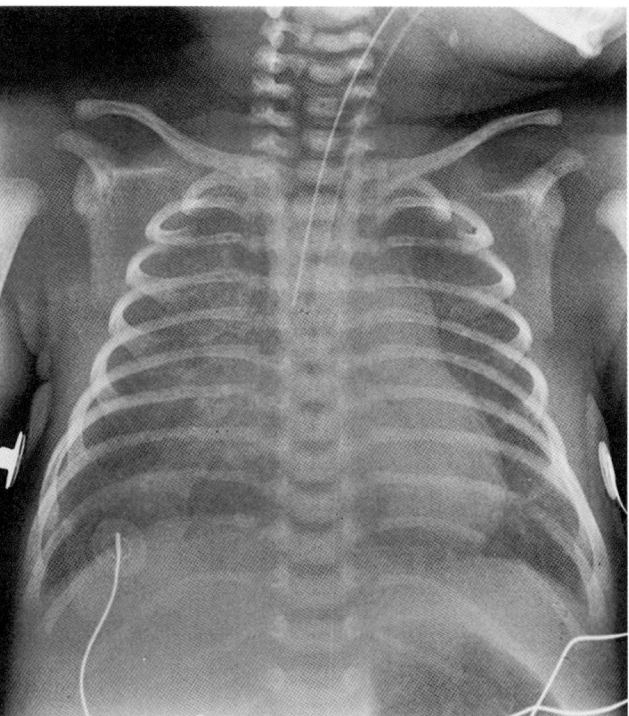

Figure 10-7. *Chest radiograph of a patient with total anomalous pulmonary venous return (obstructed), demonstrating pulmonary venous congestion and pulmonary edema.*

is typically mild. As the pulmonary resistance falls, the pulmonary blood flow increases significantly, and the infant presents with poor feeding and congestive heart failure. The cardiac examination findings are notable for a prominent right ventricular impulse, a widely split second heart sound, a systolic ejection murmur at the left upper sternal border, and, often, a diastolic rumble. All of these findings are secondary to the excessive pulmonary blood flow and mimic the findings of a large atrial septal defect. The ECG demonstrates RVH and right atrial enlargement; the chest radiograph reveals cardiac enlargement and increased pulmonary blood flow.

Infracardiac TAPVR requires prompt diagnosis and surgical repair, because postponing surgery provides no advantages. While awaiting surgery, the infant may improve with intubation and positive pressure ventilation. In the critically ill infant awaiting surgery, PGE₁ may have some positive benefits (i.e., dilatation of the ductus venosus); however, this is generally avoided because it may further increase pulmonary blood flow and increase pulmonary venous obstruction. Infants with other forms of TAPVR can be scheduled electively for surgical repair; these infants may respond to digoxin and diuretic therapy.

The long-term outcome of infants with TAPVR is generally good, although in rare cases, infants with infracardiac TAPVR have associated pulmonary vein stenosis. The results of reoperation in this setting are uniformly poor.

Truncus Arteriosus

Truncus arteriosus is an uncommon form of congenital heart disease, in which a single great artery exits from the heart and gives rise to the coronary, pulmonary, and systemic arteries (Fig. 10-8). The "common trunk" straddles the ventricular septum and communicates with both ventricles through a large ventricular septal defect (VSD). The pulmonary arteries usually arise unobstructed from the left lateral aspect of the truncus; this results in excessive pulmonary blood flow, minimal cyanosis, and severe congestive heart failure in infancy.

Approximately 30% to 50% of infants with truncus arteriosus also have velocardiofacial syndrome. This syndrome is caused by a microdeletion of the long arm of chromosome 22 and is detectable by molecular testing (fluorescent in situ hybridization). The size of the deletion may be a marker of the severity of associated anomalies. Features include wide-set eyes, protuberant ears, preauricular pits or tags, a prominent nose, palatal defects, hypocalcemia, T-cell immune deficiency, and neurodevelopmental problems.

Cardiac examination is notable for a hyperdynamic precordium with a single loud second heart sound. Truncal valve stenosis and insufficiency are common, giving rise to a to-fro systolic-diastolic murmur at the base of the heart. Pulses are often bounding, and the pulse pressure is widened. The ECG reveals biventricular hypertrophy, and the chest radiograph reveals cardiac enlargement with increased pulmonary blood flow. A right aortic arch can be seen in 30% of patients. Two-dimensional echocardiography is diagnostic.

Complete repair of truncus arteriosus is generally performed in early infancy because intractable heart failure is common and there is a risk of early development of pulmonary vascular obstructive disease. The repair includes VSD closure so that all of the left ventricular blood is directed into the truncal artery. The pulmonary arteries are removed and attached to a conduit, which is proximally inserted into the anterior right ventricle. Long-term problems include the development of conduit stenosis and insufficiency; multiple conduit replacements can be expected as the child grows. The development of human valve tissue in vitro may be an excellent replacement for these porcine or human cryopreserved conduits.

Hypoplastic Left Heart Syndrome

In its extreme form, hypoplastic left heart syndrome is characterized by aortic and mitral valve atresia, along with marked underdevelopment of the ascending aorta and left ventricle (Fig. 10-9). With prenatal echocardiography, it is known that this can be a progressive disease in utero, at times related to premature closure of the foramen ovale with limited forward flow into the left ventricle, resulting in poor left ventricular growth. After birth, affected infants are critically dependent on patency of the foramen ovale and ductus arteriosus. If spontaneous closure occurs, death ensues, with an average untreated life expectancy of 2 weeks. Hypoplastic left heart syndrome is more common in boys and is the most common cause of neonatal death from congenital heart disease.

The presenting symptoms are quite variable. If the infant is diagnosed prenatally, delivery should be arranged at a tertiary care facility, where the infant can be stabilized and treated before the onset of symptoms. If the infant is not recognized to have heart disease in the newborn nursery, the infant may be sent home, only to return at 2 days of age with tachypnea, acidosis, and poor pulses as spontaneous ductal closure occurs. When immediate severe cyanosis is noted just after birth, the foramen ovale may be closed or severely restrictive, causing pulmonary venous congestion and marked respiratory distress.

Cardiac examination typically reveals a prominent right ventricular impulse with a single second heart sound. Pulses are diffusely diminished, because the patent ductus arteriosus supplies both the upper and lower extremities. The ECG demonstrates striking RVH, and the chest radiograph often reveals cardiac enlargement with active and passive pulmonary congestion. Echocardiography is diagnostic and focuses on the adequacy of the interatrial communication.

Many affected infants require an initial period of stabilization and recovery, because they often present with severe acidosis, low cardiac output, and renal/hepatic insufficiency. Seizures are common in this setting and may play a role in the long-term neurologic outcome of these patients. The initial management includes treatment with PGE₁ to maintain ductal patency. Some infants with excessive

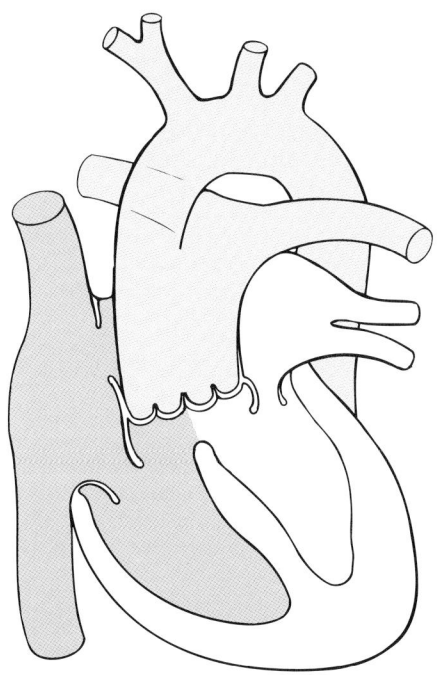

Figure 10-8. Illustration of the anatomic features and blood flow patterns in truncus arteriosus. Deoxygenated blood (*shaded*) returns to the right side of the heart and is ejected by the right ventricle into the truncal root. The truncal root gives rise to both the ascending aorta and pulmonary arteries. Mixing occurs through a large ventricular septal defect, which results in systemic desaturation.

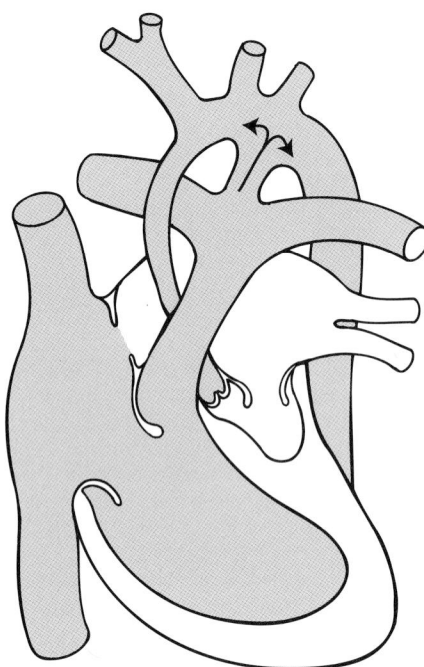

Figure 10-9. Illustration of the anatomic features and blood flow patterns in hypoplastic left heart syndrome. Oxygenated blood (*not shaded*) returns to the left atrium and must pass into the right atrium through an atrial septal defect, which results in complete mixing of systemic and pulmonary venous return in the right side of the heart. The right ventricle supplies the pulmonary circulation as well as the systemic circulation through the patent ductus arteriosus.

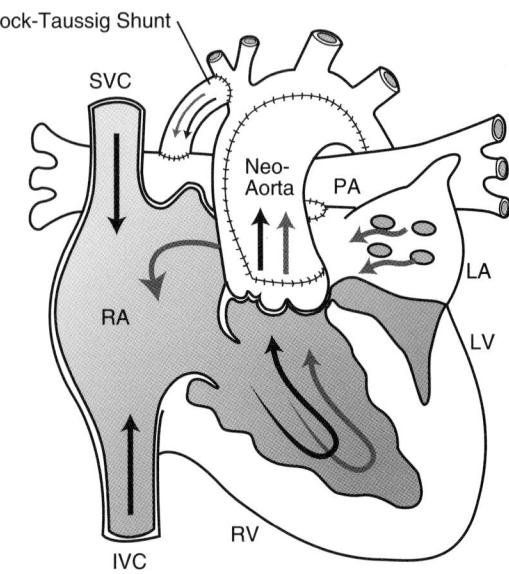

Figure 10-10. Illustration of the modified Norwood procedure for treatment of hypoplastic left heart syndrome. The proximal main pulmonary artery has been divided, and the distal main pulmonary artery has been oversewn. The hypoplastic aorta has been carefully incised, and a large patch augments the aortic arch and is attached to the main pulmonary artery to create a "neoaorta." The atrial septum is completely resected, and pulmonary blood flow is established by placement of a Blalock-Taussig shunt from the innominate artery to the right pulmonary artery. IVC, inferior vena cava; LA, left atrium; LV, left ventricle; PA, pulmonary artery; RA, right atrium; RV, right ventricle; SVC, superior vena cava. (From May LE [ed]: Pediatric Heart Surgery: A Ready Reference for Professionals. Milwaukee, Wis, Maxishare, 1999, p 42.)

pulmonary flow and a large atrial-level shunt may require intubation and mechanical ventilation to better control the pulmonary vascular resistance. Conversely, infants with an inadequate atrial defect can be severely cyanotic with a marked elevation in pulmonary vascular resistance; these infants require either surgical or interventional decompression of the left atrium before any definitive therapy.

The surgical therapy is controversial, but at many centers, Norwood palliation is the treatment of choice. This provides relief of systemic outflow obstruction by creation of a "neoaorta" and, at the same time, provides restriction of pulmonary blood flow by creation of an aortopulmonary shunt (Fig. 10-10). The postoperative management is difficult, with a hospital mortality rate of 10% to 20%. Because these infants have only a functional single right ventricle, the Norwood operation is followed by a bidirectional cavopulmonary shunt (superior vena cava to pulmonary artery anastomosis) at 4 to 6 months of age and a complete Fontan procedure is performed at 2 to 3 years of age. This latter procedure connects the inferior vena cava directly to the pulmonary arteries without a pump. Long-term complications are anticipated to include single right ventricular dysfunction and arrhythmias, with the possibility of the need for cardiac transplantation in young adulthood.

Because of the significant morbidity and mortality rates associated with the Norwood procedure, some centers advocate cardiac transplantation as the initial surgical therapy of choice. The major obstacle in this setting is a shortage of neonatal donor hearts; many affected infants die from complications while awaiting transplantation. If cardiac transplantation is performed, the 5-year survival rate is as high as 90%. Because these therapies are at best palliative with unclear long-term outcome, some families choose only supportive care. It is important to recognize that lesions such as hypoplastic left heart syndrome tend to have a high recurrence rate (10%) in subsequent

pregnancies, and a high-risk fetal echocardiogram should be performed with subsequent pregnancies.

LESIONS WITH DIMINISHED PULMONARY BLOOD FLOW

Lesions with diminished pulmonary blood flow have obstruction of flow to the pulmonary artery. If pulmonary flow is obstructed, systemic venous flow must reach the left side of the heart by means of a right-to-left shunt at the atrial, ventricular, or arterial levels.

Tetralogy of Fallot

Tetralogy of Fallot is the most common cyanotic cardiac defect. The age at presentation is quite variable and dependent on the degree of right ventricular outflow tract obstruction. The four classic anatomic features include a large outlet VSD, pulmonary stenosis (subvalvar, valvar, or supravalvar), aortic override, and right ventricular hypertrophy (Fig. 10-11). All of these features are related to one embryologic abnormality: anterior and superior displacement of the infundibular septum.

Approximately 15% of babies with tetralogy of Fallot have associated extracardiac abnormalities. These may occur in isolation, or in association with a described syndrome (e.g., de Lange syndrome, Goldenhar syndrome, and VACTERL [vertebral abnormalities, anal atresia, cardiac abnormalities, tracheoesophageal fistula and/or esophageal atresia, renal agenesis and dysplasia, and limb defects]). Most infants are referred for cardiac evaluation secondary to a murmur present at birth; some infants are also noted to be mildly cyanotic. The severity of symptoms is related to the degree of

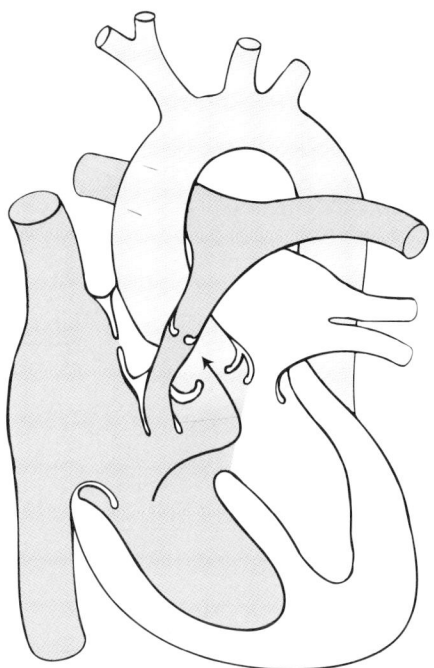

Figure 10-11. Illustration of the anatomic features and blood flow patterns in tetralogy of Fallot. Deoxygenated blood (*shaded*) returning to the right heart enters both the stenotic pulmonary artery and the aorta through a large ventricular septal defect to mix with oxygenated blood (*not shaded*), which results in systemic desaturation.

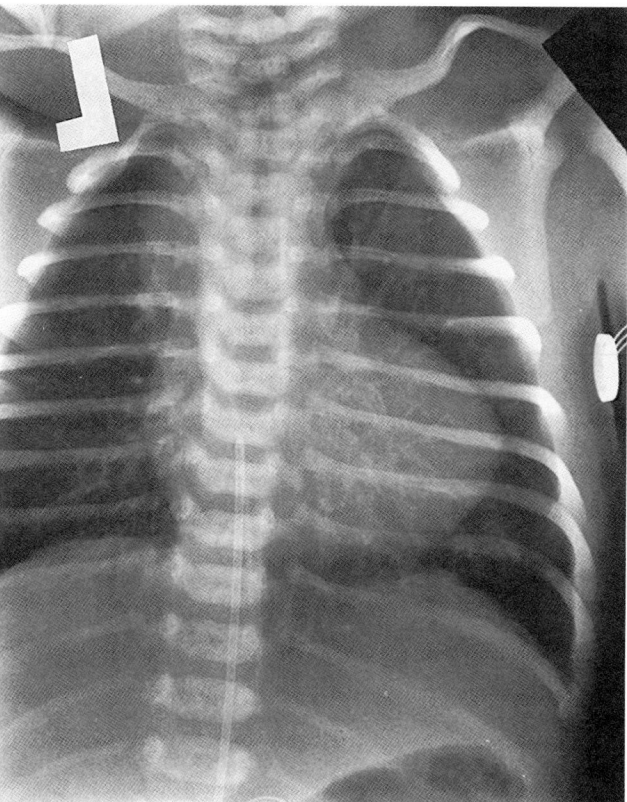

Figure 10-12. Chest radiograph of a patient with tetralogy of Fallot, demonstrating diminished pulmonary blood flow, right ventricular predominance, and absence of main pulmonary segment (boot-shaped heart). Also, note that the film is misplaced or reversed, inasmuch as there is also dextrocardia as determined by the "L," which is correctly placed over the patient but reversed on the view box.

pulmonary stenosis, whereas the constancy of the symptoms is determined by whether the stenosis is fixed or dynamic. Physical findings include a prominent right ventricular impulse with a systolic ejection murmur at the left upper sternal border. The second heart sound is single, composed only of aortic valve closure. The ECG is notable for persistent RVH. Classically, the chest radiograph demonstrates a "boot-shaped heart," with a normal heart size, an upturned cardiac apex, and decreased pulmonary vascular markings (Fig. 10-12). In addition, 25% of affected patients have a right-sided aortic arch. Echocardiography is diagnostic and focuses on the site and degree of right ventricular outflow tract obstruction. Cardiac catheterization can provide additional information regarding the branch pulmonary arteries and coronary artery anatomy; this information is critical for planning a complete surgical repair.

Surgical management of these patients is somewhat controversial; primary complete repair is considered if the operation can be performed at low risk and with a reasonable expectation of a good result. In a newborn with severe cyanosis and hypoplastic branch pulmonary arteries, most centers would elect to perform a palliative aortopulmonary shunt (Blalock-Taussig shunt) procedure because complete repair in this setting can be associated with significant rates of morbidity and mortality. This shunt connects the subclavian artery to the pulmonary artery. For the older asymptomatic infant, many centers advocate elective repair at 6 to 12 months of age.

Hypercyanotic spells can occur in the infant with unrepaired tetralogy of Fallot, and are characterized by a marked increase in cyanosis, irritability, and hyperpnea. This is secondary to an acute increase in the degree of right ventricular outflow tract obstruction, with increased right-to-left shunting through the VSD. Most infants respond to calming and placement in a knee-chest position (which increases systemic vascular resistance and promotes left-to-right shunting through the VSD); some require supplemental oxygen and/or sedation with morphine sulfate. Onset of these spells is an indication for surgical intervention.

The long-term prognosis in these patients is generally very good, although late complications include right ventricular dysfunction related to pulmonary insufficiency as well as ventricular arrhythmias related to residual right ventricular hypertension or the right ventriculotomy.

Tricuspid Atresia

Tricuspid atresia is a rare cardiac disorder consisting of an imperforate tricuspid valve and variable degrees of right ventricular hypoplasia. There is an obligate right-to-left atrial-level shunt, with complete mixing of systemic and pulmonary venous return in the left atrium and left ventricle. The great arteries are usually normally related, and the amount of pulmonary blood flow is dependent on the size of the VSD and the degree of right ventricular outflow tract obstruction (Fig. 10-13). If the great arteries are transposed (30% of affected patients), systemic blood flow is often compromised, and surgical palliation is much more difficult.

Infants with tricuspid atresia have a variable presentation, dependent on the associated cardiac anomalies. The newborn with tricuspid atresia and a very restrictive VSD may become severely cyanotic with ductal closure; the infant with tricuspid atresia and a large VSD may present later with congestive heart failure. Most affected infants present in the first month of life with some degree of cyanosis and a heart murmur. These infants are otherwise healthy without associated abnormalities. Cardiac examination reveals a prominent left ventricular impulse and a systolic ejection murmur at the left upper sternal border. The chest radiograph findings are

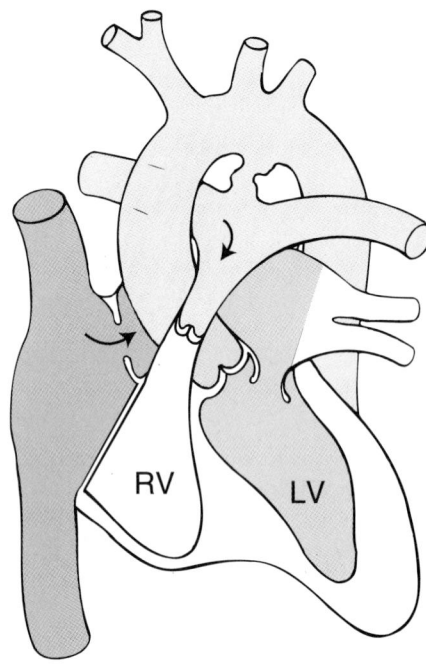

Figure 10-13. Illustration of the anatomic features and blood flow pattern in tricuspid atresia. Deoxygenated blood (*shaded*) returning to the right side of the heart mixes with oxygenated blood through a patent foramen ovale or an atrial septal defect. Tricuspid atresia is often associated with right ventricular hypoplasia and pulmonic valve atresia. LV, left ventricle; RV, right ventricle.

Lateral Tunnel Fontan

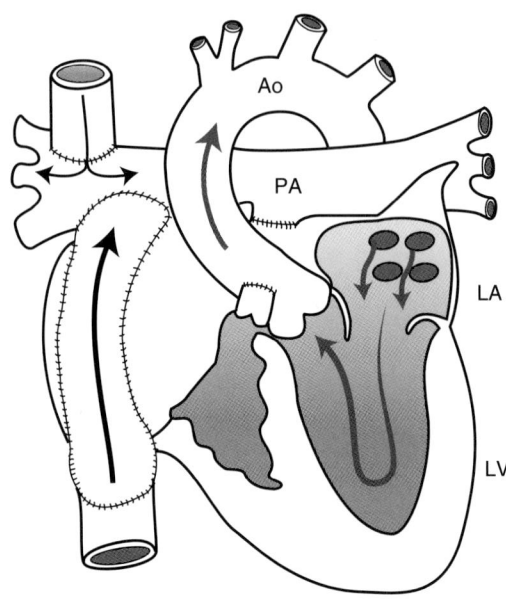

Figure 10-14. Illustration of the Fontan procedure for tricuspid atresia. The superior vena cava and inferior vena cava have been anastomosed to the confluent pulmonary arteries, allowing deoxygenated blood (*black arrows*) to flow passively to the lungs, relieving cyanosis. A small hole or fenestration can be made in the Fontan circuit to lower central venous pressure and augment cardiac output in the early post-operative period. Ao, aorta; LA, left atrium; LV, left ventricle; PA, pulmonary artery. (From May LE [ed]: Pediatric Heart Surgery: A Ready Reference for Professionals. Milwaukee, Wis, Maxishare, 1999, p 65.)

variable and are correlated with the clinical symptoms. The ECG can be quite helpful because there is left axis deviation and left ventricular hypertrophy, a distinctly unusual finding in the infant with cyanotic congenital heart disease. Echocardiography is diagnostic and focuses on the associated cardiac abnormalities.

Because of the atretic tricuspid valve and underdevelopment of the right ventricle, a Fontan procedure, or "right-sided heart bypass," is the treatment goal for these patients (Fig. 10-14). This procedure connects the systemic venous return (superior and inferior venae cavae) directly to the pulmonary arteries without a pump; the single left ventricle then pumps only oxygenated blood to the body. The success of the Fontan procedure is dependent on well-developed pulmonary arteries and low pulmonary vascular resistance. At the time of birth, a long-term treatment plan must be conceptualized for each affected baby, dependent on the individual's anatomy. Typically an infant with tricuspid atresia may undergo an initial surgical palliation with an aortopulmonary shunt, followed by a bidirectional Glenn shunt (superior vena cava–to–right pulmonary artery anastomosis) at 6 months of age, and completion of the Fontan (inferior vena cava–to–pulmonary artery anastomosis) at 3 years of age.

Late postoperative complications include the development of atrial arrhythmias and single ventricular dysfunction, as well as a protein-losing enteropathy related to the chronic systemic venous congestion.

Ebstein Malformation of the Tricuspid Valve

Ebstein malformation (Fig. 10-15) is unusual and has many manifestations, including cyanosis. There is redundancy of the tricuspid leaflets and adherence of the leaflets to the walls of the right ventricle, so that the valve apparatus is "drawn downward" into the right ventricular cavity. There is usually significant tricuspid regurgitation, and when this is severe, there may be limited antegrade flow

across the right ventricular outflow tract to the pulmonary artery, especially during the first days of life when pulmonary vascular resistance is high. In extreme cases, there is complete atresia of the pulmonic valve. The concomitant elevation of right atrial pressure from impaired right ventricular filling and significant tricuspid incompetence leads to right-to-left shunting across the patent foramen ovale and to cyanosis. The cyanosis in neonates with Ebstein malformation often improves during the first weeks of life as pulmonary vascular resistance falls. A pansystolic murmur of tricuspid incompetence is often heard at the lower left sternal border, and a diastolic rumble is present because of turbulent flow across the tricuspid valve during diastole. There may also be multiple clicks related to opening or closure of the redundant valve leaflets.

The chest radiograph typically shows an enlarged heart with a particularly large right-sided heart border caused by right atrial enlargement. The mediastinum is usually narrow because output from neither great vessel is significantly increased. Pulmonary vascular markings are diminished. This is the most common congenital heart defect associated with preexcitation and the Wolff-Parkinson-White syndrome; this ECG finding should suggest this diagnosis in the cyanotic infant. Often, only medical management during infancy is required.

Pulmonary Atresia with Intact Ventricular Septum or with Ventricular Septal Defect (Tetralogy of Fallot with Pulmonary Atresia)

Pulmonary atresia constitutes the second most common form of cyanotic heart disease in the neonate. There is complete atresia of the pulmonic valve and no antegrade pulmonary blood flow. Pulmonary artery perfusion depends completely on the presence of

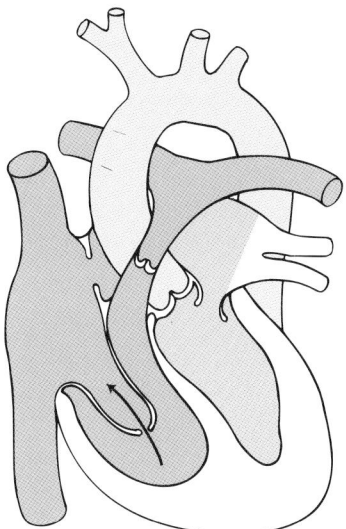

Figure 10-15. Illustration of the anatomic features and blood flow in Ebstein malformation of the tricuspid valve. Deoxygenated blood (*shaded*) returns to the right side of the heart. Significant tricuspid regurgitation occurs (*arrow*). Right-to-left shunting occurs across the patent foramen ovale.

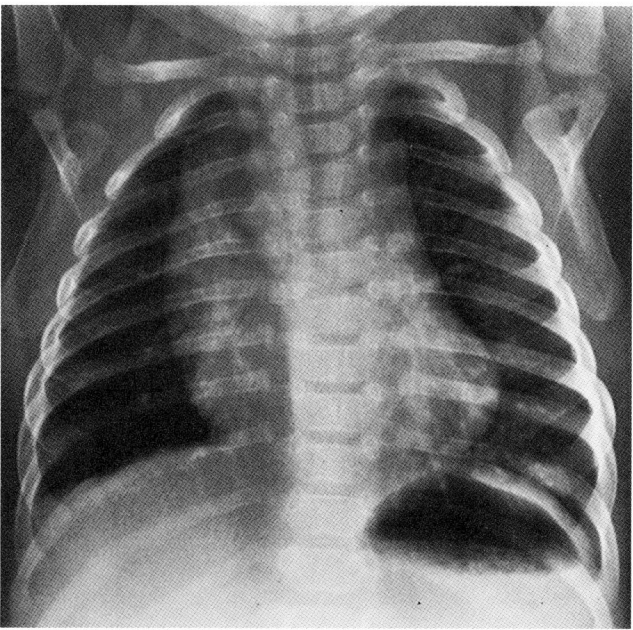

Figure 10-16. Chest radiograph of a patient with pulmonary atresia with intact ventricular septum, demonstrating decreased pulmonary vascular markings.

a patent ductus arteriosus. Systemic venous return to the right atrium cannot enter the right ventricle and be adequately ejected into the pulmonary artery. Instead, it must pass from right to left across an atrial septal defect or a VSD to reach the aortic circulation.

Because there is no antegrade flow across the pulmonic valve, there is no associated murmur except for the murmur of a patent ductus arteriosus. Infants with pulmonary atresia usually become severely cyanotic during the first day of life as the patent ductus closes. The chest radiograph usually shows markedly diminished pulmonary vascular markings (Fig. 10-16). The ECG often shows mild left axis deviation, because of the relative absence of right ventricular forces, and peaked P waves in lead II, because of right atrial enlargement. The arterial PO_2 is usually less than 50 mm Hg on room air and with 100% oxygen.

Initial stabilization includes institution of PGE_1 to maintain ductal patency. If the foramen ovale is restrictive, catheterization and balloon atrial septostomy are performed. Initial surgical treatment depends on the sizes of the tricuspid valve, the right ventricle, and the pulmonary arteries and may include pulmonary valvotomy, a Blalock-Taussig shunt, or both.

Persistent Pulmonary Hypertension of the Newborn

PPHN is defined as persistence of the fetal circulatory pattern with right-to-left shunting across the patent ductus arteriosus and patent foramen ovale as a result of high pulmonary vascular resistance. It typically occurs in full-term and post-term infants; the cause is probably multifactorial. Precipitating factors include meconium aspiration, birth asphyxia, sepsis, metabolic derangements (hypoglycemia), pulmonary hypoplasia, and congenital diaphragmatic hernia.

Infants become ill shortly after birth and are profoundly hypoxic, with little response to 100% oxygen. These infants often exhibit differential cyanosis secondary to the right-to-left ductal shunting. Intubation and mechanical ventilation with induction of controlled alkalosis may be beneficial. Improvements in the postductal saturation occur, and there is often a dramatic increase in the arterial PO_2. Infants with PPHN can have a dramatic increase in oxygenation with inhaled nitric oxide. If progressive deterioration occurs in these

infants despite hyperventilation and nitric oxide, extracorporeal membrane oxygenation is life-saving. PPHN can be clearly distinguished from cyanotic congenital heart disease by echocardiography.

THE OLDER INFANT AND TODDLER

Cyanosis in infancy may be caused by pulmonary, hematologic, or cardiac disease. As in the neonatal period, the general cause of cyanosis may often be discerned from the history, physical examination, and chest radiograph. Pulmonary causes (pneumonia, asthma, pneumothorax, pulmonary hemorrhage, empyema) are the most common in older children. Respiratory distress with possible CO_2 retention can be documented. The chest radiograph (lung fields) is usually abnormal (see Chapter 3).

Multiple pulmonary venous malformations may cause a significant right-to-left shunt at the pulmonary level. In contrast to systemic venous malformations, the pulmonary arteriovenous malformation (AVM) is often not associated with a bruit or murmur. When the pulmonary AVM is solitary, large, and in a lower lobe of the lung, the degree of right-to-left shunting through the lesion may vary with body position, particularly when the child is standing or reclining. Increased cyanosis while the child is supine is referred to as *orthodeoxia* or *orthocyanosis*. The diagnosis may be suggested by a parenchymal opacification on the chest radiograph. A contrast echocardiogram may demonstrate the presence of an intrapulmonary right-to-left shunt. Pulmonary AVMs may be associated with similar malformations of the skin or intestinal tract (Osler-Weber-Rendu syndrome). They may also occur in the presence of long-standing hepatic cirrhosis.

Certain cardiac diseases may manifest with cyanosis several weeks or months after birth. In most cases, the lesions involve abnormal connections with significant mixing of saturated and desaturated blood within the heart or obstructive lesions with milder pulmonary outflow obstruction.

The most common cyanotic heart defect to manifest after 1 month of age is tetralogy of Fallot (see previous discussion). In these older infants, the degree of right ventricular outflow tract obstruction progresses with time, leading to the development of right-to-left ventricular-level shunting and cyanosis. The older infant with undiagnosed tetralogy of Fallot can also present with a hypercyanotic spell. Other congenital heart defects that manifest later in infancy include nonobstructed forms of TAPVR and complex forms of single ventricle with pulmonary stenosis.

CYANOSIS IN LATER CHILDHOOD AND ADOLESCENCE

In childhood and adolescence, cyanosis is rarely an isolated clinical symptom or sign. Chronic cyanosis is almost always associated with long-standing respiratory disease (see Chapter 2). Hematologic or cardiac causes of cyanosis manifesting in childhood and adolescence are rare.

METHEMOGLOBINEMIA

Congenital or acquired methemoglobinemia may manifest at any time during infancy and childhood. Mild forms of congenital methemoglobinemia may manifest with cyanosis and symptoms of inadequate oxygen delivery during infections or with exposures to precipitating agents. The most common congenital forms of methemoglobinemia are abnormalities of hemoglobin (hemoglobin M), which preferentially bind the ferric (Fe^{+3}) ion, or abnormalities of enzymes (e.g., methemoglobin reductase deficiency), which otherwise keep the iron bound to hemoglobin in the ferrous (Fe^{+2}) state. Hemoglobin M is an autosomal dominant disorder in which hemoglobin is more easily oxidized to methemoglobin. This may manifest at birth, but therapy is rarely required. Methemoglobin reductase deficiency is an autosomal recessive disorder. Patients are susceptible to precipitous drops in oxygen saturation and increases in methemoglobinemia resulting from various drugs and agents (Table 10-6). Treatment is intravenous methylene blue.

Acquired methemoglobinemia may occur as a result of intestinal diarrheal infections with certain bacteria, exposure to nitrates and nitrites in well water, or exposure to oxidizing agents in dyes and medications.

Table 10-6. Agents that Oxidize Hemoglobin

I. Direct oxidation
　Ferricyanide
　Copper
　Hydrogen peroxide
　Hydroxylamine
　Others: Chromate, chlorate, nitrogen trifluoride,
　　　　tetranitromethane, quinones, dyes
II. Interaction with oxygen
　Nitrites, nitroglycerin
　Hydrazines
　Thiols
　Others: Arsine, aminophenols, arylhydroxylamines,
　　　　N-hydroxyurethane, phenylenediamines
III. Requiring biochemical transformation
　Aniline, dyes (diaper and laundry inks, red wax crayons)
　Sulfonamides
　Procaine derivatives
　4, 4′-Diaminodiphenylsulfone (dapsone)
　8-Aminoquinolines: primaquine and pamaquine
　N-Acylarylamines: acetanilid, phenacetin

Adapted from Kiese M: Methemoglobinemia: A Comprehensive Treatise. Boca Raton, Fla, CRC Press, 1974.

The diagnosis of methemoglobinemia is suspected in cyanotic patients with no predisposing pulmonary or cardiac disease who have acute cyanosis and metabolic acidosis. The cyanotic coloration is often slate gray. The blood is more brown than burgundy and does not become redder when exposed to oxygen in room air. The arterial PO_2 is normal or high if the patient is receiving oxygen; the saturation is low: cyanosis with a normal PO_2.

The diagnosis is confirmed by obtaining a methemoglobin level. The normal level is 1% to 3%, and a level above 15% is usually associated with symptoms. Because pulse oximetry is not correlated closely with the actual saturation of oxygen in the blood, the oxygen saturation should be measured directly by cooximetry. The oxygen saturation reported on the blood gas analysis is factitiously high because this value is calculated from the measured PO_2 with an algorithm that applies only to normal hemoglobin.

PRIMARY PULMONARY ARTERY HYPERTENSION

Primary pulmonary artery hypertension is defined as a mean pulmonary artery pressure of more than 25 mm Hg at rest or more than 30 mm Hg during exercise. Causes of secondary pulmonary hypertension need to be excluded (e.g., congenital heart disease, airway obstruction, pulmonary thromboembolism). Although the mechanisms (drugs, genetics) responsible for the development of primary pulmonary artery hypertension are incompletely understood, endothelial cell injury may have a central role.

Primary pulmonary artery hypertension is generally a disease of young women; the symptoms can be fairly nonspecific. The patient may initially complain of fatigue and exercise intolerance; as the disease progresses, there may be syncope, angina, and the development of right-sided heart failure. Cardiac findings include a prominent right ventricular impulse, a loud single second heart sound, and possibly a murmur of tricuspid or pulmonary insufficiency. Mild cyanosis may be present if there is a patent foramen ovale with right-to-left shunting. Echocardiography often reveals a dilated right ventricle with diminished contractility and Doppler evidence of pulmonary hypertension. Structural causes of pulmonary hypertension such as mitral stenosis or pulmonary vein stenosis should be carefully excluded. Cardiac catheterization is essential for establishing the severity of the disease and the response to vasodilator therapy. There is no known cure for this disease, but therapy with intravenous prostacyclin, anticoagulants, calcium channel blockers, or bosentan (a nonspecific endothelial receptor antagonist) have improved the outcome. In patients with progressive disease and a poor response to vasodilators, lung transplantation remains an option.

EISENMENGER SYNDROME

Cardiac causes of cyanosis in the adolescent are rare but can be seen in the setting of a patient with unrepaired or unrecognized congenital heart disease. These patients usually develop irreversible pulmonary vascular changes from a high-flow/high-pressure lesion (e.g., large VSD or patent ductus arteriosus), and typically present in the second decade of life with cyanosis, digital clubbing, and polycythemia (Eisenmenger syndrome). Cardiac examination may reveal a right ventricular heave, a loud single second heart sound, and an early high-pitched diastolic murmur caused by pulmonary insufficiency. The ECG reveals right axis deviation and RVH; a chest radiograph may show a large heart with "pruning" of the pulmonary vascular markings. Echocardiography demonstrates significant right ventricle enlargement, with Doppler evidence of pulmonary artery hypertension. Surgical treatments have included lung transplantation with anatomic correction of the defect, as long as native cardiac function is thought to be reasonable, or heart-lung transplantation.

RED FLAGS

The initial manifestation of cyanosis usually constitutes a diagnostic emergency. In the neonate, congenital heart disease or a pulmonary disorder is the most likely reason. Normal lungs on chest radiograph suggest a cardiac cause of the cyanosis. Acrocyanosis must be distinguished from generalized cyanosis. Asymmetric or absent pulses must be noted. Noncardiac anomalies need to be recognized so that a syndrome might be considered and other anomalies identified. In older infants and children, noncardiac causes are more common, and lung disease, infection, and methemoglobinemia must be considered. In the older child, digital clubbing should strongly suggest a chronic cardiac or pulmonary disorder. The sudden onset of cyanosis in an older child might suggest pulmonary disease (pneumothorax, pulmonary embolism, pulmonary hemorrhage) or acquired methemoglobinemia.

REFERENCES

Cyanosis in the Newborn

DiMaio AM, Singh J: The infant with cyanosis in the emergency room. Pediatr Clin North Am 1992;39:987.

Driscoll DJ: Evaluation of the cyanotic newborn. Pediatr Clin North Am 1990;37:1.

Franklin RCG, Spiegelhalter DJ, Macartney FJ, et al: Evaluation of a diagnostic algorithm for heart disease in neonates. BMJ 1991;302:935.

Frommelt, PC: Congenital heart disease. In Rakel R (ed): Conn's Current Therapy 2000. Philadelphia, WB Saunders, 2000.

Fyler DC (ed): Nadas' Pediatric Cardiology. Philadelphia, Hanley and Belfus, 1992.

Garson A, Bricker JT, McNamara DG (eds): The Science and Practice of Pediatric Cardiology. Malvern, Pa, Lea & Febiger, 1990.

Grifka RG: Cyanotic congenital heart disease with increased pulmonary blood flow. Pediatr Clin North Am 1999;46:405.

Lees MH, King DK: Cyanosis in the newborn. Pediatr Rev 1987;9:36.

Linday LA, Ehlers KH, O'Loughlin, et al: Noninvasive diagnosis of persistent fetal circulation versus congenital cardiovascular defects. Am J Cardiol 1983;52:847.

Rudolph AM: Congenital Diseases of the Heart. Chicago, Year Book Medical Publishers, 1974.

Siassi B, Goldberg SJ, Emmanouilides GC, et al: Persistent pulmonary vascular obstruction in newborn infants. J Pediatr 1971;78:610.

Tweddell JS, Litwin SB, Thomas JP, et al: Recent advances in the surgical management of the single ventricle pediatric patient. Pediatr Clin North Am 1999;46:465.

Waldman JD, Wernly JA: Cyanotic congenital heart disease with decreased pulmonary blood flow in children. Pediatr Clin North Am 1999;46:385.

Yabek S: Neonatal cyanosis. Am J Dis Child 1984;138:880.

Cyanosis in the Older Infant and Child

Barst RJ: Primary pulmonary hypertension in children. In Rubin LJ, Rich S (eds): Primary Pulmonary Hypertension: Lung Biology in Health and Disease. New York, Marcel Dekker, 1996.

Emmanouilides GC, Riemenschneider TA, Allen HD, et al (eds): Moss and Adams Heart Disease in Infants, Children and Adolescents Including the Fetus and Young Adult, 5th ed. Baltimore, Williams & Wilkins, 1995.

Margolis PA, Ferkol TW, Marsocci S, et al: Accuracy of the clinical examination in detecting hypoxemia in infants with respiratory illness. J Pediatr 1994;124:552.

Nadas AS: Hypoxemia. In Fyler DC (ed): Nadas' Pediatric Cardiology. Philadelphia, Hanley and Belfus, 1992.

Vongpatanasin W, Brickner ME, Hillis LD, et al: The Eisenmenger syndrome in adults. Ann Intern Med 1998;128:745.

Methemoglobinemia

Feig SA: Methemoglobinemia. In Nathan DG, Oski FS (eds): Hematology of Infancy and Childhood. Philadelphia, WB Saunders, 1974.

Jaffe ER: Methemoglobinemia in the differential diagnosis of cyanosis. Hosp Pract 1985;20:92.

Watcha MF, Connor MT, Hing AV: Pulse oximetry in methemoglobinemia. Am J Dis Child 1989;143:845.

Pulse Oximetry

Hay WW Jr, Brockway JM, Eyzaquirre M: Neonatal pulse oximetry: Accuracy and reliability. Pediatrics 1989;83:717.

Meier-Strauss P, Bucher HU, Hurlimann R, et al: Pulse oximetry used for documenting oxygen saturation and right-to-left shunting immediately after birth. Eur J Pediatr 1990;149:851.

11 Heart Sounds and Murmurs

Andrew N. Pelech

Cardiac murmurs are audible turbulent sound waves in the range of 20 to 20,000 Hz emanating from the heart and vascular system. Heart murmurs are common in neonates, infants, and children. Whereas only 0.8% to 1% of the population has structural congenital cardiac disease, as many as 80% to 85% of the population has a heart murmur sometime during childhood. Most heart murmurs are normal or innocent, and they must be distinguished from pathologic murmurs of congenital or acquired cardiac diseases. The causes of cardiac murmurs are often influenced by the age of the patient at presentation (Table 11-1). The causes of congenital heart disease are varied and may include genetic (gene or chromosomal) disorders, syndrome complexes (Table 11-2), metabolic disorders, or teratogenesis. The causes of acquired heart diseases in children include rheumatic fever, endocarditis, and cardiac injury caused by systemic illnesses.

THE SCIENCE OF CARDIAC AUSCULTATION

A cardiac murmur is the perception of sound created by vibrations or turbulence. When a guitar string is plucked, it vibrates. By moving back and forth, the string alternately pushes and pulls the surrounding air

molecules. Sound waves arise from compression or rarefaction of molecules within a medium. This results in waves of pressure that travel to the ear, where they deflect the tympanic membrane. Sound waves have three dimensions: intensity, frequency, and timbre or quality.

INTENSITY OR LOUDNESS

The crest of a pressure wave has a given height or amplitude. This amplitude determines our perception of loudness. There is a large range of amplitudes over which sounds can be heard. Sound intensity or the subjective perception of loudness varies with the square of the sound amplitude. Sound intensity is measured by comparing it to some reference value (usually the softest sound intensity that humans can hear). Sound intensity is measured in decibels (dB).

FREQUENCY OR PITCH

The distance from the crest of one pressure wave to the next is the wavelength. The number of pressure waves transmitted per second is the frequency and is measured in Hertz (Hz). With shorter wavelengths,

---

Table 11-1. Cause of Heart Murmurs

Neonate*	Infant	Older Child
Transient patency of ductus arteriosus	Congenital heart disease (L→R shunt or R→L shunt)†	Congenital valvular obstruction
Peripheral pulmonic stenosis	Ejection murmurs (normal)	Ejection murmurs (normal)
Cyanotic congenital heart disease	Anemia	Repaired congenital heart disease
		Anemia
		Mitral valve prolapse
		Venous hum
Congenital valvular obstruction	Arteriovenous malformation	Bacterial endocarditis
Arteriovenous malformation (CNS, hepatic, pulmonary)	Infective endocarditis	Rheumatic fever
Anemia		Marfan syndrome
		Prosthetic valves
	Kawasaki disease	Obstructive (hypertrophic) cardiomyopathy (subaortic stenosis)
Asphyxia myocardial ischemia (transient TI or MI)	Hunter-Hurler syndrome	Carotid or abdominal bruit
	Fabry syndrome	Tumor (atrial myxoma)
		Thyrotoxicosis
		Systemic lupus erythematosus
		Pericardial friction rub

*Common causes of congenital heart disease in low-birth-weight infants include PDA, VSD, tetralogy of Fallot, coarctation of the aorta–interrupted aortic arch, hypoplastic left heart syndrome, heterotaxias, and dextrotransposition of the great arteries, in that order. Common causes of congenital heart disease in term infants include VSD, dextrotransposition of the great arteries, tetralogy of Fallot, coarctation of the aorta, pulmonary stenosis, hypoplastic left heart syndrome, and PDA; other causes represent a smaller percentage.

†The relative percentages of congenital heart lesions are VSD (25%-30%); ASD (6%-8%); PDA (6%-8%); coarctation of aorta (5%-7%); tetralogy of Fallot (5%-7%); pulmonary valve stenosis (5%-7%); aortic valve stenosis (5%-7%); dextrotransposition of great arteries (3%-5%); and hypoplastic left ventricle, truncus arteriosus, total anomalous venous return, tricuspid atresia, single ventricle, and double-outlet right ventricle representing 1%-3% each. Other and more complex lesions (heterotaxias) together represent 5%-10% of all lesions.

ASD, atrial septal defect; CNS, central nervous system; L, left; MI, mitral insufficiency; PDA, patent ductus arteriosus; R, right; TI, tricuspid insufficiency; VSD, ventricular septal defect.

Table 11-2. Syndromes or Syndrome Complexes Associated with Congenital Heart Disease

Syndrome	Dominant Cardiac Defect
Alagille (arteriohepatic disease)	Peripheral pulmonary stenosis
Asplenia	Complex cyanotic heart disease, anomalous veins, pulmonary atresia
Carpenter	Patent ductus arteriosus, ventricular septal defect
Cat-eye	Total anomalous pulmonary venous return
Char	Patent ductus arteriosus
CHARGE	Ventricular, atrioventricular, and atrial septal defects
de Lange	Tetralogy of Fallot, ventricular septal defect
DiGeorge*	Aortic arch anomalies, conotruncal defects, tetralogy of Fallot
Down	Artioventricular septal defects, ventricular septal defect, patent ductus arteriosus
Ellis–van Creveld	Single atrium, endocardial cushion defects
Fanconi	Patent ductus arteriosus, ventricular septal defect
Fetal alcohol	Ventricular septal defect, atrial septal defect, tetralogy of Fallot
Fragile X	Mitral valve prolapse, aortic root dilation
Goldenhar	Tetralogy of Fallot
Holt-Oram	Atrial or ventricular septal defect
Hydantoin	Atrial or ventricular septal defect, coarctation of aorta
Infant of diabetic mother	Hypertrophic cardiomyopathy, ventricular septal defect
Laurence-Moon-Biedl	Tetralogy of Fallot, ventricular septal defect
Marfan	Aortic root dissection, mitral valve prolapse
Mulibrey nanism	Pericardial thickening, constrictive pericarditis
Multiple lentigines (leopard)	Pulmonary stenosis
Noonan	Pulmonic stenosis (dysplastic valve), atrial septal defect
PHACE	Coarctation of aorta, ventricular septal defect, patent ductus arteriosus
Pierre Robin	Coarctation of aorta
Polycystic kidney disease	Mitral valve prolapse
Polysplenia	Complex acyanotic lesions, azygous continuation
Rubella	Patent ductus arteriosus, peripheral pulmonary stenosis
Rubinstein-Taybi	Patent ductus arteriosus
Scimitar	Hypoplasia of the right lung, anomalous pulmonary drainage
Smith-Lemli-Opitz	Ventricular septal defect, patent ductus arteriosus
Thrombocytopenia–absent radius (TAR)	Atrial septal defect, tetralogy of Fallot, ventricular septal defect
Trisomy D	Ventricular septal defect, patent ductus arteriosus, atrial septal defect
Trisomy E	Ventricular septal defect, patent ductus arteriosus, atrial septal defect
Turner	Coarctation of aorta, bicuspid aortic valve
VACTERL (VATER)	Ventricular septal defect, tetralogy of Fallot
Valproate effects	Coarctation of aorta, hypoplastic left heart syndrome
Velocardiofacial	Ventricular septal defect, right aortic arch
Williams (7q11 deletion)	Supravalvular aortic stenosis, peripheral pulmonary stenosis
Wolf	Atrial septal defect, ventricular septal defect

*Also called CATCH 22 (cardiac defects, abnormal facial features, thymus underdevelopment, cleft palate, and hypocalcemia caused by chromosome 22 defect) or deletion 22q11 syndrome.

CHARGE, coloboma, heart disease, atresia choanae, retarded growth and development or central nervous system anomalies, genital hypoplasia, and ear anomalies and/or deafness; PHACE, posterior fossa malformations, hemangiomas, arterial anomalies, coarctation of aorta, and eye abnormalities; VACTERL, vertebral abnormalities, anal atresia, cardiac abnormalities, tracheoesophageal fistula and/or esophageal atresia, renal agenesis and dysplasia, and limb defects; VATER, vertebral defects, imperforate anus, tracheoesophageal fistula, and radial and renal dysplasia.

there are more pressure waves per second and the frequencies are higher. Conversely, with longer wavelengths, the frequencies are lower. The frequency of a pressure wave determines perception of pitch; humans hear low frequencies as low pitch and high frequencies as high pitch. The pitch of most heart sounds and murmurs ranges between 5 and 800 Hz. Low frequencies are not heard as well and need larger amplitudes to sound equally loud. Note that many sounds emanating from the heart are below the threshold of audibility and consequently may be perceived by palpation.

QUALITY OR TIMBRE

When the same musical note is played on different instruments, it sounds distinctly different. The timbre, or quality, of a sound refers to the component parts of a complex waveform. Overtones (multiple secondary waveforms) differentiate a violin and piano playing the same note. Although a variety of qualitative terms have been employed to describe heart murmurs, such as rumbling, machinery, or blowing, there are only two fundamental qualities of sound: music and noise.

Harmony or Music

The individual characteristics of the sound depend on the number and relative amplitude of the overtones. When the overtones are multiples of the primary frequency, they create a pleasing sound, termed *harmony* or *music*. Knowing about harmonics and overtones helps health care professionals understand the musical quality of some cardiac murmurs.

Dissonance or Noise

When a complex sound wave is composed of many different and unrelated frequencies, a dissonant, rough noise is perceived. Noise can originate from variable amounts of turbulent flows of gases and fluids. Water rushing through pipes or blood being ejected from the heart across a stenotic valve causes noise.

THE THORAX

Sounds travel through the heart and appear on the chest surface; chambers are in close contact with the chest wall. Knowing the location of the heart chambers and valves within the thorax helps in the interpretation of heart sounds (Fig. 11-1).

The left atrium is located posterior, close to the spine. The right atrium and right ventricle are located anterior, immediately beneath the sternum. The outflow tract of the right ventricle, which contains the pulmonary valve, rises to the left of the sternum. The parts of the left side of the heart that are close to the chest wall include the left ventricular apex and the ascending aorta as it passes up to the right of the sternum. In other areas, lung tissue lies between the heart and chest wall. This may diminish or distort the intensity of heart sounds.

THE STETHOSCOPE

The stethoscope is the most widely used instrument in the diagnoses of problems related to the heart and lungs. The stethoscope transmits sounds from the patient to the examiner (Fig. 11-2). The components of the stethoscope include the following:

1. The *earpiece* should be soft, pliable, and large enough to occlude the external ear canal and yet not be too small to cause discomfort. The earpieces can be tested by lifting the bell off of the skin. A popping sensation, indicating a proper seal and fit, should be felt.
2. The *binaurals* are the metal tubes that connect to the earpieces. They should be on the same plane as the ear canals and thus should be angled slightly forward.
3. The metal *brace* connects to the binaurals and provides necessary inward pressure.
4. *Tubing* may be single or double, either plastic or rubber, and should be of the shortest practical length.
5. The *chest piece* should consist of a bell and diaphragm. The bell should extend across an intercostal space. It should be of good

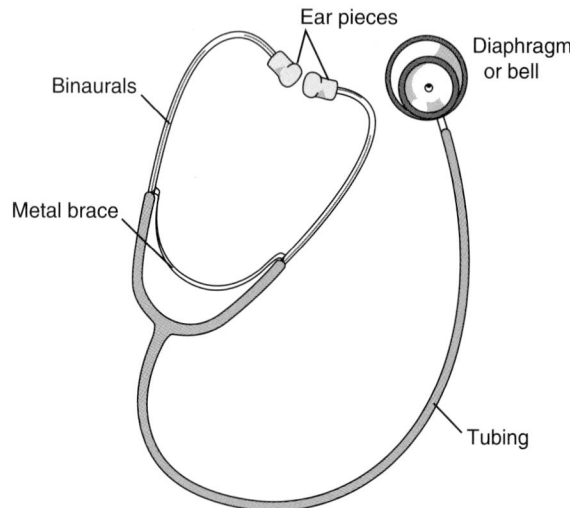

Figure 11-2. The components of the standard stethoscope. The size of the diaphragm or bell affects the examiner's ability to localize sounds. It is important that the earpieces be soft and fit comfortably in the examiner's external auditory canal, providing an airtight seal.

depth and encircled by a rubber ring to enable a tight seal. The bell must be applied very lightly to emphasize low-frequency sounds. The diaphragm should have a diameter small enough to permit localization of sounds (approximately 30 mm in a child and 45 mm in an adult). The diaphragm serves as a high-pass filter to attenuate sounds below 100 Hz. Both the bell and diaphragm should be used.

A good stethoscope should include both a shallow bell for low frequencies and a thin stiff diaphragm for high frequencies. The diaphragm is subject to damage, and regular maintenance is required. The tubing should not be of excessive length because this reduces the sound.

ORIGINS OF THE HEART SOUNDS

Normal heart sounds originate from vibrations of heart valves when they close and from heart chambers when they fill or contract rapidly. Like a door that bangs shut, the pressure that forces the valve closure influences the intensity of a heart sound. Other mechanical factors such as valve stiffness, thickness, and excursion have less effect on sound intensity.

Cardiac murmurs are the direct result of blood flow turbulence. The amount of turbulence and consequently the intensity of a cardiac murmur depend on

- the pressure difference or gradient across a narrowing or defect
- the blood flow or volume across the site

As sound radiates from its source, sound intensity diminishes with the square of the distance. Consequently, heart sounds should be loudest near the point of origin. However, other factors influence this relationship. Sound passage through the body is affected by the transmission characteristics of the tissues. Fat has a more pronounced dampening effect on higher frequencies than does more dense tissue such as bone. If the difference in tissue density is significant—for example, between the heart and lungs—more sound energy is lost. Only the loudest sounds may be heard when lung tissue is positioned between the heart and chest wall.

In contrast to intensity, the frequency of a cardiac murmur is proportional to pressure difference or gradient across a narrowing alone.

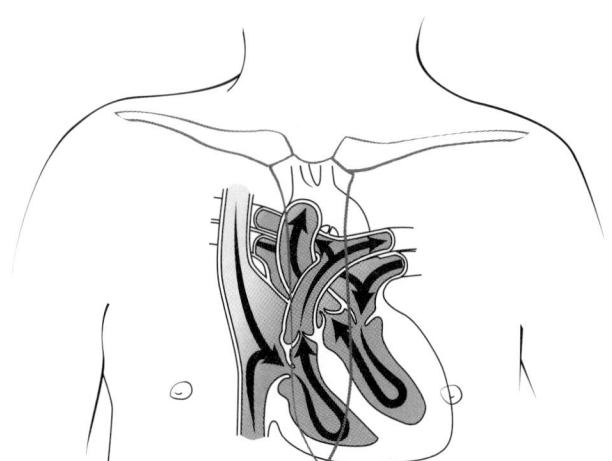

Figure 11-1. Location of the heart within the thorax. The right atrium and right ventricle lie immediately beneath the sternum. The left atrium lies posteriorly against the spine. The left ventricle extends laterally toward the chest wall, whereas the left ventricular outflow tract extends to the right side of the sternum, going upward toward the cardiac base.

THE CARDIAC CYCLE

Cardiac sounds and murmurs that arise from turbulence or vibrations within the heart and vascular system may be innocent (ejection) or pathologic. It is important to understand the timing of events in the cardiac cycle as a prerequisite to understanding heart murmurs. The relationship between the normal heart cycle and that of the heart sounds is noted in Figure 11-3.

The cardiac cycle begins with *atrial systole,* the sequential activation and contraction of the two thin-walled chambers. This is followed by the delayed contraction of the more powerful lower chambers, termed *ventricular systole.* Ventricular systole has three phases:

1. isovolumic contraction: the short period of early contraction when the pressure builds within the ventricle but has yet to rise sufficiently to permit ejection
2. ventricular ejection: when the ventricles eject blood to the body (via the aorta) and to the lungs (via the pulmonary artery)
3. isovolumic relaxation: the period of ventricular relaxation when ejection ceases and pressure falls within the ventricles

During ventricular contraction, the atria begin to relax (*atrial diastole*) and receive venous blood from both the body and the lungs. Then, in *ventricular diastole,* the lower chambers relax, allowing initial passive filling of the thick-walled ventricles and emptying of the atria. Later, during the terminal period of ventricular relaxation, the atria contract. This atrial systole augments ventricular filling just before the onset of the next ventricular contraction.

The sequence of contractions generates pressure and blood flow through the heart. The relationship of blood volume, pressure, and

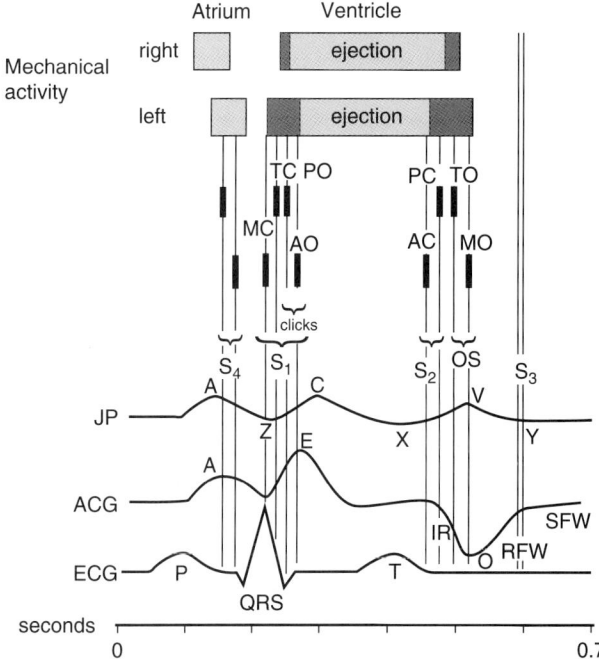

Figure 11-3. The cardiac cycle. Relationship among electrical and mechanical events, valvular motion, heart sounds (S_1, S_2, S_3, and S_4), the jugular pulse wave (JP), and the apexcardiogram (ACG). AC and AO, aortic component and opening; ECG, electrocardiogram; IR, isovolumic (isochronic) relaxation wave; MC and MO, mitral component and opening; O, opening of mitral valve; OS, opening snap of atrioventricular valves; PC and PO, pulmonic component and opening; RFW, rapid-filling wave; SFW, slow-filling wave; TC and TO, tricuspid component and opening. (From Tilkian AG, Conover MB: Understanding Heart Sounds and Murmurs: With an Introduction to Lung Sounds, 3rd ed. Philadelphia, WB Saunders, 1993.)

flow determines opening and closing of heart valves and generates characteristic heart sounds and murmurs. For example, valve closure at higher pressure creates louder heart sounds.

CHANGES IN THE CIRCULATION AT BIRTH

An understanding of the fetal, transitional, and neonatal adaptations of the circulation is important in the evaluation of the pediatric cardiovascular system, because many organic heart diseases are evident in association with the circulatory changes occurring at birth. The majority of significant structural congenital heart disease are recognized in the first few weeks of life. The age at recognition or referral often dictates the nature of the cardiac anomaly and the urgency with which assessment is necessary.

In the fetus (Fig. 11-4), oxygen is derived from the placenta and returns via the umbilical vein and through the ductus venosus to enter the inferior vena cava and right atrium. Preferentially, flow is directed across the foramen ovale to enter the left atrium and, subsequently, the left ventricle. Deoxygenated blood returning from the superior vena cava and upper body segment is preferentially directed by the flap of the eustachian valve to enter the right ventricle and then, via the ductus arteriosus, to enter the descending aorta to return via the umbilical arteries to the placenta. The pressures within both ventricles are essentially equal, inasmuch as both chambers pump to the systemic circulation. However, in utero, the right ventricle does the majority of the work, pumping 66% of the combined cardiac output. At transition (see Fig. 11-4B), with the first breath, pulmonary arterial resistance begins to fall as the lungs begin the process of respiration. Pulmonary venous return to the left atrium closes the flap of the foramen ovale. Through mechanical and chemical mechanisms, the ductus arteriosus begins to close. In the normal full-term infant, this is accomplished by 10 to 15 hours after birth. Intermittent right-to-left atrial level shunting through the foramen ovale may occur, particularly if pulmonary vascular resistance fails to drop. In addition, structural cardiac abnormalities necessitating patency of the ductus arteriosus for maintenance of either pulmonary blood flow (pulmonary atresia) or systemic blood flow (hypoplastic left heart syndrome) most often manifest within the first few days of life. Thus, the time when a pediatric patient presents for evaluation is influenced by the spectrum of heart diseases. Duct-dependent abnormalities, such as pulmonary atresia, transposition of the great arteries, coarctation of the aorta, hypoplastic left heart syndrome, or significant outflow obstructions (e.g., critical aortic valve stenosis) manifest in the first few days after birth. In the absence of an associated anomaly, hemodynamically significant ventricular septal defects (VSDs) seldom manifest before 2 to 4 weeks after birth. Atrial septal defects (ASDs) are seldom symptomatic in infancy.

NORMAL INTRACARDIAC PRESSURES

In the child after birth and successful transition, resistance to flow in the pulmonary circuit is much lower than in the systemic circuit. Therefore, the pressures in the right-sided chambers are lower than those in the left-sided chambers. The higher values (see Fig. 11-4C) reflect pressures during ventricular systole in a normal heart. Pressure in the great vessels during the systole is identical to that in the ventricles. This changes if there is outflow obstruction. In ventricular diastole, the semilunar valves (aortic and pulmonary) close. Resistance to blood flow in the vascular bed determines the diastolic pressures in the great arteries. The thin-walled atria generate much lower pressures than do the ventricles, both during the phase of passive atrial filling (v wave) and during atrial contraction (a wave). Only the mean (m) or average atrial pressure is shown in Figure 11-4C. During ventricular relaxation, the diastolic pressures are lower than those in the atria, enabling filling. Knowledge of the cardiac cycle is important in understanding the more complicated hemodynamics and flow patterns of specific cardiac abnormalities.

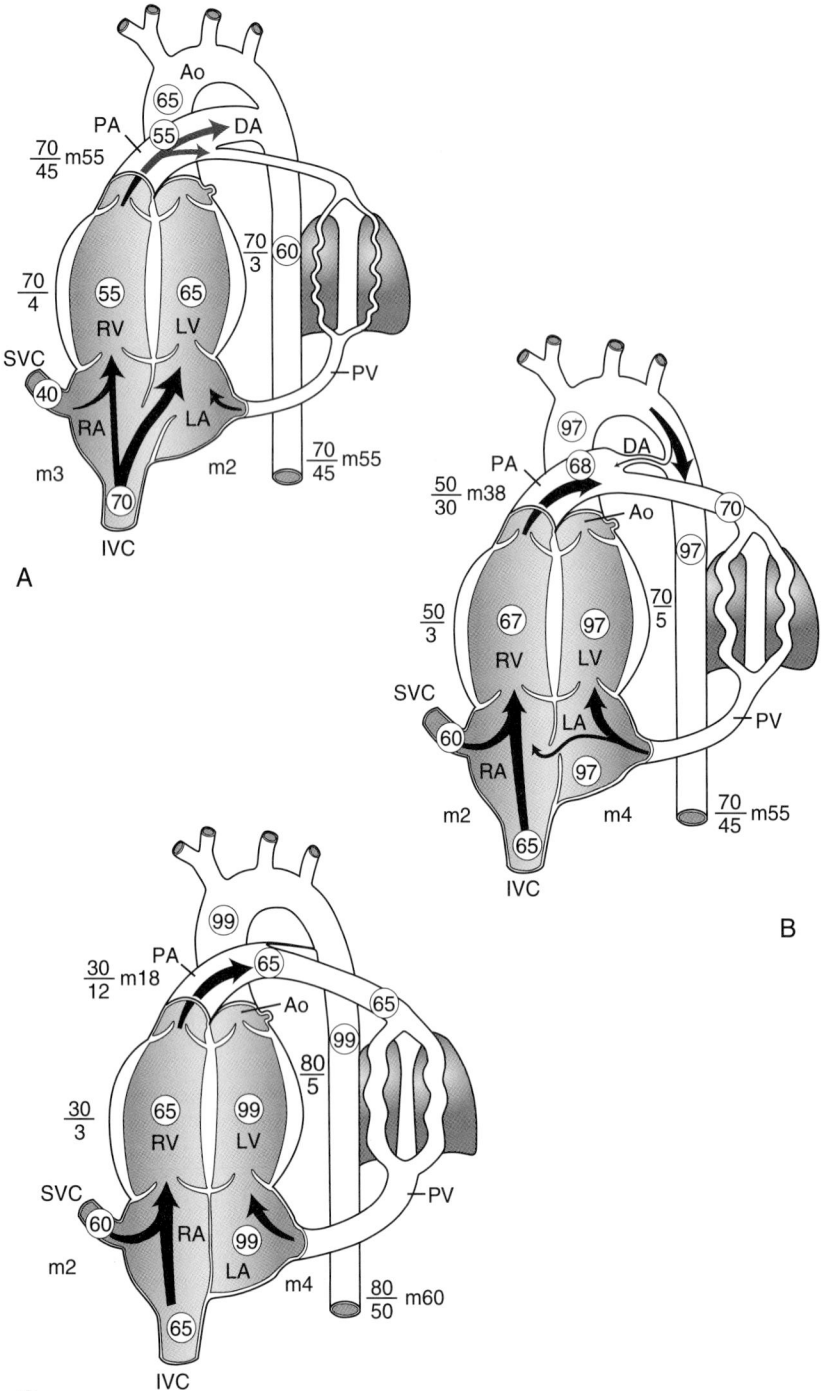

A

B

C

Figure 11-4. Fetal, transitional, and neonatal circulations. The course of the circulation in the heart and great arteries of the late-gestation fetal lamb, within a few hours of delivery and as a newborn, are presented. The figures in the circles within the chambers and vessels represent percent oxygen saturation. The numbers alongside the chambers and vessels are pressures in mm Hg related to amniotic fluid pressure as zero. Ao, aorta; DA, ductus arteriosus; IVC, inferior vena cava; LA, left atrium; LV, left ventricle; m, mean; PA, pulmonary artery; PV, pulmonary vein; RA, right atrium; RV, right ventricle; SVC, superior vena cava. (Adapted from Rudolph AM: Chapters 2 and 3. In Congenital Disease of the Heart. Chicago, Year Book Medical, 1974.)

PEDIATRIC CARDIOVASCULAR EVALUATION

The evaluation of the cardiovascular system must include a thorough history and physical examination. The history should include a detailed and chronologic assessment of symptoms, a comprehensive family history, and an assessment of cardiorespiratory system function.

The cardiovascular physical examination should include assessment of the overall appearance, growth, development, and measurement of vital signs, as well as a sequential evaluation of arterial pulses and perfusion, venous pulses, hepatic contour and size, precordial palpation, and auscultation.

In children, flexibility is the key. There is no rule against auscultating first if conditions allow listening to a sleeping or quiet infant, often in the mother's arms. There is, however, a tendency to neglect or omit important aspects of the cardiovascular examination if an orderly routine is not followed. Additional studies might include chest radiography, electrocardiography, and echocardiography.

HISTORY

Historical assessment of the pediatric patient referred for evaluation of a cardiac murmur should include questions about the family history, the pregnancy, and perinatal course, in addition to questions about symptoms of cardiovascular disease. An index of exercise or play capacity should be sought, as should an assessment of growth and development. The presence of congenital abnormalities of other major organ systems is associated with additional structural cardiac problems in as many as 25% of patients.

Structural heart disease is frequently seen in association with recognizable syndromes (see Table 11-2). Children with clearly definable chromosomal disorders known to have a significant incidence of structural cardiac abnormalities, such as Down or Turner syndrome, are usually referred for further diagnostic evaluation. Family history of sudden unexplained death, rheumatic fever, sudden infant death syndrome, or a structural cardiac abnormality in a first-degree relative may be relevant. Hypertrophic cardiomyopathy in a first-degree relative is associated with a high incidence of inheritance, and this condition is sufficiently subtle that echocardiographic screening is mandatory.

A maternal history of gestational diabetes mellitus may be associated with a transient hypertrophic cardiomyopathy in as many as 30% of infants of these mothers, as well as with definable congenital structural abnormalities. Additional relevant pregnancy history may include the presence of chronic or acute maternal illness, congenital infections, or drug use, any of which may be associated with significant structural heart disease. Unexplained fever, lethargy, or additional symptoms arising after recent dental work should arouse suspicion of possible endocarditis.

SYMPTOMS AND SIGNS OF HEART DISEASE

The general health of a child with a suspected cardiac malformation is important. Particularly relevant are the rate of growth, development, and history of past illnesses. Although symptoms of failure to thrive are nonspecific, patterns of growth reflect duration and severity of the disease and effectiveness of treatment (see Chapter 13). In an infant, feeding difficulties are often the first evidence of congestive heart failure (see Chapter 8). Heart failure occurs in 30% of infants and children with congenital heart disease. Feeding problems are common manifestations of cardiac disease and may be evidenced as disinterest, excessive fatigue, long feeding duration, diaphoresis, or a change in the pattern of respiration, tachypnea, or dyspnea. It is important to obtain a measure of caloric intake by quantitating number and/or volume of feedings. Some index of exertional tolerance should be sought in all children as an index of cardiovascular fitness and a sign of functional capability. This index should be age relevant and, in an infant, might include assessment of the vigor and duration of feeding and the time period of interactive play. In a toddler, the index might include ability to keep up with peers, climb stairs, or walk for extended periods. In an older child, a comparison with peer sporting interactions, level of function in physical education, and an index of aerobic ability should be sought.

Respiratory rates should be assessed in the quiet infant (Table 11-3). The rate and pattern of breathing should be assessed for a full minute, because rates may vary considerably with activity and feeding. Tachypnea may occur as a consequence of increased pulmonary blood flow. With increasing pulmonary congestion, particularly obstruction to pulmonary venous drainage, dyspnea is manifested as an anxious look with grunting, flaring of the alae nasi, and intercostal, suprasternal and subcostal retractions. Cardiac asthma or exercise-inducible reactive airway disease may occur as a consequence

of passive or active pulmonary congestion (see Chapter 3). Compression of airways by plethoric vessels may contribute to stasis of secretions and atelectasis that predisposes to respiratory tract infections.

Cyanosis in association with a cardiac murmur suggests a structural lesion with restriction to pulmonary blood flow (see Chapter 10) (Table 11-4). Cyanosis, or a blue discoloration of the skin and mucous membranes is a consequence of reduced hemoglobin (>5 g/dL), and is evident in one third of infants with potentially lethal congenital heart disease. Central cyanosis is distinguished from acrocyanosis or peripheral cyanosis by involvement of the warm mucous membranes, including the tongue and buccal mucosa. Acrocyanosis or peripheral cyanosis is generally confined to the perioral and perinasal regions, extremities, or nail beds and occurs in the child who is cold, vasoconstricted, or at rest. A distinctive feature is that central cyanosis generally worsens with activity and increasing cardiac output, whereas acrocyanosis generally improves or resolves with increased activity.

PHYSICAL EXAMINATION

In each routine examination, it is important that signs be critically evaluated so that when an abnormality arises, it is readily recognized. Examination of the toddler may be best performed with the child on the parent's lap. In the older patient, it is often best to allow a few minutes in conversation with the parents and child to gain the child's confidence.

Overall Appearance

Height and weight should be measured and plotted on a growth chart. An assessment of the child's overall growth, appearance, and state of distress serves as a guide to the urgency of further investigation and management. The sick infant often appears anxious, fretful, diaphoretic, pale, or breathless and is seldom consolable. Observe for evidence of cyanosis, pallor, digital clubbing, pattern of respiration, and possible dysmorphic features, which may suggest specific structural cardiac anomalies.

Vital Signs

Vital signs should be recorded on each patient. Normal resting heart rates and respiratory rate values for age are presented in Table 11-3. Appropriate-size cuffs, in which the width of the inflatable bag covers two thirds of the full length of the arm or in which just enough room is left for application of head of the stethoscope, should be used to ensure accurate blood pressure measurement. Blood pressures obtained by palpation or the flush technique are significantly less accurate. The blood pressure cuff should be applied snugly, because higher pressure may have to be applied to occlude arterial flow with a loose-fitting cuff. The systolic pressure is recorded as the first audible Korotkoff sound; the diastolic pressure is correlated best with the muffling phase or fourth Korotkoff sound. Automated oscillometric methods providing digital printouts of systolic, mean, and diastolic pressures are often employed for blood pressure measurements. The reliability of this method is generally good, although inaccuracies can occur with movement. Every child should have a comparison of upper and lower blood pressures on at least one occasion. This is

Table 11-3. Normal Values of Respiratory and Heart Rates in Infants and Children

	Age				
	Birth-6 Weeks	*6 weeks-2 Years*	*2-6 Years*	*6-10 Years*	*Older than 10 Years*
Respiratory rate	45-60/min	40/min	30/min	25/min	20/min
Heart rate	125±30/min	115±25/min	100±20/min	90±15/min	85±15/min

Table 11-4. Categories of Cyanotic Heart Lesions in the Neonate

Group	Heart Size	Pulmonary Blood Flow	Low Cardiac Output	Respiratory Distress	Examples
I	Small	Reduced	No	None	Hypoplastic RV with pulmonary atresia Hypoplastic RV with tricuspid atresia Tetralogy of Fallot (severe)
II	Small or slight cardiomegaly	Increased	No	Moderate	Transposition of great arteries with intact ventricular septum
III	Large	Increased	Yes	Yes	Complicated coarctation of aorta with VSD, hypoplastic LV
IV	Small	Pulmonary venous congestion	Yes	Yes	Obstructed total anomalous pulmonary veins

Modified from Gillette PC: The cardiovascular system. In Behrman RE, Kliegman RM (eds): Nelson Essentials of Pediatrics, 2nd ed. Philadelphia, WB Saunders, 1994, p 503.
LV, left ventricle; RV, right ventricle; VSD, ventricular septal defect.

generally performed by cuff application to the upper leg and Doppler assessment of the popliteal systolic pressure. Because of the artifact of reflectance waves or filtering of the lower frequency components of the complex arterial pulse waveform, the lower limb systolic blood pressure is normally 10 mm Hg higher in older children than the upper limb pressure. On occasion, the subclavian arteries may arise aberrantly beyond the site of ductal ligament insertion. Therefore, both upper limb pressures should be measured and compared with the lower limb pressure. Normal values for blood pressure in children are presented in Figure 11-5.

Respiratory Assessment

Respiratory distress may suggest cardiac disease (see Chapters 3 and 10). In addition to noting the rate, depth, and effort of respiration, the inspection should include observation for evidence of air trapping, increased chest diameter, or the presence of subcostal Harrison sulci as an indication of chronic upper airway obstruction. An allergic malar facies may also suggest upper airway obstructive disease with predisposition to hypercapnia and pulmonary hypertension. Although crackles in the lungs in infants and even young children

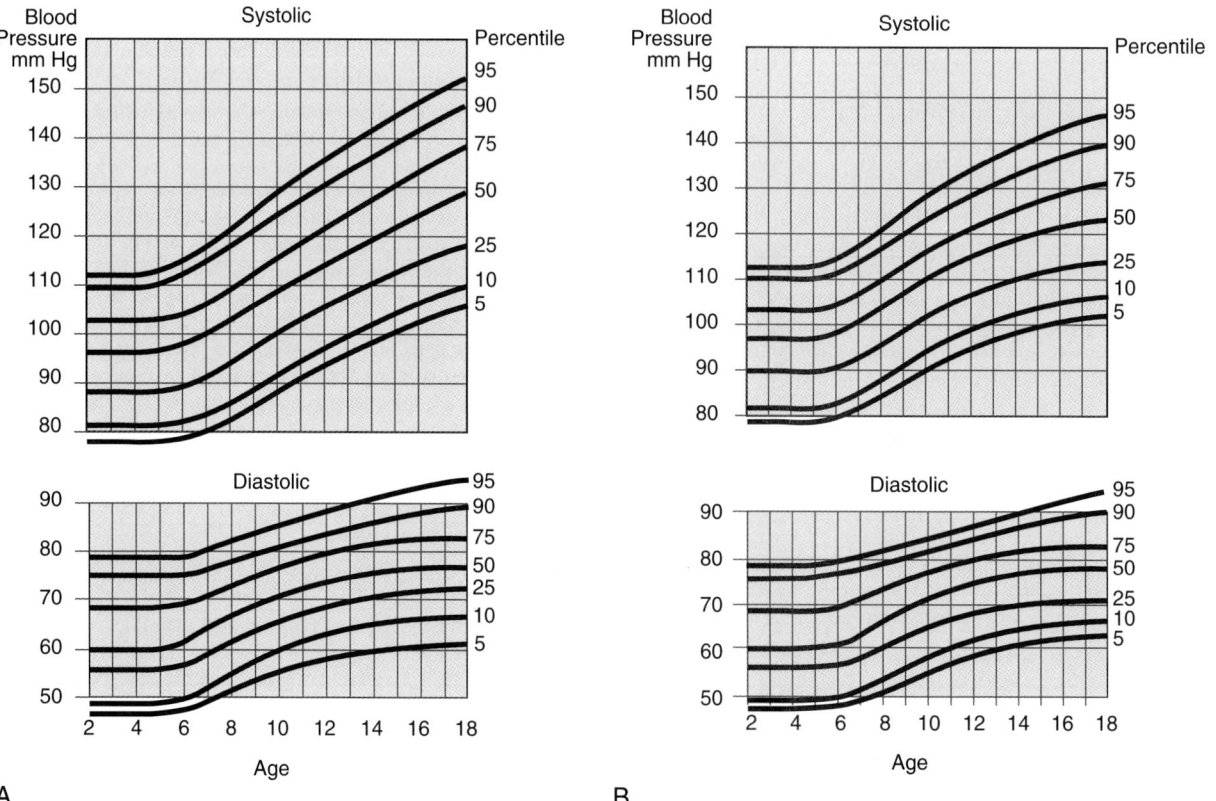

Figure 11-5. Normal blood pressure percentiles for boys (**A**) and girls (**B**), aged 2 to 18 years. The Korotkoff IV sound is used for diastolic blood pressure. (Adapted from the National Heart, Lung, and Blood Institute: Report of the second task force on blood pressure control in children, 1987. Pediatrics 1987;79:1.)

usually indicate infection, pulmonary edema should also be a consideration.

CARDIOVASCULAR ASSESSMENT

Arterial Examination

Pulses should be assessed for rate, rhythm, volume, and character. The dynamic character of the pulse may provide information about the cardiac output. A clinical index of cardiac output includes the warmth of the digits and measured capillary refill time. This is obtained by blanching the nail beds or digits and estimating the time to full reperfusion, which is normally less than 2 to 3 seconds. Initially, the radial and brachial pulses should be assessed simultaneously in the upper limb. By palpating the pulse at two sites and altering the pressure applied by the palpating fingers, a more accurate assessment of the rate of rise, volume, and contour may be obtained. Assessment of the femoral pulse requires that the infant be quiet. Palpating parallel to the inguinal crease and allowing the leg to continue to flex is generally more effective than extending the leg. Blood pressures in the arm and leg should be assessed, and the radial and femoral pulses should be palpated simultaneously. Whenever possible, the radial pulse should be brought in close apposition to the femoral pulse to compare for any delay. This enables a more accurate appreciation of any temporal delay and enables more accurate detection of the presence of coarctation of the aorta. The presence of a palpable femoral pulse is by itself an inadequate screen for coarctation because a widely patent ductus arteriosus (PDA) or collateral vessels (particularly in the older patient) may provide delayed perfusion. Previous arterial instrumentation, injury, or congenital variability may account for reduction in palpable peripheral pulses.

Venous Examination

Assessment of the jugular venous pulse as an index of right atrial pressure elevation is generally difficult in infants and young children. In infants and young children, the liver character and size offer more reliable indicators of systemic congestion. The position, size, and consistency of the liver should be assessed. Abdominal examination is best performed in an unhurried manner. By gently palpating for the tone of the rectus muscles, the lateral margin in the midclavicular line can be located. The liver edge can be located and felt by uplifting of the fingers with each quiet inspiration. The character of the normal liver margin is generally likened to that of the cartilage of the external pinna, and the margin should be sharp and angulated. In the newborn, the liver may be normally palpable at 1.5 to 2.5 cm below the right costal margin in the midclavicular line. This distance decreases to approximately 1 to 2 cm by 1 year of age and remains just palpable until school entrance age. In the presence of congestive heart failure, the liver enlarges and distends downward. The congested liver margin becomes rounded and firm and is often more difficult to feel. An enlarged liver may be tender, and aggressive palpation may cause discomfort and tensing of the abdominal musculature, making accurate assessment difficult. A transverse liver is suggestive of a heterotaxia syndrome with abnormal abdominal organ location (situs abnormalities) and complex congenital heart lesions. The spleen should always be sought; enlargement suggests endocarditis in the patient with a heart murmur. Splenic enlargement in association with congestive heart failure is unusual (see Chapter 19).

Precordial Examination

Inspection of the chest may suggest the presence of a precordial bulge of long-standing right ventricular volume overload. The examiner's entire palm and hand should be warmed and then fully applied to the patient's chest wall to maximize ability to detect thrills

or heaves. Whereas the examiner's fingertips are best utilized to localize an abnormality, the palmar surface of the metacarpals and first phalanges are more sensitive for the detection of low-frequency events. The fingertips should be used to localize the most lateral displacement of the apical impulse. In patients of all ages, the apical impulse should be confined to one intercostal interspace and would be described as diffuse, if equally dynamic, in two or more interspaces. In the neonate, a right ventricular impulse may be felt close to the sternum. Later in life, the same degree of parasternal activity is likely to suggest pulmonary hypertension, right-sided heart volume overload, or right ventricular outflow obstruction. The lateral displacement of the apex, normally located in the midclavicular line, should be compared to existing landmarks. A dynamic or thrusting character to an apical impulse may be detected in association with an elevated cardiac output or various forms of obstruction to left ventricular outflow. On occasion, an apical filling impulse, coinciding with an audible S_3, may be detected normally, particularly in the adolescent or athlete with a relative bradycardia and increased stroke volume.

A thrill is a palpable murmur and should be sought in the precordial and suprasternal areas. The palmar surface of the examiner's hand is most sensitive in detection of a thrill; however, only the tips of the digits fit in the patient's suprasternal notch. In rare cases, a palpable second heart sound (S_2), indicative of a significant level of pulmonary hypertension, may be detected as a sharp or distinctive impulse in the pulmonary outflow.

Auscultation

Thorough auscultation in the cooperative patient may take as long as 5 to 10 minutes and should include listening in the principal areas of the precordial auscultation (tricuspid, pulmonary, mitral, and aortic) with both the bell and diaphragm of the stethoscope, with the patient in the supine, sitting, and standing positions. Four areas serve as a guide to auscultation of the heart (Fig. 11-6). These are the optimal sights for listening to sounds that arise within the chambers and great vessels:

1. The tricuspid area is represented by the fourth and fifth intercostal spaces along the left sternal edge but often extends to the right of the sternum as well as downward to the subxiphisternal area.
2. The pulmonary area is the second intercostal space along the left sternal border. Murmurs that are best heard in this area may also extend to the left infraclavicular area and often lower, along the left sternal edge to the third intercostal space.
3. The mitral area involves the region of the cardiac apex and generally is at the fifth intercostal space in the midclavicular line. This area may also extend medially to the left sternal edge and laterally to the region of the axilla.
4. The aortic area, although centered at the second right intercostal space, may extend to the suprasternal area, to the neck, and inferiorly to the third left intercostal space. The margins of these areas are ill defined, and auscultation should not be limited to these sites; it may extend to the axillae, neck, back, or infraclavicular areas.

A step-by-step auscultation—first for heart sounds, subsequently for systolic murmurs, and then separately for diastolic murmurs—is essential. The ability to clearly characterize the S_2 is perhaps more crucial than for any other sound; the effects of respiration are important. The components of the S_2 in childhood are normally split with inspiration and become single on expiration. A loud pulmonary closure sound should suggest the possibility of pulmonary artery hypertension. The S_2 may be widely split and/or fixed in association with right ventricular volume overload or delayed right ventricular conduction. Normal inspiratory splitting of the S_2 should be sought and established in all patients, but this may be difficult. In the infant with a rapid respiratory rate, the presence of splitting at any time during the respiratory cycle may be accepted as normal.

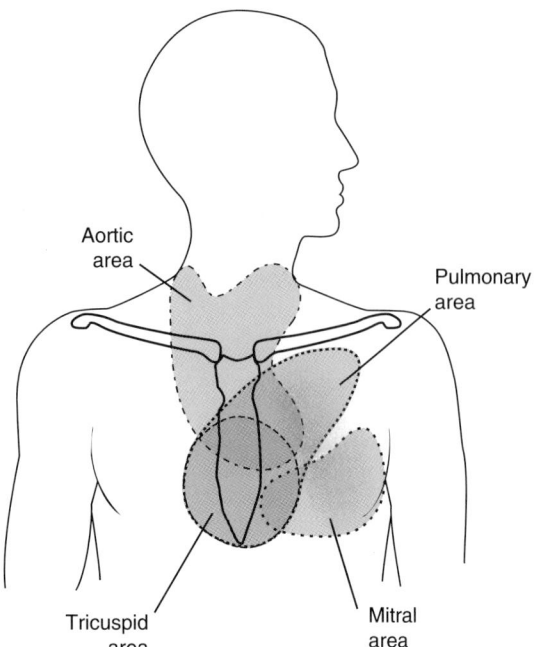

Figure 11-6. The four primary areas of auscultation represent the general regions where heart sounds and murmurs of the four cardiac valves are often best heard and defined. Note that the areas overlap considerably and that sounds and murmurs are not limited to these sites; they often extend to the lateral chest wall, abdomen, and back. (From Pelech AN: The cardiac murmur. Pediatr Clin North Am 1998;45:107-122.)

The right ventricle is normally just beneath the sternum. This proximity generally makes sounds emanating from the right heart louder and less diffuse. In addition, right heart sounds and murmurs are more influenced by the effects of respiration.

Heart Sounds

First direct the examination to the normal heart sounds in sequence. Appreciate the effects of inspiration and expiration on the heart sounds. Then address additional heart sounds and murmurs. Describe any variability that occurs with a change of body position.

The First Heart Sound

The first heart sound (S_1) (see Fig. 11-3) arises from closure of the atrioventricular (mitral and tricuspid) valves in early isovolumic ventricular contraction and, consequently, is best heard in the tricuspid and mitral valve areas. Mitral valve closure occurs slightly in advance of tricuspid valve closure, and, on occasion, near the lower left sternal edge, two components (splitting) of the S_1 may be heard. There is usually a single sound. The S_1 is most easily heard when the heart rate is slow because the interval between the S_1 and S_2 is shorter than the interval between the S_2 and subsequent S_1. The intensity of the S_1 is influenced by the position of the atrioventricular valve at the onset of ventricular contraction. If the valve leaflets are far apart, the increased excursion to accomplish valve closure increases the intensity of the S_1.

The Second Heart Sound

Shortly after the onset of ventricular contraction, the semilunar valves (aortic and pulmonary) open and permit ventricular ejection. This opening does not usually generate any sound. The atrioventricular valves remain tightly closed during ventricular ejection. As ventricular ejection nears completion, the pressure begins to fall within the ventricles, and the semilunar valves snap closed. This prevents regurgitation from the aorta and pulmonary artery back into the heart. The closure of the semilunar valves generates the S_2 (see Fig. 11-3). The S_2 usually consists of a louder and earlier aortic valve closure sound (A_2), followed by a later and quieter pulmonary valve closure sound (P_2). Normal physiologic splitting or variability is appreciated most easily in the pulmonary area during or near the end of inspiration. During expiration, the aortic and pulmonary valves close almost synchronously and produce a single or narrowly split S_2. Normal splitting of S_2 is caused by (1) increased right-sided heart filling during inspiration because of increased blood volume returning via the venae cavae; and (2) diminished left-sided heart filling because blood is retained within the small blood vessels of the lungs when the thorax expands. During inspiration, when the right ventricle is filled more than the left, it takes slightly longer to empty. This causes the noticeable inspiratory delay in P_2 in relation to A_2. Splitting of the S_2 during inspiration is a normal finding and should be sought in all patients.

The aortic and pulmonary pressure in diastole closes the semilunar valves. Many forms of congenital or acquired heart disease have an impact on the pulmonary circulation and, consequently, often affect the S_2. Thus, the *higher* the pulmonary artery diastolic pressure, the more intense and earlier the P_2 is. Pulmonary hypertension in children is suggested when the P_2 is palpable, loud, and narrowly split or cannot be separated from A_2. In adults but not in children, if P_2 is heard at the apex, pulmonary hypertension is likely. A single or narrow split S_2 may also be noted in patients with severe pulmonic or aortic valve stenosis, tetralogy of Fallot, truncus arteriosus, pulmonary atresia, hypoplastic left heart syndrome, tricuspid valve atresia, or Eisenmenger syndrome with a VSD. In the presence of pulmonic stenosis, there is low pulmonary artery diastolic pressure. The pulmonary valve closure is therefore delayed and of decreased intensity and is occasionally inaudible.

The S_2 may be widely split and/or fixed in association with right ventricular volume overload or delayed right ventricular conduction.

The Third Heart Sound

The third heart sound (S_3) (see Fig. 11-3), which is of very low frequency, occurs about a third of the way into diastole, at the time of the most rapid filling of the ventricles. It is most likely caused by sudden tension of the ventricles, enough to produce sound vibrations within the myocardial wall. Vibrations in the atrioventricular valve itself, as well as in the chordae, may also contribute to the sound. The amplitude of S_3 increases with an increased ventricular filling rate, but the frequency of the sound also increases with increased end-diastolic pressure (which perhaps makes the sound easier to hear). When heard at the apex, S_3 is considered left ventricular in origin, and when heard at the lower left sternal border, S_3 is likely to be right ventricular in origin. An apical S_3 of soft to moderate intensity is readily heard in most children and young adults. An S_3 gallop may also be caused by lesions associated with left or right ventricular diastolic overload or diminished ventricular compliance.

The Fourth Heart Sound

The fourth heart sound (S_4) (see Fig. 11-3) is also of low frequency and can be both left-sided and right-sided in origin. It occurs with atrial contraction against a high resistance and is therefore heard just before S_1. It is more difficult to hear than is S_3, particularly in children, in whom the PR interval is usually shorter than that in the adult. The S_4 may be caused by a forceful atrial contraction against a poorly compliant left ventricle (e.g., as in diastolic overload). The sound is readily heard in adults with significant chronic hypertension or left ventricular cardiomyopathy and, except for its timing, sounds much like an S_3. In a young baby with total anomalous pulmonary venous return, low pulmonary vascular resistance, and significantly increased right ventricular and pulmonary blood flow, a loud right ventricular S_4 (as well as S_3) may be heard as part of a quadruple rhythm at the lower left sternal border. An intermittent S_4 may be heard in children with complete atrioventricular block, whereas an S_3 may be heard in a normal adolescent; this may be physiologic. The S_4 always occurs in a pathologic condition.

Ejection Click

An audible ejection click (see Fig. 11-3) is abnormal and is either related to the hemodynamics associated with a dilated root of the aorta (aortic ejection click) or a dilated root of the pulmonary artery (pulmonary ejection click) or the effects of a thickened and immobile semilunar valve. The sound is sharp and of very high frequency. The pulmonary ejection click is best heard at the upper left sternal border, whereas the aortic ejection click is usually best heard at the apex. It may also be heard at the upper right sternal border, but if so, it is always louder at the apex or the lower left sternal border. The click arises either from sudden tension of the semilunar valve or from sudden distention with lateral pressure at the root of the aorta or pulmonary artery. The sound is present in aortic or pulmonary valve stenosis. In such cases, the rapid movement of the stenotic valve is suddenly checked. An aortic ejection click may be heard in the presence of a normal aortic valve (as in severe tetralogy of Fallot with a large aortic root); a pulmonary ejection click may be heard with a normal pulmonic valve (as in Eisenmenger syndrome with a large pulmonary root).

The aortic ejection click, best heard at the apex, does not vary with respirations. However, the pulmonary ejection click, best heard at the upper left sternal border, is better heard on expiration than inspiration.

An ejection click or a sharp sound present at the upper left sternal border, louder with expiration or heard only on expiration, is characteristic of pulmonary valve stenosis. The ejection click follows the period of isovolumic contraction and occurs as a consequence of restricted semilunar (aortic or pulmonary) valve excursion at the onset of ventricular ejection. When the ejection sound occurs at the upper right sternal border or at the apex, a bicuspid or stenotic aortic valve disease is suggested. In contrast to ejection clicks, right-sided cardiac murmurs are accentuated with inspiration. Note that left-sided heart auscultatory abnormalities vary little with the respiratory cycle.

In the case of the aortic ejection click, the sound is usually very well separated from S_1. However, the pulmonary ejection click is usually closer to S_1 than is an aortic click. In some moderate to severe cases, the pulmonary ejection click occurs at the same time as S_1. The intensity of S_1 is normally very low at the upper left sternal border. When a loud S_1 is present, a careful analysis may reveal that this loud S_1 is maximal on expiration, which indicates that the loudness is because of a prominent pulmonary ejection click occurring at the same time as a normally soft S_1.

Opening Snap

The opening snap, present only in rheumatic mitral valve stenosis when the anteromedial leaflet is immobile, is heard early in diastole, usually above the apex, and is of medium frequency. Because the leaflets are fused, the downward movement of the opening valve is suddenly checked, resulting in the opening snap. This sound is often confused with an S_3. The frequency is somewhat higher and the timing is earlier than those of an S_3.

Non-ejection Click

Non-ejection clicks are heard at the apex and occur one third to half of the way between S_1 and S_2. Thus, they are commonly called

midsystolic clicks. The sounds are of medium to high frequency. The sound is caused by the sudden tensing of the posterior mitral valve leaflet as it prolapses into the left atrium; in rare cases, there may be multiple midsystolic clicks. The clicks may be loud, but they may also be soft and easily missed.

CLASSIFICATION OF CARDIAC MURMURS

Heart murmurs are the consequence of turbulent blood flow. Turbulence may arise as a result of

- high flow through abnormal or normal valves
- normal flow through narrow or stenotic valves or vessels
- backward or regurgitant flow through incompetent leaky valves
- flow through congenital or surgical communications
- anemia with high flows and discrete decreased blood viscosity

Not all cardiac murmurs indicate heart problems.

The clinician should be able to determine and describe the following characteristics of heart murmurs:

timing: the relative position within the cardiac cycle relative to S_1 and S_2
intensity or loudness: murmurs are graded as
- grade I: heard only with intense concentration
- grade II: faint but heard immediately
- grade III: easily heard, of intermediate intensity
- grade IV: easily heard and associated with a thrill (a palpable vibration on the chest wall)
- grade V: very loud, with a thrill present, and audible with only the edge of the stethoscope on the chest wall
- grade VI: audible with the stethoscope off the chest wall

location: on the chest wall with regard to
- area where the sound is loudest (point of maximal intensity)
- area over which the sound is audible (extent of radiation)

duration: the length of the murmur from beginning to end
configuration: the dynamic shape of the murmur
pitch: the frequency range of the murmur, generally described as low, medium, or high-pitched
quality: aspect that relates to the presence of harmonics and the overtones
physiologic effects: of different positions, manipulations, or maneuvers

PEDIATRIC MURMUR EVALUATION

After the neonatal period, an innocent murmur may be detected at some time in the majority of children before school age. The clinical diagnosis of a normal ejection or innocent murmur should occur in the setting of an otherwise normal history, physical examination, and appearance (Table 11-5).

Table 11-5. Innocent Murmurs of Childhood

Systolic murmurs
1. Vibratory Still murmur
2. Pulmonary flow murmur
3. Peripheral pulmonary arterial stenosis murmur
4. Supraclavicular systolic murmur
5. Aortic systolic murmur

Continuous murmurs
1. Venous hum
2. Mammary arterial soufflé

Thorough auscultation in the cooperative patient should include listening in the principal areas (tricuspid, pulmonary, mitral, and aortic) of the precordium with both the bell and diaphragm of the stethoscope and with the patient in the supine, sitting, and standing positions.

SYSTOLIC MURMURS

Systolic murmurs begin with or follow the S_1 and end before the S_2 (Fig. 11-7).

Holosystolic murmurs, beginning abruptly with S_1 and continuing at the same intensity to S_2 that is graphically shown as a rectangle. This murmur occurs when there is a regurgitant atrioventricular valve (tricuspid or mitral) or in the majority of VSDs.

Ejection murmurs are crescendo-decrescendo or diamond-shaped murmurs that may arise from narrowing of the semilunar valves or outflow tracts. The rising-and-falling nature of the murmur reflects the periods of low flow at the beginning and end of ventricular systole.

Innocent murmurs are almost exclusively ejection systolic in nature (see Table 11-5). They are generally soft, are never associated with a palpable thrill, and are subject to considerable variation with positioning changes.

Early systolic murmurs start abruptly with S_1 but taper and disappear before the S_2 and are exclusively associated with small muscular VSDs.

Midsystolic to late systolic murmurs begin midway through systole and are often heard in association with the midsystolic clicks and insufficiency of mitral valve prolapse.

DIASTOLIC MURMURS

Diastole, the period between closure of the semilunar valves (S_2) and subsequent closure of the atrioventricular valves (S_1), is normally silent because of relatively low flow through large valve orifices. Regurgitation of the semilunar valves, stenosis of the atrioventricular valves, or increased flow across the atrioventricular valves all cause turbulence and may produce diastolic heart murmurs (Fig. 11-8).

Early diastolic murmurs are decrescendo in nature and arise from either aortic or pulmonary valve insufficiency (regurgitation).

Mid-diastolic murmurs are diamond-shaped and occur because of either (1) increased flow across the normal tricuspid or mitral valve or (2) normal flow across an obstructed or stenotic tricuspid or mitral valve.

Late diastolic or *crescendo murmurs* are created by stenotic or narrowed atrioventricular valves and occur during atrial contraction.

CONTINUOUS MURMURS

Flow through vessels, channels, or communications beyond the semilunar valves is not confined to systole and diastole. Thus, there may be turbulent flow throughout the cardiac cycle (Fig. 11-9). The resulting murmur extends beyond the S_2. The continuous murmur can be heard through part or all of diastole. Continuous murmurs are generally pathologic; the venous hum is an exception.

MURMURS IN CHILDREN WITH NORMAL HEARTS

Definition of "Innocence"

"Innocent" murmurs occur in the absence of structural or physiologic cardiac disease. Innocent murmurs have been called functional,

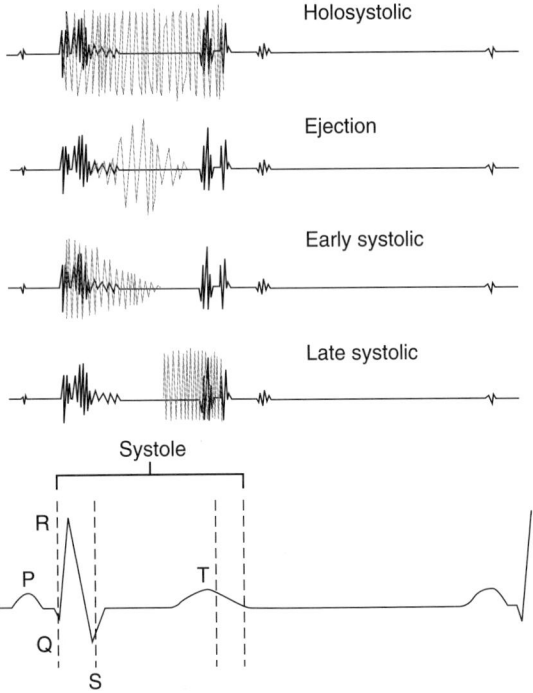

Figure 11-7. Four types of systolic heart murmurs. The holosystolic or pansystolic murmur begins abruptly with the first heart sound (S_1) and proceeds at the same intensity to the second heart sound (S_2). The ejection systolic or crescendo-decrescendo murmur begins with the onset of volume ejection from the heart. As the flow increases, the murmur varies both in intensity and frequency and subsequently tapers as the period of ejection ceases, before the S_2. The early systolic murmur begins, as does the holosystolic murmur, abruptly with S_1 but terminates in midsystole with the cessation of shunt flow. The late systolic murmur begins well after S_1, commencing in mid- to late systole in association with the development of valve insufficiency and proceeds at this intensity to S_2. (From Pelech AN: The cardiac murmur. Pediatr Clin North Am 1998;45:107-122.)

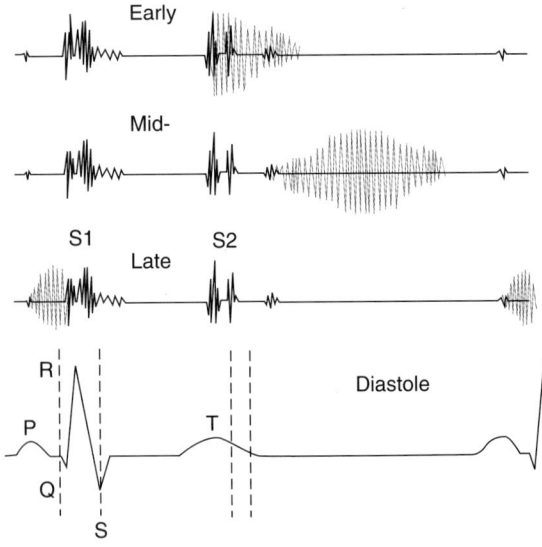

Figure 11-8. Diastolic murmurs. The early diastolic or decrescendo murmur occurs in association with closure of the semilunar valves (second heart sound) and tapers through part or all of diastole. The mid-diastolic murmur rises and falls in intensity with atrial volume entering the ventricle. The late systolic or crescendo diastolic murmur occurs late in diastole with atrial contraction, before systole, and ascends to the first heart sound. (From Pelech AN: The cardiac murmur. Pediatr Clin North Am 1998;45:107-122.)

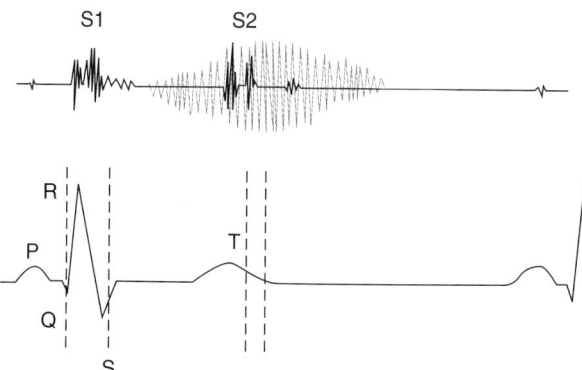

S1   S2

R
P
Q
S
T

Figure 11-9. Continuous murmur. The continuous murmur begins in systole and proceeds up to and through the second heart sound, proceeding through part or all of diastole. (From Pelech AN: The cardiac murmur. Pediatr Clin North Am 1998;45:107-122.)

benign, innocuous, or physiologic but are perhaps best termed *normal* to accurately convey to parents the favorable impression and outcome that should accompany the diagnosis. After the neonatal period, a normal murmur may be detected in the majority of children at some time before school age.

The clinical diagnosis of an innocent (normal) murmur should occur in the setting of an otherwise normal history, physical examination, and appearance.

Innocent Murmurs of Childhood

Normal murmurs of childhood are composed of five systolic and two continuous types but are never solely diastolic (see Table 11-5). The intensity or loudness of the murmur is grade III or less and consequently is never associated with a palpable thrill. The majority of all murmurs, both innocent and organic, are accentuated by fever, anemia, or increased cardiac output.

The Vibratory Still Murmur

The most common innocent murmur in children is the vibratory systolic murmur described by Sir George Still. The murmur is typically audible in children between ages 2 and 6 years, but may be present as late as adolescence or as early as infancy. The murmur is low to medium in pitch, confined to early systole, generally grade II (range I-III), and maximal at the lower left sternal edge and extending to the apex. The murmur is loudest when the patient is in the supine position and often changes in character, pitch, and intensity with upright positioning.

The most characteristic feature of the murmur is its vibratory quality described as a twanging sound, very like that made by twanging a piece of tense string. The quality of the murmur can thus never be described as "noisy" or "rough." Quite characteristically, the intensity of the murmur diminishes and the pitch changes with upright positioning; it seldom disappears.

The origins of the murmur are obscure. Its origins have been ascribed to vibration of the pulmonary valves during systolic ejection, vibrations arising from the shift in blood mass in the dynamically contracting ventricle, physiologic narrowing of the left ventricular outflow tract, and the presence of ventricular false tendons. Phonocardiographic recordings have shown the innocent murmur to arise from either the right ventricular or left ventricular outflow tracts.

The Pulmonary Flow Murmur

An innocent pulmonary outflow tract murmur may be heard in children, adolescents, and young adults. The murmur is a crescendo-decrescendo, loudest in early- to mid-peaking ejection systolic murmur confined to the second and third interspaces at the left sternal border. It is of low intensity (grades II to III) and transmits to the pulmonary area. It is rough and dissonant without the vibratory musical quality of the Still murmur. The murmur is best heard in the supine position and is exaggerated by the presence of a pectus excavatum, a straight back, or kyphoscoliosis, which results in compression or approximation of the right ventricular outflow tract to the chest wall. The murmur is augmented in full exhalation while the patient is supine, rarely resulting in the perception of a palpable thrill, and is diminished by upright positioning and held inspiration.

The murmur of an ASD is attributable to increased flow through the pulmonary outflow tract and may be indistinguishable from the innocent pulmonary flow murmur. However, the hyperdynamic right ventricular impulse, wide splitting of the pulmonary component of the S_2, and presence of a mid-diastolic flow rumble should enable distinction.

The murmur of pulmonary valve stenosis may be distinguished from the innocent pulmonary flow murmur by the frequent presence of a systolic thrill, higher pitch, longer duration, and/or presence of an ejection click. The presence of an ejection click signifies improper opening of a semilunar valve and is usually of pathologic origin. In pulmonary stenosis, the S_2 may be widely split and the P_2, when audible, is of diminished intensity.

Peripheral Pulmonary Arterial Stenosis Murmur

A common murmur heard frequently in newborns and in infants younger than 1 year is the audible turbulence of peripheral branch pulmonary arterial stenosis, angulation, or narrowing. These ejection character murmurs are typically grade I or II, are low to moderate in pitch, begin in early to middle systole, and extend up to and occasionally just after the S_2. These murmurs are most often present in normal newborns but may be associated with viral lower respiratory tract infections and reactive airway disease in older infants. In the fetus, the pulmonary trunk is a relatively dilated, domed structure because it receives the majority of combined cardiac output from the high-pressure right ventricle. Right and left pulmonary artery branches arise from this major trunk as comparatively small lateral branches that receive little intrauterine flow because of high pulmonary artery pressure. When the lungs expand at birth, the relative disparity transiently persists. The branches also arise at comparatively sharp angles from the main pulmonary trunk, accounting for turbulence and a recognized physiologic drop in pressure from the main trunk to the proximal branch pulmonary arteries. In association with a respiratory tract infection, regional vascular reactivity and pulmonary blood flow redistribution may account for the reappearance of the murmur after the neonatal period.

The murmurs are often best heard peripherally in the axillae and back with both regional and temporal variability. Because of the rapid respiratory rate of infants, similar sound frequency composition of breath sounds, and peripheral location of the murmurs, these murmurs are often overlooked. They are often most evident in the recovery phase of a respiratory illness. Of importance is that the murmur of peripheral branch stenosis changes with heart rate variability, increasing in intensity with heart rate slowing as the stroke volume increases and, conversely, diminishing with tachycardia and reduction in stroke volume.

The normal peripheral branch stenosis murmur may be indistinguishable from the peripheral murmur of significant stenosis of the branch pulmonary vessels seen in Williams or rubella syndrome or from accompanying hypoplasia or narrowing of the pulmonary arteries. Murmurs of significant anatomic narrowing may be distinguished by their higher pitch and extension after the S_2 in children after the first few months of life. The pulmonary flow murmur of an ASD may mimic this murmur but is not heard in this age group. Proximal pulmonary valve or right ventricular outflow obstruction may also closely resemble this murmur, but these obstructions are often of louder intensity, possibly associated with an ejection click, and heard maximally lower along the left sternal border.

The Supraclavicular or Brachiocephalic Systolic Murmur

A supraclavicular systolic crescendo-decrescendo murmur may be heard in children and young adults. This systolic murmur is audible maximally above the clavicles and radiates to the neck but may be present to a lesser degree on the superior chest. The murmur is low to medium in pitch, of abrupt onset, brief, and maximal in the first half or two thirds of systole. High pitch or extension into diastole is unusual and suggests significant vascular obstruction.

The murmur is present in both supine and sitting positions but varies with hyperextension of the shoulders. The shoulders can be hyperextended with the elbows brought behind the back until the shoulder girdle is taut. When this maneuver is done rapidly, the murmur diminishes or disappears altogether. Supraclavicular systolic murmurs are thought to originate from the major brachiocephalic vessels as they arise from the aorta.

The Aortic Systolic Murmur

Innocent systolic flow murmurs may arise from the outflow tract in older children and adults. The murmurs are ejection in character, confined to systole, and audible maximally in the aortic area. In children, these murmurs may arise secondarily to extreme anxiety, anemia, hyperthyroidism, fever, or any condition of increased systemic cardiac output.

In trained athletes, slower heart rates with increased stroke volume may give rise to short crescendo-decrescendo murmurs of low to medium pitch. Physical examination may suggest a relatively displaced thrusting apex and a physiologic S_3.

These murmurs must be distinguished from the systolic murmur of hypertrophic cardiomyopathy and additional fixed obstructions of the left ventricular outflow tract. The presence of a family history for hypertrophic cardiomyopathy or a family history of unexplained death in a young individual, particularly if associated with activity, is suggestive of hypertrophic cardiomyopathy. A systolic murmur that gets louder with performance of the Valsalva maneuver is considered almost diagnostic of hypertrophic cardiomyopathy with systolic anterior motion of the mitral valve. A reduction in venous return results in closer apposition of the septum and mitral valve and dynamic narrowing of the left ventricular outflow tract. In contrast, rapid squatting improves venous return; the left ventricular chamber size is enlarged, the mitral valve and septum are farther apart, and the murmur of hypertrophic cardiomyopathy gets softer. It is often difficult to be certain of the cause of this type of aortic murmur, and further investigations may be indicated.

Normal Continuous Murmurs

The Venous Hum

The most common type of continuous murmur heard in children is the innocent cervical venous hum, which is most audible on the low anterior part of the neck just lateral to the sternocleidomastoid muscle but often extends to the infraclavicular area of the anterior chest wall. The murmur is generally louder on the right than on the left, is louder when the patient is sitting than when lying down, and is accentuated in diastole. Intensity varies from faint to grade III; patients are occasionally aware of a loud hum. The murmur is quite variable in character, often described as whining, roaring, or whirring.

The venous hum is best accentuated or elicited with the patient in a sitting position and looking away from the examiner. The murmur often resolves or changes in character with lying down and may be eliminated or diminished by gentle compression of the jugular vein or turning the head toward the side of the murmur. The murmur is thought to arise from turbulence at the confluence of flow as the internal jugular and subclavian veins enter the thoracic inlet or perhaps from angulation of the internal jugular vein as it courses over the transverse process of the atlas.

The Mammary Arterial Soufflé

The mammary arterial soufflé occurs most frequently late in pregnancy and in lactating women but may occur in rare cases in adolescence. The murmur arises in systole but may extend well into diastole, being audible maximally on the anterior chest wall over the breast. There is usually a distinct gap between the S_1 and the origin of the murmur; this gap is thought to relate to the delayed arrival of cardiac stroke volume at the peripheral vasculature. The murmur is generally high pitched and has an unusual superficial character but may vary considerably from day to day. Firm pressure with the stethoscope or digit pressure on the chest wall occasionally abolishes the murmur. The murmur is thought to be arterial in origin, arising from the plethoric vessels of the chest wall. The murmur must be distinguished from the continuous high-pitched murmur of an arteriovenous fistula or a PDA. Characteristically, the mammary arterial soufflé varies significantly from day to day, is present in a most distinctive patient population, and resolves with termination of lactation.

PHYSICAL EXAMINATION OF COMMON LESIONS WITH LEFT-TO-RIGHT SHUNT

ATRIAL SEPTAL DEFECTS

The most common form of ASD (Fig. 11-10) is the ostium secundum defect in the floor of the fossae ovalis. Blood flow through an ASD in the low-pressure atria is inaudible. The auscultatory findings in ASD are related to the consequences of increased blood volume that enters the right side of the heart. The right ventricular volume overload is associated with right ventricular overactivity and a right ventricular parasternal tap.

The right atrium and ventricle receive the blood returning from the body plus the blood shunted from left to right through the ASD. This causes a prolongation of right-sided heart emptying. The P_2 of the S_2 is often widely split and fixed (no respiratory variation).

Two types of murmur may be audible:

1. The typical pulmonary flow murmur is ejection systolic in character, generally of low intensity (grade II or III), and of low pitch. The crescendo-decrescendo murmur begins shortly after the S_1 and ends well before the S_2.
2. In patients with a large atrial shunt, there is typically a well-localized, low-pitched mid-diastolic flow rumble in the tricuspid area because of increased flow across the tricuspid valve.

ASDs may lead to pulmonary hypertension in the second and third decades of life. Treatment is surgical or by device closure during cardiac catheterization.

PATENT DUCTUS ARTERIOSUS

In this condition, the connection between the aorta and pulmonary artery that exists prenatally remains open after birth (Fig. 11-11).

The amount of shunt flow is dependent not only on the size of the ductus communication but also on the differential resistances of the systemic and pulmonary circulations. In some children, the PDA

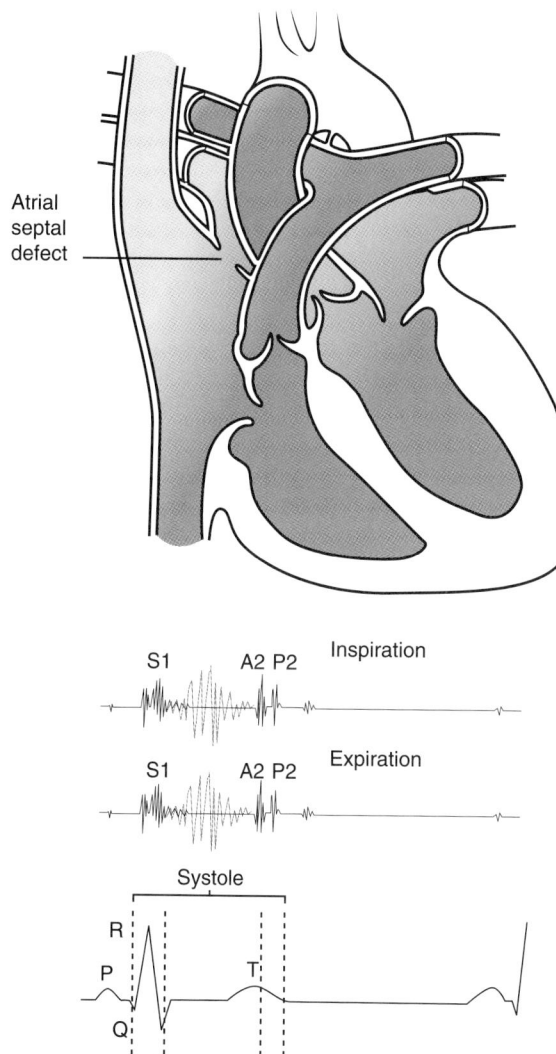

Figure 11-10. Atrial septal defects. The most common type of defect, the secundum atrial septal defect, is shown. Characteristically, in association with a large left-to-right shunt, wide and fixed splitting of the second heart sound occurs. The murmur is that of increased flow through the right ventricular outflow tract. The shunt flow through the defect, which occurs at low pressure, is inaudible.

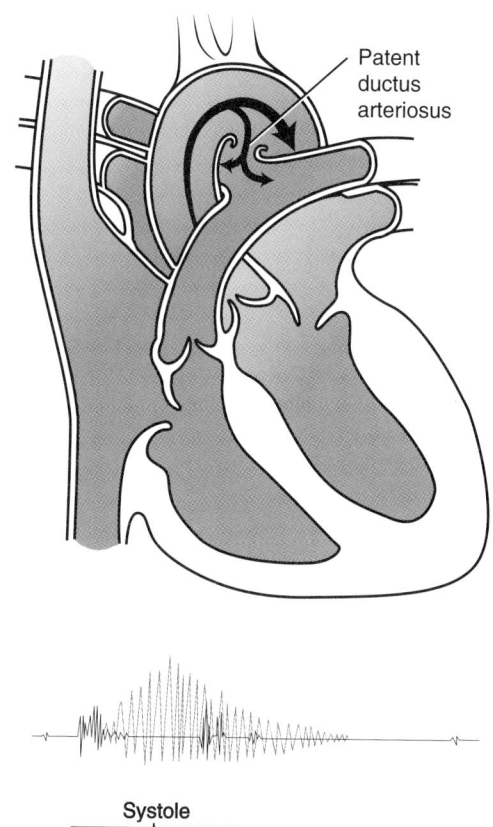

Figure 11-11. The patent ductus arteriosus consists of residual patency of a fetal communication between the two great arteries. Because the shunt occurs outside the heart, the murmur is continuous and is high pitched if the defect is restrictive and the pulmonary artery pressures are low.

may produce significant left-sided heart volume overload and signs of high-output congestive heart failure.

The peripheral pulses associated with significant diastolic runoff to the pulmonary vascular area are bounding. Palpation may reveal a thrill in systole at the upper left sternal edge (when the murmur is grade IV); an abnormal left ventricular impulse; and, if the left-to-right shunt is large, a hyperdynamic and displaced apical impulse. The majority of patients have an asymptomatic murmur.

Premature infants often have persistence of ductal patency after birth. Initially, in the presence of neonatal lung disease and elevated pulmonary vascular resistance, the shunt volume is not large. After the lung disease improves, the presence of a PDA becomes apparent through the detection of a cardiac murmur and bounding pulses. Preterm infants with a PDA may show signs of heart failure, pulmonary edema, a hyperdynamic precordium, and difficulty in weaning from the respirator. Treatment in preterm infants includes intravenous indomethacin or ibuprofen and fluid restriction; if these measures are unsuccessful, surgical ligation is indicated.

The PDA causes a continuous machine-like murmur, best heard in the pulmonary area. The murmur is generally high pitched, peaks in late systole, and continues well through the S_2. If the PDA is large, a mid-diastolic flow rumble may be heard at the apex because of relative mitral valve stenosis. Beyond the neonatal period, treatment is surgical ligation or device closure during cardiac catheterization.

VENTRICULAR SEPTAL DEFECTS

These common developmental or, more rare, acquired communications between the two ventricles (Fig. 11-12) may be classified as

- perimembranous
- muscular
- atrioventricular or inlet
- subarterial or outlet

The acoustic findings depend on five factors:

1. size
2. location
3. shunt or defect flow
4. pulmonary hypertension
5. associated anomalies

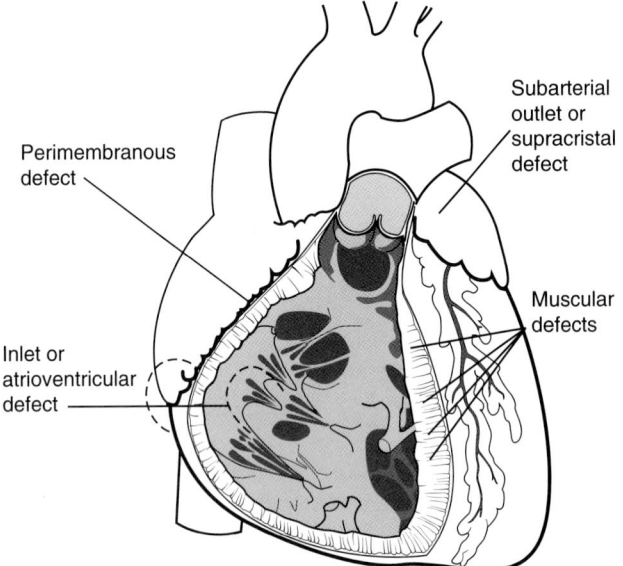

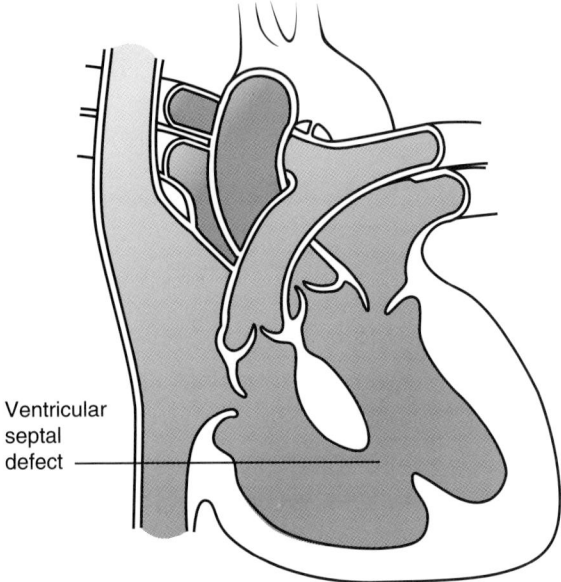

Figure 11-12. Anatomic types of ventricular septal defects. The four types of defects of the ventricular septum are shown. The most common type is the muscular defect, which commonly occurs in the anterior trabecular area of the septum. The perimembranous (often called membranous) defect occurs in the regions of the pars membranacea, or the embryonic bulboventricular foramina. The subarterial outlet, or supracristal defect, extends to the fibrous ring of the semilunar valves. The inlet or atrioventricular septal defect is that of the atrioventricular canal or embryonic atrioventricular communis.

All these factors need to be addressed in the clinical description of a VSD.

The VSD (Fig. 11-13) causes a left-to-right shunt or, in rare cases, a right-to-left shunt, depending on the resistance to the flow of blood leaving the ventricles. The turbulence and thus the intensity of the murmur are directly proportional to the flow and pressure difference between the ventricles.

Size

A moderate-sized VSD that is restrictive (i.e., a pressure difference exists between the ventricles) causes a harsh blowing holosystolic murmur, which is often very loud and frequently associated with a palpable thrill.

The very restrictive or small VSD creates a high-pitched systolic murmur and causes little or no physiologic disturbance. Muscular defects may close in midsystole, which then stops shunt flow and murmur before S_2.

In an unrestrictive or large VSD, no pressure difference exists between the two ventricles. This results in less turbulence and therefore a reduced intensity of the murmur.

Location

The perimembranous defect is best heard at the left sternal edge in the third left intercostal space. Muscular defects are heard variably from the sternal edge to the apex. Outlet or subarterial defects are best heard higher along the sternum.

Shunt Flow

If the volume of flow through the VSD (shunt flow) is large (i.e., more than two to three times normal ventricular outflow), a low-pitched, mid-diastolic flow rumble may be heard in the mitral area.

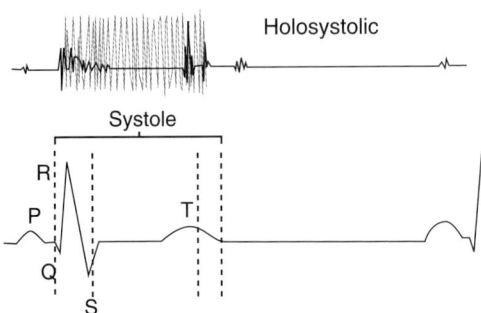

Figure 11-13. Ventricular septal defects. A ventricular septal defect is a communication between the high-pressure left ventricle and the lower pressure right ventricle. The shunt flow begins with the onset of ventricular contraction before the period of ejection (isovolumic contraction) and consequently gives rise to a holosystolic murmur that obscures the first and often the second heart sound. The murmur is high pitched if the defect is restrictive, and the right-sided heart pressures are low; however, the murmur may be low pitched or even inaudible if the defect is large or if the pulmonary artery pressures are high, as occurs in the newborn.

The extra volume of blood returning from the pulmonary circulation to the left side of the heart creates this murmur of "relative" (not true anatomic) mitral valve stenosis.

Pulmonary Hypertension

High pressure in the pulmonary artery limits left-to-right shunt flow and murmur intensity. The pulmonary closure sound is louder and is either narrowly split or single.

Associated Anomalies

Frequently there are anomalies associated with a VSD, such as right- or left-sided heart outflow obstruction or aortic insufficiency. This may affect the character of the murmur.

Of importance is that the VSD murmur begins very early with the onset of left ventricular contraction, which may precede right ventricular contraction because the left ventricle is activated earlier. The murmur commences during the period of isovolumic contraction and, if it is loud (grade III or greater), often obscures the S_1. Blood is ejected from the left ventricle to the right ventricle throughout systole, giving rise to a classical full-length, or "holosystolic," murmur. On occasion, VSD murmurs may not be full length. This may occur in a small muscular VSD that coapts or closes in midsystole or, in rare cases, in the presence of heart failure with diminished systolic function.

Analysis of the S_2 in VSD is very important and, in conjunction with precordial palpation, enables estimation of the pulmonary artery pressure. The larger the defect, the higher the pulmonary artery pressure and the earlier and louder the P_2 are. Thus, the split of S_2 may become very narrow, or the S_2 may even become single, a finding of great concern. In large defects, a balance exists between delayed P_2, caused by large pulmonary blood flow, and early P_2 caused by high pulmonary artery pressure. The wider the split of S_2, the less the concern is, because pulmonary vascular resistance is then likely to be low.

The intensity or loudness of a murmur relates to the combination of both flow and gradient across the defect. Pitch or frequency relates to gradient alone. Thus, very small defects with small left-to-right shunt flow may have a soft, high-pitched murmur. In moderate-sized defects, the murmur is loud, often associated with a palpable thrill. In large defects with no restriction between the right and left ventricle, the murmur is low pitched and less intense as the pulmonary artery and right-sided heart pressures equate with the left-sided heart pressure.

In many children, the VSD spontaneously closes, as noted, and the murmur becomes softer and softer until it disappears with defect closure. In patients who develop increased pulmonary vascular resistance and a reduction in shunt flow and who are at risk for progressing to Eisenmenger syndrome (irreversible pulmonary vascular disease and cyanosis with right-to-left ventricular level shunt), the murmur also becomes quieter. Thus, a diminishing VSD murmur may be evolving into a good or bad outcome. The treatment of a VSD includes management of heart failure and surgery (see Chapter 8).

COMPLETE ATRIOVENTRICULAR SEPTAL DEFECTS

There is great variation in the anatomy of atrioventricular septal defects (AVSDs). AVSDs (Fig. 11-14) occur in complete, partial, and intermediate forms. In the complete AVSD, the intracardiac defect extends between both the atria and ventricles. The atrial or ventricular extent of the defect may be the primary level of shunt flow; consequently, the defect may manifest primarily as either a VSD or an ASD. Often the defects are large and unrestrictive. In addition, a common accompaniment of AVSD is a cleft in the left-sided atrioventricular valve, which may cause varying degrees of valve insufficiency. Approximately half of the children born with Down syndrome have congenital heart disease, the most common abnormality of which is complete AVSD. Maturation of the pulmonary arteries and small muscular arteries is delayed in children with Down syndrome, and elevated pulmonary vascular resistance early in life is common. Therefore, the lesion may be missed early in life because signs of congestive heart failure may not occur. In patients with complete AVSDs, the electrocardiogram demonstrates an abnormally counterclockwise superior vector. If this finding is present, an echocardiogram should be obtained. In other forms of AVSDs, the intermediate or partial forms, Down syndrome is less often present.

In the partial form of AVSD, absence of the lower part of the interatrial septum, the *ostium primum,* is the major component of the abnormality. In such patients, the manifestation and examination are similar to those described for a secundum type of ASD. Often, mitral regurgitation is present and is apparent as an apical holosystolic murmur that obscures S_1. If the amount of mitral valve insufficiency is large, a mid-diastolic flow rumble of increased filling may be heard.

The manifestation and consequently the clinical signs in patients with AVSD vary considerably, depending on the patient's age, pulmonary vascular resistance, size and level of the defects, amount of

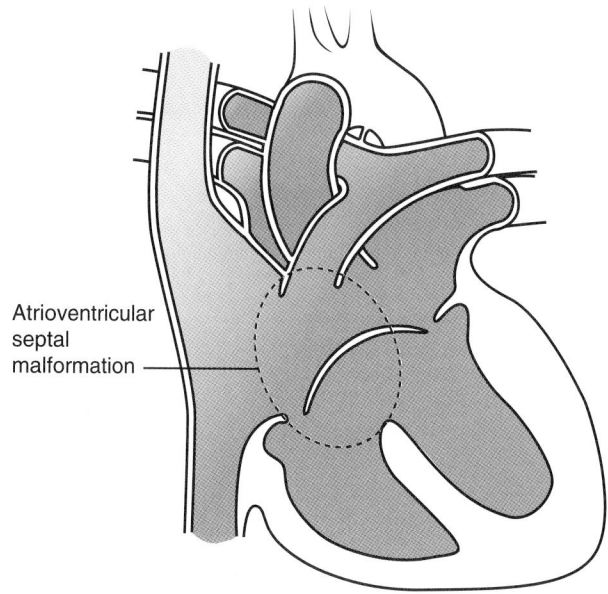

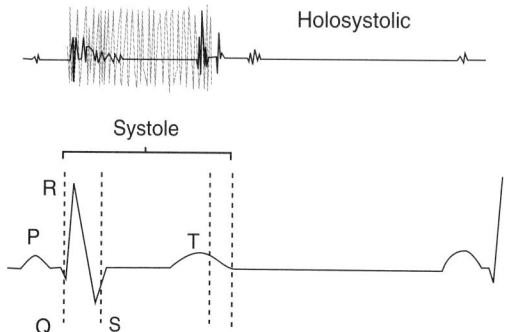

Figure 11-14. Complete atrioventricular septal malformation. The atrioventricular septal malformations vary markedly between a large atrial component with a restrictive ventricular communication to a large unrestrictive inlet ventricular septal defect. Consequently, their clinical manifestation also varies from that of an atrial septal defect to that of an unrestrictive ventricular septal defect.

valve insufficiency, and ventricular function. Patients with an AVSD often manifest the signs of congestive heart failure early in infancy. Surgical repair provides definitive treatment.

PHYSICAL EXAMINATION OF COMMON LESIONS WITH RIGHT-TO-LEFT SHUNT: CYANOSIS (see Chapter 10)

TETRALOGY OF FALLOT

The tetralogy (Fig. 11-15) has four anatomic features:

1. VSD
2. pulmonary stenosis
3. dextroposition or rightward position of the aorta
4. right ventricular hypertrophy (see Chapter 10).

The functional significance of this anomaly is related to the degree of right ventricular outflow tract obstruction. There is a harsh

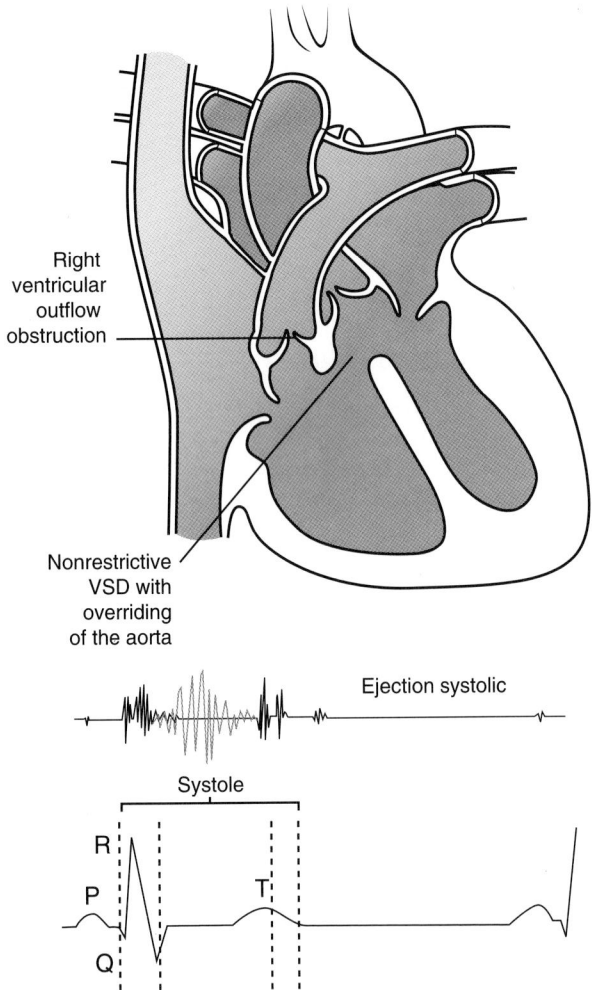

Figure 11-15. Tetralogy of Fallot. The four anatomic malformations seen in association with tetralogy of Fallot include an unrestrictive perimembranous ventricular septal defect (VSD), overriding of the aorta, right ventricular hypertrophy, and an obstructive right ventricular outflow tract. The cardiac murmur in tetralogy, a harsh loud ejection systolic murmur, arises from the turbulence generated in the right-sided heart outflow. Because the VSD is unrestrictive and the right- and left-sided heart pressures are equal, the VSD generates no sound. The pulmonary closure sound is often soft or inaudible.

ejection systolic murmur, heard best in the pulmonary area but also widely transmitted through the chest. The right ventricular outflow obstruction is most frequently a combination of muscular, annular, and valvular narrowing. Consequently, the P_2 is soft and delayed and is often inaudible. The VSD is typically large and not restrictive. The prominent systolic murmur in tetralogy of Fallot is therefore not caused by the septal defect.

Patients with tetralogy of Fallot may present with moderate to severe degrees of right ventricular outflow obstruction, right-to-left ventricular level shunting and varying degrees of cyanosis. Alternatively, the outflow obstruction may be mild, providing a predominant left-to-right shunt and causing the "acyanotic" or "pink" form of tetralogy of Fallot. In these patients, the degree of outflow obstruction becomes progressive; bidirectional flow develops and, finally, a dominant right-to-left shunt.

One aspect of tetralogy physiology is the variable degree of desaturation that may occur as a consequence of the reactive nature of the right ventricular outflow obstruction. The sudden development of severe reactive obstruction in response to temperature, illness,

dehydration, or intense crying may precipitate a *hypercyanotic* or *tetralogy spell.* Either increased infundibular reactivity or decreased systemic vascular resistance is responsible for the diminished pulmonary blood flow. This life-threatening event manifests as profound cyanosis, tachypnea, and dyspnea, progressing to acidosis, unconsciousness, and death. During a spell, the outflow tract murmur disappears with the diminution in pulmonary blood flow. Treatment of this condition includes placing the child in a knee-chest position to increase venous return and to increase systemic vascular resistance; administration of oxygen, volume (normal saline), sodium bicarbonate, morphine, and propranolol; and administration of α-adrenergic agonists (phenylephrine or methoxamine) to increase systemic vascular resistance without increasing inotropy. Inotropic agents are contraindicated because they cause contraction of the infundibulum, thus worsening outflow obstruction of the right ventricle.

Tetralogy of Fallot is a consequence of developmental anterior displacement of the conal or outlet septum and failure to adjoin with the muscular trabecular interventricular septum. Because conal tissue is needed for closure of the membranous ventricular septum, the anterior displacement and hypoplasia of the conus results in a VSD, which is characteristically nonrestrictive. The aorta extends more to the right, which results in overriding of the aorta.

In cases in which there is a predominant left-to-right shunt, the murmur is a long, loud ejection systolic murmur and may obscure the S_1. The murmur extends up the left sternal border (pulmonary area) and throughout both lung fields. The right ventricle is at systemic pressure, and the pitch of the murmur is quite high. There is a right ventricular parasternal impulse and often a palpable thrill in the pulmonary outflow region.

In cyanotic tetralogy of Fallot, the loudness or intensity of the murmur diminishes as the pulmonary blood flow decreases. The systolic murmur remains high pitched, harsh, and ejection in shape. The S_1 remains loud or normal; the S_2 is single.

In the most severe form of tetralogy, pulmonary atresia with VSD, there is no pulmonary outflow murmur at all. Definitive corrective treatment of tetralogy of Fallot is surgical.

TRICUSPID VALVE ATRESIA

In tricuspid valve atresia (Fig. 11-16) (see Chapter 10), the tricuspid valve does not develop, and in its place there may be an imperforate membrane or a thick muscle wedge. The right ventricle is usually very small; the left ventricle compensates and is large. A dynamic diffuse left ventricular cardiac impulse is palpable. All systemic venous blood returning to the right atrium must pass across at atrial septal level to enter the left atrium and then the left ventricle. Pulmonary blood flow occurs most often as a consequence of a VSD or, in rare cases, is dependent on the ductus arteriosus. The electrocardiogram reveals an abnormally superior left axis. Examination reveals a VSD murmur. The softer and shorter the murmur, the less the pulmonary blood flow is, so that, just as in tetralogy of Fallot, the softer the murmur, the more severe the cyanosis is. If there is enough pulmonary blood flow, both P_2 and A_2 may be heard. Palliative surgery is required.

PULMONARY ATRESIA WITH INTACT VENTRICULAR SEPTUM

There are two forms of pulmonary valve atresia (see Chapter 10). The first is pulmonary atresia with VSD and generally a long fibrous or muscular outflow atresia, which is the most severe malformation on the spectrum of tetralogy of Fallot. The second form occurs in association with an intact interventricular septum (Fig. 11-17), and right-sided heart hypoplasia is usually present.

The cardiac impulse in hypoplastic right ventricle with pulmonary atresia may be right ventricular even though the dominant ventricle is the left. In contrast to tricuspid valve atresia, a VSD is not

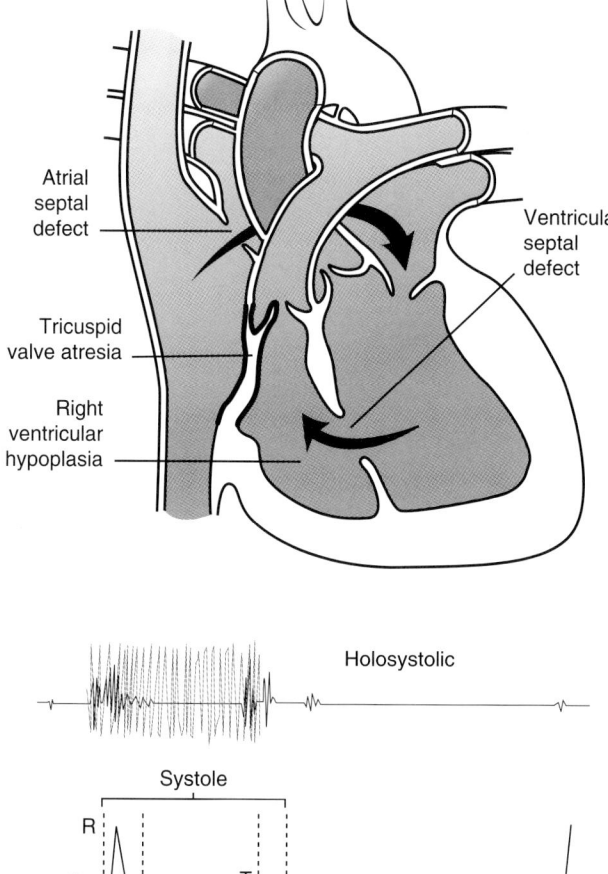

Figure 11-16. Tricuspid valve atresia. In this condition, the murmur most often detected is a holosystolic murmur of a communicating ventricular septal defect or an ejection systolic murmur related to an obstructing pulmonary outflow.

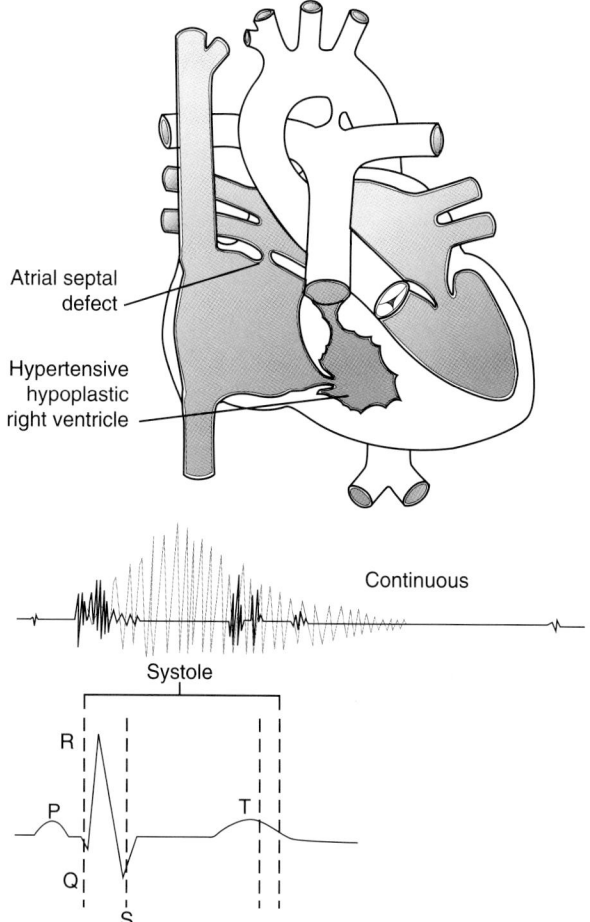

Figure 11-17. Pulmonary atresia with intact septum. Characteristically, the defect manifests in the cyanotic neonate. Most often, a continuous murmur of a patent ductus arteriosus is audible. Less often, a high-pitched murmur of tricuspid valve insufficiency may be heard.

part of this lesion. The source of the pulmonary blood flow in the neonate is a ductus arteriosus with left-to-right shunt. A murmur from this ductus may be audible. There is a single S_2 (aortic closure). On occasion, there is tricuspid valve regurgitation, which may be confused with a VSD murmur. The murmur is high pitched, because the right ventricular pressures are very high. The electrocardiogram helps differentiate tricuspid valve and pulmonary atresia. In both disorders, left ventricular hypertrophy is present, but in pulmonary atresia, there is a normal inferior vector. Echocardiography confirms the diagnosis. There is usually profound cyanosis.

Intravenous prostaglandin therapy is required to ensure ductal patency and pulmonary blood flow in the neonatal period (see Chapter 10). Complications of prostaglandin therapy include apnea, fever, seizures, thickened pulmonary secretions, and rash.

Surgical repair is usually palliative.

TRANSPOSITION OF THE GREAT ARTERIES

In transposition of the great arteries (Fig. 11-18), the aorta arises from the morphologic right ventricle, and the pulmonary artery arises from the morphologic left ventricle (see Chapter 10). In transposition of the great arteries, desaturated systemic venous blood

returns to the right atrium, passes to the right ventricle, and is returned to the aorta and thus to the systemic circulation. Any oxygenation occurring in this setting is the result of mixing of blood with the pulmonary circulation at the ductal, atrial, or ventricular level.

Transposition of the great arteries with an intact ventricular septum manifests in the neonatal period with profound cyanosis in an infant whose saturations do not improve with oxygen administration; this is the so-called hyperoxic test. There is a pronounced right ventricular impulse, and the A_2 is loud because it is anterior. There may be a faint soft short ejection murmur that is audible along the left sternal border as a result of increased pulmonary blood flow. However, there are often no murmurs. Heart failure is not expected. The P_2 is often not heard.

If there is a VSD, the patient may not present in the neonatal period. The minimal cyanosis may be difficult to detect. Such infants usually become ill at 2 to 3 weeks of age as a result of congestive heart failure rather than hypoxia. The examination findings are very different, because both ventricles are very hyperdynamic. The heart is large; there is often a palpable thrill and a loud systolic murmur.

Treatment consists of corrective surgical switching of the great vessels.

HYPOPLASTIC LEFT HEART SYNDROME

Hypoplastic left heart syndrome (Fig. 11-19) consists of varying degrees of left-sided heart (mitral valve, left ventricle, aortic valve,

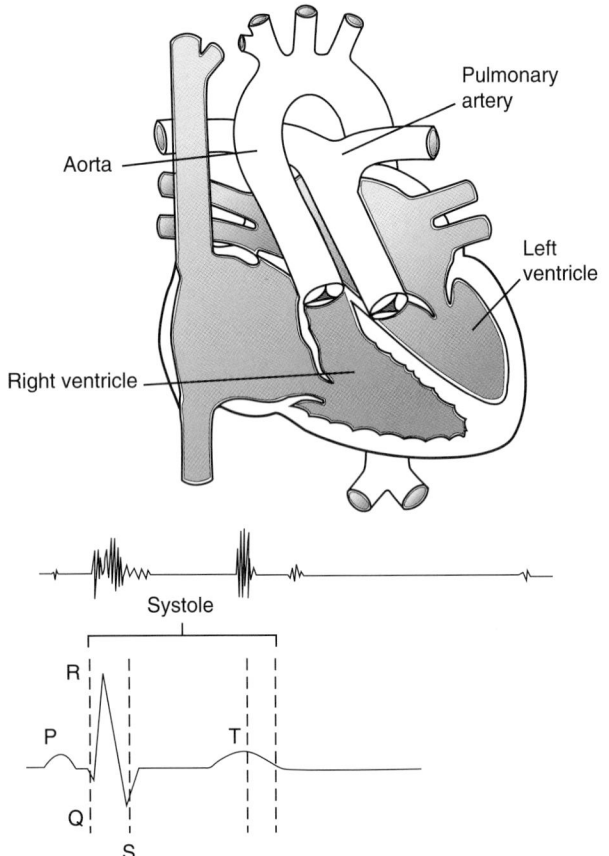

Figure 11-18. Transposition of the great arteries. The aorta in this condition arises anteriorly, giving rise to a loud, single second heart sound. Many profoundly cyanotic full-term newborns with no audible murmur have transposition of the great arteries.

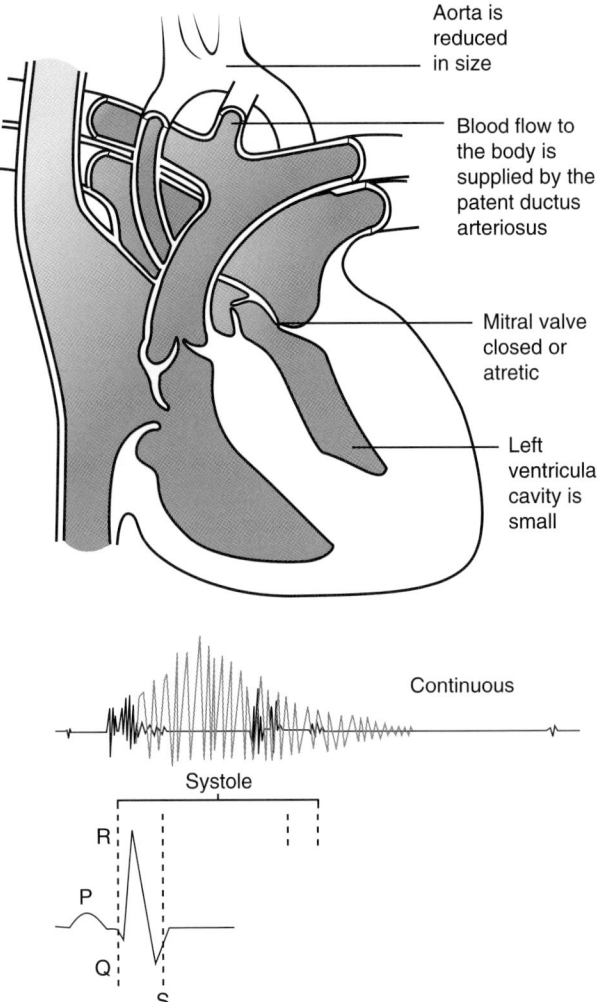

Figure 11-19. Hypoplastic left heart syndrome. In this condition, the systemic circulation is supplied from the right ventricle via the ductus arteriosus. The continuous murmur of ductal flow that may be heard is generally low pitched as a result of equal pulmonary and aortic pressures.

or arch) hypoplasia or atresia such that the left ventricle cannot support the systemic circulation (see Chapter 10). In the first day or two after birth, the neonate may not be recognized as being ill if the ductus arteriosus remains open and the right ventricular output contributes to the systemic output. When the ductus begins to close, perfusion deteriorates, the pulses are diminished, acidosis develops, and death ensues.

The affected infant is often tachypneic, gray, and poorly perfused. There may be considerable pulmonary blood flow and a dynamic right ventricle impulse. An ejection systolic murmur may be audible in the pulmonary area. The heart function may be very poor, and the precordial and auscultatory examination findings may be quiet. A significantly restrictive ASD may cause profound pulmonary venous congestion and poor oxygenation.

After intravenous prostaglandin E_1 has been given, causing opening of the ductus arteriosus, a reasonable systemic output and palpable pulses should return.

Treatment includes the staged Norwood palliative repair to single-ventricle Fontan operation or heart transplantation.

PHYSICAL EXAMINATION OF COMMON LESIONS WITH SIMPLE OBSTRUCTION

In areas of obstruction, the gradient or pressure difference across an obstruction relates to the severity of the narrowing, the flow across the narrowing and the pressure able to be generated (i.e., the cardiac function).

PULMONARY VALVE STENOSIS

The hemodynamic abnormality in pulmonary valve stenosis (Fig. 11-20) is attributable to increased pressure within a right ventricle that is attempting to eject through a narrowed or obstructed valve. The more severe the stenosis, the higher the intraventricular pressure is until cardiac failure occurs.

This condition is characterized by an ejection systolic murmur, heard best in the pulmonary area. The murmur is diamond-shaped. With increasing valvular obstruction, the murmur becomes louder and higher pitched and peaks later in systole. The P_2 is very helpful because the more severe the pulmonary valve stenosis, the more delayed and less intense the P_2 is.

An ejection click, caused by abrupt arrest of leaflet excursion in early systole, frequently precedes the ejection systolic murmur. The more severe the pulmonary valve stenosis, the earlier and softer the pulmonary ejection click is. In other forms of right ventricular out-flow obstruction such as supravalvar stenosis and subvalvar stenosis, or in the setting of a dysplastic or malformed pulmonary valve, an ejection click is not audible.

In newborns with very severe critical pulmonic stenosis and low cardiac output, the examination findings may be quite different.

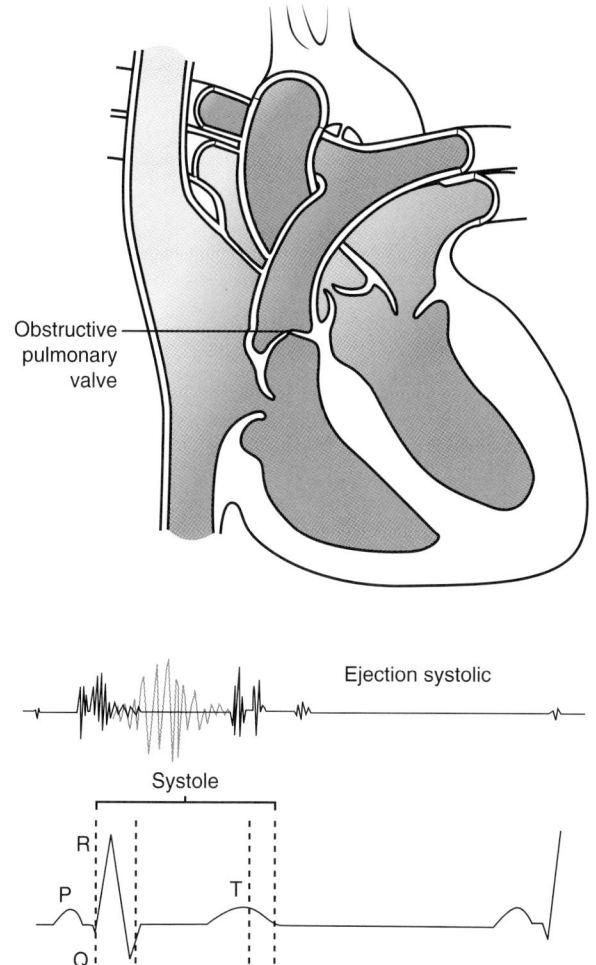

Figure 11-20. Pulmonary valve stenosis. Pulmonary valve stenosis gives rise to a rough ejection systolic murmur that is most prominent in the pulmonary area and radiates equally to both lung fields. The presence of an ejection click distinguishes valve obstruction from subvalvular or supravalvular stenosis.

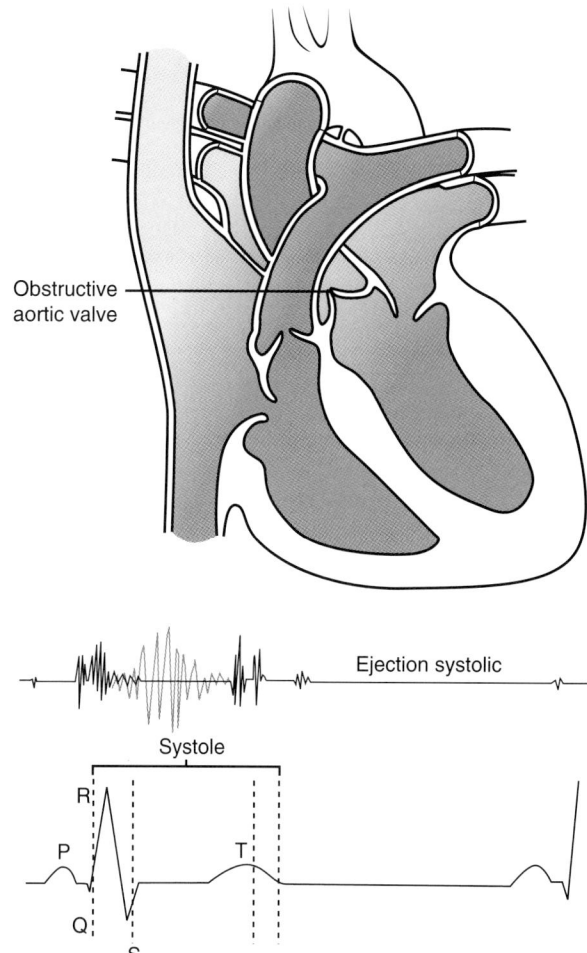

Figure 11-21. Aortic valve stenosis. The ejection systolic murmur from aortic valve stenosis is audible both at the apex and in the aortic area. The aortic area extends up to the carotid arteries. There is often a palpable thrill in the suprasternal notch. The pitch and peaking of the murmur allows estimate of the severity of stenosis. Note that a quiet and low-pitched murmur may suggest poor ventricular function and low output.

There may be no pulmonary ejection click, and the murmur may be very short, soft, or both.

Palpation in pulmonic valve stenosis may reveal a palpable thrill in the pulmonary area and an abnormal right ventricular impulse (except in mild cases).

Treatment is transcatheter balloon valve dilatation.

AORTIC VALVE STENOSIS

The hemodynamic impact of aortic valve stenosis (Fig. 11-21) is an increased pressure in the left ventricle. The more severe the stenosis, the higher the left ventricular pressure is.

The apex beat is of a thrusting character and is not displaced in the absence of left-sided heart failure. Palpation, except in very mild cases, reveals a suprasternal notch thrill and often a carotid systolic thrill. If the murmur is grade IV or greater, a precordial thrill is also palpable at the upper right sternal border (aortic area).

The murmur of aortic stenosis is a rough, harsh, diamond-shaped ejection systolic murmur. It is heard best in the aortic area but often extends into the neck and throughout the precordium.

A soft, short ejection murmur that peaks in systole indicates a mild degree of valve obstruction, whereas a loud, long, and late-peaking murmur, often associated with a palpable thrill, reflects more severe stenosis.

An ejection click often precedes the murmur and is heard best at the apex. The click intensity is inversely proportional to the severity of the valve narrowing. A loud aortic valve ejection click is often present in patients with a two-leaflet or bicuspid aortic valve even if there is no valve stenosis.

The splitting of the S_2 is normal. The paradoxical split, occurring when there is a large delay of A_2, is quite rare in children and young adults; it is seen in older people with calcific aortic valve stenosis and a failing left ventricle.

In newborns with severe or *critical aortic stenosis* and low cardiac output, the examination findings may be very different. There is often no aortic ejection click, and, strikingly, the murmur may be short, soft, or both. Significant heart failure and poor perfusion are present in such neonates.

Two other major types of aortic stenosis exist: subvalvular and supravalvular. Neither has an aortic ejection click. In *supravalvular aortic stenosis* (the major cardiac lesion associated with Williams syndrome), the murmur is usually in the aortic area, whereas in *subvalvular aortic stenosis,* the murmur position may extend to the left sternal border or the apex.

The bicuspid aortic valve is the most common of all congenital malformations of the heart. It is found in almost 2% of the general population. The normal aortic valve has three leaflets of equal size. The bicuspid valve has two functional leaflets, one generally larger than the other. The bicuspid aortic valve is often only mildly stenotic or is often unobstructed. The anomaly is recognized from the presence of an aortic ejection click. Asymmetric stresses on the valve leaflets predispose to calcification, dysfunction, and deterioration after many years. The valve is also at risk for the development of infective endocarditis.

Treatment of aortic valve stenosis may include surgical or balloon valvotomy or eventually valve replacement.

COARCTATION OF THE AORTA

Coarctation, meaning "to draw together to make tight," occurs in association with congenital cardiac anomalies or in isolation. There are fundamentally two forms of coarctation (Fig. 11-22). The more common form has been termed *juxtaductal* or *adult coarctation*

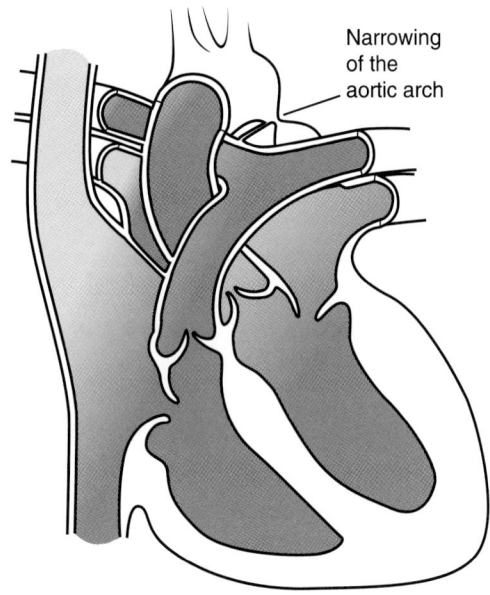

Narrowing of the aortic arch

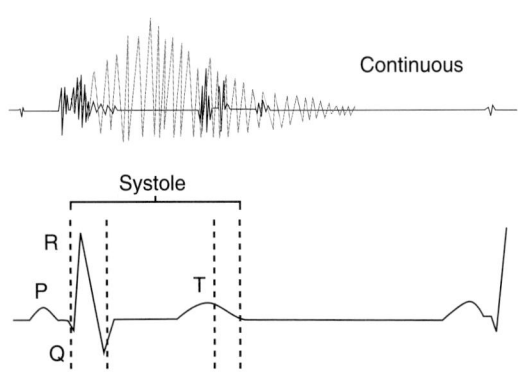

Continuous

Systole

R

P

T

Q

S

Figure 11-22. Coarctation of the aorta. The murmur of coarctation is often audible both anteriorly and posteriorly between the scapulae. It is a continuous murmur extending well into diastole.

and is typically a discrete area of aortic narrowing or indentation of ductal tissue in relationship to the ductus arteriosus or ligamentum. The second type of coarctation has been termed *infantile coarctation* and includes varying degrees of transverse and isthmic aortic arch hypoplasia.

The hemodynamic abnormality caused by a coarctation of the aorta is a high systolic pressure proximal to the area of narrowing, in the ascending aorta, the brachiocephalic vessels, and the left ventricle.

The diagnosis of coarctation of the aorta is made from recognition of systemic hypertension in the right arm and decreased arterial pulsation in the femoral arteries and the dorsalis pedis in comparison with that in the brachial arteries. The femoral pulses may be absent, or they may be diminished and delayed. In some cases, the left brachial pulse may be diminished as a result of involvement of the left subclavian artery in the site of narrowing. In rare cases, the right subclavian artery may arise aberrantly below the level of the coarctation, causing the pulse in this arm to be diminished. Therefore, brachial pulses must be felt on both sides and compared with the femoral pulses. The blood pressure must be obtained in both arms as well as in one leg. If only one arm pressure is obtained, it should be that of the right arm.

There is seldom any significant or consistent alteration in the heart sounds unless there is associated aortic valve disease. In approximately 30% to 40% of patients with juxtaductal coarctation of the aorta, there is an associated bicuspid aortic valve, usually without stenosis. In these cases, there is an aortic ejection click. More complicated heart disease, often unrestrictive VSDs or AVSDs, are seen in association with isthmic arch hypoplasia.

The murmur of coarctation is of the ejection or continuous type, is rarely louder than grade III, starts well after S_1, and may peak late in systole or extend into diastole. The point of maximal cardiac activity is very variable and is most often palpable in the fifth or sixth intercostal space, extending out to the axillary line. The murmur of coarctation extends to and is often loudest in the interscapular area posteriorly.

As with aortic stenosis and obstruction of the left heart outflow, the newborn with coarctation may present with signs of low output and heart failure. Prostaglandins have proved useful in this circumstance, alleviating the obstruction by dilating reactive muscle in the aortic wall, which may have extended from the ductus or with opening of the ductus itself, enabling right-to-left ductal flow to the lower body and relieving associated pulmonary hypertension.

Treatment in the neonate is surgical. However, after infancy, aortic coarctation angioplasty with balloon or stent may be considered, as may surgery.

MITRAL VALVE STENOSIS

Congenital mitral valve stenosis (Fig. 11-23) is uncommon; when it occurs, it is usually in association with additional left-sided heart obstructive abnormalities, particularly coarctation of the aorta, which is termed the *Shone complex.* The most common type of significant stenosis is caused by a single or "parachute" papillary muscle. In its most severe form, it is part of the hypoplastic left ventricle syndrome, in which the valve is small, very stenotic, or atretic. In affected patients, cyanosis, heart failure, and poor perfusion are evident within the first few days after birth.

The leaflets in congenital stenosis are very immobile, and there is seldom the accentuation of the S_1 or an opening snap, which is characteristic of acquired or rheumatic mitral valve stenosis.

The murmur of mitral valve stenosis arises from the increased velocity of blood flow across the relatively immobile mitral leaflets during diastolic filling of the left ventricle. This causes a characteristic low-pitched mid-diastolic flow rumble best heard in the mitral area.

Rheumatic mitral valve stenosis is common in many areas of the world but is uncommon in the United States. As a consequence of

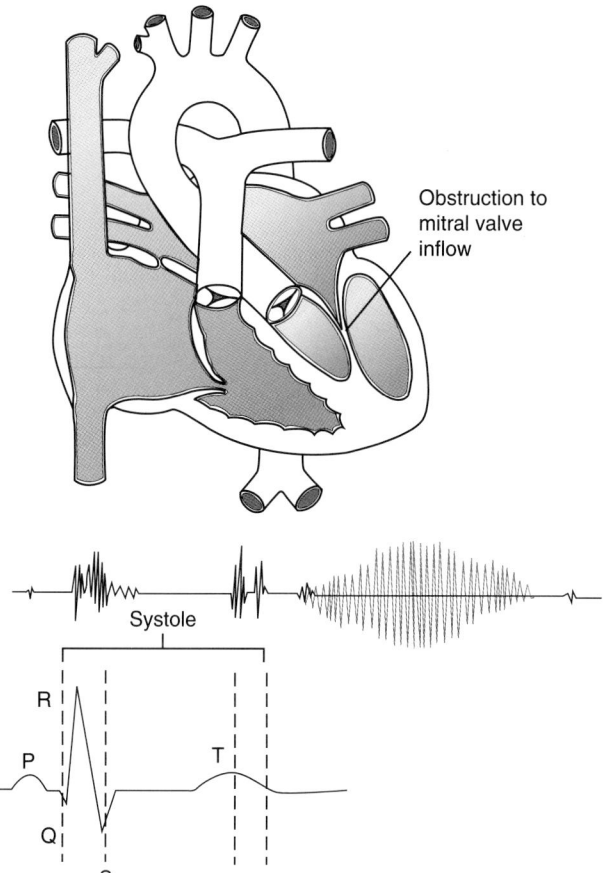

Figure 11-23. Mitral valve stenosis. The murmur of mitral valve stenosis occurs during the period of passive and active filling of the ventricle as turbulence occurs across the obstructive mitral valve. Pulmonary hypertension often arises as a consequence of the downstream obstruction.

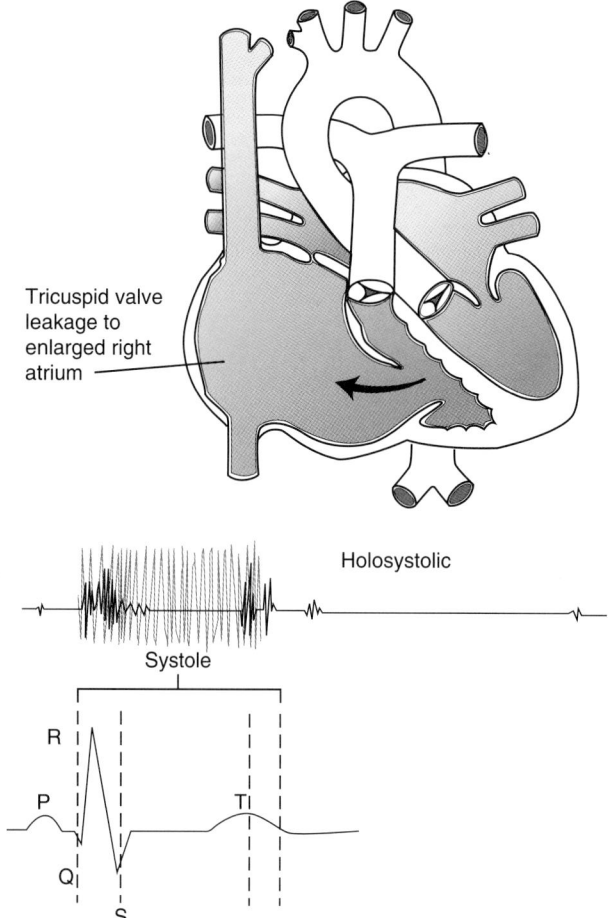

Figure 11-24. Tricuspid valve insufficiency. The holosystolic murmur of tricuspid valve insufficiency is low pitched in the absence of any pulmonary outflow obstruction. This makes tricuspid valve insufficiency very challenging to hear.

mitral obstruction, the left atrial and pulmonary venous pressures are elevated. Often there is a reflex or secondary elevation of pulmonary artery pressures caused by thickening or constriction of small muscular pulmonary arteries. The features of pulmonary hypertension, including a prominent right ventricular tap, single loud or palpable S_2, and high-pitched pulmonary insufficiency may be apparent.

Excursion of the thickened leaflets often causes an early diastolic high-pitched opening snap before the onset of the murmur. In severe stenosis, strong atrial contraction late in diastole may create a late diastolic crescendo murmur. A loud S_1 is often heard in this condition.

ATRIOVENTRICULAR VALVE AND SEMILUNAR VALVE INSUFFICIENCY

Tricuspid Valve Regurgitation

Tricuspid valve regurgitation (insufficiency) (Fig. 11-24) is uncommon in childhood in the absence of additional abnormalities. It may be a consequence of pulmonary artery hypertension, in which the high-pressure right ventricle contributes to a high-pitched holosystolic murmur at the lower left or lower right sternal border (tricuspid area).

Less often, tricuspid valve insufficiency may occur in association with a displaced and malformed tricuspid valve (*Ebstein anomaly*), in which case the pulmonary arterial and right ventricular pressures are not elevated and the holosystolic murmur is low pitched. The

features of right-sided cardiac murmurs vary much more with the respiratory cycle than do left-sided heart murmurs. There may be signs of right-sided heart failure: an enlarged pulsatile liver and, in the older child, a prominent V wave pulsation in the neck veins.

Mitral Valve Insufficiency

Mitral valve insufficiency (Fig. 11-25) is associated with a diffuse and dynamic apical impulse. If the volume of regurgitant flow is great, a bifid or double apical impulse of a palpable S_3 may be apparent.

The insufficiency jet of blood from the powerful left ventricle to the thin-walled left atrium causes a high-pitched blowing holosystolic murmur that has an abrupt onset. This murmur is heard best with the diaphragm of the stethoscope placed anteriorly in the mitral area. The systolic murmur radiates to the axillae.

The S_1 is usually of normal to increased intensity, but if the valve abnormality is rheumatic in origin, it may be sufficiently deformed that S_1 is quite soft. If the mitral regurgitation is quite significant, an S_3 filling sound is heard, often associated with a mid-diastolic flow rumble of "relative" mitral valve stenosis. Mitral valve insufficiency may be seen as a congenital lesion, in response to dilated annulus secondary to heart failure, during acute rheumatic fever or as part of the mitral valve prolapse spectrum.

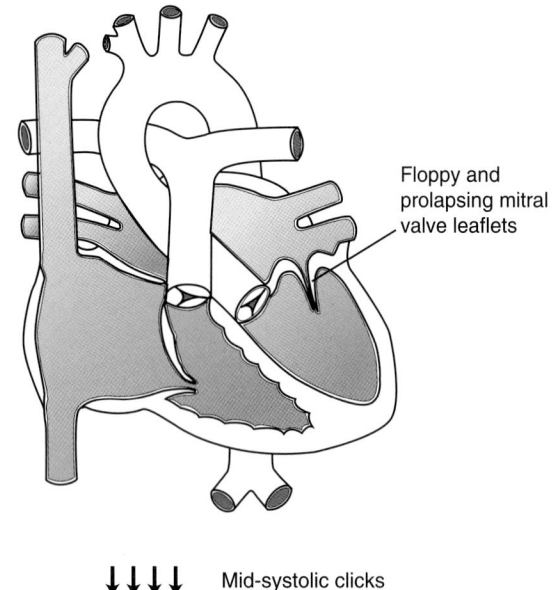

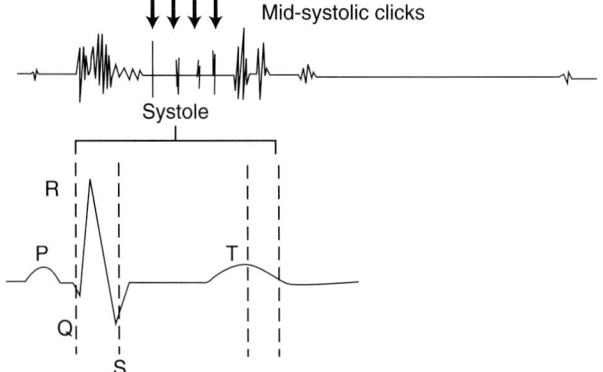

Figure 11-25. Mitral valve prolapse. The auscultatory examination findings can be very distinctive, with one or more sharp clicks being heard throughout systole. A late systolic high-pitched murmur may arise if mitral valve insufficiency occurs.

Mitral Valve Prolapse

This common condition of adolescents and young adults manifests as laxity of the mitral valve and results in slippage or displacement of the valve leaflets backward into the left atrium during systole (see Fig. 11-25).

The sudden tensing of the mitral valve often causes a midsystolic click or sometimes multiple clicks that can be heard best in the mitral area. The click is frequently followed by a late high-pitched systolic murmur of mitral valve insufficiency. The timing of the click or clicks and the intensity of the murmur often vary with body position. When the patient is sitting up (and even more so during standing), the murmur gets louder or may be heard even when no murmur was heard when the patient was lying down. This is because the left ventricular architecture changes in the upright position. In rare cases, the position change may result in a late systolic murmur's becoming full length, although with late accentuation. The electrocardiogram often shows unusually anterior and superior T waves with prominent U waves, which suggests papillary muscle dysfunction.

Mitral valve prolapse does not usually progress in childhood, but it may be associated with supraventricular tachycardia, chest pain, and possibly endocarditis or cerebrovascular embolism. Ventricular tachycardia and fibrillation may occur in adults, but sudden cardiac death is very unusual during childhood and adolescence. Thickening of the valve in addition to prolapse increases the risk of these complications.

Pulmonary Valve Insufficiency

Pulmonary valve insufficiency (Fig. 11-26) rarely if ever occurs in isolation. Most often, congenital regurgitation of the pulmonic valve occurs in association with a pulmonary outflow obstruction such as in the absent pulmonary valve syndrome.

When the pulmonary arterial pressure is low, valve insufficiency is recognized by a very low- to medium-pitched early diastolic murmur that starts with P_2. This is heard best in the pulmonary area and extends for a short distance down the left sternal edge.

The more common types of pulmonary regurgitation are acquired, commonly after surgery for severe pulmonary valve stenosis, as occurs with tetralogy of Fallot, when the pulmonary outflow patch is placed and the valve leaflets are deficient or absent. Because no P_2 exists, the murmur often appears to start significantly after S_2. Because these patients often have surgically acquired right bundle branch block, the pulmonary valve closure would be well separated from aortic valve closure if the sound could be heard. The diastolic decrescendo murmur begins at that time.

Pulmonary hypertension, particularly when associated with a high pulmonary vascular resistance, is a common cause of secondary pulmonary insufficiency. Often, a pulmonary ejection click may be present because of the dilated pulmonary root. The S_2 is narrowly split or single because the high pulmonary artery diastolic pressure closes the valve early. A diastolic decrescendo murmur then begins with pulmonary valve closure and is high in frequency because the pulmonary artery pressure is high.

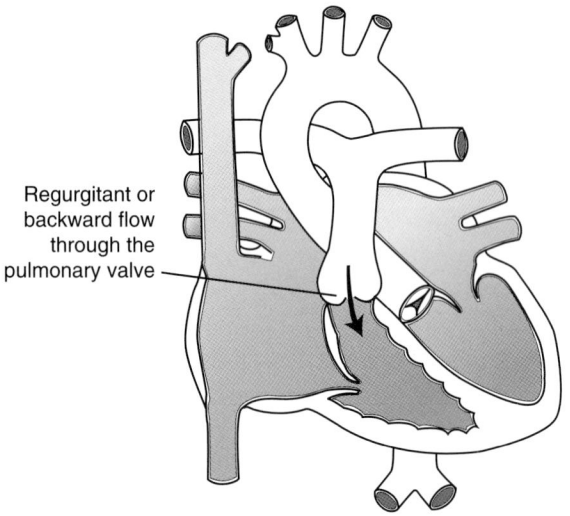

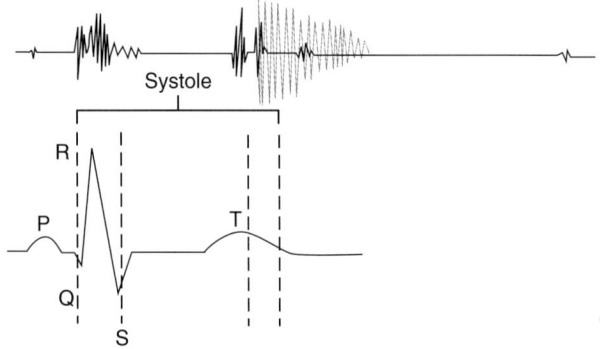

Figure 11-26. Pulmonary valve insufficiency. A low-pitched early diastolic murmur is heard just after the second heart sound. The murmur characteristically tapers into diastole.

Aortic Valve Insufficiency

Congenital insufficiency of the aortic valve (Fig. 11-27) is rare and is usually mild and may not be audible. The valve may or may not be bicuspid. There is usually an aortic ejection click that is well separated from S_1, does not vary with respiration, and is usually best heard at the apex. The S_2 split is normal, although the A_2 may be loud and may have a "tambour" quality.

After closure of the aortic valve (A_2), regurgitation of leakage at this site creates the high-pitched, early diastolic decrescendo murmur of aortic insufficiency. This murmur is heard best at the third left or right intercostal space while the patient is sitting. The pulse pressure is normal if the leak is mild.

A rare form of congenital aortic regurgitation results from a tunnel between the aorta just distal to the valve and the left ventricle just proximal to the valve. This type of aortic regurgitation is usually not associated with an aortic ejection click and is likely to be very severe and to have a very wide pulse pressure.

The most common form of aortic insufficiency is acquired, most often as a consequence of severe *rheumatic carditis,* and can be present in both acute rheumatic fever and chronic rheumatic heart disease. In acute insufficiency, there is usually no aortic ejection click. The left ventricular impulse is abnormal and hyperdynamic, and a wide pulse pressure is present.

A long, low-frequency musical diastolic rumble beginning one third of the time into diastole may occur, especially in the left lateral decubitus position in patients with significant valve insufficiency. This is called the *Austin Flint murmur.* It is related to regurgitant aortic flow passing across the anterior mitral valve and fluttering of the leaflet in conjunction with mitral valve inflow.

MISCELLANEOUS CARDIAC ANOMALIES

PERICARDIAL DISEASE

Many infectious and noninfectious diseases may cause inflammation of the pericardial sac and surrounding structures. The presence of fluid in the pericardial sac may compromise cardiac filling and result in life-threatening impairment of cardiac output, "pericardial tamponade." The auscultatory findings in these cases often include friction rubs.

These variable sounds are high pitched, superficial, and scratching noises. They occur in synchrony with cardiac movement and are heard during the early period after myocardial infarction and after cardiac surgery (see Chapter 9).

PULMONARY HYPERTENSION

After the neonatal period, pressures in the pulmonary circulation are normally low (approximately 25 mm Hg systolic, or about one fourth of the pressure in the systemic circulation or aorta). Many diseases have profound effects on the pulmonary circulation and can elevate pressures within the pulmonary arteries (see Chapter 10). These include diseases of lung, pulmonary vasculature, heart, or liver; collagen vascular diseases; and obstruction of the upper airways.

One consistent physical finding detected in pulmonary hypertension is an active right ventricular parasternal tap with a distinctive, sharp palpable P_2. The P_2 is of increased intensity, and there is a single or narrowly split S_2. There may be no audible murmur; a high-pitched murmur of pulmonary valve insufficiency or a high-pitched systolic murmur of tricuspid valve insufficiency may be present.

Recognition of pulmonary hypertension warrants a diligent search for the underlying cause. If the reason for the elevated pulmonary artery pressure remains unclear, the disorder is referred to as *primary pulmonary hypertension.* If an etiology can be found, the disorder is termed *secondary pulmonary hypertension.*

APPROACH TO CONGENITAL HEART
DISEASE (see Chapter 10)

Congenital heart disease may produce an asymptomatic murmur, heart failure, cyanosis, cyanosis with heart failure, or severe cardiogenic shock (Fig. 11-28). Malformations associated with profound and fixed cyanosis without heart failure are usually associated with right-sided obstructive lesions and a right-to-left shunt (pulmonary atresia, tetralogy of Fallot). Transposition of the great arteries with intact ventricular septum also manifests with profound and fixed hypoxia, with mild tachypnea, and with no heart failure. Malformations associated with cyanosis and heart failure have a large mixing lesion (single ventricle, truncus arteriosus, transposition plus a VSD), in which pulmonary oxygenated venous return mixes with desaturated systemic venous return before ejection to the systemic arterial circulation. In addition, obstructed total anomalous pulmonary veins may produce severe cyanosis, pulmonary venous engorgement, and pulmonary hypertension. Lesions associated with left-sided obstruction (critical aortic stenosis, interrupted aortic arch, hypoplastic left heart syndrome) produce significant cardiogenic shock, poor perfusion, and profound lactic acidosis.

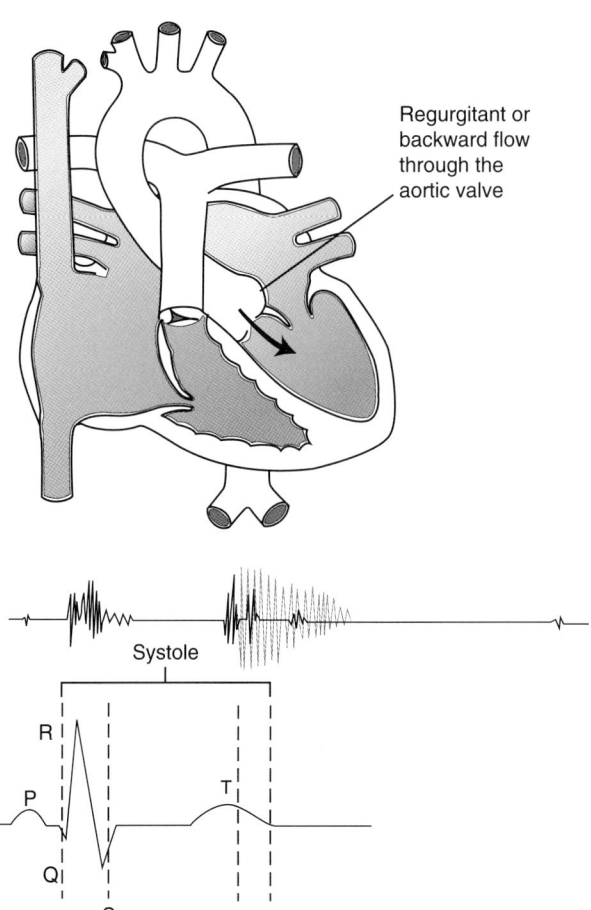

Regurgitant or
backward flow
through the
aortic valve

Systole

R

P

T

Q

S

Figure 11-27. Aortic valve insufficiency. In contrast to the low-pressure murmur of pulmonary valve insufficiency (in the absence of pulmonary hypertension), the murmur of aortic valve insufficiency is high pitched and audible from the aortic area extending to the apex. The peripheral pulses and the intensity and length of the murmur provide clinical quantification of the magnitude of regurgitant flow.

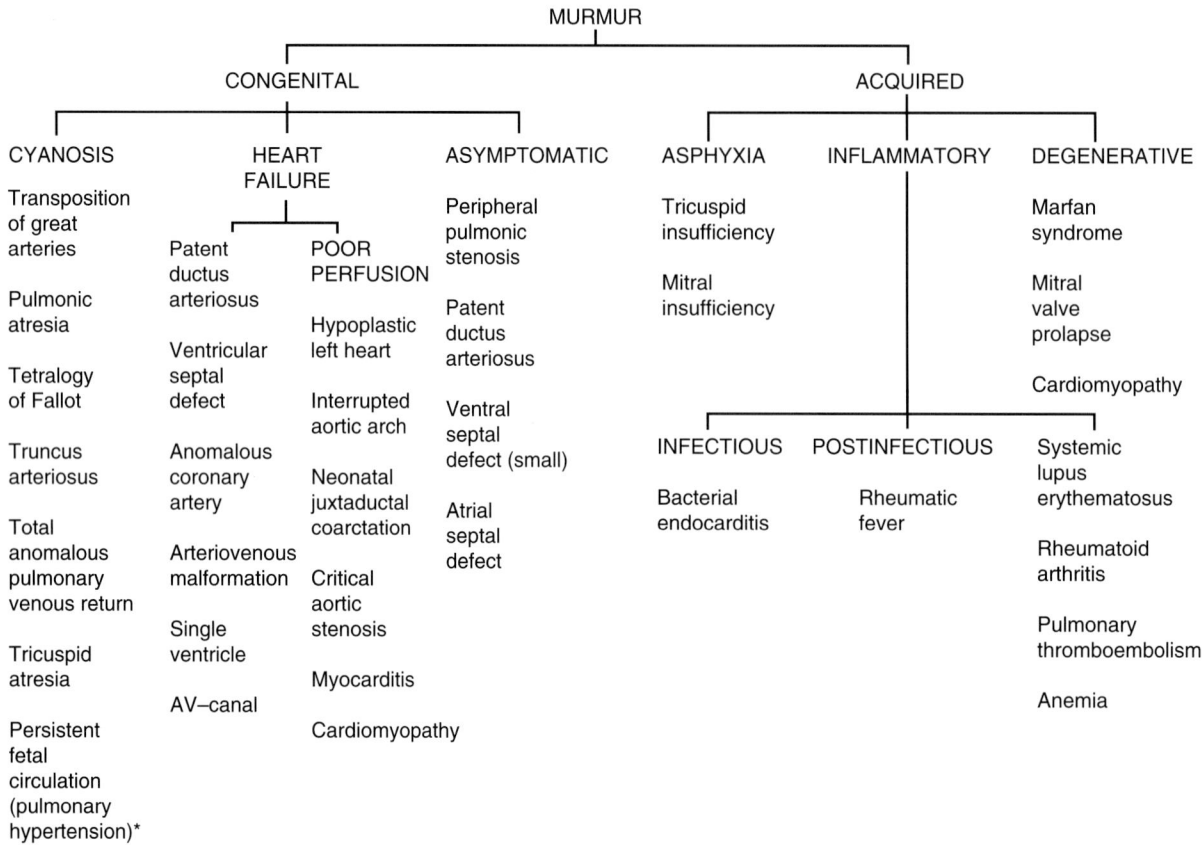

*Murmur represents tricuspid insufficiency (usually no murmur in persistent fetal circulation).

Figure 11-28. Algorithmic approach to the child with a heart murmur. AV, atrioventricular.

The *chest roentgenogram* may provide helpful clues to the cause of the lesion, depending on the paucity (pulmonary atresia) or plethora (obstructed total anomalous pulmonary venous return) of the pulmonary vascular markings; the left- or right-sided (tetralogy of Fallot, truncus arteriosus) position of the aorta; the configuration of the heart (boot-shaped, as in tetralogy of Fallot; egg-shaped, as in transposition of the great arteries; or massive enlargement, as in Ebstein anomaly); or the side of the chest (risk of heart disease is higher with dextrocardia, especially if the stomach bubble is on the left side of the abdomen or if the liver is midline). The chest roentgenogram is of some help in distinguishing heart disease from congenital pneumonia, respiratory distress syndrome, pneumothorax, and congenital diaphragmatic hernia.

The *electrocardiogram* in infancy is of help in discriminating atrial and ventricular enlargement or hypertrophy and very helpful when there is an abnormal superior vector (complete atrioventricular canal, tricuspid atresia).

Two-dimensional real-time color Doppler echocardiography is most useful in identifying the anatomy of congenital heart lesions. The echocardiogram can depict the four chambers, the interconnecting valves, the great arteries, the pulmonary venous return (the most difficult to visualize), and the anatomic relationships between these structures. Furthermore, color Doppler flow studies can determine the presence, direction, and magnitude of right-to-left or left-to-right shunts. Echocardiography has replaced cardiac catheterization for all but the most complex congenital heart lesions.

The therapy for congenital heart disease depends on the specific nature of the congenital anomaly (Tables 11-6 and 11-7). Certain lesions necessitate immediate palliative therapy (see Table 11-6)

with subsequent complete repair when the neonate becomes older and bigger (see Table 11-7). Other lesions undergo complete repair in the neonatal period (see Table 11-7). Both before and after surgery, most lesions heighten the risk for endocarditis, and prophylaxis is required for high-risk procedures (see later discussion).

ACUTE RHEUMATIC FEVER AND RHEUMATIC HEART DISEASE

The incidence of acute rheumatic fever is increasing in the United States; it remains very common in many areas of the world. Rheumatic fever is a postinfection, immunologically mediated inflammatory disease (caused by group A streptococcus) of the heart, joints, brain, and skin. Valvulitis, as manifested by specific and new heart murmurs, is often part of the initial clinical picture. The specific heart murmurs are three: mitral regurgitation, aortic regurgitation, and the Carey-Coombs murmur, a mid-diastolic rumble at the apex. Pericarditis, usually associated with valvulitis, may produce a friction rub.

After the acute rheumatic fever has run its course, any remaining murmurs become part of chronic rheumatic heart disease. If the patient has continued permanent reliable penicillin prophylaxis, the severity of the mitral regurgitation often disappears; this happens less commonly with aortic regurgitation. The development of mitral valve stenosis is part of the natural history of severe repeated episodes of acute rheumatic fever. Pure aortic stenosis does not develop, although in the presence of long-standing rheumatic heart

Table 11-6. Palliative Therapy for Congenital Heart Disease

Procedure	Lesion	Comments
Blalock-Taussig Gortex tube graft or shunt (subclavian artery to ipsilateral pulmonary artery, usually right-sided)	TOF, pulmonary valve atresia	Improves pulmonary blood flow; most common shunting procedure
Balloon atrial septostomy (Rashkind procedure)	TGA, tricuspid atresia	Improves oxygenation with increased atrial mixing
Catheter ballon–dilating valvotomy (balloon angioplasty)	Pulmonary valve stenosis; aortic valve stenosis	Increases valve patency
Operative valvotomy	Same as for balloon plus pulmonary atresia	Increased valve patency; resultant pulmonary valve insufficiency enhances RV growth
Prostaglandin E$_1$ infusion	Pulmonary atresia, tricuspid atresia, TOF, coarctation of aorta, HLHS, interrupted aortic arch	Maintains pulmonary blood flow via PDA
Pulmonary artery banding	Single ventricle, complicated VSD	Decreases pulmonary blood flow, prevents heart failure
Device occlusion (embolization, umbrella); correction/closure	PDA, VSD, ASD, arteriovenous malformations	Done at cardiac catheterization

From Gillette PC: The cardiovascular system. In Behrman RE, Kliegman RM (eds): Nelson Essentials of Pediatrics, 2nd ed. Philadelphia, WB Saunders, 1994, p 503.

ASD, atrial septal defect; HLHS, hypoplastic left heart syndrome; PDA, patent ductus arteriosus; RV, right ventricular; TGA, transposition of the great arteries; TOF, tetralogy of Fallot; VSD, ventricular septal defect.

disease with severe aortic regurgitation, some aortic stenosis may be present. In some very severe cases, tricuspid valve regurgitation has been documented, but it is rare.

The diagnosis of acute rheumatic fever is suggested (although not definitively confirmed) by application of the modified Jones criteria, last edited in 1992 (Table 11-8). In addition, evidence of a group A streptococcal pharyngitis must be present, which may include a positive throat culture, positive streptococcal antigen or antistreptococcal antibody, or a history of prior episodes of rheumatic fever. Some authors would also include echocardiographic evidence of subclinical carditis (no audible murmur) by demonstrating significant mitral regurgitation with a regurgitant jet seen in two planes with chaotic flow and holosystolic extending 1 cm into the left atrium. Criteria for subclinical significant echocardiographic aortic regurgitation include its being seen in two imaging planes, being holodiastolic, and extending 1 cm into the ventricle. The differential diagnosis is limited in the presence of carditis and arthritis (see Chapter 44) but includes systemic lupus erythematosus.

Treatment of acute carditis includes salicylate if mild, steroids if severe carditis is present, and standard therapy for heart failure (see Chapter 8). Valvular scarring and progression of carditis may be avoided by prevention of repeated episodes of group A streptococcal infections. Daily penicillin V, 250 mg taken orally twice a day (or, if patient is allergic to penicillin, sulfisoxazole, 1 g if patient

Table 11-7. Corrective Procedures for Congenital Heart Disease

Procedure	Lesion	Effect
Repair of septal defects (patching)	ASD, VSD, endocardial cushion defects	Complete repair
Valve repair, replacement	Aortic, mitral, pulmonic valve disease, Ebstein anomaly	Repair, prosthetic valve complications
Ross aortic graft repair	Aortic valve disease	Growth potential in young children
Aortic graft or subclavian flap angioplasty	Interrupted arch, coarctation of aorta	Repair, but possible late recoarctation
Total correction possible	TOF, anomalous venous return, PDA	Complete repair
Mustard or Senning procedure (atrial switch by an intraatrial baffle)	TGA	RV remains systemic ventricle
Jatene procedure (arterial switch)*	TGA	Anatomic correction
Fontan procedure (right atrium–to–pulmonary artery anastomosis)	Tricuspid atresia, single ventricle, pulmonary atresia	Alleviates shunting, enhances pulmonary blood flow; atrium functions as right ventricle
Norwood procedure	Hypoplastic left heart syndrome	Three stage procedure with variable success
Heart transplantation	Hypoplastic left heart syndrome Failed Fontan procedure	Normal heart with risk of immune rejection, premature atherosclerosis
Heart-lung transplantation	Eisenmenger syndrome; cor pulmonale?	Normal organs with risk of rejection

*Preferred procedure.

Modified from Gillette PC: The cardiovascular system. In Behrman RE, Kliegman RM (eds): Nelson Essentials of Pediatrics, 2nd ed. Philadelphia, WB Saunders, 1994, p 503.

ASD, atrial septal defect; PDA, patent ductus arteriosus; RV, right ventricle; TGA, transposition of the great arteries; TOF, tetralogy of Fallot; VSD, ventricular septal defect.

Table 11-8. Major Criteria in the Jones System for Acute Rheumatic Fever*†

Sign	Comments
Polyarthritis	Most common. Swelling, limited motion, very tender, erythema; migratory (may be aborted by anti-inflammatory agents): involves large joints (knees, ankles, wrists, elbows) but rarely small or unusual joints, such as vertebrae. Universally benign long-term joint prognosis. Robust response to salicylate within 48 hr.
Carditis	Common. Pancarditis, valvulitis, pericarditis, myocarditis; tachycardia greater than that explained by fever; new murmur of mitral or aortic insufficiency; Carey-Coombs mid-diastolic murmur; heart failure. Echocardiographic findings without auscultatory findings do not count as a major criterion.
Chorea (Sydenham disease)	Uncommon. Manifests long after infection has resolved; may be associated with antineuronal antibody.
Erythema marginatum	Uncommon. Evanescent pink macules on trunk and proximal extremities, evolving to serpiginous border with central clearing; elicited by application of local heat; nonpruritic.
Subcutaneous nodules	Uncommon. Associated with repeated episodes and severe carditis; present over extensor surface of elbows, knees, knuckles, and ankles or scalp and spine; firm, nontender, painless.

*Minor criteria include fever (101°–102° F [38.2°–38.9° C]), arthralgias, previous rheumatic fever, leukocytosis elevated erythrocyte sedimentation rate/C-reactive protein, prolonged P-R interval.

†One major plus two minor criteria, or two major criteria with evidence of recent group A streptococcal disease (scarlet fever, positive throat culture, or elevated antistreptolysin O or other antistreptococcal antibodies), strongly suggest the diagnosis of acute rheumatic fever.

Exceptions to these recommendations include chorea (which may occur too late after other signs or laboratory tests are not useful), some cases of recurrent carditis that may not fulfill the criteria, and indolent carditis or late stenotic or regurgitant murmurs far removed in time from the original episode of rheumatic fever. Isolated reactive post-streptococcal arthritis has been considered by some authorities to be in the spectrum of rheumatic fever. Nonetheless, this has not been met with uniform agreement.

weighs > 60 pounds or 0.5 g if patient weighs < 60 pounds, taken orally once a day) or long-acting penicillin, 1,200,000 U injected intramuscularly every 28 days, prevents most cases of new group A streptococcal diseases and recurrent rheumatic fever. Prophylaxis is continued for at least 5 years and at least until age 21 years (some authorities believe prophylaxis should be for life); prophylaxis is life long in patients with documented rheumatic heart disease.

INFECTIVE ENDOCARDITIS

An acute or subacute infection of the cardiac valves produces infective endocarditis. Infection may involve a native, previously normal heart valve, a valve or structure (e.g., PDA, VSD opposite an endocardial wall that is subjected to a jet stream) that is anomalous as a result of congenital heart disease (most common sites), or a prosthetic device (e.g., valve, conduit, patch, graft, shunt, or pacemaker).

Endocarditis may affect congenital heart lesions (most commonly, tetralogy of Fallot, VSD, aortic stenosis, PDA, transposition of the great arteries), valves affected by rheumatic heart disease, and mitral valve prolapse. Endocarditis may develop in congenital heart anomalies in the unoperated and the postoperative state. Furthermore, 10% to 30% of cases of infective endocarditis occur on previously normal native valves.

Endocarditis is the result of a bacteremia, which in a normal host is usually transient, asymptomatic, and without sequelae. The presence of a damaged valve, a jet stream–injured endocardium, or a foreign body (e.g., central catheter, graft, shunt, or patch) creates a nidus of infection that permits the bacteria to bind, proliferate, and remain sequestered from normal host defense mechanisms. Transient and predisposing bacteremias occur during dental procedures that induce bleeding (even dental cleaning); tonsillectomy or adenoidectomy; intestinal (e.g., gall bladder), urinary (e.g., catheterization, dilatation), prostatic (e.g., cystoscopy), or respiratory surgery; esophageal manipulation (e.g., sclerotherapy, dilatation), incision and drainage of infected tissue; and gynecologic procedures (e.g., vaginal hysterectomy, vaginal delivery).

Bacterial vegetations grow and produce cardiovascular, embolic, or immune complex–mediated signs and symptoms (Table 11-9). Responsible bacteria are noted in Table 11-10; *Staphylococcus aureus*, α-hemolytic oral mucosa–derived streptococci, and enterococcus are the dominant pathogens in native normal and unoperated anomalous valves. *Staphylococcus epidermidis* and *S. aureus* are common pathogens in the postoperative patient and in patients with prosthetic devices.

The definitive diagnosis of infective endocarditis includes recovery of a microorganism from culture or histologic study of a heart, an embolized vegetation, or an intracardiac abscess. Vegetations may be demonstrated by the sensitive technique of transesophageal echocardiography but are usually seen on transthoracic echocardiography. In the absence of direct definitive evidence, the following are important diagnostic factors: persistently positive blood cultures with a pathogen compatible with the diagnosis (see Table 11-10); echocardiographic evidence of an intracardiac mass, vegetations, perivalvular abscess, or new partial dehiscence of a prosthetic valve; and a new valvular murmur (regurgitation, or worsening or changing of a preexisting murmur). Blood cultures are helpful if two or more drawn 12 hours apart are positive or if a majority (e.g., three of four) of separate cultures drawn in 1 hour are positive. More than 85% of first blood cultures are positive; the yield approaches 95% with the second blood culture. Sufficient blood must be inoculated into the media to detect the low-grade bacteremia of infective endocarditis; excessive blood inoculation may inhibit bacterial growth by continued activity of leukocytes unless the technique involves centrifugation lysis. The cultures should be incubated for more than the routine 72 hours (often 1 to 2 weeks), and the laboratory should be notified of the possible diagnosis so that laboratory personnel can enrich the media to encourage the growth of fastidious nutrient-dependent organisms.

Additional criteria for diagnosing infective endocarditis include fever; predisposing heart lesions and procedures (many patients have undergone no identifiable procedure); vascular phenomena (embolism, Janeway lesions, petechiae, septic pulmonary infarcts, intracranial hemorrhage); immune lesions (glomerulonephritis, Roth spots, Osler nodes); a suggestive but not definitive echocardiogram;

Table 11-9. Manifestations of Infective Endocarditis

History

Prior congenital or rheumatic heart disease
Preceding dental, urinary, or intestinal procedure
Intravenous drug use
Central venous catheter
Prosthetic heart valve

Symptoms

Fever
Chills
Chest and back pain
Arthralgia/myalgia
Dyspnea
Malaise
Night sweats
Weight loss
CNS manifestations (stroke, seizures, headache, confusion)

Signs

Elevated temperature
Tachycardia
Embolic phenomena (Roth spots, petechiae, splinter nailbed
   hemorrhages, Osler nodes, CNS or ocular lesions)
Janeway lesions
New or changing murmur
Splenomegaly
Arthritis
Heart failure
Arrhythmias, heart block, conduction disturbances
Metastatic infection (arthritis, meningitis, mycotic arterial
   aneurysm, pericarditis, abscesses, septic pulmonary emboli)
Digital clubbing

Laboratory

Positive blood culture
Elevated erythrocyte sedimentation rate; may be low with
   heart or renal failure
Elevated C-reactive protein level
Anemia
Leukocytosis
Immune complexes
Hypergammaglobulinemia
Hypocomplementemia
Cryoglobulinemia
Rheumatoid factor
Hematuria
Azotemia, high creatinine level (glomerulonephritis)
Echocardiographic evidence of valve vegetations, prosthetic
   valve dysfunction or leak, or myocardial abscess

Modified from Behrman RE (ed): Nelson Textbook of Pediatrics, 14th ed. Philadelphia, WB Saunders, 1992.

CNS, central nervous system.

Table 11-10. Bacterial Agents in Pediatric Infective Endocarditis

Common: Native Valve

Streptococcus viridans group (e.g., *Streptococcus mutans,
   Streptococcus sanguis, Streptococcus mitis*)
Staphylococcus aureus
Group D streptococcus (enterococcus) *(Streptococcus bovis,
   Streptococcus faecalis)*

Uncommon: Native Valve

Streptococcus pneumoniae
Haemophilus influenzae
Group A or B streptococci
Staphylococcus epidermidis
Coxiella burnetii (Q fever)
Neisseria gonorrhoeae
Brucella species*
*Chlamydia psittaci**
*Chlamydia trachomatis**
*Chlamydia pneumoniae**
HACEK group†
*Streptobacillus moniliformis**
*Pasteurella multocida**
Campylobacter fetus
Polymicrobial
Fungal
Culture negative (5% of cases)

Prosthetic Valve

S. epidermidis
S. aureus
Viridans streptococci
Pseudomonas aeruginosa
Serratia marcescens
Diphtheroids
Legionella species*
HACEK group†
Fungi‡

Modified from Behrman RE (ed): Nelson Textbook of Pediatrics, 14th ed. Philadelphia, WB Saunders, 1992.

*These fastidious bacteria plus some fungi and pretreatment with antibiotics may produce culture-negative endocarditis. Detection may require special media, incubation for more than 7 days, or serologic study.

†HACEK group includes *Haemophilus* species (*Haemophilus paraphrophilus, Haemophilus parainfluenzae, Haemophilus aphrophilus*), *Actinobacillus actinomycetemcomitans, Cardiobacterium hominis, Eikenella corrodens,* and *Kingella* species.

‡*Candida* species, *Aspergillus* species, *Pseudallescheria boydii, Histoplasma capsulatum.*

and microbiologic criteria (positive blood culture but not as defined earlier; serologic evidence of active infection).

The treatment of presumed infective endocarditis with no known cause and the treatment of proven bacteriologic infective endocarditis are noted in Table 11-11. With appropriate therapy, the blood should be culture negative within 72 to 96 hours, and fever should subside in 1 to 2 weeks. Persistent fever should suggest the presence of resistant organisms, metastatic foci of infection, an infected clot, a myocardial abscess, pulmonary emboli, a nosocomial infection, and drug fever. Persistent infection, severe refractory heart failure,

intracardiac abscess, recurrent emboli, and possible fungal infective endocarditis are indications for surgical intervention.

To prevent infective endocarditis, high-risk patients, procedures, and factors that predispose to bacteremia need to be identified (Tables 11-12 and 11-13). Patients needing infective endocarditis prophylaxis include those with intracardiac foreign bodies (prosthetic valve, grafts), prior episodes of infective endocarditis, most congenital heart defects (except isolated secundum ASD, a repaired secundum ASD, VSD, or PDA after 6 months of operation, and pulmonary valve stenosis), hypertrophic cardiomyopathy, rheumatic or other acquired valve disease, and mitral valve prolapse with regurgitation.

Table 11-11. Treatment of Infective Endocarditis

Etiologic Agent	Drug	Dose	Route	Duration of Therapy (wk)
Streptococcus viridans, Streptococcus bovis (minimal inhibitory concentration [MIC] ≤ 0.1 µg/mL)	(1) Penicillin G *or*	200,000-300,000 U/kg/24 hr q4h, not to exceed 20 million U/24 hr	IV	4-6
	(2) Penicillin G	Same as for No. 1	IV	2-4
	plus gentamicin	3-7.5 mg/kg/24 hr q8h, not to exceed 240 mg/24 hr	IV	2
Streptococcus viridans, S. bovis (MIC ≥ 0.1 µg/mL)	(3) Penicillin G	Same as for No.2	IV	4-6
	plus gentamicin	Same as for No.2	IV	2
S. viridans or enterococci (*S. bovis* or *Streptococcus faecalis*) (MIC > 0.5 µg/mL)	(4) Penicillin G	Same as for No 2	IV	4-6
	or ampicillin	300 mg/kg/24 hr q4-6h, not to exceed 12 g/24 hr	IV	4-6
	plus gentamicin	Same as for No. 2	IV	4-6
*S. viridans, S. bovis** (penicillin allergy)†	(5) Vancomycin plus	40-60 mg/kg/24 hr q8-12h, not to exceed 2 g/24 hr	IV	4-6
	(6) gentamicin if resistant*	Same as for No. 2	IV	4-6
Staphylococcus aureus	(7) Nafcillin *or* oxacillin plus optional gentamicin	200 mg/kg/24 hr q4-6h, not to exceed 12 g/24 hr	IV	6-8
		Same as for No. 2	IV	1-2
S. aureus (methicillin-resistant) (penicillin allergy)	(8) Vancomycin plus optional trimethoprim-sulfamethoxazole	Same as for No. 5	IV	6-8
		12 mg/kg/24 hr trimethoprim q8h, not to exceed 1 g/24 hr	IV, PO	4-8
S. aureus (with prosthetic device, methicillin-sensitive)‡	(9) Nafcillin	Same as for No. 7	IV	6-8
	plus gentamicin	Same as for No. 2	IV	2
	plus optional rifampin	10-20 mg/kg/24 hr q12h, not to exceed 600 mg/24 hr	PO	≥6
S. aureus (with prosthetic device, methicillin-resistant)	(10) Vancomycin	Same as for No. 5	IV	6-8
	plus gentamicin	Same as for No. 9	IV	2
	plus optional rifampin	Same as for No. 9	PO	≥6
Staphylococcus epidermidis	(11) Vancomycin	Same as for No. 5	IV	6-8
	plus optional rifampin	Same as for No. 9	PO	6-8
Haemophilus species	(12) Ampicillin	Same as for No. 4	IV	4-6
	plus optional gentamicin	Same as for No. 2	IV	2-4
Unknown Postoperative	(13) Vancomycin	Same as for No. 5	IV	6-8
	plus gentamicin	Same as for No. 2	IV	2-4
Nonoperative	(14) Nafcillin *or* vancomycin	Same as for No. 7	IV	6-8
		Same as for No. 5	IV	6-8
	plus gentamicin	Same as for No. 2	IV	2-4
	plus optional ampicillin	Same as for No. 4	IV	6-8

From Behrman RE, Kliegman RM, Jenson HB (ed): Nelson Textbook of Pediatrics, 16th ed. Philadelphia, WB Saunders, 2000.

*Add gentamicin for relatively resistant organisms. Monitor vancomycin peaks 1 hr after infusion (30-45 µg/mL). Adjust dose according to vancomycin levels.

†Desensitization should be considered for patients who are allergic to penicillin. Cephalosporins are not recommended.

‡May require valve (device) replacement.

IV, intravenous; PO, oral.

Table 11-12. Procedures and Endocarditis Prophylaxis

Endocarditis Prophylaxis Recommended*	Endocarditis Prophylaxis Not Recommended‖
Dental	**Dental**
Tooth extractions	Restorative dentistry‡ (operative and prosthodontic) with or without retraction cord§
Periodontal procedures, including surgery, scaling and root planing, probing, and recall maintenance	Local anesthesia injections (nonintraligamentary)
Dental implant placement and reimplantation of avulsed teeth	Intracanal endodontic treatment; after placement and build-up
Endodontic (root canal) instrumentation or surgery only beyond the apex	Placement of rubber dams
Subgingival placement of antibiotic fibers or strips	Postoperative suture removal
Initial placement of orthodontic bands but not brackets	Placement of removable prosthodontic or orthodontic appliances
Intraligamentary local anesthesia injections	Taking of oral impressions
Prophylactic cleaning of teeth or implants when bleeding is anticipated	Fluoride treatments
	Taking of oral radiographs
	Orthodontic appliance adjustment
	Shedding of primary teeth
Respiratory Tract	**Respiratory Tract**
Tonsillectomy or adenoidectomy, or both	Endotracheal intubation
Surgical operations that involve respiratory mucosa	Bronchoscopy with a flexible bronchoscope, with or without biopsy§
Bronchoscopy with a rigid broncoscope	Tympanostomy tube insertion
Gastrointestinal Tract†	**Gastrointestinal Tract**
Sclerotherapy for esophageal varices	Transesophageal echocardiography§
Esophageal stricture dilation	Endoscopy with or without gastrointestinal biopsy§
Endoscopic retrograde cholangiography with biliary obstruction	**Genitourinary Tract**
Biliary tract surgery	Vaginal delivery§
Surgical operations that involve intestinal mucosa	Cesarean section
Genitourinary Tract	In uninfected tissue:
Cystoscopy	Urethral catheterization
	Uterine dilation and curettage
	Therapeutic abortion
	Sterilization procedures
	Insertion or removal of intrauterine devices
	Other
	Cardiac catheterization, including balloon angioplasty
	Implanted cardiac pacemakers, implanted defibrillators, and coronary stents
	Incision or biopsy of surgically scrubbed skin
	Circumcision

From Behrman RE, Kliegman RM, Jenson HB (eds): Nelson Textbook of Pediatrics, 16th ed. Philadelphia, WB Saunders, 2000.

*Prophylaxis is recommended for patients with high- or moderate-risk heart conditions.

†Prophylaxis is recommended for high-risk patients; optional for medium-risk patients.

‡This includes restroration of decayed teeth (filling cavities) and replacement of missing teeth.

§Prophylaxis is optional for high-risk patients.

‖Clinical judgment may indicate antibiotic use in selected circumstances that may create significant bleeding.

RED FLAGS AND THINGS NOT TO MISS

Murmurs may be caused by cardiac or noncardiac lesions and may be congenital or acquired. Murmurs in the neonatal period are often transient, as a result of the changing hemodynamics of the transitional circulation between fetal and neonatal life, or as a result of the common occurrence of a small VSD, which usually closes in the first 1 to 5 years of life. Most murmurs at all ages are not caused by cardiac disease and are not associated with symptoms or increased risk for disease.

Red flags in the neonatal period include cyanosis; fixed, profound hypoxia; heart failure; and other congenital anomalies or syndromes, such as trisomy 21. Such syndromes often manifest with multiple congenital anomalies, including those involving the cardiovascular, gastrointestinal, and central nervous systems. In the neonatal period, things not to miss include ductus-dependent lesions, in which systemic blood flow (as in interrupted aortic arch, hypoplastic left heart syndrome) or pulmonary blood flow (as in pulmonary atresia) is through the PDA. Sudden deterioration, cyanosis, or heart failure with increasing metabolic acidosis and a reduction in the murmur suggests closure of the ductus arteriosus. Another thing not to miss is the murmur associated with an arteriovenous malformation, such as the cerebral vein of Galen malformation, which manifests with heart failure and a cranial bruit. Finally, obstructed total anomalous venous return may be confused with persistent fetal circulation, and it may be difficult to establish the diagnosis. Total anomalous venous return is associated with fixed, profound cyanosis

Table 11-13. Recommendations of the American Heart Association for Prophylaxis against Bacterial Endocarditis

Dental and Oral Procedures or Surgery of the Upper Respiratory Tract or Esophagus		Gastrointestinal and Genitourinary Tract Surgery and Instrumentation	
For most patients	Oral amoxicillin Adults: 2.0 g; children: 50 mg/kg Given 1 hr before the procedure	High-risk patients	IM or IV ampicillin Adults: 2.0 g; children: 50 mg/kg *plus* IM or IV gentamicin 1.5 mg/kg (maximum dose 120 mg) Given within 30 min before the procedure *plus 6 hr later* IM or IV ampicillin or oral amoxicillin Adults: 1.0 g; children: 20 mg/kg
For patients unable to take oral medication	IM or IV ampicillin Adults: 2.0 g; children: 50 mg/kg Given within 30 min before the procedure		
Ampicillin- and amoxicillin-allergic patients	Oral clindamycin Adults: 600 mg; children: 20 mg/kg Given 1 hr before the procedure *or* Oral cephalexin* or cefadroxil* Adults: 2.0 g; children: 50 mg/kg Given 1 hr before the procedure *or* Oral azithromycin *or* clarithromycin Adults: 500 mg; children: 15 mg/kg Given 1 hr before the procedure	High-risk patients allergic to ampicillin and amoxicillin	IV vancomycin Adults: 1.0 g; children: 20 mg/kg Given over 1-2 hr *plus* IM or IV gentamicin 1.5 mg/kg (maximum dose, 120 mg) Complete injection/infusion within 30 min before starting the procedure
Ampicillin- and amoxicillin-allergic patients unable to take oral medications	IV clindamycin Adults: 600 mg; children: 20 mg/kg Given within 30 min before the procedure *or* IV cefazolin Adults: 1.0 g; children: 25 mg/kg Given within 30 min before the procedure	Moderate-risk patients	Oral amoxicillin Adults: 2.0 g; children: 50 mg/kg 1 hr before the procedure *or* IM or IV ampicillin Adults: 2.0 g; children: 50 mg/kg Given within 30 min before the procedure
		Moderate-risk patients who are allergic to ampicillin and amoxicillin	IV vancomycin Adults: 1.0 g; children: 20 mg/kg Given over 1-2 hr; complete infusion within 30 min of starting the procedure

*Cephalosporins should not be used in patients with immediate-type hypersensitivity reaction to penicillins.

High-risk patients: Prosthetic heart valves (including homografts), previous endocarditis, complex cyanotic congenital heart disease (e.g., transposition of the great arteries, tetralogy of Fallot, single ventricle), systemic-to-pulmonary artery shunts or conduits.

Moderate-risk patients: Most other congenital heart diseases (other than those specifically listed previously or further on), acquired valve dysfunction (e.g., rheumatic heart disease), hypertrophic cardiomyopathy.

Negligible-risk patients (prophylaxis not recommended): Isolated secundum ASD, surgical repair of ASD, VSD, or PDA (without residua and beyond 6 months after repair), previous coronary artery bypass surgery, functional heart murmurs, previous Kawasaki disease or rheumatic fever without valve dysfunction, cardiac pacemakers, implantable defibrillators.

The risk for mitral valve prolapse is controversial. The latest American Heart Association recommendations categorize mitral valve prolapse with regurgitation or thickened leaflets, or both, as a moderate risk; mitral valve prolapse without regurgitation is categorized as a negligible risk (for further details, see the reference).

ASD, atrial septal defect; IM, intramuscularly; IV, intravenously; PDA, patent ductus arteriosus; VSD, ventricular septal defect.

Adapted from Dajani AS, Taubert KA, Wilson W, et al: Prevention of bacterial endocarditis. Recommendations by the American Heart Association. JAMA 1997;277:1794.

(PaO_2 < 35 mm Hg), severe pulmonary venous congestion, and a small heart.

Acquired murmurs or symptomatic murmurs that change in quality should suggest acute (recurrent) rheumatic fever or infective endocarditis. Systemic symptoms and peripheral signs associated with these disorders are suggestive of the diagnosis. Arthritis (associated with rheumatic fever or endocarditis-induced immune complexes), fever, anemia, leukocytosis, cutaneous manifestations (erythema marginatum and subcutaneous nodules in rheumatic fever; Osler nodes, Janeway lesions, petechiae, and splinter hemorrhages in infective endocarditis), and evidence of prior infection (streptococcal antibodies) or current infection (positive blood cultures) help identify the nature of the acquired heart disease. Finally, heart murmurs in a normal heart may be caused by hemodynamic factors, such as severe anemia or thyrotoxicosis.

REFERENCES

Introduction

Boneva RS, Botto LD, Moore CA, et al: Mortality associated with congenital heart defects in the United States: Trends and racial disparities, 1979-1997. Circulation 2001;103:2376-2381.

Day INM, Wilson DI: Genetics and cardiovascular risk. BMJ 2001;323:1409-1412.

Goldmuntz E: The epidemiology and genetics of congenital heart disease. Clin Perinatol 2001;28:1-10.

Karl TR: Neonatal cardiac surgery: Anatomic, physiologic, and technical considerations. Clin Perinatol 2001;28:159-185.

The Science of Auscultation

American Heart Association: Physiologic Principles of Heart Sounds and Murmurs (Monograph No. 46). New York: American Heart Association, 1975.

Constant J: The stethoscope. In Bedside Cardiology. London, Little, Brown, 1993, p 122.

Selig MB: Stethoscopic and phono-audio devices: Historical and future perspectives. Am Heart J 1993;126:262-268.

Zoneraich S, Spodick DH: Bedside science reduces laboratory art. Circulation 1995;91:2089-2092.

Origins of Heart Sounds

Glover DD, Murrah RL, Olsen CO, et al: Mechanical correlates of the third heart sound. J Am Coll Cardiol 1992;19:450-457.

Nitta M, Ihenacho D, Hultgren HN: Prevalence and characteristics of the aortic ejection sound in adults. Am J Cardiol 1988;61:142-145.

Shaver JA, O'Toole JD: The second heart sound: Newer concepts, part I: Normal and wide physiological splitting. Mod Concepts Cardiovasc Dis 1977;46:7-12, 13-17.

Tilkian AG, Conover MB: Understanding Heart Sounds and Murmurs, With an Introduction to Lung Sounds, 3rd ed. Philadelphia, WB Saunders, 1993.

Zoneraich S: Evaluation of century-old physical signs, S_3 and S_4, by modern technology. J Am Coll Cardiol 1992;19:458-459.

Cardiovascular Assessment

Gessner IH: Evaluation of the infant and child with a heart murmur. In Gessner IH, Victoria BE (eds): Pediatric Cardiology: A Problem Oriented Approach. Philadelphia, WB Saunders, 1993.

Liebman J: Diagnosis and management of heart murmurs in children. Pediatr Rev 1982;321-329.

McNamara DG: Value and limitations of auscultation in the management of congenital heart disease. Pediatr Clin North Am 1990;37:93-113.

Pelech AN: The Cardiac Murmur. Pediatr Clin North Am 1998;45:107-122.

Poskitt EME: Failure to thrive in congenital heart disease. Arch Dis Child 1993;68:158-160.

Silove ED: Assessment and management of congenital heart disease in the newborn by the district paediatrician. Arch Dis Child 1994;70: F71-F74.

Murmurs in Children with Normal Hearts

Canent RV: Recognizing common innocent heart murmurs in infants and children. Mo Med 1986;83:621-625.

Etchells E, Bell C, Robb K: Does this patient have an abnormal systolic murmur? JAMA 1997;277:564-571.

Lembo N, Dell'Italia L, Crawford M, et al: Bedside diagnosis of systolic murmurs. N Engl J Med 1988;318:1572-1578.

Rosenthal A: How to distinguish between innocent and pathologic murmurs in childhood. Pediatr Clin North Am 1984;31:1229-1240.

Rosenthal A: Office maneuvers for evaluating children's heart murmurs. Consultant 1986;26:147-160.

Stein PD, Sabbah HN: Aortic origin of innocent murmurs. Am J Cardiol 1977;39:665-671.

Vibratory Still Murmur

Martins L, Van Zeller P, Roch-Goncalves F, et al: Morphology, prevalence and clinical significance of left ventricular false tendons in adults. Acta Cardiologica 1988;93:245.

Perry LW, Ruckman RN, Shapiro SR, et al: Left ventricular false tendons in children: Prevalence as detected by 2-dimensional echocardiography and clinical significance. Am J Cardiol 1983;52:1264.

Shiekh MV, Lee WR, Mills RJ, et al: Musical murmurs: Clinical implications, long term prognosis, and echo-phonocardiographic features. Am Heart J 1984;108:377-386.

Peripheral Pulmonary Arterial Stenosis

Danilowicz DA, Rudolph AM, Hoffman JI, et al: Physiologic pressure differences between the main and branch pulmonary arteries in infants. Circulation 1972;45:410.

The Supraclavicular Murmur

Kawabori I, Stevenson JG, Dooley TK, et al: The significance of carotid bruits in children. Am Heart J 1979;98:160.

Nelson WP, Hall RJ: The innocent supraclavicular arterial bruit-utility of shoulder maneuvers in its recognition. New Engl J Med 1968;278:778.

Aortic Systolic Murmur

Stein PD, Sabbah HN: Aortic origin of innocent murmurs. Am J Cardiol 1977;39:665.

Venous Hum

Cutforth R, Wiseman J, Sutherland RD: The genesis of the cervical venous hum. Am Heart J 1970;80:488.

Potain SC: Des mouvements et des bruits qui se passent dans les veines jugulaires. Bull Mem Soc Med Hop Paris 1867;4:3.

Mammary Arterial Soufflé

Tabatznik B, Randall TW, Hersch C: The mammary souffle of pregnancy and lactation. Circulation 1960;22:1069.

Congenital Heart Disease

Brickner ME, Hillis LD, Lange RA: Congenital heart disease in adults. N Engl J Med 2000;342:256-263.

Driscoll DJ: Left-to-right shunt lesions. Pediatr Clin North Am 1999;46: 355-368.

Fedderly RT: Left ventricular outflow obstruction. Pediatr Clin North Am 1999;46:369-384.

Grifka RG: Cyanotic congenital heart disease with increased pulmonary blood flow. Pediatr Clin North Am 1999;46:405-425.

Karl TR: Neonatal cardiac surgery: Anatomic, physiologic, and technical considerations. Clin Perinatol 2001;28:159-185.

Ovaert C, McCrindle BW, Nykanen D, et al: Balloon angioplasty of native coarctation: Clinical outcomes and predictors of success. J Am Coll Cardiol 2000;35:988-996.

Pihkala J, Nykanen D, Freedom RM, et al: Interventional cardiac catheterization. Pediatr Clin North Am 1999;46:441-464.

Waldman JD, Wernly JA: Cyanotic congenital heart disease with decreased pulmonary blood flow in children. Pediatr Clin North Am 1999;46: 385-404.

Acute Rheumatic Fever and Rheumatic Heart Disease

Figueroa FE, Fernandez MS, Valdes P, et al: Prospective comparison of clinical and echocardiographic diagnosis of rheumatic carditis: Long term follow up of patients with subclinical disease. Heart 2001;85: 407-410.

Marcus RH, Sareli P, Pocock WA, et al: The spectrum of severe rheumatic mitral valve disease in a developing country. Correlations among clinical presentation, surgical pathologic findings, and hemodynamic sequelae. Ann Intern Med 1994;120:177-183.

Special Writing Group of the Committee on Rheumatic Fever, Endocarditis, and Kawasaki Disease of the Council on Cardiovascular Disease in the Young of the American Heart Association: Guidelines for the diagnosis of rheumatic fever. Jones criteria, 1992 update. JAMA 1992;268:2069-2073.

Stollerman GH: Variation in group A streptococci and the prevalence of rheumatic fever: A half-century vigil. Ann Intern Med 1993;118: 467-469.

Stollerman GH: Rheumatic fever in the 21st century. Clin Infect Dis 2001;33:806-814.

Veasy LG: Time to take soundings in acute rheumatic fever. Lancet 2001;357:1994-1995.

Veasy LG, Tani LY, Hill HR: Persistence of acute rheumatic fever in the intermountain area of the United States. J Pediatr 1994;124:9-16.

Wald ER: Acute rheumatic fever. Curr Probl Pediatr 1993;23:264-270.

Infective Endocarditis

Awadallah SM, Kavey REW, Byrum CJ, et al: The changing pattern of infective endocarditis in childhood. Am J Cardiol 1991;68:90-94.

Baltimore RS: Infective endocarditis in children. Pediatr Infect Dis J 1992;11:907-913.

Bayer AS, Ward JI, Ginzton LE, et al: Evaluation of new clinical criteria for the diagnosis of infective endocarditis. Am J Med 1994;96: 211-218.

Bouza E, Menasalvas A, Munoz P, et al: Infective endocarditis: A prospective study at the end of the twentieth century. Medicine 2001;80: 298-307.

Brook MM: Pediatric bacterial endocarditis: Treatment and prophylaxis. Pediatr Clin North Am 1999;46:275-287.

Carpenter JL: Perivalvular extension of infection in patients with infectious endocarditis. Rev Infect Dis 1991;13:127-138.

Dajani AS, Taubert KA, Wilson W, et al: Prevention of bacterial endocarditis: Recommendations by the American Heart Association. JAMA 1997;277:1794-1801.

Hansen D, Schmiegelow K, Jacobsen JR: Bacterial endocarditis in children: Trends in its diagnosis, course, and prognosis. Pediatr Cardiol 1992;13:198-203.

Mylonakis E, Calerwood SB: Infective endocarditis in adults. N Engl J Med 2001;345:1318-1330.

Saiman L, Prince A, Gersony WM: Pediatric infective endocarditis in the modern era. J Pediatr 1993;122:847-853.

Tolan RW, Kleiman MB, Frank M, et al: Operative intervention in active endocarditis in children: Report of a series of cases and review. Clin Infect Dis 1992;14:852-862.

12 Hypertension

Sharon Bartosh

Blood pressure determination during routine pediatric examinations has revealed significant asymptomatic hypertension secondary to a previously undetected disorder and has also confirmed that mild elevations in blood pressure during childhood are more common than previously recognized, particularly in adolescents. The prevalence of hypertension is approximately 2% in children aged 10 to 15 years.

BLOOD PRESSURE MEASUREMENT IN CHILDREN

The American Medical Association's Task Force on Blood Pressure Control in Children recommends recording blood pressures in all children older than 3 years during both health maintenance visits and emergency visits; blood pressure should also be monitored in infants at high risk for hypertension.

Blood pressure in children is most conveniently measured with a standard clinical sphygmomanometer. The mercury-gravity manometer has the advantage of not needing any calibration while still providing accurate and reliable blood pressure readings. Its reservoir must be properly filled with mercury and be kept dust free. The aneroid type of manometer, which works by means of a metal bellows, can also give accurate readings, but it requires calibration against a mercury manometer fairly regularly: at least yearly, depending on the frequency of use. The stethoscope bell is placed over the brachial artery pulse, proximal and medial to the cubital fossa and below the bottom edge of the cuff, which is approximately 2 cm above the cubital fossa. Correct measurement of blood pressure in children requires the use of a cuff that is appropriate to the size of the child's upper right arm. The right arm is preferred for consistency and comparison with standard tables. The equipment necessary to measure blood pressure in children 3 years of age to adolescence includes three pediatric cuffs of different sizes and the standard adult cuff, a large adult cuff, and a thigh cuff for leg blood pressure measurement. The appropriate cuff should have a bladder width that is approximately 40% of the child's arm circumference when measured at a point midway between the olecranon and the acromion. The cuff bladder usually covers 80% to 100% of the circumference of the arm. If two cuffs are close in size to the measured width of the arm, the larger cuff should be selected; slightly larger cuffs do not usually mask true hypertension, whereas the use of small cuffs often leads to elevated readings. Blood pressure should be measured when the patient is in a controlled environment after 3 to 5 minutes of rest in the seated position, with the cubital fossa supported at heart level. Infants and toddlers may be supine for their blood pressure measurement. The cuff should be inflated to a pressure of 20 to 30 mm Hg above systolic blood pressure, and the cuff deflation rate should be 2 to 3 mm Hg/second. Blood pressure should be recorded at least twice on each occasion, and the average of each systolic and diastolic measurement should be used.

Oscillometric techniques of measurement determine systolic blood pressure and mean arterial pressure by detecting transmitted arterial pulsations. Diastolic blood pressure is calculated from the two measured values. True diastolic blood pressure is not accurately assessed by indirect methods used by automated devices. The use of an automated device is acceptable for pediatric blood pressure measurement in newborns and infants in whom auscultation is difficult, as well as in the intensive care setting, in which frequent blood pressure measurement is needed. There is good reliability of recording blood pressure with some of these instruments in comparison with direct radial artery pressures; however, because of the need for frequent calibration of automated devices and the lack of established reference standards, the recommended method of blood pressure measurement in children is auscultation.

Systolic blood pressure is determined by the onset of the "tapping" Korotkoff sounds. The definition of the diastolic blood pressure is controversial. The muffling of the Korotkoff sounds (the fourth Korotkoff sound) was previously taken as the diastolic pressure in children younger than 13 years. With the evaluation of more children, addition of blood pressure data, and reanalysis of the entire database, it has been determined that the fifth Korotkoff sound can be used to define diastolic blood pressure in children and adults, thereby providing a uniform designation of diastolic blood pressure for all ages. The American Heart Association established the disappearance of sounds (the fifth Korotkoff sound) as the diastolic pressure in children of all ages. In some children, Korotkoff sounds can be heard at 0 mm Hg. This occurrence excludes diastolic hypertension.

Tables 12-1 and 12-2 are the 90th and 95th percentiles of blood pressure readings for boys and girls, respectively, aged 1 to 17 years by percentiles of height. Standards for systolic and diastolic blood pressure for infants younger than 1 year of age are available in the Second Task Force Report (Fig. 12-1). The average systolic blood pressure at 1 day of age in full-term infants is 70 mm Hg, and it increases to 85 mm Hg by 1 month of age. Blood pressure in premature infants is considerably lower and is related more closely to weight than to age. Blood pressure increases at a greater rate in premature infants than in full-term infants during the first year of life; there is a possible inverse relationship between birth weight and risk of hypertension in adulthood. In children younger than 1 year, systolic blood pressure has been used to define hypertension.

Blood pressure measurements in children vary with age, height, cuff bladder size, type of sphygmomanometer used, patient position, time of day, changes in physical activity, emotional stress, and season during which the measurements are taken. This variability can make the diagnosis of hypertension difficult. The definition of hypertension in children is somewhat arbitrary. Because blood pressure values in children are normally distributed, values greater than two standard deviations above the mean are chosen as an arbitrary cutoff point for hypertension. This is based on experience and consensus; there are no studies to confirm that these cutoff points present a significant cardiovascular risk or that they are levels at which antihypertensive treatment is necessary. *Normal blood pressure* is defined as systolic and diastolic blood pressure less than the 90th percentile for age and gender; *high-normal blood pressure* is defined as an average systolic or diastolic blood pressure at the 90th

Table 12-1. Blood Pressure Levels for the 90th and 95th Percentiles of Blood Pressure for Boys Aged 1 to 17 Years by Percentiles of Height

Age (yr)	Blood Pressure Percentile*	Systolic Blood Pressure by Percentile of Height (mm Hg)†							Diastolic Blood Pressure by Percentile of Height (mm Hg)†						
		5%	10%	25%	50%	75%	90%	95%	5%	10%	25%	50%	75%	90%	95%
1	90th	94	95	97	98	100	102	102	50	51	52	53	54	54	55
	95th	98	99	101	102	104	106	106	55	55	56	57	58	59	59
2	90th	98	99	100	102	104	105	106	55	55	56	57	58	59	59
	95th	101	102	104	106	108	109	110	59	59	60	61	62	63	63
3	90th	100	101	103	105	107	108	109	59	59	60	61	62	63	63
	95th	104	105	107	109	111	112	113	63	63	64	65	66	67	67
4	90th	102	103	105	107	109	110	111	62	62	63	64	65	66	66
	95th	106	107	109	111	113	114	115	66	67	67	68	69	70	71
5	90th	104	105	106	108	110	112	112	65	65	66	67	68	69	69
	95th	108	109	110	112	114	115	116	69	70	70	71	72	73	74
6	90th	105	106	108	110	111	113	114	67	68	69	70	70	71	72
	95th	109	110	112	114	115	117	117	72	72	73	74	75	76	76
7	90th	106	107	109	111	113	114	115	69	70	71	72	72	73	74
	95th	110	111	113	115	116	118	119	74	74	75	76	77	78	78
8	90th	107	108	110	112	114	115	116	71	71	72	73	74	75	75
	95th	111	112	114	116	118	119	120	75	76	76	77	78	79	80
9	90th	109	110	112	113	115	117	117	72	73	73	74	75	76	77
	95th	113	114	116	117	119	121	121	76	77	78	79	80	80	81
10	90th	110	112	113	115	117	118	119	73	74	74	75	76	77	78
	95th	114	115	117	119	121	122	123	77	78	79	80	80	81	82
11	90th	112	113	115	117	119	120	121	74	74	75	76	77	78	78
	95th	116	117	119	121	123	124	125	78	79	79	80	81	82	83
12	90th	115	116	117	119	121	123	123	75	75	76	77	78	78	79
	95th	119	120	121	123	125	126	127	79	79	80	81	82	83	83
13	90th	117	118	120	122	124	125	126	75	76	76	77	78	79	80
	95th	121	122	124	126	128	129	130	79	80	81	82	83	83	84
14	90th	120	121	123	125	126	128	128	76	76	77	78	79	80	80
	95th	124	125	127	128	130	132	132	80	81	81	82	83	84	85
15	90th	123	124	125	127	129	131	131	77	77	78	79	80	81	81
	95th	127	128	129	131	133	134	135	81	82	83	83	84	85	86
16	90th	125	126	128	130	132	133	134	79	79	80	81	82	82	83
	95th	129	130	132	134	136	137	138	83	83	84	85	86	87	87
17	90th	128	129	131	133	134	136	136	81	81	82	83	84	85	85
	95th	132	133	135	136	138	140	140	85	85	86	87	88	89	89

From Report of the Second Task Force on Blood Pressure Control in Children—1987. Task Force on Blood Pressure Control in Children, National Heart, Lung, and Blood Institute, Bethesda, Maryland. Pediatrics 1987;79:1-25.

*Blood pressure percentile was determined by a single measurement.

†Height percentile was determined by standard growth curves.

percentile or greater but less than the 95th percentile; and *hypertension* is defined as an average systolic or diastolic blood pressure at the 95th percentile or greater for age and gender, measured on at least three separate occasions.

AMBULATORY BLOOD PRESSURE MONITORING

Ambulatory blood pressure (AMBP) monitoring is superior to intermittent blood pressure measurements in the identification of the hypertensive adult and in predicting which adults will have end-organ damage. It is considered useful for distinguishing constant blood pressure elevation from "white coat hypertension." In children, no studies have identified precisely the degree of increase in casual office blood pressure measurements that is associated with an increased risk of end-organ damage.

Mean AMBP measurements are higher than casual blood pressure measurements, although a significant correlation exists. In comparison with mercury manometers, AMBP monitors appear to be accurate for use in children, with systolic measurements 4 to 6 mm Hg higher than those obtained with simultaneous mercury manometry. Oscillometric mean AMBP values in healthy children are found in Table 12-3. The 95th percentile is usually considered the upper limit of normal for ambulatory blood pressure, but this value is arbitrary.

RACIAL DIFFERENCES

Blood pressure is higher in black children than in white children; however, the differences are not thought to be clinically relevant. The reference standards for children do not distinguish among racial or ethnic groups.

Aside from body size and sexual maturation, other potential mechanisms may contribute to racial differences in blood pressure. Black children demonstrate greater pressor reactivity to both mental and physical stress than do white children. Because black children tend to have lower sympathetic tone than do white children,

Table 12-2. Blood Pressure Levels for the 90th and 95th Percentiles of Blood Pressure for Girls Aged 1 to 17 Years by Percentiles of Height

Age (yr)	Blood Pressure Percentile*	Systolic Blood Pressure by Percentile of Height (mm Hg)[†]							Diastolic Blood Pressure by Percentile of Height (mm Hg)[†]						
		5%	10%	25%	50%	75%	90%	95%	5%	10%	25%	50%	75%	90%	95%
1	90th	97	98	99	100	102	103	104	53	53	53	54	55	56	56
	95th	101	102	103	104	105	107	107	57	57	57	58	59	60	60
2	90th	99	99	100	102	103	104	105	57	57	58	58	59	60	61
	95th	102	103	104	105	107	108	109	61	61	62	62	63	64	65
3	90th	100	100	102	103	104	105	106	61	61	61	62	63	63	64
	95th	104	104	105	107	108	109	110	65	65	65	66	67	67	68
4	90th	101	102	103	104	106	107	108	63	63	64	65	65	66	67
	95th	105	106	107	108	109	111	111	67	67	68	69	69	70	71
5	90th	103	103	104	106	107	108	109	65	66	66	67	68	68	69
	95th	107	107	108	110	111	112	113	69	70	70	71	72	72	73
6	90th	104	105	106	107	109	110	111	67	67	68	69	69	70	71
	95th	108	109	110	111	112	114	114	71	71	72	73	73	74	75
7	90th	106	107	108	109	110	112	112	69	69	69	70	71	72	72
	95th	110	110	112	113	114	115	116	73	73	73	74	75	76	76
8	90th	108	109	110	111	112	113	114	70	70	71	71	72	73	74
	95th	112	112	113	115	116	117	118	74	74	75	75	76	77	78
9	90th	110	110	112	113	114	115	116	71	72	72	73	74	74	75
	95th	114	114	115	117	118	119	120	75	76	76	77	78	78	79
10	90th	112	112	114	115	116	117	118	73	73	73	74	75	76	76
	95th	116	116	117	119	120	121	122	77	77	77	78	79	80	80
11	90th	114	114	116	117	118	119	120	74	74	75	75	76	77	77
	95th	118	118	119	121	122	123	124	78	78	79	79	80	81	81
12	90th	116	116	118	119	120	121	122	75	75	76	76	77	78	78
	95th	120	120	121	123	124	125	126	79	79	80	80	81	82	82
13	90th	118	118	119	121	122	123	124	76	76	77	78	78	79	80
	95th	121	122	123	125	126	127	128	80	80	81	82	82	83	84
14	90th	119	120	121	122	124	125	126	77	77	78	79	79	80	81
	95th	123	124	125	126	128	129	130	81	81	82	83	83	84	85
15	90th	121	121	122	124	125	126	127	78	78	79	79	80	81	82
	95th	124	125	126	128	129	130	131	82	82	83	83	84	85	86
16	90th	122	122	123	125	126	127	128	79	79	79	80	81	82	82
	95th	125	126	127	128	130	131	132	83	83	83	84	85	86	86
17	90th	122	123	124	125	126	128	128	79	79	79	80	81	82	82
	95th	126	126	127	129	130	131	132	83	83	83	84	85	86	86

From Report of the Second Task Force on Blood Pressure Control in Children—1987. Task Force on Blood Pressure Control in Children, National Heart, Lung, and Blood Institute, Bethesda, Maryland. Pediatrics 1987;79:1-25.

*Blood pressure percentile was determined by a single measurement.

[†]Height percentile was determined by standard growth curves.

the stress-associated adrenergic stimulation may lead to a greater proportional increase in peripheral vascular resistance. In addition, black children have lower dopamine β-hydroxylase levels, lower renin levels, slower heart rates, greater peripheral resistance, higher insulin levels, reduced blood glucose levels, and reduced potassium excretion. These racial differences may explain the relative intolerance by black Americans of high dietary sodium intake.

With the known excess prevalence, morbidity, and mortality of essential hypertension among adult black Americans, it is advisable to be vigilant in monitoring blood pressure and to encourage healthy diet, exercise, and weight control behaviors, especially in the presence of a family history of hypertension. This approach seems prudent for other groups such as Asian American adolescents, in whom elevated blood pressures have also been documented.

ESSENTIAL HYPERTENSION

Approximately 25% of the adult population in the United States have hypertension; 90% are classified as having essential hypertension. Before the age of 10 years, essential hypertension is an unusual cause of hypertension; however, it accounts for 30% to 35% of cases of hypertension in children 12 to 18 years of age. Ample evidence supports the concept that the roots of essential hypertension extend into childhood. Often there are other cardiovascular risk factors, such as obesity, a family history of hypertension, and an ethnic predisposition to hypertension.

With increasing age during the preschool years, blood pressure follows a pattern. Children at a given percentile of blood pressure distribution tend to maintain that approximate value ("track") in relation to their peer group as they grow older. This pattern continues from adolescence to adult life. It appears that children with blood pressure measurements that are less than the 50th percentile have

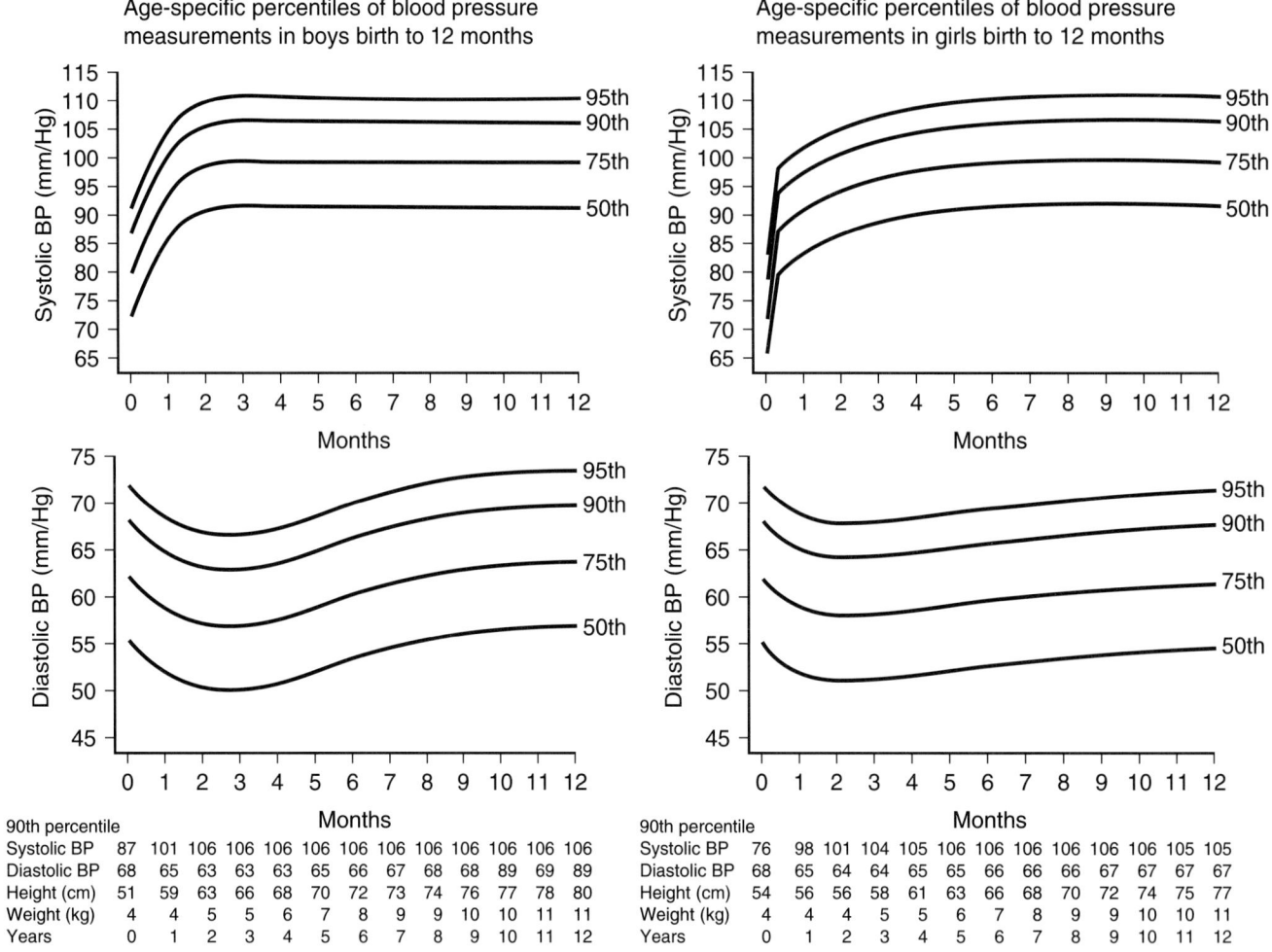

Figure 12-1. Age-specific percentiles for blood pressure in boys and girls from birth to 12 months of age. (From Report of the Second Task Force on Blood Pressure Control in Children—1987. Task Force on Blood Pressure Control in Children, National Heart, Lung, and Blood Institute, Bethesda, Maryland. Pediatrics 1987;79:1-25.)

little risk of having blood pressure measurements in the 90th percentile or higher as young adults. Children from families with hypertension tend to have higher blood pressure than do children from normotensive families. Siblings of children with high blood pressure have significantly higher blood pressure than do siblings of normotensive children. Significant correlations in blood pressure and cardiovascular risk factors exist between parents and their children. These correlations have been observed as early as in the neonatal period.

The causes of essential hypertension may include an altered "reset" point for blood pressure control of sodium excretion; a renal leak of calcium, which leads to decreased ionized serum calcium and increased parathyroid hormone production; insulin resistance; and primary defects in the renin-angiotensin system. Factors that may contribute to the risk of essential hypertension include reactivity of vascular smooth muscles, the interaction of the renin-angiotensin system, cardiac index, obesity, and hormonal and environmental factors. Univariate analysis suggests that a significant proportion of the variability of systolic and diastolic blood pressure is under genetic control. Multivariate analysis demonstrates that in adolescents, genetics and body mass index appear to influence systolic but not diastolic blood pressures. There is a link between the angiotensinogen gene locus on chromosome 1 and essential hypertension.

Several factors known to be associated with essential hypertension in adults have also been correlated with higher blood pressure

in children and adolescents. A direct relationship between weight and blood pressure has been documented as early as 5 years of age and is more prominent in the second decade. The association of obesity and hypertension is believed to be a causal one, wherein obesity not only contributes to higher blood pressure in children and adolescents but also has predictive value for its association with other cardiovascular risk factors such as cholesterol levels and serum lipoprotein ratios. Between 13% and 36% of 12- to 17-year-old adolescents are obese. Depending on gender and race, 4% to 12% may be considered excessively (morbidly) obese.

Environmental factors that interact with genes may have potential effects on blood pressure in young populations; these factors include dietary sodium, potassium, and calcium. Although decreases in dietary sodium intake may lower blood pressure in adults with established hypertension, this effect is less clear in studies of infants and adolescents. The blood pressure response to sodium seen in obese adolescents is correlated with higher fasting plasma insulin concentrations, higher aldosterone levels, and increased activity of the sympathetic nervous system. Sodium sensitivity is linked to race, family history, and obesity. A sustained reduction in sodium intake over years could possibly have an effect on blood pressure. Potassium intake has an inverse relationship with both systolic and diastolic blood pressure in children. Potassium plays a role in the regulation of blood pressure by its induction of natriuresis and suppression of renin production and release. Dietary potassium and

Table 12-3. Oscillometric Mean Ambulatory Blood Pressure Values in Healthy Children: Summary for Clinical Use

Height* (cm)	Percentile for 24-hr period		Daytime percentile[†]		Nighttime percentile[‡]	
	50th	*95th*	*50th*	*95th*	*50th*	*95th*
Boys						
120 (33)	105/65	113/72	112/73	123/85	95/55	104/63
130 (62)	105/65	117/75	113/73	125/85	96/55	107/65
140 (102)	107/65	121/77	114/73	127/85	97/55	110/67
150 (108)	109/66	124/78	115/73	129/85	99/56	113/67
160 (115)	112/66	126/78	118/73	132/85	102/56	116/67
170 (83)	115/67	128/77	121/73	135/85	104/56	119/67
180 (69)	120/67	130/77	124/73	137/85	107/56	122/67
Girls						
120 (40)	103/65	113/73	111/72	120/84	96/55	107/66
130 (58)	105/66	117/75	112/72	124/84	97/55	109/66
140 (70)	108/66	120/76	114/72	127/84	98/55	111/66
150 (111)	110/66	122/76	115/73	129/84	99/55	112/66
160 (156)	111/66	124/76	116/73	131/84	100/55	113/66
170 (109)	112/66	124/76	118/74	131/84	101/55	113/66
180 (25)	113/66	124/76	120/74	131/84	103/55	114/66

From Soergel M, Kirschstein M, Busch C, et al: Oscillometric twenty-four-hour ambulatory blood pressure values in healthy children and adolescents: A multicenter trial including 1141 subjects. J Pediatr 1997;130:178-184.

*Numbers in parentheses are numbers of children studied.

[†]Daytime: 8 AM to 8 PM.

[‡]Nighttime: midnight to 6 AM.

the ratio of potassium to sodium may be more important than dietary sodium alone in its relationship to systolic blood pressure. In addition, there may be an inverse correlation between dietary calcium with blood pressure in children. Salt-sensitive patients or those with low plasma renin activity may be more responsive to calcium supplements.

CARDIOVASCULAR EFFECTS OF HYPERTENSION

Hypertension is the most potent antecedent of cardiovascular disease. In adults, elevated blood pressure accelerates the development of coronary artery disease and contributes significantly to the pathogenesis of cerebrovascular accidents, heart failure, and renal failure. Autopsy studies in children have shown significant associations between blood pressure measurements and the degree of vascular atherosclerotic involvement.

In addition, children and adolescents have shown cardiac ventricular and hemodynamic changes consistent with an adverse effect of mild hypertension. Left ventricular wall thickness and the ratio of left ventricular thickness to chamber size are correlated with systolic blood pressure in children. Neither parameter is correlated with diastolic blood pressure. Left ventricular wall thickness increases throughout the entire systolic blood pressure distribution, which indicates that even within the "normal" range of blood pressure in healthy children, higher systolic blood pressure is associated with increased left ventricular size. The adverse effect of hypertension on cardiovascular function is also compounded by obesity. Left ventricular hypertrophy caused by obesity begins in childhood.

Cardiovascular risk factors tend to aggregate and usually appear in combination. Such combinations are present in childhood and persist into early adulthood. Multiple risk factors increase the probability of cardiovascular events because cardiovascular risk factors tend to reinforce each other in their influence on morbidity and mortality.

EVALUATION

When hypertension manifests in a child, a thorough diagnostic evaluation should be undertaken. Secondary hypertension accounts for 5% to 15% of cases of persistent hypertension in children and adolescents. The likelihood of identifying a secondary cause of hypertension is directly related to the degree of blood pressure elevation and inversely related to the age of the child. The most common causes of hypertension seen in children of varying ages are found in Table 12-4. A more complete list of potential secondary causes of hypertension is found in Table 12-5. Most children with secondary hypertension have renal parenchymal or renovascular disease; coarctation of the aorta and endocrine disorders are the next most common causes.

The Task Force on Blood Pressure Control in Children offers an excellent algorithm for guiding the evaluation of the hypertensive child after a thorough history and physical examination (Fig. 12-2). The hypertension-oriented historical information is found in Table 12-6. Guidelines for the hypertension-focused physical examination are found in Table 12-7. The evaluation occurs in steps or phases (Table 12-8 and Fig. 12-3), starting with basic screening studies and progressing to more intricate and invasive studies if warranted. A stepwise evaluation is not appropriate in children with very severe blood pressure elevations and in very young children with persistent hypertension. Phasing of the evaluation is intended to proceed most quickly in the young child and more slowly in the older child, especially if the child has no signs of end-organ (brain, eye, renal, heart) dysfunction. Phase I investigations should include electrolyte and renal function determination, urine culture, and urinalysis, as well as measurement of serum uric acid, hematocrit, and serum lipid profile (particularly if essential hypertension is suspected). The renal ultrasound study, including Doppler blood flow determination, is a simple and informative noninvasive test that is appropriate early in the evaluation of the hypertensive child. Phase II and III evaluations are designed to identify particular diagnoses.

Severe elevations of blood pressure, regardless of age, warrant aggressive evaluation. Approximately 60% to 80% of secondary

Table 12-4. **Common Basic Etiologies of Hypertension**

Newborn
Renal artery thrombosis
Renal artery stenosis
Renal venous thrombosis
Congenital renal abnormalities
Coarctation of the aorta
Bronchopulmonary dysplasia (less common)
Patent ductus arteriosus (less common)
Intraventricular hemorrhage (less common)
Endocrine causes (less common)

First Year
Coarctation of the aorta
Renovascular disease
Renal parenchymal disease

Ages 1 to 6 Years
Renal parenchymal disease
Renovascular disease
Coarctation of the aorta
Endocrine causes (less common)
Essential hypertension (less common)

Ages 6 to 12 Years
Renal parenchymal disease
Renovascular disease
Essential hypertension
Coarctation of the aorta
Endocrine causes (less common)
Iatrogenic causes (less common)

Ages 12 to 18 Years
Essential hypertension
Iatrogenic causes
Renal parenchymal disease
Renovascular disease (less common)
Endocrine causes (less common)
Coarctation of the aorta (less common)

Interpretation of the results is based on the normal renin activity for the age of the child, the norms for the laboratory being used, and the conditions of the sampling.

In all young children with hypertension, renovascular disease should be strongly suspected. The initial evaluation includes assessment of renal anatomy and blood flow. Although the "gold standard" for the evaluation of renovascular disease is renal arteriography with segmental renal vein renin sampling, the inherent difficulties in performing these studies in young children have led to the evaluation of alternative techniques. Doppler ultrasound studies may identify main renal artery stenosis but not intrarenal lesions and are thus insufficient to replace angiography in all hypertensive children believed to be at high risk for renovascular disease. Other diagnostic techniques include the captopril challenge test, captopril-enhanced radionuclide scans, color Doppler sonography with or without contrast or ACE inhibition, digital subtraction angiography, computed tomographic spiral angiography, and magnetic resonance arteriography. The choice of test is often determined by local experience and equipment.

The evaluation of a hypertensive child includes identifying a cause and determining target organ dysfunction. The target organ arm of the assessment should include funduscopy and echocardiography, which assist in determining the chronicity and the severity of the hypertension. Funduscopy rarely discloses hemorrhages or exudates but may reveal arteriolar narrowing and arteriovenous nicking. Echocardiography is more sensitive than electrocardiography for detecting early left ventricular hypertrophy secondary to hypertension.

TREATMENT

The goals of treatment of hypertension in children are to reduce the blood pressure below the 95th percentile and to prevent long-term organ effects of persistent hypertension. The available means of treatment include nonpharmacologic and pharmacologic methods.

NONPHARMACOLOGIC THERAPY

Nonpharmacologic therapy should be used as initial treatment for children with blood pressure exceeding the 90th percentile for age, gender, and height. These include the prevention and treatment of obesity, decreasing excessive sodium intake, and performing exercise. Nonpharmacologic interventions may be used in the initial treatment of mild pediatric hypertension, in the absence of end-organ damage, or they may also be adjuncts to drug therapy in early primary hypertension.

Improvement in physical fitness is correlated inversely with blood pressure in young children. Obese adolescents demonstrate reductions in blood pressure with weight loss; the effect is enhanced when exercise is incorporated into the weight-loss program. In children with borderline hypertension, treatment should include lifestyle changes with careful and frequent monitoring of blood pressure. If a child's blood pressure is in the high-normal category (between the 90th and 95th percentiles for age and height) and if a child is considered obese, a trial of weight loss is first recommended with continued monitoring of blood pressure. If high-normal blood pressure readings cannot be accounted for by weight, the child should be monitored closely, at least every 6 months (see Fig. 12-2).

Exercise, particularly aerobic activity, has been shown to have beneficial effects on blood pressure in hypertensive adolescents. Adolescents should participate in aerobic exercise for at least 30 minutes three to four times per week.

In contrast to adults, in whom an association between dietary salt intake and blood pressure has been well established, the importance of sodium intake on blood pressure in children is less clear. Because daily sodium intake often dramatically exceeds recommended

hypertension in childhood is caused by renal parenchymal disease. Adolescents with mild hypertension do not require an extensive workup. The diagnostic tests should focus on excluding renal disease. In the first year of life, virtually all hypertension is secondary, and affected infants in whom no cause is found are still suspected of having secondary hypertension.

Renovascular disease is one of the most common and important identifiable causes of childhood hypertension and is amenable to treatment or cure. Approximately 5% to 25% of children with secondary hypertension have renovascular disease. Children younger than 5 years are four times more likely than adolescents to have renal artery stenosis. Among neonates, the prevalence of renal artery stenosis as a cause of severe hypertension exceeded 90% in one series. Fibromuscular dysplasia is the most frequent cause of renovascular hypertension in childhood. Clues to the presence of renal vascular disease include a normal urinalysis and normal blood urea nitrogen and creatinine measurements, as well as the presence of café au lait spots, an abdominal bruit, normal upper and lower extremity blood pressures, and a positive family history of youth-onset hypertension. Patients with renal artery stenosis often have high circulating or selective renal vein renin levels. Peripheral plasma renin activity is influenced by a variety of blood volume–related and hormonal factors, as well as by dietary salt intake and many medications. It is critical to obtain an initial plasma renin activity value before the administration of a diuretic or first dose of an angiotensin-converting enzyme (ACE) inhibitor.

Table 12-5. Secondary Causes of Hypertension

Endocrine Causes

Hyperthyroidism (systolic only)
Congenital adrenal hyperplasia
Primary aldosteronism
Hyperparathyroidism
17-hydroxylase deficiency
Cushing syndrome
Hypercalcemia
Conn syndrome
11-hydroxylase deficiency
Pseudohypoaldosteronism type II
Liddle syndrome
Pheochromocytoma

Renal Causes

Acute nephritis (idiopathic and postinfectious)
Acute tubular necrosis
Interstitial nephritis
Familial nephritis
Diabetic nephropathy
Anaphylactoid purpura (Henoch-Schönlein purpura)
Collagen vascular disease
Hemolytic uremic syndrome
Renal trauma
Acute obstruction
Page kidney (fibrous encapsulation of kidney)
Reflux nephropathy
Obstructive uropathy
Multicystic-dysplastic kidney
Tuberous sclerosis
Polycystic kidney disease
Congenital nephrotic syndrome
Chronic renal failure
Renal transplantation (related to rejection, medications, renal artery stenosis)

Pulmonary Causes

Bronchopulmonary dysplasia
Pneumothorax

Renovascular Causes

Renal artery disease: intrinsic (e.g., fibromuscular dysplasia) or extrinsic
Renal artery or vein thrombosis
Congenital rubella syndrome
Neurofibromatosis
Idiopathic arterial calcification in infants
Posttrauma hematoma
Retroperitoneal fibrosis
Lymphadenopathy
Inflammatory stenosis (e.g., Takayasu arteritis; moyamoya and Kawasaki syndromes; sarcoidosis; aortitis)

Cardiac/Vascular Causes

Coarctation of aorta
Patent ductus arteriosus
Coarctation repair
Hypoplasia of abdominal aorta
Takayasu arteritis
Subacute bacterial endocarditis

Central and Autonomic Nervous System Causes

Increased intracranial pressure
Guillain-Barré syndrome
Familial dysautonomia (Riley-Day syndrome)
Burns
Posterior fossa lesions
Poliomyelitis
Encephalitis
Porphyria
Subdural hematoma
Seizures
Pain
Sleep apnea

Medications/Intoxications

Theophylline
Caffeine
Phenylephrine
Amphetamines
Ephedrine
Lead
Mercury
Cadmium
Cyclosporine
Tacrolimus
Oral contraceptives
Glucocorticoids and mineralocorticoids
Cocaine
Maternal heroin
Phencyclidine
Reserpine overdose
Vitamin D intoxication in infancy
Antihypertensive withdrawal (clonidine, methyldopa, propranolol)
Thallium
Licorice (glycyrrhizic acid)
Pancuronium

Neoplasia

Wilms tumor
Nephroblastoma
Leukemic infiltration of kidney
Pheochromocytoma
Ovarian tumor
Neuroblastoma
Mesoblastic nephroma
Lymphoma

Miscellaneous

Leg traction with stretching of femoral nerve
Cyclic vomiting with dehydration
Stevens-Johnson syndrome
Polycythemia
Anemia (systolic only)
Abdominal wall defect closure in infants
Extracorporeal membrane oxygenation

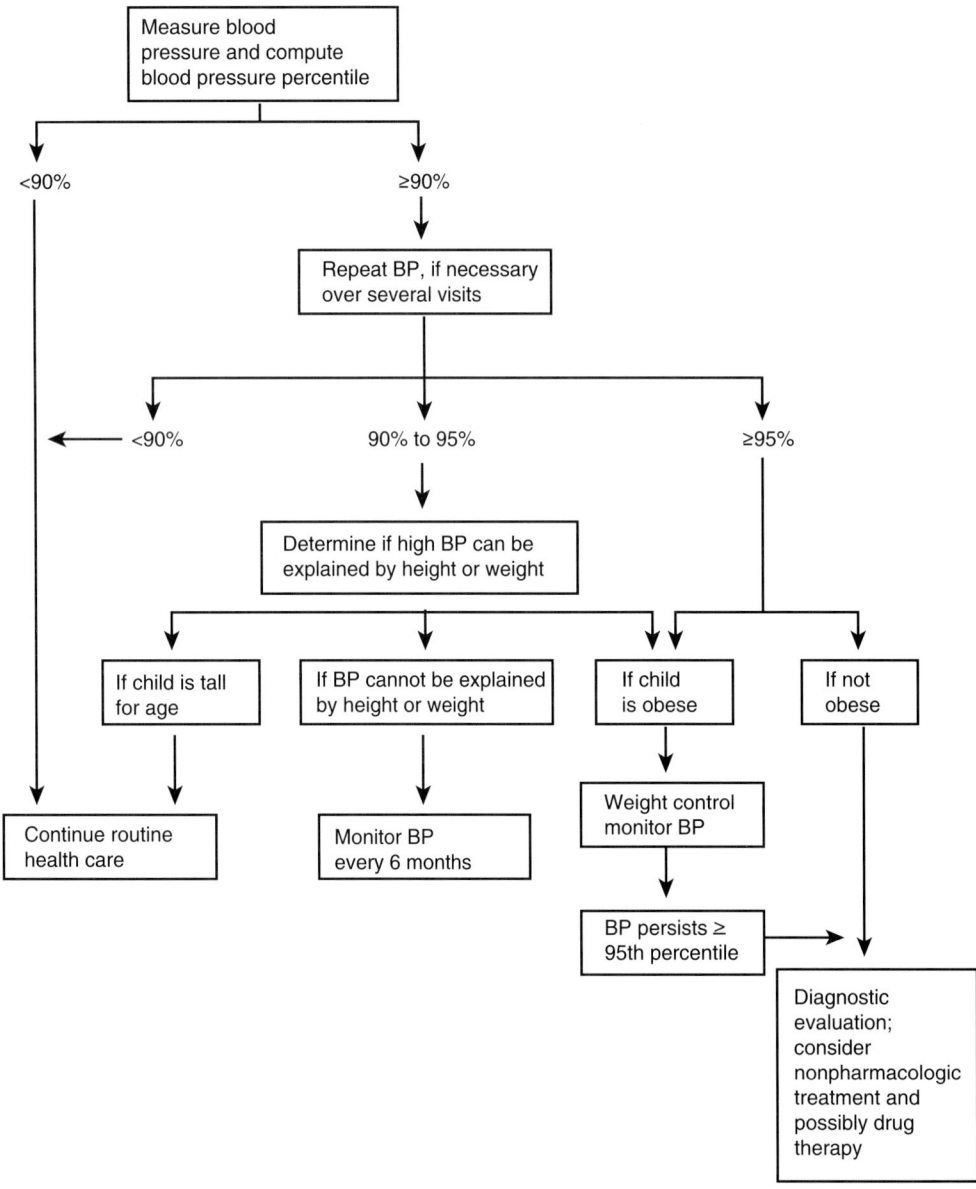

Figure 12-2. Algorithm for detecting and treating hypertension in children. BP, blood pressure. (Modified from Report of the Second Task Force on Blood Pressure Control in Children—1987. Task Force on Blood Pressure Control in Children, National Heart, Lung, and Blood Institute, Bethesda, Maryland. Pediatrics 1987;79:1-25.)

amounts because of dietary modification in the obese child, a moderate reduction in dietary sodium can be beneficial. Salt restriction has been said to be of benefit in 25% of hypertensive adolescents. Sodium intake should be reduced to no more than 2 g per day.

PHARMACOLOGIC THERAPY

Pharmacologic therapy should be administered to children who have severe hypertension, have evidence of end-organ damage, or do not respond to nonpharmacologic measures. A "stepped care" approach in the pharmacologic treatment of hypertension is recommended. It begins with a low dose of a single antihypertensive agent, followed by an increase in the dosage until blood pressure levels are controlled, the maximum dosage is reached, or adverse effects appear. If blood pressure is not lowered to an adequate level, the next step is either to replace the first drug or to add a second drug, proceeding as with the initial step. If a combination of two drugs fails to control blood pressure, a secondary cause should be more rigorously sought. It is advisable that a pediatric specialist skilled in treating refractory forms of hypertension be consulted before a third drug is added to the regimen.

Calcium Channel Blockers

Calcium channel blockers inhibit inward flux of calcium via voltage-dependent slow channels in the cellular membrane. They reduce blood pressure by dilating peripheral arterioles in a dose-dependent manner. They cause modest increases in heart rate and cardiac output shortly after initiation of therapy. In infants, they may have a severe negative inotropic effect and cause heart failure or shock. This class of drugs is preferred in patients with impaired renal function, because most of them are almost completely metabolized in the liver. Side effects include headache, flushing, and tachycardia. Gingival hyperplasia and lower extremity edema are two adverse effects unique to calcium channel blockers. Gingival hyperplasia has been reported with amlodipine, felodipine, nifedipine, and verapamil.

Nifedipine, amlodipine, isradipine, nicardipine, and felodipine are the most commonly prescribed calcium channel blockers in children. Although numerous case reports document therapy with these agents in children, few controlled studies are available for defining optimal dosages and long-term safety and efficacy.

Nifedipine is absorbed rapidly when the immediate-release form is taken sublingually or swallowed. It is important to note that during

Table 12-6. Historical Information to Elicit in the Diagnostic Evaluation of Hypertension

Information	Potential Relevance
Symptoms Referable to Hypertension	
Headaches, epistaxis, dizziness, chest pain, visual disturbances	Nonspecific
Failure to thrive, vomiting, lethargy or irritability, respiratory disturbances	Nonspecific in neonates
Questions Referable to a Renal Cause	
Gross hematuria, edema	Nephritis
UTIs, dysuria, frequency, urgency, enuresis	Pyelonephritic scarring
Flank or abdominal pain, gross hematuria	Polycystic kidney disease, obstruction, renal calculi
Polyuria, polydipsia	Tubulointerstitial disease
Use of umbilical catheter in nursery	Renal vessel thrombosis/stenosis
Rashes, weight loss, fevers, joint symptoms, oral ulcers	Connective tissue disease and/or other forms of nephritis
Questions Referable to an Endocrine Cause	
Weight loss, failure to gain weight with good appetite, sweating, flushing, fevers, palpitations, diarrhea	In combination, symptoms suggest pheochromocytoma
Weight loss, palpitations, diarrhea	Hyperthyroidism
Muscle cramps, weakness, constipation	Hypokalemia, hyperaldosteronism
Age at onset of menarche, sexual development	Hydroxylase deficiencies
Family History	
Hypertension, preeclampsia, renal disease, tumors	Essential hypertension, inherited renal disease and some endocrine diseases (e.g., familial pheochromocytoma with multiple endocrinopathy II), neurofibromatosis, tuberous sclerosis
Drugs	
Prescription and over-the-counter drugs, contraceptives, illicit drugs	Drug-induced hypertension

UTI, urinary tract infection.

"sublingual" administration, in reality, no absorption of the drug occurs in the mouth itself; rather, it is likely that all absorption occurs in the gastrointestinal tract after swallowing. The short duration of action and the unpredictable hypotensive effects of the short-acting preparation limit its usefulness for long-term treatment. When nifedipine is given sublingually to an infant or young child, the liquid is drawn up from the capsule into a large bore needle and squirted under the tongue. Each 10-mg capsule of nifedipine contains 0.34 mL of drug. The extended-release formulation is preferred in children who can swallow tablets. This form should not be cut or crushed, and the large pill size limits its use in younger children.

Amlodipine has the longest duration of action of any of the drugs of this class and once-daily administration is effective in adults. Published studies in children taking amlodipine have suggested that twice-daily dosing may be necessary in some children to achieve adequate blood pressure control. Because of the long half-life of amlodipine, dosage adjustments should be 5 to 7 days apart. Reported dosages in children have varied widely, and children seem to require higher doses of amlodipine on a per kilogram basis than those recommended for adults; the youngest children require the highest doses. Adverse effects include fatigue, headache, dizziness, abdominal pain, peripheral edema, flushing, and chest pain. With the potential for once-daily dosing, good effectiveness, and lack of reflex tachycardia, it has distinct advantages over nifedipine in pediatric patients. Infants and small children can receive doses either in crushed tablets or in a suspension made in the pharmacy.

One of the shortest-acting agents in this class is isradipine. Administration is required every 6 to 8 hours. Isradipine is available in powder-filled capsules that can be opened to prepare an oral suspension, which has been shown to be stable for up to 30 days.

Angiotensin-Converting Enzyme Inhibitors

ACE inhibitors are used to treat chronic pediatric hypertension because of their ease of administration and the relative lack of severe adverse effects. They decrease blood pressure by inhibiting formation of angiotensin II, a major vasoconstrictor in most vascular beds and a primary stimulus to aldosterone production, and by inactivating the kinases that degrade bradykinin, a potent vasodilator. They also have positive benefits on cardiac function, peripheral vasculature tone, and renal function. ACE inhibitors reduce proteinuria and preserve renal function in patients with renal disease, probably as a result of a decrease in glomerular capillary pressure. Side effects include neutropenia and agranulocytosis, rashes and angioedema of the face, persistent cough, and a taste disturbance. ACE inhibitors should be avoided during pregnancy.

Captopril is the most widely studied ACE inhibitor in children. It reduces both systemic vascular resistance and left ventricular pressure, and it causes negative inotropic and chronotropic effects. Captopril is generally given two to three times per day. ACE inhibitors do not have a dose-response effect. Blood pressure tends to fall gradually until the converting enzyme is inhibited by 90%, at which time a precipitous drop in blood pressure may occur. It is reasonable to begin captopril therapy at 0.3-0.5 mg/kg/dose in children 6 months of age or older. Neonates and infants have an increased response and a longer duration of action after administration of captopril than do older children. The International Collaborative Study Group recommends 0.02 to 2 mg/kg/day in premature infants and those up to 6 months of age.

Enalapril has a longer half-life that allows once-daily dosing, and its efficacy is similar to that of captopril in controlling blood pressure.

Table 12-7. Findings to Look For on Physical Examination

Physical Findings	Potential Relevance
General	
Pale mucous membranes, edema, growth retardation	Chronic renal disease
Elfin facies, poor growth, retardation	Williams syndrome
Webbing of neck, low hairline, widespread nipples, wide carrying angle	Turner syndrome
Moon face, buffalo hump, hirsutism, truncal obesity, striae	Cushing syndrome
Habitus	
Thinness	Pheochromocytoma, renal disease, hyperthyroidism
Virilization	Congenital adrenal hyperplasia
Rickets	Chronic renal disease
Skin	
Café au lait spots, neurofibromas	Neurofibromatosis, pheochromocytoma
Tubers, "ash-leaf" spots	Tuberous sclerosis
Rashes	SLE, vasculitis (HSP), impetigo with acute nephritis
Pallor, evanescent flushing, sweating	Pheochromocytoma
Needle tracks	Illicit drug use
Bruises, striae	Cushing syndrome
Eyes	
Extraocular muscle palsy	Nonspecific, chronic, severe
Fundal changes	Nonspecific, chronic, severe
Proptosis	Hyperthyroidism
Head and Neck	
Goiter	Thyroid disease
Cardiovascular Signs	
Absent or diminished femoral pulses, low leg pressure relative to arm pressure	Aortic coarctation
Heart size, rate, rhythm; murmurs; respiratory difficulty, hepatomegaly	Aortic coarctation, congestive heart failure
Bruits over great vessels	Arteritis or arteriopathy
Rub	Pericardial effusion secondary to chronic renal disease
Pulmonary Signs	
Pulmonary edema	Congestive heart failure, acute nephritis
Picture of bronchopulmonary dysplasia (BPD)	BPD-associated hypertension
Abdomen	
Epigastric bruit	Primary renovascular disease or in association with Williams syndrome, neurofibromatosis, fibromuscular dysplasia, or arteritis
Abdominal masses	Wilms tumor, neuroblastoma, pheochromocytoma, polycystic kidneys, hydronephrosis
Neurologic Signs	
Neurologic deficits	Chronic or severe acute hypertension with stroke
Genitalia	
Ambiguous, virilized	Congenital adrenal hyperplasia

HSP, Henoch-Schönlein purpura; SLE, systemic lupus erythematosus.

β-Adrenergic Blockers

β-Adrenergic receptor–blocking agents are not as widely advocated for treatment of pediatric hypertension as are calcium channel blockers or ACE inhibitors, probably because of concerns related to their long-term effects on lipid profiles, their tendency to cause drowsiness, and the inability to use this class of drugs comfortably in patients with asthma. These drugs decrease cardiac output, inhibit renin secretion, and reduce peripheral vascular resistance. Agents used in children include propranolol, atenolol, metoprolol, and labetalol. Propranolol has been used extensively; adverse effects include bradycardia, hypoglycemia, asthma, night terrors, and heart block.

Cardioselective agents such as atenolol and metoprolol may be used, although at higher dosages, cardioselectivity may be lost. Metoprolol blunts the systolic blood pressure and heart rate response to aerobic exercise and mental stress. Metoprolol is not associated with limitation in endurance capacity as measured by exercise stress tests; heart rates increase to maximal levels, which suggests that this agent may be effective in the athletic child.

Labetalol is a β-adrenergic blocker that also has α-blocking properties in a 4:1 ratio. Experience with this drug in treating pediatric chronic hypertension is limited, but its lack of effect on lipid concentrations and exercise tolerance make it potentially useful

Table 12-8. Stepped Approach to Evaluation of Pediatric Hypertension

Phase I

Careful history and physical examination
Complete blood cell count
Urinalysis
Urine culture (if secondary hypertension suspected)
Blood urea nitrogen, creatinine measurements (estimate glomerular infiltration rate)
Electrolyte, glucose, calcium, uric acid measurements
Lipid profile (if primary hypertension suspected)
Thyroid studies (if clinically indicated)
Renal ultrasonography and Doppler flow study
Echocardiography
Funduscopic examination

Phase II

Voiding cystography
Renal radionuclide scan
Non-invasive renovascular imaging
Plasma renin activity and aldosterone measurements
Abdominal ultrasonography or computed tomography for nonrenal imaging
Urine catecholamine and metabolite measurements
Plasma catecholamine measurements with/without clonidine suppression
Urinary aldosterone and electrolyte measurements with/without salt loading
Other urine and/or plasma hormone (e.g., free cortisol, 18-hydroxycorticosterone) measurements
Captopril challenge
Renin profiling (with/without loop diuretic)

Phase III

Arteriography (conventional or digital subtraction angiography)
Renal vein renin sampling
Metaiodobenzylguanidine scans of adrenal glands
Vena caval sampling for catecholamines
Renal biopsy

for treating adolescents. A major therapeutic indication for labetalol is in the treatment of hypertensive crises.

Diuretics

Diuretics are not first-line agents in treating hypertension. Diuretics reduce plasma volume, decrease peripheral vascular resistance, and reduce systemic blood pressure. They may be useful if multidrug treatment is required or if sodium and water retention are present. Thiazide diuretics are often given to treat mild hypertension and are the diuretics of choice in patients with normal glomerular filtration rates; they are ineffective when the glomerular filtration rate is less than 30% of normal (with the exception of metolazone). Spironolactone is the only potassium-sparing diuretic commonly given to children. Its principal indication is for hypertension caused by mineralocorticoid excess. It does not appear to be as effective as loop or thiazide diuretics in treating other forms of hypertension. Furosemide is the most commonly prescribed loop diuretic and is very effective in patients with hypertension caused by renal disease.

Diuretics are generally well tolerated in children but should be avoided in patients with salt-wasting nephropathies or adrenal insufficiency and in athletic adolescents because of the possibility of cramps and dehydration. Side effects include hyperuricemia, hyperlipidemia, and hypokalemia.

Other Agents

α-Adrenergic agonists such as clonidine, α-adrenergic antagonists such as prazosin, and vasodilators such as minoxidil and hydralazine are available for treatment of hypertension necessitating multiple drugs.

In general, drug use should be individualized to each patient, depending on the severity of hypertension, adverse effects, and medical history. Available medications and their pediatric doses are found in Table 12-9. ACE inhibitors and calcium channel blockers have become primary agents for the management of pediatric hypertension. Potential side effects of antihypertensive drugs are found in Table 12-10. Contraindications to the use of various antihypertensive medications are found in Table 12-11.

HYPERTENSIVE CRISES

Severe hypertension represents a threat to life or to the vital function of organs; disruptions in organ function may manifest as cardiac failure, renal failure, or neurologic dysfunction. *Severe hypertension* is defined as blood pressure exceeding the 99th percentile for age. The cause of severe hypertension in childhood is, in the majority of cases, some form of underlying renal disease. Other possible causes include renovascular disease and illicit drug abuse.

A *hypertensive emergency* refers to hypertension of such an extreme degree (1.3 to 1.5 times the 95th percentile) that it is associated with evidence of end-organ damage or dysfunction, such as cerebral infarction, pulmonary edema, hypertensive encephalopathy, or cerebral hemorrhage. Hypertensive crises in children are most likely secondary to drug abuse, collagen-vascular disease, acute glomerulonephritis, renovascular hypertension, or head trauma.

Hypertensive urgency describes blood pressure that is markedly increased but without accompanying end-organ damage. In hypertensive urgency, blood pressure can be gradually reduced within a few days to avoid serious sequelae. Chest radiography, head computed tomography, and electrocardiography or echocardiography may be indicated to establish whether the situation is a hypertensive emergency or urgency.

The pathogenesis of hypertensive crises may involve failure in cerebral autoregulation with secondary cerebral edema. If a hypertensive patient presents with severe headache or clouding of the sensorium, with or without a convulsion, rapid decrease in blood pressure is mandatory. The lowering of blood pressure, however, should not occur so rapidly as to cause further damage. Long-standing hypertension may lead to subintimal cellular proliferation, which may be sufficient to occlude the lumina and has important implications in terms of the ischemic complications that can be seen in severely hypertensive situations when blood pressure is lowered too rapidly. Furthermore, markedly increased blood pressure affects the autoregulatory mechanism that maintains adequate blood flow to viscera across wide ranges of arterial pressures. This is particularly relevant to the cerebral circulation. In patients with long-standing hypertension, the range is reset upward. Such individuals may be less able to compensate for sudden falls in pressure, which, at a level well tolerated with normal autoregulation, might cause cerebral infarction, transverse ischemic myelopathy, or blindness when watershed vascular beds become compromised with a decline in pressure. Too-rapid lowering of blood pressure is quite dangerous, and for that reason, rapid-acting agents such as diazoxide should be considered only when other modalities are not available.

There is wide variability among patients with regard to tolerance of high blood pressure. Signs and symptoms of severe hypertension in children vary considerably and include seizures, visual symptoms, retinopathy, altered mental status, hemiplegia, facial nerve palsy, headache, vomiting, epistaxis, papilledema, and left-sided heart failure. Differentiating neurologic symptoms caused by hypertension from hypertension that is secondary to neurologic disease with increased intracranial pressure may be difficult, although in patients

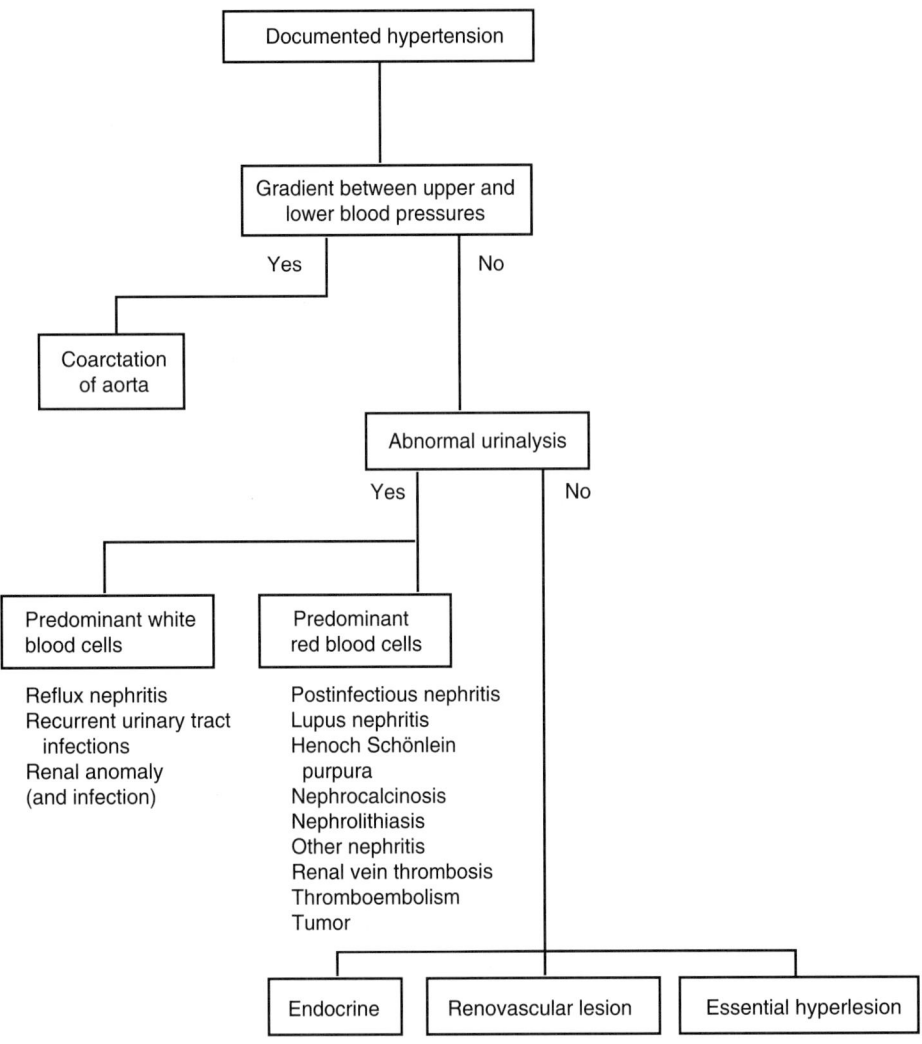

Figure 12-3. Initial diagnostic algorithm in the evaluation of hypertension.

with increased intracranial pressure, the rise in blood pressure is primarily systolic, and bradycardia and irregular respirations may also be present. Diastolic hypertension tends to occur fairly late in the course of the disease when secondary to intracranial hypertension. Similarly, children with seizures may have a secondary increase in blood pressure. Differentiating hypertension as the cause of a seizure from hypertension secondary to a seizure may be possible on the basis of the magnitude of increase of blood pressure in the postictal period. Among children with severe systemic hypertension, hypertensive retinopathy occurs in 27%, encephalopathy in 25%, seizures in 25%, left ventricular hypertrophy in 12%, visual symptoms in 9%, facial palsy in 13%, and hemiplegia in 8%. In neonates, common clinical manifestations of hypertension include tachypnea, cardiomegaly, congestive heart failure, lethargy, seizures, retinopathy, and failure to thrive. Even in the presence of severe hypertension, some neonates remain asymptomatic.

The goal of treatment in severe hypertension is to prevent hypertension-related adverse events by a controlled reduction of blood pressure, allowing preservation of target end-organ function and minimizing complications of therapy. Rapid reduction is not recommended, because of the risk of sudden hypotension, failure of autoregulatory mechanisms, and the possibility of cerebral and visceral ischemia. A reduction of the blood pressure in the first 6 hours by one third of the amount to be reduced, followed by another third over the next 24 to 36 hours and the last third by the final 48 to 72 hours,

appears prudent, although there are no universal recommendations addressing the optimal rate of reduction. Careful attention to pupillary responses, vision, level of consciousness, and neurologic examination is necessary. The therapeutic agents available for managing severe, life-threatening hypertension are most frequently administered intravenously in an intensive care unit with continuous blood pressure monitoring. These drugs should ideally have short half-lives, which allow for careful but swift modification of therapy according to response. Labetalol, sodium nitroprusside, and nicardipine are used for this purpose. Alternative intravenous agents that have been recommended include hydralazine, esmolol, and enalaprilat (Table 12-12).

Sodium nitroprusside is a vasodilator, acting equally on arteries and veins. It increases renal blood flow with minimal direct effects on cardiac output. Onset of action is instantaneous, and blood pressure returns to previous levels within 30 to 60 seconds after the infusion is discontinued. Because of the lower frequency of hypotension-induced ischemia, it is safer than bolus injections of diazoxide. The recommended starting dose of nitroprusside in pediatric patients is 0.3 to 0.5 µg/kg/minute, with stepwise increases up to 8 µg/kg/minute. If sodium nitroprusside is utilized for more than a few days, monitoring of blood cyanide or plasma cyanate levels is necessary. Neurologic symptoms secondary to an accumulation of thiocyanate include vomiting, nausea, disorientation, hallucination, and anorexia. Inhibition of oxidative phosphorylation at the cellular

Table 12-9. Pharmacologic Treatment of Chronic Hypertension in Children

Drug	Dosage	Comments
Diuretics		
Hydrochlorothiazide	1-3 mg/kg/day PO in divided doses q12h (max, 200 mg/day)	Monitor for ↓ K,↑ glu, ↑ uric acid
Chlorothiazide	Neonates: 20-40 mg/kg/day PO in divided doses q12h (max, 375 mg/day) Children > 6 months: 20 mg/kg/day PO in divided doses q12h (max, 1 g/day)	Monitor for ↓ K,↑ glu, ↑ uric acid
Chlorthalidone	0.5-2 mg/kg PO q24h	Longer lasting than thiazides; monitor for ↓ K, ↑ glu, ↑ uric acid
Furosemide	1-3 mg/kg/day PO in divided doses q6-12h	Loop diuretic; monitor for ↓ K,↑ glu, ↑ uric acid, hypercalciuria, ototoxicity
Ethacrynic acid	1-3 mg/kg/day PO in divided doses q6-12h	Loop diuretic; monitor for ↓ K, ↑ glu, ↑ acid, ototoxicity
Bumetanide	0.02-0.3 mg/kg/day PO in divided doses q6-24h (max, 10 mg/day)	Loop diuretic; monitor for ↓ K, ↑ glu, ↑uric acid
Spironolactone	1-3 mg/kg/day PO in divided doses q6-24h	Aldosterone antagonist
Triamterene	2-6 mg/kg/day PO in divided doses q12-24h (max, 300 mg/day)	Distal tubule blocker of Na:K exchange
Metolazone	0.1-0.3 mg/kg/day PO in divided doses q12-24h	Inhibits Na reabsorption
Vasodilators		
Hydralazine	0.75-7.5 mg/kg/day PO in divided doses q6-8h (max, 200 mg/day)	↑ Heart rate; headache, lupus-like syndrome (rare in pediatric patients)
Minoxidil	0.1-1 mg/kg/day PO in divided doses q12-24h	Salt and water retention, hirsutism
α-Adrenergic Antagonists		
Prazosin	0.01-0.4 mg/kg/day PO in divided doses q8-12h (max 15 mg/day)	First dose is given with patient supine
Calcium Channel Blockers		
Nifedipine (extended release)	0.25-3 mg/kg/day PO in divided doses q12-24h (max, 180 mg/day)	↑ Heart rate, flushing, headache, dizziness, fluid retention; tablet must be swallowed whole
Amlodipine	0.1-0.6 mg/kg/day PO in divided doses q12-24h (max, 20 mg/day)	Dosage adjustments 5-7 days apart; suspension can be compounded; ↑ cyclosporine levels
Diltiazem	1.5-3.5 mg/kg/day PO in divided doses q6-8h (max, 360 mg/day)	↑ Cyclosporine levels
Felodipine (extended release)	0.1-0.6 mg/kg/day PO in divided doses q12-24h (max, 20 mg/day)	Tablet must be swallowed whole; ↑ cyclosporine levels
Isradipine	0.1-0.8 mg/kg/day PO in divided doses q6-8h (max, 20 mg/day)	Rapidly acting; suspension may be compounded for infants and toddlers
Verapamil	3-8 mg/kg/day PO in divided doses q8h (max, 480 mg/day)	Avoid concomitant administration of β-adrenergic blockers; ↑ cyclosporine levels
β-Adrenergic Antagonists		
Propranolol	0.5-8 mg/kg/day PO in divided doses q6-12h	Avoid in patients with asthma or CHF; may cause hypoglycemia
Atenolol	0.8-2 mg/kg/day PO in divided doses q12-24h	↓ Bronchospasm and bradycardia; few published reports of use in children
Labetalol	Start at 1-4 mg/kg/day PO in divided doses q6-12h	α and β blockade in 1:4 ratio; few pediatric data available
α-Adrenergic Agonists		
Clonidine	5-25 μg/kg/day PO in divided doses q6-12h (max, 0.9 mg/day)	Initial drowsiness; rebound hypertension with abrupt discontinuation
Angiotensin-Converting Enzyme Inhibitors		
Captopril	0.02-2 mg/kg/day PO in divided doses q6-12h (neonates) 0.5-6 mg/kg/day PO in divided doses q6-12h (children)	↓ GFR, ↑ K, ↓ platelets, ageusia, angioedema, neutropenia, cough; use with caution in renal artery stenosis
Enalapril	0.1-0.5 (?) mg/kg/day PO in divided doses q12-24h (max, 40 mg/day)	↓ GFR, ↑ K, ↓ platelets, ageusia, angioedema, neutropenia, cough; use with caution in renal artery stenosis
Angiotensin Receptor Inhibitors		
Losartan	No pediatric data	Angioedema, headache, cough, dizziness

CHF, congestive heart failure; glu, glucose; GFR, glomerular filtration rate; K, potassium; PO, by mouth.

↑, increase in; ↓, decrease in.

Table 12-10. Potential Side Effects of Antihypertensive Drugs

Diuretics	β Blockers	Vasodilators	Central Sympatholytics	ACE Inhibitors	CCB
Hypokalemia	Bradycardia	Headache	Sedation	Renal insufficiency	Peripheral edema
Volume depletion	Syncope	Palpitations	Dry mouth	Hyperkalemia	Dizziness
Hypotension	Sleepiness	Tachycardia	Depression	Do *not* use in bilateral	Light-headedness
Hypomagnesemia	Visual disturbances	Flushing	Vivid dreams	renal artery stenosis	Headache
Hypercalcemia	Vivid dreams	Fluid/sodium	Nightmares	Neutropenia	Flushing
Glucose intolerance*	Weakness	retention	Hallucination	Hypotension	Weakness
Hyperlipidemia*	Fatigue		Rebound	Orthostatic hypotension	Transient hypotension
Hyperuricemia	Depression		hypertension†	Rash	Constipation
Gastric irritation	Bronchospasm		Impotence†	Dry cough	
Cramping	Impotence†			Bronchospasm	
Impotence†				Taste alteration	
				Angioedema	

From Feld LG, Waz, WR: Treatment of hypertension. In Barratt TM, Avner ED, Harmon WE (eds): Pediatric Nephrology, 4th ed. Baltimore, Lippincott Williams & Wilkins, 1999, p 1043.

*Only with thiazide diuretics.

†Patient incidence < 2%.

ACE, angiotensin-converting enzyme; CCB, calcium channel blocking agents.

level results in metabolic acidosis. Cyanate levels are rarely elevated unless nitroprusside is given over several days or in the presence of renal failure.

Labetalol can lower blood pressure within 5 to 10 minutes after intravenous administration. It blocks β-adrenergic and α-adrenergic receptors peripherally, causing a reduction in cardiac output as well as peripheral vasodilation. It can be given as a bolus or continuous infusion and does not cause the reflex tachycardia or increased cardiac output that is associated with nitroprusside or diazoxide. Labetalol can be given intravenously as a bolus of 0.2 to 1 mg/kg every 10 minutes with a maximum bolus dose of 20 mg. Dosages of 0.25 to 2 mg/kg/hour by intravenous infusion are recommended in children. Because it is metabolized by the liver, labetalol is effective in patients with significant renal disease. It may have limited efficacy when the mean arterial pressure is significantly elevated. Labetalol has a limited role in patients with asthma, chronic lung disease, or myocardial dysfunction because of the possibility of increased airway reactivity and its negative inotropic and chronotropic effects. Unlike direct-acting vasodilators, labetalol does not increase intracranial pressure or interfere with hypoxic pulmonary vasoconstriction.

Nicardipine is effective in rapidly controlling blood pressure in children in perioperative, intensive care, and emergency room settings. It is administered intravenously and produces its effect by dilating peripheral arteries, thus reducing peripheral vascular resistance. Its advantages include lack of decreased cardiac output and limited effects on the chronotropic and dromotropic function of the heart. A starting dosage of 5 μg/kg/minute and a maintenance dose of 1-3 μg/kg/minute may be effective. Because it increases intracranial pressure, it should not be given to patients with space-occupying intracranial lesions.

Intravenous agents such as esmolol and enalaprilat are used in treating hypertensive crises in children. Esmolol is an ultra–short-acting β-adrenergic antagonist, which may induce bronchospasm. Loading doses of 100-500 μg/kg as a bolus over 1 to 2 minutes have been used. The usual maintenance dosage is 50-300 μg/kg/minute. The ACE inhibitor enalaprilat has variable effectiveness in a hypertensive crisis. Children most likely to respond are those with high renin levels, renal artery stenosis, or a mass lesion in the kidney.

Table 12-11. Contraindications to the Use of Various Antihypertensive Medications

Angiotensin-Converting Enzyme Inhibitors
Pregnancy
Bilateral renal artery stenosis
Unilateral renal artery stenosis in a solitary kidney
Acute renal failure

Calcium Channel Blockers
Left ventricular dysfunction (verapamil and diltiazem)
Sick sinus syndrome, second- or third-degree atrioventricular block (verapamil and diltiazem)
Atrial flutter or atrial fibrillation (verapamil and diltiazem)
Neonates (verapamil and diltiazem)

β-Adrenergic Antagonists
Asthma
Insulin-dependent diabetes mellitus
Raynaud phenomenon
Congestive heart failure
Atrioventricular conduction disturbances (other than first-degree heart block)

Diuretics
Thiazides: neonates with hyperbilirubinemia
Loop diuretics: patients with hypercalciuria/nephrocalcinosis
Potassium-sparing diuretics: patients with hyperkalemia, diabetic nephropathy

Direct Vasodilators
Hydralazine: coronary artery disease, cerebrovascular disease, mitral valve disease
Minoxidil: pheochromocytoma, congestive heart failure, recent myocardial infarction
Diazoxide: cerebral hemorrhage, dissecting aortic aneurysm, acute myocardial infarction, aortic coarctation
Nitroprusside: coarctation of the aorta, increased intracranial pressure

From Feld LG, Waz, WR: Treatment of hypertension. In Barratt TM, Avner ED, Harmon WE (eds): Pediatric Nephrology, 4th ed. Baltimore, Lippincott Williams & Wilkins, 1999, p 1046.

Table 12-12. Pharmacologic Therapy for Hypertensive Emergencies in Children

Drug	Dosage	Onset of Action	Duration of Action	Comments
Sodium nitroprusside	0.3-8 µg/kg/min IV	Seconds	Seconds to minutes	May cause reflex tachycardia; thiocyanate toxicity when used >48 hours or in renal failure; increase in cerebral blood flow and ICP
Labetalol	0.2-1 mg/kg/dose (max, 20 mg) IV q10min, or 0.25-2 mg/kg/h MTN bolus or continuously	5-10 min	2-3 hr	Relative contraindications: heart failure, asthma, and BPD
Nicardipine	0.5-5 µg/kg followed by 1-3 µg/kg/min IV continuous	Minutes	10-15 min	Reflex tachycardia, increase in cerebral blood flow and ICP
Esmolol*	100-500 µg/kg IV load over 1-2 min, then 50-300 µg/kg/min continuously	Minutes	10-20 min	Not compatible with NaHCO₃; heart failure and asthma are contraindications
Hydralazine	0.1-0.2 mg/kg/dose IV q4-6h (max, 20 mg/dose)	10-30 min	4-12 hr	Reflex tachycardia, headaches, flushing, fluid retention
Enalaprilat	0.005-0.01 mg/kg/dose IV q8-24h	15 min	12-24 hr	Avoid if severe renal artery stenosis or bilateral stenosis is present or suspected
Nifedipine	0.15-0.5 mg/kg/dose (max, 10 mg) SL/PO	10-30 min	Up to 6 hr	Increases cerebral blood flow; hypotensive effect unpredictable; cautious use without IV access; flushing, headache, nausea
Minoxidil	0.1-0.2 mg/kg/dose PO	30 min	1-2 days	Reflex tachycardia, Na and water retention
Captopril	Neonates: 0.01-0.5 mg/kg/dose PO Children: 0.1-0.3 mg/kg/dose PO	15 min	6-12 hr	May abruptly decrease BP; may cause acute renal failure in patients with renovascular disease and in infants
Phentolamine mesylate	0.05-0.1 mg/kg/dose IV (max, 5 mg/dose)	Seconds	30-60 min	α-Adrenergic blocker useful in pheochromocytoma
Diazoxide	1-3 mg/kg/dose IV over 10-30 sec (max, 150 mg/dose)	Minutes	8-24 hr	Abrupt drop in BP, Na and water retention, hyperglycemia, reflex sympathetic stimulation

*Limited pediatric data available.

BP, blood pressure; BPD, bronchopulmonary dysplasia; ICP, intracranial pressure; IV, intravenously; max, maximum; MTN, maintenance; PO, by mouth; SL, sublingual.

Onset of action is 15-60 minutes even though it is given intravenously, which thus limits its use in hypertensive emergencies. The pediatric dose is 0.005-0.01 mg/kg every 8 to 24 hours.

The use of minoxidil, diazoxide, and hydralazine has decreased because of the availability of more effective agents with fewer adverse effects. Diazoxide, a potent peripheral vasodilator, can be given as a bolus or continuous infusion. As a bolus, it has been recommended to be administered over 10-30 seconds, because 90% of infused diazoxide binds to albumin and its hypotensive effect depends on free drug reaching smooth muscle receptors. Diazoxide can cause hyperglycemia, hyperuricemia, cardiac arrhythmias, headache, tachycardia, and flushing. Use of diazoxide in the hypertensive child is not recommended.

Hydralazine is a direct arteriolar vasodilator given as an intravenous bolus to treat hypertensive crises. It is less effective than diazoxide and sodium nitroprusside in reducing blood pressure and may cause reflex tachycardia. The effective dose for treating pediatric hypertensive crises is 0.1-0.2 mg/kg intravenously. Minoxidil is a potent, long-acting oral vasodilator that can be used for pediatric patients with hypertensive urgency. The usual starting dose in children is 0.1 to 0.2 mg/kg every 24 hours. The onset of action is within 30 minutes with 1 to 2 days' duration. Reflex tachycardia and fluid retention are major limiting side effects.

Oral nifedipine administered sublingually has also been recommended. Nifedipine can be either given sublingually or swallowed. It reduces blood pressure within 5 to 30 minutes, with maximum effects in 60 to 90 minutes. There is concern about the unpredictability of response after nifedipine administration. Despite these concerns, oral nifedipine continues to be used widely by pediatric nephrologists in the setting of acute severe hypertension in asymptomatic individuals with a 10% incidence of serious adverse consequences. The use of sublingual nifedipine in severe hypertension, administered without intravenous access, cannot be recommended.

Captopril is used for severe hypertension. Because children have a more active renin-angiotensin system and a higher incidence of renal artery stenosis as a cause of severe hypertension than do adults, use of an ACE inhibitor as first-line treatment is contraindicated when the underlying cause and disease duration are unknown.

Special circumstances may necessitate different approaches in the acute management phase. Patients with *pheochromocytoma* may require phenoxybenzamine, possibly in conjunction with a β blocker. Children with renin-dependent causes may need ACE inhibitors, but caution is necessary if main renal artery stenosis or bilateral stenosis is considered to be present. Patients with apparent mineralocorticoid excess or *Liddle syndrome*, both examples of low-renin, low-aldosterone hypertension, can present with life-threatening severe hypertension and may not respond adequately to any therapy other than specific agents that act on the collecting tubules of the kidneys (i.e., the potassium-sparing diuretics triamterene or amiloride).

In the treatment of the severely hypertensive neonate, it is important to appreciate the dramatic increases in systolic and diastolic blood pressure that are normal maturational events occurring over the first few months of life. Many infants, including some with very severe hypertension, may be asymptomatic. Symptoms, when they occur, are usually cardiorespiratory and neurologic. The newborn infant, especially the premature infant, has a richly perfused germinal matrix and is at risk for intracranial hemorrhages associated with hypertension, hypotension, or marked fluctuations in blood pressure; therefore, judicious lowering of the blood pressure is mandatory.

NEONATAL HYPERTENSION

The incidence of hypertension in neonates is low, ranging from 0.2% to 3%. Routine blood pressure determination is not advocated for otherwise healthy full-term infants. Among premature and otherwise high-risk newborns, the incidence of hypertension is 0.8%. Approximately 9% of infants with bronchopulmonary dysplasia, patent ductus arteriosus, or intraventricular hemorrhage or those who had indwelling umbilical arterial catheters develop hypertension.

Hypertension is a relatively infrequent clinical problem that is primarily confined to the neonatal intensive care unit.

Blood pressure in neonates increases with both gestational and postconceptual age, as well as with birth weight (Fig. 12-4). On the basis of these data, neonatal hypertension must be defined on the basis of the upper limit of the 95% confidence interval for infants of similar gestational or postconceptual age and size. For older infants, the percentile curves in Figure 12-1 are useful. According to serial blood pressure measurements from nearly 13,000 infants, hypertension in this age group is defined as an elevation above the 95th percentile based on age, size, and gender.

Common causes of hypertension in neonates include thromboembolic events related to umbilical catheterization, congenital problems such as aortic coarctation, structural renal malformations, renovascular disease, and certain medications. A more extensive list of potential causes of hypertension in the neonate is found in Table 12-13.

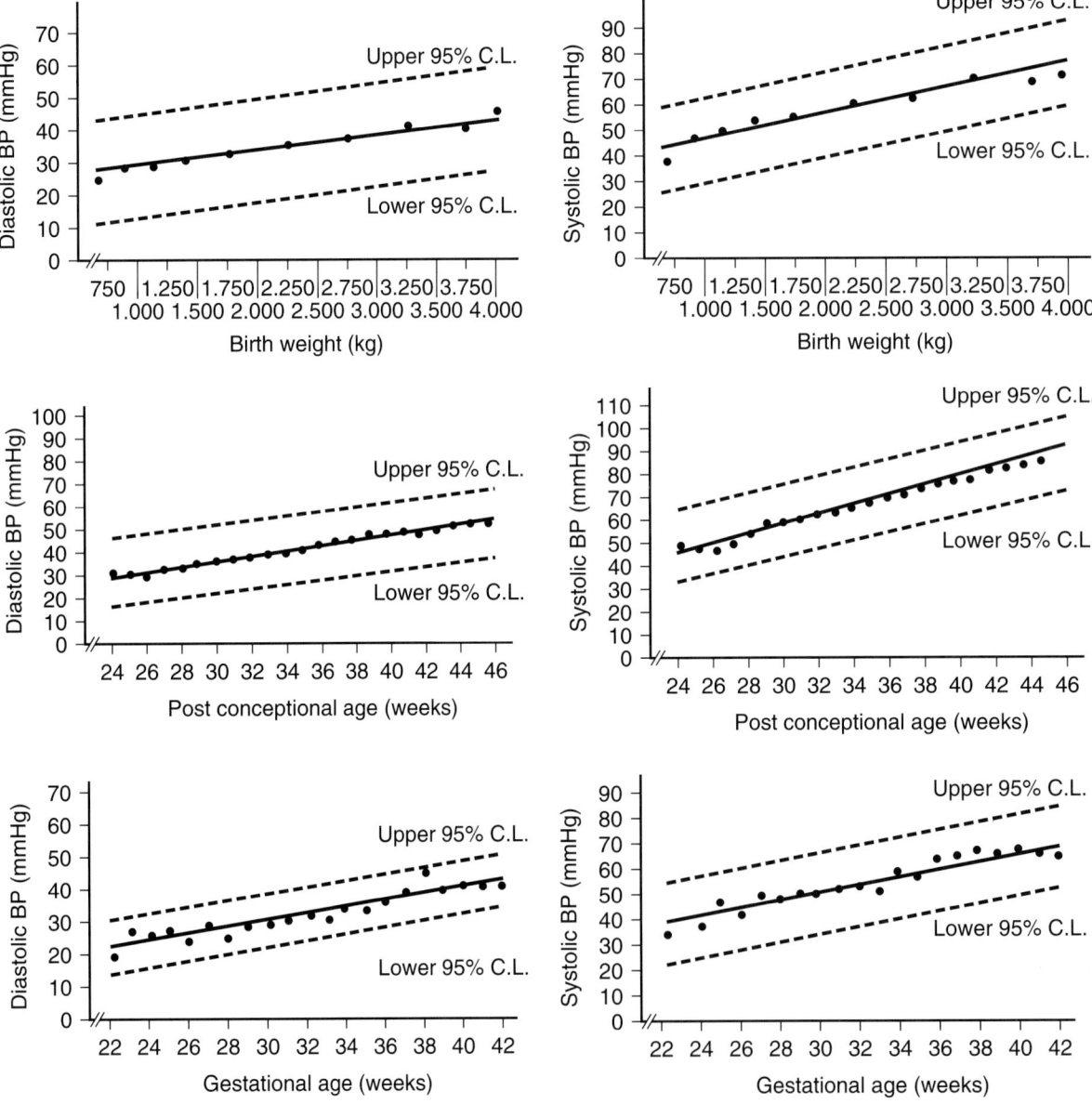

Figure 12-4. Linear regression of mean systolic and diastolic blood pressures (BP) by birth weight, postconceptual age, and gestational age on day 1 after birth, with 95% confidence limits (CL). (From Zubrow AB, Hulman S, Kushner H, et al: Determinants of blood pressure in infants admitted to neonatal intensive care units: A prospective multicenter study. J Perinatol 1995;15:470-479.)

Table 12-13. Causes of Neonatal Hypertension	
Renovascular	**Medications/Intoxications**
Thromboembolism	Infants
Renal artery stenosis	Dexamethasone
Midaortic coarctation	Adrenergic agents
Renal venous thrombosis	Vitamin D intoxication
Compression of the renal artery	Theophylline
Idiopathic arterial calcification	Caffeine
Congenital rubella syndrome	Pancuronium
	Phenylephrine
Renal Parenchymal Disease	Maternal
Polycystic kidney disease	Cocaine
Multicystic/dysplastic kidney	Heroin
Tuberous sclerosis	**Neoplasia**
Ureteropelvic junction obstruction	Wilms tumor
Unilateral renal hypoplasia	Mesoblastic nephroma
Mesoblastic nephroma	Neuroblastoma
Acute tubular necrosis	
Cortical necrosis	**Neurologic**
Interstitial nephritis	Pain
Hemolytic uremic syndrome	Intracranial hypertension
Obstruction secondary to stone or tumor	Seizures
	Familial dysautonomia
Pulmonary	Subdural hematoma
Bronchopulmonary dysplasia	**Miscellaneous**
Pneumothorax	Total parenteral nutrition
Cardiac	Closure of abdominal wall defect
Thoracic aortic coarctation	Adrenal hemorrhage
	Hypercalcemia
Endocrine	Traction
Congenital adrenal hyperplasia	ECMO
Hyperaldosteronism	Birth asphyxia
Hyperthyroidism	
Pseudohypoaldosteronism type II	

From Flynn JT: Neonatal hypertension: Diagnosis and management. Pediatr Nephrol 2000;14:322-341.

ECMO, extracorporeal membrane oxygenation.

Between 25% and 81% of normotensive infants with umbilical artery catheters have evidence of thrombus formation. Thromboembolism may then lead to hypertension in some neonates, at times days to weeks after the umbilical artery catheter was removed. Renal vein thrombosis classically manifests in the neonate with the triad of hypertension, gross hematuria, and an abdominal flank mass. Fibromuscular dysplasia leading to renal arterial stenosis, idiopathic arterial calcification, renal artery stenosis secondary to congenital rubella infection, and mechanical compression of one or both renal arteries by tumors, hydronephrotic kidneys, or other abdominal masses may also produce hypertension in the neonate.

Renal parenchymal abnormalities leading to neonatal hypertension include autosomal recessive and dominant polycystic kidney disease, unilateral multicystic dysplastic kidneys, ureteropelvic junction obstruction, unilateral renal hypoplasia, acute tubular or cortical necrosis, interstitial nephritis, congenital nephrotic syndrome, and hemolytic uremic syndrome.

The incidence of hypertension among infants with bronchopulmonary dysplasia is 43% and is correlated with severity of the pulmonary disease and with the use of theophylline and corticosteroids.

The evaluation of neonates with hypertension is usually straightforward. The history should focus on perinatal exposures, as well as to the particulars of the infant's course in the neonatal intensive care unit. Procedures such as umbilical catheter placement should be reviewed, and the current medication list should be scrutinized. The physical examination should include four extremity blood pressure measurements and the general appearance of the infant (particularly the presence of dysmorphic features); a careful cardiac and abdominal examination as well as the presence of a flank mass or epigastric bruit may be helpful. Table 12-14 lists the common diagnostic tests that are utilized in the evaluation of a hypertensive infant.

TREATMENT OF NEONATAL HYPERTENSION

For the majority of acutely ill infants, particularly those with severe hypertension, continuous intravenous infusions are the most appropriate approach to preventing too rapid a reduction in blood pressure, a situation that may lead to cerebral ischemia and hemorrhage, a problem for which premature infants in particular are already at increased risk because of the immaturity of their periventricular circulation. Infusions of nicardipine may be particularly useful in this population. Other drugs that have been successfully used in neonates include esmolol, labetalol, and nitroprusside. Intermittently administered intravenous agents such as hydralazine or labetalol may have a role in the therapy of infants with mild to moderate hypertension who are not yet candidates for oral therapy because of gastrointestinal dysfunction.

Enalaprilat, the intravenous ACE inhibitor, although reported to be useful in the treatment of neonatal renovascular hypertension, should be used with caution because even dosages at the lower end of published ranges may lead to significant, prolonged hypotension and oliguric acute renal failure. Captopril is a particularly useful oral

Table 12-14. Diagnostic Testing in Neonatal Hypertension

Generally Useful	Useful in Selected Infants
Urinalysis (± culture)	Thyroid studies
CBC and platelet count	Urine VMA/HVA
Electrolytes	Aldosterone
BUN, creatinine	Cortisol
Calcium	Echocardiogram
Plasma renin	Abdominal/pelvic ultrasound
Chest x-ray	VCUG
Renal ultrasound with	Aortography
Doppler	Renal angiography
	Nuclear renal scan

From Flynn JT: Neonatal hypertension: Diagnosis and management. Pediatr Nephrol 2000;14:322-341.

BUN, blood urea nitrogen; CBC, complete blood cell count; HVA, homovanillic acid; VCUG, voiding cystourethrography; VMA, vanillylmandelic acid.

agent for infants with less severe hypertension or for those ready to transition from intravenous therapy. For infants whose blood pressure cannot be controlled by captopril alone, addition of a diuretic is frequently helpful.

Other oral drugs found to be useful in infants include hydralazine, minoxidil, and isradipine. Isradipine has the advantage of being able to be compounded into a suspension. Nifedipine is contraindicated because it may cause rapid, profound, and short-lived drops in blood pressure and cardiac output.

RECOMMENDATIONS FOR ATHLETIC PARTICIPATION AND EXERCISE TESTING IN THE HYPERTENSIVE ADOLESCENT

During exercise, the local vascular beds in skin and muscle dilate, resulting in a reduction of vascular resistance. Because cardiac output increases to a greater degree than resistance is reduced, systolic blood pressure increases. Because of the dilation of the vascular beds, the diastolic blood pressure increases only slightly during exercise. In some normal individuals, vasodilation with exercise may even cause the blood pressure to decrease or remain unchanged. The systolic blood pressure normally increases with progressive workloads. During exercise, maximum systolic blood pressure in children rarely exceeds 200 mm Hg. Even in healthy children and adolescents whose systolic blood pressure reaches 250 mm Hg during exercise, no evidence of risk is available. The magnitude of the increase of peak blood pressure values during exercise increases with age and size. Because boys and men have a higher maximum stroke volume than do girls and women, they routinely have a higher systolic blood pressure response. During dynamic exercise, in which large muscles are in cyclic repetitive contractions, systolic blood pressure increases linearly as workload increases; diastolic blood pressure seldom increases. Systolic, mean arterial, and diastolic blood pressures increase significantly during static exercise, in contrast to dynamic exercise, whereas total peripheral resistance remains unchanged. In isometric exercise, the rises in systolic and diastolic blood pressure are in proportion to the percentage of maximal contractions of the muscle group involved, no matter how large or small that muscle group may be. As the muscle contraction is maintained over time, blood pressure continues to increase; no steady state is achieved as in dynamic exercise. Although limited evidence shows no greater risk with highly static exercise, experts are more cautious about allowing athletes with severe hypertension to participate in this

activity. Table 12-15 lists common athletic activities and their static classification.

In hypertensive patients, the increase in blood pressure during exertion is higher than expected, in view of the degree of work. Hypertension is the most common cardiovascular condition seen in people who engage in competitive athletics. Sudden death during sporting events has not been reported in hypertensive athletes, as in athletes with hypertrophic cardiomyopathy or cardiac arrhythmias. Some reports of sudden death in athletes have noted a finding of "idiopathic left ventricular hypertrophy" on autopsy. Because of the lack of data, the current approach to the hypertensive athlete is controversial. The current recommendations for athletic participation of children and adolescents with hypertension are as follows:

Significant hypertension (95th to 99th percentiles) with no target organ damage: No limitation for competitive athletics. Check blood pressure every 2 months.

Severe hypertension (>99th percentile): Restriction from competitive sports and highly static activity until blood pressure is under control with no target organ damage.

Young athlete with hypertension: Patients should be strongly encouraged to adopt healthy lifestyle behaviors: that is, avoidance of exogenous androgens, growth hormone, drugs of abuse (especially cocaine), tobacco (all routes), and high sodium intake.

Because cardiovascular conditioning may be less strenuous than competitive athletics, complete restriction of exercise may not be necessary for athletes with severe hypertension.

Exercise stress testing in adolescents may not be particularly useful in the short-term prognosis of hypertension but can be helpful in reassuring the patient with mild to moderate hypertension that he or she may safely participate in strenuous physical activities or competitive sports. Findings that warrant concern during exercise testing are ischemia, arrhythmia, and low working capacity.

Endurance training for at least 3 months usually reduces systolic and diastolic blood pressure. Resistance training by itself does not lead to baseline blood pressure change, but if it occurs after endurance training, it may lead to sustained blood pressure reductions.

When antihypertensive medications are indicated in the athletic adolescent, ACE inhibitors or dihydropyridine calcium channel blockers (nifedipine, nicardipine, isradipine, felodipine, amlodipine) effectively lower blood pressure without significant adverse effects on cardiac output or contractility, intravascular volume, or other effects that might impair athletic performance.

SUMMARY AND RED FLAGS

Regular and accurate monitoring of blood pressure should begin in childhood. Elevated blood pressure, when discovered, should be appropriately investigated, the evaluation being tailored to the age of

Table 12-15. Sports that Have a High Static Component

Low Dynamic	Moderate Dynamic	High Dynamic
Bobsledding	Bodybuilding	Boxing
Field events	Downhill skiing	Canoeing/
(throwing)	Wrestling	kayaking
Gymnastics		Cycling
Karate/judo		Decathlon
Luge		Rowing
Sailing		Speed skating
Rock climbing		
Water skiing		
Weight lifting		
Windsurfing		

the child and to the severity of the blood pressure elevation. Investigation should focus not only on a search for a cause but also on target organ effects. Timely recognition of abnormal blood pressure and appropriate interventions are necessary to prevent the future development of cardiovascular and renal morbidity and mortality.

Red flags include extreme elevation of blood pressure, end-organ dysfunction (encephalopathy, cardiomyopathy, retinopathy, nephropathy), renal failure, younger age at onset, intermittent and exercise-induced hypertension (pheochromocytoma), a family history of hypertension or tumors, growth failure, an abdominal mass or bruit, and poorly palpable femoral pulses.

REFERENCES

General

Bartosh SM, Aronson AJ: Childhood hypertension: An update on etiology, diagnosis and treatment. Pediatr Cardiol 1999;46:235-252.

Brouhard BH: Hypertension in children and adolescents. Cleve Clin J Med 1995;62:21-28.

Fernandes E, McCrindle BW: Diagnosis and treatment of hypertension in children and adolescents. Can J Cardiol 2000;16:801-811.

Lane PH, Belsha CW, Plummer J, et al: Relationship of renal size, body size, and blood pressure in children. Pediatr Nephrol 1998;12:35-39.

National Heart, Lung, and Blood Institute: Update on the Task Force (1987) on High Blood Pressure in Children and Adolescents: A Working Group from the National High Blood Pressure Education Program. Pediatrics 1996;98:649-658.

Report of the Second Task Force on Blood Pressure Control in Children—1987. Task Force on Blood Pressure Control in Children, National Heart, Lung, and Blood Institute, Bethesda, Maryland. Pediatrics 1987;79:1-25.

Sinaiko AR, Gomez-Marin O, Prineas RJ: Prevalence of "significant" hypertension in junior high school-aged children: The Children and Adolescent Blood Pressure Program. J Pediatr 1989;114:664-669.

Sorof JM: White coat hypertension in children. Blood Press Monit 2000;5:197-202.

Sorof JM: Systolic hypertension in children: Benign or beware? Pediatr Nephrol 2001;16:517-525.

Ambulatory Blood Pressure Monitoring

Belsha CW: Ambulatory blood pressure monitoring and hypertensive target-organ damage in children. Blood Press Monit 1999;4:161-164.

Nishibata K, Nagashima M, Tsuji A, et al: Comparison of casual blood pressure and twenty-four-hour ambulatory blood pressure in high school students. J Pediatr 1995;127:34-39.

Soergel M: Development of normative ambulatory blood pressure data in children. Arbeitsgruppe Pädiatrische Hypertonie. Blood Pressure Monitoring 1999;4:121-126.

Soergol M, Kirschstein M, Busch C, et al: Oscillometric twenty-four-hour ambulatory blood pressure values in healthy children and adolescents: A multicenter trial including 1141 subjects. J Pediatr 1997;130:178-184.

Racial/Ethnic Differences

Daniels SR, Obarzanek E, Barton BA, et al: Sexual maturation and racial differences in blood pressure in girls: The National Heart, Lung, and Blood Institute Growth and Health Study. J Pediatr 1996;129:208-213.

Harshfield GA, Treiber FA: Racial differences in ambulatory blood pressure monitoring–derived 24 h patterns of blood pressure in adolescents. Blood Press Monit 1999;4:107-110.

Hohn AR, Dwyer KM, Dwyer JH: Blood pressure in youth from four ethnic groups: The Pasadena Prevention Project. J Pediatr 1994;125:368-373.

Target Organ Damage

Finta KM: Cardiovascular manifestations of hypertension in children. Pediatr Clin North Am 1993; 40:51-59.

Yoshinaga M, Yuasa Y, Hatano H, et al: Effect of total adipose weight and systemic hypertension on left ventricular mass in children. Am J Cardiol 1995;76:785-787.

Essential Hypertension

Gillman MW, Cook NR, Rosner B, et al: Identifying children at high risk for the development of essential hypertension. J Pediatr 1993;122:837-846.

Lauer RM, Burns TL, Clarke WR, et al: Childhood predictors of future blood pressure. Hypertension 1991;18(Suppl I):174-181.

Nelson MJ, Ragland DR, Syme SL: Longitudinal prediction of adult blood pressure from juvenile blood pressure levels. Am J Epidemiol 1992;136:633-645.

Schieken RM: Genetic factors that predispose the child to develop hypertension. Pediatr Clin North Am 1993;40:1-11.

Shear C, Burke G, Freedman D, et al: Value of childhood blood pressure measurements and family history in predicting future blood pressure status: Results from 8 years of follow-up in the Bogalusa Heart Study. Pediatrics 1986;77:862-869.

Sorof JM, Forman A, Cole N, et al: Potassium intake and cardiovascular reactivity in children with risk factors for essential hypertension. J Pediatr 1997;131:87-94.

Renovascular Hypertension

Deal JE, Snell MF, Barratt TM, et al: Renovascular disease in children. J Pediatr 1992;121:378-384.

Hiner LB, Falkner B: Renovascular hypertension in children. Pediatr Clin North Am 1993;40:123-140.

Nonpharmacologic Therapy

Alpert BS: Exercise as a therapy to control hypertension in children. Int J Sports Med 2000;21(Suppl 2):S94-S97.

Falkner B, Michel S: Blood pressure response to sodium in children and adolescents. Am J Clin Nutr 1997;65(Suppl):618S-621S.

Rocchini AP, Key J, Bondie D, et al: The effect of weight loss on the sensitivity of blood pressure to sodium in obese adolescents. N Engl J Med 1989;321:580-585.

Sinaiko A, Gomez-Marin O, Prineas R: Effect of low sodium diet or potassium supplementation on adolescent blood pressure. Hypertension 1993;21:989-994.

Pharmacologic Therapy

Bunchman TE, Lynch RE, Wood EG: Intravenously administered labetalol for treatment of hypertension in children. J Pediatr 1992;120:140-144.

Flynn JT, Pasko DA: Calcium channel blockers: Pharmacology and place in therapy of pediatric hypertension. Pediatr Nephrol 2000;15:302-316.

Gouyon JB, Geneste B, Semama DS, et al: Intravenous nicardipine in hypertensive preterm infants. Arch Dis Child 1997;76:F126-F127.

Hirschl MM, Binder M, Bur A, et al: Clinical evaluation of different doses of intravenous enalaprilat in patients with hypertensive crisis. Arch Intern Med 1995;155:2217-2223.

Johnson CE, Jacobson PA, Song MH: Isradipine therapy in hypertensive pediatric patients. Ann Pharmacother 1997;31:704-707.

Khattak S, Rogan JW, Saunders EF, et al: Efficacy of amlodipine in pediatric bone marrow transplant patients. Clin Pediatr 1998;37:31-36.

MacDonald JL, Johnson CE, Jacobson P: Stability of isradipine in an extemporaneously compounded oral liquid. Am J Hosp Pharm 1994;51:2409-2411.

Rogan JW, Lyszkiewicz DA, Blowey D, et al: A randomized prospective crossover trial of amlodipine in pediatric hypertension. Pediatr Nephrol 2000;14:1083-1087.

Sinaiko AR: Treatment of hypertension in children. Pediatr Nephrol 1994;8:603-609.

Soergel M, Verho M, Wühl E, et al: Effect of ramipril on ambulatory blood pressure and albuminuria in renal hypertension. Pediatr Nephrol 2000;15:113-118.

Strauser LM, Groshong T, Tobias JD: Initial experience with isradipine for the treatment of hypertension in children. South Med J 2000;93:287-293.

Tallian KB, Nahata MC, Turman MA, et al: Efficacy of amlodipine in pediatric patients with hypertension. Pediatr Nephrol 1999;13:304-310.

Treluyer JM, Hubert P, Jouvet P, et al: Intravenous nicardipine in hypertensive children. Eur J Pediatr 1993;152:712-714.

Hypertensive Emergencies

Adelman RD, Coppo R, Dillon MJ: The emergency management of severe hypertension. Pediatr Nephrol 2000;14:422-427.

Deal JE, Barratt TM, Dillon MJ: Management of hypertensive emergencies. Arch Dis Child 1992;67:1089-1092.

Fivush B, Neu A, Furth S: Acute hypertensive crises in children: Emergencies and urgencies. Curr Opin Pediatr 1997;9:233-236.

Neonatal Hypertension

Flynn JT: Neonatal hypertension: Diagnosis and management. Pediatr Nephrol 2000;14:332-341.

Georgieff MK, Mills MM, Gómez-Marin O, et al: Rate of change of blood pressure in premature and full term infants from birth to 4 months. Pediatr Nephrol 1996;10:152-155.

Sports Participation

American Academy of Pediatrics Committee on Sports Medicine and Fitness: Athletic participation by children and adolescents who have systemic hypertension. Pediatrics 1997;99:637-638.

Washington RL, Bricker T, Alpert BS, et al: Guidelines for exercise testing in the pediatric age group. From the Committee on Atherosclerosis and Hypertension in Children, Council on Cardiovascular Disease in the Young, the American Heart Association. Circulation 1994;90:2166-2179.

GASTROINTESTINAL DISORDERS

13 Failure to Thrive and Malnutrition

Virginia Keane   Susan Feigelman

Calories from food provide energy for the body's maintenance functions of repair, regulation, metabolic functions, replacement of losses, and daily activity. Children have additional caloric requirements because they must also grow. Children whose caloric needs are not met do not grow according to published norms and are said to *fail to thrive* or to have *failure to thrive* (FTT). FTT raises serious concerns. It is important to have a systematic, stepwise approach to the diagnosis and management of poor growth in young children.

The term *failure to thrive* is used to describe growth failure that accompanies many pathologic conditions, including psychosocial causes. Differentiation between organic (biomedical) and non-organic (psychosocial/environmental) causes is the initial step in the diagnostic process; many studies document the high prevalence of environmental causes of poor growth. One clinical approach to FTT is to admit the infant to the hospital for an exhaustive laboratory evaluation while the infant is simultaneously fed; this results in weight gain, which confirms the environmental cause for poor growth. Nonetheless, studies have demonstrated a poor yield from exhaustive laboratory evaluations. In addition, children with biomedical and psychosocial causes of FTT may or may not gain weight in institutional settings, and this short-term outcome is not always diagnostic. Children may have a combination of psychosocial and biomedical problems, and a strict differentiation between organic and inorganic causes may be difficult. The role of infant behavior and the interaction between the child and the caregiver may result in dysfunctional feeding patterns.

NORMAL GROWTH

Newborns typically lose up to 10% of their birth weight during the first few days of life and regain this weight by the age of 2 weeks. They then gain weight at a steady pace of 20 to 30 g per day for the first 3 months; gain at half to two-thirds that rate for the next 3 months; and half to two-thirds again for the next 6 months. This results in a doubling of birth weight by the age of 4 to 6 months and a tripling before 1 year. Height and head circumference grow at similar well-defined rates. These three growth parameters should be plotted on National Center for Health Statistics (NCHS) growth charts and monitored for adherence to standard growth rates. Children grow in a stepwise manner, but on average their growth pattern follows the nationally accepted curves.

Size at birth depends on maternal factors and intrauterine environment. Between the ages of 1 to 3 years, the child's growth adjusts to the genetic potential. Ultimate height is determined by additional factors, among them rate of bone maturity and rate of pubertal development. Considerable energy from ingested food is required to achieve this growth. The energy balance can be described by the following equation, in which E equals energy:

$$E_{(ingested)} - E_{(feces)} - E_{(urine\ loss)} - E_{(insensible\ loss)}$$
$$= E_{(basal\ metabolic\ rate)} + E_{(activity)} + E_{(growth)}$$

Any imbalance in this energy equation (losing or using more calories than are ingested) results in abnormal growth patterns. Weight is usually affected first, followed by height and finally head circumference if the energy imbalance is severe and prolonged.

DEFINITIONS

FTT is a sign, not a diagnosis, with several definitions. FTT is generally used to describe children younger than 3 years who meet the following criteria:

1. grow at less than the fifth or third percentile on NCHS growth charts (<3% = less than three standard deviations below mean)
2. have weight for height that is less than the 5th or 10th percentile
3. have growth patterns that have crossed two major percentiles on the growth charts within 6 months
4. have growth velocity less than normal for age

There are inherent problems with these definitions: Three percent of the population is at or below the third percentile, and so those who are growing appropriately per their genetic potential must be differentiated from those with growth problems. The child who has been obese and is now approaching normal weight for height, crossing major weight percentiles in the process, should not be considered a child with FTT. Some children are naturally slim. The clinician must exercise considerable judgment before raising the concern of poor growth.

INTERPRETATION OF GROWTH CHARTS

The evaluation includes a careful analysis of growth charts. The more points on the growth chart, the better; this information may not be available because of lack of prior medical care or change of medical setting. The accuracy of the data should be confirmed. Measurements of length are the most susceptible to error. Possible errors in weight, head circumference, date of birth, or plotting on the growth chart should all be considered. Once the correct data are available, the charts should be examined to answer the following questions:

- Are the measurements of length, weight, and head circumference proportionate?
- Is the child a thin infant?
- Has the head grown proportionately?
- How severe are the deficits of each measurement, relative to what is expected (in units of normal developmental age, standard deviation, or percentile)?
- What is the chronology of the development of deficits?
- When did the problem start and progress?
- Is the problem acute or chronic?
- What environmental factors were present at the start of this process (weaning, introduction of new foods)?

Although weight is usually the most readily available measurement, measurement of length is particularly critical, because it serves as the point of reference for other measurements. The best way to obtain accurate length measurements is to use a specially constructed device (e.g., a reclining stadiometer). In the absence of such a device, the examiner can use a table or desk with the infant's head pressed against the wall and a firm square box or thick textbook for the sliding footer. Measurements obtained with the infant lying on a mattress and marked with a pen on the sheet are not accurate (see Chapter 60).

The choice of growth curves is important; reliable age and sex-specific growth charts based on data from the NCHS are widely available. Conventions differ in whether to plot age in relation to actual birth date or to use corrected gestational age. The difference is greatest for very young infants. Beyond the equivalent of 40 weeks of gestation, it really does not matter which method is used, as long as it is used consistently and as long as the interpretation takes into account the method used.

Because infants with FTT no longer follow their growth curves, the usual convention of expressing growth measurements in relation to normal percentiles is not always useful. The first step in interpretation should be to look at the length. The examiner must determine the percentile (or how many standard deviations below or above the median, 50%) of the length and the age at which the infant's actual length corresponds to the median (the "length age"). Next, the actual weight should be related to the expected weight for length. The expected weight for length can be determined by either of two methods: on the weight/age graph, this is the median (50%) of weight for the length age; on the direct graph of length and weight independent of age (which is included with most current versions of infant growth charts), this is the median weight for length. The difference between actual weight and expected weight for length can then be expressed as a percentage (or percentile, if within two standard deviations). A 10% variation in weight for length is within the normal range for infants. Some conventions classify the severity of wasting or "malnutrition" by the weight deficit. If this is done, it should be clear whether the examiner is comparing actual weight with expected weight for age or expected weight for length (the latter is recommended). Loss of about 40% of expected weight for length (actual weight divided by expected weight for length <60%) is the extreme of wasting that is compatible with survival. Therefore, 80% to 90% actual weight divided by expected weight for length corresponds to mild, 70% to 80% is moderate, and 60% to 70% is severe. These calculations are critical for planning nutritional rehabilitation and therefore essential to the overall diagnostic and treatment processes.

Measurements of head circumference can also be best interpreted if the measurements are expressed in relation to length age. In other words, it makes sense to express the actual head circumference as a "head-circumference age," which can then be compared with the length age. If a child's head has grown proportionately with length, these developmental "ages" will be the same. It is important to note the following points:

1. Infants who are small but have grown proportionately should be considered to have primary growth problems, including various endocrine and skeletal disorders (see Chapter 60).
2. Infants who have had inadequate feeding or assimilation or chronic illness are likely, at some point, to be abnormally thin. If the problem developed at some time after birth, weight would be expected to drop off before growth in length or head circumference.
3. Infants with disproportionately small heads may have primary neurologic problems affecting brain growth, because head growth is the last to be affected by primary malnutrition and is not characteristic of primary skeletal growth problems.

Several examples of how these patterns may be interpreted are presented in Figures 13-1 to 13-4.

New growth charts, published by the Centers for Disease Control and Prevention in 2001, combine data across geographic and ethnic populations. They include norms for body mass index (BMI) for children age two and older. The primary purpose of the BMI is to screen for children who are at risk for obesity. However, low BMI may become a new standard for defining FTT in older children. In special populations (trisomy 21, skeletal dysplasias), growth must be addressed in these diseases or definable population-based curves (Zulu vs. Pygmy tribes).

EPIDEMIOLOGY

Some studies have shown that a slightly higher proportion of children of low socioeconomic status than of other socioeconomic populations have growth failure. However, underweight children are seen in all socioeconomic groups. FTT accounts for up to 5% of all hospitalizations; up to 10% of children may have FTT at some time. Most affected children acquire this diagnosis before the age of 3 years.

CLINICAL PRESENTATION

Parents often voice concerns about their young child's weight gain. They may complain that their child is a picky eater or seems not to drink enough formula, or they worry that breast milk supplies are poor. Very commonly, parents complain that their child is not as big as a similar-aged child or a sibling at that age. Many such children are growing normally. Plotting the child's growth and reviewing it with the parent is usually reassuring, or it may serve to confirm the parents' concerns. When families raise concerns about growth, regardless of whether the concern is supported, the child and the weight have often already become a focus for that family. They may have already put a great deal of effort into changing the eating patterns of their child. The child's real or perceived weight or appetite problem is often causing conflict between family members and interfering with family relationships. In this setting, conversations about the child's growth may carry a high emotional charge.

When poor growth exists, it is often the physician who is first to raise concerns. These suspicions can be confirmed by carefully plotting the growth parameters. The clinician must then prioritize the clinical issues and decide whether the FTT should be addressed immediately or deferred for evaluation and management at another time in the very near future. In rare cases, the growth failure is so severe (child is less than 60% of ideal body weight for height) that immediate hospitalization must be instituted to begin nutritional rehabilitation. In this case, the evaluation can take place over several days, while therapeutic nutritional interventions are ongoing.

DIFFERENTIAL DIAGNOSIS

Clinicians have classified FTT in two broad categories: organic and inorganic. Although this dichotomy can be useful in helping organize an approach to evaluation and diagnosis, the experienced clinician knows that the distinctions are often blurred. Many children with FTT, particularly those with chronic diseases, have a mixed pattern of increased needs or losses attributable to organic causes, along with environmental causes of calorie deprivation.

There are several growth conditions that result in smaller than normal size but that are not due to calorie insufficiency. Children with constitutional delay usually grow normally over the first year, but weight and height decelerate to near or below the fifth percentile, and then the children continue to grow at normal rates along their new curve (see Chapter 60). The symmetric deceleration of height and weight is a clue that the child does not have calorie insufficiency. Infants who are born small for gestational age and are symmetrically small are believed to have a reduced number of somatic cells in

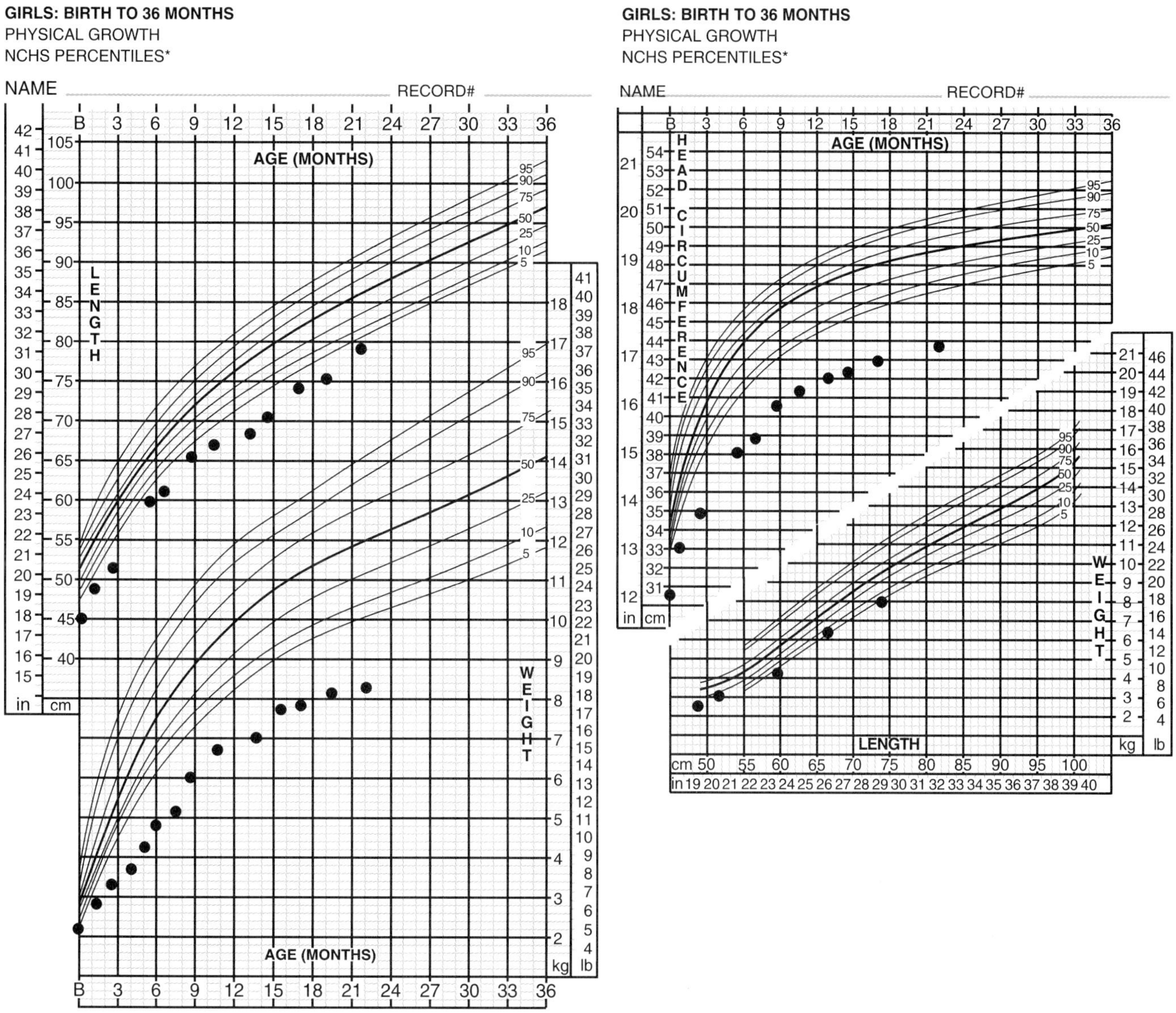

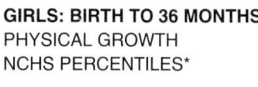

GIRLS: BIRTH TO 36 MONTHS
PHYSICAL GROWTH
NCHS PERCENTILES*

Figure 13-1. Growth curve of an infant girl with unexplained chronic failure to thrive, which affected weight and head growth more than length, which suggested an organic disorder. Intrauterine growth retardation without postnatal catch-up growth is demonstrated (see Chapter 60). (Adapted from National Center for Health Statistics: NCHS Growth Charts, 1976. Monthly Vital Statistics Report, Vol. 25, No. 3, Suppl [HRA] 76-1120. Rockville, Md, Health Resources Administration, June 1976. Data from The Fels Research Institute, Yellow Springs, Ohio. © 1976, Ross Laboratories.)

relation to their normal-sized peers as a result of an early intrauterine event. They will probably remain small for their lifespan; nutritional enhancement may not alter their ultimate size. Infants who are asymmetrically small for gestational age, with sparing of the head circumference and possibly length, probably suffered a late intrauterine event, such as poor maternal nutrition or placental insufficiency. These infants often eat voraciously and experience catch-up growth early in life. Children with genetic short stature have low weight and short height for age. Bone age is consistent with chronologic age. Other family members, particularly the parents, are usually short.

Children with FTT caused by calorie insufficiency typically have decreased weight gain, at first with sparing of height and head circumference (wasting). Long-standing calorie insufficiency results in height deceleration (stunting). Only in the worst, long-standing cases is head growth decreased. This typical pattern suggests calorie insufficiency and gives the clinician an idea of the chronicity of the problem.

There are several approaches to the differential diagnosis. The functional approach determines whether there is a problem with increased calorie requirement, increased calorie loss, or decreased calorie intake or utilization (Table 13-1). The systems approach focuses on the identification of the organ system or systems that might be responsible for the poor growth. A careful history can point the clinician toward a particular system to consider for further diagnostic evaluation (Table 13-2).

Another approach is to consider the age at onset and the conditions likely to manifest at that age. The causes of prenatal growth problems include environmental toxins, maternal drug and alcohol use, prenatal infection, congenital syndromes, placental insufficiency, and poor prenatal nutrition. Poor growth immediately after birth can be associated with maternal postpartum depression, bonding and attachment disorders, incorrect formula preparation, failed breast feeding, and congenital anomalies or metabolic conditions. In children older than 1 year, issues of separation and autonomy may result in power struggles over eating and in insufficient intake.

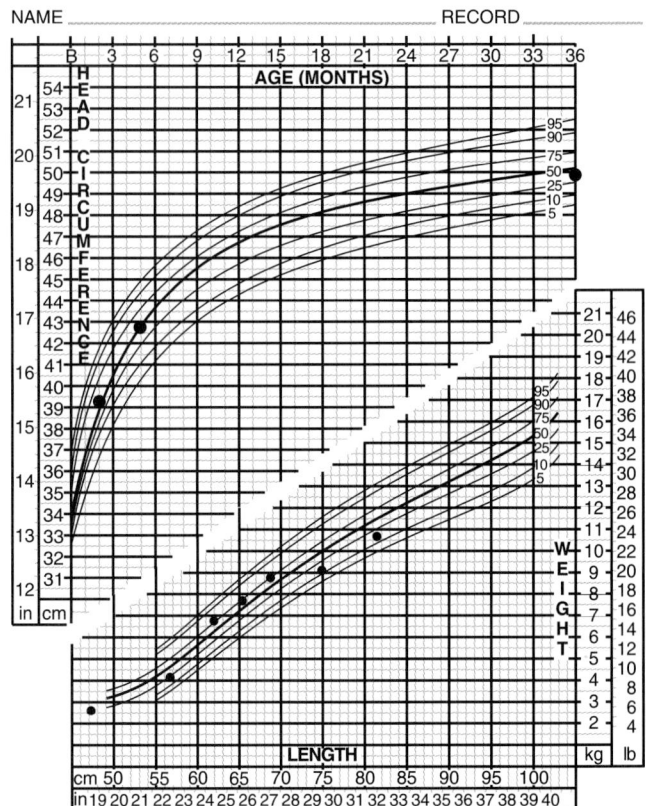

BOYS: BIRTH TO 36 MONTHS
PHYSICAL GROWTH
NCHS PERCENTILES*

BOYS: BIRTH TO 36 MONTHS
PHYSICAL GROWTH
NCHS PERCENTILES*

Figure 13-2. Growth curve of an infant boy with untreated growth hormone deficiency. Note that weight and length remain proportionate, whereas head growth is less affected. (Adapted from National Center for Health Statistics: NCHS Growth Charts, 1976. Monthly Vital Statistics Report, Vol. 25, No. 3, Suppl [HRA] 76-1120. Rockville, Md, Health Resources Administration, June 1976. Data from The Fels Research Institute, Yellow Springs, Ohio. © 1976, Ross Laboratories.)

For toddlers, poor food choices (empty calories found in juice drinks and snack foods), dysfunctional feeding interaction (the child's not being allowed to feed himself or herself or eating alone), and distraction (chaotic home environment, television) may interfere with adequate food intake.

HISTORY

The history is the most important part of the evaluation of the child with FTT.

HISTORY OF THE PRESENT ILLNESS

If poor growth is first noted by the clinician, the clinician should identify whether the family perceives a problem. What is the family members' perception of the child's food intake? When, if ever, did they first notice a problem? What changes have they made to address the problem? Asking these questions in a nonjudgmental manner will reassure the family members that the clinician regards them as partners in the task of improving the child's growth.

Are there sources of calorie loss? Does the child vomit or spit up frequently? What is the stool pattern, and what is the quality of the stools? What are the pattern and frequency of urination? Does urination seem excessive or inadequate? Affirmative answers may indicate a gastrointestinal, metabolic, or renal problem.

Are there sources of increased calorie need? Has the child been sick? Has the child had fevers? Does the child tire when feeding? Is there decreased activity? Are there any chronic conditions?

What is the child's usual daily pattern of activity? Who prepares the food and feeds the child? Is there more than one caregiver? How do the parents know what the alternative caregiver has fed the child, or if the child has vomited or defecated while in the care of another adult? Is there a difference in how the child eats or eliminates when the child is with the parents in comparison to other caretakers?

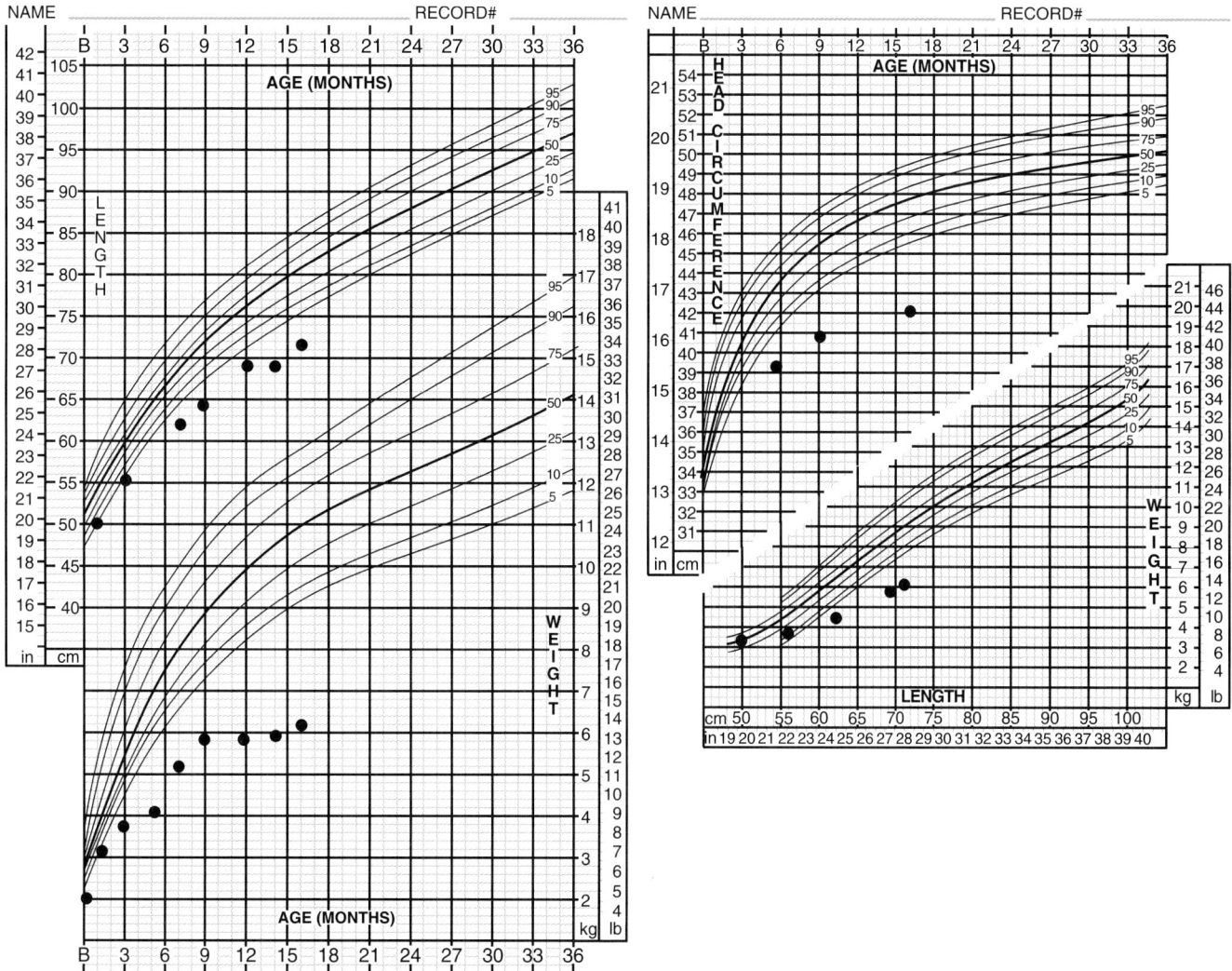

Figure 13-3. Growth curve of an infant boy with severely impaired head growth, poor weight gain, and less impairment of length. Most obvious is the marked microcephaly associated with developmental delay, suggestive of an underlying neurologic disorder. (Adapted from National Center for Health Statistics: NCHS Growth Charts, 1976. Monthly Vital Statistics Report, Vol. 25, No. 3, Suppl [HRA] 76-1120. Rockville, Md, Health Resources Administration, June 1976. Data from The Fels Research Institute, Yellow Springs, Ohio. © 1976, Ross Laboratories.)

Sometimes parents do not realize that their child is underfed while out of their care.

A detailed feeding history should start with infant feeding, and dietary sources and growth patterns should be chronologically reviewed. Was the child breast-fed or formula-fed? If the child was breast-fed, were there any problems with milk sufficiency? How did each parent feel about breast-feeding? Did the mother feel emotionally supported in her choice to breast-feed? If the child was formula-fed, what was the formula; how was it mixed; was there ever any reason to change formula and, if so, why; and how was it changed? Was feeding a pleasurable or a difficult experience for the parent and child? These questions may give insight into early parent-child interaction problems.

If the child is beyond infancy, when and how were solid foods introduced? Were there any specific food refusals, which might indicate an allergy or intolerance? How did the child accept solids? What are the child's food preferences? When did the child start to self-feed? Where does the child eat? Is there a high chair or secure place

to eat? Are there family meals, or does the child eat alone? What is going on in the immediate environment when the child is eating? These questions can reveal dysfunctional eating behaviors that can affect the child's nutrition.

Does the child have any unusual eating habits? Is there pica? This may indicate nutritional deficiencies, such as iron deficiency (Table 13-3).

Does the child have difficulty taking or manipulating food in the mouth? Is there frequent choking on food? Does the child drool? If the response to any of these questions is confirmatory, consider difficulty with oral-motor control. This is common among children with neurologic problems.

A careful dietary history is imperative. The 24-hour recall is standard, although some authorities question its validity. The clinician asks the parent to remember everything the child ate in the past 24 hours and whether that was a typical day. It is helpful to start with the present and work backward. Alternatively, the parent may keep a 3-day food diary. The diary should be

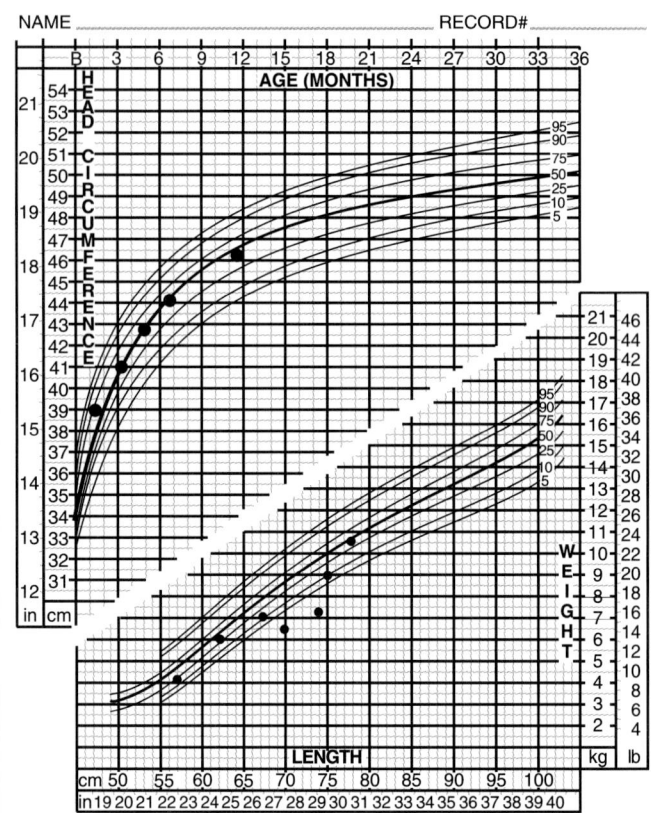

BOYS: BIRTH TO 36 MONTHS
PHYSICAL GROWTH
NCHS PERCENTILES*

Figure 13-4. Growth curve of an infant boy with acute weight loss and catch-up weight gain. Before the age of 4½ months, there was normal growth while he was breast-feeding. After a change to an inadequate weaning diet, severe weight loss developed, but less impairment of length occurred. Head size was not affected. An acute episode of diarrhea led to multiple dietary changes that resulted in further weight loss. With a proper diet history, nutritional rehabilitation with a balanced diet resolved this child's problem. This may also be a pattern of a child with celiac disease. (Adapted from National Center for Health Statistics: NCHS Growth Charts, 1976. Monthly Vital Statistics Report, Vol. 25, No. 3, Suppl [HRA] 76-1120. Rockville, Md, Health Resources Administration, June 1976. Data from The Fels Research Institute, Yellow Springs, Ohio. © 1976, Ross Laboratories.)

structured so that the type of food, quantity, method of preparation, and amount eaten are recorded; beverages should be included. The caregiver should receive prior instruction regarding how to estimate portions and to include only what the child actually eats.

Diet review is a good opportunity to explore parental beliefs about food and the feeding of children (e.g., children must drink water, they need lots of milk, juice is good for them, fats should be restricted to prevent obesity and heart disease). It may be useful to explore feeding issues of ethnic origin in the parents' families. Parents who base their assumptions about foods on their childhood experiences may not be selecting foods appropriately. The parent who sees the child as a "vulnerable child" may be overanxious and rigid about food intake. Cultural norms may dictate certain food choices, which may not provide optimal nutrition. Vegetarian diets may provide insufficient protein, vitamin B_{12}, and iron.

MEDICAL HISTORY

The prenatal and perinatal history should begin with the mother's age and general health. The number of pregnancies and children should be ascertained. Was this child the result of a planned pregnancy? What was the mother's reaction to the pregnancy? What was the reaction of the father and of the mother's family and friends? How did she feel about having a child? Was she emotionally prepared? When did she start her prenatal care? How much weight did she gain? Were there any complications during the pregnancy? Was prenatal testing for syphilis and human immunodeficiency virus obtained, and what were the results? Did the mother have any emotional problems during or before her pregnancy? What was her alcohol, tobacco, and drug intake during her pregnancy? Was she hoping for a boy or a girl?

Table 13-1. Differential Diagnosis by Functional Category
Excessive Calorie Needs
Diabetes mellitus
Cystic fibrosis
Chronic respiratory (BPD) or cardiovascular disease (CHF)
Hyperthyroidism
Cerebral palsy/spasticity
Chronic infection
Inadequate Calorie Intake
Family education and mental health: maternal depression, psychosis, substance abuse, lack of parental knowledge of child nutrition needs
Parent-child interaction: parental emotional distance, parental anxiety, mealtime distractions (i.e., television), lack of family mealtime, overindulgent or overcontrolling parent, parental inability to read hunger and satiety cues
Poor food choices: allows grazing, excessive juice intake
Child factors: neuromuscular disease, poor oral/motor coordination, chronic disease with easy tiring and failure to complete meals, difficult temperament, hyperactivity, inability to display hunger cues
Economic factors: family not able to afford adequate food, diluting formula, early conversion from formula to cow's milk
Increased Calorie Loss/Failure to Incorporate Ingested Calories
Diabetes mellitus
Malabsorption syndromes (celiac disease, lactose intolerance, cystic fibrosis, other causes of pancreatic insufficiency, chronic cholestasis)
Metabolic disorders
Chronic diarrhea
Gastroesophageal reflux and other conditions with chronic vomiting, eosinophilic gastroenteritis

BPD, bronchopulmonary dysplasia; CHF, congestive heart failure.

The perinatal history includes problems with labor, method of delivery, and the newborn's growth parameters at birth (i.e., appropriate, small, or large for gestational age). Was the delivery difficult? Did the baby have any problems in the nursery? How long did the baby stay in the hospital? Did the baby have feeding problems after birth? Was breast-feeding begun immediately?

The child's medical history should be reviewed for chronic conditions and recurrent, acute conditions, such as recurrent emesis, constipation, neurologic symptoms, or recurrent infections that suggest an organic process. Hospitalizations, surgical procedures, medications, and allergies should also be explored. Immunization status should be ascertained because delays could be associated with social dysfunction or neglect. It is essential to document neurodevelopmental progress, because motor or cognitive delays could be associated with neurologic dysfunction that increases calorie requirements and/or decreases feeding efficiency.

FAMILY HISTORY

The clinician should ascertain the growth of siblings and other family members. Are there patterns of growth in the family that might result in a child's growing less than expected in the early years? What, if any, differences do the parents notice between this child and their other children? What were the growth patterns and ultimate sizes of the parents and grandparents? What

was the age at menarche and puberty in parents and siblings? Creating a two-generation genogram that includes the height and weight of each family member may provide clues to the growth potential of the patient.

Is there any history of heart disease, renal disease, or gastrointestinal disease in the family? Have there been any early childhood deaths? Is there any sickle cell disease or other anemic condition? Are there any family members with genetic or metabolic conditions? Is there a family history of mental illness that might affect the child or the caretakers? Is there consanguinity?

SOCIAL HISTORY

Many cases of FTT are diagnosed as nonorganic or social in nature, and thus the social history is vital. The examiner should start with the family constellation and who takes care of the child. What is the relationship of the adults in the household, and how do they get along? How do the parents get along? Are the parents working, and if they work simultaneously, who takes care of the child? Does the family income allow the family to have food security? Do they have any difficulty purchasing food for the child? Are food stores accessible? Do they believe they have adequate storage and refrigeration? Are there adequate eating facilities and implements? Are there siblings who might eat the child's food? Is the child enrolled in the Women, Infants, and Children program? What is the cultural context of food selection and eating behavior?

More difficult social issues must be approached carefully, with a statement to the family that all patients with this problem are asked these routine questions. Is there any substance abuse in the home that might result in use of food dollars for tobacco, alcohol, or drugs? Have the child protection authorities ever been involved with the family?

Is the child in group day care, or has the family traveled to an area where a chronic infection might have been acquired? The child who was growing fine until he or she returned from vacation in the tropics may have acquired an infestation that is causing FTT.

Although the social history can be the most revealing part of the history, it can be the most difficult to elicit. Often the clinician must establish trust with the family before they can reveal the source of their inability to meet their child's nutritional needs.

REVIEW OF SYSTEMS

A thorough review of systems can help to reveal organic conditions. A few areas merit special attention:

Constitutional: The examiner should ask whether there are any fevers, night sweats, or changes in activity or sleep.

Gastrointestinal: The examiner should inquire about choking, swallowing, vomiting, and spitting up. Night waking and coughing may indicate reflux. Diarrhea, constipation, abdominal pain, distention, or discomfort may indicate organic disease.

Cardiopulmonary: The examiner should ask about coughing, wheezing, night waking, shortness of breath, exercise intolerance, and early tiring during feeding.

Renal: The examiner should inquire about dysuria, hematuria, increased urinary frequency or volume, secondary enuresis, and urine that seem unusually dilute.

PHYSICAL EXAMINATION

The examination should start with accurate measurement of height or length, weight, and head circumference, and these parameters should be plotted on a standard growth curve. Weight for height or BMI should also be plotted. Historic events should be obtained and plotted to identify patterns of growth.

Table 13-2. Failure to Thrive: Differential Diagnosis by System

Psychosocial/Behavioral

Inadequate diet because of poverty/food insufficiency, errors in food preparation
Poor parenting skills (lack of knowledge of sufficient diet)
Child/parent interaction problems (autonomy struggles, coercive feeding)
Food refusal
Parental cognitive or mental health problems
Child abuse or neglect

Neurologic

Oral motor dysfunction
Spasticity
Psychomotor retardation
Increased intracranial pressure

Renal

Urinary tract infection
Renal tubular acidosis
Renal failure

Endocrine

Diabetes mellitus
Hypothyroidism/hyperthyroidism
Growth hormone deficiency
Adrenal insufficiency

Genetic/Metabolic/Congenital

Cystic fibrosis
Sickle cell disease
Inborn errors of metabolism (organic acidosis, hyperammonemia, storage disease)
Fetal alcohol syndrome
Skeletal dysplasias
Chromosomal disorders
Multiple congenital anomaly syndromes (VATER, CHARGE)

Gastrointestinal

Pyloric stenosis
Gastroesophageal reflux
Malrotation
Malabsorption
Celiac disease
Milk intolerance: lactose, protein
Pancreatic insufficiency syndromes
Chronic cholestasis
Inflammatory bowel disease
Chronic congenital diarrhea states
Pseudoobstruction

Cardiac

Cyanotic heart lesions
Congestive heart failure

Pulmonary/Respiratory

Severe asthma
Cystic fibrosis; bronchiectasis
Chronic respiratory failure
Bronchopulmonary dysplasia
Adenoid/tonsillar hypertrophy
Obstructive sleep apnea

Miscellaneous

Collagen-vascular disease
Malignancy
Primary immunodeficiency
Transplantation

Infections

Perinatal infection
Occult/chronic infections
Parasitic infestation
Tuberculosis
Human immunodeficiency virus

CHARGE, coloboma, heart disease, atresia choanae, retarded growth and retarded development and/or central nervous system anomalies, genital hypoplasia, and ear anomalies and/or deafness; VATER, vertebral defects, imperforate anus, tracheoesophageal fistula, and radial and renal dysplasia.

As part of a complete physical examination, the following signs should be sought:

general: degree of emaciation, state of fat distribution and muscle mass, dysmorphic features
head, eyes, ears, nose, and throat: fontanelle size, evidence of chronic ear infections, allergic stigmata
cardiorespiratory: respiratory rate and effort, upper airway obstruction, tachypnea and tachycardia, edema
gastrointestinal: organomegaly, abdominal distention, rectal fissures or prolapse
genitourinary: renal masses, Tanner staging
musculoskeletal: joint swelling, bone deformities
skin: hydration, evidence of chronic inflammation, bruising or scarring, rashes, hair quality and distribution, nails
neurologic: muscle tone, coordination, swallowing and drooling, strength, level of consciousness

Abnormalities associated with pathologic biomedical conditions should prompt a search for a specific diagnosis (see Table 13-2). On occasion, growth failure, as well as other physical findings, can be associated with specific nutrient deficiencies (Table 13-4; see Table 13-3).

LABORATORY EVALUATION

Because almost any serious chronic illness may result in FTT, the examiner must have a broad diagnostic screening approach and simultaneously consider the more likely possibility that nonmedical processes are the cause. In most cases of chronic illness, there is probably some clue in the history, physical examination, or selected standard diagnostic laboratory screening tests. The few cases of organic FTT not detected by these screening tests may become evident when the infant does not respond to nutritional rehabilitation. If, however, the examiner attempts to pursue every conceivable diagnostic test for organic causes of FTT before implementing vigorous nutritional rehabilitation, he or she is likely to run out of time, patience, and resources and to come to no conclusion. Some unusual cases may take months or years to determine.

The choice of the appropriate initial laboratory tests should include several general screening tests (complete blood count, urinalysis, serum electrolyte levels, blood urea nitrogen level) to detect treatable conditions. A complete blood cell count can reveal clinically inapparent anemia, which, although usually secondary to the poor nutritional state, can sometimes contribute to the poor dietary intake or suggest anemia of chronic disease. A urinalysis and urine culture can reveal evidence of an occult urinary tract infection

Table 13-3. Characteristics of Mineral Deficiencies

Mineral	Function	Manifestations of Deficiency	Comments	Sources
Iron	Heme-containing macromolecules (e.g., hemoglobin, cytochrome, myoglobin)	Anemia, spoon nails, reduced muscle and mental performance	History of pica, cow's milk, gastrointestinal bleeding, excessive milk in diet	Liver, eggs, grains
Copper	Redox reactions (e.g., cytochrome oxidase)	Hypochromic anemia, neutropenia, osteoporosis, hypotonia, hypoproteine-mia, poor growth	Inborn error, Menkes kinky hair syndrome	Liver, oysters, meat, nuts, grains, legumes, chocolate
Zinc	Metalloenzymes (e.g., alkaline phosphatase, carbonic anhydrase, DNA polymerase; wound healing)	Acrodermatitis enteropathica; poor growth, acroorificial rash, alopecia, delayed sexual development, hypogeusia, infection	Protein-calorie malnutrition; weaning; malabsorption syndrome	Meat, grains, cheese, nuts
Selenium	Antioxidant Glutathione peroxidase	Keshan cardiomyopathy in China, poor growth	Endemic areas; long-term TPN	Meat, vegetables
Chromium	Insulin cofactor	Poor weight gain, glucose intolerance, neuropathy	Protein-calorie malnutrition, long-term TPN	Yeast, breads
Fluoride	Strengthens dental enamel	Caries	Supplementation during tooth growth, narrow therapeutic range, fluorosis may cause staining of the teeth	Seafood, water
Iodine	Thyroxine, triiodothyronine production	Simple endemic goiter Myxedematous cretinism: congenital hypothyroidism Neurologic cretinism: mental retardation, deafness, spasticity, normal T_4 level at birth	Endemic in New Guinea, the Congo; endemic in Great Lakes area before iodized salt available	Seafood, iodized salt, most food in nonendemic areas

From Tershakovec AM. Stallings VA: Pediatric nutrition and nutritional disorders. In Behrman RE, Kliegman RM (eds): Nelson Essentials of Pediatrics, 2nd ed. Philadelphia, WB Saunders, 1994, p 81.

T_4, thyroxine; TPN, total parenteral nutrition.

or renal tubular acidosis. An erythrocyte sedimentation rate may provide evidence of chronic inflammation or infection. The examiner may need to test for celiac disease, in which poor weight gain may be the only symptom for many years. Other specific tests are directed by the history and physical examination (Table 13-5). For example, for a child with developmental delay and FTT, a blood lead test, metabolic screening tests, a karyotype, imaging of the head, human immunodeficiency virus screening, or a lumbar puncture may be necessary, whereas a child with apparent malabsorption is evaluated completely differently (such as for cystic fibrosis or celiac disease).

OVERALL APPROACH

The evaluation of a child with FTT should proceed in a stepwise manner (Fig. 13-5). Once the clinician has arrived at a working diagnosis, treatment can be instituted. It is important to develop a therapeutic alliance with family members. Parents whose children are not growing according to expectation may already be feeling guilty or may have a sense of failure. A nonjudgmental approach, avoiding the assignment of blame, is important. Although the clinician can make suggestions, it is the family that must feel empowered to implement the plan.

Providing specific information that can be easily implemented in the family's home environment will be more successful than giving general advice. Suggestions that a parent feed more food to a child may be disregarded, particularly when the family members believe they are already doing their best. It also may increase caregiver guilt and frustration if the child does not grow as expected.

Even with the strong suspicion of a biomedical cause, it is reasonable to give specific advice on enhancing calorie intake while further evaluation and treatment is ongoing. If the condition is chronic, the child needs long-term nutritional supplementation. If the condition is acute and treatable, such as a urinary tract infection, the child needs extra calories for catch-up growth.

STEPS TO IMPROVE CALORIE INTAKE

MEALTIME BEHAVIOR

A pleasant, safe setting should be created for mealtime. An infant seat is appropriate for the first several months. Once a child can sustain a sitting position, a high chair is advantageous. This allows the child to feel safe from falling, frees up his or her hands for feeding, and keeps the child confined in one place to focus on the meal. A bib prevents the need for frequent changes of clothing. For an older child, a booster seat or a child-size table and chair are useful, along with child-size utensils. Parents who feed an infant or toddler while holding the child in their laps find that the meal is a struggle; this prevents the child from developing the skills needed for self-feeding.

To promote the important social aspect of mealtime, family members should be seated and eating with all children whenever possible. This should make the meal enjoyable and allows older

Table 13-4. Characteristics of Vitamin Deficiencies

Vitamin	Function	Manifestations of Deficiency	Comments	Sources
Water-Soluble				
Thiamine (B$_1$)	Coenzyme in ketoacid decarboxylation (e.g., pyruvate → acetyl-CoA transketolase reaction)	Beri-beri: polyneuropathy, calf tenderness, heart failure, edema, ophthalmoplegia	Inborn errors of lactate metabolism; boiling milk destroys B$_1$	Liver, meat, milk, cereals, nuts, legumes
Riboflavin (B$_2$)	FAD coenzyme in oxidation-reduction reactions	Anorexia, mucositis, anemia, cheilosis, nasolabial seborrhea	Photosensitizer	Milk, cheese, liver, meat, eggs, whole grains, green leafy vegetables
Niacin (B$_3$)	NAD coenzyme in oxidation-reduction reactions	Pellagra: photosensitivity, dermatitis, dementia, diarrhea, death	Tryptophan is a precursor	Meat, fish, liver, whole grains, green leafy vegetables
Pyridoxine (B$_6$)	Cofactor in amino acid metabolism	Seizures, hyperacusis, microcytic anemia, nasolabial seborrhea, neuropathy	Dependency state; deficiency secondary to drugs	Meat, liver, whole grains, peanuts, soybeans
Pantothenic acid	Coenzyme A in Krebs cycle	None reported	—	Meat, vegetables
Biotin	Cofactor in carboxylase reactions of amino acids	Alopecia, dermatitis, hypotonia, death	Bowel resection, inborn errors of metabolism, and ingestion of raw eggs	Yeast, meats; made by intestinal flora
B$_{12}$	Coenzyme for 5-methyl-tetrahydrofolate formation; DNA synthesis	Megaloblastic anemia, peripheral neuropathy, posterior lateral column disease, vitiligo	Vegans; fish tapeworm; transcobalamin or intrinsic factor deficiencies	Meat, fish, cheese, eggs
Folate	DNA synthesis	Megaloblastic anemia	Goat milk deficient; drug antagonists; heat inactivates	Liver, greens, vegetables, cereals, cheese
Ascorbic acid (C)	Reducing agent; collagen metabolism	Scurvy: irritability, purpura, bleeding gums, periosteal hemorrhage, aching bones	May improve tyrosine metabolism in preterm infants	Citrus fruits, green vegetables; cooking destroys it
Fat-Soluble				
A	Epithelial cell integrity; vision	Night blindness, xerophthalmia, Bitot spots, follicular hyperkeratosis, poor growth	Common with protein-calorie malnutrition; malabsorption	Liver, milk, eggs, green and yellow vegetables, fruits
D	Maintains serum calcium, phosphorus levels	Rickets: reduced bone mineralization, poor growth	Prohormone of 25- and 1,25-vitamin D	Fortified milk, cheese, liver
E	Antioxidant	Hemolysis in preterm infants; areflexia, ataxia, ophthalmoplegia	May benefit patients with G6PD deficiency	Seeds, vegetables, germ oils, green leafy vegetables
K	Posttranslation carboxylation of clotting factors II, VII, IX, and X and proteins C, S	Prolonged prothrombin time; hemorrhage; elevated PIVKA (protein induced in vitamin K absence)	Malabsorption; breast-fed infants	Liver, green vegetables; made by intestinal flora

Modified from Tershakovec A, Stallings VA: Pediatric nutrition and nutritional disorders. In Behrman RE, Kliegman RM (eds): Nelson Essentials of Pediatrics, 2nd ed. Philadelphia, WB Saunders, 1994, p 74.

FAD, flavin adenine dinucleotide; G6PD, glucose-6-phosphate dehydrogenase; NAD, nicotinamide adenine dinucleotide.

children or adults to model eating behaviors for the younger children. Toddlers and older infants are usually interested in the food served to other family members, and this encourages experimentation with new foods. There should be conversation during the meal, but the child's food intake should not be the focus of the conversation.

Distractions should be minimized during meals. The television set should be off. There should not be other commotion in the kitchen. However, for the infant, a small washable toy on the tray or table may help keep attention on the food.

Parents should understand that experimenting with food is part of the natural curiosity of older infants and toddlers. If the parent is constantly wiping the child and berating him or her for getting messy, the child cannot learn that eating can be a fun experience. If a parent has particular difficulty with messiness, the examiner can suggest spreading newspaper or a plastic sheet under the high chair. Another simple technique is the "two-spoon method" of feeding the child. If a parent insists that feeding goes only in one direction—that is, the parent feeds the child—the child will resist. The parent should

Table 13-5. Some Causes of Failure to Thrive and Screening Tests

Cause	Screening Tests
Environmental and Psychosocial*	
Inadequate caloric intake	History; observation in hospital
Emotional deprivation and disruptions	History; observation in hospital
Rumination; chronic diarrhea, gastroesophageal reflux	History; observation in hospital
Anorexia nervosa and bulimia	History; examination
Secondary to impact of organic disease	History and observation
Organic	
Central nervous system abnormalities, infection	Neurodevelopmental assessment; brain MRI
Gastrointestinal system	
Malabsorption, cystic fibrosis, inflammatory bowel disease, parasites, aganglionic megacolon; liver disease; food intolerance; celiac disease; gastroesophageal reflux	Examination of stools: stool fat, sweat test, stool ova and parasites; antigliadin and antiendomysium antibodies; liver function tests; barium swallow, erythrocyte sedimentation rate, food challenge, intestinal biopsy
Partial cleft palate	Physical examination; observation of feeding
Chronic heart failure	Physical examination; chest roentgenography; echocardiography
Endocrine disorders	Growth chart; thyroid function tests; bone age, cortisol level
Pulmonary disease	
Bronchopulmonary dysplasia; bronchiectasis; cystic fibrosis	Physical examination; chest roentgenography; tuberculin test, pulmonary function tests, sweat test
Renal disease	
Anomalies; infection; renal failure; renal tubular disorder	Urinalysis; blood urea nitrogen; ultrasonography; urinary amino acid screen; urine pH
Chromosomal disorders or syndromes	Chromosomal analysis; identification of peculiar facies or multisystem defects, skeletal radiographs
Turner syndrome	
Skeletal dysplasias	
Other metabolic or inborn errors	Urine and blood amino and organic acids, mitochondrial DNA, specific gene probes
Chronic infection	
Tuberculosis, mycotic, congenital, AIDS	Tuberculin test; appropriate laboratory identification of infectious agent, PCR
Chronic inflammation	
Juvenile rheumatoid arthritis, SLE	Physical examination; erythrocyte sedimentation rate; CBC, ANA
Immunodeficiency disease	
DiGeorge syndrome; combined immunodeficiency	History of rash and diarrhea; thymus size; tonsil size; skin tests; complete blood count, cell markers, FISH for DiGeorge syndrome
AIDS or AIDS-related complex	HIV test
Malignancies (kidney, hematologic, adrenal, brain)	Roentgenography (CT, ultrasonography) of abdomen, chest; brain CT or MRI, bone marrow scan
Congenital syndromes caused by alcohol, Dilantin, drugs, infection	Physical examination; history, TORCH evaluation

Modified from Barbero GJ: Failure to thrive. In Behrman RE (ed): Nelson Textbook of Pediatrics, 14th ed. Philadelphia, WB Saunders, 1992, p 215.

*Nonorganic may also be combined with organic.

AIDS, acquired immunodeficiency syndrome; ANA, antinuclear antibodies; CBC, complete blood cell count; CT, computed tomography; FISH, fluorescent in situ hybridization; HIV, human immunodeficiency virus; MRI, magnetic resonance imaging; PCR, polymerase chain reaction; SLE, systemic lupus erythematosus; TORCH, toxoplasmosis, other, rubella, cytomegalovirus, herpes simplex.

provide a spoon to the child to dip into the food, and the parent has the second spoon, which does the bulk of the feeding.

Once the child has communicated that the meal is finished, the parent can offer one or two more bites but then should accept that the child is no longer hungry, and the meal should be ended. The duration of the meal for a toddler is typically not more than 15 or 20 minutes. Food should not be brought out until the next regular meal or snack.

BEVERAGES

Milk intake should be the exclusive nutritional source for infants from birth to the age of 4 to 6 months. Formula-fed infants should be held during a feeding until they are able to sit on their own and hold the bottle. Bottles should never be propped. Whole cow's milk should be consumed between the ages of 1 and 2 years. Two-percent milk or whole milk may be used after the age of 2 years. The volume of formula or whole cow's milk consumed should be 32 ounces or less per day. If a child is drinking an excessive amount of formula, review the preparation procedures to ensure that the responsible caregiver can read and understand instructions for proper dilution.

All children naturally enjoy sweet foods. However, if they are introduced early or used instead of more nutritionally complete foods, children may develop a preference for sweets, especially juices. In particular, toddlers who are allowed to have bottles with sweetened juices throughout the day eat little at mealtime. Controversy exists as to whether excessive juice affects weight or even height. What is likely is that these children are poorly nourished, because of limited intake of other foods. In addition, because of limited absorption of dietary sugars, particularly in juices with high fructose-to-glucose ratios (such as apple and pear juice), children with excessive juice intake may suffer from bloating, excessive flatulence, abdominal pain, and chronic diarrhea because of undigestible carbohydrate malabsorption. The American Academy of Pediatrics suggests that juice not be introduced until after children

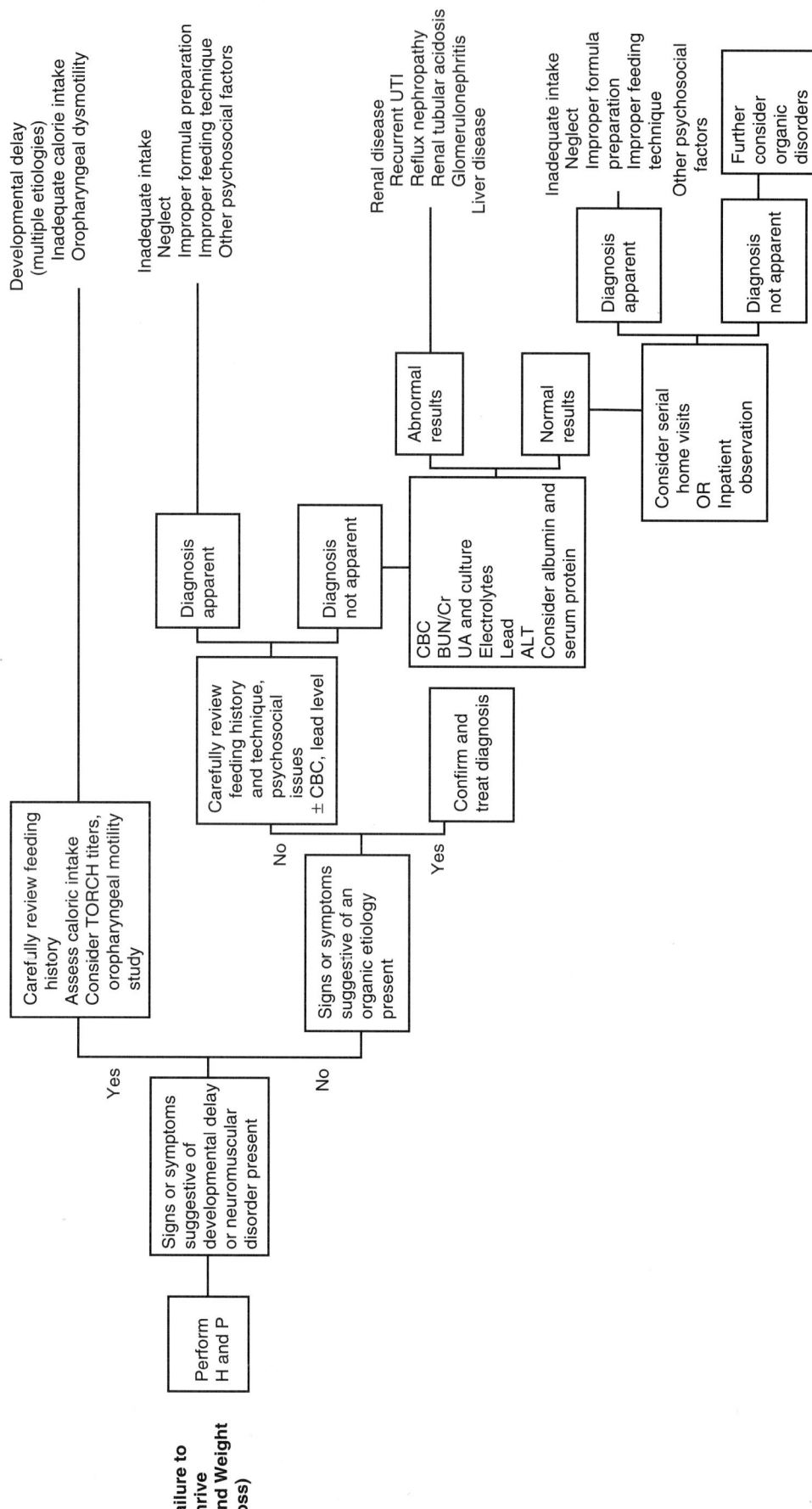

Figure 13-5. Flow chart for the stepwise evaluation of a child with failure to thrive (and weight loss). (Modified from Pomeranz AJ, Busey SL, Sabnis S, et al [eds]: Pediatric Decision-Making Strategies to Accompany Nelson Textbook of Pediatrics. Philadelphia, WB Saunders, 2002, p 313.

are 6 months of age. When introduced, juice should be offered only in a cup. Children should drink only 100% fruit juice. Intake should be limited to 4 to 6 ounces per day for children aged 1 to 6 years and to 8 to 12 ounces per day for older children and adolescents.

Various methods are available to enhance the calorie density of infant dietary beverages for nutritional supplementation. Formulas can be made with less water. Polycose and vegetable oils can be added. Pumped/expressed breast milk can be enhanced with breast milk fortifier.

FOOD SELECTION

For older toddlers and preschool-aged children, it is appropriate to allow food selection from two or three choices. Providing choices allows the child to assume some control over the feeding. Each choice must be nutritionally sound and acceptable to the parent. Parents should not become bound by social constraints when it comes to foods served at certain meals.

Infants and young toddlers may have preferences for certain food textures, temperatures, and presentations. These preferences are often short-lived. Normal children may become "picky" eaters in the second and third years of life. New foods should routinely be introduced but not forced on the child. With repetition and modeling, children will try new foods. Food preferences may be strong and cyclic. For example, a child may go through a cycle in which he or she requests peanut butter and jelly sandwiches for nearly every meal. If a variety of fruits or vegetables are given along with the sandwich, this may be a reasonable compromise.

Although it is the caregiver's responsibility to provide appropriate food, it is the child's responsibility to decide on the quantity of food to be eaten. "Force feeding" will convince the child only that mealtime is something to be feared. Parents must learn to read a child's cues for hunger and satiety.

DAILY ROUTINES AND SNACKS

Once children are receiving solid foods, they should be on a regular schedule of meals that are served at predictable times during the day. This may mean three meals and two or three snacks per day for infants and toddlers. The practice of "grazing"—having food available to the child throughout the day—should not be allowed. Small, frequent meals allow the child to be satiated, which prevents the completion of standard meals, and the ultimate outcome is that the child does not fulfill daily requirements for growth. Snacks afford the opportunity to supplement the child's diet with high-quality foods with good nutritional content. For toddlers and preschool-aged children, solids should be given at the beginning of the meal. Only after a good portion of the meal has been eaten should liquids be introduced.

CALCULATING CALORIC NEED

In order to calculate the minimal daily caloric requirements needed for catch-up growth, the examiner should determine the weight age (age at which current weight would be at 50%) and recommended calories for weight age (Table 13-6). The ideal weight for current height (50% weight for current height) should also be determined as follows:

$$\frac{(\text{kcal/kg for weight age}) \times (\text{ideal weight for height in kilograms})}{\text{actual weight in kilograms}}$$

For most children, calories needed for catch-up growth can be easily calculated as

$$\frac{(120 \text{ kcal/kg}) \times (\text{ideal weight for height in kilograms})}{\text{actual weight in kilograms}}$$

Table 13-6. Normal Calorie Requirements by Age

Age	Calorie Requirement (kcal/kg/day)	Weight Gain (g/day)
Premature	150	20-40
Full-term to 6 months	100-120	20-30
7 to 12 months	90-100	10-15
Toddler	75-85	7-9

Most infants do well on 160 to 180 kcal/kg/day. Some infants may need considerably more, up to 1.5 to 2 times the daily requirements for catch-up. Caloric intake can be estimated from the diet history.

NUTRITIONAL SUPPLEMENTATION FOR THE OLDER INFANT AND CHILD

Several products are available for nutritional supplementation. The complete liquid drinks are excellent products; very similar nutritional value can be found in packaged instant breakfast drinks when mixed with whole milk, at much lower cost. These nutrient-dense beverages should supplement the child's diet, not supplant other foods.

Many additives (powdered milk, margarine, cheese, wheat germ, peanut butter) are available. Determine which foods are familiar to the caregiver and are acceptable to the child. Attention should be paid to maximizing protein intake needed for growth.

If a child does not seem to be taking an adequate variety of foods, a supplement with multivitamins with minerals may be indicated. Particularly during periods of rapid catch-up growth, additional vitamins and minerals can be beneficial. Iron and zinc deficiencies may impede normal growth (see Table 13-3). Zinc supplementation has been shown to enhance catch-up growth in malnourished children.

REFERRAL RESOURCES AND OTHER OPTIONS

THE INTERDISCIPLINARY TEAM

Children with FTT have complex medical and psychosocial issues. As a result, a biomedical model of care may be insufficient for managing the child and family. An interdisciplinary approach may be beneficial in complicated cases by relieving the medical provider of the responsibilities of investigating the home situation, investigating the family's finances and resources, and observation of mealtime.

The multidisciplinary team could include a physician, social worker, psychologist, nutritionist, nurse, child life specialist, and home visitor. Each team member evaluates the patient and family according to his or her discipline. The team then discusses the case and develops a plan for ongoing management. Children treated by teams have been found to have better outcomes than do children receiving routine care in a primary care setting.

The psychologic evaluation may identify children with developmental delays and can assess the stressors and help identify strengths and weaknesses in the family. In some families, the child may be the indicator that there is a greater disturbance, such as depression or marital stress. The psychologist can also offer support and reassurance as the family goes through a difficult period caused by potential long-term nutritional rehabilitation of the child. In addition, the psychologist can help the caregiver understand that improving the feeding situation takes a great effort on the part of the parent as well as the child and that new strategies are required for successful weight gain.

The nutritionist's expertise is essential for a through evaluation and follow-up plan. When taking a complete nutritional history, the nutritionist can analyze the nutritional and caloric values of the foods eaten. Alternative meal plans can then be developed to maximize calories and nutritional content.

A social worker's contribution to the team is an assessment of the child's environment and factors that may be contributing to the child's state. Areas for investigation include social supports, housing conditions (crowding, space for food storage, proper refrigeration), and financial hardships. Families may need assistance with arranging work leave, rearranging work schedules, transportation, or respite care. Families can be directed to community support services that focus both on social/emotional and material/financial issues. If child maltreatment is suspected, the social worker assists with communication with the appropriate social service agency.

When feasible, home observation provides a wealth of information to the clinician about the environment in which the child resides and eats meals. Does the child have an appropriate place in which to eat? Is there a supply of appropriate foods in the home? What are the other environmental factors that may be impeding the child's growth? Studies of home interventions have had mixed success. There is some evidence that for the youngest children, developmental outcomes are improved by home intervention.

VIDEOTAPING OR DIRECT OBSERVATION

Observation or videotaping of a meal provides an opportunity to assess the child's willingness and ability to participate in the meal, the parenting style, and the interaction between the child and parents. Parent and child strengths should be pointed out to the parent. Problematic communication, both verbal and nonverbal, should be reviewed. Parents should be able to respond to the cues that their child provides. Difficulties that are observed should be discussed and become the basis for further intervention.

INVOLVEMENT OF SOCIAL SERVICE AGENCIES

Clinicians caring for children with FTT often find themselves working in conjunction with other agencies, including social service agencies. Children who are refused food or are abused in any way must be reported. It may, however, be difficult to determine what is neglectful care. Families that are disorganized and overwhelmed, have other pressing social issues, or refuse to follow recommendations, with the result of lack of sufficient progress in the child's growth, must be reported to the local agency. This reporting includes parents with cognitive deficits or mental health problems. It is important for all agencies to work together and articulate a plan, so that the families involved do not receive conflicting instructions and messages.

NON-ORAL ENTERAL FEEDING

For some children, maximizing oral intake may nonetheless provide insufficient calories for catch-up growth. The clinician may consider enteral feeding that bypasses the mouth. This intervention is needed if, despite all other attempts to maximize oral feeding, the child's growth is falling further below the fifth percentile or if the child is showing signs of severe malnourishment (e.g., hypoalbuminemia or low prealbumin levels).

Initially, nasogastric feeding can be used for night feedings. The child should be encouraged to eat orally during the day. If the need for the nasogastric tube is extended for a longer duration (some authorities use 3 months), then a referral should be made for placement of a percutaneous gastrostomy tube. This is used for supplemental nutrition for most children and is not a substitute for oral intake. Children receiving supplemental alimentation should be monitored very closely. Once the weight for height is near the 50th percentile, the supplement should be adjusted to prevent obesity. The tube is removed when the child can sustain an adequate growth rate through oral alimentation without the use of the tube.

It is very important that some oral stimulation continue even if the gastrostomy tube is the main source of nutrition. If children are denied the chance to develop competence in age-appropriate feeding behaviors, they are likely to develop food aversions. This makes reintroduction of oral intake extremely difficult.

CRITERIA FOR HOSPITALIZATION

Decisions about when to hospitalize an infant with FTT are inevitably influenced by practical considerations of the availability and quality of hospital services, cost, and distance from the family. The medical issues are whether hospitalization will facilitate further diagnostic steps and whether the affected child is malnourished enough to create a sense of urgency about nutritional rehabilitation. Loss of more than 30% of the average weight for length (to less than 70% of expected weight for length) constitutes severe malnutrition, which most physicians would be reluctant to treat on an outpatient basis unless there is no satisfactory alternative. In addition, hospitalization is indicated if there is a concern about Munchausen syndrome by proxy. In this situation, a parent may be purposefully manipulating the child in order to produce FTT or other symptoms.

Most children with FTT gain weight in the hospital within 1 to 2 weeks, but obtaining a weight gain in a short amount of time does not prove that the home environment was the problem. Alternatively, even a 1- to 2-week hospitalization in a child without an organic cause of the growth failure may not produce a sustainable weight gain. The foreign surroundings and lack of familiar faces might prevent the child from eating appropriately. Parents may not be able to remain with the child in the hospital if they have other small children to attend to at home.

Sufficient time must be anticipated in the hospital for substantial recovery; in severe cases, full recovery requires about 6 weeks. After initial stabilization and reassurance that the infant is doing well, the child can spend much of this recovery period in a less expensive, nonintensive supervised medical care facility that emphasizes nutritional support and psychosocial stimulation. Creative approaches to well-organized outpatient day programs or frequent home visiting by properly trained health care workers may provide an attractive alternative to hospitalization.

MONITORING

Long-term follow-up is required to ensure that initial weight gains are sustained. At the follow-up visits, the 24-hour diet recall is assessed, or a 3-day diet history is brought by the family. At all visits, the child's growth parameters must be plotted. Dividing weight gained by the number of days since the last measurement provides a mean growth rate. This can be compared with the normal growth rate in children by age group, which is calculated by using the fifth percentile on the standard growth charts (see Table 13-6). A child in need of catch-up growth should exceed the expected growth rate for normal children. Periodically, the family can be observed or videotaped during a feeding session to determine improvement from prior sessions.

LONG-TERM OUTCOMES

Children with early FTT may suffer long-term consequences in growth, cognitive development, and social functioning. Outcomes depend on cause, age at intervention, and associated risk factors and may not be as ominous as early studies suggested. Parental self-perceived competence and child adaptability have been associated with good outcomes.

Children with FTT who experience other social stressors are at higher risk for adverse outcomes. Poverty and associated family and environmental problems may exacerbate the negative effects of FTT. Children with FTT who experience neglect are more likely to have poor outcomes.

FTT may have long-term effects on growth. It may affect ultimate stature and possibly brain growth and development. Children in whom the FTT has an organic cause that can be successfully managed often do well. For those with undetermined causes or persistent FTT, outcome can be poor. Growth may continue to be delayed. Ultimate stature may be shorter than that predicted from mean parental heights. Of interest is that with long-term follow-up, some children have been observed to develop obesity.

Poor developmental and cognitive outcomes have been found in many children with FTT. However, studies of these children have multiple confounding factors, and it is difficult to ascribe outcomes solely to the nutritional deficiencies. Some of the children who fare poorly may have had initial mild deficits that were undetected. Those who were symmetrically small for gestational age and those with microcephaly are particularly at risk for diminished cognitive potential. Home intervention by child development specialists may lessen the impact of FTT on cognitive skills. Children should be referred for early intervention services as soon as deficits are detected. Better success will be achieved if intervention is started early.

Children with FTT may manifest behavioral problems, even after the nutritional issues appear to be resolved. If the behaviors are particularly difficult to manage, the services of a psychologist or behavior specialist are warranted.

SUMMARY AND RED FLAGS

FTT is a complex condition encompassing biomedical and psychosocial causes. In the United States, it is most often associated with various psychosocial attributes of the parents, family, or child. The keys to determining the cause are a thorough history and physical examination. In addition, the growth pattern is critical. Red flags include refusal to eat, poor response to feedings, an inappropriately small head size, and physical signs incompatible with malnutrition. Clinicians should be vigilant in identifying chronic disease as well as indicators of child abuse and neglect. Episodes of recurrent emesis, altered mental status, metabolic acidosis and hypoglycemia should raise suspicions of an inborn error of metabolism. Microcephaly, seizures, developmental delay or developmental regression, and hypotonia or hypertonia should lead to suspicions of a chronic neurologic problem. Identifying and treating the biomedical and psychosocial causes while enhancing calorie intake can result in good outcomes.

REFERENCES

Reviews

Gahagan S, Holmes R: A stepwise approach to evaluation of undernutrition and failure to thrive. Pediatr Clin North Am 1998;45:1.
Kessler DB, Dawson P: Failure to Thrive and Pediatric Undernutrition: A Transdisciplinary Approach. Baltimore, Brookes, 1999.

Mascarenhas MR: Failure to thrive and malabsorption. In Altschuler SM, Liacouras CA (eds): Clinical Pediatric Gastroenterology. Philadelphia, Churchill Livingstone, 1998, pp 71-80.
Schwartz ID: Failure to thrive: An old nemesis in the new millennium. Pediatr Rev 2000;21:8.
Zenel J: Failure to thrive: A general pediatrician's perspective. Pediatr Rev 1997;18:11.

Diagnosis and Laboratory Evaluation

Berwick D: Failure to thrive: Diagnostic yield of hospitalization. Arch Dis Child 1982;57:347-351.
Black MM: Failure to thrive: Strategies for evaluation and intervention. School Psychol Rev 1995;24:171-185.
Centers for Disease Control and Prevention: CDC growth charts: United States. www.cdc.gov/growthcharts/
Committee on Nutrition, American Academy of Pediatrics: The use and misuse of fruit juice in pediatrics. Pediatrics 2001;107:1210-1213.
Drotar D, Eckerle D, Satola J, et al: Maternal interactional behavior with nonorganic failure-to-thrive infants: A case comparison study. Child Abuse Negl 1990;14:41-51.
Dubowitz H, Black M, Starr RH, Zuravin S: A conceptual definition of child neglect. Crim Justice Behav 1993;20:8-26.
Homer C, Ludwig S: Categorization of etiology of failure to thrive. Am J Dis Child 1981;135:848-851.
Sills RH: Failure to thrive: The role of clinical and laboratory evaluation. Am J Dis Child 1978;132:967-969.
Spitz R: Hospitalism: An inquiry into the psychiatric conditions of early childhood. Psychoanal Study Child 1945;1:53-74.
Spitz R: Hospitalism: A follow-up report. Psychoanal Study Child 1946;2:113-117.

Nutrient Deficiencies

Balint J: Physical findings in nutritional deficiencies. Pediatr Clin North Am 1998;45:1.
Committee on Nutrition, American Academy of Pediatrics: Pediatric Nutrition Handbook, 4th ed. Elk Grove Village, Ill, American Academy of Pediatrics, 1998.

Treatment and Outcomes

Bithoney WG, McJunkin J, Michalek J, et al: The effect of a multidisciplinary team approach on weight gain in nonorganic failure to thrive in children. J Dev Behav Pediatr 1991;12:254-258.
Bithoney WG, Van Sciver MM, Foster S, et al: Parental stress and growth outcome in growth-deficient children. Pediatrics 1995;96:707-711.
Black MM: Failure to thrive: Strategies for evaluation and intervention. School Psychol Rev 1995;24:171-185.
Black MM, Dubowitz H, Hutcheson J, et al: A randomized clinical trial of home intervention for children with failure to thrive. Pediatrics 1995;95:807-814.
Black MM, Feigelman S, Cureton PL: Evaluation and treatment of children with failure-to-thrive: An interdisciplinary perspective. J Clin Outcomes Manage 1999;6:60-73.
Boddy J, Skuse D, Andrews B: The developmental sequelae of nonorganic failure to thrive. J Child Psychol Psychiat 2000;41:1003-1014.
Westwood M, Kramer MS, Munz D, et al: Growth and development of full-term nonasphyxiated small-for-gestational-age newborns: Follow-up through adolescence. Pediatrics 1983;71:376-382.

14 Acute and Chronic Abdominal Pain

Robert M. Kliegman*

Abdominal pain is common and is a diagnostically and therapeutically challenging complaint. At least 20% of children seek attention for abdominal pain by the age of 15 years. Only 5% require hospitalization, and fewer undergo surgical intervention. The primary care physician, pediatrician, emergency physician, and surgeon must be able to distinguish serious and potentially life-threatening diseases from more benign problems (Table 14-1). Abdominal pain may be a single acute event (Tables 14-2 and 14-3), a recurring acute problem, or a chronic problem (Table 14-4). The differential diagnosis is lengthy, differs from that in adults, and varies by age group. Although some disorders occur throughout childhood (constipation, gastroenteritis, lower lobe pneumonia, urinary tract infections), others are more common in a specific age group (e.g., intussusception in infancy) (see Table 14-2).

The clinician must have an organized evaluation of the child with abdominal pain; history and physical examination are the keys to an accurate diagnosis. Laboratory and radiologic tests are supportive and usually do not change the clinical diagnosis.

PATHOPHYSIOLOGY OF ABDOMINAL PAIN

Abdominal pain results from stimulation of nociceptive receptors and afferent sympathetic stretch receptors. The pain is classified as *visceral* or *parietal* (somatic).

VISCERAL PAIN

Visceral pain is initiated when nociceptors are stimulated by excessive contraction, stretching, or tension of the walls of hollow viscera (intestinal obstruction, appendiceal inflammation or fecalith, biliary or urinary stone), of the capsule of a solid organ (liver, spleen, kidney), or of the mesentery. In addition, extremes of temperature or tissue release of inflammatory mediators may stimulate visceral pain. Increased contraction of the smooth muscle of hollow viscera may be caused by infection, toxins (bacterial or chemical agents), ulceration, inflammation, or ischemia. Increased hepatic capsule tension may be secondary to passive congestion (heart failure, pericarditis) or inflammation (hepatitis).

Visceral pain is often of gradual onset; is poorly localized relative to the internal anatomy as a result of multisegmental and bilateral innervation of the viscera; is generally of a dull, cramping, burning, gnawing, or sickening quality; and is often accompanied by secondary manifestations, such as pallor, perspiration, emesis, nausea, and restlessness. Although localization may be imprecise with visceral pain, some general rules may be helpful (Fig. 14-1).

PARIETAL PAIN

Parietal pain arises from direct noxious (usually inflammation) stimulation of the contiguous parietal peritoneum (e.g., right lower quadrant at the McBurney point, appendicitis) or the diaphragm (splenic rupture, subdiaphragmatic abscess). Parietal pain is usually sharp, is exacerbated by movement or cough, is accompanied by tenderness over the site of irritation, and lateralizes to one of four quadrants (Fig. 14-2). Because of the relative localization of the noxious stimulation to the underlying peritoneum and the more anatomically specific and unilateral innervation (peripheral-nonautonomic nerves) of the peritoneum, it is usually easier to identify the precise anatomic location that is producing parietal pain (see Fig. 14-2).

ACUTE ABDOMINAL PAIN

The clinician evaluating the child with abdominal pain of acute onset must decide quickly whether the child has a "surgical abdomen" (a serious medical problem necessitating treatment and admission to the hospital) or a process that can be managed on an outpatient basis. Even though surgical diagnoses are fewer than 10% of all causes of abdominal pain in children, they can be life-threatening if untreated. Approximately 55% of children evaluated for acute abdominal pain have a specific medical diagnosis; in another 35%, the cause is never defined.

HISTORY

Obtaining an accurate history is critical for making an accurate diagnosis but is dependent both on the ability and willingness of the child to communicate and on the skill of the parent or guardian as an observer. The person providing an infant's care is the best source of information about the current illness. Children 4 years of age and older may contribute to the history. Some young children may give an accurate account of their illness. Some older children may be totally unwilling to communicate or may be completely silenced by fear, pain, or a talkative parent. The examining physician should try to elicit as much information from the child as possible.

Some children give a good account of their illness when they are simply asked to describe it; however, most children must be asked specific, nonleading questions. To determine the presence of anorexia, the physician must ask questions about food intake, the time the food was eaten, and how that behavior compares to the child's normal intake. The answers are often quite different from the responses to the more general questions "Are you hungry?" and "Have you eaten today?" The child's (and parents') vocabulary, especially for body parts and functions, is not a medical vocabulary. The clinician should use terms the child understands and should not be reluctant to ask what terms the child does know.

The history should be obtained in as relaxed and nonthreatening a setting as is possible. During the history taking, the child should remain in the parent's arms, at play, or comfortably seated beside the parent, as appropriate for the child's age. Many children become quite upset by being made to remove their clothes. While the history is obtained, there is no particular reason why the child should be undressed. The clinician must resist distraction or the urge to speed

*This chapter is an updated and edited version of the chapter by Ellen Hrabovsky that appeared in the first edition.

Table 14-1. **Distinguishing Features of Abdominal Pain in Children**

Disease	Onset	Location	Referral	Quality	Comments
Functional: irritable bowel syndrome	Recurrent	Periumbilical	None	Dull, crampy, intermittent, duration 2 hr	Caused by unknown physiologic factors; diarrhea/constipation are symptoms
Gastroenteritis	Acute or gradual	Periumbilical, rectal, tenesmus	None	Crampy, dull, intermittent	Emesis, fever, watery diarrhea or dysentery (mucus and blood)
Esophageal reflux	Recurrent, after meals, bedtime	Substernal	Chest	Burning	Sour taste in mouth, Sandifer syndrome
Duodenal ulcer	Recurrent, before meals, at night	Epigastric	Back	Severe burning, gnawing	Relieved by food, milk, antacids, family history
Pancreatitis	Acute	Epigastric/ hypogastric	Back	Constant, sharp, boring	Nausea, emesis, marked tenderness
Intestinal obstruction	Acute or gradual	Periumbilical– lower abdomen	Back	Alternating cramping (colic) and painless periods	Distention, obstipation, bilious emesis, increased bowel sounds
Appendicitis	Acute or gradual (1-2 days)	Initially periumbilical or epigastric; later localized to right lower quadrant	Back or pelvis if retrocecal	Sharp, steady	Nausea, emesis, local tenderness with/ without fever; patient is motionless
Meckel diverticulitis (mimics appendicitis)	Recurrent or constant	Generalized diffuse with perforation: periumbilical– lower abdomen	None	Sharp	Hematochezia: painless unless intussusception, diverticulitis, or perforation
Inflammatory bowel disease	Recurrent	Depends on site of involvement		Dull cramping, tenesmus	Fever, weight loss, with/ without hematochezia
Intussusception	Acute	Periumbilical– lower abdomen	None	Cramping, with painless periods	Guarded position with knees pulled up, "currant jelly" stools
Lactose intolerance	Recurrent with milk products	Lower abdomen	None	Cramping	Distention, gaseousness, diarrhea
Urolithiasis	Acute, sudden	Back	Groin	Severe colicky pain	Hematuria; calcification on KUB x-ray study, CT scan
Pyelonephritis	Acute, sudden	Back	None	Dull to sharp	Fever, costochondral tenderness, dysuria, pyuria, urinary frequency
Cholecystitis/ cholelithiasis	Acute	Right upper quadrant	Right shoulder, scapula	Severe colicky pain	Hemolysis with/without jaundice

Adapted from Andreoli TE, Carpenter CJ, Plum F, et al: Cecil Essential of Medicine. Philadelphia, WB Saunders, 1994, p 326.

Reprinted and modified from Behrman R, Kliegman R: Nelson Essentials of Pediatrics, 2nd ed. Philadelphia, WB Saunders, 1994, p 396.

CT, computed tomography; KUB, kidney, ureter, and bladder.

things up by examining the child while taking the history. On occasion, when seeing a seriously ill child, the physician may need to abbreviate the diagnostic process, but taking short cuts may lead to inaccurate conclusions.

Essential Components of the History

Time of Onset of Pain. The time of onset of the pain is important. Pain of less than 6 hours' duration is accompanied by nonspecific findings, and observation is often needed to determine the nature of the illness. Pain lasting from 6 to 48 hours is more apt to have a cause that warrants surgery, although delays in presentation

and diagnosis in children are not unusual. Timing of the progression of symptoms must be detailed.

Location of Pain. The location of the pain at its onset and any change in location are very important (Table 14-5; see also Table 14-1). As stated by Apley, "The further the pain from the umbilicus, the more likely there is to be an underlying organ disorder."

Most intraperitoneal visceral pain is a response to stimulation of stretch fibers in the bowel wall and is mediated through the spinal nerves at T10. This pain is sensed as a deep, aching periumbilical pain. Pain caused by inflammation of the parietal peritoneum (acute appendicitis) is localized to the area of the inflamed organ or is

Table 14-2. Causes of Acute Abdominal Pain by Age Group

Neonate	Child (2-11 yr)	Adolescent (12-19 yr)
Necrotizing enterocolitis*	Appendicitis*	Appendicitis*
Obstruction*	Gastroenteritis*†	Pelvic inflammatory disease*
Malrotation with volvulus*	Trauma*	Trauma*
Idiopathic or drug (indomethacin, steroid)–induced intestinal perforation	Henoch-Schönlein purpura	Tuboovarian abscess
	Hemolytic uremic syndrome	Fitz-Hugh–Curtis syndrome
	Hepatitis	Labor (pregnancy)
Infant (<2 yr)	Peptic ulcer disease	Hepatitis
Intussusception*	Sickle cell anemia: vasoocclusive crisis	Pancreatitis (any cause)
Incarcerated hernia*	Pancreatitis	Ectopic pregnancy
Urinary tract infection*	Pneumonia (lower lobe)	Crohn disease
Gastroenteritis*†	Abdominal tumors	Ovarian cyst/mittelschmerz*
Intestinal obstruction	Pyelonephritis/cystitis	Sickle cell crisis
Malrotation with volvulus	Testicular torsion	Peptic ulcer disease
Trauma (e.g., abuse)	Torsed cryptorchid testis	Omental torsion
Pneumonitis (lower lobe)	Incarcerated hernia	Psoas abscess or hemorrhage
Hirschsprung disease	Typhlitis	Mesenteric adenitis
Aerophagia	Pharyngitis/tonsillitis	Urinary tract infection
Spontaneous bacterial peritonitis	Meckel diverticulitis	Muscle strain (exercise, coughing)
Gastroesophageal reflux	Superior mesenteric artery syndrome	DKA
	Mesenteric adenitis	Testicular torsion
	Spontaneous bacterial peritonitis	Idiopathic*
	DKA	
	Streptococcal pharyngitis	
	Idiopathic*	

*Most commonly seen problem.

†*Gastroenteritis* indicates intestinal infection with viral, bacterial, protozoal, or parasitic agents. Giardiasis and cryptosporidiosis are particularly common and may produce acute or chronic pain.

DKA, diabetic ketoacidosis.

diffuse if the inflammation is extensive and involves more of the peritoneal cavity. Pain resulting from obstruction of an organ is localized to the area of that organ and radiates to the commonly innervated region (e.g., stones in the ureter cause intense flank pain with radiation into the groin). Pain that is migratory or fleeting in location is rarely suggestive of a problem requiring operative intervention. It is more likely to accompany gastroenteritis, constipation, or colic.

Character of Pain. The character of the pain is often difficult for the child to describe. Some older children may be able to differentiate cramping, aching, and burning sensations, but most children do not do this well. Children can relate whether the pain comes and goes or is unrelenting. The character of the pain is usually unknown

in the toddler and infant, although the parent can determine whether the discomfort is constant, cramping, or intermittent. If the child intermittently draws the legs up in a flexed position and cries, the clinician can assume that intermittent pain is present, as in intussusception.

Child's Activity Level. The effect of the pain on the child's activities is an important indicator of the severity of the underlying disease. If the pain is sufficiently severe to awaken the child from a sound sleep, it is of much more significance than pain that occurs only at school and never on weekends. If a child has had to avoid a favorite activity, the pain is more apt to have a defined organic cause. Asking whether motion worsens the pain helps differentiate peritoneal irritation or musculoskeletal diseases from more nonspecific problems. The child with acute appendicitis lies motionless, whereas the child with a renal stone, gallstone, gastroenteritis or pancreatitis may toss and turn and writhe in discomfort.

Gastrointestinal Symptoms. The presence or absence of gastrointestinal symptoms may differentiate intestinal problems (acute appendicitis, gastroenteritis, acute cholecystitis) from those arising from other intraabdominal organs (urinary tract infection, ovarian disease, abdominal wall pain).

Anorexia and *nausea* are difficult symptoms for a small child to describe. Often, if simply asked whether he or she is hungry, a child will respond in the affirmative. This may be partly because mild nausea is difficult to differentiate from hunger. Questions about recent food intake, normal eating habits, the last normal meal, and the current desirability of a favorite food often provide more accurate information about the presence or absence of anorexia and nausea than do direct questions about appetite or nausea. Anorexia and nausea may be caused by specific gastrointestinal disorders or a systemic illness (influenza).

Table 14-3. Sudden Acute Excruciating Abdominal Pain (Within Minutes)

Intestinal Perforation	Luminal Occlusion
Peptic ulcer disease	Urolithiasis
Appendicitis	Cholelithiasis
Diverticula	Strangulated hernia
Vascular Occlusion	**Intraabdominal Hemorrhage**
Midgut volvulus	Ectopic pregnancy
Emboli	Ruptured aortic aneurysm
Endocarditis	Ruptured spleen
Strangulated hernia	
Ovarian torsion	
Testicular torsion	

Table 14-4. Causes of Chronic and Recurrent Abdominal Pain by Age Group*

Infant (<2 Yr)	Child (2-11 Yr)	Adolescent (12-19 Yr)
Colic[†]	Constipation[†]	Irritable bowel syndrome[†]
Inguinal hernia	Functional pain[†]	Psychogenic factors[†]
Malabsorption[‡]	Giardiasis[†]	Dysmenorrhea[†]
Milk allergy	Peptic ulcer disease	Mittelschmerz[†]
Hirschsprung disease	Toxins (lead)	Peptic ulcer disease
Cystic fibrosis	Pancreatitis	Gallbladder disease
Rotational defects	Parasites	Pelvic inflammatory disease
Malformations	Tumors/masses	Ovarian cysts
Esophagitis	Diskitis/osteomyelitis	Diabetes mellitus
	Abdominal migraine	Inflammatory bowel disease
	Diabetes mellitus	Malignancy
	Volvulus	Giardiasis
	Intraabdominal abscess[§]	Serositis (e.g., SLE, familial Mediterranean fever)
	Choledochal cyst	Intraabdominal abscess[§]
		Hereditary angioedema

*See also Table 14-6.

[†]Most common diagnoses.

[‡]Includes lactose and sorbitol (and other fruit juice polyalcohols) intolerance.

[§]Hepatic, pancreatic, subphrenic, psoas, perinephric, renal, pelvic.

SLE, systemic lupus erythematosus.

Vomiting is usually associated with intestinal disease, such as ileus, gastroenteritis, or acute problems of the gastrointestinal tract that warrant surgery (see Chapter 16). However, vomiting may occur as a response to severe nonintestinal pain such as in testicular torsion; this vomiting is usually not recurring and is not a prominent feature. Vomiting may be a sign of increased intracranial pressure and may or may not be accompanied by associated headache or vital sign changes (bradycardia, hypertension, irregular respirations), a bulging fontanel, an altered level of consciousness, or neurologic findings (third or sixth cranial nerve palsies) (see Chapter 37). Care should be taken to determine whether the pain occurs before or after the onset of the vomiting. With acute surgical lesions (those caused by intestinal obstruction, acute appendicitis, acute cholecystitis), the pain always occurs before or during the vomiting. If the vomiting occurred *before* the onset of pain, the clinician should suspect gastroenteritis or another nonspecific problem. The appearance of the vomited material is also important. Feculent or dark green material always suggests intestinal obstruction. Dark brown or frankly bloody material indicates gastritis, Mallory-Weiss gastric tears, or peptic ulcer disease as the source of pain.

Diarrhea occurs commonly in intestinal diseases of viral, parasitic, or bacterial origin (see Chapter 15). The stool volume is large, and defecation is usually preceded by cramping pain that is alleviated by the passage of the diarrheal stool. Diarrhea may also occur in the presence of acute appendicitis or other pelvic infections (such as those resulting from pelvic inflammatory disease, tuboovarian abscess); in these cases, diarrhea is caused by inflammation and irritation of an area of colon adjacent to an inflammatory mass. The diarrhea in this instance is of small volume and is frequent. It is important to obtain an estimate of the volume of stool. Diarrhea may also occur in lesions that cause partial obstruction of the bowel, such as strictures, adhesions, and Hirschsprung disease. In this situation, the patient also has some degree of abdominal distention. Diarrhea with abdominal distention suggests intestinal obstruction.

Constipation alone can cause acute abdominal pain (see Chapter 21). Constipation may also indicate other gastrointestinal

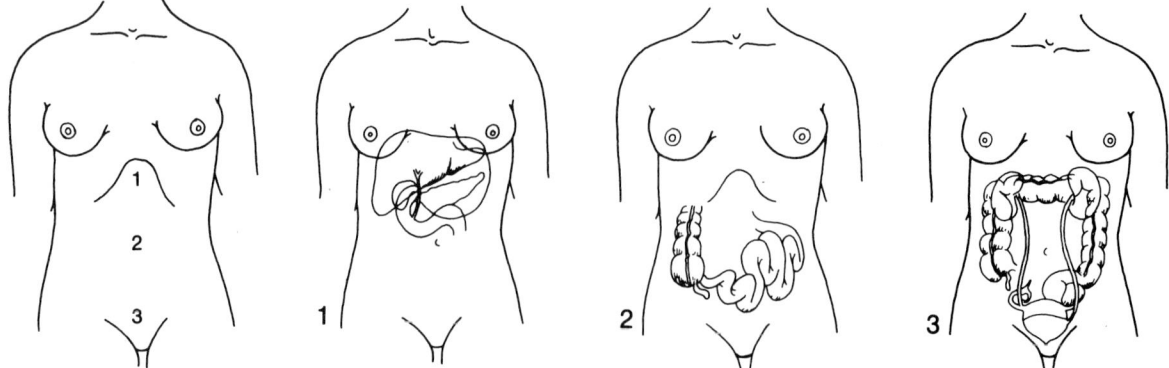

Figure 14-1. "Visceral" abdominal pain: deep, dull, diffuse. The three general localizations of midline "visceral" abdominal pain are epigastric (1), periumbilical (2), and hypogastric (3). **1,** Epigastric pain usually suggests disease of the thorax, stomach, duodenum, pancreas, liver, or gallbladder. **2,** Periumbilical pain usually implies disease of the small intestine, cecum, or both. **3,** Hypogastric pain usually implicates the large intestine, pelvic organs, or urinary system. (From Reilly BM: Abdominal pain. In Practical Strategies in Outpatient Medicine, 2nd ed. Philadelphia, WB Saunders, 1991, p 702.)

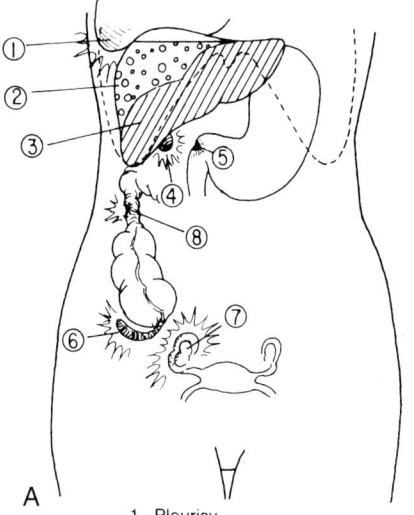

A

1. Pleurisy
2. Subdiaphragmatic abscess
3. (Peri) hepatitis
4. Cholecystitis
5. Perforated duodenal ulcer
6. Appendicitis
7. Ectopic pregnancy, tuboovarian hemorrhage, abscess, or rupture
8. Perforated colon (cancer or diverticulum)

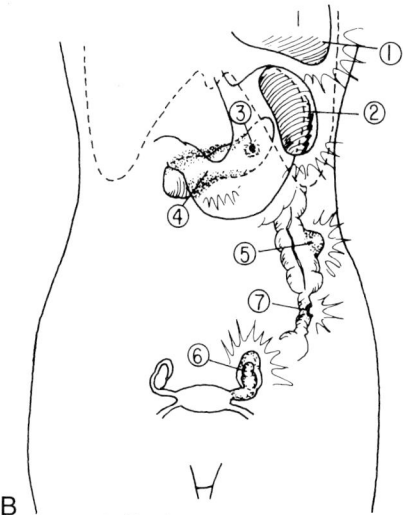

B

1. Pleurisy
2. Splenic rupture or infarct
3. Perforated gastric ulcer
4. Pancreatitis
5. Diverticulitis (splenic flexure)
6. Ectopic pregnancy, tuboovarian hemorrhage, abscess, or rupture
7. Perforated colon (carcinoma)

Figure 14-2. Common and uncommon conditions that may cause "parietal" pain and localized peritonitis in the various quadrants of the abdomen. **A,** Right upper quadrant. **B,** Left upper quadrant. **C,** Right lower quadrant. **D,** Left lower quadrant. (From Reilly BM: Abdominal pain. In Practical Strategies in Outpatient Medicine, 2nd ed. Philadelphia, WB Saunders, 1991, p 703.)

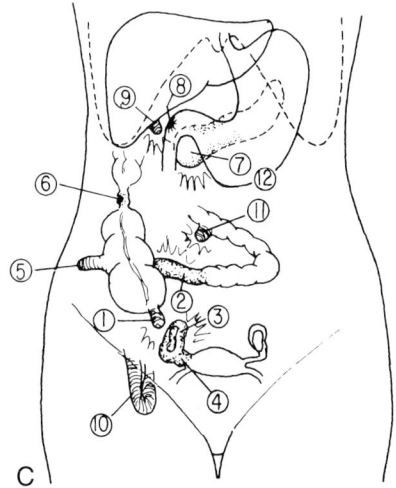

C

1. Appendicitis
2. Acute Crohn's disease
3. Ectopic pregnancy, tuboovarian abscess, or ovarian torsion/hemorrhage
4. Pelvic inflammatory disease
5. Cecal diverticulitis
6. Colon cancer (perforation)
7. Acute pancreatitis and/or pseudocyst
8. Perforated duodenal ulcer
9. Acute cholecystitis
10. Incarcerated inguinal hernia
11. Meckel's diverticulitis
12. Leaking aortic aneurysm

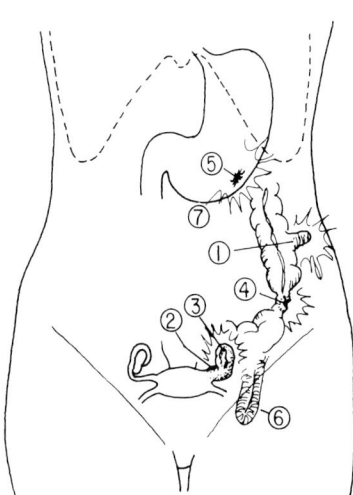

D

1. Sigmoid diverticulitis
2. Pelvic inflammatory disease
3. Ectopic pregnancy, tuboovarian abscess, or ovarian torsion / hemorrhage
4. Perforated sigmoid carcinoma
5. Perforated gastric ulcer
6. Incarcerated inguinal hernia
7. Leaking aortic aneurysm

Table 14-5. Localization of Abdominal Pain: Referred or Radiated

Referred

Extraabdominal lesion pain referred to abdomen	*Intraabdominal extraperitoneal origin*
Thorax	Pancreas
Spine	Kidney
Hips	Ureters
Pelvis	Great vessels
	Pelvic organs
	Retroperitoneal space

Radiated

Origin is primary site with simultaneously perceived pain in a secondary site

Cholecystitis radiates to subscapular area
Splenic injury radiates to shoulder
Ureteral colic (stones) radiates to testis, upper leg or groin
Pancreatitis radiates to back

---

dysfunction. Some children present with a picture very similar to that seen in acute appendicitis but have a large amount of stool filling the entire colon. The pain often disappears after enemas and a brief period of bowel rest. The "gas-stoppage sign" is a sensation of fullness that suggests the need for a bowel movement in patients with appendicitis but is not relieved by attempts at defecation.

Systemic Symptoms. The presence of headache, sore throat, and other generalized aches and pains moves the examiner away from a diagnosis of an acute problem warranting surgery and strongly suggests a viral flulike syndrome. Asking the child where the worst pain is sometimes results in the child's pointing a finger to the head or throat. The examiner must be careful to remember the whole child and not to focus on the abdomen just because that is the area of the presenting complaint. Many systemic diseases directly or indirectly

produce abdominal pain and must be considered in the differential diagnosis (Table 14-6).

Family History and Personal Medical History. Viral gastroenteritis, other viral syndromes, and food poisoning may affect the patient's family or schoolmates; it is important to ask whether other family members, classmates, or playmates have recently had similar symptoms. Certain systemic and inherited diseases, such as sickle cell anemia, diabetes mellitus, spherocytosis, familial Mediterranean fever, and porphyria, are associated with episodes of abdominal pain. The family must be asked about familial diseases and any previous episodes of pain in the child (see Table 14-6). Previous intraabdominal operations may result in adhesions that can cause pain, intestinal obstruction, or both. A history of such procedures suggests the possibility of bowel obstruction. Some specific medical illnesses result in identifiable or predictable causes of abdominal pain (Table 14-7).

PHYSICAL EXAMINATION

The physical examination begins when the clinician enters the room. Observing the child's activity and demeanor while obtaining the history is the first step of the physical examination. Does the child appear ill? Is the patient lethargic, rolling about in discomfort, alert but lying very still, or bouncing all over the room?

Each of these activities conveys a message. The listless, lethargic child may be in shock, dehydrated, and very ill. The child who is crying out loudly and generally dominating the scene probably does not have a problem that warrants surgery and may have gastroenteritis with cramping abdominal pain. The child who seems only mildly ill but moves with great care, if at all, is assumed to have an inflammatory process until it is proven otherwise (acute appendicitis or an incarcerated hernia).

The child should be asked to get onto the examination table with as little assistance as possible. If the child does this easily, the probability of an intraabdominal inflammatory process is quite low. Outer bulky clothing should be removed, but the child does not need to be completely undressed, especially if being undressed seems

---

Table 14-6. Systemic Causes of Acute Abdominal Pain

Metabolic, Hematologic	Neurologic	Infectious, Inflammatory
Acute porphyria	Abdominal epilepsy	Acute rheumatic fever
Familial Mediterranean fever	Abdominal migraine	Infectious mononucleosis
Hereditary angioneurotic edema	Brain tumor	Rocky Mountain spotted fever
Sickle cell crisis	Multiple sclerosis	Measles
Leukemia	Radiculopathy	Mumps
Acute hemolytic states	Neuropathy	Pneumonia (lower lobe)
Diabetic ketoacidosis	Herpes zoster	Pericarditis
Hemolytic uremic syndrome	Dysautonomia (Riley-Day syndrome)	Pharyngitis
Addison disease		Epididymitis/orchitis
Uremia	**Drugs, Toxins**	Henoch-Schönlein purpura
Electrolyte disturbances	Heavy metal poisoning	Hemolytic uremic syndrome
Hyperparathyroidism-hypercalcemia	Lead	Systemic lupus erythematosus
(urolithiasis, pancreatitis)	Arsenic	Endocarditis
Hypertriglyceridemia (pancreatitis)	Mercury	Anaphylaxis
	Mushroom ingestion	
Musculoskeletal	Narcotic withdrawal	**Other**
Arthritis/diskitis	Black widow spider bite	Pneumothorax
Osteomyelitis		Pulmonary embolism
Thoracic nerve root dysfunction		Functional
Trauma/child abuse		Aerophagia
Hernia		
Psoas abscess or hemorrhage		

Table 14-7. **Current or Past Aspects of Medical History that May Suggest Cause of Abdominal Pain**

Historical Factor	Cause of Pain
Cystic fibrosis	Pancreatitis, diabetes mellitus, meconium ileus equivalent, appendicitis, intussusception, biliary or urinary stones
Sickle cell anemia	Vasoocclusive crisis, cholelithiasis, hepatitis, hemolytic crisis, renal infarction, splenic sequestration
Diabetes mellitus	Pancreatitis, gastric neuropathy
Cirrhosis, nephrotic syndrome	Primary bacterial peritonitis
SLE, other autoimmune disorders	Vasculitis, pancreatitis, serositis, infarction
Corticosteroids	Gastric ulceration, pancreatitis
NSAID	Ileal perforation, gastric ulceration, renal-papillary necrosis
HIV	Gastroenteritis, hepatitis, pancreatitis, esophagitis, lymphoma
Mononucleosis	Hepatitis, splenic rupture
Henoch-Schönlein purpura	Mucosal hemorrhage, intussusception
Hemolytic-uremic syndrome	Colitis
Upper respiratory tract infection	Pneumonia, mesenteric adenitis
Pneumonia	Mesenteric adenitis
Prior surgery	Abscess, adhesions, obstruction, stricture, pancreatitis, ectopic pregnancy
Inborn errors of metabolism, hypertriglyceridemia, hypercalcemia	Pancreatitis
Drugs (valproic acid)	Pancreatitis

HIV, human immunodeficiency virus; NSAID, nonsteroidal antiinflammatory drug; SLE, systemic lupus erythematosus.

distressing to the child. Clothing can be rearranged to allow good exposure of the abdomen without the child's having to feel completely vulnerable.

The examination must be performed in a relaxed, friendly manner with attention fully focused on the child. An accurate examination depends on the child's trust and cooperation. A conversation with the child about family, friends, pets, school, sports, music, or other specific interests of that child diverts attention from the examination and increases cooperation. The examiner should never surprise the child and should never lie. The first surprise or untruth, such as the statement "This won't hurt," destroys any trust that has developed.

Low-grade fever (<101°F) is seen in early appendicitis but is also common in many other diseases. The absence of fever does not exclude the diagnosis of acute appendicitis or other problems necessitating surgical intervention. If the patient has been given an antipyretic just before the visit, the temperature may be suppressed. Tachycardia may reflect only anxiety or may be caused by dehydration, shock, or fever. Tachypnea suggests a metabolic acidosis (shock, diabetes mellitus, toxic ingestion), an intrapulmonary process, sepsis, or fever. The vital signs must be viewed in context but may be the first clue to a serious illness.

Examination of the head, neck, chest, and extremities should precede the abdominal examination, and any uncomfortable parts of the examination should be deferred. In infants, otitis media is sufficiently painful to cause striking restlessness and may be confused with abdominal pain. In children too young to describe the location of the pain, a careful examination of the ears is very important but can be performed after the rest of the examination. Streptococcal pharyngitis or mononucleosis is sometimes accompanied by severe abdominal pain. Affected children have a significant fever, appear ill, and have tender cervical adenopathy and an obvious tonsillitis, pharyngitis, or both.

Decreased breath sounds and/or rales in a lower lung lobe, especially on the right side, may indicate pneumonia. Children with lower lobe bacterial pneumonia present with severe abdominal pain, high fever, tachypnea, and, on occasion, vomiting. Such children appear quite ill. This presentation may mimic that of a child with peritonitis from a perforated acute appendicitis. However, the abdominal findings are not consistent with the diagnosis of an acute intraabdominal process, and examination of the lungs should demonstrate the pneumonia.

The *abdominal examination* should be performed systematically and with the child as comfortable as possible. Before the examiner actually touches the child's abdomen, he or she should observe it, looking for distention, inguinal masses, peristaltic waves, and scars from old injuries or surgical incisions. Inguinal and femoral hernias are an overlooked but common cause of abdominal pain. Next, the child should be asked to indicate with one finger the point of greatest pain. The point may be a vague circle in the area of the umbilicus, but if the child specifies a defined spot, the examiner should avoid that area until the remainder of the abdomen has been palpated.

Gentleness is essential to successful palpation of the abdomen. The examiner must warm both hands and the stethoscope before touching the patient. The stethoscope is an excellent tool for palpation of the abdomen. Auscultation of the chest can simply be extended to the abdomen, with the examiner assuring the child that the stethoscope did not hurt on the chest. The initial examination of the abdomen with the stethoscope should be just for listening, with no pressure exerted, so that no discomfort results.

Bowel sounds are usually nonspecific in most children with abdominal pain; however, in certain processes, they are helpful. High-pitched tinkling sounds or rushes are usually associated with an obstructive process. Bowel sounds in gastroenteritis are ordinarily very active and loud but may be normal. Acute appendicitis is accompanied by normal sounds in the early stages, but bowel sounds disappear with diffuse peritonitis.

Watching the child's reaction to the auscultation may be a valuable clue to areas of true tenderness. Most children do not expect the auscultation to be uncomfortable, so they are not guarding in anticipation of pain. As the examiner continues to listen over the entire anterior abdomen, the pressure on the head of the stethoscope increases until the examiner is, in fact, palpating with the stethoscope. This often is a much more reliable method of eliciting true tenderness and guarding than is the palpating hand. If the child is cooperative, stethoscope palpation may not be needed and the examiner can proceed to manual palpation of the abdomen.

Palpation is begun as *far away* from the area of pain identified by the child as possible. The examiner's hand should be softly placed flat (in parallel) on the child's abdomen. Directing fingers into the abdomen (perpendicular) as a method of palpation is unnecessary and often frightening. The clinician should watch the child's face, not the abdomen, during the palpation. Some children are extremely stoic, and only the slightest grimace betrays the discomfort they are experiencing. Attention is paid during palpation to the presence of masses or feces. Voluntary guarding usually starts before the palpation starts and can be overcome by asking the child to take deep breaths, flexing the knees and hips, or by using other distractions appropriate to the child's age and temperament. Involuntary guarding occurs when the examiner's hand encounters an area of tenderness. When encountering tenderness, the examiner should palpate only deeply enough to elicit the complaint of pain and some guarding. There is no need to bring on unnecessary pain by deep palpation. A rigid or boardlike abdomen is the result of involuntary guarding of the entire anterior abdominal wall because of diffuse intraperitoneal inflammation.

Rebound pain is an indicator of peritoneal irritation and is elicited during examination of the anterior abdominal wall. It occurs when an inflamed focus within the abdomen is compressed and the pressure is then quickly released, resulting in sudden and sometimes severe pain. The standard method to elicit rebound is to palpate deeply, then suddenly remove the palpating hand. Although this sign aids in the determination of the presence of an intraperitoneal inflammatory process, it is not necessary to cause the child this extra discomfort.

Other areas of inflammation can be detected by maneuvers that move muscles adjacent to the inflammation. The *psoas sign* occurs when elevation and extension of the leg against the pressure of the examiner's hand causes pain. An inflammatory mass, such as an inflamed appendix, a psoas abscess, or a perinephric abscess, in contact with the psoas muscle is the cause of this pain (Fig. 14-3). Likewise, the *obturator sign* is pain with flexion of the thigh at right angles to the trunk and external rotation of the same leg while the patient is in the supine position. This sign results from contact of an inflammatory mass with the obturator muscle (see Fig. 14-3).

The flanks and back must be inspected and palpated. Percussion at the costovertebral angle elicits pain in the presence of renal or perinephric inflammation. Vertebral body and disk disease may be detected by palpitation of the spine. The perineum and genitalia must be inspected and palpated as necessary. External examination of the genitalia in prepubertal girls is adequate. If a more thorough examination or an intravaginal examination is needed in prepubertal girls, it should generally be performed with the patient under anesthesia. In postpubertal girls, a pelvic examination may be valuable, regardless of the patient's sexual activity history.

The need for a rectal examination is controversial. If a diagnosis is already obvious, the rectal examination may be eliminated. If an imaging study or endoscopy is planned, a rectal examination may be unnecessary. The rectal examination, if performed, should be the last part of the physical examination and should be performed only once. The child should be relaxed and should be given an honest explanation of the procedure. The examiner should use plenty of lubricant and should perform the rectal examination very gently. If the child strongly resists, it is pointless to perform a forceful examination. This is when the rectal examination may truly be deferred. Lateralizing pain, masses, and the presence and character of stool in the rectum are assessed. The stool should always be tested for blood.

Clues to an organic and at times more serious cause of abdominal pain are noted in Table 14-8. Furthermore, peritoneal signs—which suggest a "surgical abdomen," most often caused by peritonitis—are noted in Table 14-9. In addition, the presence of shock suggests other serious diseases (see Table 14-9).

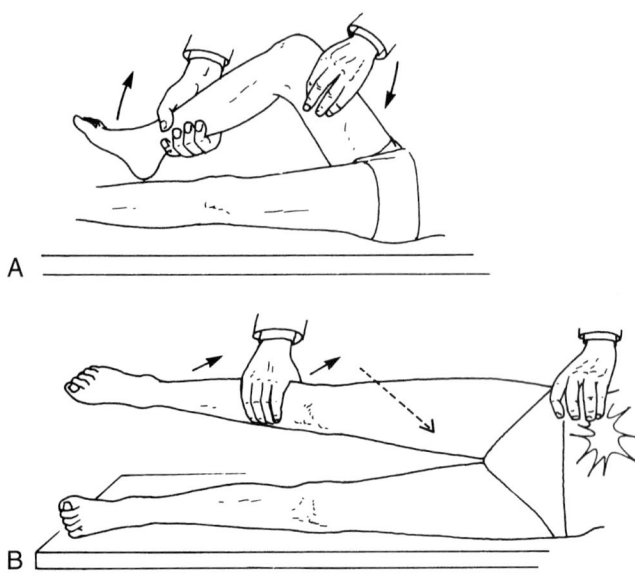

Figure 14-3. **A,** The obturator sign. Pain occurs when the hip is flexed and rotated. Internal rotation is most likely to cause pain as a result of pelvic or retroperitoneal disease or both. **B,** The psoas sign. The test may be performed passively or actively. The hip is passively extended, thus stretching the psoas muscle (*solid arrow*). The hip is actively flexed usually against resistance, thus tensing the psoas muscle (*dotted arrow*). (From Reilly BM: Abdominal pain. In Practical Strategies in Outpatient Medicine, 2nd ed. Philadelphia, WB Saunders, 1991, p 714.)

LABORATORY EVALUATION

After a careful history is obtained and thorough physical examination is performed, the diagnosis or a short list of possible diagnoses should be apparent. Laboratory data are supportive in confirming or ruling out suspected disease.

Complete Blood Cell Count

The hemoglobin and hematocrit levels can reveal anemia caused by acute or chronic blood loss (as with ulcers, inflammatory bowel disease, Meckel diverticula) or the anemia of chronic disease (as with systemic lupus erythematosus, inflammatory bowel disease). The white blood cell count indicates the possibility of infection or blood dyscrasias. In uncomplicated acute appendicitis, the white blood cell count ranges from normal values to 15,000 to 16,000. A very high white blood cell count (>18,000) indicates intestinal gangrene, perforation, peritonitis, or abscess formation, but this count may also be high in acute bacterial gastroenteritis, streptococcal diseases, pyelonephritis, pelvic inflammatory disease, hemolytic uremic syndrome, and pneumonia.

The differential cell count may also be helpful. In studies of children with acute appendicitis, 95% had neutrophilia, but only half had leukocytosis in the first 24 hours. If the child's history and physical examination findings are highly suggestive of appendicitis, a normal or mildly elevated white blood cell count should not dissuade the clinician from that diagnosis. However, a striking lymphocytosis may suggest gastroenteritis or a systemic illness. Overreliance on the complete blood count can cause delay in reaching the correct diagnosis.

Urinalysis

The *urinalysis* is an important and useful laboratory test in the evaluation of abdominal pain. The presence of ketones and a high

Table 14-8. Red Flags and Clues to an Organic Cause of Abdominal Pain

Age less than 4 years of old
Localized pain in nonperiumbilical site
Referred pain
Pain awakes child from sleep
Sudden onset of excruciating pain
Crescendo nature of pain
Sudden worsening of pain
Fever (high fever >39.4°C suggests pneumonia, pyelonephritis, dysentery, cholangitis, more than perforation or abscess)
Jaundice
Distention*
Dysuria
Emesis (especially bilious)
Anorexia
Weight loss
Positive family history (metabolic disorders, peptic ulcer disease)†
Change in urine or stool color (blood, acholic) or frequency
Vaginal discharge
Sexual activity
Delayed sexual development (chronic pain)
Anemia
Elevated erythrocyte sedimentation rate
Specific physical findings (hepatomegaly, absent bowel sounds, adnexal tenderness, involuntary guarding, focal or diffuse tenderness, positive rectal examination results, perianal disease, joint swelling)

*Consider 5 Fs: fat, feces, flatus (aerophagia, obstruction), fluid (ascites, hydronephrosis, cysts), fetus (pregnancy or fetal-like abnormal growth [e.g., tumors]).

†Family history is also positive for dysfunctional pain syndromes (constipation, irritable bowel, dysmenorrhea, and lactase deficiency).

Table 14-9. Peritoneal Signs of a "Surgical Abdomen"

Severe pain
Patient's eyes anxiously open during examiner's palpation
Patient is motionless
Absent bowel sounds
Extreme tenderness to palpation or percussion
Voluntary guarding with gentle palpation
Involuntary guarding: boardlike rigidity
Rebound tenderness (do not intentionally elicit)
Pain with movement or cough

If shock is present, consider:

Severe pancreatitis
Trauma: intraabdominal hemorrhage
Ruptured spleen (trauma, mononucleosis)
Spontaneous peritonitis
Secondary peritonitis (appendicitis, intussusception, perforated ulcer)
Urosepsis
Associated severe gastrointestinal bleeding
Rupture of fallopian tube from ectopic pregnancy
Pulmonary embolism
Aortic dissection
Volvulus
Child abuse
Addisonian crisis (adrenal insufficiency)

specific gravity suggest poor food intake and dehydration. Large amounts of glucose and ketones in the urine indicate diabetic ketoacidosis. A pregnancy test should be performed on postpubertal girls, regardless of sexual activity history. The presence of both white cells and bacteria indicates a urinary tract infection; either finding alone may not be sufficient for that diagnosis (see Chapter 23). White blood cells may be present in the urine from irritation caused by an inflammatory mass adjacent to the bladder or ureter; hematuria may be seen with nephrolithiasis.

Other Laboratory Tests

Other laboratory tests, such as measurement of serum electrolytes, amylase, and lipase; liver function studies; and arterial blood gases should be ordered on the basis of the differential diagnosis after a thorough history and physical examination are completed.

IMAGING EVALUATION

A multitude of imaging studies are available; none should be obtained until the patient has been examined.

Plain Radiography

Plain radiographs, especially kidney-ureter-bladder (KUB) films, with or without upright lateral views of the chest and abdomen, are routinely obtained in most emergency departments as part of the evaluation of acute abdominal pain. The chest film helps assess the presence of a lower lobe pneumonia, which often causes severe abdominal pain, especially in small children. However, early in the disease, the physical examination may be more helpful. Often, if the KUB-abdominal radiographic study includes the lower lobes, the chest radiographic study can be deferred and performed only if the KUB demonstrates lung abnormalities.

Only approximately 10% of abdominal radiographic results are positive when they are obtained as part of the routine workup for abdominal pain. Of those that are limited to patients with serious illness, 46% of the results are positive. Used to confirm the presence of intestinal obstruction, renal or biliary tract calculi, calcified fecaliths, or intestinal perforation (pneumoperitoneum-free air), plain abdominal radiographs may be helpful. These studies detect bowel distention (air-fluid levels on upright views), calcification, free air, and large masses but are not helpful in detecting most other diseases. If free air or intestinal obstruction is suspected, the abdominal films must include a flat and upright or decubitus view of the abdomen to demonstrate the air-fluid interface.

In acute appendicitis, a calcified appendicolith may be seen (Fig. 14-4). This finding automatically makes the diagnosis of appendiceal dysfunction and confirms the need for appendectomy. The absence of an appendicolith (appendiceal fecalith) does not rule out appendicitis. More often, the noncalcified appendicolith may obstruct the appendix; ultrasonographic or computed tomographic (CT) imaging is necessary to visualize this lesion. If an inflammatory mass lies near the iliopsoas muscle, mild lumbar scoliosis may be present as a result of spasm of the muscle.

Radiographic studies are not always necessary. If the diagnosis is already obvious, specific therapy is indicated. In some situations, other types of imaging studies are more useful, and plain radiographs are not prerequisite.

Ultrasonography

Ultrasonographic examination is ideal for children. It is usually painless, emits no radiation, requires no intravenous contrast material, and can be performed without sedation. It is usually readily available and, in selected patients, can be extremely helpful.

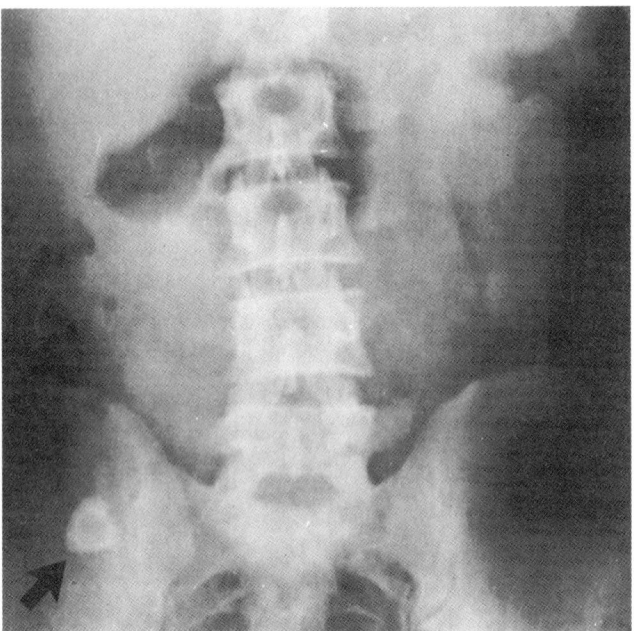

Figure 14-4. The patient described the gradual onset of anorexia, nausea, and vague periumbilical abdominal pain. Twenty-four hours later, the pain was much more severe in the right lower quadrant, where localized peritoneal signs were apparent. The radiographic film of the abdomen reveals a huge calcified density in the right lower quadrant; it proved to be an appendiceal fecalith at surgery. (From Reilly BM: Abdominal pain. In Practical Strategies in Outpatient Medicine, 2nd ed. Philadelphia, WB Saunders, 1991, p 16.)

Lower abdominal gynecologic pain in girls, especially in adolescent girls, can be confused with appendicitis. Pelvic ultrasonography demonstrates pathologic processes of the ovaries and fallopian tubes, the size of the uterus, and the presence of free fluid in the pelvis. An enlarged, inflamed appendix can also be visualized (Fig. 14-5). Any girl with abdominal pain in whom the diagnosis is not obvious should undergo an ultrasonographic examination.

Gallstones, a dilated thick-walled gallbladder, or a dilated common bile duct can be visualized by ultrasonography; all three support the diagnosis of biliary disease. Edema and enlargement of the pancreas are seen in acute pancreatitis. Ultrasonography also details the character of abdominal masses, differentiating cystic from solid masses, and can be helpful in demonstrating free fluid or abscesses. The anatomy of the urinary tract is well defined by ultrasonography; nephromegaly may be seen with pyelonephritis. Ultrasonography is very operator dependent; the choice of ultrasonography versus CT is

dependent on the expertise of the regional imaging center. Abdominal ultrasonography is an excellent screening method for detecting intussusception and midgut volvulus. If an ileus or intestinal obstruction is present, interpretation of the ultrasonographic examination becomes difficult because of the multiple air-filled loops of intestine.

Contrast Studies

In some situations, certain bowel lesions are best delineated with a contrast medium placed in the bowel, either in an upper gastrointestinal series or by enema. If a colonic obstruction is suspected, such as in Hirschsprung disease, the appropriate contrast material is a barium enema. If the presence of a perforation is possible, as in a perforated duodenal ulcer, a water-soluble agent is the contrast medium of choice.

Malrotation of the midgut with a volvulus in infants and older children is often seen on ultrasonography but can be diagnosed by an upper gastrointestinal study. The barium enema study was once the favored method, but confusion about the position of the cecum, as a result of either reflux of barium into the ileum or the mobile nature of the cecum in infants, led to inaccurate conclusions. In the infant who presents with an acute abdomen and bilious vomiting and in the older child who manifests chronic abdominal pain and intermittent vomiting, the oral barium contrast study is highly reliable. The significant findings include incomplete obstruction of the duodenum caused by compression or volvulus of the intestine and abnormal position of the duodenojejunal junction (position of the ligament of Treitz).

Intussusception is both diagnosed and treated by means of barium enema. Initial diagnosis is possible with ultrasonography. The sudden onset of severe, diffuse pain, evidence of blood in the stool, and the suggestion of a soft, nontender mass in the right upper quadrant of the abdomen in a previously well young child constitute the classical picture of intussusception. The plain films may be nonspecific, may show evidence of intestinal obstruction, or may show a mass. A high index of suspicion is all that is needed to justify the barium enema study; some centers now use air rather than barium. Sedation with morphine is helpful for comforting the child and for performing a useful study. The weight of the barium column often completely reduces the intussusception, eliminating the need for surgical intervention. Brisk reflux of contrast into the terminal ileum signifies a complete reduction. This study should always be performed in consultation with a surgeon and with the child prepared to go to the operating room in case of failure of reduction or perforation of the colon. Successful hydrostatic reduction of the intussusception is accomplished in 50% to 75% of cases. Contraindications for reduction enemas include perforation and signs of peritonitis. Patients beyond the usual age range (3 months to 6 years) for intussusception often have an anatomic lead point (polyp, Meckel diverticulum, lymphoma); successful hydrostatic reduction may not

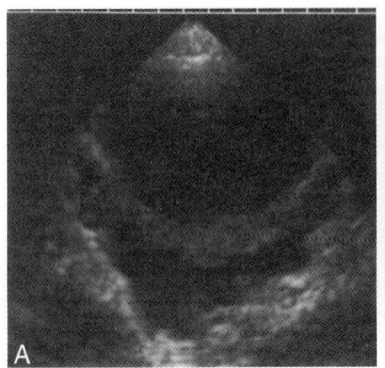
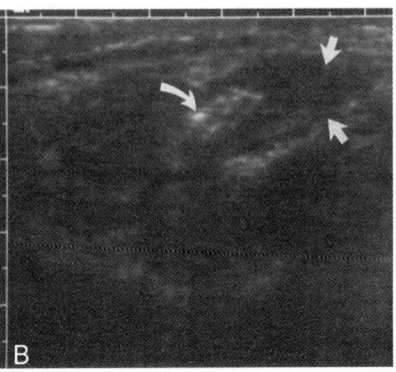

Figure 14-5. A transverse scan of the pelvis shows free fluid pooling behind the bladder (**A**). The longitudinal scan of the right lower quadrant (**B**) shows a shadowing appendicolith (*curved arrow*) in a thick-walled appendix, typical of appendicitis. *Straight arrows* outline the appendiceal tip, which looks ready to perforate. Free fluid in the pelvis always increases the suspicion of appendicitis. (From Teele R, Share J: Appendicitis and other causes of intra-abdominal inflammation. In Ultrasonography of Infants and Children. Philadelphia, WB Saunders, 1991, p 349.)

be possible in these situations. In the presence of pneumoperitoneum, peritonitis, or unsuccessful hydrostatic reduction, surgical intervention is indicated. Recurrences occur in 5% of patients treated with reduction enemas.

A mass from appendicitis that is pressing against the cecum or thickening of the cecal wall may be seen on the barium enema study, but ultrasonography and CT scanning with oral contrast media are much more reliable. Contrast studies of the bowel are quite useful in the patient with suspected *inflammatory bowel disease* or *polypoid lesions* of the colon and small intestine.

Computed Tomography

CT scanning is quite valuable in the evaluation of acute-onset abdominal pain. If a study is needed, it is the imaging study of choice for suspected appendicitis. CT is also very useful in the initial evaluation of abdominal trauma and in the determination of the extent of abdominal masses. Intravenous and gastrointestinal contrast must be used in CT of the abdomen to obtain the most information especially if inflammatory bowel disease is suspected. CT is also useful in the evaluation of chronic pain or persistent undefined inflammatory processes.

MANAGEMENT

Numerous diseases cause acute abdominal pain (see Tables 14-1 and 14-2). It is necessary to be aware of the multiple etiologic factors; however, many are rare "zebras" and deserve little initial attention unless there is a family history or other specific clues (see Tables 14-6 and 14-7). The immediate concern is the differentiation of serious surgical and medical problems from the more common but less serious causes of abdominal pain (see Tables 14-1, 14-3, 14-8, and 14-9). In fact, nonspecific findings and no specific diagnosis are what are usually found. A guide to the treatment of the child with acute-onset abdominal pain is noted in Figure 14-6.

An obvious diagnosis leads promptly to appropriate consultation and management. Mild, nonspecific illness is easily treated on an outpatient basis, with follow-up by telephone or in the office. However, the child who appears ill but in whom a specific diagnosis is not apparent presents a problem. Such a child should be examined by a surgeon to be sure that no correctable intraabdominal disease is present. If the diagnosis is still not apparent, the child should be admitted for active observation, which includes no oral food or liquid, appropriate intravenous fluids, hourly vital signs, and frequent examinations. If the abdominal examination is difficult because of poor cooperation, sedation or, more likely, analgesia is appropriate. Morphine therapy has not reduced the accuracy of the diagnosis of appendicitis by experienced physicians. Such an agent permits an adequate abdominal examination but does not eliminate the tenderness caused by an inflammatory process. The examination should be repeated 2 to 3 hours later. About 10% of children admitted for observation go on to show obvious signs of a process warranting surgery in the first few hours. In approximately 50% of the observed children, a specific diagnosis, such as constipation or gastroenteritis, becomes apparent. The other patients improve with this management and are discharged with no specific cause being found for the pain. CT imaging (or ultrasonography) is valuable in most circumstances when the diagnosis is uncertain or the examination is equivocal.

SPECIFIC CAUSES OF ACUTE ABDOMINAL PAIN

Appendicitis

Appendicitis is an acute inflammation of the appendix that may be initiated by luminal obstruction by a fecalith, lymphoid hyperplasia (secondary to viral infections), inflammation, or, in rare cases, parasites (pinworm, *Ascaris* species). Obstruction with ongoing distal secretion of mucus causes distention of the appendix, increased luminal pressure, and subsequent arterial obstruction and ischemia.

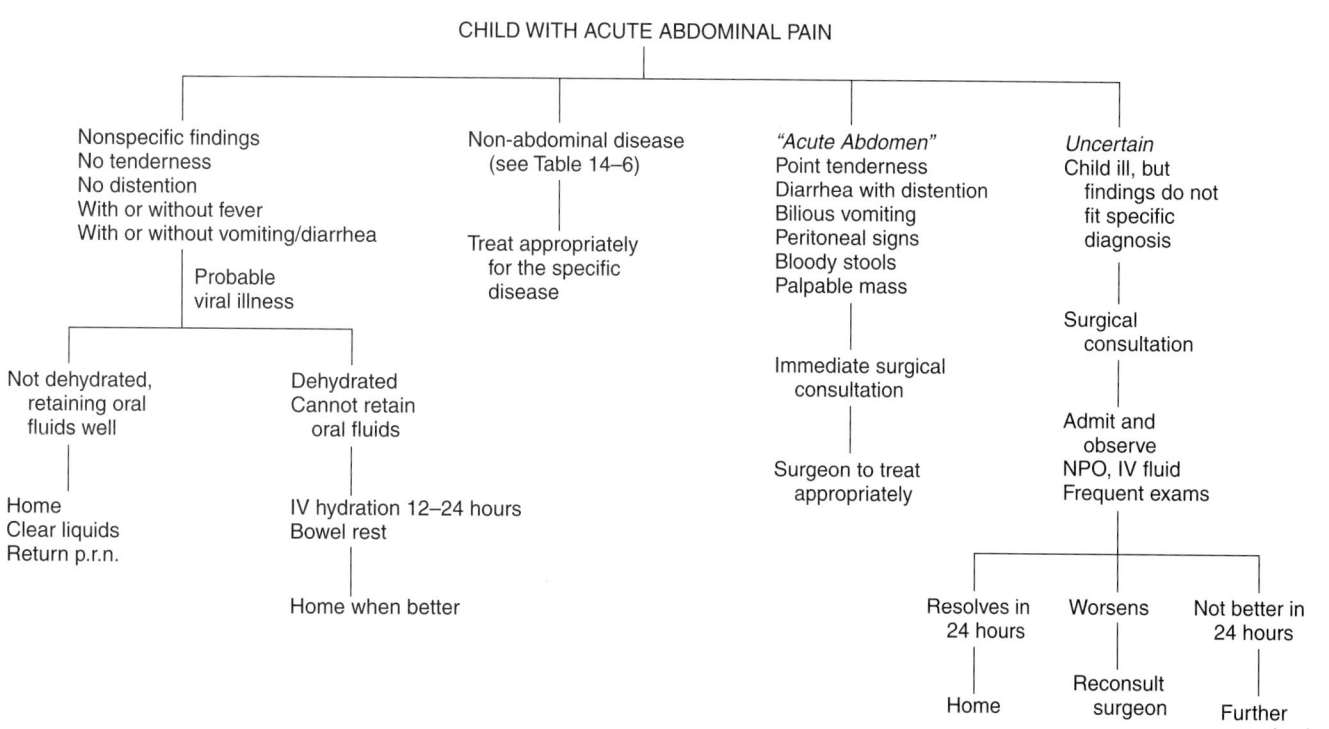

Figure 14-6. Algorithm for evaluating acute abdominal pain. IV, intravenous; NPO, nil per os (no oral intake); p.r.n., as needed.

Mucosal ulceration, fibropurulent serosal exudates, and bacterial infection lead to gangrene (from arterial obstruction) and rupture. On occasion, the greater omentum may seal over a ruptured appendix, producing a right lower quadrant mass and periappendiceal abscess.

Appendicitis may be *simple* (focal inflammation, no serosal exudate), *suppurative* (obstructed, inflamed, edematous, increased local peritoneal fluid with omental and mesenteric containment, or walled off), *gangrenous* (like suppurative, plus gray-green or red-black areas of gangrene, with or without microperforations, and purulent peritoneal fluid), *ruptured* (gross perforation, usually on antimesenteric side; peritonitis present), and *abscessed* (development of pus from rupture into right ileal fossa, lateral to cecum or retrocecal, subcecal, or pelvic). The bacteriologic components of appendicitis include normal intestinal flora, such as enterococci, *Escherichia coli*, *Pseudomonas* species, *Klebsiella* species, and anaerobic bacteria, such as *Clostridium* and *Bacteroides* species.

Appendicitis affects approximately 60,000 children each year in the United States; it primarily affects adolescents and young adults but may develop at any age, even in neonates. The disease is particularly severe in young children, often because of a delay in diagnosis with subsequent perforation. Appendicitis in young children is difficult to diagnose because of atypical manifestations and the clinician's inability to obtain an accurate history. The thinness of the appendix and the paucity of the omentum in younger children may result in rapid, unimpeded spread of intraabdominal infection after rupture.

Diagnosis

An accurate and early diagnosis is critical for avoiding rupture and peritonitis and for excluding other causes of abdominal pain. Appendicitis usually manifests initially with a gradual onset of periumbilical (occasionally epigastric) pain, which may begin as a dull ache but becomes constant (or, less often, colicky) and of mild to moderate intensity. This is then followed by anorexia, nausea, and a few episodes of emesis. Emesis preceding the pain is more typical of gastroenteritis. There may be constipation and the sensation that a bowel movement will improve the condition ("gas-stoppage sensation"). On occasion, an inflamed appendix irritates the colon, producing diarrhea. Furthermore, the appendix may irritate the bladder, causing urinary frequency and dysuria. Pain may transiently stop, or, as local peritonitis develops, the pain may continue and shift to the right lower quadrant. (The McBurney point is defined by placing the little finger of one hand in the umbilicus and the thumb on the anterior superior ileal spine. The index finger, if extended perpendicularly to the abdominal wall, identifies the McBurney

point.) The shifting of pain from the periumbilical area to the right lower quadrant area may take 12 to 36 hours but usually occurs in 2 to 8 hours and may not yet be evident in an acute onset of less than 4 to 6 hours. Unfortunately, the appendix is not always in its classic position; thus, appendicitis may produce pain in the pelvis, in the retrocecal area (back or flank pain, psoas muscle spasm with limp), or elsewhere (Fig. 14-7). With these locations, the psoas or obturator sign may be positive (see Fig. 14-3).

Patients with unperforated appendicitis have a low-grade fever (<38.5°C), are anxious while watching where examiners place their hands, are motionless, walk slowly, get on the examining table with difficulty, and exhibit a nondistended but tender abdomen with voluntary guarding, reduced bowel sounds, and point tenderness in any area overlying the appendix. Rectal examination may reveal right-sided or diffuse tenderness and a mass.

Perforation (rupture) or extensive gangrene should be suspected in the presence of progression for more than 36 to 48 hours; high fever; diffuse abdominal pain and tenderness; a rigid, boardlike abdomen; leukocytosis; a right lower quadrant mass; and other signs of generalized peritonitis (see Table 14-9).

Laboratory and Radiographic Testing

The use of laboratory and radiographic tests in determining the differential diagnosis of acute abdominal pain has been discussed previously. Ultrasonography has been of benefit in the diagnosis of appendicitis and in excluding other important disease processes (Table 14-10). It is particularly helpful in girls when gynecologic disorders or pregnancy must be considered. Helpful ultrasonographic features suggestive of appendicitis include a noncompressible appendix, an inability to visualize an appendix (ruptured), the presence of periappendiceal fluid, and the presence of an appendicolith (Figs. 14-8 and 14-9). Ultrasonography helps define other disease processes, such as mesenteric adenitis (Fig. 14-10) and gynecologic processes. These conditions must be considered in all female patients. Ectopic pregnancy is a particularly serious condition that must not be missed (Fig. 14-11). Nonetheless, gastroenteritis is one of the more common conditions to be considered in the differential diagnosis (Table 14-11). In boys and nonpregnant girls, CT scanning is the imaging study of choice.

Treatment

Appendicitis is treated by surgical appendectomy and ligation of the stump by open or by laparoscopic methods. If an abscess mass is

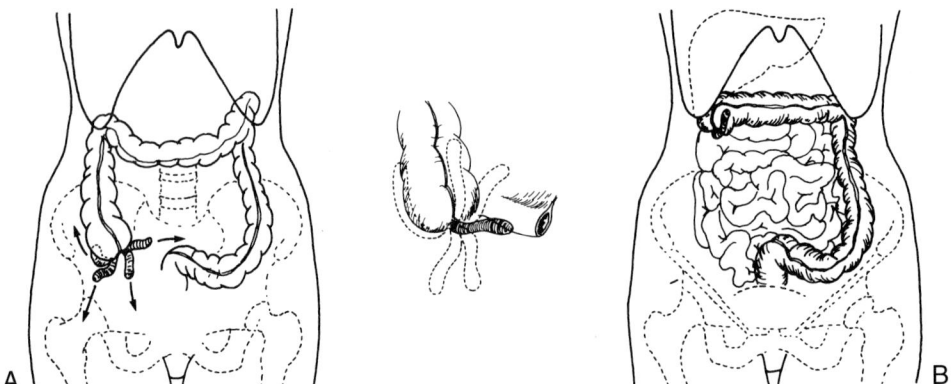

Figure 14-7. The appendix. **A,** The appendix may be located anteriorly, medially, or retrocecally or in the pelvis. **B,** The location of the appendix depends on the location of the cecum. Because the bowel may be quite mobile in some patients, the appendix may be located in many different sites in the abdomen. In this figure, the appendix is in the right upper quadrant. (From Reilly BM: Abdominal pain. In: Practical Strategies in Outpatient Medicine, 2nd ed. Philadelphia, WB Saunders, 1991, p 728.)

Table 14-10. Final Diagnoses in Cases of Clinically Suspected Appendicitis

Appendicitis	Gastroenteritis
Pelvic inflammatory disease	Urinary tract infection
Ovarian cyst: torsion	Meckel diverticulitis
Ectopic pregnancy	Pancreatitis
Mesenteric adenitis	Primary peritonitis
Perforated peptic ulcer	Cholecystitis

present in the right lower quadrant and the patient demonstrates few signs of toxicity, elective nonurgent appendectomy may be delayed for 4 to 8 weeks to permit preoperative rehydration and antibiotic therapy. In appendicitis, parenteral antibiotics (usually ampicillin, gentamicin, and clindamycin) are given before surgery and are continued postoperatively only in the presence of frank contamination (gangrenous or perforated appendicitis). The duration of antibiotic therapy is determined by the presence of infectious complications. If the appendix appears normal, other intraabdominal sources of pain, such as Meckel diverticulitis, should be sought during the surgery.

Complications of appendicitis are uncommon but include sepsis, intraabdominal abscess formation, wound infections, hepatic abscesses, ileus, and peritoneal adhesion formation, and there is subsequent risk for intestinal obstruction and tubal infertility in girls.

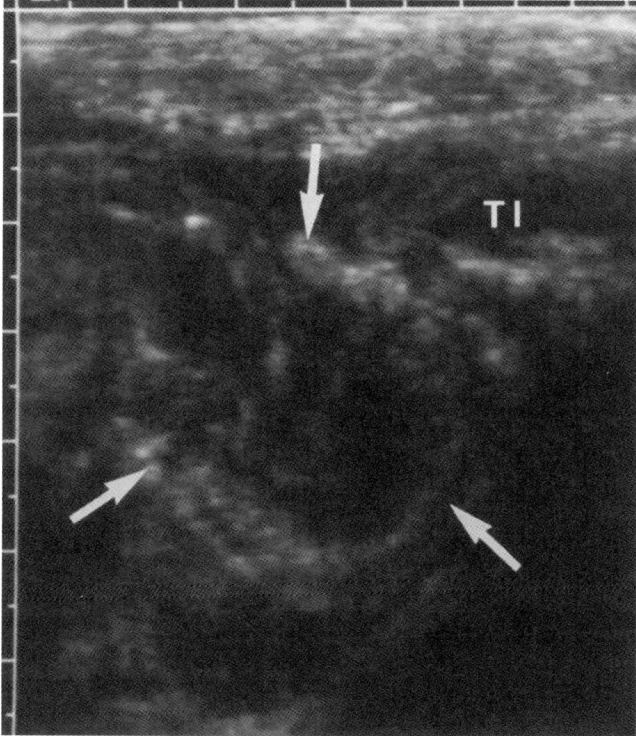

Figure 14-8. An ultrasound scan of the right lower quadrant in a 6-year-old girl, demonstrating a thick-walled cecum (*arrows*) outlined by echogenic fluid. No appendix was found in spite of careful ultrasonographic searching. During surgery, the patient was found to have a perforated appendix and early periappendiceal abscess. TI, terminal ileum. (From Teele R, Share J: Appendicitis and other causes of intraabdominal inflammation. In: Ultrasonography of Infants and Children. Philadelphia, WB Saunders, 1991.)

Pancreatitis

Pancreatitis is an acute inflammatory condition of the pancreas and is often a result of obstruction of the pancreatic duct. Release and activation of pancreatic digestive enzymes subsequently result in extensive destruction (autodigestion) and necrosis of pancreatic and, if severe, adjacent tissue. Proteolysis, fat necrosis, and hemorrhage are noted in severe or fatal cases of pancreatitis, which is often complicated by multiorgan dysfunction syndrome (e.g., hypotension, acute respiratory distress syndrome, acute tubular necrosis, cardiogenic shock).

Pancreatitis is less common in children than in adults, in whom the cause is often alcohol ingestion or gallstones. The etiologic factors in childhood encompass a broad differential diagnosis (Table 14-12) but often include passage of biliary sludge (microlithiasis), drugs (valproate), multisystem diseases (Reye syndrome, hemolytic uremic syndrome, cystic fibrosis), trauma (including abuse), biliary or pancreatic anatomic anomalies, infections, and metabolic conditions (hypercalcemia, hypertriglyceridemia).

Manifestations

Manifestations of acute pancreatitis include intense epigastric abdominal pain that is steady, boring, constant, achelike, knifelike, and exacerbated by recumbency and may radiate to the back, the upper abdominal quadrants, or the scapula. Emesis is common, often protracted, and occasionally bilious. Fever is usually low to moderate grade; high fever (>39° to 40°C) suggests the presence of a primary infectious process with or without secondary pancreatitis or bacterial superinfection and pancreatic abscess formation. The patient often assumes a hunched-over or knee-chest lateral fetal posture and may manifest epigastric tenderness; bowel sounds may be reduced or absent. Signs of peritonitis suggest more extensive necrosis, as do signs of spreading hemorrhage, such as blue-green discoloration of the flanks (Grey Turner sign) or of the periumbilical region (Cullen sign). Intravascular fluid depletion, cardiogenic shock, hemorrhagic shock, hypocalcemic tetany, or systemic inflammatory response syndrome with multiorgan system failure may ensue. Pain may last for 3 to 10 days.

The diagnosis is confirmed by an elevated serum amylase and/or lipase level (lipase levels may be elevated initially with normal amylase values) (Table 14-13). In addition, ultrasonography and CT scanning are helpful in identifying the acutely inflamed pancreas (Fig. 14-12), the degree of necrosis, and the later development of a pancreatic pseudocyst (Fig. 14-13).

Adverse prognostic factors in severe acute pancreatitis include the presence of leukocytosis (white blood count > 16,000/mm³), hyperglycemia (glucose level > 200 mg/dL), a high lactic dehydrogenase level (>350 U/L), and a high aspartate aminotransferase level (>250 U/L) on admission and a decrease in hematocrit value (>10%), an increase in blood urea nitrogen level (>5 mg/dL), a low calcium level (<8 mg/dL), hypoxia (<60 mm Hg), acidosis (base deficit > 4 mmol/L), or severe dehydration (>6 L in adults) by 48 hours of hospitalization. The degree of pancreatic necrosis may be determined from the failure of CT scans to depict intravenous contrast parenchymal enhancement; severe pancreatitis is associated with more than 50% necrosis of the gland.

Complications

Complications of pancreatitis include local tissue necrosis with or without superinfection (pancreatic abscess), fistulization (to colon), left-sided pleural effusion, gastrointestinal hemorrhage (ulceration, vascular rupture, splenic rupture), shock, coagulopathy, acute tubular necrosis, myocardial depression, acute respiratory distress syndrome, hyperglycemia, hypocalcemia, subcutaneous nodules (fat necrosis), hypoalbuminemia, mental changes, and retinopathy.

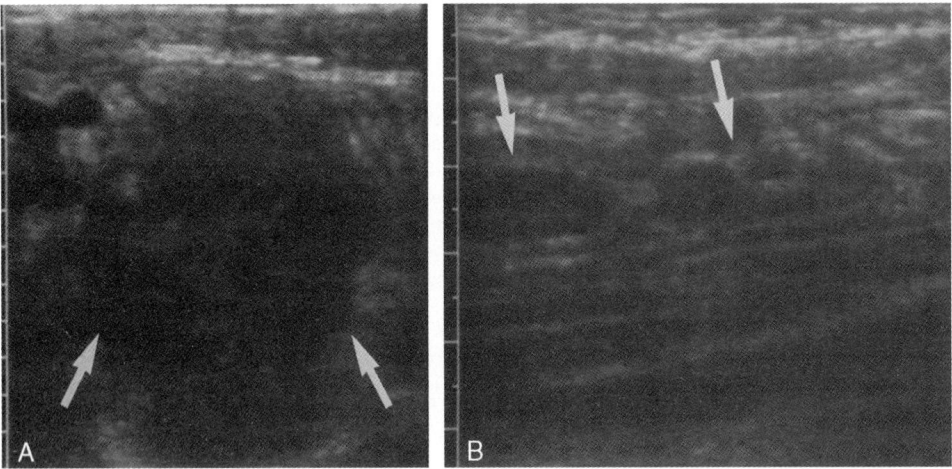

Figure 14-9. An 11-year-old girl presented with fever, diarrhea, and vomiting. Ten days before admission to the hospital, she was seen by a physician because of abdominal pain. She had been partially treated with antibiotics for a presumed "strep throat" in the interim. When she presented to the hospital, she again had pain in the right lower quadrant, especially when the ultrasound transducer was pressed over the area. **A,** The right lower quadrant abscess (*arrows*) was quickly identified. The appendix could not be visualized. **B,** In scans along the psoas, multiple lymph nodes (*arrows*) were apparent. The child's appendix had ruptured 1 week before admission, but her symptoms had been masked by the antibiotics that she had been given. (From Teele R, Share J: Appendicitis and other causes of intra-abdominal inflammation. In: Ultrasonography of Infants and Children. Philadelphia, WB Saunders, 1991, p 348.)

Management

The management of acute pancreatitis consists of supportive care, such as nasogastric tube decompression for patients with an ileus or severe emesis, administration of intravenous fluids, administration of narcotics (meperidine) for pain, and therapy for accompanying complications (e.g., shock, adult respiratory distress syndrome, and acute tubular necrosis). Endoscopic sphincterotomy by endoscopic retrograde cholangiopancreatography (ERCP) is of benefit if gallstones and, possibly, microlithiasis are present. Nonetheless, this procedure has its own risks, which include the induction of pancreatitis.

Enteral alimentation should be initiated as soon as possible, even with a partial ileus. This is usually possible when the pain is

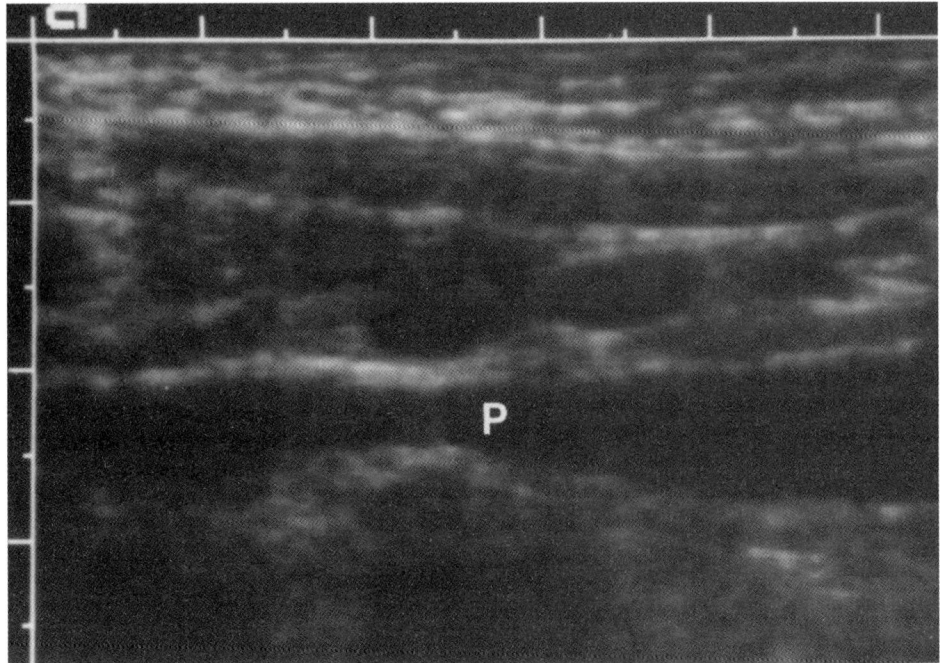

Figure 14-10. This longitudinal scan of the right lower quadrant shows lymph nodes arranged in a line along the psoas muscle (P). These are nodes enlarged from mesenteric adenitis. The patient did not have appendicitis. (From Teele R, Share J: Appendicitis and other causes of intra-abdominal inflammation. In Ultrasonography of Infants and Children. Philadelphia, WB Saunders, 1991.)

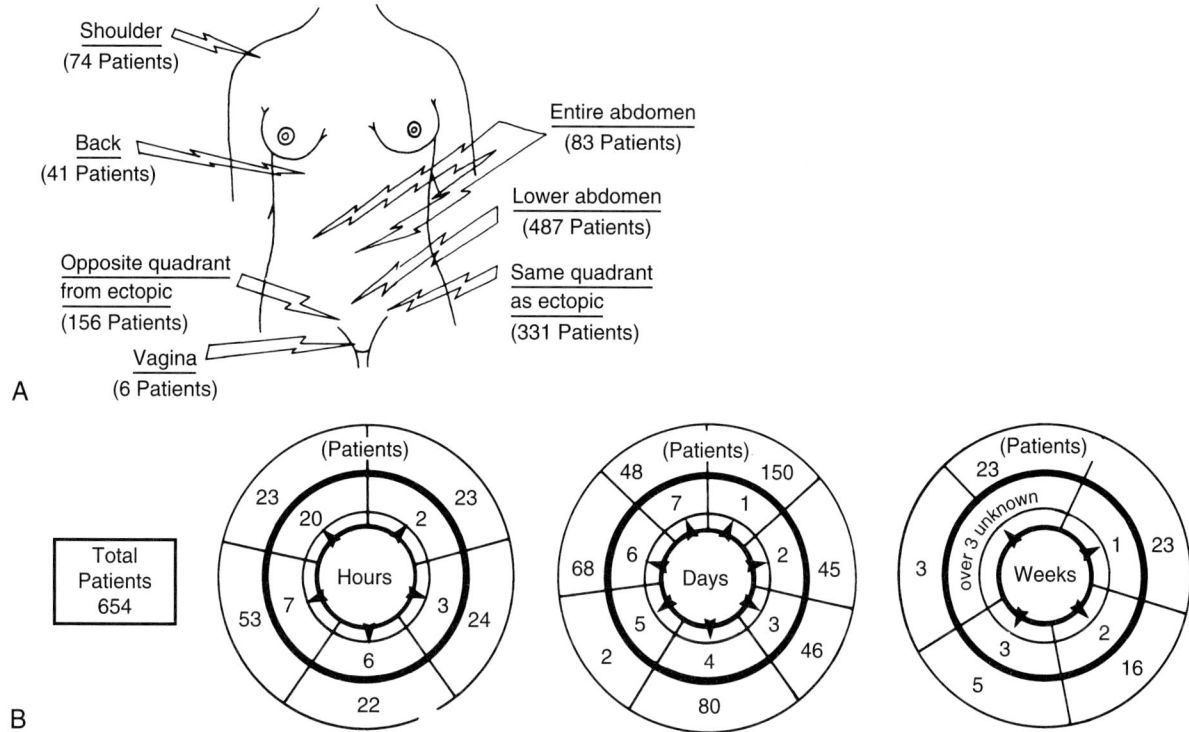

Figure 14-11. Ectopic pregnancy. **A,** Anatomic location of pain in 654 patients with ectopic pregnancy. **B,** Duration of abdominal pain before the diagnosis of ectopic pregnancy was confirmed among 654 patients. (Adapted from Breen JL: A 21-year survey of 654 ectopic pregnancies. Am J Obstet Gynecol 1970;106:1004-1019.)

Table 14-11. Comparison of Gastroenteritis and Appendicitis

	Gastroenteritis	Appendicitis
Pain	Diffuse, cramps, intermittent	Periumbilical shifting to RLQ; constant Exacerbated by movement, coughing
Vomiting	With or before pain	Follows pain
Diarrhea	Frequent, large volume	Can occur; small volume (from irritation of bowel); may be watery, too
Fever	Variable	Low grade, goes up with gangrene or perforation
Course	Intermittently improves	Worsens with time
Systemic symptoms	Variable: headache, malaise, myalgia, arthralgia, sore throat	Rare
Physical examination	General: fussy, restless, frequent motion Abdomen: soft, mild, diffuse tenderness, hyperactive bowel sounds	Quiet, discomfort with movement Abdomen: RLQ tenderness, guarding peritoneal signs, with/without rectal tenderness/mass, absent bowel sounds
Laboratory values	WBC count: variable, may be quite high Urine: nonspecific	WBC count: mild elevation, early left shift; becomes high only with gangrene or perforation Urine: may have WBCs and/or RBCs if bladder irritated, ketosis if vomiting is prolonged
Imaging studies	Abdominal films: nonspecific ileus Ultrasonography: not indicated	Abdominal films: often nonspecific, with/without fecalith, with/without loss of psoas definition, with/without scoliosis caused by inflammation in RLQ Ultrasonography: enlarged appendix, peritoneal fluid, RLQ abscess, absent appendix, fecalith

RBC, red blood cell; RLQ, right lower quadrant; WBC, white blood cell.

Table 14-12. Causes of Acute Pancreatitis in Children

Drugs and Toxins	Infections	Systemic Disease
Alcohol	Coxsackie B virus	α_1-Antitrypsin deficiency
Acetaminophen	Epstein-Barr virus	Cystic fibrosis
Azathioprine	Hepatitis A, B	Diabetes mellitus
L-Asparaginase	HIV	Henoch-Schönlein purpura
Cimetidine	Influenza A	Hemochromatosis
Corticosteroids	Leptospirosis	Hemolytic uremic syndrome
Didanosine	Measles	Hyperlipidemia types I, IV, and V
Estrogens	Mumps	Hyperparathyroidism
Furosemide	Mycoplasma	Hypothermia
Gila monster bite	Rubella	Kawasaki syndrome
6-Mercaptopurine	Reye syndrome	Systemic lupus erythematosus
Methyldopa	**Obstructive**	Malnutrition
Organophosphates		Organic acidemias
Pentamidine	Ascariasis	Periarteritis nodosa
Scorpion bites	Biliary sludge	Peptic ulcer
Spider bites	Biliary tract malformation	Post–pancreatic transplantation
Sulfonamides	Cholelithiasis	Refeeding after malnutrition
Tetracycline	Crohn disease	Reye syndrome
Thiazides	Duplication cyst	Uremia
Valproic acid	Pancreatic pseudocyst	**Traumatic**
Hereditary Pancreatitis	Pancreas divisum	Blunt injury
	Postoperative	Child abuse
SPINK1	Sphincter of Oddi dysfunction	Post-ERCP
CFTR	Tumor	Surgical trauma
Cationic trysinogen		Total body cast

Adapted from Behrman RE (ed): Nelson Textbook of Pediatrics, 14th ed. Philadelphia, WB Saunders, 1992, p 999.

CFTR, cystic fibrosis transmembrane conductance receptor; ERCP, endoscopic retrograde cholangiopancreatography; HIV, human immunodeficiency virus; SPINK1, serine protease inhibitor Kazal type 1.

Table 14-13. Differential Diagnosis of Hyperamylasemia

Pancreatic Pathology

Acute or chronic pancreatitis
Complications of pancreatitis (pseudocyst, ascites, abscess)
Factitious pancreatitis
Complication of ERCP

Salivary Gland Pathology

Parotitis (mumps, *Staphylococcus aureus*, CMV, HIV, EBV)
Sialadenitis (calculus, radiation)
Eating disorders (anorexia nervosa, bulimia)

Intraabdominal Pathology

Biliary tract disease (cholelithiasis)
Peptic ulcer perforation
Peritonitis
Intestinal obstruction
Appendicitis

Systemic Diseases

Metabolic acidosis (diabetes mellitus, shock)
Renal insufficiency, transplantation
Burns
Anorexia-bulimia
Pregnancy
Drugs (morphine)
Head injury
Cardiopulmonary bypass

Adapted from Behrman RE (ed): Nelson Textbook of Pediatrics, 14th ed. Philadelphia, WB Saunders, 1992, p 999.

CMV, cytomegalovirus; EBV, Epstein-Barr virus; ERCP, endoscopic retrograde cholangiopancreatography; HIV, human immunodeficiency virus.

---

subsiding and biochemical signs of inflammation are improving. Alimentation usually occurs within a few days of onset and may be by oral, nasogastric or nasojejunal routes. The nasojejunal tube should be placed distal to the ligament of Treitz to avoid pancreatic stimulation.

Additional therapies include prophylactic antibiotics in acute necrotizing pancreatitis. Infected necrotic tissue must be removed surgically; large persistent pseudocysts are managed by CT-guided drainage or surgical drainage.

Cholelithiasis

Gallstones (see Chapter 20) are uncommon in children, but they complicate chronic diseases, such as hemolytic anemia (sickle cell anemia, spherocytosis), cholestatic jaundice in which total parenteral nutrition is given, and other cholestatic diseases; it may result from prematurity or drug intake (furosemide, ceftriaxone), or it may be idiopathic. Biliary obstruction (stone in cystic or common bile duct) often results in jaundice; sudden onset of severe, sharp right upper quadrant pain; localized deep tenderness in the right upper quadrant (superficial tenderness suggests an associated cholecystitis); and emesis. The pain is episodic and colicky (but often constant, superimposed with waves of more intense pain) and may radiate to the angle of the scapula, the back, or other areas of the abdomen or chest. Patients frequently move about to find a comfortable position. There is associated diaphoresis, pallor, tachycardia, weakness, nausea, and lightheadedness. There may be a round or pear-shaped, slightly tender mass palpated in the right upper quadrant of the abdomen if the gallbladder is distended. The pain may be diurnal, with increased intensity at night. Many patients with single or multiple gallstones (without obstruction) are asymptomatic.

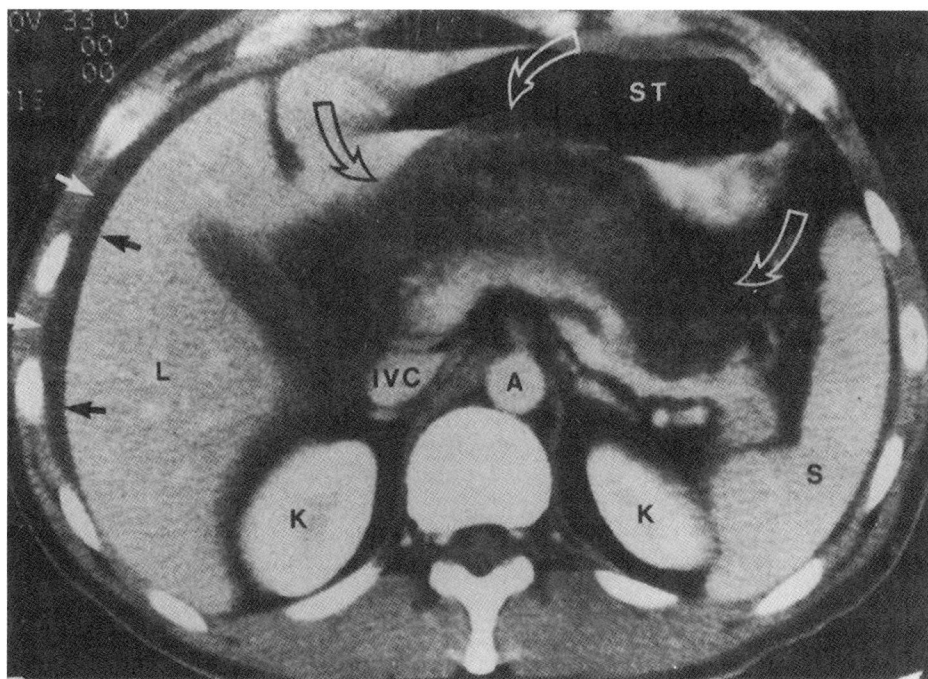

Figure 14-12. Acute pancreatitis. Computed tomographic (CT) scan through the body of the pancreas demonstrates a halo of decreased attenuation around the pancreas that represents a peripancreatic zone of edema and fluid (*curved arrows*). Note the pancreatic ascites, most obvious lateral to the liver (*small arrows*). If intravenous contrast were administered before the CT scan, the inflamed pancreas would appear more dense (whiter). A, aorta; IVC, inferior vena cava; K, kidney; L, liver; PV, portal vein; S, spleen; ST, stomach. (From Freeny P, Lawson T: In Putman CE, Ravin CE [eds]. Textbook of Diagnostic Imaging. Philadelphia, WB Saunders, 1988.)

Acute cholecystitis is caused by inflammation of the gallbladder wall (as a result of duct obstruction [calculus] or nonobstructing [acalculous] conditions) and is manifested by fever, mild jaundice, severe abdominal pain, emesis, nausea, and leukocytosis. Pain may be similar to that in cholelithiasis and radiates to the right scapula, shoulder, or chest. The *Murphy sign* is demonstrated by palpating an acutely inflamed gallbladder, which causes the patient to halt respiration and feel the pain. Fever of greater than 39.5°C suggests perforation or gallbladder gangrene, whereas a high direct bilirubin

level (>4 mg/dL) suggests a common duct stone. Pain may last for 5 to 10 days. Passage of stones or microlithiasis (sludge) may also produce acute pancreatitis. Intolerance (pain) to fatty foods is, unfortunately, a nonspecific observation.

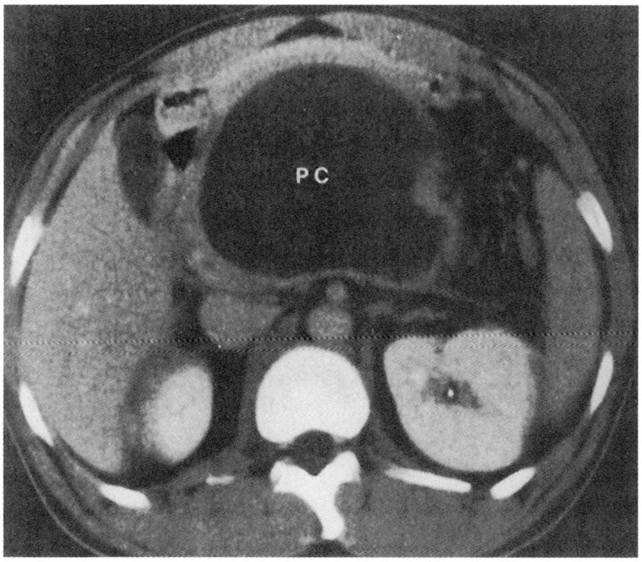

Diagnosis

The diagnosis is confirmed by ultrasonography that demonstrates acalculous or calculus-induced cholecystitis or acute duct obstruction by a stone (Fig. 14-14).

Treatment

Treatment of obstructing stones may include endoscopic open or laparoscopic cholecystectomy. Many patients may go directly to surgery. However, medical management may include ursodeoxycholic acid for stone dissolution. Meperidine is used for pain relief, and broad-spectrum antibiotics are indicated for cholecystitis or cholangitis.

Peptic Ulcer Disease

Peptic ulceration is becoming recognized in children with increasing frequency. Risk factors for peptic ulcer disease (see Chapter 17), including gastritis, include a positive family history of ulcer disease, presence of *Helicobacter pylori,* treatment with nonsteroidal antiinflammatory agents and corticosteroids, cigarette smoking, and severe injury (burns, head injury, shock). Manifestations include pain, gastrointestinal bleeding (melena, hematemesis, anemia), emesis, and, in rare cases, perforation. Nocturnal pain, pain relieved by food, and a family history of peptic ulcer disease are often present in older affected children. The pain is often chronic, recurrent, and located in the epigastrium; tenderness may be localized to the epigastric region, but this is an inconsistent finding.

Acute perforation is characterized by sudden worsening of pain or a new abrupt onset of excruciating epigastric pain. There is associated pallor, faintness, weakness, syncope, diaphoresis, and a rigid abdomen. Corticosteroids may mask some of the signs of perforation.

Figure 14-13. Pseudocyst. Follow-up computed tomographic scan (same patient as in Fig. 14-12) 5 months after the episode of acute pancreatitis demonstrates a large pseudocyst (PC). This large pseudocyst will probably not resolve spontaneously and may need drainage. (From Freeny P, Lawson T: In Putman CE, Ravin CE [eds]. Textbook of Diagnostic Imaging. Philadelphia, WB Saunders, 1988.)

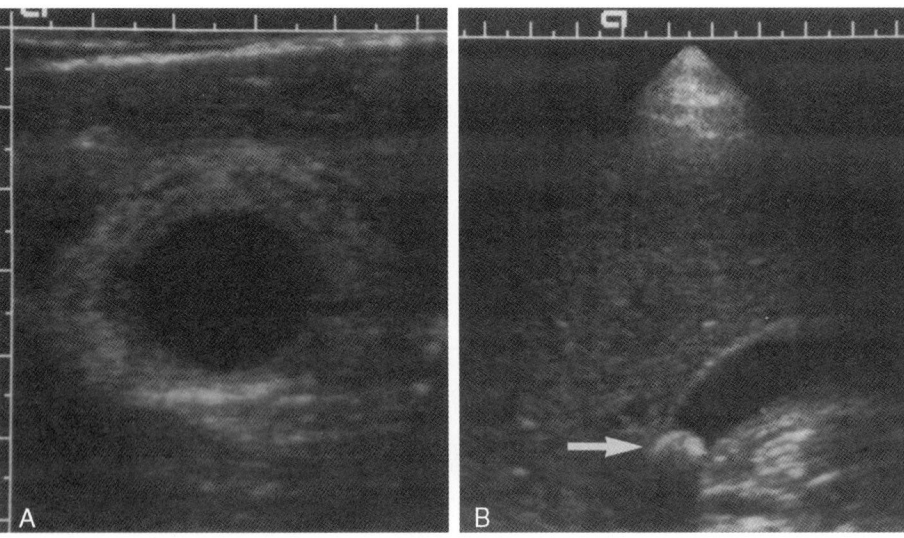

Figure 14-14. Transverse scan with linear array transducer shows pericholic edema in a teenaged boy, who presented with severe pain in the right upper quadrant from acute cholecystitis (**A**). A longitudinal scan of the right upper quadrant (**B**) shows a stone (*arrow*) that was thought to be impacted in the neck of the gallbladder because it did not change at all with position. The patient had severe pain with palpation over the gallbladder. (From Teele R, Share J: The liver. In: Ultrasonography of Infants and Children. Philadelphia, WB Saunders, 1991.)

CHRONIC AND RECURRENT ABDOMINAL PAIN

Chronic abdominal pain refers to recurrent (at least three episodes) or persistent bouts of pain that occur over a minimum of 3 months and that usually compromise normal daily activities. An estimated 10% to 15% of school-aged children experience recurring abdominal pain at some point (see Table 14-4). This general category of disease is often referred to as *recurrent abdominal pain.* The "functional" nature of this pain does not mean that the pain is imaginary or that it may not interfere with the child's daily activities. Recurrent abdominal pain may be organic or psychologic but is most often functional. Functional pain is localized to the periumbilical area, is self-limited, is unrelated to meals or activities, and rarely wakes the child from sleep. *Irritable bowel syndrome* is defined as pain relieved by defecation, a change in stool frequency when the pain begins, altered stool form, passage of mucus, and bloating with distention. Constipation or diarrhea may dominate the clinical manifestations of irritable bowel syndrome.

Organic pain originates from a specific organ, which may be intraabdominal or extraabdominal in location. The cause of organic abdominal pain may be inflammation, obstruction, the presence of masses, or peritoneal irritation.

Functional pain is real and quite perceivable and arises from normal physiologic processes that become uncomfortable, such as alteration of bowel motility, excessive luminal pressure (distention) or muscle (muscularis) contraction (spasms), colic, and mittelschmerz. A very high percentage of children with chronic or recurrent abdominal pain have dysfunctional pain. The pain is real, but a specific diagnosis (e.g., ulcer) may not be identifiable.

Psychogenic pain is pain experienced in the absence of physical stimuli. It may be associated with headache, muscle pain, depression, or poor school performance.

Chronic or recurring abdominal pain may begin with an acute episode, which is evaluated in the manner already described. The initial episode may be attributed to gastroenteritis, or no diagnosis may be made. Diseases that should not be missed include peptic ulcer disease, inflammatory bowel disease, recurrent intestinal obstruction, biliary or urinary stones, esophagitis, carbohydrate intolerance, giardiasis and infection with other parasites, physical or sexual abuse, and genitourinary tract disease. Helpful clues for identifying organic conditions are noted in Tables 14-7 and 14-8. Patients with recurrent abdominal pain experience real pain and should not be considered to be faking it or to be not experiencing it at all.

If the evaluation has been thorough and no cause for the complaints have been found, referral to a specialist may be necessary to provide reassurance to both the family and the clinician that nothing has been missed. The clinician seeing the child in referral must be careful to support the conclusions of the primary care clinician if the workup has been appropriate and no organic cause for the pain can be found. Reassurance that the primary care physician has done a fine job is often enough to enable the family to work together with their physician to monitor and support the child.

If the original complaints of pain were not completely investigated, however, the referral might be time to start again and search for possible organic or nonorganic causes of the pain. If the history includes any aberration in bowel function, upper and/or lower gastrointestinal radiologic studies, followed by upper or lower endoscopy (if indicated by radiologic studies), should be pursued. Contrast CT scans are often helpful and are readily accepted by the family. Evidence of malabsorption syndromes (e.g., lactase deficiency, celiac disease) would be suggested by cramping pain, weight loss, and diarrhea.

Complaints of abdominal pain with absolutely no gastrointestinal symptoms should lead to a thorough evaluation of the urinary tract, a search for inguinal or femoral hernias, and, in rare cases, a neurologic evaluation, including electroencephalography. Abdominal migraines and abdominal epilepsy are unusual causes of recurring pain. Musculoskeletal problems, such as costochondritis, muscle sprain, or nerve root irritation, may cause abdominal wall pain.

The evaluation of the child with chronic or recurring abdominal pain requires the integration of history, objective findings, and laboratory data. The history should be detailed and, in most instances, obtained separately from the parents and the child. A private conversation with each often provides better insight into all factors affecting the child. In addition to covering the historical information already detailed, the clinician should pay attention to factors in the child's environment, family, school, and social interactions that may be sources of undue stress. Stress has been an inconsistent cause of recurrent abdominal pain. Furthermore, little convincing evidence suggests that patients with recurrent abdominal pain have specific or generalized psychologic disturbances. Just because stress exists (e.g., marital discord, school problems) does not mean that stress is the cause of the pain until all other reasonable diagnoses have been investigated. The incidence of life stresses is relatively high among children, and the clinician must not assume, on the basis of poor school performance or perceived psychologic dysfunction, that chronic pain is not organic.

Functional abdominal pain (nonorganic, recurrent abdominal pain) is described as dull and in the periumbilical area, but it may be colicky or burning. Onset often occurs between 4 and 14 years of age. It is rare in children younger than 4 years. There may be a family history of irritable bowel disease and occasionally a personal history of sleepwalking, infant colic, enuresis, or nightmares. There is no consistent duration, frequency, or periodicity. The pain is usually brief (<1 hour); pain-free intervals range from days to weeks. When asked to point to the site of pain, the child may place the entire hand over the umbilicus or, less often, the epigastrium. There is usually no radiation to other sites.

Laboratory studies may not be specific but should include a complete blood cell count, erythrocyte sedimentation rate measurement, urinalysis, stool assessment for ova and parasites (particularly *Giardia* species) and for occult blood, and, if indicated, a breath hydrogen test (for lactose malabsorption). Anemia, leukocytosis, an elevated sedimentation rate, and abnormal serum protein levels are some of the data that may indicate organic disease.

Once the evaluation, including the history, physical examination, and appropriate screening laboratory tests, has been completed and findings are normal, a search for nonorganic sources of pain is appropriate. Many disorders can cause chronic abdominal pain, but only 10% or fewer of all children with chronic complaints of abdominal pain have an organic cause as the source of the pain. Other systemic symptoms, such as headache, nausea, pallor, sleepiness, diarrhea, and dizziness, may be present in patients with functional abdominal pain. In patients with functional recurrent abdominal pain, alterations in bowel habits are common. Growth and development are normal in patients with functional pain.

The child with functional pain may improve once the child and the family understand the nature of the pain. Knowing that there is no serious organic disease and that the sensations are not imaginary is usually welcome information to the family. Simple treatment strategies, such as stool softeners for the constipated child or dietary manipulation for the child who seems to have a lactose (or sorbitol) intolerance, often provide relief sufficient that the child can resume a more normal life.

When there is neither an organic source nor a dysfunctional origin for the pain, a more in-depth examination of psychologic factors is needed. Referral to a mental health professional may trigger more anxiety than it relieves in many families. Examiners must gather positive evidence of emotional maladaptation, such as symptoms of depression, recent academic deterioration, maladaptive coping, or serious family discord, before referring for mental health evaluation. When a child is responding to environmental stresses, the primary physician is usually in the best position to evaluate and counsel.

On occasion, specific medical (organic) conditions may mimic recurrent abdominal pain of functional etiology.

Peptic ulcer disease in children (see Chapter 17) often manifests with abdominal pain that may be atypical from the classic description given by adults. Peptic ulcer disease should be considered if there is chronic pain that is present at night (awakens the patient) or in the morning or before meals (and is relieved by food). There may be recurrent emesis after meals and a positive family history of ulcers. Anemia and occult or gross gastrointestinal blood loss (hematochezia, melena, or hematemesis) may also be present.

Gastroesophageal reflux and peptic esophagitis may manifest with recurrent abdominal pain in the epigastric or substernal area (see Chapter 16). Classic signs of retrosternal pain (odynophagia) or discomfort (dysphagia) and water brash (dyspepsia) are often absent. Patients may respond to antireflux precautions and antacids or H_2-receptor blocking agents.

Carbohydrate malabsorption or intolerance from lactose or sorbitol or related polyalcohol sugars (fruit juices) may produce ingestion-related pain that responds to dietary elimination of the offending sugar (see Chapter 15). Additional conditions to consider include inflammatory bowel disease (see Chapter 15), pancreatitis, intestinal obstruction (see Chapter 16), and genitourinary tract diseases (see Chapters 23 to 29). Persistent, unrelieved, escalating, debilitating pain with associated fever, night sweats, and weight loss should suggest more serious disorders, such as a malignancy (lymphoma, hepatoblastoma, neuroblastoma) or infection (abscesses).

Sometimes, despite diligent evaluation by the most skilled and patient clinician, symptoms persist. In such cases, the following guidelines can help:

- Assure the parents and the child that no major illnesses are present.
- Identify any red flags that might arise, and pursue an appropriate investigation (see Table 14-8).
- Avoid emotional or psychologic labels arrived at by a process of elimination.
- Assure the child and the family that the pain is real and not imaginary.
- See the child regularly to monitor the symptom or symptoms.
- Have the family document the episodes of pain, and review this diary at the patient's regular office visit.
- Do not feel pressured to make a specific diagnosis before the situation is clarified.
- Avoid making a pseudodiagnosis, such as "allergy" or "virus" or "nervous bowel."
- During return office visits, allow time to speak with the child alone and with the parents alone.
- Obtain consultation, especially when the family does not seem completely satisfied with the current situation.
- Try to normalize the child's life by encouraging school attendance and participation in all other regular activities.

Pharmacologic therapy with antispasmodic, anticholinergic, anticonvulsant, or antidepressant agents has not consistently proved effective in children with functional recurrent abdominal pain. Such therapy has sometimes been effective in young adults with irritable bowel syndrome but is not recommended for younger children. If reassurance and time do not result in improvement in children with recurrent abdominal pain, a high-fiber diet may be effective. Ten grams of corn fiber each day, introduced slowly, may benefit as many as 50% of patients.

Managing recurring abdominal pain can be a severe test of the physician's endurance, tenacity, and patience, but in most circumstances, the long-term support of these children and their families can be most satisfying. In as many as 30% to 50% of appropriately diagnosed cases, improvement may be seen within 2 to 6 weeks. An undetermined number of children continue to have abdominal or other pain syndromes (headache) into adulthood. Poor prognostic features include coming from a "pain-identifying" family, male gender, onset of pain before 6 years of age, and duration of pain for more than 6 months before therapy.

COLIC

Colic is defined as fussiness and crying for 3 hours a day, 3 days per week, lasting at least 3 weeks. Some authorities do not use the 3-week criteria. It usually begins in the first month (in rare cases, the first week) after birth and begins to abate by the age of 3 to 6 months. It is unknown whether colic and the crying associated with it are caused by pain, although the parents believe that their child is experiencing pain.

The differential diagnosis includes gastroesophageal reflux (see Chapter 16) and conditions associated with the irritable child (see Chapter 34). Therapy includes hypoallergenic formula and low-allergen diets.

REFERENCES

Apley J: The Child with Abdominal Pains, 2nd ed. Oxford, Blackwell Scientific, 1975.
Harberg FJ: The acute abdomen in childhood. Pediatr Ann 1989;18:169-178.

Hatch EI: The acute abdomen in children. Pediatr Clin North Am 1985;32:1151-1164.

John SD: Imaging of acute abdominal emergencies in infants and children. Curr Prob Pediatr 2001;31:315-358.

Acute Abdominal Pain

Alford BA, McIlhenny J: The child with acute abdominal pain and vomiting. Radiol Clin North Am 1992;30:441-453.

Barr RG, Levine MD, Watkins JB: Recurrent abdominal pain of childhood due to lactose intolerance. N Engl J Med 1979;300:1449-1451.

Bonadio WA: Clinical features of abdominal painful crisis in sickle cell anemia. J Pediatr Surg 1990;25:301-302.

Buchert GS: Abdominal pain in children: An emergency practitioner's guide. Emerg Med Clin North Am 1989;7:497-517.

Byrne WJ, Arnold WC, Stannard MW, et al: Ureteropelvic junction obstruction presenting with recurrent abdominal pain: Diagnosis by ultrasound. Pediatrics 1985;76:934-937.

Daneman A, Navarro O: Intussusception. Pediatr Radiol 2003;33:79-85.

Grey DWR, Dixon MD, Collin J: The closed eye sign: An aid to diagnosing non-specific abdominal pain. BMJ 1988;297:836-837.

Helms M, Vastrup P, Gerner-Smidt P, et al: Short and long term mortality associated with foodborne bacterial gastrointestinal infections: Registry based study. BMJ 2003;326:357-360.

Henrikson S, Blane CE, Koujok K, et al: The effect of screening sonography on the positive rate of enemas for intussusception. Pediatr Radiol 2003;33:190-193.

Jeddy TA, Vowles RH, Southam JA: "Cough sign": A reliable test in the diagnosis of intra-abdominal inflammation. Br J Surg 1994;81:279-281.

Katz JA, Wagner ML, Gresik MV, et al: Typhlitis: An 18-year experience and postmortem review. Cancer 1990;65:1041-1047.

Kim MK, Strait RT, Sato TT, et al: A randomized clinical trial of analgesia in children with acute abdominal pain. Acad Emerg Med 2002;9:281-287.

Leahy AL, Fogarty EE, Fitzgerald RJ, et al: Discitis as a cause of abdominal pain in children. Surgery 1984;95:412-414.

Lebenthal E, Rossi TM, Nord KS, et al: Recurrent abdominal pain and lactose absorption in children. Pediatrics 1981;67:828-832.

Moustaki M, Zeis PM, Katsikari M, et al: Mesenteric lymphadenopathy as a cause of abdominal pain in children with lobar or segmental pneumonia. Pediatr Pulmonol 2003;35:269-273.

Murphy TV, Gargiullo PM, Massoudi MS, et al: Intussusception among infants given an oral rotavirus vaccine. N Engl J Med 2001;344:564-572.

Soltero MJ, Bill AH: The natural history of Meckel's diverticulum and its relation to incidental removal. Am J Surg 1976;132:168-173.

Thomas SH, Silen W: Effect on diagnostic efficiency of analgesia for undifferentiated abdominal pain. Br J Surg 2003;90:5-9.

Towne BH, Mahour GH, Woolley MM, et al: Ovarian cysts and tumors in infancy and childhood. J Pediatr Surg 1975;10:311-320.

Peptic Ulcer Disease

Chiang B-L, Chang M-H, Lin M-I, et al: Chronic duodenal ulcer in children: Clinical observation and response to treatment. J Pediatr Gastroenterol Nutr 1989;8:161-165.

Colin-Jones DG: Acid suppression: How much is needed? Adjust it to suit the condition. BMJ 1990;301:564-565.

Drumm B, Rhoads JM, Stringer DA, et al: Peptic ulcer disease in children: Etiology, clinical findings, and clinical course. Pediatrics 1988;82:410-414.

Gormally S, Drumm B: Helicobacter pylori and gastrointestinal symptoms. Arch Dis Child 1994;70:165-166.

Hosking SW, Ling TKW, Chung SCS, et al: Duodenal ulcer healing by eradication of Helicobacter pylori without anti-acid treatment: Randomised controlled trial. Lancet 1994;343:508-510.

Huang JQ, Sridhar S, Hunt RH: Role of Helicobacter pylori infection and non-steroidal anti-inflammatory drugs in peptic-ulcer disease: A meta-analysis. Lancet 2002;359:14-22.

Murphy MS, Eastham EJ, Jimenez M, et al: Duodenal ulceration: Review of 110 cases. Arch Dis Child 1987;62:554-558.

Suerbaum S, Michetti P: Helicobacter pylori infection. N Engl J Med 2002;347:1175-1186.

Appendicitis

Benjamin IS, Patel AG: Managing acute appendicitis. BMJ 2002;325:505-506.

Doraiswamy NV: Leukocyte counts in the diagnosis and prognosis of acute appendicitis in children. Br J Surg 1979;66:782-784.

Flum DR, Morris A, Koepsell T, et al: Has misdiagnosis of appendicitis decreased over time? JAMA 2001;286:1748-1754.

Jones DJ: Appendicitis. BMJ 1992;305:44-48.

Knight PJ, Vassy LE: Specific diseases mimicking appendicitis in childhood. Arch Surg 1981;116:744-746.

Lee SL, Walsch AJ, Ho HS: Computed tomography and ultrasonography do not improve and may delay the diagnosis and treatment of acute appendicitis. Arch Surg 2001;136:556-562.

Murch SH: Diarrhoea, diagnostic delay, and appendicitis. Lancet 2000;356:787.

Neilson IR, Laberge J-M, Nguyen C: Appendicitis in children: Current therapeutic recommendations. J Pediatr Surg 1990;25:1113-1116.

Oestreich AE, Adelstein EH: Appendicitis as the presenting complaint in cystic fibrosis. J Pediatr Surg 1982;17:191-194.

Paulson EK, Kalady MF, Pappas TN: Suspected appendicitis. N Eng J Med 2003;348:236-242.

Tate JJT, Dawson JW, Chung SCS, et al: Laparoscopic versus open appendicectomy: Prospective randomized trial. Lancet 1993;342:633-637.

Pancreatitis

Beckingham IJ, Bornman PC: Acute pancreatitis. BMJ 2001;322:595-598.

Bornman PC, Beckingham IJ: Chronic pancreatitis. BMJ 2001;322:660-663.

Fernandez-del Castillo C, Rattner DW, Warsha AL: Acute pancreatitis. Lancet 1993;342:475-479.

Kahler SG, Sherwood WG, Woolf D, et al: Pancreatitis in patients with organic acidemias. J Pediatr 1994;124:239-243.

Lee SP, Nicholls JF, Park HZ: Biliary sludge as a cause of acute pancreatitis. N Engl J Med 1992;326:589-593.

Mitchell RMS, Byrne MF, Baillie J: Pancreatitis. Lancet 2003;361:1447-1455.

Munoz-Bongrand N, Panis Y, Soyer P, et al: Serial computed tomography is rarely necessary in patients with acute pancreatitis: A prospective study in 102 patients. J Am Coll Surg 2001;193:146-152.

Rabeneck L, Feinstein AR, Horwitz RI, et al: A new clinical prognostic staging system for acute pancreatitis. Am J Med 1993;95:61-70.

Steinberg W, Tenner S: Acute pancreatitis. N Engl J Med 1994;330:1198-1210.

Weizman Z, Durie PR: Acute pancreatitis in childhood. Pediatrics 1988;113:24-29.

Williamson RCN: Endoscopic sphincterotomy in the early treatment of acute pancreatitis. N Engl J Med 1993;328:279-280.

Yazdani K, Lippmann M, Gala I: Fatal pancreatitis associated with valproic acid. Medicine 2002;81:305-310.

Hepatobiliary Tract Disease

Cuschieri A: Management of patients with gallstones and ductal calculi. Lancet 2002;360:739-740.

De Caluwe D, Akl U, Corbally M: Cholecystectomy versus cholecystolithotomy for cholelithiasis in childhood: Long-term outcome. J Pediatr Surg 2001;36:1518-1521.

Debray D, Pariente D, Gauthier F, et al: Cholelithiasis in infancy: A study of 40 cases. J Pediatr 1993;122:385-391.

Indar AA, Beckingham IJ: Acute cholecystitis. BMJ 2002;325:639-644.

Johnston DE, Kaplan MM: Pathogenesis and treatment of gallstones. N Engl J Med 1993;328:412-421.

Kim SH: Choledochal cyst: Survey by the surgical section of the American Academy of Pediatrics. J Pediatr Surg 1981;16:402-407.

Krige JEJ, Beckingham IJ: Liver abscesses and hydatid disease. BMJ 2001;322:537-540.

Reif S, Sloven DG, Lebenthal E: Gallstones in children. Am J Dis Child 1991;145:105-108.

Chronic Abdominal Pain

Barr RG: Changing our understanding of infant colic. Arch Pediatr Adolesc Med 2002;156:1172-1174.

Castile RG, Telander RL, Cooney DR, et al: Crohn's disease in children: Assessment of the progression of disease, growth and prognosis. J Pediatr Surg 1980;15:462-469.

Garrison MM, Christakis DA: Infant colic. Pediatr Case Rev 2001;1:19-24.

Horwitz BJ, Fisher RS: The irritable bowel syndrome. N Engl J Med 2001;344:1846-1850.

Levine MD, Rappaport LA: Recurrent abdominal pain in school children: The loneliness of the long distance physician. Pediatr Clin North Am 1984;31:969-991.

Liebman WM: Recurrent abdominal pain in children: A retrospective survey of 119 patients. Clin Pediatr 1978;17:149-153.

Mamula P, Telega GW, Markowitz JE, et al: Inflammatory bowel disease in children 5 years of age and younger. Am J Gastroenterol 2002;97: 2005-2010.

Murphy MS: Management of recurrent abdominal pain. Arch Dis Child 1993;69:409-415.

Silverberg M: Chronic abdominal pain in adolescents. Pediatr Ann 1991;20:179-185.

Talley NJ, Spiller R: Irritable bowel syndrome: A little understood organic bowel disease? Lancet 2002;360:555-564.

Thiessen PN: Recurrent abdominal pain. Pediatr Rev 2002;23:39-46.

Wade S, Kilgour T: Infant colic. BMJ 2001;323:437-440.

15 Diarrhea

Subra Kugathasan*

Childhood diarrhea is one of the most common reasons for a sick visit to a health care provider. In the United States, 220,000 hospital admissions occur annually because of diarrhea; these account for 10% of all hospitalizations of young children. About 300 deaths occur from diarrhea and its complications each year in the United States; worldwide, an estimated 5 to 18 million children die each year from diarrhea.

It is important to distinguish acute from chronic diarrhea because the causes and differential diagnoses are very different. Acute diarrhea is usually a self-limited illness that lasts for 2 weeks or less. Chronic diarrhea is defined as diarrhea that persists for more than 2 or 3 weeks. Diarrhea in adults is usually defined as a stool volume output of more than 200 mL each day. In children, a stool output that exceeds 10 mL/kg/day is considered diarrhea. A more practical definition is that diarrhea is present when stools increase in frequency, fluidity (water content), or volume, in comparison with the previously established "normal" pattern. Wide variability exists in normal bowel patterns from child to child; age-related changes occur. Breast-fed infants may pass a loose or seedy stool with each nursing. In older infants or children, stool frequency may vary from several times each day to once every several days. The differential diagnosis of acute and chronic childhood diarrhea is presented in Table 15-1; the epidemiology is outlined in Table 15-2.

PATHOPHYSIOLOGY OF DIARRHEA

Diarrhea is often subdivided into four main categories: secretory, osmotic, increased motility, and inflammation. In simple terms, diarrhea results from a relative increase in secretion, a decrease in intestinal absorption, or both. Differentiating between osmotic and secretary diarrhea is clinically necessary (Tables 15-3 and 15-4). The mechanisms of diarrhea among the various causes are illustrated in Table 15-5.

ACUTE DIARRHEA

VIRAL GASTROENTERITIS

Viral agents account for most cases of acute gastroenteritis (Table 15-6; see Table 15-2). Stools are watery and do not usually contain white or red blood cells. A short incubation period of 2 to 5 days is followed by inflammation of the intestinal lamina propria and varying degrees of villous and microvillous shortening. There are often contacts with diarrhea. Systemic features, such as low-grade fever, vomiting, and respiratory symptoms often accompany the diarrhea. Infants in particular are susceptible to dehydration.

Rotavirus

Rotavirus is the most common cause of diarrhea in childhood. Person-to-person transmission of this virus occurs via the fecal-oral route, although respiratory transmission has been suggested. Household spread, transmission at day care centers and schools, and nosocomial infection are common. Children younger than 2 years are most susceptible, but infection occurs in all age groups. In temperate climates, the disease displays seasonal distribution: Infection is most common during the cooler months (November through May). Affected children are usually ill for 2 to 8 days, after a 1- to 3-day incubation period. Symptomatic infections are common in newborns and older individuals. Acute diarrhea in the young child, occurring during winter and associated with vomiting, low-grade fever, and dehydration, probably represents rotavirus infection. Confirmation may be obtained with enzyme-linked immunosorbent assay (ELISA) and latex agglutination assays for rotavirus detection in stool. Chronic infection does not occur in immune-competent hosts, but after severe infection, the small intestinal mucosa may require 3 to 8 weeks to recover its absorptive ability; this possibly leads to a chronic, postinfectious enteropathy in some individuals.

Norwalk Virus

Norwalk agent is the second most common cause of viral gastroenteritis in children. Affected children are older than those with rotavirus infection; a seasonal pattern of infection is not consistently recognized. In addition to diarrhea and vomiting, headache, myalgia, and malaise are common. Epidemic outbreaks of infection are common, although sporadic cases also occur. Diagnostic tests for the Norwalk virus are not available.

Numerous other viruses are associated with childhood diarrhea (see Tables 15-2 and 15-6), the clinical features of which may be indistinguishable from those of the more common viral agents. Viral gastroenteritis is best managed with oral electrolyte-carbohydrate rehydration solutions. In the absence of severe dehydration (shock, tachycardia, hypotension [Table 15-7]), most infants can be treated with 24 hours of oral rehydration therapy, followed by reinitiation of standard formula. If unstable vital signs or refractory emesis is present, intravenous fluid therapy is indicated. Nonetheless, most infants with emesis can be treated with small-volume, frequent oral rehydration solution feeding; those in shock can be resuscitated parenterally and then given oral rehydration solutions.

BACTERIAL DIARRHEA

Bacterial infections of the intestine cause diarrhea through a variety of mechanisms (Table 15-8; see Table 15-5): direct invasion of intestinal mucosa, followed by intraepithelial cell multiplication or invasion of lamina propria; production of cytotoxin, which disrupts cell function; production of enterotoxin, which alters cellular electrolyte and water balance; and adherence to the mucosal surface, with resultant flattening of the microvilli and disruption of normal cell functioning. The epidemiology of common bacterial pathogens is noted in Table 15-2. Differentiation from viral causes of diarrhea may be difficult (Table 15-9).

---

*This chapter is an updated and edited version of the chapter by Jonathan Flick that appeared in the first edition.

Table 15-1. Differential Diagnosis of Diarrhea

	Infant	Child	Adolescent
Acute			
Common	Gastroenteritis Systemic infection Antibiotic associated Overfeeding	Gastroenteritis Food poisoning Systemic infection Antibiotic associated	Gastroenteritis Food poisoning Antibiotic associated
Rare	Primary disaccharidase deficiency Hirschsprung toxic colitis Adrenogenital syndrome Neonatal opiate withdrawal	Toxic ingestion	Hyperthyroidism
Chronic			

Common	Postinfectious secondary lactase
	  deficiency
	Cow's milk/soy protein intolerance
	Chronic nonspecific diarrhea of infancy
	Excessive fruit juice (sorbitol) ingestion
	Celiac disease
	Cystic fibrosis
	AIDS enteropathy
		Postinfectious secondary
		  lactase deficiency
		Irritable bowel syndrome
		Celiac disease
		Lactose intolerance
		Excessive fruit juice
		  (sorbitol) ingestion
		Giardiasis
		Inflammatory bowel disease
		AIDS enteropathy
			Irritable bowel syndrome
			Inflammatory bowel disease
			Lactose intolerance
			Giardiasis
			Laxative abuse (anorexia nervosa)
			Constipation with encopresis

Rare	Primary immune defects
	Glucose-galactose malabsorption
	Microvillus inclusion disease
	  (microvillus atrophy)
	Congenital transport defects
	  (chloride, sodium)
	Primary bile acid malabsorption
	Munchausen syndrome by proxy
	Hirschsprung disease
	Shwachman syndrome
	Secretory tumors
	Acrodermatitis enteropathica
	Lymphangiectasia
	Abetalipoproteinemia
	Eosinophilic gastroenteritis
	Short bowel syndrome
	Intractable diarrhea syndrome
	Autoimmune enteropathy
		Acquired immune defects
		Secretory tumors
		Pseudoobstruction
		Sucrase-isomaltase deficiency
		Eosinophilic gastroenteritis
			Secretory tumor
			Primary bowel tumor
			Parasitic infections and venereal
			  diseases
			Appendiceal abscess
			Addison disease

Adapted from Kirschner BS, Black DD: The gastrointestinal tract. In Behrman RE, Kliegman RM (eds): Nelson Essentials of Pediatrics, 2nd ed. Philadelphia, WB Saunders, 1994, p 399.
AIDS, acquired immunodeficiency syndrome.

Salmonellosis

Salmonella infection is estimated to cause 1 to 2 million annual gastrointestinal infections in the United States. The attack rate is highest in infancy; the incidence of symptomatic infections is lower in patients older than 6 years. *Salmonella* infection may cause an asymptomatic intestinal carrier state (rare in children), enterocolitis with diarrhea, or bacteremia without gastrointestinal manifestations but with subsequent local infections (meningitis, osteomyelitis). *Salmonella* infection is usually spread through contaminated water supplies or food (meat, chicken, eggs, raw milk, and fresh produce). Most infections in the United States are sporadic rather than epidemic. Although an infected food handler may contaminate food sources, the farm animals are often infected. Cats, turtles, lizards, snakes, and iguanas may also harbor *Salmonella* organisms. Outbreaks may occur among institutionalized children; outbreaks in day care centers are rare.

After a 12- to 72-hour incubation period, gastroenteritis develops and is characterized by the sudden onset of diarrhea, abdominal cramps and tenderness, and fever. The diarrhea is watery, with stools containing polymorphonuclear leukocytes and, on occasion, blood. Symptoms slowly resolve within 3 to 5 days. Excretion of the organism may persist for several weeks. The peripheral blood white blood cell count is usually normal. The organism is readily isolated from stool culture or rectal swab. Owing to the increased risk of developing the carrier state, antimicrobial therapy of uncomplicated cases of *Salmonella* infection is not recommended. Treatment is indicated for children at increased risk for bacteremia and disseminated disease, including infants younger than 3 months and immunocompromised patients (Table 15-10). For others, treatment is directed at maintaining adequate hydration. Treatment with antiperistaltic drugs is thought to be contraindicated in cases of invasive bacterial dysentery because it may lead to more severe symptoms or intestinal perforation.

Table 15-2. Epidemiology of Infectious Agents Causing Diarrhea in the United States

	Percentage of Cases of Diarrhea	Epidemiology
Viruses		
Rotavirus	15-35	Person-to-person spread; winter months; infants
Enteric adenovirus	5-15	Types 40, 41; person-to-person spread; all ages
Norwalk-like viruses (Snow Mountain, Hawaii, Ditchling)	5-15	Foodborne and waterborne common source, person-to-person spread; all ages
Astrovirus (Marin County agent)	1-5	Nosocomial, foodborne, and waterborne; epidemics; all ages
Calicivirus	1-2	Year round, sporadic and epidemic cases; infants
Coronavirus	<1	Pathogenicity uncertain
Bacteria		
Campylobacter jejuni	5-15	Source: wild and domestic animals, poultry, water, raw milk; fecal-oral spread; infants and adolescents
Salmonella enteritidis	3-5	May be underreported; source: poultry, meat, eggs, milk, pigs, turtles; fecal-oral spread; infants, young children
Shigella species (*sonnei, flexneri*)*	3-5	Person-to-person transmission, summer-fall season, dysentery; young children (1-3 yr)
Escherichia coli 0157:H7*	1-3	Person-to-person spread, foodborne (milk, water, meat); all ages
Enterotoxigenic *E. coli*	1-3	Most common cause of traveler's diarrhea
Yersinia enterocolitica	1-3	Source: animals, raw milk, tofu, bean sprouts, chitterlings, diarrhea in infants, mesenteric adenitis in adolescents
Clostridium difficile	1-2	Antibiotic associated: person-to-person nosocomial spread
Staphylococcus aureus	1	Toxin-mediated food poisoning, common source
Clostridium perfringens	1	Toxin-mediated food poisoning, common source
Aeromonas hydrophila	<1	Waterborne: shellfish, sewage, vegetables
Plesiomonas shigelloides	<1	Shellfish, foreign travel
Vibrio cholerae	<1	Gulf of Mexico, shellfish, water
Vibrio parahaemolyticus	<1	Gulf of Mexico, shellfish
Bacillus cereus	<1	Toxin-mediated food poisoning, common source
Parasites		
Giardia lamblia	High incidence in day care centers, residential facilities	Most common parasitic cause of diarrhea, person-to-person, fecal-oral, waterborne spread; all ages
Cryptosporidium species	Unknown; common in day care centers	Waterborne, animal-human, person-to-person, AIDS spread; infants, older if AIDS is a factor
Entamoeba histolytica	<1	Person-to-person spread, southwestern United States
Balantidium coli	<1	Pig contact, contaminated water
Strongyloides stercoralis	<1	Eosinophilia, urticaria

Modified from Behrman RE (ed): Nelson Textbook of Pediatrics, 14th ed. Philadelphia, WB Saunders, 1992, p 664.

AIDS, acquired immunodeficiency syndrome.

*E. coli 0157:H7 and, less often, *Shigella* species are associated with the hemolytic-uremic syndrome.

Table 15-3. Differential Diagnosis of Osmotic versus Secretory Diarrhea

	Osmotic Diarrhea	Secretory Diarrhea
Volume of stool	<200 mL/24 hr	>200 mL/24 hr
Response of fasting	Diarrhea stops	Diarrhea continues
Stool Na+	<70 mEq/L	>70 mEq/L
Reducing substances*	Positive	Negative
Stool pH	<5	>6

From Ghishan FK: Chronic diarrhea. In Behrman RE, Kliegman RM, Jenson HB (eds): Nelson Textbook of Pediatrics, 16th ed. Philadelphia, WB Saunders, 2000, p 1173.

*Sucrose is not a reducing agent. Add 5 drops of 0.1 N HCl to a stool sample before adding reducing agent (Clinitest tablet).

Shigellosis

Most *Shigella* infections in the United States occur in young children, 1 to 4 years of age, with a peak incidence in late summer and early autumn. The organism is transmitted via the fecal-oral route, most often by hands. It may also be the most common bacterial cause of outbreaks of diarrhea in day care settings. During a 12- to 72-hour incubation period, patients may develop a non-specific prodrome characterized by fever, chills, nausea, and vomiting. A colitis affecting predominantly the rectosigmoid region develops and results in abdominal cramps and watery diarrhea. In more severe infections (bacillary dysentery), blood and mucus are passed in small, very frequent stools. High fever in young infants may induce a febrile seizure (see Chapter 39). The association of seizures with shigellosis was attributed to neurotoxic effect of *Shigella* toxin. The seizures may represent a subgroup of common febrile seizures. Stool culture provides the only definitive means of differentiating this organism from other pathogens. Unlike *Salmonella*-caused gastro-enteritis, antibiotic treatment is indicated in shigellosis because it

Table 15-4. Causes of Osmotic Diarrhea

Ingestion of Poorly Absorbable Solutes

Magnesium sulfate, sodium sulfate, citrate-containing
  laxatives
Some antacids: $Mg(OH)_2$
Mannitol, sorbitol (chewing gum, diet candy)

Maldigestion

Disaccharidase deficiencies (lactose, sucrose-isomaltose,
  trehalose intolerance)
Gastrocolic fistula, jejunoileal bypass, short-bowel syndrome
Lactulose therapy

Mucosal Transport Defects

Glucose-galactose malabsorption
Chloridorrhea
Congenital sodium diarrhea
General malabsorption in diffuse disease of small-bowel
  mucosa

Adapted from Krejs GJ: Diarrhea. In Wyngaarden JB, Smith LH, Bennett JC (eds): Cecil Textbook of Medicine, 19th ed. Philadelphia, WB Saunders, 1992, p 682.

shortens the duration of diarrhea, prevents further spread of the organism, and decreases the secondary attack rate, inasmuch as humans provide the only reservoir for this organism (see Table 15-10).

Campylobacter Infection

Many animal species, including poultry, farm animals, and household pets, serve as reservoirs of *Campylobacter jejuni*. Transmission occurs through ingestion of contaminated food, especially undercooked food, and through person-to-person spread via the fecal-oral route. The disease is common in infants and adolescents. Day care and college outbreaks have been reported. Asymptomatic carriage is uncommon. *Campylobacter* infection may cause disease ranging from mild diarrhea to frank dysentery. The organism causes diffuse, invasive enteritis that includes the ileum and colon. Fever, cramping, abdominal pain, and bloody diarrhea are characteristic and may mimic those of acute appendicitis or inflammatory bowel disease (IBD). Fever and diarrhea usually resolve after 5 to 7 days; prolonged illness or relapse occasionally occurs. *Campylobacter* infection is also known to cause meningitis, abscesses, pancreatitis, and pneumonia. Guillain-Barré syndrome has been reported after *Campylobacter* infection. Culture of the organism from fecal specimens is routinely accomplished in many laboratories. Supportive treatment alone is sufficient in most cases. Treatment is recommended only in severe cases. Antibiotic treatment eradicates the organism from the stool and may therefore prevent person-to-person spread; it may also shorten the period of clinical illness if it is started early in the disease process.

Table 15-5. Mechanisms of Diarrhea

Primary Mechanism	Defect	Stool Examination	Examples	Comment
Secretory	Decreased absorption, increased secretion, electrolyte transport	Watery, normal osmolality; osmoles = $2 \times (Na^+ + K^+)$	Cholera, toxigenic *E. coli*; carcinoid, VIP, neuroblastoma, congenital chloride diarrhea, *Clostridium difficile*, cryptosporidiosis (AIDS)	Persists during fasting; bile salt malabsorption also may increase intestinal water secretion; no stool leukocytes
Osmotic	Maldigestion, transport defects, ingestion of unabsorbable solute	Watery, acidic, and reducing substances; increased osmolality; osmoles $>2 \times (Na^+ + K^+)$	Lactase deficiency, glucose-galactose malabsorption, lactulose, laxative abuse	Stops with fasting; increased breath hydrogen with carbohydrate malabsorption; no stool leukocytes
Increased motility	Decreased transit time	Loose to normal-appearing stool, stimulated by gastrocolic reflex	Irritable bowel syndrome, thyrotoxicosis, postvagotomy dumping syndrome	Infection also may contribute to increased motility
Decreased motility	Defect in neuro-muscular unit(s) Stasis (bacterial overgrowth)	Loose to normal appearing stool	Pseudoobstruction, blind loop	Possible bacterial overgrowth
Decreased surface area (osmotic, motility)	Decreased functional capacity	Watery	Short bowel syndrome, celiac disease, rotavirus enteritis	May require elemental diet plus parenteral alimentation
Mucosal invasion	Inflammation, decreased colonic reabsorption, increased motility	Blood and increased WBCs in stool	*Salmonella*, *Shigella*, infections; amebiasis; *Yersinia*, *Campylobacter* infections	Dysentery evident in blood, mucus, and WBCs

From Behrman RE, Kliegman RM, Jenson HB (eds): Nelson textbook of pediatrics, 16th ed, Philadelphia, WB Saunders, 2000.

AIDS, acquired immunodeficiency syndrome; VIP, vasoactive intestinal peptide; WBC, white blood cell.

Table 15-6. Viral Enteric Pathogens

	Predominant Age Group Affected	Seasonality	Duration of Symptoms
Rotavirus	6-24 months	↑ in winter months	2-8 days
Norwalk virus	Older children, adults	Winter and summer	12-48 hours
Enteric adenovirus	<2 years	↑ in summer months	Up to 14 days
Calcivirus	3 months–6 years	Unknown	2-8 days
Astrovirus	1-3 years	Unknown	1-4 days

From Laney DW Jr, Cohen MB: Infectious diarrhea. In Wylie R, Hyams JS (eds): Pediatric Gastrointestinal Diseases: Pathophysiology, Diagnosis, Management, Philadelphia, WB Saunders, 1993, p 613.

Table 15-7. Assessment of Degree of Dehydration

	Mild	Moderate	Severe
Infant	5%	10%	15%
Adolescent	3%	6%	9%
Signs and Symptoms			
General appearance and condition			
Infants/young children	Thirsty; alert; restless	Thirsty; restless or lethargic but irritable or drowsy	Drowsy; limp, cold, sweaty, cyanotic extremities; may be comatose
Older children	Thirsty; alert; restless	Thirsty; alert (usually)	Usually conscious (but at reduced level), apprehensive; cold, sweaty, cyanotic extremities; wrinkled skin on fingers/toes; muscle cramps
Tachycardia	Absent	Present	Present
Palpable pulses	Present	Present (weak)	Decreased
Blood pressure	Normal	Orthostatic hypotension	Hypotension
Cutaneous perfusion	Normal	Normal	Reduced/mottled
Skin turgor	Normal	Slight reduction	Reduced
Fontanel	Normal	Slightly depressed	Sunken
Mucous membrane	Moist	Dry	Very dry
Tears	Present	Present/absent	Absent
Respirations	Normal	Deep, may be rapid	Deep and rapid
Urine output	Normal	Oliguria	Anuria/severe oliguria

From Lewy JE: Nephrology: Fluids and electrolytes. (Adapted from World Health Organization Guide.) In Behrman RE, Kliegman RM (eds): Nelson Essentials of Pediatrics, 2nd ed. Philadelphia, WB Saunders, 1994, p 582.

Yersinia Infection

Yersinia infection may cause various clinical syndromes, including gastroenteritis, mesenteric adenitis, pseudoappendicitis, and post-infectious reactive arthritis. The organism is present in animals and may be spread to humans by consumption of undercooked meat (especially pork), unpasteurized milk, and other contaminated foods. Person-to-person spread also occurs. Young children are particularly susceptible to disease, and the frequency of infections is increased during the summer months.

The organisms may be cultured from rectal swab or stool specimens, but selective media are required, and the organism may not be identified for several weeks. The microbiology laboratory should be notified if *Yersinia* infection is suspected. Antibiotics are not effective in alleviating symptoms of *Yersinia* infection or in shortening the period of its excretion. Patients with extraintestinal infection

Table 15-8. Bacterial Pathogens Grouped by Pathogenic Mechanism

Invasive	Cytotoxic	Toxigenic	Adherent
Shigella species	*Shigella* species	Shigella species	Enteropathogenic *Escherichia coli*
Salmonella species	Enteropathogenic *E. coli*	Enterotoxigenic *E. coli*	Enterohemorrhagic *E. coli*
Yersinia enterocolitica	Enterohemorrhagic *E. coli*	*Yersinia enterocolitica*	Enteroaggregative *E. coli*
Campylobacter jejuni	*Clostridium difficile*	*Aeromonas* species	Diffuse-adherent *E. coli*
Vibrio parahaemolyticus		*Vibrio cholerae* and non-01 *Vibrio* species	

Modified from Cohen MB: Etiology and mechanisms of acute infectious diarrhea in infants in the United States. J Pediatr 1991; 118:S34-S43.

Table 15-9. Differentiation of Bacterial and Viral Causes of Gastroenteritis

Variable	Bacterial	Viral
Temperature >39.0° C	Yes	Unusual
Abdominal pain, tenesmus	Yes	Unusual
>8 bowel movements/24 hr	Yes	Unusual
Emesis	Yes, less common	Yes
Duration >5 days	Yes	No
Erythrocyte sedimentation rate	Elevated	Normal
Leukocytosis	Yes	No
Stool leukocytes and mucus present	Yes (*Shigella, Salmonella, Yersinia, Campylobacter* species; invasive *Escherichia coli; Plesiomonas* species)	Unusual
Stool leukocytes absent: secretory diarrhea	Yes (*Vibrio cholerae,* toxigenic *E. coli, Aeromonas* species)	No
Hematochezia	Yes (*Shigella, Salmonella, Yersinia, Campylobacter* species; enterohemorrhagic *E. coli,* pseudomembranous colitis due to *Clostridium difficile; Plesiomonas* species)	No, except rotavirus in preterm infants
History of shellfish consumption	Yes (*E. coli, V. cholerae, Vibrio parahaemolyticus, Campylobacter* species)	Yes (Norwalk agent)
Traveler's diarrhea	Yes (toxigenic *E. coli; Salmonella, Shigella* species)	Unusual (Norwalk agent and rotavirus)
Single-source outbreak	Yes (*Salmonella, Shigella* species; *Staphylococcus aureus; Bacillus cereus; Clostridium perfringens; Yersinia* species; *E. coli*)	Yes (Norwalk agent)
Seasonal epidemics	Unusual (*Campylobacter* species)	Yes (rotavirus)

From Behrman RE (ed): Nelson Textbook of Pediatrics, 14th ed. Philadelphia, WB Saunders, 1992, p 665.

should receive therapy (see Table 15-10). Most *Yersinia* organisms are susceptible to aminoglycosides, third-generation cephalosporins, chloramphenicol, and trimethoprim-sulfamethoxazole.

Escherichia coli Infection

Although *E. coli* is the predominant normal flora in the colon, some strains are pathogenic. Diarrhea caused by *E. coli* can be watery, inflammatory, or bloody, depending on the strain involved (Table 15-11). These diarrheogenic *E. coli* strains are currently classified, on the basis of serogrouping or pathogenic mechanisms, into five major groups: (1) Enteropathogenic *E. coli* (EPEC), an important cause of diarrhea in infants; (2) enterotoxigenic *E. coli* (ETEC), a cause of diarrhea in infants and a cause of traveler's diarrhea; (3) enteroinvasive *E. coli,* which causes watery ETEC-like illness or, less commonly, a dysentery-like illness; (4) enterohemorrhagic *E. coli,* which causes hemorrhagic colitis and hemolytic uremic syndrome (HUS); and (5) enteroaggregative *E. coli,* which along with EPEC has been implicated as a cause of persistent diarrhea. Enteric infections with *E. coli* are acquired via the fecal-oral route. Enterohemorrhagic strains are the only diarrhea-producing *E. coli* strains that are common in the United States and have been associated with foodborne epidemic outbreaks transmitted by undercooked meat.

EPEC is a well-established cause of infantile diarrhea, especially in developing countries. Asymptomatic carriage is common. At least two separate mechanisms are responsible for diarrhea: adherence to intestinal epithelial cells, leading to villous injury and mucosal inflammation, and production of a toxin similar to that of *Shigella* organisms. Chronic infection with failure to thrive may also occur. ETEC is the major cause of traveler's diarrhea; occasional nosocomial outbreaks have also occurred in hospitalized infants. At least three different types of *E. coli* enterotoxins (heat-labile, heat-stable toxin A, and heat-stable toxin B) have been identified. Definitive diagnosis requires enterotoxin identification, and this method is not widely available.

Prophylactic antibiotics are effective in reducing the incidence of traveler's diarrhea but are not recommended for use in young children.

Enterohemorrhagic *E. coli* produces a Shiga-like cytotoxin and causes diarrhea, hemorrhagic colitis, and, in about 20% of infected persons, results in HUS. Both epidemic and sporadic cases have been recognized. Infection is more common in the summer and fall. A particular serotype, *E. coli* 0157:H7, has been isolated in several outbreaks associated with undercooked beef and has been linked to the development of HUS in young children. The most common manifestation of enterohemorrhagic *E. coli* infection begins with severe abdominal cramps and watery diarrhea, followed by grossly bloody stools and emesis. Fever is uncommon. Fecal leukocytes are absent or few. Other manifestations include asymptomatic infection and watery diarrhea without progression to hemorrhagic colitis. *E. coli* 0157:H7 is cleared from the stool in 5 to 12 days. HUS develops in a smaller number of children in the week after the onset of diarrhea. HUS manifests with renal failure, microangiopathic hemolytic anemia, thrombocytopenia, and diarrhea. There is no role for antimicrobial therapy in enterohemorrhagic *E. coli* disease. Antibiotics neither shorten the duration of disease nor prevent progression to HUS; they may predispose to HUS.

Clostridium difficile Infection

C. difficile causes acute and chronic diarrhea in children when the normal colonic flora is disrupted. Pseudomembranous colitis is the most severe form of this infection, occurring as a result of a severe inflammatory response to the *C. difficile* toxins.

Epidemiology. The prevalence of carrier status for *C. difficile* in healthy, asymptomatic outpatients is reported to be up to 70% in healthy infants, 3% in children, and 2% in adults and as many as 20% of asymptomatic hospitalized patients. The organism grows rapidly when other intestinal pathogens are suppressed by antibiotic therapy; it can be spread rapidly from patient to patient.

Table 15-10. Antibiotic Therapy for Diarrhea

Organism	Treatment*	Comment
Salmonella typhi	Ampicillin,[†] chloramphenicol,[†] trimethoprim/ sulfamethoxazole, cefotaxime, ciprofloxacin[‡]	Invasive, bacteremic disease
Other *Salmonella* species	Usually none; amoxicillin, ampicillin, trimethoprim/sulfamethoxazole, cefotaxime, ciprofloxacin[‡]	Treatment indicated if patient is younger than 3 months or if malignancy, sickle cell anemia, AIDS, or evidence of nongastrointestinal foci of infection is present
Shigella species	Trimethoprim/sulfamethoxazole, ampicillin	Amoxicillin not recommended; treatment reduces infectivity and improves outcome
Escherichia coli		
Toxigenic	Usually none if endemic; trimethoprim/ sulfamethoxazole or ciprofloxacin[‡] for traveler's diarrhea	Prevention of traveler's diarrhea with bismuth subsalicylate, doxycycline, or ciprofloxacin[‡]
Invasive or pathogenic	Trimethoprim/sulfamethoxazole, neomycin	No treatment if HUS is suspected
Campylobacter species	Mild disease necessitates no treatment; erythromycin or azithromycin for diarrhea; aminoglycoside, meropenem, or imipenem for systemic illness	If started early (days 1-3), treatment reduces symptoms and fecal organisms
Yersinia species	None for diarrhea; gentamicin, chloramphenicol, trimethoprim/sulfamethoxazole, or cefotaxime for systemic illness	Value of treatment of mesenteric adenitis with antibiotics is not established
Vibrio cholerae	Tetracycline, trimethoprim/sulfamethoxazole	Fluid maintenance is critical
Clostridium difficile	Oral vancomycin, metronidazole[§]	*C. difficile* is agent of antibiotic-associated diarrhea and pseudomembranous colitis
Giardia lamblia	Quinacrine, furazolidone, metronidazole[§]	Furazolidone is only preparation available in liquid form
Cryptosporidium species	None; azithromycin or paromomycin and octreotide in AIDS	A serious infection in immunocompromised patients (AIDS)
Entamoeba histolytica	Metronidazole,[§] tinidazole followed by iodoquinol	

From Behrman RE, Kliegman RM, Jenson HB (eds): Nelson Textbook of pediatrics, 16th ed. Philadelphia, WB Saunders, 2000, p 476.

*All treatment is predicated on knowledge of antimicrobial sensitivities.

[†]Organism is often resistant to this drug.

[‡]Ciprofloxacin is not indicated for children with growing bones and uncomplicated infections.

[§]The safety of metronidazole in children is unknown.

AIDS, acquired immunodeficiency syndrome; HUS, hemolytic-uremic syndrome.

Transmission occurs through person-to-person contact and environmental contamination. Environmental contamination occurs through the spores formed by *C. difficile,* which retain viability for up to 1 week on dry surfaces. *C. difficile* and its toxin have been identified in the feces of healthy infants in concentrations similar to those found in adults with pseudomembranous colitis. The apparent resistance of infants to *C. difficile* and its toxin is caused by a developmental absence of the toxin-binding site in the immature intestine.

Clinical Features. *C. difficile* infection is highly associated with recent antibiotic exposure, particularly to broad-spectrum antibiotics. These drugs disrupt the endogenous colonic flora that inhibits the growth of *C. difficile.* Other risk factors for C. difficile diarrhea include gastrointestinal surgery or procedures and chemotherapy.

C. difficile infection should be considered in patients in whom diarrhea develops during or within several weeks of antibiotic therapy. Illness associated with this organism varies from a mild,

Table 15-11. Enteric *Escherichia coli* Infections

Type	Mechanism	Clinical Syndrome	Stools
Enterotoxigenic	Enterotoxin(s); adherence	Traveler's diarrhea; nursery outbreaks	Watery; no blood or polys
Enteropathogenic	Adherence; Shiga-like toxin	Infantile diarrhea; asymptomatic carriage	Watery ± blood; no polys
Enterohemorrhagic*	Shiga-like toxin	Hemorrhagic colitis	Bloody; rare polys
Enteroadherent	Adherence	Chronic childhood diarrhea; traveler's diarrhea	Chronic watery; no blood or mucus
Enteroinvasive	Shiga-like toxin	Dysentery	Blood, polys, mucus in stools
Enteroaggregative	Toxin (?)	Persistent diarrhea in developing countries	Watery with or without blood

*Associated with hemolytic-uremic syndrome.

polys, polymorphonuclear leukocytes.

self-limited, nonbloody diarrhea to severe hemorrhagic colitis, protein-losing enteropathy, toxic megacolon, colonic or cecal perforation, peritonitis, sepsis, shock, and death. In rare cases, manifestations of *C. difficile* infection include fever or abdominal pain without diarrhea or diarrhea in the absence of recent antibiotic use.

C. difficile–associated colitis is caused by potent toxins produced by this organism: toxin A, a lethal enterotoxin, causes hemorrhage and fluid secretion in the intestines, and toxin B is a cytotoxin detectable by its cytopathic effects in tissue culture. Both toxins play a role in disease production, although toxin A may be more important.

Diagnosis. The diagnosis of *C. difficile* infection is made from detection of toxin A and/or toxin B in stool samples. Sigmoidoscopy or colonoscopy reveals pseudomembranes in 30% to 50% of cases, typically in association with more severe disease.

Treatment. The offending antibiotic is discontinued, and oral metronidazole or vancomycin therapy is initiated. Parenteral metronidazole therapy is used for severe ileus, toxic megacolon, or impending intestinal perforation (see Table 15-10).

Aeromonas Infection

Aeromonas species are gram-negative organisms that may cause a mild, self-limited diarrheal illness in children. The most common manifestation is a watery, nonbloody, nonmucoid diarrhea seen during the late spring, summer, and early fall. More severe infections may resemble ulcerative colitis, with chronic bloody diarrhea and abdominal pain. Treatment with trimethoprim-sulfamethoxazole is indicated in these severe cases.

Plesiomonas Infection

Plesiomonas shigelloides is a *Vibrio*-like organism that is sometimes implicated in childhood diarrhea. It has been linked to consumption of shellfish and travel to Mexico and Asia.

DIARRHEA CAUSED BY PARASITES

Giardia Infestation

Giardia lamblia is a flagellated protozoan that can cause many different symptoms, such as diarrhea, malabsorption, abdominal pain, and weight loss. It spreads through contaminated food and water as well as through person-to-person contact via the fecal-oral route. The latter mode of transmission is responsible for outbreaks of diarrhea in day care centers and residential facilities. Infection is often asymptomatic. Symptomatic illness usually develops 1 to 3 weeks after exposure and may mimic acute gastroenteritis with fever, nausea, vomiting, and watery diarrhea. In some patients, a chronic illness develops, characterized by intermittent, foul-smelling diarrhea, abdominal bloating, nausea, abdominal pain, and weight loss. The stool should be examined for cysts or trophozoites on at least three fresh specimens, because excretion of the organism is only intermittent. An ELISA-based *Giardia* antigen test is a more sensitive means of detecting infection and should be performed, if available. All infected persons should be treated. Many agents are available (see Table 15-10). Metronidazole (20-40 mg/kg/day t.i.d. for 5 days) is highly effective. Furazolidone (5 mg/kg four times a day for 7 days) is less effective but is better tolerated and is available in liquid form.

Entamoeba histolytica Infestation

This organism is acquired in warm climates (Mexico, southwestern United States) by ingestion of cysts in fecally contaminated material. Infected individuals are often asymptomatic. Amebic dysentery

may occur, but hepatic abscess and other remote infections are uncommon. Because cysts are shed in the stool on an intermittent basis, examination of several fecal specimens may be required for identification. Asymptomatic or mild infections may be treated with a luminal amebicide, such as diiodohydroxyquin; more severe infections (invasive intestinal or extraintestinal) are treated with metronidazole.

Cryptosporidium Infestation

This protozoan causes watery diarrhea in both immunocompetent and immunocompromised hosts. It is an important cause of severe diarrhea in individuals infected with the human immunodeficiency virus. It has also been recognized as an occasional cause of self-limited diarrhea in travelers, as well as in children in day care centers and persons in residential institutions. The mechanisms by which these organisms cause diarrhea are unknown. Special techniques are required for identifying the oocysts in fecal specimens and should be requested if *Cryptosporidium* infestation is suspected. Antimicrobial therapy is not indicated in immunocompetent hosts.

OTHER CAUSES OF ACUTE DIARRHEA

Parenteral Secondary Diarrhea

Acute diarrhea may accompany infections outside of the gastrointestinal tract (so-called parenteral diarrhea). Thus, upper respiratory tract and urinary tract infections may be associated with increased bowel movement frequency or stool water. The mechanism is unclear but may involve alterations in bowel motility, changes in diet, or effects of antibiotic treatment.

Drugs

Various prescription and over-the-counter drugs may cause acute diarrhea. The most commonly implicated agents are antibiotics, acting through mechanisms other than *C. difficile*. Several other medications are also associated with diarrhea in children (Table 15-12).

Table 15-12. Medications Associated with Diarrhea in Children

Agent	Mechanism
Stimulant laxatives (senna, phenolphthalein, bisacodyl)	Increased intestinal secretion
Antacids	Osmotic effect (Mg^{2+})
Prokinetic agents (metoclopramide, bethanechol, cisapride)	Increased peristalsis
Measles-mumps-rubella vaccine	Unknown
Thyroid hormone	Increased peristalsis
Monosodium glutamate	Unknown
Chemotherapeutics	Intestinal mucosal injury
Mushrooms	Multiple mechanisms
Heavy metals	Toxic effect
Organophosphates	Cholinergic effects
Diuretics	Unknown
Digitalis	Unkown
Colchicine	Unknown
Indomethacin	Prostaglandin synthesis inhibition
Theophylline	Increased peristalsis

Food Poisoning (Table 15-13)

Staphylococcal food poisoning results from ingestion of preformed enterotoxin, produced in contaminated food that has incubated at or above room temperature for a suitable period. Staphylococcal food intoxication is suggested by the sudden onset of vomiting followed, usually within 4 to 6 hours after ingestion of the contaminated food, by explosive diarrhea. The illness is self-limited and usually resolves within 12 to 24 hours. The diagnosis is made on the basis of a characteristic clinical picture. Treatment is supportive; antibiotics are not indicated.

Bacillus cereus, a gram-positive, spore-forming organism found in soil, is usually associated with contamination of refried rice or vegetables. Two food poisoning syndromes can occur. A short-incubation disease (1 to 6 hours) results from ingestion of preformed toxin and is characterized by nausea, vomiting, and diarrhea, similar to staphylococcal food poisoning. A long-incubation period disease (8 to 16 hours) is caused by in vivo production of an enterotoxin and is characterized by abdominal pain, tenesmus, and profuse watery diarrhea. Vomiting is usually absent. Both syndromes resolve spontaneously within 24 hours and are managed with supportive care.

Clostridium perfringens food poisoning has been associated with ingestion of contaminated beef and poultry. The disease results from production and release of an enterotoxin into the lower bowel 8 to 24 hours after ingestion of the vegetative form of the organism. Onset is sudden, with abdominal pain and watery diarrhea. Fever and vomiting are absent.

Other causes of food poisoning are noted in Table 15-13.

CHRONIC DIARRHEA

Chronic diarrhea is defined as diarrhea lasting longer than 2 or 3 weeks. Causes of chronic diarrhea are numerous and vary markedly with age (Table 15-14). In the small infant, this disorder is known as intractable diarrhea of infancy (Table 15-15).

Chronic diarrhea needs to be distinguished from various malabsorption states, which are classified by the nutrient that is malabsorbed (Table 15-16). Initial screening and stepwise testing for malabsorption are noted in Table 15-17 and explained in Table 15-18. Common causes of malabsorption are noted in Table 15-19. Clues to the presence of malabsorption are noted in Table 15-20. Therapy depends on the primary disease and includes treatment of that process plus replacement of the malabsorbed nutrient.

CHRONIC DIARRHEA IN INFANCY

Prolonged Infection and Postinfectious Enteropathy

Chronic intestinal infections occur only occasionally, particularly in infants with preexisting malnutrition and in those children with immunologic deficiencies. More commonly, persistent diarrhea after acute enteritis is caused by a postinfectious enteropathy. Predisposing factors include age younger than 6 months, malnutrition, and feeding with formula rather than breast milk. Pathophysiologic mechanisms include damage to the small intestinal villi with loss of disaccharidase activity and reduction in the mucosal surface absorptive area. Small-bowel bacterial overgrowth and absorption of potentially antigenic proteins may aggravate the malabsorptive state. Patients with mild involvement may do well on a non–lactose-containing formula. More severely affected infants may require a protein hydrolysate formula, whereas the most severely affected infants may not tolerate any enteral feedings and must be placed on parenteral nutrition. Recovery usually occurs over 4 to 6 weeks, provided that the child is supplied with adequate nutrition.

Milk and Soy Protein Intolerance

Formula protein (cow's milk and/or soy protein) intolerance is caused by sensitization to dietary proteins that are absorbed intact through the intestinal mucosa. Two syndromes are most commonly seen: an *enterocolitis,* with inflammatory changes in the small bowel and colon, usually manifesting with bloody diarrhea in the first 3 months of life, and a less common *protein-losing enteropathy,* associated with diarrhea, occult intestinal blood loss, and hypoproteinemia, most often seen in infants older than 6 months.

The diagnosis of formula protein intolerance is based on exclusion of infectious causes and response to withdrawal and later repeated challenge with the suspected antigen. Skin and radio-immunosorbent test results are usually negative. This is a non–immunoglobulin E–mediated illness. There is a significant cross-reactivity between cow's milk and soy protein allergy (20% to 40%); therefore, use of a protein-hydrolysate formula is indicated.

CHRONIC DIARRHEA IN TODDLERS

Chronic Nonspecific Diarrhea

Chronic nonspecific diarrhea, also known as "toddler's diarrhea," typically affects children between 1 and 3 years of age and is characterized by the passage of several watery and unformed stools each day. Frequently, the stools are relatively well formed in the morning but become looser as the day progresses. The stools often appear to contain undigested vegetable matter but are without blood, mucus, or excessive fat. Children with chronic nonspecific diarrhea, if offered a normal diet, continue normal weight gain. In an attempt to treat the diarrhea, however, many children are placed on diets with restrictions of milk, other fats, and occasionally starches (wheat); such restrictions lead to failure to thrive.

The pathophysiology of chronic nonspecific diarrhea may involve abnormal intestinal motility with decreased mouth-to-anus transit time. This disorder is thought to be a variant of irritable bowel syndrome (IBS), and it is common with such patients to find a family history of IBS. Excessive fruit juice intake, which is common among affected children, may also contribute to the diarrhea by overwhelming the carbohydrate absorptive capacity of the gut. Because chronic nonspecific diarrhea is a benign and self-limited condition, usually resolving by age 3 to 4 years, drug therapy is neither indicated nor effective. Parents should be encouraged to place the child on a regular, unrestricted diet to provide adequate calories. The diarrhea often improves with removal of prior dietary restrictions and limitations in fruit juice intake.

FAT MALABSORPTION CAUSED BY PANCREATIC INSUFFICIENCY

Fat malabsorption must be suspected in any infant with chronic diarrhea and failure to thrive (see Chapters 2 and 13). Cystic fibrosis is the most common cause of fat malabsorption resulting from exocrine pancreatic deficiency in children. The diagnosis is often made through neonatal screening in most of the United States. Rare forms of exocrine pancreatic insufficiency include Shwachman-Diamond syndrome (see Table 15-14).

CELIAC DISEASE

Celiac disease (celiac sprue, gluten-sensitive enteropathy) is defined as a disease of the proximal small intestine, characterized by an abnormal small intestinal mucosa, and is caused by a permanent intolerance to gluten. If untreated, it results in a lifelong inflammation of the small intestine in genetically susceptible individuals. Complete avoidance of gluten from the diet leads to disappearance of clinical symptoms and restoration of the small intestinal mucosa to normal.

Table 15-13. Foodborne Gastrointestinal Illnesses

Cause	Incubation Period	Clinical Clues	Common Vehicle	Diagnosis
Monosodium glutamate	Minutes to 2 hours	Chinese restaurant syndrome Burning in abdomen, neck, chest, extremities Lightheadedness, chest pain	Chinese food	Large amount of monosodium glutamate found in incriminated food
Heavy metals (copper, zinc, cadmium, tin)	Minutes to 2 hours	Metallic taste, diarrhea Vomiting prominent No fever	Carbonated or acidic beverages in metal containers	Chemical study of incriminated beverage
Mushroom toxin*	Minutes to 2 hours	Altered mental status with visual disturbance (encephalopathy) Hepatitis	Noncommercially obtained mushrooms	Identify mushroom and/or toxic chemical (e.g., muscarine, psilocybin)
Fish/shellfish* Scombrotoxin	Minutes to 2 hours	Histamine reaction: flushing, headache, dizziness, burning of throat and mouth	Tuna, mackerel, bonito, skipjack, mahi-mahi	
Paralytic shellfish toxin	Minutes to 2 hours	Paresthesias, dizziness Sometimes paralysis "Red tide" in incriminated water	Mussels, clams, oysters, scallops	Identify fish and/or chemical toxin (ciguatoxin, tetrodotoxin, histamine, etc.)
Puffer fish toxin	Minutes to 2 hours	Paresthesias	Puffer fish	
Ciguatoxin	2-24 hours	Paresthesias, cramps Itching, arthralgias, metallic taste, visual disturbances "Loose" painful teeth	Barracuda, red snapper, grouper, amberjack, mackerel	
Norwalk virus	24-48 hours	Epidemic watery diarrhea	Clams, oysters	Radioimmunoassay
Staphylococcus aureus†	2-8 hours	Prominent vomiting No fever Duration less than 24 hours	Ham, poultry, pastries (cream-filled), mixed salads, egg salad	Isolate 10⁵ organisms from food Preformed toxin
Bacillus cereus Emetic form: short incubation	2-8 hours	Prominent vomiting No fever Duration less than 48 hours	Fried rice Macaroni/cheese	Isolate 10⁵ organisms from food Preformed toxin
Diarrhea form: long incubation	8-14 hours	Abdominal cramps Severe diarrhea No fever Duration less than 48 hours	Fried rice, vegetables Macaroni/cheese	Isolate 10⁵ organisms from food and/or stool In vivo toxin production
Clostridium perfringens†	8-14 hours	Abdominal cramps Severe diarrhea No fever Duration less than 48 hours	Meat, poultry, gravy	Isolate 10⁵ organisms from food and/or stool In vivo toxin production
Enterotoxigenic *Escherichia coli*	12 hours to several days	Abdominal cramps, watery diarrhea May be prolonged (up to 1 week)	Incomplete data (rarely reported)	Isolate organism and test for enterotoxin production
Vibrio cholerae	12 hours to days	Abdominal cramps, watery diarrhea May be prolonged (up to 1 week)	Incomplete data (very rare in United States)	Isolate organism in stool and/or food
Invasive *E. coli*	12 hours to days	Prolonged febrile diarrhea and/or dysentery	Incomplete data	Isolate organism in stool and test for enteroinvasiveness
Shigella species	12 hours to days	Prolonged febrile diarrhea and/or dysentery	Fish, mixed salads	Stool culture (or food culture)
Vibrio parahaemolyticus	12 hours to days	Prolonged febrile diarrhea and/or dysentery	Seafood	Stool culture (or food culture)
Campylobacter species	12 hours to days	Prolonged febrile diarrhea and/or dysentery	Unpasteurized milk Poultry, meat	Stool culture (or food culture)
Clostridium botulinum†	12 hours to days	Diarrhea, constipation Cranial nerve palsies, paralysis, respiratory failure	Home-canned foods, fish, honey	Botulinum toxin in food, stool, and serum
Yersinia enterocolitica	Uncertain	Prolonged diarrhea and/or dysentery	Milk, pig intestine	Stool culture

Adapted from Reilly BM; Practical Strategies in Outpatient Medicine, 2nd ed. Philadelphia, WB Saunders, 1991, p 888.

*Potentially dangerous; observation in hospital often required.

†*Salmonella* species (23%), *S. aureus* (18%), *C. perfringens* (8%), and *C. botulinum* (8%) are the most common causes of food poisoning.

Table 15-14. Causes of Chronic Diarrhea

Intraluminal Factors	Mucosal Factors
Pancreatic Disorders	**Altered Integrity**
Cystic fibrosis	Infections: bacterial, viral,
Shwachman-Diamond	fungal
syndrome	Infestations: parasitic
Johannson-Blizzard	Cow's milk and soy protein
syndrome	intolerance
Isolated pancreatic enzyme	Inflammatory bowel disease
deficiencies	(ulcerative colitis,
Chronic pancreatitis	microscopic colitis, Crohn
Pearson syndrome	disease)
Bile Acid Disorders	**Altered Immune Function**
Chronic cholestasis	Autoimmune enteropathy
Terminal ileum resection	Eosinophilic
Bacterial overgrowth	gastroenteropathy
Chronic use of bile acid	AIDS
sequestrants	Combined
Primary bile acid	immunodeficiency
malabsorption	Immunoglobulins A and
	G deficiencies
Intestinal Disorders	**Altered Function**
Intraluminal osmolarity	Defects in Cl^-/HCO_3,
Carbohydrate	Na^+/H^+, bile acids, acro-
malabsorption	dermatitis enteropathica,
Congenital and acquired	selective folate deficiency,
sucrase, lactase	abetalipoproteinemia
deficiencies	
Congenital and acquired	**Altered Digestive Function**
monosaccharide	Enterokinase deficiency
deficiency	Glucoamylase deficiency
Excessive carbonated fluid	**Altered Surface Area**
intake	Celiac disease, post-
Excessive intake of	gastroenteritis syndrome
sorbitol, $Mg(OH)_2$, and	Microvillus inclusion
lactulose	disease
	Short bowel syndrome
	Altered Secretory
	Function
	Enterotoxin-producing
	bacteria
	Tumors secreting vasoactive
	peptides
	Altered Anatomic
	Structures
	Hirschsprung disease
	Partial small bowel
	obstruction
	Malrotation

From Ghishan FK: Chronic diarrhea. In Behrman RE, Kliegman RM; Janson HB (eds): Nelson Textbook of Pediatrics, 16th ed. Philadelphia, WB Saunders, 2000, p 1173.

AIDS; acquired immunodeficiency syndrome.

Table 15-15. Causes of Protracted Diarrhea

Idiopathic

Disorders of Intestinal Epithelial Structure or Function
Congenital microvillus atrophy
Tufting enteropathy
Congenital transport defects
   Congenital glucose-galactose malabsorption
   Congenital chloride diarrhea
   Congenital sodium diarrhea
   Primary bile salt malabsorption
Hormonally mediated secretory diarrhea
Mitochondrial disease

Infectious, Inflammatory, and Immunologically Based Disorders
Infection
Cow's milk– and soy protein–sensitive enteropathy
Celiac disease
Immunodeficiency
   X-linked agammaglobulinemia
   T cell and combined T and C cell immunodeficiencies
   Human immunodeficiency virus infection
   Miscellaneous immunodeficiencies associated with
      protracted diarrhea
Autoimmune enteropathy

Miscellaneous Disorders
Hirschsprung disease

From Wyllie R, Hyams JS (eds): Pediatric Gastrointestinal Disease, 2nd ed. Philadelphia, WB Saunders, 1999, p 288.

Pathogenesis

Celiac disease is an autoimmune enteropathy resulting from an inappropriate T cell–mediated immune response against the gliadin fraction of wheat gluten and against similar proteins in rye and barley that are responsible for the intestinal damage. The toxicity of oats has been questioned because both in vivo challenges and in vitro immunologic studies suggest that oats can be safely ingested. Rice and corn are nontoxic. The disease is associated with human leukocyte antigen (HLA) alleles DQA10501 or DQB10201. The typical intestinal damage is characterized by loss of absorptive villi (flattening) and hyperplasia of the crypts, which result in malabsorption.

Clinical Manifestation

Children frequently present with diarrhea, malabsorption and steatorrhea, failure to thrive, vomiting, poor appetite, muscle wasting, signs of hypoproteinemia (including edema and ascites), and general irritability. Adult manifestations include anemia, infertility, and osteoporosis. A wide range of vague abdominal symptoms is also possible. Children may present with associated conditions such as insulin-dependent diabetes mellitus, in which 6% to 8% of patients have concomitant celiac disease. Other conditions include cerebral calcification and thyroid disease. Celiac disease should also be considered in children with unexplained folic acid, iron, and vitamin B_{12} deficiencies; hypoalbuminemia; and osteopenia.

Diagnosis

The mainstay of diagnosis is an endoscopic intestinal biopsy demonstrating damage to the normal villous structure with a decreased ratio of villous height to crypt depth and increased lymphocytic infiltration of the mucosa. Serologic tests are very useful for screening

Epidemiology

Celiac disease was once thought to be a disease of childhood; manifestation in adults is increasingly recognized. The prevalence varies between 1:152 to 1:300 in Ireland, the United Kingdom, Italy, and Sweden. The prevalence in the United States is approximately 1:250.

Table 15-16. Specific Defects of Digestive-Absorptive Function Occurring in Children

Disease	
Intestinal	
Fat	Abetalipoproteinemia
Protein	Enterokinase deficiency
	Amino acid transport defects (cystinuria, Hartnup disease, methionine malabsorption, blue diaper syndrome)
Carbohydrate	Disaccharidase deficiencies (congenital: sucrase-isomaltase, lactase; developmental; lactase, acquired)
	Glucose: galactose malabsorption (congenital, acquired)
Vitamin	Vitamin B_{12} malabsorption (juvenile pernicious anemia, transcobalamin II deficiency, Immerslund syndrome)
Ions, trace elements	Chloride-losing diarrhea
	Congenital sodium diarrhea
	Acrodermatitis enteropathica (zinc deficiency)
	Menkes syndrome (copper malabsorption)
	Vitamin D–dependent rickets
	Primary hypomagnesemia
Drug-induced	Sulfasalazine (folic acid malabsorption)
	Cholestyramine (calcium, fat malabsorption)
	Phenytoin (Dilantin) (calcium malabsorption)
Pancreatic	Specific enzyme deficiencies
	Lipase
	Trypsinogen

From Behrman RE (ed): Nelson Textbook of Pediatrics, 14th ed. Philadelphia, WB Saunders, 1992, p 974.

Table 15-17. Diagnostic Studies in the Evaluation of Maldigestion and Malabsorption

Initial Studies

Stool examination for blood, leukocytes, reducing substances, and *Clostridium difficile* toxin; stool examination for ova and parasites and cultures for infectious bacterial pathogens
Complete blood count
Serum electrolytes, blood urea nitrogen, creatinine, calcium, phosphorus, albumin, total protein
Urinalysis and culture

Second-Phase Studies

Sweat chloride test
Breath analysis
D-Xylose test
Serum carotene, folate, B_{12}, and iron levels
Fecal α_1-antitrypsin level
Fecal fat studies or coefficient of fat absorption studies
Fatty test meal, Lundh test meal

Third-Phase Studies

Fat-soluble vitamin levels: A, 25-hydroxy D, and E
Contrast radiographic studies: upper gastrointestinal series or barium enema
Small intestinal biopsy for histology and mucosal enzyme determination
Bentiromide excretion test

Specialized Studies

Schilling test
Serum/urine bile acid determination
Endoscopic retrograde pancreatography
Provocative pancreatic secretion testing

From Wyllie R, Hyams JS (eds): Pediatric Gastrointestinal Disease, 2nd ed. Philadelphia, WB Saunders, 1999, p 283.

patients who have nonspecific symptoms or an associated condition. Measurement of immunoglobulin A (IgA) antiendomysial antibodies is the best serologic test for celiac disease, with a sensitivity of 97% to 100% and a specificity of 98% to 99%. Because 2% to 3% of individuals with celiac disease have selective IgA deficiency, IgA levels should also be measured. Measurement of antigliadin is not the best approach, because the specificity and sensitivity are low in comparison with those of antiendomysial antibody. The enzyme tissue glutaminase is the antigen for the antiendomysial antibody. The tissue glutaminase assay is a promising new test, but the usefulness of this serologic test has not been well validated in children.

Treatment

The cornerstone of treatment is a lifelong gluten-free diet. Patients should omit wheat, rye, and barley from their diet. Oats may be permitted, although the majority of commercially available oat flour is contaminated with wheat gluten. Although increased risk of small bowel lymphoma had been reported in celiac disease, this has been doubted. It is advisable for patients and families to join a celiac disease group that publishes lists of locally available gluten-free products.

CHRONIC DIARRHEA IN OLDER CHILDREN AND ADOLESCENTS

Irritable Bowel Syndrome

Patients with IBS usually present with a constellation of symptoms, including abdominal pain and changes in bowel habits. Patients report alternating bouts of diarrhea and constipation, with one symptom predominant during one episode. Abdominal distention and a sense of incomplete evacuation are also common. The diagnosis of IBS is based on the presence of a number of subjective clinical symptoms. A thorough history, including a positive family history, history of infantile colic, and psychologic factors as possible inciting events, should be explored. The physical examination findings in most patients with IBS are normal. No laboratory tests are diagnostic for IBS, but several routine laboratory studies are used as a general screen to aid in the exclusion of other diseases.

Inflammatory Bowel Disease

IBD comprises two principal categories: Crohn disease and ulcerative colitis. Crohn disease is a transmural, usually patchy inflammation that may affect any part of the gastrointestinal tract from the mouth to the anus. Its most common distributions are the small bowel alone, the colon alone, and both large and small bowel simultaneously. Ulcerative colitis is a diffuse mucosal inflammation limited to the colon; it invariably affects the rectum and may extend proximally in a symmetric, uninterrupted pattern to involve part or all of the large intestine.

Epidemiology. The incidence of Crohn disease and, to a lesser extent, that of ulcerative colitis have been rising since the early 1960s. The incidence of IBD is variable in different countries. In Scandinavia, the incidence of Crohn disease in children is 5.3 per 100,000. The incidence of ulcerative colitis in persons younger than

Table 15-18. Tests for Malabsorption

Test	Normal Values	Comments Relevant to Patients with Malabsorption
Screening Tests		
Serum carotene	>0.06 mg/dL	Decreased, very good test if poor oral intake has been excluded
Serum calcium	9.0-10.5 mg/dL	Decreased, not very sensitive
Serum cholesterol	150-250 mg/dL	Decreased, not very sensitive
Serum albumin	4.0-5.2 mg/dL	Decreased, not very sensitive
Serum magnesium	1.7-2.0 mEq/L	Decreased, not very sensitive
Prothrombin time	Control value	Increased, not very sensitive
Qualitative stool fat	No fat globules per hpf	Numerous fat globules per hpf; part 1 for neutral fats, part 2 for split fats
Specific Tests		
Serum iron	80-150 µg/dL	Malabsorbed in proximal small-bowel disease
Serum folate	5-21 ng/mL	Decreased in proximal small-bowel disease, may be increased in bacterial overgrowth
Serum cobalamin (vitamin B_{12})	200-900 pg/mL	Malabsorbed in distal small-bowel disease, pernicious anemia, bacterial overgrowth, chronic pancreatitis
Urinary D-xylose	>5 g/5 hr	Decreased in small-bowel disease and bacterial overgrowth, normal in pancreatic disease
Bentiromide test	Arylamine excretion >57% in 6 hr	A value of <50% is diagnostic of pancreatic insufficiency
Serum trypsin–like immunoreactivity	29-80 ng/mL	A value of <20 ng/mL is specific for pancreatic insufficiency
Secretin test	HCO_3^- concentration >80 mEq/L Volume >1.8 mL/kg/hr	Most sensitive test of pancreatic function
^{57}Cyanocobalamin urinary excretion test	>8%/ 24 hr	Decreased in pernicious anemia, chronic pancreatitis, bacterial overgrowth, ileal disease
Urine 5-HIAA	1.7-8.0 mg/24 hr	Markedly elevated in carcinoid syndrome, minimally elevated in any kind of malabsorption
Breath tests		
^{14}C-xyclose	<0.0013% of administered dose as breath $^{14}CO_2$ at 30 min	Elevated in bacterial overgrowth
Cholyl-1-^{14}C-glycine	<1% of administered dose as breath $^{14}CO_2$ at any interval over 4 hr	Elevated in bacterial overgrowth or bile acid malabsorption
Lactulose H_2	<10 ppm rise in breath H_2 over baseline at any interval for 120 min	Elevated in bacterial overgrowth; increase in fasting breath H_2 suggests bacterial overgrowth; up to 27% of patients may not have flora that produces H_2
Lactose H_2	<20-ppm rise in breath H_2 over baseline at any interval for 180 min	Elevated in lactase deficiency
Small intestinal culture	≤10^5organisms per mL jejunal secretions	>10^5organisms per mL jejunal secretions indicates bacterial overgrowth
Small intestinal biopsy		Morphologic study of villus atrophy; bacteriology; enzyme assays

Adapted from Toskes PP: Malabsorption. In Wyngaarden JB, Smith LH, Bennett JC (eds): Cecil Textbook of Medicine, 19th ed. Philadelphia, WB Saunders, 1992, p 691.

hpf, high-power field; 5-HIAA, 5-hydroxyindoleacetic acid; ppm, parts per million.

20 years is approximately 1.5 to 2 per 100,000 in Scotland. In England, the incidence of IBD in persons younger than 16 years is 5.2 per 100,000. IBD affects boys and girls equally.

Etiopathogenesis. The precise cause of IBD is unknown. No infectious agents have been associated with the development of IBD. The greatest known risk factor for the development of IBD is having a first-degree relative with IBD, although IBD is not inherited in a simple mendelian manner. Mutations in the *NOD2* gene on chromosome 16 have been seen in 30% of patients.

The immune system appears to play a significant role in the pathogenesis of IBD. Evidence supporting this association includes the histopathologic findings of intestinal lesions with marked mononuclear cell infiltration, the response of these diseases to immunosuppressive therapy, and multiple immunologic laboratory abnormalities. An antigen of dietary or infectious origin may stimulate the normally rich immune system of the intestinal mucosa. Activated immune cells present in the intestinal mucosa secrete a number of soluble mediators of inflammation, including cytokines. Imbalance of the cytokine milieu in the mucosa results in cell injury and pathologic inflammation. No specific immune aberration in children has been found.

Clinical Manifestation of Crohn Disease. The diagnosis of IBD is frequently delayed, especially for Crohn disease, in which symptoms can be insidious. The presenting symptoms of Crohn disease are variable, often depending on the particular sites of involvement. Common features at presentation include abdominal pain, weight loss, and diarrhea (Table 15-21). The abdominal pain tends to be particularly severe and frequently wakes the sleeping child. Fever

Table 15-19. Generalized Malabsorptive States in Childhood

Site	More Common	Less Common
Exocrine pancreas	Cystic fibrosis Chronic protein-calorie malnutrition	Shwachman-Diamond syndrome Chronic pancreatitis
Liver, biliary tree	Biliary atresia	Other cholestatic states (including Alagille syndrome, familial neonatal hepatitis)
Intestine		
Anatomic defects	Massive resection Stagnant loop syndrome	Congenitally short gut
Chronic infection	Giardiasis	Immune deficiency
Others	Celiac disease Dietary protein intolerance (cow's milk, soy)	Topical sprue Idiopathic diffuse mucosal lesions

From Ulshen M: Malabsorptive disorders. In Behrman RE, Kliegman RM, Jenson HB (eds): Nelson Textbook of Pediatrics, 16th ed. Philadelphia, WB Saunders, 2000, p 1159.

Table 15-21. Presenting Clinical Features of Crohn Disease

Feature	Percentage Affected
Abdominal pain	75
Diarrhea	65
Weight loss	65
Growth retardation	25
Nausea/vomiting	25
Perirectal disease	25
Rectal bleeding	25
Extraintestinal manifestations	25

From Wyllie R, Hyams JS (eds): Pediatric Gastrointestinal Disease, 2nd ed. Philadelphia, WB Saunders, 1999, p 406.

may be low grade and persist for extended periods before a diagnosis is made. Perirectal inflammation with fissures or tags develops in approximately 30% of affected children and may be misdiagnosed as hemorrhoids or condylomata. Extraintestinal manifestations and complications of Crohn disease are well recognized and seen in 25% to 30% of pediatric patients (Table 15-22). Failure to thrive without diarrhea or a fever of unknown origin may also occur.

Table 15-20. Symptoms and Signs of Malabsorption

History	Pathophysiology	Physical Examination	Pathophysiology
Diarrhea	Increased secretion and impaired absorption of water and electrolytes, unabsorbed dihydroxy bile acids, unabsorbed fatty acids	Pallor	Anemia secondary to iron, folate, or cobalamin deficiency
Greasy, bulky, malodorous stools that are difficult to flush	Increased fat in stool	Glossitis, stomatitis, cheilosis	Iron, folate, cobalamin, and other vitamin deficiencies
Oil seeping from rectum	Unabsorbed triglyceride (pancreatic insufficiency)	Ecchymosis, purpura	Vitamin K malabsorption
Weight loss despite good appetite	Loss of calories from malabsorption	Acrodermatitis	Zinc and fatty acid deficiency
Excessive flatus	Fermentation of unabsorbed carbohydrates by colonic bacteria	Dehydration, hypotension	Water and electrolyte malabsorption
Diffuse abdominal pain	Inflammation or infiltration of tissue (pancreatic insufficiency, Crohn disease, lymphoma)	Edema	Protein malabsorption (decreased serum albumin)
Postprandial (30 minutes after eating) midabdominal pain	Intestinal ischemia	Peripheral neuropathy	Cobalamin, thiamine, vitamins E and B_6 deficiencies
Abnormal bruisability	Vitamin K malabsorption		
Weakness and fatigue	Protein, electrolyte, fat, iron, folate, cobalamin malabsorption		
Milk intolerance	Lactase deficiency		
Bone pain	Calcium and protein malabsorption		
Tetany, paresthesias	Calcium and magnesium malabsorption, cobalamin deficiency (paresthesias only)		
Night blindness	Vitamin A malabsorption		
Nocturia	Delayed absorption of water, hypokalemia		
Amenorrhea	Protein malabsorption		

Modified from Toskes PP; Malabsorption. In Wyngaarden JB, Smith LH, Bennett JC (eds): Cecil Textbook of Medicine, 19th ed. Philadelphia, WB Saunders, 1992, p 691.

Table 15-22. Extraintestinal Complications of Inflammatory Bowel Disease

Musculoskeletal
Peripheral arthritis (colitic arthritis)
Granulomatous monoarthritis
Granulomatous synovitis
Rheumatoid arthritis
Sacroiliitis
Ankylosing spondylitis
Digital clubbing and hypertrophic osteoarthropathy
Periosteitis
Osteoporosis, osteomalacia
Rhabdomyolysis
Pelvic osteomyelitis
Relapsing polychondritis
Skin and Mucous Membranes
Oral lesions
Cheilitis
Apthous stomatitis, glossitis
Granulomatous oral Crohn disease
Inflammatory hyperplasia fissures and cobblestone mucosa
Peristomatitis vegetans
Dermatologic
Erythema nodosum
Pyoderma gangrenosum
Sweet syndrome
Metastatic Crohn disease
Psoriasis
Epidermolysis bullosa acquisita
Perianal skin tags
Polyarteritis nodosa
Ocular
Conjunctivitis
Uveitis, iritis
Episcleritis
Scleritis
Retrobulbar neuritis
Chorioretinitis with retinal detachment
Crohn keratopathy
Posterior segment abnormalities
Retinal vascular disease
Bronchopulmonary
Chronic bronchitis with bronchiectasis
Chronic bronchitis with neutrophilic infiltrates
Fibrosing alveolitis
Pulmonary vasculitis
Reduced CO_2 diffusing capacity
Small airway disease and bronchiolitis obliterans
Eosinophilic lung disease
Interstitial lung disease (sulfa-containing drugs)
Granulomatous lung disease
Tracheal obstruction
Cardiac
Pleuropericarditis
Cardiomyopathy
Endocarditis
Myocarditis
Malnutrition
Decreased intake food: IBD, dietary restriction
Malabsorption: IBD, bowel resection, bile salt depletion, bacterial overgrowth
Intestinal losses: electrolytes, minerals, nutrients
Increased caloric needs: inflammation, fever
Drug interference: corticosteroids, sulfasalazine, cholestyramine

Hematologic
Anemia: iron deficiency (blood loss)
Vitamin B_{12} (ileal disease or resection, bacterial overgrowth, folate deficiency)
Heinz body, anemia of chronic inflammation
G6PD deficiency
Anaphylactoid purpura (Crohn disease)
Hyposplenism
Autoimmune hemolytic anemia
Coagulation abnormalities
  Increased activation of coagulation factors
  Activated fibronolysis
  Anticardiolipin antibody
  Increased thrombin generation and fibrinogen monomers
  Decreases or alteration in anticlotting protein: C, S, factor V Leiden
  Increased risk of arterial and venous thrombosis with cerebrovascular stroke, myocardial infarction, peripheral arterial and venous occlusions
  Takayasu arteritis
  Wegener arteritis
Renal and Genitourinary
Metabolic: urinary crystal formation (nephrolithiasis, uric acid, oxalate)
Hypokalemic nephropathy
Inflammation: retroperitoneal abscess, fibrosis with ureteral obstruction, fistula formation
Glomerulitis
Membranonephritis
Renal amyloidosis, nephrotic syndrome
Drug nephrotoxicity: cyclosporine, sulfasalazine, aminosalicylates
Pancreatitis
Secondary to medications (sulfasalazine, 6-mercaptopurine, azathioprine, parenteral nutrition)
Ampullary Crohn disease
Granulomatous pancreatitis
Decreased pancreatic exocrine function
Sclerosing cholangitis with pancreatitis
Pancreatic autoantibodies to acinar cells
Hepatobiliary
Primary sclerosing cholangitis (PSC)
Small duct PSC (pericholangitis)
Carcinoma of the bile ducts
Fatty infiltration of the liver
Cholelithiasis
Autoimmune hepatitis
Primary bilary cirrhosis (PBC) (?)
Endocrine and Metabolic
Growth failure, delayed sexual maturation
Thyroiditis
Osteoporosis, osteomalacia
Neurologic
Peripheral neuropathy
Meningitis
Vestibular dysfunction
Pseudotumor cerebri
Undernutrition, malnutrition

From Kirsner JB: Inflammatory bowel disease, II. Clinical and therapeutic aspects. Disease-a-Month 1991;37:669.

G6PD, glucose-6-phosphate dehydrogenase; IBD; inflammatory bowel disease.

Table 15-23. Symptoms at Diagnosis of Ulcerative Colitis

Symptoms and Signs	Diagnoses 1970-1978 (*N* = 87)		Diagnoses Before 1967 (*N* = 125)	
	No. of Patients	*% of Population*	*No. of Patients*	*% of Population*
Hematochezia	84	96	107	86
Diarrhea	82	94	116	93
Abdominal pain	77	88	107	86
Anorexia	44	50	—	—
Nocturnal diarrhea	43	49	—	—
Weight loss	37	42	64	51
Fever	12	13	46	37
Vomiting	10	11	53	42

From Wyllie R, Hyams JS (eds): Pediatric Gastrointestinal Disease, 2nd ed. Philadelphia, WB Saunders, 1999, p 422.

Clinical Manifestation of Ulcerative Colitis. Diarrhea, with or without blood and often associated with tenesmus, low-grade fever, weight loss, and mild anemia, is a very common manifestation of ulcerative colitis (Table 15-23). As in Crohn disease, extraintestinal manifestations are also common (see Table 15-22).

Table 15-24. Comparison of Clinical and Pathologic Features of Crohn Disease and Ulcerative Colitis

Feature	Crohn Disease	Ulcerative Colitis
Clinical		
Smoker	++	+/–
Malaise, fever	++	+
Rectal bleeding	++	+++
Abdominal tenderness	+++	+
Abdominal mass	++	–
Abdominal pain	+++	+
Perianal disease	+++	–
Risk of cancer	+	++
Endoscopic		
Rectal disease	+	+++
Diffuse, continuous symmetric involvement	+	+++
Aphthous or linear ulcers	+++	–
Cobblestoning	++	–
Friability	++	+++
Radiologic		
Continuous disease	+	+++
Ileal involvement	++	–
Asymmetry	+++	–
Strictures	++	+
Fistulas	++	–
Pathologic		
Discontinuity	++	–
Transmural involvement	+++	+/–
Lymphoid aggregates	+++	–
Crypt abscesses	+++	+++
Granulomas	++	–
Sinus tract/fistula	+++	–

Adapted from Hanauer SB: Inflammatory bowel disease. In Wyngaarden JB, Smith LH, Bennett JC (eds): Cecil Textbook of Medicine, 19th ed. Philadelphia, WB Saunders, 1992, p 705.

+++, always; ++, common; +, occasional; –, never.

Diagnosis. The diagnosis of IBD is based on clinical, laboratory, radiologic, and endoscopic findings (Table 15-24). The differential diagnosis is noted in Tables 15-25 and 15-26. Examination of the colon should be performed early in the evaluation of any child with chronic bloody diarrhea. The findings of aphthous lesions with intervening normal appearing mucosa is highly suggestive of Crohn disease, whereas diffuse inflammation that begins at the anal verge and progresses proximally suggests ulcerative colitis. Mucosal biopsies taken to detect histopathologic abnormalities are still the most sensitive test for differentiating among Crohn disease, ulcerative colitis, and infectious colitides. Severity may be judged by the features in Table 15-27.

Treatment. Current medical and surgical treatments are directed toward controlling symptoms, treating complications, and preventing recurrent or worsening disease. The approach to therapy in Crohn disease is rapidly changing with the addition of more potent, mucosal healing properties of immunomodulator drugs and biologic agents (Table 15-28). Steroids are not considered the mainstay of therapy in IBD, but they are used in patients with active severe disease. The relapse rate after discontinuation of steroids may be as high as 70% within 1 year.

Sulfasalazine and its analogues (mesalamine) are used in mild to moderate Crohn colitis and ulcerative colitis. These agents have been shown to facilitate discontinuation of steroids and may reduce the relapse rate afterward. Despite the efficacy of salicylate preparations, many children cannot be maintained in remission without the use of steroids. Because long-term use of steroids can lead to numerous steroid-related complications, immunomodulatory agents are first-line treatment in moderate to severe Crohn disease. The two most commonly used agents are azathioprine and 6-mercaptopurine. Both appear to maintain remission while allowing reduction in steroid dosage. In addition, 6-mercaptopurine is effective in the healing of perineal fistulas. The use of cyclosporine and tacrolimus in the treatment of severe refractory disease has been disappointing. Antibiotics, particularly metronidazole, are effective in healing certain perineal lesions in Crohn disease but are not beneficial in the general management of Crohn colitis and ileocolitis.

Nutritional therapy, both as primary treatment and as adjunctive support for drug treatment, is critical for children with IBD, particularly those with Crohn disease. Weight loss occurs in 87% of children presenting with Crohn disease and is often accompanied by impaired linear growth, decreased bone mineralization, and delayed sexual maturation. Undernutrition is multifactorial, including poor intake caused by anorexia, meal-related cramping, and diarrhea, as well as malabsorption from small-bowel involvement and increased metabolic demands from the chronic inflammatory process. Nutritional support can be provided by either the enteral or

Table 15-25. Differential Diagnosis of Presenting Symptoms of Crohn Disease

Primary Presenting Symptom	Diagnostic Considerations
Right lower quadrant abdominal pain, with or without mass	Appendicitis, infection (e.g., *Campylobacter, Yersinia* species, lymphoma, intussusception, mesenteric adenitis, Meckel diverticulum, ovarian cyst
Chronic periumbilical or epigastric abdominal pain	Irritable bowel syndrome, constipation, lactose intolerance, peptic disease
Rectal bleeding, no diarrhea	Fissure, polyp, Meckel diverticulum, rectal ulcer syndrome
Bloody diarrhea	Infection, hemolytic-uremic syndrome, Henoch-Schönlein purpura, ischemic bowel, radiation colitis
Watery diarrhea	Irritable bowel syndrome, lactose intolerance, giardiasis, *Cryptosporidium* infection, sorbitol, laxatives
Perirectal disease	Fissure, hemorrhoid (rare), streptococcal infection, condyloma (rare)
Growth delay	Endocrinopathy
Anorexia, weight loss	Anorexia nervosa
Arthritis	Collagen vascular disease, infection
Liver abnormalities	Chronic hepatitis

From Hyams JS: Crohn's disease. In Wyllie R, Hyams JS (eds): Pediatric Gastrointestinal Diseases. Pathophysiology, Diagnosis, Management. Philadelphia, WB Saunders, 1993, p 754.

Table 15-26. Infectious Agents Mimicking Inflammatory Bowel Disease

Agent	Manifestations	Diagnosis	Comments
Bacterial			
Campylobacter jejuni	Acute diarrhea, fever, fecal blood and leukocytes	Culture	Common in adolescents, may relapse
Yersinia enterocolitica	Acute → chronic diarrhea, right lower quadrant pain, mesenteric adenitis—pseudoappendicitis, fecal blood and leukocytes	Culture	Common in adolescents as FUO, weight loss, abdominal pain
	Extraintestinal manifestations		Mimics Crohn disease
Clostridium difficile	Postantibiotic onset, watery diarrhea, pseudomembrane on sigmoidoscopy	Culture and cytotoxin	May be nosocomial Toxic megacolon possible
Escherichia coli 0157:H7	Colitis, fecal blood, abdominal pain	Culture and typing	Hemolytic-uremic syndrome
Salmonella species	Watery → bloody diarrhea, fecal leukocytes, cramps	Culture	Usually acute; foodborne
Shigella species	Watery → bloody diarrhea, fecal leukocytes, fever, pain, cramps	Culture	Dysentery symptoms
Edwardsiella tarda	Bloody diarrhea, cramps	Culture	Ulceration on endoscopy
Aeromonas hydrophila	Cramps, diarrhea, fecal blood	Culture	May be chronic From contaminated drinking water
Plesiomonas species	Diarrhea, cramps	Culture	Shellfish source
Tuberculosis	Rarely bovine, now *Mycobacterium tuberculosis* Ileocecal area, fistula formulation	Culture, PPD, biopsy	May mimic Crohn disease
Parasites			
Entamoeba histolytica	Acute bloody diarrhea and liver abscess, colic	Trophozoite in stool, colonic mucosal flask ulceration, serologic findings	Acquired during travel to endemic area
Giardia lamblia	Foul-smelling, watery diarrhea, cramps, flatulence, weight loss; no colonic involvement	"Owl" – like trophozoite and cysts in stool; rarely duodenal intubation	May be chronic
AIDS-Associated Enteropathy			
Cryptosporidium species	Chronic diarrhea, weight loss	Stool microscopy	Mucosal findings not like IBD
Isospora belli	As in *Cryptosporidium* infection		Tropical location
Cytomegalovirus	Colonic ulceration, pain, bloody diarrhea	Culture, biopsy	

From Behrman RE (ed): Nelson Textbook of Pediatrics, 14th ed. Philadelphia, WB Saunders, 1992, p 968.

→, progressing to; AIDS, acquired immunodeficiency syndrome; FUO, fever of unknown origin; IBD, inflammatory bowel disease; PPD, purified protein derivative.

Table 15-27. Inflammatory Bowel Disease: Severity Criteria*

	Mild	Severe	Fulminant/Toxic
Bowel frequency	<4/day	>6/day	>10/day
Blood in stool	Occasional/never	Common	Continuous
Fever	Normal	>37.5° C	>37.5° C
Pulse	Normal	>90/min	>90/min
Hemoglobin	Normal	<75% of normal	Transfusion required
Erythrocyte sedimentation rate	<30 mm/hr	>30 mm/hr	>30 mm/hr
Abdominal radiograph	Normal	Colonic edema, thumb-printing, air-fluid levels	Dilated colon or small bowel
Clinical sign		Abdominal tenderness	Rebound tenderness, distention, diminished bowel sounds

From Hanauer SB: Inflammatory bowel disease. In Wyngaarden JB, Smith LH, Bennett JC (eds): Cecil Textbook of Medicine, 19th ed. Philadelphia, WB Saunders, 1992, p 705.

*Criteria are based on adolescent and adult norms (e.g., pulse).

parenteral route; use of the patient's intestine is optimal. Even patients with severe inflammation can often tolerate an enteral liquid formula.

Surgery. Crohn disease cannot be cured by surgery because the postoperative recurrence rate at 10 years is high, up to 80%. Surgery for Crohn disease is therefore reserved for the management of certain complications of the disease, such as intestinal perforation, obstruction, bleeding, and abscess and occasionally for growth failure in the prepubertal child with a delayed bone age. In contrast, surgical resection for ulcerative colitis can be very useful in patients with severe, acute complications or persistent disease that is unresponsive to medical therapy.

Table 15-28. Medical Therapeutic Options for Treating Inflammatory Bowel Disease in Children

Anti-inflammatory Agents
Corticosteroids
   Prednisone, prednisolone, hydrocortisone
   Budesonide
5-Aminosalicylates
   Sulfasalazine
   Olsalazine
   Mesalamine
   Balsalazide

Immunomodulators
6-Mercaptopurine
Azathioprine
Cyclosporine
Tacrolimus
Methotrexate

Biologic Therapy
Infliximab

Nutritional therapy
Polymeric or elemental liquid diet
ω-3 fatty acids (fish oil)

SUMMARY AND RED FLAGS

Acute diarrhea is a common childhood illness (Fig. 15-1). For most children, the etiologic agent is of no therapeutic significance. Exceptions are giardiasis, pseudomembranous colitis, or dysentery suggestive of *Shigella* infection, amebiasis, or *Campylobacter* infection, all of which necessitate specific treatment. Of greater importance are the secondary complications associated with fluid and electrolyte losses and the reduced oral fluid intake, which may result in shock and its multiorgan system complications.

Red flags for acute diarrhea are the manifestations of dehydration (see Table 15-7). Young age (<6 months) is associated with a greater risk of dehydration, as are 10 or more stools a day and frequent emesis and fever.

Chronic diarrhea may be benign or may signify a more serious illness associated with malabsorption, inflammation, or congenital defects. Red flags include onset of diarrhea in the neonatal period, weight loss, growth stunting, digital clubbing, poor growth, anorexia, fever, fatty stools, blood in stools, extraintestinal manifestations associated with intestinal disease, history of travel to countries with poor sanitation and water supply, and specific nutritional deficiencies associated with malabsorption.

REFERENCES

General, Bacterial, Parasitic

Blake PA, Ramos S, MacDonald KL, et al: Pathogen-specific risk factors and protective factors for acute diarrheal disease in urban Brazilian infants. J Infect Dis 1993;167:627-632.

Cohen MB: E. coli 0157:H7 infections: A frequent cause of bloody diarrhea and hemolytic uremic syndrome. Adv Pediatr 1996;43:171-207.

Craven D, Brick D, Morrisey A, et al: Low yield of bacterial stool culture in children with nosocomial diarrhea. Pediatr Infect Dis J 1998;17:1040-1044.

de la Morena ML, Van R, Singh K, et al: Diarrhea associated with Aeromonas species in children in day care centers. J Infect Dis 1993;168:215-218.

Doyle MP: Foodborne illness. Pathogenic Escherichia coli, Yersinia enterocolitica and Vibrio parahaemolyticus. Lancet 1990;336:1111-1115.

Huskins WC, Griffiths JK, Faruque ASG, et al: Shigellosis in neonates and young infants. J Pediatr 1994;125:14-22.

Kader HA, Piccoli D, Jawad AF, et al: Single toxin detection is inadequate to diagnose Clostridium difficile diarrhea in pediatric patients. Gastroenterology 1998;115:1329-1334.

Lengerich EJ, Addiss DG, Juranek DD: Severe giardiasis in the United States. Clin Infect Dis 1994;18:760-763.

MacKenzie WR, Hoxie NJ, Proctor ME, et al: A massive outbreak in Milwaukee of Cryptosporidium infection transmitted through the public water supply. N Engl J Med 1994;331:161-167.

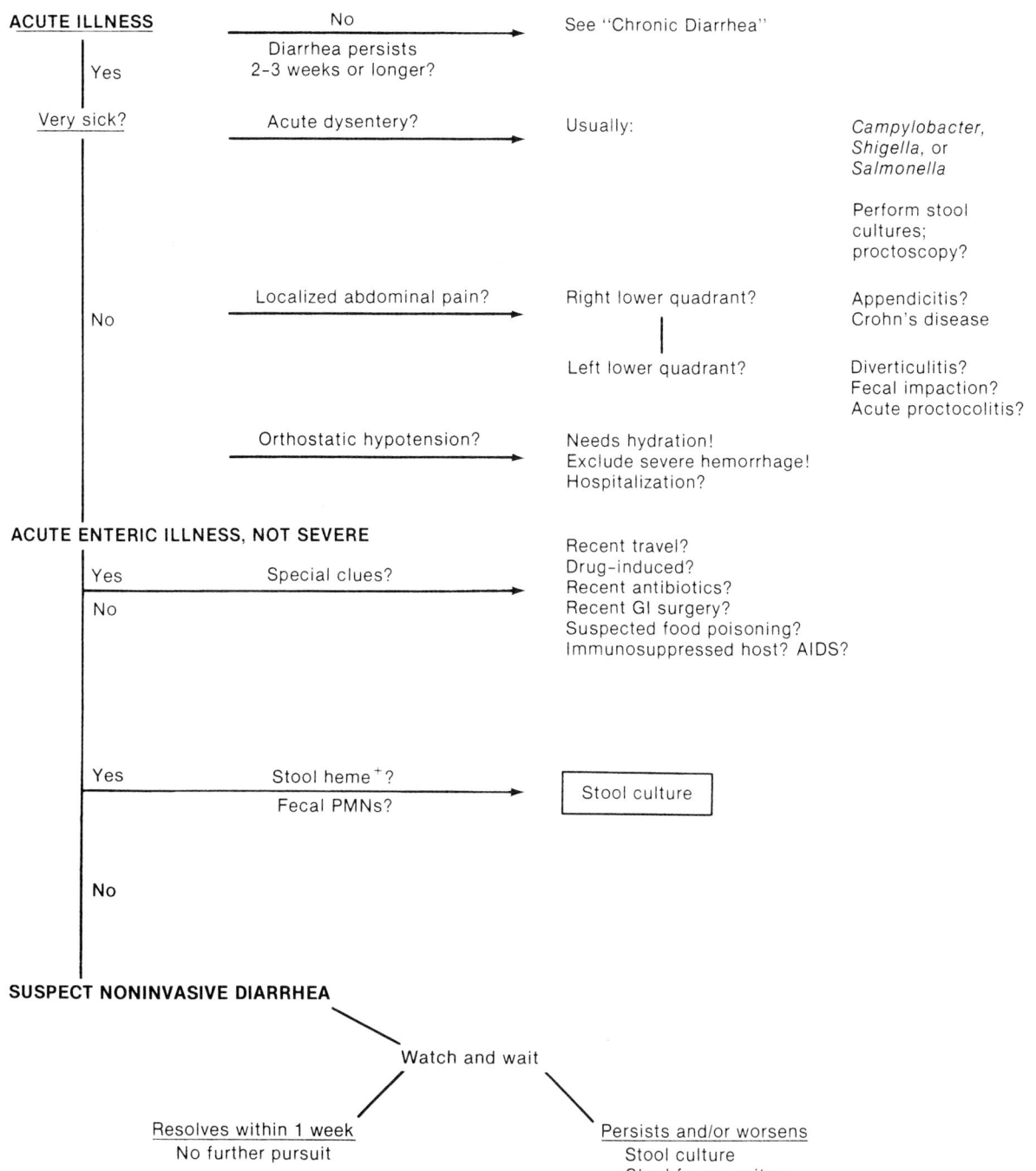

Figure 15-1. Acute diarrhea. AIDS, acquired immunodeficiency syndrome; GI, gastrointestinal; PMNs, polymorphonuclear leukocytes. (From Reilly BM: Diarrhea. In Practical Strategies in Outpatient Medicine, 2nd ed. Philadelphia, WB Saunders, 1991, p 854.)

Murphy GS, Bodhidatta L, Echeverria P, et al: Ciprofloxacin and loperamide in the treatment of bacillary dysentery. Ann Intern Med 1993;118: 582-586.

Naqvi SH, Swierkosz EM, Gerard J, et al: Presentation of *Yersinia enterocolitica* enteritis in children. Pediatr Infect Dis J 1993;12:386-389.

Pablo Caeiro J, Mathewson JJ, Smith MA, et al: Etiology of outpatient pediatric non-dysenteric diarrhea: A multicenter study in the United States. Pediatr Infect Dis J 1999;18:94-97.

Scheidler MD, Giannella RA: Practical management of acute diarrhea. Hosp Pract 2001;7:49-56.

Schiller LR: Diarrhea. Med Clin North Am 2000;84:1259-1273.

Surawicz CM, McFarland LV: Pseudomembranous colitis: Causes and cures. Digestion 1999;60:91-100.

Waites WM, Arbuthnott JP: Foodborne illness: An overview. Lancet 1990;336:722-725.

Wood RC, MacDonald KL, Osterholm MT: *Campylobacter* enteritis outbreaks associated with drinking raw milk during youth activities: A 10-year review of outbreaks in the United States. JAMA 1992;268: 3228-3230.

Wurtz R: *Cyclospora:* A newly identified intestinal pathogen of humans. Clin Infect Dis 1994;18:620-623.

Viral

Graham DY, Jiang X, Tanaka T, et al: Norwalk virus infection of volunteers: New insights based on improved assays. J Infect Dis 1994;170:34-43.

Haffejee IE: Neonatal rotavirus infections. Rev Infect Dis 1991;13: 957-962.

Kapikian AZ: Viral gastroenteritis. JAMA 1993;269:627-630.

Mitchell DK, Van R, Morrow AL, et al: Outbreaks of astrovirus gastroenteritis in day care centers. J Pediatr 1993;123:725-732.

Treatment

Armon K, Stephenson AK, MacFaul R, et al: An evidence and consensus based guideline for acute diarrhoea management. Arch Dis Child 2001;85:132-142.

Bang A: Towards better oral rehydration. Lancet 1993;342:755-756.

Burks AW, Vanderhoof JA, Mebra S, et al: Randomized clinical trial of soy formula with and without added fiber in antibiotic-induced diarrhea. J Pediatr 2001;139:578-582.

Fayad IM, Hashem M, Duggan C, et al: Comparative efficacy of rice-based and glucose-based oral rehydration salts plus early reintroduction of food. Lancet 1993;342:772-775.

Nataro JP: Treatment of bacterial enteritis. Pediatr Infect Dis 1998;17: 420-421.

Celiac Disease

Carlsson AK, Axelsson IRM, Borulf SK, et al: Serological screening for celiac disease in healthy 2.5-year-old children in Sweden. Pediatrics 2001;107:42-45.

Catassi C, Ratsch I-M, Fabiani E, et al: Coeliac disease in the year 2000: Exploring the iceberg. Lancet 1994;343:200-203.

Fasano A: Celiac disease: The past, the present, the future. Pediatrics 2001;107:768-770.

McMillan SA, Haughton DJ, Biggart JD, et al: Predictive value for coeliac disease of antibodies to gliadin, endomysium, and jejunum in patients attending for jejunal biopsy. BMJ 1991;303:1163-1165.

Rossi TM, Albini CH, Kumar V: Incidence of celiac disease identified by the presence of serum endomysial antibodies in children with chronic diarrhea, short stature, or insulin-dependent diabetes mellitus. J Pediatr 1993;123:262-264.

Inflammatory Bowel Disease

Fiocchi C: Inflammatory bowel disease: Etiology and pathogenesis. Gastroenterology 1998;115:182-205.

Greenberg GR, Feagan BG, Martin F, et al: Oral budesonide for active Crohn's disease. N Engl J Med 1994;331:836-841.

Greenberger NJ, Miner PB: Is maintenance therapy effective in Crohn's disease? Lancet 1994;344:900-901.

Hanauer SB: Medical therapy of ulcerative colitis. Lancet 1993;342:412-417.

Hyams JS, Markowitz J, Wyllie R: Use of infliximab in the treatment of Crohn's disease in children and adolescents. J Pediatr 2000;137: 192-196.

Langholz E, Munkholm P, Davidsen M, et al: Course of ulcerative colitis: Analysis of changes in disease activity over years. Gastroenterology 1994;107:3-11.

Sands BE: Biologic therapy for inflammatory bowel disease. Inflamm Bowel Dis 1997;3:95-113.

Sawczenko A, Sandhu BK, Logan RFA, et al: Prospective survey of childhood inflammatory bowel disease in the British Isles. Lancet 2001;357:1093-1094.

Chronic Diarrhea

Bisset WM, Stapleford P, Long S, et al: Home parenteral nutrition in chronic intestinal failure. Arch Dis Child 1992;67:109-114.

Drossman DA, Grant Thompson W: The irritable bowel syndrome: Review and a graduated multicomponent treatment approach. Ann Intern Med 1992;116:1009-1016.

Fell JM, Miller MP, Finkel Y, et al: Congenital sodium diarrhea with a partial defect in jejunal brush border membrane sodium transport, normal rectal transport, and resolving diarrhea. J Pediatr Gastroenterol Nutr 1992;15:112-116.

Girault D, Goulet O, Le Deist F, et al: Intractable infant diarrhea associated with phenotypic abnormalities and immunodeficiency. J Pediatr 1994;125:36-42.

Johnston KR, Govel LA, Andritz MH: Gastrointestinal effects of sorbitol as an additive in liquid medications. Am J Med 1994;97:185-191.

Orenstein SR: Enteral versus parenteral therapy for intractable diarrhea of infancy: A prospective randomized trail. J Pediatr 1986;109:277-286.

Phillips AD, Schmitz J: Familial microvillous atrophy: A clinicopathological survey of 23 cases. J Pediatr Gastroenterol Nutr 1992;14:380-396.

Smith LJ, Szymanski W, Foulston C, et al: Familial enteropathy with villous edema and immunoglobulin G2 subclass deficiency. J Pediatr 1994;125:541-548.

Treem WR: Chronic nonspecific diarrhea of childhood. Clin Pediatr 1992;31:413-420.

16 Vomiting and Regurgitation

Susan R. Orenstein   John M. Peters

Vomiting in its most ominous forms accompanies catastrophic, life-threatening disorders; in contrast, vomiting can also be a physiologic behavior in young infants. Determining the cause of vomiting in a child and treating it appropriately are thus of major importance. It is critical to remember that vomiting may be caused by gastrointestinal disease or by more systemic disturbances, including inborn errors of metabolism, intracranial pathologic processes, nongastrointestinal infection, or systemic poisoning.

PATHOPHYSIOLOGY

DEFINITIONS

Vomiting is a protective reflex that removes toxic material from the body or relieves pressure in hollow organs distended by distal obstruction. In this context, the term *vomiting* encompasses all retrograde ejection of gastrointestinal (or esophageal) contents from the mouth. Strictly speaking, however, vomiting is subdivided according to its forcefulness; thus, effortless, or nearly effortless, regurgitation is distinguished from true vomiting, which is propelled both by forceful abdominal wall contractions and by retrograde intestinal peristalsis (Table 16-1).

True vomiting is often accompanied by nausea and retching. *Nausea* is an unpleasant, vaguely epigastric or abdominal sensation accompanied by a variety of autonomic changes: decreases in gastric tone, contractions, secretion, and mucosal blood flow; increases in salivation, sweating, pupil diameter, and heart rate; and changes in respiratory rhythm. During nausea, retrograde peristalsis from the small intestine to the gastric antrum or generalized simultaneous contractions of antrum and duodenum may produce duodenogastric reflux.

Retching is defined as strong, involuntary efforts to vomit, which may be seen as preparatory maneuvers to vomiting. These efforts consist of spasmodic contractions of the diaphragm and abdominal wall at the same time that the lower esophageal sphincter relaxes. This sphincter is also pulled cephalad by contraction of the longitudinal muscles of the upper esophagus and may herniate through the diaphragmatic hiatus, preventing the increased intraabdominal pressure from augmenting the sphincter pressure. During retching, gastric material is moved into the esophagus by the combination of increased abdominal pressure and decreased intrathoracic pressure, but this material may be returned to the stomach by secondary (non-swallow) esophageal peristalsis.

Vomiting (emesis) differs from retching in that material is expelled from the mouth. This is fostered by relaxation of the diaphragm and reversal of intrathoracic pressure from negative to positive. The upper esophageal sphincter also relaxes, perhaps in response to the increase of intraluminal pressure in the esophagus.

Regurgitation is considered a form of gastroesophageal reflux and, as such, is caused predominantly by lower esophageal sphincter dysfunction. Although apparently effortless, it may be propelled by contraction of abdominal wall musculature; this propulsion perhaps

distinguishes regurgitant from nonregurgitant reflux, which remains in the esophagus.

Rumination is similar to regurgitation in its effortless appearance and its probable propulsion by somatic muscle contraction. However, ruminated material is usually reswallowed rather than ejected from the mouth, and psychological or behavioral problems are considered the cause.

NEUROANATOMY OF VOMITING

The stereotypical motor response of vomiting is mediated by efferent fibers in the vagal, phrenic, and spinal nerves. Input to these nerves rise from the brainstem "vomiting center." There is probably no single anatomic structure identifiable as the vomiting center, but the final common pathway for this centrally programmed complex reflex is through medullary interneurons in the solitary tract nucleus and a variety of sites in the nearby reticular formation. These interneurons receive input from the cortex, the vagus, the vestibular system, and the area postrema. The area postrema, the "chemoreceptive trigger zone," is located on the dorsal surface of the floor of the fourth ventricle, outside the blood-brain barrier, and has been identified as a crucial source for neural input that causes vomiting, particularly as a response to circulating drugs and toxins. Brain tumors, other central nervous system disease, and emotional stress, in contrast, cause vomiting via cortical afferent nerves, whereas intraabdominal disease, such as luminal obstruction or distention, causes vomiting via vagal afferent nerves. Vomiting may be classified by the origin of the afferent nerves (Table 16-2).

When vomiting is a result of intraabdominal disease, it is useful to define whether obstruction, dysmotility, inflammation, or ischemia is the mechanism.

DATA TO GUIDE THE DIAGNOSIS

HISTORY

Demographics

The child's age is a major determinant of the diagnostic possibilities (Table 16-3). Affected neonates present with congenital disorders and, in particular, structural abnormalities of the gastrointestinal tract or severe metabolic diseases. Sepsis is also an important neonatal consideration.

Older infants with vomiting may have less severe structural or metabolic disorders, or they may have common acquired disorders such as gastroenteritis, mild systemic infections, gastroesophageal reflux, or allergies. Some metabolic disorders first manifest in older infants when dietary changes expose them to provocative foods for the first time, and gastroenteritis and other infections are important considerations in these relatively immunocompromised younger patients.

Toddlers frequently experience gastroenteritis, because they are repeatedly exposed to organisms to which they have no immunity;

Table 16-1. Force of Vomiting

Force	Cause	Example
None	Esophageal emptying	Achalasia; some reflux
Minimal	Regurgitation	Regurgitant reflux; rumination
Moderate	Vomiting	Most vomiting diseases
Severe	Projectile vomiting with retching	Obstructions; metabolic; poisons

this age group also presents with acquired obstructive gastrointestinal disorders such as intussusception or volvulus or with vomiting caused by ingested poisons.

Throughout childhood and adolescence, a wide variety of acquired disorders become symptomatic, and some subtle congenital malformations may also first become evident at these older ages. Metabolic disorders continue to be an important but infrequent cause of recurrent vomiting throughout childhood. In adolescents, pregnancy, drug ingestion, and eating disorders are added to the diagnostic considerations.

Characteristics of the Vomiting

The contents (Table 16-4) and forcefulness (see Table 16-1) of the vomitus narrow the diagnostic possibilities. Hematemesis and bilious vomiting, in particular, are approached in a manner very different from that of vomiting without these characteristics, and they represent more serious underlying disorders.

Associated Symptoms

Vomiting must be characterized as acute, chronic, or recurrent. Temporal associations of chronic or recurrent vomiting are important (Table 16-5). Associated symptoms must be described (Table 16-6); they are crucial, for example, in distinguishing life-threatening intracranial and metabolic disorders (Table 16-7). Abdominal pain is a central symptom that, if present, narrows the diagnosis. Vomiting associated with neurologic symptoms requires very careful evaluation. Post-tussive emesis is not usually confused with vomiting of other causes; it should direct diagnostic attention to the cause of the cough itself (see Chapter 2). Regurgitation in an infant with apnea may signal reflux-associated apnea, although many infants with reflux-associated apnea have minimal regurgitation (see Chapter 6) Additionally, infant regurgitation is so common that it is quite nonspecific.

Table 16-2. Differential Diagnosis of Vomiting by Anatomic Locus of Stimulus

I. **Stimulation of Supramedullary Receptors**
   A. Psychogenic vomiting
   B. Increased intracerebral pressure (subdural effusion or hematoma, cerebral edema or tumor, hydrocephalus, meningoencephalitis, Reye's syndrome)
   C. Vascular (migraine, severe hypertension)
   D. Seizures
   E. Vestibular disease, "motion sickness"

II. **Stimulation of Chemoreceptive Trigger Zone**
   A. Drugs: opiates, ipecac, digoxin, anticonvulsants
   B. Toxins
   C. Metabolic products (acidemia, ketonemia, hyperammonemia, uremia, etc.):
      Acidemia, ketonemia (diabetic ketoacidosis, lactic acidosis, phenylketonuria, renal tubular acidosis)
      Aminoacidemia (tyrosinemia, hypervalinemia, hyperglycinemia, lysinuria, maple syrup urine disease)
      Organic acidemia (methylmalonic acidemia, propionic acidemia, isovaleric acidemia)
      Hyperammonemia (Reye's syndrome, urea cycle defects)
      Uremia (renal failure)
      Other (hereditary fructose intolerance, galactosemia, fatty acid oxidation disorders, diabetes insipidus, adrenal insufficiency, hypercalcemia, hypervitaminosis A)

III. **Stimulation of Peripheral Receptors and/or Obstruction of the Gastrointestinal Tract**
   A. Pharyngeal: gag reflex (sinusitis secretions, post-tussive, self-induced, rumination)
   B. Esophageal:
      Functional: reflux, achalasia, other esophageal dysmotility
      Structural: stricture, ring, atresia, etc.
   C. Gastric:
      Peptic ulcer disease (including Zollinger-Ellison syndrome), infection, dysmotility/gastroparesis
      Obstruction (e.g., bezoar, pyloric stenosis, web, chronic granulomatous disease, eosinophilic gastroenteritis)
   D. Intestinal:
      Infection, enteritis, enterotoxin, appendicitis
      Dysmotility (e.g., metabolic or diabetic neuropathy; intestinal pseudoobstruction)
      Nutrient intolerance (e.g., cow's milk, soy, gluten, eosinophilic enteropathy)
      Obstruction (e.g., atresia, web, stenosis, adhesions, bands, volvulus, intussusception, superior mesenteric artery syndrome, duplication, meconium plug, meconium ileus, Hirschsprung disease, distal intestinal obstruction syndrome in cystic fibrosis)
   E. Hepatobiliary, pancreatic: hepatitis, cholecystitis, pancreatitis, cholelithiasis
   F. Cardiac: intestinal ischemia
   G. Renal: pyelonephritis, hydronephrosis, renal calculi, glomerulonephritis
   H. Respiratory: pneumonia, otitis, pharyngitis, sinusitis, common cold
   I. Miscellaneous: peritonitis, sepsis, pregnancy; improper feeding techniques

Modified from Orenstein SR: Dysphagia and vomiting. In Wyllie R, Hyams JS (eds): Pediatric Gastrointestinal Disease: Pathophysiology, Diagnosis, Management. Philadelphia, WB Saunders, 1983, p 147.

Table 16-3. Differential Diagnosis of Vomiting by Age

I. Newborn
  A. Congenital obstructive gastrointestinal malformations:
    Atresias or webs of esophagus or intestine
    Meconium ileus or plug; Hirschsprung disease
  B. Inborn errors of metabolism:
    Organic acidemias, amino acidemias,
      hyperammonemias (urea cycle), adrenogenital
      syndromes
II. Infant
  A. Acquired or milder obstructive lesions:
    Pyloric stenosis, malrotation and volvulus,
      intussusception
  B. Metabolic diseases, inborn errors of metabolism
  C. Nutrient intolerances
  D. Functional disorders:
    Gastroesophageal reflux
  E. Psychosocial disorders:
    Rumination, injury from child abuse
III. Child
  Most causes in Table 16-6
IV. Adolescent
  Most childhood causes, plus pregnancy, drugs (of abuse,
    suicide), eating disorders

Modified from Orenstein SR: Dysphagia and vomiting. In Wyllie R, Hyams JS (eds): Pediatric Gastrointestinal Disease: Pathophysiology, Diagnosis, Management. Philadelphia, WB Saunders, 1993, p 147.

Medical, Family, and Social History

Previous surgery, hospitalizations, and medications may provide important clues. A family history of fetal or neonatal deaths suggests a genetic or metabolic cause; similar illness in family members or other contacts may suggest infections or common toxic exposures. Psychosocial stressors may be found in adolescents with bulimia, peptic ulcer disease, or intentional self-poisonings.

PHYSICAL EXAMINATION

Although vomiting is a "gastrointestinal" symptom, it can be a manifestation of disease in multiple systems of the body. A complete physical examination is thus critical. Vital signs identify fever, which is important in narrowing the differential diagnosis, and shock (tachycardia, hypotension), which is important in determining the urgency of evaluation. Kussmaul breathing (deep, slow respirations with a prolonged expiratory phase) represents respiratory compensation for metabolic acidosis. It is an important clue in vomiting illness

because acidosis is seen only with vomiting from metabolic causes or poisoning or with vomiting associated with marked diarrhea or shock. Examination of the fundi is often inappropriately neglected. The absence of venous pulsations or sharp optic disk margins may be the only evidence of a brain tumor or other intracranial lesion causing vomiting.

Abdominal Examination

Simple observation of scars may suggest the possibility of obstruction from adhesions, and visible distention may represent ascites caused by liver disease or intraluminal distention caused by intestinal obstruction or ileus. The order of the examination is important because auscultation performed after stimulation of intestinal motility by palpation may artifactually change the auscultatory findings. An important distinction in the vomiting child is whether bowel sounds are increased, as in gastroenteritis or in bowel obstructions, or absent, as in ileus caused by peritonitis or in pseudoobstruction. Increased bowel sounds resulting from luminal obstruction are often characterized by intermittent "rushes" of high-pitched sounds that are coordinated with episodes of colicky pain.

Abdominal pain and tenderness associated with vomiting often represent disorders necessitating surgery (see Chapter 14). Vague periumbilical pain is quite nonspecific, but the localized, very sharp pain signifying inflammation of the peritoneum requires immediate attention. Initial luminal obstruction may progress to later ileus as peritonitis intervenes. Localization of nonperiumbilical pain or tenderness helps a great deal in determining the diseased intra-abdominal organ (see Table 16-6).

Abdominal pain often represents luminal obstruction, ischemia, or perforation (surgical disease), but nonsurgical diseases must also be considered (see Chapter 14). These disorders include nonobstructive inflammatory diseases (infectious gastroenteritis, pancreatitis), metabolic crises (e.g., adrenal crisis), and poisonings (e.g., lead, narcotics, insecticides).

Rectal Examination

A rectal examination should be performed in the vomiting child. This examination is, however, often inappropriately neglected in children.

Preparation of the child depends on the age, but all verbal children benefit from a description of the examination. Even preschool children can usually be examined without discomfort if they are properly prepared. The physician should ascertain whether they have ever had a rectal examination. Even if they have had one that hurt them, they can be reassured and examined atraumatically. For young children, the description can be something like this: "I will put this glove on my hand and some of this goo on my finger, and then I will put my finger in your bottom, where your poops come

Table 16-4. Contents of Emesis

Material	Source	Examples
Undigested food	Esophageal	Stricture, achalasia
Digested food: curds	Gastroduodenal	Pyloric stenosis, bezoar
Bile: green/yellow	Postampullary	Small bowel obstruction
Blood: red/brown	Lesion above ligament of Treitz	See Tables 16-11 and 16-12
Feculent: malodorous	Bacterial overgrowth	Stasis syndrome
	Colon	Gastrocolic fistula
	Necrotic bowel	Ischemic injury, peritonitis
Acid: clear (voluminous)	Gastric outlet obstruction	Pyloric stenosis
	Increased gastric secretion	Zollinger-Ellison syndrome
Mucus	Gastric, respiratory mucus	Sinusitis, eosinophilic esophagitis

Table16-5. Temporal Associations of Chronic or Recurrent Vomiting

Temporal Associations	Diagnosis	Other Clues
Time of day: early morning	Increased intracranial pressure	Headache, papilledema
	Sinusitis with postnasal mucus	Sinus tenderness
	Pregnancy	Secondary amenorrhea
	Uremia	
During or after meals		
Any meals	Peptic ulcer disease, reflux	Epigastric pain, heartburn
Specific foods		See Tables 16-7, 16-13, 16-14
Fructose	Hereditary fructose intolerance	
Galactose	Galactosemia	
High protein	Metabolic inborn error	Hyperammonemia, acidosis
Specific protein		
Cow, soy	Cow's or soy milk intolerance	
Gluten	Gluten-sensitive enteropathy (celiac)	Failure to thrive
Various (especially egg, wheat, fish, nut, chocolate, strawberry)	Miscellaneous allergic, eosinophilic gastroenteropathies	History of asthma, hives, ↑ eosinophils, family history of allergies
After fasting		
Food vomited	Gastric stasis/obstruction	Distention, tympany
Food not vomited	Metabolic disease	See Tables 16-7, 16-13, 16-14
Other precipitants		
Cough	Post-tussive	Respiratory disease
Infections	Metabolic	See Tables 16-7, 16-13, 16-14
	Recurrent gastroenteritis	
Vestibular stimulation	Motion sickness	Nystagmus
	Ménétrier's disease	Vertigo
Hyperhydration	Ureteropelvic junction obstruction ("beer-drinker's kidney," Dietl crisis)	Spontaneous resolution with normal hydration
Menses	Dysmenorrhea-associated vomiting	Relief with NSAIDs
	Acute intermittent porphyria	Nonperitonitis pain, distention, tachycardia, constipation
	Pelvic inflammatory disease	Vaginal discharge
Medications, toxins	Medication side effect: pancreatitis, hepatitis	Opiate withdrawal
	Acute intermittent porphyria	
	Steroid withdrawal: Addison disease	
	Poisonings; NSAID stricture; laxative, etc.	
	Ipecac abuse in anorexia nervosa	
Episodic/cyclic	Abdominal migraine, abdominal epilepsy	
	Pheochromocytoma	
	Porphyria	
	Familial dysautonomia	
	Metabolic inborn error	
	Familial Mediterranean fever	
	Malrotation and intermittent volvulus	
	Intermittent intussusception	
	Self-induced	
	Cyclic vomiting	

NSAIDs, nonsteroidal antiinflammatory drugs.

from. It doesn't hurt. The only time it would hurt is if you get scared and squeeze your muscles back there, so if you feel that happening, you just say 'stop,' and I will stop right away. When your muscles get soft again, you can say 'go,' and we'll go further. You're in charge." Children between about 12 and 24 months of age generally object to the examination in any case; with these patients, the examiner can briefly describe it and proceed gently but firmly. Examination is easiest in infants, and adolescents respond much as adults if their sensitivity and privacy are respected.

The rectal examination is simpler to perform with the patient recumbent. The patient is placed with his or her head toward the examiner's left; most children are examined lying on their left side, but it may be easiest to examine the infant prone or supine. Children older than 2 years are appropriately draped. Before starting, it is important to get the child's hips and knees flexed maximally, thus preventing gluteal contraction from interfering with the examination. The buttocks are spread, and the anus is carefully observed for presence and patency in the newborn and for tags or fistulas that suggest inflammatory bowel disease in the older child. The lubricated finger is inserted with gentle, persistent pressure into the anus. (The index finger is the most sensitive and may be used by many examiners in most children; the examiner can mentally compare the size of the finger to the usual diameter of the child's stools.)

A common mistake is to hurry the examination, thus causing spasm of the external anal sphincter and associated discomfort. The child's trust that the examiner will stop when he or she says "stop"

Table 16-6. Clues to the Diagnosis and Localization of the Cause of Emesis

Associated Symptoms	Diagnoses to Consider
Local abdominal pain	See Chapter 14
Epigastric	Peptic ulcer disease, reflux, pancreatitis
Periumbilical	Nonspecific or small intestinal obstruction
Pelvic	Cystitis, pelvic inflammatory disease, ovarian torsion
Right upper quadrant	Hepatitis, pancreatitis, cholecystitis, biliary colic, duodenal hematoma/ulcer, right pyelonephritis, pneumonia
Left upper quadrant	Peptic ulcer disease, pancreatitis, splenic torsion, left pyelonephritis, pneumonia
Right lower quadrant	Appendicitis, right tuboovarian disease
Left lower quadrant	Left tuboovarian disease, sigmoid disease
Right flank	UPJ/renal obstruction or infection, biliary obstruction, adrenal hemorrhage
Left flank	UPJ/renal obstruction or infection, adrenal hemorrhage
Other pain	
Headache	Increased intracranial pressure
	Sinusitis with postnasal mucus
	Migraine
Chest pain, dysphagia	Esophagitis, achalasia
	Pneumonia
Joint pain	SLE, FMF, IBD
Diarrhea	Partial intestinal obstruction
	Infectious enteritis
	Poison, inborn error of metabolism
Constipation	Intestinal obstruction or dysmotility (pseudoobstruction)
	Hypercalcemia, hypokalemia, porphyria, lead poisoning
Jaundice	Hepatitis, cholecystitis
	Hepatobiliary obstruction
	Metabolic disease
	Urinary obstruction or infection, pyloric stenosis (neonate)
Neurologic	Metabolic, toxic (lead), central nervous system disease, porphyria, hepatic failure
Vertigo	
Visual changes	
Abnormal tone, seizure	
Full fontanelle	
Cardiac	
Valvular disease	Mesenteric arterial thrombosis (or embolism)
Hypotension	Mesenteric thrombosis, intestinal ischemia
Hypertension	Pheochromocytoma
Respiratory	Pneumonia, otitis, aspiration of vomitus
Urinary	Pyelonephritis, hydronephrosis, calculi, renal hypertension, cholestasis, porphyria
Gynecologic	
Menstrual irregularity	Pregnancy, ectopic pregnancy
Vaginal discharge	Pelvic inflammatory disease
Menses-associated	Porphyria, endometriosis, dysmenorrhea

FMF, familial Mediterranean fever; IBD, inflammatory bowel disease; SLE, systemic lupus erythematosus; UPJ, ureteropelvic junction.

helps the sphincter to relax receptively; if the sphincter is tightening but the child does not say "stop," it is useful to stop anyway and allow the sphincter to relax. The examiner should not withdraw the finger but, rather, simply wait until the child consents to continuing. In young children, the sensation of losing control of feces, often provoked by the examination, produces anxiety; it helps to reassure them that although it feels as though they are going to defecate, they will not. The finger is inserted to the metacarpal joint, the walls of the rectum are explored by rotating the hand, and then the finger is withdrawn. In adolescents, a gynecologic examination and bimanual examination may be useful.

The presence and consistency of rectal stool are determined. Simple fecal impaction occasionally causes vomiting in children, whereas liquid stools may suggest gastroenteritis. Pelvic masses and tenderness identified rectally may represent appendicitis, ovarian torsion, or pelvic inflammatory disease. The stool should always be tested for blood and should be considered for testing for pH, reducing substances, fat, leukocytes, and infectious organisms, depending on the situation.

LABORATORY DATA

Well-appearing infants with typical regurgitant reflux usually require no laboratory evaluation, except probably an upper gastrointestinal study if they do not respond readily to conservative therapy (see later discussion). Similarly, a single, brief episode of mild vomiting with

Table 16-7. When to Consider Metabolic Work-up*

Nutritional abnormalities	Failure to thrive, anorexia
Dietary provocations	Fructose, galactose, protein, fasting
Neurologic abnormalities	Lethargy, coma
	Tone ↑ or ↓, developmental delay
	Seizures
Liver abnormalities	Hepatosplenomegaly
	Jaundice
Respiratory abnormalities	Apnea
	Hyperpnea (caused by metabolic acidosis)
Odd odors (breath, urine, ear wax)	Maple syrup: maple syrup urine disease
	Cabbage: tyrosinemia
	Sweaty feet: isovaleric acidemia
	Musty: phenylketonuria, hepatic coma (fetor hepaticus)
	Fruity: ketones (many, nonspecific)
	Other: 3-methylcrotonyl-CoA carboxylase deficiency
	Multiple carboxylase deficiency
	Acyl-CoA dehydrogenase deficiency
	Putrid: sinusitis
	Alcohol: alcohol ingestion
Miscellaneous abnormalities	Eye abnormalities (cataracts)
	Hair abnormalities (fragile)
	Pigmentation of skin ("tan") and mucosa
	Adrenal calcifications
	Ambiguous genitalia
	Cardiomyopathy
	Family history of fetal or neonatal deaths; consanguinity
Screening study abnormalities	Metabolic acidosis
	Hypoglycemia (hyperketonuric or hypoketonuric)
	Hyperkalemia (with hyponatremia)
	Hyperammonemia
	Hypertransaminasemia
	Anemia, leukocytopenia, thrombocytopenia
	Urinary non–glucose reducing substance
	Urinary Fanconi syndrome

*See also Tables 16-13 and 16-14.

CoA, coenzyme A; ↑, hypertonia; ↓ hypotonia.

a clear etiology and no suggestion of dehydration or other complications may necessitate no laboratory studies. Most other children—those with severe acute vomiting or with chronic or recurrent vomiting—should have screening studies of blood or urine (Table 16-8). Blood and urine screening for several metabolic disorders are positive only *during* an actual vomiting episode; therefore, attempts to obtain specimens at these times may increase the diagnostic yield. Examples include measuring serum lactate, serum and urine carnitine (possible fatty acid oxidation defect), and urine δ-aminolevulinic acid and porphobilinogen (possible acute intermittent porphyria).

RADIOGRAPHIC AND PROCEDURE DATA

If the history and physical examination suggest the possibility of abdominal disease, endoscopic evaluation or abdominal plain films (including a second image such as an upright film) are usually warranted (Table 16-9). Endoscopy is particularly useful in hematemesis, in suspected peptic ulcer disease, or when tissue is needed for histologic study (e.g., establishing a diagnosis of *Helicobacter pylori* gastritis or of eosinophilic gastroenteropathy). Radiographic testing is useful in most other situations. Further evaluation, such as contrast studies, ultrasonography, computed tomography (CT), or magnetic resonance imaging, is tailored to the suspected diagnoses. In rare cases, manometric evaluation is prompted by the suggestion of motor dysfunctions, such as achalasia and chronic intestinal pseudoobstruction.

DIFFERENTIAL DIAGNOSIS

GENERAL APPROACH

Cardinal symptoms or signs accompanying the vomiting direct the differential diagnosis. Abdominal pain, which frequently accompanies vomiting, can suggest both the type of disorder (luminal obstruction, inflammation, ischemia, or peritonitis) and the organ involved (see Table 16-6). Hematemesis leads to the considerations indicated in Tables 16-10 and 16-11 (see Chapter 17). Symptoms referable to nongastrointestinal organ systems direct attention to those systems. For example, accompanying neurologic symptoms direct attention to central nervous system disorders, metabolic disease, poisonings, or psychobehavioral disease.

GASTROINTESTINAL OBSTRUCTION (Table 16-12)

Esophageal Obstruction

Esophageal lesions produce welling up or drooling of oropharyngeal secretions or esophageal contents rather than actual vomiting; the material is, of course, undigested. Respiratory symptoms from aspiration may be prominent.

Esophageal Atresia. Infants with esophageal atresia present at birth with a prenatal history of polyhydramnios and intolerance of even the initial feeding. The esophageal atresia is accompanied by a distal tracheoesophageal fistula in 85% of cases, by a proximal fistula in a small percentage, and by no fistula in the remainder (Fig. 16-1). Esophageal atresia is associated with other anomalies in 15% to 50% of patients; cardiac, anorectal, and genitourinary defects are most common. Ten percent of all esophageal atresia patients, and 25% of those without a fistula, have the VATER or VACTERL (vertebral, anorectal, cardiac, tracheoesophageal, renal, radial, limb) association. As many as 33% of affected infants are premature. Diagnosis can usually be made by plain films after passage of an opaque rubber catheter, which coils in the upper pouch (Fig. 16-2). Treatment is surgical. Many infants experience reflux and reactive airway disease in the postoperative period.

Esophageal Stenosis. Persons with esophageal stenoses present in later infancy and occasionally as late as adulthood. Stenoses are divided into tracheobronchial rings that often contain cartilage, fibromuscular stenoses, and membranous webs. Diagnosis is by contrast radiography and may require pressure injections of contrast material if the stenosis is not tight. Tracheobronchial rings generally necessitate surgery, membranous webs can be treated with endoscopic dilation, and muscular stenoses may respond to dilation or may necessitate surgery.

Esophageal Strictures. Esophageal strictures are acquired lesions that are usually caused by reflux esophagitis but sometimes result from caustic ingestions (acid, alkali) or other causes (Fig. 16-3). The strictures are best demonstrated with contrast radiography; endoscopic biopsies are used to diagnose the cause as reflux.

Table 16-8. Diagnostic Tests: Blood and Urine

	Findings	Possible Significance
Blood Test		
CBC		
Hct/Hb	↑	Dehydration: general vomiting
	↓	Hematemesis; metabolic; chronic malnutrition; hypersplenism; hemolysis (e.g. sickle cell)
WBC (PMNs, bands)	↑	Sepsis; inflammatory/ischemic lesions
	↓	Metabolic; sepsis; viral; hypersplenism; malnutrition
Eosinophils	↑	Allergic (eosinophilic gastroenteropathy), parasitic
Platelets	↑	Inflammatory (e.g., inflammatory bowel disease)
	↓	Hematemesis; metabolic; hypersplenism
Electrolytes		
Na	↓ (↓)	Adrenal insufficiency; general vomiting
	↑	Salt poisoning, dehydration
K	↓	General vomiting
	↑	Adrenal insufficiency; uremia; bleeding; digitalis; diuretics (e.g., spironolactone)
Cl	↓ (↓)	Adrenal insufficiency; general vomiting
	↑	Salt poisoning, hypernatremic dehydration
Bicarbonate	↑ (pH ↑)	General vomiting, pyloric stenosis
	↓ (pH ↓)	Metabolic; adrenal insufficiency; poison; renal tubular acidosis; severe diarrhea; shock
Glucose	↑	Metabolic: diabetic ketoacidosis
	↓	Metabolic, toxins
BUN	↑	Dehydration, hematemesis
Creatinine	↑	Dehydration, renal failure
Calcium	↑	Hypercalcemia
Blood gas	↓ pH, ↓ PCO_2	Metabolic disease; adrenal insufficiency; poison; severe diarrhea; shock
ALT, AST	↑	Heptatitis; metabolic
GGT, ALP	↑	Biliary obstruction
Bilirubin	↑	Heptatitis; metabolic; hemolysis (e.g., sickle cell)
Conjugated	↑	Biliary obstruction
Amylase, lipase	↑	Pancreatitis
NH_4	↑	Metabolic, liver failure, *Proteus* urinary infection
Ketones	↑	Metabolic, fasting/starvation
Amino acids	↑	Metabolic
Organic acids	↑	Metabolic
IgE, RAST (especially foods)	↑	Allergic enteropathies
PT, PTT	↑	Hematemesis, coagulopathy, liver failure, poisoning
Toxicology	+	Drug; poison
Culture	+	Sepsis; ischemic/perforated bowel
Urine Test		
pH	↑	General vomiting
WBC	+	Urinary tract infection
Protein, casts	+	Renal disease
Blood	+	Urinary tract infection or bleeding
Bilirubin	+	Liver disease, hemolysis
Electrolytes		
Na	↓	General vomiting
K	↑	General vomiting
Cl	↓	General vomiting
Bicarbonate	↑	General vomiting
Ketones	+	Metabolic, fasting/starvation
Reducing substance		
Glucose	+	Diabetic ketoacidosis
Nonglucose	+	Galactosemia
Fanconi syndrome	+	Metabolic
FeCl	+	Metabolic
Amino acids	↑	Metabolic
Organic acids	↑	Metabolic
Toxicology	+	Drug; poison
Culture	+	Urinary tract infection; sepsis

ALP, alkaline phosphatase; ALT, alanine aminotransferase; AST, aspartate aminotransferase; BUN, blood urea nitrogen; CBC, complete blood count; Cl, chloride; FeCl, iron chloride; GGT, γ-glutamyltransferase; Hct/Hb, hematocrit/hemoglobin; IgE, immunoglobulin E; K, potassium; metabolic, inborn error of metabolism; Na, sodium; NH_4, ammonium; PCO_2, partial pressure of carbon dioxide; PMNs, polymorphonuclear neutrophils; PT, prothrombin time; PTT, partial thromboplastin time; RAST, radioallergosorbent test; WBC, white blood cell count; +, present; ↑, increased; ↓, decreased; (↓), may or may not be decreased.

Table 16-9. Other Diagnostic Tests

Test	Findings	Possible Significance
Imaging		
Routine	Isolated/distended loops	Obstruction, ischemia
Plain abdomen	"Ladder" pattern	Small-bowel obstruction
	"Inverted U" pattern	Distal colon obstruction
	Double bubble	Duodenal atresia
	Calcifications	Biliary, renal stones, appendicitis
	Free air	Intestinal perforation
	Free fluid	Ascites
	Foreign bodies	Foreign body
	Organomegaly, masses	Organomegaly, masses
Upright abdomen	Air-fluid levels	↑ Secretion: gastroenteritis
		Obstruction
Laterals, decubitus	Free air	Perforation
Chest film	Heart or lung disease; free air	Heart or lung disease; perforation
Barium		
Upper fluoroscopy	Malrotation; obstructions	Volvulus; obstructing lesions
Enteroclysis	Distal obstructions	Distal small bowel lesions
Lower fluoroscopy	Mass, obstruction, intussusception	Therapeutic: intussusception
Gastrografin		
Upper fluoroscopy		
Lower fluoroscopy		Therapeutic: meconium ileus, DIOS
Ultrasonography	Mass, cyst, abscess; pyloric stenosis; hepatobiliary, pancreatic, urinary, gynecologic lesions; blood flow in vessels	
CT/MRI abdomen	Mass, cyst, inflammatory lesions; hepatobiliary, pancreatic, urinary, gynecologic lesions	
MRI/CT head	CNS lesions	Neurogenic vomiting
Endoscopy		
Upper		
Diagnostic	Diagnosis: obstruction, hemorrhage, *Giardia* or *Helicobacter pylori* infection	Obstruction, hemorrhage
Therapeutic		Therapeutic: hematemesis
Lower		
Diagnostic	Diagnosis: distal obstruction, infection	Obstruction, infection
Therapeutic		Therapeutic: sigmoid volvulus
Manometry		
Esophagus	Failure sphincter relaxation	Achalasia
	Dysmotility	Pseudoobstruction
Small bowel	Dysmotility	Pseudoobstruction
Rectum/colon	Failure sphincter relaxation	Hirschsprung disease
	Dysmotility	Pseudoobstruction

CNS, central nervous system; CT, computed tomography; DIOS, distal intestinal obstruction syndrome: cystic fibrosis; MRI, magnetic resonance imaging.

Adequate treatment of the gastroesophageal reflux that has produced a stricture generally requires fundoplication; endoscopic dilation of the stricture is performed repeatedly with balloons or bougies until the strictured site remains patent.

Pyloric Stenosis

Pyloric stenosis manifests with nonbilious projectile vomiting beginning at 2 to 3 weeks of age and increasing during the next month or so, usually in a firstborn male child. The vomitus may contain some blood, and propulsive gastric waves can be seen on the abdominal wall. Dehydration, poor weight gain, metabolic alkalosis, and mild jaundice are sometimes evident. A palpable "olive" in the epigastrium (felt best after a feeding) represents the hypertrophied pyloric muscle.

Gastric distention is seen on the plain film, and a contrast study shows the "string sign" of contrast passing through the narrowed

pyloric channel. Ultrasound diagnosis is less invasive (Fig. 16-4). Eosinophilia, eosinophilic infiltration of endoscopic antral biopsy specimens, and an excellent response to treatment with a casein hydrolysate "hypoallergenic" formula are suggestive of an allergic or idiopathic eosinophilic gastroenteropathy and not pyloric stenosis.

In older children, gastric outlet obstruction may result from ulceration, chronic granulomatous disease, foreign bodies, and bezoars. Bezoars may be caused by hair, vegetable matter, milk curds, or medications. Long-acting formulated oral medications may also become bezoars in the distal intestine and cause obstruction.

Intestinal Obstruction

Rushes of bowel sounds associated with cramping and colic often indicate intestinal obstruction. Vomiting is a cardinal sign of intestinal obstruction, being more prominent in high small-bowel obstruction

Table 16-10. Hematemesis

Source of Blood	Lesion	Clues Regarding Source
Nasopharynx, respiratory	Epistaxis	Nosebleed history
	Hemoptysis	Cough, other respiratory symptoms
Esophageal	Varices	Copious; splenomegaly
	Esophagitis, Barrett ulcer	Heartburn
	Foreign body erosion	Foreign body history
	Aortoesophageal fistula	Copious; esophageal intubation
	Duplication	
Gastroduodenal	Mallory-Weiss tear	Emesis before hematemesis
	Peptic ulcer disease	History: smoking, alcohol, NSAIDs, pain, relation to meals
	Gastritis, ulcer	
	Duodenitis, ulcer	
	Stress ulcer	
	Dieulafoy ulcer	
	Vascular malformation	Recurrent (may have negative endoscopy)
	Aortoenteric fistula	"Herald bleed," arterial graft or aneurysm
	Duplication	
	Pyloric stenosis, web	
	Hemobilia	Trauma, gallstones, pain, jaundice
Extrinsic		
Maternal	Intrapartum	Apt test*
	Mastitis, cracked nipples	Maternal history, Apt test*
Factitious	Psychological	Affect, secondary gain
Nonblood	Red or brown food or medicine	Guaiac-negative

*See Chapter 17.

NSAIDs, nonsteroidal antiinflammatory drugs.

than in low small-bowel or colon obstruction. With high obstructions, vomiting is not feculent, the onset is often acute, and crampy pain may occur at frequent intervals; abdominal distention is minimal. With low obstructions, in contrast, the vomiting may be feculent and less acute in onset, the interval between cramping is longer, and distention is more notable. Identification of the site of obstruction is aided by the plain film and by other radiographic studies (see Table 16-9).

Obstructions may be categorized by type and site. Intraluminal lesions (e.g., tumors; intussusceptions; or extrinsic material such as feces, foreign bodies, bezoars, and gallstones) can be differentiated from bowel wall lesions (strictures, stenoses, atresias) and from extraluminal lesions (adhesions, congenital bands, tumors, volvulus). Again, radiographic studies are useful, beginning with the plain film and progressing to ultrasonography or CT. Fluoroscopy with contrast material such as barium or diatrizoate (Gastrografin) is very helpful

Table 16-11. Hematemesis: Causes Not to Miss and Red Flags

Finding	Etiology	Physical Examination and Laboratory Studies: Clues Regarding Source
Coagulopathy (PT ↑, PTT ↑)	Vitamin K deficiency	Newborn, antibiotics, fat malabsorption
	Genetic coagulopathies	Specific factor deficiencies
	Liver failure	Liver disease, factor VIII normal
	DIC	Sepsis, factor VIII ↓
	Drug	Drug history
	Warfarin (Coumadin)	
	Heparin	
Thrombocytopenia (platelets ↓)	Hypersplenism	Splenomegaly (Hct ↓, WBC ↓)
	Chemotherapy	Chemotherapy history (Hct ↓, WBC ↓)
	DIC	Sepsis (PT ↑, PTT ↑)
Platelet dysfunction (bleeding time ↑)	Drug	Drug history
	Salicylates/NSAIDs	
	Antibiotics	
Portal hypertension	Varices; gastritis	Splenomegaly
		Abdominal veins; angiomas
		Ascites
		Clubbing; palmar erythema

DIC, disseminated intravascular coagulation; Hct, hematocrit; NSAIDs, nonsteroidal antiinflammatory drugs; PT, prothrombin time; PTT, partial thromboplastin time; WBC, white blood cell count.

Table16-12. Causes of Gastrointenstinal Obstruction	
Esophagus	
Congenital	Esophageal atresia (with or without fistula)
	Isolated esophageal stenosis
	Duplication
	Vascular ring
Acquired	Caustic agent esophageal stricture
	Peptic stricture
	Chagas disease
	Collagen-vascular disease
Stomach	
Congenital	Antral webs
Acquired	Pyloric atresia*
	Bezoars/foreign body
	Pyloric stenosis
	Pyloric stricture (ulcer)
	Crohn disease
	Eosinophilic gastroenteropathy
	Prostaglandin-induced pyloric stenosis
	Chronic granulomatous disease
Small Intestine	
Congenital	Duodenal atresia
	Annular pancreas
	Malrotation/volvulus
	Malrotation/Ladd bands
	Ileal atresia, stenosis
	Duplications
	Meconium ileus
	Inguinal hernia
	Gastroschisis
Acquired	Postsurgical adhesions or strictures
	Crohn disease (stricture)
	Intussusception
	Duodenal hematoma (abuse, trauma)
	Meconium ileus equivalent
Colon	
Congenital	Meconium plug
	Hirschsprung disease
	Colonic atresia, stenosis
	Imperforate rectum/anus
	Rectal stenosis
	Malrotation/volvulus
	Small left colon syndrome (IDM)
Acquired	Ulcerative colitis (toxic megacolon)†
	Crohn disease (stricture)
	Chagas disease
	Stricture post-NEC

From Behrman R, Kliegman R: Nelson Essentials of Pediatrics, 2nd ed. Philadelphia, WB Saunders, 1994, p 407.

*Often associated with epidermolysis bullosa.

†Produces an ileus.

IDM, infant of diabetic mother; NEC, necrotizing enterocolitis.

in identifying both the site and the type of obstruction, but the decision to introduce contrast into an intestine that may perforate or be operated on must be made with surgical and radiologic consultation. Often the decision to operate can be made without certain identification of the lesion, and contrast studies are unnecessary.

Infantile bilious vomiting is an important symptom of intestinal obstruction, which often signals a congenital gastrointestinal anomaly, particularly intestinal obstruction below the ampulla of Vater. Surgical consultation is needed early in these infants, because they often require emergency therapy (see Table 16-12).

Duodenal Atresia, Stenosis, and Web; Annular Pancreas. The juxtaampullary duodenum is susceptible to a cluster of obstructing congenital anomalies. Infants with complete duodenal obstruction, most commonly atresia, present with bilious vomiting and a radiographic "double-bubble" sign (Fig. 16-5). Associated prematurity (and polyhydramnios) or anomalies, including renal, cardiac, and vertebral defects, occur in approximately 75% of infants; trisomy 21 is seen in about 50%. Double atresias, duplications, and malrotations are frequently seen.

Infants with a partial duodenal obstruction caused by a stenosis or web may have such mild symptoms that they do not come to medical attention until regurgitation produces esophagitis or until a foreign body or bezoar is trapped at the obstruction. Treatment is surgery.

Duodenal Hematoma. Blunt abdominal trauma (seat belt injury, child abuse), or even endoscopic biopsies in the context of a coagulopathy, can produce an obstructing duodenal hematoma. Therapy is symptomatic; parenteral nutrition may be required as the problem resolves.

Jejunal Atresia, Ileal Atresia, and Ileal Stenosis. Patients with these congenital lesions present with bilious vomiting and more abdominal distention than those with duodenal lesions. The atresias are readily suspected and diagnosed in the neonatal period. Stenotic lesions may require radiography for diagnosis. Treatment is surgical.

Intestinal Strictures. Strictures produce partial obstruction of the gastrointestinal tract and may be located from the esophagus to the anus. They may occur postsurgically (anastomotic), may follow necrotizing enterocolitis, may be caused by Crohn disease, or may result from ingestion of nonsteroidal antiinflammatory medications or high-dose pancreatic enzymes.

Some patients may be treated with endoscopic dilatation, but many require surgical stricturoplasty (opening the bowel longitudinally and closing it transversely) or resection.

Adhesions. Obstructive symptoms in the child with a history of prior abdominal surgery may be caused by adhesive bands.

Duplications. These uncommon lesions may cause vomiting by extrinsic obstruction of the intestine or by intussusception. An abdominal mass may be palpable.

Meconium Ileus and Distal Intestinal Obstruction Syndrome. Ten percent of infants with cystic fibrosis present in the newborn period with failure to pass meconium, caused by meconium ileus (Fig. 16-6). The inspissated meconium may be treated by diatrizoate (Gastrografin) enema, but some infants require surgery, particularly if they have a perforated viscus, which occurs prenatally in 10% and produces a calcified meconium peritonitis. Virtually all infants with meconium ileus have cystic fibrosis; the diagnosis should be confirmed by sweat test or DNA analysis. Older children with cystic fibrosis who stop defecating and have abdominal pain and occasionally vomiting are said to have distal intestinal obstruction syndrome (DIOS), formerly termed meconium ileus equivalent.

The sticky, poorly hydrated intestinal mucus plays a role. Initial treatment with intestinal lavage and enemas may be successful, but, if not, diatrizoate (Gastrografin) enemas (at times mixed with N-acetylcysteine) are nearly always successful. Surgery is rarely required. Close attention to fluid and electrolyte balance is vital in all infants and children treated with a hypertonic contrast medium such as diatrizoate (Gastrografin).

Incarcerated Hernia. Whenever vomiting is accompanied by signs of obstruction, sites of potential herniation should be examined

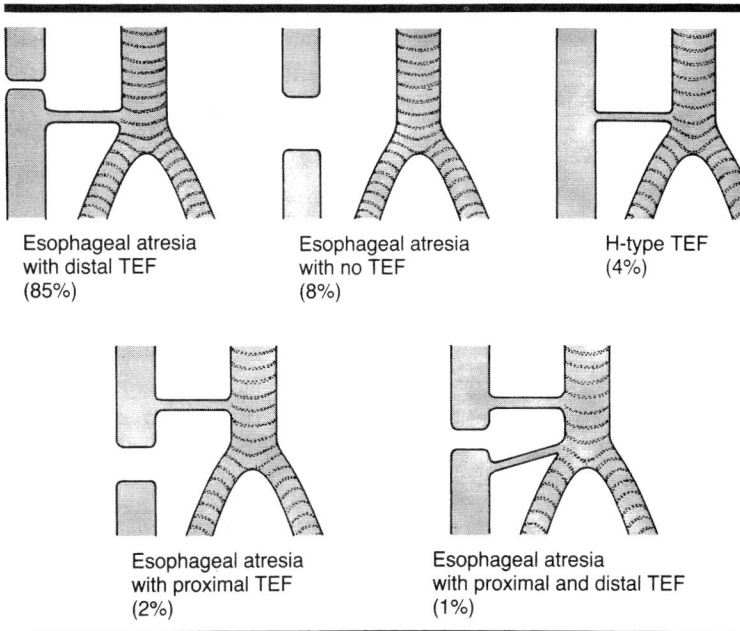

Esophageal atresia
with distal TEF
(85%)

Esophageal atresia
with no TEF
(8%)

H-type TEF
(4%)

Esophageal atresia
with proximal TEF
(2%)

Esophageal atresia
with proximal and distal TEF
(1%)

Figure 16-1. Various types of tracheoesophageal fistulas (TEF) with relative frequency (%). (From Kirschner BS, Black DD: The gastrointestinal tract. In Behrman RE, Kliegman RM [eds]: Nelson Essentials of Pediatrics, 2nd ed. Philadelphia, WB Saunders, 1994, p 413.)

for incarceration of a loop of bowel (Fig. 16-7). Inguinal incarceration is most common, but other types of hernias are femoral, obturator, spigelian, umbilical (1 in 1500 incarcerate), epigastric, and postoperative incisional hernias.

Inguinal hernias are often reduced by gentle, firm, constant pressure that is directed through the scrotum toward the inguinal canal. Sedation and the Trendelenburg position may facilitate reduction (see Chapter 28).

Malrotation and Volvulus. Volvulus is the twisting of a loop of bowel on the mesentery. Midgut volvulus occurs most often in the context of congenital intestinal malrotation, in which the small intestine is not normally fastened in place (Fig. 16-8). More than half of patients found to have malrotation present symptomatically (the rest of such cases are discovered incidentally), and about half of the symptomatic patients present in the neonatal period with bilious vomiting caused by volvulus. Those presenting later often do not have bilious vomiting; the vomiting may be intermittent for years.

Volvulus is an *extremely hazardous* obstructing lesion. The luminal obstruction is closed at both ends, which leads to sepsis from rapidly proliferating and translocating bacteria. There is also vascular obstruction in which the root of the mesentery is twisted, which quickly produces ischemia of the small intestine. Even if volvulus is diagnosed and repaired promptly, massive intestinal resection may be necessary; this produces short bowel syndrome. Because volvulus may be intermittent, it may produce episodic or chronic intermittent vomiting or nonspecific abdominal pain before a lethal event.

Upper intestinal contrast radiographs should be considered in the intermittently regurgitating infant, and surgery must be performed if a malrotation is found (i.e., if the ligament of Treitz is not to the left of the spine), even if volvulus is not present at the time of the examination. In an infant in whom an ongoing volvulus is suspected, an abdominal flat plate may show a "double bubble with distal air" or a "volvulus/corkscrew" pattern. In the sick infant or child in whom volvulus seems likely, surgery without contrast studies may be preferred. Surgery deals both with the malrotation and with the often-accompanying, potentially obstructing Ladd bands.

Other types of volvulus not associated with malrotation include cecal, sigmoid, and transverse colonic volvulus. They are less common in children and less apt to produce short bowel syndrome, but they,

too, may manifest with vomiting and result in death if untreated. Sigmoid volvulus is sometimes treated nonoperatively.

Meckel Diverticulum. Meckel diverticula may cause obstructive vomiting by intussusception (Fig. 16-9) or by intestinal volvulus around a fibrous band. They may also cause vomiting by inflammatory changes, and they may bleed. This fibrous remnant of the omphalomesenteric duct is a small intestinal diverticulum. The "rule of 2s" identifies characteristic findings: These diverticula are present in 2% of the population; the male-female ratio is 2:1; the diverticula occur within 2 feet of the ileocecal valve and are 2 inches long; there are two major types of heterotopic mucosa (50% of patients have gastric mucosa, and a minority have pancreatic mucosa; in rare cases, colonic mucosa is present); the condition is confused with two diseases (appendicitis and peptic ulcer); and there are two complications (hemorrhage occasionally with perforation or intussusception).

Diagnosis of the ectopic gastric mucosa is by Meckel scan (technetium 99m pertechnetate); it has imperfect sensitivity, which may be improved by pentagastrin, glucagon, and cimetidine. Treatment is surgical.

Intussusception. The normal function of the intestine is to constrict above and relax below an intraluminal bolus. When such a bolus (a "lead point") is attached to the intestinal wall, the propulsive activity of the intestine produces telescoping of proximal intestine (intussusceptum) into distal intestine (intussuscipiens), causing both luminal obstruction and mesenteric vascular compromise. Abdominal pain occurs in nearly all children with intussusception, whereas vomiting results in about 65% and "currant-jelly stools" (from mucosal hemorrhage) occur in fewer than 20%. The pain is severe, crampy, and often contemporaneous with the vomiting. Between cramps, the child may be listless, may sleep, or may even play. Vomiting and bloody stools are more common in younger infants and in those with longer duration of symptoms. An abdominal mass is palpable in about 25% of patients.

The lead point of the intussusception is usually ileal, with the intussusception ileocecal or ileocolonic. It is probable that prominent ileal lymphoid nodules provide the lead point for most young children presenting with intussusception, 66% of whom are younger than 2 years, with a peak incidence late in the first year of life. Other

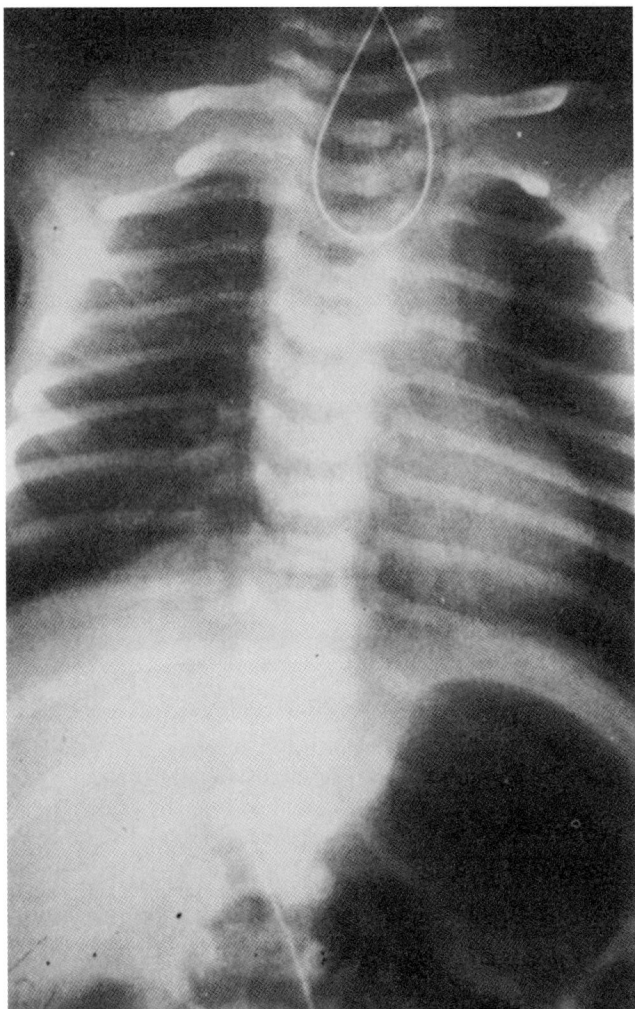

Figure 16-2. Tracheoesophageal fistula (TEF). Coiled radiopaque nasogastric tube in blind upper pouch. Note the air in the gastrointestinal tract, indicating a distal TEF. In rare cases, the TEF is so big that a large amount of air enters the stomach, and preliminary gastrostomy is necessary to avoid gastric perforation. (From Ein SH: Esophageal atresia and tracheoesophageal fistula. In Wyllie R, Hyams JS [eds]: Pediatric Gastrointestinal Disease: Pathophysiology, Diagnosis, Management. Philadelphia, WB Saunders, 1993, p 320.)

lead points (Meckel diverticulum [see Fig. 16-9], appendix, duplication, polyp, lymphoma, hematoma from trauma or from Henoch-Schönlein purpura) or disorders (cystic fibrosis) must be considered in the very young or older child presenting with intussusception (see Chapter 14).

Visualization may be by ultrasonography if the diagnosis is uncertain but is more often by radiographic studies, inasmuch as radiologic reduction enemas are usually curative in infants.

Treatment is by hydrostatic reduction with barium; rectal insufflation of air has also been used but may be less able to document a lead point that necessitates surgical resection. Contraindications to reduction by hydrostatic enemas include the presence of symptoms for longer than 48 to 72 hours, peritonitis, and intestinal perforation. Approximately 10% of patients experience recurrences.

Superior Mesenteric Artery Syndrome. Superior mesenteric artery (SMA) syndrome is caused by extrinsic compression of the duodenum, which is trapped between the SMA anteriorly and the aorta posteriorly as the SMA crosses over the duodenum in the root of the mesentery. The compression is usually just to the right of midline, where it produces a cutoff of the duodenum that is visible radiographically, often with proximal dilation. Synonyms include Wilkie syndrome, arteriomesenteric duodenal compression, and cast syndrome.

SMA syndrome may be suspected when bilious emesis and epigastric discomfort relieved by vomiting occur in the context of weight loss, lordosis, body casts, lengthy bed rest, or prior abdominal surgery, particularly when crampy pain is relieved by prone or knee-chest positions. Adolescents and young adults are most often affected.

Nutritional rehabilitation, either intravenously or by the enteral route, is important in SMA syndrome. The prone position may improve duodenal emptying. Surgery may be needed if there are chronic symptoms despite nutritional rehabilitation.

Constipation, Meconium Plug, and Anal Stenosis. These distal colonic problems produce obstipation primarily, but if they are severe and persistent, vomiting may result. Rectal examination provides the diagnosis.

Enemas, laxatives, dietary changes, and behavioral modification are useful in treating constipation, whereas surgery is usually necessary to treat anal atresia or stenosis (see Chapter 21). Infants with meconium plug syndrome need clinical follow-up to monitor for the presence of coexistent Hirschsprung disease.

GASTROINTESTINAL DYSMOTILITY

Achalasia

Achalasia, like esophageal stenoses and strictures, produces effortless retrograde emptying of undigested food from the esophagus.

Contrast radiography and esophageal manometry are needed for diagnosis. Calcium channel blockers such as nifedipine produce at least temporary clinical benefit in many patients. Balloon dilation or surgical myotomy produce more sustained benefit more reliably but with a somewhat higher complication rate.

Gastroesophageal Reflux

The apparently effortless regurgitation that represents gastroesophageal reflux in infants is of particular importance because (1) it is the most common cause of "vomiting" in infants; (2) physiologic reflux must be distinguished from reflux necessitating evaluation and therapy; and (3) the practitioner must be vigilant to avoid misdiagnosing other infantile vomiting diseases as reflux. Lethal malrotation with volvulus, partially obstructing duodenal web, and metabolic disorders are three examples of such misdiagnoses. Children with primary neurologic disease may be more likely to regurgitate and suffer from reflux disease; it must be remembered that many metabolic disorders manifest both as neurologic dysfunction and as regurgitation.

Infants with problematic regurgitant reflux who come to medical attention should undergo upper gastrointestinal radiography to rule out the possibility of malrotation. Reflux may cause weight deficit (resulting from regurgitation of caloric feedings, odynophagia from esophagitis, or parental reluctance to feed a recurrently spitting infant), apnea, chronic respiratory disease, hoarseness or stridor, abdominal or chest pain, infantile irritability, or Sandifer syndrome (arching of the spine and turning of the neck). Diagnostic evaluation should be tailored to the presentation: Regurgitation prompts barium contrast radiography with fluoroscopy; anorexia or infantile irritability prompts evaluation for esophagitis by endoscopy with esophageal biopsy, esophageal biopsy alone if feasible, or possibly pH probe if no response to a 2-week trial of hypoallergenic formula and/or acid suppression is noted; apnea prompts pH probe with pneumogram

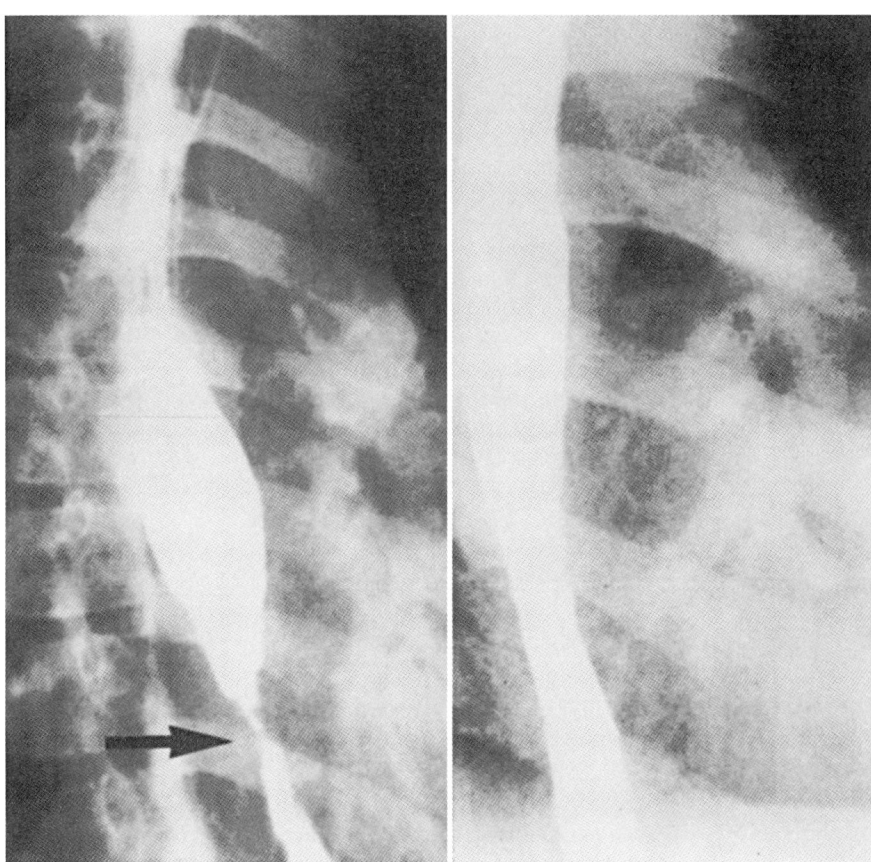

Figure 16-3. Esophageal stricture. Radiograph of a peptic esophageal stricture before and after treatment with dilatations. The patient, a 10-year-old boy, had a 6-month history of dysphagia before his stricture (*arrow*) was demonstrated by barium esophagogram (*left*). His weight had dropped to the 10th percentile, but his height was at the 50th percentile. The stricture was improved symptomatically and radiographically (*right*) by a series of bougienage dilatations, and subsequent fundoplication allowed the underlying peptic esophagitis to heal. (From Orenstein SR: Dysphagia and vomiting. In Wyllie R, Hyams JS [eds]: Pediatric Gastrointestinal Disease: Pathophysiology, Diagnosis, Management. Philadelphia, WB Saunders, 1993, p 137.)

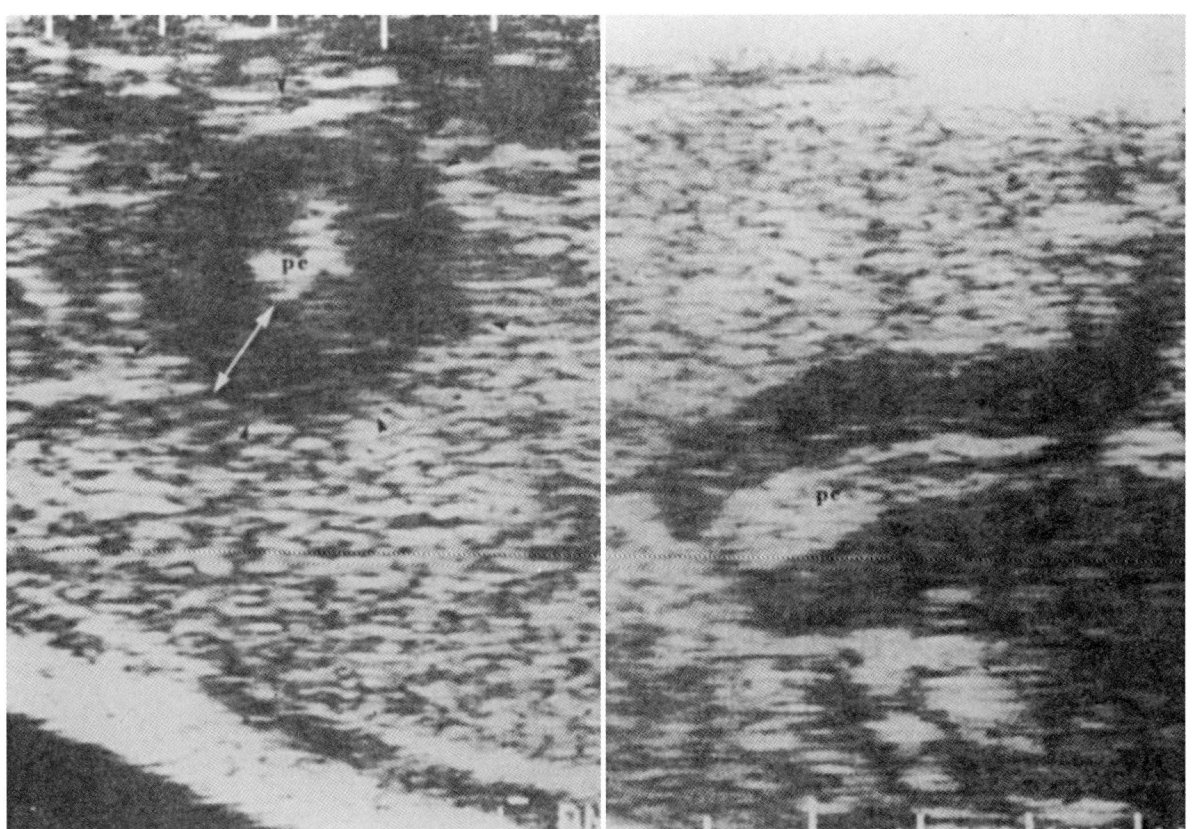

Figure 16-4. Pyloric stenosis. Cross-sectional (*left*) and transverse (*right*) sonograms of hypertrophic pyloric stenosis, showing increased thickness and length of pyloric muscle. pc, pyloric channel. (From Alexander F: Pyloric stenosis and congenital anomalies of the stomach and duodenum. In Wyllie R, Hyams JS [eds]: Pediatric Gastrointestinal Disease: Pathophysiology, Diagnosis, Management. Philadelphia, WB Saunders, 1993, p 416.)

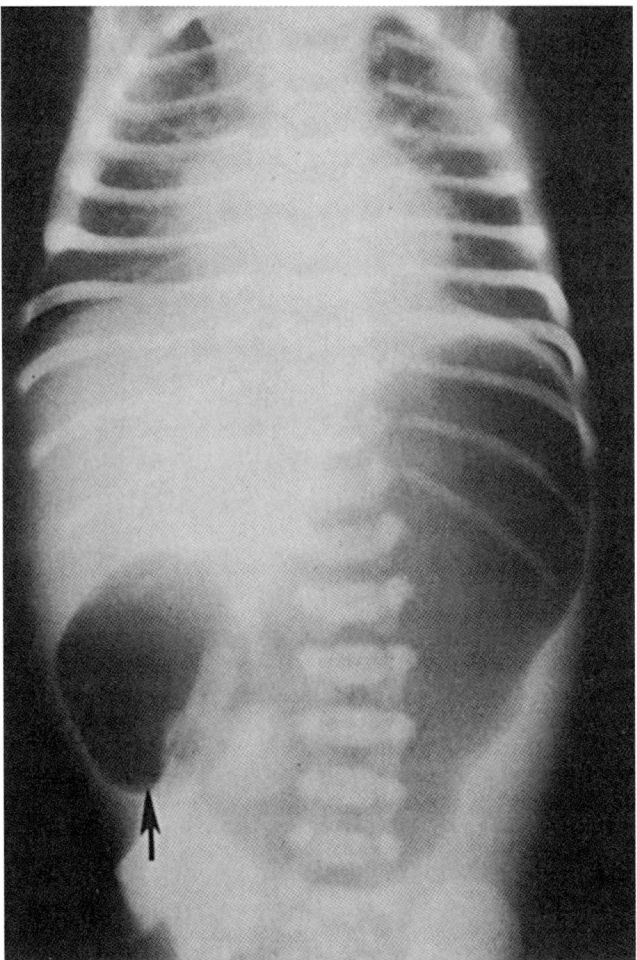

Figure 16-5. "Double-bubble" sign in duodenal obstruction. Swallowed air fills the stomach and the obstructed duodenum (*arrow*). Usually accompanied by bilious vomiting, the double-bubble sign is not specific for any of the duodenal obstructions but implies a need for surgery. (From Teplick SK, Glick SN, Keller MS: The duodenum. In Putman CE, Ravin CE [eds]: Textbook of Diagnostic Imaging. Philadelphia, WB Saunders, 1988, p 815.)

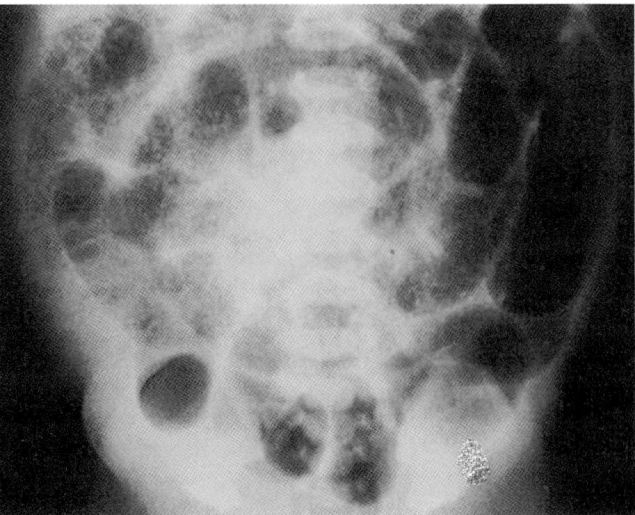

Figure 16-6. Meconium ileus. Supine radiograph shows gas-distended small bowel and mottled appearance of inspissated meconium in a newborn. (From Lappas JC, Maglinte DDT: The small bowel. In Putman CE, Ravin CE [eds]: Textbook of Diagnostic Imaging. Philadelphia, WB Saunders, 1988, p 859.)

(especially if the apnea is repetitive); hoarseness or stridor prompts laryngoscopy, endoscopy for esophageal histologic study, a modified Bernstein test (acid infusion test to reproduce symptoms), or possibly a trial of aggressive therapy that may include proton pump inhibitor (PPI) agents; heartburn prompts a 2- to 4-week trial of either histamine-blocking or PPI agents, followed by endoscopy if no response is seen or if symptoms resume as medication is tapered; Sandifer syndrome prompts endoscopy, pH probe, or modified Bernstein test. The wheezing infant or child with overt regurgitation or other symptoms of reflux merits an empirical trial of at least 3 months of aggressive acid suppressive therapy, possibly augmented by a prokinetic agent. An asthmatic child without reflux symptoms but in whom recurrent radiographic evidence of pneumonia, nocturnal wheezing, or inability to wean from frequent or continuous steroid therapy is documented should be assessed by pH probe and possibly endoscopy. If results of these studies are abnormal, medical therapy for reflux is commenced.

Treatment of regurgitant reflux in infants is initiated with avoidance of seated or supine positioning (particularly postprandially) and with thickening of the feedings with 1 tablespoon of dry rice cereal per ounce of formula. In many infants, this reduces regurgitation remarkably. Problematic regurgitation persisting during this treatment, particularly if associated with poor weight gain or other signs of

illness, necessitates upper gastrointestinal fluoroscopic evaluation and consideration of other causes for the vomiting, such as metabolic or allergic disease. A 2-week trial of a protein hydrolysate formula as empirical therapy for allergic vomiting (formula protein intolerance) may be helpful, particularly if there is a family history of allergy or if there is peripheral eosinophilia. If the diagnosis remains reflux, a prokinetic agent is frequently begun. Cisapride had previously been front-line prokinetic therapy for pediatric reflux, but since July 2000 it has been available in the United States only via a limited-access program because of concerns over the potential for cardiac arrhythmias. Metoclopramide may be used, although its efficacy in reflux never has been proved and its therapeutic margin is narrow. An oral H_2 receptor antagonist or proton pump inhibitor is added if esophagitis is suspected or documented. In view of the current limitations and uncertainties surrounding prokinetic agents, however, many infants and children may be adequately managed with aggressive acid suppression alone.

Management is reevaluated at least every 2 months for the need to increase doses, to discontinue medications, or to reevaluate the diagnosis. Infants with reflux usually improve on this management, which can usually be discontinued between 8 and 18 months of age, as symptoms resolve. The rare infant who does not improve and develops nutritional, respiratory, or peptic complications from reflux is evaluated for surgical fundoplication (Fig. 16-10).

Gastric Stasis and Gastroparesis

Gastric stasis is suggested by the vomiting of food eaten hours earlier and by the presence of food in the stomach of a fasting patient undergoing an upper gastrointestinal series. If the contrast study excludes gastric outlet obstruction, gastroparesis is likely. Diabetic gastroparesis, in which autonomic neuropathy resulting from diabetes causes gastric atony, is the classic example of this disorder but is rare in childhood. Surgical vagotomy produces similar symptoms. Other causes of generalized ileus or pseudoobstruction can involve the stomach primarily. Viral infections, perhaps including gastric cytomegalovirus, and drugs such as anticholinergics may also produce gastric stasis.

Gastric stasis may respond to the prokinetic agents, erythromycin or metoclopramide, particularly if the cause is neurogenic. These medications may have additive effects.

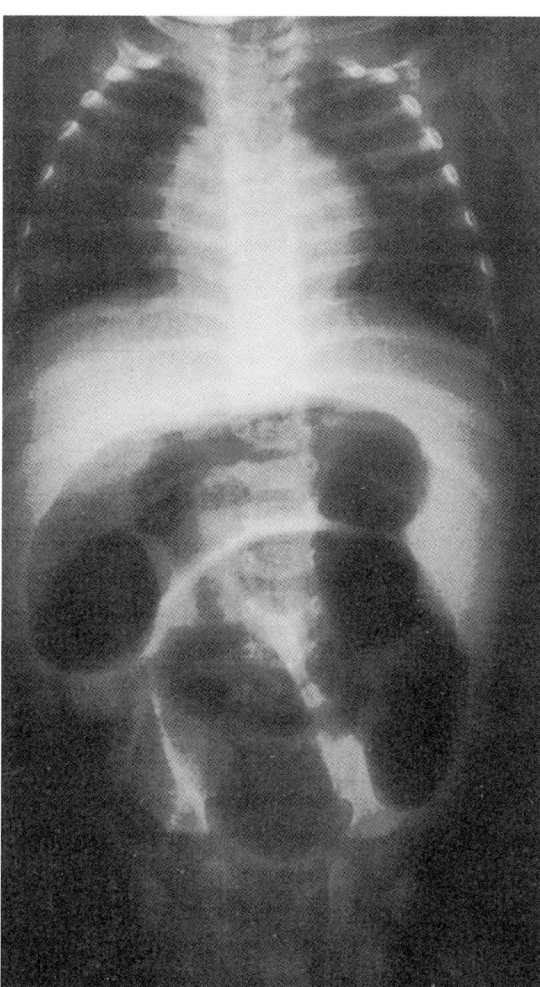

Figure 16-7. Intestinal obstruction. Plain radiograph of the abdomen reveals massive intestinal dilatation in a 4-month-old child with abdominal distention and vomiting secondary to intestinal obstruction from inguinal hernias. Note the presence of gas within the scrotum. (From Markowitz JF: Intestinal obstruction and ileus. In Wyllie R, Hyams JS [eds]: Pediatric Gastrointestinal Disease: Pathophysiology, Diagnosis, Management. Philadelphia, WB Saunders, 1993, p 246.)

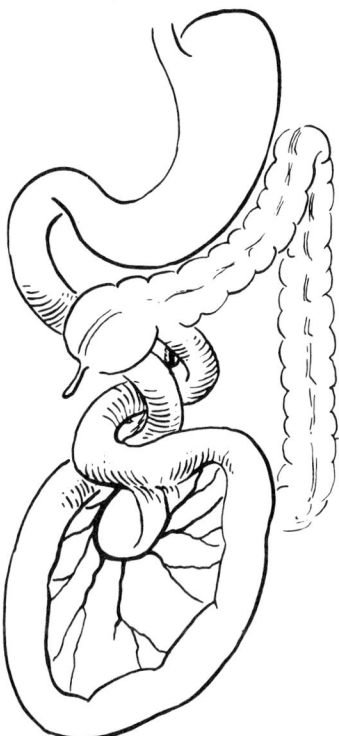

Figure 16-8. Diagram of malrotation with the mesentery twisted on its pedicle. (From Wang C, Welch CE: Anomalies of intestinal rotation in adolescents and adults. Surgery 1963;54:839-855.)

Ileus

Paralytic ileus, typified by the postoperative ileus that follows most abdominal surgery, is very common. As in intestinal obstruction, intestinal contents fail to progress, causing abdominal pain and vomiting. Typically, the bowel sounds are decreased or absent; there may be abdominal distention. Other causes of ileus include unrelieved intestinal obstruction, peritonitis, intestinal ischemia, and sepsis. Signs of ileus may follow signs of intestinal obstruction; in this context, ileus is an ominous sign. Other causes of paralytic ileus are drugs (phenothiazines, narcotics, laxative abuse, atropine), electrolyte disturbances (hypokalemia, hypercalcemia), endocrinopathies (hypothyroidism), or injuries (spinal fractures). Both chemotherapy and radiation therapy can produce reversible acute symptoms of vomiting, abdominal pain, and diarrhea within a few days to several weeks of the insult; intestinal motor disturbances are the suggested cause.

Treatment of ileus requires correction of any correctable provocative abnormalities and nasogastric tube decompression until normal peristalsis begins.

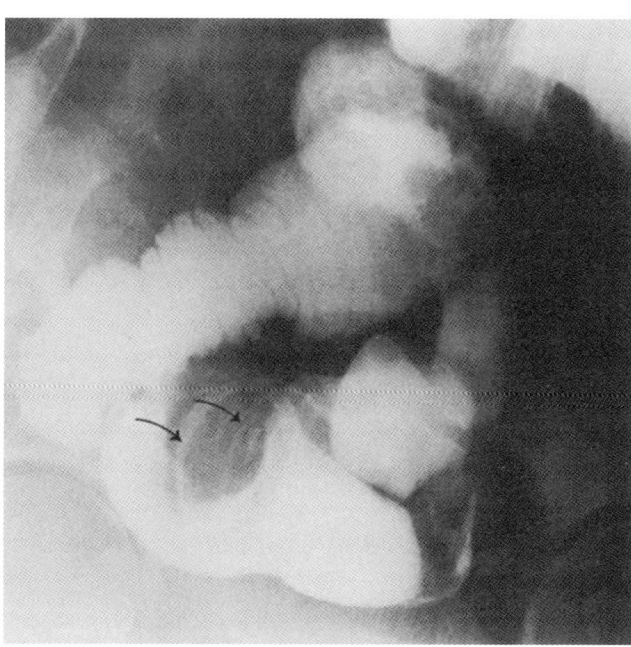

Figure 16-9. Enteroenteric intussusception. Luminal mass defect due to intussusception of a Meckel diverticulum. A coil-spring appearance has been created around the intussusceptum (*arrows*). (From Lappas JC, Maglinte DDT: The small bowel. In Putman CE, Ravin CE [eds]: Textbook of Diagnostic Imaging. Philadelphia, WB Saunders, 1988, p 858.)

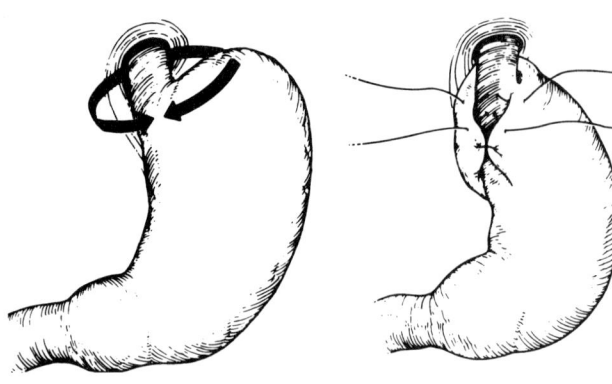

Figure 16-10. Diagrams of a Nissen fundoplication. (From Schatzlein MH, Ballantine TVN, Thirunavukkarasu S, et al: Gastroesophageal reflux in infants and children. Arch Surg 1979;114: 505-510. Copyright 1979, American Medical Association.)

Pseudoobstruction

Like ileus, intestinal pseudoobstruction represents intestinal dysmotility rather than obstruction. Pseudoobstruction, however, is a chronic illness, sometimes with remissions and relapses, and is far rarer than acute ileus. Enteroclysis radiographic studies may be necessary to confirm the absence of partial obstruction. There is a family history in 20% to 30% of patients, and nearly 50% of children with the disorder are symptomatic in the first month of life, although diagnosis is often quite delayed. Malrotation may be found in up to 40% of patients with pseudoobstruction. The disorder may involve any part or the entire luminal gastrointestinal tract and occasionally (in up to 10% of patients) involves the urinary tract. A relatively quiet abdomen or prominent borborygmi may be present, and abdominal distention (in 70% of patients) is often associated with succussion splashes when the patient moves. Vomiting occurs in 50% of patients, and constipation may be prominent (in >50%). Weight loss is caused by both vomiting of nutrients and by bacterial overgrowth–induced malabsorption.

Several causes for pseudoobstruction have been identified; they are generally classified as either neuropathic or myopathic. Familial versus nonfamilial and primary versus secondary are two other classifications. Differentiation between neuropathic and myopathic types is best made by small intestinal manometry; esophageal manometry may contribute as well. Full-thickness intestinal biopsy is sometimes useful for distinguishing specific entities causing the disorder; special silver stains of the myenteric plexus are particularly helpful. The myopathic causes (in 10% of pediatric patients, a much lower proportion than that of adults) include collagen-vascular causes of myositis or muscle fibrosis (progressive systemic sclerosis), various muscular dystrophies, megacystis-microcolon, and "familial visceral myopathies." The neuropathic causes (90%) include Hirschsprung disease, Chagas disease, diabetic and other autonomic neuropathies, autoimmune disorders producing inflammatory neurodegeneration, multiple endocrine neoplasia, and "familial visceral neuropathies." Both types of pseudoobstruction are difficult to manage; the myopathic form, representing dysfunction of the "end organ," is particularly difficult.

A third category that is sometimes included in the myopathic type is fibrotic involvement of the muscularis propria. It may follow collagen vascular diseases, radiation therapy (>6 months after), or chemotherapy by months or years, causing either myopathic pseudoobstruction or obstruction resulting from inflammatory strictures.

Functional failure of intestinal propulsion can be treated with erythromycin or metoclopramide. These medications are more apt to be useful in neurogenic disorders than in myogenic ones. Because of their different sites of action, they may have additive effects. Patients with pseudoobstruction also benefit from antibiotic treatment of bacterial overgrowth syndrome, when present, or from nutritional rehabilitation with total parenteral nutrition. Collagen vascular or autoimmune causes of pseudoobstruction may respond to steroids.

Cautious surgery is occasionally beneficial; some patients eventually require intestinal transplantation.

GASTROINTESTINAL INFLAMMATION

Esophagitis

Although esophagitis is often associated with vomiting, it is usually not the cause of vomiting. Esophagitis is caused by gastroesophageal reflux or by vomiting from various other causes.

Gastroenteritis

Gastroenteritis is a frequent cause of acute vomiting illness in childhood. The vomiting is often associated with diarrhea and sometimes with crampy abdominal pain or fever (see Chapter 15). Rotavirus, especially in infants, is notable for its prominent vomiting, which often precedes the diarrhea. "Food poisoning" also produces vomiting and diarrhea, often caused by bacterially derived toxin. The time course and symptoms suggest which organism is involved. Gastroenteritis, like regurgitant reflux, is common and often necessitates minimal diagnostic procedures and therapy; however, the examiner must constantly guard against making this diagnosis in a child who might have metabolic or surgical disease (see Table 16-20).

Treatment of acute gastroenteritis mandates attention to hydration. Oral rehydration is feasible in many children with gastroenteritis, but prominent vomiting may make intravenous rehydration necessary. A common error is to use clear liquids longer than 24 hours; this leaves nutritional needs unmet. Early refeeding in gastroenteritis is most successful when the food is low in fat and lactose and high in complex carbohydrates.

Peptic Ulcer Disease

The term *peptic ulcer disease* includes gastritis, gastric ulcer, duodenitis, and duodenal ulcer (see Chapters 14 and 17). In children, in contrast to adults, these disorders frequently cause vomiting. Defined causes for peptic ulcer disease include *H. pylori* infections, bile reflux gastritis, nonsteroidal antiinflammatory agents, and rare gastrin-secreting tumors (Zollinger-Ellison syndrome). Stress ulcers occur in the context of sepsis, burns, surgery, head trauma, and severe acute illness.

The optimal diagnostic method is endoscopy, with evaluation for *H. pylori* or elevated gastrin in appropriate cases. H_2 receptor blockade is the main treatment; supplementary antacids are sometimes useful, and proton pump inhibitors are beneficial in the patient with intractable disease. Discontinuation of tobacco smoke exposure is important. *H. pylori* infections are less apt to recur if treated with triple therapy, which includes a PPI agent and two antibiotics, such as amoxicillin, clarithromycin, or metronidazole. Zollinger-Ellison syndrome is optimally treated by tumor resection and evaluation for related endocrine tumors; PPI treatment is helpful if complete tumor resection is impossible.

Meckel's Diverticulitis

In addition to presenting as gastrointestinal obstruction, via volvulus or intussusception, Meckel's diverticula may become inflamed and mimic appendicitis.

Treatment is surgical, so preoperative distinction of Meckel's diverticulitis from other causes of an acute abdomen is not crucial (see Chapter 14).

Mesenteric Adenitis

Inflammation of lymph nodes in the mesentery is probably caused by viral (adenovirus, measles) or bacterial (*Yersinia enterocolitica*) infection, but the symptoms are similar enough to appendicitis that the diagnosis is usually not made before surgery. Ultrasonography can readily distinguish mesenteric adenitis from appendicitis (see Chapter 14).

Appendicitis

When vomiting occurs in appendicitis, it *follows* the periumbilical pain but may precede the localization of the pain to the McBurney point, two thirds of the way between the umbilicus and the right anterior iliac spine. Before perforation, there is only occasional vomiting. After perforation, the fever may be higher, the child lies still with the right hip flexed, and vomiting may be more frequent and more feculent. In appendicitis, there is later vomiting, less diarrhea, fewer bowel sounds, and more rectal or rebound tenderness than in gastroenteritis. It is also associated with less diarrhea, less fever, and less leukocytosis than is bacterial enteritis, although *Yersinia* in particular has caused right lower quadrant pain mimicking appendicitis. Crohn disease is usually more chronic than is appendicitis.

Treatment of appendicitis is discussed in Chapter 14.

Inflammatory Bowel Disease

Crohn disease, in particular, may produce vomiting on occasion, particularly when obstructing intestinal strictures develop. Other extraintestinal manifestations of Crohn disease also, in rare cases, produce vomiting (see Chapter 15).

Allergic Enteropathy, Eosinophilic Gastroenteropathy, and Eosinophilic Esophagitis

Vomiting is a frequent response to ingestion of allergens and may be seen as early as the first weeks of life in infants with allergy to cow's milk or soy and in older children as potentially allergenic foods are introduced. There may be associated diarrhea and hematochezia and, in the older child, urticaria or other systemic signs of allergy. A strong family history for allergic diathesis is very suggestive. Laboratory studies may show peripheral blood eosinophilia or an elevated serum immunoglobulin E level; positive radioallergosorbent test results to individual foods are helpful if present.

In infants, the simplest diagnostic test is a change to a protein hydrolysate formula for at least 2 weeks. If the vomiting (and other symptoms) resolve, it is generally not necessary to rechallenge for diagnosis, but empirical treatment can be continued for several months. Because infants usually outgrow these "formula protein intolerances" at between 10 and 24 months of age, a normal diet can later be gradually introduced as tolerated. Older children with vomiting that represents eosinophilic gastroenteropathy or other immunoglobulin E–mediated food allergy are less likely to lose the allergy over time. Diagnosis otherwise is by upper intestinal endoscopy with biopsies, which demonstrate an increased number of mucosal and intraepithelial eosinophils and, possibly, varying degrees of villous injury. Eosinophilic esophagitis, which may occur independently of eosinophilic gastroenteropathy, should be kept in mind, particularly with patients manifesting dysphagia or reflux symptoms poorly responsive to standard therapy. At endoscopy, the esophageal mucosa displays a ringed or furrowed appearance with granularity (Fig. 16-11).

If sensitization to particular foods is identified through radioallergosorbent or skin testing, an elimination diet is employed; patients with prohibitive numbers of food allergies may require an amino acid–based diet. Steroids may be necessary for children with negative investigation findings for food allergy or for whom compliance with a restricted diet is problematic.

GASTROINTESTINAL ISCHEMIA AND VASCULAR INSUFFICIENCY

Some of the causes of gastrointestinal ischemia can produce perforation, peritonitis, and death quite rapidly. A high degree of suspicion is useful, because the signs are nonspecific.

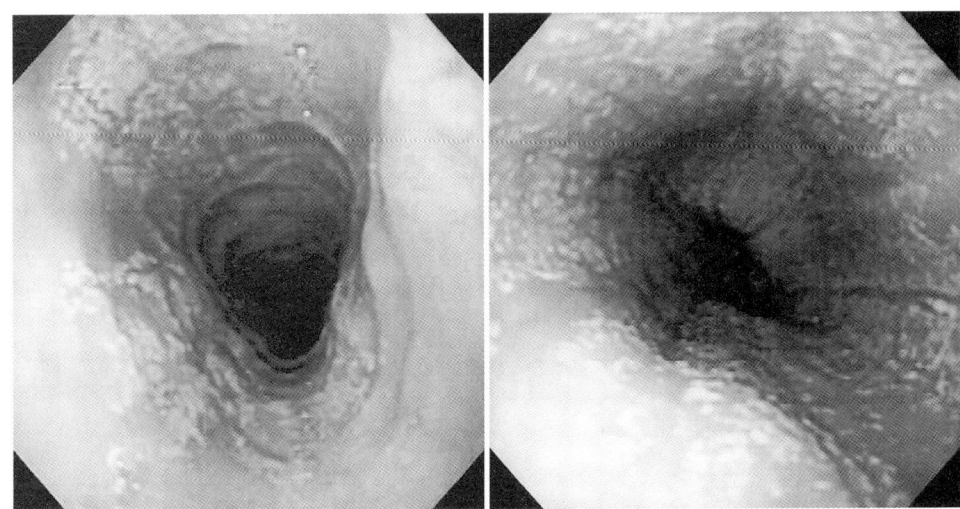

Figure 16-11. Endoscopic appearance of eosinophilic esophagitis, demonstrating concentric rings in proximal esophagus (**A**) and granularity with mucosal furrowing in digital esophagus (**B**). (Courtesy of Seema Khan, M.D.)

A   B

Abdominal Migraine

In this periodic syndrome of abdominal symptoms, epigastric or periumbilical pain may accompany nausea and vomiting. Diarrhea, fever, chills, vertigo, irritability, and polyuria have also been reported. The symptoms are probably a result of muscular constriction of the mesenteric arteries, which causes ischemia. Some pathophysiologic overlap with cyclic vomiting syndrome also has been proposed. When these abdominal symptoms coexist with head pain, which occurs in 30% to 40% of patients with migrainous headaches, the diagnosis is simpler than when they occur in isolation, which happens in about 3% of patients who later experience typical migrainous headaches. Usually, isolated abdominal migrainous attacks occur suddenly, last an hour to days, and are consistent in character within the same individual. There is usually a family history of migraine, and patients are asymptomatic between attacks. A personal history of car (motion) sickness may be present.

Symptoms of abdominal migraine often respond to prophylactic propranolol, cyproheptadine, or amitriptyline.

Vasculitis

Inflammation of the mesenteric vessels is uncommon but may cause gastrointestinal complaints, including vomiting, abdominal pain, diarrhea, and gastrointestinal bleeding. Henoch-Schönlein purpura is the most common pediatric vasculitis; systemic lupus erythematosus, dermatomyositis, polyarteritis nodosa, and other hypersensitivity vasculitides are occasional causes.

Henoch-Schönlein Purpura. The most diagnostic sign of Henoch-Schönlein purpura is the palpable purpuric rash, typically found on the buttocks, posterior legs, and feet in 97% of patients. However, because the vomiting or hematemesis and the nonspecific abdominal pain (found in nearly 90%) may precede the rash, the diagnosis may initially be obscure. Repeated examination of the skin of a child with persistent vomiting and pain is therefore useful, particularly when the gastrointestinal symptoms are accompanied by polyarthritis, which occurs in 65% of such patients.

Platelet function and coagulation studies are normal; hematuria is often present. Steroids may shorten the abdominal pain by 1 or 2 days, but they might also mask symptoms of accompanying intussusception or perforation.

Volvulus and Intussusception

Volvulus and intussusception have been discussed earlier, but, as noted, some of the symptoms and complications result from vascular obstruction and ischemia.

Mesenteric Ischemia

The mesenteric arteries may be occluded by emboli from a diseased heart or from thrombi formed locally. Nonocclusive ischemia may be caused by poor cardiac output, hypotension, dehydration, or endotoxemia. Mesenteric venous occlusion is very rare. Severe, crampy, diffuse abdominal pain may be accompanied by vomiting, diarrhea, or constipation. The crampy pain becomes continuous, and gangrene, peritonitis, sepsis, and shock supervene.

In a suggestive setting (e.g., heart disease), vomiting accompanied by diffuse severe abdominal pain should suggest the possible need for mesenteric and celiac angiography and emergency surgery. Acute arterial insufficiency may be preceded by chronic symptoms of "abdominal angina," which are episodes of several hours of crampy pain beginning about 20 minutes after meals. Such premonitory symptoms in suggestive settings should receive serious attention.

GASTROINTESTINAL PERFORATION AND PERITONITIS

Gastrointestinal perforation is often the end stage of obstructing, inflammatory, or ischemic disorders. Perforation is heralded by sudden abdominal pain, with subsequent signs of peritonitis (see Chapter 14). Perforated peptic ulcer pain may track to the right lower quadrant and mimic appendicitis, but the onset is more sudden, and the child is sicker than with appendicitis. Shock, metabolic acidosis, sepsis, and disseminated intravascular coagulopathy may ensue. Vomiting is not prominent.

When luminal obstruction leads to perforation and peritonitis, the abdominal findings change in characteristic ways. Vague, crampy, periumbilical pain becomes sharp, continuous, and localized. Rushes of increased, high-pitched bowel sounds disappear, leaving the abdomen silent. The active, sometimes writhing child becomes still. Vomiting previously associated with cramping pain is no longer present. The physical examination discloses point tenderness, abdominal rigidity, involuntary guarding, and rebound tenderness.

HEPATOBILIARY DISORDERS

Hepatitis

The presence of acute viral hepatitis (see Chapter 20) is usually suspected in patients who have jaundice, but up to 50% of patients with hepatitis A are anicteric, and even those in whom jaundice develops have a preicteric prodrome lasting up to a week. In children with acute hepatitis, therefore, the presenting symptom may be vomiting, another reason for including liver enzymes in the screening evaluation of the ill-appearing vomiting child. The vomiting is often accompanied by fatigue, fever, headache, rhinorrhea, sore throat, and cough.

The findings of serum antigens and antibodies to hepatitis viruses establish the diagnosis. Acute hepatitis with vomiting is treated symptomatically. Management also includes watching for the ominous findings of progressive encephalopathy, ascites, and coagulopathy.

Biliary Colic and Cholecystitis

Biliary obstruction (see Chapters 14 and 20) produces vomiting and abdominal pain in children; the vomiting is usually less severe and occurs later than that in pancreatitis. Biliary colic is visceral pain resulting from transient obstruction of the cystic duct, usually by a stone. In occasional patients, biliary dyskinesia causes these symptoms. Biliary colic produces several hours of steady, vaguely localized pain, often in the right upper quadrant; most patients also have vomiting. Episodes of biliary colic commonly recur at unpredictable intervals, from weeks to years. Acute cholecystitis may ensue if the obstruction persists and leads to inflammation of the gallbladder. The pain may localize more clearly to the right upper quadrant and may radiate to the back or shoulder. There may be fever or mild jaundice.

Serum alanine aminotransferase, aspartate aminotransferase, γ-glutamyl transpeptidase, alkaline phosphatase and bilirubin levels may be elevated. In both biliary colic and acute cholecystitis, abdominal films and ultrasonography may disclose stones or gallbladder thickening. Common duct stones may produce concurrent elevations of liver enzymes and pancreatic enzymes.

Recurrent biliary colic and cholecystitis are managed by cholecystectomy, which can now be performed laparoscopically in many children. Endoscopic removal of common duct stones is also possible, although it does not prevent recurrence.

PANCREATIC DISORDERS: PANCREATITIS

Pancreatitis is usually associated with epigastric abdominal pain, which may radiate to the back. Elevated serum amylase and lipase levels usually confirm the diagnosis. Pancreatitis with normal amylase but elevated lipase levels is not rare. Important causes of pancreatitis are noted in Chapter 14.

ADRENAL DISORDERS: HEMORRHAGE

Overwhelming sepsis, particularly with meningococcemia, is the most common cause of adrenal hemorrhage. Vomiting that is accompanied by shaking chills, headache, vertigo, petechial or purpuric rash, and very high or subnormal temperature characterizes the precipitous onset. Prostration, shock, and death occur quickly. Shock and fulminant sepsis can coexist without adrenal insufficiency. Adrenal hemorrhage may be identified by abdominal ultrasonography. Treatment includes appropriate antibiotics, intensive supportive care, and stress doses of steroids.

Other causes for adrenal hemorrhage are birth or other trauma, adrenal vein thrombosis, and seizures; it can also occur after excessive anticoagulation. In these settings, vomiting associated with flank or epigastric pain and hypotension should suggest acute adrenal insufficiency.

GYNECOLOGIC AND UROLOGIC DISORDERS

Pyelonephritis

High fever, chills, nausea, vomiting, and, less often, diarrhea develop rapidly. There may be symptoms of cystitis with dysuria, frequency, urgency, and suprapubic pain (see Chapter 23). Costovertebral angle tenderness focuses the diagnosis on the urinary tract.

The urinalysis shows pyuria and bacteriuria, and the hemogram shows leukocytosis. Treatment is with antibiotics.

Ureteropelvic Junction Obstruction and Hydronephrosis

Ureteropelvic junction obstruction ("beer-drinker's kidney," Dietl crisis) is caused by partial obstruction at the ureteropelvic junction and by the resulting hydronephrosis during fluid loading and diuresis. Congenital cases are usually diagnosed in the first year of life (usually on the basis of a renal hydronephrotic mass or urinary tract infection); 10% to 30% of affected older children present with flank or periumbilical pain, frequently accompanied by vomiting.

Typically, the symptoms commence in the evening after an increased fluid intake, although the hyperhydration history is often unclear. The child's pain and vomiting usually remit spontaneously in several hours, as dehydration gradually relieves the renal pelvic distention. Superimposed unilateral urinary tract infection may cause additional findings of fever, failure to thrive, and pyuria.

Ultrasonography at the time of an episode or after furosemide, or an intravenous pyelogram, provides the diagnosis; the treatment is surgical.

Renal Colic

Passage of a renal stone usually causes more pain than vomiting. Lateralized colicky pain, hematuria, and confirmatory radiologic studies assist the diagnosis.

Dysmenorrhea, Endometriosis, and Pelvic Inflammatory Disease

These gynecologic disorders manifest with lower abdominal pain but only occasionally manifest with vomiting. Association with menses or vaginal discharge aids the diagnosis. Motion of the cervix exacerbates the pain in pelvic inflammatory disease (see Chapter 29).

Ovarian Torsion

Torsion of a normal ovary occasionally occurs in girls of any age, probably caused by laxity of adnexal supports. Repeated attacks of crampy, lower abdominal pain culminates in a final acute episode with severe retching and vomiting, an enlarged ovarian mass, and eventual signs of peritonitis. Leukocytosis may be accompanied by fever.

The location of the pain suggests the diagnosis, and the treatment is surgical.

Hyperemesis Gravidarum

Pregnant adolescents may have prolonged vomiting. In parallel to the experience with ruminating infants, esophagitis has been suggested to play a role in this disease.

Testicular Torsion

Testicular torsion is a vascular emergency. It is readily diagnosed by the site of pain; surgical treatment is required (see Chapter 28).

RESPIRATORY DISORDERS

Sinusitis, Pharyngitis, and Otitis

Sinusitis may induce chronic, unexplained vomiting. The vomiting is more apt to occur in the morning and must be differentiated from serious intracranial processes. Sinus tenderness and sinus CT scans suggest the diagnosis, and a successful trial of antibiotic therapy confirms it. Less often, pharyngitis or otitis media may manifest acutely with nonspecific vomiting.

Pneumonia

Because pneumonia can also be caused by vomiting on the basis of aspiration, it is important to consider the direction of causality in children with pneumonia and vomiting. Aspiration of vomitus is particularly likely to occur in the context of obtundation or other neurologic dysfunction.

CENTRAL NERVOUS SYSTEM DISORDERS

Increased Intracranial Pressure

Various causes of increased intracranial pressure (e.g., tumors) induce vomiting, typically described as projectile but without retching. This description may be an oversimplification, but the occurrence on awakening and before eating is important information.

A careful neurologic and funduscopic examination, attention to measurement of occipitofrontal head circumference, and relevant radiologic studies (CT or magnetic resonance scans) should help the examiner make the diagnosis (see Chapter 40).

Abdominal Epilepsy

The diagnosis of abdominal epilepsy is suggested by recurrent episodes of nausea or vomiting, usually accompanied by abdominal pain and by symptoms suggesting its central nervous system origin, such as headache, dizziness, confusion, or temporary blindness. Patients may sleep after an episode.

The diagnosis is aided by neurologic consultation, electroencephalography during an episode, and response to anticonvulsant therapy.

Vestibular Disorders, Motion Sickness

Motion sickness is a nearly universal experience in some situations. Vestibular disorders produce similar symptoms (see Chapter 42).

Because of the symptoms of nausea, nystagmus, vertigo, and dizziness, the diagnosis is usually obvious. Antihistamines and anticholinergics are particularly useful for motion sickness.

Ventriculoperitoneal Shunt Complications

Occlusion or infection of a shunt may produce vomiting on a neurologic basis, whereas the intraabdominal end of the shunt may provoke intestinal obstruction by volvulus, adhesions, or loculations. These possibilities must be kept in mind for the vomiting patient with a shunt.

PSYCHOBEHAVIORAL DISORDERS

Psychogenic Vomiting

The syndrome of vomiting without organic cause illustrates the prominent influence that cortical and psychological inputs may have in stimulating nausea and vomiting. Characteristic features of psychogenic vomiting include chronicity, association with stress and with meals, suppressibility by distracting the patient, the patient's indifference toward the symptom itself, and relief by hospitalization. There may be no nausea or anorexia, and the vomiting may be self-induced.

Rumination

In the process of rumination, food is regurgitated, then mouthed or chewed and reswallowed, apparently voluntarily and pleasurably. Adults and older children may regurgitate by contracting abdominal muscles; infants may put their fingers or fists deep in their mouths in an apparent attempt to stimulate regurgitation. Whereas such apparent self-stimulation probably has a psychogenic origin in many cases, some infants cease ruminating when esophagitis is treated, which suggests that in some cases what appears to be an attempt to stimulate the gag reflex may actually be a response to pain in the throat. Thus, diagnosis of and treatment for both psychogenic causes and esophagitis should be considered.

Two types of rumination, psychogenic and self-stimulating, have been described. The former tends to occur in normal infants with a disturbed parent-child relationship; the latter occurs in mentally retarded individuals of any age and without regard to nurturing. Both positive reinforcement and negative reinforcement have been utilized in behavioral therapy.

Eating Disorders

Anorexia nervosa and bulimia are considered eating disorders primarily of psychogenic origin. However, symptoms of disordered upper gastrointestinal motility, including esophageal dysmotility, may manifest in a manner similar to these eating disorders, and patients with primary anorexia nervosa often manifest delayed gastric emptying, which may benefit from therapy with prokinetic agents.

Management

Psychiatric consultation and therapy are often needed for eating disorders, rumination, and psychogenic vomiting. Principles of behavior modification help to eliminate secondary gain from the vomiting. Nasogastric or nasojejunal feedings can be used to guarantee nutritional rehabilitation if voluntary oral nutrition is not readily reestablished; such tube feedings also provide the child with the incentive to return to oral nutrition. A prokinetic agent and H_2 receptor blocker therapy are often useful initially, both to treat esophagitis and to maximize forward movement of enteral nutrients through the gastrointestinal tract.

METABOLIC DISORDERS

Metabolic diseases that cause vomiting are difficult to diagnose because they are both rare and diverse. Their diagnosis and treatment, however, are crucial because of the severe morbidity and death they can cause and their amenability to treatment. They are also important because of their relevance to genetic counseling, inasmuch as most metabolic disorders are hereditary, on an autosomal recessive basis. Situations that should prompt consideration of metabolic diseases are listed in Table 16-7.

The history and physical examination (Table 16-13) and screening studies (Table 16-14) that help distinguish among many of the specific metabolic disorders provide useful clues. Laboratory studies should be done while the child is symptomatic. Vomiting accompanied by hyperammonemia is a particular diagnostic problem, for which a schematic is presented in Figure 16-12.

POISONINGS AND DRUGS

Most ingested poisons, and some absorbed by inhalation, skin contact, or intravenous administration, induce vomiting, which can be seen as a physiologic protection against harmful substances. Symptoms and signs of some of the most common pediatric poisonings causing vomiting are indicated in Table 16-15. Acute known poisonings, either accidental or intentional, are a management problem rather than a diagnostic one. A Poison Control Center and more complete references on poisoning (see references) should be consulted for more detail. When an acute poisoning is suspected but the agent is unknown, these resources are also useful.

Initial diagnostic evaluation can be directed by a careful search of the environment for poisonous items and by toxicology screens on blood, urine, vomitus, and stool; these materials should not be discarded. A few agents, such as lead, cause chronic poisoning, manifested by vomiting, among other symptoms. Because it may be particularly difficult to suspect and treat these poisonings, an index of suspicion of poisoning is important in the chronically vomiting child. Laboratory studies that are useful in addition to toxicology screenings are presented in Table 16-16.

HEMATEMESIS

Endoscopic evaluation (and therapy) is often needed for children with hematemesis (see Chapter 17). Before such evaluation, however, it is important to know the most likely causes (see Table 16-10). The physician should also have determined that there is no underlying coagulopathy necessitating correction (see Table 16-11) and that hematemesis is a primary symptom, not a secondary one caused by a Mallory-Weiss tear.

Peptic ulcer disease, particularly duodenal ulcer, is the most common cause of hematemesis in children; in newborns, swallowed maternal blood (uterine, breast milk), esophagitis, gastritis, and duodenal ulcers are most common; in preschool children, gastric ulcers predominate; and in older children and adolescents, duodenal ulcers are most common. Esophagitis is occasionally severe enough to cause hematemesis, as is Barrett's ulcer, a premalignant lesion superimposed on chronic esophagitis. Obstructive lesions such as pyloric stenosis and antral webs are occasionally associated with hematemesis.

Variceal bleeding is uncommon but serious. Gastric vascular malformations are rare and serious and may be difficult to diagnose. Duplications are lined by gastric mucosa in 30% of affected patients; if they are located above the ligament of Treitz, they may cause hematemesis. The metabolic and toxic (iron, salicylates, theophylline, corrosives, isopropyl alcohol, mushroom poisoning) causes of hematemesis should be kept in mind.

Therapy of hematemesis includes, as needed, correction of any abnormalities of coagulation: hemostasis, stabilization of

Table 16-13. Metabolic Disease: History and Physical Examination

	Neurologic			Liver		Gastrointestinal	Respiratory		Precipitants/ Aversions	Other
	Lethargy, Coma	Hypo-hypertonicity	Seizure	Jaundice	Hepatomegaly	Diarrhea	Tachypnea	Apnea		
Galactosemia	+			+	+	+	(+)		Galactose	Eye: cataracts (use slit lamp)
Fructose-1-phosphate aldolase ↓: HFI	+		+	+	+	+	(+)		Fructose	Absent caries (older child)
Tyrosinemia	+			+	(+)	+				Odor: cabbage; Quebe native; ↑ AFP; hepatoma
Maple syrup urine disease	+	+	+				+	+	Protein; infections	Odor: maple syrup
Hypervalinemia*	+	+								
HHH syndrome*	+	+	+		(+)				Protein	Occasional bleeding tendency
Lysinuric protein intolerance	+	+			+/spl	+			Protein; fasting; infections	Hair fragile; Finnish native ↑; ferritin ↑
Methylmalonic acidemia	+	+	(+)		(+)		+		Protein	Vitamin B₁₂ responsive or not?
Propionic acidemia	+	+	(+)		(+)		+		Protein; infections	Osteoporosis
Isovaleric acidemia*	+	(+)	+				+		Protein; infections	Odor: sweaty feet
3-Methylcrotonyl-CoA carboxylase ↓*	(+)	+				(+)	+	+	Protein; infections	Odor: cat urine; biotin unresponsive
Multiple carboxylase ↓*	+	+	+				+	+	Protein; infections	Odor: cat urine; biotin responsive; rash
Glutaric acidemia I	+	+	(+)		+		(+)		Infections	Fevers
Glutaric acidemia II	+	+			(+)		(+)		?Fasting	Odor: sweaty feet; heart; renal
Acyl-CoA dehydrogenase ↓: MCAD, etc	+		(+)		(+)		(+)	(+)	Fasting; infections	
HMG-CoA lyase ↓*	+	+	(+)		(+)		+		Protein; fasting	
Wolman disease*	+	(+)		(+)	(+)/spl	+				Adrenal calcifications; foam cells
Farber disease*	(+)	+			(+)					Skin nodules; arthritis; hoarseness
Urea cycle (AL, AS, CPS, OTC)	+	+	+		+		+	+	Protein; infections	Respiratory alkalosis; trichorrhexis (AL)
Reye syndrome ?Miscellaneous fatty acid oxidation ↓	+	+	+	No	+					Prior virus (flu, varicella); salicylates
Diabetic ketoacidosis	+						+			Odor: ketones

Continued

Table 16-13. Metabolic Disease: History and Physical Examination—cont'd

	Neurologic			Liver		Gastrointestinal	Respiratory		Precipitants/Aversions	Other
	Lethargy, Coma	Hypo-hypertonicity	Seizure	Jaundice	Hepatomegaly	Diarrhea	Tachypnea	Apnea		
Adrenal insufficiency	+					(+)				Pigment: skin, mucosa (80%–98%); salt craving (20%)
Chronic, primary: Addison disease										
Acute: adrenal crisis									Sepsis; steroid DC	Shock; abdominal pain (34%); K↑; Na↓
Congenital adrenal hyperplasia	+									M or virilized F neonate; salt-losing
RTA, Fanconi syndrome							(+)			Acidosis and urine findings
Nephrogenic diabetes insipidus									Water deprivation	Polyuria; polydipsia; dehydration
Uremia	(+)		(+)		+/spl				Protein	Odor: uremic fetor; BUN↑; BP↑
Glucose-6-phosphatase ↓ (GSD I)			+		+		+		Fasting	Doll-like face; TG-xanthomas; epistaxis

*Fewer than 100 patients with each of these disorders have been reported. Incidences of the other 11 diseases listed before Reye syndrome are 1/20,000 to 1/200,000. GSD I is ~1/200,000; diabetes is acquired in ~1/400 children; adrenal insufficiency of all causes is relatively frequent; congenital adrenal hyperplasia with salt-losing 21-hydroxylase deficiency is ~1/5000.

AFP, alpha-fetoprotein; AL, arginosuccinic acid lyase deficiency; AS, arginosuccinic acid synthase deficiency; BP, blood pressure; BUN, blood urea nitrogen; CoA, coenzyme A; CPS, carbamyl phosphate synthase deficiency; DC, discontinuation; F, female; GSD, glycogen storage disease; HFI, hereditary fructose intolerance; HHH, hyperornithinemia-hyperammonemia-homocitrullinemia syndrome; HMG, 3-hydroxy-3-methylglutaric acidemia; K, potassium; M, male; MCAD, medium-chain; acyl-CoA dehydrogenase deficiency; Na, sodium; OTC, ornithine transcarbamylase deficiency; RTA, renal tubular acidosis; spl, splenomegaly; TG, triglycerides; +, common; (+), may occur; ↓, deficiency.

Table 16-14. Metabolic Disease: Laboratory Studies

	Blood							Urine†					
	pH ↓	Glucose ↓	NH₃* ↑	LFTs ↑	CBC (Het ↓ WBC ↓ Plt ↓)	Amino Acids	Ketones	Red. Subs.	FeCl +	Fanconi Syndrome†	Amino Acids	Organic Acids	Orotate
Galactosemia	+	+		+	Lysis			+Non-glucose	?	+			
Fructose-1-phosphate aldolase ↓: HFI	+	+		+	+	+		+Non-glucose	?	+	+		
Tyrosinemia	(+)	+		+	(↑)	+	Suc-ace	+phppa	+Green	+	+	+phppa	
Maple syrup urine disease					(↑)	+	+		+Gray		+		
Hypervalinemia						+					+		
HHH syndrome			+			+					+	+	
Lysinuric protein intolerance			+	(+)	+	+					+	+	
Methylmalonic acidemia	+	+	+		+	(+)	+				(+)	+	
Propionic acidemia	+	+ No: ↑	+		+	+	+				+	+	
Isovaleric acidemia	+	+			+	+	+					+	
3-Methylcrotonyl-CoA carboxylase ↓	+	+					+					+	
Multiple carboxylase ↓	+	+	+				+					+	
Glutaric acidemia type I	+	+	+	+			No				+	+	
Ethylmalonic-adipic aciduria, etc.	+	+	(+)	(+)							+	+	
Acyl-CoA dehydrogenase ↓: MCAD, etc.	+	+	(+)	(+)			No (↓)					+	
HMG-CoA lyase ↓	+	+	(+)	(+)			No					+	
Wolman disease				+	Vacuoles								
Farber disease													
Urea cycle defects	+	No	+			+							+
Reye syndrome	+	+	+	+		+						+	
Miscellaneous fatty acid oxidation ↓												+	
Diabetic ketoacidosis	+	No:↑					+	+ Glucose	+ Red				
Adrenal insufficiency Chronic, primary: Addison disease Acute: adrenal crisis													
Congenital adrenal hyperplasia													
Renal tubular acidosis; Fanconi syndrome	(+)							(Glucose)		+			
Nephrogenic diabetes insipidus													
Uremia													
Glycogen storage disease type I	+	+			(+)								

*See Figure 16-12.

†Glucose, amino acids, phosphate.

CBC, complete blood count; CoA, coenzyme A; FeCl, iron chloride; Het, hematocrit; HFI, hereditary fructose intolerance; HHH, hyperornithinemia-hyperammonemia-homocitrullinemia syndrome; HMG, 3-hydroxy-3-methylglutaric acidemia; LFTs, liver function tests; MCAD, medium-chain acyl-CoA dehydrogenase deficiency; NH₃, ammonia; phppa, p-OH-phenylpyruvate; Plt, platelets; Red Subs, reducing substances; Suc-ace, succinylacetone; WBC, white blood cell count; (+), may occur; +, common.

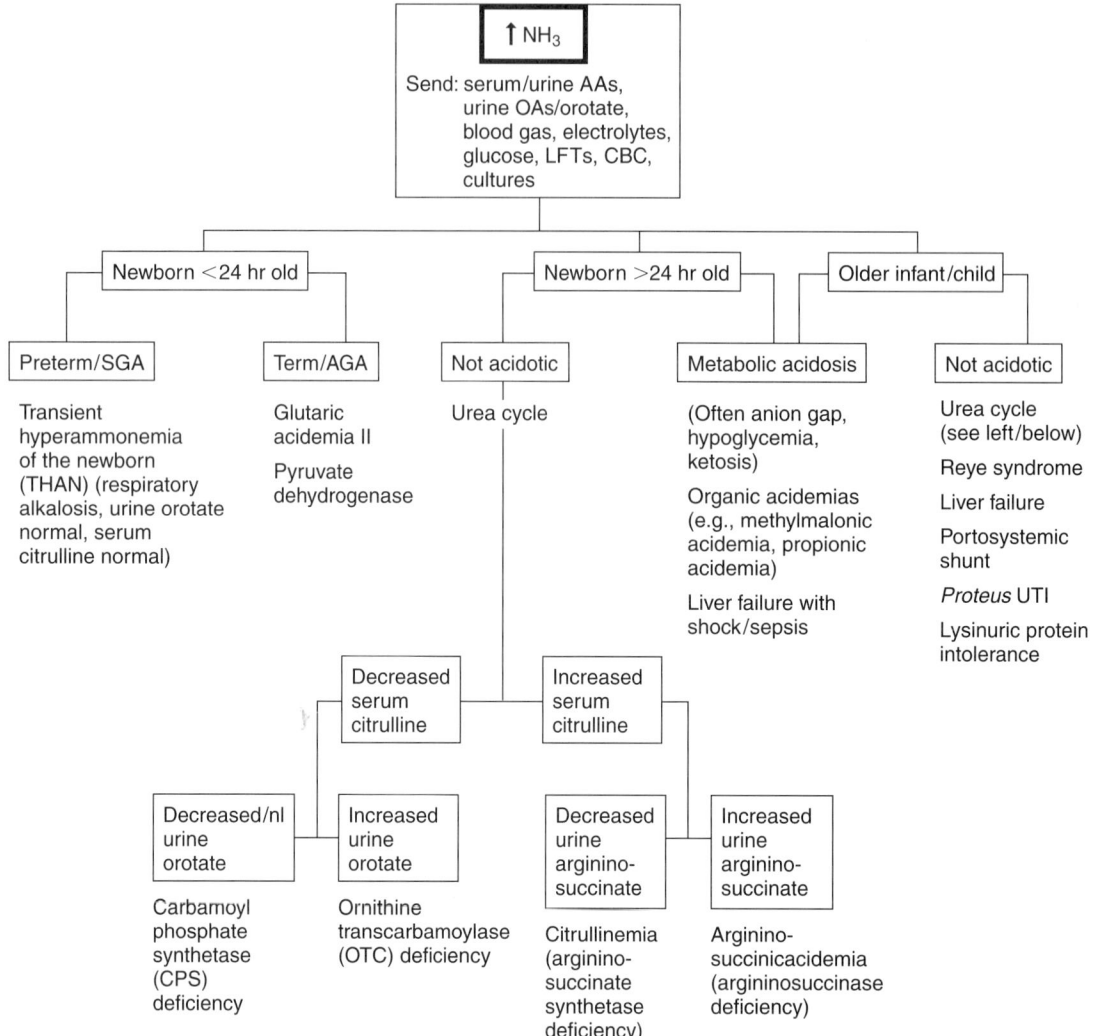

Figure 16-12. Flow diagram for evaluation of hyperammonemia in children. AAs, amino acids; AGA, appropriate for gestational age; CBC, complete blood count; LFTs, liver function tests; nl, normal; OAs, organic acids; SGA, small for gestational age; UTI, urinary tract infection.

hemodynamic status, and direct attention to the bleeding site endoscopically (e.g., heater probe, injection therapy) or surgically. Reduction of gastric acid secretion pharmacologically is useful in virtually all cases of hematemesis and carries minimal risk.

OTHER CAUSES OF VOMITING

Chemotherapy

Chemotherapy causes predictable vomiting, which is usually not a diagnostic but a management problem. It may be complicated by anticipatory vomiting. Ondansetron, high-dose metoclopramide (accompanied by diphenhydramine for prophylaxis of extrapyramidal side effects), dexamethasone, and the marijuana-related nabilone have all shown some effectiveness against chemotherapy-induced vomiting. Anxiolytics may also be beneficial as a component of combination antiemetic therapy.

Radiation Therapy

Like chemotherapy, radiation therapy may cause acute vomiting, apparently by stimulating giant retrograde peristaltic waves. Subacutely, diarrhea predominates as a complication of radiation therapy. Months to years later, vomiting may again be a result of

radiation therapy, often caused by inflammatory ulcers and strictures. These lesions are difficult to treat without surgery.

Cyclic Vomiting

Cyclic vomiting syndrome (CVS) is a chronic, potentially disabling condition marked by a history of three or more bouts of intense, acute nausea and vomiting that may last hours or days, punctuated by entirely symptom-free intervals that last weeks to months. Work-up, which may ultimately include endoscopy and imaging studies of the gastrointestinal tract and brain, reveals no evidence of significant underlying primary disease. Typically, bouts begin in children 2 to 7 years old (range, 6 months to 18 years) and occur an average of 12 times yearly (range, 1 to 70). For a particular patient, episodes tend to begin at the same time of day (usually during the night or early morning hours) and have similar durations. An inciting event such as an infection or emotional excitement can be identified in 80% of episodes. Bouts are often accompanied by pallor, intolerance of noise or light, abdominal pain, or diarrhea. The pathophysiologic process of CVS remains speculative at this time but may overlap with that of migrainous phenomena. One hypothesis purports that stress-initiated release of corticotropin-releasing hormone leads to cascading production of substances such as adrenocorticotropic hormone, antidiuretic hormone, histamine, and catecholamines, which in turn mediate the

Table 16-15. Poisoning: History and Physical Examination

	Vital Signs				Neurologic					Pupils			Skin	Odor	Other
	P ↑↓	R ↑↓	BP ↑↓	T ↑↓	Coma	Ψ	Paralysis	Ataxia	Sz	↑	↓	Nystagmus			
Ipecac															ECG changes
Salicylates	•		•	•	•	•			•				Cyanotic	Acetone	Metabolic acidosis; tinnitus; uremia; bleeding
Acetaminophen					•								Jaundiced		Ill 24 hr → better × 48 hr → liver failure
Digitalis	•		•		•	•			•						CNS and arrhythmias; vision changes
Theophylline	•	•	•		•	•			•						Hematemesis/pain; arrhythmia
Fe (Iron)	•	•	•		•	•		•	•				Jaundiced		Hematemesis/pain → liver failure; pyloric stenosis
Pb (Lead)			•		•	•	•	•	•						Constipation; HA; abdominal pain; renal
Misc. (Sb, As, Cd, Cr, Hg, Zn)					•	•			•				Jaundiced	Garlic	Diarrhea; LFTs ↑; Hct ↓; nephritis; neuritis
Metal fume fever (oxides)				•											Muscle pain/HA; WBC ↑; respiratory distress
Opiates/narcotics	•	•	•		•	•			•		•		Cyanotic		Abdominal cramping
Opiate withdrawal		•	•							•					Irritable; BS ↑/pain; reflexes ↑; sweat; tear
Insecticides (miscellaneous)		•	•		•			•			•		Miscellaneous		Wheeze; salivation; sweat; tear
Especially organophosphates	•				•				•		•			Garlic	Diarrhea/abdominal pain; vision impaired
Corrosives						•									Pain; hematemesis; respiratory distress
Methanol					•	•			•	•		•	Cyanotic	Acetone	Blindness; metabolic acidosis
Ethanol		•	•		•	•		•	•				Pink	Alcohol	Vision impaired; hypoglycemia
Isopropyl alcohol				•	•									Acetone	Hematemesis/pain; oliguria
Ethylene glycol					•		•		•	•		•	Cyanotic		Anuria
"Food poisoning"															See Chapter 15
Fish poisoning							•		•						Some seasonally poisonous; paresthesia
Shellfish: summer ingestion							•								Respiratory paralysis; paresthesia
Plants (akee, hemlock)	•		•			•			•						Respiratory; renal; shock; liver
Mushroom poisoning	•	•	•		•	•			•	•			Jaundiced		Respiratory; hepatic failure; hematemesis
Venomous bites (see Chapter 53)									•		•		Lesion		Bite history

As, arsenic; BP, blood pressure; BS, bowel sounds; Cd, cadmium; CNS, central nervous system; Cr, chromium; ECG, electrocardiographic; HA, headache; Hct, hematocrit; Hg, mercury; LFTs, liver function tests; P, pulse; R, respiration; Sb, antimony; Sz, seizure; T, temperature; WBC, white blood count; Zn, zinc; ψ, psychological manifestations; •, present.

Table 16-16. Poisoning: Laboratory Studies and Treatment

	Laboratory Studies												Treatment*	
	CBC	Electrolytes	Ca, Mg, Phos	BUN, Creat	Glucose	LFTs, Coag	ABGs	UA	Other	Level	Lavage	Charcoal and 70% Sorbitol	Diuresis? Dialysis? Other?	Specific
Ipecac														
Salicylates	•	•	•	•	•	•	•	•	ECG FeCl Purple	•	•	•	•	Fluids, electrolytes HCO₃, vitamin K
Acetaminophen	•	•				•				•				N-acetylcysteine
Digitalis		•	•	•			•		ECG	•	• (Vagal hazard)	•		Digibind, antiarrhythmics
Theophylline	•	•	•		•	•	•		ECG	•	•	No		Antiarrhythmics, antiseizure
Fe (Iron)	•				•		•		KUB	•	•	No	•	Deferoxamine, fluids
Pb (Lead)	•							•	KUB Bones	FEP				BAL-CaEDTA, fluids, succimer
Others (Sb, As, Cd, Cr, Hg, Zn, P)	•					•			KUB	•	•			
Metal fume fever (oxides)	•													
Opiates/Narcotics											•			Narcan (0.01 mg/kg)
Opiate withdrawal														Methadone, paregoric, diazepam, phenobarbital
Organophosphate cholinesterase														Atropine
Corrosives	•					•	•		CXR		No	No		Antibiotics, endoscopy
Methanol		•		•					ECG	•	•	No	•	Ethanol
Ethanol					•							No	•	Glucose/bicarbonate
Isopropyl alcohol	•			•			•				•	No	•	
Ethylene glycol				•			•					?No	•	Ethanol, ?Ca gluconate
"Food poisoning"														
Fish poisoning											•			
Shellfish: summer ingestion														
Plants (akee, castor, hemlock)	•	•		•		•		•			•	•		
Mushroom poisoning				•				•			•			Atropine?, cimetidine
Venomous bites		•	•			•		•						Antiserum

*The utility of emesis/lavage varies with the poison, the amount ingested, and the duration since ingestion. If obtunded, lavage requires endotracheal tube airway protection. Avoid charcoal/sorbitol in recent bowel surgery or ileus.

ABGs, arterial blood gases; As, arsenic; BUN, blood urea nitrogen; BAL-CaEDTA, dimercaprol–calcium ethylenediaminetetraacetic acid; Ca, calcium; CBC, complete blood count; Cd, cadmium; Coag, coagulation studies; Cr, chromium; Creat, creatinine; CXR, chest radiography; ECG, electrocardiography; FeCl, iron chloride; FEP, free erythrocyte protoporphyrin; HCO₃, bicarbonate; Hg, mercury; KUB, kidney, ureter, and bladder; LFTs, liver function tests; Mg, magnesium; P, phosphorus; Phos, phosphate; Sb, antimony; UA, urinalysis; Zn, zinc; •, present.

syndrome's signs and symptoms. Some children may harbor subclinical defects in mitochondrial fatty acid oxidation metabolism or neuronal ion channel function that heighten their susceptibility to attacks when confronted by the increased cellular energy needs created by a physiologic or emotional stressor. Although CVS is now becoming better characterized, the physician should not be lulled into missing treatable, "look-alike" organic conditions. Reported cases of organic disease mislabeled "cyclic vomiting" have included intermittent intussusception or volvulus caused by enteric duplication, diverticulum, or malrotation; increased intracranial pressure in patients with shunts who have slit ventricles; and toxic or metabolic disease. Additional considerations in the differential diagnosis include brainstem glioma, obstructive uropathy, porphyria, and familial dysautonomia.

In CVS, the patient experiences nausea and pallor during the stereotypical and characteristic episodes but is symptom-free between episodes.

Medications potentially useful in CVS prophylaxis and in treatment of acute episodes are listed in Table 16-17.

Porphyria

Acute intermittent porphyria is an autosomal dominant disorder of episodic abdominal pain (85% to 95% of patients); 40% to 90% of patients have associated vomiting. The association of neurologic symptoms such as mental symptoms (50%), muscle weakness (50%), sensory loss (20%), and convulsions (15%); the onset after puberty; and the frequent association with menses or provocative drugs (phenobarbital) are suggestive. Elevated levels of porphobilinogen and δ-aminolevulinic acid in urine are suggestive, and decreased red blood cell porphobilinogen deaminase is diagnostic.

Familial Mediterranean Fever (Benign Paroxysmal Peritonitis, Periodic Peritonitis, Polyserositis)

Episodic attacks of abdominal pain with rapid development and resolution (within 48 hours) of peritoneal signs (fever, vomiting, absent bowel sounds) occurring in a child of Israeli or North African

---

Table 16-17. Pharmacologic Therapies for Vomiting Episodes

Disease/Condition	Therapy–Drug Class: Specific Agent/Trade Name (Dose)
Reflux	Dopamine antagonist: metoclopramide (Reglan) (0.1-0.2 mg/kg q.i.d. PO/IV)
	Peripheral dopamine antagonist: domperidone (Motilium) (0.2–0.6 mg/kg t.i.d.-q.i.d. PO)
Gastroparesis	Metoclopramide, domperidone; see above
	Motilin agonist: erythromycin (2-4 mg/kg t.i.d.-q.i.d. PO/IV)
Intestinal pseudoobstruction	Stimulation of intestinal migratory myoelectric complexes: octreotide (Sandostatin) (1 μg/kg b.i.d.-t.i.d. SC)
Chemotherapy	Metoclopramide; see above (0.5-1.0 mg/kg q.i.d. IV, with antihistamine prophylaxis of extrapyramidal side effects)
	Serotoninergic 5-HT$_3$ antagonist: ondansetron (Zofran) (0.15-0.3 mg/kg t.i.d IV/PO)
	Phenothiazines: (extrapyramidal, hematologic side effects)
	prochlorperazine (Compazine) (≈0.3 mg/kg b.i.d.-t.i.d. PO)
	chlorpromazine (Thorazine) (>6 months of age: 0.5 mg/kg t.i.d.-q.i.d. PO/IV)
	Steroids: dexamethasone (Decadron) (0.1 mg/kg t.i.d. PO)
	Cannabinoids: nabilone (tetrahydrocannabinol) (0.05-0.1 mg/kg b.i.d.-t.i.d. PO)
Postoperative	Ondansetron, phenothiazines: see above
Motion sickness; vestibular disorders	Antihistamine: dimenhydrinate (Dramamine) (1 mg/kg t.i.d.-q.i.d. PO)
	Anticholinergic: scopolamine (Transderm Scōp) (adults: 1 patch/3 days)
Adrenal crisis	Steroids: cortisol (2 mg/kg bolus IV followed by 0.2-0.4 mg/kg/hr IV [± 1 mg/kg IM])
Cyclic vomiting syndrome (CVS)*	Supportive:
	Analgesic: meperidine (Demerol) (1-2 mg/kg q4-6h IV/IM)
	Anxiolytic, sedative: Lorazepam (Ativan) (0.05-0.1 mg/kg q6h IV)
	Antihistamine, sedative: diphenhydramine (Benadryl) (1.25 mg/kg q6h IV)
	Abortive:
	Serotoninergic 5-HT$_3$ antagonist:
	Ondansetron: see above
	Granisetron (Kytril) (10 μg/kg q4-6h IV)
	Nonsteroidal antiinflammatory agent (GI ulceration side effect):
	Ketorolac (Toradol) (0.5-1.0 mg/kg q6-8h IV)
	Serotoninergic 5-HT$_{1D}$ agonist: sumatriptan (Imitrex) (>40 kg; 20 mg intranasally/25 mg PO, one time only)
	Prophylactic: (if >1 CVS bout/month; taken daily)
	Antimigraine, β-adrenergic blocker: propranolol (Inderal) (0.5-2.0 mg/kg b.i.d. PO)
	Antimigraine, antihistamine: cyproheptadine (Periactin) (0.25-0.5 mg/kg/day ÷ b.i.d.-t.i.d.PO)
	Antimigraine, tricyclic antidepressant: amitriptyline (Elavil) (0.33-0.5 mg/kg t.i.d. PO, and titrate to maximum of 3.0 mg/kg/day as needed; obtain baseline ECG at start of therapy, and consider monitoring drug levels)
	Antimigraine antiepileptic: Phenobarbital (Luminal) (2-3 mg/kg q.h.s.)
	Erythromycin: see above
	Low estrogen oral contraceptives: consider for catamenial CVS episodes

*Adapted from Li BUK, Balint JP: Cyclic vomiting syndrome: Evolution in our understanding of a brain-gut disorder. Adv Pediatr 2000:47:149.

b.i.d., twice daily; ECG, electrocardiogram; GI, gastrointestinal; IM, intramuscularly; IV, intravenously; PO, orally; q4-6h, every 4 to 6 hours; q6h, every 6 hours; q6-8h, every 6 to 8 hours, q.h.s. each bedtime; SC, subcutaneously; t.i.d., three times daily; q.i.d., four times daily.

descent should suggest this autosomal recessive diagnosis. Synovitis, pleuritis, and an erysipelas-like skin lesion are also characteristic. The erythrocyte sedimentation rate is raised. Fifty percent of patients have their first attack between 1 and 10 years of age; 90%, by age 20. Amyloidosis, a possible etiologic role for C5a inhibitor deficiency, and probable response to colchicine have been described. Definitive genetic testing is now available for detection of the familial Mediterranean fever gene, which has been localized to the short arm of chromosome 16.

FAMILIAL DYSAUTONOMIA

Familial dysautonomia may manifest with episodic vomiting. It is an autosomal recessive disorder of the sensory and autonomic nervous systems affecting children of Ashkenazi Jewish descent. The gene for familial dysautonomia has been localized to the distal long arm of chromosome 9, allowing for both prenatal diagnosis and identification of carriers. Associated symptoms include disturbed swallowing, drooling, frequent pneumonias, absence of overflow tearing, erratic temperature control, skin blotching, postural hypotension, relative indifference to pain, corneal anesthesia, breath-holding spells, motor incoordination, spinal curvature, and growth retardation. Glossal fungiform papillae are also absent. The disease is diagnosed with the intradermal histamine test or the conjunctival methacholine (or pilocarpine) test.

Management is complex and requires a multidisciplinary team.

COMPLICATIONS OF VOMITING

The complications of vomiting are shown in Table 16-18. Their importance is twofold. First, these complications, particularly the metabolic, nutritional, esophagitis, and hemodynamic ones, must be treated. Second, there may be diagnostic implications. Hematemesis resulting from Mallory-Weiss tear should be distinguished from primary hematemesis caused by some other lesion. Metabolic acidosis or hyperkalemia should be recognized as atypical for vomiting illnesses and possible crucial signs of metabolic disease or severe intraabdominal disease.

METABOLIC COMPLICATIONS

Dehydration results from the inability to ingest fluid effectively, because of anorexia or nausea, as well as from the loss of secretions in the emesis. Alkalosis resulting from loss of gastric hydrogen chloride in the vomitus is exacerbated by a shift of H^+ into cells because of potassium deficiency and by contraction of the extracellular fluid because of sodium deficiency. Potassium and sodium are lost in the vomitus, and are also wasted by the kidneys, when they accompany the renal excretion of bicarbonate caused by the alkalosis. In states of marked alkalosis, urine pH is 7 or 8, and urinary sodium and potassium levels are high despite sodium and potassium depletion. Urine chloride, however, remains low, reflecting the nonrenal losses of sodium chloride and potassium chloride.

If intravenous fluid therapy is required, it must be designed with understanding of the sodium and potassium deficits. The usual metabolic alkalosis is adequately compensated by the patient's spontaneous hyperpnea and responds to fluid and electrolyte therapy.

NUTRITIONAL COMPLICATIONS

The nutritional deficits resulting from chronic vomiting and associated anorexia are obvious. Their correction must be included in the treatment plan for chronic vomiting. No more than a day or two of fluid therapy should take place without attention to nutritional needs. Frequent, small, high-carbohydrate feedings may minimize the stimulation to vomit, but continuous nasogastric feedings are sometimes needed for chronic vomiting. The presence of metabolic or allergic disease should be considered when the reintroduction of protein leads to relapse of symptoms.

MALLORY-WEISS TEAR

This linear mucosal laceration in the juxtaesophageal gastric mucosa usually occurs after prolonged forceful retching or vomiting, but it

Table 16-18. Complications of Vomiting

Complication	Pathophysiology	History, Physical Examination, and Laboratory Studies
Metabolic	Fluid loss in emesis	Dehydration
	HCl loss in emesis	Alkalosis*; hypochloremia
	Na, K loss in emesis	Hyponatremia; hypokalemia*
	Alkalosis →	
	Na into cells	
	HCO_3 loss in urine	Urine pH 7-8
	Na and K loss in urine	Urine Na ↑, K ↑
	Hypochloremia →	
	Cl conserved by kidneys	Urine Cl ↓
Nutritional	Emesis of calories and nutrients	Malnutrition; "failure to thrive"
	Anorexia for calories and nutrients	
Mallory-Weiss tear	Retching → tear at lesser curve of gastroesophageal junction	Forceful emesis → hematemesis
Esophagitis	Chronic vomiting → esophageal acid exposure	Heartburn; Hemoccult + stool
Aspiration	Aspiration of vomitus, especially in context of obtundation	Pneumonia; neurologic dysfunction
Shock*	Severe fluid loss in emesis or in accompanying diarrhea	Dehydration (accompanying diarrhea can explain acidosis?)
	Severe blood loss in hematemesis	Blood volume depletion

*If patient is acidotic, hyperkalemic, or in shock, see Table 16-20.

Cl, chloride; HCl, hydrogen chloride; HCO_3, bicarbonate; K, potassium; Na, sodium.

occasionally produces blood in the initial vomitus. Invisible radiographically, it is diagnosed endoscopically (if necessary).

Mallory-Weiss tears usually necessitate no treatment, but transfusion is occasionally necessary. Intractable cases are quite rare and may be treated with vasopressin infusion, balloon tamponade, angiographic embolization, or surgery.

PEPTIC ESOPHAGITIS

Esophagitis, similar to that resulting from gastroesophageal reflux, may result from chronic vomiting from many causes. Diagnosed endoscopically or histologically, it should be treated. The treatment of esophagitis usually includes H_2 receptor antagonists or proton pump inhibitors; prokinetic agents may also be needed. The use of antacids should be tempered by knowledge of the acid-base status of the patient.

THERAPY

Therapy of vomiting starts with treatment of the cause, treatment of complications, and treatment of behavioral aspects that may perpetuate the vomiting. General supportive and more specific pharmacologic approaches to therapy are outlined in Table 16-17 and Table 16-19. The physician should be very careful about treating the vomiting symptom without diagnosing and treating its cause. In several situations, diagnostic procedures, such as diatrizoate (Gastrografin) enema for fecal obstructions in cystic fibrosis, barium enema for intussusception, and endoscopy with sclerotherapy for variceal hematemesis, are also therapeutic.

TREATMENT OF BEHAVIORAL ASPECTS

Treatment of psychobehavioral aspects of vomiting may also be important because of the cortical influences on emesis. Such treatment may include eliminating secondary gain for vomiting and reducing anxiety about the vomiting through a confident approach to the child.

ANTIEMETIC DRUGS

In situations of persistent vomiting, antiemetic drugs are useful to reduce the metabolic and nutritional consequences and perhaps

to interrupt vicious circles in which psychogenic factors may also participate. Currently available antiemetic drugs include the prokinetic agents, metoclopramide, erythromycin, domperidone, and bethanechol as well as the other medications listed in Table 16-17. These drugs function at many sites by

- modifying central cortical input (anxiolytic agents)
- depressing the chemoreceptor trigger zone (metoclopromide, domperidone)
- reducing vestibular input
- enhancing the secretion or effects of acetylcholine from the motor neuron (cisapride, available in the United States on restricted-use protocol only)
- blocking serotonin receptors, which inhibit the function of the acetylcholine-secreting motor neuron (ondansetron)
- blocking dopamine's inhibitory effect at the neuromuscular junction (domperidone, metoclopramide)
- stimulating the motilin receptor on gastric smooth muscle (erythromycin)
- substituting for acetylcholine's stimulatory effect at the neuromuscular junction (bethanechol)

In some settings, the diverse sites of action account for the useful additive effects of these drugs. Optimal therapy for vomiting caused by chemotherapy, for example, may include several agents in order to provide blockade of the multiple receptor types in the chemoreceptive trigger zone and elsewhere. Metoclopramide and ondansetron have been the most widely used general antiemetic agents.

SUMMARY AND RED FLAGS

Vomiting and regurgitation are commonly encountered symptoms in children. Most commonly they are the result of acute, self-resolving illnesses, such as acute gastroenteritis. In infants, regurgitation caused by gastroesophageal reflux must be distinguished from other more serious causes. Symptoms suggesting vomiting emergencies are listed in Table 16-11 and Table 16-20. These are generally diseases that arise after surgery, are metabolic, or are caused by poisoning, but liver failure and neurologic disorders are also included.

Table 16-19. Supportive and Nonpharmacologic Therapies for Vomiting Episodes*	
Disease	**Therapy**
All	Treat Cause: obstruction → operate; allergy → change diet (± steroids); metabolic error → Rx defect; acid peptic disease → H_2RAs, PPIs, etc.
Complications	
Dehydration	IV fluids, electrolytes
Hematemesis	Transfuse, correct coagulopathy
Esophagitis	H_2RAs, PPIs
Malnutrition	NG or NJ drip feeding useful for many chronic conditions
Mecomium ileus	Gastrografin enema
DIOS	Gastrografin enema; balanced colonic lavage solution (e.g.,GoLytely)
Intussusception	Barium enema; air reduction enema
Hematemesis	Endoscopic: injection sclerotherapy or banding of esophageal varices; injection therapy, fibrin sealant application, or heater probe electrocautery for selected upper GI tract lesions
Sigmoid volvulus	Colonoscopic decompression
Reflux	Positioning; dietary measures (infants: rice cereal, 1 TBSP/ounce of formula)
Psychogenic components	Psychotherapy; tricyclic antidepressants; anxiolytics (e.g., diazepam: 0.1 mg/kg/t.i.d.-q.i.d. PO)

*If patient is acidotic, hyperkalemic, or in shock, see Table 16-20; adrenal crisis therapy outlined in Table 16-17.

DIOS, distal intestinal obstruction syndrome; GI, gastrointestinal; H_2RAs, histamine$_2$-receptor antagonists; IV, intravenous; NG, nasogastric; NJ, nasojejunal; PO, orally; PPIs, proton pump inhibitors; q.i.d, four times a day; TBSP, tablespoon; t.i.d, three times a day.

Table 16-20. Vomiting Emergencies*

Symptoms	Drug/Poison†	Metabolic‡	Surgical	Neurologic	Liver Failure	Further Laboratory Studies
Shock	+	+	+			
Mental status change, lethargy, coma, seizure, psychosis	++	++		+++	+++	NH_3, head CT/MRI, glucose
Severe abdominal pain/distention	++	+	+++		+	Abdominal films
Acute liver dysfunction Jaundice Anicteric	++	++	+	+	+++	NH_3, PT
Respiratory Apnea, Kussmaul's breathing	++	++	+	++	++	Blood gas; electrolytes; urinalysis, glucose
Other						
Bilious emesis		+	+++		+	Abdominal films
Silent abdomen			+++			
Hematemesis			+		++	Endoscopy

*An acutely ill child with vomiting needs:

Physical examination: especially vital signs, neurologic, funduscopic, abdominal (ausculation, peritoneal signs), rectal.

Laboratory tests: complete blood cell count, differential white blood cell count, platelets; sodium, potassium, chloride, carbon dioxide; glucose (Dextrostix); blood urea nitrogen, creatinine; liver function tests; amylase, lipase; blood gas; urinalysis.

If fever is present: cultures of blood, urine, cerebrospinal fluid (if mentation change), and stool (if diarrhea or hematochezia) are also needed.

If hematemesis is present: platelets, prothrombin time, and partial thromboplastin time also must be measured.

†See Tables 16-15, 16-16.

‡See Tables 16-13, 16-14.

CT, computed tomography; MRI, magnetic resonance imaging, NH_3, ammonia; PT, prothrombin time.

+, suggestive; ++, moderately suggestive; +++, highly suggestive.

REFERENCES

General

Li BUK, Sferra TS: Vomiting. In Wyllie R, Hyams JS (eds): Pediatric Gastrointestinal Disease: Pathophysiology, Diagnosis, Management. Philadelphia, WB Saunders, 1999, pp 14-31.

Lilien LD, Srinivasan G, Pyati SP, et al: Green vomiting in the first 72 hours in normal infants. Am J Dis Child 1986;140:662-664.

Martin TG, Burgess JL: Dreisbach's Handbook of Poisoning, 13th ed. London: Parthenon Publishing, 2001.

O'Neill JA, Rowe MI, Grosfield JL, et al: Pediatric Surgery, 5th ed. St. Louis: Mosby–Year Book, 1998.

Rollins MD, Shields MD, Quinn RJM, et al: Value of ultrasound in differentiating causes of persistent vomiting in infants. Gut 1991;32:612-614.

Scriver CR, Beaudet AL, Sly WS, et al: The Metabolic and Molecular Bases of Inherited Disease, 7th ed. New York: McGraw-Hill Information Services, 1995.

Gastrointestinal Obstruction

Caniano DA, Beaver BL: Meconium ileus: A fifteen year experience with forty-two neonates. Surgery 1987;102:699-703.

Champoux A, Del Beccaro M, Nazar-Stewart V: Recurrent intussusception: Risk features. Arch Pediatr Adolesc Med 1994;148:474-478.

Depaepe A, Dolk H, Lechat MF, et al: The epidemiology of tracheo-oesophageal fistula and oesophageal atresia in Europe. Arch Dis Child 1993;68:743-748.

Devane SP, Coombes R, Smith VV, et al: Persistent gastrointestinal symptoms after correction of malrotation. Arch Dis Child 1992;67:218-221.

Ford EG, Senac MO, Srikanth MS, et al: Malrotation of the intestine in children. Ann Surg 1992;215:172-178.

Hernanz-Schulman M: Imaging of neonatal gastrointestinal obstruction. Radiol Clin North Am 1999;37:1163-1186.

Macdessi J, Oates RK: Clinical diagnosis of pyloric stenosis: A declining art. BMJ 1993;306:553-555.

Mitchell LE, Risch N: The genetics of infantile hypertrophic pyloric stenosis. A reanalysis. Am J Dis Child 1993;147:1203-1210.

Rescorla FJ, Shedd FJ, Grosfeld JL, et al: Anomalies of intestinal rotation in childhood: Analysis of 447 cases. Surgery 1990;108:710-716.

Seashore JH, Touloukian RJ: Midgut volvulus. An ever-present threat. Arch Pediatr Adolesc Med 1994;148:43-46.

Gastroesophageal Reflux

Albanese CT, Towbin RB, Ullman I, et al: Percutaneous gastrojejunostomy versus Nissen fundoplication for enteral feeding of the neurologically impaired child with gastroesophageal reflux. J Pediatr 1993;123:371-375.

Booth IW: Silent gastro-oesophageal reflux: How much do we miss? Arch Dis Child 1992;67:1325-1326.

Brown P: Medical management of gastroesophageal reflux. Curr Opin Pediatr 2000;12:247-250.

Chidiac P, Alexander IS: Head retraction and respiratory disorders in infancy. Arch Dis Child 1990;65:567.

Grill BB: Twenty-four-hour esophageal pH monitoring: What's the score? J Pediatr Gastroenterol Nutr 1992;14:249-251.

Hoeffel JC, Nihoul-Fekete C, Schmitt M: Esophageal adenocarcinoma after gastroesophageal reflux in children. J Pediatr 1989;115:259-261.

Kiely EM: Surgery for gastro-oesophageal reflux. Arch Dis Child 1990; 65:1291-1292.

Orenstein SR: Prone positioning in infant gastroesophageal reflux: Is elevation of the head worth the trouble? J Pediatr 1990;117:184-187.

Orenstein SR: Update on gastroesophageal reflux and respiratory disease in children. Can J Gastroenterol 2000;14:131-135.

Orenstein SR, Izadnia F, Khan S: Gastroesophageal reflux disease in children. Gastroenterol Clin North Am 1999;28:947-969.

Orenstein SR, Shalaby TM, DiLorenzo C, et al: The spectrum of pediatric eosinophilic esophagitis beyond infancy: A clinical series of 30 children. Am J Gastroenterol 2000;95:1422-1430.

Rudolph CD, Mazur LJ, Liptak GS, et al: Evaluation and treatment of gastroesophageal reflux in infants and children: Recommendations of the

North American Society for Pediatric Gastroenterology and Nutrition. J Pediatr Gastroenterol Nutr 2001;32(Suppl 2):S1-S31.

Shulman RJ, Boyle JT, Colletti RB, et al: Use of cisapride in children. An updated medical position statement of the North American Society for Pediatric Gastroenterology and Nutrition. J Pediatr Gastroenterol Nutr 2000;31:232-233.

Other Etiologies

Barkin RM: Toxicologic emergencies. Pediatr Ann 1990;19:629-633.

Bray GP: Liver failure induced by paracetamol. BMJ 1993;306:157-158.

Buck ML, Grebe TA, Bond GR: Toxic reaction to salicylate in a newborn infant: Similarities to neonatal sepsis. J Pediatr 1993;122:955-958.

Duane PD, Magee TM, Alexander MS, et al: Oesophageal achalasia in adolescent women mistaken for anorexia nervosa. BMJ 1992;305:43.

Fleisher D, Matar M: Cyclic vomiting syndrome: A report of 71 cases and literature review. J Pediatr Gastroenterol Nutr 1993;17:361-369.

Forbes D: Cyclic vomiting syndrome. In Hyman PE (ed): Pediatric Functional Gastrointestinal Disorders. New York, Academy Professional Information Services, 1999, pp 5.1-5.12.

Gordon GS, Wallace SJ, Neal JW: Intracranial tumours during the first two years of life: Presenting features. Arch Dis Child 1995;73:345-347.

Harrington J, Gianos E, Stiefel M: Index of suspicion: Case 3. Diagnosis: Riley-Day syndrome (familial dysautonomia [FD]). Pediatr Rev 2000; 21:243, 246-247.

Li BUK, Balint JP: Cyclic vomiting syndrome: Evolution in our understanding of a brain-gut disorder. Adv Pediatr 2000;47:117-160.

Rasquin-Weber A, Hyman PE, Cucchiara S, et al: Childhood functional gastrointestinal disorders. Gut 1999;45(Suppl II):II60-II68.

Samuels J, Aksentijevich I, Torosyan Y, et al: Familial Mediterranean fever at the millennium: Clinical spectrum, ancient mutations, and a survey of 100 American referrals to the National Institutes of Health. Medicine 1998;77:268-297.

Therapy

Grunberg SM, Hesketh PJ: Control of chemotherapy-induced emesis. N Engl J Med 1993;329:1790-1796.

Israel DM, Hassall E: Omeprazole and other proton pump inhibitors: Pharmacology, efficacy, and safety, with special reference to use in children. J Pediatr Gastroenterol Nutr 1998;27:568-579.

Kulig K: Initial management of ingestions of toxic substances. N Engl J Med 326;25:1677-1681.

Pinkerton CR, Williams D, Wootton C, et al: 5-HT$_3$ antagonist ondansetron— An effective outpatient antiemetic in cancer treatment. Arch Dis Child 1990;65:822-825.

17 Gastrointestinal Bleeding

Francisco A. Sylvester   Jeffrey S. Hyams

Gastrointestinal bleeding in children can range from small amounts of blood in the stool, associated with milk protein allergy or anal fissure, to life-threatening hemorrhage, associated with portal hypertension or peptic ulcer disease. Fortunately, the overwhelming majority of cases are of a benign nature. However, severe bleeding is a true medical emergency and necessitates prompt diagnostic attention and appropriate management. Hemodynamic stabilization of the patient with severe bleeding should always precede diagnostic studies. An accurate history and thorough physical examination usually allow the physician to categorize the problem as mild or severe and to direct evaluation at the appropriate pace.

DEFINITIONS

Children with gastrointestinal bleeding generally present with hematemesis, hematochezia, or melena, although the clinical manifestation can be as subtle as evidence of occult blood loss. The initial diagnostic evaluation should focus on determining whether the source of the bleeding is from the upper or the lower gastrointestinal tract (Tables 17-1 and 17-2). Bleeding from the esophagus, stomach, or duodenum is an *upper gastrointestinal bleed.* Blood in vomitus confirms an upper gastrointestinal source. A *lower gastrointestinal bleed* is a site of bleeding distal to the ligament of Treitz. Blood passed per rectum can originate from either an upper gastrointestinal source or a lower one. Determining whether the site of bleeding is in the upper or lower gastrointestinal tract affects not only the differential diagnosis but also therapeutic interventions. Occult bleeding can occur from disorders at numerous sites (Table 17-3).

Hematemesis. Vomited blood can be either red or like the color of coffee grounds. Hematemesis is most commonly associated with an upper gastrointestinal bleed, although swallowed blood produces the same clinical picture. Bright red hematemesis suggests active bleeding that has not come in contact with gastric secretions. When gastric secretions have had a chance to interact with the blood, "coffee ground" emesis results.

Hematochezia and Melena. Maroon stools from the rectum are generally associated with a lower gastrointestinal bleed. The presence of melena—passage of black, tarry stools—generally results from significant blood loss proximal to the ileocecal valve. The color results from bacterial breakdown of the hemoglobin. The presence of hematochezia (bright red blood) is generally associated with colonic bleeding, although brisk upper gastrointestinal bleeding (e.g., duodenal ulcer, esophageal varices) can produce a similar clinical picture.

DIAGNOSTIC STRATEGIES

The first step is to determine whether the problem is actually gastrointestinal bleeding. Many foodstuffs and other substances may simulate blood. Punch (Kool-Aid), gelatin, food coloring, beets,

laxatives, and antibiotic syrups can mimic bright red blood. Some substances, such as iron, bismuth (Pepto Bismol), beets, licorice, spinach, and blueberries, can simulate melena. Nongastrointestinal sources of bleeding, such as epistaxis, hemoptysis, recent dental work, pharyngitis, recent tonsillectomy, or menses, can complicate the diagnosis.

TESTS FOR BLOOD

Stool guaiac and the modified guaiac (Gastroccult) tests for emesis are used to determine the presence of blood. These tests are readily available, inexpensive, and very sensitive. Red meat, vegetables, fruit high in vitamin C or rich in peroxidases, supplemental vitamin C in excess of 250 mg/day, aspirin, and antiinflammatory drugs (steroids and nonsteroidal antiinflammatory drugs [NSAIDs]) should be avoided for 3 days before testing. Although iron preparations may blacken stools, they do not lead to false-positive results. Female patients should be told not to collect test samples for 3 days after a menstrual period. To avoid potential false-positive or false-negative results, stool should be collected from diapers or from disposable collection devices rather than directly from toilet water. Finally, an Apt-Downey test should be performed when a breast-fed infant vomits bright red blood or passes bloody (red) stools, to distinguish whether maternal or fetal hemoglobin is the cause.

HISTORY

Historical information can be extremely important and should be obtained promptly. A history of vomiting, regurgitation, or abdominal pain suggests a mucosal lesion. Forceful, repeated vomiting may result in a Mallory-Weiss tear. Severe, acute abdominal pain occurs in patients with vascular compromise, such as in intussusception, midgut volvulus, and bowel ischemia (e.g., Henoch-Schönlein purpura). The presence of large amounts of blood from the mouth without the presence of significant gastric fluid suggests variceal bleeding until proven otherwise.

A previous history of jaundice, hepatitis, or blood transfusion should be obtained (see Chapter 20). Sepsis, shock, neonatal exchange transfusions, neonatal umbilical vein catheterization, and neonatal omphalitis are risk factors for portal vein thrombosis. Painless rectal bleeding suggests a Meckel diverticulum, a duplication, a polyp, or angiodysplasia. On rare occasions, painless rectal bleeding may be secondary to a deep ulceration of the right colon or terminal ileum, as in Crohn disease. Bloody diarrhea, which may or may not be associated with tenesmus, is typical of an inflammatory colitis (see Chapter 15). Infectious causes of bleeding should be sought (see Chapter 15). Information regarding travel (either by the patient or by visitors), sick contacts, day care exposure, camping, and antibiotic exposure should be obtained. Rectal bleeding in infants may be caused by milk or soy protein intolerance; dietary history is mandatory. Hirschsprung disease may manifest as enterocolitis, and often there is a history of constipation. Constipation in a well-appearing child may suggest a rectal fissure as the source of

Table 17-1. Upper Gastrointestinal Bleeding

Age Grouping	Common	Less Common
Neonates (0-30 days)	Swallowed maternal blood during delivery or from breast milk Gastritis Duodenitis	Coagulopathy Sepsis Vitamin K deficiency Vascular malformation Leiomyoma Gastric or esophageal duplication
Infants (30 days-1 year)	Gastritis/gastric ulcer Esophagitis Duodenitis	Esophageal varices Foreign body Aortoesophageal fistula Gastrointestinal duplication Leiomyoma
Children (1-18 years)	Esophagitis Esophageal varices Gastroduodenal ulcer Gastritis Mallory-Weiss tear Nasopharyngeal bleeding Prolapse gastropathy	Gastrointestinal duplication Vascular malformation Thrombocytopenia Munchausen syndrome by proxy Leiomyoma Pulmonary hemorrhage Hematobilia

Modified from Olson AD, Hillemeier AC: Gastrointestinal hemorrhage. In Wyllie R, Hymans JS (eds): Pediatric Gastrointestinal Disease. Philadelphia, WB Saunders, 1993, p 259.

Table 17-2. Lower Gastrointestinal Bleeding

Age Grouping	Common	Less Common
Neonates (0-30 days)	Swallowed maternal blood during delivery or from breast milk Milk protein allergy Anal fissure Upper gastro-intestinal bleeding	Coagulopathy Sepsis Vitamin K deficiency Vascular malformation Hirschsprung's enterocolitis Intestinal duplication Necrotizing enterocolitis Colonic stricture post-NEC Volvulus
Infants (30 days-1 year)	Anal fissure Upper gastro-intestinal bleeding Intussusception Meckel diverticulum Infectious diarrhea Milk protein allergy	Vascular malformation Volvulus Intestinal duplication Thrombocytopenia Eosinophilic colitis Perianal strepto-coccal cellulitis
Children (1-18 years)	Anal fissure Infectious diarrhea Intussusception (<3 yr) Meckel diverticulum Inflammatory bowel disease Milk allergy (<4 yr) Upper gastrointestinal bleeding Juvenile polyps	Henoch-Schönlein purpura Vascular malformation Vasculitis Nodular lymphoid hyperplasia Pseudomembranous colitis Intestinal duplication Perianal strepto-coccal cellulitis Hemorrhoids Solitary rectal ulcer Colonic or rectal varices Rectal trauma or sexual abuse

Modified from Olson AD, Hillemeier AC: Gastrointestinal hemorrhage. In Wyllie R, Hymans JS (eds): Pediatric Gastrointestinal Disease. Philadelphia, WB Saunders, 1993, p 259.

NEC, necrotizing enterocolitis.

bleeding (see Chapter 21). There may be a history of perianal pain or discomfort with bowel movements. The blood is often bright red and coats the stool rather than being mixed throughout. This can also be seen in cases of proctitis.

Information regarding chronic pulmonary disease, renal disease, bleeding disorders, and liver disease should be obtained. Patients with cystic fibrosis are at risk not only for the development of esophageal varices caused by biliary cirrhosis but also for coagulopathies from vitamin K deficiency. Hemorrhagic disease of the newborn occurs when neonates do not receive prophylactic vitamin K (see Chapter 50). In patients with renal disease, uremia causes platelet dysfunction, which may manifest as a gastrointestinal bleed. Certain medications, such as NSAIDs, are possible causes of bleeding. The family history should address the presence of bleeding disorders, peptic ulcer disease, polyps, and inflammatory bowel disease.

PHYSICAL EXAMINATION

A careful physical examination is mandatory and aids in the differential diagnosis and management (Table 17-4). Immediate attention must be given to signs of hypovolemia, anemia, or shock. An orthostatic change, such as a pulse rate increase of 20 beats per minute or a drop in systolic blood pressure of more than 10 mm Hg when the patient changes from the supine to standing positions, is a sensitive index of significant volume depletion, usually greater than 20%. Blood pressure may remain normal up to the point of circulatory collapse in children.

The child's growth curve should be reviewed. It may suggest a chronic disease such as inflammatory bowel disease, which is some-times associated with digital clubbing or failure to thrive. Cutaneous lesions should be evaluated. Hyperpigmented lesions of the oral or anal mucosa may indicate Peutz-Jeghers disease. Petechiae can indicate disseminated intravascular coagulation or another bleeding abnormality. Purpura, although not always present initially, is seen in Henoch-Schönlein purpura; it may also be seen in hemolytic uremic syndrome. Cutaneous telangiectasia and hemangiomas may indicate such diseases as Osler-Weber-Rendu syndrome and ataxia-telangiectasia, or they may simply suggest a predisposition for

Table 17-3. Causes of Occult Gastrointestinal Bleeding

Inflammatory Causes

Peptic esophagitis
Crohn disease
Ulcerative colitis
Mild enterocolitis
Celiac disease
Eosinophilic gastroenteritis
Meckel diverticulum
Solitary colon ulcer

Vascular Causes

Angiodysplasia and vascular ectasias
Gastroesophageal varices
Congestive gastropathy
Hemangiomas

Drugs

Nonsteroidal anti-inflammatory drugs

Extragastrointestinal Causes

Hemoptysis
Epistaxis
Oropharyngeal bleeding

Infectious Causes

Hookworm
Strongyloidiasis
Ascariasis
Tuberculous enterocolitis
Amebiasis

Tumors and Neoplastic Causes

Polyps
Lymphoma
Leiomyoma
Lipoma
Carcinoma

Artifactual Causes

Hematuria
Menstrual bleeding
Nonspecific test positivity

Miscellaneous Causes

Long-distance running
Coagulopathies
Factitious

Modified from Ahlquist DA: Approach to the patient with occult gastrointestinal bleeding. In Yamada T (ed): Textbook of Gastroenterology. Philadelphia, JB Lippincott, 1991, p 620.

Table 17-4. Signs and symptoms in Gastrointestinal (GI) Hemorrhage

Sign	Indication	Site of Bleeding
Splenomegaly Caput medusae Jaundice	Portal hypertension	Esophageal varices Portal gastropathy
Hemangioma Telangiectasis	Multiple hemangioma syndrome	Vascular malformation of GI tract
Hematemesis	Bleeding from above the ligament of Treitz	Upper GI tract
Melena	Bleeding from above the ileocecal valve	Upper GI tract or small intestine
Hematochezia	Colonic bleeding, massive upper GI bleeding	GI tract
Nasogastric aspirate: gross blood	Bleeding from above the ligament of Treitz	Upper GI tract
Palpable purpura	Henoch-Schönlein purpura	GI tract
Mouth ulcers, perianal fistula, or skin tags; erythema nodosum, arthritis, uveitis	Inflammatory bowel disease	Lower GI tract

Modified from Olson AD, Hillemeier AC: Gastrointestinal hemorrhage. In Wyllie R, Hyams JS (eds): Pediatric Gastrointestinal Disease. Philadelphia, WB Saunders, 1993, p 251.

vascular malformations. Jaundice or spider nevi suggest underlying liver disease; subcutaneous nodules or masses may be part of an underlying polyposis syndrome.

The abdomen is examined closely for bowel sounds and bruits before palpation of the abdomen is performed, because palpation may induce gas movement in an otherwise silent abdomen. A prominent venous pattern and an enlarged spleen or ascites suggest portal hypertension (see Chapter 19). Tenderness and guarding indicate a significant inflammatory process. A right lower quadrant abdominal mass suggests intussusception in an infant or toddler.

During the rectal examination, the anus needs to be examined closely for fissures, skin tags, or fistulas, all of which are seen in Crohn disease. Local tenderness and erythema suggests group A β-hemolytic streptococcus infection. During the digital examination, tenderness may indicate the presence of inflammation. Stool should

be checked for occult blood by a rectal examination. This procedure should be performed even if a bloody specimen is brought directly to the emergency department. Stool should be checked for the presence of white blood cells. If the stool smear shows large numbers of white blood cells, a stool culture for enteric infections, such as *Salmonella, Shigella, Yersinia,* and *Campylobacter* species and *Escherichia coli* O157:H7, is warranted (see Chapter 15).

LABORATORY AND DIAGNOSTIC EVALUATION

A complete blood cell count with differential should be performed and repeated. If the bleeding has been very recent, it may take time for the hematocrit to equilibrate to a new, lower value. The mean corpuscular volume is normal in acute bleeding but is commonly low in chronic, low-grade bleeding. An elevated differential white blood cell count suggests acute inflammation. An elevated eosinophil count may signify a hypersensitivity or an allergic process (e.g., eosinophilic gastroenteritis) or inflammatory bowel disease. Thrombocytopenia may indicate hemolytic uremic syndrome, another consumptive process, hypersplenism, or failure of bone marrow production. Prothrombin time and partial thromboplastin time should be measured to rule out a bleeding diathesis. Prothrombin time is an excellent marker of liver function and should be determined as part of screening for significant liver disease. Severe gastrointestinal hemorrhage itself can cause a prolonged prothrombin time and partial thromboplastin time. Serum creatinine, electrolytes, and blood urea nitrogen are helpful for detecting kidney disease and secondary electrolyte disturbances. Normal serum aminotransferases make the diagnosis of liver disease less likely.

Hematemesis establishes an upper gastrointestinal source. As mentioned, blood passed per rectum may originate from an upper or lower gastrointestinal source. A nasogastric tube should be placed in any child in whom the source of bleeding is not clear. The possibility of bleeding varices is not a contraindication to placement of a nasogastric tube. Some clinicians also use an indwelling nasogastric tube to monitor the activity of upper gastrointestinal bleeding during therapeutic intervention. In cases of pyloric channel or duodenal bulb lesions, the gastric lavage may be nonbloody as a result of edema and partial obstruction at the level of the lesion. The clinical history of significant vomiting and persistent high-volume drainage from the nasogastric tube should raise suspicion for these lesions.

Esophagogastroduodenoscopy (EGD) is the procedure of choice in identifying the site of upper gastrointestinal bleeding. EGD can also allow direct intervention at the bleeding site, as in the case of esophageal varices or a visible vessel in an ulcer crater. Endoscopic visualization of the stomach and duodenum should be performed even if the bleeding is thought to originate from esophageal varices. Of patients with proven esophageal varices, 50% may manifest bleeding from gastritis or peptic ulcer disease rather than the varices. Endoscopy, however, should not be performed until the patient is as hemodynamically stable as possible.

Lower gastrointestinal tract bleeding can also be evaluated endoscopically. Procedures frequently used in children include proctosigmoidoscopy and flexible colonoscopy. With the patient under appropriate sedation, exploration of the distal colon to the level of the splenic flexure can be achieved with a 60-cm flexible sigmoidoscope, and the entire colon to the terminal ileum can be explored with the flexible colonoscope. Therefore, lower gastrointestinal endoscopy allows for full exploration of the colon; identifies the presence of multiple lesions; allows for therapeutic intervention to bleeding lesions through electrocoagulation, laser therapy, or thermocoagulation; and allows for removal of bleeding lesions, such as polyps. Colonoscopy is indicated when there is melena or severe bleeding with no evidence of upper gastrointestinal lesions, when stools are guaiac-positive over a long time, and when examination of the terminal ileum is indicated to determine whether inflammatory bowel disease is present. One disadvantage is that large amounts of luminal blood obscure visualization of a lesion. Before lower gastrointestinal colonoscopy, intestinal lavage with oral administration of polyethylene glycol should be used to remove as much of the luminal blood and stool as possible. If intussusception is suspected, a contrast enema is indicated and may also be therapeutic. An upper gastrointestinal contrast study is indicated for suspected volvulus and occasionally for peptic ulcer disease. Abdominal ultrasonography is not the preferred imaging study but has at times been useful in the diagnosis of volvulus or intussusception. Scans of tagged red blood cells may help identify vascular sources of gastrointestinal bleeding.

DIFFERENTIAL DIAGNOSIS

See also Common Causes of Gastrointestinal Bleeding below.

Swallowed maternal blood is frequently misinterpreted as upper gastrointestinal bleeding in neonates after birth or in breast-fed infants. The blood may have been swallowed during delivery or through cracked, irritated nipples in breast-fed infants. Rupture of a milk duct may produce bleeding into milk without obvious features on physical examination. Diagnosis is based on obtaining an Apt test on bloody (red) fluid to confirm the presence of maternal blood. "Bleeding" does not recur once the source is eliminated and the initial swallowed blood is passed.

In infants, esophagitis, gastritis, and ulcers are the most common causes of upper gastrointestinal bleeding. Esophagitis may be associated with dysphagia, irritability, and arching with feeds (see Chapter 16). Clinical signs of gastroesophageal reflux may not be prominent. An allergic origin should be considered. Diagnosis is made by EGD, and treatment consists of gastric acid suppression if reflux is suspected or dietary intervention in cases of allergy. In children with forceful emesis, hematemesis may be the presenting feature of pyloric stenosis or other causes of gastric outlet obstruction.

Mallory-Weiss tears can occur in infants. These tears are most commonly associated with repeated forceful vomiting from a variety of causes (e.g., acute gastroenteritis). The forcefulness of the vomiting causes a tear in the distal esophagus at the level of the lower esophageal sphincter. The history is generally one of frequent nonbloody vomiting that then becomes hematemesis. *Prolapse gastropathy,* caused by prolapse of gastric mucosa into the distal esophagus, can similarly occur in infants who vomit forcefully. Diagnosis is commonly made on a clinical basis; if not, the diagnosis is made by esophagoscopy. Treatment is of the underlying cause of vomiting and, if necessary, with blood transfusion.

Causes of lower gastrointestinal bleeding in the neonate and infant are numerous. *Anal fissures* are probably the most frequent cause of streaks of bright red blood. The bleeding may be associated with hard bowel movements. There is an association with group A streptococcal perianal cellulitis and bleeding; if the perianal area is erythematous, this pathogen should be sought and treated appropriately with antibiotics. If streptococci are not present, healing generally occurs within 24 to 48 hours. Local treatment with zinc oxide is helpful. Anal fissure may also be a manifestation of milk protein allergy with resultant perianal inflammation and subsequent constipation to avoid painful defecation.

Infectious colitis causes infants to have frequent, often watery bloody bowel movements (see Chapter 15). The patient feels crampy pain before and during the bowel movement as a result of the colitis. Common pathogens include *Salmonella* and *Shigella* organisms, especially with dysentery type stools, but *E. coli* O157:H7, *Campylobacter* species, *Yersinia* species, and *Entamoeba histolytica* should also be considered. A specimen obtained by rectal swab and cultured for pathogens is the quickest means to the diagnosis. A stool culture is more likely to be positive early in the course of illness. The specimen is obtained before a rectal examination with lubricant because of the presence of bacteriostatic agents in the lubricants. Antibiotic treatment depends on the specific organism and the status of the patient with regard to age and immunocompetence (see Chapter 15).

Milk protein allergy may manifest with bloody stools. There may be a history of increasing frequency along with blood and mucus in the stool. The infant may exhibit cramping with bowel movements; this needs to be distinguished from infectious colitis. In general, the patients appear well, but vomiting may be part of the presentation. There may be peripheral eosinophilia along with mild anemia. There may be a few white blood cells in the stool and, on occasion, eosinophils. Often there is a family history of food allergies. Milk protein allergy can be seen in infants fed cow's milk– or soy protein–based formulas, as well as in breast-fed infants. On occasion, bleeding may even be seen in infants on protein hydrolysate formulas. Treatment involves the removal of the specific antigen through the change to a hypoallergenic formula. Restricting cow's milk protein and potentially other antigens in the mother's diet may result in cessation of bleeding in 30% to 40% of breast-fed infants.

Meckel diverticulum occurs in 1% to 3% of the population. It is more common in boys and often manifests by the age of 2 years. When bleeding occurs from this lesion, it is usually brisk and painless. Bleeding results from mucosal ulceration secondary to secretion of gastric acid or pepsin from ectopic gastric or pancreatic tissue, respectively, in the tip of the diverticulum. The blood ranges from dark red to bright red.

Diagnosis is made by a Meckel scan (Fig. 17-1). A positive scan has a high correlation with finding a diverticulum at the time of surgery. There have been reports of negative scans in patients with a documented Meckel diverticulum. In the presence of a negative scan and repeated bleeding episodes, the scan should be repeated. Treatment is by surgical removal.

Necrotizing enterocolitis is usually associated with rectal bleeding in sick-appearing, low-birth-weight neonates. Risk factors include prematurity, cyanotic heart disease, polycythemia, chronic diarrhea, and gastrointestinal malformations. The rectal bleeding may be preceded or accompanied by signs of illness, such as apnea, lethargy, cyanosis, bradycardia, and temperature instability. Diagnosis is confirmed by the presence of pneumoperitoneum, pneumatosis intestinalis, or hepatic portal vein gas on radiologic examination of the abdomen. Treatment consists of bowel rest, broad-spectrum antibiotics, and surgery if intestinal perforation is present.

IMAGING

RADIOGRAPHY

Radiographic studies are useful in identifying mass lesions or mucosal ulcerations. A simple flat plate of the abdomen helps exclude large abdominal masses and may indicate intestinal obstruction. Upper gastrointestinal contrast studies can discern anatomic lesions, such as strictures, stenoses, atresias, errors in rotation, large ulcerations, and masses. Most mucosal lesions in children are best evaluated with endoscopy because children cannot comply with the procedures necessary for air-contrast examination of the gastrointestinal tract. Small bowel follow-through examination allows evaluation of the small bowel from the ligament of Treitz to the

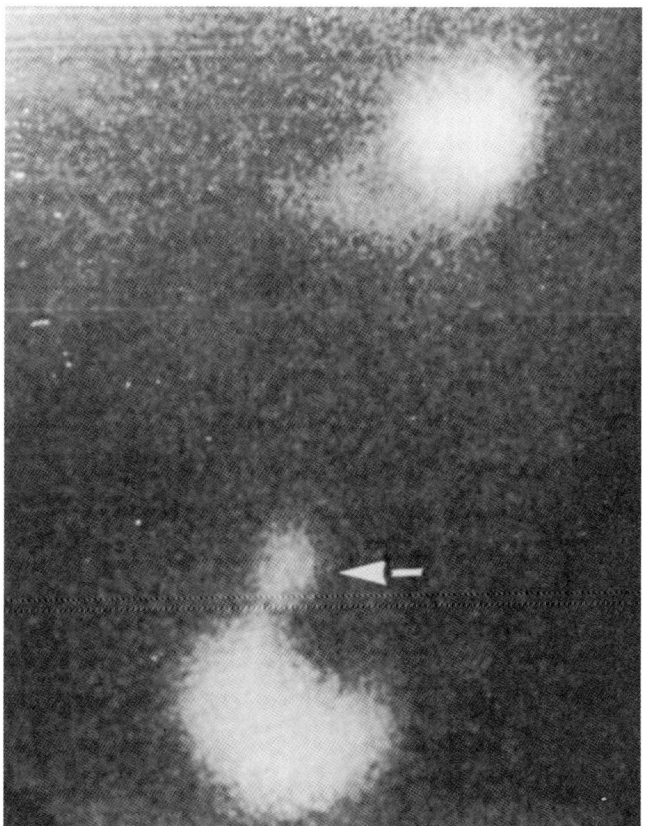

Figure 17-1. Typical appearance of a positive Meckel scan with an area of increased uptake above the area of the bladder in the lower midabdomen. (From Schwartz MZ, Smolens I: Meckel's diverticulum and other omphalomesenteric duct remnants. In Wyllie R, Hyams JS [eds]: Pediatric Gastrointestinal Disease. Philadelphia, WB Saunders, 1993, p 674.)

ileocecal valve. Areas of ulceration, mucosal thickening, and narrowing can be appreciated.

A barium (or air) enema should be performed in neonates and infants in whom there is a concern of distal intestinal obstruction, such as intussusception. In cases of intussusception, the barium enema not only aids in diagnosis but also may be therapeutic. The presence of polyps can be documented. To visualize mucosal lesions of the colon, an air-contrast barium enema is required, but the child must be very cooperative. Crohn disease and ulcerative colitis may be suggested by results of this test, but direct visualization of the colon with endoscopy allows for histologic confirmation of these diagnoses. Barium enemas are frequently used as a way to evaluate areas of the colon that cannot be examined by endoscopy.

ANGIOGRAPHY

Angiography should be considered in a child with active bleeding if fiberoptic endoscopy is inconclusive or cannot be performed. Angiography is useful in determining the extent of varices, determining the cause of portal hypertension, and excluding sources of upper gastrointestinal bleeding other than varices. In lower intestinal bleeding, the usefulness of angiography is limited because the bleeding may not be brisk enough. A rate of 0.5 mL/minute at the time of contrast injection is necessary to identify the source of bleeding. Nevertheless, angiography can identify extravasation of contrast in a Meckel diverticulum or the presence of vascular malformations of the bowel, which may be acquired or congenital. Vascular malformations may also be identified during the passage of a swallowed small encapsulated camera through the small and large bowel.

Therapeutic angiography is frequently used to control gastrointestinal bleeding. Vasopressin infusion or transcatheter embolization may directly control bleeding. The rate of complications from angiography is 2%, whether the procedure is diagnostic or therapeutic. Deep sedation or general anesthesia is required.

NUCLEAR IMAGING

Nuclear medicine can determine the site of bleeding with minimal complications; it is associated with minimal radiation exposure and requires minimal sedation. Technetium 99m (^{99m}Tc) pertechnetate is rapidly taken up by gastric mucosa, and it is useful in identifying sites of bleeding secondary to ectopic gastric mucosa. Gastric mucosa is found in 90% of bleeding Meckel diverticula, which makes this a useful test (see Fig. 17-1). The radioisotope has a short half-life, and the test itself can be done without significant preparation. False-negative results have been reported frequently because of insufficient gastric tissue mass, downstream washout of isotope, impaired blood supply, or suboptimal techniques. Repeated Meckel scans may be necessary to identify ectopic gastric tissue. Positive identification may be improved by the administration of ranitidine to prevent excretion of pertechnetate from gastric tissue. A ^{99m}Tc pertechnetate scan does not interfere with subsequent bleeding scans. A recent stannous pyrophosphate red blood cell bleeding scan may interfere with the distribution of ^{99m}Tc pertechnetate so that gastric tissue is not visualized. Thus, if a patient requires evaluation of significant gastrointestinal bleeding, a Meckel scan should be performed first.

Bleeding scans are performed by intravenously injecting technetium sulfur colloid. The agent is distributed quickly and is rapidly taken up by the reticuloendothelial system. It can detect a rate of bleeding of 0.1 mL/minute. However, because the technetium is taken up by the reticuloendothelial system, this may hinder the search for bleeding sites behind the liver or spleen. Finally, the clearance is very rapid, with a half-life of 2 minutes, which means that bleeding has to be occurring at the time of the scan.

The ^{99m}Tc pertechnetate–labeled red blood cell scan is a sensitive and accurate test for the localization of active bleeding. In cases of intermittent bleeding, a single injection of labeled cells allows repeated scans for up to 24 hours. It can detect as little blood as 0.5 mL/minute.

TREATMENT

The severity of bleeding determines the general guidelines for treatment. For severe bleeding, initial management reestablishes and maintains the intravascular volume. Subsequently, the site of blood loss must be determined and attempts made to stop the hemorrhage. Severe anemia also necessitates packed red blood cell transfusions after the intravascular volume deficit is corrected (Tables 17-5 and 17-6).

Although parents tend to overestimate the amount of blood lost by their child, a major error in the management of gastrointestinal bleeding is underestimating blood loss. The hematocrit may remain unchanged initially, despite significant blood loss, and therefore is not a good indicator of significant bleeding. If orthostatic blood pressure changes are present, the initial goal of treatment should be to hemodynamically stabilize the patient, maintain the intravascular volume, and provide adequate oxygen delivery to the tissues. To do this, large-bore intravenous (IV) lines must be started.

A second potential error is the failure to establish adequate IV access. The largest possible IV catheter must be rapidly placed in a child with active bleeding. If the blood loss is thought to be 20% or more of the intravascular volume, suggesting hypovolemic shock, two IV catheters should be placed. The size of the IV catheter inserted depends on the child's age and size. Blood loss should be replaced immediately with a crystalloid solution, such as normal saline or lactated Ringer solution. Initially, a fluid push of 20 mL/kg should be given. As this is being done, a second catheter should be in place, and coagulation studies, platelet count, and a type and cross-match study should be done. If blood loss continues and the patient appears to be at risk for hypovolemic shock, infusion of normal saline or colloid solutions (5% albumin) can be continued until blood is available. Plasma is indicated if coagulation factors are depleted. Once bleeding has stopped, transfusions of packed red blood cells should continue, to slowly raise the hematocrit to 30%. If continued blood loss necessitates multiple transfusions, fresh-frozen plasma and calcium should be given to replace coagulation factors

Table 17-5. Treatment of Patients with Hypovolemic Shock Secondary to Gastrointestinal Hemorrhage

Establish adequate intravenous (IV) access by placing IV catheters: for mild shock, one IV catheter; for moderate or severe shock, two IV catheters
Recommended catheter size:
  Infant: 20 gauge
  Child: 18 gauge
  Adolescent: 16 gauge
Rapidly infuse saline or lactated Ringer solution (10 mL/kg/10 min until vital signs normalized)
Carefully monitor pulse, blood pressure, and central venous pressure to avoid fluid overload
Monitor urine output, skin perfusion, and orthostatic changes in pulse and blood pressure for early recognition of shock
Transfuse with packed red blood cells to return oxygen-carrying capacity to normal
Carefully record all fluids transfused, and estimate and record all recognized fluids lost

Modified from Olson AD, Hillemeier AC: Gastrointestinal hemorrhage. In Wyllie R, Hyams JS (eds): Pediatric Gastrointestinal Disease. Philadelphia, WB Saunders, 1993, p 253.

Table 17-6 Pharmacotherapy in Pediatric Patients with Gastrointestinal Bleeding

Acid Reduction*	Dose
Magnesium hydroxide and aluminum hydroxide suspension (oral/NG)	0.5-1.0 mL/kg/dose every 3-6 h Titrate to gastric pH > 4
Ranitidine (H_2 receptor antagonist)	2-4 mg/kg/day continuous or divided doses (IV) 6-10 mg/kg/day divided in 2-3 doses (oral)
Omeprazole (proton-pump inhibitor)	1 mg/kg/dose (max 40 mg) every 12-24 hr (oral)
Cytoprotection	
Sucralfate	1-4 g/day in 4 divided doses (oral)
Misoprostol (prostaglandin agonist)	100-200 μg every 6-8 hr (oral)
Vasoconstriction	
Octreotide (somatostatin analog)	1-1.5 μg/kg (max, 100 μg) bolus followed by 1-2 μg/kg/hr continuously (IV) 1 μg/kg/dose (max, 100 μg) every 8-12 hr (subcutaneously)

Modified from Fox VL: Upper gastrointestinal bleeding. In International Seminars in Pediatric Gastroenterology and Nutrition. Hamilton, Ontario, BC Decker, 1999, pp 1-9.

*Treatment is optimal when maintaining gastric pH > 4.

IV, intravenous; max, maximum; NG, nasogastric.

and correct the hypocalcemia caused by the citrate in blood products. The platelet count in such patients must be monitored because thrombocytopenia may develop.

If a nasogastric tube is inserted, the tube size is determined by the child's age and size. A 12-French tube is used in infants and preschool children; a 14- or 16-French tube is appropriate for children of elementary school age or older. Gastric lavage should be undertaken with room-temperature normal saline. The color of the gastric lavage fluid gives the physician an indication of the rate of bleeding. Lavage returns that are bright red indicate significant ongoing bleeding; pink-tinged or brown flecks in the solution indicate less significant or minimal bleeding.

Maintaining a gastric pH of more than 4 is considered standard therapy for upper gastrointestinal mucosal bleeding. This can be accomplished with either H_2 receptor antagonists or proton pump inhibitors.

VASOACTIVE AGENTS

If variceal or upper gastrointestinal mucosal bleeding persists, a continuous infusion of octreotide may be started. This agent reduces splanchnic blood flow with minimal disturbance to other organs. It is much safer than vasopressin.

Customarily, a bolus of octreotide (1 to 2 μg/kg) is given over 5 to 10 minutes, and this is followed by a continuous infusion of 1 μg/kg/hour. The infusion is continued until 8 hours after cessation of bleeding and then tapered over 12 hours.

Balloon tamponade with a Sengstaken-Blakemore tube is rarely used anymore. If bleeding is coming from esophageal varices and does not respond to octreotide infusion, then variceal banding or sclerotherapy is performed.

ENDOSCOPIC MODALITIES

Variceal banding is now the preferred method for treating bleeding esophageal varices. Ideally, the banding takes place after good control of acute bleeding, affording the endoscopist an unobstructed view of the varices. Side effects of this therapy are minimal, and the procedure is repeated at monthly intervals until the varices are obliterated. *Sclerotherapy* is also effective in controlling the acute bleeding from esophageal varices and is repeated at monthly intervals until the varices are obliterated. Complications include esophageal ulceration and esophageal stricture. A number of sclerosing agents (sodium morrhuate, ethanol, tetradecyl sulfate) are efficacious in treating varices.

Injection with a diluted epinephrine solution, thermal coagulation, and laser photocoagulation can be used to stop active gastric bleeding. The bleeding site must be adequately visualized through the upper endoscope. Complications include perforation.

INTERVENTIONAL RADIOLOGY

Selective embolization during angiography can be used to treat vascular malformations and to control bleeding from ulcers. In patients with intrahepatic portal hypertension with bleeding from gastrointestinal sites inaccessible to sclerotherapy or banding, transjugular intrahepatic portosystemic shunting may be beneficial.

COMMON CAUSES OF GASTROINTESTINAL BLEEDING

INTUSSUSCEPTION

Intussusception is a common cause of lower gastrointestinal bleeding during the first 2 years of life (see Chapter 14). The hallmark of intussusception is the presence of "currant jelly" stools associated with colicky abdominal pain, lethargy, or irritability. The physical examination occasionally reveals a palpable abdominal mass in the right lower quadrant. A barium or air-contrast enema is most useful as a diagnostic modality but is also therapeutic because the hydrostatic pressure usually reduces the intussusception. If the barium enema does not reduce the intussusception, surgery is required. Lead points for the intussusception are unusual in infants but should be suspected in adolescents.

ESOPHAGEAL VARICEAL BLEEDING

Esophageal variceal bleeding in association with portal hypertension is a common cause of upper gastrointestinal bleeding in preschool- and elementary school–aged children (see Chapters 18 to 20). Extrahepatic portal obstruction may develop after neonatal omphalitis and may manifest with bleeding many years later. With the advent of liver transplantation programs nationwide, the incidence of significant liver disease resulting in portal hypertension and esophageal variceal bleeding has declined dramatically. Endoscopy is the test of choice for diagnosing variceal bleeding, and variceal banding is the best treatment.

INFLAMMATORY BOWEL DISEASE

Inflammatory bowel disease is generally accompanied by fever, weight loss, and rectal bleeding (see Chapter 15). The rectal bleeding varies from occult to frank blood in the bowel movements. Blood is present in 100% of cases of ulcerative colitis and in 30% to 50% of cases of Crohn disease. The patient may be anemic, and the erythrocyte sedimentation rate is usually elevated. Definitive diagnosis can be made by performing colonoscopy and, if small bowel disease is suspected, contrast radiography.

Table 17-7. Major Symptoms of Peptic Ulcer Disease in Children According to Age

	Neonatal Period	Infancy	Early Childhood	Late Childhood
Hematemesis	+	+	+	+
Melena	+	+	+	+
Vomiting	+	+	+	
Abdominal plain			+	+
Failure to thrive		+		
Anorexia		+	+	

Modified from Gryboski Jd, Moyer MS: Peptic ulcer in children. In Wyllie R, Hyams JS (eds): Pediatric Gastrointestinal Disease. Philadelphia, WB Saunders, 1993, p 453.

HENOCH-SCHÖNLEIN PURPURA

Henoch-Schönlein purpura is a vasculitic syndrome with the following clinical features: crampy abdominal pain, bloody stools, purpuric rash (palpable purpura), joint swelling, scalp edema (infants and toddlers), and occasionally nephritis (see Chapters 25 and 56). Treatment is generally supportive, and patients recover with

Table 17-8 Causes of Peptic Ulcers in Children

Primary Peptic Ulcers

Helicobacter pylori–associated
H. pylori–negative/idiopathic

Secondary Peptic Ulcers

Physiologic stress (decreased gastric blood flow)
Burns, sepsis, shock, hypoxemia, head injury, uremia, exercise-induced
Traumatic gastropathy
  Forceful retching, nasogastric tubes, foreign bodies
Drugs
  NSAIDs, alcohol, valproic acid, chemotherapy, potassium chloride
Immune-mediated
  Celiac gastritis, allergic gastritis, eosinophilic gastritis, graft-versus-host disease
Infections
  Cytomegalovirus, herpes simplex, anisakiasis, influenza A, *Candida albicans,* syphilis, histoplasmosis, mucormycosis, phlegmonous gastritis, emphysematous gastritis
Corrosive gastropathy
  Iron overdose, acid indigestion
Autoimmune
  Diabetes mellitus, connective tissue disease
Granulomatous gastritides
  Crohn disease, foreign body reaction, idiopathic, histiocytosis X, tuberculosis
Hypersecretory states
  Zollinger-Ellison syndrome, G-cell hyperplasia/hyperfunction, systemic mastocytosis, cystic fibrosis, short bowel syndrome, hyperparathyroidism
Vascular insufficiency
  Sickle cell disease, Henoch-Schönlein disease
Hepatic cirrhosis
Radiation gastropathy

From Hassall E: Peptic ulcer disease and current approaches to *Helicobacter pylori.* J Pediatr 2001;138:462-468.
NSAIDs, nonsteroidal antiinflammatory drugs.

Table 17-9. Gastrointestinal Polyps in Children

Syndrome	Gene Defect	Histology	Frequency	Gastrointestinal Cancer Risk
Common juvenile polyps	Unknown	Hamartoma	1:100 to 1:50	None*
FAP coli (including Gardner and Turcot variants)	APC	Adenoma	1:17,000 to 1:5000	100%
PJS	LKB1 (STK11); others (?)	Hamartoma	1:120,000	Increased
CS	PTEN; others (?)	Hamartoma	Rare	Uncertain
BRRS	PTEN; others (?)	Hamartoma	Rare	None
Juvenile polyposis	Smad4; PTEN (?); others (?)	Hamartoma	Rare	50%

From Corredor J, Wambach J, Barnard J: Gastrointestinal polyps in children: Advances in molecular genetics, diagnosis, and management. J Pediatr 2001;138:621-628.

*If solitary.

APC, adenomatous polyposis coli; BRRS, Bannayan-Riley-Ruvalcaba syndrome; CS, Cowden syndrome; FAP, familial adenomatous polyposis; PJS, Peutz-Jeghers syndrome; PTEN, protein tyrosine phosphatase and tensin homolog.

no significant morbidity. Corticosteroids have been used for children with significant abdominal pain and appear to cause a more rapid resolution of symptoms; the use of steroids is controversial.

PEPTIC ULCER DISEASE

Peptic ulcer disease is less common in children than in adults (see Chapter 14). A child with epigastric abdominal pain, early satiety, and vomiting with evidence of an upper gastrointestinal bleed should be evaluated for peptic ulcer disease. The presenting manifestations are age-dependent (Table 17-7). The differential diagnosis is noted in Table 17-8.

The diagnosis is most effectively made by upper endoscopy with biopsy. Infection with *Helicobacter pylori* (a gram-positive microaerophilic spiral organism) is a significant risk factor for development of peptic ulcer disease. If a child is to be evaluated for peptic ulcer disease, it is imperative to determine whether *H. pylori* infection is present. The gold standard for detection of *H. pylori* colonization in children is endoscopic biopsy. Serologic and urea–breath hydrogen tests are not reliable in the pediatric population. Children with peptic ulcer disease who are infected with *H. pylori* should be treated with triple therapy (omeprazole plus clarithromycin with amoxicillin or metronidazole) for 2 weeks. With good compliance, eradication rates exceed 90% with this combination.

POLYPS

The hallmark of juvenile polyps is painless rectal bleeding. Juvenile polyps are uncommon in children under 1 year of age; the incidence peaks between ages 5 and 7 years. The incidence is 1 in 50 to 1 in 100 children. Most juvenile polyps are found in the distal colon, although colonoscopy detects polyps in the right colon as well. Once polyps are identified endoscopically, they are usually removed via electrocautery. The presence of adenomatous polyps in children suggests an inherited disorder such as familial adenomatous polyposis. Affected individuals are at significant risk for the development of colonic carcinoma and require repeated colonoscopies and, eventually, prophylactic colectomy and ileoanal pouch procedures. Gastrointestinal polyp–related syndromes are noted in Table 17-9.

RED FLAGS

Any sign of volume depletion, such as orthostatic changes, is an important red flag. Blood loss may be gravely underestimated, and the bleeding may be undetected because a liter of blood can remain unobserved within the gastrointestinal tract. A normal hematocrit may provide false reassurance because reequilibration may take hours. Other red flags include signs of prior liver disease or chronic illnesses, such as cystic fibrosis, or inflammatory bowel disease.

SUMMARY

Significant gastrointestinal bleeding should be viewed in three stages and as an emergency. First, signs of hypovolemia and anemia must be sought; if detected, these conditions must be aggressively treated. Second, the site of bleeding must be determined. Third, specific therapy must be instituted if possible.

REFERENCES

Etiology

Bishop PR, Nowicki MJ, Parker PH: Vomiting-induced hematemesis in children: Mallory-Weiss tear or prolapse gastropathy? J Pediatr Gastroenterol Nutr 2000;30:436-441.

Boyle L, Lack EE: Solitary cavernous hemangioma of small intestine. Case report and literature review. Arch Pathol Lab Med 1993;117:939-941.

Chandler JC, Hebra A: Necrotizing enterocolitis in infants with very low birth weight. Semin Pediatr Surg 2000;9:63-72.

Corredor J, Wambach J, Barnard J: Gastrointestinal polys in children: Advances in molecular genetics, diagnosis, and management. J Pediatr 2001;138:621-628.

Fox VL: Gastrointestinal bleeding in infancy and childhood. Gastroenterol Clin North Am 2000;29:37-66.

Hassall E: Peptic ulcer disease and current approaches to *Helicobacter pylori*. J Pediatr 2001;138:462-468.

Lake AM: Food-induced eosinophilic proctocolitis. J Pediatr Gastroenterol Nutr 2000;30(Suppl):S58-S60.

Ng S: Necrotizing enterocolitis in the full-term neonate. J Paediatr Child Health 2001;37:1-4.

Pohl JF, Melin-Aldana H, Rudolph C: Prolapse gastropathy in the pediatric patient. J Pediatr Gastroenterol Nutr 2000;30:458-460.

Pumberger W, Pomberger G, Geissler W: Proctocolitis in breast fed infants: A contribution to differential diagnosis of haematochezia in early childhood. Postgrad Med J 2001;77:252-254.

Rodgers BM: Upper gastrointestinal hemorrhage. Pediatr Rev 1999;20:171-174.

Sicherer SH, Noone SA, Koerner CB, et al: Hypoallergenicity and efficacy of an amino acid–based formula in children with cow's milk and multiple food hypersensitivities. J Pediatr 2001;138:688-693.

St. Vil D, Brandt ML, Panic S, et al: Meckel's diverticulum in children: A 20-year review. J Pediatr Surg 1991;26:1289-1292.

Yahchouchy EK, Marano AF, Etienne JC, Fingerhut AL: Meckel's diverticulum. J Am Coll Surg 2001;192:658-662.

Diagnosis

Afshani E, Berger PE: Gastrointestinal tract angiography in infants and children. J Pediatr Gastroenterol Nutr 1986;5:173-186.

Garcia N Jr, Sanyal AJ: Portal hypertension. Clin Liver Dis 2001;5:509-540.

Lobritto SJ: Endoscopic considerations in children. Gastrointest Endosc Clin North Am 2001;11:93-109.

Navarro O, Dugougeat F, Kornecki A, et al: The impact of imaging in the management of intussusception owing to pathologic lead points in children. A review of 43 cases. Pediatr Radiol 2000;30:594-603.

Treatment

Barkun AN, Cockeram AW, Plourde V, Fedorak RN: Review article: Acid suppression in non-variceal acute upper gastrointestinal bleeding. Aliment Pharmacol Ther 1999;13:1565-1584.

Gold BD: Current therapy for *Helicobacter pylori* infection in children and adolescents. Can J Gastroenterol 1999;13:571-579.

Heyman MB, LaBerge JM: Role of transjugular intrahepatic portosystemic shunt in the treatment of portal hypertension in pediatric patients. J Pediatr Gastroenterol Nutr 1999;29:240-249.

Karrer FM, Narkewicz MR: Esophageal varices: Current management in children. Semin Pediatr Surg 1999;8:193-201.

Siafakas C, Fox VL, Nurko S. Use of octreotide for the treatment of severe gastrointestinal bleeding in children. J Pediatr Gastroenterol Nutr 1998;26:356-359.

Zellos A, Schwarz KB: Efficacy of octreotide in children with chronic gastrointestinal bleeding. J Pediatr Gastroenterol Nutr 2000;30:442-446.

18 Hepatomegaly

Frederick J. Suchy*

Hepatomegaly occurs commonly in children as a feature of primary liver disease or as a result of systemic disorders involving the liver and other organs (Table 18-1). Hepatomegaly may occur without other signs and symptoms, or it may occur with liver dysfunction (including jaundice), encephalopathy, or bleeding. Because of congenital anomalies, inborn errors of metabolism, and perinatal infections, there may be a greater number of disorders manifesting with hepatomegaly during infancy than during any other time of life (see Table 18-1). Causes of hepatomegaly associated with jaundice are discussed in Chapter 20.

EVALUATION OF LIVER SIZE

At birth, the liver constitutes approximately 4% of body weight and normally occupies a larger portion of the abdominal cavity than it does later in life. Liver weight increases twofold by the end of the first year of life, triples by age 3 years, and is increased sixfold by age 9 years. In the adult, liver weight is approximately 12 times that in the neonate.

An accurate assessment of liver size is an important initial step in evaluating a patient with possible liver disease. Considerable patience may be necessary to obtain the required information. The lower edge of the liver should be determined by palpation just lateral to the right rectus muscle. The liver is usually palpable in normal subjects with deep inspiration when it moves downwards 1 to 3 cm. In the newborn, the liver edge may be palpable 2 to 3 cm below the right costal margin, but that distance is usually less than 2 cm by 4 to 6 months of age. In older children, the liver edge is usually not more than 1 cm below the right costal margin except on deep inspiration. The liver may be normally palpable in the midline several cm below the xiphoid.

It is a common error to express liver size and to define hepatomegaly on the basis of only the liver edge felt below the right costal margin. The liver may be displaced downward in patients with pulmonary disease, particularly with hyperaeration of the lungs. Careful palpation of the liver edge along as much of the lower border as possible should be combined with percussion of the upper and lower boundaries of the liver. The upper edge of the liver is determined through percussion passing downward from the nipple line. In a liver that is not readily palpable, the examiner may also define the lower edge through light percussion, moving upward from the umbilicus toward the costal margin. The examiner should also be sure that the lower border of a massively enlarged liver is not missed by failure to palpate below the umbilicus. The anterior span of the liver is the difference between the highest and lowest points of hepatic dullness in the right midclavicular line. Table 18-2 shows normal values for liver span at various ages. Careful, direct percussion of the liver may be as accurate as ultrasonography in estimating liver span.

The consistency of the liver should be noted, including whether the liver edge is sharp, hard, or irregular. The liver edge is normally soft, fairly sharp, and nontender. It may be difficult in some cases to distinguish masses arising from the right kidney or adrenal gland from an enlarged liver. Cysts of the biliary tract may also be confused with hepatomegaly. The Riedel lobe is a downward, tonguelike projection of the right lobe. It is an anatomic variant that is more commonly found in girls. Livers enlarged because of congestive heart failure or because of acute infiltration by inflammatory cells or tumor are firm, have a somewhat rounded edge, have smooth surfaces, and are tender if the process is acute, because of distention of the liver capsule. In cirrhosis, the liver is hard and may have an irregular surface and edge. The surface of the liver should also be palpated in the epigastrium, and any irregularity or tenderness should be defined. In the Budd-Chiari syndrome or in some cases of cirrhosis, the caudate lobe may become enlarged and palpated in the epigastrium.

Hepatomegaly may resolve rapidly when congestive heart failure is controlled, obstructive jaundice is relieved, and diabetes is better controlled or in the setting of massive liver cell necrosis associated with deteriorating liver function. By auscultating over the liver, the examiner may detect increased hepatic blood flow in vascular lesions such as hemangiomas. Other signs of liver disease, including splenomegaly, ascites, or a prominent vascular pattern on the anterior abdominal wall (caput medusa), should also be noted.

PATHOPHYSIOLOGY

The pathophysiologic mechanisms underlying the sudden or gradual enlargement of the liver are complex and heterogeneous. Hepatomegaly may reflect proliferation or enlargement of one or more component cells of the liver, including hepatocytes, cholangiocytes, and Kupffer cells. Enlargement of the liver resulting from distention of hepatocytes and/or Kupffer cells with undegraded glycolipids and other abnormal material may be the first sign of lysosomal storage disease. Resident stellate cells produce collagen, leading to fibrosis and eventually cirrhosis in response to injury of liver cells from numerous causes, including infection, drug toxicity, and biliary obstruction. The liver also increases in size as a result of hepatic tumors, benign cysts, and infiltration of inflammatory or malignant cells. Distention of hepatic sinusoids in congestive heart failure or obstruction of hepatic veins as a result of drug toxicity or thrombosis can also produce hepatomegaly (Table 18-3). Several of these mechanisms may be operative in contributing to hepatomegaly.

Hepatomegaly can occur as a result of cellular infiltration by inflammatory cells. In various forms of acute and chronic viral hepatitis, as well as in autoimmune hepatitis, there may be a substantial infiltration of portal tracts with lymphocytes. Plasma cells may also be a prominent part of the infiltrate in autoimmune disease. With acute hepatitis, there may be inflammation in the lobule. Macrophages may also be observed, particularly in reaction to liver cell necrosis. The increase of liver size resulting from cellular

*This chapter is an updated and edited version of the chapter by J. Timothy Boyle that appeared in the first edition.

Table 18-1. **Causes of Hepatomegaly in Infants and Children**

Infection and Inflammation
Viral hepatitis (hepatitis A, B, C, D, E; CMV; EBV; TORCH)
Autoimmune hepatitis
Autoimmune disease
  Systemic lupus erythematosus
  Juvenile rheumatoid arthritis
Primary sclerosing cholangitis
Perinatal infections
Allograft rejection
Graft-versus-host disease
Systemic granulomatous disease
  Sarcoid
  Tuberculosis
Hepatic abscess (bacterial and parasitic)
Parasitic infection
  Visceral larva migrans
  Schistosomiasis
  Malaria
  Liver flukes
Hepatotoxicity (drugs and toxins)
Kupffer cell hyperplasia
  Sepsis
  Malignancy
Macrophage activation syndromes
Biliary obstruction
Biliary atresia
Choledochal cysts
Stricture of common bile duct

Infiltration
Extramedullary hematopoiesis
  Erythroblastosis fetalis
  Thalassemias
Metastatic tumors
  Neuroblastoma
  Wilms tumor
Leukemia
Lymphoma
Histiocytic disorders/hemophagocytic lymphohistiocytosis

Storage/Metabolic Disease
Glycogen storage disease
Gaucher disease
Niemann-Pick disease
Gangliosidoses
Galactosemia
Hereditary fructose intolerance

Storage/Metabolic Disease—cont'd
Tyrosinemia
Wilson disease
Neonatal iron storage disease
Mucopolysaccharidoses
Amyloidosis
α_1-antitrypsin deficiency
Hepatic porphyrias
Cystic fibrosis
Infants of diabetic mothers

Expansion of Extracellular Matrix
Cirrhosis
Fibrocystic disease (congential hepatic fibrosis)

Steatosis
Malnutrition
Nonalcoholic steatohepatitis (obesity)
Cystic fibrosis
Parenteral nutrition
Diabetes mellitus
Hereditary fructose intolerance
Galactosemia
Wolman disease
Cholesterol ester storage disease
Mitochondrial hepatopathies
β-oxidation defects
Drug toxicity
Tetracycline
Valproic acid
Reye syndrome

Hepatic Malignancy/Tumor
Hepatoblastoma
Hepatocellular carcinoma
Hemangioma/hemangioendothelioma
Other

Vascular Congestion
Congestive heart failure
Budd-Chiari syndrome
Venoocclusive disease

Cystic Disease
Fibrocystic disease
Autosomal dominant polycystic disease
Other

CMV, cytomegalovirus; EBV, Epstein-Barr virus; TORCH, association of toxoplasmosis, other infections, rubella, cytomegalovirus infection, and herpes simplex.

Table 18-2. **Normal Liver Span in Infants and Children**

Age	Span (cm)
Preterm infant	4-5
Full-term infant	5-6.5
1-5 years	6-7
5-10 years	7-9
10-16 years	8-10

infiltration may in fact be balanced by loss of liver cell mass from liver cell necrosis or apoptosis.

The liver is the largest reticuloendothelial organ, and Kupffer cells, which are intensely phagocytic cells that line the sinusoids, constitute 15% of all the cells in the liver. In septicemia, hepatitis, or a number of other inflammatory conditions, hepatomegaly may result from proliferation and hyperplasia of Kupffer cells. Kupffer cells are involved in the cellular response to hepatocellular destruction. The liver is particularly susceptible to injury from toxic agents such as endotoxin after activation of inflammatory cells and production of cytokines. Significant cellular infiltration may also result from toxic drug and chemical injury to the liver.

Cellular infiltration of the liver may also occur in malignant disorders such as leukemia. A number of intraabdominal malignancies

Table 18-3. Pathophysiologic Mechanisms Underlying Hepatomegaly

Cellular infiltration
Glycogen or lipid storage
Fatty infiltration
Kupffer cell hyperplasia
Fibrosis
Vascular congestion
Cyst
Tumors
Abscess

such as neuroblastoma may metastasize to the liver, producing massive hepatomegaly.

Hepatocellular injury can result in activation of stellate cells, which leads to the production of collagen and fibrosis. Depending on how long-standing and severe the reaction is, the process may evolve to cirrhosis. Although a cirrhotic liver is often small, it may be significantly enlarged during early stages of hepatic injury and formation of scar tissue. Moreover, in many cases of biliary obstruction such as biliary atresia, there may be significant hepatic enlargement, related in part to fibrosis and portal tract edema. As part of the liver's response to biliary obstruction, there may also be marked proliferation of small bile ductules that contribute to liver mass. Other conditions in which this could occur include choledochal cysts and common bile duct strictures.

Inborn errors of metabolism can be responsible for disturbances of liver structure and function and can produce hepatomegaly. The liver can be enlarged because of storage of glycogen and/or lipid within the hepatocyte. In glycogen storage disease type I, the cytoplasm of enlarged hepatocytes is filled with dense pools of glycogen particles that displace other organelles. Large lipid droplets are also a conspicuous finding, and an increase in size of mitochondria is often observed. Steatosis is a frequent finding in diabetic or obese patients and is characterized ultrastructurally by large lipid inclusions, which may almost entirely fill the cytoplasm of hepatocytes. In lysosomal storage disorders such as Gaucher disease and Niemann-Pick disease, there is marked involvement of Kupffer cells with lysosomal inclusions characteristic of each disorder. Inclusions may also be present within hepatocytes; they contribute to hepatomegaly.

Hepatomegaly can also occur as a result of structural anomalies or birth defects involving the liver. Congenital hepatic fibrosis is an inherited malformation of the liver characterized by the presence of broad bands of fibrous tissue and numerous distorted bile ducts and vascular structures. All of these abnormal components contribute to marked enlargement and hardening of the liver.

About 15% of the liver is occupied by sinusoidal and vascular structures. The liver is therefore capable of rapid and massive enlargement in association with increased venous pressure that occurs with right-sided heart failure, constrictive pericarditis, and obstruction of hepatic veins. The diagnostic picture can be confusing in these cases because passive congestion of the liver can be associated with liver dysfunction varying from mild elevation of aminotransferase levels to hepatic failure.

A variety of space-occupying lesions can lead to hepatomegaly. Cysts either isolated or communicating with the biliary tract, tumors intrinsic to the liver, and hepatic abscesses can all be associated with hepatomegaly. Each must be differentiated by clinical features and defined more precisely by imaging studies.

Splenomegaly occurs frequently with hepatomegaly and suggests several diagnostic possibilities or stages of liver disease. Hepatosplenomegaly is a common finding in advanced liver disease with portal hypertension as a result of the hyperdynamic circulation in cirrhosis and resistance to blood flow within the liver.

Splenomegaly may occur in association with systemic bacterial infections or with congenital infections. Hepatosplenomegaly is a typical finding in infants with congenital syphilis, rubella, or cytomegalovirus infection. Splenic enlargement also occurs in infiltrative disease such as histiocytosis. Many storage disorders, including Gaucher disease and Niemann-Pick disease, lead to enlargement of both liver and spleen (see Chapter 19).

EVALUATION OF THE CHILD WITH HEPATOMEGALY

Important historical or physical examination findings are noted in Tables 18-4 and 18-5.

LABORATORY STUDIES

Laboratory assessment of liver function in children with hepatomegaly is essential. Because of the large functional reserve of the liver, hepatomegaly may be the only indication of liver disease. The onset of symptoms such as jaundice and bleeding may be delayed long after laboratory evidence of disturbed liver function is evident. Patients with progressive liver disease, including those with chronic viral hepatitis, Wilson disease, or α_1-antitrypsin deficiency, may be asymptomatic for years or even decades. The pattern of liver test abnormalities may be helpful in suggesting whether the patient's liver disease is primarily hepatocellular or related to obstruction of the biliary tree. Moreover, some laboratory studies, particularly when followed sequentially, may provide information about the degree of liver injury and, to some extent, prognosis. Although these studies are often referred to as liver function tests, most of these laboratory tests do not specifically measure liver function. Elevations in serum aminotransferase levels, such as the alanine aminotransferase (ALT) level, reflect hepatocyte injury. Measurements of serum albumin, serum cholesterol, and blood glucose and the coagulation studies (prothrombin time [PT] and partial thromboplastin time [PTT]) potentially are measures of hepatic synthetic function. In a patient with hepatomegaly, initial laboratory studies should include a complete blood cell count, serum liver chemistry profiles, and a urinalysis.

Table 18-4. Historical Features in the Diagnostic Evaluation of Hepatomegaly or Hepatosplenomegaly

Symptom	Diagnosis
Failure to thrive (infancy)	Glycogen storage disease types I, III, IV, IX, X
	Hereditary fructose intolerance
	Organic acidemias
	Wolman disease
	Cystic fibrosis
	Hemophagocytic lymphohistiocytosis
Fever	Acute and chronic hepatitis
	Systemic illness
	Hepatic abscess
	Hemophagocytic lymphohistiocytosis
	Viral infection
Diarrhea	Wolman disease
Peculiar odor	Organic acidemias
	Hepatic failure
Neurologic/ psychiatric symptoms in older child	Wilson disease
	Porphyria
	Urea cycle disorders
	Drug intoxication/toxicity

Table 18-5. Physical Signs in Differential Diagnosis of Hepatomegaly

Sign	Differential Diagnosis	Sign	Differential Diagnosis
Asymmetric hepatomegaly	Tumor, cyst, abscess	Skin findings	
Abdominal mass	Congenital hepatic fibrosis/ polycystic kidneys	Papular acrodermatitis	Hepatitis B
		Eczematoid rash	Histiocytosis
	Extrahepatic tumors (neuroblastoma, Wilms tumor)	Neurodegeneration	Mucopolysaccharidoses (types IH, II, III)
	Choledochal cysts		Gaucher disease types II and III
	Hepatoma		GM_2 gangliosidosis
	Hepatoblastoma		Niemann-Pick disease types A, B, C
	Hepatocellular carcinoma		Glycoproteinoses
Hepatic bruit	Hemangioendothelioma		Mucolipidoses
Splenomegaly	Congenital infection		Disorders of protein glycosylation
	Systemic infection (viral/bacterial/fungal)		Peroxisomal disorders (Zellweger syndrome)
	Cirrhosis		Mitochondrial disorders
	Portal hypertension	Hypotonia	Glycogen storage disease type II
	Lysosomal storage disease		Peroxisomal disorders (Zellweger syndrome)
	Lymphoma		Mitochondrial disorders
Cutaneous hemangioma or telangiectasia	Hemangioendothelioma		Mucolipidoses
	Hereditary hemorrhagic telangiectasia	Malnutrition	Cystic fibrosis
	Cirrhosis (vascular spiders)		Steatosis
Coarse/dysmorphic facial features	Mucopolysaccharidoses	Virilization	Hepatoblastoma
	GM_1 gangliosidosis	Eye findings	
	Glycoproteinoses (sialidosis)	Cataracts	Galactosemia
	Mucolipidosis II	Kayser-Fleischer rings	Wilson disease
	Disorders of protein glycosylation	Telangiectasias	Hereditary hemorrhagic telangiectasia
	Glycogen storage disease type I	Iritis	Primary sclerosing cholangitis
	Alagille syndrome	Cherry red spot	Glycoproteinoses (sialidosis)
	Zellweger syndrome		GM_2 gangliosidosis
Episodic acute encephalopathy/ coma	Disorders of fatty acid oxidation		Niemann-Pick disease type B
	Mitochondrial disorders	Posterior embryotoxon	Alagille syndrome
	Some urea cycle disorders (arginosuccinic lyase deficiency)	Liver tenderness	Acute hepatitis (viral, toxic, immune)
Skeletal deformities	Sialidosis (dysostosis multiplex)		Congestion (heart failure, hepatic vein obstruction)
	Mucopolysaccharidoses (dysostosis multiplex)		Trauma (subcapsular hematoma, fracture, laceration)
	Gaucher disease (marrow infiltration, deformities, fractures)		Abscess (hepatic, subphrenic)
	Mucolipidosis II (restricted joint mobility)		Cholangitis

The concentrations of serum ALT and aspartate aminotransferase (AST) are frequently studied to assess hepatocellular injury. Abnormal levels of these enzymes are a nonspecific measure of liver cell injury and have little correlation with the specific diagnosis or prognosis. Because of the wide tissue distribution of AST, including significant amounts in muscle and brain, the physician must be careful in diagnosing liver injury solely on the basis of an AST evaluation. Hemolysis may also lead to an artifactual elevation of this enzyme. Some patients with a systemic viral illness such as influenza may have acute rhabdomyolysis, which leads to a very marked increase in serum AST. ALT is present in much lower concentration in most tissues other than the liver. Therefore, its measurement is a more specific test for liver disease than that of AST. The serum AST and ALT levels may be elevated as a result of hepatocyte necrosis induced by a number of different inflammatory disorders or by drug toxicity. Although in most cases of liver disease there is some elevation of aminotransferase values, significant liver disease may be present even when these test results are normal. Serum aminotransferase levels may be minimally elevated or even normal in some cases of hepatic steatosis, in hepatitis C infection, and in many metabolic disorders.

Serum alkaline phosphatase elevations occur commonly in both intrahepatic and extrahepatic cholestasis. The extent of the elevation does not differentiate between these conditions, nor do values differ significantly among various obstructive disorders such as choledochal cysts, bile duct strictures, or sclerosing cholangitis. Alkaline phosphatase is found in several other tissues, including bone, small intestine, placenta, and kidney. Because children have a significant proportion of serum alkaline phosphatase activity originating from bone, the determination of this test may be of less value in the assessment of pediatric liver disease. The tissue origin of alkaline phosphatase can be determined by specialized tests, but these are not routinely available.

Measurement of serum γ-glutamyltransferase (GGT) is useful in the diagnosis of cholestatic liver disorders. This enzyme is found in hepatocytes and in biliary epithelial cells. As with other microsomal enzymes, GGT activity is easily induced by many drugs, particularly anticonvulsants. The normal newborn may have very high levels of GGT, up to 10 times the upper limit of normal for adults. Values of GGT for premature babies may be higher than that for term infants during the first weeks after birth. In comparison with other standard serum assays, that of GGT may be the most sensitive indicator of hepatobiliary disease, but it is not of value in determining a specific diagnosis. Nonetheless, the highest levels of GGT are found in biliary obstruction. GGT levels may be paradoxically normal or low in several familial cholestatic syndromes, including Byler syndrome, and in some inborn errors of bile acid metabolism.

Serum bilirubin determinations are well correlated with a key clinical finding of liver dysfunction, specifically jaundice. The total, conjugated, and unconjugated serum bilirubin concentrations are frequently elevated in a variety of hepatic disorders. Because bilirubin requires conjugation with glucuronic acid in the hepatocyte and excretion across the canalicular membrane, the serum concentration of conjugated bilirubin represents a true test of liver function and excretion. High levels of unconjugated bilirubin suggest the possibility of a concurrent hemolytic disorder or may reflect inborn errors of conjugation or very disturbed liver function to the extent that bilirubin conjugation is impaired (see Chapter 20).

There are several routine assays that provide valuable information about liver synthetic function. Albumin is the principal serum protein synthesized by the liver and has a half-life in serum of approximately 20 days. A decrease in serum albumin concentration may result from decreased production by the liver caused by severe impairment of liver function or significant loss of liver parenchyma. Serum albumin may also be low because of malnutrition or because of loss into urine or the gastrointestinal tract.

The liver plays a central role in production of coagulation factors. The PT and PTT are reasonable tests of liver synthetic capacity once vitamin K deficiency has been excluded. All of the clotting factors except factor VIII are exclusively made by the hepatocyte. The half-life of several clotting factors is short (factor VII has a half life of 3 to 5 hours), and so the PT rapidly reflects changes in hepatic synthetic function and even serves as an indicator of prognosis in patients with fulminant hepatic failure. Caution should be used in interpreting a prolonged PT or PTT in patients with liver disease, because other factors such as disseminated intravascular coagulation may cause abnormalities.

The serum ammonia concentration is another index of hepatic function. Clearance of ammonia is mainly by the liver through transformation of ammonia to urea via the urea cycle. In chronic liver disease, impairment of the urea cycle can be caused by destruction of hepatocytes as well as by shunting of portal blood as a result of portal hypertension, which permits large amounts of ammonia and other toxins to bypass the liver and reach the systemic circulation.

The liver is the main site of biosynthesis and processing of lipids and chylomicrons. Liver disease may profoundly affect serum lipid and lipoprotein concentrations. A state of dyslipidemia may occur in chronic, cholestatic liver disease. In this setting, there may be extreme elevations of free cholesterol and phospholipids. These abnormalities are accompanied by the presence of an abnormal low-density lipoprotein fraction called lipoprotein X. In end-stage liver disease and acute liver failure, serum cholesterol may be low.

A number of other studies may be obtained, depending on the clinical findings (Tables 18-6 and 18-7). In a patient with vomiting and hepatomegaly, a metabolic cause of hepatomegaly should be considered. Patients with inborn errors of metabolism, including glycogen storage diseases and fatty acid β-oxidation defects, may be hypoglycemic. Blood glucose levels should be determined in patients, particularly those with alterations in their sensorium. Blood gas (and anion gap) analysis and determination of serum and urinary organic acids may also be necessary in patients with acidosis. In the presence of hypoglycemia and trace levels or absence of ketones in the urine, a fatty acid β-oxidation defect or a mitochondrial disorder should be considered. Metabolite analysis for the organic acids, acylcarnitines, and acylglycines, as well as the ratios of total and esterified to free serum carnitine concentrations, should be determined.

Normal fatty acid mobilization and oxidation are likely in a patient with large amount of ketones in the urine and hypoglycemia. In this setting, a defect in gluconeogenesis, an organic aciduria,

Table 18-6. Helpful Laboratory Abnormalities in the Evaluation of Hepatomegaly

Vacuolated white blood cells in peripheral smear	Wolman disease
	GM_1 gangliosidosis
Neutropenia	Glycogen storage disease type I
	Organic acidurias
	Shwachman syndrome
	Hemophagocytic lymphohistiocytosis
	Sepsis, leukemia, neuroblastoma
Hemolytic anemia	Wilson disease, autoimmune diseases, hemoglobinopathy
Hypophosphatemia	Glycogen storage disease type I
	Hereditary fructose intolerance
Hypertriglyceridemia	Glycogen storage disease type I
	Hemophagocytic lymphohistiocytosis
Elevated creatinine phosphokinase level	Disorders of fatty acid oxidation
	Reye syndrome
Renal tubular dysfunction	Tyrosinemia
	Glycogen storage disease type I
	Hereditary fructose intolerance
	Wilson disease
	Lactic acidurias
	Galactosemia

hepatic failure, glycogen storage disease, or hereditary fructose intolerance should be considered. Disorders of gluconeogenesis, pyruvate metabolism disorders, Krebs cycle disorders, and mitochondrial respiratory chain defects may manifest with lactic acidosis. In addition, hypoglycemia, ketonuria, hepatomegaly, and neurologic dysfunction are frequently present in patients with mitochondrial or other metabolic disorders. Serum and urinary amino acids and organic acid analyses are important for establishing a specific diagnosis in these patients. Type I or type II glycogen storage disease should be considered in patients with hepatomegaly, hypoglycemia, elevated serum lactate levels, ketonuria, hypertriglyceridemia, and hyperuricemia. Enzymatic analysis of cultured lymphocytes or

Table 18-7. Laboratory Investigation of Patients with Hepatomegaly Associated with Prominent Vomiting and Altered Sensorium

Blood

Electrolytes
Serum transaminases
Glucose
Ammonia
Lactic acid, pyruvic acid, lactate/pyruvate ratio
Uric acid
Ketone bodies
Carnitine (total, esterified/free ratio)
Acylcarnitine (esterified fraction of carnitine)
Amino acids

Urine (first voided urine at time of presentation)

Ketone bodies and/or reducing substances
Organic acids
Amino acids
Acylcarnitine
Acylglycine
Drug screen

hepatic tissue may aid in the diagnosis. Genetic diagnosis is possible in a number of these disorders. Hyperammonemia occurs in patients with inherited defects in urea cycle, organic acidemias, disorders of fatty acid oxidation, hepatic failure, portosystemic shunting, and Reye syndrome. Hyperammonemia and severe metabolic acidosis with an elevated anion gap suggest an organic acidemia. A positive diagnosis of these disorders requires careful analysis of urinary organic acids.

IMAGING STUDIES

A plain film of the abdomen may initially suggest the possibility of hepatomegaly. Focal masses in the liver may be appreciated along the liver periphery as a result of displacement of the diaphragm or of adjacent intestine. Air within the liver parenchyma can be observed and may be focal or diffuse. The air may be within the portal venous system, a late finding in bowel infarction and necrosis, intraabdominal sepsis, and associated inflammatory bowel disease. Air may also be present within the biliary tree, especially in patients who have undergone recent biliary tract surgery or who have an enterobiliary fistula. Calcifications may also be observed. Coarse calcifications may be found in hepatoblastoma and laminated calcifications in hepatocellular carcinoma. Subacute abscesses may also contain calcium, and echinococcal cysts may have so-called eggshell calcification within their walls.

Ultrasonography is often the most useful initial imaging modality. A high-frequency real-time examination can assess gallbladder size, detect gallstones and sludge in the bile ducts and gallbladder, demonstrate ascites, and define cystic or obstructive dilatation of the biliary tree. Extrahepatic anomalies may also be detected. Mass lesions in the liver, including tumors, cysts, abscesses, vascular malformations, and hematomas, can be defined. Abnormal echogenicity may suggest diffuse parenchymal liver disease, as might occur with fatty infiltration or fibrosis. The combination of real-time sonography with Doppler studies may be used to differentiate between vascular and nonvascular structures. The study may be particularly useful for assessing portal hypertension, in which portal venous flow may be decreased or reversed.

Computed tomography (CT) provides information similar to that obtained by ultrasonography but may be less useful in infants because of the paucity of intraabdominal fat for contrast and because of the need for sedation. Magnetic resonance imaging is also useful. Magnetic resonance angiography may be of value in assessing the vascularity of masses within the liver. Magnetic resonance cholangiography is commonly used to assess the biliary tract with visualization previously possible only with transhepatic or endoscopic retrograde cholangiography.

Hepatic scintigraphy can be useful for assessing the liver parenchyma and biliary tree. The most frequently performed study is hepatobiliary scintigraphy performed with a technetium 99m (^{99m}Tc)–labeled iminodiacetic acid derivative. Biliary imaging with this technique provides information about patency of the biliary tract and gall bladder. ^{99m}Tc–sulfur colloid scanning may be used in assessing a patient with a mass lesion. ^{99m}Tc–sulfur colloid accumulates in Kupffer cells. Most malignant tumors, hemangiomas, abscesses, and cysts lack Kupffer cells and appear as "cold" spots on these scans. In contrast, a nodule taking up the isotope suggests a benign lesion containing Kupffer cells, such as a regenerative nodule of cirrhosis, fatty change, or focal nodular hyperplasia.

LIVER BIOPSY

Percutaneous or open-liver biopsy remains one of the most important diagnostic steps in evaluating a child with hepatomegaly. Liver biopsy is essential in establishing a diagnosis and possibly prognosis in patients with chronic viral hepatitis, drug-induced liver disease, autoimmune hepatitis, and various metabolic disorders. Abnormal

storage of material in hepatocytes or Kupffer cells and viral inclusions may also be found. Electron microscopy and immuno-histochemical methods may aid in identification and localization of these abnormalities. Liver tissue may also be frozen for later biochemical or molecular analysis.

SPECIFIC ISSUES IN DIAGNOSIS AND TREATMENT OF HEPATOMEGALY

Table 18-5 lists some of the physical signs that may be associated with hepatomegaly and may be informative for devising the differential diagnosis. These physical signs, the age of the patient, and associated symptoms such as jaundice, progressive neurologic deterioration, and symptoms of systemic disease should direct the investigation (Table 18-8).

HEPATOMEGALY IN THE INFANT

Hepatomegaly in the neonate is commonly associated with liver dysfunction and jaundice (see Chapter 20). In infants, jaundice is a frequent presenting feature of liver disease rather than a later manifestation of advanced liver disease, as in the older child or adult. The majority of infants with cholestatic liver disease manifest the disease during the first month of life. The initial goal should be to exclude rapidly life-threatening but potentially treatable disorders such as gram-negative infection, endocrinopathies such as panhypopituitarism, galactosemia, and inborn errors of bile acid metabolism. Prompt identification of cholestatic infants is also required to minimize complications such as hemorrhage from vitamin K malabsorption. The possibility of liver or biliary tract disease must be considered in any infant with jaundice after 2 weeks of age (see Chapter 20).

A number of clinical features may provide clues about the cause of neonatal cholestasis. *Idiopathic neonatal hepatitis* occurs more commonly in boys, especially those born prematurely or those with low birth weight. There is a familial incidence of other affected relatives in approximately 10% to 15% of patients. In contrast, *biliary atresia* is more common in girls of normal birth weight; familial cases are rare. An enlarged liver with a firm or hard consistency is more commonly found in infants with extrahepatic bile duct obstruction. Congenital infection may be associated with low birth weight, hepatomegaly, microcephaly, purpura, and chorioretinitis. Dysmorphic facial features may be seen in association with chromosomal abnormalities and with *syndromic paucity of the intrahepatic bile ducts.* Congenital malformations, including cardiac anomalies, polysplenia, intestinal malrotation, and situs inversus, may be found in almost a third of infants with biliary atresia. In the *polysplenia syndrome,* a midline liver may be palpable in the hypogastrium. The spleen may also be enlarged with infection or as a result of advanced perinatal liver disease and fibrosis, but it is often of normal size early in the course of biliary tract disease. Hepatomegaly, as well as a mass in the upper quadrant, may be felt in approximately 50% of infants with a choledochal cyst.

Irritability, poor feeding, and vomiting are frequent symptoms in metabolic disorders such as galactosemia and tyrosinemia. Ascites, edema, and coagulopathy may manifest soon after feedings are initiated or may evolve rapidly during the first week of life after massive loss of hepatocytes through necrosis or apoptosis. A profound impairment of hepatic synthetic function, often in excess of that expected for the degree of cholestasis, may be an early indication of metabolic liver disease such as *neonatal iron storage disease* or *tyrosinemia.*

Infants may present with hepatomegaly and hepatic failure related to infection. Enteroviruses and parvovirus B19 are sometimes isolated from these patients. Hepatomegaly and cholestasis can also

Table 18-8. Evaluation of Patients with Hepatomegaly

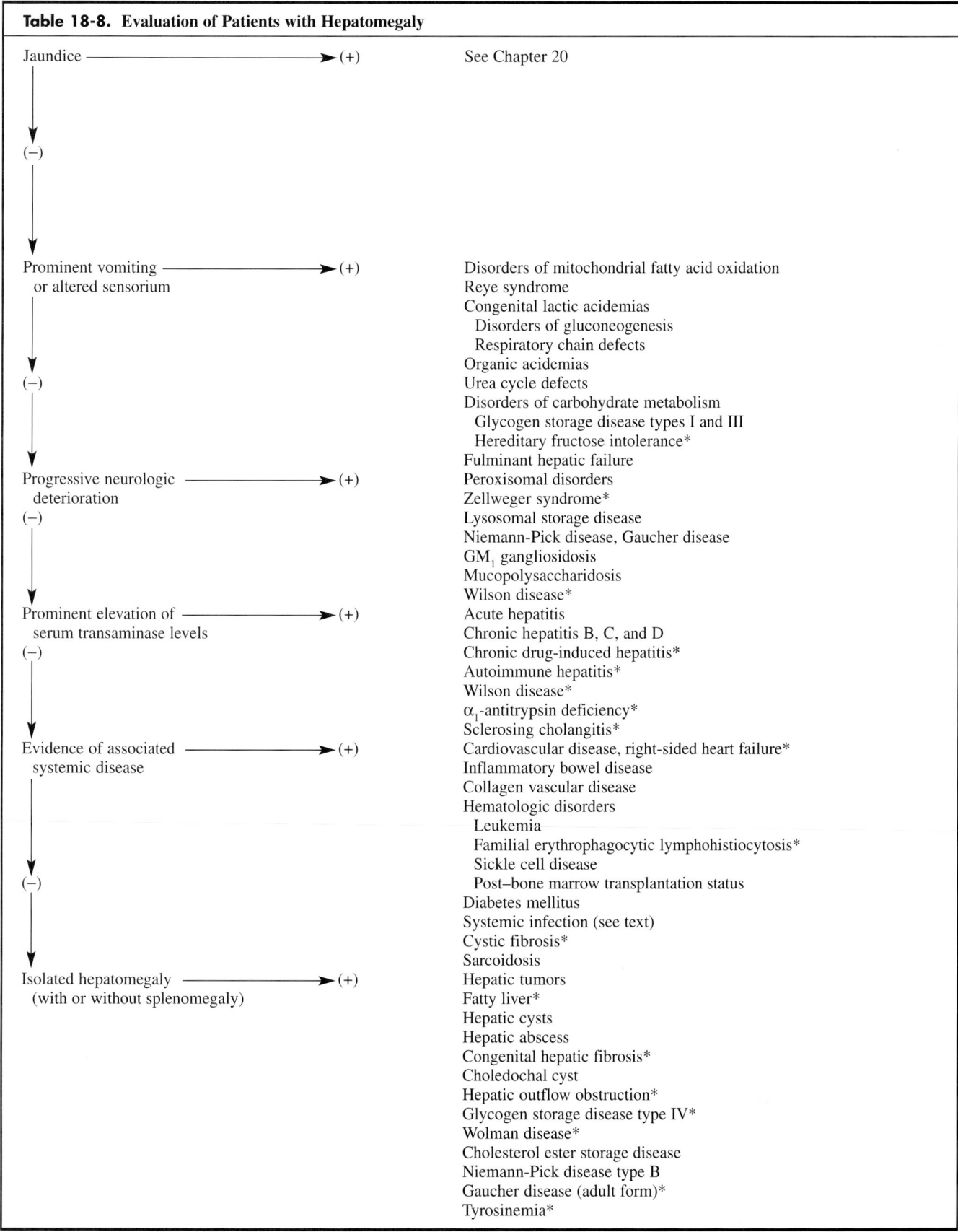

Jaundice ⟶ (+)   See Chapter 20

(−)

Prominent vomiting ⟶ (+)   Disorders of mitochondrial fatty acid oxidation
    or altered sensorium   Reye syndrome
        Congenital lactic acidemias
          Disorders of gluconeogenesis
          Respiratory chain defects
(−)   Organic acidemias
        Urea cycle defects
        Disorders of carbohydrate metabolism
          Glycogen storage disease types I and III
          Hereditary fructose intolerance*
        Fulminant hepatic failure

Progressive neurologic ⟶ (+)   Peroxisomal disorders
    deterioration   Zellweger syndrome*
(−)   Lysosomal storage disease
        Niemann-Pick disease, Gaucher disease
        GM_1 gangliosidosis
        Mucopolysaccharidosis
        Wilson disease*

Prominent elevation of ⟶ (+)   Acute hepatitis
    serum transaminase levels   Chronic hepatitis B, C, and D
(−)   Chronic drug-induced hepatitis*
        Autoimmune hepatitis*
        Wilson disease*
        α_1-antitrypsin deficiency*
        Sclerosing cholangitis*

Evidence of associated ⟶ (+)   Cardiovascular disease, right-sided heart failure*
    systemic disease   Inflammatory bowel disease
        Collagen vascular disease
        Hematologic disorders
          Leukemia
          Familial erythrophagocytic lymphohistiocytosis*
          Sickle cell disease
          Post–bone marrow transplantation status
(−)   Diabetes mellitus
        Systemic infection (see text)
        Cystic fibrosis*
        Sarcoidosis

Isolated hepatomegaly ⟶ (+)   Hepatic tumors
    (with or without splenomegaly)   Fatty liver*
        Hepatic cysts
        Hepatic abscess
        Congenital hepatic fibrosis*
        Choledochal cyst
        Hepatic outflow obstruction*
        Glycogen storage disease type IV*
        Wolman disease*
        Cholesterol ester storage disease
        Niemann-Pick disease type B
        Gaucher disease (adult form)*
        Tyrosinemia*

*Disease that may result in cirrhosis.

be associated with bacterial sepsis, tuberculosis, and toxoplasmosis. Each of these disorders necessitates specific therapy, which should lead to resolution of jaundice and hepatomegaly.

Inborn errors of metabolism must also be considered. Several of these, such as neonatal iron storage disease, may manifest with hepatic failure at birth. Patients with neonatal iron storage disease may benefit from treatment with antioxidants and may require liver transplantation. Hepatomegaly and liver failure may occur in association with mitochondrial disorders. Multiple organs may be involved in addition to the liver. Affected patients often have a profound lactic acidosis.

Infants with storage diseases affecting the liver present with hepatomegaly and may initially be otherwise asymptomatic. Splenomegaly is often present. Hepatomegaly is a regular feature of these disorders because of a pathologic accumulation of undegraded or partially degraded macromolecules in the lysosome. The mucopolysaccharidoses, the lipid storage diseases, the mucolipidoses, and the glycoprotein storage disease are examples of these disorders. The clinical features of lysosomal storage diseases are determined by where the deficient enzyme is expressed and the rate of accumulation of the abnormal material. Hepatomegaly in the neonate can occur in Gaucher disease, Niemann-Pick disease type A, and Wolman disease. Neonatal hepatosplenomegaly and jaundice may occur in Niemann-Pick disease type C. Progressive neurologic dysfunction may occur later. Hepatosplenomegaly accompanied by coarse facial features and skeletal abnormalities is present in infants with the GM_2 gangliosidoses and mucopolysaccharidoses. Significant liver disease may occur in some of these disorders, leading to chronic liver failure and cirrhosis. On the basis of clinical features and manifestation, specific enzymatic activities may be determined in peripheral white blood cell culture or in cultured skin fibroblasts to establish a precise diagnosis. Treatment options are limited for most of these disorders. Enzyme replacement with recombinant α-glucosidase is effective in treating patients with Gaucher disease but without neurologic involvement. Although of limited efficacy, bone marrow transplantation has been used in patients with several of these disorders, including the mucopolysaccharidoses and Gaucher disease.

HEPATOMEGALY IN THE CHILD AND ADOLESCENT

Hepatomegaly in the older child and adolescent suggests many additional diagnostic possibilities. Specific therapies are available for many of these disorders and must be promptly instituted if progressive liver disease is to be avoided. Hepatomegaly in the child or adolescent may be an isolated finding on a routine physical examination or may be associated with many other clinical features related to systemic disease or impaired liver function.

Fatty liver disease in the child and adolescent is associated with childhood obesity. Ten percent of children in the United States are obese, as defined by a body mass index above the 95th percentile. An increase in serum ALT value is found in 6% of overweight children and 10% of obese children. A large number of U.S. adolescents may have fatty infiltration of the liver (nonalcoholic steatohepatitis). Nonalcoholic steatohepatitis should be suspected in any obese child with hepatomegaly and/or abnormal liver test results. Many of these children have elevated serum cholesterol and triglyceride levels. The pathophysiologic mechanism of steatosis in these patients is not completely understood, but a role for oxidative stress and circulating cytokines such as tumor necrosis factor α has been defined. In children presenting with hepatomegaly and liver dysfunction, nonalcoholic steatohepatitis should be the primary diagnostic consideration, but other disorders such as autoimmune hepatitis and chronic viral hepatitis must also be considered. Imaging studies including ultrasonography and CT may suggest altered composition of the liver consistent with steatosis. Liver biopsy in patients with persistent abnormality should be considered; it may show steatosis, inflammation, and early fibrosis. Steatohepatitis can uncommonly progress to cirrhosis. The efficacy of treatment strategies is unknown. In severely obese patients, weight loss through diet and exercise is extremely important. Often, there is resolution of liver test abnormalities and hepatomegaly.

Acute Viral Hepatitis

Acute viral hepatitis should be considered in the child with hepatomegaly and liver dysfunction. The patient may be acutely ill with the sudden onset of fever, anorexia, nausea, and vomiting. Jaundice may occur, but many children with acute viral hepatitis are anicteric. On physical examination, varying degrees of tender hepatomegaly may be defined. Hepatitis is confirmed by an elevation in serum aminotransferase levels. Hepatitis may be caused by hepatitis A, B, C, D, or E or by other viral infections that can involve the liver, such as cytomegalovirus and Epstein-Barr virus. Serodiagnosis of all these infections is possible. The evaluation for various forms of hepatitis should include anti–hepatitis A virus immunoglobulin M, hepatitis B surface antigen, anti–hepatitis B core antibody, anti–hepatitis C antibody, anti–cytomegalovirus immunoglobulin M, and Epstein-Barr virus serologic profiles. There is no specific treatment for acute viral hepatitis. Hepatitis C infection becomes chronic in as many as 80% of infected patients, with the potential to develop into progressive liver disease and even liver cancer. The rate of chronicity for hepatitis B is age dependent. More than 90% of infected infants become chronic carriers if not protected by hepatitis B immunoglobulin; chronic infection develops in 5% of adolescent and adult patients after acute HBV infection.

Patients may also present with hepatomegaly, liver test abnormalities, and evidence of chronic infection with hepatitis B or C. Both of these infections have the potential to evolve to cirrhosis over many years. Table 18-9 presents the main causes of chronic hepatitis in children.

Chronic Hepatitis B

Chronic hepatitis B infection is defined by persistently elevated serum levels of hepatitis DNA and hepatitis B surface antigen, with or without hepatitis B early antigen. There are persistently elevated serum aminotransferase levels and histologic evidence of a chronic hepatitis. Several forms of therapy are possible and are most effective in patients who have an active hepatitis. Therapy with interferon α for a period of 4 to 6 months induces a remission, defined as undetectable hepatitis B virus DNA and hepatitis B early antigen levels and normal serum aminotransferase levels, in 25% to 35% of patients.

Table 18-9. Causes of Chronic Hepatitis in Children

Viral hepatitis
  Hepatitis B
  Hepatitis C
  Hepatitis D
Autoimmune hepatitis
  Type 1 (anti–smooth muscle antibody, antinuclear antibody positive)
  Type 2 (anti–liver-kidney microsomal antibody)
Primary sclerosing cholangitis (overlap syndrome with autoimmune hepatitis)
α_1-antitrypsin deficiency
Wilson disease
Drugs

Hepatitis C

Hepatitis C is an indolent infection with the potential to evolve to cirrhosis over several decades. However, some children who acquire a high viral load, particularly from human immunodeficiency virus–infected mothers at the time of birth, may have more rapidly progressive liver disease. Chronic hepatitis C infection is defined by the presence of serum anti–hepatitis C antibodies and hepatitis C RNA in serum, in addition to elevated aminotransferase levels and histologic evidence of a chronic hepatitis. Initial efforts to treat with interferon have not been satisfactory, in that most patients suffer relapse after therapy is discontinued.

All patients presenting with hepatomegaly and liver dysfunction should be questioned about recent exposure to medication or environmental toxins. Acute and chronic hepatitis can be caused by a number of different drugs such as isoniazid and methyldopa. Treatment of drug- or toxin-related liver injury is mainly supportive. Contact with the offending agent should be avoided. Corticosteroids may have a role in immune-related injury, as may occur with phenytoin. *N*-acetylcysteine therapy, by stimulating glutathione synthesis, is effective in preventing hepatotoxicity when administered within 16 hours after an overdose of acetaminophen and appears to improve survival in patients with severe liver injury even 36 hours after toxin ingestion. Liver injury in most cases is completely reversible when the hepatotoxic drug is withdrawn. With continued use of certain drugs, such as methotrexate, the effects of hepatotoxicity may proceed insidiously to cirrhosis.

There are several inborn errors of metabolism that can cause hepatomegaly and liver dysfunction. Children and adolescents with α_1-*antitrypsin deficiency* may present with manifestations of chronic liver disease or cirrhosis with evidence of portal hypertension. Liver biopsy may show a chronic hepatitis with varying degrees of fibrosis. The diagnosis is established by determination of the α_1-antitrypsin phenotype and may be confirmed by liver biopsy. Periportal hepatocytes demonstrate periodic acid–Schiff–positive diastase-resistant intracytoplasmic globules. Immunocytochemical studies confirm that this material is the abnormal α_1-antitrypsin. There is no specific treatment other than to manage the complications of cirrhosis and portal hypertension. Liver transplantation is curative.

Wilson Disease

Wilson disease is another metabolic disorder that may manifest with hepatic disease in childhood, ranging from asymptomatic hepatomegaly (with or without splenomegaly) to subacute or chronic hepatitis or fulminant hepatic failure. Initial manifestations of Wilson disease may include portal hypertension, ascites, edema, and esophageal hemorrhage. The disorder is due to mutations in a copper-transporting P-type adenosine triphosphatase, which lead to a failure of biliary copper excretion and a progressive accumulation of copper in the liver and other organs. Lipid peroxidation, particularly of mitochondrial membranes resulting from copper overload, leads to the functional alterations in liver and in brain. A low serum ceruloplasmin level suggests the diagnosis of Wilson disease. Serum copper levels may also be elevated, and urinary copper excretion is high, often up to 1000 μg or more per day. The optimal test for diagnosis is a quantitative copper determination in a liver biopsy specimen.

Treatment of Wilson disease involves chelation and urinary excretion of the excess copper. The most frequently employed agent is penicillamine. In response to chelation therapy, urinary copper excretion increases markedly, and this is associated with a gradual clinical improvement. Liver transplantation may be required for treatment of fulminant Wilson disease or in patients with decompensated cirrhosis.

Autoimmune Liver Disease

Several forms of autoimmune liver disease may also manifest with hepatomegaly during childhood and adolescence. First, autoimmune hepatitis is defined as a continuing inflammatory process manifested by elevated aminotransferase concentrations and a number of circulating autoantibodies. The severity at presentation is highly variable; affected children may have only biochemical evidence of liver disease, may have stigmata of chronic liver disease, or may present in hepatic failure. In 25% to 30% of patients with autoimmune hepatitis, particularly children, the illness may mimic acute viral hepatitis. However, in most patients, the onset is insidious. The patient may be asymptomatic or have fatigue, malaise, behavioral changes, anorexia, and amenorrhea. Months or even years may pass before a liver problem is recognized with onset of jaundice or bleeding. There is a high association with extrahepatic disorders, including arthritis, vasculitis, nephritis, thyroiditis, and Coombs-positive anemia.

Laboratory studies in autoimmune hepatitis reveal a moderate elevation, usually less than 1000 IU/L, of serum aminotransferase activities. Serum bilirubin levels are commonly 2 to 10 mg/dL. Serum alkaline phosphatase activity is normal or only slightly increased. A diagnosis of autoimmune hepatitis may initially be suggested by marked polyclonal elevations of serum gamma globulin levels. Characteristic patterns of serum autoantibodies may be present. The most common is formation of non–organ-specific antibodies such as antiactin (smooth muscle), and antinuclear antibodies. In this variant of autoimmune hepatitis, most patients are in the 10- to 20-year age range. High titers of a liver-kidney microsomal antibody can be detected in another form of autoimmune hepatitis that usually affects children between the ages of 2 and 14 years. Liver biopsy is useful in confirming the diagnosis and assessing the degree of liver damage. Cirrhosis may be present at the time of diagnosis in children.

Immunosuppressive drugs are necessary to treat autoimmune hepatitis. Corticosteroid therapy, with or without low doses of azathioprine, improves the clinical biochemical and histologic features in most patients and prolongs survival in most patients with severe disease.

Primary Sclerosing Cholangitis

Primary sclerosing cholangitis is another autoimmune disorder with the focus of injury on the biliary tract. The disorder may be difficult to distinguish from autoimmune hepatitis, and some patients have an overlap syndrome with features of both disorders. Hepatomegaly is frequently present. Patients may be asymptomatic or have jaundice, pruritus, or abdominal pain. Although serum aminotransferase levels are elevated, there is more striking elevation of serum alkaline phosphatase, 5′nucleotidase, and GGT activities. Inflammatory bowel disease occurs in 50% to 75% of patients and is manifest at any time in the course of the liver disease. Cholangiography reveals beading and irregularity of the intrahepatic and extrahepatic bile ducts. There is no definitive treatment. Ursodeoxycholic acid given in a dose of 15 mg/kg/day may lead to improvement of pruritus and a decrease in abnormal biochemical values. The course of the disorder is slowly progressive and eventually necessitates liver transplantation.

SYSTEMIC INFECTION

Acquired Immunodeficiency Syndrome

Hepatobiliary manifestations are protean in patients with acquired immunodeficiency syndrome (AIDS). Hepatomegaly may be present, caused by a heterogeneous group of problems that includes viral hepatitis, opportunistic infections, drug-induced hepatic injury, malnutrition, peliosis hepatitis, AIDS cholangiopathy, and neoplasm. Pathologic features that are most typical of pediatric AIDS include giant cell transformation and diffuse parenchymal lymphoplasmacytic infiltrates, the latter being associated with lymphoid interstitial pneumonitis. Hepatosplenomegaly and anicteric hepatitis have been reported with cat-scratch disease, typhoid, brucellosis, tularemia, syphilis, Lyme disease, leptospirosis, Rocky Mountain spotted fever, Q fever, tuberculosis, and actinomycosis.

Fitz-Hugh-Curtis Syndrome

Fitz-Hugh-Curtis syndrome is a perihepatitis associated with acute salpingitis. Symptoms and signs include acute onset of severe right upper quadrant abdominal pain, friction rub over the anterior liver surface, and physical signs of pelvic inflammatory disease on pelvic examination. The diagnosis is confirmed by isolation of *Neisseria gonorrhoeae* or *Chlamydia trachomatis* from the cervix, urethra, or rectum.

HEPATIC ABSCESS

A pyogenic, fungal, or parasitic hepatic abscess is an unusual infection in children. Common clinical findings are fever, abdominal pain, and hepatomegaly, with or without tenderness, and physical and radiographic evidence of ileus. Symptoms of respiratory infection are not uncommon, and chest radiography often reveals evidence of lower-lobe pneumonia.

Pyogenic abscesses occur most frequently in infants who have had sepsis or umbilical infections. Cases in older children are usually associated with underlying host defense defects, particularly human immunodeficiency virus, chronic granulomatous disease, and leukemia, or with occurrence of previous blunt trauma to the liver. Pyogenic abscess may follow an episode of appendicitis. Liver abscess may also occur in previously healthy children. *Staphylococcus aureus* and enteric and anaerobic bacteria are common etiologic agents. Liver function test results are commonly normal. Ultrasonography or CT scan confirms the presence and number of lesions. Echogenic debris or gas may be seen. Distal acoustic enhancement is often present, suggesting a cystic origin.

Epidemiologically, *amebiasis* occurs in clusters in the southern United States, with person-to-person transmission in association with poor sanitation and crowding. Amebic abscess follows portal invasion by the parasite. The diagnosis is established by demonstrating a positive result of enzyme-linked immunosorbent assay for antibody to *Entamoeba histolytica* or by finding trophozoites or cysts in the stool. Toxocariasis and echinococcosis are caused by abortive infection of the liver in humans with the natural parasite of dogs or cats. The diagnosis is confirmed by specific serologic profiles.

ENDOCRINE DISORDERS

Hepatomegaly and mild elevations of transaminase levels and bilirubin are common in hypothyroidism and are occasionally observed in hyperthyroidism. Clinically, an enlarged liver is often found in patients with diabetes mellitus, particularly those with severe or poorly controlled diabetes, mainly as a result of excessive glycogen deposition. An extreme, rare case of this process is represented by *Mauriac syndrome,* which is characterized by dwarfism, obesity, moon facies, hypercholesterolemia, and marked hepatomegaly. Patients with *acromegaly* can also have mild to severe hepatomegaly as part of a generalized visceromegaly associated with the disease.

HEPATIC TUMORS

Overall, hepatic neoplasms (see Chapter 22) are the third most common solid nonbrain tumors, after neuroblastoma and Wilms tumor. Hepatic metastases can also occur with many childhood neoplasms, most frequently neuroblastoma, leukemia, and lymphoma. Fortunately, the primary tumor is almost always known. An exception is stage IV-S neuroblastoma, which may manifest as hepatomegaly in an otherwise normal-appearing infant in the first few months of life. Because stage IV-S neuroblastoma metastasizes to skin and bone marrow, skin nodules should be a red flag. All patients with suspected neuroblastoma should undergo quantitative evaluation of serum ferritin and urinary catecholamine levels, including levels of homovanillic acid and vanillylmandelic acid (see Chapter 22).

Of primary hepatic tumors, benign liver tumors account for 33% of cases. Benign liver tumors include hemangioendotheliomas, mesenchymal hamartomas, focal nodular hyperplasia, and adenomas. Malignant tumors include hepatoblastoma, hepatocellular carcinoma, and undifferentiated embryonal cell sarcoma. Of all hepatic neoplasms, hepatoblastoma, hepatocellular carcinoma, and infantile hemangioendothelioma are the three most common, accounting for 65% of cases. Most hepatic tumors are asymptomatic or may manifest with abdominal distention, abdominal pain, weight loss, vomiting, or diarrhea. A given lesion may manifest with acute abdominal pain caused by hemorrhage into the tumor or peritoneal cavity.

Hemangioendotheliomas are the most common benign hepatic tumors. Nearly 95% of all hemangioendotheliomas manifest in the first year of life. Congestive heart failure may be present in 10% to 15% of cases. Hemangiomas of the skin, lungs, lymph nodes, pancreas, retroperitoneum, intestine, or bone as well as anemia suggest hemangioendothelioma. Diagnostic imaging is helpful in evaluation. After the administration of intravenous contrast, intense peripheral or diffuse enhancement of the tumor becomes evident on CT scans. Delayed CT scans may show a gradual filling of the hypodense central portion over time.

Of *mesenchymal hamartomas,* 70% manifest in the first 2 years of life. Typically, a mesenchymal hamartoma, which consists of multiple cysts filled with serous fluid separated by myxomatous stroma, has no capsule. *Hepatic adenoma* is a rare benign tumor seen primarily in teenaged girls taking oral contraceptives, in children with diabetes mellitus or glycogen storage disease, and in patients receiving androgen therapy for Fanconi anemia.

Focal nodular hyperplasia is also seen predominantly in females and may occur at all ages. Both adenomas and focal nodular hyperplasia consist primarily of well-differentiated hepatocytes arranged in cords and plates but with normal lobular pattern. The serum α-fetoprotein (AFP) level is normal in mesenchymal hamartoma, focal nodular hyperplasia, and adenoma. The diagnosis is confirmed by needle biopsy, usually with CT guidance.

Of malignant hepatic neoplasms, 68% of *hepatoblastomas* manifest before age 2 years and 90% by age 4. *Hepatocellular carcinoma,* which is associated with hepatitis B or hepatitis C infections of a chronic nature, and the less commonly seen undifferentiated embryonal sarcoma occur primarily in older children. Serum AFP is the most useful marker of malignant liver tumors; 80% to 90% of hepatoblastomas and 60% to 90% of hepatocellular carcinoma are positive. Elevation of the AFP level, calcification on CT scans, and absence of prominent cystic component on sonograms distinguish hepatoblastoma from mesenchymal hamartoma. However, the diagnosis is usually established by biopsy before results of such testing can be obtained. Hepatocellular carcinoma is associated with hereditary tyrosinemia, ataxia-telangiectasia, glycogenosis type I, chronic hepatitis B or C, and familial cholestatic cirrhosis, which thus justifies serial screening of AFP levels in these patients.

HEPATIC CYSTS

Solitary and traumatic cysts are uncommon. The origin of solitary cysts is unknown. Traumatic cysts are probably the sequelae of intrahepatic hemorrhage. *Peliosis hepatitis,* characterized by blood-filled spaces of varying sizes within the liver parenchyma, can be a complication of long-term treatment with anabolic steroids. Hepatomegaly, often with tenderness, may be present before any evidence of liver biochemical abnormality is evident.

Table 18-10. "Red Flags" Suggesting Serious Liver Disease in a Patient with Hepatomegaly

History

History of prolonged hyperbilirubinemia in infancy
Family history of liver, neurologic, or psychiatric disease
Previous blood transfusion, intravenous drug use
Past history of hepatitis
Delayed puberty
Gastrointestinal bleeding

Physical Examination

Hard or nodular liver
Firm splenomegaly
Ascites
Prominent abdominal venous pattern
Growth retardation
Muscle wasting
Digital clubbing
Palmar erythema
Spider angiomata
Arthritis
Papular acrodermatitis
Kayser-Fleischer rings
Mental status changes
Asterixis

Laboratory Test Results

Prolonged prothrombin time
Hypoglycemia
Decreased serum albumin

HEPATIC VENOUS OUTFLOW OBSTRUCTION

Hepatic venous outflow obstruction is classified into three categories on the basis of the level of obstruction:

- hepatic venous
- intrahepatic (venoocclusive disease)
- suprahepatic vena caval

Hepatic venous outflow obstruction manifests with acute ascites and tender hepatomegaly. Abdominal pain, distention, and splenic enlargement may be prominent. Minimal elevations of the transaminase or serum bilirubin level are present in the acute stage.

The pathologic hallmark of venoocclusive disease is occlusion of central and sublobular hepatic veins by intimal edema and fibrosis. The illness classically follows ingestion of plants that contain a toxic pyrrolizidine alkaloid (*Senecio, Crotalaria, Heliotropium*), the leaves of which are used in bush teas and herbal medicines or may contaminate poorly winnowed wheat. Venoocclusive disease may also occur as a hepatic response to irradiation and chemotherapy for bone marrow transplantation. A familial form of venoocclusive disease associated with immunodeficiency has also been reported.

Budd-Chiari syndrome is defined as a noncardiogenic hepatic venous outflow obstruction. It develops in a variety of conditions that predispose to thrombosis, including intake of oral contraceptives, pregnancy, previous trauma, tumor invasion, cirrhosis, inflammatory bowel disease, collagen vascular disease, protein C deficiency, sickle cell anemia, polycythemia vera, and lymphoproliferative disorders. Membranous obstruction of the suprahepatic vena cava is the most common cause of suprahepatic outflow obstruction. However, thrombosis of the suprahepatic vena cava can occur in any condition that may precipitate Budd-Chiari syndrome. Diagnostic evaluation begins with pulsed Doppler sonography of the hepatic vessels.

Liver-spleen scintigraphy may be helpful if it reveals diminished uptake in the right and left lobes and increased uptake in the caudate lobe that drains directly into the suprahepatic vena cava. Liver biopsy in hepatic outflow obstruction reveals a characteristic pattern of sinusoidal dilatation with centrilobular congestion. Cirrhosis is a poor prognostic sign.

SUMMARY AND RED FLAGS

Hepatomegaly that is persistent suggests a chronic illness, which with time may produce serious morbidity or mortality, despite an initial well appearance of the patient. It is important to determine whether the hepatomegaly is isolated as a result of a specific liver disease or whether it is part of a generalized systemic illness affecting other organs. Red flags include signs of acute hepatic failure (coma, hemorrhage), developmental delay, failure to thrive, and those noted in Table 18-10.

REFERENCES

General Review

Wolf AD, Lavine JE: Hepatomegaly in neonates and children. Pediatr Rev 2000;21:303-310.

Clinical Assessment of Liver Size

Konus OL, Ozdemir A, Akkaya A, et al: Normal liver, spleen, and kidney dimensions in neonates, infants, and children: Evaluation with sonography. AJR Am J Roentgenol 1998;171:1693-1698.
Naveh Y, Berant M: Assessment of liver size in normal infants and children. J Pediatr Gastroenterol Nutr 1984;3:346-348.
Noda T, Todani T, Watanabe Y, et al: Liver volume in children measured by computed tomography. Pediatr Radiol 1997;27:250-252.
Weisman LE, Cagle N, Mathis R, Merenstein GB: Clinical estimation of liver size in the normal neonate. Clin Pediatr (Phila) 1982;21:596-598.
Younoszai MK, Mueller S: Clinical assessment of liver size in normal children. Clin Pediatr (Phila) 1975;14:378-380.

Biochemical Studies of Liver Function and Injury

D'Agata ID, Balistreri WF: Evaluation of liver disease in the pediatric patient. Pediatr Rev 1999;20:376-390.
Rosenthal P: Assessing liver function and hyperbilirubinemia in the newborn. Natl Acad Clin Biochem Clin Chem 1997;43:228-234.

Neonatal Cholestasis

Bezerra JA, Balistreri WF: Cholestatic syndromes of infancy and childhood. Semin Gastrointest Dis 2001;12:54-65.
Fischler B, Papadogiannakis N, Nemeth A: Aetiological factors in neonatal cholestasis. Acta Paediatr 2001;90:88-92.
Jacquemin E, Hadchouel M: Genetic basis of progressive familial intrahepatic cholestasis. J Hepatol 1999;31:377-381.
Nio M, Ohi R, Hochman JA, et al: Biliary atresia. Semin Pediatr Surg 2000;9:177-186.
Suchy FJ: Approach to the infant with cholestasis. In Suchy FJ, Sokol RJ, Balistreri WB (eds): Liver Disease in Children, 2nd ed. Philadelphia, Lippincott Williams & Wilkins, 2001, pp 187-194.
Zerbini MC, Gallucci SD, Maezono R, et al: Liver biopsy in neonatal cholestasis: A review on statistical grounds. Mod Pathol 1997;10:793-799.

Viral Hepatitis

Chang MH: Natural history of hepatitis B virus infection in children. J Gastroenterol Hepatol 2000;15(Suppl):E16-E19.
Hochman JA, Balistreri WF: Viral hepatitis: Expanding the alphabet. Adv Pediatr 1999;46:207-243.
Jonas MM: Viral hepatitis. From prevention to antivirals. Clin Liver Dis 2000;4:849-877.

Metabolic Liver Disease

Gollan JL, Gollan TJ: Wilson disease in 1998: Genetic, diagnostic and therapeutic aspects. J Hepatol 1998;1:28-36.

McGovern MM, Mistry PK: The lysosomal storage diseases. In Suchy FJ, Sokol RJ, Balistreri WB (eds): Liver Disease in Children, 2nd ed. Philadelphia, Lippincott Williams & Wilkins, 2001, pp 687-700.

Perlmutter DH: Alpha-1-antitrypsin deficiency. Semin Liver Dis 1998; 18:217-225.

Rashid M, Roberts EA: Nonalcoholic steatohepatitis in children. J Pediatr Gastroenterol Nutr 2000;30:48-53.

Saudubray JM, Martin D, de Lonlay P, et al: Recognition and management of fatty acid oxidation defects: A series of 107 patients. J Inherit Metab Dis 1999;22:488-502.

Sokol RJ, Treem WR: Mitochondria and childhood liver diseases. J Pediatr Gastroenterol Nutr 1999;28:416.

Autoimmune Liver Disease

Gregorio GV, Portmann B, Karani J, et al: Autoimmune hepatitis/sclerosing cholangitis overlap syndrome in childhood: A 16-year prospective study. Hepatology 2001;33:544-553.

Roberts EA: Primary sclerosing cholangitis in children. J Gastroenterol Hepatol 1999;14:588-593.

Yachha SK, Srivastava A, Chetri K, et al: Autoimmune liver disease in children. J Gastroenterol Hepatol 2001;16:674-677.

Liver Tumors

Stocker JT: An approach to handling pediatric liver tumors. Am J Clin Pathol 1998;109:S67-S72.

Stocker JT: Hepatic tumors in children. Clin Liver Dis 2001;5:259-281.

Miscellaneous Disorders Causing Hepatomegaly

D'Agata ID, Jonas MM, Perez-Atayde AR, et al: Combined cystic disease of the liver and kidney. Semin Liver Dis 1994;14:215-228.

Gentil-Kocher S, Bernard O, Brunelle F, et al: Budd-Chiari syndrome in children: Report of 22 cases. J Pediatr 1988;113:30-38.

19 Splenomegaly

Kelly W. Maloney*

Enlargement of the spleen, or splenomegaly, is a physical sign that is common to many disorders. The spleen has multiple functions (Table 19-1); it is usually an alteration in one of these functions that leads to splenomegaly. The spleen consists of red pulp and white pulp, contains large amounts of lymphoid tissue and macrophages, and is heavily involved in immunologic reactions. Sensory innervation of the spleen is limited to the capsule; pain is characteristic of rapid enlargement with stretching of the capsule or inflammatory processes that generate cytokines that cause pain. The splenic blood supply is closely linked to the portal system, and increased pressure in the portal system is transmitted to the spleen. Splenomegaly can be caused by diseases that result in hyperplasia of the lymphoid and reticuloendothelial systems (infections, connective tissue disorders), infiltrative disorders (Gaucher disease, leukemia, lymphoma), hematologic disorders (thalassemia, hereditary spherocytosis), and conditions that cause distention of the sinusoids whenever there is increased pressure in the portal or splenic veins (portal hypertension) (Table 19-2).

A challenge to the clinician is the decision of whether a mildly enlarged spleen can be carefully observed or whether it requires a more immediate evaluation. Careful determination of additional systemic signs and symptoms is helpful in the decision to evaluate a patient.

Palpable spleens in children and adolescents are not always indicative of disease. Up to 30% of full-term neonates and 5% to 15% of children have palpable spleens. In one study, 3% of college freshmen were found to have palpable spleens, and one third of these subjects had persistently palpable spleens for at least 3 years. The finding of palpable spleens could not be explained by body habitus or infectious mononucleosis. In 10-year follow-up of these patients, there was no evidence of an increase in lymphoreticular malignancy, and, other than an increased frequency of infections and physician office visits, their health was no different from that of the control group.

An organized approach to the evaluation of the child/adolescent with splenomegaly with a detailed history, physical examination, and laboratory evaluation often identifies the diagnosis.

HISTORY

HISTORICAL FEATURES

Many of the common causes of splenomegaly are elucidated by the personal and family histories. Key elements to determine are exposure to drugs and infectious agents, results of previous physical examinations and laboratory tests, and ethnic background of the family.

CHIEF COMPLAINT

It is crucial to determine whether the enlargement of the spleen is acute or chronic and whether it is directly related to the child's symptoms. Incidental splenic enlargement is much more likely to represent a more chronic process than is splenomegaly noted as part of an evaluation for an acute illness. Symptoms referable to the left upper quadrant, such as fullness or pain (often referred to the left shoulder), indicate that the splenic capsule is being stretched, which is causing symptoms. Asymptomatic splenic enlargement noted at a well-child examination in a 5-year-old child is more likely to be caused by a storage disease than by acute leukemia; pain on palpation of a spleen implies that the capsule has been stretched acutely and suggests the presence of acute infection or hemolysis rather than a chronic process, such as a storage disease.

Nonspecific symptoms, or symptoms referable to other organ systems, suggest diagnoses in which the splenomegaly is a secondary, rather than a primary, process. Bone pain, fevers, lethargy, and bruising suggest bone marrow infiltration (acute leukemia); jaundice and ascites suggest primary liver disease.

MEDICAL HISTORY

In the neonatal period, placement of umbilical catheters may induce thrombosis and persistent obstruction in a number of blood vessels, particularly the extrahepatic portal vein, which may lead to congestive splenomegaly. Exchange transfusion through an umbilical venous catheter is usually also performed for hematologic indications (hemolysis) that may independently lead to splenomegaly (hereditary spherocytosis).

Certain previous infections may be followed by splenomegaly. These infections include hepatitis, mononucleosis, and malaria. Drugs that may cause liver disease may lead to portal hypertension, which may in turn lead to splenomegaly.

Past surgical procedures that may provide clues to the cause of splenomegaly include abdominal procedures, especially in the upper abdomen, or any hepatic procedures and cardiac surgery, which may be followed by blood-borne infections (hepatitis, cytomegalovirus), thrombosis, portal hypertension, or congestive heart failure.

Abdominal trauma may acutely produce a splenic hematoma (Fig. 19-1) or may be followed by development of a chronic splenic pseudocyst.

FAMILY HISTORY

Both ethnic background and medical histories of specific family members must be elicited to identify potential patterns of inheritance. Frequently, family members may not be aware of the specific diagnosis, and a history of anemia, transfusions, early biliary stones, cholecystectomy (for hemolytic anemia–associated bilirubin biliary stones), and splenectomy (for hemolytic anemia) may be known instead. Identification of Mediterranean (thalassemia, glucose-6-phosphate dehydrogenase [G6PD] deficiency), African (sickle cell anemia, G6PD deficiency), southern Asian (thalassemia, G6PD deficiency), or Ashkenazi Jewish (storage disease) ancestry in patients with splenomegaly is helpful in identifying an inherited process.

Red blood cell membrane disorders, such as hereditary spherocytosis, may occur in any ethnic group, whereas hereditary elliptocytosis

*This chapter is an updated and edited version of the chapter by Susan B. Shurin that appeared in the first edition.

Table 19-1. Functions of the Spleen

Filtration
  Destruction of erythrocytes and other blood cells
  Removal and remodeling of cell membranes
Reservoir for platelets, red blood cells, granulocytes, and iron
Site and control of hematopoiesis
Immunologic
  Trapping circulating antigens and processing antigens
  Inducing antibody formation
  Lymphocyte transformation and proliferation
  Macrophage activation

and hereditary pyropoikilocytosis occur in persons of African descent. *Red blood cell enzyme disorders* are associated with splenomegaly only when hemolysis is chronic. Pyruvate kinase deficiency is found primarily in persons of northern European descent (Irish, English, German). It is an autosomal recessive disorder; parental consanguinity greatly increases the probability. Severe G6PD deficiency is associated with chronic hemolysis and splenomegaly in persons of Mediterranean and southern Asian descent. G6PD deficiency is X-linked, and so boys are more often affected. Mild G6PD deficiency may not cause chronic hemolysis and may not be associated with splenomegaly.

Hemoglobinopathies frequently have associated splenomegaly. β-Thalassemia intermedia and major occur in persons of Mediterranean, Middle Eastern, southern Asian, and African descent. Hemoglobin E occurs with a gene frequency of up to 50% in some areas of Southeast Asia. Sickle cell variants, especially hemoglobin SC and S-thalassemia, are seen primarily in persons of African descent but occur in Mediterranean populations as well. The spleen is usually palpable in young infants with sickle cell disease (hemoglobin SS), but the spleen autoinfarcts by 12 to 15 months of age. Sudden onset of splenomegaly should suggest acute splenic sequestration crisis (see Chapter 48).

Ashkenazi Jewish heritage raises the question of Gaucher disease and other storage diseases. Osteopetrosis is an autosomal recessive disorder without ethnic patterns of inheritance and is associated with extramedullary hematopoiesis in the spleen.

REVIEW OF SYSTEMS

Systemic symptoms, such as fever and weight loss, are seen in many disorders that manifest splenomegaly, particularly infections, malignancies, and inflammatory or granulomatous processes, such as histiocytosis and sarcoid. A careful drug history is also important. Exposure to infectious agents or a travel history that might result in exposure to infectious agents unusual for the patient's community (malaria, leishmaniasis, schistosomiasis, trypanosomiasis for U.S. citizens with a travel history to an endemic country) should be determined. Social and behavioral issues of parents, children, and adolescents heavily affect certain risks and exposures. Chief among these issues are homosexual intercourse, promiscuous sexual behavior regardless of sexual orientation, or intravenous and illicit drug exposure, all of which may expose patients to hepatitis, cytomegalovirus, and human immunodeficiency virus (HIV). Sexual abuse may place even young children at risk, and it may be extremely difficult to elicit accurate histories (see Chapter 36).

SKIN

Pallor suggests anemia (hemolysis, bone marrow infiltration, hypersplenism); purpura and petechiae suggest thrombocytopenia (bone marrow failure, autoimmune disorder, hypersplenism, bone marrow infiltration); and jaundice suggests hemolytic anemia, liver dysfunction, or both. Itching may also suggest liver disease. Rashes caused by a variety of acute and chronic infections, systemic lupus erythematosus (SLE), rheumatoid arthritis, infective endocarditis, histiocytosis, and hemangiomata that are part of a systemic process involving the spleen may provide cutaneous clues to splenic disease.

HEAD, EYES, EARS, NOSE, AND THROAT

Conjunctival icterus may be easier to appreciate than cutaneous jaundice. Cherry-red retinal spots or cloudy corneas suggest storage diseases (see Chapter 43).

CARDIOVASCULAR SYSTEM

Dyspnea, orthopnea, and fatigue suggest anemia or congestive heart failure. A previously identified murmur or a changing murmur raises the suspicion of infective endocarditis (see Chapter 11).

RESPIRATORY SYSTEM

Dyspnea, cough, and tachypnea suggest associated respiratory disease, such as infection, Langerhans cell histiocytosis, and sarcoid. Dyspnea and orthopnea can also be associated with lymphoma, particularly Hodgkin disease.

GASTROINTESTINAL SYSTEM

Diarrhea caused by *Salmonella* infection or inflammatory bowel disease may be accompanied by splenic enlargement. Abdominal pain may be caused by gallstones, hepatitis, trauma, or acute splenomegaly. A history of hepatitis raises the question of portal hypertension.

GENITOURINARY SYSTEM

Sexually transmitted diseases in patients and transplacentally transmitted infections, especially congenital syphilis, are often associated with splenic enlargement.

EXTREMITIES

Arthritis resulting from SLE, rheumatoid arthritis, septic arthritis, and other autoimmune inflammatory diseases may also be associated with splenomegaly. Bone pain is a feature of bone marrow infiltrative processes, particularly leukemia or neuroblastoma.

NEUROLOGIC SYSTEM

Poor vision in an infant with splenomegaly suggests osteopetrosis (with deafness) or uveitis-iritis (sarcoidosis, rheumatoid arthritis) (see Chapter 44). Loss of developmental milestones occurs with storage diseases (see Chapter 32). Myasthenia gravis may in rare cases be accompanied by splenomegaly.

PHYSICAL EXAMINATION

Proper attention must be paid to techniques of the physical examination because an enlarged spleen may be missed, particularly in a struggling child who does not lie down quietly. Careful physical assessment requires that the patient be supine or in the right recumbent position, that the examiner be on the patient's right side (Fig. 19-2). Creative play is sometimes necessary, with the use of pacifiers or bottles; a child is frequently more relaxed on a parent's

Table 19-2. Differential Diagnosis of Splenomegaly by Pathophysiology

Anatomic Lesions

Cysts, pseudocysts
Hamartomas
Polysplenia syndrome
Hemangiomas and lymphangiomas
Hematoma or rupture (traumatic)

Hyperplasia Caused by Hematologic Disorders

*Acute and Chronic Hemolysis**

Hemoglobinopathies (sickle cell disease in infancy with or
  without sequestration crisis and sickle variants, thalassemia
  major, unstable hemoglobins)
Erythrocyte membrane disorders (hereditary spherocytosis,
  elliptocytosis, pyropoikilocytosis)
Erythrocyte enzyme deficiencies (severe G6PD deficiency,
  pyruvate kinase deficiency)
Immune hemolysis (autoimmune and isoimmune hemolysis)
Paroxysmal nocturnal hemoglobinuria

Chronic Iron Deficiency

Extramedullary Hematopoiesis

Severe hemolytic anemias
Myeloproliferative diseases: chronic myelogenous leukemia
  (CML), juvenile CML, myelofibrosis with myeloid
  metaplasia, polycythemia vera
Osteopetrosis
Patients receiving granulocyte and granulocyte-macrophage
  colony-stimulating factors

Infections†

Bacterial

Acute sepsis: *Salmonella typhi, Streptococcus pneumoniae,
  Haemophilus influenzae* type b, *Staphylococcus aureus*
Chronic infections: infective endocarditis, chronic
  meningococcemia, brucellosis, tularemia, cat-scratch disease
Local infections: splenic abscess (*S. aureus*, streptococci, less
  often *Salmonella* species, polymicrobial species), pyogenic
  liver abscess (anaerobic bacteria, gram-negative enteric
  bacteria), cholangitis

*Viral**

Acute viral infections, especially in children
Congenital cytomegalovirus (CMV), herpes simplex, rubella
Hepatitis, A,B, and C; CMV
Epstein-Barr virus (EBV)
Psittacosis
Viral hemophagocytic syndromes: CMV, EBV, HHV-6
Human immunodeficiency virus (HIV)

Spirochetal

Syphilis, especially congenital syphilis
Lyme disease
Leptospirosis

Rickettsial

Rocky Mountain spotted fever
Q fever
Typhus

Fungal/Mycobacterial

Miliary tuberculosis
Disseminated histoplasmosis
South American blastomycosis
Systemic candidiasis (in immunosuppressed patients)

Parasitic

Malaria
Toxoplasmosis, especially congenital
Toxocara canis, Toxocara cati (visceral larva migrans)
Leishmaniasis (kala-azar)
Schistosomiasis (hepatic-portal involvement)
Trypanosomiasis
Fascioliasis

Immunologic and Inflammatory Processes

Collagen vascular diseases
Systemic lupus erythematosus
Rheumatoid arthritis
Mixed connective tissue disease
Systemic vasculitis
Serum sickness
Drug hypersensitivity, especially to phenytoin
Graft-versus-host disease
Sjögren syndrome
Cryoglobulinemia
Amyloidosis
Inflammatory bowel disease
Myasthenia gravis
Sarcoidosis
Large granular lymphocytosis and neutropenia
Histiocytosis syndromes
Hemophagocytic syndromes (nonviral, familial)
Graves disease
Hashimoto thyroiditis

Malignancies

Primary: leukemia (acute, chronic), lymphoma, angiosarcoma,
  Hodgkin disease
Metastatic

Storage Diseases

Lipidosis (Gaucher disease, Niemann-Pick disease, infantile
  GM_1 gangliosidosis)
Mucopolysaccharidoses (Hurler, Hunter-type)
Mucolipidosis (I-cell disease, sialidosis, multiple sulfatase
  deficiency, fucosidosis)
Defects in carbohydrate metabolism: galactosemia, fructose
  intolerance
Sea-blue histiocyte syndrome
Amyloidosis

Congestive

Congestive heart failure
Intrahepatic cirrhosis
Extrahepatic portal (thrombosis), splenic, and hepatic vein
  obstruction (thrombosis, Budd-Chiari syndrome)

*Common

†Chronic or recurrent infection suggests underlying immunodeficiency.

G6PD, glucose-6-phosphate dehydrogenase; HHV-6, human herpesvirus 6.

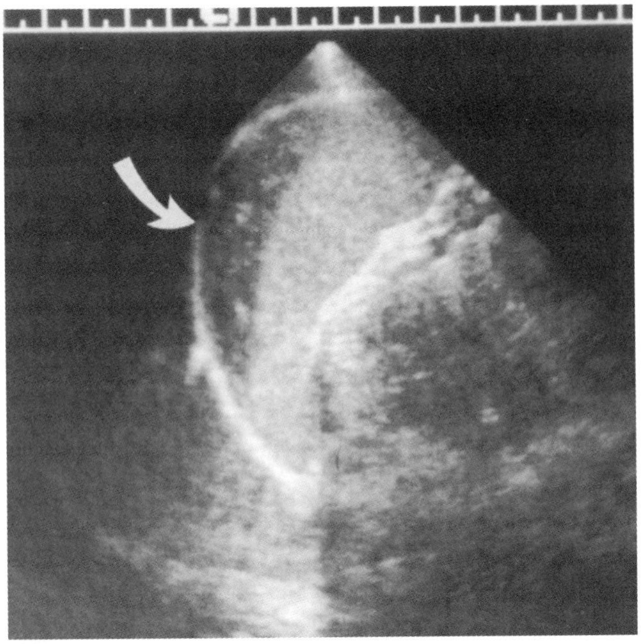

Figure 19-1. The subcapsular hematoma (*arrow*) in a 15-year-old boy, who had been in an automobile accident, was best seen on coronal scans through the left intercostal spaces. (From Teele RL, Share JC: Ultrasonography of Infants and Children. Philadelphia, WB Saunders, 1991, p 406.)

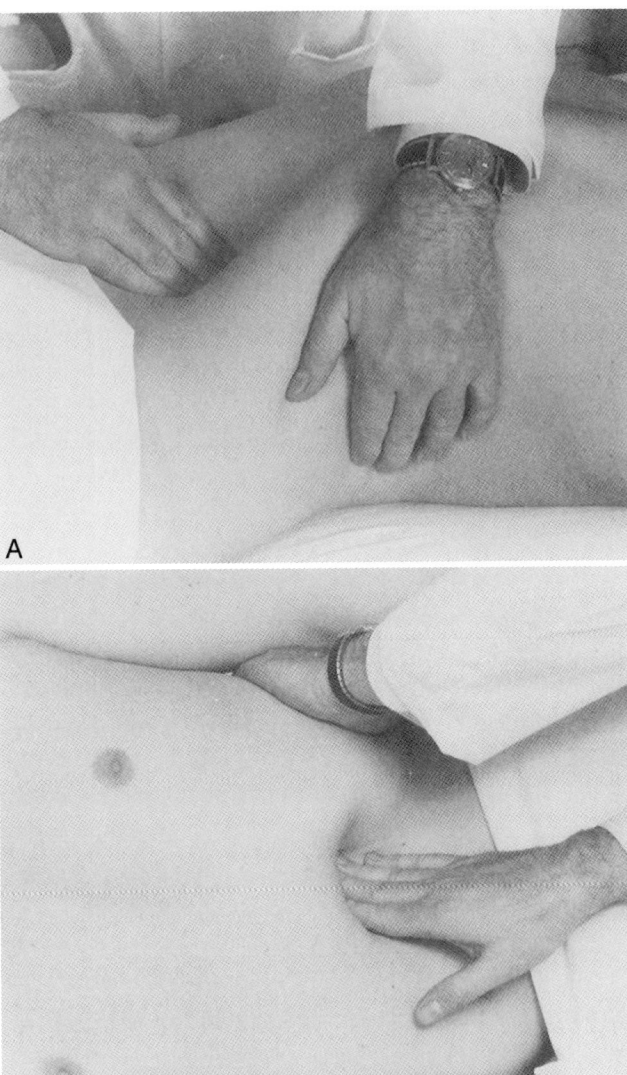

Figure 19-2. A, B, Techniques for splenic palpation. (From Swartz MH: Textbook of Physical Diagnosis: History and Examination. Philadelphia, WB Saunders, 1989, p 345.)

lap than on the examining table. A very enlarged spleen is frequently visible, with fullness of the left side of the abdomen.

Beginning in the patient's right iliac fossa (to avoid missing a grossly enlarged spleen or liver with extension of the left hepatic lobe into the splenic area in the left upper quadrant), the examiner's right hand should move toward the patient's left upper quadrant to find the spleen's lower pole or medial border. The examiner's left hand is placed in the patient's left flank, and gentle displacement of the thoracic cage toward the examiner's right hand often displaces the spleen forward enough to make it appreciable. The spleen should move downward with inspiration. It is equally important for the examiner to palpate the spleen as it is for the spleen to "touch" the examiner during its descent with inspiration. Overaggressive palpation may push the spleen away, whereas gentle or light palpation permits the examiner to feel the spleen's edge passively. The characteristic notch in the medial or inferior border may not be palpable when the spleen is enlarged only a few centimeters, but the notch's presence usually clearly distinguishes an enlarged spleen from other abdominal masses on the examination alone. Because the extent to which the spleen extends below the costal margin depends heavily on the patient's position, the extent of the spleen below the costal margin should be measured with the patient supine. Measurement from the left costal margin to the lower pole of the spleen defines the splenic axis. Ordinarily, the long axis of the spleen is along the length of the 10th rib. As it enlarges, it extends medially and downward.

Percussion over the lower ribs may detect splenomegaly that is not evident on palpation, especially if splenic dullness extends medially beyond the left anterior axillary line.

Masses in the left upper quadrant, especially left renal masses, may be difficult to distinguish from an enlarged spleen (see Chapter 22). In general, the presence of the splenic notch helps identify the mass as a spleen, but nodular masses, such as Wilms tumor of the kidney, neuroblastoma, and retroperitoneal teratomas may masquerade as splenomegaly. Imaging studies, such as ultrasonography and computed tomography (CT), usually resolve such questions.

Many enlarged spleens are not palpable on physical examination because of their relationship to other organs and the thoracic cage. Hyperinflation of lungs (as occurs in asthma, bronchiolitis, ipsilateral pneumothorax) may make a normal-sized liver or spleen palpable. Some spleens that are repeatedly palpable are not affected by any pathologic process. Nonetheless, a persistently enlarged spleen should be considered potentially affected with significant disease.

Isolated splenomegaly has very different implications from splenomegaly accompanied by evidence of systemic disease.

Physical examination findings associated with specific diseases, when present, may help elucidate the cause of the splenomegaly.

GENERAL

Nutritional status and growth provide clues to disorders that affect the patient's metabolic state and tissue oxygenation. Poor nutrition (as evidenced by such problems as weight loss and failure to thrive) in a child with splenomegaly suggests malignancy, chronic hemolysis, chronic infection, a metabolic disorder, or liver disease.

SKIN

Pallor, petechiae, purpura, icterus, hemangiomata, septic emboli to the skin, infiltrative lesions (leukemia cutis, solid tumors), seborrhea, or eczema (as occurs in histiocytosis and immunodeficiency) should be noted.

HEAD, EYES, EARS, NOSE, AND THROAT

Conjunctival pallor, cloudy corneas, scleral icterus, fundal hemorrhages or cherry-red spots, evidence of sinus infection or otitis media, condition of gingivae, and evidence of salivary gland enlargement should be noted.

CARDIOVASCULAR SYSTEM

The clinician should look for signs of heart failure or murmurs, which suggest valvular or other structural heart disease or endocarditis.

RESPIRATORY SYSTEM

Any distress, rales, rhonchi, or suggestions of pneumonia or asthma should be noted.

ABDOMEN

Distention, prominent veins on the abdomen, hepatomegaly, fluid wave, tenderness, or rebound should be noted, as should specific characteristics of the spleen itself: texture (hard or soft), nodularity, and the size of the spleen in centimeters.

EXTREMITIES

Arthritis, splinter hemorrhages, and poor bone growth (as occurs in storage diseases and osteopetrosis) should be noted.

LYMPH NODES

Size, texture, mobility, tenderness, and distribution (see Chapter 47) should be noted. Enlarged (>1 cm), firm, fixed lymph nodes are suggestive of lymphoma or leukemia. Tender, enlarged lymph nodes are suggestive of more common infections.

NEUROLOGIC SYSTEM

Poor development suggests chronic infection, immunodeficiency, or storage diseases.

APPROACH TO THE CHILD WITH SPLENOMEGALY

The most common cause of splenomegaly in childhood is viral infection, which should induce only moderate splenomegaly (<5 cm below the left costal margin) that is transient, lasting less than 4 to 6 weeks. The approach to the child with splenomegaly is affected by several key factors, each of which indicates the probability of significant disease necessitating diagnosis and intervention.

AGE

A palpable spleen (≤2 cm below the left costal margin) is a normal finding in a child younger than 3 years and may be a normal finding in an older child. Combinations of the following other factors are necessary to determine whether any evaluation other than repeat examination is indicated.

ETHNICITY

In persons of African ancestry, hemoglobinopathies, especially sickle syndromes, are suggested by historical features of pain; swelling of hands and feet (dactylitis); and physical findings of poor physical growth, pallor, and jaundice. Splenic sequestration crisis should be considered in a child younger than 4 years with sickle cell disease or thalassemia who has a spleen that is palpable more than 2 cm below the left costal margin. This manifestation is important to identify, because it is a cause of preventable death. Close observation, red blood cell transfusion, and splenectomy (if the condition is recurrent) are often indicated (see Chapter 48).

In persons of Mediterranean descent (including North Africa and the Middle East), Indian descent, and Southeast Asian ancestry, hemoglobinopathies, especially thalassemia and hemoglobin E, are suggested by historical features of prominent abdomen or poor exercise tolerance and by physical findings of failure to thrive, abdominal distention, characteristic facial features, pallor, and jaundice. In persons of Ashkenazi Jewish ancestry, storage diseases, especially Gaucher disease and Niemann-Pick disease, should be considered.

FEVER

Fever suggests three processes: infection, inflammation, and malignancy. When fever is acute in onset, infection is most likely. Chronic fever, often gradual in onset and not associated with chills, is more likely to be caused by inflammatory processes (SLE, juvenile rheumatoid arthritis, sarcoid, Langerhans cell histiocytosis) or tumors (lymphomas, especially Hodgkin disease, or leukemia).

OTHER SYSTEMIC SYMPTOMS

Symptoms such as weight loss, lethargy, easy bruising, adenopathy, diarrhea, respiratory difficulties, jaundice, and rashes should direct evaluation to specific organ systems or processes involving those organs.

DEGREE OF SPLENOMEGALY

A spleen that is more than 5 cm below the left costal margin is usually not transient and represents significant disease. A hard or nodular spleen suggests malignancy or chronic hemolysis. A tender spleen suggests either acute enlargement or infection or both.

DURATION OF SPLENOMEGALY

Acute onset of splenomegaly is most characteristic of an acute infection or a rapidly progressive malignancy (acute leukemia, lymphoma). Chronic splenomegaly (present for ≥1 month) is much more likely to represent a chronic process, such as storage diseases; congestive processes (portal hypertension, congestive heart failure); hemolysis; chronic infection; or inflammation.

LABORATORY INVESTIGATION

Once a list of probable processes has been derived from the history and physical examination, laboratory investigation is directed by the processes or diagnoses that are suspected. Table 19-3 summarizes laboratory investigations for suspected diagnosis.

COMPLETE BLOOD CELL COUNT

A complete blood cell count is the first test indicated in all patients with undiagnosed splenomegaly. This count provides extensive information about hematologic, infectious, and inflammatory

Table 19-3. Summary of Laboratory Investigations for Suspected Diagnosis

Suspected Diagnosis	Tests to Be Performed
Hemolysis	CBC, reticulocyte count, blood smear, serum bilirubin measurement, Coombs test, osmotic fragility study, RBC enzyme assays, hemoglobin electrophoresis
Infection	CBC, differential, blood cultures, viral studies (EBV, CMV, HIV), toxoplasmosis, TB test, malaria test
Liver disease	Liver function tests, albumin measurement, prothrombin time, α_1-antitrypsin, serum copper, ceruloplasmin
Portal hypertension	Liver function tests; albumin measurement; prothrombin time; ultrasonography/CT of portal veins, liver, and spleen
Immunologic and inflammatory disease	ESR; C3, C4, antinuclear antibody, rheumatoid factor measurements; urinalysis; blood urea nitrogen, serum creatinine, and immunoglobulins measurements
Infiltrative disease	Bone marrow aspiration, CT, enzyme assay for Gaucher disease, tests as indicated for other storage diseases

CBC, complete blood count; CMV, cytomegalovirus; CT, computed tomography; EBV, Epstein-Barr virus; ESR, erythrocyte sedimentation rate; HIV, human immunodeficiency virus; RBC, red blood cell; TB, tuberculosis.

processes, and the result may be abnormal in patients with hypersplenism caused by portal hypertension.

Leukocyte Count and Differential

Elevation or decrease in the number of total white blood cells (WBCs), the neutrophil count, and the lymphocyte count and the presence of abnormal cells (atypical lymphocytes, blasts) should be noted. Viral infection is the most common cause of splenomegaly in children, and atypical lymphocytosis may be a clue. Viral infections may be associated with an increased WBC count (early) or a decreased WBC count. Most significant bacterial infections produce neutrophilia and reactive changes in the neutrophils. Infections with intracellular bacteria or some viruses may produce neutropenia. Leukemia can manifest with an increased or decreased total WBC count. The presence of blasts is confirmatory, but they are not always present in this disease.

Hemoglobin, Erythrocyte Morphology, and Reticulocyte Count

Hemolytic anemia may be unsuspected without examination of the blood smear and the reticulocyte count. Malarial parasites may be seen on the blood smear but may be missed unless a thick preparation is examined. Clues found on the blood smear include spherocytes (present in hereditary spherocytosis and hemolytic anemias); elliptocytes (present in hereditary elliptocytosis); polychromasia, poikilocytes, and fragmented cells (present in hemolytic anemias); sickled cells with target cells, spherocytes, and nucleated red blood cells (present in sickle cell anemia and variants); and microcytosis, hypochromia (present in thalassemias), and Howell-Jolly bodies (present in splenic dysfunction).

Platelet Count

Thrombocytopenia ($<150,000$ platelets/mm^3) may be caused by decreased platelet production or increased platelet destruction. Production is diminished in conditions characterized by bone marrow infiltration (leukemia, neuroblastoma). Increased destruction accompanies immunologic processes, drug reactions, histiocytoses, and viral infections. Thrombocytosis ($>400,000$ platelets/mm^3) often accompanies iron deficiency or acute infection as an acute-phase reactant.

Pancytopenia

Pancytopenia implies bone marrow dysfunction, bone marrow infiltration, or portal hypertension with hypersplenic destruction (increased sequestration and lysis by splenic macrophages) of all of the formed elements of the blood. A bone marrow aspiration and biopsy should be performed in any child with splenomegaly and pancytopenia. Tests of liver function, including prothrombin time and albumin, are indicated.

Erythrocyte Sedimentation Rate

Elevation of erythrocyte sedimentation rate (ESR) is nonspecific but suggests infection, especially bacterial, mycobacterial, or fungal infection, or an inflammatory process, such as rheumatoid arthritis or SLE. The ESR may be normal despite significant inflammation. The C-reactive protein level may be elevated when the ESR is normal.

LIVER FUNCTION TESTS

Liver function tests are indicated if splenomegaly is significant (>2 cm) or persists longer than 1 month. Portal hypertension is often asymptomatic until hepatic fibrosis is far advanced. Liver synthetic function (albumin, prothrombin time, fibrinogen), direct bilirubin levels, and transaminase enzyme levels should be assessed.

IMMUNOLOGIC EVALUATION

Immunologic evaluation is needed when autoimmune disorders (rheumatoid arthritis, SLE) or immunodeficiency disorders (inherited or acquired) are suspected. This assessment includes measurements of antinuclear antibody titer, immunoglobulin levels, and immunoglobulin subclass levels; tests of neutrophil function; and measurements of T cell subclasses. Repeated infections stimulate the immune system and may cause splenomegaly.

VIRAL ANTIBODY TITERS

Viral antibody titers should be obtained when a mononucleosis syndrome is present, especially when splenomegaly persists. The results of these tests rarely affect management but may permit a presumptive diagnosis of a self-limited process to be made, and they may preclude more invasive tests (imaging, bone marrow examination) and allay both parental and physician anxiety. Epstein-Barr viral antibody panels may need to include more than antibody to viral capsid antigen alone if persistent Epstein-Barr virus infection is suspected. Cytomegalovirus and toxoplasmosis may also cause a mononucleosis syndrome. Primary infection with HIV frequently causes splenomegaly. HIV nucleic acid detection by polymerase chain reaction of DNA from peripheral blood mononuclear cells is the preferred test for diagnosis. Other tests include HIV RNA polymerase chain reaction, viral culture, detection of p24 antigen, and detection of HIV antibody. It is important to make this diagnosis, because it does affect management. Because acute infection may not be accompanied by positive antibody titers, follow-up titers 3 to 6 months after the initial evaluation may be needed.

CULTURES

Bacterial, fungal, and other cultures may be necessary and are dictated by the suspected infection.

BONE MARROW EXAMINATION

Bone marrow examination is appropriate for diagnosing infiltrative processes (acute leukemia, histiocytosis, other malignancies), storage disorders (Gaucher disease, Niemann-Pick disease, sea-blue histiocyte syndrome), virus-associated hemophagocytic syndromes, and some infections that may be difficult to diagnose from other tissues (disseminated histoplasmosis, miliary tuberculosis, bacterial endocarditis, and other chronic infections, especially in immunocompromised patients).

IMAGING

Imaging of the spleen should be performed selectively. It is definitely required when these questions are unanswered:

1. Are there other masses (e.g., hepatic, lymph node) that suggest more widespread involvement by tumor?
2. Is there silent portal hypertension?

The choice of imaging depends on the questions to be asked. Ultrasonography has been the preferred method of imaging. It is used to assess size and to visualize cysts and other lesions. Guidelines are available for the upper limit of normal splenic length (measured as the greatest longitudinal distance between the dome of the spleen and the tip). Doppler-flow ultrasonography can detect portal hypertension.

Spiral CT shortens the scanning time and provides optimal enhancement. Spiral CT allows for reconstruction capabilities that can improve lesion characterization without increasing radiation exposure. Spiral CT of the spleen can define focal lesions (Fig. 19-3) and nonfocal enlargement, as well as evaluating the splenic and portal veins and the vasculature of the spleen.

Less common in children than in adults, splenic cysts and pseudocysts may manifest with palpable spleens (Fig. 19-4). Both CT and ultrasonography identify such cysts well, and they image the pancreas as well. Pancreatitis is a common cause of splenic cysts. Subcapsular hematoma can also be visualized by ultrasonography (see Fig. 19-1). Splenic lacerations are seen well on CT (Fig. 19-5).

Persistent splenomegaly after systemic infections may be caused by splenic abscesses, which are visualized with ultrasonography (Fig. 19-6). CT is an alternate imaging procedure for each of these problems.

SUMMARY AND RED FLAGS

Splenomegaly is often a manifestation of acute and benign common viral infections in children. Red flags include chronicity, a positive family or travel history, pancytopenia, and signs of disease in addition to splenomegaly (weight loss, pallor, jaundice, fever, malaise, petechiae) that may or may not be caused by hypersplenism or another primary disease and trauma.

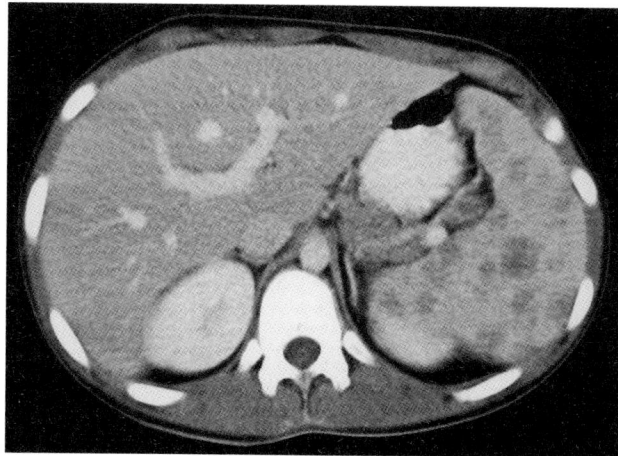

Figure 19-3. Abdominal computed tomographic scan of a 15-year-old with fever, weight loss, and orthopnea. The diagnosis was Hodgkin disease. The spleen shows hypoechoic lesions, typical of lymphoma.

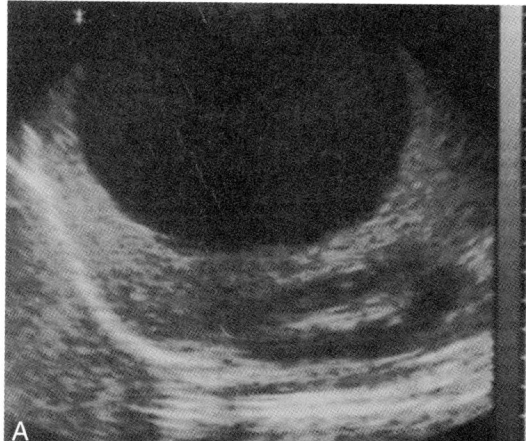
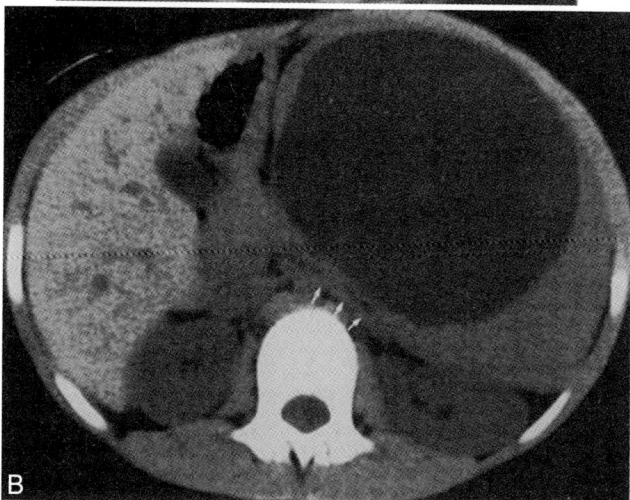

Figure 19-4. The large epidermoid cyst of the spleen in a boy, shown on ultrasonography **(A)**, is shown by computed tomographic scan **(B)** to compress the left renal vein (*arrows*). The boy presented with varicocele. (From Teele RL, Share JC: Ultrasonography of Infants and Children. Philadelphia, WB Saunders, 1991, p 412.)

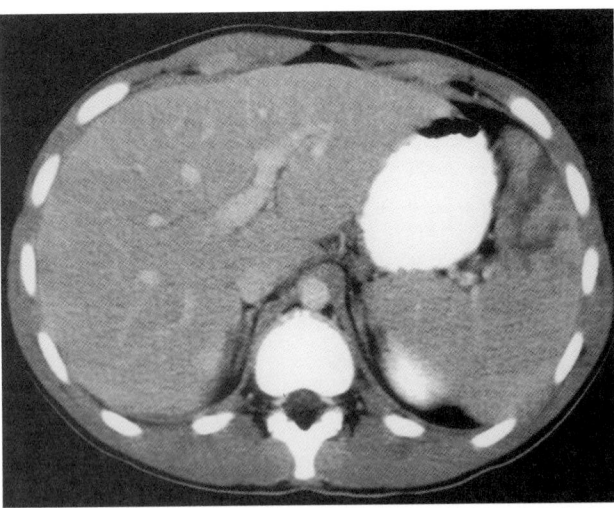

Figure 19-5. Splenic laceration that resulted from trauma in a 15-year-old boy.

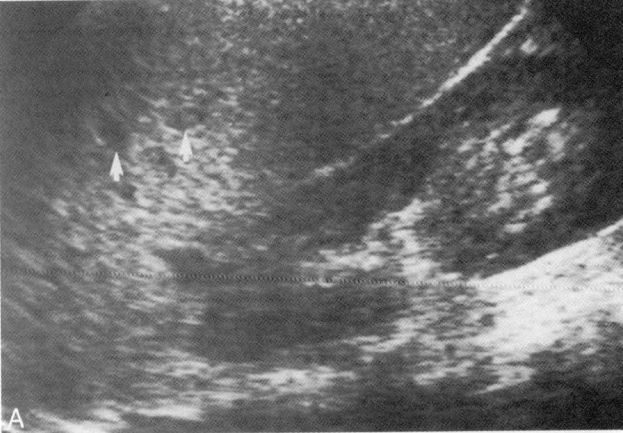

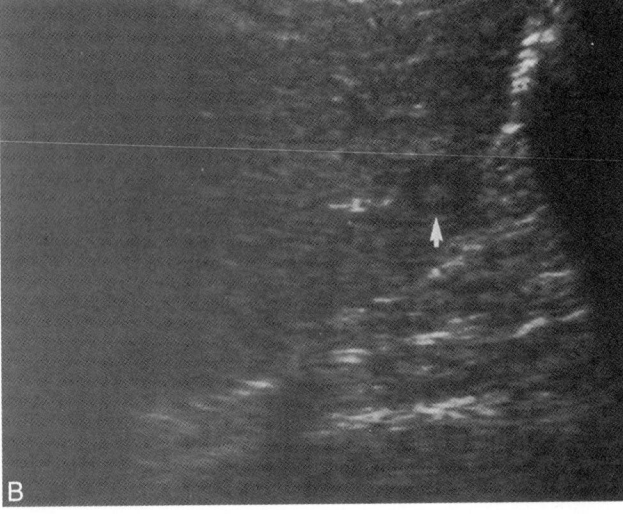

Figure 19-6. A 10-year-old girl had been treated for acute myelogenous leukemia. She had taken multiple antibiotics for recurrent infections. Unremitting fevers then developed. Candidiasis was strongly suspected, and ultrasonography was requested. Two weeks after the clinical suspicion of candidiasis was raised, obvious focal defects (*arrows*) could be seen within the spleen **(A)** and liver **(B)**. (From Teele RL, Share JC: *Ultrasonography of Infants and Children.* Philadelphia, WB Saunders, 1991, p 408.)

REFERENCES

Andrews MW: Ultrasound of the spleen. World J Surg 2000;24:183-187.

Bohnsack JF, Brown EJ: The role of the spleen in resistance to infection. Annu Rev Med 1986;37:49-98.

Donnelly LF, Foss JN, Frush DP, et al: Heterogeneous splenic enhancement patterns on spiral CT images in children: Minimizing misinterpretations. Radiology 1999;210:493-497.

Ebaugh FG Jr, McIntyre OR: Palpable spleen. A ten year follow-up. Ann Intern Med 1979;90:130-131.

Emond AM, Collis R, Darville D, et al: Acute splenic sequestration in homozygous sickle cell disease: Natural history and management. J Pediatr 1985;107:201-206.

Klopfenstein KJ, Grossman NJ, Fishbein M, et al: Cavernous transformation of the portal vein: A cause of thrombocytopenia and splenomegaly. Clin Pediatr 2000;39:727-730.

McIntyre OR, Ebaugh FG Jr: Palpable spleens in college freshmen. Arch Intern Med 1967;66:301-306.

Munolini F, Merlob J, Ashkenazi S, et al: Palpable spleens in newborn term infants. Clin Pediatr 1985;24:197-198.

Rogers DW, Vaidya S, Sergeant GR: Early splenomegaly in homozygous sickle cell disease: An indicator of susceptibility to infection. Lancet 1978;2:963-965.

Rosenberg HK, Markowitz RI, Kolberg H, et al: Normal splenic size in infants and children: Sonographic measurements. AJR Am J Roentgenol 1991;157:119-121.

Sheth S, Ruzal-Shapiro C, Piomelli S, et al: CT imaging of splenic sequestration in sickle cell disease. Pediatr Radiol 2000;30:830-833.

Tamato SG, Rickman LS, Mathews WC, et al: Examiner dependence on physical diagnostic tests for the detection of splenomegaly: A prospective study with multiple observers. J Gen Intern Med 1993;8:69-75.

Urban BA, Fishman EK: Helical CT of the spleen. AJR Am J Roentgenol 1998;170:997-1003.

Wang ML, Maller E: A case of hepatosplenomegaly. Pediatr Case Rev 2002;2:7986.

20 Jaundice

Jane P. Balint

Jaundice, the yellow discoloration of skin and sclerae, results when the serum level of bilirubin, a pigmented compound, is elevated. Jaundice is not evident until the total serum bilirubin is at least 2 to 2.5 mg/dL.

Bilirubin is formed from the degradation of heme-containing compounds, particularly hemoglobin (Fig. 20-1). Microsomal heme oxygenase, located principally in the reticuloendothelial system, catabolizes heme to biliverdin, which is then reduced to bilirubin by biliverdin reductase. This *unconjugated bilirubin* (UCB) is a nonpolar, lipid-soluble compound. It cannot be eliminated via the kidney because of its insolubility in water. UCB, bound primarily to albumin, is transported in the plasma to the liver for metabolism and excretion. A receptor on the hepatocyte surface facilitates bilirubin uptake. Bilirubin is then bound to glutathione S-transferase B and transported to the endoplasmic reticulum, where conjugation with glucuronic acid by bilirubin uridine diphosphate glucuronosyltransferase (UDPGT) occurs. UDPGT can be induced by a variety of drugs (e.g., narcotics, anticonvulsants, and contraceptive steroids) and by bilirubin itself. Enzyme activity is decreased by restriction of calorie and protein intake.

Conjugated bilirubin (CB) is a polar, water-soluble compound that exists primarily as a diglucuronide. It is excreted from the hepatocyte to the bile canaliculi, through the biliary tree, and into the duodenum. Once CB reaches the colon, hydrolysis by bacterial β-glucuronidase converts CB to urobilinogen. A small amount of urobilinogen is reabsorbed and returned to the liver (i.e., enterohepatic circulation) or excreted by the kidneys. The remainder is converted to stercobilin and excreted in feces. In neonates, β-glucuronidase in the intestinal lumen hydrolyzes CB to UCB, which is then absorbed and returned to the liver via the enterohepatic circulation.

Hyperbilirubinemia can result from alteration of any step in this process. Hyperbilirubinemia can be classified as conjugated (direct) or unconjugated (indirect), depending on the concentration of CB in the serum. *Conjugated* and *unconjugated* are more accurate terms, because "direct" and "indirect" refer to the *van den Bergh reaction,* used for measuring bilirubin. In this assay, the unconjugated fraction is determined by subtracting the direct fraction from the total and, therefore, is an indirect measurement. The direct fraction includes both conjugated bilirubin and Δ bilirubin, an albumin-bound bilirubin glucuronide. Normal bilirubin values vary by laboratory; however, the total serum bilirubin concentration is generally less than 1.5 mg/dL. Conjugated hyperbilirubinemia exists when more than 20% of the total bilirubin or more than 2 mg/dL is conjugated. If neither criterion is met, the hyperbilirubinemia is classified as unconjugated.

Unconjugated hyperbilirubinemia can be caused by any process that results in increased production, decreased delivery to the liver, decreased hepatic uptake, decreased storage, decreased conjugation, or increased enterohepatic circulation of bilirubin. The primary concern in patients with high levels of unconjugated bilirubin is *kernicterus,* the neurotoxicity that results from diffusion of UCB across the blood-brain barrier and deposition in the basal ganglia, pons, or cerebellum. This is a concern primarily in neonates.

Conjugated hyperbilirubinemia can occur with either hepatocellular or cholestatic disease. In cholestatic disease, there is an impairment of bile flow from either a mechanical or a functional block in any one of the steps involved in the secretion and drainage of bile into the duodenum.

DIAGNOSTIC STRATEGIES

The causes of jaundice in the neonate and older infant are not the same as the causes of jaundice in the older child or adolescent (Figs. 20-2 and 20-3). The approach to the problem varies with age. Some basic laboratory and radiologic studies are useful in all age groups.

BILIRUBIN

In any patient with jaundice, the total serum bilirubin should be fractionated, as the differential diagnosis of unconjugated hyperbilirubinemia is distinct from that of conjugated hyperbilirubinemia (see Figs. 20-2 and 20-3). On occasion, hemolysis interferes with some assays and may result in a falsely elevated conjugated fraction. This can be problematic with specimens obtained by heel stick or finger stick. If the clinical picture is consistent with unconjugated hyperbilirubinemia, the assay should be repeated with a venous sample.

AMINOTRANSFERASES

The serum levels of aspartate aminotransferase (AST)/glutamate oxaloacetate transaminase and alanine aminotransferase (ALT)/ glutamate pyruvate transaminase are increased to varying degrees in the presence of liver injury. Levels of both are markedly elevated (>5- to 10-fold normal) with hepatocellular injury caused by viral hepatitis, toxin- or drug-induced injury, or ischemia. Because AST also resides in many other tissues, including red blood cells and muscle, AST levels are increased with hemolysis and with cardiac or skeletal muscle damage. Because ALT is less abundant in nonhepatic tissue, an increased ALT level is more suggestive of liver disease. If AST levels are elevated in excess of ALT, a source of injury outside the hepatobiliary system should be sought. AST and ALT levels are generally only mildly elevated with intrahepatic or extrahepatic obstruction. With acute biliary obstruction, however, there can be initial sharp increases in ALT and AST levels and a rapid decline in 12 to 72 hours. With hepatocellular injury, ALT and AST levels tend to remain elevated longer, except in hepatic failure. A rapid decline in ALT and AST levels, with worsening coagulopathy and a decrease in liver size after hepatocellular injury, suggests severe liver failure and poor resolution of the disease process; treatment should be sought promptly.

There is usually no correlation between the severity of the liver disease and the degree of elevation of ALT and AST levels. However, relative changes in serum levels are useful in monitoring disease

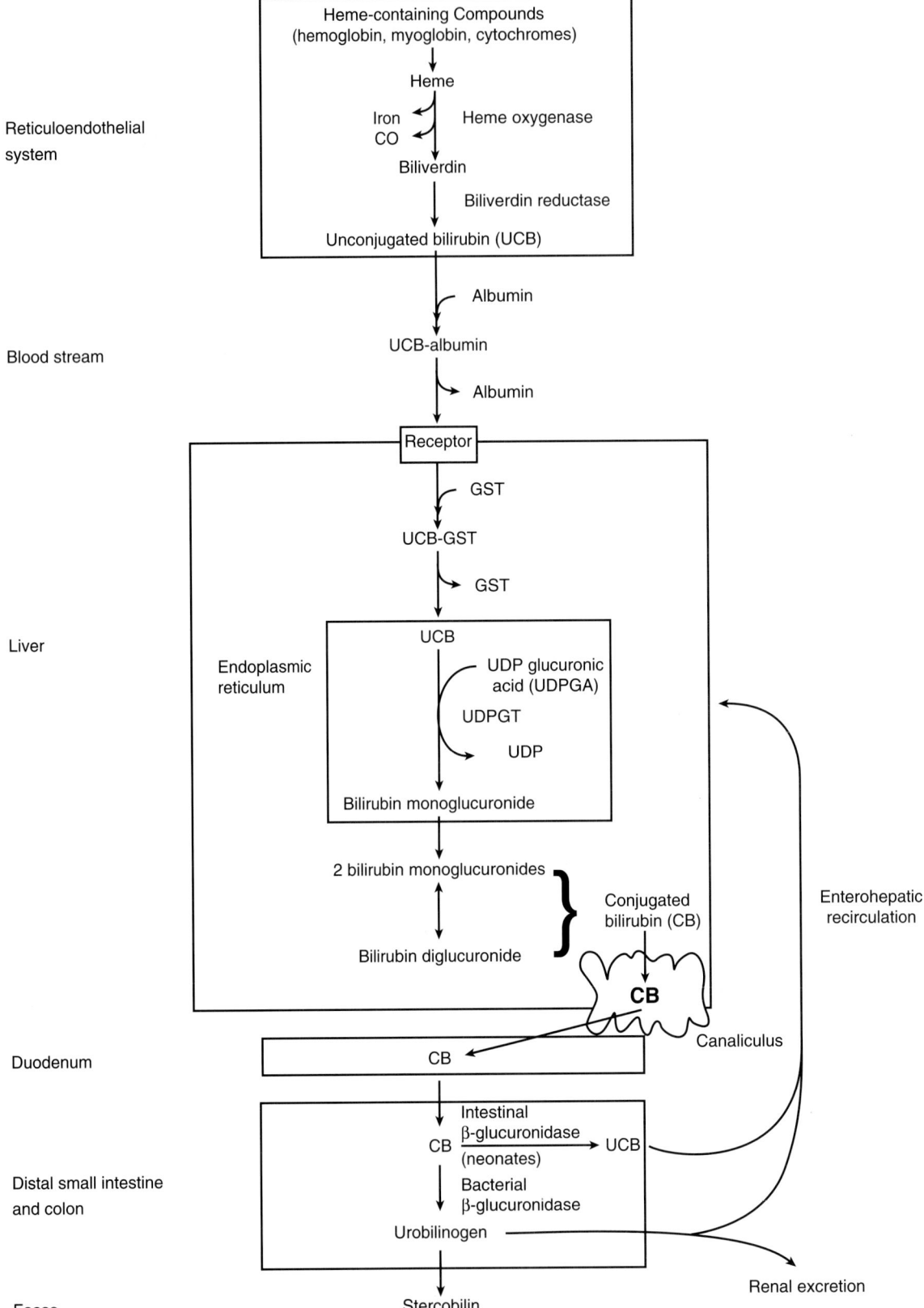

Figure 20-1. Bilirubin production and metabolism. CB, conjugated bilirubin; CO, carbon monoxide; GST, glutathione S-transferase B; UCB, unconjugated bilirubin; UDP, uridine diphosphate; UDPGA, uridine diphosphate glucuronic acid; UDPGT, uridine diphosphate glucuronosyltransferase. (Modified from Gourley GR: Jaundice. In Wyllie R, Hyams JS [eds]: Pediatric Gastrointestinal Disease: Pathophysiology, Diagnosis, Management, 2nd ed. Philadelphia, WB Saunders, 1999, p 89.)

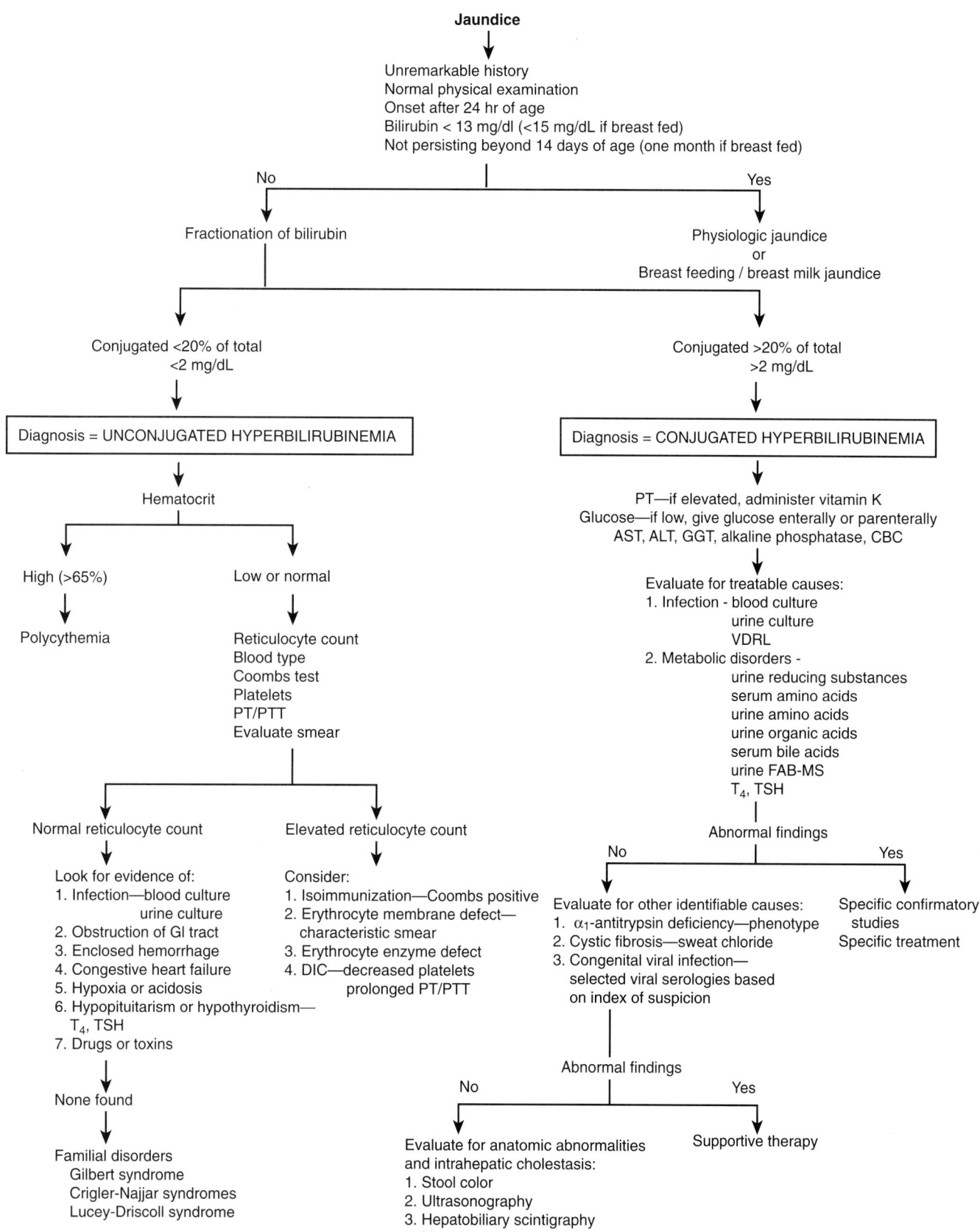

Figure 20-2. Diagnostic approach to the neonate or infant with hyperbilirubinemia. ALT, alanine aminotransferase; AST, aspartate aminotransferase; CBC, complete blood cell count; DIC, disseminated intravascular coagulation; FAB-MS, fast atom bombardment mass spectrometry; GGT, γ-glutamyltransferase; GI, gastrointestinal; PT, prothrombin time; PTT, partial thromboplastin time; T_4, thyroxine; TSH, thyroid-stimulating hormone; VDRL, Venereal Disease Research Laboratory.

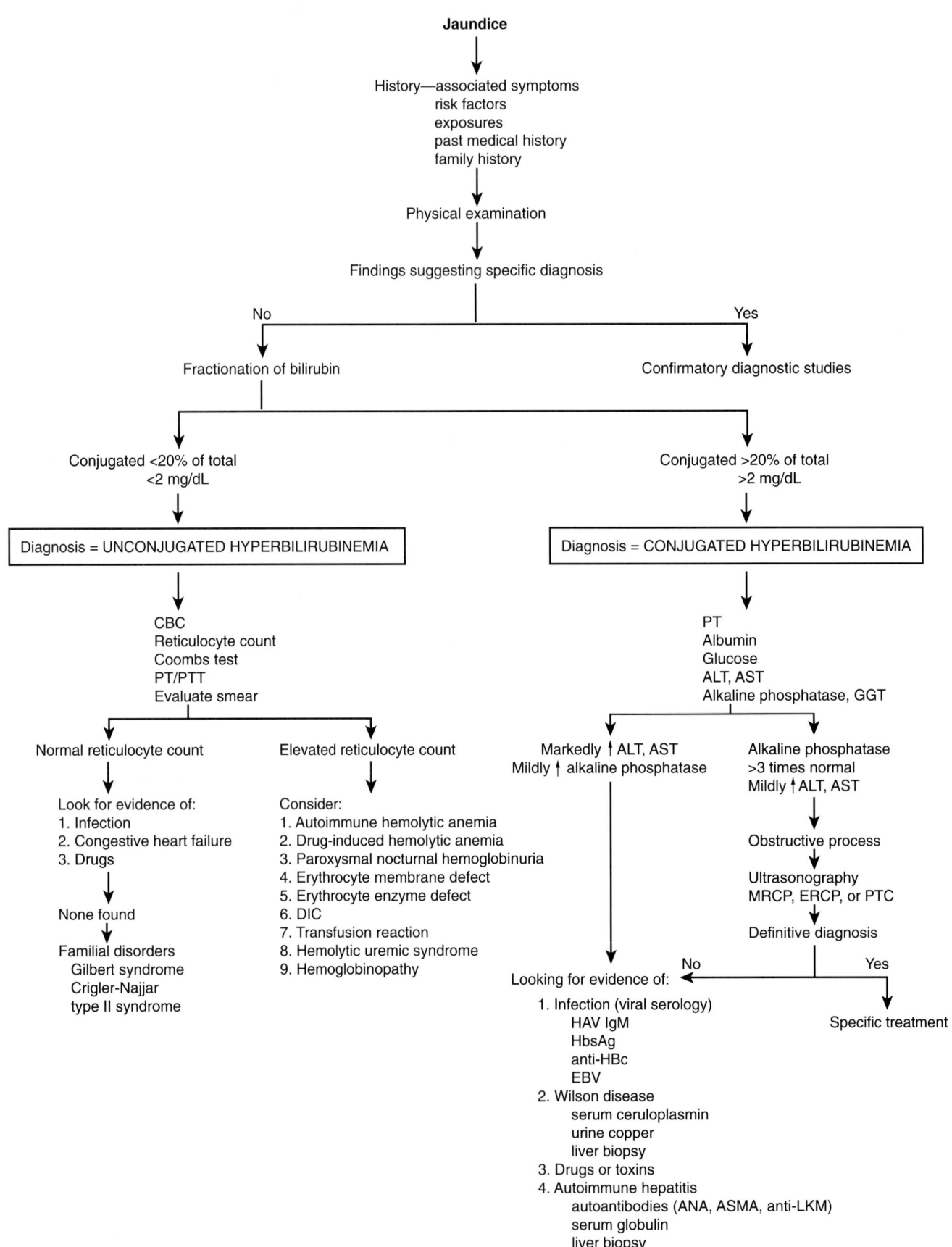

Figure 20-3. Diagnostic approach to the child or adolescent with hyperbilirubinemia. ALT, alanine aminotransferase; ANA, antinuclear antibody; ASMA, antismooth muscle antibody; AST, aspartate transaminase; CBC, complete blood cell count; DIC, disseminated intravascular coagulation; EBV, Epstein-Barr virus; ERCP, endoscopic retrograde cholangiopancreatography; GGT, γ-glutamyltransferase; HAV, hepatitis A virus; HBc, hepatitis B core; HBsAg, hepatitis B surface antigen; IgM, immunoglobulin M; LKM, liver-kidney microsomal; MRCP, magnetic resonance cholangiopancreatography; PT, prothrombin time; PTC, percutaneous transhepatic cholangiography; PTT, partial thromboplastin time.

activity for chronic problems such as chronic viral and autoimmune hepatitis.

ALKALINE PHOSPHATASE

Alkaline phosphatase is an enzyme found in liver, bone, intestine, placenta, and tumors. Elevations in the serum alkaline phosphatase level occur with normal growth, healing fractures, bone disease, pregnancy, malignancy, and hepatobiliary disease. Fractionation of the enzyme sample can help to determine its site of origin. A mild increase can be seen transiently in normal individuals. In the evaluation of conjugated hyperbilirubinemia, an alkaline phosphatase level of greater than three times normal indicates cholestasis; a milder elevation is more consistent with hepatocellular disease.

γ-GLUTAMYLTRANSFERASE

The γ-glutamyltransferase (GGT) level is more specific for biliary tract disease than are ALT and AST levels. However, GGT elevations are inducible by alcohol and certain drugs, including phenytoin and phenobarbital. GGT is found in a variety of tissues and can be elevated in chronic pulmonary disease, renal failure, and diabetes mellitus. The GGT concentration is most helpful in confirming that an elevated alkaline phosphatase level is a result of liver disease rather than bone disease and in differentiating familial cholestatic syndromes.

BILE ACIDS

Serum bile acids are a very sensitive measure of cholestatic disease. Bile acid levels may be elevated before an increase in bilirubin. Levels are generally very high with obstructive disease but only mildly increased (more than twice normal) in hepatocellular disease.

ALBUMIN

Albumin is produced in the liver, and levels can reflect hepatic synthetic function. Serum albumin levels can be useful in monitoring progression of chronic liver disease and in discriminating an acute illness from a previously unrecognized chronic disorder. *Hypoalbuminemia* can also be secondary to poor nutrition, renal disease, or a protein-losing enteropathy (see Chapter 15).

PROTHROMBIN TIME

Prothrombin time (PT) is a useful marker of hepatic synthetic function, as the vitamin K-dependent clotting factors are produced in the liver. It is important not only to measure the PT but also to document the response to parenteral administration of vitamin K. With severe hepatocellular injury, there is little improvement in the PT. In cholestatic disease, the PT should improve if the coagulopathy is secondary to inadequate enteral absorption of this fat-soluble vitamin from malabsorption. A consumptive process, such as disseminated intravascular coagulation, should not be overlooked as the cause of a prolonged PT.

ULTRASONOGRAPHY

Ultrasound studies are useful, noninvasive, relatively inexpensive diagnostic tools for the evaluation of liver disease. Ultrasonography provides information on the size and consistency of the liver and spleen and can identify dilatation of the biliary tree, gallstones, and hepatic masses such as cysts, tumors, or abscesses. Dilated intrahepatic ducts indicate extrahepatic obstruction; however, the absence of dilatation on ultrasonography cannot exclude obstruction, and further studies are required for definitive diagnosis. The utility of ultrasonography is limited in obese patients and in patients with excessive bowel gas. Ultrasonography is preferred over computed tomography and magnetic resonance (MR) imaging because it is less expensive and does not involve radiation. Doppler ultrasonography also demonstrates dynamic flow in hepatic blood vessels and the portal vein.

SCINTIGRAPHY

Hepatobiliary scintigraphy can be helpful in discriminating primarily hepatocellular damage from biliary obstruction. In the normal person, hepatic uptake and excretion of the radionuclide via the biliary system are prompt. When there is injury to the hepatocyte, the uptake of radionuclide by the liver is diminished; however, the tracer should eventually be visualized in the intestinal tract. With obstructive processes, such as biliary atresia, uptake should be relatively normal unless the problem has been present long enough to have caused hepatocellular injury; however, there is no excretion into the intestinal tract. Administration of phenobarbital (5 mg/kg/day) for 5 days before the study may increase bile flow and thus can increase the diagnostic accuracy. Unfortunately, even with this, a significant percentage of patients with intrahepatic cholestasis and neonatal hepatitis do not demonstrate biliary excretion, and further evaluation is needed.

COMPUTERIZED TOMOGRAPHY

Computerized tomography is useful for identifying mass lesions within the liver and when there are technical problems with ultrasonography.

MAGNETIC RESONANCE

MR imaging can demonstrate storage of heavy metals, such as iron in neonatal iron storage disease. MR angiography is useful in studying the vascular system, including the vascular supply of tumors. MR cholangiopancreatography (MRCP), used to evaluate abnormalities of the intrahepatic and extrahepatic biliary tree, is also quite useful in evaluating the pancreatic-biliary duct system. Unlike endoscopic retrograde cholangiopancreatography (ERCP) or percutaneous transhepatic cholangiography (PTC), MRCP is noninvasive.

ENDOSCOPIC RETROGRADE CHOLANGIOPANCREATOGRAPHY

ERCP is performed for evaluation of biliary anatomy. Unlike MRCP, ERCP is both diagnostic and potentially therapeutic for common duct stones and for strictures. It can be used to define the anatomy of the biliary tree in sclerosing cholangitis. Complications of the procedure include cholangitis and pancreatitis.

PERCUTANEOUS TRANSHEPATIC CHOLANGIOGRAPHY

PTC can be used as an alternative to ERCP as a diagnostic and therapeutic tool in evaluating the biliary tree. Under ultrasound guidance, a needle is passed through the liver and into the biliary tree, and contrast material is injected. If obstruction is identified, biliary drainage, if required, can be performed at the same time. PTC is contraindicated if there is marked ascites or irreversible coagulopathy. The complications of PTC include bleeding, pneumothorax, infection, and bile leakage.

LIVER BIOPSY

Liver biopsy is often necessary to determine the cause of conjugated hyperbilirubinemia. In some instances, a specific pattern of injury, such as paucity of bile ducts or bile duct proliferation, may be evident. In other cases, specific markers of disease may be identified (the distinctive inclusions in α_1-antitrypsin deficiency) or measured (metabolic enzyme activity). There can be sampling error with a percutaneous biopsy if a relatively small amount of tissue has been provided. An open biopsy may be necessary when a large sample of tissue is needed or when there are contraindications to the percutaneous approach, such as ascites or coagulopathy. The complications of liver biopsy are the same as those for PTC.

JAUNDICE IN THE NEONATE AND INFANT

HISTORY

The first step in treating the infant with jaundice is a thorough history, including age at onset and duration of jaundice (see Fig. 20-2). In the neonate, the causes of jaundice range from a benign, self-limited process associated with immaturity of hepatic excretory function (physiologic jaundice) to life-threatening metabolic disorders (galactosemia, fructosemia, tyrosinemia) or anatomic disorders (biliary atresia). In older infants, there are fewer benign explanations for jaundice. For example, physiologic jaundice generally resolves by 1 to 2 weeks of age, and jaundice associated with breast milk usually resolves by the time the infant is 1 month old.

Clues to the diagnosis of hyperbilirubinemia are often found in the prenatal and perinatal history (Table 20-1). Maternal infections that can be transmitted to the fetus or neonate, such as syphilis, toxoplasmosis, cytomegalovirus (CMV), hepatitis B, enterovirus, herpes simplex, and human immunodeficiency virus, are rare causes of cholestatic liver disease in the neonate. Intrauterine growth retardation is a manifestation of some congenital infections, such as CMV, rubella, and toxoplasmosis. Premature infants are prone to higher bilirubin levels and more prolonged hyperbilirubinemia; they are also more likely to have delayed enteral feedings, require parenteral nutrition, and have perinatal insults with hypoxia and acidosis.

Delay of feeding can contribute to both conjugated and unconjugated hyperbilirubinemia. Breast-feeding is associated with higher levels of unconjugated bilirubin and a longer duration of jaundice than is formula-feeding. Galactosemia does not manifest in the infant who receives a lactose-free formula. Hereditary fructose intolerance is not clinically apparent until the infant ingests fluids or solids containing fructose or sucrose. Infants with metabolic disorders often present with a history of vomiting, lethargy, and poor feeding. Vomiting may also be a symptom of intestinal obstruction.

Acholic stools, which are never normal, usually indicate obstruction of the biliary tree; however, nonpigmented stools can be seen with severe hepatocellular injury. The center of the stool should be examined, because the outside may be lightly pigmented from sloughed jaundiced cells of the intestinal tract. Delayed passage of meconium may be secondary to cystic fibrosis or Hirschsprung disease. Delayed passage of stools, by itself, can lead to increased enterohepatic circulation of bilirubin.

The family history can often provide direction to the evaluation, particularly with some of the less common hereditary disorders. This can include most of the metabolic disorders, hemolytic diseases, and disorders associated with intrahepatic cholestasis (Tables 20-2 and 20-3).

PHYSICAL EXAMINATION

With increasing levels of bilirubin, neonatal icterus becomes more extensive, spreading in a cephalopedal direction. When the serum bilirubin level is approximately 5 mg/dL, only the head and neck are icteric. With an increase to 10 mg/dL, jaundice extends to the trunk.

Table 20-1. Diagnostic Clues in the Evaluation of the Infant with Jaundice

Clue	Possible Diagnosis
Maternal Infection	
Syphilis	Syphilis
Toxoplasmosis	Toxoplasmosis
Cytomegalovirus	Cytomegalovirus
Hepatitis B	Hepatitis B
Herpes simplex	Herpes simplex
Enterovirus	Enterovirus
Human immunodeficiency virus	Human immunodeficiency virus
Polyhydramnios	Intestinal atresia
In utero growth retardation	Cytomegalovirus; rubella; toxoplasmosis
Vomiting/poor feeding	Metabolic disorders
Delayed passage of meconium	Cystic fibrosis; Hirschsprung disease
Constipation, hypotonia, hypothermia	Hypothyroidism
Characteristic Facies	
Narrow cranium, prominent forehead, hypertelorism, epicanthal folds, large fontanelle	Zellweger syndrome
Triangular face with broad forehead, hypertelorism, deep-set eyes, long nose, pointed mandible	Alagille syndrome
Microcephaly	Congenital viral infections
Ophthalmologic Findings	
Cataracts	Galactosemia; rubella
Chorioretinitis	Congenital infections
Nystagmus with hypoplasia of optic nerve	Hypopituitarism with septo-optic dysplasia
Posterior embryotoxon	Alagille syndrome
Microphallus	Hypopituitarism

When the level reaches 15 mg/dL, the lower extremities become involved. Pallor may indicate hemolytic disease. Petechiae alert the clinician to possible sepsis, congenital infections, or severe hemolytic disease.

The facies can provide clues to chromosomal disorders or inherited disorders, such as Zellweger syndrome or Alagille syndrome (see Table 20-1). The characteristic facies of Alagille syndrome may not be recognizable until later in childhood. Microcephaly that accompanies jaundice is associated with congenital viral infections.

An ophthalmologic examination can demonstrate a variety of abnormalities. Cataracts are seen in galactosemia and rubella. Chorioretinitis accompanies congenital infections (toxoplasmosis, syphilis, rubella, CMV, herpes simplex virus). Nystagmus with hypoplasia of the optic nerve suggests hypopituitarism associated with septooptic dysplasia. Posterior embryotoxon is found in Alagille syndrome.

A heart murmur may be caused by underlying congenital heart disease, which may be associated with Alagille syndrome, one of the trisomies, and some forms of biliary atresia (polysplenia syndrome). Heart disease that results in ischemia or congestion can be a cause of conjugated or unconjugated hyperbilirubinemia.

Hepatomegaly, splenomegaly, and ascites are nonspecific findings but are not associated with physiologic or breast milk jaundice.

Microphallus can be associated with septooptic dysplasia and hypopituitarism.

Table 20-2. Differential Diagnosis of Unconjugated Hyperbilirubinemia in Neonates and Infants

Physiologic Jaundice

Breast-Feeding/Breast Milk Jaundice

Polycythemia
Diabetic mother
Fetal transfusion (maternal, twin)
Intrauterine hypoxemia
Delayed cord clamping
Congenital adrenal hyperplasia
Neonatal thyrotoxicosis

Hemolysis
Isoimmune
   Rh incompatibility
   ABO incompatibility
   Other (M, S, Kidd, Kell, Duffy)
Erythrocyte membrane defects
   Hereditary spherocytosis
   Hereditary elliptocytosis
   Infantile pyknocytosis
Erythrocyte enzyme defects
   Glucose-6-phosphate dehydrogenase
   Pyruvate kinase
   Hexokinase
   Other
Hemoglobinopathy
   Thalassemia
Sepsis
Hemangioma
Congenital erythropoietic porphyria

Infection

Intestinal Obstruction
Pyloric stenosis
Intestinal atresia
Hirschsprung disease
Cystic fibrosis

Enclosed Hematoma (Cephalohematoma, Ecchymoses)

Congestive Heart Failure

Hypoxia

Acidosis

Hypothyroidism or Hypopituitarism

Drugs/Toxins
Maternal oxytocin
Vitamin K
Antibiotics
Phenol disinfectants
Herbs

Familial Disorders of Bilirubin Metabolism
Gilbert syndrome
Crigler-Najjar syndrome types I and II
Lucey-Driscoll syndrome

Modified from Balistreri WF: Liver disease in infancy and childhood. In Schiff ER, Sorrell MF, Maddrey WC (eds): Schiff's Diseases of the Liver, 8th ed. Philadelphia, Lippincott-Raven, 1999, p 1364.

DIFFERENTIAL DIAGNOSIS

When a neonate has jaundice, a thorough history, including the obstetric history, and physical examination should provide most of the information necessary to determine whether the condition represents physiologic jaundice or breast milk jaundice or whether further investigation (see Fig. 20-2) is needed. A total and fractionated bilirubin measurement may help in this decision.

Physiologic and Breast Milk Jaundice

A number of factors are responsible for production of jaundice in the normal neonate. Increased bilirubin production is caused by the normally increased neonatal red blood cell mass and the decreased life span of the red blood cell (80 versus 120 days). Albumin binding is decreased because of lower albumin concentrations and diminished binding capacity, which results in decreased transport of UCB to the liver with increased deposition in tissues. Uptake of bilirubin by the hepatocyte is defective. Low levels of glutathione S-transferase B decrease intracellular binding, which may impede transport of UCB to the endoplasmic reticulum. Conjugation is impaired by decreased activity of UDPGT. Secretion into the canaliculi is impaired. There is increased enterohepatic circulation of unconjugated bilirubin as a result of increased concentrations of β-glucuronidase in the intestinal lumen and as a result of decreased intestinal bacterial flora, leading to diminished urobilinogen formation (see Fig. 20-1).

These features contribute in varying degrees to physiologic jaundice, characterized by a peak bilirubin level of less than 13 mg/dL on postnatal days 3 to 5, a decrease to normal by 2 weeks of age, and a conjugated fraction of less than 20%. In premature, breast-fed, infants of diabetic mothers and in Asian and Native American infants, the peak is higher and lasts longer.

Breast-feeding has been associated with an increased incidence of unconjugated hyperbilirubinemia outside the expected range (>13 mg/dL). Jaundice of this level may occur in 10% to 25% of breast-fed infants, in contrast to 4% to 7% of formula-fed infants. It can occur within the first 5 days of life and is referred to as "early" or "breast-feeding" jaundice. Breast-feeding jaundice is seen in infants who are not feeding adequately and may be dehydrated or malnourished. In a second group of breast-fed infants, the jaundice develops slowly, occurring after the first week of life, and peaks between the second and third weeks of life at 10 to 20 mg/dL. This is referred to as "late" or "breast milk" jaundice. The precise cause of increased bilirubin levels in this latter setting has not been established; alternative theories include inhibition of glucuronosyltransferase activity and increased enterohepatic circulation of UCB. Kernicterus appears to be very rare but has been reported in association with breast-feeding. No treatment is necessary for physiologic jaundice. Practices that support breast-feeding, such as rooming in on the maternity ward and frequent feedings, decrease the risk for breast-feeding jaundice. If the bilirubin exceeds 20 mg/dL in the breast-fed infant, discontinuing breast-feeding for 24 hours results in a decreased bilirubin level. Phototherapy or exchange transfusion may also be needed.

If there are any red flags (Table 20-4) or if treatment is being considered, the hyperbilirubinemia should be investigated further, including fractionation of the bilirubin. Any abnormality identified by history or physical examination is a matter of concern.

Unconjugated Hyperbilirubinemia

The differential diagnosis of unconjugated hyperbilirubinemia in the neonate and infant is presented in Table 20-2. Unless abnormalities in the history and physical examination direct the evaluation more specifically, hematologic evaluation, which may identify causes of increased bilirubin production, should be performed. This includes a complete blood cell count with examination of the smear, a reticulocyte count, a direct Coombs test, and blood typing (mother and infant).

Polycythemia

Neonatal polycythemia, defined as a hematocrit greater than 65% by venipuncture, is caused by maternal diabetes, maternal-fetal or

Table 20-3. Differential Diagnosis of Conjugated Hyperbilirubinemia in Infants

Infections

Bacterial (gram negative) sepsis
Urinary tract infection
Listeriosis
Syphilis
Toxoplasmosis
Tuberculosis
Cytomegalovirus
Herpesvirus (herpes simplex, herpes zoster, human
  herpesvirus 6)
Rubella virus
Hepatitis B virus
Human immunodeficiency virus (HIV)
Coxsackievirus
Echovirus
Parvovirus B19
Adenovirus

Metabolic Disorders

α_1-Antitrypsin deficiency
Cystic fibrosis
Neonatal hemochromatosis (neonatal iron storage disease)
Endocrine disorders
  Panhypopituitarism
  Hypothyroidism
Disorders of carbohydrate metabolism
  Galactosemia
  Hereditary fructose intolerance (fructosemia)
  Glycogen storage disease type IV
Disorders of amino acid metabolism
  Tyrosinemia
  Hypermethionemia
Disorders of lipid metabolism
  Wolman disease
  Cholesterol ester storage disease
  Niemann-Pick disease
  Gaucher disease
Disorders of bile acid synthesis and metabolism
  Primary enzyme deficiencies
    3β-Hydroxy-Δ^5-C$_{27}$-steroid dehydrogenase/isomerase
    Δ^4-3-oxosteroid 5β-reductase
    Oxysterol 7α-hydroxylase
  Secondary (peroxisomal disorders)
    Zellweger syndrome (cerebrohepatorenal syndrome)
    Infantile Refsum disease
    Other enzymopathies
Mitochondrial disorders (respiratory chain)

Obstructive/Anatomic Disorders

Biliary atresia
Choledochal cyst
Caroli disease (cystic dilatation of intrahepatic ducts)
Congenital hepatic fibrosis
Neonatal sclerosing cholangitis
Bile duct stenosis
Spontaneous bile duct perforation
Anomalous choledochopancreaticoductal junction
Cholelithiasis
Inspissated bile or mucous
Mass or neoplasia

Intrahepatic Cholestasis

Alagille syndrome (arteriohepatic dysplasia)
Nonsyndromic paucity of intrahepatic bile ducts
Progressive familial intrahepatic cholestasis (PFIC)
  Type 1: Byler disease
  Type 2: defect in the bile salt export pump
  Type 3: defect in canalicular phospholipid transporter
Benign recurrent intrahepatic cholestasis
Greenland familial cholestasis (Nielsen syndrome)
North American Indian cirrhosis
Hereditary cholestasis with lymphedema (Aagenaes syndrome)

Toxin- or Drug-Related

Cholestasis associated with total parenteral nutrition
Chloral hydrate
Home remedies/herbal medicines
Venoocclusive disease

Miscellaneous

Idiopathic neonatal hepatitis
Shock or hypoperfusion (including cardiac disease)
Intestinal obstruction
Langerhans cell histiocytosis
Neonatal lupus erythematosus
Dubin-Johnson syndrome
Navajo neuropathy
Trisomies (18, 21)
Donahue syndrome (leprechaunism)
Arthrogryposis, cholestatic pigmentary disease, renal
  dysfunction syndrome
Familial erythrophagocytic lymphohistiocytosis

Modified from Balistreri WF: Liver disease in infancy and childhood. In Schiff ER, Sorrell MF, Maddrey WC (eds): Schiff's Diseases of the Liver, 8th ed. Philadelphia, Lippincott-Raven, 1999, p 1370; and Suchy FJ: Approach to the infant with cholestasis. In Suchy FJ, Sokol RJ, Balistreri WF (eds): Liver Disease in Children, 2nd ed. Philadelphia, Lippincott Williams & Wilkins, 2001, p 188.

twin-twin transfusion, intrauterine hypoxemia, endocrine disorders, and delayed cord clamping (see Table 20-2). Polycythemia results in increased bilirubin production because of the increased red blood cell mass.

Hemolytic Disorders

Reticulocytosis and an increased nucleated red blood cell count, with either a low or normal hematocrit, suggest hemolysis. This can result from isoimmunization; erythrocyte membrane, hemoglobin, or enzyme defects; or sepsis with disseminated intravascular coagulation. Some causes of isoimmunization have low reticulocyte counts because

the antibody binds to these precursor cells. Rarer causes of hemolysis include hemangiomas and congenital erythropoietic porphyria.

Isoimmune Hemolytic Disease. In this group of disorders, maternal antibodies (immunoglobulin G) to the infant's erythrocytes cross the placenta, resulting in red blood cell destruction. The administration of anti-D gamma globulin (Rh$_O$[D] immune globulin [RhoGAM]) after delivery to women who are Rh-negative has reduced the incidence of Rh sensitization and erythroblastosis fetalis. If a woman has been sensitized, the fetus can be monitored with serial amniocenteses. If necessary, intrauterine transfusion can then be performed to prevent the sequelae of severe hemolysis,

Table 20-4. Red Flags in the Evaluation of the Infant with Jaundice

Onset

<24 hr of age
>2 wk of age

Course

Increases by >5 mg/dL/day
Persists beyond 14 days of age

Prenatal History

Maternal infection
Maternal diabetes mellitus
Maternal drug use
Polyhydramnios
Intrauterine growth retardation

Delivery

Prematurity
Perinatal asphyxia
Small for gestational age

Feeding

Delayed enteral feeding
Vomiting
Poor feeding
Associated with change in formula

Stools

Acholic
Delayed passage of meconium

Family History

Jaundice
Anemia
Liver disease
Splenectomy
Cholecystectomy

Physical Examination

Ill-appearing
Pallor
Petechiae
Hematoma or ecchymoses
Chromosomal stigmata
Abnormal facies
Microcephaly
Cataracts
Chorioretinitis
Nystagmus
Optic nerve hypoplasia
Posterior embryotoxon
Heart murmur
Hepatosplenomegaly (or isolated hepatomegaly or
  splenomegaly)
Ascites
Acholic stools
Dark urine
Microphallus

Bilirubin

Total
  >13 mg/dL formula-fed
  >14-15 mg/dL breast-fed
Conjugated
  >20% of total or >2 mg/dL

which include fetal and neonatal anemia, edema, hepatosplenomegaly, and circulatory collapse or stillbirth of an infant with hydrops fetalis. If the problem has not been recognized prenatally, the infant with Rh incompatibility presents with pallor, hepatosplenomegaly, and rapidly developing jaundice.

The diagnosis is confirmed by demonstrating that the infant is Rh-positive, that the direct Coombs test result is positive, and that maternal antibody is coating the infant's red blood cells. These test results are modified with in utero transfusions with Rh-negative cells. Depending on the degree of hemolysis, postnatal phototherapy and/or exchange transfusion may be required.

ABO blood type incompatibility causes a less severe form of isoimmune hemolytic disease with a less rapid development of jaundice. It is more common in infants with blood type A or B who are born to mothers with blood type O. Hemolysis develops in 50% of sensitized infants; of these infants, 50% have a bilirubin level greater than 10 mg/dL. In addition to showing anemia, reticulocytosis, and spherocytes on the smear, the direct Coombs test result is weakly positive, and the indirect Coombs test result is positive. In rare cases, other minor blood group antibodies can also cause hemolysis.

Erythrocyte Membrane Defects. Red blood cell membrane defects are relatively uncommon causes of unconjugated hyperbilirubinemia. There is often a family history of hemolysis, transfusions, cholecystectomy for bilirubin stones, or splenectomy. Hemolysis results from fragility of the red blood cell membrane. When the defect is present in infancy, there are anemia, jaundice, and splenomegaly, and the smear is often characteristic (e.g., spherocytosis or elliptocytosis). Spherocytes are also seen with ABO incompatibility. All membrane defects yield negative results of the Coombs tests.

Erythrocyte Enzyme Defects (see Chapter 48). Glucose-6-phosphate dehydrogenase (G6PD) deficiency is common. Jaundice is seen more frequently in persons with a Mediterranean or Far Eastern ancestry who have complete absence of the enzyme. In these individuals, hemolysis can occur without a precipitant. In African-American patients, the disease is generally less severe, and hemolysis is rare without exposure to a drug, toxin, or infection that causes an oxidant stress. G6PD deficiency can manifest as neonatal jaundice on day 2 or 3 after birth; alternatively, it may not manifest until later in childhood, when jaundice is associated with an acute hemolytic crisis. Of note, G6PD deficiency has been associated with significant neonatal jaundice even without evidence of hemolysis. The reason for this may be an associated Gilbert disease. The diagnosis of G6PD deficiency is confirmed by documenting deficiency of the enzyme in red blood cells.

Numerous deficiencies of enzymes in the glycolytic pathway have been identified. Pyruvate kinase deficiency is the most common of these rare disorders. Most of these disorders are thought to have an autosomal recessive mode of transmission and have been identified in only a small number of individuals. They all result in hemolysis. The time of manifestation depends on the degree of hemolysis.

Other Considerations

If the hematocrit is normal and there is no evidence of hemolysis or a consumptive process, other explanations for unconjugated hyperbilirubinemia should be sought. Blood and urine cultures rarely identify infectious etiologic agents if the patient is otherwise clinically normal. Obstruction of the gastrointestinal tract should be evident on clinical grounds when vomiting, abdominal distention, and delayed passage of meconium are present. Obstruction should be confirmed with plain abdominal roentgenograms and contrast studies. Clinical examination should also identify cephalohematoma, ecchymoses, heart failure, hypoxia, and acidosis. Thyroxine and thyroid-stimulating hormone levels should be obtained or checked from the state neonatal screening program to look for evidence of hypothyroidism or hypopituitarism.

Drugs, administered to either mother or neonate, and toxins should be identified by careful record review. Examples include oxytocin, excess vitamin K in premature infants, some antibiotics, and phenol disinfectants used in nurseries. Use of herbal remedies should also be investigated.

In the evaluation process, it is important to remember that the division of causes into hemolytic and nonhemolytic is an arbitrary one. For example, drugs, infection, and G6PD deficiency can contribute to both hemolytic and nonhemolytic neonatal jaundice. In addition, the cause of jaundice can be multifactorial.

Familial Disorders

Final consideration should be given to the familial disorders of bilirubin metabolism.

Gilbert Syndrome. Gilbert syndrome is a benign condition that occurs in up to 8% of the population. A familial incidence is reported in 15% to 40% of cases. Gilbert syndrome is a heterogeneous group of disorders that have in common at least a 50% decrease in UDPGT activity as a result of a defect in the gene responsible for this enzyme. In 20% to 30% of individuals with Gilbert syndrome, there is also a decrease in hepatocyte bilirubin uptake. Affected individuals are generally asymptomatic and may not present with jaundice until the second or third decade of life. Gilbert syndrome may be responsible for some cases of neonatal jaundice. Mild jaundice with a bilirubin level up to 7 mg/dL can occur transiently with fatigue, exercise, fasting, febrile illness, and alcohol ingestion. Except for showing an increased indirect bilirubin level, all laboratory studies are normal. The diagnosis is generally a clinical one but can be confirmed by documenting a twofold to threefold rise in unconjugated bilirubin during a 24-hour fast.

Crigler-Najjar Syndrome. Crigler-Najjar syndrome types I and II (also known as Arias syndrome) are rare autosomal recessive conditions caused by mutations (different alleles from those of Gilbert syndrome) in the gene coding for UDPGT. Crigler-Najjar syndrome type I is characterized by marked hyperbilirubinemia (20 to 40 mg/dL) in the neonatal period in an otherwise healthy infant. Among untreated infants, kernicterus is universal, and affected individuals usually die with severe neurologic problems. Because UDPGT is undetectable, there is no conjugated bilirubin in the bile or serum, and the bile is colorless. There is no decrease in serum UCB levels during phenobarbital administration. The only therapies are exchange transfusion, intensive phototherapy, and liver transplantation. Hepatocyte transplantation has been reported, and gene therapy may be a future option.

The onset of Crigler-Najjar syndrome type II is usually at birth, although it can be in late childhood. There is less than 5% of the normal UDPGT activity. Bile contains bilirubin monoglucuronides. Bilirubin levels, generally 8 to 25 mg/dL, respond to phenobarbital administration with a significant decrease. Neurologic disease is rare.

Lucey-Driscoll Syndrome. Lucey-Driscoll syndrome is a transient familial neonatal hyperbilirubinemia that appears in the first few days of life and resolves by 2 to 3 weeks of age. This results from inhibition of UDPGT by a substance that has been found in both maternal and infant serum. The bilirubin level can rise to greater than 60 mg/dL in untreated infants, resulting in severe neurotoxicity. The condition is treated with exchange transfusion.

Therapy

Treatment of unconjugated hyperbilirubinemia depends on the degree of elevation of bilirubin. Considerable controversy exists over which level is toxic and when treatment should be initiated. Because it is lipid soluble, unconjugated bilirubin can diffuse into the central nervous system, which results in neurologic toxicity. Most authorities agree that kernicterus does not occur below a bilirubin level of 20 to 25 mg/dL in the healthy, full-term infant without evidence of hemolysis. Kernicterus may occur at lower bilirubin levels in premature or sick neonates.

Treatment options include phototherapy and exchange transfusion. Phototherapy produces a reduction of bilirubin by 1 to 2 mg/dL in 4 to 6 hours by causing the photoisomerization and photodegradation of unconjugated bilirubin to more water-soluble forms that are more readily excreted in bile and urine. Potential complications include retinal damage, diarrhea, and dehydration. Phototherapy is begun at levels below that for exchange transfusion (~5 mg/dL less) or during preparations for an exchange transfusion.

Exchange transfusion with blood cross-matched against that of the mother is indicated for severe hyperbilirubinemia. This decision must be based not only on the bilirubin level but also, as important, on the infant's age and clinical condition. In full- or near-term infants (>2000 g in weight) with evidence of hemolysis, exchange transfusion is indicated if the serum unconjugated bilirubin level is higher than 20 mg/dL or if the bilirubin level does not rapidly respond to phototherapy. Signs of kernicterus (i.e., a high-pitched cry, gaze paralysis, fever, lethargy, and opisthotonic posture) warrant exchange transfusion, no matter what the bilirubin level is.

Neonatal Conjugated Hyperbilirubinemia

Potential causes of conjugated hyperbilirubinemia in the neonate and infant are extensive (see Table 20-3). It is important to first evaluate the infant for potentially treatable problems (Tables 20-5 and 20-6) and institute specific therapy that prevents significant morbidity and may be life-saving. Figure 20-2 outlines a diagnostic approach when the clinical presentation has not suggested a likely diagnosis.

Common to all of these conditions is the potential for hypoprothrombinemia. If the PT is prolonged, the infant should be treated with intravenous vitamin K to avoid spontaneous hemorrhage, particularly intracranial. Depending on the degree of hepatocellular damage, vitamin K may not correct the PT. This is very worrisome and mandates prompt evaluation for the underlying cause. Even with a normal PT at the outset, infants with conjugated hyperbilirubinemia should be on oral vitamin K until their cholestasis resolves.

Hypoglycemia is another danger that is associated with diseases that cause severe hepatic dysfunction as well as with hypopituitarism. The infant may be relatively asymptomatic despite significant hypoglycemia. The serum glucose level can be measured before a feeding. If hypoglycemia is present, the infant should receive frequent feedings, continuous feedings, or intravenous dextrose infusions.

Serum levels of aminotransferases, GGT, and alkaline phosphatase, in addition to a complete blood cell count, should be included in the initial evaluation.

Treatable Infections

Bacterial Infection. An infant may, in rare cases, appear clinically well, with jaundice as the only sign of bacterial infection. Blood and urine specimens for culture should be obtained in infants with unexplained conjugated hyperbilirubinemia. Infection is less likely to be missed in the symptomatic infant who presents with poor feeding, lethargy, vomiting, temperature instability, apnea, bradycardia, or shock. *Escherichia coli* is the most common organism identified in either sepsis or urinary tract infection (often with bacteremia) when jaundice is present. The hyperbilirubinemia may be caused by endotoxin-mediated canalicular dysfunction. Less often, other gram-negative bacilli or *Listeria, Staphylococcus,* or *Streptococcus* species may be identified as the causative agent. Although sepsis accounts

Table 20-5. Conditions Not to Miss in the Infant with Conjugated Hyperbilirubinemia

Hypoprothrombinemia
Hypoglycemia
Infections
  Sepsis
  Urinary tract infection
  Syphilis
  Toxoplasmosis
  Herpes simplex virus
Endocrine disorders
  Hypopituitarism
  Hypothyroidism
Metabolic disorders
  Galactosemia
  Hereditary fructose intolerance (fructosemia)
  Tyrosinemia
  Neonatal hemochromatosis
  Bile acid abnormalities
Extrahepatic biliary atresia
Choledochal cyst
Intestinal obstruction
Heart disease
Toxins

for only a small percent of the cases of neonatal cholestasis, it is easily diagnosed and treated.

Syphilis. Congenital syphilis remains a problem despite maternal screening. With severe infection, the infant has fever, a diffuse macular-papular rash, hepatosplenomegaly, edema, anemia, and periostitis, in addition to jaundice. Nontreponemal serologic tests (Venereal Disease Research Laboratory) may be routinely performed on cord blood. If the result is positive, the diagnosis should be confirmed on serum from the infant. Confirmation requires a positive specific test for syphilis such as the immunoglobulin M (IgM) or immunoglobulin G fluorescent treponemal antibody. Treatment is with intravenous penicillin for 10 to 14 days.

Herpes Simplex. Herpes simplex causes a severe neonatal infection that usually manifests at 7 to 14 days of age with lethargy,

Table 20-6. Frequency of Causes of Conjugated Hyperbilirubinemia in Infants*

Biliary atresia	31%
Idiopathic neonatal hepatitis	30%
α_1-Antitrypsin deficiency	13%
Alagille syndrome	5%
All others	20%

Based on 65 cases from Balistreri WF: Neonatal cholestasis. In Lebenthal E (ed): Textbook of Gastroenterology and Nutrition in Infancy. New York, Raven Press, 1981; 171 cases from Danks DM, Campbell PE, Jack I, et al: Studies of the aetiology of neonatal hepatitis and biliary atresia. Arch Dis Child 1977;52:360-367; 1086 cases from Mieli-Vergani G, Howard ER, Mowat AP: Liver disease in infancy: A 20 year perspective. Gut 1991;32:S123-S128; 130 cases from Pretorius PJ, Roode H: Obstructive jaundice in early infancy: Aetiological, clinical and prognostic aspects. S A Med J 1974;48:811-815; and 164 cases from Stormon MO, Dorney SFA, Kanath KR, et al: The changing pattern of diagnosis of infantile cholestasis. J Paediatr Child Health 2001;37:47-50.

*A large percentage of cases were seen at a referral center and thus may not be representative of the general population. In addition, parenteral nutrition associated cholestasis was specifically excluded in some series.

poor feeding, a vesicular rash (in 60% to 70% of patients), jaundice, hepatomegaly, temperature instability, encephalitis, and a coagulopathy. The diagnosis is made by identification of the virus in skin lesions through direct fluorescent antibody staining or enzyme immunoassay detection of herpes antigens, cell culture, or polymerase chain reaction of herpes simplex DNA. Treatment is with intravenous acyclovir. Among infants with disseminated infection, the mortality rate is 15% to 35%.

Enteroviruses. Maternal infection at the time of delivery may result in severe enteroviral disease in the infant within 1 to 7 days of birth. Manifestations are similar to that of herpes simplex virus except a macular rash, rather than the vesicular rash of herpes simplex virus, is seen. Severe hepatitis, carditis, or encephalitis or a sepsis picture may develop. Diagnosis is made through polymerase chain reaction or viral culture. Treatment is with pleconaril.

Toxoplasmosis. If toxoplasmosis is suspected on clinical grounds, IgM titers should be obtained, or the placenta should be examined histologically. Most infected infants are asymptomatic. Infants with severe congenital infection may have hydrocephaly or microcephaly, intracranial calcifications, chorioretinitis, aseptic meningitis, jaundice, purpura, and hepatomegaly. Postnatal treatment consists of pyrimethamine and sulfadiazine; folinic acid is added to prevent folate deficiency.

Treatable Metabolic Disorders

There are several useful screening modalities: urine-reducing substances (galactosemia), serum and urine amino acids, urine organic acids, quantitative serum bile acids, qualitative analysis of urinary bile acids by fast atom bombardment mass spectrometry, the thyroxine level, and the thyroid-stimulating hormone level. Some of these (e.g., galactosemia and thyroid) are included in state neonatal screening programs.

Hypothyroidism and Hypopituitarism. Jaundice can be a manifestation of both hypothyroidism and hypopituitarism. Hypopituitarism may manifest with hypoglycemia, microphallus, and signs of hypothyroidism in addition to jaundice. Wandering nystagmus is present when hypopituitarism is associated with septooptic dysplasia. Treatment of the underlying endocrinopathy leads to resolution of the liver disease.

Galactosemia and Hereditary Fructose Intolerance. Although rare, galactosemia, a life-threatening disorder, can easily be detected. It is an autosomal recessive disorder with deficiency of galactose-1-phosphate uridyltransferase, which is required for conversion of galactose to glucose. As a result, galactose-1-phosphate accumulates; this compound is thought to be hepatotoxic. Once lactose (glucose-galactose) is introduced in the infant's diet, vomiting, diarrhea, jaundice, hepatomegaly, and cataracts develop. Affected infants often present with *E. coli* sepsis in the first weeks of life.

Laboratory evaluation may demonstrate elevations of aminotransferase levels, a prolonged PT, hemolytic anemia, and aminoaciduria. The urine yields positive findings for reducing substances (galactose) if the infant is receiving a lactose-containing formula or breast milk. The diagnosis can be confirmed by documenting deficiency of the enzyme in erythrocytes or leukocytes. Transfusions may cause false-negative results. Treatment consists of eliminating galactose from the diet.

Hereditary fructose intolerance (fructosemia) is an uncommon disorder; it can manifest with hepatic failure in an infant exposed to fructose or sucrose in formula, juice, fruit, or medications. A thorough diet history in relation to the onset of jaundice is often the key to this diagnosis. Prompt removal of fructose, sucrose, and sorbitol from the diet is essential.

Tyrosinemia and Inborn Errors of Bile Acid Metabolism.
Also rare but readily identifiable are tyrosinemia and inborn errors of bile acid metabolism. Tyrosinemia is diagnosed from serum and urine amino acid levels and urine organic acid levels. Elevated urinary succinylacetone is pathognomonic. Treatment involves dietary restriction of phenylalanine, methionine, and tyrosine and the use of 2-(2-nitro-4-trifluoromethylbenzoyl)-1,3-cyclohexanedione) to prevent formation of toxic metabolites. Liver transplantation may still be required. Disorders of bile acid metabolism can be detected by FAB-MS analysis of urine. Treatment consists of oral bile acid therapy.

Other Identifiable Infectious and Metabolic Causes of Cholestasis

α_1-Antitrypsin Deficiency.
An α_1-antitrypsin phenotype can detect α_1-antitrypsin deficiency, which is the most common inherited cause of neonatal cholestasis. Deficiency occurs in 1 in 1600 to 2000 live births. α_1-Antitrypsin is a protease inhibitor that is synthesized in the liver and inactivates neutrophil proteases. The normal protease inhibitor phenotype, MM, is found in 80% to 90% of the population. There are numerous allelic variants. Liver disease is associated with the ZZ phenotype and sporadically with other variants. The exact mechanism of liver injury is unclear, and there is variability in expression, so that clinically significant liver disease develops in only 10% to 15% of individuals with the ZZ phenotype. There is also great variability in manifestation. Commonly, the disorder manifests in early infancy with prolonged conjugated hyperbilirubinemia, failure to thrive, acholic stools, hepatomegaly, and possibly ascites. However, it may not manifest until later childhood or even adulthood. Manifestations in the older individual include jaundice, hepatosplenomegaly, ascites, portal hypertension with varices, chronic hepatitis, cryptogenic cirrhosis, or, rarely, hepatocellular carcinoma. The diagnosis is established by serum phenotyping (ZZ). Treatment is supportive. Some individuals do very well with minimal liver dysfunction. Others have progressive liver disease, requiring transplantation. The progression may be rapid or slow. All individuals with α_1-antitrypsin deficiency should be aware of the potential for lung disease when they are older.

Cystic Fibrosis.
As many as one third of infants with cystic fibrosis may have evidence of liver involvement, frequently cholestasis. The incidence is increased among infants with meconium ileus. The diagnosis can be confirmed with a sweat chloride test or by detecting the abnormal gene. Although the cholestasis resolves, the infant with cystic fibrosis often has additional hepatobiliary problems later in childhood. These problems may include focal biliary cirrhosis, multilobular cirrhosis, fatty liver, obstruction of the common duct secondary to pancreatic duct sludge or pancreatic fibrosis, cholelithiasis, sclerosing cholangitis, and, rarely, cholangiocarcinoma.

Congenital Viral Infections.
A number of viral infections have been associated with neonatal cholestasis, but routine toxoplasmosis, other infections, rubella, CMV, and herpes (TORCH) titers are not indicated. Selected serologic or viral studies should be performed only if there is a high index of suspicion on the basis of the history or physical examination.

Cytomegalovirus Infection.
CMV infection is common, but 90% of affected infants are asymptomatic at birth. In the severely affected infant with vertical transmission, CMV can manifest within the first 24 hours after birth with intrauterine growth retardation, conjugated hyperbilirubinemia, hemolytic anemia, thrombocytopenic purpura, and hepatosplenomegaly. Often an infant with low birth weight presents with microcephaly, periventricular calcifications, and chorioretinitis. The diagnosis can be made by obtaining urine specimens for culture.

Treatment includes use of ganciclovir and possibly CMV immunoglobulin. The liver disease resolves in most patients, but neurologic sequelae are common. Postnatal acquisition from CMV-positive blood transfusion may produce a sepsis syndrome and hepatitis.

The findings of CMV in a cholestatic infant without other features of congenital CMV infection should not stop the search for other causes of cholestasis, particularly biliary atresia.

Rubella.
Congenital infection with rubella is rare because of immunization. Jaundice is present in only 15% to 20% of cases. Other manifestations include low birth weight, cataracts, heart disease (patent ductus arteriosus), hepatosplenomegaly, and thrombocytopenic purpura. The diagnosis is made by viral isolation. There is no proven therapy. The liver disease usually resolves completely; the infant is left with other organ sequelae, such as deafness and microcephaly.

Hepatitis B.
Hepatitis B infection manifests with jaundice in fewer than 5% of perinatal infections. Perinatal transmission is high when mothers are chronic carriers who are seropositive for hepatitis B e antigen or when they acquire acute infection in the last trimester. Most infants are asymptomatic, but there is a high incidence of subsequent chronic infection. Perinatal infection can be prevented with hepatitis B immune globulin and vaccination. It is important to identify mothers who are seropositive for hepatitis B surface antigen (HBsAg); identification requires universal screening.

Obstructive/Anatomic Abnormalities, Idiopathic Cholestasis, and Idiopathic Neonatal Hepatitis

Biliary Atresia.
Biliary atresia accounts for approximately 30% of cases of neonatal cholestasis seen at major referral centers (see Table 20-6). It occurs in 1 in 8000 to 15,000 live births. This condition is the result of a progressive inflammatory process leading to obliteration of the lumen of the extrahepatic duct. It is the leading indication for liver transplantation in the pediatric population. Infants are less often icteric from birth and more often develop jaundice at 2 to 6 weeks of age. Infants are usually full term and initially appear healthy except for jaundice, dark urine, and acholic stools. The family history is negative. There appear to be two forms of biliary atresia:

1. In the "embryonic" or "fetal form," which occurs in 15% to 30% of cases, there is no jaundice-free period. There are often associated defects, including cardiac defects, polysplenia, malrotation, and situs inversus.
2. In the "perinatal form," there is a jaundice-free interval after the normal physiologic jaundice and there are no associated anomalies.

At the time of presentation, infants with biliary atresia have an enlarged, firm liver. Pruritus, splenomegaly, and ascites often develop.

Diagnostic workup includes exclusion of other identifiable causes of neonatal cholestasis. The workup should be performed expeditiously; it is important to identify biliary atresia early because the success of surgical establishment of drainage is correlated with early age at surgery. Surgery performed before the infant is 2 months old carries an approximately 80% rate of success in terms of obtaining some bile flow. This rate decreases to about 20% for surgery performed in patients older than 3 months. An ultrasound study helps exclude other treatable anatomic abnormalities, such as a choledochal cyst. The gallbladder is usually absent in infants with biliary atresia. Some centers utilize hepatobiliary scintigraphy, which demonstrates uptake of tracer but no excretion into the duodenum if biliary atresia is present. Characteristic findings on liver biopsy are portal and perilobular edema and fibrosis, bile duct proliferation, and bile duct plugs.

The diagnosis is confirmed by intraoperative cholangiography at the time of surgery. The surgical procedure, a hepatoportoenterostomy, is that initially described by Kasai. The porta hepatis is transected, and a loop of intestine is brought up to drain the bile ducts. In a small percentage of patients (5% to 15%), a discrete distal lesion is identified and the surgery is curative. Those in whom bile drainage is not established require early liver transplantation. In the remainder, surgery is palliative, allowing time before liver transplantation is needed. The primary postoperative complication is bacterial cholangitis.

Intrahepatic Paucity of Bile Ducts. This condition is defined as the absence or marked reduction in the number of interlobular bile ducts. Jaundice may have its onset in the neonatal period or may not appear until later in childhood. There is a syndromic form known as arteriohepatic dysplasia, or Alagille syndrome. This is characterized by unusual facies (a triangular face with broad forehead, widely spaced and deep-set eyes, a long nose, and a pointed mandible), vertebral arch defects (butterfly vertebrae, hemivertebrae, decreased interpedicular distance), posterior embryotoxon (ocular), and cardiac anomalies (ranging from peripheral pulmonic stenosis to complex congenital heart disease), in addition to cholestasis secondary to paucity of ducts. Renal anomalies and growth retardation are also often present. This appears to be a progressive phenomenon and may not be readily recognizable in neonates. By age 4 to 6 months, pruritus develops and can be severe. Xanthomas appear in association with a markedly elevated cholesterol level. Alagille syndrome has an autosomal dominant transmission with highly variable expression. Often other family members are recognized as being affected when an infant is brought to medical attention. There is a high proportion of sporadic cases (up to 70%) with de novo mutations in the Jagged-1 gene responsible for this syndrome.

The diagnosis is confirmed by liver biopsy. Symptoms often improve over time. There is a 20% to 25% rate of mortality from serious cardiac or liver disease.

There is a nonsyndromic form with cholestasis caused by bile duct paucity but not the other features. The prognosis for this form is less favorable.

Choledochal Cysts. Manifestations include conjugated hyperbilirubinemia with jaundice, vomiting, acholic stools, and hepatomegaly in the neonate. Alternatively, choledochal cysts can manifest with jaundice, abdominal pain, and a right upper quadrant mass in the older child. There are five types of cystic dilatations of the extrahepatic or intrahepatic bile ducts. The diagnosis is made by ultrasound studies and confirmed by intraoperative cholangiography. Treatment involves surgical excision. Cholangitis may occur postoperatively. If the cyst is not fully excised, carcinoma can develop in the residual cyst tissue.

Idiopathic Neonatal Hepatitis. Idiopathic neonatal hepatitis is a descriptive term rather than a specific disease entity. The diagnosis is made by exclusion of other causes of cholestasis, particularly biliary atresia. The infant with neonatal hepatitis is more likely to be premature or small for gestational age. Acholic stools are uncommon but can occur when the hepatitis is severe. In 5% to 15% of cases, there is a familial incidence. Hepatobiliary scintigraphy demonstrates delayed uptake, but there is usually excretion into the duodenum unless the hepatitis is severe. In this case, intraoperative cholangiography may be required. Biopsy findings include panlobular disarray indicative of severe hepatocellular disease, inflammatory infiltrate in the portal areas, focal hepatocellular necrosis, multinucleated giant cells, and increased extramedullary hematopoiesis.

Treatment is supportive. The outcome is variable and is better for infants with sporadic (nonfamilial) cases; of such infants, approximately 60% recover, 10% have chronic liver disease, and 30% die without liver transplantation. The percentages for recovery and death are reversed—30% and 60%, respectively—in familial cases.

Progressive Familial Intrahepatic Cholestasis

Progressive familial intrahepatic cholestasis (PFIC) was originally described in an Amish kindred (Byler disease). Several distinct types are known. The molecular defects for three PFIC types appear to involve defective hepatocyte transporters for either bile acids or phospholipids. PFIC is inherited in an autosomal recessive manner and results in progressive cholestasis and pruritus, leading to cirrhosis and end-stage liver disease. PFIC type I was first described in the Byler family. This type of PFIC has low or normal serum γ-glutamyl transpeptidase (GGTP) and cholesterol levels and high serum concentrations of bile acids. The defect in Byler disease is in gene *FICI,* which encodes a P-type adenosine triphosphatase that may be involved in the transport of amino phospholipids in the hepatocyte. Several homozygous mutations in the *FICI* gene have been identified in children with PFIC type 1. This same gene appears to be defective in a milder form of cholestatic liver disease, benign recurrent intrahepatic cholestasis. Patients with PFIC type 2 also exhibit cholestasis, normal serum GGTP and cholesterol levels, and high levels of serum bile acids. These patients are unrelated to the Byler family and have a defect in an adenosine triphosphate–dependent canalicular bile acid transporter or bile salt export pump. Several mutations of the gene for this transporter have been identified. Patients with PFIC type 3 have high serum GGTP and cholesterol levels. They demonstrate symptoms later in life and reach end-stage liver disease at a later age. PFIC type 3 is caused by a defect in the *MDR3* gene, which encodes a phospholipid transporter in the canalicular membrane and results in low biliary phospholipid levels. Except in cases necessitating liver transplantation, chronic biliary diversion and ursodeoxycholic acid therapy may reduce pruritus and improve liver function.

Treatment of Cholestasis

Some interventions are essential for all infants with cholestasis. Malabsorption of fats and fat-soluble vitamins occurs as a result of a decreased concentration of bile salts in the intestinal lumen. Affected infants should be given a formula containing medium-chain triglycerides, which are digested and absorbed without bile salts. Even with the use of special formulas, such infants have some degree of malabsorption and require extra calories for growth. Some affected infants require supplemental nasogastric feedings. Supplemental vitamins A, D, E, and K are given to prevent visual problems, rickets, neuropathy, and coagulopathy, respectively. A water-soluble vitamin E preparation, d-α-tocopheryl-polyethylene glycol-1000 succinate (TPGS), forms micelles without bile salts and is therefore readily absorbed. Mixing vitamins A and D with TPGS promotes their absorption.

Ascites can be managed with sodium restriction and diuretics. Pruritus is often severe and is not readily treatable. Several medications have been tried, including ursodeoxycholic acid, antihistamines, cholestyramine, phenobarbital, and rifampin. Ursodeoxycholic acid is beneficial in some infants with cholestasis and helps to improve bile excretion, thus reducing serum bile acid levels. Biliary diversion has been effective in some cases.

In summary, there are often clues in the history or physical examination that guide the workup for conjugated hyperbilirubinemia in infants and preclude the need for extensive testing. In addition, there are a limited number of disorders that can be ameliorated by early diagnosis and treatment. As long as these are excluded and appropriate supportive care is given, there is time to make a more definitive diagnosis. Supportive care should include removal of potential toxins from the diet (such as galactose and fructose), provision of supplemental vitamin K, avoidance of hypoglycemia, and early referral to a transplantation center for the infant with worsening hepatic dysfunction.

JAUNDICE IN THE CHILD AND ADOLESCENT

HISTORY

The individual with hepatocellular disease generally feels ill. Fatigue, anorexia, myalgias, nausea, vomiting, and fever are often seen in patients with viral hepatitis or autoimmune hepatitis. Acute biliary obstruction is signaled by right upper quadrant pain, vomiting, fever, and acholic stools in addition to jaundice. Neurologic and psychiatric symptoms may be among the manifestations of Wilson disease. Autoimmune hepatitis may be accompanied by manifestations of other autoimmune disorders.

The child's age at the onset of symptoms may be helpful. For example, Wilson disease commonly manifests in preadolescents and adolescents.

A thorough history should include past and present use of prescription, over-the-counter (e.g., acetaminophen), and street drugs. Many medications have been associated with hepatobiliary damage; others, with hemolysis. Drug abuse is a risk factor for viral hepatitis and human immunodeficiency virus. Other risk factors for viral hepatitis include homosexual activity, obtaining tattoos, and a history of blood transfusions or dialysis. Adolescents in particular should be asked about alcohol use.

Information about exposure to viral hepatitis, either by travel to an endemic area or during an outbreak, should be pursued. There is a high transmission rate in day care centers.

The patient's medical history should be reviewed because some chronic illnesses are associated with specific hepatobiliary complications. These include acquired immunodeficiency syndrome, cystic fibrosis, heart disease, hemolytic disorders, hemoglobinopathies, and inflammatory bowel disease.

A family history of inheritable disorders, such as Wilson disease or spherocytosis, is informative. Less specific but still useful clues are a history of jaundice, anemia, cholecystectomy, or splenectomy in other family members.

PHYSICAL EXAMINATION

Some patients present with previously unidentified chronic liver disease. Evidence of chronicity includes spider angiomas, palmar erythema, dilated abdominal veins, cutaneous excoriation as evidence of pruritus, xanthomas, clubbing of digits, ascites, and splenomegaly with a small liver. Splenomegaly is also a characteristic finding in hemolytic disorders and in some oncologic disorders (see Chapter 19). A large, tender liver is suggestive of acute viral hepatitis or congestive heart failure. A small liver may be found in patients with severe hepatitis or cirrhosis. A tender gallbladder is indicative of choledocholithiasis. Abnormal neurologic findings, including tremor, fine motor incoordination, clumsy gait, and choreiform movements, suggest Wilson disease. A slit-lamp examination should be included to look for the Kayser-Fleischer rings (a brownish discoloration at the periphery of the cornea) of Wilson disease.

DIFFERENTIAL DIAGNOSIS

A specific diagnosis may seem highly likely, on the basis of the clinical presentation. In such a case, laboratory evaluation should first be directed at confirming the suspected diagnosis. If no clear diagnosis is readily apparent, the evaluation should proceed as outlined in Figure 20-3. Just as with the infant, an initial step in the diagnosis of jaundice in the older child should be fractionation of the bilirubin to discriminate unconjugated from conjugated hyperbilirubinemia.

Unconjugated Hyperbilirubinemia

Most causes of unconjugated hyperbilirubinemia in the child and adolescent are secondary to hemolysis (Table 20-7) (see Chapter 48). A complete blood cell count with evaluation of the smear, reticulocyte count, and Coombs test can differentiate hemolytic from nonhemolytic disorders.

Erythrocyte membrane defects (spherocytosis) and enzyme defects (pyruvate kinase deficiency, G6PD) may not be apparent until childhood or adolescence. Acquired autoimmune hemolytic anemia is characterized by pallor, abdominal pain, fever, and dark urine in addition to jaundice. Laboratory studies document anemia and reticulocytosis. The direct Coombs test result is positive. Hemolytic anemia can be associated with infection, immunodeficiency, malignancy, hemolytic uremic syndrome, or other autoimmune disorders, such as systemic lupus erythematosus, rheumatoid arthritis, thyroid disorders, and autoimmune hepatitis. Most autoimmune hemolytic anemia is idiopathic.

Most of the nonhemolytic causes of unconjugated hyperbilirubinemia are identified during the initial assessment. Congestive heart failure and infection should be suspected from physical examination.

Table 20-7. Differential Diagnosis of Unconjugated Hyperbilirubinemia in Childhood and Adolescence

Increased Bilirubin Production
Autoimmune hemolytic anemia
  Idiopathic
  Secondary
    Infection (viral, mycoplasma)
    Diseases with autoantibody production
    Immunodeficiency
    Malignancy
Drug-induced hemolytic anemia
Paroxysmal nocturnal hemoglobinuria
Erythrocyte membrane defects
  Hereditary spherocytosis
  Hereditary elliptocytosis
Erythrocyte enzyme defects
  Glucose-6-phosphate dehydrogenase
  Pyruvate kinase
  Hexokinase
  Other
Hemoglobinopathy
  Sickle cell disease
  Thalassemia
Hemolytic uremic syndrome
Sepsis with disseminated intravascular coagulation
Reabsorption of hematoma
Transfusion reaction

Decreased Uptake, Storage, or Metabolism
Congestive heart failure
Sepsis
Acidosis
Gilbert syndrome
Crigler-Najjar syndrome type II
Prolonged fasting
Drugs
Portacaval shunt

The child or adolescent with infection severe enough to cause jaundice has other signs of sepsis. If no other explanation is found, Gilbert syndrome or Crigler-Najjar syndrome type II should be considered.

Conjugated Hyperbilirubinemia

In the child with conjugated hyperbilirubinemia, the PT and the albumin, glucose, AST, ALT, GGT, and alkaline phosphatase levels should be measured. Albumin and PT determinations provide evidence of hepatocyte synthetic function. Hypoglycemia is another marker of severity of hepatocellular damage. This is important in considering how quickly the evaluation should proceed or how closely the patient should be monitored. For example, the child who has a classic presentation for hepatitis A but also a prolonged PT or hypoglycemia may be in that small group who develop fulminant hepatic failure; these children should be admitted to the hospital and observed very closely. An attempt should be made to correct the PT to differentiate hepatocellular from cholestatic disease. Hypoglycemia should be corrected with frequent meals or intravenous dextrose.

Obstruction

The relative elevation of AST/ALT and alkaline phosphatase levels in the context of the clinical picture determines the likelihood of an obstructive cause. Although obstructions occur less commonly in children than in adults, it is important not to miss correctable causes of obstruction that, if left untreated, can cause hepatocellular damage. These patients usually have markedly elevated alkaline phosphatase and minimally elevated AST and ALT levels. They should be evaluated promptly with ultrasonography and possibly with MRCP, ERCP, or PTC. The possible causes of obstruction are listed in Table 20-8.

Gallstones. Gallstones are particularly common in children with hemolytic disorders, such as sickle cell disease, thalassemia, erythrocyte membrane defects, erythrocyte enzyme defects, and autoimmune hemolytic anemia. The mean age at presentation is 12 years. Gallstones are also associated with anatomic abnormalities of the biliary tract, cystic fibrosis, ileal dysfunction, obesity, parenteral nutrition, sepsis, prematurity, and pregnancy. Stones may be found incidentally on abdominal radiographs or ultrasound studies in

---

Table 20-8. Differential Diagnosis of Conjugated Hyperbilirubinemia in Childhood and Adolescence

Obstructive	Drug or Toxin
Gallstones	Drugs*
Primary sclerosing cholangitis	Chlorpromazine
Choledochal cyst	Hormones (estrogens, androgens)
Bile duct stenosis	Antibiotics (amoxicillin-clavulanate, dicloxacillin,
Anomalies of the choledochopancreaticoduodenal junction	erythromycin, sulfonamides, tetracycline)
Pancreatitis	Anticonvulsants (carbamazepine, phenytoin, valproate)
Caroli disease	Acetaminophen
Congenital hepatic fibrosis	Alcohol
Tumor	Halothane
Hepatic	Isoniazid
Biliary	Antineoplastics
Pancreatic	Toxins
Duodenal	*Amanita phalloides* (mushroom)
	Insecticides
Infection	Carbon tetrachloride
Non–A-E hepatitis	Phosphorus
Hepatitis A	Herbal teas
Hepatitis B	Total parenteral nutrition
Hepatitis C	
Hepatitis D	**Autoimmune Hepatitis**
Hepatitis E	
Epstein-Barr virus	**Intrahepatic Cholestasis**
Cytomegalovirus	Benign recurrent intrahepatic cholestasis
Human herpesvirus 6	Progressive familial intrahepatic cholestasis type 3
Herpes simplex virus	
Varicella zoster virus	**Miscellaneous**
Human immunodeficiency virus	Dubin-Johnson syndrome
Leptospirosis	Rotor syndrome
Sepsis/shock	Indian childhood cirrhosis
Liver abscess	Cardiovascular
	Ischemia
Metabolic Disorders	Congestive heart failure
Wilson disease	Cardiomyopathy
Cystic fibrosis	Oncologic
Cholesterol ester storage disease	Leukemia
Alpers syndrome	Lymphoma
α_1-antitrypsin deficiency	Graft-versus-host disease
	Veno-occlusive disease
	Sickle cell disease with intrahepatic sickling
	Heat stroke
	Navajo neuropathy

*Many other drugs have been implicated in the etiology of conjugated hyperbilirubinemia; these are the most commonly cited.

asymptomatic individuals. Alternatively, gallstones may manifest with nausea, vomiting, right upper quadrant or nonspecific abdominal pain, and jaundice. Ultrasonography is a very sensitive diagnostic test. Treatment for symptomatic patients is cholecystectomy. ERCP can be used to remove common bile duct stones.

Primary Sclerosing Cholangitis. Primary sclerosing cholangitis is characterized by focal dilatation and stenosis of the intrahepatic or extrahepatic bile ducts with surrounding fibrosis resulting from an inflammatory process. It can manifest from early childhood through adulthood. In adults, it is frequently associated with inflammatory bowel disease, especially ulcerative colitis. It may precede the onset of inflammatory bowel disease by many years (see Chapter 15). It has also been found in association with Langerhans cell histiocytosis and immunodeficiency states. There is an overlap syndrome with features of both sclerosing cholangitis and autoimmune hepatitis. It can occur in the absence of any underlying condition. The onset may be insidious. Symptoms include diarrhea, abdominal pain, fever, and jaundice.

Diagnostic evaluation includes ultrasound studies, which may show dilated ducts, and cholangiography (MRCP, ERCP, or PTC), which demonstrates the characteristic beading of bile ducts. The disorder can progress to cirrhosis with ultimate liver failure. Cholangiocarcinoma has occurred in 10% to 15% of adults. There is no documented efficacy of any therapy except transplantation.

Other Causes. If an obstructive process has been excluded or is less likely, according to a combination of the clinical picture and aminotransferase levels that are more elevated than the alkaline phosphate and GGT levels, the evaluation should focus on infectious, metabolic, toxic, and autoimmune causes.

Infection

Infections are a common cause of jaundice in the child and adolescent. To diagnose acute hepatitis, the following studies should be obtained: hepatitis A IgM, HBsAg, and hepatitis B core IgM (anti-HBc). If HBsAg is positive, it may be useful to measure hepatitis D antibodies as well. Epstein-Barr virus titers may also be useful.

Hepatitis A. Hepatitis A virus (HAV) infection is usually anicteric or asymptomatic in children younger than 5 years of age. However, in almost 66% of infected patients between 5 and 17 years of age, a symptomatic illness with jaundice develops. Two to 7 days before the onset of jaundice, there is a flulike illness with symptoms that can include malaise, headache, myalgias, anorexia, vomiting, diarrhea, right upper quadrant pain, and fever. Some children present with cough and coryza. The urine becomes dark, and jaundice and pale or acholic stools develop. Aminotransferase levels are 10 to 100 times normal.

The diagnosis is confirmed by HAV IgM study. Children generally recover within 2 weeks. On occasion, fulminant hepatitis develops from HAV infection. Small percentages develop either a relapsing or protracted cholestatic illness lasting up to 8 months. There is no carrier state or chronic illness.

HAV is an enterovirus of the picornavirus group. Transmission is by the fecal-oral route, which may include contaminated water and food, especially shellfish. The greatest fecal excretion is before the onset of jaundice, when the disease has not yet been recognized (Fig. 20-4). Transmission rates are high in day care centers and institutions for the mentally retarded. The incubation period is 15 to 40 days. After exposure, infection can be prevented in 85% to 90% of cases by giving intramuscular immunoglobulin to contacts within 2 weeks of exposure. Hepatitis A vaccine is available for long-term prophylaxis.

Hepatitis B. Hepatitis B virus (HBV) infection has a more insidious onset than does HAV infection, but it produces the same symptoms. In addition, there may be evidence of arthritis, polyarteritis, urticaria, and nephritis from circulating immune complexes. As with HAV, HBV infection may be asymptomatic.

There are a number of serologic markers of HBV infection. HBsAg is the first antigenic marker to appear; it disappears after 1 to 3 months if HBV resolves (Fig. 20-5). Hepatitis B surface antibody (anti-HBs) levels help document recovery and immunity. In patients whose infections resolve, there is a window of 2 to 6 weeks between the disappearance of HBsAg and the appearance of anti-HBs. During this window, anti-HBc may be the only evidence of infection with HBV. Hepatitis B e antigen (HBeAg) correlates with viral replication and thus is a marker of the degree of infectivity. HBV DNA is a measure of viral replication. The diagnosis of acute infection is made with HBsAg and anti-HBc.

Although acute HBV infection is rarely a severe illness, fulminant hepatic failure develops in up to 1% of patients.

Chronic infection, defined as the persistence of HBsAg for at least 6 months, occurs in 90% of infected neonates, 25% to 50% of infected children younger than 5 years, and 5% to 10% of infected adults. HBV is a DNA virus that is transmitted through blood products, shared needles, and sexual contact; vertically during childbirth; and from occupational exposure. Risk of vertical infection in the infant is greatest in the presence of maternal HBeAg. Infection is prevented by administration of hepatitis B immunoglobulin within 12 hours of birth and a series of three hepatitis B vaccinations.

Hepatitis C. Acute hepatitis C virus (HCV) infection is often mild and may be subclinical. Jaundice is unusual but can be seen in severe HCV infection, which resembles HAV and HBV infections clinically. HCV is a rare cause of fulminant hepatic failure. Chronic infection occurs in 40% to 60% of affected children, in contrast with up to 80% of infected adults, and can progress to cirrhosis. It is currently diagnosed by anti-HCV antibodies. The utility of anti-HCV is limited by the fact that titers may be undetectable in early

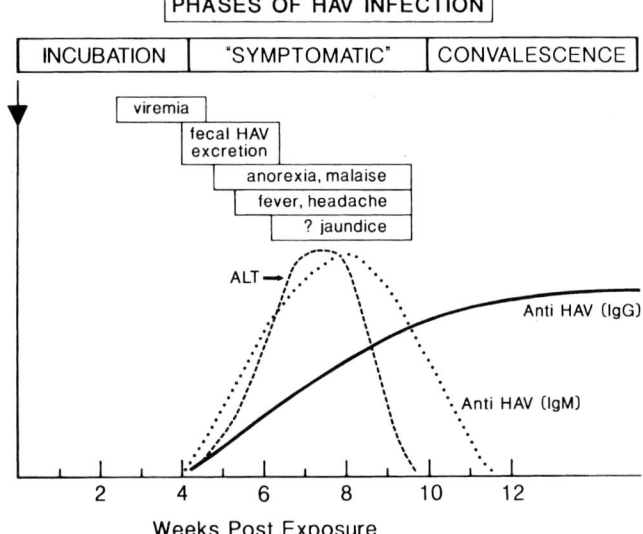

Figure 20-4. Typical course of hepatitis A virus (HAV) infection. ALT, alanine aminotransferase; IgG, immunoglobulin G; IgM, immunoglobulin M. (From Balistreri WF: Viral hepatitis. Pediatr Clin North Am 1988;35:640.)

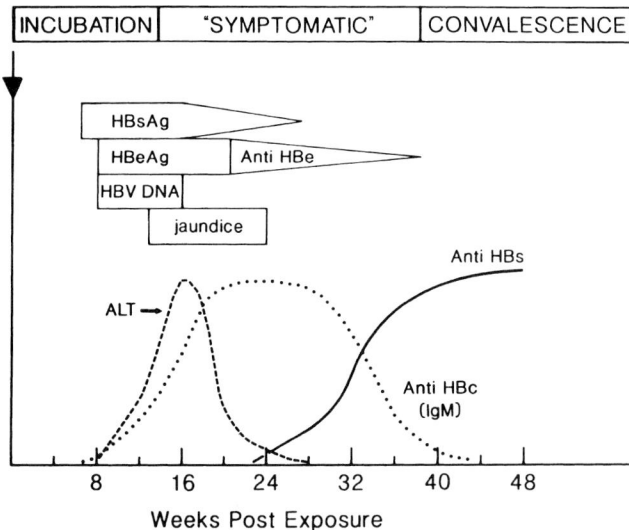

Figure 20-5. *Typical course of acute hepatitis B virus (HBV) infection. ALT, alanine aminotransferase; HBc, hepatitis B core; HBe, hepatitis B e; HBeAg, hepatitis B e antigen. HBs, hepatitis B surface; HBsAg, hepatitis B surface antigen; IgM, immunoglobulin M. (From Balistreri WF: Viral hepatitis. Pediatr Clin North Am 1988;35:647.)*

infection (before 16 weeks) and in immunosuppressed individuals. In these circumstances, polymerase chain reaction should be used to look for HCV RNA. Transmission may be parenteral or, rarely, vertical.

Hepatitis D. Hepatitis D virus (HDV) infection can occur only in the presence of HBV as either a coinfection or a superinfection. Its route of transmission is parenteral. As with HBV, it can become chronic. The diagnosis is confirmed by the presence of HDV antibody.

Hepatitis E. Hepatitis E (HEV) infection is similar to HAV in its manifestation and mode of transmission. It is a self-limited illness with no chronic state. However, fulminant hepatitis may occur in up to 20% of cases. Serologic diagnosis can be made by finding antibodies to HEV.

Epstein-Barr Virus. Epstein-Barr virus infection can mimic HAV, HBV, or HCV infection. Often there is an exudative pharyngitis and lymphadenopathy. Fatal hepatic necrosis can occur. This is rare, but it is of particular concern in the immunocompromised host. The diagnosis is confirmed by elevation of Epstein-Barr virus IgM titers.

Other Viruses. Other viruses, including herpes simplex, human herpesvirus 6, and CMV, can also cause hepatitis, particularly in the immunosuppressed patient.

Wilson Disease

Wilson disease, an inborn error of copper metabolism with autosomal recessive transmission, can manifest in a variety of ways (see Chapter 18). The hepatic manifestation predominates in childhood; a neuropsychiatric manifestation becomes more common later, in adolescence and adulthood. The liver involvement may manifest as acute hepatitis, fulminant hepatic failure, chronic hepatitis, cirrhosis, or asymptomatic elevation of serum aminotransferases. Neurologic symptoms, such as dysarthria, clumsiness, and tremor, may be present in addition or can be the only manifestations. As a result of defective metabolism, copper cannot be excreted and it accumulates in the liver, which causes hepatic necrosis. Copper is then released into the circulation and is ultimately deposited in the central nervous system, kidneys, and cornea. In the kidney, the result is tubular dysfunction; in the cornea, the result is Kayser-Fleischer rings.

The diagnosis is supported by documenting a low serum ceruloplasmin level, high urinary copper excretion, and increased hepatic copper concentrations on liver biopsy. Effective treatment is provided by administration of D-penicillamine, which chelates copper, and by dietary restriction of copper, unless the patient presents in fulminant hepatic failure. In this case, liver transplantation is the only therapy.

Drugs and Toxins

Numerous drugs and toxins are associated with hepatic injury (see Table 20-8) and should be considered in the evaluation of jaundice. The reaction can be idiosyncratic or dose related. In the latter case, this may be associated with either accidental or purposeful overdose. The manifestation can be that of acute hepatitis, fulminant hepatic failure, or cholestatic disease, depending on the drug.

Autoimmune Hepatitis

Autoimmune hepatitis often manifests acutely with malaise, anorexia, nausea, vomiting, and jaundice; it can also manifest with evidence of chronic liver disease (see Chapter 18). There may be associated autoimmune problems, such as arthritis, thyroiditis, vasculitis, nephritis, hemolytic anemia, or diabetes mellitus. Autoimmune hepatitis may be associated with inflammatory bowel disease. Laboratory studies demonstrate elevated aminotransferase levels, mild hyperbilirubinemia, and hypergammaglobulinemia. Children may have anti–liver-kidney microsomal antibodies, antinuclear antibodies, or anti–smooth muscle antibodies.

Liver biopsy is required for diagnosis. Characteristic findings are an inflammatory infiltrate expanding the portal area and moderate to severe piecemeal necrosis. Treatment consists of steroids and often azathioprine.

In evaluating the older child or adolescent with jaundice, it is important to determine whether the condition represents a hepatobiliary problem, a hematologic disorder, or a systemic illness. If there is conjugated hyperbilirubinemia, it is essential to evaluate for synthetic dysfunction (prolonged PT, hypoglycemia) suggestive of serious hepatocellular injury, which could progress to worsening hepatic failure or an obstructive process, both of which mandate early intervention. Causes of acute hepatic failure are listed in Table 20-9. Unfortunately, there are no reliable criteria on which to base prognosis in a child with acute hepatic failure.

RED FLAGS

Red flags suggesting serious liver dysfunction in children with conjugated hyperbilirubinemia include altered mental status (hepatic encephalopathy), coagulopathy (prolonged PT unresponsive to parenteral vitamin K), hypoglycemia, ascites, gastrointestinal bleeding, hypoalbuminemia, rising bilirubin with falling ALT and AST levels, cerebral edema, anuria, metabolic acidosis, and at-risk drug levels after acetaminophen poisoning. In patients with severe liver dysfunction, early referral should be made to a center with expertise in caring for such children.

Table 20-9. Etiologic Considerations for Hepatic Failure

Neonate

Infectious
  Herpes virus
  Hepatitis B virus
  Echovirus
  Adenovirus
  Epstein-Barr virus
  Parvovirus
  Human immunodeficiency virus
  Leptospirosis
Metabolic
  α_1-Antitrypsin deficiency
  Neonatal hemochromatosis
  Galactosemia
  Hereditary fructose intolerance
  Tyrosinemia
  Niemann-Pick disease
  Bile acid metabolic disorders
  Zellweger syndrome
  Mitochondrial disorders
Miscellaneous
  Familial erythrophagocytic lymphohistiocytosis
  Shock or hypoperfusion (including cardiac disease)

Older Child and Adolescent

Infectious
  Hepatitis A
  Hepatitis B
  Hepatitis C
  Hepatitis D
  Hepatitis E (especially if pregnant)
  Non–A-E hepatitis
  Herpes virus
  Varicella
  Cytomegalovirus
  Epstein-Barr virus
  Paramyxovirus
  Parvovirus
  Sepsis
Drugs
  Acetaminophen
  Isoniazid
  Valproate
  Carbamazepine
  Phenytoin
  Tetracycline
  Salicylate
  Halothane
  Cocaine
  Ecstasy
Chemical toxins
  Carbon tetrachloride
  Phosphorus
  Amanita phalloides
Miscellaneous
  Autoimmune hepatitis
  α_1-Antitrypsin deficiency
  Hereditary fructose intolerance
  Wilson disease
  Ischemia/hypotension
  Leukemia/lymphoma
  Mitochondrial disorder
  Erythropoietic protoporphyria

REFERENCES

General

Kelly DA (ed): Diseases of the liver and biliary system in children. Oxford, United Kingdom: Blackwell Science, 1999.

Suchy FJ, Sokol RJ, Balistreri WF (eds): Liver disease in children, 2nd ed. Philadelphia, Lippincott Williams & Wilkins, 2001.

Diagnostic Strategies

Batres LA, Maller ES: Laboratory assessment of liver function and injury in children. In Suchy FJ, Sokol RJ, Balistreri WF (eds): Liver Disease in Children, 2nd ed. Philadelphia, Lippincott Williams & Wilkins, 2001, pp 155-169.

Gubernick JA, Rosenberg HK, Ilaslan H, Kessler A: US approach to jaundice in infants and children. Radiographics 2000;20:173-195.

Jaw T-S, Kuo Y-T, Liu G-C, et al: MR cholangiography in the evaluation of neonatal cholestasis. Radiology 1999;212:249-256.

Rosenthal P: Assessing liver function and hyperbilirubinemia in the newborn. Clin Chem 1997;43:228-234.

Neonatal Jaundice

Andres JM: Neonatal hepatobiliary disorders. Clin Perinatol 1996;23:321-352.

Balistreri WF: Liver disease in infancy and childhood. In Schiff ER, Sorrell MF, Maddrey WC (eds): Schiff's Diseases of the Liver, 8th ed. Philadelphia, Lippincott-Raven, 1999, pp 1357-1512.

Dennery PA, Seidman DS, Stevenson DK: Neonatal hyperbilirubinemia. N Engl J Med 2001;344:581-590.

Gourley GR: Jaundice. In Wyllie R, Hyams JS (eds): Pediatric Gastrointestinal Disease: Pathophysiology, Diagnosis, Management, 2nd ed. Philadelphia, WB Saunders, 1999, pp 88-103.

Jacquemin E, Lykavieris P, Chaoui N, et al: Transient neonatal cholestasis: Origin and outcome. J Pediatr 1998;133:563-567.

Alagille Syndrome

Alagille D, Odievre M, Gautier M, et al: Hepatic ductular hypoplasia associated with characteristic facies, vertebral malformations, retarded physical, mental, and sexual development, and cardiac murmur. J Pediatr 1975;86:63-71.

Crosnier C, Lykavieris P, Meunier-Rotival M, Hadchouel M: Alagille syndrome: The widening spectrum of arteriohepatic dysplasia. Clin Liver Dis 2000;4:765-778.

Shneider BL: Genetic cholestasis syndromes. J Pediatr Gastroenterol Nutr 1999;28:124-131.

α_1-Antitrypsin Deficiency

Francavilla R, Castellaneta SP, Hadzic N, et al: Prognosis of alpha-1-antitrypsin deficiency–related liver disease in the era of paediatric liver transplantation. J Hepatol 2000;32:986-992.

Perlmutter DH: Alpha-1-antitrypsin deficiency. Semin Liver Dis 1998;18:217-225.

Biliary Atresia

Chardot C, Carton M, Spire-Bendelac N, et al: Prognosis of biliary atresia in the era of liver transplantation: French national study from 1986 to 1996. Hepatology 1999;30:606-611.

Chardot C, Carton M, Spire-Bendelac N, et al: Is the Kasai operation still indicated in children older than 3 months diagnosed with biliary atresia? J Pediatr 2001;138:224-228.

McKiernan PJ, Baker AJ, Kelly DA: The frequency and outcome of biliary atresia in the UK and Ireland. Lancet 2000;355:25-29.

Crigler-Najjar Syndromes

Fox IJ, Chowdhury JR, Kaufman SS, et al: Treatment of the Crigler-Najjar syndrome type I with hepatocyte transplantation. N Engl J Med 1998;338:1422-1426.

Hardikar W: Genes for jaundice. J Paediatr Child Health 1999;35:522-524.

Cystic Fibrosis

Shapira R, Hadzic N, Francavilla R, et al: Retrospective review of cystic fibrosis presenting as infantile liver disease. Arch Dis Child 1999;81:125-128.

Erythrocyte Enzyme Defects

Kaplan M, Hammerman C: Severe neonatal hyperbilirubinemia: A potential complication of glucose-6-phosphate dehydrogenase deficiency. Clin Perinatol 1998;25:575-590.
Nathan DG, Orkin SH (eds): Nathan and Oski's hematology of infancy and childhood, 5th ed. Philadelphia, WB Saunders, 1998.

Gilbert Syndrome

Burchell B, Hume R: Molecular genetic basis of Gilbert's syndrome. J Gastroenterol Hepatol 1999;14:960-966.
Monaghan G, McLellan A, McGeehan A, et al: Gilbert's syndrome is a contributory factor in prolonged unconjugated hyperbilirubinemia of the newborn. J Pediatr 1999;134:441-446.

Lucey-Driscoll Syndrome

Arias IM, Wolfson S, Lucey JF, et al: Transient familial neonatal hyperbilirubinemia. J Clin Invest 1965;44:1442-1450.
Lucey JF, Arias IM, McKay RJ: Transient familial neonatal hyperbilirubinemia. Am J Dis Child 1960;100:787-789.

Physiologic and Breast Milk Jaundice

Gartner LM, Lee K-S: Jaundice in the breastfed infant. Clin Perinatol 1999;26:431-445.

Jaundice in Older Children and Adolescents

Balistreri WF: Liver disease in infancy and childhood. In Schiff ER, Sorrell MF, Maddrey WC (eds): Schiff's Diseases of the Liver, 8th ed. Philadelphia, Lippincott-Raven, 1999, pp 1357-1512.

Autoimmune Hemolytic Anemia

Ware RE, Rosse WF: Autoimmune hemolytic anemia. In Nathan DG, Orkin SH (eds): Nathan and Oski's Hematology of Infancy and Childhood, 5th ed. Philadelphia: WB Saunders, 1998, pp 499-522.

Autoimmune Hepatitis

Mieli-Vergani G, Vergani D: Immunological liver diseases in children. Semin Liver Dis 1998;18:271-279.

Drugs

Lee W: Drug-induced hepatotoxicity. N Engl J Med 1995;333:1118-1127.
Zimmerman HJ: Hepatotoxicity: The Adverse Effects of Drugs and Other Chemicals on the Liver, 2nd ed. Philadelphia, Lippincott Williams & Wilkins, 1999.

Gallstones

Rescorla FJ: Cholelithiasis, cholecystitis, and common bile duct stones. Curr Opin Pediatr 1997;9:276-282.

Hepatitis

Aach RD, Yomtovian RA, Hack M: Neonatal and pediatric posttransfusion hepatitis C: A look back and a look forward. Pediatrics 2000;105:836-842.
Balistreri WF: Viral hepatitis. Pediatr Clin North Am 1988;35:637-669.
Befeler AS, Di Bisceglie AM: Hepatitis B. Infect Dis Clin North Am 2000;14:617-632.
Cheney CP, Chopra S, Graham C: Hepatitis C. Infect Dis Clin North Am 2000;14:633-667.
Debray D, Cullufi P, Devictor D, et al: Liver failure in children with hepatitis A. Hepatology 1997;26:1018-1022.
Kemmer NM, Miskovsky EP: Hepatitis A. Infect Dis Clin North Am 2000;14:605-615.
Ryder SD, Beckingham IJ: Acute hepatitis. BMJ 2001;322:151-153.

Primary Sclerosing Cholangitis

Debray D, Pariente D, Urvoas E, et al: Sclerosing cholangitis in children. J Pediatr 1994;124:49-56.
Roberts EA: Primary sclerosing cholangitis in children. J Gastroenterol Hepatol 1999;14:588-593.
Wilschanski M, Chait P, Wade JA, et al: Primary sclerosing cholangitis in 32 children: Clinical, laboratory, and radiographic features with survival analysis. Hepatology 1995;22:1415-1422.

Wilson Disease

Loudianos G, Gitlin JD: Wilson's disease. Semin Liver Dis 2000;20:353-364.
Wilson DC, Phillips MJ, Cox DW, Roberts EA: Severe hepatic Wilson's disease in preschool-aged children. J Pediatr 2000;137:719-722.

21 Constipation

Rita Steffen   Robert Wyllie

Approximately 3% of pediatric patients have constipation or fecal soiling; 10% to 25% of patients referred to pediatric gastroenterologists experience difficulties with defecation. The number of children from birth to 9 years of age brought to a physician's attention for constipation has increased from approximately 850 per 100,000 visits to 1700 per 100,000 visits since 1970. Much of this increase involved 0- to 2-year-old patients, both sexes being equally represented.

The diagnosis of constipation requires a careful history and interpretation because the history is often obtained from the parents, reflects their observations of the child's defecation behavior, and may be influenced by their perception of what is normal. Constipation is defined by the frequency and consistency of bowel movements, straining activity in passing a stool, or pain associated with the passage of a hard stool. In view of the variable range of normal defecation patterns in children, it is difficult to assign a numeric value to normal bowel frequency. Formula-fed infants may have four to five stools per day in the first weeks of life; stool frequency gradually decreases to one to two per day by 1 year of age. Breast-fed infants usually pass softer and more frequent stools in the first few months and also show a gradual diminution in stool frequency to one to two bowel movements per day by 1 year of age. Of children aged 1 to 4 years, 85% have one to two bowel movements per day, and 96% have a range of three bowel movements per day to one bowel movement every other day.

The daily bowel habits of children are susceptible to change in routine or environment. Infants frequently experience at least transient constipation as a result of changes in their diet, such as formula changes or the addition of solid foods. Constipation is often secondary to inadequate intake of dietary fiber, fluid, or both. In general, young children in the United States have a diet that is low in fiber content and high in refined sugars. Infrequently, infectious enteritis may manifest with constipation. An infectious illness, including a diarrheal illness, may also be the initial event that causes constipation. A diaper dermatitis or an anal fissure may cause painful defecation, leading to fecal retention, constipation, and, if it is persistent, dilation of the rectal vault, with loss of normal sensation and overflow encopresis.

Patients with chronic constipation have been found to have physiologic abnormalities that can be demonstrated by anorectal manometric evaluation. The most consistent abnormality is a blunted rectal sensation, rendering the patient unable to feel the bolus of stool in the rectum. Other findings include incomplete relaxation of the internal anal sphincter and paradoxical contraction of the external sphincter during attempted defecation. A significant proportion of chronically constipated patients show contraction rather than relaxation of the external anal sphincter during attempted defecation. Patients who have paradoxical anal contraction are less likely to respond to routine medical therapy and have high rates of recurrence of constipation after routine treatment regimens are terminated. These abnormalities may slowly diminish with medical therapy, but they do not resolve; therefore, these patients are at increased risk for recurrent problems, especially if treatment for constipation is withdrawn.

Many children develop constipation at one time in their lives; in most such children, it is transient. If problems with defecation persist, an individualized plan of management is successful in most patients.

PHYSIOLOGY OF NORMAL DEFECATION

Normal defecation patterns and behavior depend on a host of factors, including the following:

1. The abdominal musculature and the diaphragm allow intra-abdominal pressure to build during the Valsalva maneuver.
2. Innervation of the smooth muscle in the colonic wall results in peristalsis, which is necessary to propel the fecal mass to the anorectum.
3. The normal rectum is distensible and can act as a reservoir for the bolus of stool until it can be expelled.
4. The internal anal sphincter is under involuntary, tonic autonomic control, maintaining the anal canal closed at rest and maintaining continence. Arrival of a bolus of stool in the anorectum causes the internal anal sphincter to reflexively relax, thus allowing the stool to be expelled.
5. The external anal sphincter and the levator ani muscles work in concert. Voluntary contraction of these muscles causes the anus to close and be lifted, thus decreasing the rectoanal angle and delaying defecation. Relaxation of these muscles allows the rectoanal angle to increase or straighten, facilitating the passage of stool into the anal canal.
6. Transitional epithelium in the anorectal area enables the awareness of the urge to defecate and allows discrimination between the sensations caused by solid, liquid, and gas.

Anomalies in any of these structures can result in significant difficulties in defecation, as well as in the colonic transit time. Mean colonic transit times increase with age from approximately 8.5 hours at 1 to 3 months of age to 26 hours at 3 to 13 years of age. Ninety percent of children have total colonic transit times of within 33 hours. Children who show delayed transit have fecal retention in the distal colon, which suggests that the problem is that of expulsion of stool from the distal rectum or voluntary retention of the stool. Delayed transit in the small bowel or other parts of the colon is uncommon in children. A special test reserved for difficult cases is a "marker study," in which the child swallows small plastic radiopaque markers. An abdominal radiograph is taken 5 days later to demonstrate the distribution of markers in the colon. Patterns help separate subgroups of patients with pelvic outlet obstruction, total or segmental colonic inertia, and functional constipation.

DATA COLLECTION AND ASSESSMENT

HISTORY

Obtaining a thorough and accurate history is of paramount importance because much of the initial evaluation and management decision making is based on the presenting history. The differential diagnosis of constipation varies with age at the onset of symptoms. Constipation in the newborn or very young infant or a history of constipation since infancy suggests a diagnosis of Hirschsprung disease

Table 21-1. Causes of Constipation during the Neonatal Period

Meconium plug (rule out cystic fibrosis)
Meconium ileus (rule out cystic fibrosis)
Hirschsprung disease
Intestinal pseudoobstruction
Anatomic anomalies
  Anteriorly displaced anus
  Ectopic anus
  Anal stenosis
  Imperforate anus
Hypothyroidism
Hypercalcemia
Spina bifida
Neuronal intestinal dysplasia types A and B
Medications (opioids, paralytic agents, magnesium)

(Tables 21-1 and 21-2). The severity and duration of the constipation should be noted, with the frequency, the pattern, and the volume of bowel movements as well as any associated signs and symptoms, such as abdominal pain, intermittent diarrhea alternating with the constipation, blood in the stool, soiling, and changes in appetite or activity level.

Abdominal pain is a common complaint in constipated patients; when present, it is often mild, nonspecific, and periumbilical. Older children may describe discomfort in the lower abdomen and a history of relief of pain after a stool is passed. Appetite is often diminished. A diary recording the passage of stools, the timing of meals, and the onset of abdominal pain over a period of several days to a few weeks can aid in the diagnosis of constipation and in monitoring of therapy. The personal medical history and the family history are important because constipation can be associated with many other illnesses and conditions (Table 21-3).

The child's behavior during defecation should be noted. A history of straining, as an index of difficulty in defecation, can be misinterpreted by parents, who often view a child's efforts to withhold stool as efforts to pass a bowel movement. Parents often describe a toddler who hides in a corner, with stiffened straight legs, or who may lean into the wall or hold onto a table while "straining." The likely events leading up to this situation are simple to describe to the parents. The young child, having become constipated for many reasons, passes a painful stool. Passage of a large, painful stool may be associated with a fissure. If a fissure is present, a small amount of blood is usually passed with the stool. The child associates the passage of stools with pain and tries to prevent further painful episodes by withholding fecal matter. This behavior results in the formation of even larger, harder stools, which are painful to pass, thus establishing a link between pain and defecation that perpetuates the cycle. Children with stool retention may go 3 to 5 days without defecating. They may pass small, pellet-like stools or large, bulky stools. Enuresis and soiling of underwear may occur.

PHYSICAL EXAMINATION

Typically, the child who presents with the chief complaint of constipation (not caused by Hirschsprung disease) is healthy, with normal growth and development. Abnormal growth patterns should alert the physician to the possibility of underlying organic disease. Abdominal examination is usually benign. Stool may be palpable in the sigmoid and descending colon through the abdominal wall. On occasion, a large, firm fecal mass extends from the symphysis pubis to the umbilicus, which raises concerns of an abdominal malignancy. The abdomen is not tender to palpation; there may be some mild tenderness in the left lower quadrant on palpation of a segment of bowel that is full of stool.

Table 21-2. Distinguishing Features of Hirschsprung Disease and Functional (Acquired) Constipation

	Functional Constipation	Hirschsprung Disease*
History		
Gender of patients	Male	Male
Onset of constipation	After 2 yr of age	At birth
Prevalence	1%-3% of boys	1:5000-1:15000
Encopresis	Common	Very rare
Forced bowel training	Usual	None
Stool size	Very large	Small, ribbon-like
Enterocolitis	None	Possible
Abdominal pain	Common	Rare except with obstruction, toxic megacolon, or enterocolitis
Failure to thrive	Uncommon	Common
Examination		
Abdominal distention	Variable	Common
Poor growth	Rare	Common
Anal tone	Patulous	Tight
Rectal examination	Stool in ampulla	Ampulla empty
Malnutrition	Absent	Possible
Laboratory		
Barium enema	Massive amounts of stool, no transition zone	Transition zone, delayed evacuation (>24 hr)
Rectal biopsy	Normal	No ganglion cells; ↑ acetylcholinesterase staining
Anorectal manometry	Distention of the rectum causes relaxation of the internal sphincter	No sphincter relaxation

Adapted form Behrman RE (ed): Nelson Textbook of Pediatrics, 16th ed. Philadelphia; WB Saunders, 2000, p 1140.
*Note that ultrashort-segment Hirschsprung disease may have clinical features of functional (acquired) megacolon (e.g., constipation).

Table 21-3. Causes of Constipation in Infants and Children

Functional

Faulty diet (poor fiber intake, excessive cow's milk, inadequate nutrition)
Inadequate fluid intake
Symptoms of irritable bowel syndrome
Situational
Depression
Familial-constitutional

Anatomic

Anterior anal displacement
Ectopic anus
Anal stenosis
Malrotation
Colonic anomalies (rectocele, duplications)
Stricture (postsurgical, sequelae of inflammatory disorders)
Painful anorectal lesions (fissures, dermatitis, abscess)
Abnormal abdominal musculature (prune belly, gastroschisis)
Intestinal neoplasm, extraintestinal pelvic mass (teratoma)

Endocrine

Hypothyroidism
Panhypopituitarism
Diabetes mellitus

Metabolic

Hypercalcemia
Metal intoxication (lead, arsenic, mercury)
Dehydration
Cystic fibrosis: meconium ileus equivalent
Hypokalemia
Acute intermittent porphyria
Blue diaper syndrome
Hereditary coproporphyria

Infectious

Typhoid

Abnormal Innervation

Aganglionosis
  Congenital: Hirschsprung disease
  Acquired: Chagas disease
Neural dysgenesis (pseudoobstruction syndromes)
Hyperganglionosis

Spinal Cord Lesions

Spina bifida and spina bifida occulta
Tethered cord
Spinal cord tumors
Traumatic lesions

Neurologic

Infant botulism
Myotonic dystrophy
Cerebral palsy

Psychologic Illness

Anorexia nervosa
Depression

Drugs

Anticonvulsants
Antacids (aluminum and calcium)
Iron
Barium
Opiates (codeine, diphenoxylate–atropine sulfate [Lomotil], loperamide [Imodium])
Antidepressants
Anticholinergics
Phenothiazines
Vincristine
Calcium channel blockers
Bismuth
Clonidine
Antihistamines
Diuretics

Other

Milk protein–induced anal inflammation and fissure formation
Collagen vascular disease (SLE, mixed connective tissue disease, scleroderma)
Amyloidosis
Rubinstein-Taybi syndrome
Williams syndrome (hypercalcemia)

SLE, systemic lupus erythematosus.

The spine and sacral area should be examined closely: A tuft of hair, a dimple, or a palpable defect or mass in this area should prompt an evaluation to rule out spina bifida occulta or a tethered spinal cord. The perianal area should be examined for evidence of fissures, which suggests the passage of large, hard stools. The examination is facilitated if an assistant gently spreads the patient's buttocks apart while the examiner illuminates the area. Soiling in the underwear may indicate fecal impaction with overflow encopresis. The anus in relation to the other perineal structures should be located to rule out anatomic or structural anomalies, such as anterior displacement of the rectum. The presence of a normal anal wink, as elicited by gentle stroking of the perianal skin with a sharp object, such as a wooden tongue blade or the corner of a small package of lubricant, gives evidence of intact sacral innervation.

Digital examination can identify such anomalies as anal stenosis. A dilated rectal vault with a large fecal mass is usually seen in chronic constipation. In most patients with Hirschsprung disease, retained fecal material is not encountered within the first few centimeters of the anal canal.

LABORATORY EVALUATION

Routine laboratory evaluation is usually not helpful in the evaluation of constipation. Analysis is indicated if a metabolic abnormality is suspected on the basis of the history or physical examination. Endocrinologic disturbances, such as hypothyroidism, can be associated with constipation. Stool studies may be obtained to rule out infectious agents, if the patient's history indicates that infection may be present (Figs. 21-1 and 21-2).

A rectal motility evaluation is often helpful in the diagnosis and management of chronic constipation. Anorectal manometry can be used to evaluate the integrity of the muscles and the innervation of the defecatory mechanism. The determination of sensory threshold can give clues to the projected length of therapy. Patients who cannot detect a balloon filled with 120 mL of air usually have encopresis. Hirschsprung disease is ruled out if a reflex relaxation of the internal anal sphincter occurs in the presence of rectal distention. Manometry and electromyography document the presence of paradoxical contraction of the external anal sphincter on attempted defecation. Anorectal manometry can also be used as a therapeutic modality in

DELAYED PASSAGE OF MECONIUM

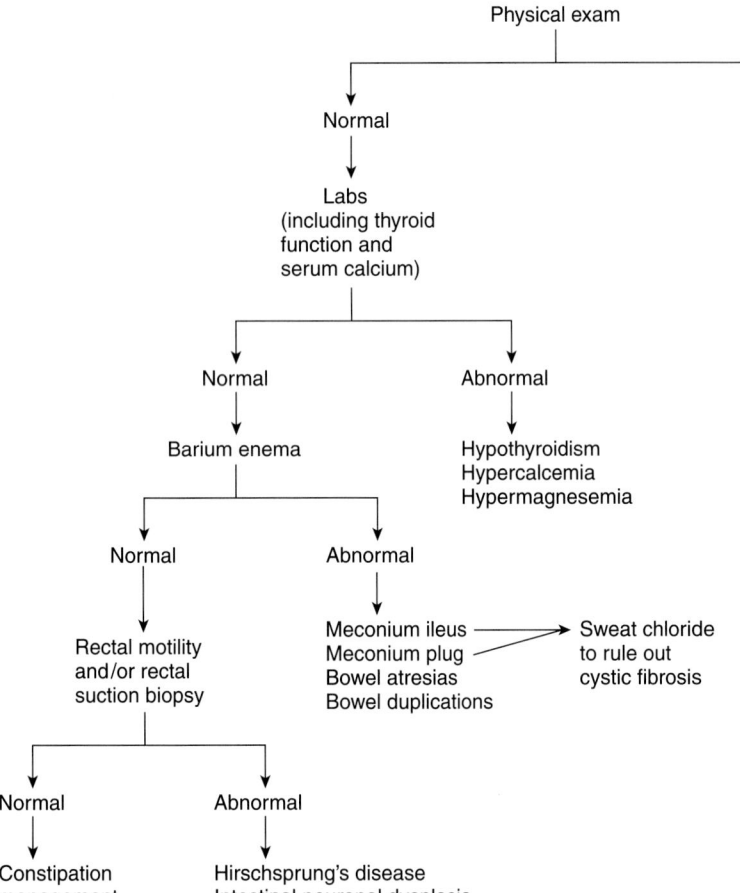

Figure 21-1. Algorithmic approach to the differential diagnosis of delayed passage of meconium.

biofeedback therapy in patients with constipation and encopresis and in patients with paradoxical external anal sphincter contraction. Total colonic motility is performed by placing a catheter in the colon to monitor pressures from the rectum to the cecum. Motility tracings reveal information about the function of the colon that is useful in diagnosis and treatment, particularly if surgical options need to be explored.

IMAGING

Plain films of the abdomen are rarely necessary, but if they are obtained, they may demonstrate stool in the large bowel. This information is occasionally useful in the case of a child with complaints of diarrhea who suffers from fecal impaction and overflow of liquid stools. If Hirschsprung disease is to be evaluated by radiologic studies, the examination of choice is the "unprepped" barium enema. In some older children, defecography may provide useful information on the dynamics of defecation and may allow measurement of the rectoanal angle at rest and during straining.

DIFFERENTIAL DIAGNOSIS
(See Tables 21-2 and 21-3)

ANATOMIC LESIONS

Hirschsprung Disease

Congenital aganglionic megacolon, or Hirschsprung disease, is a common cause of neonatal intestinal obstruction. It occurs in

approximately 1:5000 to 1:15,000 live births, with a male-to-female ratio of about 4:1. The disease is rare in premature births, may be familial, and is associated with trisomy 21, Waardenburg syndrome, multiple endocrine neoplasia type 2A syndrome, and piebaldism. The absence of ganglion cells in both the Meissner (submucosal) plexus and the Auerbach (myenteric) plexus results in an inability of the involved segment of bowel to relax in response to distention from the presence of stool. In the newborn, passage of meconium is often delayed beyond the usual 24 or 48 hours after birth. Most such conditions are diagnosed during infancy; 50% are diagnosed in the first months of life, 75% by 3 months, and 80% by the end of the first year. Diagnosis may be delayed into childhood and, in rare cases, into adolescence or even adulthood in some patients with ultrashort-segment disease. These patients complain of constipation; manifestations usually start in infancy.

The lesion begins at the internal anal sphincter and extends continuously into the rectum or the rectosigmoid in 75% to 80% of cases. In 10% of cases, there is total colonic aganglionosis; in another 10%, there is variable involvement of the small intestine in addition to total colonic disease. Delayed passage of meconium is the most common manifestation in the neonate, followed by lower intestinal obstruction (distention, bile-stained emesis), obstipation, failure to thrive, or, in rare cases, intestinal perforation. Meconium plug syndrome may also be present. In addition, if stool is passed immediately after a rectal examination is performed in an obstipated (no stools) or constipated patient, Hirschsprung disease should be suspected.

Anorectal manometry is a valuable diagnostic procedure. Normal internal anal sphincter relaxation with transient rectal distention

CONSTIPATION

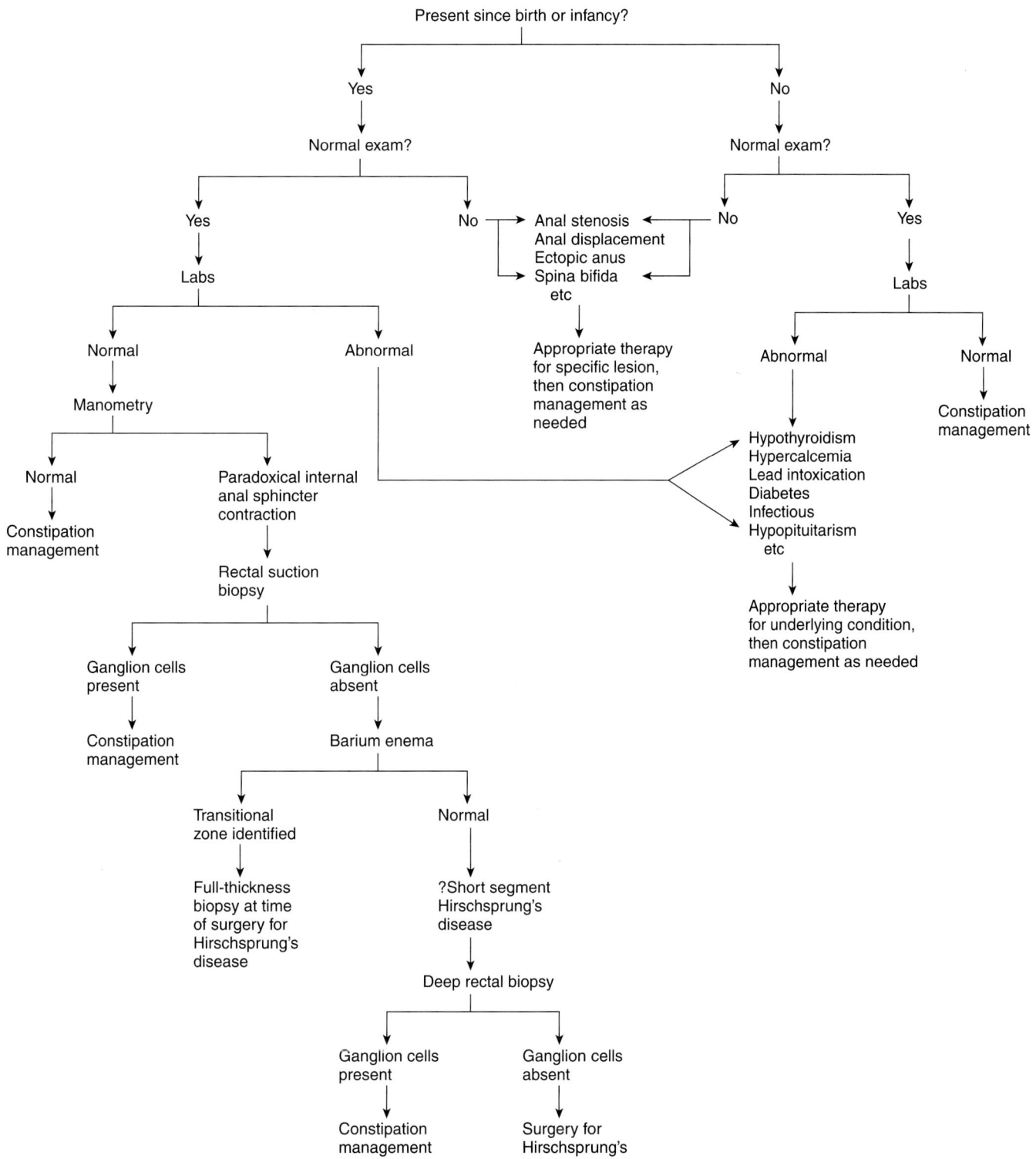

Figure 21-2. Algorithmic approach to the diagnosis of constipation.

rules out Hirschsprung disease. Paradoxical contraction of the internal anal sphincter suggests an absence of ganglion cells and is most common in Hirschsprung disease. Absence of relaxation has been noted in premature infants, in neonates with infection or sepsis, and in one baby with thyroid aplasia; normal function is seen after

appropriate therapy. The sensitivity and specificity of this test varies somewhat among the different age groups (children versus infants versus neonates). This test has a sensitivity that ranges from 0.79 to 0.90, a specificity ranging from 0.97 to 1.00, and a positive predictive value of 0.94 to 1.00.

A plain abdominal film occasionally reveals distention of the normally innervated bowel proximal to the affected segment. The most useful radiographic test is the "unprepped" barium enema, which usually demonstrates a small-caliber rectum with a transition in the rectosigmoid to the dilated, obstructed, normal proximal colon. A delayed lateral radiograph 24 hours after the barium enema aids in identifying a transition zone in the sigmoid colon.

A definitive diagnosis of Hirschsprung disease requires histologic confirmation of the absence of ganglion cells; such confirmation may be accomplished by a simple submucosal suction biopsy, which may be performed in the physician's office. Suction biopsy excludes the diagnosis if ganglion cells are present. However, there may be a 10% false-negative rate. A full-thickness rectal biopsy procedure is reserved for infants with bowel obstruction and for older children with abnormal rectal motilities and suction biopsies in which ganglion cells have not been identified. In patients with undiagnosed Hirschsprung disease, acute toxic megacolon or an infectious enterocolitis may develop (caused by *Staphylococcus aureus, Clostridium difficile*). Therapy for these complications includes correcting electrolyte abnormalities (hypokalemia), broad-spectrum parenteral antibiotics, bowel rest, rectal tube placement, and if needed, emergency cecostomy or colectomy. Treatment for Hirschsprung disease is surgical resection of the affected segment of bowel and various strategies for an ileal or colonic rectal pull-through procedure. Red flags to indicate Hirschsprung disease are noted in Table 21-2. Diseases that may mimic Hirschsprung disease and necessitate biopsy diagnosis include other abnormalities of intestinal innervation such as pseudoobstruction (neural dysgenesis) and hyperganglionosis.

Chronic Intestinal Pseudoobstruction

This disorder is characterized by manifestations of intestinal obstruction but without an identifiable anatomic lesion and may be secondary to an intestinal neuropathy or myopathy. Congenital cases may be sporadic or inherited (autosomal dominant or recessive).

Congenital disease is often manifested in the first months of life. Patients may be premature and may have an associated malrotation. Manifestations include abdominal distention, emesis, constipation, growth failure, and pain; diarrhea is less common. The diagnosis is based on the clinical manifestations in the absence of an anatomic obstruction and motility studies. Intestinal biopsy increases the risk of postoperative adhesions and an acquired obstruction.

Therapy includes parenteral nutrition, combined if possible with oral feedings, plus prokinetic agents. Bacterial overgrowth from stasis must be treated aggressively with antibiotics. Constipation is managed with enemas, stool softeners, or suppositories. If the colon is the only involved site, colectomy is curative.

Anterior Anal Displacement

The position of the anus may be described in terms of the anogenital index: that is, the ratio of the distance from the posterior aspect of the vagina or scrotum to the anus, divided by the full distance to the tip of the coccyx. Among individuals with a normally placed anus, this value is greater than 0.34 in girls and greater than 0.45 in boys. There are two forms of displacement of the anus. In the *anterior ectopic* anus, the anal canal and the internal anal sphincter as a unit are displaced anteriorly in the perineum and are separated from the external anal sphincter, which remains posterior in its usual position. On physical examination, it may be possible to elicit an external sphincter anal wink in the usual location, posterior to the opening of the anal canal. Rectal examination often reveals a sharp posterior angulation in the anal canal. In the *anteriorly located* anus, the entire normal anal unit is located in the anterior perineum (Fig. 21-3). Both of these entities are found more commonly in girls. Symptoms of constipation often begin in the neonatal period and are related to the difficulty in expelling stool through a canal that is angled anteriorly. If the displacement is severe enough to cause symptoms, surgical correction may be necessary to relocate the anus and relieve the obstruction.

Anal Stenosis

The diagnosis of anal stenosis may be delayed beyond the neonatal period, especially if the degree of stenosis is not severe. Any portion of the anal canal or the entire canal may be involved. The diagnosis can be made by digital examination or by endoscopy. Constipation is caused by fecal retention secondary to outlet obstruction. Treatment is by dilatation or anorectal myectomy.

Imperforate Anus

Imperforate anus is usually diagnosed in the neonatal nursery. Passage of meconium is delayed or is noted to take place through an abnormal location as a result of the presence of a fistula (rectovaginal, rectovesicular, or rectoperineal). Treatment is surgical; the actual procedure depends on the level and the extent of the defect.

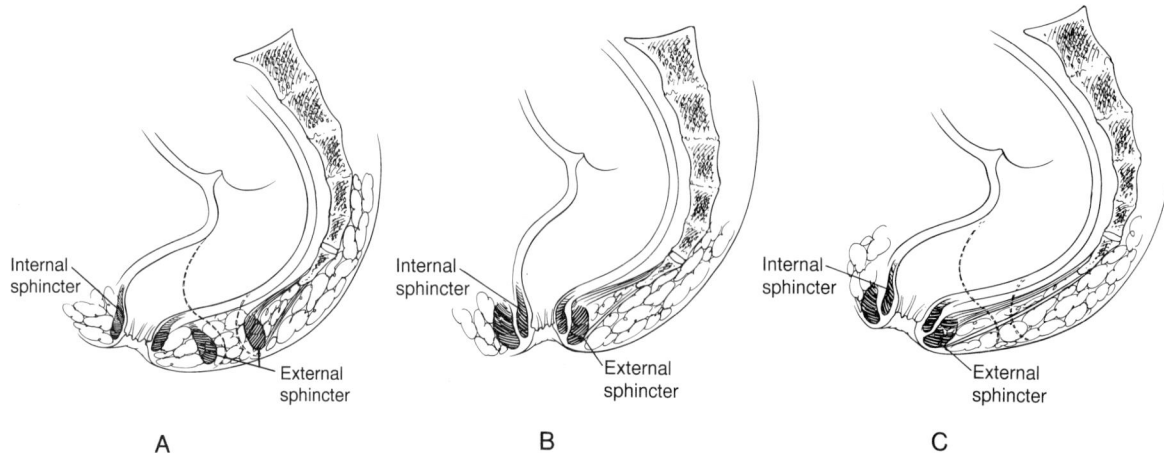

Figure 21-3. A, Anterior ectopic anus. B, Normal anal anatomy. C, Anterior anal displacement.

Spina Bifida and Spina Bifida Occulta

Defecation disturbances, most frequently constipation, are common in patients with spina bifida and spina bifida occulta, especially if the defect involves the lumbosacral spine. The spinal and nerve root injury results in poor functioning of the terminal bowel. Voluntary external sphincter control and rectoanal sensation are most often diminished or absent, and the degree of difficulty with defecation is related to the degree and the extent of the injury.

Anticipatory management and education are very important in these patients. Most patients can achieve an acceptable level of continence when they are given a bowel regimen that is individualized to their needs. Dietary fiber, stool softeners, suppositories, and enema continence catheters are treatment options. Biofeedback and pudendal nerve stimulation have been reported to be successful in some patients. In most patients, a combination of treatment modalities allows social continence to be achieved and dramatically improves the patients' quality of life. Treatment of patients with spinal or nerve injury or dysfunction from other causes is similar.

METABOLIC DISEASES

The appropriate laboratory tests should be performed to rule out the various metabolic and endocrinologic conditions that may manifest with constipation (see Table 21-3). The most important of these conditions is hypothyroidism. In routine neonatal screening, hypothyroidism manifesting solely with constipation is rarely seen. It should be suspected in any infant presenting with constipation and a history of prolonged neonatal jaundice.

NEUROLOGIC DISEASES

The neurologically impaired child often has constipation for many reasons, including poor intestinal motility, lack of dietary fiber, and poor awareness of rectal vault distention with stool retention. Any illness affecting the spinal cord or sacral nerves, degenerative muscle diseases, cerebral palsy, and demyelinating diseases can result in constipation.

PHARMACOLOGIC SIDE EFFECTS

A complete list of any drugs being taken by the patient should be obtained because many classes of drugs can cause constipation (see Table 21-3).

ENCOPRESIS

Idiopathic constipation is much more common than Hirschsprung disease. Long-standing constipation leads to encopresis, the deposition of stools in the undergarments or other unorthodox locations that persists or occurs beyond the age of formal bowel training. This definition is flexible in that the age by which a child should be toilet trained for feces varies in different cultures. In some cultures, delayed bowel training up to the age of 6 years is normal. It is generally accepted in the United States that healthy children should be bowel trained by the age of 4 years.

Encopresis is thought to be the end result of chronic withholding of stool. As the fecal mass accumulates, it causes rectal distention, increases rectal compliance, and eventually results in blunted or absent sensitivity of the rectum to the presence of liquid stool passing around a firm fecal mass. Children with encopresis usually pass small stools and do not completely empty the rectum. Periodically, they pass huge stools, which may block the toilet. It is important to specifically question the patient or parents regarding these massive stools because this information is frequently not volunteered.

Encopresis has been incorrectly considered a symptom or manifestation of psychiatric illness. It was thought that the patient retained stools either consciously or subconsciously as a way to rebel against, please, or anger caretakers. Although encopresis may be seen in association with emotional and behavioral problems, it is usually the result of painful defecation followed by a pattern of stool withholding, leading to chronic constipation, overflow encopresis, and possibly poor relations with peers as a result of fecal soiling. In the few patients in whom encopresis is truly a manifestation of psychiatric disease, there is often no stool retention, and the prognosis for fecal continence with therapy is poor.

Idiopathic constipation with or without encopresis may compress the bladder by a dilated rectum, thus causing stasis and urinary tract infections.

MANAGEMENT

The treatment of chronic constipation must be individualized (Table 21-4). Medical therapy is usually protracted, lasting from several weeks to months. The cooperation and compliance of the patient and the family are of paramount importance. Providing the family with information on the physiology of constipation and encopresis is essential to ensure compliance. Frequent office visits are needed initially, with the initial follow-up either by telephone or in the physician's office 1 to 2 weeks after therapy is initiated. Once therapy is well under way, follow-up can be performed at longer intervals.

An assessment must be made of the degree of constipation present. Adequate bowel cleansing must be accomplished before stool softeners are given, because softeners increase the frequency of

---

Table 21-4. Management of Constipation and Encopresis

Initial Evaluation

Appropriate studies to rule out underlying disease
Rectal manometry if clinically indicated
Education

Initial Bowel Evacuation (1-4 days)

Mineral oil large doses (15 mL per year of age or 5 mL/kg of body weight) initially to complete evacuation
In severe cases, one or more enemas may be needed to empty the bowel
A balanced electrolyte colonic lavage solution may also be given orally or via nasogatric tube, if needed

Maintenance

Mineral oil titrated to effect (very soft stool without excessive leakage of oil), starting at 5 mL/kg of body weight (not indicated in patients at risk for aspiration or in infants <6 months of age)
Alternatively, lactulose may be used in cases in which mineral oil is contraindicated or not tolerated; doses must be tailored to individual patient; some guidelines for initial doses:
  <10 kg (to 1 year): 1 teaspoonful PO b.i.d.
  10-20 kg: 1 tablespoonful PO b.i.d.
  >20 kg: 2 tablespoonful PO b.i.d.
Recommend increased fiber and fluid intake
Toilet training: sitting on toilet for 5-10 minutes b.i.d. after meals
Gradual reduction of lubricant over several weeks to months once symptoms have resolved

b.i.d., twice a day; PO, orally.

encopresis in the child with fecal impaction. Some patients object to enemas; many do not require one. A patient who has fecal impaction may require an enema in the physician's office and at home before treatment is initiated. The administration of a balanced electrolyte colonic lavage solution either orally or by gavage may be necessary in selected patients with severe impaction.

Once the bowel is emptied, the patient begins taking sufficient doses of mineral oil or lactulose. Both of these agents have proved to be effective. Mineral oil is more palatable if it is served very cold, and it can be mixed with any food or liquid to aid in administration. It should not be used if the patient is at increased risk of vomiting or aspiration. Lactulose is a nonabsorbable sugar that is usually well tolerated. Both agents have been found to be safe for use in the treatment of constipation. No nutritional deficiencies have been reported with the use of mineral oil over a 6-month course of therapy. Some practitioners supplement the patient's diet with vitamins.

The child should attempt defecation twice daily, sitting on the toilet with proper foot support for approximately 5 to 10 minutes shortly after meals (breakfast and dinner) to try to take advantage of the gastrocolic reflex. The goal of therapy is for the child to pass one soft stool at least every day. The stools should be soft enough not to cause pain. Eventually, the patient loses the fear of pain with the passage of stool. Regular evacuation of the rectum allows the rectum to return to normal caliber, with improved compliance and sensory threshold. The addition of dietary fiber as a maintenance measure helps to maintain regular defecation habits and may help to prevent acute recurrences. The efficacy of bulking agents depends on an adequate fluid intake. Manipulation of the diet to increase fiber content is difficult with children, especially toddlers.

Children who have paradoxical external anal contraction during attempted defecation can greatly benefit from biofeedback therapy. The child must be old enough to understand directions and to cooperate with the exercises. As few as two to three 1-hour sessions can be curative. Additional booster sessions are occasionally needed.

SUMMARY AND RED FLAGS

Constipation is a common concern in infants and young children. A detailed history of the child's bowel patterns identifies children with normal bowel movements whose parents need reassurance. The history should also include a review of all medications and a search for an associated chronic disease, such as a metabolic or neurologic disease. This complete history, combined with a careful physical examination, including the spine and sacral area, location of the anus and a digital rectal examination, should alert the physician to the need for further evaluation. Red flags include onset in the neonatal period, growth failure, and prolonged jaundice in the neonatal period. Distinguishing features associated with Hirschsprung's disease are listed in Table 21-2.

REFERENCES

Constipation

American Gastroenterological Association medical position statement: Guidelines on constipation. Gastroenterology 2000;119:1761-1778.

American Gastroenterological Association medical position statement on anorectal testing techniques. Gastroenterology 1999;116:732-760.

Baker SS, Liptak GS, Colletti RB, et al: Constipation in infants and children: Evaluation and treatment. A medical position statement of the North American Society for Pediatric Gastroenterology and Nutrition. J Pediatr Gastroenterol Nutr 1999;29:612-626.

Bampton PA, Dinning PG, Kennedy ML, et al: Prolonged multi-point recording of colonic manometry in the unprepared human colon: Providing insight into potentially relevant pressure wave parameters. Am J Gastroenterol 2001;96:1838-1848.

Brooks RC, Copen RM, Cox DJ, et al: Review of the treatment literature for encopresis, functional constipation, and stool-toileting refusal. Ann Behav Med 2000;22:260-267.

Gold DM, Levine J, Weinstein TA, et al: Frequency of digital rectal examination in children with chronic constipation. Arch Pediatr Adol Med 1999;153:377-379.

Heyman S, Wexner SD, Vickers D, et al: Prospective, randomized trial comparing four biofeedback techniques for patients with constipation. Dis Colon Rectum 1999;42:1388-1393.

Imaji R, Kubota Y, Hengel P, et al: Rectal mucosal biopsy compared with laparoscopic seromuscular biopsy in the diagnosis of intestinal neuronal dysplasia in children with slow-transit constipation. J Pediatr Surg 2000; 35:1724-1727.

Kiristioglu I, Akbunar T, Kilic N, et al: Quantification of defecation function using radionuclide artificial stool in children with chronic constipation. Eur J Pediatr Surg 2000;10:383-386.

Patel H, Law A, Gouin S: Predictive factors for short-term persistence in children after emergency department evaluation for constipation. Arch Pediatr Adol Med 2000;154:1204-1208.

Solzi G, Di Lorenzo C: Are constipated children different from constipated adults? Dig Dis 1999;17:308-315.

Staiano A: Use of polyethylene glycol solution in functional and organic constipation in children. Ital J Gastroenterol Hepatol 1999;31:S260-S263.

Wheatley JM, Hutson JM, Chow CW, et al: Slow-transit constipation in childhood. J Pediatr Surg 1999;34:832-833.

Hirschsprung Disease

Coran AG, Teitelbaum DH: Recent advances in the management of Hirschsprung's disease. Am J Surg 2000;180:382-387.

Di Lorenzo C, Solzi GF, Flores AF, et al: Colonic motility after surgery for Hirschsprung's disease. Am J Gastroenterol 2000;95:1759-1764.

Miele E, Tozzi A, Staiano A, et al: Persistence of abnormal gastrointestinal motility after operation for Hirschsprung's disease. Am J Gastroenterol 2000;95:1226-1230.

Minkes RK, Langer JC: A prospective study of botulinum toxin for internal anal sphincter hypertonicity in children with Hirschsprung's disease. J Pediatr Surg 2000;35:1733-1736.

Reid JR, Buonomo C, Moreira C, et al: The barium enema in constipation: Comparison with rectal manometry and biopsy to exclude Hirschsprung's disease after the neonatal period. Pediatr Radiol 2000;30:681-684.

Teitelbaum DH, Cilley RE, Sherman NJ, et al: A decade of experience with the primary pull-through for Hirschsprung disease in the newborn period: A multicenter analysis of outcomes. Ann Surg 2000;232:372-380.

van der Zee DC, Bax KN: One-stage Duhamel-Martin procedure for Hirschsprung's disease: A 5-year follow-up study. J Pediatr Surg 2000; 35:1434-1436.

Encopresis

Borowitz SM, Cox DJ, Sutphen JL: Differences in toileting habits between children with chronic encopresis, asymptomatic siblings, and asymptomatic nonsiblings. J Dev Behav Pediatr 1999;20:145-149.

Buttross S: Encopresis in the child with a behavioral disorder: When the initial treatment does not work. Pediatr Ann 1999;28:317-321.

Catto-Smith AG, Nolan TM, Coffey CM: Clinical significance of anismus in encopresis. J Gastroenterol Hepatol 1998;13:955-960.

Fennig S, Fennig S: Management of encopresis in early adolescence in a medical-psychiatric unit. Gen Hosp Psychiatry 1999;21:360-367.

Fonkalsrud EW, Dunn JC, Kawaguchi AI: Simplified technique for antegrade continence enemas for fecal retention and incontinence. J Am Col Surg 1998;187:457-460.

Griffiths P, Dunn S, Evans A, et al: Portable biofeedback apparatus for treatment of anal sphincter dystonia in childhood soiling and constipation. J Med Eng Tech 1999;23:96-101.

Issenman RM, Filmer RB, Gorski PA: A review of how bowel and bladder control development in children: How gastrointestinal and urologic conditions relate to problems in toilet training. Pediatrics 1999;103: 1346-1352.

Kuhn BR, Marcus BA, Pitner SL: Treatment guidelines for primary nonretentive encopresis and stool toileting refusal. Am Fam Physician 1999;59:2171-2178.

Loening-Baucke V: Clinical approach to fecal soiling in children. Clin Pediatr 2000;39:603-607.

Loening-Baucke V: Toilet tales: Stool toileting refusal, encopresis and fecal incontinence. J Wound Ostomy Continence Nurs 1998;25:304-313.

Nolan T, Catto-Smith T, Coffey C, et al: Randomised controlled trial of biofeedback training in persistent encopresis with anismus. Arch Dis Child 1998;79:131-135.

Smith L, Smith P, Lee SK: Behavioral treatment of urinary incontinence and encopresis in children with learning disabilities: Transfer of stimulus control. Dev Med Child Neurol 2000;42:276-279.

Staiano A, Ciarla C: Pelvic floor syndromes: Infant dyschezia, functional fecal retention, and nonretentive soiling. In Hyman PE (ed): Pediatric Functional Gastrointestinal Disorders 10. New York: Academy Professional Information Services, 1999.

Steffen R, Loening-Baucke V: Constipation and encopresis. In Wyllie R, Hyams JS (eds): Pediatric Gastrointestinal Disease: Pathophysiology, Diagnosis, Management 4. Philadelphia: WB Saunders, 1999.

van Ginkel R, Benninga MA, Blommaart P, et al: Lack of benefit of laxatives as adjunctive therapy for functional nonretentive fecal soiling in children. J Pediatr 2000;137:808-813.

Varea Calderon V, Delgado Carbajal L, Camacho Diaz E, et al: Role of manometry, defecography and anal endosonography in the evaluation of colorectal disorders. Rev Esp Enferm Dig 2000;92:147-159.

22 Abdominal Masses

Michael W. L. Gauderer   John C. Chandler

The discovery of an abdominal mass or abdominal swelling in a child is of great concern to parents and physicians. Most masses are not observed until late in their development. Often, the parents note changes in the abdominal contour of the child or accidentally discover a mass while bathing or dressing the child. Abdominal masses may arise from hollow or solid intraabdominal or retroperitoneal viscera, or they may arise from the abdominal wall (Figs. 22-1 and 22-2). The mass may be life-threatening, as in the case of a highly malignant neoplasm; it may have been present since birth and gradually evolved, as in the case of a mesenteric cyst; or it may be caused by something less foreboding, such as functional constipation. A child with an abdominal mass usually requires hospitalization and a prompt, accurate, and cost-effective workup.

DIAGNOSTIC STRATEGIES

CLINICAL HISTORY

The clinical history helps to identify the most likely tumor category (Table 22-1). The nature of the mass is also related to the age and gender of the child (Table 22-2). The duration and character of the symptoms should be noted. It is important to know whether the child has general systemic symptoms such as fatigue, fever, or weight loss. In addition, gastrointestinal, urogenital, or pulmonary symptoms as well as any complaints of chronic or acute pain should be identified. Abdominal trauma (hematoma of liver or spleen, pancreatic pseudocyst) or infectious disease may lead to the formation of a cyst, lymphadenopathy, or an abscess. Some systemic diseases, genetic abnormalities, and genetic anomalies are associated with intraabdominal tumors (aniridia with Wilms tumor; hemihypertrophy with neuroblastoma and Wilms tumor). A family history is also pertinent, as is a sexual history, particularly in adolescent girls.

PHYSICAL EXAMINATION

Special attention should be paid to the general condition of the child and to signs of possible metastatic disease. The patient's blood pressure must be determined and may be elevated in patients with Wilms tumor, neuroblastoma, or pheochromocytoma. Any enlarged lymph nodes and their locations should be noted, the skin inspected, and the lungs and heart auscultated. In addition, a neurologic examination may reveal signs of nervous system involvement.

To successfully perform abdominal palpation in a child, the physician must approach the patient with the greatest care, gentleness, and respect. It is important that the child cooperates and is able to relax. The various locations in the abdomen should be examined systematically (Table 22-3; see Figs. 22-1 and 22-2). With the patient in the supine position, the shape of the abdomen should be inspected and any visible masses or the presence of ascites observed. The position of the umbilicus and the presence of any hernias should be assessed. The mass should be localized, and its size, shape, texture, motility, tenderness, and relation to the midline noted. Signs of

peritoneal irritation must be sought. If there is any suspicion of obstipation or urinary retention, the patient should be reexamined after voiding or defecating.

Approximately half of abdominal masses in older children are caused by enlargement of the liver (see Chapter 18) or spleen (see Chapter 19) or both. The liver is normally palpated in the right upper quadrant and epigastrium, 1 to 2 cm below the costal margin. It has a sharp edge, is usually nontender, and moves with respiration. The spleen is located in the left upper quadrant and is nonpalpable in most healthy children. It has a rounded edge, moves with respiration, and is more superficial than a renal mass. Next to enlargement of the liver and spleen, lateral flank masses are the most common, particularly in neonates and children. Renal masses usually extend downward and do not move with respiration. They rarely cross the midline.

Lower abdominal masses may be caused by constipation or urinary retention. These may be functional or caused by spinal cord disease. A perforated appendix with resulting abscess formation can cause a right lower quadrant mass. Ovarian or uterine tumors occasionally develop into huge abdominal masses. A rectal examination must be considered for any case in which it would provide information, and examination of the external genitalia is indicated in girls with a lower abdominal mass, to check for imperforate hymen.

LABORATORY AND IMAGING STUDIES

Laboratory data, including complete blood count with white blood cell differential and erythrocyte structure, measurements of serum electrolytes and serum amylase, urinalysis, and analysis for tumor markers (Table 22-4), should be obtained. Liver and kidney function tests should be obtained when appropriate.

Plain abdominal radiographs may reveal tumor calcifications, organomegaly, or any displacement of intraabdominal organs, such as the intestines. Contrast studies can help identify such displacement or diagnose masses within the gastrointestinal tract (Fig. 22-3). Ultrasonography is an excellent screening imaging modality. It is noninvasive, is not painful, and can give detailed information on the location and nature of the tumor and adjacent structures (Fig 22-4). The most widely used imaging techniques are computed tomography (CT), with or without contrast (Fig. 22-5), and magnetic resonance imaging (MRI). Arteriography is used infrequently.

NEUROBLASTOMA

Neuroblastoma is the most common extracranial solid malignancy in childhood. It is of embryonic origin, arising from primitive sympathetic system cells derived from the neural crest. The malignant growth may develop wherever sympathetic tissue is found, but 75% of the tumors are abdominal, and 65% of these originate in the adrenal glands. Neuroblastoma is an unusual tumor in that its behavior is not always predictable: Well-advanced lesions may regress spontaneously or mature into benign tumors, whereas others

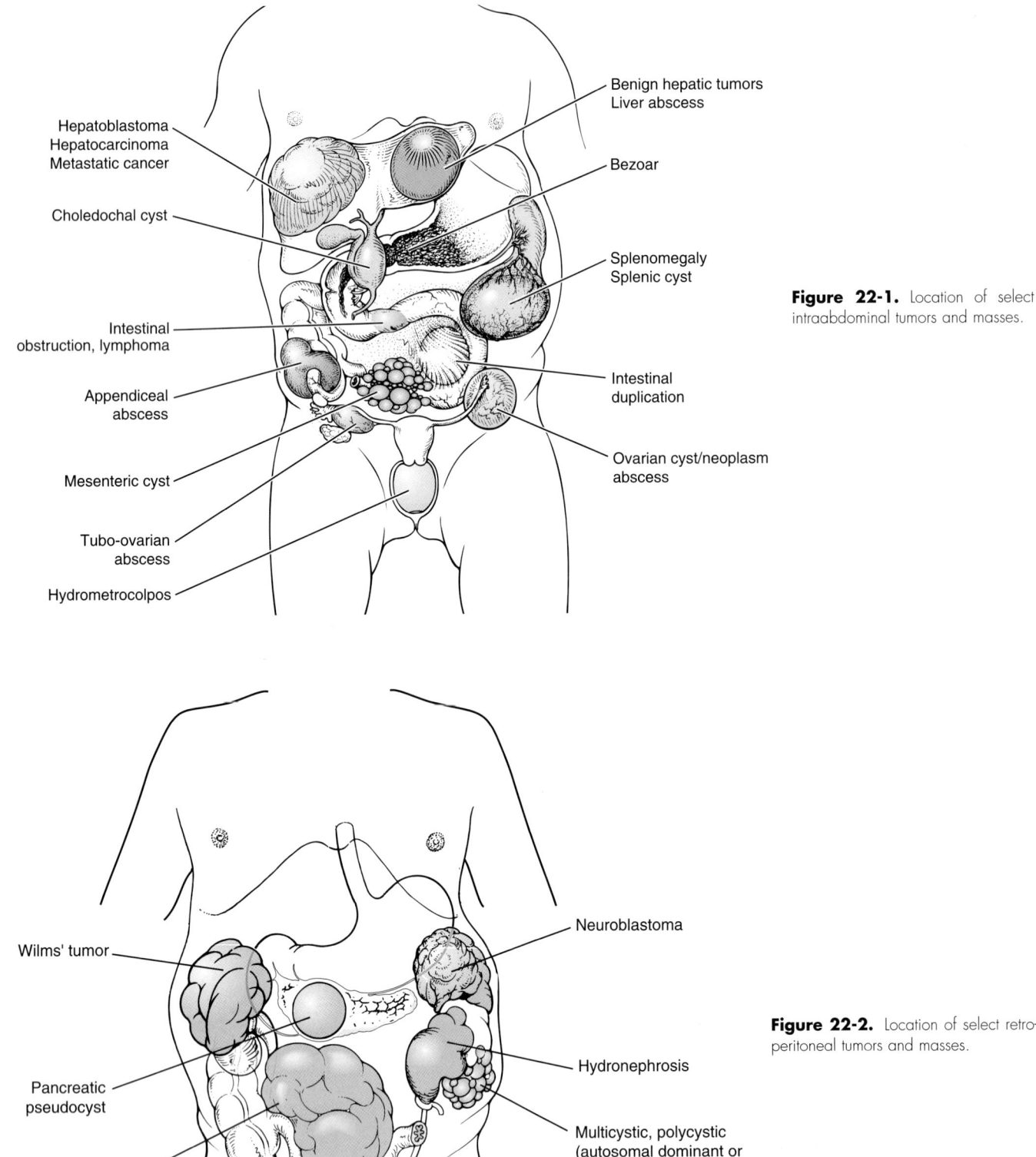

Figure 22-1. Location of select intraabdominal tumors and masses.

Hepatoblastoma
Hepatocarcinoma
Metastatic cancer

Choledochal cyst

Intestinal obstruction, lymphoma

Appendiceal abscess

Mesenteric cyst

Tubo-ovarian abscess

Hydrometrocolpos

Benign hepatic tumors
Liver abscess

Bezoar

Splenomegaly
Splenic cyst

Intestinal duplication

Ovarian cyst/neoplasm
abscess

Figure 22-2. Location of select retroperitoneal tumors and masses.

Wilms' tumor

Pancreatic pseudocyst

Lymphoma

Neuroblastoma

Hydronephrosis

Multicystic, polycystic
(autosomal dominant or
recessive) renal disease

Table 22-1. Stepwise Evaluation of an Abdominal Mass

Clinical History

Age and gender
General symptoms
Pain
Gastrointestinal symptoms
Urogenital symptoms
Pulmonary symptoms
Family history
Sexual history
Weight loss
Travel

Physical Examination

General condition
Lymph nodes
Associated physical findings
Cachexia

Abdominal Palpation

Quadrant of the abdomen
Organ most likely to be affected
Characteristics (soft or hard, mobile or nonmobile, crosses
  midline, moves with respiration, tender)

Ultrasonography

Location
Solid or cystic

**Depending on the Clinical Suspicion, Evaluation can be
Continued with One or More of the Following:**
Laboratory studies: CBC, urinalysis, tumor markers
Imaging studies: plain radiography of chest and abdomen,
  contrast radiography of the gastrointestinal tract,
  computed tomography, magnetic resonance imaging,
  angiography, scintigraphy

Table 22-2. Age-Related Etiology of Abdominal Masses

Age	Benign	Malignant
Neonate (0-1 month)	Congenital hydronephrosis	Neuroblastoma
	Cystic kidney disease	
	Intestinal duplication	
	Mesenteric/omental cyst	
	Neurogenic bladder	
	Ovarian cyst	
	Renal vein thrombosis	
	Choledochal cyst	
	Mesoblastic nephroma	
	Meconium ileus	
	Hematoma (adrenal, hepatic, splenic)	
Infant (0-1 year)	Intestinal duplication	Neuroblastoma
	Mesenteric/ omental cyst	Hepato-blastoma
	Ovarian cyst	Wilms tumor (rare)
	Mesoblastic nephroma	Teratoma
	Liver hamartomas	
	Hepatic cavernous hemangioma	
	Liver hemangioen-dothelioma	
	Teratoma	
	Intussusception	
	Hepatosplenomegaly	
	Choledochal cyst	
	Megacolon	
Child (2-10 years)	Mesenteric/omental cyst	Neuroblastoma
	Choledochal cyst	Hepato-blastoma
	Appendiceal abscess	Wilms tumor
		Leukemia
		Lymphoma
Adolescent (11-16 years)	Bezoar	Neuroblastoma
	Hematocolpos	Hepato-carcinoma
	Hydrometrocolpos	Ovarian neoplasm
	Pregnancy	Lymphoma
	Inflammatory bowel disease	
	Retroperitoneal hematoma (hemophilia)	

with similar histologic features rapidly progress in spite of intensive therapy. This tumor has unique biochemical properties (produces catecholamines) and immune properties that can aid in the diagnosis but that also produce adverse symptoms and a variable response to treatment.

The incidence of neuroblastoma is approximately 1 in 10,000 children and is more common in boys than in girls (1.2:1). The tumor affects primarily children younger than 8 years, and more than 50% occur in children older than 2 years of age.

Neuroblastoma usually manifests with an abdominal mass or abdominal discomfort. The mass is solid, is often fixed and painful, and may cross the midline. Its position does not change with respiration. Catecholamine production by the tumor occasionally results in flushing, sweating, and irritability, and vasoactive intestinal polypeptides, also produced by the tumor, may in rare cases cause secretory diarrhea. A variety of neurologic symptoms (opsoclonus-myoclonus) may also be seen, as may weight loss and anorexia. Many patients have metastases at the time of diagnosis, mainly to regional and distant lymph nodes, bone marrow and bone cortex, the orbit, the liver, and occasionally the lungs. Symptoms related to metastases include bone pain and pancytopenia.

The purposes of the diagnostic studies are to find the exact location and size of the tumor and to determine regional invasion, metastatic disease, and histologic features. A plain radiograph shows finely stippled tumor calcifications in 50% of cases and also reveals displacement of bowel gas. Ultrasonography distinguishes a solid mass from a cystic mass and determines its position in relation to the kidney. CT further demonstrates calcifications of the tumor and determines the exact position in relation to other intraabdominal and

retroperitoneal organs (Fig. 22-6). It also reveals any intraspinal or intracranial (if a cervical primary) extension of the tumor or its metastases. Bone marrow metastases are detected by bone marrow aspiration. Plain radiographs or isotope bone scans can be used to detect cortical bone lesions. In 90% of patients, the tumor excretes high levels of catecholamines and their metabolites. Homovanillic acid and vanillylmandelic acid urine levels aid in the assessment of the patient. Twenty-four-hour urine collections show no benefit over random samples. Other tumor markers include lactate dehydrogenase, ferritin, and neuron-specific enolase.

Surgical resection is the primary treatment of localized neuroblastoma. Adjuvant chemotherapy and radiotherapy are added to the therapy, depending on the stage of the disease and the age of the patient. If the tumor is considered unresectable, a diagnostic open biopsy or a needle biopsy is performed. Bone marrow

Table 22-3. Location and Nature of Abdominal Masses

Organ	Congenital	Benign	Malignant	Acquired
Liver and biliary tract	Hemangioma Choledochal cyst	Hemangioendothelioma Hamartoma	Hepatoblastoma Lymphoma Leukemia Hepatocarcinoma	Abscess Hematoma Parasitic disease Hydrops of the 　gallbladder
Spleen		Cyst	Sarcoma	Splenomegaly 　(e.g., mononucleosis)
Kidney	Hydronephrosis Cystic disease Duplication		Wilms tumor	Hematoma
Adrenal gland	Neuroblastoma		Neuroblastoma	Hematoma
Stomach	Duplication Teratoma	Leiomyoma Inflammatory pseudotumor	Leiomyosarcoma Adenocarcinoma	Bezoar
Intestines	Duplication Megacolon	Lymphangioma Hemangioma	Carcinoma Lymphoma	Appendiceal abscess Intussusception Obstipation
Mesentery		Mesenteric/omental cyst		Inflammatory bowel 　disease Parasitic disease Tuberculosis
Pancreas		Cyst	Carcinoma	Pseudocyst
Uterus	Hydrometrocolpos	Myoma	Rhabdomyosarcoma	Pregnancy
Ovaries	Cyst Teratoma	Cyst Cystic teratoma Cystic adenoma Granulosa cell tumor	Yolk sac tumor Embryonal carcinoma Dysgerminoma Choriocarcinoma	Tuboovarian abscess
Bladder	Urachal cyst Urethral valve	Inflammatory pseudotumor	Rhabdomyosarcoma	Urinary retention
Retroperitoneum	Presacral teratoma Anterior 　myelomeningocele	Ganglioneuroma	Neuroblastoma	Psoas abscess Aortic aneurysm
Abdominal wall	Hernia Omphalocele Gastroschisis	Hemangioma	Rhabdomyosarcoma	Hematoma Rectus sheath hematoma Abscess

aspiration findings may also demonstrate classic small, round cells forming rosettes. To control the disease, the child may be given chemotherapy and radiotherapy before attempted resection. In some, high-dose chemotherapy is followed by bone marrow transplantation. The use of differentiating agents, such as retinoic acid, is occasionally indicated.

Staging is based on the regional extension of the tumor, the level of metastatic disease, and the degree of resectability. The outcome of the patient is determined primarily by the child's age and tumor stage. Children younger than 1 year, especially neonates, have the best prognosis; about 75% of these patients survive. However, for children older than 2 to 3 years, the outlook is guarded. In fact, neuroblastomas diagnosed in these two age groups may represent different disease processes. This possibility is underscored by mass screening programs in some countries that detect many tumors that would probably mature or resolve, leaving the patient asymptomatic, but do not affect the incidence of disease discovered at later ages, which generally has a poorer prognosis.

Histologic features also play a part in prognosis. N-myc gene amplification portends aggressive clinical behavior. Deletions of the short arm of chromosome 1 are probably associated with the loss of a tumor-suppressor gene. Hyperploid DNA is associated with a lower stage and better prognosis (contrary to most other tumors).

RENAL MASSES

The most common causes of a renal mass are congenital hydronephrosis (often bilateral), congenital multicystic-dysplastic kidney (often unilateral), and, in older infants, Wilms tumor (nephroblastoma). Ultrasonography immediately reveals whether the mass is solid or cystic, thus directing further investigation. An ectopic or horseshoe midline kidney can also be palpable, in which case the renal mass is found in an unexpected location.

Table 22-4. Tumor Markers

Tumor	Tumor Markers
Neuroblastoma	Urinary catecholamines LDH Ferritin Neuron-specific enolase
Wilms tumor	Erythropoietin
Hepatoblastoma, 　pancreatoblastoma, yolk 　sac tumors	α-Fetoprotein
Germ cell tumors	β-hCG

hCG, human chorionic gonadotropin; LDH, lactate dehydrogenase

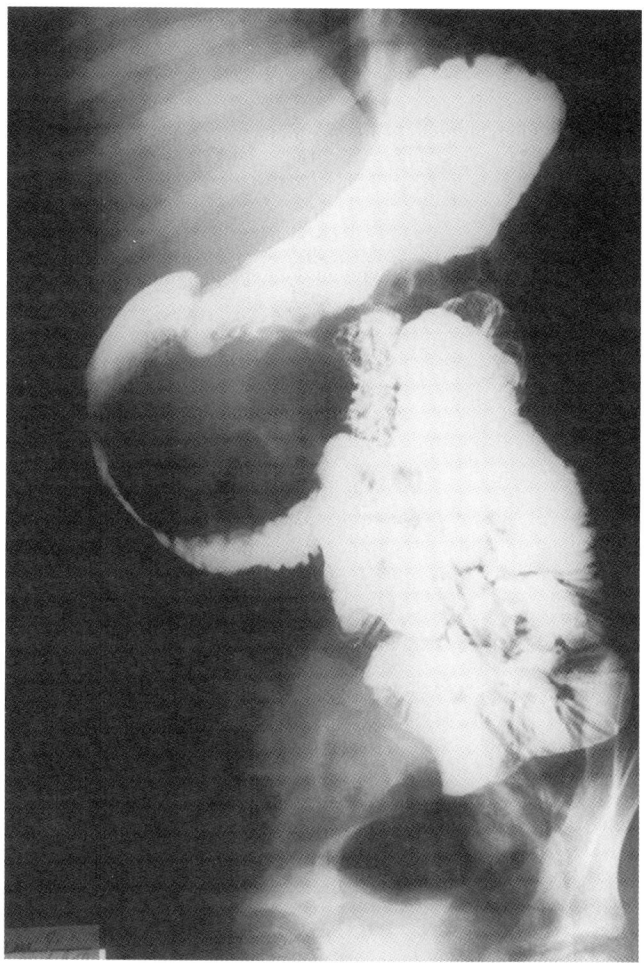

Figure 22-3. A contrast study of the upper gastrointestinal tract shows anterior displacement of the stomach and duodenum by a pancreatic pseudocyst.

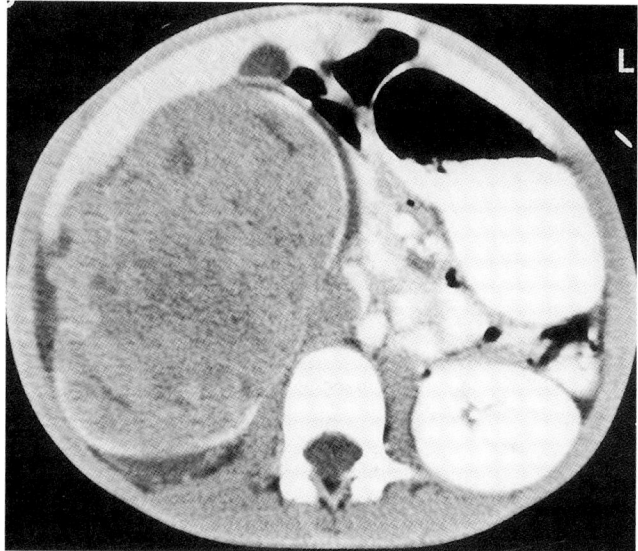

Figure 22-5. Computed tomogram revealing a large Wilms tumor replacing the right kidney. Notice that the renal cortex, enhanced by contrast medium, is splayed out around the mass. This characteristic helps differentiate Wilms tumor from neuroblastoma, which would displace a normal-appearing kidney.

CONGENITAL HYDRONEPHROSIS

Hydronephrosis secondary to ureteropelvic obstruction may result in a flank mass discovered in the neonatal period or in later childhood. An aberrant renal artery or adhesions kinking the ureter can also cause the obstruction. Hydronephrosis is found mainly in young children. It is more common in boys and on the left side. The most common presenting symptom in infants is an abdominal mass or urinary tract infection. In older children, distention of the renal pelvis may cause intermittent pain; hematuria can be seen as a result of minor abdominal trauma.

The diagnosis is confirmed with ultrasonography and, occasionally, intravenous pyelography. Diuretic renal scintigraphy demonstrates the degree of obstruction and relative function, and a voiding cystourethrogram excludes ureterovesical reflux and posterior

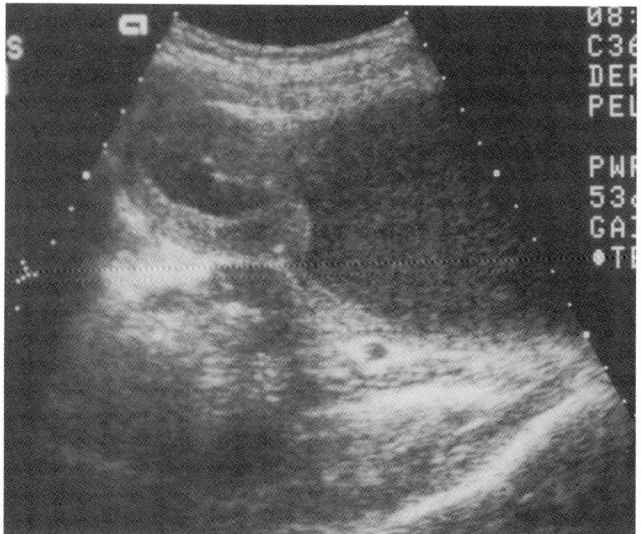

Figure 22-4. An ultrasonic longitudinal view of the pelvis reveals hydrometrocolpos. The uterus and cervix are readily seen superior to the large collection of fluid in the vagina located at the right of the image.

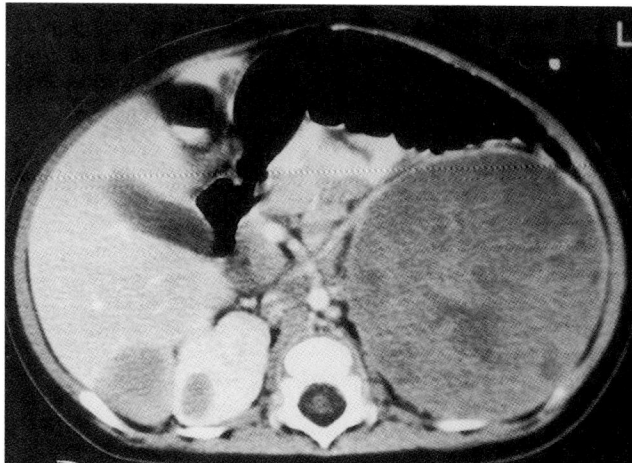

Figure 22-6. Computed tomogram of a left adrenal neuroblastoma reveals metastatic disease in the right kidney and liver. The patient, in whom the disease was diagnosed before 1 year of age, died of the disease.

urethral valves (in boys). Treatment consists of pyeloplasty with resection of the obstruction and, if necessary, parts of the distended renal pelvis.

With fetal ultrasonography, hydronephrosis can be detected and treated antenatally (Fig. 22-7). The management of asymptomatic neonates remains controversial, because it has been demonstrated that unilateral neonatal hydronephrosis may improve without operative intervention.

CYSTIC ABNORMALITIES OF THE KIDNEY

A unilateral multicystic-dysplastic kidney usually manifests as a flank mass in the newborn. Ultrasonography, intravenous pyelography, or CT demonstrates a cystic kidney with absence of renal parenchyma and decreased function. The contralateral kidney should be carefully evaluated for cysts or other abnormalities. Treatment usually consists of surgical excision, because a dysplastic kidney increases the child's risk for hypertension, urinary tract infection, tumor, or pain. Alternatively, select patients without recurrent infection or hypertension and with small lesions may be managed nonoperatively with long-term follow-up.

In the more serious case of *autosomal recessive infantile polycystic disease,* both kidneys are affected. The kidneys are filled with thousands of small cysts derived from the collecting tubules. The clinical manifestation varies, depending on the degree of renal failure. Unfortunately, almost 50% of patients experience severe renal insufficiency before the age of 15 years. The neonatal form is fatal without renal transplantation. Abdominal ultrasonography discloses the cystic nature of the condition, and pyelography may show very poor function. Besides supportive treatment (dialysis), the only therapeutic option available at this time is renal transplantation.

WILMS TUMOR (NEPHROBLASTOMA)

Wilms tumor is an embryonal renal neoplasm, one of the most common childhood abdominal malignancies. The estimated incidence is close to 1 in 15,000 live births, with a male-to-female ratio of 0.9:1. The mean age at diagnosis is 3.5 years, and at least 90% of the patients present before the age of 8 years. Between 4% and 10% of children with Wilms tumor have bilateral disease; the mean age in bilateral cases is 2.5 years. Associated conditions include aniridia, hemihypertrophy, genitourinary anomalies, and Beckwith-Wiedemann syndrome.

The origin of Wilms tumor remains unclear, but evidence of a genetic component is emerging. Some patients have other types of malignant renal tumors (no longer classified as Wilms tumor), such as rhabdoid tumors and sarcoma.

Most asymptomatic abdominal masses are discovered accidentally by the child's parents or by a physician during routine examination. Microscopic hematuria is present in about 30% of patients. In rare cases, occlusion of the left renal vein may obstruct the left spermatic vein and thus cause left-sided varicocele. Other, less common symptoms or signs include anemia, polycythemia, weight loss, hypertension, or frank hematuria after rupture of the tumor secondary to minor abdominal trauma.

Diagnostic imaging techniques include one or more of the following: plain radiography, ultrasonography, CT or MRI, and, less often, intravenous pyelography (Fig. 22-8). The location, size, and resectability of the tumor; the presence of local tumor invasion; and infiltration of the renal vein and inferior vena cava are assessed. Metastatic or bilateral disease must be ruled out. Differentiation of Wilms tumor from neuroblastoma on CT or intravenous pyelography is based on whether the renal pelvis is splayed by an intrinsic renal mass or simply displaced by a suprarenal mass. In Wilms tumor, lung metastases from renal vein and inferior vena cava infiltration may be present, whereas bone metastases are rare; these features distinguish this from neuroblastoma. Chest CT offers no benefit over plain radiograph of the chest for the assessment of metastatic disease.

Treatment includes a transabdominal nephrectomy with early ligation of the renal vein to avoid tumor mobilization. Postoperatively, a team of oncologists, surgeons, pathologists, and radiotherapists decides on further treatment. Chemotherapy and radiotherapy are added, depending on the stage and histologic features of the tumor. Trials are under way to confirm that adjuvant therapy after surgical resection is not required for stage 1 tumors with favorable histology. For very large or complex tumors, especially those with extension of tumor into the renal vein, inferior vena cava, and right atrium, preoperative chemotherapy has been employed in selected patients. Preresection percutaneous biopsy, although practiced in other

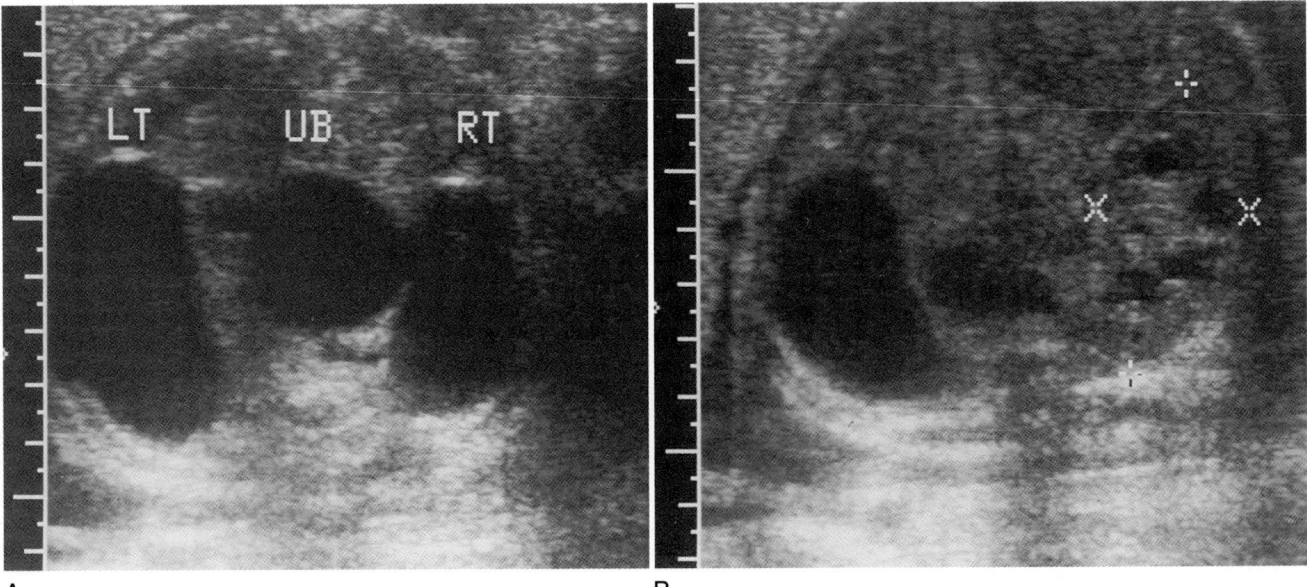

A   B

Figure 22-7. Fetal ultrasonography showing bilateral hydronephrosis. **A,** The urinary bladder (UB) is seen between the two dilated renal pelvises (LT and RT). **B,** The renal cortex is seen on the right side of the same fetus, between the two Xs.

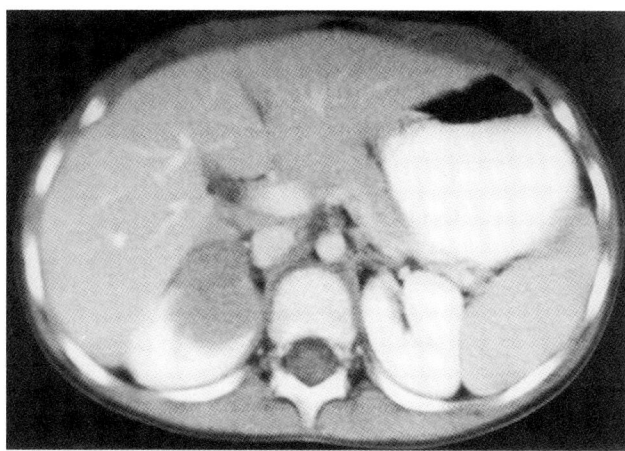

Figure 22-8. An exophytic Wilms tumor noted incidentally on a computed tomogram obtained for trauma.

countries, is generally avoided in the United States because of differences in opinion regarding the adequacy of the tissue obtained. In some cases of bilateral disease, partial resection with nephron-sparing surgery is employed. For children with excessive loss of functional renal parenchyma, transplantation is an option.

Tumor staging is based on radiographic evaluation (metastatic disease) and intraoperative findings (tumor size, extrarenal extension of the tumor, tumor spillage, status of local lymph nodes). The stage determines the prognosis and treatment of the disease. Survival depends on the prognostic factors, the success of treatment, the histologic features of the tumor, and the age of the patient. Younger patients have a better prognosis. Most children have either stage I or stage II disease (regional extension of the tumor but complete surgical removal), and most cases of Wilms tumor have favorable histologic features. Overall, the survival rate currently approaches 90%. The late complications of therapy for Wilms tumor include the development of acute myelogenous leukemia, short stature, and congestive heart failure.

LIVER TUMORS

Hepatomegaly (diffuse enlargement of the liver) or a hepatic mass may be caused by infections (hepatitis, abscess, cyst), as well as by benign or malignant lesions. Primary liver tumors are uncommon in children, but about 66% of them are malignant. Hepatoblastomas predominate, followed by hepatocellular carcinoma, mesenchymoma, and, rarely, sarcoma.

Hepatic abscesses are caused by pathogens such as *Staphylococcus aureus,* anaerobic bacteria, or *Escherichia coli.* Certain conditions, such as chronic granulomatous disease or a previous appendicitis, may predispose the child to this complication. Amebic infection of the liver caused by *Entamoeba histolytica* and parasite infestation with *Echinococcus* species may also lead to abscess formation in tropical climates. Abscesses are treated with appropriate antibiotics and surgical or percutaneous drainage.

Benign tumors can be of either mesenchymal or epithelial origin. Mesenchymal tumors include disorders such as hamartomas, cavernous hemangiomas, and infantile hemangioendotheliomas in young children. These conditions manifest as asymptomatic abdominal masses. Hemangiomas, particularly diffuse ones, may be difficult to resect and should be managed nonoperatively unless complications develop. Hamartomas, which usually manifest in the first year of life, should be resected. Epithelial lesions include focal nodular hyperplasia, hepatic adenoma, and nonparasitic solitary or multiple cysts.

For liver masses, initial radiographic evaluation should include plain abdominal radiography, to detect calcifications and the mass effect, and ultrasonography, to determine the origin, size, and echogenicity of the tumor. In addition, an abdominal CT or MRI scan can be obtained to define the exact localization and extent of the tumor (Fig. 22-9). Angiography is occasionally useful for determining resectability. Chest radiography or CT is used to determine the presence of pulmonary metastases.

HEPATOBLASTOMA

Hepatoblastoma is usually found in children younger than 5 years of age; more than half of the cases are diagnosed during the first 2 years of life. It is twice as common in boys as in girls. The most common presentation is a child with a palpable abdominal mass, occasionally associated with anemia, nausea, vomiting, weight loss, or abdominal pain. An unusual manifestation is precocious puberty resulting from tumor secretion of human chorionic gonadotropin. Elevated levels of serum α-fetoprotein are seen in about 90% of cases, and this feature is helpful in the posttherapy monitoring of disease activity. Ultrasonography, CT, and, on occasion, MRI are used to image the lesion (Fig. 22-10).

The tumor is usually solitary and located predominantly in the right hepatic lobe. If it is deemed resectable after radiographic evaluation (no portal vein or extrahepatic invasion, limited to one lobe) and there are no metastases, complete surgical removal in combination with chemotherapy is the primary treatment. A significant number of tumors are not resectable at diagnosis. These are treated with preoperative chemotherapy in hopes of converting the

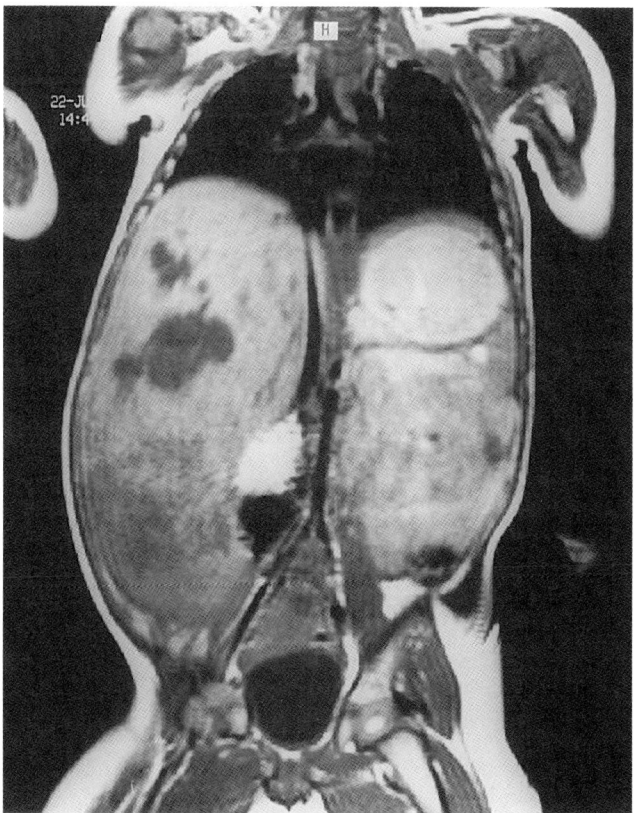

Figure 22-9. Magnetic resonance image showing a liver hamartoma in a 13-month-old boy. Note the excellent visualization of the blood vessels. The child presented with abdominal distention, poor appetite, and decreased activity. The liver was nontender and was palpated 15 cm below the costal margin. Operative resection was successful.

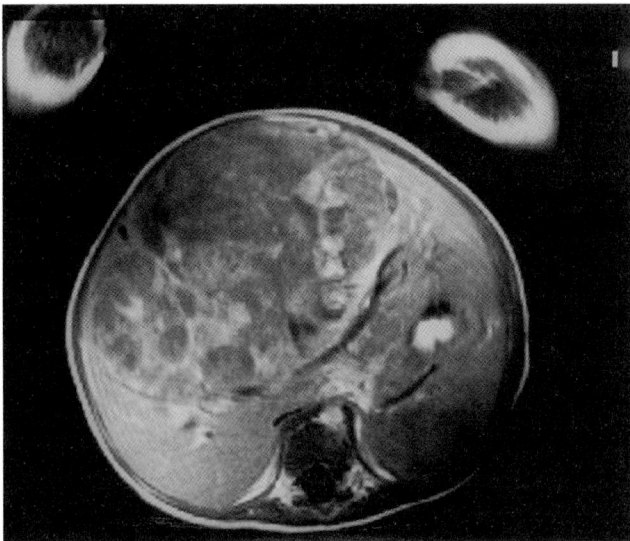

Figure 22-10. Computed tomogram of a hepatoblastoma in an 8-month-old girl. The child presented with hepatomegaly, increased abdominal girth, weight loss, and lethargy. The voluminous tumor occupies a large part of the upper abdominal cavity.

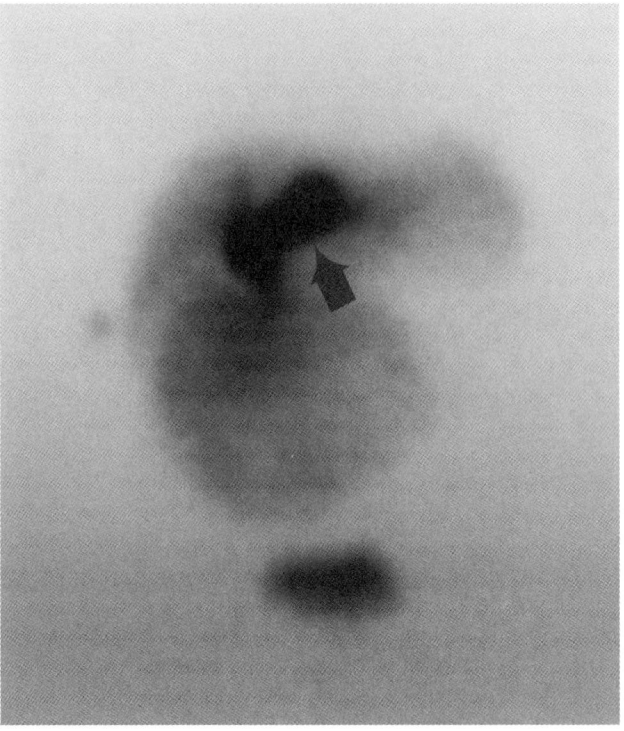

Figure 22-11. Hepato-iminodiacetic acid (HIDA) scan revealing a large choledochal cyst, marked by the *arrow*. The liver and urinary bladder are also outlined.

tumor to a resectable one. Irradiation is an additional but less desirable option. Approximately 80% of patients with completely resected tumors survive, whereas those with incompletely resected lesions have a poor prognosis. Pretreatment variables associated with survival are the extent of the tumor and the presence of metastases.

HEPATOCARCINOMA

Hepatocarcinoma, the adult type of liver tumor, usually occurs in an already diseased liver, such as that found after hepatitis B or C virus infection, tyrosinemia, galactosemia, biliary atresia, or cirrhosis. It is rare in younger children and has a peak incidence between the ages of 10 and 15 years. The tumor manifests as a painful abdominal mass; in more than 65% of patients, it is not resectable. The diagnostic evaluation, staging, and treatment of hepatocarcinoma are similar to those of hepatoblastoma.

CONGENITAL DILATATION OF THE BILE DUCTS

Any congenital cystic dilatation of the bile ducts is commonly called choledochal cyst. There are several anatomic varieties of this condition, and the cause remains unknown. The classic choledochal cyst is seen when the common bile duct is grossly dilated. However, the size varies, and the child may remain asymptomatic for many years. About 20% of patients present with the classic triad of jaundice, pain, and a right upper quadrant abdominal mass. The jaundice is of the obstructive type with associated pruritus, dark urine, and acholic stools.

Ultrasonography reveals the location, size, and nature of the cyst. If there is any doubt about its origin, a HIDA scan (Fig. 22-11) can be used to outline the biliary tract and help differentiate it from other lesions such as duodenal duplication. Treatment consists of resection of the cyst and drainage of the hepatic duct into an intestinal segment (Fig. 22-12). Incomplete resection of at least the mucosa of the affected portion of the biliary tree predisposes to the development of cancer.

INTESTINAL AND PANCREATIC MASSES

APPENDICEAL PHLEGMON AND ABSCESS

Either delayed manifestation (walled off by mesentery) or delayed diagnosis of acute appendicitis may enable the development of a right lower quadrant mass after perforation as the inflamed tissues amalgamate into a phlegmon (see Chapter 14). Further maturation of this process may lead to an abscess. Diagnosis is often facilitated by the history, which can differentiate from many other causes of abdominal mass by the recent (days to weeks) history of fever associated with abdominal pain and nausea. Antibiotic therapy may mask the diagnosis of appendicitis. CT scan is warranted in this circumstance because of the desirability of treating an abscess by percutaneous aspiration and antibiotics (Fig. 22-13). Interval appendectomy in a noninflamed field is performed 6 to 8 weeks later. This approach is not appropriate for either suspected uncomplicated acute appendicitis or for diffuse peritonitis.

BEZOAR

Emotionally disturbed or developmentally delayed children occasionally eat their own hair or other indigestible material. Ninety percent of these patients are girls, usually in their teens. A trichobezoar (hair) or a phytobezoar (vegetable matter) forms in the stomach and causes partial gastric outlet obstruction. Gastric bezoars may extend into the small intestine. If hair manages to pass the stomach, it collects in the duodenum and causes biliary tract obstruction; if it collects in the ileum, it may lead to intestinal obstruction.

The clinical picture is characterized by poor appetite, vague abdominal discomfort, and intolerance to solid foods. Physical examination reveals loss of hair on the scalp and a movable mass in the epigastrium. The diagnosis is confirmed with upper gastrointestinal contrast radiography. The bezoar is usually removed at

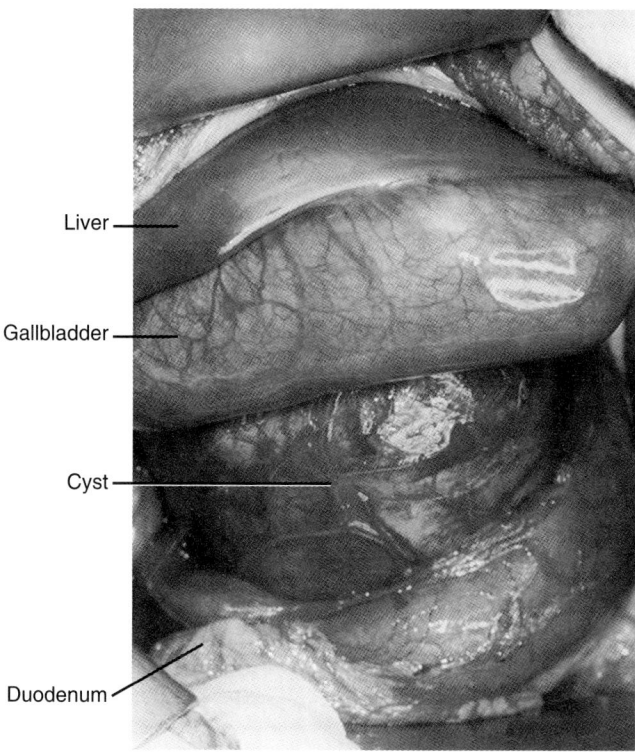

Figure 22-12. Operative photograph of a choledochal cyst between the gallbladder and the duodenum, displacing both.

endoscopy, but operative removal is indicated if the bezoar is large or if endoscopy is not successful.

DUPLICATIONS

Duplications of the gastrointestinal tract occur anywhere from the esophagus to the anus and are either cystic or tubular. The more common cystic duplications are lined with endothelium and are enclosed in a muscular wall common with the adjacent intestinal segment. Tubular duplications are located on the mesenteric side of the bowel and are either blind or in communication with the bowel. The lining is usually that of the adjacent intestine but may be heterotopic, such as gastric mucosa in a duplication of the small bowel.

Most duplications are diagnosed during the first years of childhood. The manifestations depend on the size and location of the malformation. Many intraabdominal duplications manifest as an asymptomatic, palpable mass but may also cause pain, intestinal obstruction, hemorrhage, or volvulus. Ultrasonography differentiates the cystic nature of duplications from solid tumors and also demonstrates the intimate association between the duplication and the bowel wall. Treatment consists of resection of the duplication alone or, more commonly, along with the part of the gut from which the duplication arose, depending on the anatomic location and amount of shared wall and blood supply (Fig. 22-14).

NEOPLASMS OF THE GASTROINTESTINAL TRACT

Neoplasms of the gastrointestinal tract of children are rare. The symptoms are often nonspecific, and diagnosis tends to be delayed. A gastric teratoma may appear as an epigastric mass, while gastric leiomyosarcomas or leiomyomas manifest with bleeding.

Non-Hodgkin lymphoma is the most common malignant tumor of the small intestine and may act as a leading point for an intussusception. Other malignant tumors of the small intestine include leiomyosarcoma, angiosarcoma, and carcinoid tumor. These conditions also occur in the large intestine. Carcinoid tumors are most commonly found in the appendix, where they can cause obstruction and lead to appendicitis. The colon is the most common site for the rare adenocarcinoma of the gastrointestinal tract in children.

Benign neoplasms of the small and large intestine include hemangiomas, lymphangiomas, leiomyomas, and polyps. All malignant neoplasms and most benign neoplasms should be resected.

MESENTERIC AND OMENTAL CYSTS

Cysts located in the omentum or mesentery are benign, are unilocular or multilocular, and contain clear serous fluid. They arise from a developmental abnormality of the lymphatic system that results in lymphatic obstruction. Most of these cysts are diagnosed during the first 5 years of life. They may be asymptomatic for a long period or manifest with a distended abdomen, abdominal mass, intestinal

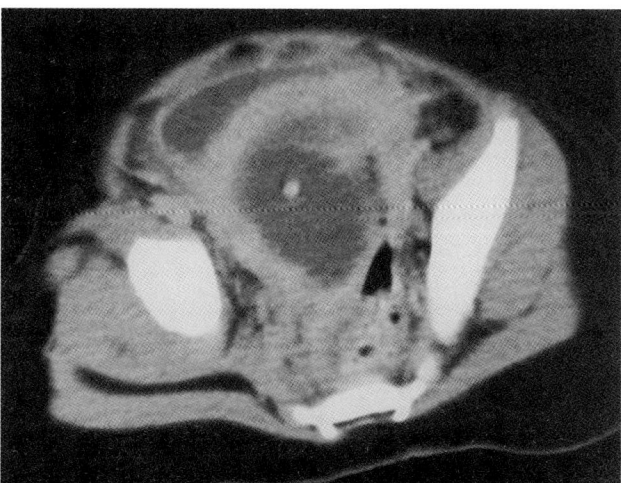

Figure 22-13. A large appendiceal abscess with a calcified fecalith. The abscess was drained percutaneously and treated with antibiotics. Interval appendectomy was performed 8 weeks later.

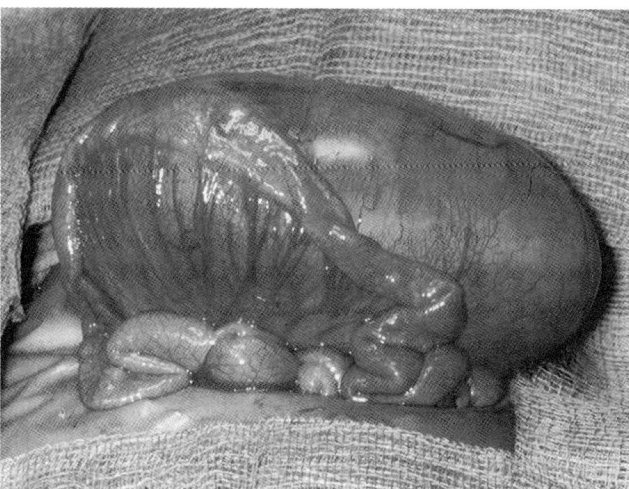

Figure 22-14. Operative photograph of the typical appearance of an intestinal duplication.

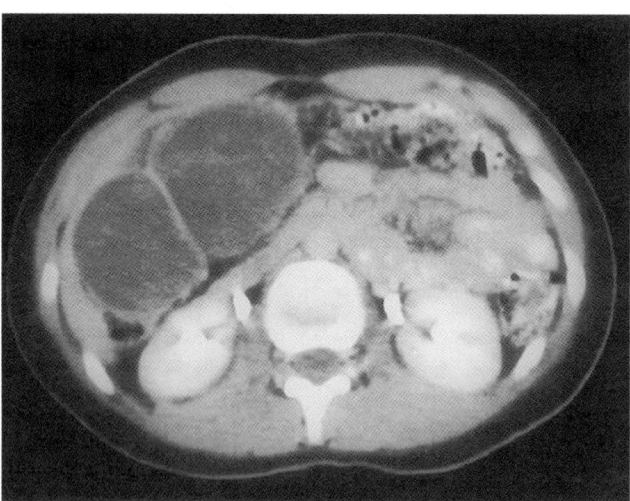

Figure 22-15. Computed tomographic scan of the abdomen in an 11-year-old boy, showing a mesenteric cyst in the transverse mesocolon.

obstruction, volvulus, or abdominal pain. The abdomen is usually nontender with a mobile mass. In contrast to ascites, the flanks do not bulge when a child with an abdominal cyst is in the supine position.

A plain abdominal radiograph shows intestinal gas displaced forward in the case of a mesenteric cyst and backward in the case of an omental cyst. Small amounts of calcification may be seen in the wall of the cyst. Ultrasonography or CT further elucidates the nature, size, and location of the cyst (Fig. 22-15). An ovarian, pancreatic, or choledochal cyst or an intestinal duplication may be difficult to differentiate from a mesenteric or omental cyst. On occasion, cerebrospinal fluid from a ventriculoperitoneal shunt fails to be resorbed because of scarring of the peritoneum, leading to a "CSFoma" (Fig. 22-16), which also may be mistaken for a mesenteric or omental cyst. Treatment consists of surgical removal. Often, bowel has to be removed together with a mesenteric cyst because of its intimacy with enteric vessels.

PANCREATIC PSEUDOCYST AND NEOPLASMS

Pancreatic tumors are rare in children and are cystic or solid, benign or malignant. Functional neoplasms arise from the islet cells, and the clinical manifestation is not of an abdominal mass but rather is characterized by the effects of the endocrine substances secreted by the tumor (hypoglycemia caused by insulinoma). Tumors arising from the acinar or ductal parts of the pancreas are nonfunctional and usually manifest as an abdominal mass. They may be benign (cystadenoma) or malignant (adenocarcinoma). Metastases are common.

Diagnosis is made by ultrasonography and CT and, in cases of suspected endocrine tumors, by measurements of active hormones. Both benign and malignant tumors should be surgically resected. The outlook for pediatric patients with pancreatic neoplasms may be better than for affected adults.

A pancreatic pseudocyst lacks epithelial lining and is the result of pancreatitis or pancreatic blunt trauma. Often, there is a symptom-free interval of several weeks or months between the trauma and the appearance of symptoms. Typical signs and symptoms are nausea, abdominal pain, and an epigastric mass (see Chapter 14). Ultrasonography and upper gastrointestinal contrast radiography locate the cyst and identify any displacement of the bowel. The cysts usually resolve spontaneously; however, if they do not, they should be drained externally percutaneously or internally to the gastrointestinal tract .

OVARIAN TUMORS

Ovarian tumors in children are uncommon, with an incidence of about 25 in 100,000 children's hospital admissions. They must be considered in any girl with lower abdominal pain, an abdominal mass, or precocious puberty. They manifest at any age from birth to adulthood but occur slightly more frequently in children older than 8 years of age. The risk of malignancy increases with age. Cystic tumors are more common than solid tumors, and the majority of masses are benign. An ovarian lesion may also be the presenting

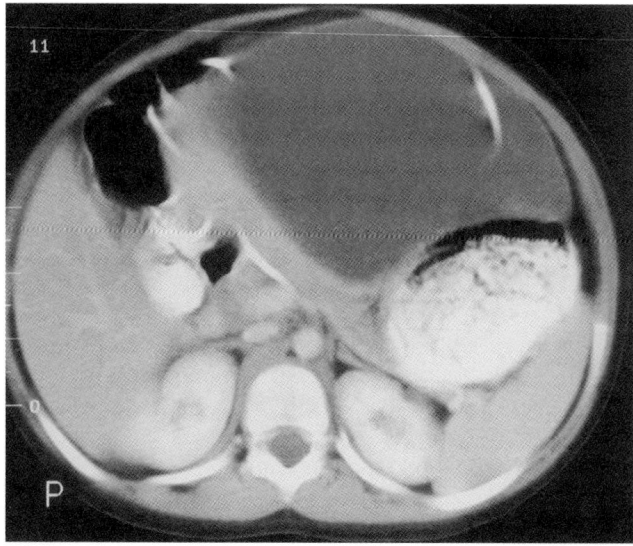

Figure 22-16. A large fluid collection associated with a ventriculoperitoneal shunt ("CSFoma").

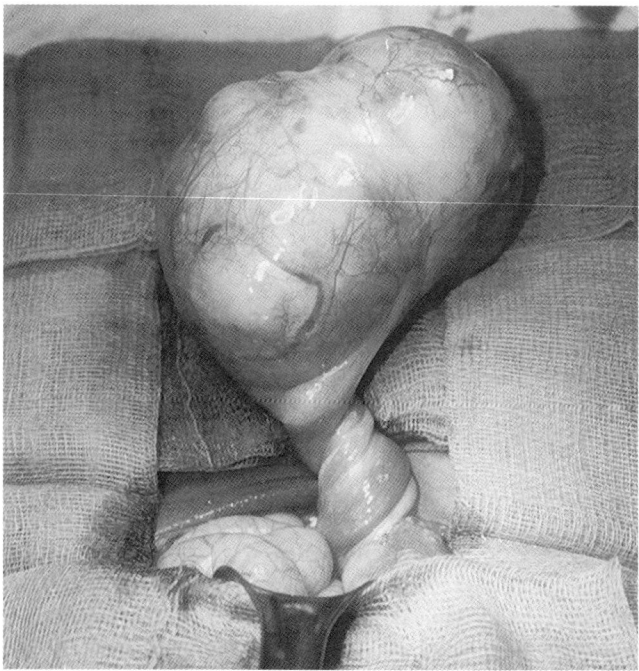

Figure 22-17. Torsion of an ovarian teratoma in a 5-year-old girl. The child presented with acute abdominal pain and a movable mass. A preoperative radiograph showed calcified material in the mass.

Table 22-5. Red Flags
1. Lower Abdominal Mass in Girls
May be indication of pregnancy, imperforate hymen, torsion of ovarian tumor, tuboovarian abscess
2. Appendiceal Abscess
Can often appear as a small bowel obstruction in younger children, in whom the diagnosis is often missed
3. Nonmobile Mass
Is suggestive of malignancy
4. Skeletal Pain or Pathologic Fracture
Is suggestive of metastatic disease (neuroblastoma) or lymphoma
5. Sudden Increase in Size of Clothing
May represent a mass or ascites
6. Left-Sided Varicocele
May be a consequence of a left-sided Wilms tumor
7. Systemic Signs of Weight Loss, Fever, Night Sweats, Anorexia, Petechiae, Anemia
Should trigger concern for malignancy, inflammatory bowel disease, or atypical infections

manifestation of other metastatic diseases, such as neuroblastoma or rhabdomyosarcoma. Malignant gonadal tumors (dysgerminoma, gonadoblastoma) are common in girls with gonadal dysgenesis (see Chapter 31) and boys with cryptorchidism. Other causes of lower abdominal mass in a girl include pregnancy and imperforate hymen, which leads to hydrocolpos or hydrometrocolpos.

Diagnosis is made by ultrasonography, which provides information on the size, consistency, location, and wall characteristics of the tumor. Abdominal radiography may reveal calcifications. CT can locate local or distant metastases. Because endocrinopathies are present in 5% to 10% of children with ovarian tumors, elevated levels of tumor markers, such as α-fetoprotein or human chorionic gonadotropin, should be investigated.

A simple cyst may appear in a neonate as a mobile abdominal mass or may even be detected incidentally by ultrasonography. Small cysts (generally less than 4 cm) can be monitored with ultrasonography and should spontaneously disappear. Larger cysts should be excised, because they can undergo torsion. The symptoms of ovarian torsion in an older child simulate those of appendicitis or ectopic pregnancy (Fig. 22-17) (see Chapter 14).

All other tumors of the ovaries should be excised, whether benign (cystic teratoma, cystic adenoma, granulosa cell tumor) or malignant (endodermal sinus tumor, yolk sac tumor, embryonal carcinoma, malignant teratoma, adenocarcinoma, dysgerminoma, choriocarcinoma). Great care should be taken to spare as much of the adnexa as possible to preserve future fertility. Depending on the histologic appearance and stage, most malignant lesions should be treated postoperatively with chemotherapy. Survival depends on the nature of the lesion; however, with the exception of highly malignant tumors such as endodermal sinus tumors and embryonal carcinoma, the prognosis is good.

SUMMARY AND RED FLAGS

Although the discovery of an abdominal mass in a child is of great concern, there is good reason for the physician to reassure the parents. The prognoses of most congenital masses are excellent, and with modern diagnostic techniques and advanced multimodal therapy, the prognoses for malignant tumors continue to improve. Red flags are listed in Table 22-5.

REFERENCES

Neuroblastoma

Haase GM, Perez C, Atkinson JB: Current aspects of biology, risk assessment, and treatment of neuroblastoma. Semin Surg Oncol 1999; 16:91-104.
LaQuaglia MP: Surgical management of neuroblastoma. Semin Pediatr Surg 2001;10:132-139.
Lukens JN: Neuroblastoma in the neonate. Semin Perinatol 1999;23: 263-273.
Maris JM, Matthay KK: Molecular biology of neuroblastoma. J Clin Oncol 1999;17:2264-2279.
Nagabuchi E, Ziegler MM: Neuroblastoma. In Oldham KT, Colombani PM, Foglia RP (eds): Surgery of Infants and Children: Scientific Principles and Practice. Philadelphia, Lippincott-Raven, 1997.

Renal Masses

Farmer DL: Urinary tract masses. Semin Pediatr Surg 2000;9:109-114.
Feldenberg LR, Siegel NJ: Clinical course and outcome for children with multicystic dysplastic kidneys. Pediatr Nephrol 2000;14:1098-1101.
Ulman I, Jayanthi VR, Koff SA: The long-term follow-up of newborns with severe unilateral hydronephrosis initially treated nonoperatively. J Urol 2000;3:1101-1105.

Wilms Tumor

Blakely ML, Ritchey ML: Controversies in the management of Wilms' tumor. Semin Pediatr Surg 2001;10:127-131.
Graf N, Tournade MF, de Kraker J: The role of preoperative chemotherapy in the management of Wilms' tumor. The SIOP studies. International Society of Pediatric Oncology. Urol Clin North Am 2000;27:443-454.
Green DM, Breslow NE, Beckwith JB, et al: Treatment with nephrectomy only for small stage I/favorable histology Wilms' tumor: A report from the National Wilms' Tumor Study Group. J Clin Oncol 2001;19: 3719-3724.
Neville HL, Ritchey ML: Wilms' tumor. Overview of National Wilms' Tumor Study Group results. Urol Clin North Am 2000;27:435-442.
Ritchey ML: Wilms' tumor. In Andrassey RJ (ed): Pediatric Surgical Oncology. Philadelphia, WB Saunders, 1998.

Liver Tumors

Carceller A, Blanchard H, Champagne J, et al: Surgical resection and chemotherapy improve survival rate for patients with hepatoblastoma. J Pediatr Surg 2001;36:755-759.
Newman KD: Hepatic tumors in children. Semin Pediatr Surg 1997;6:38-41.
Raney B: Hepatoblastoma in children: A review. J Pediatr Hematol Oncol 1997;19:418-422.

Congenital Dilatation of the Bile Ducts

Fu M, Wang Y, Zhang J: Evolution in the treatment of choledochus cyst. J Pediatr Surg 2000;35:1344-1347.
Imazu M, Iwai N, Tokiwa K, et al: Factors of biliary carcinogenesis in choledochal cysts. Eur J Pediatr Surg 2001:11:24-27.

Intestinal and Pancreatic Masses

Swenson O: Foreign bodies in the gastrointestinal tract. In Raffensperger JG (ed): Swenson's Pediatric Surgery, 5th ed. Norwalk, Conn, Appleton & Lange, 1990.

Duplications

Wrenn EL, Hollabaugh RS: Alimentary tract duplications. In Ashcraft KW, Murphy JP, Sharp RJ, et al (ed): Pediatric Surgery, 3rd ed. Philadelphia, WB Saunders, 2000.

Neoplasms of the Gastrointestinal Tract

Takano H, Smith WL: Gastrointestinal tumors of childhood. Radiol Clin North Am 1997;35:1367-1389.
Zinzani PL, Magagnoli M, Pagliani G, et al: Primary intestinal lymphoma: Clinical and therapeutic features of 32 patients. Haematologica 1997;82:305-308.

Mesenteric and Omental Cysts

Egozi EI, Ricketts RR: Mesenteric and omental cysts in children. Am Surg 1997;63:287-290.

Kosir MA, Sonnino RE, Gauderer MWL: Pediatric abdominal lymphangiomas: A plea for early recognition. J Pediatr Surg 1991; 26:1309.

Pancreatic Pseudocyst and Neoplasms

Johnson PR, Spitz L: Cysts and tumors of the pancreas. Semin Pediatr Surg 2000;9:209-215.

Ovarian Tumors

Brown MF, Hebra A, McGeehin K, et al: Ovarian masses in children: A review of 91 cases of malignant and benign masses. J Pediatr Surg 1993; 28:930.

Dolgin SE: Ovarian masses in the newborn. Semin Pediatr Surg 2000;9: 121-127.

Rescorla FJ: Pediatric germ-cell tumors. In Andrassy RJ (ed): Pediatric Surgical Oncology. Philadelphia, WB Saunders, 1998.

SECTION FOUR

GENITOURINARY DISORDERS

23 Dysuria

Candice E. Johnson

Dysuria is a symptom of urethral irritation that is usually associated with urinary frequency. Children with severe dysuria may refuse to voluntarily void, but more commonly they have frequent, urgent urination, and may become enuretic. The main cause of dysuria in children is bacterial infection of the urethra, bladder, and kidneys. Viruses play a minor role in causing dysuria; chlamydial urethritis, which is rare in young children, suggests possible sexual abuse (see Chapter 36). Causes of mechanical irritation are uncommon. Among young women and adolescent girls, urinary tract infection (UTI) is the explanation for dysuria in only 50% of cases. The other 50% of patients have vaginitis or urethritis caused by sexually transmitted pathogens, including *Chlamydia* species (see Chapter 29).

Dysuria (and the associated UTI) is an important symptom in children because it may be the first indication of an anatomic lesion, such as obstruction of the urinary tract or vesicoureteral reflux (VUR). Recurrent or persistent UTI in such children can cause kidney damage, leading to end-stage renal disease. Even simple UTIs not accompanied by obstruction or reflux can recur so often that the parents perceive the child as chronically ill. Much attention has been directed at the localization of the site of urinary infection to the upper or lower tract (pyelonephritis versus cystitis) in the hope that the site would determine the long-term prognosis.

Pyelonephritis refers to upper UTIs, as defined by the presence of fever, flank pain, or both. No other markers of inflammation (elevated C-reactive protein, erythrocyte sedimentation rate, or leuko-cyte count) are superior to these clinical symptoms in children. Not all cases of pyelonephritis produce fever in adults, but it is generally believed that afebrile pyelonephritis is uncommon in children. A renal scan is the "gold standard" for localizing the infection to the kidney or kidneys.

Cystitis is defined as an afebrile infection without flank pain or tenderness but including dysuria, frequency, or both. *Urethritis* is dysuria accompanied by pyuria but without significant bacteriuria or bacteria cultured from the urine. *Asymptomatic bacteriuria* is coloni-zation of the bladder (often chronically) with bacteria in amounts exceeding 10^5/mL and, by definition, is not accompanied by dysuria, urinary frequency or urgency, or daytime enuresis. *VUR* is the retro-grade flow of urine from the bladder toward the kidney. It is graded I through V, on the basis of the appearance of the calyces and ureter on voiding cystourethrography (VCUG). This is the most common and serious predisposing factor for pyelonephritis identified in children with UTIs.

HISTORY AND PHYSICAL EXAMINATION

NEONATES

A history that is suggestive of urinary infection in the neonate is the same as that for suspected sepsis. A mother whose vaginal culture is positive for group B streptococci or who presents with fever, pro-longed rupture of the amniotic membranes (>18 to 24 hours), uterine tenderness, or preterm labor is at increased risk for delivering a premature baby with pyelonephritis as part of the neonatal sepsis syndrome. A maternal urinary infection at or near term may increase the risk for neonatal pyelonephritis. The siblings of children with known VUR also have a significant risk of reflux, with or without infection, and they should be screened with radionuclide cystog-raphy within 4 weeks of birth. Neonates may also present with jaundice, vomiting, or abdominal distention. Palpation of kidney masses helps identify obstructive lesions and cystic kidneys.

INFANTS

Because infants cannot report dysuria, a UTI should be suspected in any boy younger than 6 months with unexplained fever, especially if he is uncircumcised. For all infant girls with unexplained fever, a urinalysis should be performed; a catheterized specimen should be obtained if pyuria is present. Data from Sweden suggest that the United States and Great Britain underdiagnose UTIs in the first year of life.

TODDLERS

A UTI should be suspected in toddlers with a delayed onset of daytime toilet mastery. However, because of the large variability in the time of achievement of daytime dryness (15 months to 4 years), this symptom is unreliable. Nocturnal enuresis is rarely a sign of UTI, but urine cultures should probably be obtained in children who do not stay dry at night by 5 years of age. A more significant symptom in toddlers is the acute onset of daytime enuresis after a period of continence. Boys who present with a history of dribbling rather than a strong urine stream should be suspected of having posterior urethral valves; a standard VCUG must be obtained. Girls who present with episodes of squatting or curtseying to stop urination may have a UTI. This behavior arises from uncontrolled bladder contractions against a closed bladder sphincter. Some terms for this are *bladder dyssynergia, unstable bladder, uninhibited bladder,* and *persistence of the infantile bladder.* Because many of these children develop VUR and infection, it is important to ask about the voiding pattern in dysuric children.

Both urine and stool withholding have a role in causing UTI in young children. Constipation is associated with large residual urine volumes after voiding. The treatment of constipation leads to a reduction in UTIs.

Uncircumcised boys, patients with neurogenic bladders (spina bifida), and patients with renal anomalies (cysts, obstructed hydronephrosis, double collecting systems, ectopic ureter, horseshoe kidney, VUR) are at increased risk for UTI.

OLDER CHILDREN

Most children with a UTI present with dysuria, frequency, or fever. It is worthwhile to ask about any urine color change, which suggests the presence of hematuria. A history of anal pruritus is suggestive of pinworms, which may also irritate the urethral area. The child should be questioned about the frequency, character, and size of his or her bowel movements. Bulky stools associated with constipation may predispose the child to a UTI; stool softeners, such as mineral oil or fiber, may be indicated (see Chapter 21).

ADOLESCENTS

In the adolescent, a detailed sexual history is mandatory, focusing on cystitis from sexual intercourse or vaginitis. Herpes simplex, infections with *Trichomonas* and *Chlamydia* species, and gonorrhea all cause urethritis. The most likely time for this to appear is within 1 month of beginning a relationship with a new sexual partner. Because the use of a diaphragm for contraception is associated with an increased risk of UTI, adolescents experiencing recurrent UTIs should be offered an alternative form of birth control. Similarly, adolescent girls should be questioned about voiding before or after intercourse, because studies have shown a reduction of UTI with postintercourse urination.

Pelvic examination to exclude vaginitis is essential in all sexually active adolescent girls when pyuria is absent or when vaginal discharge is reported. Conversely, adolescents with dysuria and pyuria may be assumed to have a UTI if the urinalysis is free of contaminating squamous epithelial cells. The presence of more than rare epithelial cells suggests contamination of the urine with vaginal white cells and bacteria. The pelvic examination should include cervical cultures for *Neisseria gonorrhoeae* and *Chlamydia* species because both organisms can cause urethritis. *Trichomonas* species and clue cells should be checked with a saline preparation, and any lesions suggestive of herpes simplex should be cultured (see Chapter 29).

A cause for dysuria may be found in 90% of young women. About 10% may have vaginitis, whereas about 50% have more than 10^5 bacteria/mL in a midstream urine sample. The remaining 40% of women with fewer than 10^5 bacteria/mL were once considered to have "urethral syndrome" and were believed not to have true bacteriuria. However, according to direct bladder sampling, half had positive bacterial cultures of the usual pathogens, one third had positive *Chlamydia* cultures from the bladder, and 10% had no cause for dysuria. This last group probably had mechanical or chemical irritation of the urethra, from either sexual intercourse or bath soaps.

Boys and men with dysuria may also have penile pain or dysuria as a result of phimosis, paraphimosis, balanitis, urethral trauma, epididymitis, or meatal stenosis. *Phimosis* is a scarring or narrowing of the preputial opening and manifests as failure to retract the foreskin (the foreskin is normally difficult to retract in neonates, but by 3 years of age it is easily retracted). *Paraphimosis,* an emergent disease, is an incarceration of the prepuce behind the glans. Edema, pain, and swelling are present. *Balanitis* is an infection of the prepuce (by *Streptococcus* species, *Candida* species, mixed flora, *Trichomonas* species); it may be recurrent and warrants circumcision.

METHODS OF OBTAINING URINE CULTURES

A properly obtained urine specimen for urinalysis and culture is critical for accurate treatment. Numerous studies have shown that more than 50% of all positive cultures obtained from a "bagged" specimen are skin contaminants. In the non–toilet-trained toddler, urine should be obtained by a bag only if treatment is not planned that day, and a confirmatory culture may be done the next day. The confirmatory culture may be either a suprapubic aspiration or a catheterized urine specimen. Because aspiration requires a full bladder and infants void every 1 to 2 hours, it is often impractical to wait. Catheterization is more efficient, but it does carry approximately a 1% risk of introducing infection into the bladder. Uncircumcised infants with a nonretractile foreskin should have a suprapubic aspiration.

In the toilet-trained child, a clean-void urine specimen is adequate. There are several exceptions to this rule. Uncircumcised boys have a contamination rate of 5% to 9%, depending on whether soap cleansing was used. Therefore, if treatment is needed urgently in such boys, two urine samples should be cultured, or a suprapubic aspiration should be performed. Adolescent girls may also fail to cleanse adequately, as may obese younger girls. The urine sample should be examined for squamous epithelial cells and should be discarded if such cells are present.

The gold standard for a UTI is a positive culture, by the criterion of 10^5 bacteria/mL; nonetheless, lower colony counts are present in a significant number of patients. Lower colony counts occur in boys, in diluted urine, in specimens from suprapubic or catheterized samples, and in infections with certain pathogens (for *Staphylococcus saprophyticus,* colony counts may be as low as 10^2/mL). About 33% of women have true cystitis with colony counts of less than 10^5 bacteria/mL; therefore some investigators have suggested a criterion of 10^2 bacteria/mL for dysuric women. In children, the use of colony counts as low as 10^2 bacteria/mL results in overdiagnosis, which is a problem because it may lead to unnecessary radiologic evaluation of the urinary tract. Of children with positive suprapubic tap results, 90% have at least 10^4 bacteria/mL; therefore, this seems a reasonable criterion for defining infection on clean-void urine samples. For symptomatic children with less than 10^4 bacteria/mL, a second specimen must be analyzed before treatment. Table 23-1 summarizes the recommended colony counts to define UTI in children. *Escherichia coli* is the dominant pathogen causing UTI in all ages; less common pathogens include *Klebsiella* species, *Proteus* species, *S. saprophyticus,* and *Enterococcus* species.

Mixed urine cultures do not always signify a contaminated specimen. Mixed coliform infections were noted in women (19% of all positive cultures) who were catheterized to avoid contamination. Mixed infections are also seen in children, but a catheterized specimen is necessary to confirm the infections.

Urinalysis should be performed both microscopically and by the dipstick method to detect the presence of nitrites, hematuria, and leukocyte esterase (Fig. 23-1). Decisions on treatment are usually based on the urinalysis results, not urine culture results, which require 18 to 24 hours of incubation. Fortunately, the sensitivity and specificity of the combination of the presence of leukocyte esterase and nitrite are very high in older children (Table 23-2). The accuracy of these tests in young infants and neonates is much lower. In these patients, presumptive therapy is often begun for presumed sepsis before confirmation of infection from urine, blood, or other cultures.

Microscopic evaluation of the urine for white blood cells and bacteria improves the diagnostic accuracy of the urinalysis (see Table 23-2). Therefore, in the evaluation of older children, a dipstick test for the presence of nitrites and leukocyte and a microscopic evaluation should be performed. The presence of leukocytes and bacteria, even with a negative nitrite test result, suggests a diagnosis of a UTI. The presence of only leukocytes indicates a diagnosis of vaginitis or *Chlamydia, Mycoplasma hominis,* or *Ureaplasma*

Table 23-1. Criteria for Urinary Infection in Children

Suprapubic aspiration	Any growth significant
Catheterization*	$\geq 10^3$ bacteria/mL
Clean-void urine (CVU) in symptomatic patient	$\geq 10^4$ bacteria/mL
CVU in asymptomatic patient	$>10^5$ bacteria/mL in 2 samples

*The exception is the uncircumcised neonate with a nonretractile foreskin. If colony count is <10^5 bacteria/mL, a suprapubic aspiration should be performed.

Dipstick Testing

Store strips at proper humidity and temperature
Test fresh urine (bilirubin and urobilinogen are light - and heat-sensitive)
Mix urine thoroughly (red blood cells will settle to bottom)
Compare reagent strips carefully, under good lighting
Read strip at proper time

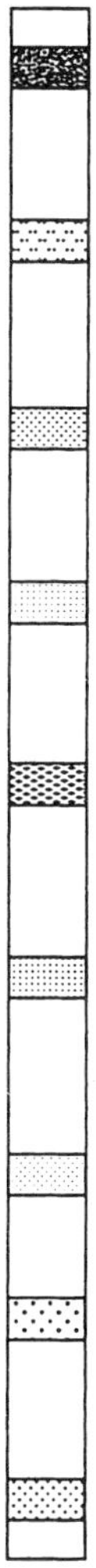

Finding		Normal Result	Method	Source of Error
Leukocytes		Negative (60–120 seconds)	Leukocyte esterase enzyme assay	Possible false-negatives with phenazopyridine HCl (Pyridium), vitamin C, nitrofurantoin
Nitrite		Negative (30 seconds)	Use first morning specimen since reaction may take 4 hours	Bacteriuria will cause positive results; vitamin C, acid pH may cause false-negative results
pH		5 to 7 (immediate)	Methyl red and bromthymol blue indicators for pH 5–9	Bacteriuria increases pH by converting urea to ammonia
Protein		Negative (30–60 seconds)	More sensitive to albumin than globulin; can detect as little as 60 mg/liter of protein	False-positives may be due to very alkaline urine, radiographic dyes
Glucose		Negative (60 seconds)	Glucose oxidase is specific for glucose	False-negatives occasionally seen resulting from tetracycline, aspirin, L-dopa, and vitamin C
Ketones		Negative (60 seconds)	Sodium nitroprusside forms violet dye with acetone, acetoacetate (not beta hydroxybutyrate)	False-positives may be seen with L-dopa, methyldopa (Aldomet), captopril, phenylketones
Urobilinogen		Negative (10–30 seconds)		Many possible false-positives and false-negatives
Bilirubin		Negative (30–60 seconds)		Vitamin C, nitrates may cause false-negatives; rifampin, chlorpromazine may cause false-positives
Blood		Negative (60 seconds)	Red blood cells cause stippling; free hemoglobin, or myoglobin causes diffuse pigment change	Nonspecificity of diffuse pigment change for hemoglobin, myoglobin, and others

Figure 23-1. Dipstick testing. Strips are stored at proper humidity and temperature. Fresh urine is tested (bilirubin and urobilinogen are light sensitive and heat sensitive). The urine is mixed thoroughly (red blood cells settle to the bottom). Reagent strips are compared carefully, under good lighting. The strip is read at the proper time. (From Reilly BM: Practical Strategies in Outpatient Medicine, 2nd ed. Philadelphia, WB Saunders, 1991, p 983.)

urealyticum urethritis if the patient is an adolescent. Alternatively, sterile pyuria may suggest prior treatment with antibiotics, renal abscess, viral cystitis, appendicitis, inflammatory bowel disease, Kawasaki disease, Stevens-Johnson syndrome, tuberculosis, analgesic nephropathy, sarcoidosis, interstitial nephritis, heavy metal toxicity, acute tubular necrosis, Reiter syndrome, renal transplant rejection, use of nephrotoxic drugs, or nephrolithiasis. The presence of only bacteria with or without a positive nitrite test result may still indicate a UTI because the sensitivity of leukocytes on urinalysis is only 80% to 85%. Neonates and infants may have a UTI in the absence of pyuria or other laboratory evidence other than a positive urine culture. The "gold standard" for a UTI in a child remains the quantitative urine culture.

Table 23-3 offers clues found in the urinalysis that point to the correct diagnosis. Although microscopic hematuria is common in all UTIs, gross hematuria is more common with cystitis, glomerulonephritis, and renal calculi (see Chapter 25). The presence of red blood cell casts suggests glomerulonephritis, whereas the presence of white blood cell casts suggests pyelonephritis. The combination of proteinuria and a UTI should suggest infection in a child with reflux nephropathy or a urologic anomaly, such as polycystic kidney disease. Urate crystals may move as a result of brownian motion and resemble motile rods, but they dissolve with gentle heating of the test tube or slide. Finally, breast-fed neonates often produce salmon-colored patches in the urine that are caused by urate crystals filtered on the diaper.

Table 23-2. Urinalysis Methods in Children

Method	Sensitivity (%)	Specificity (%)	Positive Predictive Value (%)	Negative Predictive Value (%)
Dipstick*				
Leukocyte esterase	79	73	34	95
Nitrite	37	100	100	90
Leukocyte and/or nitrite	83	72	34	96
Microscopy of sediment*				
Leukocytes (>5/hpf)	80	84	47	96
Bacteria (any)	99	71	37	100
Leukocytes and/or bacteria	99	65	33	100
Unspun urine in counting chamber†				
>5 motile bacteria/mm³	96	89	75	99
>5 WBC/mm³	64	92	70	88

*Adapted from Lohr JA, Portilla MG, Geuder TG, et al: Making a presumptive diagnosis of urinary tract infection by using a urinalysis performed in an on-site laboratory. J Pediatr 1993;122:22-25.

†Adapted from Corman LI, Horbison RW: Simplified urinary microscopy to detect significant bacteriuria. Pediatrics 1982;70:133-135.

hpf, high-power field; WBC, white blood cell.

DIFFERENTIAL DIAGNOSIS OF DYSURIA

After the history and physical examination, a list of probable diagnoses should be developed. This list determines which laboratory tests or radiologic studies are needed and cost effective. Table 23-4 outlines the differential diagnosis of dysuria, regardless of patient age.

NEONATES

UTI in the first month of life has different epidemiologic characteristics than does UTI in later infancy and childhood. It affects more boys than girls at a 5:1 ratio; about 5% of these infant boys have obstructive uropathy (Fig. 23-2). It was once thought that all these infections were hematogenous, but the high incidence of VUR and obstructive uropathy suggests that many of these infections are ascending from the bladder to the kidney. In addition, the rate of UTI in the first year of life is 11 times higher among uncircumcised boys than among circumcised boys, which suggests that infection originates in the prepuce. Furthermore, the rate of UTI is lower in the first 72 hours after birth than afterward. In the first 72 hours, 90% of the urinary infections were accompanied by bacteremia, which suggests the presence of disseminated sepsis. Thereafter, the rate of accompanying bacteremia is 10% to 20%.

In a prospective screening study of 1762 infants admitted to a neonatal intensive care nursery, 2.4% of patients were bacteriuric, of whom 1.9% had symptomatic bacteriuria and 0.5% had asymptomatic bacteriuria. Of 43 UTIs, only 6 were associated with bacteremia. Radiologic anomalies were found in 44% of the symptomatic neonates, including three children with hydronephrosis. In another study, hydronephrosis caused by obstructive lesions was seen in about 5% of neonates, and severe (grade IV or V) VUR in about 19% of neonates with symptomatic UTI. Many neonates with a UTI require urologic follow-up.

When uncircumcised infant boys are evaluated for sepsis, a suprapubic aspiration yields a much lower contamination rate than does a catheter specimen. The bladder is a more superficial abdominal organ until the end of infancy and is readily accessible with a 1½-inch-long, 22-gauge needle, inserted perpendicular to the abdominal wall, 1 to 2 cm above the symphysis pubis in the midline. Negative pressure is applied while the needle is advanced slowly until urine is obtained. No anesthetic or sterile gloves are necessary, but the infant's perineum and genitals should be cleansed with an antiseptic solution and should not have voided for 1 hour before the procedure is performed, to ensure that the bladder is full.

Obstructive uropathy can also cause neonatal UTI and sepsis. In many affected neonates, it is diagnosed by prenatal ultrasonography; therefore, antibiotic prophylaxis or immediate surgical correction can prevent sepsis and renal injury (see Chapter 22). Any neonate with bilateral hydronephrosis should undergo VCUG before discharge to rule out posterior urethral valves or bladder neck obstruction. If VUR is found, antibiotic prophylaxis should be started. Neonates with the more common diagnoses of ureteropelvic junction obstruction and unilateral multicystic dysplastic kidney do not usually need prophylaxis; subspecialty consultation should be obtained.

Table 23-3. Clues on Urinalysis that Point to the Correct Diagnosis for Dysuria

1. *Gross hematuria* suggests
   a. Glomerulonephritis, especially Berger disease (IgA nephropathy)
   b. Cystitis
   c. Renal calculi
   d. Trauma
   e. Tumor (rare)
2. *White blood cell casts* suggest pyelonephritis but are rarely seen in children; *red blood cell casts* suggest acute glomerulonephritis.
3. *Proteinuria* and yellow urine suggest glomerular damage; reflux nephropathy and polycystic kidney disease may produce a UTI and proteinuria.
4. *Proteinuria* in pink or red urine may indicate hemolysis or rhabdomyolysis.
5. *Urate* crystals resemble bacteria but may be dissolved by heating the slide or test tube.
6. *Alkaline pH* in the presence of pyuria suggests a urease-producing bacterium, such as *Proteus* species.
7. *Salmon-colored urine* in neonates is urate crystals, not blood. It is not a sign of UTI but rather of concentrated urine.

UTI, urinary tract infection.

Table 23-4. Differential Diagnosis of Dysuria

Urinary Tract Infections*
Urethritis
Cystitis
Pyelonephritis
Adenoviral hemorrhagic cystitis
Schistosomiasis

Vaginitis*
Candida albicans
Trichomonas vaginalis
Nonspecific vaginitis with clue cells
Group A streptococci
Proteus species, *Escherichia coli*, and other enteric
pathogens
Sexual abuse: gonorrhea, chlamydia, and herpes simplex
Foreign body in vagina
Herpes simplex

Tumor-Related Dysuria
Passage of blood clots from kidney tumors (Wilms)
Chemotherapy-related hemorrhagic cystitis
(cyclophosphamide)
Rhabdomyosarcoma of bladder
Urethral polyps or diverticula
Fibromas of the bladder
Hemangiomas

Mechanical Irritation of the Urethra

Boys
Water injection or foreign body insertion
Hypercalciuria or frank calculi
Balanitis or penile ulcers
Urethral stricture
Posterior urethral valves
Masturbation

Girls
Hypercalciuria
Bubble bath or detergent
Pinworms
Labial adhesions
Urethral prolapse
Sexual abuse

Other
Dysfunctional voiding syndrome
Appendicitis
Inflammatory bowel disease

*Common.

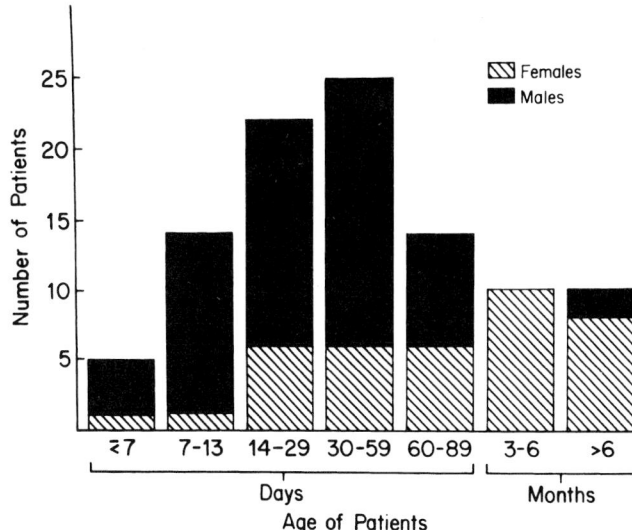

Figure 23-2. Distribution by age and sex of 100 infants with urinary tract infections. (From Ginsburg CM, McCracken GH Jr: Urinary tract infections in young infants. Pediatrics 1982;69:409-412.)

bacteriuria should not be treated because of the excellent prognosis for spontaneous clearing of the infection.

Several prospective studies have shown that about 5% of febrile infants have a UTI. Among infants younger than 3 months, UTI is more common in boys. After 3 months of age, UTIs were uncommon in infant boys in one study of predominantly uncircumcised infant boys (see Fig. 23-2). Nonetheless, in other studies, some infant boys with UTIs present as late as 1 year of age. Bacteremia is less common in patients with UTIs after the neonatal period (rates range from 6% to 31% in various studies), but fever is seen in most patients. Because pyuria is seen in only about 50% of all infants with UTIs, it is important for a catheterized or suprapubic urine specimen to be obtained from all infants in whom the source of fever cannot be identified. It is impossible to confirm a suspicious urine culture obtained with a urine bag after antibiotic therapy has begun. Therefore, all febrile infants younger than 12 months (and possibly those <24 months) of age require a urinalysis and culture if no other definite source of fever is found.

Should circumcision be recommended in all newborn boys? Boys who are uncircumcised have a 10-fold increased risk of UTI in infancy. At present, clinicians should leave the decision for circumcision up to the family, unless there is a family history of VUR, in which case circumcision should be recommended to the family.

PRESCHOOL- AND SCHOOL-AGED CHILDREN

The preschool years are when the child usually begins toilet training, which may cause dysfunctional voiding patterns, such as urine retention and contractions against a closed sphincter. In boys, such problems may not be identified, because the length of the male urethra and meatal position are protective against ascending infection. Girls readily become infected, and bladder edema may then intensify the voiding problems. Children with daytime incontinence after 4 years of age need a urine culture and possibly cystography. Attempting to void with the sphincter closed generates high intravesicular pressures and may cause VUR, even in the absence of congenital reflux. Urodynamic studies are extremely difficult to perform in toddlers; most investigators recommend a 6-month trial of therapy before cystometric tests are attempted. Anticholinergic therapy, timed voiding programs, and antibiotic prophylaxis are useful for children who have recurrent infections, urgency, and frequency.

INFANTS (YOUNGER THAN 12 MONTHS)

About 0.9% of infant girls and 2.5% of infant boys may have asymptomatic bacteriuria. An additional 1.2% of both boys and girls may develop symptomatic UTI before the age of 12 months. UTI is one of the most common bacterial causes of fever without a focus in children younger than 2 years of age. Nonetheless, the high background rate of asymptomatic bacteriuria may explain why many studies in febrile infants show apparent UTI with no pyuria. These infants may have another source of fever (viral infection) and coincident asymptomatic bacteriuria. Because no laboratory test can distinguish asymptomatic bacteriuria from pyelonephritis in a febrile infant, all such infants must be treated as if they are infected and should subsequently be evaluated radiologically. True asymptomatic

Tumors of the kidney or ureters can cause dysuria by passive bleeding that produces clots. Hemorrhagic cystitis, whether caused by chemotherapy or by adenoviral infection, is very painful. Tumors of the bladder are quite rare in children but can produce urinary retention or dysuria. Fibromas, rhabdomyosarcomas, and hemangiomas may occur. Congenital urethral polyps occur in young boys and may prolapse. In prepubertal girls, the urethra may prolapse and bleed. Labial adhesions are a common problem of unknown cause that may produce either dysuria or a true UTI.

Mechanical irritation of the male urethra may result from water injection, foreign body insertion, renal calculi, or masturbation. In the uncircumcised male, balanitis or penile ulcers may cause dysuria. In infants, recurrent diaper dermatitis may lead to a urethral stricture that necessitates surgery. Urethral stenosis is no longer believed to cause UTIs in girls or women; because of that earlier belief, thousands of unfortunate women underwent urethral dilatations in the past.

In young children, the incidence of asymptomatic bacteriuria is approximately 1% in girls and 0% in boys. Symptomatic infection is also uncommon in boys; hence, when it occurs, a complete radiologic evaluation for anomalies or reflux should be performed.

Sexual abuse frequently causes dysuria but less often causes a UTI. Although 10% of abuse victims aged 1 to 16 years had dysuria or urinary frequency in one study, only two (0.5%) had pyuria and a UTI. However, urine cultures for *Chlamydia* organisms were not performed in this study. Urine cultures for *Chlamydia* species should be obtained in any abused child with pyuria, as should the standard vaginal and rectal cultures for gonorrhea.

Vaginitis can cause dysuria in girls and women. In prepubertal girls in whom a UTI is ruled out, a careful examination of the introitus for discharge or foreign body should be made. Cultures for enteric pathogens, group A streptococci, gonorrhea, *Chlamydia* species, and *Candida* species should be obtained if a discharge is seen. A digital rectal examination may palpate foreign bodies in the vagina, and ultrasonography may visualize the foreign body. However, it is often necessary to perform an examination with the patient under anesthesia if a foreign body is suspected but is not felt or seen.

Ascending bacterial infection of the urinary tract causes most instances of dysuria. About 80% of infections are caused by *E. coli*, 10% by *Klebsiella* or *Proteus* species, and 5% by *S. saprophyticus*. These infections originate in the fecal reservoir and spread to the introitus and urethra and finally into the bladder.

Table 23-5 is a stepwise evaluation scheme for children who are dysuric but have fewer than 10^4 bacteria/mL on a clean-void urine culture. First, a complete history and physical examination should be performed. If vaginitis is present, appropriate specimens for culture should be obtained. If anal pruritus is present, a pinworm tape slide should be sent home with the patient for early morning testing. If no vaginitis or anal excoriation is present, one of two strategies is possible: A first morning urine or a catheterized urine specimen can be obtained. The decision of which strategy is used should be based on the severity of the symptoms. Commonly, symptoms are mild and self-limited and do not necessitate catheterization. A 24-hour urine sample for calcium may be ordered (>4 mg/kg/day defines hypercalciuria). Hypercalciuria may cause dysuria (see Chapter 25). If no diagnosis is reached after these steps, the severity and duration of dysuria should guide the clinician. Referral to a urologist for cystoscopy may be necessary to diagnose the extremely rare occurrence of a bladder tumor in a child.

ADOLESCENTS

In adolescent boys, lack of circumcision increases the risk of UTI about threefold, in comparison with that in those who are circumcised. Because the risk of UTI is so low in boys of this age group, this is a poor argument in favor of late circumcision. It is useful to obtain a urine culture as well as cultures for *Chlamydia* species (EIA on urine sediment or EIA or DFA on a urethral swab) and *N. gonorrhoeae* in all dysuric adolescent boys. Careful examination of the scrotum for signs of epididymitis is indicated (see Chapter 28).

Among adolescent girls, cystitis and urethritis are more common in those who are sexually active, especially those using barrier contraception. Diaphragm, spermicide and foam, and condom users have a much higher rate of bacteriuria than do those taking birth control pills. Pyelonephritis occurs in nonsexually active adolescents only rarely and should suggest the possibility of (1) neglected UTI symptoms for days to weeks or (2) VUR. Table 23-6 provides guidelines for evaluating the adolescent with dysuria.

Pitfalls in the diagnosis of dysuria are noted in Table 23-7.

Table 23-5. Stepwise Evaluation Strategy for Children with Urinary Frequency and/or Dysuria and <10^4 Pathogens per Milliliter

1. Check for bubble bath or harsh detergent use in the bath water
2. Ask about masturbation or foreign body insertion into the penile urethra
3. If vaginitis is present, obtain cultures for gonorrhea, *Candida, Chlamydia,* and bacteria (group A streptococci, *Escherichia coli*)
4. Examine for pinworms with a tape slide of perianal region
5. Check for dysfunctional voiding patterns: enuresis, urgency, curtsying, encopresis
6. Obtain a second urine for culture
   a. First A.M. urine or
   b. Catheterized urine sample (>10^3 pathogens/mL indicate urinary tract infection)
7. Obtain a 24-hour urine specimen for calcium
8. Treat for 3 days with an antibiotic for presumed urethritis

---

Table 23-6. Adolescent History and Physical Examination for Dysuria

Differential Diagnosis

Urinary tract infection (UTI)
Vaginitis caused by *Candida* species, herpes simplex, or nonspecific anaerobic overgrowth
Cervicitis caused by gonorrhea or chlamydia
Chemical irritation (e.g., from douches, bubble bath)

History

Blood pressure and temperature
New sexual partner in past month (suggests sexually transmitted diseases)
Hematuria (suggests UTI)
Use of a diaphragm with spermicide (predisposes to UTI)
Personal history of UTIs
Family history of vesicoureteral reflux (suggests UTI)

Physical Examination

Pelvic examination with wet preparation and cultures
Perianal examination for pinworms or group A streptococcal proctitis

Laboratory Studies

Urinalysis, both dipstick and microscopic
Vaginal wet preparation for trichomonas and clue cells
Cultures of urine and cervix (gonorrhea, chlamydia, herpes)

Table 23-7. Common Pitfalls in the Correct Diagnosis of Dysuria

Neonates

Assume that significant bacteriuria in a bagged urine specimen is a true UTI, and treat before a confirmatory culture is obtained

Fail to obtain a urine culture in a neonate older than 3 days and miss obstructive uropathy with a secondary infection

Toddlers and School-Aged Children

Trust a urine culture from a bagged urine specimen

Accept a laboratory report of "no significant growth" on urine, without knowing that the laboratory reports only $>5 \times 10^4$ CFU/mL as "significant"

Fail to label a urine as "catheterized specimen," so that the laboratory can plate 0.1 mL as well as 0.01 mL

Fail to obtain a cystogram after the first infection, trusting to see reflux on sonogram or intravenous pyelogram

Adolescents

Fail to ask about sexual history suggestive of vaginitis, such as a new sexual partner and condom or other birth control device use

Treat pyuria as a UTI in a sample contaminated with vaginal leukocytes

CFU, colony-forming unit; UTI, urinary tract infection.

ASYMPTOMATIC BACTERIURIA

It was once believed that asymptomatic bacteriuria could lead to silent renal damage and ultimate renal failure. The completion of several long-term prospective studies of school-aged girls with asymptomatic bacteriuria has put such fears to rest. The incidence of asymptomatic bacteriuria in females is about 1.5%. About 33% of girls with asymptomatic bacteriuria have VUR, and as many as 10% to 25% may have renal scarring. However, the long-term prognosis is excellent, even in patients with ongoing bacteriuria. Treatment with short courses of antibiotics may lead to more episodes of pyelonephritis in comparison with no treatment. It is strongly recommended that no prophylaxis be administered; treatment is indicated for symptomatic episodes.

For these reasons, it is best not to screen for asymptomatic bacteriuria. When the condition is found incidentally, the family should be counseled with regard to its favorable outcome. Radiologic studies are not indicated unless a symptomatic UTI subsequently develops. The physician may wish to repeat a urine culture in 3 to 6 months because most cases of asymptomatic bacteriuria clear spontaneously, and the family can be reassured.

Knowledge of asymptomatic bacteriuria may be beneficial when an affected woman becomes pregnant. During pregnancy, asymptomatic bacteriuria increases the risk of pyelonephritis, preterm labor, and the possibility of sepsis in the infant.

TREATMENT

CYSTITIS

Treatment of afebrile UTIs in children differs significantly from treatment in adults. This is because until radiologic evaluation has ruled out VUR and other abnormalities, it may be assumed that the child may have occult pyelonephritis and is at risk of renal scarring. Therefore, the first afebrile UTI should be treated with 10 days of antibiotics, followed by prophylaxis until radiologic studies are completed. Subsequent UTIs without fever can then be treated similarly to those in adults, with brief courses of 3 to 7 days of antibiotics. Single-dose therapy has a high failure rate. Culture and sensitivity testing are desirable but not mandatory in adolescents with cystitis, inasmuch as antibiotics are highly concentrated in the bladder urine. For adolescents and adults with recurrent UTIs, providing a 3-day supply of an antibiotic for episodes of dysuria that occur on weekends or while traveling is a good plan.

The choice of antibiotic depends on the rate of resistance of *E. coli* in any geographic area. Amoxicillin resistance rates exceed 40% worldwide, but trimethoprim-sulfamethoxazole resistance rates vary, being highest in the western United States (30%) and lowest in the eastern states (10%). For adults in the western states, a fluoroquinolone for 3 days is preferred. Alternative drugs are cefdinir and cefuroxime. Nitrofurantoin may be used for cystitis but not for pyelonephritis. Adolescents may be treated with fosfomycin for cystitis but it is not approved for those younger than 12 years of age. There is a guideline for treatment of adults by the Infectious Disease Society of America, which is updated every 2 years (http://www.idsociety.org).

PYELONEPHRITIS

Infants Younger than 3 Months

Because of the higher risk of bacteremia and renal scarring in infants younger than 3 months, management of pyelonephritis is best started on an inpatient basis. About 66% of bacteremic children with a UTI are younger than 3 months; these infants have higher rates of anatomic obstruction of the urinary tract. If the blood culture remains negative after 48 to 72 hours and the child is doing well, the child may complete therapy as an outpatient with an oral antibiotic.

Children Older than 3 Months

Oral therapy with a second- or third-generation cephalosporin to which *E. coli* is rarely resistant may be effective and safe in children older than 3 months. Resistance rates to amoxicillin and trimethoprim-sulfamethoxazole exceed 10%; neither drug should be used empirically to treat pyelonephritis. There may be a trend toward more renal scarring in infants receiving only oral antibiotics. About 83% of U.S. pediatricians treat pyelonephritis patients as outpatients, despite the fact that only 30% of U.S. nephrologists recommend doing so. Outpatient therapy is contraindicated if the child is unable to take oral antibiotics or appears septic or there is concern about the family's reliability. If there is any concern, the initial 24 hours of therapy should be administered intravenously.

Adolescent Girls and Women

Outpatient management is common in this group, again assuming that there is no contraindication such as toxic appearance or inability to take oral medication because of emesis. Ciprofloxacin is a good choice because of the low rate of antibiotic resistance.

FOLLOW-UP MONITORING AND PROPHYLAXIS AFTER A URINARY TRACT INFECTION

A follow-up urine culture (proof of cure) is not necessary if the patient is receiving an appropriate antibiotic, unless there is an underlying urologic condition or the response to therapy is poor. Periodic telephone or office follow-up is appropriate for any child who is receiving outpatient management for pyelonephritis.

If a child has had three or more afebrile UTIs in a year, or more than one febrile UTI, oral antimicrobial prophylaxis at bedtime for 6 months is a cost-effective method of preventing a new UTI. For sexually active adolescents, an alternative method is to recommend

Table 23-8. Prophylactic Antibiotics for Childhood Urinary Infections

	Dose	Timing	Side-Effects
Trimethoprim-sulfamethoxazole (TMP-SMX)	2 mg/kg of TMP component (up to 40 mg) (½ tablet)	Bedtime	Rash in 6%, Stevens-Johnson (rare)
Nitrofurantoin	1-2 mg/kg/day up to 100 mg	Bedtime	GI intolerance, pulmonary fibrosis (rare)
Trimethoprim	2 mg/kg up to 40 mg	Bedtime	Rash in 1%

GI, gastrointestinal.

one tablet of trimethoprim-sulfamethoxazole after each episode of sexual intercourse. Drugs appropriate for prophylaxis are shown in Table 23-8. It is not appropriate to use amoxicillin or cephalosporins for prophylaxis, because they alter bowel flora and may select resistant organisms. An exception is made for neonates (<1 month), in whom sulfonamides may displace bilirubin from albumin-binding sites and cause kernicterus. Low doses of the three drugs listed in Table 23-8 are concentrated in urine and vaginal secretions and reduce the relapse rate to fewer than 0.1 infections/patient/year. The use of trimethoprim-sulfamethoxazole for several years in children with VUR is highly effective in preventing UTI and allowing resolution of VUR without surgery.

Prophylactic strategies in sexually active adolescent girls and women include the use of low-dose antibiotics for 6 months to 5 years. It is also useful to recommend changing contraception to avoid spermicides and a diaphragm, to recommend voiding after intercourse, and to recommend increasing fluid intake. Unfortunately, data on cranberry juice as prophylaxis are limited. There are data showing that poor hygiene plays no role in causing UTIs.

RADIOLOGIC EVALUATION OF URINARY TRACT INFECTIONS

LONG-TERM OUTCOME OF CHILDHOOD URINARY TRACT INFECTIONS AND REFLUX

Figure 23-3 shows the probable mechanisms by which renal scarring (also called reflux nephropathy) develops. Figure 23-4 shows progressive renal scarring, as well as four grades of VUR. VUR is the major cause of renal scarring but not the only cause. Children born with renal dysplasia, which may be caused by in utero reflux, are clearly the group at highest risk of scarring. However, normal kidneys, even without VUR, may develop renal scarring. The factors that contribute to this are shown in Table 23-9. The main factor under the control of the primary care physician is prompt diagnosis and treatment of the UTI. The second controllable factor is identification of VUR with obstruction and appropriate referral to a specialist. Table 23-10 shows that the risk of renal scarring rises from 5% to

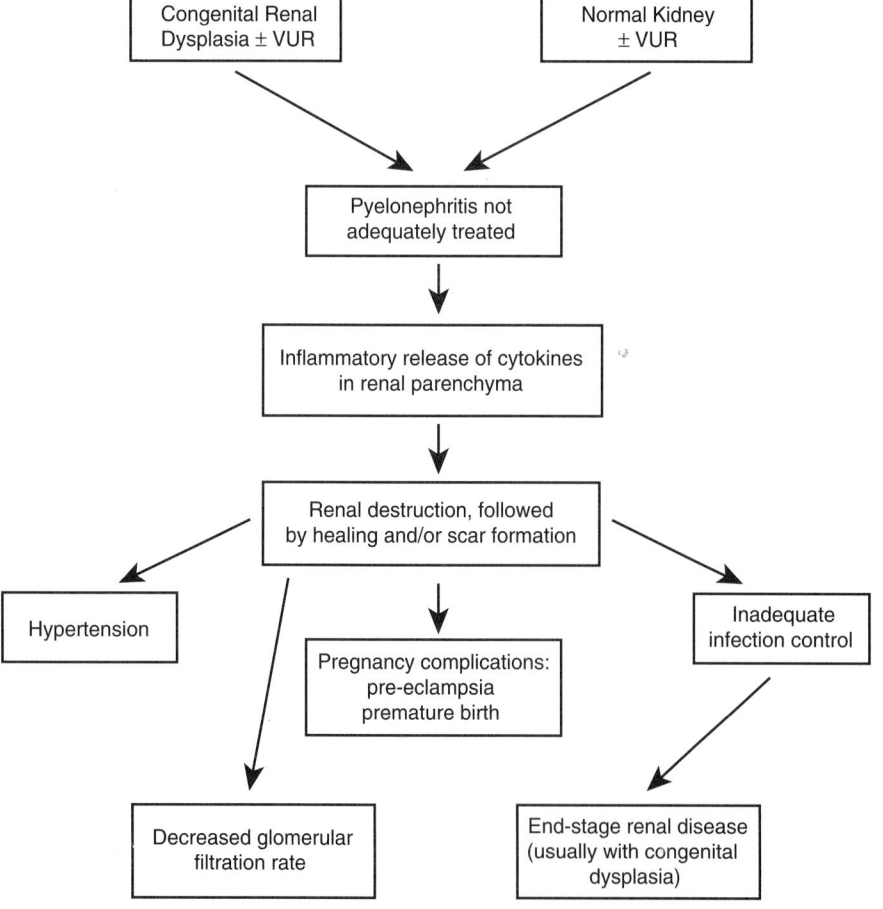

Figure 23-3. Renal scarring and the role of childhood urinary tract infection.

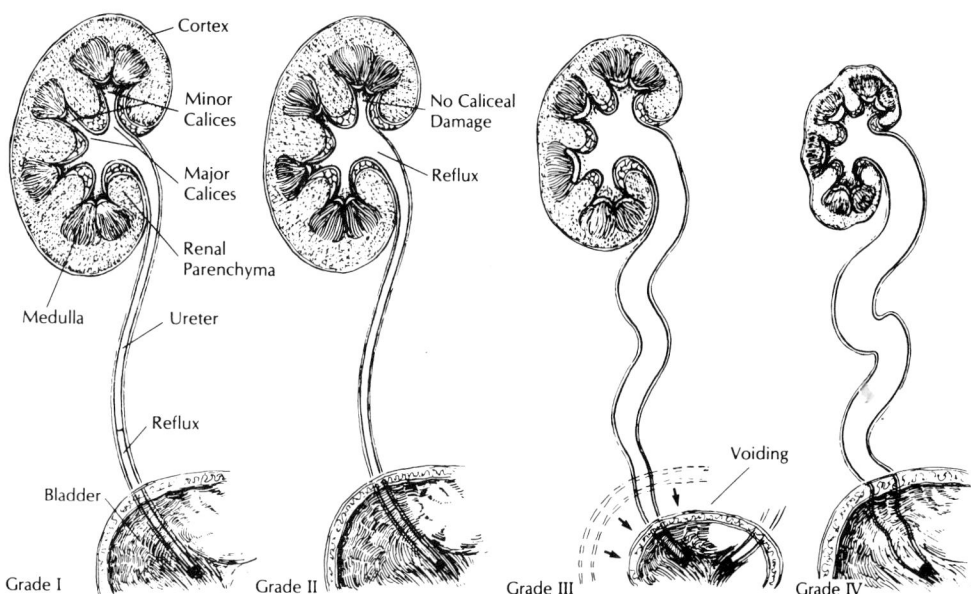

Figure 23-4. Renal scarring progression associated with vesicoureteral reflux (VUR) and grades of VUR from I to IV. (From Hodson CJ, Cotran RS: Reflux nephropathy. Hosp Pract 1982; 133-156. Copyright © Enid Hatton, with permission.)

66% with the grade of reflux; therefore, grading reflux helps predict the risk of scarring. The third way to prevent scarring is to use judicious prophylaxis in the boys with VUR who are younger than 2 years and the girls with VUR who are younger than 5 years. Table 23-11 shows that the risk of scarring increases from 9% after one pyelonephritis episode to 58% after more than four episodes. Prophylaxis should help prevent pyelonephritis, although this has never been proved in a randomized trial, because of ethical concerns.

The long-term consequences of recurrent pyelonephritis, shown in Figure 23-3, include hypertension, decreased glomerular filtration rate, complications of pregnancy such as preeclampsia, and end-stage renal disease (uncommon in developed countries) (Table 23-12). The 10- to 40-year follow-up of adults who as children had recurrent UTI shows 7% with sustained hypertension, 4% with labile hypertension, and 8% with abnormal plasma creatinine levels (see Table 23-12). In a prospective Swedish study by Martinell and colleagues, all patients had well-preserved renal function, but a similar Swedish study by Jacobson published 7 years earlier showed that 10% of patients had impaired renal function and 23% had sustained hypertension. It is speculated that because the index infections in the latter study occurred a decade earlier, the advances in diagnosis and treatment in Sweden may have improved the long-term outcome. Three factors

are correlated with progressive renal scarring: (1) grade of reflux, (2) number of episodes of pyelonephritis, and (3) young age at the time of the first UTI. Long-term low-dose prophylaxis is most important in young children; older children may be treated only with acute infections. Postcoital prophylaxis may also benefit women. In summary, long-term studies support early identification of children at risk of renal scarring and close medical management throughout childhood and pregnancy.

The practitioner should be aware that arguments against identifying VUR include the belief that virtually all renal scars are congenital, not acquired. If this were true, early identification would be without value. There is, however, a large body of evidence showing that scars are acquired. In one study, only 4 of the 51 women with scarred kidneys had evidence of possible congenital scarring. Nevertheless, it is possible that more boys than girls have congenital scarring and are therefore more likely to progress to end-stage renal disease than are girls.

ULTRASONOGRAPHY VERSUS INTRAVENOUS PYELOGRAPHY

Renal ultrasound studies are the least invasive method for studying the kidney and the most acceptable to parents and children. Ultrasonography evaluates the gross anatomy of the kidney and the collecting system for obstruction; its resolution for parenchymal

---

Table 23-9. Risk Factors for Permanent Renal Scarring in Children

Febrile UTI (pyelonephritis) compared with afebrile UTI
Age <12 months, but can occur at any age up to puberty; risk declines with age
Vesicoureteral reflux; higher grades have higher scarring rates: grade 1, 9%; grade 2, 15%; grade 3, 35%; grade 4 or 5, 58%
Dysfunctional voiding with high bladder pressures (Hinman syndrome; often associated with encopresis)
Delay in initiating antibiotic therapy (exact time is unknown)
Recurrent UTIs in a child with scarring
Congenital renal dysplasia

UTI, urinary tract infection.

Table 23-10. Renal Scarring in Relation to Grade of Vesicoureteral Reflux (VUR) in 444 Children with First-Time Acute Pyelonephritis

Grade of VUR	Children (*n*)	No. with Renal Scarring	% with Renal Scaring
No reflux	278	15	5
I	29	3	10
II	99	17	17
≥ III	38	25	66
Total	444	60	14

From Jodal U: The natural history of bacteriuria in childhood. Infect Dis Clin North Am 1987;1:713-729.

Table 23-11. Renal Scarring in Relation to the Number of Pyelonephritic Attacks in 664 Children

Attacks (*n*)	Children (*n*)	No. with Renal Scarring	% with Renal Scarring
0	141	7	5
1	366	32	9
2	98	15	15
3	35	12	35
≥ 4	24	14	58
Total	664	80	12

From Jodal U: The natural history of bacteriuria in childhood. Infect Dis Clin North Am 1987;1:713-729.

scarring is poor. It does not show acute density changes of pyelonephritis as well as does dimercaptosuccinic acid (DMSA) scanning, computed tomography, or gallium scanning. Its two advantages over DMSA scanning are that it shows the collecting system well and it demonstrates a nonfunctional pole of a duplex kidney. Intravenous pyelography, once the "gold standard" for renal scarring, is rarely used and has been replaced by DMSA scanning. It surpasses renal sonography in the detection of renal scars, and it demonstrates the width and path of the ureter.

DIMERCAPTOSUCCINIC ACID SCANS

Technetium 99m–labeled DMSA scintigraphy provides a renal image that is based on glomerular filtration and intrarenal blood flow. The isotope is given intravenously, and the child is then scanned about 90 to 120 minutes later. Image quality is very sensitive to motion artifacts, but sedation is usually not required unless more extensive computed tomography (single photon emission computed tomography) is performed. Interpretation of images may be difficult, with as low as 35% agreement between radiologists in some studies. Radiation to the gonads is low.

DMSA scans have two potential uses: first, to localize infection to the kidney and, second, to visualize permanent renal damage. Early imaging is recommended by some authorities to differentiate upper tract from lower tract UTI; one study found positive DMSA scans in only 42% of febrile children younger than 6 years. In this study, the scan was done at a median of 13 days after the onset of symptoms, and the authors show that the incidence of an abnormal scan declined from 60% on day 2 to 35% on day 14. Another significant finding was that an elevation of the C-reactive protein level was 95% sensitive for DMSA abnormalities. Because a C-reactive protein test costs less than 10% of a DMSA scan, it is not currently cost effective to perform an acute scan.

The need to perform a delayed DMSA scan to document renal scarring, as well as congenital damage, remains controversial. This scan should be obtained at least 6 months after acute UTI, to avoid

overdiagnosis of perfusion defects that will heal. This is a long time for parents to wait, and they should be continuing prophylaxis if DMSA scanning instead of cystography is performed. In a mobile society such as the United States, early cystography is probably preferable, with DMSA scans used only in patients with VUR.

Finally, the long-term prognosis for the small renal scars seen on DMSA but not on an intravenous pyelogram is not yet known. It is possible that the DMSA scan is too sensitive and that only the larger scars seen on intravenous pyelogram carry a high risk for renal damage. Until better long-term data are available, the decision on whether DMSA scanning or intravenous pyelography should be performed is best made in consultation with the child's urologist and the local radiologist.

VOIDING CYSTOGRAPHY

Renal ultrasonography, intravenous pyelography, and DMSA scanning may all miss significant degrees of VUR. Reflux is graded I through V (see Fig. 23-4) on standard contrast cystograms. Because standard cystography requires placement of a urinary catheter, many physicians and parents are reluctant to obtain this study after only one UTI. Several studies have reported that this study is seldom carried out until two or more UTIs occur or the child is hospitalized. To increase parental acceptance, *indirect radionuclide cystography* was developed. In this procedure, isotope is injected intravenously, and images are made after the child's bladder is filled. Unfortunately, this method may miss 61% of grade II VUR and even 12% of grade IV VUR.

Direct radionuclide cystography is very sensitive for VUR. This method requires urinary catheterization, but usually no sedation is needed. The radiation to the gonads is much less than with standard cystography, and the sensitivity for lower grades of VUR may surpass that of the standard study. It is difficult with this study to grade reflux except into low grade (II and III) and high grade (IV and V). The main drawback of direct radionuclide cystography is the poor resolution of the posterior urethra, which makes it unsuitable for the diagnosis of posterior urethral valves. Most clinicians prefer to use standard cystography for the first study after a UTI, even in girls, to allow accurate grading of VUR and to detect ureteroceles, ectopic ureters, and ureteral diverticula.

To avoid the problems associated with catheter placement, several approaches may be used. First, midazolam (Versed) sedation has been used in toddlers with excellent results. Second, a Child Life worker may prepare the child older than 3 years. The presence of a parent during the procedure is also reassuring to most children.

RECOMMENDATIONS FOR RADIOLOGIC EVALUATION

The 1999 Practice Parameters of the American Academy of Pediatrics could not agree on whether evidence supports a lower tract study in children younger than 2 years. The compromise was to "strongly encourage" a lower tract study but to acknowledge that the strength of evidence was only "fair."

Table 23-12. Long-Term Studies of the Consequences of Renal Scarring Associated with Childhood Urinary Tract Infection

Reference	No. of Patients	Follow-up Duration (yr)	Hypertension (%)	Impaired Renal Function*	Study Design
Jacobson et al, 1989	30 scarred	27	23	10	Retrospective
Smellie et al, 1994	52	1-12	8	8	Retrospective
Martinell et al, 1996	107 (54 scarred)	15	6	0	Prospective
Smellie et al, 1998	226 (85 scarred)	10-41	7	8	Retrospective
Wennerstrom et al, 2000	108 (57 scarred)	16-26	Not reported	7	Prospective

*Definition: glomerular filtration rate (GFR) < 30 for Jacobson et al and Smellie et al 1994, GFR < 80 for Wennerstrom et al. Abnormal plasma creatinine for Smellie et al, 1998.

Table 23-13. Radiologic Examinations for Childhood Urinary Tract Infection, in Order of Preference

	Advantages	Disadvantages
Upper Tract Studies		
Dimethylsuccinic acid–^{99m}Tc (DMSA) scan	Decreased gonadal radiation in comparison with IVP or cystography	Cost is higher than IVP or sonography
	Only method useful in defining acute kidney infection	IV route may be difficult or painful
	Much more sensitive for renal scarring than IVP or sonography	May not be available in all hospitals
Renal sonography	Readily available	Cannot detect small renal scars, but the technology improves every year
	Painless	
	Radiation free	Cannot document progression of renal scars over years
	Rapidly diagnoses renal obstruction	
IVP	Available at all hospitals and easily read	Requires a bowel preparation to see scars
	Inexpensive	Painful IV route
		Risk of allergic reactions
Lower Tract Studies for Vesicoureteral Reflux		
Contrast voiding cystogram	Defines the penile urethra, for posterior urethral valves	Up to 20 times more gonadal radiation than an isotopic study
	Readily available	
Isotopic voiding cystogram	Low gonadal radiation	Cannot grade reflux as I-V, only as mild, moderate, or severe
		May miss small ureteroceles or duplex kidneys
		Does not visualize the penile urethra

IV, intravenous; IVP, intravenous pyelography; ^{99m}Tc, technetium 99m.

The goal of evaluation is to identify children at risk for renal scarring, which can lead to future hypertension, pregnancy complications, and, in rare cases, end-stage renal disease. In the past, renal scarring was believed to occur only in children with VUR, but evidence with DMSA imaging has shown that scars develop in febrile UTIs without VUR, particularly those occurring in children with the risk factors shown in Table 23-9. The advantages and disadvantages of the various studies are outlined in Table 23-13. Local radiologic preferences should be determined before the examiner chooses how to evaluate a child.

Parents often ask the yield of treatable abnormalities found with an evaluation, because they wish to minimize the child's discomfort, radiation exposure, and expense incurred. Figures 23-5 and 23-6 show the results of a prospective study of 215 children younger than 13 years in a nonreferral primary care clinic in Cleveland, Ohio. Children younger than 5 years with a febrile UTI had a 33% risk of a treatable abnormality, consisting primarily of grade II, III, or IV VUR. In countries where prenatal ultrasonography is standard, obstructive lesions such as posterior urethral valves or ureteropelvic junction obstruction are usually diagnosed and treated before the child gets a UTI. In children younger than 5 years without fever, there was a 10% risk of a treatable problem. Because children in this age group are at high risk of scarring, most United States experts

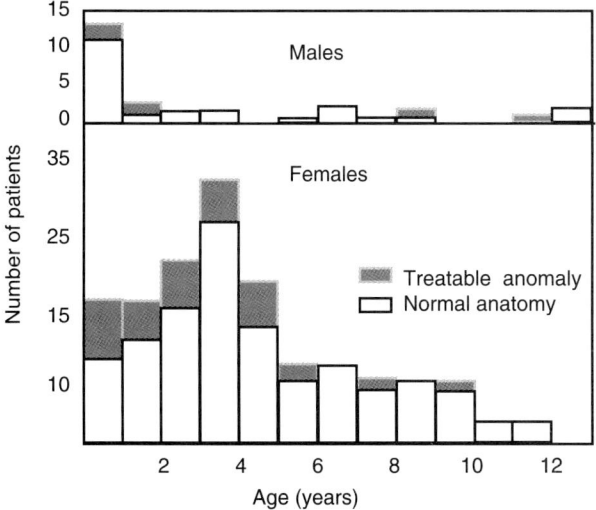

Figure 23-5. Incidence of treatable abnormalities in 215 children younger than 13 years of age with first-time urinary tract infection, classified by age and sex. (From Johnson CE: New advances in childhood urinary tract infections. Pediatr Rev 1999;20:335-342.)

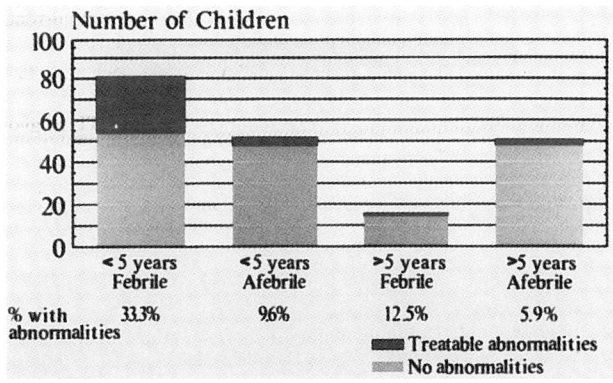

Figure 23-6. Incidence of treatable abnormalities found by radiologic evaluation 4 to 6 weeks after urinary tract infection in children 2 weeks to 13 years old, classified by age at evaluation and presence of fever of at least 38° C rectally or 37° C orally. (From Johnson CE: New advances in childhood urinary tract infections. Pediatr Rev 1999;20:335-342.)

believe they merit full radiologic evaluation. In children aged 5 to 13 years, the risk of treatable abnormalities is less than 10%, and it seems reasonable to obtain a sonogram but to defer cystography unless there is a second UTI or a history of voiding dysfunction. In Sweden, 97% of all children were evaluated with a renal sonogram and VCUG, and 36% of girls and 24% of boys were found to have VUR.

Figure 23-7 is an algorithm developed by expert consensus in the United States for evaluating the child with a UTI. An alternative algorithm, taken from a publication in 1999 by U. Jodal and U. Lindberg, is shown in Figure 23-8. This guideline was the consensus of the Swedish Medical Research Council. Many of the Council's principles are also incorporated into the first algorithm (see Fig. 23-7), especially with regard to DMSA renal scans.

Children are hospitalized for UTI treatment if they are younger than 3 months, appear extremely ill, are unable to take oral medication and fluids, or are likely to be noncompliant with the treatment regimen. If hospitalized, a renal sonogram is desirable in the first 24 to 48 hours to rule out obstruction. If the diagnosis in a febrile infant is in doubt, an acute DMSA scan is highly sensitive for pyelonephritis, if done in the first week. All hospitalized children merit a VCUG, which can be done during the hospitalization; there is no benefit in delaying the study. Because more than 30% of

children may fail to return for this study as outpatients, it is wise to obtain the study as early as day 3 or 4 of hospitalization. If the cystography is done on an outpatient basis, continuous prophylaxis must be given until the result is known. If VUR is found, prophylaxis should be continued and a DMSA renal scan scheduled 6 months after the UTI. A referral to a pediatric nephrologist or urologist is appropriate for children with renal scarring or with dilating reflux (grades III, IV, and V), and is optional for grades I and II reflux without scarring.

In outpatients, to minimize costs, a VCUG may be the first study, followed by sonography if no VUR is seen. If VUR is seen, a DMSA scan 6 to 12 months later reveals renal scarring. Alternatively, the evaluation of children older than 2 years with a febrile UTI may omit cystography and proceed to early sonography, and a DMSA scan may be obtained 6 to 12 months later. This approach is cost efficient, because children need only one upper tract study; however, there is a danger that children may become unavailable for follow-up before the DMSA scan is performed.

Figure 23-8 is the algorithm published in Sweden and differs in the following ways: (1) no evaluation for lower tract UTIs in children over 1 year of age, (2) sonography as the initial study in all children, and (3) cystography for all children younger than 2 years but only a DMSA scan for those older than 2 years. Swedish investigators have

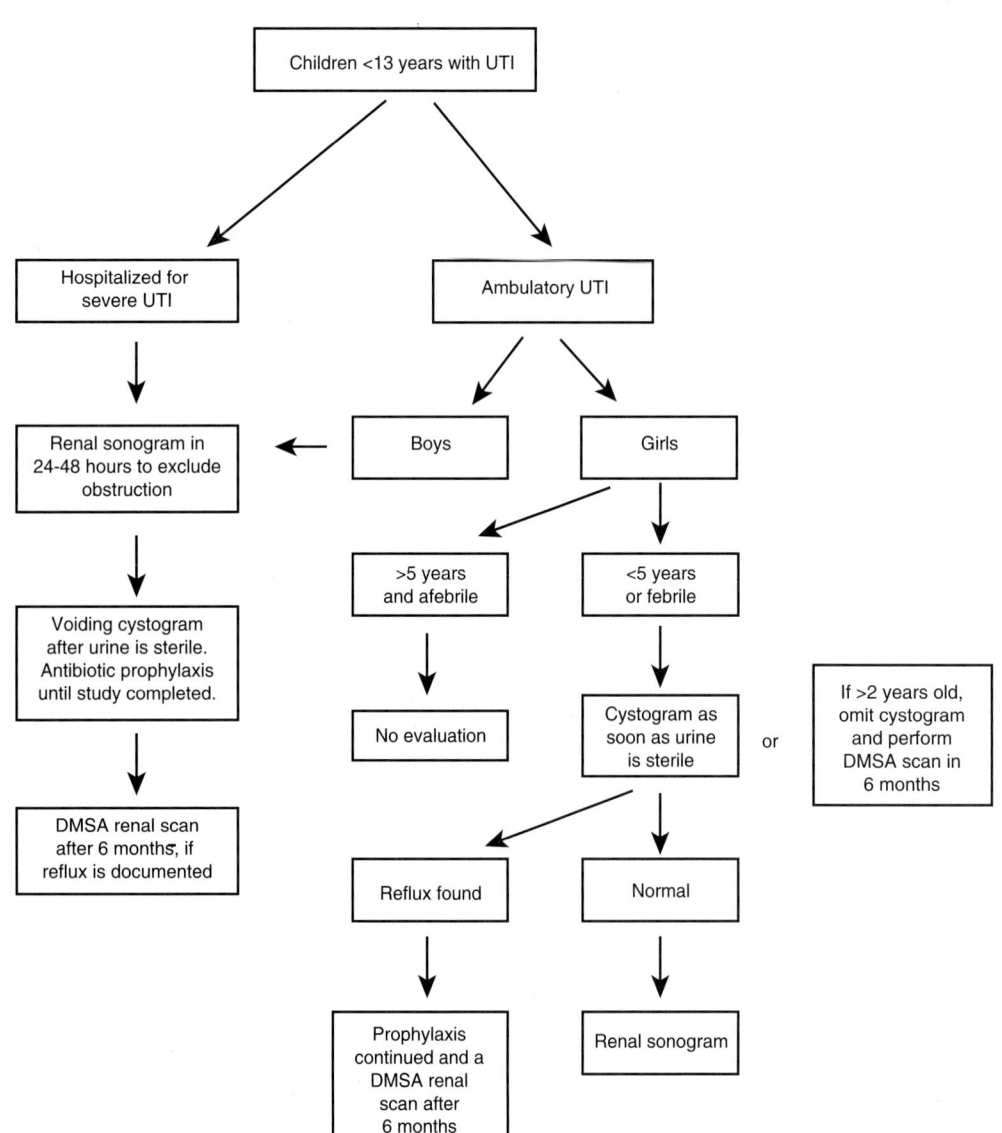

Figure 23-7. Radiologic evaluation of childhood urinary tract infection (UTI), based on U.S. practices. Scarring on sonogram or dimercaptosuccinic acid (DMSA) scan, or grade III, IV, or V reflux even without scarring are indications for referral to nephrology or urology specialists.

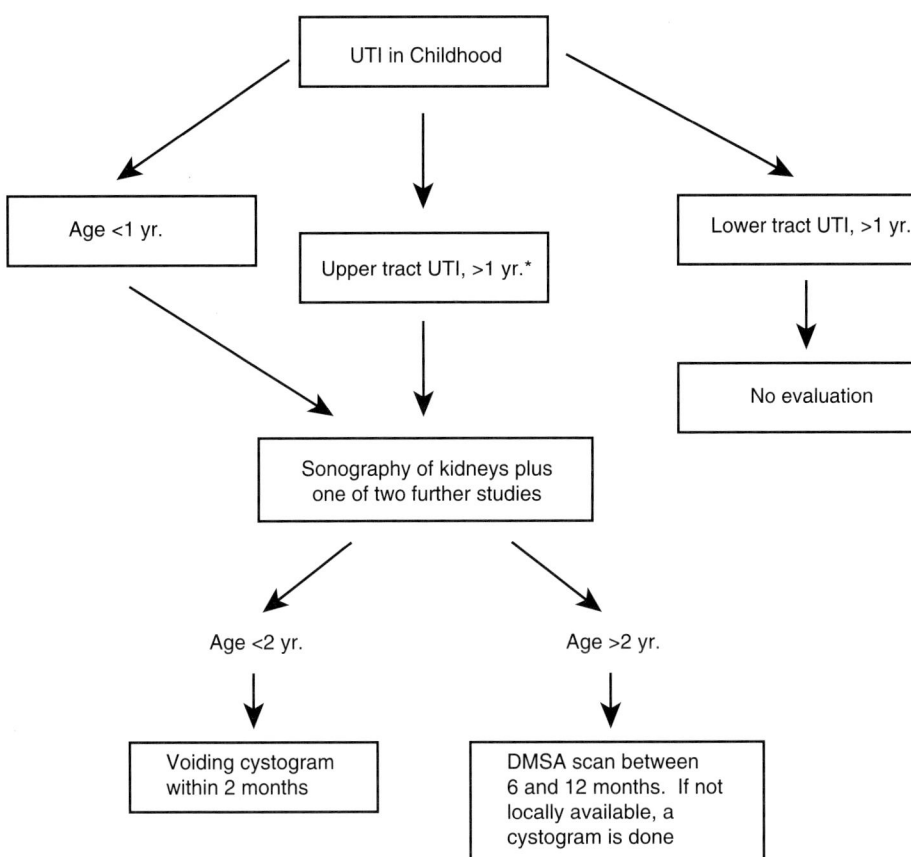

Figure 23-8. Recommendations for radiologic evaluation of childhood urinary tract infection (UTI) by Swedish Medical Research Council in 1999 (Jodal and Lindberg). DMSA, dimercaptosuccinic acid.

performed many studies on localization of UTIs to the kidney or bladder, and they have found the presence of fever with temperature higher than 38.5° C, back or loin pain, or a C-reactive protein level exceeding 20 mg/L to be very reliable in identifying upper tract infection. Many U.S. experts are skeptical and would prefer to use age as the major decision factor in whom to evaluate.

Finally, the issue of evaluation of adolescents must be addressed. There is general agreement that recurrent cystitis needs no evaluation unless stones are present or a *Proteus* species is isolated. Adolescents with pyelonephritis should undergo sonography and cystography after the second episode, if they fail to respond promptly, or if a history of multiple earlier UTIs before puberty is elicited.

MANAGEMENT OF VESICOURETERAL REFLUX

1. After identifying VUR, parents need education about risks and the importance of rapid treatment of UTIs.
2. All children with dilating reflux (grades III to V) or scarring need referral to a pediatric urologist or pediatric nephrologist. Those with grades I and II reflux may be referred as well, depending on the experience of the primary care practitioner.
3. The American Urological Association published guidelines on surgery for VUR in 1997. Immediate surgery is limited to those with bilateral grade V disease after 1 year of age, grade V unilateral disease after 6 years of age, and bilateral grades III and IV after 6 years of age.

4. If surgery is needed, the transabdominal route is standard for care, but endoscopic correction is available at some centers.
5. Children with breakthrough pyelonephritis, especially if taking prophylaxis, need referral for possible surgery.
6. Prophylaxis with low-dose bedtime antibiotics is recommended for grade III and higher VUR by the 1999 Swedish guidelines. They recommend discontinuing prophylaxis at 2 years in boys and 10 years in girls, regardless of the grade of VUR. Alternatively many U.S. nephrologists recommend prophylaxis to all with VUR until age 5 to 6 years and longer if UTIs continue to occur.
7. Blood pressure and urinary protein should be measured yearly. Children with significant scarring should have creatinine measurements.
8. Dysfunctional voiding needs to be corrected if present because it perpetuates VUR. Girls in particular seem to develop detrusor-sphincter dyscoordination (i.e., attempting to void with a closed sphincter). This may explain the peak in UTIs among girls at ages 3 to 4 years, which is often during toilet training. Most of these children have enuresis in the daytime, and some have encopresis or constipation. Referral to a pediatric urologist is indicated for all children with UTIs who have these symptoms. A noninvasive urine flow study and measurement of residual urine are performed. Treatment may involve oxybutynin (Ditropan), to reduce bladder spasms; antibiotic prophylaxis; and timed voiding.
9. Finally, pregnancy in adolescent girls or women with VUR needs monitoring by a high-risk obstetric team. This applies even if the woman has undergone reimplantation of her ureters. Pregnant women with VUR and scarring are candidates for antibiotic prophylaxis.

Table 23-14. Red Flags for Referral to a Pediatric Urologist or Nephrologist after a Urinary Tract Infection
Dilating VUR (grade III, IV, or V)
Renal scarring detected on sonography and IVP or a DMSA scan obtained >6 months after the UTI
Urinary obstruction seen on a sonogram or IVP
Voiding dysfunction (enuresis, frequency, "curtsy" to stop voiding)
Breakthrough UTI in the child with VUR receiving prophylaxis
Elevated serum creatinine level
Hypertension
Antenatal hydronephrosis that is confirmed after day 3 after birth

DMSA, dimercaptosuccinic acid; IVP, intravenous pyelography; UTI, urinary tract infection; VUR, vesicoureteral reflux.

SUMMARY

Dysuria in children who are prepubertal is usually a symptom of UTI. The differential diagnosis expands greatly in adolescents, in whom a sexually transmitted disease may be the cause. Because children younger than 2 years cannot verbalize complaints, the presence of a UTI is often overlooked. It is precisely these infants and toddlers who may suffer the most renal damage from a febrile UTI. Awareness by medical providers that both boys and girls have relatively high rates of UTI in the first year will help prevent renal damage.

The second step in preventing renal scarring is to evaluate children radiologically after the first febrile UTI. There remains considerable disagreement among experts on the most cost-effective and painless way to accomplish this. The key point is to obtain a VCUG and/or a DMSA renal scan on each child; a sonogram alone is an inadequate evaluation that does not rule out renal scarring or VUR.

Finally, close medical supervision of children with VUR and/or renal scarring is needed throughout childhood and pregnancy. The medical community finally agrees that surgical intervention is rarely necessary for VUR, but that puts more responsibility on the medical provider to monitor for infection, hypertension, and renal insufficiency.

Table 23-14 shows red flags for referral to a pediatric urologist or nephrologist.

REFERENCES

General Review Articles

American Academy of Pediatrics Subcommittee on Urinary Tract Infection: Practice Parameter: The diagnosis, treatment, and evaluation of the initial urinary tract infection in febrile infants and young children. Pediatrics 1999;103:843-852.

Hansson S, Bollgren I, Esbjorner E, et al: Urinary tract infections in children below two years of age: A quality assurance project in Sweden. Acta Paediatr 1999;88:270-274.

Hellerstein S: Urinary tract infections—Old and new concepts. Pediatr Clin North Am 1995;42:1433-1451.

Johnson CE: New advances in childhood urinary tract infections. Pediatr Rev 1999;20:335-342.

Kunin CM: Perspectives of a long-time observer. J Infect Dis 2001;183 (Suppl 1):S9-S11.

Rushton HG: Urinary tract infections in children—Epidemiology, evaluation, and management. Pediatr Clin North Am 1997;44:1133-1169.

Bladder Dysfunction

Austin PF, Ritchey ML: Dysfunctional voiding. Pediatr Rev 2000;21: 336-341.

Farhat W, McLorie G: Urethral syndromes in children. Pediatr Rev 2001; 22:17-20.

Sillen U: Bladder dysfunction in children with vesico-ureteric reflux. Acta Paediatr Suppl 1999;431:40-47.

Diagnosis of Urinary Tract Infection

Bachur R, Harper MB: Reliability of the urinalysis for predicting urinary tract infections in young febrile children. Arch Pediatr Adolesc Med 2001;155:60-65.

Lin D-S, Huang F-Y, Chiu N-C, et al: Comparison of hemocytometer leukocyte counts and standard urinalysis for predicting urinary tract infections in febrile infants. Pediatr Infect Dis J 2000;19:223-227.

Poole C: The use of urinary dipstix in children with high-risk renal tracts. Br J Nurs 1999;8:512-516.

Treatment of Urinary Tract Infection

Hoberman A, Wald ER, Hickey RW, et al: Oral versus initial intravenous therapy for urinary tract infections in young febrile children. Pediatrics 1999;104:79-86.

Honkinen O, Jahnukainen T, Mertsola J, et al: Bacteremic urinary tract infection in children. Pediatr Infect Dis J 2000;19:630-634.

Talan DA, Stamm WE, Hooton TM, et al: Comparison of ciprofloxacin (7 days) and trimethoprim-sulfamethoxazole (14 days) for acute uncomplicated pyelonephritis in women—A randomized trial. JAMA 2000;283:1583-1590.

Warren JW, Abrutyn E, Hebel JR, et al: Guidelines for antimicrobial treatment of uncomplicated acute bacterial cystitis and acute pyelonephritis in women. Clin Infect Dis 1999;29:745-758.

Prophylaxis of Urinary Tract Infections

Bollgren I: Antibacterial prophylaxis in children with urinary tract infection. Acta Paediatr Suppl 1999;431:48-52.

Circumcision

Christakis DA, Harvey E, Zerr DM, et al: A trade-off analysis of routine newborn circumcision. Pediatrics 2000;105:246-249.

Schoen EJ, Colby CJ, Ray GT: Newborn circumcision decreases incidence and costs of urinary tract infections during the first year of life. Pediatrics 2000;105:789-793.

Radiologic Evaluation and Sonograms

Barry BP, Hall N, Cornford E, et al: Improved ultrasound detection of renal scarring in children following urinary tract infection. Clin Radiol 1998; 53:747-751.

Craig JC, Knight JF, Sureshkumar P, et al: Vesicoureteric reflux and timing of micturating cystourethrography after urinary tract infection. Arch Dis Child 1997;76:275-277.

Sixt R, Stokland E: Assessment of infective urinary tract disorders. Q J Nucl Med 1998;42:119-125.

Dimercaptosuccinic Acid Scans

Smellie JM: Technetium-99m–dimercaptosuccinic acid studies and urinary tract infection in childhood. Acta Paediatr 1998;87:132-133.

Stokland E, Hellstrom M, Jacobsson B, et al: Evaluation of DMSA scintigraphy and urography in assessing both acute and permanent renal damage in children. Acta Radiol 1998;39:447-452.

Stokland E, Hellstrom M, Jakobsson B, Sixt R: Imaging of renal scarring. Acta Paediatr Suppl 1999;431:13-21.

Renal Scarring and Long-Term Outcomes

Bukowski TP, Betrus GG, Aquilina JW, Perlmutter AD: Urinary tract infections and pregnancy in women who underwent antireflux surgery in childhood. J Urol 1998;159:1286-1289.

Jacobson SH, Hansson S, Jakobsson B: Vesico-ureteric reflux: Occurrence and long-term risks. Acta Paediatr Suppl 1999;431:22-30.

Martinell J, Lidin-Janson G, Jagenburg R, et al: Girls prone to urinary infections followed into adulthood. Indices of renal disease. Pediatr Nephrol 1996;10:139-142.

Smellie JM, Prescod NP, Shaw PJ, et al: Childhood reflux and urinary infection: A follow-up of 10-41 years in 226 adults. Pediatr Nephrol 1998;12:727-736.

Wennerstrom M, Hansson S, Jodal U, et al: Renal function 16 to 26 years after the first urinary tract infection in childhood. Arch Pediatr Adolesc Med 2000;154:339-345.

Vesicoureteral Reflux Management

Decter RM: Vesicoureteral Reflux. Pediatr Rev 2001;22:205-209.

Elder JS, Peters CA, Arant BS, et al: Pediatric vesicoureteral reflux guidelines panel summary report on the management of primary vesicoureteral reflux in children. J Urol 1997;157:1846-1851.

Jodal U, Lindberg U: Guidelines for management of children with urinary tract infection and vesico-ureteric reflux. Recommendations from a Swedish state-of-the-art conference. Acta Paediatr Suppl 1999;431:87-89.

Smellie JM, Barratt TM, Chantler C, et al: Medical versus surgical treatment in children with severe bilateral vesicoureteric reflux and bilateral nephropathy: A randomised trial. Lancet 2001;357:1329-1333.

24 Proteinuria

Robert J. Cunningham III

An evaluation of the pediatric patient with proteinuria requires a consideration of age, gender, the presence of edema, the presence of hypertension, and a measure of renal function. In many cases, the diagnostic workup is brief; it is unusual for a pediatric patient to require a renal biopsy as part of the initial evaluation. Proteinuria may be an inconsequential finding or a manifestation of a more serious disease (Table 24-1).

The workup and differential diagnosis in a child with proteinuria depends on the presence or absence of *nephrotic syndrome*. The four defining features of nephrotic syndrome are proteinuria, hypoalbuminemia, edema (with or without ascites), and hyperlipidemia. Nephrotic syndrome may be a result of many primary etiologic factors, with varying renal pathologic processes and long-term consequences. Most cases of nephrotic syndrome in children are caused by *minimal change nephrotic syndrome,* defined as normal histologic features of the kidney according to light microscopy and immune stains. Proteinuria that causes edema is always clinically significant, although not all edema is secondary to proteinuria (Table 24-2). All children with nephrotic syndrome must be evaluated, and most require treatment. In contrast, the workup of *asymptomatic proteinuria,* often a benign condition, is done in a staged manner, and treatment is usually not necessary.

There are well-accepted definitions of proteinuria (Table 24-3). Children with nephrotic syndrome invariably have "nephrotic-range" proteinuria. In rare cases, a child with asymptomatic proteinuria has nephrotic-range proteinuria. If there is concomitant hypoalbuminemia and hyperlipidemia, the workup proceeds as if the child presented with nephrotic syndrome, despite the absence of edema. Even without hypoalbuminemia and hyperlipidemia, nephrotic-range proteinuria is less likely to be benign than is less marked asymptomatic proteinuria.

NEPHROTIC SYNDROME IN YOUNG CHILDREN

MINIMAL CHANGE DISEASE

Preschool-aged children constitute the age group in which minimal change nephrotic syndrome is most common. Patients often present with asymptomatic edema, which may manifest as swollen or puffy eyes on awakening in the morning; increasing abdominal girth (increased waist or belt size) from ascites; pedal or leg edema, which causes difficulty in putting on their regular-sized shoes, especially after being upright during the daytime; or swelling in other sites, such as the scrotum, penis, vulva, and scalp. Tense edema or ascites is occasionally painful.

The initial evaluation of a patient with proteinuria is presented in Table 24-4. Indications for a referral to a pediatric nephrologist are described in Table 24-5. If there is obvious edema with proteinuria, the diagnostic evaluation noted in Table 24-4 advances directly to the second phase and, if necessary, to the third phase. A biopsy may or may not be indicated, and it is usually avoided until the response to therapy is noted to be poor (Table 24-6).

Differential Diagnosis

The evaluation requires that the examiner consider the causes of nephrotic syndrome in early childhood. The data in Table 24-7 are from the International Study of Kidney Disease in Children (ISKDC); three diseases constitute 92% of all cases of nephrotic syndrome in children older than 1 year of age but younger than 17: minimal change disease (the most common); focal segmental sclerosis (also called focal glomerular sclerosis), seen in 8.5%; and membranoproliferative glomerulonephritis (MPGN) (7.5%).

The features of these three common disorders producing nephrotic syndrome are noted in Table 24-8, and they are compared with membranous nephropathy, a common cause of nephrosis in young adults. Nephrotic syndrome in membranous disease may be primary or secondary to other diseases (e.g., hepatitis or systemic lupus erythematosus [SLE]) or toxins and drugs such as gold, mercury, bismuth, silver, D-penicillamine, trimethadione, probenecid, and captopril.

Systemic diseases also cause childhood nephrotic syndrome but account for 10% of cases. The three foremost considerations include SLE, anaphylactoid purpura (Henoch-Schönlein purpura), and hemolytic-uremic syndrome.

These diseases have extrarenal manifestations in addition to the proteinuria and must be considered in any child who presents with systemic illness and significant proteinuria.

Minimal change nephrotic syndrome is slightly more common in boys than in girls. The hallmark of this disease is total clearing of the proteinuria with a 1-month course of daily oral prednisone therapy. A common misconception is that neither hematuria nor hypertension is present in children with minimal change disease. As demonstrated in Table 24-8, hematuria and hypertension are present in up to 20% of children who have minimal change disease. The blood urea nitrogen (BUN) or serum creatinine level may also be elevated in up to 30% of the cases, although an elevation of creatinine above 1 to 1.5 mg/dL is rarely seen. Serum complement studies, specifically C3, are invariably normal. Older age, hematuria, hypertension, and azotemia may occur with minimal change nephrotic syndrome, but the combination suggests another disease.

Diagnosis

Studies that would help confirm that a patient with nephrotic syndrome has minimal change disease include urinalysis, serum C3 level, serum cholesterol determination, serum albumin level, BUN level, and serum creatinine level.

The urinalysis would be expected to show 3+ to 4+ protein, which is correlated with a urine concentration of 300 to 2000 mg/dL. The urine may also yield positive results for hemoglobin. Microscopic examination of the urine sediment often shows oval fat bodies and/or refractile granular casts, which are seen when there is significant lipiduria. Red blood cells might also be present, but it is unusual to see red blood cell casts. Their presence would suggest a diagnosis of poststreptococcal glomerulonephritis or other causes of nephritis (see Chapter 25).

Table 24-1. Classification of Proteinuria

Nonpathologic Proteinuria
Postural (orthostatic)
Febrile
Exercise

Pathologic Proteinuria
Tubular
Hereditary
  Cystinosis
  Wilson disease
  Lowe syndrome
  Proximal renal tubular acidosis
  Galactosemia
Acquired
  Analgesic abuse
  Vitamin D intoxication
  Hypokalemia
  Antibiotics
  Interstitial nephritis
  Acute tubular necrosis
  Sarcoidosis
  Cystic diseases
  Homograft rejection
  Penicillamine
  Heavy metal poisoning (mercury, gold, lead, bismuth, cadmium, chromium, copper)
Glomerular
Persistent asymptomatic
Nephrotic syndrome
  Idiopathic
    Minimal change
    Mesangial proliferation
    Focal segmental glomerulosclerosis
    Membranous
    Membranoproliferative
    Immunoglobulin A (IgA)
  Secondary
    Glomerulonephritis
    Alport syndrome
    Collagen-vascular disease
    Henoch-Schönlein purpura
    Cancer
    Congenital

Adapted from Behrman RE (ed): Nelson Textbook of Pediatrics, 16th ed. Philadelphia, WB Saunders, 2000, p 1591.

The C3 complement level is normal in minimal change disease and is depressed in poststreptococcal glomerulonephritis and some other causes of nephritis (see Chapter 25). If hematuria is not present by microscopic examination or dipstick, postinfectious glomerulonephritis is unlikely, and C3 determinations are unnecessary.

The serum cholesterol values are elevated in minimal change nephrotic syndrome and are usually higher than 250 mg/dL; levels in the range of 500 to 600 mg/dL may occur. The serum albumin concentration is invariably less than 2.5 and often less than 2.0 g/dL. Studies that are not of help include complete blood cell counts and a 24-hour urinary protein determination. A renal biopsy is not immediately indicated because most patients (>90%) with minimal change disease respond to prednisone, a response that is considered diagnostic.

Treatment

With a presumptive diagnosis of minimal change nephrotic syndrome, it is recommended that patients be placed on a therapeutic

Table 24-2. Causes of Edema

Kidney Diseases
Acute glomerulonephritis
Nephrotic syndrome
Acute renal failure
Chronic renal failure

Heart Failure
Liver Failure
Nutritional and Gastrointestinal Disorders
Protein-calorie malnutrition
Protein-losing enteropathy
Nutritional edema (especially on refeeding)

Endocrine Disorders
Hypothyroidism
Mineralocorticoid excess

Miscellaneous
Hydrops fetalis
Venocaval obstruction
Capillary leak syndrome (systemic inflammatory response syndrome)
Turner syndrome (lymphedema)
Allergic reaction (periorbital edema)

course of prednisone, 2 mg/kg/day for 4 weeks, followed by a dose of 1.5 mg/kg given every other morning for another 4 weeks. In most patients, there is total resolution of proteinuria within 10 to 21 days of initiating therapy. Patients who do not respond to prednisone therapy should be considered candidates for a renal biopsy (see Table 24-6). There are no data to suggest that more prednisone therapy increases the response rate. A longer duration of prednisone treatment increases the side effects without concomitant benefit. Therefore, if there is no response, prednisone should be discontinued after the 2-month course and a renal biopsy performed to guide further therapy.

Total clearing of proteinuria in response to prednisone is an excellent prognostic sign. Very few patients progress to renal failure, although many patients who initially respond to prednisone therapy

Table 24-3. Definition of Significant Proteinuria

Qualitative
1+ (30 mg/dL) on dipstick examination of two of three random urine specimens collected 1 week apart if urine specific gravity < 1.015
or
2+ (100 mg/dL) on similarly collected urine specimens if urine specific gravity > 1.015

Semiquantitative
Urine protein-to-creatinine ratio (mg/dL:mg/dL) of > 0.2 on an early morning urine specimen

Quantitative
Normal: <100 mg/m^2/day in a timed 12- to 24-hour urine collection
Abnormal: 100-1000 mg/m^2/day in a timed 12- to 24-hour urine collection
Nephrotic range: >1000 mg/m^2/day in a timed 12- to 24-hour urine collection

Modified from Norman ME: An office approach to hematuria and proteinuria. Pediatr Clin North Am 1987;34:545-561.

Table 24-4. Workup of a Child with Proteinuria

Pediatrician's Workup: Phase I

Early morning urinalysis to include examination of the
sediment
Ambulatory and recumbent urinalyses for dipstick protein
testing

Pediatrician's Workup: Phase II

Blood electrolytes, BUN, creatinine, serum proteins,
cholesterol
ASLO titer, C_3 complement, ANA
Timed 12-hour urine collections, recumbent and ambulatory
Renal ultrasonography, IVP, voiding cystourethrography

Pediatric Nephrologist's Workup: Phase III

Renal biopsy
Management of established renal disease

Modified from Norman ME: An office approach to hematuria and proteinuria. Pediatr
Clin North Am 1987;34:545-562.

ANA, antinuclear antibody; ASLO, antistreptolysin O; BUN, blood urea nitrogen; IVP,
intravenous pyelography.

Table 24-6. When to Consider Renal Biopsy in a Child
with Proteinuria

Strong family history of chronic nephritis or unexplained
renal failure
Unexplained failure to thrive
Coexistent hypertension and nephrotic syndrome, or evidence
of a systemic inflammatory process
Coexistent significant hematuria (≥10 erythrocytes/hpf) with
or without erythrocyte casts in the spun sediment
Nephrotic-range proteinuria with poor response to prednisone
Renal glomerular insufficiency
Biochemical evidence of renal tubular dysfunction
(e.g., renal tubular acidosis, Fanconi syndrome)

Modified from Norman ME: An office approach to hematuria and proteinuria. Pediatr
Clin North Am 1987;34:545-561.

hpf, high-power field.

with total clearing of proteinuria may have relapses and require
intermittent prednisone therapy for many years. Approximately 18%
of patients treated with prednisone for minimal change nephrotic
syndrome respond to therapy and never experience a relapse.

Patients with recurrent nephrotic syndrome are subgrouped into
those who experience *frequent* and *infrequent* relapses. A patient
with infrequent relapse has fewer than two relapses in any 6-month
period; a person with frequent relapse has two or more relapses
within 6 months. Prednisone should be reinitiated at a dose of
2 mg/kg/day and continued until the urine test results are negative for
protein for 4 consecutive days. After that, alternate-day prednisone is
given at a dose of 1.5 mg/kg in the morning for another 2 weeks and
then discontinued altogether. Relapses are frequent during the
influenza virus seasons; any minor upper respiratory infection may
trigger a relapse of nephrotic syndrome. Patients who suffer infrequent
relapses may be treated with prednisone alone. If there are three
relapses a year and clearing of proteinuria in 10 to 12 days after
beginning prednisone therapy, a patient would receive approximately
45 days of daily prednisone in a 1-year interval. The patient would
also receive 8 weeks of prednisone administered on an alternate-
morning schedule. Most patients have few long-term side effects
when given this amount of prednisone.

Patients with frequently relapsing nephrotic syndrome respond
with total clearing of proteinuria after daily prednisone therapy but
experience relapse more frequently than four times a year and may

require constant daily prednisone therapy to maintain a remission.
Because constant daily prednisone has significant untoward side
effects (growth failure, cushingoid facies, osteoporosis, cataracts,
opportunistic infections, hypertension, and glucose intolerance),
other therapies need to be considered.

Four strategies are employed in the treatment of patients with
frequent-relapse but steroid-responsive minimal change nephrotic
syndrome: alternate-day prednisone, cyclophosphamide (Cytoxan),
chlorambucil, and cyclosporine.

Prednisone

On occasion, it is possible to maintain the patient in remission on a
low dose of alternate-day prednisone therapy. This is well tolerated
with minimal toxicity and is the first method employed in an attempt
to maintain the patient in remission and avoid the long-term side
effects of daily steroids. In many cases, however, patients relapse
while receiving alternate-day prednisone therapy, and other therapies
need to be considered.

Cyclophosphamide and Chlorambucil

Cyclophosphamide and chlorambucil are given on a daily basis for
approximately 8 weeks. After the use of either agent, patients have a
70% chance of long-term remission (2½ to 3 years in duration).
Patients require no prednisone therapy. Unfortunately, after this

Table 24-5. When to Refer the Child with Proteinuria
to a Nephrologist

Persistent nonorthostatic proteinuria
A family history of glomerulonephritis, chronic renal failure,
or kidney transplantation
Systemic complaints such as fever, arthritis or arthralgias,
and rash
Hypertension, edema, cutaneous vasculitis, or purpura
Coexistent hematuria with or without cellular casts in the
spun sediment
Elevated blood urea nitrogen (BUN) and creatinine levels or
unexplained electrolyte abnormalities
Increased parental anxiety

Modified from Norman ME: An office approach to hematuria and proteinuria. Pediatr
Clin North Am 1987;34:545-561.

Table 24-7. Distribution of Unselected Patients with
Nephrotic Syndrome

Histology	No. of Patients	(%)
Minimal change disease	398	(76.5)
Focal segmental sclerosis	44	(8.5)
Membranoproliferative glomerulonephritis (MPGN)	39	(7.5)
Mesangial proliferation	12	(2.3)
Proliferative glomerulonephritis	12	(2.3)
Membranous nephropathy	8	(1.5)
Chronic glomerulonephritis	3	(0.6)
Unclassified	4	(0.8)
Total	520	100

Adapted from a report of the International Study of Kidney Disease in Children.

Table 24-8. Summary of Primary Renal Diseases that Manifest as Idiopathic Nephrotic Syndrome

| | Minimal Change Nephrotic Syndrome (MCNS) | Focal Segmental Sclerosis | Membranoproliferative Glomerulonephritis (MPGN) | | Membranous Nephropathy |
			Type I	Type II	
Frequency*					
Children	75%	10%	10%	10%	<5%
Adults	15%	15%	10%	10%	50%
Clinical Manifestations					
Age (yr)	2-6, some adults	2-10, some adults	5-15	5-15	40-50
Sex	2:1 male	1.3:1 male	Male-female	Male-female	2:1 male
Nephrotic syndrome	100%	90%	60%	60%	80%
Asymptomatic proteinuria	0	10%	40%	40%	20%
Hematuria	10%-20%	60%-80%	80%	80%	60%
Hypertension	10%	20% early	35%	35%	Infrequent
Rate of progression to renal failure	Does not progress	10 yr	10-20 yr	5-15 yr	50% in 10-20 yr
Associated conditions	Allergy? Hodgkin disease, usually none	None	None	Partial lipodystrophy	Renal vein thrombosis, cancer, SLE, hepatitis B virus
Laboratory Findings	Manifestations of nephrotic syndrome ↑ BUN in 15%-30%	Manifestations of nephrotic syndrome ↑ BUN in 20%-40%	Low C1, C4, C3-C9	Normal C1, C4; low C3-C9	Manifestations of nephrotic syndrome
Immunogenetics	HLA-B8, -B12 (3.5)[†]	Not established	Not established	C3 nephritic factor Not established	HLA-DRW3 (12-32)[†]
Renal Pathology					
Light microscopy	Normal	Focal sclerotic lesions	Thickened GBM, proliferation, lobulation		Thickened GBM, spikes
Immunofluorescence	Negative	IgM, C3 in lesions	Granular IgG, C3	C3 only	Fine granular IgG, C3
Electron microscopy	Foot process fusion	Foot process fusion	Mesangial and subendothelial deposits	Dense deposits	Subepithelial deposits
Response to Steroids	90%	15%-20%	Not established	Not established	May be slow progression

Modified from Couser WG: Glomerular disorders. In Wyangaarden JB, Smith LH, Bennett JC (eds): Cecil Textbook of Medicine, 19th ed. Philadelphia, WB Saunders, 1992, p 560.

*Approximate frequency as a cause of idiopathic nephrotic syndrome. About 10% of cases of adult nephrotic syndrome are caused by various diseases that usually manifest with acute glomerulonephritis.

†Relative risk.

BUN, blood urea nitrogen; C, complement; GBM, glomerular basement membrane; HLA, human leukocyte antigen; Ig, immunoglobulin; SLE, systemic lupus erythematosus; ↑, elevated.

time, relapses often recur, and further courses of prednisone therapy are required.

Toxic effects of the two drugs differ; the choice of agent is determined by the toxicity profile. Both are equally efficacious in generating long-term remission, and the relapse rates are similar.

Cyclophosphamide. The major toxic effects of cyclophosphamide include hair loss, hemorrhagic cystitis, leukopenia, sterility (particularly in men), and possible predisposition to future neoplasia.

Hair Loss. Hair loss is the side effect that most often disturbs the patient. It is short-lived, and hair growth returns to normal.

Cystitis. Hemorrhagic cystitis is more dangerous and can be difficult to control. It is not the drug itself but rather a hepatic metabolite that is toxic to bladder epithelial cells. The resulting irritation may in rare cases necessitate surgical intervention to control the bleeding. Considering the risk of hemorrhagic cystitis, it is recommended that patients increase their fluid intake by an additional 500 to 1000 mL each day. This medication should be given in the morning. If a patient forgets to take a morning dose, the medication should not be taken in the evening. The rationale is that after ingestion, the drug is metabolized by the liver and excreted by the kidney. A dose given in the evening may cause the metabolites to remain in contact with the bladder epithelium overnight, which may increase the risk of mucosal bleeding.

Leukopenia. Leukopenia is unusual at the recommended doses; nonetheless, white blood cell counts need to be checked every 2 weeks while patients are receiving the drug.

Sterility. Sterility can be a side effect of cyclophosphamide therapy. Postpubertal men taking the drug at 2 mg/kg/day have very low sperm counts. Studies of long-term toxicity of cyclophosphamide therapy have shown that 5 years after completion of the therapeutic course, 20% of men still demonstrate abnormally low sperm counts. Ten years after completion of therapy, 10% still have abnormally low sperm counts, but this percentage approaches that of the normal male population who has not received any chemotherapy. The question as to the effect of cyclophosphamide therapy on the prepubertal testes has not been studied thoroughly; however, cyclophosphamide has been used for the treatment of nephrotic syndrome since 1960, and there are multiple reports of patients who have normal fertility and who have fathered children many years after a cyclophosphamide course. Although this remains a concern that must be discussed with parents, it appears to be more of a theoretical risk than a documented one.

Risk of Neoplasia. The risk of neoplasia must be discussed with parents because it has been shown that low-dose cyclophosphamide therapy given to experimental animals increases the incidence of neoplasia. However, cancer has not been reported in any patient treated with a course of cyclophosphamide therapy for nephrotic syndrome.

Chlorambucil. The efficacy of chlorambucil parallels that of cyclophosphamide, but the toxic effects differ. There is no evidence that chlorambucil causes hair loss, but leukopenia is a prominent problem. The white blood cell counts need to be checked every 2 weeks while patients are taking the drug, and the drug should be discontinued if the absolute neutrophil count falls below 1000/mm³. Hemorrhagic cystitis does not occur with chlorambucil. The risk of sterility appears to be similar to that of cyclophosphamide, although studies have not been as detailed and the follow-up for patients treated with chlorambucil has not been as long as for those treated with cyclophosphamide.

The one major concern has been reports of lymphoma after chlorambucil treatment of nephrotic syndrome in childhood. Most of the affected children were treated in France, and the doses of chlorambucil were higher than those given today. Patients who developed lymphoma had received a total dose of chlorambucil of greater than 14 mg/kg. Current guidelines would keep the total chlorambucil dose between 8 and 10 mg/kg. Cancer has not been reported when this drug is given in accordance with these recommendations.

Cyclosporine

Cyclosporine is an immunosuppressive agent developed to prevent solid organ transplant rejection; patients with nephrotic syndrome who respond to prednisone therapy also respond to cyclosporine. For the patient who has frequent relapses of nephrotic syndrome and who has significant steroid toxicity, cyclosporine offers another choice of therapy. Patients require treatment with 5 to 7 mg/kg/day given in divided doses on a 12-hour schedule.

Many children tolerate cyclosporine therapy for years with minimal toxicity. The major side effects of cyclosporine are nephrotoxicity, hypertension, hirsutism, and tremor. Therefore, the blood pressure and renal function (creatinine, BUN) need to be monitored.

Complications of Nephrotic Syndrome

Even in patients with the frequent-relapse variant of minimal change disease, the incidence of renal failure is only 1%. The reported mortality rate remains higher, at approximately 5%.

Infection

The major cause of death in nephrotic syndrome is overwhelming infection, usually secondary to spontaneous bacterial peritonitis, which develops in as many as 10% of patients with nephrotic syndrome at some point in the course of illness. Such infection is most frequent in patients who are edematous with significant ascites. Peritoneal fluid interferes with macrophage function, whereas ascitic fluid may dilute local complement or immunoglobulin levels, altering host defense mechanisms in the peritoneum.

The most common pathogen is *Streptococcus pneumoniae*. *Escherichia coli* and *Staphylococcus aureus* are other etiologic agents that may cause spontaneous peritonitis in patients with minimal change disease. Before 1940, the rate of mortality from nephrotic syndrome was approximately 60%. With the use of antibiotics, mortality dropped rapidly to 10% to 15% because penicillin offered an effective treatment for peritonitis. Infections remain the major cause of mortality, and any child with nephrotic syndrome in relapse with evidence of ascites needs to be evaluated quickly if either abdominal pain or fever develops. A blood specimen and paracentesis (Gram stain, culture, neutrophil count, measurement of glucose and protein level) should be obtained and the patient started on intravenous cefotaxime (or ceftriaxone) and an aminoglycoside without further delay.

Thrombosis

A second serious complication of nephrotic syndrome is spontaneous thrombosis, pulmonary embolus, or both. The blood of patients with nephrotic syndrome is hypercoagulable, and there is an increased incidence of thrombotic phenomena in these children. Children have lost parts of their lower limbs because of arterial thrombosis, and a number of deaths in children with nephrotic syndrome have resulted from pulmonary emboli. The renal vein is another possible site of thrombosis. Use of streptokinase or urokinase has allowed for more effective treatment of thrombotic complications.

Hyperlipidemia

Hyperlipidemia is treated by some authorities with statins to lower the serum cholesterol levels and possibly reduce vascular pathologic processes.

OTHER FORMS OF NEPHROTIC SYNDROME

FOCAL SEGMENTAL SCLEROSIS

Diagnosis

Inspection of the clinical criteria outlined in Table 24-8 does not always allow clinicians to differentiate minimal change disease from focal segmental sclerosis before completion of a course of prednisone therapy. Inability to clear proteinuria completely during prednisone therapy may be the first indication of focal segmental sclerosis. Patients who respond to prednisone initially with clearing of proteinuria but do not respond to a subsequent course of steroids should also be considered to have focal segmental sclerosis. Such patients represent about 7% of those who have an initial response to prednisone therapy. A patient who does not respond to prednisone with total clearing of proteinuria should undergo renal biopsy. Focal segmental sclerosis may be primary or secondary to reflux nephropathy, sickle cell nephropathy, reduced renal mass (single kidney), opiate or analgesic abuse, chronic bacteremia (endocarditis), renal transplant rejection, or nephropathy resulting from human immunodeficiency virus infection.

Treatment of Focal Segmental Sclerosis

Results of treatment of focal segmental sclerosis have usually been uniformly poor. Patients have severe and unremitting proteinuria despite treatment with prednisone, chlorambucil, or cyclophosphamide. None of these agents is warranted for treatment of a child once the diagnosis of focal segmental sclerosis is established. The long-term outcome has been poor; 33% are in renal failure approximately 10 years after diagnosis, and nearly 100% are in renal failure 20 years after diagnosis. There is an alarming trend in that the incidence of focal segmental sclerosis appears to be increasing, particularly in the African American population.

Patients with focal segmental sclerosis present two difficult problems. First, renal function may be maintained reasonably well for years, but massive proteinuria persists. Hence, patients are often edematous for months or years, and stigmata of protein malnutrition may develop as a result of large protein losses. Symptomatic therapy with a low-sodium diet and judicious use of diuretics is sometimes effective. Dietary manipulation of protein intake is ineffective; increasing dietary protein intake is accompanied by a concomitant increase in urinary protein excretion. There is no evidence that protein restriction either modifies serum proteins or prevents progression to renal insufficiency.

The second problem occurs when affected patients progress to end-stage renal failure. Recurrence of the disease in transplanted kidneys occurs in 25% to 30% of recipients. Therefore, many patients undergo a long period of dialysis before receiving a kidney transplant in an effort to diminish the frequency of recurrent disease.

Some patients respond to cyclosporine with total clearing of their proteinuria. There may be no progression to renal insufficiency. It is unknown what percentage of patients with focal segmental sclerosis respond to cyclosporine; it is estimated that between 25% and 60% initially respond.

MEMBRANOPROLIFERATIVE GLOMERULONEPHRITIS

Major diagnostic considerations in patients with hypertension, hematuria, older age, and mild to moderate edema should be MPGN and SLE (see Table 24-8). Both diseases are more common in girls and occur during adolescence. There may be proteinuria or nephrotic syndrome accompanying hematuria. In both diseases, cholesterol levels may be normal or minimally elevated in the presence of proteinuria and hypoproteinemia; serum C3 is often reduced. SLE is diagnosed by the presence of anti-DNA antibodies (particularly anti–double-stranded DNA). MPGN is a renal disease without multisystem involvement, whereas SLE affects other organ systems (skin, joints, mucous membranes, bone marrow, serous surfaces, heart, lungs, and brain).

It is important to identify patients with possible MPGN because daily prednisone therapy is contraindicated for these individuals; in a number of cases, malignant hypertension has developed after its use. Therefore, if MPGN is suspected, a renal biopsy is indicated before therapy is initiated.

The preadolescent patient is a more likely candidate for renal biopsy than preschool-aged children. Although 80% of the patients with minimal change disease are younger than age 6, MPGN and focal segmental sclerosis increase in frequency with aging. At age 6 years, only 6% of the renal biopsies show lesions other than minimal change disease. At age 10 years, the probability of other lesions increases to 28%.

The treatment of MPGN includes low-dose, alternate-day prednisone; the antiplatelet agents dipyridamole (Persantine) and aspirin; and angiotensin-converting enzyme (ACE) inhibitors, which may reduce glomerular hyperfiltration and thus improve proteinuria. Few studies have confirmed the efficacy of any therapy. Few patients progress to renal failure within 5 years, but a large percentage progress slowly, with renal insufficiency developing over 10 to 20 years.

NEPHROTIC SYNDROME IN INFANTS YOUNGER THAN 1 YEAR

Nephrotic syndrome that manifests very early in life is a much more serious entity, and the prognosis is guarded. The outlook is poorest in younger infants (<6 months of age) and improves as the age at presentation approaches 1 year. Minimal change disease is rarely seen in infants younger than 6 months of age. It is more common in infants who present at 6 to 8 months. By 1 year, it is the most common cause of nephrotic syndrome.

The conditions that result in nephrotic syndrome in infants differ markedly from those seen in older children. Secondary causes are more prominent and need to be considered, particularly in newborns or very young infants (Table 24-9).

It is especially important to test for syphilis because early institution of penicillin therapy may lead to resolution of the renal disease and may mitigate the involvement of other organ systems as well. Congenital toxoplasmosis is also treatable with the combination of steroids and pyrimethamine–sulfadiazine–folinic acid. Other congenital infections offer less opportunity for treatment to influence outcome; extrarenal manifestations of these infections are much more serious than the kidney disease.

Primary renal disease causing nephrotic syndrome in early infancy is most often caused by either congenital nephrotic syndrome or diffuse mesangial sclerosis. In both diseases, prognosis for survival is poor unless aggressive supportive therapy and kidney transplantation are undertaken.

CONGENITAL NEPHROTIC SYNDROME

Congenital nephrotic syndrome is an autosomal recessive disorder resulting from mutations in the gene encoding the protein nephrin.

Table 24-9. Causes of Nephrotic Syndrome in Infants Younger than 1 Year

Secondary Causes
Infections
Syphilis
Cytomegalovirus
Toxoplasmosis
Rubella
Hepatitis B
Human immunodeficiency virus
Malaria
Drug reactions
Toxins
Mercury
Systemic lupus erythematosus
Syndromes with associated renal disease
Nail-patella syndrome
Lowe syndrome
Nephropathy associated with congenital brain malformation
Drash syndrome–Wilms tumor
Hemolytic uremic syndrome

Primary Causes
Congenital nephrotic syndrome
Diffuse mesangial sclerosis
Minimal change disease
Focal segmental sclerosis
Membranous nephropathy

Adapted from Mauch TJ, Vernier RL, Burk BA, et al: Nephrotic syndrome in the first year of life. In Holiday MA, Barratt TM, Avner ED, et al (eds): Pediatric Nephrology. Baltimore, Williams & Wilkins, 1994, p 791.

Infants with congenital nephrotic syndrome are often premature, with a low birth weight, placentomegaly, increased amniotic fluid α-fetoprotein levels, and hypogammaglobulinemia (decreased immunoglobulin G levels).

Ascites and edema, caused by massive proteinuria, are usually present in affected infants during the first few weeks after birth. Patients do not respond to steroids or cytotoxic therapy. Infections and thrombosis are the two major complications; they cause considerable morbidity and mortality. Because of the massive proteinuria, patients fail to thrive; they require nasogastric feeding with a high-calorie, high-protein formula. Nephrectomy and peritoneal dialysis are often necessary to control protein losses and allow for adequate growth and control of uremia so that the infant can reach a size and nutritional state sufficient for renal transplantation.

DIFFUSE MESANGIAL SCLEROSIS

Diffuse mesangial sclerosis is the other diagnostic entity seen in infants. This disease is similar to congenital nephrotic syndrome, but it often results in less severe protein losses. Patients are often full term and of normal birth weight. The amniotic fluid α-fetoprotein is normal, and onset of edema (1 week to 33 months) is later than in congenital nephrotic syndrome (birth to 3 months). The patients have hypertension, hematuria, and renal insufficiency at presentation. When diffuse mesangial sclerosis is seen in association with a female phenotype, chromosome typing is recommended to look for patients with Drash syndrome (XY gonadal dysgenesis, nephropathy, and Wilms tumor). When this syndrome is present, bilateral nephrectomy and gonadectomy are recommended because the potential for malignancy is very high.

Treatment is as in patients with congenital nephrotic syndrome and eventually requires renal transplantation. The major goal is to help these infants achieve the growth and good nutrition necessary for successful renal transplantation. Nephrotic syndrome occasionally

occurs after transplantation for congenital nephrotic syndrome, probably secondarily to an autoimmune reaction to nephrin.

ASYMPTOMATIC PROTEINURIA DISORDERS

Many patients have proteinuria, but there is no edema, the blood pressure is normal, and serum protein levels are normal. The extent of the workup must be tailored to the seriousness of the problem (see Tables 24-1, 24-3, and 24-4). Whether an evaluation should be performed depends on whether the proteinuria is both persistent and nonorthostatic. The proteinuria that appears in two of four urinalyses is not significant, and the patient would be labeled as having transient proteinuria. There is no renal pathologic process in patients who occasionally have proteinuria but at other times have urine free of protein.

The more common situation involves a teenager who demonstrates orthostatic proteinuria. Some patients have protein in their urine when they are standing or sitting but have no protein in their urine when they are recumbent. The simplest way of evaluating the presence of protein is to obtain a first morning urine specimen and compare it with specimens obtained later in the day. The first morning urine specimen is often free of protein, and subsequent urinalysis during the day demonstrates increasing levels of protein. Individuals who have proteinuria only in the upright position do not have serious disease. There is no increased incidence of renal disease or hypertension in later life. It is critical to determine that the proteinuria is both persistent and orthostatic before any further evaluation is pursued. Protein should be present in three consecutive urinalyses before an evaluation for isolated proteinuria is initiated. The first step in evaluation is to check for orthostatic proteinuria; a protocol is described in Figure 24-1 and Table 24-10. The five urine samples are collected in separate containers, and qualitative analysis can then be performed. Typically observed in patients with

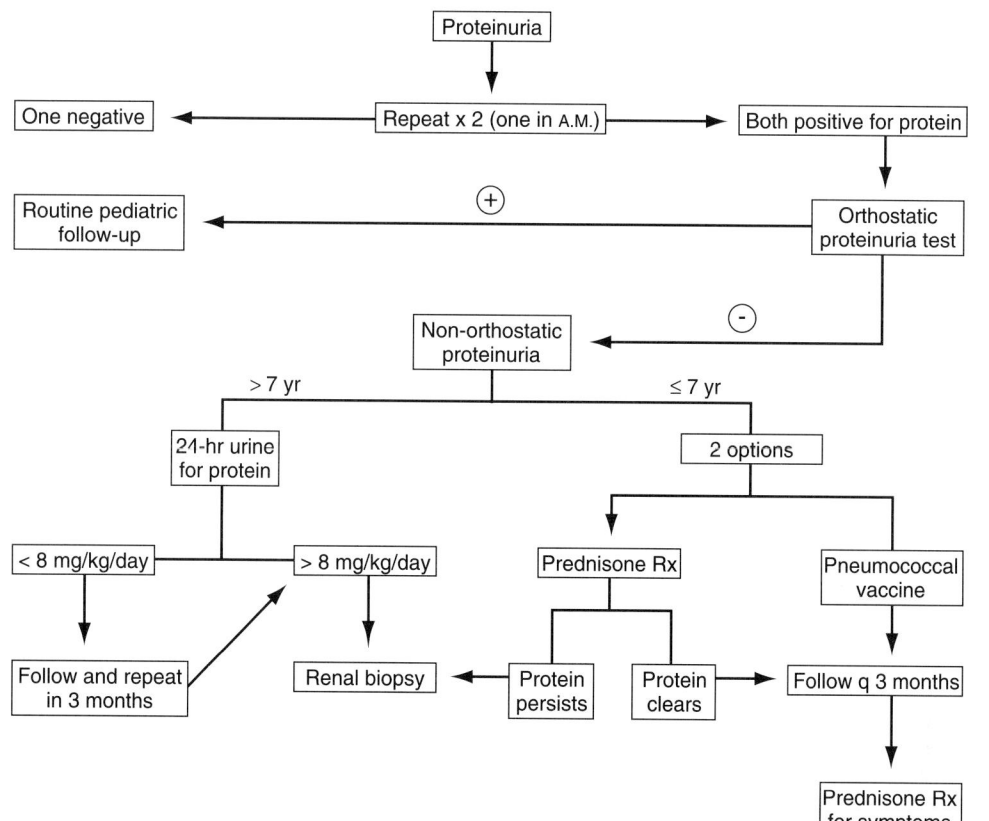

Figure 24-1. Protocol for the evaluation of orthostatic proteinuria.

Table 24-10. **Test for Orthostatic Proteinuria**

1. Have patient void before bedtime 9:00-10:00 P.M and save specimen in a labeled container. Dipstick urine for protein, and record result.
2. Patient should then go to bed and lie *flat*. At midnight, patient should void into a container (while in bed and remaining flat). Again, put the urine specimen in a container and label it. Dipstick for protein, and record result.
3. Patient should void again 5:00-6:00 A.M. (remaining in bed and flat). Again, place specimen in labeled container. Dipstick for protein and record result.
4. Repeat procedure at 7:00-7:30 A.M. (patient still in bed, still lying flat). Record protein result, and place urine in a labeled container.
5. Patient may then rise. Obtain another urine specimen at 9:00-9:30 A.M. The specimen may be obtained with the patient in the standing or sitting position. Place the specimen in a labeled container. Urine should be tested for protein and the result recorded. Patients should bring urine sample to the next clinic visit (all five specimens in separate containers).

Note: It is difficult and seemingly silly to have to urinate while lying flat in bed. This is, however, a very important part of the test.

orthostatic proteinuria is a pattern of positive samples at 9 P.M. and 12 A.M. The urine excreted at midnight was probably filtered at the glomerular level before urination at 9 P.M. If the specimen is again positive for protein only when the patient is standing, no further evaluation is necessary.

For a patient with persistent proteinuria that is nonorthostatic, further evaluation depends on the child's age. An overview of the approach to such a patient is outlined in Figure 24-1.

For the child younger than 7 or 8 years of age who has persistent proteinuria, with normal total protein and serum albumin levels, normal complement, and no other signs of renal disease, there are two options.

One option is to observe the patient carefully with repeated urinalyses every 3 to 6 months and to counsel the parents with regard to swelling and/or ascites, which may develop in association with influenza or an upper respiratory infection. If there is evidence of overt nephrotic syndrome with edema, a decrease in serum albumen, and an increase in serum cholesterol, a trial of daily prednisone therapy is indicated. It is good practice to give the pneumococcal vaccine to patients who have persistent proteinuria but no evidence of edema or nephrotic syndrome, because of the risk of pneumococcal peritonitis if nephrotic syndrome develops.

The other option involves instituting prednisone therapy to document that proteinuria has disappeared; this confirms the suspicion that the patient has steroid-responsive nephrotic syndrome.

The rationale for withholding prednisone unless symptoms develop is that the natural history of minimal change disease is to remit; this may occur with or without prednisone administration. If the patient has a more serious lesion, symptoms will develop, at which time evaluation and therapy may be undertaken.

In a patient older than 8 or 9 years, once the presence of persistent and nonorthostatic proteinuria is established, the next step is to quantify the amount of protein in a 24-hour specimen. If urinary protein excretion is greater than 8 mg/kg/day, a renal biopsy is indicated. The choice of 8 mg/kg/day of proteinuria is arbitrary; the ISKDC definition of proteinuria is 8 mg/m²/hour, and nephrotic syndrome is defined as 40 mg/m²/hour. Hence, for an average 8-year-old patient who weighs 30 kg and is 1 m² tall, proteinuria by these definitions is a level of 96 mg/day, and nephrotic syndrome is a level of 960 mg/day. Renal biopsy is recommended at a level of 240 mg/day of proteinuria. This guideline helps avoid a biopsy for the patient with minimal proteinuria but does not require full-blown nephrotic syndrome to develop before a definitive workup is initiated. Because the patient has isolated proteinuria, MPGN or SLE is an unlikely possibility. However, the incidence of focal segmental sclerosis is much higher in adolescents than in younger children. With the possibility of treatment with cyclosporine and/or ACE inhibitors preventing future renal failure, aggressive evaluation is warranted to identify patients who might benefit from these therapies.

It has become evident that the presence of protein in the urine increases the risk of renal insufficiency regardless of its cause. This has led to therapies that reduce proteinuria, thereby decreasing the risk of progressive loss of renal function. The traffic of protein across the glomerular capillary membrane appears to stimulate a cascade of inflammatory events that cause interstitial fibrosis. ACE inhibitors result in efferent arteriolar vasodilatation, leading to a decrease in intraglomerular pressure, which in turn leads to a decreased transport of protein across the glomerular filter. Patients who are treated with ACE inhibitors are less likely to increase their level of proteinuria and are less likely to lose their renal function than are patients who are not treated with these agents. This was first apparent in the treatment of diabetic nephropathy, but there is evidence that ACE inhibitors offer advantages to patients with other nephropathies as well. Angiotensin II blockers offer another avenue for accomplishing a decrease in intraglomerular pressures, and these also decrease proteinuria when used alone or in conjunction with an ACE inhibitor. ACE inhibitors and angiotensin II blockers may be useful for patients with proteinuria either as a first step or as adjunctive therapy for those who fail to respond to other medications.

SUMMARY AND RED FLAGS

Asymptomatic proteinuria may be associated with nonspecific febrile benign illnesses, postural mechanisms, and glomerular or tubular dysfunction. Significant proteinuria with edema suggests the nephrotic syndrome, which in most children suggests minimal change nephrotic syndrome. An age younger than 1 year or older than 10 years plus significant hematuria, azotemia, and hypertension is a red flag that suggests a cause of nephrosis other than the more benign minimal change disease. Additional red flags include a poor response to prednisone therapy and signs of multiple organ system involvement by a primary systemic disease, such as SLE. Fever and abdominal pain in a patient with nephrotic syndrome should suggest spontaneous primary bacterial peritonitis.

REFERENCES

Bergstein JM: A practical approach to proteinuria. Pediatr Nephrol 1999;13:697-700.
Bonilla-Felix M, Parra C, Dajani T, et al: Changing patterns in the histopathology of idiopathic nephrotic syndrome in children. Kidney Int 1999;55:1885-1890.
Chesney RW: The idiopathic nephrotic syndrome. Curr Opin Pediatr 1999;11:158-161.
Durkan A, Hodson E, Willis N, et al: Non-corticosteroid treatment for nephrotic syndrome in children. Cochrane Database Syst Rev 2001; (4):CD002290.
Gorensek MJ, Lebel MH, Nelson JD: Peritonitis in children with nephrotic syndrome. Pediatrics 1988;81:849.
Greenstein SM, Delrio M, Ong E, et al: Plasmapheresis treatment for recurrent focal sclerosis in pediatric renal allografts. Pediatr Nephrol 2000;14:1061-1065.
Hodson EM, Knight JF, Willis NS, et al: Corticosteroid therapy for nephrotic syndrome in children. Cochrane Database Syst Rev 2001;(1):CD001533.
Hogg RJ, Portman RJ, Milliner D, et al: Evaluation and management of proteinuria and nephrotic syndrome in children: Recommendations from a pediatric nephrology panel established at the National Kidney

Foundation Conference on Proteinuria, Albuminuria, Risk, Assessment, Detection, and Elimination (PARADE). Pediatrics 2000:105:1242-1249.

Homberg C, Jalanko H. Tryggvason K, Rapola J: Congenital nephrotic syndrome. In Barratt TM, Avner ED, Harmon WE (eds): Pediatric Nephrology. Baltimore, Lippincott Williams & Wilkins, 1999, p 765-777.

Korbet SM: Clinical picture and outcome of primary focal segmental glomerulosclerosis. Nephrol Dial Transplant 1999;14:68-73.

Leung AK, Robson WL: Evaluating the child with proteinuria. J R Soc Health 2000;120:16-22.

Lin CY, Sheng CC, Chen CH, et al: The prevalence of heavy proteinuria and progression risk factors in children undergoing urinary screening. Pediatr Nephrol 2000;14:953-959.

McBryde KD, Kershaw DB, Smoyer WE: Pediatric steroid-resistant nephrotic syndrome. Curr Probl Pediatr Adolesc Health Care 2001; 31:280-307.

Nephrotic syndrome in children: Prediction of histopathology from clinical and laboratory characteristics at time of diagnosis. A report of the International Study of Kidney Disease in Children. Kidney Int 1978;13:159-165.

The primary nephrotic syndrome in children: Identification of patients with minimal change nephrotic syndrome from initial response to prednisone. A report of the International Study of Kidney Disease in Children. J Pediatr 1981;98:561-564.

Remuzzi G, Ruggenenti P, Benigni A: Understanding the nature of renal disease progression. Perspective in Clinical Nephrology. Kidney Int 1997;51:2-15.

Roth KS, Amaker BH, Chan JC: Nephrotic syndrome: Pathogenesis and management. Pediatr Rev 2002;23:237-248.

Ruggenenti P, Perna A, Gherardi G, et al: Renoprotective properties of ACE-inhibition in non-diabetic nephropathies with non-nephrotic proteinuria. Lancet 1999;53:359-364.

Rytand DA, Spreiter S: Prognosis in postural (orthostatic) proteinuria. N Engl J Med 1981;305:618.

Trompeter RS, Lloyd BW, Hicko J, et al: Long-term outcome for children with minimal change nephrotic syndrome. Lancet 1985;1:368.

Vehaskari VM, Rapola J: Isolated proteinuria: Analysis of a school-age population. J Pediatr 1982;101:661.

Yashikawa N, Kitagawa K, Ohta K, et al: Asymptomatic constant isolated proteinuria in children. J Pediatr 1991;119:375.

25 Hematuria

Ben H. Brouhard

Hematuria is a common urinary complaint in childhood. The presence of blood in the urine by itself rarely indicates a serious or an immediately life-threatening illness. Because of this, screening for asymptomatic hematuria, or the aggressive evaluation of hematuria in general, may be overly deemphasized. Conversely, the anxiety provoked by blood in the child's urine may cause physicians to perform extensive and costly evaluations.

INITIAL APPROACH TO HEMATURIA

Some general guidelines can be listed for all cases of hematuria, regardless of whether it is gross or microscopic, symptomatic, or asymptomatic. Historically, it is important to inquire about the results of previous urinalyses and about any abnormalities of the urine that might have been present (proteinuria, leukocyturia). Differentiating between acute and chronic hematuria is useful diagnostically. For children with gross hematuria, the number of episodes, how long they last, and the circumstances surrounding the episodes may provide clues to the diagnosis. A history of hypertension suggests a chronic kidney disease. Because a number of familial disorders may manifest with hematuria, documentation of the family history should focus on kidney abnormalities, hypertension, nephrolithiasis, hematuria, deafness, and renal failure (specifically with regard to dialysis and kidney transplantation).

The physical examination may be unrevealing in patients with renal disease but must include determining the blood pressure and careful palpation of the abdomen, the flank regions, the back, and the suprapubic region. The initial evaluation must include the urinalysis: the "physical examination of the kidneys." The color of the urine should be noted. A reagent strip may reveal the presence of proteinuria and may also suggest the presence of blood and leukocytes. Heme-positive findings on a reagent strip must be confirmed by microscopic examination for the presence of red blood cells. Other elements to be particularly noted on microscopic examination are white blood cells, casts, and crystals (see Fig. 23-1).

Hematuria is categorized as (1) gross hematuria (blood in the urine visible to the naked eye) or (2) microscopic hematuria (red blood cells found only on microscopic examination of the urine). It is also useful to categorize gross hematuria as symptomatic or asymptomatic. Another useful point to consider is whether the blood is originating from the kidney or the lower urinary tract. These categories provide a framework for the evaluation and the differential diagnosis. However, a specific entity may have variable manifestations. For example, acute postinfectious nephritis may manifest with asymptomatic microscopic hematuria with or without proteinuria; the more classical manifestation is gross hematuria, usually with proteinuria.

Regardless of whether the blood is gross or microscopic, it must be determined that red blood cells are present in the urine. Red or brown urine does not always indicate gross hematuria. Table 25-1 indicates causes of urine discoloration that may be mistaken for gross hematuria. Pink stains in the diapers of infants can be mistaken for blood; these stains represent urate crystals, which disappear from the urine when acid is added.

Even the reagent strip may not accurately reflect the presence of red blood cells in the urine. The reagent strip, which is impregnated with orthotolidine peroxide and enhanced with 6-methoxyquinolone, turns blue in the presence of hemoglobin or myoglobin (Table 25-2; see also Fig. 23-1). False-negative results for hemoglobin are unusual but have been reported in the presence of high concentrations of ascorbic acid. False-positive results occasionally occur in urine infected with bacteria that produce peroxidase. With a positive reagent strip result, it is important to determine whether there are red blood cells in the urine or whether this result is caused by free hemoglobin or myoglobin, indicating another disease process and not necessarily disease of the urinary tract. Hemoglobinuria occurs in the setting of brisk hemolysis (often caused by glucose-6-phosphate dehydrogenase deficiency or autoimmune hemolysis) and may be accompanied by pallor, tachycardia, dyspnea, and reduced exercise tolerance (see Chapter 48). Myoglobinuria frequently follows rhabdomyolysis secondary to viral myositis (influenza, enterovirus) in the setting of tender muscles and weakness. Rhabdomyolysis may also occur in patients with inborn errors of energy metabolism affecting the muscle and is often noted in these patients after exercise. Both hemoglobin and myoglobin may produce renal tubular injury and thus produce elevated serum blood urea nitrogen and creatinine levels, giving the false impression of primary renal disease. Forced diuresis is indicated in hemoglobinuria and myoglobinuria.

When red blood cells are present, a positive reagent strip result is correlated with more than two to five red blood cells per high-power field (hpf) on fresh centrifuged urine. A result of more than five red blood cells/hpf in centrifuged urine is abnormal.

UPPER VERSUS LOWER TRACT BLEEDING

Once the presence of red blood cells is documented, the differential diagnosis is simplified if the abnormality can be categorized into upper or lower tract bleeding. The color of the urine should be noted: Brown, smoky, or tea-colored urine indicates an upper urinary tract source of the bleeding; acidic urine changes hemoglobin to hematin, producing brown coloration. It is also important to determine whether protein is in the urine samples. The presence of protein may localize the origin of the blood to the glomerulus. Grossly bloody urine coming from the lower urinary tract rarely contains significant amounts of protein. Bright red blood is more likely to be originating from the lower urinary tract. Blood noted at the beginning or end of the stream also indicates lower tract bleeding. The presence of clots points to the lower urinary tract as the source of the blood. Microscopic hematuria provides no clue as to the source of the bleeding, unless proteinuria is present; microscopic hematuria and proteinuria are highly suggestive of glomerular disease.

Another method used to localize the bleeding is determination of the red blood cell structure. Dysmorphic cells indicate disruption of

Table 25-1. Conditions Other than Gross Hematuria that Cause Urine Discoloration

Pink, Red, Cola-Colored, Burgundy

Disease-Associated; Multiple Causes

Gross hematuria	Myoglobinuria
Hemoglobinuria	Porphyrinuria

Associated with Drug/Food Ingestion

Aminopyrine	Nitrofurantoin
Anthrocyanin	Phenazopyridine
Azo dyes	Phenolphthalein
Beets	Pyridium
Blackberries	Red food coloring
Chloroquine	Rifampin
Deferoxamine mesylate	Rhodamine B
Ibuprofen	Sulfasalazine
Methyldopa	Urates

Dark Brown, Black

Disease-Associated

Alkaptonuria	Methemoglobinemia
Homogentisic aciduria	Tyrosinosis
Melanin	

Associated with Food/Drug Ingestion

Alanine	Resorcinol
Cascara	Thymol

From Travis LB, Brouhard BH, Kalia A: An approach to the child with hematuria. In Cornfeld D, Silverman B (eds): Dialogues in Pediatrics Management. East Norwalk, Conn, Appleton-Century-Crofts, 1985.

Table 25-2. Hemoglobinuria without Hematuria

Disease States

Hemolytic anemias: all types
Hemolytic-uremic syndrome
Septicemia
Paroxysmal nocturnal hemoglobinuria

Drugs/Chemicals

Aspidium
Betanaphthol
Carbolic acid
Carbon monoxide
Chloroform
Fava beans
Mushrooms
Naphthalene
Pamaquine
Phenylhydrazine
Potassium chlorate
Quinine
Snake venom (and occasionally spider venom)
Sulfonamide

Miscellaneous

Cardiopulmonary bypass
Drowning (freshwater)
Mismatched blood transfusions

From Travis B, Brouhard BH, Kalia A: An approach to the child with hematuria. In Cornfeld D, Silverman B (eds): Dialogues in Pediatric Management. East Norwalk, Conn, Appleton-Century-Crofts, 1985.

cell membrane integrity after passing through the glomerular basement membrane, whereas isomorphic cells indicate an origin below the glomerulus. These studies are performed with a phase-contrast microscope. The distinction between dysmorphic and isomorphic red blood cells has a great deal of overlap; it has been proposed that for a diagnosis of upper tract bleeding, at least 75% of the cells should be dysmorphic, whereas for a diagnosis of lower tract hematuria, no more than 17% should be dysmorphic. Other methods that have been proposed include measurement of mean corpuscular volume of the urinary red blood cells or use of the red blood cell distribution width, which would be abnormally high in upper tract bleeding.

GROSS HEMATURIA

SYMPTOMATIC HEMATURIA

Symptoms can be divided into two groups: those that originate from the kidney itself and those that are associated with systemic illnesses that affect the kidney secondarily (Table 25-3).

Nephrolithiasis can occur at any age and may cause the symptoms of renal colic, manifested as intense, episodic flank pain that often radiates to the groin. In young infants, renal colic may manifest as generalized irritability or abdominal pain. The episode of hematuria, which has been reported in 28% of patients with nephrolithiasis, may begin abruptly without a history of hematuria. The physical examination may be unrevealing; the urinalysis may contain crystals, in addition to red blood cells. The family history may suggest the diagnosis because up to 70% of children with hypercalciuria have a family history of stone disease. The medical history of furosemide administration to premature neonates, especially those with bronchopulmonary dysplasia, may suggest nephrolithiasis or nephrocalcinosis with gross hematuria. A high-resolution CT scan is the best radiologic test for confirming the presence of a stone.

Table 25-3. Differential Diagnosis of Symptomatic and Asymptomatic Hematuria

Confirm the Presence of Red Blood Cells

Symptomatic

Renal symptoms
　Urinary tract infections
　Nephrolithiasis
　Urethrorrhagia
Systemic symptoms
　Henoch-Schönlein purpura
　Tuberous sclerosis

Asymptomatic

Cystic disease
Obstruction
Vascular
Arteriovenous malformation
Thrombosis
Trauma
Tumor
Hemoglobinopathies
Coagulopathies
Exercise-induced hematuria
Benign familial hematuria (thin basement membrane)
Glomerulonephritis
Acute postinfectious nephritis
Immunoglobulin A nephropathy
Henoch-Schönlein purpura

Children with nephrolithiasis should undergo a workup to search for a metabolic explanation for their predisposition to form kidney stones. This begins with a 24-hour urine collection for calcium, urate, citrate, oxalate, cystine, and creatinine. *Cystinuria,* a hereditary cause of stone formation in childhood, results from a defect in the reabsorption of cystine and other dibasic amino acids in the proximal tubule. *Primary hyperoxaluria type I* and *primary hyperoxaluria type II* are autosomal recessive disorders that cause a metabolic overproduction of oxalate. The clinical manifestation ranges from severe nephrocalcinosis and renal failure in infancy to recurrent nephrolithiasis in late childhood or even later. Hyperoxaluria may be secondary to excessive intake or excessive absorption in intestinal disorders such as inflammatory bowel disease. Patients with nephrolithiasis may have decreased excretion of citrate, which promotes the crystallization of calcium salts. This commonly occurs in patients with chronic diarrhea or renal tubular acidosis. Uric acid stones, which are radiolucent, may result from high uric acid production in patients with lymphoma or leukemia. On occasion, uric acid stones from overproduction are the initial complaint in *Lesch-Nyhan syndrome.* Uric acid stones occur in children on a ketogenic diet, presumably because of the decreased solubility of uric acid in highly acidic urine. The determination of creatinine excretion is important to ensure that an adequate collection has been obtained (10 to 15 mg/kg/24 hours).

Hypercalciuria is the most common metabolic abnormality found in children with nephrolithiasis. Furthermore, hypercalciuria (defined as urinary calcium levels of 4 mg/kg/day) without an overt stone can manifest as gross hematuria with abdominal or flank pain. Indeed, 2.0% to 9.1% of normal children may have hypercalciuria, and 1.8% have hyperuricosuria. Hypercalciuria can be idiopathic or secondary to another disease, such as renal tubular acidosis (Table 25-4). Hypercalciuria is a frequent cause of hematuria,

and it increases the risk for future nephrolithiasis. Therapy depends on the cause of the hypercalciuria or the type of stone present.

Urinary tract infection is a common cause of symptomatic gross hematuria (see Chapter 23). In this circumstance, the infection is usually confined to the bladder; the blood is bright red rather than brown and may contain clots. As many as 25% of children presenting with gross hematuria have a documented symptomatic urinary tract infection; an additional 35% have a suspected but unproven infection. The urine culture is the sine qua non for a diagnosis of urinary tract infection.

Symptoms of *urethritis* with gross hematuria and a negative urine culture in boys suggest *urethrorrhagia.* The most common complaint is bloodstained underwear. The symptoms tend to occur at intervals several months apart and may persist for up to 10 years. Cystoscopy does not show a treatable lesion and may be contraindicated because of the possibility of producing a stricture. Low-dose, long-term antibiotic treatment may help in some cases. The condition appears to be benign and self-limited; reassurance is the treatment of choice.

Gross hematuria with systemic symptoms may be indicative of a generalized process in which the kidney is involved. The triad of abdominal pain, joint pain, and lower extremity purpuric rash with gross hematuria (with or without proteinuria) suggests *anaphylactoid purpura,* also known as *Henoch-Schönlein purpura* (HSP). HSP affects children between the ages of 3 and 10 years, and more boys than girls are affected. In 60% of cases, an upper respiratory tract infection precedes the onset of the disease by 1 to 3 weeks. There is a seasonal variation, with a peak around November to January in the northern hemisphere. The rash is an acute symmetric erythematous maculopapular purpuric vasculitic rash that characteristically starts around the malleoli but extends to the dorsal surface of the legs, the buttocks, and, less commonly, the ulnar side of the arms. These lesions may coalesce into large patches or ecchymoses (palpable purpura) and may persist for up to 2 weeks.

Joint pain is present in about 60% to 75% of children with HSP. The arthralgia or periarticular swelling of HSP affects the knees and ankles most commonly. Abdominal pain, occurring in about 50% of cases, consists of severe colicky abdominal pain with melena or bloody diarrhea; in rare cases, intussusception develops. Between 50% and 70% of children have hematuria with mild to moderate proteinuria. It is not known how many children with HSP have gross hematuria. Usually, the other symptoms cause the child to visit the physician. No pathognomonic laboratory test exists for HSP; 50% of children have elevated serum immunoglobulin A (IgA) concentrations. No specific therapy exists, and 5% to 10% of children eventually develop renal failure. These children tend to be more severely affected, with gross hematuria and nephrotic range proteinuria, and show severe lesions on renal biopsy, in addition to IgA deposits in the glomerulus.

Classic findings in *tuberous sclerosis,* an autosomal dominant disorder, include epilepsy, developmental delay, and skin manifestations (see Chapter 56). Hematuria in such patients suggests a diagnosis of renal cysts and/or angiomyolipomas that have bled. The former are uncommon, but the latter occur in 50% to 80% of patients, increasing in size and number with time. These tumors are histologically benign and consist of smooth muscle, adipose tissue, and vascular elements. Symptomatic renal tumors are more common in affected adults. Hematuria, retroperitoneal hemorrhage, and abdominal or flank pain may be present. Ultrasonography suggests the diagnosis, and histologic features are diagnostic.

Table 25-4. Causes of Hypercalciuria

Physiologic Stimuli to Calcium Excretion

Sodium excretion
Acidosis
Hypophosphatemia

Increased Filtered Load

Hypercalcemia (hyperparathyroidism, dietary, vitamin D excess)
Excess calcium administration

Impaired Renal Tubular Reabsorption of Calcium

Loop diuretics
Selective tubular defects
Bartter syndrome
Hereditary hypophosphatemic rickets with hypercalciuria
Syndrome of hypercalciuria, normocalcemia, growth retardation, polyuria, and proteinuria (Dent disease)
Renal tubular acidosis
Fanconi syndrome

Idiopathic Hypercalciuria

Absorptive
Renal leak

Hypercalciuria of Unknown Cause

Medullary sponge kidney
Diabetes mellitus
Syndrome associated with total parenteral nutrition

From Milliner DS, Stickler GB: Hypercalcemia, hypercalciuria and renal disease. In Edelmann CM (ed): Pediatric Kidney Disease, 2nd ed. Boston, Little, Brown, 1992, pp 1661-1687.

ASYMPTOMATIC HEMATURIA

Gross hematuria is often asymptomatic. The presence of brown or smoky urine or significant proteinuria indicates upper tract bleeding, whereas bright red urine or blood denotes lower tract bleeding.

Postinfectious Nephritis

Gross hematuria appearing 4 days to 3 weeks after a febrile illness suggests a diagnosis of acute *postinfectious nephritis,* the most common form of acute nephritis in childhood. The classical findings are hematuria, oliguria, edema, and hypertension. Microscopic hematuria is present in virtually all cases; gross hematuria is present in about 30%. The urine is characteristically described as smoky or tea-colored to cola-colored. The gross hematuria usually disappears in 3 to 5 days, proteinuria disappears in several weeks, and microscopic hematuria resolves in months to 1 year. Group A streptococcal infection is the most well-defined cause, having occurred in 80% of patients with postinfectious nephritis; however, other causes have also been documented, ranging from other bacteria to viruses. The usual age at involvement is school age, and the streptococci usually come from cutaneous infection (impetigo) in the southern United States and the pharynx in the northern United States.

It is important to document the time of appearance of the hematuria after the infection. It should be between 4 days and 3 weeks; a shorter time may suggest IgA nephropathy or exacerbation of a preexisting nephritis. Laboratory confirmation consists of identifying the streptococcal cause and noting the decrease in serum C3 concentration and variable decreases in C4 levels. Determinations of serum creatinine concentration should also be performed because a rapidly progressive decline in renal function can occur. This situation should also suggest additional diseases (the differential diagnosis is noted in Tables 25-5 and 25-6).

Differential Diagnosis

Important diseases manifesting as an acute proliferative glomerulonephritis include postinfectious nephritis, systemic infections, IgA nephropathy, and HSP. Infectious agents producing postinfectious nephritis other than group A streptococci have included viridans group streptococcus, *Streptococcus pneumoniae, Staphylococcus aureus, Staphylococcus epidermidis, Corynebacterium* species, *Mycoplasma* species, meningococci, *Leptospira* species, varicella virus, rubella virus, cytomegalovirus, Epstein-Barr virus, *Toxoplasma* species, *Trichinella* species, and *Rickettsia* species. Less common causes of childhood-onset acute proliferative glomerulonephritis include membranoproliferative glomerulonephritis, systemic lupus erythematosus (SLE), familial nephritis, endocarditis, and shunt nephritis; uncommon causes include Wegener granulomatosus and polyarteritis nodosa.

Glomerulonephritis may also be classified by its histologic appearance. In *crescentic glomerulonephritis,* there is a proliferation in the Bowman space. This disorder is usually a problem of adolescents who have hypertension, anemia, hypocomplementemia, hematuria (gross in 50% to 80%), proteinuria, and edema. Primary renal diseases include anti–glomerular basement membrane disease, immune complex disease, IgA nephropathy, and membranous and membranoproliferative glomerulonephritides. Systemic illnesses producing crescentic glomerulonephritis include postinfectious disease, shunt nephritis (infected ventriculoatrial shunts for hydrocephalus), endocarditis, SLE, HSP, polyarteritis, cryoglobulinemia, and Wegener granulomatosus.

Membranoproliferative glomerulonephritis is categorized into three types:

Type I manifests as nephritis-nephrosis, hypocomplementemia, subendothelial glomerular deposits, mesangial proliferation, and deposition of immunoglobulins and complement; it is rarely asymptomatic.

Type II is similar to type I except that the deposits are in the lamina densa, the basement membrane demonstrates dense deposits, the mesangial cell proliferation is milder, and only C3 is deposited.

Table 25-5. Classification of Rapidly Progressive (Crescentic) Glomerulonephritis (RPGN)

Type of RPGN	Frequency
Anti-GBM Antibody–Mediated RPGN	20%
Goodpasture syndrome	
Idiopathic anti-GBM nephritis	
Membranous nephropathy with crescents	
RPGN-Associated with Granular Immune Deposits	40%
Postinfectious	
Poststreptococcal glomerulonephritis	
Bacterial endocarditis	
"Shunt" nephritis	
Visceral abscesses, other nonstreptococcal infections	
Noninfectious	
Systemic lupus erythematosus	
Henoch-Schönlein purpura	
Mixed cryoglobulinemia	
Solid tumors	
Primary Renal Disease	
Membranoproliferative glomerulonephritis	
IgA nephropathy	
Idiopathic "immune complex" nephritis	
RPGN Without Glomerular Immune Deposits	40%
Vasculitis	
Polyarteritis	
Hypersensitivity vasculitis	
Wegener granulomatosis	
Idiopathic RPGN	

Modified from Couser WG. Glomerular disorders. In Wyngaarden JB, Smith LH, Bennett JC (eds). Cecil Textbook of Medicine, 19th ed. Vol 1. Philadelphia, WB Saunders, 1992, p 552.

GBM, glomerular basement membrane; IgA, immunoglobulin A.

Type III differs in that asymptomatic hematuria or proteinuria may be present at first, nephritis-nephrosis is unusual at presentation, and deposition of C3 and C5 with few immunoglobulins occurs within the glomerular basement membrane.

Membranoproliferative glomerulonephritis is usually idiopathic, but it may be secondary to immune complex disease (SLE, HSP, hereditary complement deficiencies, other collagen vascular diseases), infections (bacteremia, human immunodeficiency virus), malignancy (lymphoma), chronic liver disease (hepatitis, cirrhosis, α_1-antitrypsin deficiency), or other lesions (hemolytic-uremic syndrome, sickle cell anemia, partial lipodystrophy, renal graft rejection).

Membranous glomerulopathy involves the glomerular basement membrane in stages with increasing severity of deposits: scant discrete subepithelial deposits (stage I); larger, confluent, diffuse, electron-dense subepithelial deposits (stage II); large deposits in an irregularly thickened glomerular basement membrane surrounded by projection spikes of the glomerular basement membrane (stage III); and a thickened glomerular basement membrane with intramembranous deposits and an electron-lucent pattern (stage IV). Membranous glomerulopathy may be idiopathic (primary) or associated with infectious diseases (hepatitis B, congenital syphilis, malaria, filariasis), immune-mediated diseases (SLE, Crohn disease, pemphigus, enteropathy), drug intake (penicillamine), malignancy (neuroblastoma,

Table 25-6. Summary of Primary Renal Diseases that Manifest as Acute Glomerulonephritis

Diseases	Poststreptococcal Glomerulonephritis (PSGN)	IgA Nephropathy	Goodpasture Syndrome	Idiopathic Rapidly Progressive Glomerulonephritis (RPGN)
Clinical manifestations				
Age and sex	All ages, mean 7 yr, 2:1 male	15-35 yr, 2:1 male	15-30 yr, 6:1 male	Mean 58 yr, 2:1 male
Acute nephritic syndrome	90%	50%	90%	90%
Asymptomatic hematuria	Occasionally	50%	Rare	Rare
Nephrotic syndrome	10%-20%	Rare	Rare	10%-20%
Hypertension	70%	30%-50%	Rare	25%
Acute renal failure	50% (transient)	Very rare	50%	60%
Other	Latent period of 1-3 weeks	Follows viral syndromes	Pulmonary hemorrhage; iron deficiency anemia	None
Laboratory findings	↑ ASO titers (70%) Positive streptozyme (95%) ↓ C3-C9; normal C1, C4	↑ Serum IgA (50%) IgA in dermal capillaries	Positive anti-GBM antibody	Positive ANCA in some
Immunogenetics	HLA-B12, D "EN" (9)*	HLA-Bw 35, DR4 (4)*	HLA-DR2 (16)*	None established
Renal pathology				
Light microscopy	Diffuse proliferation	Focal proliferation	Focal → diffuse proliferation with crescents	Crescentic GN
Immunofluorescence	Granular IgG, C3	Diffuse mesangial IgA	Linear IgG, C3	No immune deposits
Electron microscopy	Subepithelial humps	Mesangial deposits	No deposits	No deposits
Prognosis	95% resolve spontaneously 5% RPGN or slowly progressive	Slow progression in 25%-50%	75% stabilize or improve if treated early	75% stabilize or improve if treated early
Treatment	Supportive	Uncertain (options include steroids, fish oil, and ACE inhibitors)	Plasma exchange, steroids, cyclophosphamide	Steroid pulse therapy

Modified from Couser WG: Glomerular disorders. In Wyngaarden JB, Smith LH, Bennett JC (eds). Cecil Textbook of Medicine, 19th ed. Vol 1. Philadelphia, WB Saunders, 1992, p 552.

*Relative risk.

ACE, angiotensin-converting enzyme; ANCA, antineutrophil cytoplasm antibody; ASO, anti–streptolysin O; GBM, glomerular basement membrane; GN, glomerulonephritis; HLA, human leukocyte antigen; Ig, immunoglobulin.

Wilms tumor, gonadoblastoma), or other diseases (renal transplant graft, Fanconi syndrome, sickle cell anemia, anti–glomerular basement membrane/anti–alveolar basement membrane antibodies, thrombocytopenia with microangiopathic anemia, α_1-antitrypsin deficiency). This disorder rarely manifests with macroscopic hematuria; microscopic hematuria is present in 70% of patients. Renal failure and hypocomplementemia are rare, whereas nephrotic syndrome occurs in 70% of patients (see Chapter 24).

Treatment

Therapy for postinfectious nephritis is symptomatic, with particular attention to the hypertension that may be present; the acute morbid conditions result principally from hypertension and may include seizures, hypertensive encephalopathy, and congestive heart failure. Renal failure is uncommon. The prognosis of postinfectious nephritis is excellent. The rate of early mortality is 0.5% to 0.8%. The long-term outlook is for complete recovery in 95% of patients. Recurrence caused by streptococcal disease has been documented in fewer than 5% of cases. Early treatment of streptococcal disease does not, however, prevent postinfectious nephritis or recurrences (see Chapter 1). Recurrent hematuria and proteinuria can occur in patients who have a nonspecific upper respiratory tract febrile illness within 6 weeks of the original episode.

Immunoglobulin A Nephropathy

IgA nephropathy is a common cause of nephropathy, and its manifestations vary from gross hematuria (30%), nephrotic syndrome (6%), acute nephritis (10%), and malignant hypertension (8%) to chronic (6%) and acute renal failure (6%). Although IgA nephropathy is usually asymptomatic, loin pain has been reported in some patients. There is a male predominance, with a peak incidence in late childhood and early adult life. Gross hematuria appears within 48 hours of an upper respiratory tract infection. Between episodes, the urine may be free of blood or may show microscopic hematuria. No pathognomonic laboratory tests exist for IgA nephropathy; however, the serum IgA concentration may be increased during episodes of gross hematuria. The diagnosis can be made with certainty only with renal biopsy when mesangial deposits of IgA are noted, usually in association with the presence of C3 and immunoglobulin G. No specific therapy exists for IgA nephropathy; alternate-day steroid therapy may be useful for patients with nephrotic-range proteinuria. The prognosis is not necessarily benign.

Thirty percent of adults and 10% of children progress to end-stage renal disease.

Other Causes of Asymptomatic Hematuria

Asymptomatic gross hematuria occurring after exercise is known as *stress hematuria*. It is characterized by gross hematuria immediately or a few hours after exercise. The episodes are usually of short duration and painless. The blood may be bright red or a darker color. Proteinuria does not occur. No laboratory or radiographic abnormalities exist. An extensive investigation is not warranted. With a decrease in exercise, the hematuria disappears.

Two less common, familial syndromes can produce asymptomatic gross hematuria: *progressive familial nephritis (Alport syndrome)* and *polycystic kidney disease.* A family history of renal disease, deafness, hematuria, or renal failure suggests a diagnosis of Alport syndrome. The first symptoms of hematuria may occur early in life, especially in boys. Approximately 72% of affected children are symptomatic before 6 years of age, and hematuria is the most common sign. Like the renal disease, the hearing loss is progressive. The only definitive method of diagnosis is renal biopsy, which shows the characteristic electron microscopic appearance of attenuation, disruption, and lamellation of the glomerular basement membrane. Although no specific therapy exists, genetic counseling is needed. In most cases, the inheritance is X-linked, although an autosomal recessive variant also exists.

Some patients with a more common form of familial hematuria demonstrate persistent microscopic and recurrent gross hematuria without deterioration of renal function. This is called *benign familial hematuria,* an autosomal dominant disorder. Evidence of disease can also be obtained when urinalyses are performed on family members. An autosomal dominant pattern of inheritance has been proposed. Renal biopsy demonstrates normal light and immunofluorescent microscopic findings; electron micrographs show attenuation and disruption of the glomerular basement membrane (thin basement membrane disease).

Autosomal dominant polycystic kidney disease has been documented in children—in rare cases, as early as birth. Gross hematuria may be the first manifestation of this disorder and occurs in 50% of patients; minimal trauma produces hematuria as a result of stretching of the vessels surrounding the cyst. The usual presenting manifestations of the disease (hematuria, hypertension, abdominal mass, and uremia in adults) are seldom seen in children. Adults tend to demonstrate symptoms not seen in children, which include acute and chronic pain (60%), urinary tract infection, and nephrolithiasis (20%). With the use of ultrasonography, it is more common to detect the disease when the children are asymptomatic. The cysts are bilateral and may involve other organs, the liver most commonly. There are no specific laboratory findings and no specific therapy except genetic counseling and control of hypertension if present.

The mechanism of hematuria in cystic disease may occur in other conditions that produce dilatation of the upper urinary tract. *Hydronephrosis* caused by ureteropelvic junction obstruction or vesicoureteral reflux may also result in hematuria when the dilated areas are subjected to even minimal trauma.

Coagulation abnormalities and *hemoglobinopathies* are rarely found in patients with gross hematuria. Sickle cell disease and sickle cell trait are hemoglobinopathies that cause asymptomatic gross hematuria (see Chapter 48). A combination of low oxygen tension, reduced blood flow, low pH, and high osmolality in the medulla induces sickling and sludging of erythrocytes, resulting in areas of infarction and hemorrhage. The bleeding commonly comes from the left kidney, for unknown reasons. Conventional therapy consists of hydration and rest; intravenous desmopressin therapy may also be useful.

Renal tumors are a rare cause of gross hematuria in children. Wilms tumor, the most common pediatric renal malignancy, usually manifests as a flank mass (see Chapter 22). Adenocarcinoma is rarely found in children but has been reported in older children and may manifest as gross hematuria. The diagnosis is suspected radiographically through ultrasonography or computed tomography and is confirmed at the time of surgery.

Bladder tumors are a rare cause of asymptomatic gross hematuria. These can be detected with ultrasonography of the bladder.

Gross hematuria in the neonate (Table 25-7) can originate from thrombotic events associated with an umbilical artery catheter, trauma, hypercoagulable states, or disseminated intravascular coagulation and may result from thrombosis of the renal vein or renal artery. Thrombosis can be caused by catastrophic events at the time of delivery that cause trauma or hypotension and decreased perfusion to the kidney. The incidence of renal vein thrombosis ranges from 0.26% to 0.70% of autopsies; infants younger than 1 year of age account for up to 90%. A male predominance (2:1) has been reported. Infants of diabetic mothers are more prone to renal vein thrombosis, possibly as a result of polycythemia, dehydration, trauma, or a hypercoagulable state. Along with hematuria, the physical examination may demonstrate a palpable enlarged kidney on the affected side.

Another group of children who are susceptible to thrombotic events with gross hematuria are children with nephrotic syndrome (associated with a hypercoagulable state). The diagnosis of renal vein thrombosis can be suspected from the patient's history and can be confirmed with a Doppler flow study or an isotope scan. A spectrum of therapies has been advocated, ranging from watchful waiting with careful attention to hemodynamic status, hydration, and electrolyte abnormalities to reduction of blood pressure, anticoagulation, and treatment of the underlying abnormality with thrombolytic agents. Nephrectomy, which had been advocated in the past, has been abandoned with the expectation of recovery of renal function without surgery. Follow-up studies have reported that 60% to 80% of patients demonstrate renal atrophy, with 8% to 12% of the patients developing hypertension.

Bleeding from *arteriovenous malformations* of the kidney can manifest as asymptomatic gross hematuria. The blood may be bright

Table 25-7. **Causes of Hematuria in Neonates and Children**

Common	Rare
Neonates	
Thrombosis (renal vein or artery)	Mesoblastic nephroma
	Factitious causes
Nephrolithiasis (including hypercalciuria)	
Obstruction	
Reflux	
Cystic disease	
Syphilis (congenital)	
Children	
Glomerulonephritis	Wilms tumor
Postinfectious nephritis	Arteriovenous malformations
Immunoglobulin A nephropathy	Factitious causes
Henoch-Schönlein purpura	
Systemic lupus erythematosus	
Familial nephritis (Alport syndrome)	
Nephrolithiasis (including hypercalciuria)	
Cystic disease, reflux	
Interstitial nephritis	

red as a result of the rapid transit of the blood and urine down the ureter. The blood can be localized to one kidney with cystoscopy; angiography is indicated when the bleeding is so severe that surgery for the malformation would be considered. Hemangiomas of the bladder can also be detected with the use of cystoscopy.

Gross hematuria can occur from direct injury to the bladder epithelium from *cyclophosphamide*. This problem results from prolonged contact with the toxic metabolites of this drug. Prevention includes increased hydration to ensure adequate urine flow and the use of mesna, a drug that coats the bladder to prevent contact of the metabolites with the bladder mucosa.

Many affected children present with gross hematuria without history or physical findings that suggest a cause. Laboratory data should then be obtained, including determinations of serum creatinine concentration, complement levels (low in postinfectious glomerulonephritis, SLE, serum sickness, endocarditis, membranoproliferative glomerulonephritis, and hypocomplementemic vasculitis), and a 24-hour urine collection for calcium. The initial radiographic study should be ultrasonography of the entire urinary tract. If all of these results are normal, then cystoscopy can be considered to localize the bleeding to the urethra, bladder, or one or both ureters. If these results are normal or suggest that only one kidney is the source of the bleeding, renal angiography should be considered to detect an arteriovenous malformation. Renal biopsy is seldom indicated for gross hematuria with no other signs or symptoms.

MICROSCOPIC HEMATURIA

WITHOUT PROTEINURIA

School-screening data demonstrate a high prevalence of isolated, often intermittent, asymptomatic microscopic hematuria. The rate varies by sex, age, and definition of hematuria. More girls than boys have microscopic hematuria. Half of the children screened had no blood in the urine after the initial positive results of urinalysis. When yearly urinalyses are performed, the disappearance rate of hematuria is 30%. Children with more than 20 red blood cells/hpf of spun urine are more likely to have persistent hematuria. It is imperative that the urinalysis be repeated over the course of 2 to 3 months in patients with isolated asymptomatic microscopic hematuria. Isolated asymptomatic hematuria usually follows a benign course in the absence of proteinuria or hypertension and if there are fewer than 20 red blood cells/hpf.

If isolated asymptomatic hematuria persists after two to three examinations over 2 to 3 months, then further evaluation is indicated (Table 25-8). The evaluation is similar to that for patients with asymptomatic gross hematuria because the same disease entities can produce microscopic hematuria and gross hematuria. It is important to document whether there have been episodes of gross hematuria with persistent microscopic hematuria between episodes, as well as whether there has been a prior viral or streptococcal illness. Screening of siblings of patients with classic post-streptococcal glomerulonephritis demonstrated that 30% could have asymptomatic disease. The diagnosis of postinfectious nephritis should be considered even if the usual symptoms are not present.

Other causes of asymptomatic gross hematuria can also manifest as asymptomatic microscopic hematuria, including HSP, IgA nephropathy, cystic disease (polycystic or multicystic), obstructive uropathy, Alport syndrome, benign familial hematuria, and hypercalciuria (see Tables 25-5 to 25-7).

Loin-pain hematuria syndrome consists of microscopic hematuria (with or without proteinuria) with incapacitating pain. The pain is of such severity that it often leads to narcotic dependency. Nephrectomy with or without autotransplantation is the only treatment. This is an uncommon idiopathic disorder and is a diagnosis of exclusion.

If no cause can be ascertained from the history of the current illness, family history, or physical examination (including urinalyses),

Table 25-8. Differential Diagnosis of Hematuria with or without Proteinuria*

Proteinuria	No Proteinuria
<40 mg/m²/hr	
Acute postinfectious nephritis	Hypercalciuria
IgA nephropathy	Acute postinfectious nephritis
Henoch-Schönlein purpura and other vasculitides	IgA nephropathy
Hereditary nephritis (Alport)	Benign familial hematuria
Systemic lupus erythematosus	Factitious conditions
Interstitial nephritis	Juvenile rheumatoid arthritis
	Loin pain/hematuria
	Exercise
	Other vasculitides
	Coagulopathies
	Hemoglobinopathies
≥40 mg/m²/hr; Nephrotic Syndrome	
Minimal change disease	
Focal segmental glomerulosclerosis	
Membranoproliferative	
Membranous	

*Remember to first confirm the presence of red blood cells.
IgA, immunoglobulin A.

the laboratory evaluation should focus on two areas: renal function and renal anatomy. Thus, serum creatinine concentration should be determined as a measure of renal function, and serum complement concentrations could be obtained to document any decreases that would suggest postinfectious nephritis or asymptomatic SLE. A 24-hour urine sample should be analyzed to test for hypercalciuria. The normal value is less than 4 mg/kg/day.

If all results are normal but the hematuria persists, the clinician may consider factitious hematuria, which is a form of *Munchausen syndrome by proxy* (see Chapter 36). This diagnosis can be confirmed by comparing the red blood cell antigens in the urine with those of the patient's blood. A difference proves the diagnosis.

Renal ultrasonography should be performed to define the presence of hydronephrosis, cysts, or tumor (although rare, the latter is a concern to parents). If all results are normal but hematuria persists, renal biopsy may be considered. This test provides a morphologic diagnosis. However, therapy is unlikely to be found for asymptomatic isolated hematuria; most nephrologists would propose close observation with semiannual or annual reevaluations. If there is an increase in the number of red blood cells, if the character of the hematuria changes (microscopic to gross), if proteinuria appears, if hypertension emerges, or if serum creatinine concentration increases, then biopsy is indicated.

Neither cystoscopy nor renal angiography is indicated for children with asymptomatic isolated microscopic hematuria.

WITH PROTEINURIA

When the child has blood and protein in the urine, it is important to document the amount of protein. Proteinuria can be determined qualitatively with a dipstick. If the proteinuria is persistent at or above 1+, then quantitation should be undertaken. Proteinuria is defined as a protein level of 4 mg/m²/hour; nephrotic-range proteinuria is defined by values greater than 40 mg/m²/hour. Proteinuria suggests glomerular disease. Causes of glomerular disease include

IgA nephropathy, HSP, and postinfectious nephritis (see Tables 25-5, 25-6, and 25-8 and Chapter 24).

Differential Diagnosis

Systemic Lupus Erythematosus

A butterfly rash on the face, fever, mouth ulcers, and joint pain suggest a diagnosis of SLE. Cutaneous lesions (butterfly rash, discoid rash, vasculitis, alopecia, photosensitivity, Raynaud phenomenon) occur in most patients with SLE. Fever occurs in 60% to 70%, weight loss in 30% to 40%, and arthritis (morning stiffness) in 40% to 80% of children. Renal manifestations of SLE occur in more than 50% of children. These manifestations range from hematuria (microscopic with some proteinuria), to hypertension, nephrotic syndrome, rapidly progressive glomerulonephritis (see Table 25-5), and acute renal failure. Various glomerular lesions have been associated with SLE, including minimal or mesangial disease, focal proliferative nephritis, diffuse proliferative nephritis, and membranous nephritis. Laboratory confirmation rests with the finding of antibodies to DNA, usually with a decrease in serum complement concentration.

The mainstay of therapy for SLE is corticosteroids. Other agents that have been used as adjuncts include azathioprine, cyclophosphamide, and mycophenolate mofetil. The prognosis depends on the renal lesion. Diffuse proliferative glomerulonephritis is the most severe renal lesion and can lead to end-stage renal disease. Treatment for SLE nephritis includes the usual therapy for SLE, such as pulsed steroids and renal transplantation for end stage renal disease.

Previously discussed causes of isolated hematuria—IgA nephropathy, HSP, and postinfectious nephritis—can also manifest with hematuria and proteinuria.

Tubulointerstitial Nephritis

Tubulointerstitial nephritis (TIN) is the term applied to a heterogeneous group of diseases that primarily affect the tubules and interstitial structure of the kidney. Acute TIN is characterized by an abrupt clinical onset with infiltration of the renal interstitium by inflammatory cells. Acute TIN may be an entity unto itself or a part of another process, such as SLE. TIN has been commonly associated with the use of antibiotics, especially penicillins (methicillin, penicillin) and cephalosporins. Antibiotic-associated TIN is associated with high-dose, long-term antibiotic therapy. The clinical picture is characterized by fever, rash, and eosinophilia, with pyuria, eosinophiluria, hematuria, proteinuria, and nonoliguric renal failure. Hematuria is present in more than 90% of patients with TIN, but casts are rarely seen. With discontinuation of the drug, the presumed hypersensitivity reaction rapidly remits, and renal function returns toward baseline. Other drugs commonly associated with TIN include sulfonamides, rifampin, and tetracyclines. Nonsteroidal agents can produce renal disease both by inhibiting prostaglandin synthesis and by the development of TIN. Diuretics, such as furosemide and the thiazides, have also been incriminated, as have *cis*-platinum, methyllomustine, and lithium. Heavy metals, such as cadmium and lead, can also result in interstitial nephritis.

Miscellaneous Disease

Other systemic diseases that have renal manifestations with hematuria (usually microscopic) and proteinuria are the *systemic vasculitides.* These diseases have characteristic systemic signs and symptoms. Renal involvement can be very severe in Wegener granulomatosus and usually includes hematuria and proteinuria; acute or chronic renal failure may occur. Seventy percent to 80% of patients with polyarteritis nodosa demonstrate renal involvement. Other diseases in this category include allergic granulomatosis (Churg-Strauss syndrome), Takayasu arteritis, and giant cell arteritis.

The patient's history and physical examination findings should help define the cause of hematuria in these syndromes.

Systemic infections can affect the kidneys and produce hematuria. *Bacterial endocarditis* can be associated with hematuria and proteinuria; the hematuria may be gross or microscopic. In *shunt nephritis,* an infected shunt (ventricular-atrial for hydrocephalus) or an infected central catheter leads to glomerulonephritis, characteristically with hematuria and proteinuria. Congenital syphilis in infants can cause a glomerulonephritis. All of these systemic infections produce an immune complex–mediated glomerulonephritis, usually with depressed complement levels.

Nephrotic Syndrome (see Chapter 24)

A number of primary disorders generally manifest with nephrotic syndrome, with variable degrees of hematuria (see Table 25-8). The most common cause of nephrotic syndrome in childhood is minimal change disease. It has been estimated that 20% of children with this disorder have microscopic hematuria and 2% have gross hematuria. The second most common cause of nephrotic syndrome in childhood is *focal segmental glomerulosclerosis,* in which the frequency of hematuria is 50%.

The classic disease causing nephrotic syndrome with gross hematuria, microscopic hematuria, or both is membranoproliferative glomerulonephritis. Affected children are usually teenagers; the disease is rare among children younger than 6 years. Edema, gross hematuria, and hypertension are the predominant symptoms at the time of diagnosis. Laboratory features include an elevated serum creatinine concentration and depressed serum complement (C3) concentrations. Treatment is controversial, but alternate-day low-dose prednisone has been reported to offer some long-term benefit.

Membranous nephropathy is a rare cause of nephrotic syndrome in children. It usually manifests with edema and nephrotic syndrome. Microscopic hematuria has been found in rare cases. Biopsy is the only method for establishing the diagnosis.

Almost any cause of glomerulonephritis can potentially cause nephrotic syndrome, almost invariably with hematuria. Common causes in children include SLE, HSP, postinfectious nephritis, and occasionally IgA nephropathy.

Most children with nephrotic syndrome have minimal change disease and receive empirical treatment with corticosteroids (see Chapter 24). Gross hematuria is possible in minimal change disease but increases the likelihood of an alternative diagnosis. Gross hematuria with nephrotic syndrome is usually an indication for a kidney biopsy. Other factors that may support undertaking a kidney biopsy in a child with nephrotic syndrome include hypertension, renal insufficiency, and hypocomplementemia. All children with a poor response to empirical corticosteroids should undergo a kidney biopsy.

SUMMARY AND RED FLAGS

Blood in the urine is a great concern to the child, the parents, and the physician. Blood can originate from any place along the urinary tract. Parents are always concerned that hematuria is a manifestation of a tumor; this should be addressed initially with reassurance that hematuria as the initial manifestation of a urinary tract tumor is very rare. The history of the current illness and the family history, as well as associated signs or symptoms, can usually direct the appropriate evaluation. If no diagnosis is readily apparent, then, depending on whether the hematuria is gross or microscopic, further studies may be indicated. Invasive studies, such as cystoscopy, angiography, and renal biopsy, are rarely indicated.

Red flags include absence of red blood cells in the urine (which suggests hemoglobinuria or myoglobinuria), hypertension, azotemia, pain, and a palpable mass. The presence of proteinuria is a red flag that almost always indicates the presence of glomerular disease. A kidney biopsy is usually indicated unless the patient has a probable acute postinfectious glomerulonephritis.

REFERENCES

Belman AB, King LR, Kramer SA (eds): Clinical Pediatric Urology, 4th ed. London, Martin Dunitz, 2002.

Boineau FG, Lewy JE: Office evaluation of the child with hematuria. Compr Ther 1997;23:583-588.

Diven SC, Travis LB: A practical primary care approach to hematuria in children. Pediatr Nephrol 2000;14:65.

Edelmann CM: Pediatric Kidney Disease, 2nd ed. Boston: Little, Brown, 1992.

Patel HP, Bissler JJ: Hematuria in children. Pediatr Clin North Am 2001;48:1519-1537.

Localization

Angulo JC, Lopez-Rubio M, Guil M, et al: The value of comparative volumetric analysis of urinary and blood erythrocytes to localize the source of hematuria. J Urol 1999;162:119-126.

Hyodo T, Kumano K, Sakai T: Differential diagnosis between glomerular and nonglomerular hematuria by automated urinary flow cytometer. Kitasato University Kidney Center criteria. Nephron 1999;82:312-323.

Symptomatic Gross Hematuria

Furth SL, Casey JC, Pyzik PL, et al: Risk factors for urolithiasis in children on the ketogenic diet. Pediatr Nephrol 2000;15:125-128.

Pietrow PK, Pope JC 4th, Adams MC, et al: Clinical outcome of pediatric stone disease. J Urol 2002;167:670-673.

Polito C, La Manna A, Cioce F, et al: Clinical presentation and natural course of idiopathic hypercalciuria in children. Pediatr Nephrol 2000;15: 211-214.

Santos-Vicario M, Brouhard BH, Cunningham RJ: Renal stone disease in children. Clin Pediatr 1998;37:383.

Shukla AR, Hoover DL, Homsy YL, et al: Urolithiasis in the low birth weight infant: The role and efficacy of extracorporeal shock wave lithotripsy. J Urol 2001;165:2320-2323.

Smergel E, Greenberg SB, Crisci KL, et al: CT urograms in pediatric patients with ureteral calculi: Do adult criteria work? Pediatr Radiol 2001;31: 720-723.

Asymptomatic Gross Hematuria

Abarbanel J, Benet AE, Lask D, et al: Sport hematuria. J Urol 1990;143:887.

Bruno D, Wigfall DR, Zimmerman SA, et al: Genitourinary complications of sickle cell disease. J Urol 2001;166:803-811.

Klein AJ, Kozar RA, Kaplan LJ: Traumatic hematuria in patients with polycystic kidney disease. Am Surg 1999;65:464-466.

Parekh DJ, Pope JC 4th, Adams MC, Brock JW 3rd: The association of an increased urinary calcium-to-creatinine ratio, and asymptomatic gross and microscopic hematuria in children. J Urol 2002;167:272-274.

Pham PT, Pham PC, Wilkinson AH, et al: Renal abnormalities in sickle cell disease. Kidney Int 2000;57:1-8.

Roth KS, Amaker BH, Chan JC: Pediatric hematuria and thin basement membrane nephropathy: What is it and what does it mean? Clin Pediatr (Phila) 2001;40:607-613.

Saulsbury FT: Henoch-Schönlein purpura in children. Report of 100 patients and review of the literature. Medicine (Baltimore) 1999;78:395-409.

Microscopic Hematuria

Bircan Z, Kervancioglu M, Demir F, et al: Frequency of microscopic hematuria in acute poststreptococcal glomerulonephritis. Pediatr Nephrol 1999;13:269-270.

Brown SL, Haas C, Dinchman KH, et al: Radiologic evaluation of pediatric blunt renal trauma in patients with microscopic hematuria. World J Surg 2001;25:1557-1560.

Hisano S, Kwano M, Hotae K, et al: Asymptomatic isolated microhematuria: Natural history of 136 children. Pediatr Nephrol 1991;5:578.

Praga M, Alegre R, Hernandez E, et al: Familial microscopic hematuria caused by hypercalciuria and hyperuricosuria. Am J Kidney Dis 2000;35: 141-145.

Hematuria with Proteinuria

Andreoli SP: Renal manifestations of systemic diseases. Semin Nephrol 1998;18:270-279.

Mahan JD, Turman MA, Mentser MI: Evaluation of hematuria, proteinuria and hypertension in adolescents. Pediatr Clin North Am 1997;44:1573.

McLean RH: Complement and glomerulonephritis—An update. Pediatr Nephrol 1993;7:226.

Niaudet P: Treatment of lupus nephritis in children. Pediatr Nephrol 2000;14:158-166.

Yalcindag A, Sundel R: Vasculitis in childhood. Curr Opin Rheumatol 2001;13:422-427.

Yoshikawa N, Ito H, Sakai T, et al: A controlled trial of combined therapy for newly diagnosed severe childhood IgA nephropathy. The Japanese Pediatric IgA Nephropathy Treatment Study Group. J Am Soc Nephrol 1999;10:101-109.

26 Renal Failure

Daniel W. McKenney

Acute renal failure (ARF) is a rapid loss of normal renal function, typically associated with azotemia (elevation of serum urea and creatinine) and oliguria or anuria, although urine output is occasionally normal or elevated (Tables 26-1 and 26-2). Oliguria and azotemia may be the result of intravascular volume depletion, one of the more common causes of renal dysfunction in children. In this case, prompt fluid resuscitation often results in improved urine output, resolution of azotemia, and little or no kidney damage. In contrast, if hypoperfusion is persistent or severe, tubular damage may have occurred, leading to more prolonged renal dysfunction. In this instance, continued aggressive fluid resuscitation in an oliguric patient can have deleterious consequences.

In the child with ARF, the initial challenge is to identify the underlying cause. For many patients, supportive care is the only treatment. In other patients, disease specific therapy is necessary to reverse the underlying ARF and prevent the potential development of chronic renal failure (CRF).

DIFFERENTIAL DIAGNOSIS

The causes of renal failure in children are diverse, although a few causes account for most of the cases. The likely cause of renal failure at the time of presentation (e.g., hemolytic uremic syndrome or severe dehydration) differs from that of renal failure that develops during the course of hospitalization (e.g., after treatment with nephrotoxic agents or after surgery). Clinically, it is helpful to classify the causes of ARF into three categories on the basis of pathogenesis: prerenal azotemia, intrinsic renal azotemia, and postrenal or obstructive azotemia (Table 26-3). In addition, it is important to consider the possibility that a patient has CRF and is only now coming to medical attention.

PRERENAL AZOTEMIA

A common cause of prerenal azotemia is vomiting and diarrhea from acute gastroenteritis (see Chapter 15). Intravascular volume depletion is secondary to gastrointestinal losses and poor fluid intake. Physiologic compensatory mechanisms attempt to maintain adequate circulation and glomerular filtration. Renal autoregulatory mechanisms allow the glomerular filtration rate (GFR) to remain normal despite decreased renal perfusion pressure. The mechanisms that maintain GFR include glomerular afferent arteriolar vasodilatation, from the production of vasodilator prostaglandins and kallikrein-kinins, and efferent arteriolar vasoconstriction from the effects of angiotensin II. Therefore, early in the course of dehydration, GFR is typically maintained in children with previously normal renal function. Increased tubular reabsorption of water and sodium helps maintain the intravascular volume and produces concentrated urine (high specific gravity and osmolality) with a very low concentration of sodium (decreased fractional excretion of sodium; see later discussion). The urine volume is low. The increased fluid reabsorption in the renal tubules decreases urea clearance because of passive tubular

reabsorption; the serum blood urea nitrogen (BUN) level can increase dramatically. Although creatinine clearance also decreases, the effect is much less dramatic than that of BUN, and therefore the ratio of BUN to creatinine is often high (>20). Because urea is a breakdown product of protein, this ratio can be deceptively low in a child who has had poor protein intake. Appropriate fluid resuscitation increases the urine output and allows the BUN and creatinine levels to normalize.

Although dehydration from gastrointestinal losses is the most common cause of prerenal azotemia in children, there are many other causes of prerenal azotemia (see Table 26-3). Volume depletion can be secondary to excessive urinary losses (see Chapter 62), skin losses or hemorrhage. Inadequate renal perfusion and secondary prerenal azotemia also occurs in patients with normal or even increased total body volume. A patient with heart failure may be grossly edematous but may nonetheless have inadequate renal perfusion (see Chapter 8). Similarly, intravascular volume depletion is a potential complication in patients with sepsis, nephrotic syndrome, cirrhosis, or postoperative third space fluid losses.

Typically, renal compensatory mechanisms are adequate to maintain glomerular filtration until effective circulatory volume can be restored. However, a prolonged period of renal hypoperfusion or the addition of another insult may damage renal tissue, causing intrinsic renal azotemia. For example, in a child with dehydration, the administration of a nonsteroidal antiinflammatory drug (NSAID), which prevents prostaglandin synthesis, may adversely affect the autoregulatory ability of the kidneys to maintain GFR, precipitating intrinsic renal azotemia. Medications such as aminoglycosides or substances such as intravenous radiocontrast are more likely to cause intrinsic renal azotemia when the urine is highly concentrated as a result of prerenal azotemia.

INTRINSIC RENAL AZOTEMIA

Intrinsic renal azotemia is due to damage of the renal parenchyma. Intrinsic renal azotemia in children frequently occurs from prolonged prerenal azotemia, resulting in ischemic (hypotensive) acute tubular necrosis (ATN). The cause of ATN is often multifactorial; intravascular volume depletion is often associated with the administration of nephrotoxic medications. Many affected children are brought to the intensive care unit with multiorgan system failure.

There are a large number of potential causes of intrinsic ARF that often overlap, although for diagnostic and therapeutic purposes, it is helpful to categorize the causes on the basis of the area of parenchymal damage: the tubules, glomeruli, interstitium, or vasculature (see Table 26-3). Damage to the renal vessels may occur in hypercoagulable states, as with renal vein thrombosis in the stressed neonate or renal infarction caused by indwelling umbilical arterial catheters. Damage to the renal microvasculature occurs with hemolytic uremic syndrome and vasculitis. Acute glomerular damage and renal failure may result from glomerulonephritis, as seen in postinfectious glomerulonephritis, rapidly progressive glomerulonephritis, or lupus nephritis (see Chapter 25). Treatment of some of these causes may

Table 26-1. Differential Diagnosis of Increased Blood Urea Nitrogen and Creatinine

Increased Blood Urea Nitrogen

Decreased circulatory volume
Renal insufficiency or failure
Gastrointestinal bleeding
Excessive protein intake
Catabolic states (burns, infection, postsurgery)
Medications: corticosteroids, nonsteroidal antiinflammatory agents, tetracyclines, β blockers, diuretics, angiotensin-converting enzyme inhibitors, and others

Increased Creatinine

Decreased circulatory volume
Renal insufficiency or failure
Muscle injury
Drugs: cimetidine, trimethoprim, methyldopa, cephalosporins, and others

require aggressive use of immunosuppressive medications. Renal tubular damage and necrosis may be caused by renal ischemia, infection, or nephrotoxins, including medications or endogenous compounds such as myoglobin from rhabdomyolysis, hemoglobin from hemolytic anemia, or uric acid and cellular breakdown products with tumor lysis syndrome. Damage to the renal interstitium may occur as a consequence of the vascular, glomerular, or tubular diseases just noted, or it may be direct, as with interstitial nephritis caused by infection or medications, tumor infiltration, or granulomatous infiltration (e.g., sarcoidosis). The differential diagnosis of ARF includes undiagnosed CRF and global parenchymal damage progressing to end-stage renal disease.

Renal tubular epithelial cell damage results in the release of vasoactive compounds, including angiotensin II, adenosine, and endothelin. The resultant afferent and efferent glomerular arteriolar vasoconstriction compromises renal perfusion and function, particularly in patients with decreased effective circulatory volume. Tubular cell breakdown causes accumulation of cell products (casts) in the renal tubules and intratubular obstruction. Renal vasoconstriction and intratubular obstruction contribute to oliguria and anuria seen in many patients. Damage to renal tubular epithelial cells is associated with loss of polarity of sodium-dependent adenosine triphosphatases that are critical for normal tubular reabsorptive processes. Loss of tubular cells and damage to basement membrane can result in "backleak" of filtrate into the circulation.

Clinically, with intrinsic renal failure, oliguria may or may not occur, depending on the degree of renal vasoconstriction, the extent of tubular cell injury, and the degree of tubular obstruction. Renal

Table 26-2. Differential Diagnosis and Definitions of Oliguria

Differential Diagnosis

Decreased fluid intake
Decreased circulatory volume
Renal or cardiac failure
Syndrome of inappropriate secretion of antidiuretic hormone
Urinary tract obstruction

Definitions

Premature infant	<2 mL/kg/hr
Full-term infant	<1 mL/kg/hr
Child	<1 mL/kg/hr
Adolescent	<0.5 mL/kg/hr or <400 mL/day

disease affecting primarily the vasculature and glomeruli, such as acute glomerulonephritis or the onset of hemolytic uremic syndrome, may result in low urine output because of intact tubular function. In these situations, the tubules avidly retain sodium and water because of breakdown in the normal systems that control tubular reabsorption on the basis of intravascular volume status. This partially explains the edema and hypertension that commonly complicate postinfectious glomerulonephritis despite relatively mild decreases in GFR.

POSTRENAL FAILURE

Postrenal failure is defined as renal dysfunction caused by obstruction of urine flow in the urinary collecting system. A typical pediatric patient is the boy with bladder outlet obstruction resulting from posterior urethral valves (PUVs). The diagnosis of PUVs is often made on a prenatal ultrasound by the detection of hydronephrosis, bladder dilation, and oligohydramnios. However, the presentation of children with PUVs varies, depending on the severity of the obstruction. Children may present with Potter sequence at delivery (renal failure, typical facies, and pulmonary hypoplasia caused by severe oligohydramnios) or with normal respiratory function but with abdominal distention and oliguria in the neonatal period. Children with partial obstruction may present later in infancy or childhood with a poor urinary stream, urinary tract infection, ARF, or CRF.

Except in the case of a solitary kidney, proximal obstruction of a single kidney, as with ureteropelvic junction obstruction or a kidney stone, is not expected to cause a significant change in renal function or urine output. Other causes of urinary outflow obstruction include bladder dysfunction, caused by a neurogenic bladder, and urethral obstruction (tumor, calculus, ureterocele, fungus ball, or blocked urinary catheter).

Obstruction of the distal urinary tract results in increased pressure transmitted proximally to the upper urinary tracts. Dilatation of the collecting system (hydronephrosis, hydroureteronephrosis) often occurs. Renal vasoconstriction occurs early with acute obstruction and results in decreased filtration, azotemia, and either oliguria or anuria. Persistent obstruction eventually results in intrinsic renal failure with renal tubular damage and loss of normal tubular function.

CHRONIC RENAL FAILURE

There are many causes of CRF in children (Table 26-4). CRF may also be a sequela of ARF. This is uncommon with ATN, but may occur in severe cases, especially if the patient develops cortical necrosis. All glomerular diseases can progress to CRF, although this is very uncommon with postinfectious glomerulonephritis. Most glomerular diseases are diagnosed before the development of CRF. Focal segmental glomerulosclerosis, one of the most common causes of CRF in children, usually is detected because of symptoms of nephrotic syndrome (see Chapter 24) before renal failure. Other glomerular diseases are detected because of hematuria (see Chapter 25), proteinuria (see Chapter 24), or hypertension (see Chapter 12).

Other causes of renal failure may be more insidious. This is especially true of anatomic disorders such as PUVs and other obstructive diseases, renal dysplasia, and juvenile nephronophthisis. Certain features are useful in differentiating ARF and CRF (Table 26-5). Some patients may have undiagnosed CRF with an acute insult that dramatically worsens renal function (PUVs with a urinary tract infection or acute obstruction).

HISTORY

The initial history and physical examination of the child with renal failure help guide the laboratory evaluation and management. A review of the prenatal history, medical history, family history,

Table 26-3. Differential Diagnosis of Acute Renal Failure in Children

Prerenal

Hypovolemia
  Gastrointestinal losses: vomiting, diarrhea, or ostomies
  Excessive urinary losses: diabetes insipidus, diabetes mellitus, diuretics, adrenal disease, or renal salt-wasting disease
  Skin losses: burns, prematurity, cystic fibrosis
  Inadequate intake
  Blood loss: gastrointestinal bleeding, trauma, placental abruption, twin-twin transfusion
Altered distribution of body fluids
  Sepsis syndromes
  Third space losses: postsurgical losses, capillary leak syndrome, ascites, pancreatitis
  Nephrotic syndrome or protein-losing enteropathy
  Hepatic dysfunction
Decreased cardiac output
  Congestive heart failure
  Cardiac tamponade
Medications or substances causing renal vasoconstriction
  NSAID
  Angiotensin-converting enzyme inhibitors
  Cyclosporine or tacrolimus
  Radiocontrast

Intrinsic Renal

Acute tubular necrosis
  Ischemic or hypoxic insult
  Nephrotoxin
    Medications (e.g., aminoglycosides, cisplatin)
    Exogenous toxins (e.g., ethylene glycol, heavy metals)
    Endogenous toxins (e.g., myoglobin, hemoglobin)
Glomerular disease
  Postinfectious glomerulonephritis
  Membranoproliferative glomerulonephritis

IgA nephropathy; Henoch-Schönlein purpura
  Lupus nephritis
  Idiopathic rapidly progressive glomerulonephritis
  Wegener granulomatosis
  Goodpasture syndrome
Tubulointerstitial disease
  Interstitial nephritis (medications, infections or idiopathic)
  Malignancy
  Sarcoidosis
Vascular disease
  Hemolytic uremic syndrome or thrombotic thrombocytopenic purpura
  Vasculitis: systemic lupus erythematosus, Wegener granulomatosis
  Renal artery thrombosis
  Renal vein thrombosis
Infection
  Pyelonephritis
  Sepsis
Uric acid nephropathy (e.g., tumor lysis syndrome)

Postrenal

Developmental/anatomic
  Urethral obstruction (e.g., posterior urethral valves)
  Bilateral ureteropelvic or ureterovesical junction obstruction
  Obstruction of a solitary kidney: ureteropelvic or ureterovesical junction obstruction, ureteral stricture, ureterocele, kidney stone
Neurologic
  Neurogenic bladder (e.g., trauma, meningomyelocele)
Extrinsic
  Mass, tumor
  Obstructing bladder mass
  Improperly placed or obstructed urinary catheter, fungus ball, stone, clots or tumor

IgA, immunoglobulin A; NSAID, nonsteroidal antiinflammatory drug.

infectious and environmental exposures, and medications, and a complete review of systems is often essential for establishing a diagnosis as well as providing clues to the complications of renal failure that will necessitate therapy (Table 26-6). Also, there should be a thorough review of intake (fluid, dietary), output (number of voids, diaper changes, stool output, other losses) and changes in weight if available to assist in addressing hydration status and management. Certain historical features point toward a diagnosis of CRF (see Table 26-5).

NEONATES

Maternal health history before delivery, including prenatal exposures (medications, infections) and lack of prenatal care, is important in evaluating the neonate with renal failure. Maternal diabetes mellitus is associated with an increased incidence of urinary tract anomalies and spontaneous renal vein thrombosis. Certain medications (e.g., angiotensin-converting enzyme [ACE] inhibitors) and illicit drugs (e.g., cocaine) have been associated with oliguria and malformation of the urinary tract, respectively, and with renal failure in neonates. Congenital and perinatal infections may also cause ARF in the neonate. Prenatal ultrasonography may provide clues to congenital urinary tract anomalies. Findings may include absence of one or both kidneys, hydronephrosis (ureteropelvic junction obstruction or PUVs),

renal cysts (one or both multicystic dysplastic kidneys), distended bladder (PUVs or ureterocele), large kidneys (autosomal recessive polycystic kidney disease), small kidneys (renal dysplasia), or decreased amniotic fluid, which is an indicator of low prenatal urine output. Perinatal events of importance include eclampsia or preeclampsia, premature rupture of membranes, placental abruption, and perinatal asphyxia, which may predispose the neonate to hypoxic-ischemic ARF. Neonates with complications of prematurity, including sepsis, hypotension, respiratory distress, necrotizing enterocolitis, intraventricular hemorrhage, and patent ductus arteriosus, are at increased risk of ARF because of the conditions themselves or because of the medications (e.g., indomethacin) and interventions (indwelling umbilical catheters, surgery) used to monitor and treat these patients. Glomerulonephritis in neonates and young infants is rare.

PREVIOUSLY HEALTHY INFANTS AND CHILDREN

As the origin of ARF in this population of children is most commonly prerenal because of dehydration, the history should include a review of any recent illnesses that may cause poor or suboptimal fluid intake and excessive volume loss, such as gastroenteritis with vomiting and diarrhea. A history of fever indicates increased insensible fluid losses, whereas treatment of fever with an NSAID may precipitate ATN in the dehydrated child.

Table 26-4. Causes of Chronic Renal Failure in Children

Common

Focal segmental glomerulosclerosis
Posterior urethral valves
Renal dysplasia
Cortical or tubular necrosis
Eagle-Barrett syndrome
Pyelonephritis and reflux nephritis
Lupus erythematosus
Congenital nephrotic syndrome
Cystinosis
Juvenile nephronophthisis
Autosomal recessive polycystic kidney disease
Hemolytic uremic syndrome

Less Common

Wegener granulomatosus
Henoch-Schönlein purpura
Membranoproliferative glomerulonephritis
Goodpasture syndrome
IgA nephropathy
Membranous glomerulonephritis
Alport syndrome
Autosomal dominant polycystic kidney disease
Hyperoxaluria
Drash syndrome
Uteropelvic junction obstruction (bilateral or in a single kidney)
Trauma
Renal vascular disease
Bilateral renal vein thrombosis
Hypertension
HIV infection
Sickle cell disease
Wilms tumor and other malignancies
Interstitial nephritis

HIV, human immunodeficiency virus; IgA, immunoglobulin A.

One of the most common causes of intrinsic ARF in previously healthy children is diarrhea-associated hemolytic uremic syndrome. The history may reveal exposure to sick contacts or other potential sources of infection with *Escherichia coli* O157:H7, including undercooked meats or uncleaned fruits and vegetables, toddler wading pools, petting zoos, and fairs. The incubation period is approximately 3 to 8 days before the onset of gastrointestinal symptoms.

Table 26-5. Clues for Differentiating Acute and Chronic Renal Failure

Acute	Chronic
Previously healthy	Poor growth
Gross hematuria	Family history of renal disease
Large kidneys	Chronic illness
	History of hypertension
	History of abnormal urinalysis
	Hypertensive retinopathy
	Anemia
	Bone disease
	Small kidneys
	Broad waxy casts

A history of gastrointestinal symptoms, including vomiting, diarrhea that is often mucoid and bloody, and abdominal pain, are typical of the acute colitis phase of hemolytic uremic syndrome. The child is often brought to medical attention for these symptoms as well as for dehydration. However, whereas most children with typical gastroenteritis respond to rehydration with resolution of azotemia, children with hemolytic uremic syndrome may have persistent oliguria and progressive azotemia and may develop symptoms of volume overload with hypertension and edema. Hemolytic anemia and thrombocytopenia are important clues to the diagnosis. Pneumococci may also be a cause of hemolytic uremic syndrome and should be considered in the child with pneumonia or sepsis and ARF.

A history of possible tick exposure in endemic areas in association with symptoms of headache, fever, rash, or abdominal symptoms suggests rickettsial infections such as Rocky Mountain spotted fever, which causes acute renal insufficiency in 25% of affected patients. A history of constitutional symptoms, rash, fatigue, and arthralgia may occur with rheumatologic disease, such as systemic lupus erythematosus (SLE) or vasculitis. Henoch-Schönlein purpura (HSP), the most common vasculitis in childhood, produces a purpuric rash of the lower extremities and buttocks. Variable features include abdominal pain, arthritis, and glomerulonephritis.

Medications (such as penicillins, cephalosporins, or sulfonamides) prescribed for common illnesses may cause interstitial nephritis. Exposure to excessive heat, trauma, or intense physical exercise and a history of myalgia raise the possibility of rhabdomyolysis. Influenza myositis is the most common infectious cause of rhabdomyolysis.

HOSPITALIZED OR PREVIOUSLY ILL CHILDREN

A large number of potential factors, often coinciding, may result in ARF in ill or hospitalized children. The initial evaluation should include not only a history of the presenting illness but also a very thorough review of all hospital events, medications, and procedures. Important events include hypotension, hypoxia, cardiorespiratory arrest, infection or sepsis, radiologic procedures with intravenous contrast material, and surgical procedures. Daily body weights, fluid intake and fluid output from all sources, and hemodynamic parameters before and during the hospitalization should be reviewed. Medications, which should be evaluated for appropriate dosing and drug interactions, are potential causes of direct tubular injury and interstitial nephritis.

PHYSICAL EXAMINATION

The initial examination should assess the adequacy of the airway, breathing, and circulation. Fever may be associated with infectious or rheumatologic disorders and results in increased insensible fluid losses. Tachycardia may be present with fever, decreased intravascular volume, or vasodilatory states predisposing to renal failure. Hypotension may be seen with sepsis, bleeding, or severe dehydration. Hypertension may be caused by increased intravascular volume and may be associated with renal failure caused by glomerulonephritis, hemolytic uremic syndrome, or vasculitis. Tachypnea and hyperpnea may be seen with volume overload, pulmonary hemorrhage (SLE, Wegener granulomatosis, Goodpasture syndrome), or acidosis. Pallor of nail beds and mucous membranes may be noted with anemia of chronic renal insufficiency and may also be seen with hemolytic anemia (e.g., hemolytic-uremic syndrome [HUS]).

Short stature may be evidence of CRF or renal tubular acidosis. An acute decrease in weight suggests dehydration, whereas an increase in weight may be secondary to edema from renal failure or nephrotic syndrome.

Table 26-6. History and Review of Systems of Children with Renal Failure

Historical Finding	Significance
Medical History	
Abnormal prenatal ultrasonogram	Congenital renal disease
	Urinary tract obstruction (e.g., posterior urethral valves or neurogenic bladder)
Perinatal distress	Hypoxic-ischemic renal failure
	Renal vascular thrombosis
	Congenital renal disease, urinary tract obstruction
Genitourinary abnormalities	Congenital renal disease
Gastrointestinal abnormalities (i.e., imperforate anus)	
Cardiovascular disease	
Spina bifida	Urinary tract obstruction
	Neurogenic bladder
Sickle cell disease, trait	Rhabdomyolysis
	Papillary necrosis
Diabetes mellitus	Prerenal failure caused by dehydration from osmotic diuresis
Diabetes insipidus, central or nephrogenic	Excessive urine losses, prerenal failure
Family History	
Hereditary kidney disease, dialysis, transplantation, hypertension, proteinuria, hematuria, deafness	Polycystic kidney disease (autosomal dominant and recessive)
	Hereditary nephropathy (Alport disease)
	Congenital renal disease
Environmental Exposure	
Infant warmers, phototherapy, excessive heat, hyperthermia, sweating	Dehydration, prerenal failure
	Rhabdomyolysis
Heavy metals: lead, mercury	Heavy metal nephropathy
Trauma	Hemorrhage
	Rhabdomyolysis
	Obstructive uropathy
Burns	Decreased intravascular volume, prerenal failure
Day care; exposure to sick contacts	Infectious agents; hemolytic uremic syndrome
Travel	Endemic infections
Tick exposure	Rocky Mountain spotted fever
Pets; animal exposures; petting zoos	Hemolytic uremic syndrome
	Leptospirosis
Dietary: undercooked meats, unpasteurized ciders; uncleaned raw fruits and vegetables	Hemolytic uremic syndrome
Poisons, Ingestions	
Medications in household	Nephrotoxic ATN
Ethylene glycol (antifreeze)	Oxalate nephropathy
Medication History	
NSAIDs, ACE inhibitors, cyclosporine	Prerenal failure
Chemotherapeutic agents, antibiotics, other medications	Nephrotoxic ATN
	Interstitial nephritis
Surgical History	
Cardiac surgery: aortic clamping, congestive heart failure	Prerenal failure and ischemic acute renal failure
Abdominal surgery	Third-space fluid losses, nonreplaced losses from surgical drains, prerenal failure
Surgical drains	
Blood loss	Prerenal failure
Hypotension	Ischemic acute renal failure
Review of Systems	
General	
Failure to thrive, short stature	Chronic renal failure
	Renal tubular acidosis
	Renal osteodystrophy
Constitutional symptoms: fever, weight loss, fatigue, malaise, anorexia	Infection
	Vasculitis, SLE
	Uremia
	Anemia of renal failure

Continued

Table 26-6. **History and Review of Systems of Children with Renal Failure—cont'd**

Historical Finding	Significance
General—cont'd	
Edema	Volume overload
	Nephrotic syndrome
Neurologic	
Headaches	Hypertension
Seizures	Hypertensive encephalopathy, hypocalcemia
Irritability	Uremia
Obtundation, confusion	HUS
Respiratory	
Cough	Pneumonia, sepsis
Labored breathing	Acidosis
Hemoptysis	Pulmonary edema
	Pleural effusions
	Goodpasture syndrome
	Wegener granulomatosis
	SLE
History of upper respiratory infection; sore throat	Postinfectious glomerulonephritis
Neonatal respiratory distress	Pulmonary hypoplasia due to oligohydramnios
Cardiovascular	
Hypertension	Renal vascular lesions
Palpitations, arrhythmia	Renal scarring
	Glomerulonephritis
	Electrolyte abnormalities
Gastrointestinal	
Vomiting, diarrhea	Gastroenteritis, dehydration
Bloody diarrhea	HUS
Poor feeding, decreased intake	HSP
	Pyelonephritis
	Uremia
Abdominal pain	HUS
	HSP
Genitourinary	
Genitourinary abnormalities	Congenital urinary tract abnormalities
Dysuria, suprapubic pain, flank pain, dysfunctional voiding, urinary retention, staccato voiding	Urinary tract infection
	Congenital urinary tract abnormalities
Red or brown urine	Glomerulonephritis
	HUS
	Renal vascular thrombosis
	Hemoglobinuria, myoglobinuria
Dermatologic	
Rash	Vasculitis; SLE
	HSP
	Infection
Impetigo, pyoderma in past 4-6 weeks	Post-streptococcal glomerulonephritis
Musculoskeletal	
Arthralgia	Vasculitis
Muscle aches	Rhabdomyolysis
Muscle cramps	Electrolyte abnormalities
Hematologic	
Heavy menstrual flow	Bleeding with acute and chronic renal failure

ACE, angiotensin-converting enzyme; ATN, acute tubular necrosis; HSP, Henoch-Schönlein purpura; HUS, hemolytic uremic syndrome; NSAIDs, nonsteroidal antiinflammatory drugs; SLE, systemic lupus erythematosus.

An assessment of circulatory status includes skin perfusion and capillary refill, quality of central and peripheral pulses, and the presence or absence of edema. Signs of decreased intravascular volume in infants include sunken fontanelle, sunken eyes, and decreased skin turgor with tenting and lack of rebound after the skin of the abdominal wall is pinched. Periorbital or peripheral edema suggests increased intravascular volume, although there may be decreased effective circulatory volume in conditions with edema caused by nephrotic syndrome, liver failure, cardiac failure, or capillary leak syndromes. The periorbital edema from glomerulonephritis may be subtle and is seen most often after the patient wakes in the morning; the parent may be the most reliable observer to comment on the change from baseline.

Neurologic symptoms and signs associated with renal failure may be secondary to uremia, hypertension, volume depletion, or electrolyte disturbances. The risk of uremic symptoms is increased when the BUN level is higher than 100 mg/dL or when there is a rapid rise in BUN. Uremic manifestations include anorexia, nausea, emesis, lethargy, confusion, agitation, coma, asterixis, hyperreflexia, and seizures. Hypertension may cause irritability, headache, seizures, coma, or focal neurologic signs (e.g., cortical blindness). Funduscopic examination may reveal features of retinopathy, including arteriolar narrowing and tortuosity and cotton-wool spots. Neurologic signs are also common because of the vasculitis associated with HUS or thrombotic thrombocytopenic purpura (TTP). Hypocalcemia from renal insufficiency may be severe, potentially causing tetany or seizures. Obtundation, irritability, and seizures may occur with hypernatremic or hyponatremic dehydration or result from hyponatremia caused by renal failure and volume overload.

On pulmonary examination, tachypnea and decreased basilar breath sounds may be present with pleural effusion or pulmonary edema secondary to volume overload or heart failure. Pleural effusions may also be present with nephrotic syndrome, vasculitis, and SLE. Heart murmurs occur with underlying cardiac disease and are also common with anemia-induced flow murmurs (see Chapter 11) associated with renal failure. Distended neck veins and hepatomegaly may be present with congestive heart failure resulting from primary cardiac disease or with volume overload resulting from renal insufficiency. A pericardial effusion (volume overload) and pericarditis (uremia, SLE) may be suggested by the finding of diminished heart sounds or a pericardial friction rub.

Abdominal distention may be caused by ileus (sepsis or intra-abdominal infection) or abdominal masses (urinary tract obstruction and hydronephrosis or renal vein thrombosis) (see Chapter 22). Lax or absent abdominal musculature and tone are seen with Eagle-Barrett syndrome (also known as prune belly syndrome). Pain on palpation may be caused by peritonitis (nephrotic syndrome), vasculitis (HSP), or colitis (HUS). HUS has also been associated with toxic megacolon, bowel wall necrosis, and pancreatitis, all of which may cause abdominal pain and distention. Flank pain may result from obstruction of the urinary tracts or pyelonephritis.

Hepatomegaly may be present with certain infections (e.g., Rocky Mountain spotted fever), heart failure, sepsis with disseminated intravascular coagulation, and HUS. Genital abnormalities such as hypospadias and cryptorchidism may be associated with other urologic abnormalities.

Examination of the skin may reveal rashes associated with vasculitis and SLE; purpuric lesions of the buttocks and lower extremities, which are associated with HSP; drug eruptions, which may be associated with interstitial nephritis; and petechiae, seen with infection or thrombocytopenia caused by sepsis, HUS, or thrombotic thrombocytopenic purpura.

LABORATORY EVALUATION

The laboratory evaluation of the child with renal failure focuses on both finding a cause for the renal dysfunction and identifying potential complications, some life-threatening, that will necessitate intervention.

BLOOD UREA NITROGEN AND CREATININE

There are various causes of elevations in BUN and creatinine levels (see Table 26-1). In general, the creatinine level is a more reliable indicator of renal function because of the multiple other factors that affect BUN level. The creatinine level may be deceptively elevated as a result of disease (e.g., muscle injury) or laboratory error (ketoacids in diabetic ketoacidosis). Normal creatinine levels vary dramatically with age; a 1-year-old with a creatinine level of 1.0 mg/dL has significant renal insufficiency. In addition, a child with markedly decreased muscle mass has a very low baseline creatinine. In neonates, the serum creatinine level within the first 4 days of life reflects the maternal serum creatinine level. However, a rising serum creatinine level within the first week of life, or a serum creatinine level that fails to fall to normal levels beyond the first 2 weeks of life, is consistent with renal insufficiency.

A high BUN-to-creatinine ratio (>20:1) is suggestive of prerenal failure. This is explained by the avid tubular reabsorption of urea that occurs with intravascular volume depletion. A high ratio may be secondary to the other causes of a high BUN level listed in Table 26-1. Gastrointestinal bleeding, excessive catabolism, and administration of corticosteroids are the most common causes in clinical practice. A normal BUN-to-creatinine ratio can exist with prerenal failure if the child's intake of protein has been poor.

URINARY INDICES

A patient with oliguria may have prerenal failure or intrinsic renal failure. Urinary indices may be helpful in distinguishing between these two possibilities (Table 26-7). Children with early prerenal

Table 26-7. Urinary Indices in Children with Renal Failure

| Index | Prerenal | Intrinsic Renal | | | | Postrenal |
		ATN	Interstitial Nephritis	GN	HUS	Obstruction
Urine osmolality (mOsm/L)	>500	<350	<350	<500	Variable	<350 (variable)
(Neonate)	(>350)	(<300)				
Urine Sodium (mEq/L)	<10	>30	>30	<10	Variable	>30 (variable)
FE_{Na} (%)*	<1%	>2%	>2%	<1%	Variable	>2% (variable)
(Neonate)	(<2.5%)	(>2.5%)				(Variable)

*FE_{Na} (%) = [(Urine$_{Na}$)/(Plasma$_{Na}$)] ÷ [(Urine$_{Cr}$)/(Plasma$_{Cr}$)] × 100. Note: FE_{Na} is also high with glucosuria and after administration of diuretics or bicarbonate.

ATN, acute tubular necrosis; FE_{Na}, fractional excretion of sodium; GN, glomerulonephritis; HUS, hemolytic uremic syndrome.

failure have intact renal tubular function with maximal reabsorption of sodium and concentration of the urine. This leads to a low urine sodium, a high urine osmolality and low fractional excretion of sodium (FE_{Na}). In contrast, ATN leads to tubular dysfunction, with a consequent inability to reabsorb sodium and water, producing a relatively high urine sodium level and FE_{Na} for a patient with oliguria. The FE_{Na} calculation, which requires simultaneous measurement of urine and plasma sodium and creatinine, is the most useful test for distinguishing between prerenal failure and ATN:

$$FE_{Na}\,(\%) = [(Urine_{Na})/(Plasma_{Na})] \div [(Urine_{Cr})/(Plasma_{Cr})] \times 100$$

The FE_{Na} in children with glomerulonephritis may also be low when tubular function remains intact. Urinary indices are variable in children with obstructive renal failure, depending on the duration of obstruction and degree of renal involvement. The FE_{Na} is low early in obstruction but increases with prolonged obstruction as tubular function deteriorates. Neonates, because of immature tubular function, have less of an ability to retain sodium during dehydration than do older children; therefore, an FE_{Na} of less than 2.5% may still be consistent with prerenal failure.

URINALYSIS

A dipstick urinalysis may be performed with commercially available reagent strips with indicators to measure specific gravity, urine pH, the presence of leukocyte esterase, nitrites, protein, glucose, ketones, blood, and hemoglobin. Specific gravity is higher than 1.015 in children with prerenal failure and is also high with significant proteinuria caused by nephrotic syndrome and with glucosuria with diabetic ketoacidosis. A positive test result for leukocyte esterase is nonspecific; it may be seen with glomerulonephritis, interstitial nephritis, or urinary tract infection. A positive test result for nitrites is more specific for urinary tract infection although not very sensitive. Low- to moderate-grade proteinuria is common in prerenal failure with concentrated urine specimens, obstructive uropathy, or intrinsic renal failure resulting from a number of causes, including ATN, interstitial nephritis, and glomerulonephritis. Moderate- to high-grade proteinuria on urine dipstick tests may be further assessed with semiquantitative (random urine protein-to-creatinine ratio) or quantitative (timed urine specimen) methods. Nephrotic-range proteinuria (see Chapter 24) is suggestive of glomerular disease. Glucosuria and ketonuria may be present with diabetic ketoacidosis. Glucosuria may also be caused by renal tubular dysfunction with decreased renal tubular reabsorption of glucose; the serum glucose level is normal. Ketonuria resulting from poor nutritional intake occurs with prerenal failure. Urine dipstick reagents for hemoglobin are very sensitive and can detect the presence of less than 5 red blood cells per high-power field. The dipstick test for hemoglobin is positive without red blood cells in the presence of hemoglobin (with hemolytic anemias) or myoglobin (in rhabdomyolysis); a positive test result for hemoglobin must always be confirmed by microscopic examination of the urine for the presence of red blood cells.

Microscopic urinalysis may be unremarkable in prerenal failure and obstructive uropathy, although hyaline and granular casts may be noted in dehydration. Segmented white blood cells may be seen with urinary tract infection and glomerulonephritis. Eosinophils may be seen with interstitial nephritis, and lymphocytes may be present with viral infections and renal transplant dysfunction with rejection. Red blood cells may be present because of trauma from bladder catheterization and may also be seen with infection, obstructive uropathy, and most causes of intrinsic renal failure. Epithelial and mixed cellular casts are common in ATN; white blood cell casts may be seen with pyelonephritis and glomerulonephritis. Red blood cell casts are seen with acute glomerulonephritis. Pigmented casts are noted with hemoglobinuria and myoglobinuria, as well as with ischemic ARF. Crystalluria may be seen with certain medications (e.g., acyclovir) or toxic ingestions (e.g., ethylene glycol), which suggests the cause of the renal failure.

SPECIFIC TESTS

Other laboratory studies are indicated on the basis of the suspected cause. A child with bloody diarrhea may have HUS. The stool should be sent for culture of *E. coli* O157:H7. The complete blood cell count in HUS is remarkable for thrombocytopenia, a rapidly falling hematocrit, and a peripheral smear finding consistent with a microangiopathic hemolytic anemia (e.g., schistocytes). The lactate dehydrogenase level is usually markedly elevated as a result of hemolysis. Complement levels are helpful in children with suspected glomerulonephritis. The C3 level is low, and the C4 level is normal in postinfectious glomerulonephritis. Further support for this diagnosis is obtained through a throat culture and measurement of antibodies that suggest a recent streptococcal infection (Streptozyme, anti–deoxyribonuclease B, antihyaluronidase, anti–streptolysin O). Patients with SLE usually have low C3 and low C4 levels, along with a positive antinuclear antibody and a positive antibody to double-stranded DNA (anti-dsDNA). A patient with suspected SLE and glomerulonephritis needs a renal biopsy to confirm the diagnosis and to stage the nephritis.

A child with glomerulonephritis and rapid loss of renal function may have rapidly progressive glomerulonephritis. A renal biopsy is urgently necessary. Blood studies should include tests for anti-glomerular basement membrane antibody (Goodpasture syndrome), cytoplasmic antineutrophil cytoplasmic antibody (elevated in Wegener granulomatosus), perinuclear antineutrophil cytoplasmic antibody (elevated in various vasculitides), antinuclear antibody and anti-dsDNA (elevated in SLE), and C3 and C4 levels (may be low in postinfectious glomerulonephritis, SLE, and membranoproliferative glomerulonephritis).

Sarcoidosis is an unusual cause of renal insufficiency in children. Diagnostic studies should include measurement of ACE (angiotensin-converting enzyme) level, renal biopsy, and a chest radiograph. Patients with suspected infection should have appropriate cultures and serologic profiles. Creatinine kinase and urine myoglobin are useful tests in patients with possible myoglobinuria. Children with hemoglobinuria should have a workup for hemolytic anemia (see Chapter 48).

Children with suspected CRF may have significant anemia. In addition, an elevated serum alkaline phosphatase level suggests renal osteodystrophy caused by CRF. This is confirmed by the presence of an elevated serum parathyroid hormone level.

Along with CRF, severe anemia may result from hemolysis (as in HUS), pulmonary hemorrhage (as in SLE, Wegener granulomatosus, and Goodpasture syndrome), or traumatic hemorrhage. Mild dilutional anemia is a common consequence of volume overload in renal failure.

RADIOLOGIC STUDIES

Renal imaging is useful in selected children with renal failure. A renal ultrasonogram identifies obstruction (hydronephrosis) and gross structural lesions (small kidneys in dysplasia, cysts in polycystic kidney disease or multicystic dysplasia, malignancy). Doppler examination of the major renal vessels may provide an assessment of appropriate vascular flow. In children with a clear history for prerenal failure, the renal ultrasonogram typically provides little diagnostic or therapeutic information. In HUS, acute glomerulonephritis, ischemic ATN, and renal failure resulting from infectious causes, the kidneys may appear enlarged with echogenic cortices and loss of corticomedullary differentiation as a result of interstitial edema. When the duration or chronicity of renal failure is questionable, the finding of small echogenic kidneys on renal ultrasonography is suggestive of preexisting CRF.

Examination of the major renal vessels and Doppler ultrasonography is also beneficial in selected children. Vascular thrombi or obstruction to venous or arterial flow may be demonstrated in neonates with indwelling umbilical catheters or renal vein thrombosis. The renal vessels should be imaged for diagnosis in children at risk for renal vein thrombosis who develop gross hematuria, abdominal mass, hypertension, or thrombocytopenia. In HUS and ATN, increased resistive indices or increased resistance to flow in the renal vasculature may be noted, but this finding is of questionable clinical importance.

In the neonate presenting with renal failure and abdominal distention on examination, the renal ultrasonogram may demonstrate findings consistent with bladder outlet obstruction caused by PUVs, including bilateral hydronephrosis, hydroureter, thickened bladder with trabeculations, and dilation of the posterior urethra. Bladder obstruction from fungal debris or an obstructing ureterocele may also be seen on ultrasonography. In neonates with ATN, loss of corticomedullary differentiation may be seen, as in older children with ATN, although marked echogenicity of the renal pyramids resembling nephrocalcinosis may also be seen.

Voiding cystourethrography is the definitive diagnostic test in PUVs. If a renovascular origin, such as renal infarction caused by thromboembolism, is suspected, magnetic resonance imaging with gadolinium may be useful. Otherwise, further studies are seldom indicated and of little benefit in children with most causes of renal failure. Intravenous contrast studies, including excretory urography, are relatively contraindicated in children with ARF because of the high osmotic load and risk of further tubular toxicity. For children who fail to recover normal function after ischemic ATN, renal ultrasonography and cortical nuclear scans may suggest regions of cortical necrosis of prognostic importance.

Chest roentgenography may be helpful in evaluation of volume overload (heart size, pulmonary edema), pulmonary infiltrates from infectious causes or pulmonary-renal syndromes, pleural and pericardial effusions, and adenopathy. A plain film of the hand or knees is useful for identifying rachitic changes that support a diagnosis of CRF.

RENAL BIOPSY

For most causes of renal failure with a definable origin, a renal biopsy provides little diagnostic or prognostic information. Unless there is an atypical manifestation or clinical course, the diagnoses of diarrhea-associated HUS and postinfectious glomerulonephritis are made by clinical manifestation and laboratory studies without the need for renal biopsy. A renal biopsy is indicated for patients with renal failure of unclear origin, suspected lupus nephritis, atypical hemolytic uremic syndrome or thrombotic thrombocytopenic purpura, HSP, and rapidly progressive glomerulonephritis.

ELECTROLYTE COMPLICATIONS IN RENAL FAILURE

Abnormalities of sodium are typically reflective of fluid status. Hyponatremia is common in ARF because of increased water intake in relation to solute and inability to excrete a volume load (see Chapter 27). Hyponatremia may also be seen with hyponatremic dehydration, increased capillary permeability caused by infection or sepsis, nephrotic syndrome, diabetic ketoacidosis, and sodium losses caused by obstructive uropathy and tubulopathies. Hypernatremia may result from hypernatremic dehydration, inappropriate fluid administration in relation to urine output, and increased urinary water losses resulting from diabetes insipidus or diabetes mellitus.

Hyperkalemia is common in renal failure because of decreased urinary potassium excretion, particularly in the presence of continued dietary and intravenous potassium intake (see Chapter 27). Factors that contribute to hyperkalemia and its toxicity in patients with renal failure include acidosis, insulin resistance, and hypocalcemia. Acidosis and insulin deficiency result in decreased intracellular

uptake of potassium, and hypocalcemia increases the risk of cardiac toxicity associated with hyperkalemia. Because potassium is primarily an intracellular ion, an increase in serum potassium level is seen with cell lysis syndromes (hemolysis, tumor lysis, and rhabdomyolysis). Hypokalemia may be seen with renal failure in association with diarrhea, poor oral intake, or renal tubular toxicity secondary to medications, including ifosfamide, aminoglycosides, and amphotericin B.

Hyperphosphatemia is common in renal failure because of decreased urinary phosphate excretion, again particularly with continued dietary or intravenous phosphorus intake. As with hyperkalemia, hyperphosphatemia may also be seen with cell lysis syndromes. The increased phosphate complexes with calcium, contributing to hypocalcemia. Parathyroid hormone resistance and decreased renal synthesis of 1,25-dihydroxycholecalciferol also contribute to hypocalcemia. Other factors that may contribute to hypocalcemia include hypomagnesemia and citrate administration with blood products. Hypocalcemia may cause tetany, seizures, or cardiac dysrhythmias.

Serum magnesium levels are often elevated in renal failure because of decreased excretion, although this is usually not of clinical significance. Decreases in serum magnesium levels may be caused by diarrhea, primary tubular disorders, or tubular damage from medications, including cyclosporine, cisplatinum, amphotericin B, and aminoglycosides.

Metabolic acidosis is common in renal failure because of increased acid production related to the primary illness, increased catabolism, and decreased renal buffering capacity and acid excretion, particularly with oliguric or anuric renal failure (see Chapter 27). Poor peripheral perfusion, as occurs in severe dehydration or sepsis, may result in increased lactate production and decreased clearance, which may exacerbate acidosis. Parenteral nutrition with high protein intake also exacerbates the metabolic acidosis with renal failure.

MANAGEMENT

The treatment of ARF is mostly supportive with the following goals:

1. treatment of the underlying cause of the renal failure
2. careful attention to fluid management during initiation, maintenance, and recovery phases of renal failure
3. anticipation and treatment of electrolyte abnormalities
4. provision of adequate nutrition
5. recognition of the indications for renal replacement therapy

SPECIFIC MANAGEMENT OF ACUTE RENAL FAILURE

Prerenal Failure

In children with prerenal failure caused by dehydration, aggressive fluid resuscitation and replacement of fluid deficits, as well as provision of maintenance fluid and replacement of ongoing losses, often results in resolution of azotemia and oliguria within 24 to 48 hours. Medications that contribute to prerenal failure, including NSAIDs and ACE inhibitors, should be discontinued or reduced. Children with maldistribution of circulatory volume as a result of shock or sepsis syndromes may require significant volume replacement, ideally in an intensive care unit setting. Prerenal failure associated with infection is treated with appropriate antibiotics; antibiotic dosages are adjusted for the degree of renal dysfunction.

Intrinsic Renal Failure

For most patients, management of intrinsic renal failure is largely supportive. There are no proven specific therapies for HUS caused by *E. coli* O157:H7. Patients receive blood transfusions as needed, with anticipation of ongoing hemolysis. Platelet infusions are usually reserved for active bleeding or in preparation for invasive procedures. Plasma exchange appears beneficial in the treatment of renal failure for some patients with atypical non–diarrhea-associated or familial HUS and thrombotic thrombocytopenic purpura.

Early treatment with corticosteroids may decrease the risk of chronic renal insufficiency in children with HSP who have significant renal involvement. Immunosuppressive therapy, typically corticosteroids and cyclophosphamide, is life-saving in children with Wegener granulomatosus. Immunomodulating agents, particularly corticosteroids, are beneficial in the treatment of certain types of glomerulonephritis manifesting with ARF, including idiopathic, rapidly progressive glomerulonephritis; SLE; and membranoproliferative glomerulonephritis. There is no role for the use of corticosteroids in the treatment of postinfectious glomerulonephritis. Goodpasture syndrome is treated with a combination of plasma exchange, cyclophosphamide, and corticosteroids.

Discontinuation of the offending agent is the primary treatment of medication-induced acute interstitial nephritis. Corticosteroid therapy with either high-dose intravenous methylprednisolone or oral prednisone is reported to aid in recovery of renal function when given early in the disease course, before the development of interstitial fibrosis. Interstitial nephritis caused by infectious agents necessitates appropriate antibiotic therapy. Sarcoidosis may cause renal failure with granulomatous interstitial nephritis that is also responsive to treatment with corticosteroids; recurrence of disease is common, necessitating a long tapering schedule and the possible addition of other medications, including methotrexate. An idiopathic form of acute tubulointerstitial nephritis associated with uveitis occurs in adolescents; it may respond to a short course of corticosteroids.

The initial goal of the management of cell lysis syndromes—myoglobinuria, hemoglobinuria and tumor lysis—is the prevention of the electrolyte complications from cell breakdown (hyperkalemia, hyperphosphatemia, hyperuricemia, acidosis) and the prevention of progressive renal failure from the nephrotoxicity of myoglobin, hemoglobin, and uric acid. An initial fluid challenge of 10 to 20 mL/kg of isotonic fluid in combination with furosemide (initial dose, 2 mg/kg intravenously, increased to 5 mg/kg if there is no response in 2 to 3 hours) may initiate diuresis. If diuresis occurs with fluid challenge and furosemide, the goal of therapy is to maintain urine output of at least 2 and preferably up to 4 mL/kg/hour with vigorous hydration. Alkalinization of the urine to a pH of 6.5 to 8 increases the solubility and decreases the toxicity due to these tubular toxins. In children with tumor lysis syndrome, rasburicase is extremely effective at reducing serum uric acid concentrations and therefore decreases the risk of nephrotoxicity from hyperuricosuria. Volume status and serum electrolytes must be closely monitored. If renal failure is well established and diuresis fails to occur, urgent dialysis may be necessary to control hyperkalemia.

Treatment of ATN is supportive, although minimizing nephrotoxic medications and careful maintenance of intravascular volume are helpful conservative measures.

Postrenal Failure

Treatment for postrenal failure is relief of the obstruction. Bladder outlet obstruction caused by PUVs may be temporarily relieved by placement of an indwelling catheter, with eventual definitive repair by transurethral ablation of the valves. With other causes of obstruction, such as with ureteral stenosis in a child with a solitary kidney, urinary diversion (e.g., ureterostomies or pyelostomies) may be indicated, depending on the level of obstruction. If a child with an indwelling urinary catheter develops oliguria or anuria, the catheter should be flushed and successfully aspirated to ensure patency; if oliguria persists, a bladder sonogram may be helpful for checking proper catheter placement and bladder urine volume.

SUPPORTIVE MANAGEMENT OF RENAL FAILURE

Supportive care of renal failure includes careful fluid management, monitoring for and treatment of electrolyte problems, treatment of hypertension, and, in some cases, dialysis. Patients often need cardiac monitoring because of the risk of arrhythmias caused by electrolyte disturbances. Infection is common in renal failure and is a major cause of morbidity and mortality in patients with renal failure. Invasive monitoring procedures, including arterial and venous access and bladder catheterization, significantly increase the risk for infection. Sources of infection should be sought in patients with fever, clinical deterioration, hypotension, persistent catabolic state, or acidosis despite therapy. Medication dosages must be reviewed and adjusted for renal insufficiency. In addition, patients should receive adequate nutrition.

Fluid Management

Children with ARF present with a wide range of fluid states, ranging from severe dehydration to severe volume overload. Fluid management depends on the volume status at presentation, sources of ongoing fluid administration (e.g., nutrition, blood products) or fluid loss, and the amount of urine output. The main goal of fluid management is to maintain a normal intravascular volume. In some children, such as those with capillary leak syndrome or congestive heart failure, there may be total body fluid overload and edema, despite intravascular volume depletion. In children with volume depletion, the initial goal of therapy is correction of intravascular volume, albeit judiciously if renal failure is present. Oliguric children with prerenal failure may respond to a fluid bolus and volume replacement alone. Patients with prerenal failure should receive an initial fluid challenge of 10 to 20 mL/kg of isotonic fluid (e.g., 0.9% normal saline). Patients with severe dehydration or maldistribution of circulatory volume as a result of shock or sepsis may require repeated fluid boluses. On the other hand, in patients with volume overload, particularly in association with hyponatremia, hypertension, pulmonary edema, or congestive heart failure, fluid restriction is indicated and fluid removal with diuretics or renal replacement therapy may be necessary.

When the patient reaches a normal volume status, fluid management depends on carefully balancing intake and output. The patient should receive fluid to balance insensible losses, typically estimated to be about one third of standard maintenance fluids. In addition, ongoing losses (e.g., diarrhea, nasogastric, urine) should be replaced milliliter per milliliter with an appropriate replacement solution. Patients with ATN or after relief of urinary obstruction may enter a polyuric phase, with extremely high urine output. Provision of urine replacement to these patients is critical for preventing dehydration.

Fluid status should be carefully monitored and therapy adjusted appropriately. Monitoring includes physical examination for signs of volume depletion or volume overload, strict measurement of all intake and output, and daily weighings. Central venous pressure monitoring may be indicated in children with questionable intravascular volume status.

There is no evidence that use of diuretics alters the outcome in ARF. In some cases, however, diuretics are useful for addressing volume overload. A loop diuretic, such as furosemide, can be very effective in children with postinfectious glomerulonephritis, in which hypertension caused by fluid overload may be severe. In other instances, a loop diuretic is helpful in the management of hyperkalemia (see later discussion). In contrast, if a patient has not responded to a high dosage of a loop diuretic, then further dosing is usually futile and only exposes the patient to unnecessary toxicity.

Electrolyte Management

A variety of electrolyte problems can occur in patients with renal insufficiency. These may cause considerable morbidity and even mortality. Consequently, the patient should have regular monitoring, the frequency depending on the severity of the renal dysfunction, the underlying disease process, and the presence of electrolyte abnormalities, especially those that are imminently dangerous.

Sodium

Hyponatremia is more common in renal failure than is hypernatremia. Hyponatremia, which is usually mild, results from a decreased ability to excrete water. It is especially common in the patient with volume overload, and the primary treatment is fluid restriction. In rare instances, severe hyponatremia, especially if associated with symptoms such as seizures or obtundation, necessitates treatment with hypertonic saline (see Chapter 27). Overly rapid correction of hyponatremia may cause central pontine myelinosis.

Potassium

Hyperkalemia in renal failure is a consequence of decreased renal excretion of potassium. It may be especially severe in patients with tumor lysis syndrome, rhabdomyolysis, or hemolysis because of release of intracellular potassium. On occasion, patients with renal insufficiency have hypokalemia because of excessive potassium losses or poor intake. High losses may occur from the gastrointestinal tract (diarrhea or emesis) or urine (e.g., osmotic diuresis in diabetic ketoacidosis). Even when a patient with renal insufficiency has a normal or low serum potassium level, it is important to consider measures to prevent hyperkalemia. This should include restriction of oral and intravenous potassium, and discontinuation or judicious use of medications that may cause hyperkalemia (e.g., potassium-sparing diuretics, ACE inhibitors, succinylcholine). Blood transfusions can be a significant source of exogenous potassium. Washing the cells before transfusion can reduce the potassium load.

Hyperkalemia may cause symptoms such as muscle weakness, twitching and cramping, ascending paralysis, and cardiac rhythm disturbances. Some patients may be asymptomatic but still have potentially lethal changes on electrocardiography, which emphasizes the importance of cardiac monitoring. Peaked T waves are the classic initial electrocardiographic abnormality, but this may be followed by a prolonged PR interval and widening of the QRS complex. The end result can be ventricular fibrillation or asystole.

The two goals in treating hyperkalemia are acute prevention of arrhythmias and removal of potassium from the body (Table 26-8). A patient with a significant elevation in potassium or an abnormal electrocardiogram should receive the measures for acute prevention of arrhythmias. These measures are just temporizing, and must be followed by efforts to eliminate potassium.

Table 26-8. Treatment of Hyperkalemia

Acute Prevention of Arrhythmias
Membrane stabilization
  Calcium chloride or calcium gluconate
Shift potassium intracellularly
  Sodium bicarbonate
  Insulin plus glucose
  Nebulized albuterol

Removal of Potassium from the Body
Sodium polystyrene (Kayexalate), oral or rectal
Loop diuretic
Dialysis

Phosphorus

Hyperphosphatemia occurs in renal failure as a result of decreased renal excretion. Hyperphosphatemia causes calcium and phosphate to precipitate in tissues. The most important immediate consequence is hypocalcemia, but if this is severe or long-standing, it leads to dangerous tissue calcification. Treatment focuses on minimizing phosphorus intake and the use of oral phosphorus binders, which complex with phosphorus in food to prevent its absorption. Binders, such as calcium carbonate, work best if given with food, although there is some effect even in patients without oral intake. Recalcitrant hyperphosphatemia, especially if associated with hypocalcemia, can be treated with dialysis.

Calcium

Hypocalcemia is common in renal failure as a result of poor absorption of intestinal calcium because of the lack of 1,25-dihydroxyvitamin D, which is synthesized in the kidneys. In addition, hyperphosphatemia, as detailed previously, can further exacerbate hypocalcemia. Hypocalcemia may cause paresthesias, tetany, seizures, and electrocardiographic abnormalities, including prolongation of the QT interval, heart block, and ventricular fibrillation. Treatment focuses on control of hyperphosphatemia and administration of calcium (oral or intravenous) and 1,25-dihydroxyvitamin D (oral or intravenous).

Acid-Base Balance

A metabolic acidosis frequently occurs in renal failure as a result of decreased acid excretion. In addition, underlying conditions, such as diabetic ketoacidosis or sepsis causing a lactic acidosis, may exacerbate the problem. The initial therapeutic focus should be correction of underlying problems (e.g., volume depletion) that may be contributing to the acidosis. Normally, the kidneys respond to an acidosis by increasing acid excretion. Because this cannot occur in many patients with renal failure, therapy also usually requires administration of base, either intravenously or orally. Dialysis is another effective therapy for acidosis.

Hypertension

Hypertension associated with renal failure may be caused by the primary disease or by intravascular volume overload. Although hypertension is defined as blood pressure elevation greater than the 90th to 95th percentiles for age and stature, the level of blood pressure elevation that defines severe hypertension is not as well established (see Chapter 12). For the purpose of management, severe hypertension may be defined as systolic or diastolic blood pressure significantly (>20 mm Hg) above the 95th percentile, or symptomatic hypertension. The goal of treatment is to attain a safe and gradual decrease in blood pressure to within the normal range. An abrupt decrease in blood pressure should be avoided because of the risk of cerebral hypoperfusion, hypotension, and worsening renal perfusion. For children with severe hypertension or hypertensive crisis, one third of the blood pressure reduction should be accomplished in the first 6 hours of therapy and the remaining two thirds in 36 to 72 hours. Severe or symptomatic hypertension is best managed in an intensive care unit setting, in which blood pressure and medication response can be closely monitored; however, it is often necessary to initiate therapy in the emergency department or hospital ward.

In addition to medications, the management of hypertension associated with volume overload and complications of congestive heart failure and pulmonary edema should include volume restriction, diuretics, and possibly dialysis for the anuric or oliguric patient. Various medications are available for acute and chronic management of hypertension (see Chapter 12).

Table 26-9. Indications for Renal Replacement Therapies for Children with Renal Failure

Volume Management

Symptoms of volume overload, including congestive heart failure, pulmonary edema, hypertension

Oliguria or anuria with anticipated need for significant infusion of volume, including medications, parenteral nutrition, and blood products

Anticipation of prolonged course of renal failure that limits nutritional intake because of protein and fluid restrictions

Management of Electrolyte and Metabolic Disturbances

Symptomatic hyperkalemia refractory to medical therapy

Symptomatic hyponatremia caused by volume overload

Hypocalcemia with severe hyperphosphatemia

Symptomatic uremia, rapidly rising BUN, or BUN > 100 mg/dL

Anticipation of continued potassium or phosphorus loading caused by tissue injury, tumor lysis, or rhabdomyolysis

Management of Acid/Base Balance

Severe metabolic acidosis necessitating significant bicarbonate therapy

Toxin Removal (e.g., Ethylene Glycol)

BUN, blood urea nitrogen.

Renal Replacement Therapy

There are various indications for renal replacement therapy (Table 26-9). Many children and adolescents with renal failure can be treated conservatively with judicious fluid and electrolyte management without the need for dialysis. However, ultrafiltration and dialysis therapies play a significant role in the management of ARF for selected patients. Acute dialysis and ultrafiltration therapy can be life-saving in the treatment of symptomatic hyperkalemia, significant volume overload, and severe uremia and in the removal of certain toxins. Several key concepts are important in understanding the indications for specific renal replacement therapies. Therapies available for pediatric patients include peritoneal dialysis, intermittent

hemofiltration, intermittent hemodialysis (IHD), and the continuous renal replacement therapies, which include continuous venovenous hemofiltration, and continuous venovenous hemofiltration with dialysis (CVVHD). Dialysis is the removal of solutes down concentration gradients by diffusion and convection across semipermeable membranes. An artificial membrane filter serves as the membrane in hemodialysis therapies (intermittent hemodialysis, CVVHD), whereas the highly vascular peritoneal membrane is used with peritoneal dialysis. Ultrafiltration is the net removal of fluid from the patient and can be accomplished by hydrostatic pressure (from pump-generated pressure gradients with hemofiltration, intermittent hemodialysis, continuous venovenous hemofiltration, and CVVHD) or by the use of hyperosmolar solutions with peritoneal dialysis. Solutes may also be removed by convection, which is the drag of solvent that accompanies fluid removal. Significant removal of solute can also be attained by convection with ultrafiltration therapy alone when a large amount of fluid is removed with the simultaneous intravenous infusion of physiologically appropriate replacement fluid.

The choice of therapy depends on the indication for renal replacement therapy, the size and condition of the patient, and the experience and expertise of the physicians and nursing staff (Table 26-10). In general, solute and fluid removal is most efficient and can be regulated more tightly with hemodialysis and hemofiltration therapies than with peritoneal dialysis. However, these therapies require vascular access with relatively large-bore catheters, which carry inherent risks of inadequate flow, thrombosis, anticoagulation, and infection. Other potential risks include hemolysis, thrombocytopenia, electrolyte abnormalities, hypothermia, and acute hypotension. Intermittent hemodialysis typically is performed over 3 to 4 hours; the fluid and solute removal required in this time frame to obtain and maintain a euvolemic state may be substantial and may be poorly tolerated by some patients, particularly infants, small children, and critically ill or hypotensive patients. The continuous renal replacement therapies allow gradual removal of fluid and solute throughout the day, allowing better maintenance of homeostasis and avoiding potentially significant shifts of volume and electrolytes.

In contrast, peritoneal dialysis entails relatively easy access with the possibility of placement of an acute dialysis catheter at the patient's bedside or surgical placement of a cuffed catheter tunneled through subcutaneous tissue into the peritoneal space. There is an increased risk of catheter leak and infection with bedside catheter placement. Peritoneal dialysis can be safely performed in patients of

Table 26-10. Renal Replacement Therapies for Children with Renal Failure

Therapy (Description)	Advantages	Disadvantages	Typical patients
Peritoneal dialysis (dialysis with ultrafiltration)	Continuous therapy Relatively easy access and procedure	Less precise control of solute and fluid removal Contraindicated with acute abdomen	Small infants and children Patients with difficult vascular access
Intermittent hemofiltration (ultrafiltration without dialysis)	Removal of volume over short time interval	Vascular access Anticoagulation Acute fluid shift	Relatively stable children with volume overload
Intermittent hemodialysis (dialysis with or without ultrafiltration)	Quick and efficient therapy Rapid correction of fluid and electrolyte abnormalities	Vascular access Anticoagulation Acute fluid and electrolyte shifts	Relatively stable older children
Continuous venovenous hemofiltration (ultrafiltration without dialysis)	Prevents significant fluid shifts Fluid removal adapted hourly to patient need	Vascular access Anticoagulation Immobilization of patient Intensive nursing care	Critically ill children
Continuous venovenous hemofiltration and dialysis (dialysis with or without ultrafiltration)	Fluid and electrolyte homeostasis maintained continuously	Vascular access Anticoagulation Immobilization of patient Intensive nursing care	Critically ill children

all ages, including premature infants of very low birth weight. Peritoneal dialysis can be performed continuously, with frequency of dialysate exchanges and osmolality of dialysate tailored to the volume status, BUN level, and electrolyte status of the patient. Hourly exchanges are often initiated for critically ill, hypervolemic, and hyperkalemic patients; exchanges are needed less frequently for more stable patients. Peritoneal dialysis may not be possible in infants and children with acute abdominal processes, including necrotizing enterocolitis. Abdominal distention with dialysate may also compromise the respiratory status of children with respiratory failure.

CLINICAL COURSE AND PROGNOSIS

In children with prerenal failure, fluid resuscitation with correction of the underlying causes and appropriate supportive therapy often results in recovery of renal function and normal urine output within 24 to 48 hours. Once ARF is established, the course and prognosis are the same as those for intrinsic renal failure.

The clinical course of intrinsic renal failure depends on the cause and degree of parenchymal damage. The initiation phase of ATN is typically followed by a maintenance phase of renal failure lasting from several days up to weeks, with possible complete recovery of renal function. As in renal recovery after relief of obstruction, a period of significant diuresis may occur until the integrity of damaged tubular epithelium is restored. The recovery phase with repair and regeneration of tubular epithelium is a particularly vulnerable period during which interruption of renal recovery with further ischemia, hypotension, hypovolemia, or nephrotoxic agents may result in irreversible damage. Progression to end-stage renal disease is associated with the development of cortical necrosis. Reported mortality rates (5% to 45%) vary considerably because of definitions of renal failure (e.g., need for dialysis), and differences in the population of patients studied. Increased mortality rates are associated with renal failure caused by sepsis, shock, hypotension, multisystem organ failure, cancer, respiratory failure, and cardiac disease, whereas children with primary renal disease as the cause of ARF have a relatively low risk of mortality. However, most children with ARF recover normal renal function. Follow-up of children who have recovered from ARF is recommended, because 5% to 10% of children may develop chronic renal dysfunction over time.

Oliguria and renal failure associated with HUS typically lasts from several days to several weeks. Although renal failure persisting beyond 4 weeks is associated with a worse prognosis, renal recovery has been reported in a few children requiring dialysis for up to 6 months. Eighty-five percent to 90% of children with diarrhea-associated HUS have full recovery of renal function. In contrast, only 50% to 65% of children with atypical or non–diarrhea-associated HUS recover renal function. Long-term follow-up is recommended because studies have demonstrated persistent urinary abnormalities, renal scarring, and alteration of renal function in up to 25% of children who had renal recovery after HUS.

For children with renal failure caused by obstruction, renal recovery is highly dependent on the duration and severity of the obstruction and the extent of renal parenchymal damage. Prolonged obstruction of the urinary tract during fetal development, as with PUVs, often results in irreversible renal scarring and dysplasia. Its clinical course is highly variable, ranging from recovery of normal renal function to progression to end-stage renal disease. Acute diuresis after the relief of obstruction is common and results from improvement in renal vascular flow and glomerular filtration beyond the reabsorptive capacity of the damaged tubular epithelium. If significant renal parenchymal damage has been established, initial improvement in renal function after repair of the obstruction is often followed by progression to end-stage renal disease over a period of several months or gradual progression over a number of years.

Table 26-11. Red Flags and Appropriate Actions

Red Flag	Action
Glomerulonephritis with rapidly deteriorating renal function	Biopsy and probable immuno-suppressive therapy
Renal failure caused by tumor lysis or rhabdomyolysis	Aggressive fluid management and a low threshold for initiating dialysis
Symptomatic hypertension	Control of blood pressure, usually in an intensive care unit
Prerenal failure caused by volume depletion	Volume resuscitation
Postrenal failure	Relief of obstruction

SUMMARY AND RED FLAGS

The child with renal failure should be evaluated for prerenal, intrinsic renal, and postrenal causes. It is also important to consider the possibility that the first visit represents the initial manifestation of CRF. Management is mostly supportive, although there are important red flags indicating the need for urgent, specific therapy (Table 26-11).

REFERENCES

Acute Renal Failure

Badr KF, Ichikawa I: Prerenal failure: A deleterious shift from renal compensation to decompensation. N Engl J Med 1988;319:623-629.
Brady JR, Singer GG: Acute renal failure. Lancet 1995;346:1533-1540.
Breen D, Bihari D: Acute renal failure as a part of multiple organ failure: The slippery slope of critical illness. Kidney Int 1998;53:S25-S33.
Flynn JT: Causes, management approaches, and outcome of acute renal failure in children. Curr Opin Pediatr 1998;10:184-189.
Moghal NE, Brocklebank JT, Meadow SR: A review of acute renal failure in children: Incidence, etiology, and outcome. Clin Nephrol 1998;49:91-95.
Rossi R, Kleta R, Ehrich JH: Renal involvement in children with malignancies. Pediatr Nephrol 1999;13:153-162.
Siegel NJ, Van Why SK, Devarajan P, et al: Pathogenesis of acute renal failure. In Barratt TM, Avner ED, Harmon WE (eds): Pediatric Nephrology, 4th ed. Baltimore, Lippincott Williams & Wilkins, 1999, pp 1109-1118.
Stewart CI, Kaskel FJ, Fine RN: Acute renal failure in children and newborns: Pathophysiology, clinical patterns, and therapeutic approach. In Ronco C, Bellomo R (eds): Critical Care Nephrology. Dordrecht, The Netherlands, Kluwer Academic, 1998, pp 821-829.
Thadhani R, Pascual M, Bonventre JV: Acute renal failure. N Engl J Med 1996;334:1448-1460.
Toth-Heyn P, Drukker A, Guignard JP: The stressed neonatal kidney: From pathophysiology to clinical management of neonatal vasomotor nephropathy. Pediatr Nephrol 2000;14:227-239.

Creatinine Clearance

Schwartz GJ, Brion LP, Spitzer A: The use of plasma creatinine concentration for estimating glomerular filtration in infants, children, and adolescents. Pediatr Clin North Am 1987;34:571.

Specific Causes

Hawkins EP, Berry PL, Silva FG: Acute tubulointerstitial nephritis in children: Clinical, morphologic, and lectin studies. Am J Kidney Dis 1989;14:466-471.
Jones DP, Mahmoud H, Chesney RW: Tumor lysis syndrome: Pathogenesis and management. Pediatr Nephrol 1995;9:206-212.

Schaller S, Kaplan BS: Acute nonoliguric renal failure in children associated with nonsteroidal anti-inflammatory agents. Pediatr Emerg Care 1998;14:416-418.

Zager RA: Rhabdomyolysis and myohemoglobinuric acute renal failure. Kidney Int 1996;49:314-326.

Hemolytic Uremic Syndrome

Kaplan BS, Meyers KE, Schulman SL: The pathogenesis and treatment of hemolytic uremic syndrome. J Am Soc Nephrol 1998;9:1126-1133.

Neild GH: Hemolytic uremic syndrome/thrombotic thrombocytopenic purpura: Pathophysiology and treatment. Kidney Int 1998;53: S45-S49.

Siegler RL: Spectrum of extrarenal involvement in postdiarrheal hemolytic-uremic syndrome. J Pediatr 1994;124:511-518.

Siegler RL: The hemolytic uremic syndrome. Pediatr Clin North Am 1995;42:1505-1529.

Trachtman H, Christen E: Pathogenesis, treatment, and therapeutic trials in hemolytic uremic syndrome. Curr Opin Pediatr 1999;11:162-168.

Management

Andreoli SP: Management of acute renal failure. In Barratt TM, Avner ED, Harmon WE (eds): Pediatric Nephrology, 4th ed. Baltimore, Lippincott Williams & Wilkins, 1999, pp 1119-1133.

Better OS, Stein JH: Early management of shock and prophylaxis of acute renal failure in traumatic rhabdomyolysis. N Engl J Med 1990;322: 825-829.

Conger JD: Interventions in clinical acute renal failure: What are the data? Am J Kidney Dis 1995;26:565-576.

Gouyon JB, Guignard JP: Management of acute renal failure in newborns. Pediatr Nephrol 2000;14:1037-1044.

Niaudet P, Habib R: Methylprednisolone pulse therapy in the treatment of severe forms of Schönlein-Henoch purpura. Pediatr Nephrol 1998;12: 238-243.

Hyperkalemia

Ohlsson A, Hosking M: Complications following oral administration of exchange resins in extremely low birth weight infants. Eur J Pediatr 1987;146:571-574.

Rodriguez-Soriano J: Potassium homeostasis and its disturbances in children. Pediatr Nephrol 1995;9:364-374.

Hypertension

Fivush B, Neu A, Furth S: Acute hypertensive crises in children: Emergencies and urgencies. Curr Opin Pediatr 1997;9:233-236.

Flynn JT, Mottes TA, Prophy PD, et al: Intravenous nicardipine for treatment of severe hypertension in children. J Pediatr 2001;139:7-9.

Sinaiko AR: Hypertension in children. N Engl J Med 1996;335:1968-1973.

Tenney F, Sakarcan A: Nicardipine is a safe and effective agent in pediatric hypertensive emergencies. Am J Kidney Dis 2000;35:E20.

Update on the 1987 Task Force Report on High Blood Pressure in Children and Adolescents: A working group report from the National High Blood Pressure Education Program. National High Blood Pressure Education Program Working Group on Hypertension Control in Children and Adolescents. Pediatrics 1996;98:649-658.

Renal Replacement Therapy

Bunchman TE, Maxvold NJ, Kershaw DB, et al: Continuous venovenous hemodiafiltration in infants and children. Am J Kidney Dis 1995;25:17-21.

Chadha V, Warady BA, Blowey DL, et al: Tenckhoff catheters are superior to Cook catheters in pediatric acute peritoneal dialysis. Am J Kidney Dis 2000;35:1111-1116.

Donckerwolcke RA, Bunchman TE: Hemodialysis in infants and small children. Pediatr Nephrol 1994;8:103-106.

Lowrie LH: Renal replacement therapies in pediatric multiorgan dysfunction syndrome. Pediatr Nephrol 2000;14:6-12.

Maxvold NJ, Smoyer WE, Gardner JJ, et al: Management of acute renal failure in the pediatric patient: Hemofiltration vs. hemodialysis. Am J Kidney Dis 1997;30:S84-S88.

Reznick VM, Griswold WR, Peterson, RA, et al: Peritoneal dialysis for acute renal failure in children. Pediatr Nephrol 1991;5:715-717.

Outcome

Arora P, Kher V, Rai PK, et al: Prognosis of acute renal failure in children: A multivariate analysis. Pediatr Nephrol 1997;11:153-155.

Blowey DL, McFarland K, Alon U, et al: Peritoneal dialysis in the neonatal period: Outcome data. J Perinatol 1993;13:59-64.

Gallego N, Perez-Caballero C, Gallego A, et al: Prognosis of patients with acute renal failure without cardiopathy. Arch Dis Child 2001;84:258-260.

Goldstein SL, Currier H, Graf C, et al: Outcome in children receiving continuous venovenous hemofiltration. Pediatrics 2001;107:1309-1312.

Small G, Watson AR, Evans JH, et al: Hemolytic uremic syndrome: Defining the need for long-term followup. Clin Nephrol 1999;52:352-356.

27 Acid-Base and Electrolyte Disturbances

Vimal Chadha   Uri S. Alon

Acid-base and electrolyte disorders are commonly seen in pediatric practice. The presence of such a disorder may explain a patient's symptoms or may lead to a specific diagnosis.

ACID-BASE DISORDERS

The hydrogen ion concentration is measured in pH units. The pH is the negative logarithm of H^+ concentration ($pH = -\log_{10} [H^+]$). The normal systemic arterial pH is maintained within a narrow limit of 7.35 to 7.45 (venous blood has a slightly lower pH: 7.31 to 7.41) to ensure normal physiologic functioning of enzymes and other cellular processes. Because bicarbonate/carbonic acid is the most abundant buffer system in the body, the body pH is determined by the ratio of bicarbonate to carbonic acid and is expressed by the Henderson-Hasselbalch equation as follows:

$$pH = 6.1 + \log_{10}\left[\frac{HCO_3^- \text{ (conjugate base)}}{0.03 \times PCO_2 \text{ (carbonic acid)}}\right]$$

Because carbonic acid is not measured routinely, and because its concentration is directly proportional to the partial pressure of CO_2 (PCO_2) multiplied by its solubility coefficient (0.03), this buffer system is practically characterized in terms of the HCO_3^-/PCO_2 relationship.

Alterations in hydrogen ion concentration cause the clinical problems of acid-base disorders. A $[H^+]$ exceeding 45 nmol/L ($pH < 7.35$) is defined as acidosis, and a $[H^+]$ of less than 35 nmol/L ($pH > 7.45$) is defined as alkalosis. These disorders are further classified as either metabolic or respiratory in origin, on the basis of primary change in HCO_3^- or PCO_2, respectively.

In order to maintain body homeostasis, changes in $[H^+]$ are resisted by a complex system of body defense mechanisms, which include extracellular and intracellular chemical buffers, respiratory compensation by the lungs, and metabolic compensation by the kidneys.

Chemical buffering is the first line of defense. In metabolic disorders, mainly extracellular buffers (bicarbonate) rapidly titrate the addition of strong acids or bases. Intracellular buffers chiefly accomplish the buffering of respiratory disorders. Secondary respiratory compensation (change in ventilation) for metabolic acid-base disorders begins within minutes and is usually complete in 12 to 24 hours. In contrast, secondary metabolic compensation for respiratory disorders occurs more slowly, beginning within hours but requiring 2 to 5 days for completion. The kidneys increase net acid excretion in response to a primary respiratory acidosis; renal net acid excretion also increases during a metabolic acidosis if the kidneys themselves are not the cause of the metabolic acidosis. The expected compensation for primary acid-base disorders is shown in Table 27-1. These compensatory mechanisms, however, never return the pH back to normal (except occasionally in the case of respiratory alkalosis) until the underlying disease process has subsided or has been effectively treated.

When only one primary acid-base abnormality occurs and its compensatory mechanisms are activated, the disorder is classified as a simple acid-base disorder. When a combination of acid-base disturbances occurs, the disorder is classified as a mixed acid-base disorder. The latter should be suspected if the compensation in a given patient differs from the predicted values shown in Table 27-1.

Interpretation of data in infants and young children requires caution. Crying results in hyperventilation and can quickly change PCO_2 and consequently pH.

MANIFESTATION OF ACID-BASE DISORDERS

Acid-base disturbances are usually detected on routine blood investigations in a sick patient. The signs and symptoms associated with acid-base abnormality are generally nonspecific or are dominated by the features of the underlying disease. Metabolic acidosis results in increased respiratory work because of respiratory compensation. In severe acidosis ($pH < 7.20$), the respiratory pattern is characterized by deep and rapid breaths (Kussmaul respiration). Severe acidosis may also lead to hypotension, pulmonary edema, and, ultimately, asystole; its harmful effects are accentuated in the presence of hypoxia. Chronic metabolic acidosis leads to growth retardation and causes hypercalciuria and bone disease as bone buffering leads to marked mineral losses.

Similarly, there are no pathognomonic symptoms or signs of metabolic alkalosis. Careful examination of the child may detect hypoventilation. Severe alkalosis ($pH > 7.55$) can lead to tissue hypoxia, mental confusion, obtundation, muscular irritability, tetany, and an increased risk of seizures and cardiac arrhythmias. Some of these signs and symptoms are related to decreased concentration of serum ionized calcium as a result of its increased binding to protein in the presence of alkalosis.

RENAL REGULATION OF ACID-BASE BALANCE

The kidneys are the principal regulator of bicarbonate homeostasis. The renal regulation of HCO_3^- can be divided into two processes: (1) reclamation of filtered HCO_3^-, which occurs mostly in the proximal tubule, and (2) excretion of H^+ and, as a consequence, generation of new bicarbonate, which takes place primarily in the distal tubule and collecting duct. The excretion of acid by the kidneys is necessary because of normal endogenous acid production.

Most (80% to 90%) of the filtered HCO_3^- is reabsorbed in the proximal tubule. Bicarbonate reabsorption at this site is increased by contraction of the extracellular fluid (ECF) volume, activation of the renin-angiotensin system (mainly through the effect of angiotensin II), an elevated PCO_2, and hypokalemia. Conversely, HCO_3^- reabsorption is decreased when there is expansion of the ECF volume, inhibition of angiotensin II, a fall in PCO_2, and an elevation of the parathyroid hormone level.

The distal tubule and collecting duct regenerate bicarbonate via H^+ ion secretion into the tubular lumen by a H^+–adenosine triphosphatase (H^+-ATPase) pump in the luminal membrane. This active secretion can generate a H^+ ion gradient of 1000:1 between tubular fluid and cells, permitting the urine pH to fall to as low as 4.5.

Table 27-1. Expected Compensation for Primary Acid-Base Disorders*

Disorder	Primary Event	Compensation	Degree of Compensation
Metabolic acidosis	$\downarrow$ [HCO$_3^-$]	$\downarrow$ PCO$_2$	For 1 mEq/L $\downarrow$ [HCO$_3^-$], PCO$_2$ $\downarrow$ 1-1.5 mm Hg
Metabolic alkalosis	$\uparrow$ [HCO$_3^-$]	$\uparrow$ PCO$_2$	For 1 mEq/L $\uparrow$ [HCO$_3^-$], PCO$_2$ $\uparrow$ 0.5-1 mm Hg
Respiratory acidosis			
Acute (<12-24 hr)	$\uparrow$ PCO$_2$	$\uparrow$ [HCO$_3^-$]	For 10 mm Hg $\uparrow$ PCO$_2$, [HCO$_3^-$] $\uparrow$ 1 mEq/L
Chronic (3-5 days)	$\uparrow$ PCO$_2$	$\uparrow\uparrow$ [HCO$_3^-$]	For 10 mm Hg $\uparrow$ PCO$_2$, [HCO$_3^-$] $\uparrow$ 4 mEq/L
Respiratory alkalosis			
Acute (<12 hr)	$\downarrow$ PCO$_2$	$\downarrow$ [HCO$_3^-$]	For 10 mm Hg $\downarrow$ PCO$_2$, [HCO$_3^-$] $\downarrow$ 1-3 mEq/L
Chronic (1-2 days)	$\downarrow$ PCO$_2$	$\downarrow\downarrow$ [HCO$_3^-$]	For 10 mm Hg $\downarrow$ PCO$_2$, [HCO$_3^-$] $\downarrow$ 2-5 mEq/L

From Brewer ED: Disorders of acid-base balance. Pediatr Clin North Am 1990;37:429-447.

*Normal serum [HCO$_3^-$] is 24 mEq/L, and normal arterial partial pressure of carbon dioxide (PCO$_2$) is 40 mm Hg.

$\downarrow$, decrease; $\downarrow\downarrow$, greater decrease; $\uparrow$, increase; $\uparrow\uparrow$, greater increase.

The active H$^+$ secretion is significantly influenced by the luminal electronegativity caused by active Na$^+$ reabsorption in the cortical collecting duct. Thus, in the cortical collecting duct, H$^+$ excretion is influenced by distal Na$^+$ delivery and reabsorption. In contrast, in the outer medullary portion of the collecting duct, aldosterone stimulates the H$^+$ excretion independently of Na$^+$ delivery or reabsorption. Some of the H$^+$ secreted is consumed in reclaiming the small amount of HCO$_3^-$ that escaped reabsorption at proximal sites; the rest of the H$^+$ is excreted in the urine. The ability to excrete large amount of H$^+$ ions is dependent on the presence of buffers. The H$^+$ ions are buffered by phosphates and, to a lesser extent, by other nonreabsorbable anions. The other very important urinary buffer is ammonia (NH$_3$), which combines with a secreted H$^+$ to generate an ammonium ion (NH$_4^+$). The proximal tubular cells generate ammonia through the metabolism of the amino acid glutamine. For every H$^+$ that is finally excreted, a HCO$_3^-$ is added to the ECF compartment. Metabolic acidosis by itself enhances NH$_4^+$ production and excretion. Ammonia genesis by proximal tubular cells is also stimulated by hypokalemia, whereas hyperkalemia inhibits ammonia genesis. The ability of the kidney to produce ammonia is markedly decreased in conditions such as chronic renal failure, as a result of reduced renal mass, and in some types of renal tubular acidosis (RTA).

The amount of bicarbonate that is generated daily is equal to the net acid excretion by the kidneys and, in healthy people, equals the amount of net endogenous production of nonvolatile acids. Nonvolatile acids cannot be converted to CO$_2$, and their elimination from the body is solely dependent on the kidneys. Their generation rate in adults is about 1 mEq per kilogram of body weight per day, and in children it is higher (1-3 mEq/kg/day) because of growth-associated metabolism.

Under normal physiologic conditions, approximately two thirds of net acid is excreted as ammonium. During sustained metabolic acidosis, ammonium excretion increases progressively to 6 to 10 times its baseline value and reaches its maximum by the fifth day. The ability to lower urine pH and increase net acid excretion in response to an acid load is achieved as soon as 4 to 6 weeks of age.

METABOLIC ACIDOSIS

A metabolic acidosis can result from addition of H$^+$ to the body, failure to excrete H$^+$, or loss of HCO$_3^-$. The differential diagnosis of metabolic acidosis is simplified by classifying the causes into those associated with a normal anion gap (also known as a hyperchloremic metabolic acidosis) and those associated with an increased anion gap. The various causes of a metabolic acidosis are shown in Table 27-2.

The anion gap is easily calculated: Na$^+$ − (Cl$^-$ + HCO$_3^-$). The anion gap, which is normally 8 to 16 mEq/L, is schematically represented in Figure 27-1. Whenever a strong acid (e.g., lactic acid) is added to or produced in the body, hydrogen ions are neutralized by bicarbonate,

HCO$_3^-$ is consumed by the H$^+$, and the bicarbonate concentration falls. The accompanying anion, such as lactate, is a new unmeasured anion, which increases the anion gap. The increase in the anion gap is usually proportional to the fall in serum [HCO$_3^-$]. In contrast, when HCO$_3^-$ is lost from the body, no new anion is generated. In this situation, there is a reciprocal increase in the serum Cl$^-$ to maintain electroneutrality. The anion gap does not change; the rise in [Cl$^-$] is proportional to the fall in [HCO$_3^-$].

Normal Anion Gap (Hyperchloremic) Metabolic Acidosis

Renal Tubular Acidosis

RTA is a group of disorders characterized by impairment of renal HCO$_3^-$ reabsorption and/or H$^+$ excretion in the presence of a relatively normal glomerular filtration rate (GFR). On the basis of

Table 27-2. Causes of Metabolic Acidosis

Normal Anion Gap (Hyperchloremic Acidosis)

Renal loss of bicarbonate
  Renal tubular acidosis
  Carbonic anhydrase inhibitor
  Potassium-sparing diuretics
Gastrointestinal loss of bicarbonate
  Diarrhea
  Fistulas or drainage of the small bowel or pancreas
  Ureteral sigmoidostomy
  Rectourethral fistula
  Use of anion exchange resins
Miscellaneous causes
  Recovery from ketoacidosis
  Dilutional acidosis
  Addition of HCl, NH$_4$Cl, arginine, or lysine hydrochloride
  Parenteral alimentation

Increased Anion Gap

Increased acid production
  Diabetic ketoacidosis
  Lactic acidosis of prematurity
  Inborn errors of metabolism
  Late metabolic acidosis of prematurity
  Poisonings (e.g., salicylate, ethylene glycol)
Failure of acid excretion
  Acute renal failure
  Chronic renal failure

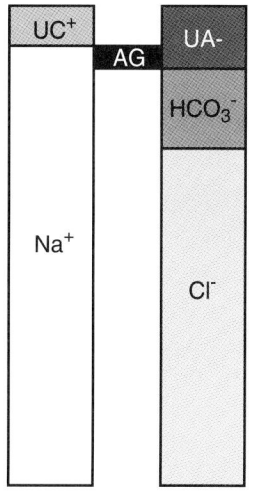
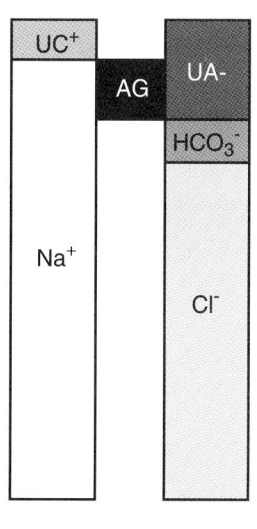
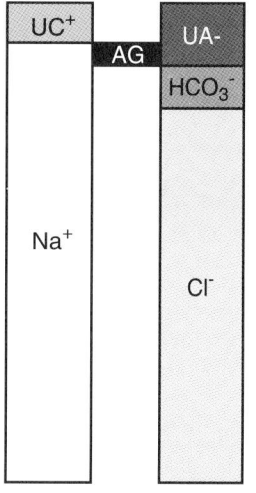

Normal

Increased anion-gap metabolic acidosis

Hyperchloremic normal anion-gap metabolic acidosis

Figure 27-1. Anion gap under conditions of normal acid-base balance and during metabolic acidosis. The increased anion gap with an elevated anion gap metabolic acidosis is secondary to an increase in unmeasured anions (e.g., lactate in lactic acidosis). Note that in cases with increased anion gap, serum chloride levels remain unchanged. AG, anion gap; UA^- = unmeasured anions; UC^+ = unmeasured cations.

the distinctive pathophysiologic features, three types of RTA—type I (distal or classic), type II (proximal or bicarbonate wasting), and type IV (hyperkalemic)—are recognized. The differentiating features of the three types of RTA are shown in Table 27-3.

Proximal RTA is caused by an impairment of HCO_3^- reabsorption in the proximal tubule and is characterized by a decreased renal HCO_3^- threshold. Because the distal acidification mechanisms are intact, these patients can lower the urine pH to less than 5.5 and can excrete adequate amounts of NH_4^+ when the serum HCO_3^- is below the threshold. Hence, their acidosis is usually less profound than that which occurs in distal RTA. However, when serum HCO_3^- is normalized by administration of alkali, a large fraction of HCO_3^- reaches the distal nephron, leading to an elevated urine pH. When the serum bicarbonate level is normalized, the fractional excretion of bicarbonate is increased (>15%). Associated with this increased HCO_3^- loss is an obligate loss of Na^+ and K^+ to maintain the urine electroneutrality. Therefore, polyuria and hypokalemia are quite common. In some patients, there may be an increase in urinary

calcium excretion, but because citrate excretion is normal, nephrocalcinosis is uncommon. Proximal RTA may in rare cases occur as an isolated defect, but it usually coexists with other defects in proximal tubule function. Fanconi syndrome is the combination of multiple defects in proximal tubule reabsorption and, in addition to type II RTA, includes excessive urinary losses of glucose, amino acids, phosphate, and uric acid. The excessive losses of phosphate often cause hypophosphatemic rickets. There are many causes of proximal RTA (Table 27-4).

Distal RTA is caused by the inability to secrete H^+ in the distal tubule and is characterized by a more profound acidosis than in proximal RTA and by the tendency to develop nephrocalcinosis and nephrolithiasis. This development results from the excretion of large quantities of calcium, combined with an alkaline urine pH and hypocitraturia. In addition to the deficient H^+ secretion, these patients are unable to increase ammonia genesis. The patient's urine pH remains alkaline (>5.5) despite extreme systemic metabolic acidosis. With normalization of serum HCO_3^- with alkali therapy,

Table 27-3. Differential Features of Various Types of Renal Tubular Acidosis in Children

Feature	Type I (Distal)	Type II (Proximal)	Type IV (Hyperkalemic)
Urine pH during acidosis	>5.5	<5.5	<5.5
Urine anion gap	Positive	Negative	Positive
$Fe_{HCO_3^-}$ at normal serum HCO_3^-	<5%*	>15%	<15%
Urine-to-blood PCO_2	<20 mm Hg	>20 mm Hg	<20 mm Hg
Serum potassium	Normal or ↓	Normal or ↓	↑
Calcium excretion	↑	Normal or ↑	Normal (?)
Citrate excretion	↓	Normal	Normal
Nephrocalcinosis	Common	Rare	Absent
Associated tubular defects	Rare	Common	Rare
Rickets	Rare	Common	Absent
Daily alkali requirement (mEq/kg/day)	1-4†	10-15	2-3
Potassium supplementation	No	Yes	No

Modified from Alon U, Chan JCM: Inherited forms of renal tubular acidosis. In Fernandes J, Sandubray JM, Tada K (eds): Inborn Metabolic Diseases: Diagnosis and Treatment. Berlin, Springer-Verlag, 1990.

*Losses are higher during infancy.

†Dosages are higher for infants.

Table 27-4. Clinical Spectrum of the Three Types of Renal Tubular Acidosis (RTA)

Proximal RTA	Distal RTA	Type IV RTA
Isolated	**Primary**	**Mineralocorticoid Deficiency**
Sporadic, transient in infancy	Transient in infancy	Aldosterone disorders ($\downarrow$ A, $\uparrow$ R)
Hereditary	Persistent	Addison disease
	Incomplete	Congenital adrenal hyperplasia
Fanconi Syndrome	Adult type	Primary hypoaldosteronism
Primary	With nerve deafness	Hyporeninemic hypoaldosteronism ($\downarrow$ A, $\downarrow$R)
Secondary	With bicarbonate wasting	
Inherited		**Other**
Cystinosis	**Secondary**	Obstructive uropathy
Wilson disease	Interstitial nephritis	Pyelonephritis
Lowe syndrome	Obstructive uropathy	Interstitial nephritis
Leigh syndrome	Reflux nephropathy	Nephrosclerosis
Galactosemia	Pyelonephritis	Diabetes mellitus
Glycogen storage disease type I	Transplant rejection	Chloride shunt syndrome ($\downarrow$ A, $\downarrow$ R)
Hereditary fructose intolerance	Lupus nephritis	Pseudohypoaldosteronism ($\uparrow$ A, $\uparrow$ R)
Tyrosinemia	Sickle cell nephropathy	Transient in infancy (normal A, normal R)
Mitochondrial cytopathies	Nephrocalcinosis	Unilateral kidney diseases
Metachromatic leukodystrophy	Medullary sponge kidney	Idiopathic
Medullary cystic disease		
Carbonic anhydrase II deficiency	**Other Causes**	
Acquired	Carbonic anhydrase II deficiency	
Heavy metals	Chronic active hepatitis	
Outdated tetracycline	Ehlers-Danlos syndrome	
Nephrotic syndrome	Elliptocytosis	
Interstitial nephritis	Osteopetrosis	
Hyperparathyroidism		
Vitamin D deficiency rickets	**Toxin or Drug Induced**	
Gentamicin	Lithium	
Cyclosporine	Amphotericin B	
	Analgesics	
	Toluene	

Modified from Bergstein JM: Renal tubular acidosis. In Behrman RE, Kliegman R, Jenson HB (eds): Nelson Textbook of Pediatrics, 16th ed. Philadelphia, WB Saunders, 2000.

A, aldosterone; R, renin; $\downarrow$, decreased; $\uparrow$, increased.

loss of bicarbonate in the urine varies with age; in children and adults, it is less than 3%; in infants, it might reach up to 15%, because of the greater role of bicarbonate reabsorption in the distal tubule during infancy. Hypercalcemia has been observed in some infants with distal RTA, but its mechanism remains unclear. Distal RTA may occur as an isolated condition or may develop secondary to several diseases, medications, or toxins (see Table 27-4).

Some patients have an incomplete distal RTA. They are able to maintain normal plasma HCO_3^- and systemic pH under most circumstances but do not respond appropriately to an acid challenge.

A syndrome with features of failure to thrive, RTA, osteopetrosis, and cerebral calcifications caused by deficiency of carbonic anhydrase II isoenzyme (the intracellular carbonic anhydrase) has been described. This condition is a mixed RTA. Usually the distal RTA is most apparent, but there are varying degrees of bicarbonate losses as a result of the proximal tubule involvement. Affected patients lack carbonic anhydrase II activity in their red blood cells.

Type IV RTA results from low circulating aldosterone concentrations or from partial or complete end-organ resistance to aldosterone. The various causes of mineralocorticoid deficiency are listed in Table 27-4. The lack of aldosterone effect impairs the establishment of the lumen negative electrochemical gradient that is favorable to H^+ ion secretion in the collecting duct. In addition, because of the lack of aldosterone effect, affected patients develop hyperkalemia, which is the most characteristic feature of type IV RTA and differentiates it from the other two types.

All forms of RTA are associated with growth failure. Associated symptoms may include vomiting, polyuria, and dehydration. Patients with full-blown Fanconi syndrome have severe rickets/osteomalacia

and malnutrition. Laboratory workup in all patients with RTA shows metabolic acidosis with hyperchloremia and a normal anion gap.

The urine pH always exceeds 5.5 in type I RTA but can be less than 5.5 in type II and type IV RTA. It should be measured on a fresh urine sample with a pH meter.

The amount of urine acid excretion can be measured indirectly by evaluating urinary net charge. Urine net charge (or urine anion gap = $Na^+ + K^+ - Cl^-$) is used as an indirect estimation of urinary NH_4^+ excretion. This test is valid only for the evaluation of hyperchloremic acidosis and should be conducted before acidosis is treated. The main cations in the urine are Na^+ and K^+ (Ca^{2+} and Mg^{2+} are present in small quantities). Ammonium is normally the other major cation present. In states of hyperchloremic acidosis, Cl^- is the only anion present in significant amount (phosphate, sulfate, and organic acids are present in small and relatively fixed quantities). When the acidification mechanism is intact, urinary Cl^- concentration exceeds that of Na^+ plus K^+ by an amount that is directly proportional to the amount of NH_4^+ in the urine (the urine net charge is negative). Conversely, the urine anion gap is positive (e.g., in distal RTA) when the urinary acidification mechanisms are abnormal and not enough NH_4^+ is excreted in response to the acidosis, and consequently less Cl^- is found in the urine.

Measuring the urine-to-blood PCO_2 gradient can help assess hydrogen ion secretion. In contrast to urine net charge, this test is performed in the presence of an alkaline urine (urine pH > 7.4, urine $HCO_3^- > 80$ mEq/L). The urine can be made alkaline by administering either exogenous alkali or acetazolamide. Acetazolamide (carbonic anhydrase inhibitor) prevents the proximal tubular reabsorption of HCO_3^-, thereby increasing its urinary concentration. The H^+ secreted into the collecting duct lumen combines with the

HCO_3^- to form H_2CO_3. Because carbonic anhydrase is absent in the lumen of this segment, the conversion to CO_2 and H_2O is slow and occurs largely in the urinary collecting system (renal pelvis, ureters, and urinary bladder). The ratio of surface area to volume at these sites is unfavorable for any significant CO_2 absorption, and as a result, CO_2 is trapped in the urine. In the presence of a normal distal H^+ secretion, the urine PCO_2 is greater than the blood PCO_2 by more than 20 mm Hg. Failure to achieve this gradient suggests impaired distal H^+ excretion. The sample for urine PCO_2 should be collected fresh, either under oil or in a narrow air-free syringe, and immediately analyzed in the laboratory for pH and PCO_2.

Because of the common occurrence of nephrocalcinosis, ultrasonography of the kidneys should be routinely included in the workup of patients with suspected RTA. Ultrasonography is also necessary in children with type IV RTA to exclude obstruction as a potential cause. A skeletal survey to look for rickets should also be done, especially in cases of proximal RTA. Patients with Fanconi syndrome should be evaluated for cystinosis, the most common cause of Fanconi syndrome in children. Some patients with inherited distal RTA have sensorineural deafness; therefore, infants and children with established distal RTA need routine audiograms.

In all forms of RTA, the cornerstone of therapy is adequate alkali administration. In patients with proximal RTA, very large quantities (10 to 15 mEq/kg/day) of base are required, and in some of these patients, achievement of normal serum bicarbonate concentration by oral alkali therapy alone is impossible. The treatment is complicated, inasmuch as increased alkali intake results in massive bicarbonaturia, which further aggravates the urinary potassium losses and hypokalemia. Therefore, at least half of the alkali should be in the form of potassium salts. Patients with Fanconi syndrome also require supplementation with phosphate, calcium, vitamin D, and, at times, thiazides and prostaglandin-synthetase inhibitors. In patients with secondary proximal RTA, treatment should be aimed at the primary disorder.

The alkali requirement of patients with distal RTA is significantly lower (1 to 4 mEq/kg/day) and is based on the sum of daily urine bicarbonate excretion plus 2 mEq/kg needed to buffer the daily endogenous acid production. The total daily dose might reach up to 15 mEq/kg during infancy when an element of bicarbonaturia exists. In contrast to the situation in patients with proximal RTA, little or no potassium supplementation is required during treatment of distal RTA. Most children with primary distal RTA have a permanent defect and require lifelong treatment.

Treatment of patients with type IV RTA depends on the primary cause. In patients with aldosterone deficiency, treatment with a mineralocorticoid, such as fludrocortisone (Florinef Acetate), corrects the acidosis and hyperkalemia as well as the salt wasting. Patients with chloride shunt syndrome require treatment with a thiazide diuretic. Patients with pseudohypoaldosteronism require treatment with large quantities of sodium chloride and sodium bicarbonate. The critical period is during infancy, and there is a relative gradual decline in the required dose of sodium chloride and sodium bicarbonate with advancing age. Patients who have partial end-organ resistance with no salt loss require only sodium bicarbonate.

Additional Causes of Renal Loss of Bicarbonate

Carbonic anhydrase inhibitors such as acetazolamide inhibit the carbonic anhydrase present in the proximal tubule, thus preventing the reabsorption of HCO_3^-. The net effect is similar to that of proximal RTA.

Potassium-sparing diuretics such as spironolactone or amiloride can impair H^+ secretion by the distal nephron by blocking Na^+ absorption in this segment.

Gastrointestinal Loss of Bicarbonate

In pediatric practice, *diarrhea* is the most common cause of hyperchloremic metabolic acidosis. The acidosis is secondary to loss of stool bicarbonate (which can be as high as 30 to 50 mEq/L). The expected body response is lowering of urine pH to less than 5.5. However, in the event of associated dehydration, the Na^+ delivery to the distal renal tubules can be markedly diminished, resulting in impaired acidification of the urine. This can lead to an unnecessary diagnostic workup for RTA. The results of the urine net charge ($Na^+ + K^+ - Cl^-$) can be misleading in the presence of dehydration, which causes a decrease in urinary sodium excretion. In addition, the secondary compensation by the kidneys (increased ammonia genesis) is slow to develop. The urinary findings in this situation should be interpreted with caution. The dehydration should be corrected and adequate urinary Na^+ concentration (>10 mEq/L) ensured before further studies to investigate RTA are conducted. Once proper precautions have been taken, the urine net charge is negative and urine-blood PCO_2 is higher than 20 mm Hg, if the acidosis is caused by increased gastrointestinal losses of HCO_3^-. In distal RTA, however, the urine net charge is positive and urine-blood PCO_2 is lower than 20 mm Hg.

The loss of fluid from the gastrointestinal tract from duodenum onward, either by drainage or through *fistulas,* causes acidosis by the same mechanisms as discussed previously. The drainage of urine into the colon (through ureterosigmoidostomy, rectourethral fistula) can result in metabolic acidosis caused by bowel mucosal secretion of HCO_3^-, which is then exchanged for Cl^-. *Anion exchange resins* can cause acidosis by exchanging Cl^- for HCO_3^-.

Miscellaneous Causes of Hyperchloremic Acidosis

Recovery from Ketoacidosis. During recovery from diabetic ketoacidosis (DKA), many patients may eliminate the organic anions (through increased renal clearance and utilization) faster than their acidosis resolves. The clinical picture can resemble normal anion gap acidosis.

Dilutional Acidosis. The rapid expansion of ECF volume with fluids that do not contain HCO_3^- leads to a dilution of HCO_3^- and mild metabolic acidosis. In addition, the expansion of ECF volume by itself promotes urinary HCO_3^- loss, possibly contributing to the dilutional acidosis.

Parenteral Alimentation. Amino acid infusions without concomitant administration of alkali (or alkali-generating precursors) may produce a normal anion gap acidosis in a manner similar to that of addition of HCl. This can be avoided by replacing the chloride salt of these amino acids with an acetate salt.

Increased Anion Gap Acidosis

Increased Acid Production

Diabetic Ketoacidosis. In DKA, the lack of insulin and excess of glucagon shunts free fatty acids into ketone body formation. The rate of formation of these ketone bodies, principally β-hydroxybutyrate and acetoacetate, exceeds the capacity for their peripheral utilization and renal excretion. Accumulation of these ketoacids (both of which are relatively strong acids and dissociate rapidly into H^+ and the ketoacid anions) results in metabolic acidosis. Acetone is formed by nonenzymatic conversion of acetoacetate and is responsible for the fruity odor of the patient's breath.

Patients with DKA typically present with altered sensorium, deep respirations, and severe increased anion gap metabolic acidosis with pH values that may be lower than 7.0. Initially, the increase in the anion gap is in proportion to the decrease in HCO_3^-, but once the patients start recovering with successful management, the kidneys clear the ketoacid anions, and the increase in the anion gap becomes less than the fall in HCO_3^-. The loss of ketoacid anions in urine increases the urinary losses of Na^+ and K^+ as the accompanying cations.

The diagnosis of DKA is made by the combination of increased anion gap metabolic acidosis, hyperglycemia, and demonstration of serum (or urine) ketoacid anions. During the phase of severe acidosis, the Acetest used to detect ketoacid anions can underestimate their actual content, because Acetest is relatively insensitive to β-hydroxybutyrate, which is the dominant ketoacid anion present in severe acidosis.

The therapy for DKA includes insulin, volume repletion, and correction of electrolyte disturbances. Most patients with DKA present with considerable total body deficits of potassium, magnesium, and phosphorus, even though serum levels, particularly of potassium, may actually be high on presentation. The role of bicarbonate buffer therapy in the management of DKA is controversial. The potential hazards associated with this therapy are discussed later in the section on acute therapy for metabolic acidosis.

Lactic Acidosis. Carbohydrates, through the glycolytic pathway, are metabolized to pyruvate, which then undergoes oxidative metabolism within the mitochondria. Under anaerobic conditions, pyruvate is converted to lactate. Under normal conditions, lactate is formed in relatively small amounts and is further metabolized by the liver. Pathologic conditions associated with either local or systemic hypoxia or ischemia, hypotension (shock), impaired oxidative metabolism, or impaired hepatic clearance can cause significant lactic acidosis.

The diagnosis of lactic acidosis must be considered in all forms of increased anion gap metabolic acidosis, because this is a very common cause of acidosis in sick patients. The diagnosis can be confirmed by measuring the serum lactate level. Treatment must be directed at the underlying pathophysiologic process. Buffer therapy with sodium bicarbonate has not been found to be effective and may be deleterious. Some studies have reported usefulness of dichloroacetate, a buffer that stimulates lactate metabolism.

Inborn Errors of Metabolism. Most patients with inborn errors of metabolism that cause a metabolic acidosis present in the neonatal period or shortly thereafter. Organic acidemias, aminoacidopathies, disorders of fatty acid oxidation, mitochondrial disorders, and defects in carbohydrate metabolism are associated with acidosis. Associated presenting signs and symptoms may include vomiting, failure to thrive, lethargy, seizures, developmental abnormalities, hepatomegaly, and elevated blood or urine levels of a particular metabolite. Urea cycle disorders during the first few days of life manifest with *respiratory alkalosis* because of stimulation of the respiratory center by increased ammonia levels.

Poisonings. A variety of toxic agents may be associated with increased anion gap metabolic acidosis. Some examples include salicylate intoxication, ethylene glycol (a component of antifreeze), and methanol. Carbon monoxide, cyanide poisoning, or methemoglobinemia induces hypoxic acidosis.

Classically, salicylate intoxication is described as causing respiratory alkalosis (stimulation of the respiratory center), followed by increased anion gap metabolic acidosis (accumulation of salicylic acid itself and lactic acidosis as a result of uncoupling of mitochondrial oxidative phosphorylation). However, children may present with simple increased anion gap metabolic acidosis. Nausea, tinnitus, noncardiogenic pulmonary edema, and prolonged prothrombin time are other associated features.

Alkalization of the blood and urine with sodium bicarbonate is beneficial despite the potential problems associated with its use in acute metabolic acidosis. Alkalization of the plasma decreases the diffusion of salicylate into the central nervous system, and alkaline urine improves renal excretion. In severe poisoning, hemodialysis is quite effective at removing salicylate from the body. In cases of poisonings, dialysis serves the dual purposes of removing the poison (if dialyzable) and correcting the acid-base and electrolyte abnormalities.

Failure of Acid Excretion

In both *acute* and *chronic renal failure,* the kidneys fail to excrete the acid produced from normal daily metabolism. Both H^+ and anions accumulate in the body, resulting in slow consumption of bicarbonate stores. However, the acidosis is generally not severe unless a markedly catabolic state occurs or other associated conditions coexist. In acute renal failure, there is abrupt and complete shutdown of acid excretion, whereas in chronic renal failure, there initially is enhanced ammonia genesis by the remaining nephrons. As renal failure progresses, excretion of both NH_4^+ and phosphate declines. In addition, the secondary hyperparathyroidism seen with chronic renal failure decreases proximal tubular HCO_3^- reabsorption and adds a component of hyperchloremic acidosis to the increased anion gap acidosis.

Treatment of Metabolic Acidosis

The morbidity and mortality caused by metabolic acidosis are determined not only by the severity of acidosis but also by the amenability of the underlying disorder to medical management. During treatment of metabolic acidosis, the primary effort should focus on the management of the underlying condition. The recommendations and goals of buffer therapy differ for acute acidotic disorders such as DKA and for chronic acidotic states such as RTA. The role of buffer therapy for acute metabolic acidosis is very limited; many studies have failed to demonstrate any beneficial effect of such therapy, and there may be some harmful side effects. In some situations, base therapy is definitely indicated. For example, correction of the metabolic acidosis in salicylate intoxication increases renal salicylate excretion and protects the brain. In renal insufficiency, the metabolic acidosis is never corrected unless base is administered. In some inborn errors of metabolism, base therapy is also recommended.

During the correction of acute metabolic acidosis, particular attention should be paid to ensure an appropriate potassium balance. During an episode of metabolic acidosis, potassium moves from the intracellular space to the extracellular space in exchange for H^+, and thus the presence of a total body potassium deficit may not be appreciated. Hypokalemia may become evident only as the pH increases and potassium returns to the intracellular space.

Chronic metabolic acidosis slows linear growth and interferes with bone mineralization. In chronic metabolic acidosis, there is a need for alkali therapy.

METABOLIC ALKALOSIS

Metabolic alkalosis (pH > 7.45) occurs as a result of a primary increase in the serum HCO_3^-, which may occur as a result of (1) net loss of H^+, (2) net gain of HCO_3^- (or its precursors), or (3) loss of fluid with more Cl^- than HCO_3^-. Normally functioning kidneys can excrete large amounts of HCO_3^- and should offset any increase in serum HCO_3^- resulting from these causes. Therefore, factors that prevent the kidneys from excreting HCO_3^- also must be present to maintain the metabolic alkalosis.

Factors Initiating Metabolic Alkalosis

1. The H^+ can be lost externally, either through the gastrointestinal tract or through the kidneys. For every H^+ lost at these sites, the body gains one HCO_3^- ion. This is because H^+ production at both these sites (gastric parietal cell and renal tubular cells) is associated with generation of an equivalent number of HCO_3^- molecules. H^+ can also be "lost" internally, by shifting into the intracellular compartment. This occurs in states of severe potassium depletion (H^+ moves in, whereas K^+ exits the cell, to maintain electroneutrality).
2. The administration of HCO_3^- or its precursors (such as lactate, citrate, and acetate), at a rate greater than normal metabolic production of acid can lead to net gain of HCO_3^- by the body.

3. External loss of fluid (gastric fluid) containing more Cl^- than HCO_3^- raises the concentration of HCO_3^- in the body. One of the factors responsible for this type of alkalosis is the associated volume contraction, which leads to increased bicarbonate reabsorption by the proximal tubule of the kidney.

Factors Responsible for Sustaining Alkalosis

1. Decrease in effective blood volume and kidney perfusion causes increased Na^+ reabsorption, in both the proximal tubule (angiotensin II effect) and the distal renal tubule (mineralocorticoid effect), thereby increasing H^+ excretion.
2. Increased mineralocorticoid directly increases H^+ secretion in the outer medullary collecting duct.
3. Chloride depletion increases HCO_3^- reabsorption in the proximal tubule. This effect is independent of ECF volume status.
4. Potassium depletion stimulates ammonia genesis in the proximal tubular cells. Metabolic alkalosis and hypokalemia exist in a state of a vicious cycle and exacerbate each other.
5. Hypercapnia induces a state of intracellular acidosis, which increases H^+ secretion. Although PCO_2 increases as a normal compensatory response to metabolic alkalosis, the elevated PCO_2 prevents the renal correction of alkalosis.

Differential Diagnosis of Metabolic Alkalosis

The causes of a metabolic alkalosis can be subdivided on the basis of the urinary chloride level and the patient's blood pressure (Table 27-5). There is a small group of patients who do not fit into this classification scheme.

Urinary Chloride Level Lower than 10 mEq/L

Chloride-Deficient Diet. Although currently uncommon, the ingestion of milk formula with low chloride content has been shown to result in hypochloremic metabolic alkalosis and failure to thrive in infants and to result in later neurodevelopmental abnormalities in childhood.

Gastric Losses. The gastric fluid has a high H^+ concentration; loss of gastric fluid by vomiting or by nasogastric drainage leads to a net gain of HCO_3^- in the body. Although this is the initiating factor, the alkalosis is sustained by concomitant Cl^- and K^+ losses. Secondary hyperaldosteronism, resulting from volume contraction, promotes further urinary potassium and H^+ excretion, worsening the hypokalemia and alkalosis. In fact, urine is the source of most of the potassium losses caused by emesis. The degree of metabolic alkalosis associated with vomiting is generally mild except in conditions in which gastric secretions are greatly stimulated (e.g., Zollinger-Ellison syndrome) or there is protracted vomiting (e.g., pyloric stenosis).

Metabolic alkalosis can also be seen in newborns of mothers with eating disorders (bulimia). The baby reflects the electrolyte changes of the mother and sustains alkalosis because of the Cl^- deficiency.

Chloride Diarrhea. This is a rare congenital syndrome characterized by a defect in small- and large-bowel chloride absorption that leads to a chronic diarrhea with high chloride losses in the stool. The ongoing chloride depletion leads to a sustained metabolic alkalosis.

Diuretic Therapy. Loop and thiazide diuretics cause a metabolic alkalosis. The alkalosis is sustained because of hypochloremia, hypokalemia, and volume contraction with resultant secondary hyperaldosteronism. The urinary Cl^- may be high if the diuretics have been ingested recently. The metabolic derangements caused by

Table 27-5. Differential Diagnosis of Metabolic Alkalosis
Urinary Chloride < 10 mEq/L
Low chloride intake
Gastric losses (e.g., vomiting, nasogastric suctioning)
Intestinal losses (e.g., congenital chloride diarrhea, colonic adenoma)
Diuretic therapy (prolonged)
Contraction alkalosis
Posthypercapnia
Cystic fibrosis
Urinary Chloride > 20 mEq/L
With Hypertension
High renin, high aldosterone
Renal artery stenosis
Renin-secreting tumors
Low renin, high aldosterone
Primary hyperaldosteronism (adenoma or hyperplasia)
Dexamethasone suppressible hyperaldosteronism
Low renin, low aldosterone
Congenital adrenal hyperplasia variants
11-β-Hydroxylase deficiency
17-α-Hydroxylase deficiency
Exogenous mineralocorticoids
Liddle syndrome
With Normal Blood Pressure
Bartter syndrome
Gitelman syndrome
Diuretic therapy (recent)
Miscellaneous Causes
Gastrocystoplasty
Excessive alkali administration with renal failure
Hypoparathyroidism, hypercalcemia
Massive blood transfusion
Recovery from organic acidosis
Glucose ingestion after starvation

loop diuretics are virtually identical to those seen in Bartter syndrome.

Posthypercapnia. Chronic hypercapnia, as seen in bronchopulmonary dysplasia or cystic fibrosis, leads to an elevated serum bicarbonate concentration from metabolic compensation. The increase in bicarbonate is balanced by a decrease in chloride. Affected patients have chloride depletion, which may be worsened by concomitant diuretic use. With resolution of the hypercapnia, the bicarbonate concentration remains high until the chloride depletion is corrected.

Cystic Fibrosis. Metabolic alkalosis develops from marked losses of Cl^- in the sweat, which has relatively little HCO_3^-. The alkalosis is aggravated and sustained by accompanying volume depletion and possibly compensation of hypercapnia.

Urinary Chloride Level Higher than 20 mEq/L with Hypertension

The disorders of mineralocorticoid excess are characterized by volume expansion and hypertension (see Table 27-5). The mineralocorticoid excess stimulates the renal excretion of H^+ and K^+, resulting in metabolic alkalosis and hypokalemia. The various causes can be differentiated by evaluating the renin-aldosterone axis. Treatment is aimed at removing or correcting the source of the mineralocorticoid excess.

Urinary Chloride Level Higher than 20 mEq/L
with Normal Blood Pressure

Bartter Syndrome and Gitelman Syndrome. These uncommon autosomal recessive disorders result from defects in various ion transporters within the nephron. Bartter syndrome is a severe disorder that is characterized by urinary chloride wasting, hypokalemia, metabolic alkalosis, and increased serum levels of aldosterone and renin. Hypercalciuria is also common and leads to nephrocalcinosis in some patients. Urinary prostaglandin levels are elevated, especially in the more severe neonatal Bartter syndrome. Affected patients present with a history of failure to thrive, polyuria, polydipsia, and an easy tendency for dehydration. In neonatal Bartter syndrome, there is usually a history of polyhydramnios and premature delivery. Gitelman syndrome, in contrast, is a milder disorder characterized by hypokalemia, metabolic alkalosis, and hypomagnesemia caused by urinary magnesium wasting; calcium excretion is normal. The growth retardation is not as severe. Children with Gitelman syndrome, however, are more prone to febrile seizures and tetanic episodes.

Miscellaneous Causes of Metabolic Alkalosis. *Gastrocystoplasty,* urinary bladder augmentation with part of the stomach, can result in metabolic alkalosis caused by acid secretion from the gastric mucosa and its loss in the urine. The administration of excessive alkali in the presence of renal failure when the kidneys are unable to excrete HCO_3^- can cause metabolic alkalosis. Hypercalcemia resulting from nonparathyroid causes (e.g., sarcoidosis, malignancy) can cause mild metabolic alkalosis by inhibiting parathyroid hormone secretion; hypoparathyroidism is another cause of metabolic alkalosis.

Treatment of Metabolic Alkalosis

Treatment focuses on correcting the underlying disorder and depends on the pathophysiologic mechanisms of the alkalosis. Patients with a chloride-responsive metabolic alkalosis (urine Cl^- < 10 mEq/L) respond to volume repletion; both sodium and potassium chloride are necessary. In rare cases, if alkalosis persists despite chloride supplementation, the carbonic anhydrase inhibitor acetazolamide can be used to increase urinary bicarbonate losses. In patients undergoing persistent gastric drainage, administration of either an H_2 blocker or H^+ pump inhibitor can be beneficial by decreasing the gastric H^+ secretion.

Treatment of chloride-resistant metabolic alkalosis with hypertension (urinary Cl^- > 20 mEq/L) generally mandates interference with the mineralocorticoid (or mineralocorticoid-like substance) that is maintaining renal H^+ losses. This can sometimes be accomplished pharmacologically (e.g., with spironolactone or with other distal potassium-sparing diuretics such as amiloride).

The management of Bartter syndrome involves potassium chloride supplementation, but this alone usually does not normalize serum potassium concentration, and addition of a potassium-sparing diuretic (i.e., spironolactone, amiloride, or triamterene) is usually necessary. Nonsteroidal antiinflammatory agents, because of their ability to decrease prostaglandin synthesis, are helpful in patients with Bartter syndrome and are the cornerstone of therapy in children with neonatal Bartter syndrome. In patients with Gitelman syndrome, potassium supplementation is invariably necessary. Magnesium supplementation may diminish urinary losses of sodium, potassium, and chloride. Amiloride and triamterene are also useful in these patients because they are potassium- and magnesium-sparing diuretics.

When an elevated systemic pH becomes life-threatening because of the development of seizures and ventricular arrhythmias, rapid reduction in systemic pH may be accomplished by controlled mechanical ventilation or dialysis. Although administration of either HCl or its congeners (e.g., arginine chloride or ammonium chloride)

has historically been advocated to correct metabolic alkalosis, they must be used cautiously because of significant potential complications.

RESPIRATORY ACIDOSIS

Respiratory acidosis results when there is a primary increase in PCO_2 that is secondary to impaired pulmonary ventilation. The nonbicarbonate intracellular buffers attenuate the initial decrease in pH. Renal compensation starts in 12 to 24 hours and reaches maximum in 3 to 5 days. The management of respiratory acidosis is directed toward improving alveolar ventilation and treating the underlying disorder (see Chapter 3).

RESPIRATORY ALKALOSIS

Respiratory alkalosis occurs when there is a primary decrease in PCO_2 as a result of pulmonary hyperventilation. In a spontaneously breathing child, this can result from fever, sepsis, mild bronchial asthma, or central nervous system disorders. In the intensive care unit, the most common cause is mechanical overventilation of an intubated child. The initial alkalosis is acutely titrated by the intracellular buffers, and metabolic compensation by the kidneys returns pH toward normal within 1 to 2 days. Interestingly, this is the only simple acid-base disorder in which, at least in the adult, the pH may be completely normalized by the compensatory mechanisms. The treatment is management of the underlying process.

MIXED ACID-BASE DISORDERS

Mixed acid-base disorders occur when two or even three primary events act to alter the acid-base state at the same time. The deviations in pH are more marked when two primary events block the compensation of each other, such as the combination of a metabolic acidosis and a respiratory acidosis seen in a patient with shock and respiratory failure. In contrast, in the presence of two opposing primary events, the pH may be normal or only minimally abnormal, as can be seen with combined vomiting and diarrhea. A mixed acid-base disorder is commonly seen when neonates with respiratory acidosis caused by chronic lung disease also receive diuretics, which can cause a metabolic alkalosis.

The diagnosis of mixed acid-base disorder should be suspected in the following situations:

1. if the compensation for the primary event is absent or is out of the expected range
2. if the deviation in anion gap and/or serum Cl^- is out of proportion to the change in HCO_3^-
3. if the anion gap is significantly increased in the presence of a near-normal pH

POTASSIUM DISORDERS

Potassium is the major intracellular cation; less than 2% is present in the ECF at a concentration of 3.5 to 5.5 mEq/L (during the early neonatal period, the upper limit of normal can be up to 6.0 mEq/L). The differential distribution of potassium between the intracellular (150 mEq/L) and extracellular compartments, sustained by the action of the Na^+,K^+-ATPase pump, is the chief determinant of the resting membrane potential. Not surprisingly, both hyperkalemia (serum K^+ > 5.5 mEq/L) and hypokalemia (serum K^+ < 3.5 mEq/L) have a profound effect on the excitability of the neuromuscular tissue, especially the cardiac tissue. As a result, fatal cardiac arrhythmias are possible sequelae of hypokalemia and hyperkalemia. Perturbations in serum K^+ homeostasis also affect the smooth and striate muscles. In contrast, changes in the concentration of intracellular K⁺ do not result in significant alterations of excitability of neuromuscular tissue.

Almost all dietary potassium is absorbed. The kidney is the major organ responsible for K⁺ excretion, eliminating more than 90% of the daily K⁺ intake. However, after an acute ingestion of K⁺, the kidneys excrete only half of it over the first 4 to 6 hours; the remainder is transiently redistributed intracellularly before the kidneys eventually excrete it. This intracellular redistribution has a very important role in offsetting acute changes in serum K⁺, but it has a limited capacity to do so. Redistribution of a very small fraction (1% to 2%) of intracellular K⁺ into the ECF can easily increase serum K⁺ to a dangerous level. A number of factors affect the distribution of K⁺ between the intracellular space and the ECF (Table 27-6). The colonic excretion of K⁺ is of no significance under normal conditions, but in patients with chronic renal failure, it becomes an important route of K⁺ elimination, when colonic excretion increases substantially.

Because the kidney is the major route of potassium elimination from the body, a disturbance in renal potassium handling can be the cause of excessive loss or retention.

RENAL POTASSIUM HANDLING

The filtered K⁺ is extensively (up to 75%) reabsorbed in the proximal tubule, and the thick ascending limb reabsorbs another 15% of the filtered K⁺. Under normal circumstances, urinary K⁺ excretion is determined primarily by K⁺ secretion or reabsorption along the distal nephron. In the cortical collecting duct, active K⁺ secretion occurs, which at times can increase to the point at which the amount of K⁺ in the luminal fluid exceeds the amount that was originally filtered. Reabsorption of K⁺ is never complete; there is always an obligatory urinary loss of 4 to 5 mEq/L of K⁺ (this is in contrast to Na⁺, which can be almost completely reabsorbed).

The principal cells secrete potassium in the distal nephron. Potassium from the blood enters the principal cells through the basolateral membrane via the Na⁺,K⁺-ATPase pump. The associated extrusion of Na⁺ results in a low intracellular Na⁺ concentration, which facilitates the inward movement of Na⁺ from the luminal fluid. This Na⁺ absorption, when unaccompanied by an anion, generates a negative charge in the lumen. The development of a negative charge in the lumen is necessary for K⁺ secretion and fails to develop if (1) the Na⁺ delivery to the distal nephron is decreased (e.g., because of low flow as observed during volume depletion), (2) the Na⁺ conductance channels in the luminal membrane are blocked (e.g., by a potassium-sparing diuretic such as amiloride), or (3) an equimolar or increased amount of anion accompanies Na⁺ reabsorption (e.g., as in excessive Cl⁻ absorption, as seen in chloride shunt syndrome).

Aldosterone or hyperkalemia increases K⁺ secretion by the principal cells. Anions other than Cl⁻ (such as SO_4^{2-} and HCO_3^-) in the distal nephron can greatly augment K⁺ losses. During a metabolic alkalosis, urinary K⁺ excretion increases because of increased Na⁺ and decreased Cl⁻ delivery to the distal nephron. During an episode of metabolic acidosis, urinary K⁺ losses are usually decreased; the important exceptions are type I and type II RTA and DKA.

Spironolactone, amiloride, and triamterene decrease K⁺ excretion. Whereas spironolactone is an aldosterone antagonist, amiloride and triamterene block the Na⁺ conductance channels present in the principal cell luminal membrane. The antimicrobial trimethoprim prevents K⁺ secretion by the same mechanism as amiloride.

During evaluation of potassium disorders, it is important to determine the appropriateness of the renal response, because it aids in establishing the differential diagnosis of both hypokalemia and hyperkalemia. The appropriateness of the renal response can be checked by determining 24-hour potassium excretion (expected value < 15 mEq during hypokalemia and > 200 mEq during hyperkalemia), ratio of K⁺ to creatinine (expected value < 1 mmol/mmol during hypokalemia and > 20 mmol/mmol during hyperkalemia), and fractional excretion of K⁺ (expected values depend on GFR and require a nomogram). However, all these three methods have their drawbacks. The transtubular potassium gradient (TTKG) is currently regarded as the most useful test, because it is based on the physiologic processes of K⁺ excretion.

The TTKG reflects the driving force for K⁺ secretion. Theoretically, it is the ratio of the K⁺ in the collecting duct (distal nephron) to the K⁺ in the peritubular vessels. None of these values can be directly measured. Collecting duct K⁺ is indirectly calculated from urine K⁺ and from serum and urine osmolalities: namely, collecting duct K⁺ = $[K^+]_{urine}$/(urine/plasma)$_{osmolality}$. This calculation is permitted only when the urine osmolality is greater than the serum osmolality. This estimated collecting duct K⁺ is then divided by serum K⁺, which approximates peritubular vessel K⁺:

$$TTKG = [K]_{urine}/[K]_{plasma} \times (plasma\ osmolality/urine\ osmolality),$$

where $[K]_{urine}$ is the urine potassium concentration and $[K]_{plasma}$ is the plasma potassium concentration.

To calculate the TTKG, urine and blood samples for K⁺ and osmolality should be obtained simultaneously. The TTKG in a healthy person varies from 5 to 15. During hypokalemia of nonrenal origin, the expected TTKG should be lower than 2; a value higher than 6 indicates inappropriate renal potassium losses. During hyperkalemia of nonrenal origin, the expected TTKG should exceed 10; a value lower than 5 suggests inadequate renal potassium excretion.

HYPOKALEMIA

Hypokalemia (Table 27-7) may result from (1) increased renal losses, (2) increased extrarenal losses, (3) redistribution, or (4) prolonged decreased intake of potassium. When interpreting cases of hypokalemia, the clinician should pay careful attention to blood pressure and obtain laboratory data concerning acid-base status, electrolytes, osmolality of blood and urine, and the renin-aldosterone axis. These investigations should be done before any intervention is undertaken.

Increased Renal Losses (TTKG > 6) with Hypertension

Mineralocorticoid Excess

The presence of excess mineralocorticoid hormone, regardless of its source, results in stimulation of potassium secretion by the distal tubular cells of the nephron. Mineralocorticoid excess can result from *primary hyperaldosteronism,* rare forms of *congenital adrenal hyperplasia* (17-α-hydroxylase or 11-β-hydroxylase deficiency), and *Cushing syndrome.* The hypokalemia in these conditions is associated with increased sodium chloride retention, causing hypertension. The expansion of the extracellular volume eventually leads to the suppression of Na⁺-retaining mechanisms, but the K⁺ losses continue unabated. Metabolic alkalosis develops as a result of

Table 27-6. Factors Affecting Potassium Distribution between Extracellular Fluid and Intracellular Fluid

Insulin	Excess causes hypokalemia
	Deficiency causes hyperkalemia
Catecholamines	β agonists cause hypokalemia
	β antagonists cause hyperkalemia
Acid-base status	Metabolic alkalosis causes hypokalemia
	Metabolic acidosis (especially inorganic) causes hyperkalemia
Tissue injury	Causes hyperkalemia

Table 27-7. **Differential Diagnosis of Hypokalemia**
Increased Renal Losses (TTKG > 6)
With Hypertension
Mineralocorticoid excess
Primary aldosteronism
Congenital adrenal hyperplasia
17-α Hydroxylase deficiency
11-β Hydroxylase deficiency
Hyperreninemic hyperaldosteronism
Glucocorticoid-suppressible hyperaldosteronism
Exogenous mineralocorticoid
Cushing syndrome
Liddle syndrome
With Normal Blood Pressure
With Acidosis
Renal tubular acidosis
Diabetic ketoacidosis
With Alkalosis
Vomiting
Diuretics
Congenital chloride diarrhea
Bartter syndrome
Gitelman syndrome
Magnesium depletion
Normotensive hyperaldosteronism
With Normal Acid-Base
Recovery from acute tubular necrosis
Postobstructive diuresis
Drugs (penicillins, amphotericin B)
Extrarenal Losses (TTKG < 2)
Diarrhea/GI fistulas
Laxative abuse
Profuse sweating
Redistribution
Alkalosis
β-adrenergic agonists
Barium intoxication
Familial hypokalemic periodic paralysis

GI, gastrointestinal; TTKG, transtubular potassium gradient.

enhanced proximal ammonium production secondary to potassium depletion.

Liddle Syndrome

This is a rare cause of hypokalemia; it is characterized by a primary increase in sodium reabsorption in the collecting tubule and is usually associated with increased potassium secretion. The sodium reabsorption is increased through activation of the amiloride-sensitive renal sodium channel. Because serum aldosterone levels are low, spironolactone is ineffective, but amiloride or triamterene, which block the sodium channel, decrease potassium losses and help ameliorate the hypokalemia and the hypertension.

Increased Renal Losses (TTKG > 6) with Normal Blood Pressure

The hypokalemia associated with Bartter syndrome, Gitelman syndrome, RTA, DKA, and vomiting are discussed in the section on acid-base disorders.

Hypomagnesemia of any cause can lead to K^+ depletion, and correction of hypokalemia is not possible until magnesium balance is restored. These effects are believed to be secondary to magnesium's affect on aldosterone secretion and K^+ channels. Magnesium replacement in this situation should be done with magnesium oxide, because the sulfate ion of magnesium sulfate can increase the urinary K^+ losses.

The polyuric recovery phase of *acute tubular necrosis* and the postobstructive diuresis after relief of urinary tract obstruction are commonly encountered clinical conditions that may be associated with excess urine potassium losses. Penicillins can increase urinary K^+ losses by increased delivery of sodium and nonabsorbable anions to the distal nephron. Amphotericin B enhances urinary K^+ loss by increasing the tubular K^+ permeability and also by causing type I RTA.

Increased Extrarenal Losses (TTKG < 2)

Diarrhea is a very common cause of hypokalemia in pediatric practice. Profuse sweating is a much less frequent cause of hypokalemia.

Redistribution

Alkalosis causes potassium to enter cells in exchange for H^+ (this principle is utilized in the management of hyperkalemia; see later discussion). β-Adrenergic agonists increase intracellular movement of potassium.

Familial hypokalemic periodic paralysis is a rare disorder characterized by recurring transient episodes of net K^+ transfer from ECF to intracellular fluid (ICF). The autosomal dominant form manifests between the ages of 10 and 19 years. Another variant appears later in life (30 to 40 years) and is associated with thyrotoxicosis. The dominant finding is muscle weakness, which may advance to paralysis. Episodes typically occur after large carbohydrate-rich meals, strenuous exercise, or insulin administration. Therapy is largely symptomatic; empirical treatment with acetazolamide has yielded some results.

Consequences of Hypokalemia

Hypokalemia produces functional alterations in skeletal muscle, smooth muscle, and the heart. The cardiac effects are the most serious consequence of hypokalemia. The characteristic electrocardiographic (ECG) changes include flattening of the T wave with appearance of the U wave. Skeletal muscular weakness usually starts in the limbs before involving the trunk and respiratory muscles. Paralytic ileus and gastric dilatation reflect smooth muscle dysfunction. Rhabdomyolysis is a dramatic and serious complication of hypokalemia. Hypokalemia is particularly dangerous in patients taking digoxin.

In the kidney, potassium deficiency may result in vacuolar changes in the tubular epithelium. The renal concentrating capacity is decreased, causing polyuria. Prolonged and sustained hypokalemia leads to systemic alkalosis.

Treatment of Hypokalemia

The immediate objective of potassium replacement is to prevent life-threatening cardiac and muscular complications. The ultimate goal is to replenish total body potassium stores. There is no method of determining the potassium deficit, because there is no definite correlation between the plasma potassium concentration and body potassium stores. A decrease of 1 mEq/L in serum potassium concentration secondary to potassium loss generally corresponds to a loss of approximately 10% to 30% of body potassium. In conditions with associated acidosis and/or hyperosmolality (e.g., RTA, DKA), the plasma potassium concentration may underestimate potassium stores, and correction of acidosis with bicarbonate in these conditions may rapidly lower the serum potassium concentration.

The safest route to administer potassium is by mouth, but in states of severe symptomatic hypokalemia or when there are gastrointestinal problems, potassium must be given intravenously. The usual concentration of potassium in intravenous fluid solutions is up to 40 mEq/L. Higher concentrations of up to 60 to 80 mEq/L can be given in a central vein under continuous ECG monitoring. Dextrose should be avoided in the initial fluids, because its administration with secondary increased insulin secretion may result in further lowering of the plasma potassium concentration. The choice of potassium salt depends on the clinical situation. Under most circumstances, when hypovolemia coexists, potassium chloride is appropriate. Potassium bicarbonate (or, more often, other salts such as citrate and acetate, which generate bicarbonate) can be given in the presence of coexistent metabolic acidosis. If there is an associated phosphate deficiency (as in DKA), potassium phosphate can be used. It is important to remember that correction of total body potassium deficits can take days to weeks.

HYPERKALEMIA

Moderate (6.1 to 7.0 mEq/L) to severe (>7.0 mEq/L) hyperkalemia, especially if it develops acutely, can lead to grave consequences and requires prompt treatment. *Pseudohyperkalemia* can occur as result of release of intracellular potassium (e.g., hemolysis caused by mechanical trauma during venipuncture), and it can also be seen in conditions with marked leukocytosis and thrombocytosis. It can be avoided by minimizing trauma and hand clenching during venipuncture, by rapidly separating red blood cells, and by using plasma rather than serum for potassium measurements. An unexpected elevated potassium level should be repeated.

Hyperkalemia can be caused by (1) reduced urinary potassium excretion, (2) increased potassium intake, (3) release of intracellular potassium, and/or (4) impaired cellular potassium uptake (Table 27-8).

Reduced Urinary Potassium Excretion (TTKG < 5)

Renal potassium excretion decreases when the GFR is decreased or when there is a defect in tubular potassium excretion resulting from lack of aldosterone, medications, or a primary defect in tubular potassium excretion.

Renal Failure

Potassium excretion is decreased in both acute and chronic renal failure. Severe hyperkalemia occurs more commonly in acute renal failure. In contrast, in patients with chronic renal failure, hyperkalemia does not occur unless the GFR is lower than 10 mL/minute or some other factor predisposing to hyperkalemia is present. In patients with chronic renal failure, potassium balance is maintained by increased K^+ secretion per functioning nephron and also by enhanced excretion of K^+ through the gastrointestinal tract.

Hypoaldosteronism

Low levels or absence of aldosterone may result from a variety of conditions (Addison disease, congenital adrenal hyperplasia [deficiency of 21-hydroxylase], and hyporeninemic hypoaldosteronism). In *pseudohypoaldosteronism* there is a lack of response to aldosterone, despite high aldosterone levels. In addition to hyperkalemia, hyponatremia and hyperchloremic metabolic acidosis are the associated features in these disorders. The diagnosis can be confirmed by measurement of renin activity and aldosterone levels.

Table 27-8. Differential Diagnosis of Hyperkalemia
Pseudohyperkalemia
Hemolysis
Thrombocytosis
Leukocytosis
Reduced Urinary Potassium Excretion (TTKG < 5)
Renal Failure
Acute
Chronic
Hypoaldosteronism
Addison disease
Hereditary adrenal enzyme defects
21-Hydroxylase deficiency
Hyporeninemic hypoaldosteronism
Pseudohypoaldosteronism
Drugs
ACE inhibitors
Potassium-sparing diuretics
Spironolactone
Amiloride
Triamterene
Cyclosporine
Trimethoprim
Heparin
Nonsteroidal antiinflammatory agents
Primary Tubular Defects
Postrenal transplantation
Lupus nephritis
AIDS
RTA type IV (chloride shunt)
Increased Intake/Tissue Release (TTKG > 10)
Intravenous/oral administration
Hemolysis (endogenous or transfused blood)
Rhabdomyolysis
Tumor lysis
Redistribution
Acidosis
Insulin deficiency (diabetes)
Familial hyperkalemic periodic paralysis
Digitalis toxicity
β-adrenergic blockade
Succinylcholine

ACE, angiotensin-converting enzyme; AIDS, acquired immunodeficiency syndrome; RTA, renal tubular acidosis; TTKG, transtubular potassium gradient.

Drugs

Several drugs are known to be associated with hyperkalemia; they can either impair renin-aldosterone secretion or action (angiotensin-converting enzyme inhibitors, spironolactone, cyclosporine, or heparin) or impair renal tubular potassium secretion (amiloride, triamterene, trimethoprim, or cyclosporine).

Primary Tubular Defects

In some patients, hyperkalemia occurs as a result of low urinary K^+ excretion despite normal renin and aldosterone levels. The presence of a selective defect in K^+ secretion has been described in subjects with renal transplant rejection and lupus nephritis. A selective defect of K^+ secretion is also seen in patients with chloride shunt syndrome.

This syndrome is characterized by enhanced Cl^- absorption in the distal nephron, which decreases the electrical gradient necessary for K^+ secretion in the collecting duct (see previous discussion).

Increased Potassium Intake/Tissue Release (TTKG > 10)

Acute increases in potassium intake, usually through parenteral administration, may result in hyperkalemia. The hyperkalemia is typically transient, inasmuch as normal kidneys have a large capacity for excreting potassium. Sustained hyperkalemia is seen only when renal excretory mechanisms are impaired.

In *tumor lysis syndrome* and *rhabdomyolysis,* massive amounts of K^+ are released from the intracellular compartment, but hyperkalemia does not usually occur unless acute renal failure supervenes. Similarly, trauma, intravascular hemolysis, transfusion of stored blood, and catabolic states such as infection or high fever are associated with release of K^+ from the cells; however, hyperkalemia is uncommon as long as renal function is normal and normal to high urine output is maintained with fluid therapy.

Redistribution

Acidosis and insulin deficiency result in egress of intracellular potassium (as discussed previously). *Familial hyperkalemic periodic paralysis* is a rare hereditary disorder characterized by episodes of muscular weakness and hyperkalemia (movement of K^+ from ICF to ECF) resulting from mutations in cellular sodium channels. β_2-Receptor blockers, digitalis (by inhibiting the Na^+, K^+-ATPase pump), and succinylcholine (by inhibiting cellular repolarization) cause hyperkalemia by impairing cellular potassium uptake.

Consequences of Hyperkalemia

Overt clinical manifestations are uncommon with hyperkalemia, but cardiac arrhythmias are potentially life-threatening. Generalized muscular weakness and paralysis can occur. The characteristic ECG findings seen with increasing $[K^+]$ are tall, peaked T waves; widening of the QRS complex; decreased amplitude of the P wave; and fusion of the QRS complex with the T wave, forming a sine wave. This can be rapidly followed by atrioventricular dissociation and ventricular tachycardia or fibrillation. Cardiac arrest is more common with hyperkalemia than with hypokalemia.

Treatment of Hyperkalemia

The treatment of hyperkalemia depends on the magnitude of the hyperkalemia, the severity of ECG changes, and the anticipated future rise in $[K^+]$. The specific therapy should always focus on the underlying cause. However, a plasma potassium concentration higher than 7.0 mEq/L or marked ECG changes are potentially life-threatening and necessitate immediate treatment. A normal ECG result should not lead to a more casual approach, because significant ECG changes can appear over a short period of time. All potassium intake (parenteral nutrition, medications with potassium salt) and medications that cause hyperkalemia, such as potassium-sparing diuretics, angiotensin-converting enzyme inhibitors, and trimethoprim, should be discontinued. The treatment modalities usually belong to the following three categories: (1) antagonism of membrane excitability, (2) shifting of potassium into the intracellular compartment, and (3) elimination of excess potassium (Table 27-9).

Calcium protects the heart from fatal arrhythmias caused by hyperkalemia by normalizing the difference between the resting and threshold potentials. This protective effect is quite rapid but relatively short-lived; therefore, other measures to reduce the concentration of serum potassium are necessary.

Potassium can be shifted from the extracellular to the intracellular compartment by administration of sodium bicarbonate, glucose and insulin, and β_2-adrenergic agonists, as detailed in Table 27-9. Although the intracellular shift of potassium can be accomplished rather quickly, this is only a temporary measure, and further steps should be taken to establish a negative potassium balance.

Loop or thiazide diuretics increase renal potassium excretion. In patients with aldosterone deficiency, fludrocortisone increases renal potassium excretion. Alkalinizing the urine through systemic base administration can further enhance urinary potassium losses.

Cation exchange resins actually remove potassium from the body and are effective in acute situations, particularly when poor renal function is present. Dialysis is needed in patients with severe hyperkalemia, especially in the presence of advanced renal failure or when accompanied by a hypercatabolic state or severe tissue necrosis. For urgent potassium removal, hemodialysis is more effective than continuous hemodiafiltration or peritoneal dialysis.

SODIUM DISORDERS

Sodium is the principal cation of the ECF compartment, and total body sodium content is the major determinant of ECF volume. A normal ECF volume is essential for maintaining an adequate circulating blood volume. Being the chief determinant of ECF osmolality, the sodium concentration determines cell volume by directing water movement between the ECF compartment and the intracellular compartment. An increase in ECF osmolality causes water to move out of cells, and a decrease in ECF osmolality causes water to move into cells. Sodium homeostasis is coupled with water homeostasis; therefore, disorders of sodium homeostasis usually occur as a result of imbalances of both sodium and water rather than an isolated imbalance of either sodium or water.

Table 27-9. Treatment of Hyperkalemia

Antagonism of Membrane Excitability

Calcium gluconate 10% (elemental calcium, 0.45 mEq/mL), 0.5-1.0 mL/kg body weight (maximum = 10 mL), injected intravenously and slowly over 5-10 min, with continuous monitoring of heart rate)

Shift of Potassium into the Intracellular Compartment

Sodium bicarbonate, 1-2 mEq/kg body weight intravenously over 10-20 min; usefulness is limited in patients with volume expansion

Glucose, 1 g/kg body weight, and insulin, 1 unit per every 4 g of glucose, intravenously over 20-30 min

β_2-Adrenergic agonists, such as albuterol, intravenously or by nebulizer or aerosol

Elimination of Excess Potassium

Loop/thiazide diuretics

Fludrocortisone (0.05-0.1 mg/day); should be avoided or given with great caution to hypertensive patients

Cation exchange resin, sodium polystyrene sulfonate, 1 g/kg body weight (maximum, 15 g/dose), administered orally or rectally in 20%-30% sorbitol or 10% glucose, 1 g resin/4mL (additional 70% sorbitol syrup may be given if constipation occurs)

Peritoneal dialysis, hemodialysis, or hemodiafiltration

Modified from Hellerstein S, Alon US, Warady BA: Renal impairment. In Ashcraft KW, Murphy JP, Sharp RJ, et al (eds): Pediatric Surgery, 3rd ed. Philadelphia, WB Saunders, 2000, pp 47-57.

The kidneys are pivotal regulators of sodium and water balance. Sodium excretion, which is regulated by the renin-angiotensin-aldosterone system and atrial natriuretic peptide, increases in response to an expanded intravascular volume, as may occur with a high sodium intake. In response to a decreased intravascular volume, the urine can be made virtually sodium free. Osmolality is regulated by thirst and vasopressin production, which determines renal water excretion.

A detailed history of the underlying disease, food and fluid intake, fluid losses in the form of stool, emesis, and urine should be obtained. The physical examination focuses on an evaluation of the patient's volume status, including the nature and rate of peripheral pulses, blood pressure, fullness of the fontanelle, level of consciousness, dryness of mucous membranes, coolness of extremities, and capillary refill time. Urinary sodium concentration can provide valuable information regarding the child's effective blood volume, but it can be misleading if the patient is receiving diuretics or has abnormal renal sodium handling. The clinical features associated with alterations in plasma osmolality are nonspecific. A low serum osmolality may produce lethargy and confusion, whereas a high serum osmolality may lead to irritability, a high-pitched cry, and a doughy skin texture. The determination of plasma osmolality requires a direct laboratory measurement or can be estimated from the following formula:

$$\text{Serum osmolality}_{(mOsm)} = 2[Na^+]_{mEq/L} + [\text{glucose}]_{mg/dL}/18 + [\text{urea}]_{mg/dL}/2.8$$

The ECF volume is the best indicator of body sodium balance, and the plasma osmolality reflects water balance.

HYPONATREMIA

Hyponatremia (plasma sodium < 135 mEq/L) should be differentiated from pseudohyponatremia and factitious hyponatremia. *Pseudohyponatremia* occurs in the presence of excessive amounts of plasma proteins and lipids, which decrease the percentage of plasma water and thus artificially lower the plasma sodium concentration. The measured plasma osmolality of these patients is normal, inasmuch as lipids and proteins do not contribute significantly to osmolality because of their large size. Therefore, a gap between measured and calculated osmolalities can indicate pseudohyponatremia. Many clinical laboratories now measure the serum sodium concentration by using ion-selective electrodes, which are not affected by the presence of lipids and proteins and thus eliminate the possibility of pseudohyponatremia.

Factitious hyponatremia results from high plasma concentrations of impermeable solutes such as glucose or mannitol that cause movement of water from the intracellular to the extracellular space. In contrast to pseudohyponatremia, the low plasma sodium concentration in these situations is a true value, and plasma osmolality is increased as a result of the presence of the extra solutes. The decrease in plasma sodium is approximately 1.6 mEq/L for every 100 mg/dL increase in the plasma glucose concentration.

In true hyponatremia, the plasma osmolality is low (<280 mOsm/kg), and the pathophysiologic processes are caused by (1) loss of both body sodium and water (sodium losses exceeding water losses), (2) increase in body water (without edema), or (3) increase in both body water and sodium (increase in water exceeding that of sodium). Estimating the status of the ECF volume (hypovolemia, euvolemia, or hypervolemia) is therefore useful in narrowing the differential diagnosis (Fig. 27-2).

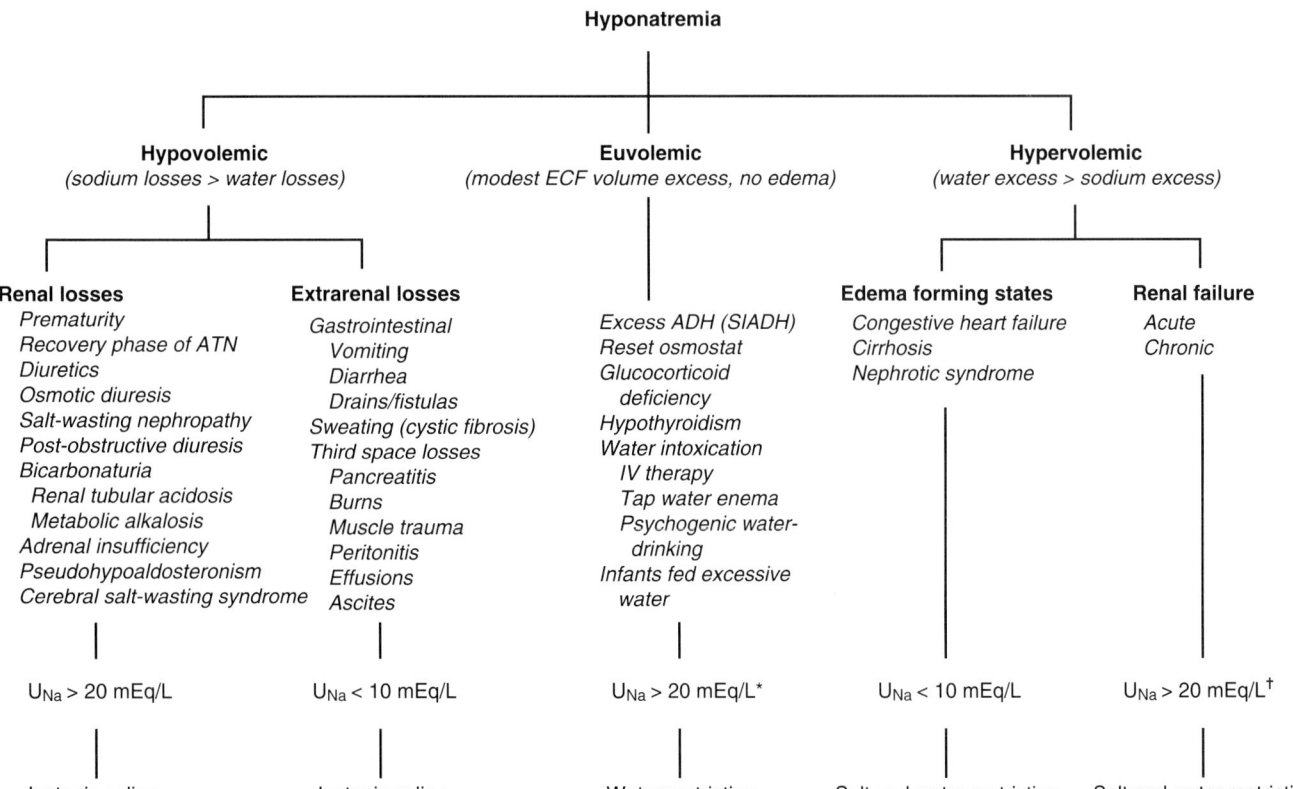

Figure 27-2. Classification, diagnosis and treatment of hyponatremic states. *In water intoxication the urine sodium is often <20 mEq/L. †Urinary sodium is < 10 mEq/L in acute renal failure secondary to glomerular disease. ADH, antidiuretic hormone; ATN, acute tubular necrosis; ECF, extracellular fluid; SIADH, syndrome of inappropriate antidiuretic hormone secretion. (Modified from Beri T, Schrier RW: Disorders of water metabolism. In Schrier RW [ed]: Renal and Electrolyte Disorders. Philadelphia, Lippincott-Raven, 1997.)

Hypovolemic Hyponatremia

These disorders occur when sodium losses exceed those of water. The two primary sources for such losses are the kidneys and the gastrointestinal tract. The sodium losses can also occur when fluids are sequestered into "third spaces" such as the peritoneal cavity and bowel lumen.

The most common cause of hypovolemic hyponatremia in children is gastroenteritis. Fistulas and various types of gastrointestinal tubes for drainage can also lead to a similar clinical picture. Uncommonly, hypovolemic hyponatremia can result from excessive sweat sodium losses in patients with cystic fibrosis or from sweating in hot climatic zones. The normally functioning kidneys respond by conserving sodium, and the urine sodium concentration is usually less than 10 mEq/L (with the exception of metabolic alkalosis associated with vomiting and bicarbonaturia).

The kidneys can be the source of excessive sodium loss in premature infants (tubular immaturity), in patients receiving diuretics, and in those having an osmotic diuresis. The presence of increased urinary bicarbonate, as seen in certain patients with metabolic alkalosis and RTA, leads to obligatory losses of sodium in the urine. The urinary sodium losses are increased during the recovery phase of acute tubular necrosis, after relief of urinary tract obstruction, and in certain renal diseases (salt-wasting nephropathies) such as medullary cystic disease, polycystic kidney disease, and tubulointerstitial diseases. All of these disorders are usually accompanied by hypokalemia. The presence of hyperkalemia and normal renal function in patients with hypovolemic hyponatremia suggests mineralocorticoid deficiency or type IV RTA.

Some children with acute or chronic central nervous system damage (closed-head trauma, surgery, tumors, or meningitis) present with excessive renal sodium losses and develop hypovolemic hyponatremia. The condition is known as *cerebral salt wasting syndrome* and occurs because of inappropriate secretion of atrial natriuretic hormone. Cerebral salt wasting is usually associated with hypovolemia and can be confused with the *syndrome of inappropriate antidiuretic hormone secretion* (SIADH) in the absence of marked hypovolemia. The two syndromes can be differentiated by measuring plasma uric acid concentration, which is increased in cerebral salt wasting syndrome and decreased in SIADH. Apart from managing the underlying condition, patients with cerebral salt wasting syndrome require complete replacement of urinary sodium and water losses.

In all patients with renal losses of sodium as a cause of hypovolemic hyponatremia the urinary sodium concentration is usually greater than 20 mEq/L, despite the presence of hypovolemia.

Euvolemic Hyponatremia

The ECF volume status of patients in this group is usually normal; some persons have a slightly increased ECF volume, but they are not edematous. Owing to slight ECF volume expansion, urinary sodium concentration is usually greater than 20 mEq/L.

The *syndrome of inappropriate antidiuretic hormone secretion* (SIADH) is a common cause of euvolemic hyponatremia. Exogenous administration of DDAVP (synthetic analogue of vasopressin) can produce a similar clinical picture. SIADH, which has multiple causes (e.g., central nervous system infections, trauma, hypoxia, and various malignancies), results from antidiuretic hormone (ADH) secretion despite the absence of increased plasma osmolality or volume depletion, the normal stimuli for ADH secretion. The diagnostic criteria are as follows:

1. hypoosmolar hyponatremia
2. urine osmolality higher than serum osmolality
3. normal renal function
4. normal adrenal and thyroid function

5. high urinary sodium concentration (this is not an absolute criterion, inasmuch as urinary sodium concentrations may be low in patients who are severely sodium depleted)
6. absence of hypovolemia or edema
7. hypouricemia

In the absence of any obvious clinical signs, the laboratory finding of hyponatremia is usually the first clue to the presence of SIADH.

Because SIADH is a problem of water retention and not of sodium depletion, the most appropriate treatment is water restriction. Attempts to correct the hyponatremia with sodium administration cause an increase in urinary sodium excretion and little change in the plasma sodium concentration. Nonetheless, sodium administration is needed if severe hyponatremia leads to neurologic symptoms.

A variant of SIADH occurs in chronically ill or malnourished children. This condition, referred to as a "reset osmostat," is characterized by downward resetting of the osmoreceptors located in the anterolateral region of the hypothalamus. As a result, ADH is released at lower levels of plasma osmolality, and affected patients have asymptomatic chronic hyponatremia. However, they respond to water loading by decreasing ADH secretion and by diluting the urine. Likewise, sodium administration results in an increase in ADH secretion and hypertonic urine. Treatment of these patients should focus on management of the underlying disease.

Glucocorticoid and thyroid hormone deficiency can cause a hyponatremic picture similar to that of SIADH. The hyponatremia resolves with appropriate hormonal replacement therapy.

Acute water intoxication is an uncommon cause of euvolemic hyponatremia in children receiving hypotonic intravenous fluids; it is likely to happen only if there is an associated impairment of free water excretion capability. Postoperative patients are at particularly increased risk because of high ADH secretion secondary to pain and emotional stress. As the free water excretion ability of infants is limited in comparison with that in older children, they are at increased risk of developing hyponatremia from excessive oral water intake. Infants younger than 1 year but more often younger than 6 months fed water without electrolytes may develop hyponatremia and associated symptoms such as lethargy, seizures, and hypothermia. Symptoms correct rapidly with water restriction.

Hypervolemic Hyponatremia

Affected patients have both total body sodium and water in great excess and present with pulmonary or peripheral edema. The edema-forming states such as congestive heart failure, cirrhosis, and nephrotic syndrome are characterized by decreased effective blood volume (despite an increased ECF) that leads to stimulation of the renin-angiotensin-aldosterone axis as well as ADH secretion. Although both sodium and water are retained, hyponatremia develops because of proportionately greater water retention. The urinary sodium is usually less than 10 mEq/L because of avid sodium reabsorption as a consequence of decreased effective blood volume and decreased renal perfusion.

Patients with oliguric acute or chronic renal failure retain sodium and water because of severely reduced GFR. The urinary sodium concentration in these patients is variable (<10 mEq/L in patients with acute renal failure caused by glomerular diseases and >20 mEq/L in those with acute tubular necrosis or chronic renal failure).

Consequences of Hyponatremia

Most patients with mild degrees of hyponatremia (plasma sodium levels, 125 to 135 mEq/L) are asymptomatic. Once the serum sodium concentration falls below 120 mEq/L, serious sequelae, especially involving the central nervous system, can follow. Cerebral edema develops because the decrease in plasma osmolality causes water to move into the cells. Cerebral overhydration can manifest with varied symptoms, such as headache, vomiting, altered consciousness, seizures, and coma. The severity of symptoms is dependent on both the magnitude and rapidity of the fall in the plasma sodium concentration. Although seizures are common with acute hyponatremia, patients with chronic hyponatremia may manifest focal neurologic deficits and ataxia. The brain is protected during chronic hyponatremia by adaptive changes involving loss of intracellular osmolytes. However, the same protective changes can be responsible for the harmful effects seen when chronic hyponatremia is corrected too rapidly (see later discussion).

Patients with hyponatremia can develop shock at lesser degrees of body water depletion in comparison with patients with normal or increased serum sodium concentration, because of the associated fluid shift from the ECF to the ICF compartment. The decrease in the intravascular volume is a stimulus for ADH secretion, which serves to perpetuate the hyponatremia by limiting renal water excretion.

Treatment of Hyponatremia

The treatment of hyponatremia depends on its severity, its duration, and the ECF volume status. The primary goal should be to treat the underlying condition giving rise to hyponatremia (e.g., management of diarrhea, mineralocorticoid deficiency, nephrotic syndrome, or congestive heart failure). However, management of hypovolemia often requires initiation of corrective therapy before the underlying disease is controlled.

Patients with severe hypovolemia should promptly receive parenteral fluids to restore the circulating blood volume and normalize tissue perfusion. Blood and urine specimens should ideally be obtained as soon as possible to assess serum electrolytes, blood urea nitrogen level, creatinine level, and urinary sodium excretion. As correction of severe hypovolemia takes precedence over normalization of osmolality, isotonic solutions can be safely administered before the blood chemistry results are available. Crystalloids are the preferred replacement fluids except if blood transfusion is required in cases of hemorrhagic shock. Isotonic crystalloids such as 0.9% saline (sodium level, 154 mEq/L) or lactated Ringer solution (sodium level, 130 mEq/L) are administered at rate of 10 to 20 mL/kg over a short period of time. Fluid boluses can be repeated as needed until clinical improvement has occurred. The correction of hypovolemia helps in reversing the pathophysiologic factors causing water retention, thus ameliorating the hyponatremia. In patients with known cardiac, renal, or pulmonary diseases, fluid should be administered with caution, and concomitant measurement of central venous pressure and respiratory function is desirable.

After correction of acute hypovolemia, the remaining fluid deficit should be corrected slowly over 24 to 48 hours; additional fluid should be given to accommodate ongoing losses.

Patients with significant symptoms attributable to severe hyponatremia should receive hypertonic (3%) saline (513 mEq/L). Central nervous system symptoms almost always lessen when the serum sodium concentration is increased by 10 mEq/L. This can be achieved by giving 12 mL/kg of 3% saline (6 mEq/kg) over 6 hours. It is recommended that the serum sodium concentration not exceed 125 mEq/L with this treatment.

Patients with SIADH require water restriction. In this group of patients, it is difficult to raise the plasma sodium concentration even with hypertonic saline, unless the ECF volume is simultaneously reduced. Whereas water restriction is enough for patients with mild hyponatremia, patients with symptoms should receive intravenous furosemide (1 to 2 mg/kg/day) followed by intravenous hypertonic saline. In chronic SIADH, demeclocycline (300 to 1200 mg/day) is effective because it diminishes the renal response to ADH.

Patients with hypervolemic hyponatremia require salt and water restriction. Any effort to increase the serum sodium concentration by saline administration causes further ECF volume expansion and may worsen the patient's condition. In cases of severe salt and water

overload associated with renal failure, dialysis is the most effective therapy.

The management of patients with chronic hyponatremia is controversial. These patients usually have very subtle symptoms because the brain has time to adapt to the disturbance with a decrease in the intracellular osmolytes. Rapid correction of hyponatremia can lead to cellular shrinkage and can cause an osmotically induced demyelination syndrome, particularly in the pons. The patients with extensive lesions can have flaccid quadriplegia, dysphagia, and dysarthria.

HYPERNATREMIA

Hypernatremia (plasma sodium level > 145 mEq/L) can occur as result of (1) loss of both body sodium and water (water losses exceeding those of sodium), (2) isolated loss of water, and (3) increase in body sodium.

The development of hypernatremia is usually prevented by thirst and renal concentrating mechanisms. Thirst is so effective that even patients with complete diabetes insipidus (DI) avoid hypernatremia by drinking. Hypernatremia develops only when hypotonic fluid losses occur in combination with a disturbance in water intake, as a result of inadequate access (as in comatose, handicapped or very young patients), or as a result of a primary abnormality of thirst mechanism (e.g., hypothalamic adipsic syndrome). As is the case with hyponatremia, establishing the differential diagnosis of hypernatremia is aided by determining the patient's ECF volume status (hypovolemia, euvolemia, or hypervolemia), as shown in Figure 27-3.

Hypovolemic Hypernatremia

Disorders associated with losses of both sodium and water but with a relatively greater loss of water lead to hypovolemic hypernatremia. Many of the common causes (e.g., diarrhea, diuretic use) are similar to those that cause hypovolemic hyponatremia. Hypernatremia in these situations develops because of failure to ingest water. Hypernatremic dehydration and failure to thrive often develop in neonates who nurse poorly, especially if the mother's breast milk has not begun flowing. If the losses are extrarenal (e.g., through diarrhea, vomiting, profuse sweating), the urinary sodium concentration is less than 10 mEq/L. The renal causes are usually associated with a urine sodium concentration higher than 20 mEq/L.

Euvolemic Hypernatremia

Pure water losses do not lead to volume contraction unless the water losses are massive; these patients therefore appear euvolemic. In addition, hypernatremia develops only when the hypotonic losses are not accompanied by appropriate water intake. Although water loss can occur through the skin or the respiratory tract, the most important disorder in this group is DI.

Patients with DI have a very low urine osmolality. Central DI is caused by a failure to secrete ADH; nephrogenic DI is secondary to a renal resistance to ADH. Acquired forms of central and nephrogenic DI are more common than the hereditary forms.

Hereditary central DI can be either autosomal dominant or, less commonly, autosomal recessive. The autosomal recessive form occurs in association with diabetes mellitus, optic atrophy, and deafness (Wolfram syndrome). The acquired causes of central DI include central nervous system trauma, infections, tumors, granulomatous infiltration, and vascular malformations.

Congenital nephrogenic DI is a rare X-linked disorder affecting mainly boys, with variable penetrance in girls. The acquired form of nephrogenic DI can be seen in association with chronic renal diseases (e.g., polycystic disease, medullary cystic disease, ureteral obstruction), electrolyte disorders (e.g., hypokalemia, hypercalcemia),

Hypernatremia

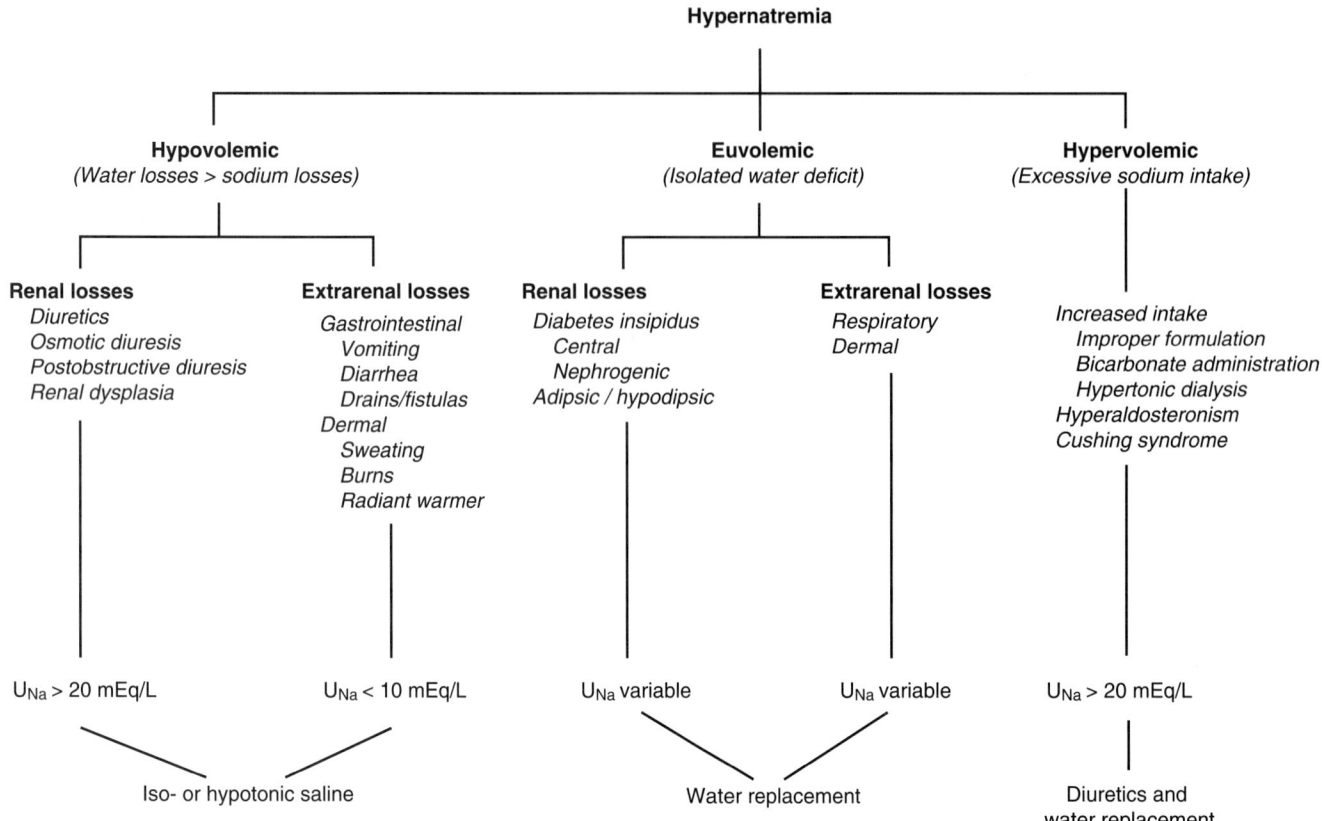

Figure 27-3. Classification, diagnosis, and treatment of hypernatremic states. (Modified from Beri T, Schrier RW: Disorders of water metabolism. In Schrier RW [ed]: Renal and Electrolyte Disorders. Philadelphia, Lippincott-Raven, 1997.)

drugs (e.g., lithium, demeclocycline, amphotericin, foscarnet), and sickle cell disease/trait.

Older children with DI have polyuria, polydipsia, and nocturia. The urine is hyposmolar and remains so even when these children develop dehydration and consequently increased serum osmolality. During infancy, DI can manifest with recurrent episodes of unexplained dehydration and fever. Repeated episodes of hypernatremic dehydration can lead to permanent neurologic sequelae.

Performing a fluid deprivation test and then determining the response to injectable vasopressin can help diagnose DI and differentiate between the central and nephrogenic forms. Primary treatment should focus on the underlying cause if possible. Central DI is managed with hormonal replacement therapy with desmopressin (DDAVP). DDAVP is administered intranasally in a dosage ranging from 2.5 to 20 μg every 8 to 12 hours. Alternatively, the oral preparation can be administered (starting dosage, 0.05 mg b.i.d.). There is considerable individual variation in the required dosage, and it is important to allow patients to revert to mild polyuria before the next dose is given, to prevent excessive water accumulation. An intravenous form of antidiuretic hormone can be used in sick and comatose patients.

Therapy for nephrogenic DI should ensure a sufficient intake of water to replace the large urinary losses. Because obligatory urinary water losses increase with increasing solute load, restriction of sodium intake reduces the urine output. Administration of diuretics, such as thiazides and amiloride, keeps these patients in a mildly dehydrated state, which leads to increased water reabsorption in the more proximal segments of the nephron, thereby decreasing urine output. Nonsteroidal anti-inflammatory drugs such as indomethacin also reduce polyuria and may be used in combination with diuretics. Careful attention should be paid to the fluid balance in these patients

when they are sick and cannot drink on their own, because they require large quantities of water replacement. Frequent monitoring of serum electrolytes is mandatory during these periods.

Adipsic/hypodipsic hypernatremia (essential hypernatremia; reset osmostat) characterizes a group of patients who have persistent hypernatremia, absence or attenuation of thirst, and often-partial DI. Many patients are obese as a result of polyphagia. These patients require regimental intake of fluids; they may need supplementation with DDAVP.

Hypervolemic Hypernatremia

This is the least common type of hypernatremia. Most of the causes are iatrogenic (administration of improperly formulated oral rehydration solution, administration of intravenous fluids, excessive bicarbonate administration during resuscitative efforts, inadvertent dialysis against a high sodium concentration dialysate, and seawater drowning). Other causes include primary hyperaldosteronism and Cushing syndrome.

Consequences of Hypernatremia

Hypernatremia causes intracellular dehydration by movement of water from the intracellular to the extracellular compartment. The consequences of intracellular dehydration are particularly marked in the brain and manifest with irritability, altered sensorium, lethargy, and hyperreflexia and eventually seizures, coma, and death. Brain hemorrhages can result from tearing of small blood vessels when the brain shrinks as a result of intracellular dehydration. Hypernatremia and dehydration may predispose to dural sinus thrombosis. During chronic hypernatremia, the brain cells adapt to the increased ECF osmolality by accumulating "idiogenic osmoles" (which are mostly amino acids, particularly taurine). They increase intracellular osmolality, consequently restoring intracellular volume. This protective response has significant implications for therapy and the speed with which hypernatremia should be corrected (see later discussion).

Treatment of Hypernatremia

The treatment of hypernatremia is guided by its severity, its chronicity, and the ECF volume status of the patient.

It is important to realize that patients with hyperosmolality maintain the ECF space at the expense of the ICF compartment, and, therefore, the degree of sodium and fluid losses may be profound before clinical signs of hypovolemia develop. As a consequence, large volumes of isotonic crystalloid may be necessary to replace the fluid deficit.

Once initial fluid resuscitation has been performed, the serum sodium concentration should be restored slowly over a minimum period of 48 hours. The total water deficit can be estimated as follows:

$$\text{Free water deficit (in liters)} = ([P_{Na\,(mEq/L)}/140] - 1) \times 0.6 \times \text{weight (kg)}$$

Hypernatremia is corrected especially slowly when it is more severe and chronic. The rate of fall in plasma sodium concentration should be less than 1 mEq/L/hour. During the correction of hypernatremia, the idiogenic osmoles that brain cells produce to prevent cellular dehydration dissipate slowly. If hypernatremia is corrected too rapidly, the increased intracellular osmolality from the idiogenic osmoles can lead to cerebral edema. In patients with hypervolemic hypernatremia, the first line of therapy is restriction of salt intake, followed by administration of diuretics.

SUMMARY AND RED FLAGS

Acid-base and electrolyte disturbances have many causes that reflect abnormalities of regulation or compensation of these systems. For many acid-base or electrolyte disturbances, the underlying condition needs to be treated before consideration of the disturbance. This is true in all causes of shock, such as dehydration, adrenal crisis, or hemorrhage. The circulating blood volume must be quickly reestablished; this is usually performed as part of the resuscitation phase of treating dehydration. Thereafter, specific acid-base or, more often, electrolyte abnormalities can be attended to during the replacement phase to correct electrolyte deficits. In general, electrolyte disturbances can and often must be corrected slowly. This is particularly true for sodium abnormalities. The major exceptions are hyperkalemia and acute hypercarbic respiratory acidosis, which must be treated immediately. Hyperkalemia can cause life-threatening arrhythmias (see Chapter 7) and cardiac arrest, whereas acute respiratory acidosis signifies impending respiratory failure and respiratory arrest (see Chapter 3).

Each of the discussed acid-base and electrolyte disturbances are red flags, but hyperkalemia remains the one of most concern and the most dangerous. Anuria, hypotension, weight loss, seizures, coma, hypoglycemia or hyperglycemia, apnea, and arrhythmias are additional red flags. Moreover, the clinician must remain vigilant in identifying the primary reason or reasons for any of these acid-base or electrolyte disturbances.

REFERENCES

Acid-Base Disorders

Adrogue HJ, Madias NE: Management of life-threatening acid-base disorders. New Engl J Med 1998;338:26.

Batlle D, von Riotte A, Schlueter W: Urinary sodium in the evaluation of hyperchloremic metabolic acidosis. New Engl J Med 1987;316:144.

Benaron DA, Yorgin PD, Lapuk S, et al: Alkalemia in a newborn infant. J Pediatr 1992;120:489.

Bergstein JM: Renal tubular acidosis. In Behrman RE, Kliegman RM, Jenson HB (eds): Nelson Textbook of Pediatrics. Philadelphia, WB Saunders, 2000.

Bettinelli A, Bianchetti MG, Girardin E, et al: Use of calcium excretion values to distinguish two forms of primary renal tubular hypokalemic alkalosis: Bartter and Gitelman syndromes. J Pediatr 1992;120:38.

Brewer ED: Disorders of acid-base balance. Pediatr Clin North Am 1990;37:429.

Fall PJ: A stepwise approach to acid-base disorders. Practical patient evaluation for metabolic acidosis and other conditions. Postgrad Med 2000;107:249.

Hanna JD, Scheinman JI, Chan JCM: The kidney in acid-base balance. Pediatr Clin North Am 1995;42:1365.

Izraeli S, Rachmel A, Frishberg Y, et al: Transient renal acidification defect during acute infantile diarrhea: The role of urinary sodium. J Pediatr 1990;117:711.

Lorenz JM, Kleinman LI, Markarian K, et al: Serum anion gap in the differential diagnosis of metabolic acidosis in critically ill newborns. J Pediatr 1999;135:751.

Mingin GC, Stock JA, Hanna MK: Gastrocystoplasty: Long-term complications in 22 patients. J Urol 1999;162:1122.

Paces R: Long-term follow-up in distal renal tubular acidosis with sensorineural deafness. Pediatr Nephrol 2000;15:63.

Rodriguez-Soriano J, Garcia-Fuentes M, Vallo A, et al: Hypercalcemia in neonatal distal renal tubular acidosis. Pediatr Nephrol 2000;14:354.

Shapiro JI, Kaehny WD: Pathogenesis and management of metabolic acidosis and alkalosis. In Schrier RW (ed): Renal and Electrolyte Disorders. Philadelphia, Lippincott-Raven, 1997.

Zelikovic I: Molecular pathophysiology of tubular transport disorders. Pediatr Nephrol 2001;16:919.

Potassium Disorders

Alon US: Renal tubular acidosis. In Finberg L (ed): Saunders Manual of Pediatric Practice. Philadelphia, WB Saunders, 1998, p 694.

Carlisle EJF, Donnelly SM, Ethier JH, et al: Modulation of the secretion of potassium by accompanying anions in humans. Kidney Int 1991;39:1206.

Chacko M, Fordtran JS, Emmett M: Effect of mineralocorticoid activity on transtubular potassium gradient, urinary [K]/[Na] ratio, and fractional excretion of potassium. Am J Kidney Dis 1998;32:47.

Halperin ML, Kamel K: Potassium. Lancet 1998;352:135.

Hellerstein S, Alon US, Warady BA: Renal impairment. In Ashcraft KW (ed): Pediatric Surgery. Philadelphia, WB Saunders, 2000.

Mandal AK: Hypokalemia and hyperkalemia. Med Clin North Am 1997;81:611.

Perazella MA: Drug-induced hyperkalemia: Old culprits and new offenders. Am J Med 2000;109:307.

Peterson LN, Levi M: Disorders of potassium metabolism. In Schrier RW (ed): Renal and Electrolyte Disorders. Philadelphia, Lippincott-Raven, 1997.

Rodriguez-Soriano J, Ubetagoyena M, Vallo A: Transtubular potassium concentration gradient: A useful test to estimate renal aldosterone bioactivity in infants and children. Pediatr Nephrol 1990;4:105.

Wilson FII, Disse-Nicodcme S, Choate KA, et al: Human hypertension caused by mutations in WNK kinases. Science 2001;293:1107.

Sodium Disorders

Abrahm WT, Schrier RW: Renal sodium excretion, edematous disorders, and diuretic use. In Schrier RW (ed): Renal and Electrolyte Disorders. Philadelphia, Lippincott-Raven, 1997.

Ball SG, Vaidja B, Baylis PH: Hypothalamic adipsic syndrome: Diagnosis and management. Clin Endocrinol 1997;47:405.

Berl T, Schrier RW: Disorders of water metabolism. In Schrier RW (ed): Renal and Electrolyte Disorders. Philadelphia, Lippincott-Raven, 1997.

Berry PL, Belsha CW: Hyponatremia. Pediatr Clin North Am 1990;37:351.

Cadnapaphornchai MA, Schrier RW: Pathogenesis and management of hyponatremia. Am J Med 2000;109:688.

Conley SB: Hypernatremia. Pediatr Clin North Am 1990;37:365.

Ganong CA, Kappy MS: Cerebral salt wasting in children. The need for recognition and treatment. Am J Dis Child 1993;147:167.

Hall RT, Simon S, Smith MT: Readmission of breastfed infants in the first 2 weeks of life. J Perinatol 2000;20:432.

Harris HW Jr: Diabetes insipidus. In Behrman RE, Kliegman RM, Jenson HB (eds): Nelson Textbook of Pediatrics. Philadelphia, WB Saunders, 2000.

Haycock GB: The syndrome of inappropriate secretion of antidiuretic hormone. Pediatr Nephrol 1995;9:375.

Jakobsson B, Berg U: Effect of hydrochlorothiazide and indomethacin treatment on renal function in nephrogenic diabetes insipidus. Acta Pediatr 1994;83:522.

Manganaro R, Mami C, Marrone T, et al: Incidence of dehydration and hypernatremia in exclusively breast-fed infants. J Pediatr 2001;139:673.

Trachtman H: Sodium and water homeostasis. Pediatr Clin North Am 1995;6:1343.

28 Acute and Chronic Scrotal Swelling

Jack S. Elder

The most serious causes of acute scrotal swelling are testicular torsion and incarcerated or strangulated inguinal hernia, both of which necessitate immediate surgical correction. Consequently, a prompt, careful approach to a painful or inflamed scrotum is essential. The differential diagnosis of scrotal swelling is extensive and varies depending on age of the patient (Tables 28-1 and 28-2). Optimal treatment requires an expeditious diagnosis. If there is any ambiguity regarding the diagnosis, a pediatric urologist should be consulted.

SCROTAL AND INGUINAL ANATOMY

INGUINAL REGION

All abdominal muscles and their aponeuroses contribute to the inguinal ligament and canal. The inguinal canal runs obliquely between the external and the internal inguinal rings. The anterior wall of the canal is formed by the external oblique aponeurosis; the floor, by the inguinal ligament; the roof, by arching fibers of the internal oblique and transversus abdominis muscles; and the posterior wall by the conjoined tendon, by the internal oblique and transversus abdominis muscles. The oblique direction of the inguinal canal allows for the posterior and anterior walls to coapt with increases in intraabdominal pressure.

TESTIS DESCENT

The testes develop in the lumbar region of the abdominal cavity between the peritoneum and the transversalis fascia at approximately 7 weeks of gestation. By the eighth week of gestation, the gubernaculum extends from the caudal end of the epididymis through the inguinal canal to insert on the internal wall of the scrotum. The processus vaginalis, a finger-like outpouching of the peritoneum, extends adjacent to the gubernaculum to form the inguinal canal. As the processus vaginalis descends into the scrotum, it carries extensions of the abdominal wall layers.

The testis normally descends through the inguinal canal into the scrotum before birth. As the testis and the spermatic cord descend through the inguinal canal, they are covered by the three concentric layers of the anterior abdominal fascia (Fig. 28-1). When the testis reaches the scrotum, the processus vaginalis is patent, leaving a connection between the scrotum and the peritoneal cavity. Normally, the processus vaginalis becomes obliterated, leaving a residual tunica vaginalis surrounding the testis. Typically, 1 to 2 mL of clear fluid is in the tunica vaginalis.

SCROTUM

The scrotum has two separate compartments, each containing a testis, epididymis, and distal spermatic cord. It comprises multiple layers that are continuous with the superficial layers of the anterior abdominal wall. The external location of the scrotum results in the temperature of the testes being 2° to 3° F below core body temperature, which allows for normal spermatogenesis.

TESTIS

The testes are the male reproductive organs and are suspended in the tunica vaginalis of the scrotum by the spermatic cords. The epididymis, attached to the testis posteriorly, consists of the caput (upper pole), corpus (body), and cauda (tail) (Fig. 28-2). The cauda epididymis is attached to the vas deferens, which can be palpated as a small, rubbery structure in the spermatic cord. The epididymis is responsible for sperm maturation and storage. Each testis relies on three arteries for its blood supply: the testicular artery, the cremasteric artery, and the deferential artery. Each enters the scrotum through the spermatic cord. The testicle receives both sympathetic and parasympathetic innervation. These autonomic nerves carry impulses that, with testicular stimulation, produce symptoms of deep visceral pain and associated nausea.

DIAGNOSTIC STRATEGIES

HISTORY

A detailed history is critical in evaluating a boy with acute or chronic scrotal swelling. If there is painful testicular or scrotal swelling, knowledge of the following characteristics is helpful:

1. *Onset of pain:* Testicular torsion and torsion of an appendix testis often occur after exercise or minor genital injury. Pain caused by these conditions may also awaken the patient from sleep.
2. *Duration of pain:* number of hours or days since onset of symptoms.
3. *Evolution of pain:* Testicular torsion tends to occur abruptly, whereas torsion of an appendix testis and epididymitis typically have an insidious onset.
4. *Associated/radiation of pain:* Inguinal discomfort suggests inguinal pathologic processes such as a hernia. If there is radiation of pain from the flank, then renal or ureteral pathologic processes, such as an obstructing ureteral calculus, should be considered in the differential diagnosis. Pain, with or without swelling of the scrotum, has a large differential diagnosis (Table 28-3).

Although sometimes nonspecific, associated manifestations are also important:

1. *General systemic:* Fever, chills, or rigors suggest an infectious cause.
2. *Abdominal signs/symptoms:* Nausea, vomiting, and abdominal or inguinal pain suggest testicular torsion or, on occasion, epididymitis. Some patients with testicular torsion initially experience severe abdominal pain as well as testicular pain.
3. *Urologic signs/symptoms:* Dysuria, urinary frequency, hematuria, or penile discharge suggests a urinary tract infection, urethritis, or epididymitis in a sexually active boy or man.

Table 28-1. Differential Diagnosis of Scrotal Masses in Young and Adolescent Boys

Painful	Painless*
Testicular torsion	Hydrocele
Torsion of testicular appendage	Inguinal hernia (reducible)
	Varicocele
Epididymoorchitis	Spermatocele
Trauma: testicular rupture, hematocele	Testicular tumor
	Paratesticular tumor
Inguinal hernia (incarcerated or strangulated)	Idiopathic scrotal edema
	Henoch-Schönlein purpura
Mumps orchitis	

*Occasionally associated with discomfort.

4. *Unusual rashes:* Henoch-Schönlein purpura may result in vasculitis of the spermatic cord with associated scrotal pain and swelling.

In addition, a thorough medical history is imperative. Significant questions include the following:

1. History of urinary tract infections, sexually transmitted diseases, or renal calculi.
2. History of any surgical procedures on the groin, scrotum, or abdomen. Often an orchiopexy performed for an undescended testis places the testis in a dartos pouch, which would prevent testicular torsion in the future.
3. History of any previous episodes of testicular pain. Previous intermittent severe pain in the same testis may be secondary to intermittent torsion of the testis.
4. Obstructive voiding pattern, such as slow, intermittent stream or incomplete bladder emptying predisposes to urinary infection, which could cause epididymitis.
5. Lower urinary tract pathologic processes, such as posterior urethral valves, urethral stricture (after trauma or hypospadias repair), or neuropathic bladder, may predispose to urinary infection, which could cause epididymitis.

PHYSICAL EXAMINATION

Examination of the scrotal contents should be routine in any boy presenting with abdominal, inguinal, or scrotal pain. Inspection, palpation, and transillumination of any mass are integral parts of a thorough physical examination.

Pubertal Development. Testicular torsion is much less common than torsion of the appendix testis in a prepubertal child (Table 28-4). Conversely, in an adolescent, testicular torsion and epididymitis (if the patient is sexually active) are most common.

Scars in the Inguinal Region. Scars imply previous surgery for hernia, hydrocele, undescended testis, or varicocele.

Table 28-2. Differential Diagnosis of Scrotal Swelling in Newborns

Hydrocele	Scrotal hematoma
Inguinal hernia (reducible)	Testicular tumor
Inguinal hernia (incarcerated)*	Meconium peritonitis
Testicular torsion*	Epididymitis*

*May be associated with scrotal inflammation.

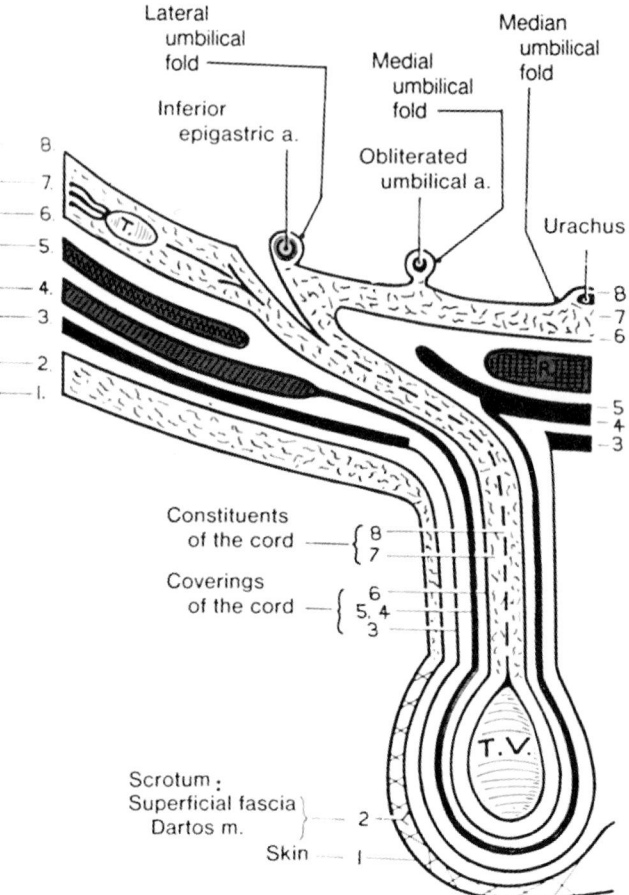

Figure 28-1. Diagram illustrating the inguinal canal and the origin of the layers of the spermatic cord. The drawing demonstrates the eight layers of the abdominal wall, the scrotal wall, and the spermatic cord. The external spermatic fascia is derived from the external oblique aponeurosis; the cremaster muscle and cremasteric fascia are derived from the external oblique and its fascia; and the internal spermatic fascia is derived from the transversalis fascia. R, rectus abdominis; T, testis; TV, tunica vaginalis. (From Moore KL: Clinically Oriented Anatomy, 2nd ed. Baltimore, Williams & Wilkins, 1985.)

Scrotal Skin Changes and Fixation. Erythema suggests an underlying inflammatory process but is nonspecific. Fixation of skin over the testis is suggestive of testicular necrosis.

Testis Position within the Scrotum. An inflamed testis positioned high in the scrotum is suggestive of testicular torsion. Palpation provides information about intrascrotal structures. The testis should be evaluated for size and consistency (soft, firm, or hard) and compared with the testis on the contralateral side. Accurate localization of pain and swelling to the testis or epididymis, or both, is important. The consistency, size, and relationship to the testis of a paratesticular mass should be noted, along with its reducibility. Any scrotal soft tissue swelling should be evaluated by transillumination. The cremasteric reflex is stimulated by gently scratching the ipsilateral medial thigh; cremasteric muscle contraction causes the scrotum to retract. The presence of a symmetric cremasteric reflex makes testicular torsion unlikely; absence of the reflex is a nonspecific finding.

LABORATORY DATA

Basic laboratory data for evaluation of acute and chronic swelling of the testis include urinalysis, urine culture, and tests for chlamydia

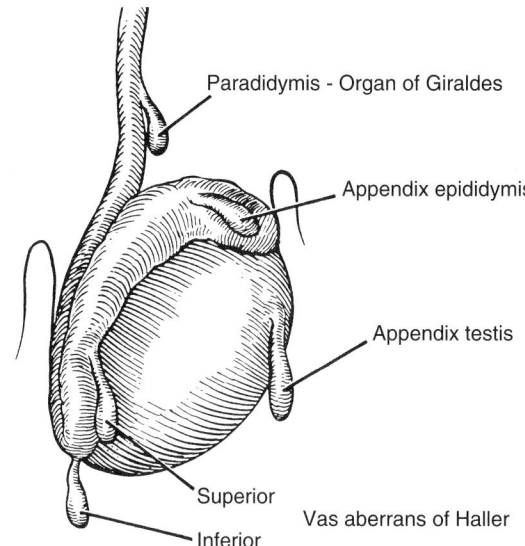

Paradidymis - Organ of Giraldes

Appendix epididymis

Appendix testis

Superior

Vas aberrans of Haller

Inferior

Figure 28-2. Lateral view of the testis showing posterior location of epididymis and appendix testes. The appendix testis is present in almost all boys, the appendix epididymis is present approximately 50% of boys, and the other appendages are rarely present. (From Kelalis PP, King LR, Belman AB [eds]: Clinical Pediatric Urology, 2nd ed. Philadelphia, WB Saunders, 1985.)

Table 28-3. **Causes of Acute Scrotal Pain**

Common

Testicular torsion
Torsion of testicular appendage
Epididymitis (gonorrhea, chlamydial infection in sexually active adolescents)*
Trauma*
Scrotal edema (Henoch-Schönlein purpura)
Pain referred to scrotum (nephrolithiasis, ureteropelvic junction obstruction, appendicitis, spinal cord tumor, immunoglobulin A [IgA] nephropathy)

Less Common

Orchitis (mumps, varicella, coxsackievirus, dengue)*
Abscess
Infarction
Malignancy: primary testicular neoplasm (e.g., seminoma), embryonal cell (usually painless mass)
Leukemia: primary or relapse (usually painless swelling)*

Uncommon

Granulomatous orchitis*
Drug-induced epididymitis (amiodarone)*
Behçet disease
Sarcoidosis
Polyarteritis nodosa*
Epididymitis (tuberculosis, brucellosis, actinomycosis, leprosy, *Salmonella* infection, fungal infection, parasitic infestation, *Nocardia* infection)
Orchitis (rickettsial, *Nocardia* infections; toxoplasmosis; cytomegalovirus)
Testicular pyocele
Fournier gangrene*

*Bilateral involvement possible.

and gonorrhea if the patient is sexually active (see Chapters 23 and 29). A complete blood cell or white blood cell count is generally not useful in establishing a diagnosis.

IMAGING STUDIES

Imaging studies are often helpful in determining the cause of acute and chronic testicular or scrotal swelling. They should not be substituted for a thorough history and careful physical examination performed by a surgical specialist. The conditions necessitating immediate surgical treatment include testicular torsion, incarcerated inguinal hernia, and testicular rupture secondary to trauma; testicular tumor mandates urgent surgical attention. Although the diagnosis of incarcerated hernia usually is straightforward, testicular torsion can be easily confused with several conditions that can be managed nonoperatively, including epididymitis and torsion of the appendix testis.

The two diagnostic studies most frequently utilized are color Doppler ultrasonography and the radionuclide scrotal (testicular flow) scan. These studies assess whether blood flow is normal or increased, observed with epididymitis and torsion of the appendix testis, or whether blood flow is absent or reduced, observed with testicular torsion. Unfortunately, neither imaging study is 100% accurate. If the clinician strongly suspects that the patient has testicular torsion, then prompt surgical exploration is recommended, without confirmation by an imaging study. If the clinician seems certain of the diagnosis (e.g., torsion of the appendix testis, simple hydrocele), then it is unnecessary to obtain the study. Ordering a color Doppler ultrasonographic study or testicular flow scan is recommended in the following situations:

1. when the clinician is relatively certain that the child does not have testicular torsion and desires confirmation.
2. if acute scrotal pain and swelling have been present for more than 48 hours, in which case the likelihood of testicular salvage with ischemia-producing testicular torsion is low.
3. if the diagnosis cannot be made with certainty from the history and physical examination.
4. if there is a hydrocele that prevents palpation of the testis (on occasion, a testis tumor may be present).

Color Doppler Ultrasonography

Sonography provides a relatively accurate image of the testis and epididymis, and color Doppler imaging assesses blood flow. It is performed by examining the normal testis first and adjusting the color flow settings to detect normal flow. The affected testis is then examined for decreased or absent flow in comparison with the normal testis. Color flow Doppler imaging is able to distinguish between the increased collateral blood flow within the scrotal skin and the decreased blood flow to the testis in patients with testicular torsion. Sonography also can differentiate testicular rupture from a scrotal hematoma. Color flow Doppler imaging is nearly 100% accurate in demonstrating increased flow resulting from torsion of the appendix testis or epididymitis, but it is usually unable to distinguish these two entities. If a tumor is present (usually the mass is hypoechoic), sonography can demonstrate that the mass arises from the testis. There are a few benign localized testicular tumors that can be excised, with sparing of the remainder of the testis.

The test is quick, easy to perform, and noninvasive. Accuracy rates of this modality are at least 95%, which compares favorably with those of scrotal scintigraphy. In addition, it is performed more rapidly than scintigraphy and is less expensive.

There are several limitations of color Doppler imaging:

1. In boys with testicular torsion of short duration and if the torsion is less than 360 degrees, there may be venous congestion without impairment of testicular blood flow; color Doppler imaging may demonstrate normal flow.

Table 28-4. Differentiation of Acute Painful Scrotal Swelling in Childhood

	Spermatic Cord Torsion	Epididymoorchitis	Torsion of Appendix Testis
Age	Usually perinatal and 10-18 yr, but any age possible	Usually adolescence, but any age possible	2-12 yr
Symptoms and signs	Abrupt onset; there may have been previous similar episodes	Gradual onset	Gradual onset
Pain	Localized to the testis and may radiate to groin and lower abdomen	Localization to epididymis; may involve entire testis after 24 hr	Localization to upper pole of testis; may involve entire testis after 24 hr
Fever	Rare	Common	Rare
Vomiting	Common	Rare	Rare
Dysuria	Rare	Common	Rare
Physical examination	Testis may be high riding, swollen, exquisitely tender; scrotal erythema may be present; cremasteric reflex is absent	Testis and epididymis are firm, tender, swollen; scrotal erythema may be present; cremasteric reflex present	Testis is normal or enlarged; firm mass may be seen or felt at upper pole, distinct from epididymis; scrotal erythema may be present; cremasteric reflex present
Pyuria, urinary infection	Rare	Common	Rare
Blood flow (color Doppler study; isotope scrotal scan)	Diminished or absent	Increased	Normal or increased

2. In the prepubertal testis, blood flow may be difficult to demonstrate, even when the testis is normal, and absence of flow may be misinterpreted for testicular torsion.
3. The color Doppler aspect of the study is user dependent.

Testicular Flow Scan

The technetium 99m–pertechnetate testicular flow scan can distinguish between inflammatory and ischemic conditions of the testis. After intravenous injection of the radionuclide, both flow studies and static images of the testes are obtained. Typically, the study takes 20 to 30 minutes. Testicular torsion appears as a "cold spot" of radionuclide deficiency secondary to diminished blood flow. In contrast, inflammatory conditions, such as epididymitis or torsion of the appendix testis, produce normal or increased uptake of ^{99m}Tc. If the testicle has been torsed for longer than 48 hours, there is often a hyperemic rim of tissue surrounding a cold spot, referred to as the "vascular rim." Accuracy rates of scrotal scintigraphy are 90% to 95%.

There are several limitations to the testicular flow scan:

1. The test is not available at all hospitals.
2. A false-positive scan (incorrectly interpreted as reduced flow, suggestive of torsion) can result from a hernia, hydrocele, or spermatocele, which may falsely decrease the radionuclide counts in the region of the testis. A false-negative scan (torsion is present but scan is read as normal) may occur in boys with late-phase testicular torsion, in which hyperemia of the scrotal wall is misinterpreted as flow to the testis.
3. If the extent of testicular torsion is 180 to 360 degrees, the scan may suggest normal flow.
4. If the patient has torsion-detorsion syndrome with only partial detorsion, the scan may demonstrate normal testicular flow.
5. No anatomic information regarding the scrotal contents is provided.
6. Although many institutions can rapidly arrange this study during weekday hours, considerable time delays may be encountered in arranging scans at night or on weekends.

DIFFERENTIAL DIAGNOSIS
(See Tables 28-3 and 28-4)

TESTICULAR TORSION

Testicular torsion is a surgical emergency because of the risk of gonadal loss. The likelihood of testicular survival depends on the duration and severity of torsion. Consequently, testicular survival depends on accurate diagnosis and expedient management.

The incidence of spermatic cord torsion is 1 in 4000 among boys and men younger than 25 years. The peak ages for testicular torsion are 10 to 18 years and the neonatal period. The pathogenesis of torsion and presentation in these two age groups are different.

In testicular torsion, the testis and spermatic cord rotate or twist within the tunica vaginalis (termed "intravaginal"), resulting in obstruction of venous drainage, followed by compromise of arterial flow and subsequent infarction (Fig. 28-3). In many older boys with torsion, there is a predisposing anatomic abnormality that increases the likelihood that the testis can rotate on the spermatic cord, termed the "bell-clapper" abnormality. The "bell-clapper" refers to horizontal positioning of the testis that results from a redundant tunica vaginalis or from an abnormal insertion of the epididymis to the testis (Fig. 28-4). The likelihood of irreversible testicular damage depends on the severity and duration of torsion. If the testicular torsion exceeds 360 degrees, then the testis may become necrotic within 6 to 12 hours. However, if testicular torsion is less than 360 degrees, then there may be continued arterial perfusion for 24 to 48 hours.

Patients typically experience the sudden onset of severe testicular pain and swelling. The event often occurs after minor trauma or exercise and may awaken the patient from sleep. Although the pain is usually localized to the affected hemiscrotum, there can be pain referred to the ipsilateral groin, and some patients also report abdominal pain. Associated symptoms may include nausea and vomiting. Thirty percent to 50% of patients describe previous episodes of severe scrotal pain that have resolved spontaneously. Patients do not have irritative voiding symptoms.

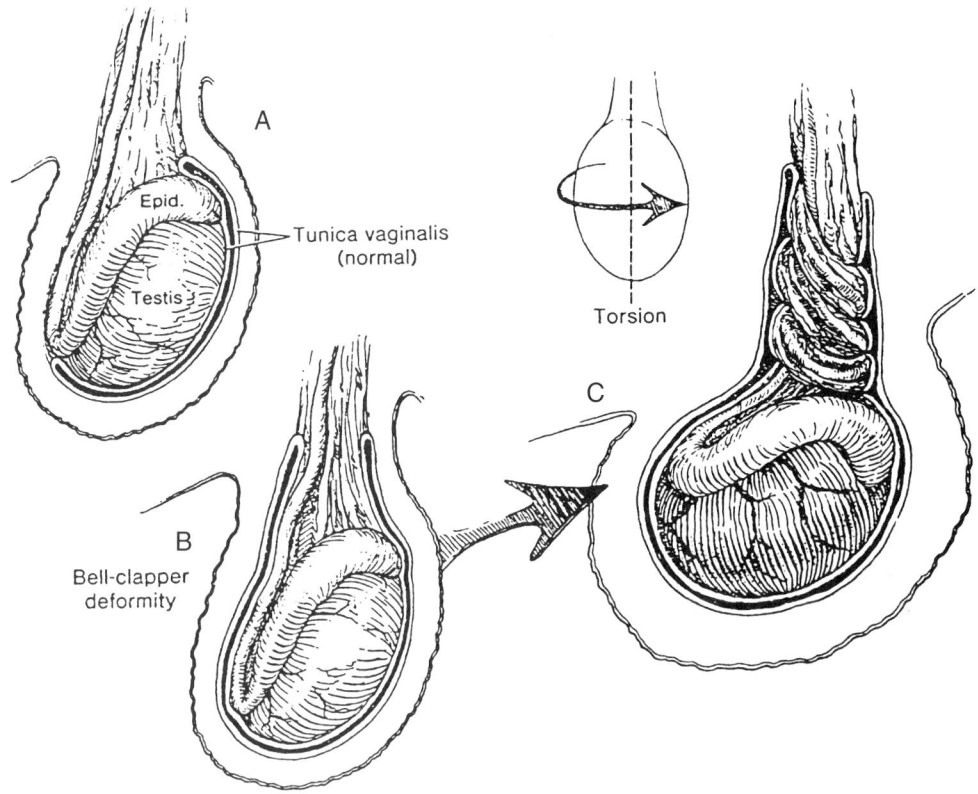

Figure 28-3. A to C, Mechanism of testicular torsion associated with the bell-clapper deformity. (From Fleisher GR, Ludwig S: Textbook of Pediatric Emergency Medicine, 3rd ed. Baltimore, Williams & Wilkins, 1993.)

On examination, the scrotum is erythematous and edematous, and the testis is enlarged and extremely tender. The relationship between the testis and the epididymis depends on the degree of testicular torsion; often the epididymis is posterior, as in normal male genitalia. If the patient has been experiencing pain for more than 24 hours, there may be too much inflammation to delineate the

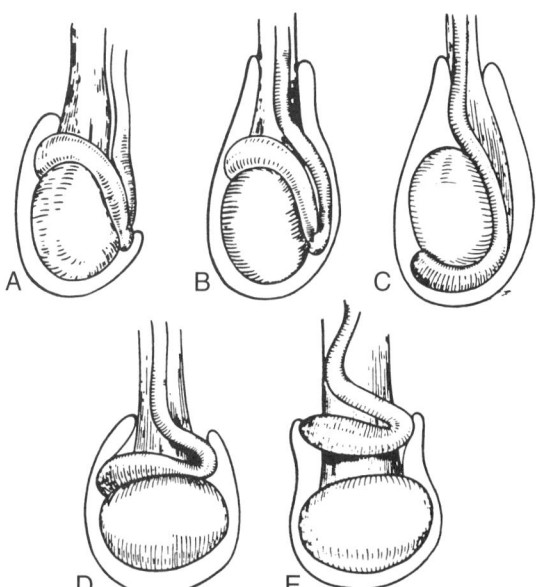

Figure 28-4. Anomalies of suspension associated with intravaginal testicular torsion. **A,** Normal. **B,** Envelopment by the tunica vaginalis. **C,** Inversion of the epididymis. **D** and **E,** Horizontal lie. Bell-clapper deformity is shown in **B** through **E.** (From Kelalis PP, King LR, Belman AB [eds]: Clinical Pediatric Urology, 2nd ed. Philadelphia, WB Saunders, 1985.)

scrotal contents. The cremasteric reflex is nearly always absent. The testis may be high in the scrotum. Urinalysis results are negative.

In most cases, the diagnosis of testicular torsion can be made from the history and physical examination. If torsion is the likely diagnosis, scrotal exploration should proceed immediately. Imaging studies such as color Doppler ultrasonography and radionuclide testicular flow scan typically demonstrate absence of blood flow. Because excessive time spent obtaining diagnostic studies can result in significant delay in therapy, these studies should be reserved for cases in which torsion is not suspected.

If the duration of symptoms is less than 4 to 6 hours, manual detorsion can be attempted. After administration of intravenous morphine (0.1 mg/kg body weight), manual detorsion can be attempted by lifting the scrotum and rotating the testis on its vascular pedicle. Usually, torsion occurs in a medial direction; therefore, the testis should be rotated outward toward the thigh. Successful detorsion is indicated by both relief of pain and a lower testicular position within the scrotum. Although successful manual detorsion may obviate emergency surgery, surgical fixation must be performed promptly because of the risk of recurrence.

Some boys present with a history of severe testicular pain that resolved in the emergency room or on the way to the hospital. In these cases, *torsion-detorsion syndrome* should be suspected, and scrotal orchiopexy should be considered.

If testicular torsion has been present more than 48 hours, the scrotum typically is severely enlarged, edematous, and erythematous, and the testis is an enlarged indurated mass. Color Doppler imaging in this situation typically reveals hyperemia in the scrotal wall with absence of testicular flow. The most appropriate term for this situation is *late-phase torsion.* Some clinicians use the inappropriate term "missed torsion." Late-phase torsion refers to a testis that has been torsed for a prolonged period of time and is necrotic.

Surgical management of testicular torsion consists of exploration, detorsion, and evaluation of testicular viability. An infarcted testicle is removed. If the testis is viable, it is fixed to the scrotal wall with nonabsorbable suture; this procedure is termed *scrotal orchiopexy.*

Contralateral scrotal orchiopexy is necessary because there is a significant risk of contralateral torsion. If torsion is detected and treated within 4 hours of the onset of symptoms, the salvage rate approaches 100%; at 8 to 12 hours, it falls to 20%; and after 24 hours, infarction is the rule.

Testicular torsion can also occur in the fetus and neonate. In these cases, torsion results from incomplete attachment of the gubernaculum to the scrotal wall and is "extravaginal." When torsion occurs in utero, often the testis is nonpalpable because it has become atrophic. If torsion occurs just before birth, the testis is typically large, firm, and nontender. Usually the ipsilateral hemiscrotum is ecchymotic. In these cases, the testis always is nonviable because torsion was a remote event. On occasion, extravaginal testicular torsion occurs after delivery, and the baby is at risk until 30 days beyond term; in these cases, the infant becomes irritable, the testis enlarges, and the scrotum becomes erythematous.

Color Doppler ultrasonography in the neonate is fairly reliable in distinguishing testicular torsion from scrotal hematoma and testicular tumor. However, testicular flow scanning is unreliable. Although testicular salvage in neonates with in utero torsion is highly unlikely, urgent exploration is recommended to confirm the diagnosis and to perform a contralateral scrotal orchiopexy to protect the solitary testis. If there is a possibility that torsion occurred after birth, there is a chance of saving the testis, and immediate exploration is therefore warranted.

TORSION OF APPENDIX TESTIS

The appendix testis is a vestigial remnant of the müllerian (mesonephric) ductal system that is attached to the upper pole of the testis. Some boys and men also have an appendage attached to the epididymis. When these appendages are long and pedunculated, they have a tendency to twist at their base, which results in ischemia and eventual infarction. This entity is most common in boys between 2 and 12 years of age and is uncommon in adolescents. Torsion of the appendix testis results in progressive inflammation and swelling of the epididymis and testis.

The onset of testicular pain and swelling is typically gradual. Usually affected boys walk into the emergency room and appear comfortable. Constitutional symptoms are usually less severe than with testicular torsion, but pain referred to the lower abdomen, nausea, and vomiting can occur. Physical examination reveals an erythematous and edematous scrotum with underlying testicular enlargement. Palpation of the testis should reveal a 3- to 5-mm tender, indurated mass on the upper pole. In some cases, the torsed appendix testis may be visible through the scrotal skin; this is termed the *blue dot sign*. As the duration of inflammation becomes longer, the cremasteric reflex is less likely to be present. Later in its clinical course, differentiation from testis torsion becomes increasingly difficult because there is associated reactive enlargement of the testis and epididymis (epididymoorchitis). A clinical diagnosis of torsion of the appendix testis should not be made unless the appendix testis is palpated or visualized.

The natural history of torsion of the appendix testis is for the inflammation to resolve gradually after infarction of the appendage. In general, the process is complete within 10 days from the onset of symptoms. Management includes bed rest for 24 to 48 hours and nonsteroidal antiinflammatory medication (e.g., ibuprofen) for 5 days to reduce inflammation and pain. The patient should be instructed to return promptly to the emergency room or physician's office if the pain worsens, because it may be an indication of testicular torsion.

Scrotal exploration and excision of the torsed appendage for pain control is unnecessary.

If the likely diagnosis is torsion of the appendix testis but the clinician desires confirmation, color Doppler sonography or a testicular flow scan may be ordered. Either of these studies should demonstrate hyperemia to the testis. However, if there is any ambiguity regarding the diagnosis, emergency scrotal exploration should be performed to be certain that the child does not have testicular torsion.

EPIDIDYMOORCHITIS

Epididymitis refers to an inflammatory process that involves the epididymis and usually results from a urethral infection that passes in a retrograde manner through the vas deferens to the epididymis (Fig. 28-5). Epididymal inflammation without infection also may be a secondary reaction to torsion of the appendix testis. Frequently, scrotal sonography in a prepubertal boy with testicular pain and swelling shows epididymal swelling indicative of a diagnosis of epididymitis, but usually it is not secondary to infection and does not necessitate antibiotic therapy. Some clinical reviews of boys with testicular pain include many with epididymitis, whereas the true origin in many of those cases is torsion of the appendix testis.

Epididymitis secondary to infection is most common during adolescence; it is rare before puberty. In most postpubertal boys, epididymitis results from a sexually transmitted disease (see Chapter 29), unless there is a preexisting abnormality of the lower genitourinary tract (neuropathic bladder, urethral stricture). Organisms responsible include *Chlamydia* species, *Mycoplasma* species, and *Neisseria gonorrhoeae*. In prepubertal boys, in contrast, epididymitis is most frequently secondary to a structural abnormality of the lower genitourinary tract, including ectopic ureter, ectopic vas deferens, rectourethral fistula associated with imperforate anus, urethral stricture, or dysfunctional voiding. If the condition is diagnosed and treated early, the testicle is not involved. In many cases, however, the inflammatory process also involves the testis and is termed *epididymoorchitis*. If the infection is bacterial (e.g., *Escherichia coli* or other gram-negative uropathogen) and is not treated for 1 to 2 weeks, testicular infarction can occur.

Epididymitis typically causes testicular pain and swelling that is insidious in onset. There may be symptoms of urinary tract infection, including dysuria, urgency, and frequency, as well as urethral discharge. Some patients report transient inguinal pain secondary to inflammation of the spermatic cord before the onset of testicular symptoms. On physical examination, fever is common, as is scrotal erythema. The epididymis is tender, enlarged, indurated, and posterior to the testis. Often the testis is also enlarged and tender. The cremasteric reflex is frequently absent. A reactive hydrocele may be present and obscures the testicular examination. If there is fixation of skin over the testis, the testis may be nonviable.

For sexually active adolescents, diagnosis focuses on *Chlamydia trachomatis* and *N. gonorrhoeae*. These patients should have a

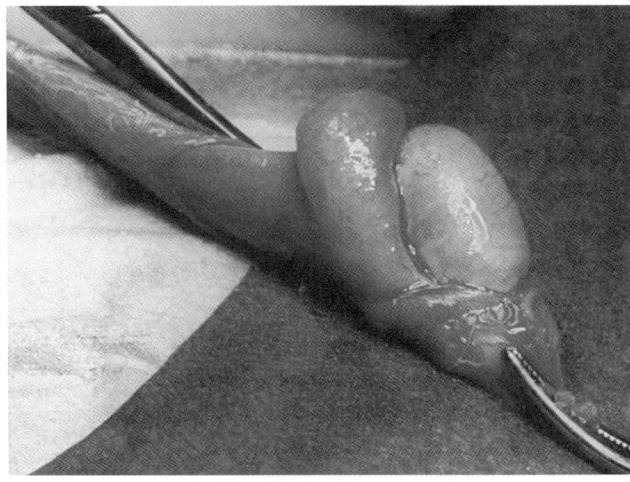

Figure 28-5. Epididymitis in a 6-year-old boy. Note the reactive orchitis as well as significant enlargement of the epididymis.

nucleic acid amplification test on either an intraurethral swab or a first-void urine sample for *N. gonorrhoeae* and *C. trachomatis*. Alternatively, a culture of intraurethral exudate can be obtained. A Gram stain smear of urethral exudate or intraurethral swab specimen confirms the diagnosis of urethritis (more than 5 polymorphonuclear leukocytes per field) and may suggest gonococcal infection (intracellular gram-negative diplococci). If the urethral Gram stain result is negative, then a culture and Gram stain test should be obtained from a first-void uncentrifuged urine specimen. Testing for syphilis and human immunodeficiency virus should be performed (see Chapter 29).

In prepubertal boys, the most important laboratory study is the urinalysis, which often shows pyuria or bacteriuria, or both (see Chapter 23). The urine should be subjected to culture. Not all prepubertal boys with epididymitis have an abnormal urinalysis result; in rare cases, boys with testicular torsion may have evidence of infection. If there is a urethral discharge, a specimen of urethral fluid should be obtained for Gram stain and culture. After treatment, these young boys should undergo voiding cystourethrography and renal ultrasonography as part of the evaluation for an underlying anatomic abnormality.

If the diagnosis is not definitive or if testicular torsion is suspected, color Doppler ultrasonography or a testicular flow scan may be helpful by showing blood flow to the testis. Sonography may also show evidence of an abscess.

Empirical treatment for sexually acquired epididymitis should include coverage for *N. gonorrhoeae* (ceftriaxone, 250 mg intramuscularly in a single dose) and *Chlamydia* species (doxycycline, 100 mg orally b.i.d. for 10 days) (see Chapter 29). Supportive measures include an ice pack, scrotal support, nonsteroidal antiinflammatory medication for analgesia, and bed rest for 48 hours. In non–sexually active children, *E. coli* is the most common cause. The patient should initially receive empirical treatment with a broad-spectrum antibiotic (gentamicin or cefotaxime). All patients should be reexamined periodically until the inflammatory process resolves completely. Approximately 15% of individuals with a testis tumor are initially treated for epididymitis.

Surgical management is reserved primarily for cases in which there is ambiguity regarding the diagnosis and testicular torsion is suspected or if there is a suspected abscess.

Orchitis as an isolated infection is uncommon in boys. Most often, it results from extension of an epididymal inflammatory process. Mumps orchitis occurs most frequently in postpubertal boys. The onset of orchitis usually occurs 4 to 6 days after the parotitis. As many as 33% of patients with orchitis develop testicular atrophy.

Treatment of orchitis includes broad-spectrum antibiotics until the urine culture result is available. If the primary infection is obviously viral, only symptomatic therapy (nonsteroidal antiinflammatory drugs, scrotal support, ice pack) is necessary.

TRAUMA AND HEMATOCELE

Blunt scrotal trauma can result in a spectrum of injuries ranging from testicular contusion to rupture of the testis (Fig. 28-6). Testicular injuries usually result from a fall, kick, or direct blow from a blunt object. A detailed history of the nature of the injury aids in recognizing the likelihood of serious testicular injury. With disruption of the tunica albuginea (capsule) of the testis, there is such significant painful scrotal swelling that the testis cannot be palpated. Often there is associated erythema or ecchymosis of the scrotal wall. In most cases of suspected testicular injury, scrotal ultrasonography is performed to assess the integrity of the testis.

In many boys with testicular torsion or torsion of the appendix testis, there is often, inexplicably, a history of recent mild scrotal trauma. Although there is no evidence that these disorders can result from blunt trauma, these diagnoses should be considered if there is not an obvious significant testicular injury, but the scrotal examination is abnormal.

Treatment of scrotal trauma is determined by the extent of the injury. Boys with a small, nonexpanding hematocele and a normal testis are managed nonoperatively with bed rest, scrotal support, and ice packs. In contrast, a ruptured testis associated with a large hematocele necessitates urgent surgical exploration and repair.

VARICOCELE

A varicocele is an abnormal dilation of the veins of the pampiniform plexus in the scrotum. Approximately 10% of adolescent boys and 15% of men have a varicocele; 15% of these men are infertile.

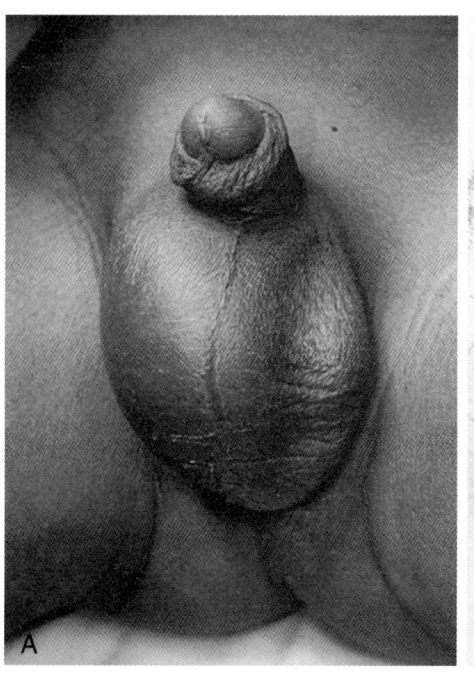
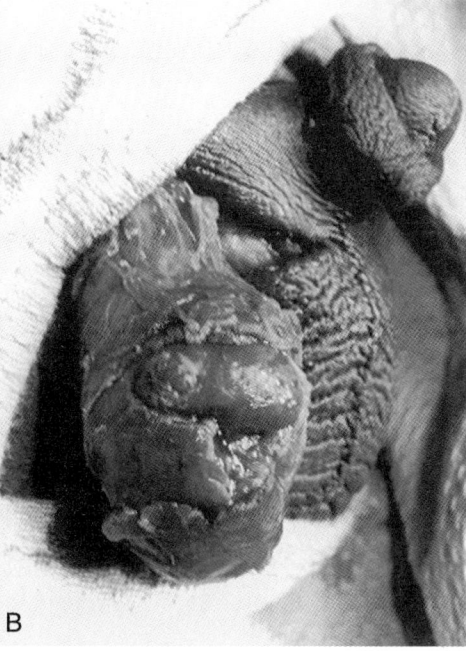

Figure 28-6. A, Appearance in an 8-year-old boy kicked in the scrotum while performing karate with his brother. Note right scrotal swelling. An ultrasound study showed scrotal hematoma and a ruptured testis. B, Scrotal exploration shows a nonviable testis. Orchiectomy was performed.

A varicocele is the most common surgically correctable cause of infertility in men. Infertility is thought to result from the effect of elevated temperature on the testis. Varicoceles are rare in boys younger than 10 years of age. The increased prevalence among adolescents is secondary to the increased testicular blood flow that occurs with puberty. More than 95% of cases involve the left testis; this involvement is secondary to multiple factors, including the long length of the left internal spermatic vein in comparison with that of the right and the absence of a venous valve at the insertion of the left internal spermatic vein into the renal vein.

A varicocele manifests as a painless, paratesticular mass often described as a "bag of worms." On occasion, patients describe a chronic, dull ache in or adjacent to the testis. Physical examination of the patient in both the supine and the upright positions, with and without the Valsalva maneuver, facilitates the diagnosis. Typically, the varicocele is decompressed when the patient is supine and prominent when standing. Varicocele size may be graded: grade I means barely palpable; grade II, easily palpable but not visible in the standing position; and grade III, easily visible in the standing position. Measurement of the volume of both testicles is important to document differences in the size of the testis. Calipers or an orchidometer may be used to assess testicular size; scrotal ultrasonography may also be used. Approximately 33% of affected boys have an associated volume loss of the left testis. If a varicocele is detected in a boy younger than 10 years old or on the right side (both red flags), abdominal ultrasonography is indicated to ascertain whether an abdominal mass is present.

Histologic studies have demonstrated pathologic testicular changes in some adolescent boys and men with varicoceles, including degeneration of germinal centers, interstitial fibrosis, and impaired spermatogenesis. The goal in treatment of a varicocele is preservation and restoration of spermatogenesis. Because the majority of testicular volume is composed of seminiferous tubules, if the left testis is significantly smaller than the right, the clinician may presume that the varicocele has affected testicular growth. Typically, after varicocelectomy in an adolescent, the testis shows catch-up growth and ultimately is similar in size to the contralateral testicle.

Indications for varicocelectomy in boys and adolescents include significant disparity in testicular size, pain, and diseased or absent contralateral testis.

Surgical repair should also be considered for very large varicoceles and if bilateral testicular growth arrest is suspected. Varicocelectomy is accomplished by ligating the dilated veins of the pampiniform plexus through a low inguinal incision or by ligating and dividing the internal spermatic vein through a high transverse inguinal incision or by a laparoscopic approach. All of these techniques may be performed on an ambulatory basis.

INGUINAL HERNIA

Hernias and hydroceles result from incomplete obliteration of the processus vaginalis. Indirect inguinal hernias result from a patent processus vaginalis that allows a loop of bowel, omentum, or other abdominal organ to pass through the internal inguinal ring. Patients usually present with nontender groin, scrotal swelling, or both, which reduce with minimal pressure (Fig. 28-7). A hernia that cannot be reduced is called an *incarcerated hernia*. A *strangulated hernia*, in which the vascular supply of the herniated bowel is compromised, is a surgical emergency. Physical signs of incarceration include inguinal or scrotal erythema, pain, signs of bowel obstruction, and inability to reduce the hernia. Infants with an incarcerated hernia have a 10% incidence of ipsilateral testicular infarction secondary to increased pressure on the spermatic cord.

If an incarcerated hernia is suspected, the child is admitted and sedated, and manual reduction of the hernia is attempted. Most hernias can be reduced successfully and should be repaired promptly. Children with an easily reducible hernia should also undergo herniorrhaphy within a reasonable time to reduce the possibility of incarceration or strangulation. Neonates and small infants with an incarcerated hernia may present with painful scrotal swelling without an inguinal mass, but this manifestation is unusual in older children.

Surgical correction involves dissection and high ligation of the hernial sac through a small inguinal incision. Elective herniorrhaphy

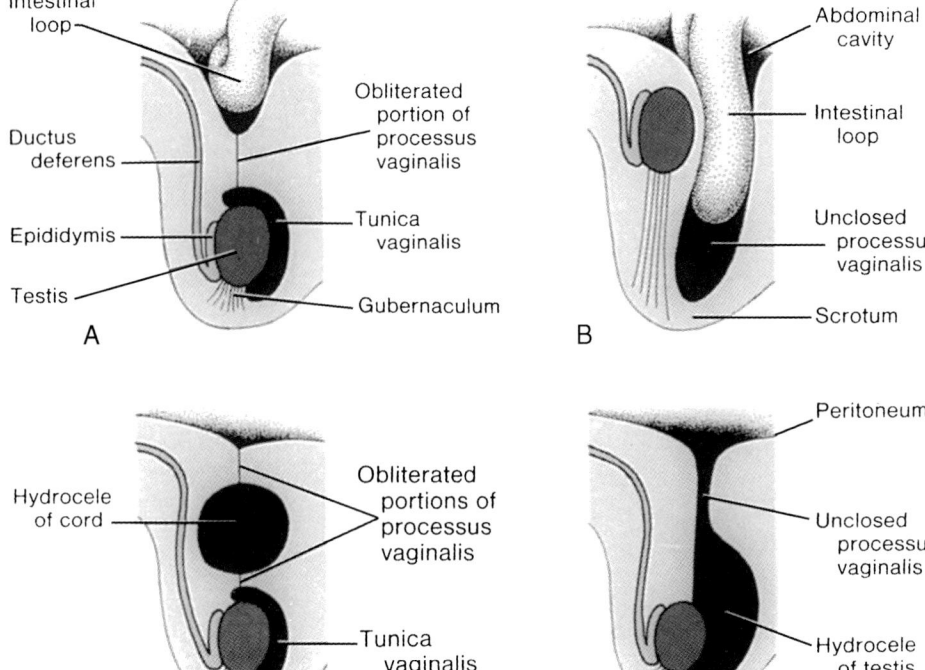

Figure 28-7. Diagrams of sagittal sections of the inguinal region. **A,** Incomplete indirect inguinal hernia, resulting from persistence of the proximal processus vaginalis. **B,** Indirect inguinal hernia into the scrotum, resulting from persistence of the entire processus vaginalis. Note the presence of an undescended testicle, which is a commonly associated malformation. **C,** Hydrocele of the cord, derived from an unobliterated portion of the processus vaginalis. **D,** Communicating hydrocele, resulting from peritoneal fluid passing through a patent processus vaginalis. (From Moore KL: Clinically Oriented Anatomy, 2nd ed. Baltimore, Williams & Wilkins, 1993, p 299.)

is usually performed as an ambulatory surgical procedure when the infant is 5 to 6 months of age.

HYDROCELE

A hydrocele is an accumulation of fluid within the tunica vaginalis. Approximately 1% to 2% of newborn boys have a hydrocele. In most of these cases, which are noncommunicating hydroceles, the fluid disappears by 1 year of age. Communicating hydroceles, defined by a patent processus vaginalis (see Fig. 28-7), tend to persist. Typically, affected boys have progressive scrotal swelling over the course of the day that decreases by morning as the hydrocele fluid returns to the abdomen during sleep. In infants who are not walking, the hydrocele usually does not change in size. In an older boy, a non-communicating hydrocele can result from an inflammatory condition within the scrotum (testicular torsion, torsion of the appendix testis, epididymitis, testis tumor). Communicating hydroceles and hernias differ by the anatomy and contents of the processus vaginalis. In communicating hydroceles, the diameter of the processus vaginalis is much smaller in relation to a hernia, allowing only fluid to pass into the scrotum.

On examination, hydroceles are smooth and nontender and can be associated with thickening of the cord structures. Bright transillu-mination of the scrotum confirms the fluid-filled nature of the mass. If compression of the fluid-filled mass eliminates the hydrocele, then the patent processus vaginalis is large, and the boy can be considered to have an inguinal hernia. Because hydroceles can be associated with testicular neoplasms, the testis should be palpated to document that it is normal. If the diagnosis is uncertain with regard to the mass, scrotal ultrasonography is advised.

A severe form of the hydrocele is the *abdominoscrotal hydrocele,* in which the hydrocele sac is tense with fluid and extends from the scrotum proximally through the inguinal canal into the abdominal cavity. On examination, these hydroceles are palpable in the inguinal canal, and an abdominal mass is often present. These hydroceles do not resolve and may cause extrinsic testicular compression; consequently, repair is recommended.

Treatment depends on several factors. Most hydroceles resolve by 12 months of age after reabsorption of the hydrocele fluid. If the hydrocele is large and tense, however, early surgical correction is recommended for two reasons: (1) It is often impossible to verify that the child does not have a hernia, and (2) large hydroceles rarely disappear spontaneously. Hydroceles persisting beyond the age of 12 to 18 months are usually communicating and thus rarely regress; hence, these hydroceles should be surgically repaired. If left untreated, most eventually progress to an inguinal hernia. Parents should be advised to watch for more severe inguinal or scrotal swelling, or both, which indicates that a hernia has developed.

Surgical repair of hydroceles is essentially identical to a herniorrhaphy. Through an inguinal incision, the spermatic cord is identified, the hydrocele fluid is drained, and a high ligation of the processus vaginalis is performed.

TESTICULAR TUMORS

Although testicular and paratesticular tumors are uncommon, they can occur at any age, even in the newborn. In men, 98% of testicular tumors are malignant. In children, however, only 35% are malignant; they include yolk sac carcinoma, rhabdomyosarcoma, and, in rare cases, leukemias. Most manifest as a painless, hard testicular or paratesticular mass that does not transilluminate. Ten percent to 15% are associated with a hydrocele. Scrotal ultrasonography should be performed to confirm the finding of a testicular mass and may help delineate the type of testicular tumor. Serum tumor markers (α–fetoprotein and human chorionic gonadotropin) should be evaluated before surgical intervention.

Definitive therapy includes surgical exploration through an inguinal incision. Radical orchiectomy involves ligation of the

spermatic cord, followed by removal of the testis and spermatic cord. If the ultrasound study or surgical exploration suggests the presence of a benign tumor, such as a teratoma or epidermoid cyst, with a significant amount of normal testicular parenchyma, excision of the mass only (testis-sparing surgery) may be performed. If the tumor is malignant, a metastatic workup, including abdominal and chest computed tomographic scan, is obtained to evaluate the most common sites of metastatic disease: the retroperitoneum and lung.

MECONIUM PERITONITIS

Antenatal peritonitis may result from intestinal perforation. Although the intestinal perforation may heal, the intraabdominal meconium may track down the patent processus vaginalis into the scrotum, resulting in the formation of an inflammatory mass. This condition can manifest as bilateral neonatal hydroceles, which eventually regress into firm, nodular masses involving either or both testicles. Scrotal sonography demonstrates multiple areas of echogenic foci suggestive of calcification. In addition, a plain film of the scrotum shows calcification.

SCROTAL WALL SWELLING

Henoch-Schönlein Purpura

Henoch-Schönlein purpura is a systemic vasculitis of unknown origin that involves the skin, gastrointestinal tract, joints, and kidneys. Most affected patients are younger than 7 years. Genitourinary manifestations may include glomerulonephritis (see Chapter 25), ureteritis, renal pelvic bleeding, and acute swelling of the scrotum and spermatic cord. Scrotal wall and testicular involvement has been reported in up to 33% of affected patients.

A maculopapular purpuric rash (palpable purpura) often begins in the lower extremities and buttock region. Later the rash may spread to the scrotum. The initial manifestation may, however, be a scrotal rash. With testicular involvement, which is relatively un-common, there is mild to moderate swelling and tenderness of the testes. Differentiation from testicular torsion can be made if the characteristic rash and associated symptoms develop before the acute enlargement of the scrotum. These two conditions can coexist; therefore, if there is any uncertainty regarding the diagnosis, color Doppler ultrasonography or scrotal scintigraphy should be performed.

Acute Idiopathic Scrotal Wall Edema

Acute idiopathic scrotal wall edema is an uncommon entity that accounts for 2% to 5% of acute scrotal swelling. The average patient is between 4 and 7 years of age. Patients typically present with the sudden onset of unilateral or bilateral scrotal wall edema associated with mild tenderness. The overlying skin is erythematous, and the edema may extend anteriorly onto the abdominal wall or posteriorly into the perineum. The testicles are easily palpable, normal in size, and nontender. The origin of this syndrome is unknown, but allergic causes have been implicated.

Therapy consists of bed rest and parental reassurance. Although treatment with antibiotics, antihistamines, and corticosteroids has been proposed, most children experience improvement within 48 to 72 hours regardless of therapy.

Idiopathic Fat Necrosis

Idiopathic fat necrosis causes acute painful swelling of the scrotum secondary to necrosis of intrascrotal fat. Examination of the under-lying testis may be hampered by inflammation within the scrotal wall. The cause of this problem is unknown but may be related to trauma with physical activity. Sonography may help differentiate this entity from an intrascrotal process.

Treatment is supportive if the diagnosis is made nonoperatively.

Fournier Gangrene

Fournier gangrene of the scrotum usually affects adults but occasionally afflicts infants and children. In children, it occurs primarily in those with severe diaper rash, in those with insect bites, after circumcision, or in those with perianal skin abscess. Other predisposing factors include diabetes mellitus, trauma, instrumentation, urethral stricture, and inguinal or perineal surgery. Symptoms of this life-threatening infection include acute scrotal swelling with tenderness, erythema, and systemic manifestations of fever, chills, and septicemia. The most common organisms identified include *Staphylococcus aureus, Streptococcus* species, *Bacteroides fragilis, E. coli,* and *Clostridium welchii.*

Treatment involves emergency débridement with the patient under anesthesia; copious irrigation; and broad-spectrum parenteral antibiotics. In some cases, hyperbaric oxygen therapy is beneficial. Despite aggressive treatment, mortality rates approach 50%.

RED FLAGS

Because testicular torsion is a surgical emergency, acute scrotal pain should be evaluated promptly. Physical examination findings suggesting testicular torsion include marked tenderness, high-riding testis, and absent cremasteric reflex. A varicocele before puberty or on the right side is a red flag; abdominal ultrasonography is indicated.

REFERENCES

Diagnostic Strategies

Burgher SW: Acute scrotal pain. Emerg Clin North Am 1998;16:781.
Galeis LE: Diagnosis and treatment of the acute scrotum. Am Fam Phys 1999;59:817.
Hawtrey CE: Assessment of acute scrotal symptoms and findings. A clinician's dilemma. Urol Clin North Am 1998;25:715.
Kadish HA, Bolte RG: A retrospective review of pediatric patients with epididymitis, testicular torsion, and torsion of testicular appendages. Pediatrics 1998;102:73.
Kass EJ, Lundak B: The acute scrotum. Pediatr Clin North Am 1997;44:1251.
Lewis AG, Bukowski TP, Jarvis PD, et al: Evaluation of acute scrotum in the emergency department. J Pediatr Surg 1995;30:277.
Marcozzi D, Suner S: The nontraumatic acute scrotum. Emerg Clin North Am 2000;19:547.

Imaging

Allen TD, Elder JS: Shortcomings of color Doppler sonography in the diagnosis of testicular torsion. J Urol 1995;154:1508.
Baker LA, Sigman D, Mathews RI, et al: An analysis of clinical outcomes using color Doppler testicular ultrasound for testicular torsion. Pediatrics 2000;105:604.
Dogra VS, Sessions A, Mevorach RA, et al: Reversal of diastolic plateau in partial testicular torsion. J Clin Ultrasound 2001;29:105.
Kravchick S, Cytron S, Leibovici O, et al: Color Doppler sonography: Its real role in the evaluation of children with highly suspected testicular torsion. Eur Radiol 2001;11:1000.
Paltiel HJ, Connolly LP, Atala A, et al: Acute scrotal symptoms in boys with an indeterminate clinical presentation: Comparison of color Doppler sonography and scintigraphy. Radiology 1998;207:223.
Weber DM, Rosslein R, Fliegel C: Color Doppler sonography in the diagnosis of acute scrotum in boys. Eur J Pediatr Surg 2000;10:235.

Testicular Torsion

Barada JH, Weingarten JL, Cromie WJ: Testicular salvage and age-related delay in the presentation of testicular torsion. J Urol 1989;142:746.
Cornel EB, Karthaus HF: Manual detorsion of the twisted spermatic cord. BJU Int 1999;83:672.
Cuckow PM, Frank JD: Torsion of the testis. BJU Int 2000;86:349.
Dunne PJ, O'Loughlin BS: Testicular torsion: Time is the enemy. Aust N Z J Surg 2000;70:441.
Pinto KJ, Noe HN, Jerkins GR: Neonatal testicular torsion. J Urol 1997; 158:1196.
Van Glabeke E, Philippe-Chomette P, Gall O, et al: Spermatic cord torsion in the newborn: Role of surgical exploration. Arch Pediatr 2000;7:1072.

Epididymoorchitis

Beard CM, Benson RC, Kelalis PP, et al: The incidence and outcome of mumps orchitis in Rochester, Minnesota, 1935 to 1974. Mayo Clin Proc 1977;52:3.
Bukowski TP, Lewis AG, Reeves D, et al: Epididymitis in older boys: Dysfunctional voiding as an etiology. J Urol 1995;154:762.
Siegel A, Snyder H, Duckett JW: Epididymitis in infants and boys: Underlying urogenital anomalies and efficacy of imaging modalities. J Urol 1987; 138:1100.

Inguinal Hernia

Puri P, Guiney EJ, O'Donnell B: Inguinal hernia in infants: The fate of the testis following incarceration. J Pediatr Surg 1984;19:44.
Stoker DL, Spiegelhalter DJ, Singh R, et al: Laparoscopic versus open inguinal hernia repair: Randomised prospective trial. Lancet 1994; 343:1243.

Other Diagnoses

Anzai AK: Fournier's gangrene: A urologic emergency. Am Fam Phys 1995; 52:1821.
Corman JM, Moody JA, Aronson WJ: Fournier's gangrene in a modern surgical setting: Improved survival with aggressive management. BJU Int 1999;84:85.
Dayanir YO, Akdilli A, Karaman CZ, et al: Epididymoorchitis mimicking testicular torsion in Henoch-Schönlein purpura. Eur Radiol 2001; 11:2267.
Diamond DA, Paltiel HJ, DiCanzio J, et al: Comparative assessment of pediatric testicular volume: Orchidometer versus ultrasound. J Urol 2000; 164:1111.
Ioannides AS, Turnock R: An audit of the management of the acute scrotum in children with Henoch-Schönlein purpura. J R Coll Surg Edinb 2001; 46:98.
Kaplan GW: Acute idiopathic scrotal edema. J Pediatr Surg 1977;12:647.
Kass EJ, Stork BR, Steinert BW: Varicocele in adolescence induces left and right testicular volume loss. BJU Int 2001;87:499.
Levy DA, Kay R, Elder JS: Neonatal testis tumors: A review of the prepubertal testis registry. J Urol 1994;151:715.
Nemoy NJ, Rosin S, Kaplan L: Scrotal panniculitis in the prepubertal male patient. J Urol 1977;118:492.
Ross J, Kay R, Elder J: Testis sparing surgery for pediatric epidermoid cysts of the testis. J Urol 1993;149:353.
Rushton HG, Belman AB, Sesterhenn I, et al: Testicular sparing surgery for prepubertal teratoma of the testis. J Urol 1990;144:726.
Sayfan J, Siplovich L, Koltun L, et al: Varicocele treatment in pubertal boys prevents testicular growth arrest. J Urol 1997;157:1456.
Thomas JC, Elder JS: Testicular growth arrest and adolescent varicocele: Does varicocele size make a difference? J Urol 2002;168:1689.
Vasavada S, Ross J, Nasrallah P, et al: Prepubertal varicoceles. Urology 1997;50:774.
Walsh C, Rushton HG: Diagnosis and management of teratomas and epidermoid cysts. Urol Clin North Am 2000;27:509.
Yeh ML, Chang CJ, MU SC: Neonatal idiopathic scrotal hemorrhage: Patient reports. Clin Pediatr 2000;39:493.

29 Sexually Transmitted Diseases

Gale R. Burstein*

Adolescents represent an age group at high risk for acquisition and transmission of sexually transmitted diseases (STDs). Most STDs are asymptomatic and are diagnosed by screening asymptomatic sexually active individuals.

A national survey of high school students demonstrated that 46% have engaged in sexual intercourse, with an increase to 61% of 12th graders. Seven percent initiated sexual intercourse before 13 years of age, and 36% had had a sexual encounter within the previous 3 months. Adolescents are likely to have multiple sexual partners over relatively short periods of time, fail to recognize the symptoms of STDs, and use condoms inconsistently. Adolescents who engage in sex for money, who are homeless, or who are involved with the juvenile justice system are at especially high risk for acquiring STDs. Young men who have sex with men are at very high risk for human immunodeficiency virus (HIV) infection, as well as other STDs.

HISTORY

The adolescent seeking medical care for evaluation of any sexual health issue, including STDs, may complain of vague symptoms and avoid discussing the actual concern. Providers should suspect a "hidden agenda" from an adolescent patient who presents for a check-up. The majority of STDs in adolescents are asymptomatic or manifest symptoms that are not recognized. Therefore, providers miss most infections by testing only patients presenting with suggestive symptoms.

The sexual history should be obtained from the adolescent patient confidentially. Interviewing the adolescent in the room alone (i.e., without a parent present) for at least a portion of the visit is the standard of care for *all* adolescent health care visits. The terms of a confidential visit should be explained to the adolescent (and parent, if present); all information disclosed by the adolescent remains confidential, unless he or she reveals a risk of rendering harm to himself or herself or to others, such as with suicidal or homicidal ideation.

Tables 29-1 and 29-2 detail important points from the history that should be discussed with the patient who is sexually active. It is critical that the provider perform a thorough history in a nonjudgmental and nonthreatening manner. Because many patients infected with STDs may be asymptomatic, gaining insight into sexual activity and orientation is most important. A history of a previous STD places the patient at high risk for future STDs.

Questions about victimization and abuse are part of the sexual history, regardless of age or gender. If the patient has been a victim of assault, a description of the assault should be obtained, and the sites of attempted or successful penetration should be noted. If possible, the offender should be identified. The time interval between the assault and evaluation is important. Any bathing, douching, urinating, defecating, tooth brushing, or gargling since the time of the assault must be documented, because such activities may interfere with specimen collection. Clinical symptoms that should specifically be noted include vaginal or rectal discharge, odor, pruritus, or pain; sore throat; local bleeding; dysuria, urgency, or frequency; abdominal pain; warts; and abnormal menstrual bleeding. A history of any known STD, voluntary sexual relationships, or previous sexual assault and relevant medical treatment should be obtained.

Although most STDs are asymptomatic among both boys and girls, certain symptoms should raise clinical suspicion. Symptomatic girls may present with vaginal discharge, genital lesions, abdominal pain, dysuria, or menstrual spotting. Boys may complain of dysuria, genital lesions, testicular pain, urethral discharge, or scrotal swelling. A variety of rashes may be noted with STDs and may be the reason for seeking medical attention. Constitutional symptoms may include fever, malaise, lymphadenopathy, and, less often, arthritis. If the patient has any constitutional symptoms, the examiner should inquire about weight loss, appetite, sleep patterns, energy level, headaches, and weakness.

Vaginal discharge in the adolescent girl is a nonspecific symptom, but its presence should lead to the consideration of bacterial vaginosis (BV), vulvovaginal candidiasis (VVC), trichomoniasis, chlamydia, and gonorrhea. BV and VVC are not sexually transmitted. In the prepubescent girl with acute onset of vaginal irritation or discharge, an *Escherichia coli* or streptococcal infection is likely, whereas nonspecific, mixed bacterial vulvovaginitis is the most likely cause of chronic vaginal symptoms in this younger age group.

Male patients who seek medical attention for a urethral discharge or urethritis may be infected with *Neisseria gonorrhoeae* or *Chlamydia trachomatis*. However, the proportion of urethritis cases caused by these organisms has been declining since the early 1990s. Boys and girls who describe genital lesions may have ulcers, vesicles, papules, or warts (Table 29-3).

Patients presenting with systemic complaints such as arthralgias, weight loss, headache, or fever may have an infection with HIV, syphilis, herpes simplex virus (HSV), disseminated gonorrhea infection, or reactive arthritis.

PHYSICAL EXAMINATION

A complete physical examination and laboratory evaluation are necessary to evaluate a symptomatic patient for STDs. Table 29-4 is a brief listing of general physical examination findings that must be sought. Tables 29-5 and 29-6 review the physical examination procedures that should be followed for a comprehensive STD evaluation in adolescent boys and girls. The complete rectal examination may not be necessary if the patient reports no anal sex or symptoms. Table 29-3 should assist the clinician in distinguishing genital lesions associated with some of the more common infectious agents. Table 29-7 offers an approach to the physical examination in the prepubertal girl who presents with vaginal irritation or discharge.

If the clinician suspects that a prepubertal child has been sexually abused, a careful general examination is performed. Anatomic

---

*This chapter is an updated and edited version of the chapter by Trina M. Anglin that appeared in the first edition. The points of view expressed in this chapter are the author's and do not necessarily reflect the opinion of the Centers for Disease Control and Prevention.

Table 29-1. Approach to Clinical Evaluation of Sexually Transmitted Diseases: Sexual History

Age at coitarche
Date of most recent sexual encounter
Duration of relationship with current partner
Numbers of current, recent (within past 3-6 months), and lifetime partners
Condom usage (overall consistency)
Contraceptive usage
Vaginal intercourse
Oral intercourse
Anal intercourse
Dyspareunia
Gender of partners
Involuntary sexual encounters (abuse, rape)
Partner's sexually transmitted disease symptoms and relevant sexual history (i.e., other sex partners)

Table 29-2. Approach to Clinical Evaluation of Sexually Transmitted Diseases: Symptoms and General Health

Symptoms (Duration, Intensity, Course)

Urinary (dysuria, urgency, frequency, hematuria)
Vaginal discharge (quantity, color, odor, consistency, pruritus, burning)
Urethral discharge (character, quantity, when it occurs)
Anorectal discharge (character, quantity, when it occurs; bowel movements)
Local pain (character; location: mucosal, abdominal, testicular, inguinal, anal)
Genital lesions (onset, quantity, appearance, pain, pruritus)

Self-Treatment

Over-the-counter medication
Douching
Antibiotic usage

Reproductive Health History

Sexually transmitted diseases
Pregnancies

Menstruation

Last menstrual period (date, duration, quantity, associated pain or cramping, comparison with usual menses)
Spotting or intramenstrual bleeding

Review of Systems

Skin (rash, pruritus, lesions)
Joints (pain, swelling, redness)
Bowel changes (diarrhea, bleeding)
Constitutional (fever, weight loss, night sweats, malaise, cough, depression)

General Health

Medical problems
Medication usage/allergies
Travel

Substance Abuse

Alcohol and illicit drug usage (self and partner)
Needle injection (self and partner)

abnormalities (trauma, lacerations, erythema, scarring) of the external genitalia and the anorectal area should be documented; colposcopic magnification and photography are standard (see Chapter 36).

LABORATORY TESTING

Adolescents who present with one STD are at high risk for having another STD. Table 29-8 provides a template for the basic diagnostic laboratory evaluation for treatable STDs that should be performed on all sexually active adolescents, regardless of presenting symptoms. Additional laboratory tests may be indicated, depending on the clinical scenario (see later discussion).

Pregnancy testing is indicated when an adolescent girl presents with symptoms of an STD. The test results may influence the treatment plan.

Table 29-9 lists the circumstances in which HIV counseling, testing, and referral should be considered for adolescents.

SEXUALLY TRANSMITTED DISEASE SYNDROMES

GENITAL ULCER DISEASE

Table 29-3 describes the clinical manifestations of various causes of genital ulcer disease. Pustules and vesicles atop an erythematous base are most often a result of HSV. Fluid from these vesicles may be sent for herpes culture. Antigen detection tests do not distinguish HSV type 1 (HSV-1) from HSV type 2 (HSV-2). Material from the ulcer or chancre associated with syphilis can be examined via dark-field microscopy for the presence of the treponeme, or the material can be air-dried on a slide and a direct fluorescent antibody test for *Treponema pallidum* can be performed (highly sensitive and specific). Lymphogranuloma venereum and chancroid are rarely seen in the United States. Laboratory evaluation of an ulcer caused by syphilis, lymphogranuloma venereum, and chancroid is complicated and usually not performed in the primary care office setting. Consultation with an infectious diseases specialist or the local health department STD clinic is recommended for these evaluations.

Two noninfectious causes of genital ulcers that can be confused with infection include inflammatory bowel disease and Behçet syndrome. Inflammatory bowel disease usually manifests with intestinal symptoms, deeper ulcers, and a longer duration of ulcerative lesions. Behçet syndrome may manifest with lesions of other mucous membranes as well as ocular, central nervous system, and joint manifestations. If the clinical diagnosis is not definitive, viral culture of the lesions is recommended.

GENITAL WARTS

Human papillomavirus (HPV) types 6 and 11 are most commonly associated with genital warts. The clinical manifestations are described in Table 29-3. Although all the HPV types causing genital warts are not likely to cause cervical cancer, they often produce abnormalities on Papanicolaou (Pap) smears, and patients may be infected simultaneously with multiple types of HPV. Annual cervical cancer screening with a Pap smear of adolescent females should begin 3 years after the onset of sexual activity. The majority of cervical cancers are associated with specific serotypes of HPV.

Patients with genital warts usually present with complaints of bumps or growths on their genitalia. On occasion, patients may complain of itching, burning sensation, pain, or bleeding. Genital warts can appear on the penis, urethral meatus, scrotum, and perianal areas in boys and on the vulvar skin and mucosa, vagina, cervix, and perianal area in girls. In general, HPV is a multifocal disease. The entire genitalia should be inspected for warts because more than one lesion and lesions on different sites are usually present.

Table 29-3. Diagnostic Characteristics of Genital Lesions

Syndrome	Appearance	Number of Lesions	Pain	Adenopathy	Occurrence in the United States
Herpes	Vesicles and superficial ulcers on erythematous base (1-2 mm)	Multiple	Often	Bilateral; inguinal; firm; movable; tender	Frequent
Syphilis	Papule and superficial or deep ulcer (5-15 mm)	Single	No	Bilateral; inguinal; firm; movable; nontender	Uncommon
Lymphogranuloma venereum	Ulcer (2-10 mm), resolves quickly	Single	Yes	Unilateral; inguinal; fluctuant; may suppurate; tender	Rare
Human papillomavirus	Anogenital exophytic warts; may resemble cauliflowers or be papular with projections	Single or multiple	No	None	Frequent
Lice or nits	Tiny (≤1 mm) insects or eggs adherent to hair shaft; excoriations	Multiple	No but pruritic	None	Common
Chancroid	Deep, purulent ulcers (2-20 mm)	Multiple	Yes	Unilateral; inguinal; fluctuant; may suppurate; tender	Rare

The four morphologic types of genital warts are

1. condylomata acuminata (cauliflower-like appearance)
2. papular warts (flesh-colored, dome-shaped papules, usually 1-4 mm in diameter)
3. keratotic warts (resemble common skin wart with thick, crustlike layer)
4. flat-topped papules (macular, slightly raised)

The differential diagnosis for genital warts includes

1. Anatomic structures: skin tags, pearly penile papules, vestibular papillae, sebaceous glands, melanocytic nevi
2. Acquired lesions: molluscum contagiosum, Crohn disease, seborrheic keratosis, lichen planus, lichen nidus, and condyloma latum.

Clinical diagnosis of exophytic condylomata caused by HPV is usually straightforward. However, it is important to distinguish them from the lesions of secondary syphilis (condylomata lata). A nontreponemal syphilis test should be performed in patients presenting with genital warts. Condylomata lata are more rounded, and the patient has a strongly positive (i.e., titer > 1:16) nontreponemal serologic syphilis test result. The lesions of molluscum contagiosum are smooth, firm, dome-shaped, and umbilicated. In rare cases, nongenital HPV types that cause common warts on the hands and feet can cause warts in the genital region.

Females with cervical lesions should be referred for colposcopy; males and females with recurrent perianal lesions, for anoscopy; and males with lesions at the distal urethral meatus and terminal hematuria or an abnormal urinary stream, for urethroscopy. Use of mild acetic acid solution to detect subclinical disease is not recommended because of its poor sensitivity and specificity.

The primary goal of treatment of visible genital warts is their removal. Without treatment, visible genital warts may resolve, remain unchanged, or increase in size or number. Treatment of warts does not eradicate the virus or its infectivity, nor does it affect the development of cervical cancer that may result from simultaneous infection with high-risk HPV types. Treatment should be guided by patient preference, provider experience, and treatment availability.

Table 29-4. Sexually Transmitted Disease Evaluation: General Physical Examination

Vital signs
Skin (rash; excoriations; location of lesions, especially palms, soles, face, trunk, extremities)
Oropharynx (inflammation, lesions, exudates, enanthem)
Nodes
Abdominal tenderness
Back (costovertebral angle tenderness)
Joints (tenderness, swelling, erythremia, warmth)

Table 29-5. Comprehensive Physical Examination of the Adolescent Female

External Genitalia
Pubic hair sexual maturation rating
Lice and nits
Mucosal estrogenization
Erythema
Edema
Lesions (erythema, ulcers, warts, fissures, excoriation)
Bartholin and Skene (periurethral) glands
Urethra
Discharge at introitus
Trauma

Speculum Examination (see Chapter 30)
Vagina (erythema, lesions, quantity/color/consistency/odor of vaginal pool)
Cervix (conformation, bleeding, erythema, friability, character of mucus, lesions)

Bimanual Examination
Uterus (size, position, mobility, tenderness, consistency)
Adnexa (tenderness, enlargement, mass)
Cervical motion tenderness

Rectal Examination
Lesions of perianal skin or anal verge
Sphincter tone
Ampulla (mass, tenderness, feces)
Stool character and Hematest

Table 29-6. Comprehensive Physical Examination of the Adolescent Male

External Genitalia

Sexual maturation ratings (pubic hair and genitalia)
Lice and nits
Skin lesions (penis, foreskin, scrotum, inguinal region, and medial thighs; ulcers, warts, papules, nodules, erythema, or excoriation)
Urethral meatus (erythema, lesions, tenderness)
Urethral discharge (quantity, color, consistency)
Scrotum/testes (tenderness, mass, edema)

Rectal Examination

Lesions of perianal skin or anal verge
Sphincter tone
Ampulla (mass, tenderness, feces)
Stool character and Hematest

Table 29-7. Approach to the Physical Examination in Prepubertal Females with Vaginal Irritation or Discharge

General Physical Examination

Skin for evidence of viral exanthem, atopic or seborrheic dermatitis, and other lesions
Evidence of acute respiratory, pharyngeal, or gastrointestinal illness
Chronic disease
Inspection of underpants for discharge

Visualization of External Genitalia and Perianal Area

Supine, lithotomy, or modified lithotomy position (includes labial separation and traction):
 Inflammation and lesions of skin and vulva mucosa
 Evidence of poor toilet hygiene
 Signs of excoriation
 Presence of discharge at introitus
 Presence of pinworms (*Enterobius vermicularis*)
 Degree of estrogenization
 Hymenal configuration
 Evidence of recent or past trauma
 Ectopic urethra
 Congenital anomalies
 Evidence of scabies

Visualization of Vagina and Cervix

Knee-chest position with traction on buttocks and use of otoscope as light source

Vaginal Specimen Collection

Saline-moistened cotton/Dacron-tipped nasopharyngeal or urethral swabs or "catheter within a catheter" technique to aspirate specimen
Normal saline preparation for microscopic examination
Potassium hydroxide preparation
Cultures for *Neisseria gonorrhoeae*, *Chlamydia trachomatis*, *Candida* species, group A streptococci, anaerobes, and gram-negative enteric bacteria
Request that laboratory identify and quantify all predominant isolates
Tape test (nonfrosted cellophane tape) for pinworms (best performed by parent before child arises in the morning; specimen of tape then applied to microscope slide and brought to laboratory)

Rectoabdominal Examination

Lithotomy or modified lithotomy position
Tenderness
Expression of vaginal discharge
Palpation of mass or firm foreign body through rectovaginal wall

Table 29-10 lists patient-applied and provider-administered treatment regimens recommended by the Centers for Disease Control and Prevention (CDC) for genital warts. All of these regimens are comparably effective.

URETHRAL DISCHARGE IN THE ADOLESCENT MALE

Urethritis, inflammation of the urethra, is more commonly diagnosed in older adolescent males and young men. *N. gonorrhoeae* and *C. trachomatis* are the clinically important bacterial pathogens of adolescent urethritis that warrant diagnostic evaluation. Nongonococcal urethritis is urethritis caused by pathogens other than *N. gonorrhoeae*. Because the proportion of cases of nongonococcal urethritis caused by *C. trachomatis* has been declining since the early 1990s, many diagnostic workups for nongonococcal urethritis do not yield an identifiable pathogen.

Objective clinical or laboratory evidence of urethral inflammation must be demonstrated to make a diagnosis of urethritis (Table 29-11). Patient complaints without objective examination or laboratory findings do not fulfill diagnostic requirements. In a patient with symptoms, stripping the urethra from the base to the meatus three or four times and examination after a long interval without voiding (i.e., at least 2 hours) increases the likelihood of a positive finding. However, highly sensitive nucleic acid amplification tests (NAATs) identify STD pathogens in boys who do not meet the diagnostic criteria for urethritis.

The CDC recommends gonorrhea and chlamydia testing of all boys who meet the diagnostic criteria for urethritis. NAATs, the most sensitive combination gonorrhea and chlamydia diagnostic test, can be performed on a single urine or urethral specimen. Tables 29-12 and 29-13 summarize advantages and disadvantages of various laboratory diagnostic tests for gonorrhea and chlamydia.

Treatment should be provided as soon as possible after diagnosis of a pathogen (Table 29-14). Empirical gonorrhea and chlamydia treatment of symptomatic patients without documentation of urethritis by examination or laboratory is recommended for males who are unlikely to return for a follow-up evaluation.

Patients should be instructed to return for evaluation if symptoms persist or recur after completion of therapy. Patients who have persistent or recurrent urethritis should be re-treated with the initial regimen if noncompliance or reexposure from an untreated partner is a possibility. If this is unlikely, a test for *Trichomonas vaginalis* should be performed, and patients should be treated for recurrent/persistent urethritis (Table 29-15).

VAGINAL DISCHARGE IN THE ADOLESCENT FEMALE

An adolescent girl presenting with complaints of vaginal discharge may have mucopurulent cervicitis (MPC), vaginitis, or both. An evaluation for both conditions should be performed.

Mucopurulent Cervicitis

MPC is characterized by mucopurulent discharge from an inflamed cervix. A test for *C. trachomatis* and *N. gonorrhoeae* should be performed. However, an infectious cause is often not identified. The adolescent with MPC may present with complaints of vaginal discharge; vaginal itching; irregular vaginal bleeding, especially after

Table 29-8. Laboratory Evaluations for Treatable Sexually Transmitted Diseases in Adolescents

Disease	Males	Females
Gonorrhea	X	X
Chlamydia	X	X
Vulvovaginal candidiasis		X
Bacterial vaginosis		X
Trichomoniasis		X
Syphilis	X	X
Human immunodeficiency virus infection	X	X

sexual intercourse; and dyspareunia. Pelvic inflammatory disease (PID) must be considered if there is a history of lower abdominal pain.

Purulent or mucopurulent discharge from the cervical os, easily induced endocervical bleeding (friability), and edema and erythema of the zone of ectopy on the cervix are found on examination. The presence of yellow mucopus collected from the endocervix and evident on a white swab is indicative of MPC. Friability alone does not constitute MPC.

Diagnoses to consider with findings of an inflamed cervix on examination include vaginitis; endometritis; PID; inflammation of an ectropion secondary to allergies; trauma; and presence of a foreign body, such as a tampon.

The "gold standard" for laboratory diagnosis of MPC is an NAAT. Tables 29-12 and 29-13 summarize advantages and disadvantages of various laboratory diagnostic tests for gonorrhea and chlamydia.

Table 29-9. Adolescents Who Should Receive Human Immunodeficiency Virus Prevention Counseling, Testing, and Referral

- All sexually active adolescents in settings serving populations at increased behavioral or clinical HIV risk, e.g., adolescent or school-based health clinics with high STD rates, juvenile detention centers, drug or alcohol prevention and treatment programs, homeless shelters, clinics serving men who have sex with men, freestanding HIV test sites, or STD clinics
- Individual clients in setting with <1%* HIV prevalence who:
  Have clinical signs or symptoms suggesting HIV infection (e.g., fever or illness of unknown origin, opportunistic infection [including tuberculosis] without known reason for immune suppression)
  Have diagnosis suggesting increased risk for HIV infection (e.g., another STD or blood borne infection)
- Self-report HIV risks
  Diagnosis or treatment for an STD, hepatitis, or tuberculosis
  Unprotected sexual intercourse with a partner at risk for HIV (e.g., partner who has injected drugs, been diagnosed or treated for an STD or hepatitis, had multiple or anonymous sex partners, or exchanged sex for drugs or money)
  Injection drug use with needle sharing
  History of an infection related to a "weak immune system"
- Specifically request an HIV test
- All adolescents in settings with a ≥1%† HIV prevalence
- All pregnant females

Adapted from Centers for Disease Control and Prevention: Revised guidelines for HIV counseling, testing, and referral. MMWR Morb Mortal Wkly Rep 2001;50:1-57.

*Or lower than other settings in the community.

†Or higher than other settings in the community.

HIV, human immunodeficiency virus; STD, sexually transmitted disease.

Table 29-10. Treatment Regimens for Genital Warts

Patient-Applied Treatments

Podofilox, 0.5% solution or gel*
  Patients may apply with a cotton swab or finger to visible genital warts twice a day for 3 days, followed by 4 days of no therapy
  Cycle should be repeated as needed up to four times
  Provider should apply first treatment to demonstrate proper application technique and to identify which warts should be treated
Imiquimod, 5% cream*
  Patients may apply with a finger at bedtime three times per week for up to 16 weeks
  The treatment should be washed with mild soap and water 6-10 hr after application

Provider-Administered Treatments

Cryotherapy with liquid nitrogen or cryoprobe
  Applications should be repeated every 1-2 weeks
Podophyllin resin, 10%-25% in compound tincture of benzoin*
  Patients apply a small amount to each wart and allow to air dry
  Patients wash off 1-4 hr after application
  Applications may be repeated weekly if necessary
Trichloroacetic acid (TCA) or bichloracetic acid (BCA), 80%-90%
  Patients apply a small amount only to warts and allow to dry, at which time a white "frosting" develops; patients powder with talc, sodium bicarbonate, or liquid soap preparations to remove unreacted acid if an excess amount is applied
  Patients may repeat weekly if necessary
Surgical removal by tangential scissor excision, tangential shave excision, curettage, or electrosurgery

Recommended Treatments by Wart Location

Cervical warts	Consult with an expert; high-grade squamous intraepithelial lesions must be excluded before treatment is begun
Vaginal warts	Cryotherapy with liquid nitrogen (use of cryoprobe in vagina is not recommended because of risk for vaginal perforation) TCA or BCA, 80%-90%
Urethral meatal warts†	Podophyllin resin, 10%-25% in compound tincture of benzoin* Cryotherapy with liquid nitrogen
Anal warts	Management of warts on rectal mucosa should be referred to an expert Cryotherapy with liquid nitrogen TCA or BCA, 80%-90% Surgical removal
Oral warts	Cryotherapy with liquid nitrogen Surgical removal

Adapted from Centers for Disease Control and Prevention: Sexually transmitted diseases treatment guidelines 2002. MMWR Morb Mortal Wkly Rep 2002;51:1-84.

*Safety of use during pregnancy has not been established.

†Some specialists recommend podofilox and imiquimod for the treatment of distal meatal warts in certain patients.

Although no infection is identified for many cases of MPC, the CDC recommends empirical treatment for *C. trachomatis* and *N. gonorrhoeae* in populations such as adolescents that are at high risk for infection and unlikely to follow up for test results (see Table 29-14).

Table 29-11. **Diagnostic Criteria to Demonstrate Urethral Inflammation**

Observation of mucoid or purulent urethral discharge
Positive leukocyte esterase test on first-void urine
Gram stain findings of
  ≥5 White blood cells per high-powered field
                    or
  Gram-negative intracellular diplococci

Adapted from Centers for Disease Control and Prevention: Sexually transmitted diseases treatment guidelines 2002. MMWR Morb Mortal Wkly Rep 2002;51:1-80.

Vaginitis

Vaginitis is inflammation of the squamous epithelial tissues lining the vagina. Three conditions cause most cases of adolescent vaginitis: VVC, BV, and trichomoniasis. All three treatable conditions can be diagnosed by examination of vaginal secretions during an office visit.

The presence of sexual activity influences the differential diagnosis; trichomoniasis and BV are more common in sexually experienced adolescents. In non–sexually active girls, VVC is the major cause of vaginal complaints and inflammation. Local chemical or allergic irritants, bacterial infections caused by *Streptococcus* or *Staphylococcus* species, trauma, and secondary infections from foreign bodies, may also cause vaginitis. Rare causes of vaginitis include ulcerating conditions of the mucous membranes, such as toxic shock and Stevens-Johnson syndromes.

The physical examination is an important part of the diagnostic workup (Table 29-16). Thick, adherent cottage cheese–like discharge is suggestive of VVC. The clinician may also find erythema, edema, and excoriation of the vagina in a girl with VVC. Thin, homogeneous, gray-white, foul-smelling discharge is suggestive of BV. Purulent, profuse, irritating, frothy green-yellow discharge often accompanies trichomoniasis.

Table 29-16 summarizes the diagnostic workup for vaginitis. The evaluation includes description of the vaginal discharge, measurement of vaginal pH, performance of a whiff test, and microscopic examination. Care should be taken to obtain a vaginal swab that is not contaminated with alkaline cervical secretions. Rubbing the specimen over a pH paper strip and matching the resulting color to the color chart determines the vaginal pH. Diluting a sample in a drop of 10% potassium hydroxide (KOH), referred to as the whiff test, produces a "fishy" odor with BV and sometimes with trichomoniasis.

Microscopy is critical in the diagnostic process (see Table 29-16). On the wet preparation, the clinician should look for (1) an excessive number of white blood cells, which is evidence of the inflammation often found with trichomoniasis and VVC; (2) vaginal "clue cells," which are typical of BV (Fig. 29-1); (3) motile or static trichomonads (Fig. 29-2), which are diagnostic of trichomoniasis; and (4) budding yeast and pseudohyphae (Fig. 29-3), which are diagnostic of VVC. Warming the solution to body temperature may improve identification of trichomonads and pseudohyphae. Because normal vaginal bacteria may be confused with yeast forms, the clinicians should look for pseudohyphae to help identify true yeast. Adding 10% KOH solution to the vaginal fluid lyses other cells and bacteria and often improves pseudohyphae visualization.

Alternative diagnostic strategies can aid or substitute for the conventional etiologic workup. For BV, the FemExam pH and Amines TestCard and the PIP Activity TestCard (Quidel Corp, San Diego, California) can substitute for the pH paper, the whiff test, and microscopic examination on a vaginal specimen by detecting an elevated vaginal pH, trimethylamines generated by BV associated anaerobic bacteria, and an enzyme produced by *Gardnerella vaginalis*. Although rarely performed as part of an office-based vaginitis evaluation, a Gram stain of vaginal fluid can provide a quantitative assessment (Nugent score) of BV-associated organisms.

For trichomoniasis, the InPouch TV test (BioMed Diagnostics, San Jose, California) is an office-based self-contained culture kit. The clinician inoculates a culture medium–filled pouch with a vaginal fluid specimen from girls or sediment from a spun first-void urine specimen from boys and examines its contents for trichomonads by microscopy. The clinician can incubate and repeatedly examine the transparent culture pouch under the microscope for up to 5 subsequent days. The InPouch TV test can be a valuable adjunct because most clinical laboratories do not perform the standard culture technique with Diamond medium.

For offices without microscopy, a professional laboratory that offers the Affirm VP III Microbial Identification Test (Becton Dickinson, Sparks, Maryland) provides a diagnostic option. The Affirm VP III, a DNA probe performed on vaginal fluid specimens, offers the advantage of diagnosing BV, VVC, and trichomoniasis. Correlating results of this test with clinical symptoms and elevated vaginal pH is recommended.

VAGINAL DISCHARGE AND IRRITATION IN THE PREPUBERTAL FEMALE

Nonsexually transmitted vulvovaginitis in infants and prepubertal girls is common. In prepubertal girls, the vulvar mucosa is thin and susceptible to inflammation from chemicals and mechanical irritation. Because the labia are not well developed, the vulvar mucosa is

Table 29-12. **Diagnostic Laboratory Test Performances for *Neisseria gonorrhoeae***

Test	Advantages	Disadvantages
Culture	Sensitivity ≈ 85% Specificity ≈ 100% Inexpensive, not labor intensive Not technically difficult Can determine antimicrobial susceptibility	Transport in CO_2 medium Requires urethral or cervical specimens
DNA probe	Sensitivity = 85% Inexpensive Easy transport	Requires urethral or cervical specimens
Gram stain	Inexpensive Easy transport Sensitivity = 95% for urethral specimens	Requires urethral or cervical specimens Sensitivity = 55% for cervical specimens
Nucleic acid amplification	Sensitivity/specificity = 80%-90% Urine specimens	High cost

Table 29-13. Diagnostic Laboratory Test Performances for *Chlamydia trachomatis*

Test	Advantages	Disadvantages
Cell culture	Specificity ≈ 100%	Sensitivity = 70% Complicated transport medium Requires urethral or cervical specimens High cost Labor intensive Technically difficult
ELISA immunoassay	Inexpensive Not technically difficult	Sensitivity = 60% Requires urethral or cervical specimens
DNA probe	Sensitivity = 65% Inexpensive Easy transport	Requires urethral or cervical specimens
Nucleic acid amplification	Sensitivity/specificity = 85% Urine specimens	High cost

Adapted from Centers for Disease Control and Prevention (CDC): Take action on HEDIS. *http://www.cdc.gov/nchstp/dstd/Reports_Publications/HMOletter.pdf.* Accessed on August 26, 2002.

not anatomically shielded and is thus vulnerable to irritation. In addition, a girl's hymenal configuration may predispose to vaginitis: A high, small opening may interfere with vaginal drainage, whereas a wide, gaping hymen (e.g., "posterior rim" configuration or after episodes of sexual abuse) permits easy contamination of the vagina by urine and feces.

In the majority of cases, vulvovaginitis in prepubertal girls is a mixed, nonspecific bacterial infection secondary to contamination by urine and feces. The responsible bacteria are usually normal flora: diphtheroids, α-hemolytic streptococci, lactobacilli, and *E. coli.* Other organisms include nonhemolytic streptococci, groups B and D streptococci, β-hemolytic group A streptococci, *Staphylococcus aureus, Staphylococcus epidermidis, Klebsiella* species, *Pseudomonas* species, *Proteus* species, and *G. vaginalis.* Anaerobes, *Candida* species, *Mycoplasma hominis,* and *Ureaplasma urealyticum* have also been found.

Bloody vaginal discharge in young girls may be caused by *Shigella* species or group A streptococcal infections, a foreign body, neoplasm (such as rhabdomyosarcoma), or trauma. Retained toilet paper is a common foreign body. It can usually be flushed out of the vagina with normal saline.

Several vulvar skin disorders can be confused with vulvovaginitis. Lichen sclerosus manifests as white patches on the glabrous skin that are thinned and atrophic and are easily traumatized with resultant bullae (which may be blood-filled) in the vulvar region. Seborrheic dermatitis may manifest with inflammation and secondary infection of the intertriginous areas; the face and scalp may be involved as well. Labial or vulvar agglutination may be noted and can be secondary to previous vulvovaginitis of unestrogenized epithelia.

Other etiologic factors in premenarchal vulvovaginitis include infection (fungi, pinworms, scabies), irritation (soap, shampoo, detergent, bubble bath), systemic illness (Stevens-Johnson syndrome), and trauma (abuse, play, tight clothing, masturbation).

Finally, some young girls with emotional or behavioral problems (occasionally caused by sexual abuse) may complain of vulvar symptoms in the absence of any findings on examination. Most cases of prepubertal nonspecific vaginitis can be managed with hygiene and 10 to 14 days of antibiotics, topical premarin vaginal cream (b.i.d.), and Phisohex liquid antibacterial soap in the bath water 1 to

Table 29-14. Treatment for Uncomplicated Genital *Chlamydia trachomatis* and *Neisseria gonorrhoeae* Infections in Adolescents*

Pathogen	Treatment
C. trachomatis	Azithromycin, 1 g orally in a single dose *or* Doxycycline, 100 mg orally twice daily for 7 days
N. gonorrhoeae[†]	Cefixime,[§] 400 mg orally in a single dose *or* Ciprofloxacin,[‡] 500 mg orally in a single dose *or* Ofloxacin,[‡] 400 mg orally in a single dose *or* Levofloxacin,[‡] 250 mg orally in a single dose *or* Ceftriaxone, 125 mg intramuscularly in a single dose *plus* Treatment for *C. trachomatis* if indicated[†]

Adapted from the Centers for Disease Control and Prevention. Sexually transmitted diseases treatment guidelines 2002. MMWR Morb Mortal Wkly Rep 2002;51:1-84.

*8 years of age or older.

[†]Centers for Disease Control and Prevention recommend treating persons with a positive gonorrhea test result for both gonorrhea and chlamydia unless a negative result has been obtained with a sensitive chlamydia test.

[‡]Fluoroquinolones have not been recommended for persons younger than 18 years because they damage articular cartilage in juvenile animal models. However, among children treated with fluoroquinolones, no joint damage attributable to therapy has been observed. Quinolones should not be used to treat gonorrhea infections acquired in Asia or the Pacific islands, including Hawaii.

[§]Cefixime is no longer produced in the USA; availability is limited.

Table 29-15. Centers for Disease Control and Prevention Recommended Treatment for Recurrent/Persistent Urethritis

Metronidazole, 2 g orally in a single dose
plus
Erythromycin base, 500 mg orally 4 times a day for 7 days
or
Erythromycin ethylsuccinate, 800 mg orally 4 times a day for 7 days

Table 29-16. Clinical and Laboratory Features of Vaginitis

Infection	Symptoms	Vaginal Discharge	Whiff Test	Microscopic Findings	pH	Enhanced Diagnosis
Bacterial vaginosis	Foul smelling discharge, ↑ after intercourse	Thin Homogenous Gray-white	Positive	>20% clue cells	>4.5	Gram stain Affirm VP III
Trichomoniasis	Frothy, foul smelling discharge, pruritus, dysuria	Purulent, profuse, irritating, frothy, green-yellow	Variably positive	↑ WBCs Trichomonads	>4.5	Diamond media culture Inpouch TV test Affirm VP III
Vulvovaginal candidiasis	Pruritus, burning, discharge	Thick Adherent White	Negative	↑ WBCs Budding yeast Pseudohyphae	4-4.5	Affirm VP III

WBC, white blood cell. ↑, increased.

2 times per week. The treatment of vulvovaginitis in prepubertal girls is summarized in Tables 29-17 and 29-18.

EVALUATION AND MANAGEMENT OF SEXUALLY TRANSMITTED DISEASES AMONG SEXUALLY ABUSED CHILDREN AND ADOLESCENTS

The prevalence of STDs among prepubertal victims of sexual assault has been reported as 5%, and it is generally accompanied by symptoms. Because the STD risk is low and the risk of imparting psychological and physical discomfort with the specimen collection procedures is high, many experts recommend reserving STD screening of prepubertal children for the situations listed in Table 29-19.

The examination should be performed in compliance with expert recommendations by an experienced clinician. Table 29-20 lists recommended STD tests. Because children can acquire an STD through vertical transmission, autoinoculation, or sexual contact, STD screening should focus on likely anatomic sites. Table 29-21 lists the likelihood of an STD as evidence of sexual assault and suggested action.

Because sexually experienced adolescents may have an asymptomatic infection unrelated to the alleged event and the risk of complications of an untreated STD are high, most experts recommend empirical STD screening and treatment of postpubertal victims. STD screening should focus on likely anatomic sites.

The timing of the examination depends on the history of the assault. When the alleged assault has occurred within the previous 72 hours or when there is bleeding or acute injury, the examination should be performed immediately, and specific protocols to collect forensic evidence should be followed. To allow sufficient time for concentrations of organisms to reach detectable levels, clinicians may recommend a follow-up visit 2 weeks after the most recent sexual exposure for a repeat examination and collection of additional specimens. If syphilis,

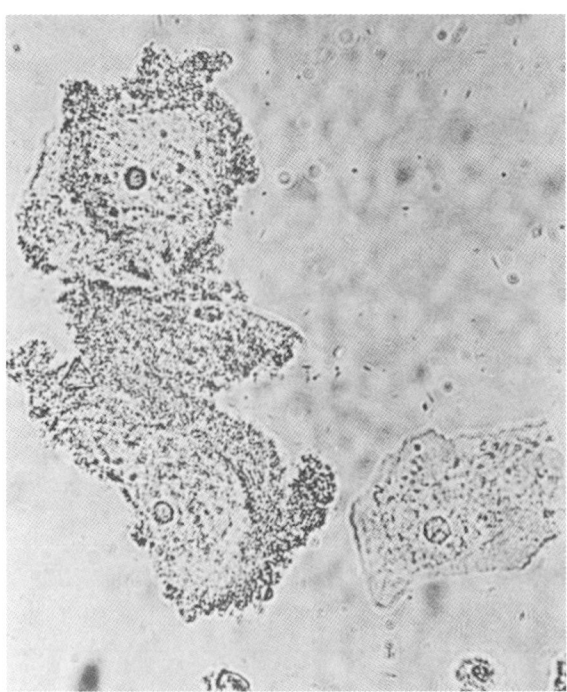

Figure 29-1. Bacteria clinging to the sides of a vaginal epithelial cell ("clue cell"). This occurrence is significant in bacterial vaginosis. (Reproduced by courtesy of Dr. Herman L. Gardner. From Huffman JW: Genitourinary infections. In Feigin RD, Cherry JD [eds]: Textbook of Pediatric Infectious Diseases, 2nd ed. Philadelphia, WB Saunders, 1992, p 570.)

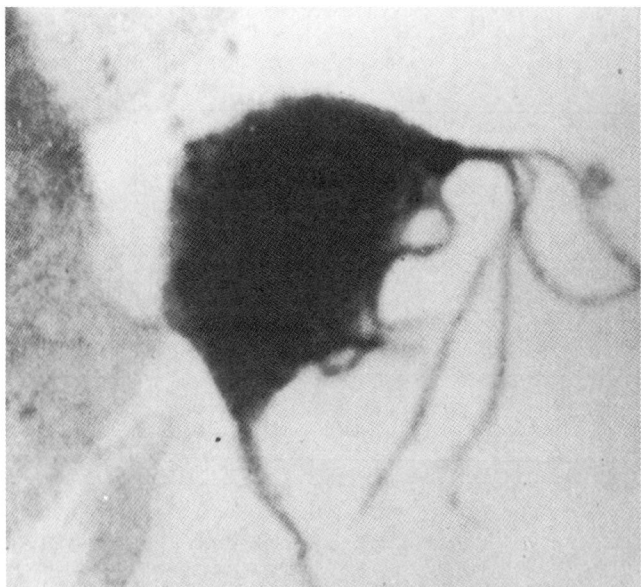

Figure 29-2. *Trichomonas vaginalis* is a triflagellated protozoan that, when motile, is easily identified in wet smears of the vaginal discharge. (From Huffman JW: Genitourinary infections. In Feigin RD, Cherry JD [eds]: Textbook of Pediatric Infectious Diseases, 2nd ed. Philadelphia, WB Saunders, 1992, p 568.)

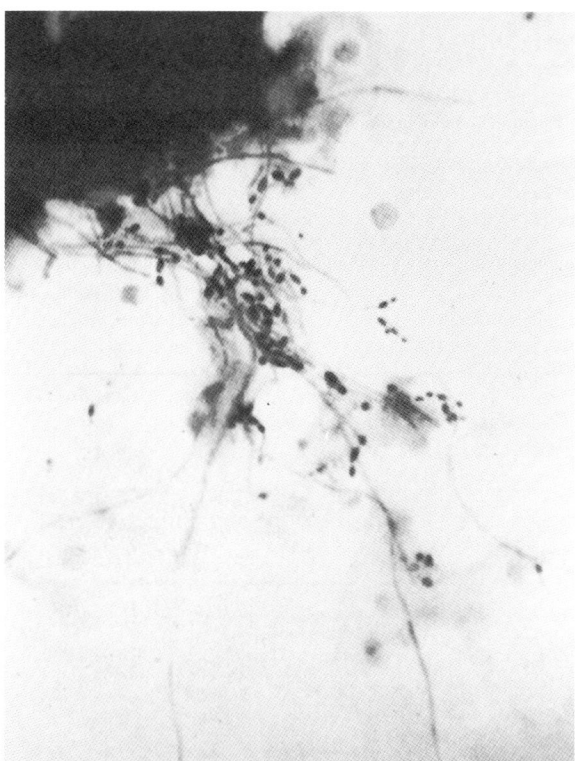

Figure 29-3. Hyphae of *Candida albicans* discovered on wet smear of vaginal discharge. (From Huffman JW: Genitourinary infections. In Feigin RD, Cherry JD [eds]: Textbook of Pediatric Infectious Diseases, 2nd ed. Philadelphia, WB Saunders, 1992, p 564.)

HIV, or hepatitis B virus transmission is of concern, another visit in 12 weeks may be necessary to collect sera for specific antibodies.

Presumptive STD treatment for children who have been sexually assaulted or abused is not routinely recommended. However, if patients or parents/guardians are concerned about the possibility of infection, providers may choose to presumptively treat after all specimens for

---

Table 29-17. Treatment of Nonspecific Vulvovaginitis in Young Females

Toilet Hygiene

Wipe in an anterior-to-posterior direction with supervision
Diaper wipes are useful
Urinate with knees spread apart

Clothing

Choose white cotton underpants
Wear loose-fitting clothing

Bathing

Take sitz baths in clear water up to four times a day
Wash gently with unperfumed soap
Do not use bubble bath or wash hair in bath
Rinse perineum with clear water, dry gently with towel
Take baths with Phisohex liquid antibacterial soap in bathwater once or twice per week for 10-14 days

Management of Inflammation and Pruritus

Premarin vaginal cream topically twice daily for 10-14 days
Hydroxyzine, 0.5-1 mg/kg/dose orally q.i.d. as needed
or
Diphenhydramine, 1.25 mg/kg/dose orally q.i.d. as needed

Table 29-18. Oral Treatment of Non–Sexually Transmitted Causes of Vulvovaginitis in Prepubertal Females

β-Hemolytic Group A Streptococci

Clindamycin, 30 mg/kg/day ÷ t.i.d. for 10-14 days
or
Penicillin VK, 25-50 mg/kg/day ÷ t.i.d. for 10-14 days
or
Erythromycin, 40 mg/kg/day ÷ t.i.d. for 10-14 days
or
Cephalexin, 25-100 mg/kg/day ÷ q.i.d. for 10-14 days

Streptococcus pneumoniae

Penicillin VK, 25-50 mg/kg/day ÷ t.i.d. for 10-14 days
or
Erythromycin, 40 mg/kg/day ÷ t.i.d. for 10-14 days
or
Cephalexin, 25-100 mg/kg/day ÷ q.i.d. for 10-14 days

Staphylococcus aureus

Dicloxacillin, 25 mg/kg/day ÷ q.i.d. for 10-14 days
or
Amoxicillin plus clavulanate, 25-45 mg/kg/day ÷ b.i.d. for 10-14 days
or
Cefpodoxime proxetil, 10 mg/kg/day daily or ÷ b.i.d. for 10-14 days
or
Cephalexin, 25-100 mg/kg/day ÷ q.i.d. for 10-14 days
or
Clindamycin, 30 mg/kg/day ÷ t.i.d. for 10-14 days
or
Cefuroxime, 30 mg/kg/day ÷ b.i.d. for 10-14 days
or
Clarithromycin, 15 mg/kg/day ÷ b.i.d. for 10-14 days

Haemophilus influenzae

Erythromycin ethylsuccinate/sulfisoxazole, 50 mg/kg/day ÷ q.i.d. for 10-14 days
or
Trimethoprim/sulfamethoxazole, 8-10 mg/kg/day ÷ b.i.d. for 10-14 days
or
Amoxicillin/clavulanate, 25-45 mg/kg/day ÷ b.i.d. for 10-14 days
or
Clarithromycin, 15 mg/kg/day ÷ b.i.d. for 10-14 days
or
Cefixime, 8 mg/kg/day daily or ÷ b.i.d. for 10-14 days*

Shigella

Trimethoprim/sulfamethoxazole, 8-10 mg/kg/day ÷ b.i.d. for 10-14 days

Candida

Nystatin vaginal cream, apply topically b.i.d. for 10-14 days

Enterobius vermicularis

Mebendazole, 100 mg as a single dose for patient and all household members, then repeated in 2 weeks

b.i.d., twice per day; t.i.d., three times per day; q.i.d., four times per day.

*Cefixime production was discontinued in the United States in July 2002; availability is limited.

Table 29-19. Sexually Transmitted Diseases Screening Indications for Sexually Victimized Children

The child has signs or symptoms of a sexually transmitted disease (STD), including genital pain, vaginal or urethral discharge, pruritus or odor, urinary symptoms, or genital ulcers or lesions.
A suspected sex offender is known to have an STD or to be at high risk for STDs
A sibling or another child or adult in the household or child's immediate environment has an STD
The patient or parent requests testing
Evidence of genital, oral, or anal penetration or ejaculation

Adapted from Centers for Disease Control and Prevention: Sexually transmitted diseases treatment guidelines 2002. MMWR Morb Mortal Wkly Rep 2002;51:1-80.

relevant diagnostic tests are collected. Adolescent sexual assault victims should be offered prophylactic treatment for STDs and pregnancy prevention. Table 29-22 lists recommended presumptive treatment.

HIV postexposure assessment and prophylaxis should be considered for abused children on a case-by-case basis, depending on the likelihood of HIV infection among the assailant or assailants (Table 29-23).

Table 29-20. Recommended Sexually Transmitted Diseases Testing in a Prepubertal Child when Sexual Abuse Is Suspected

Organism/Syndrome	Specimens
Neisseria gonorrhoeae	Rectal, throat, urethral, and/or vaginal culture(s)*
Chlamydia trachomatis	Rectal and vaginal cultures[†]
Syphilis	Darkfield examination of chancre fluid, if present; blood for serologic tests at time of abuse and 6, 12, and 24 weeks later
Trichomonas vaginalis	Wet mount and culture of vaginal discharge
Bacterial vaginosis	Wet mount and culture of vaginal discharge
Hepatitis B virus	Serum hepatitis B surface antigen test[‡]
Human papillomavirus	Biopsy of lesion
Pediculosis capitis	Identification of eggs, nymphs, and lice with naked eye or by using hand lens
Human immunodeficiency virus	Serologic test of abuser; serologic test of child at time of abuse and 12, and 24 weeks later if indicated

Adapted from American Academy of Pediatrics. Sexually transmitted diseases in adolescent and children. In Pickering LK (ed): 2003 Redbook: Report of the Committee on Infectious Diseases, 26th ed. Elk Grove Village, Ill, American Academy of Pediatrics, 2003, pp 159-167.

*Cervical specimens are not recommended. A meatal discharge specimen is an adequate substitute for an intraurethral specimen. Only standard culture systems should be used for prepubertal females.

[†]A meatal specimen should be obtained if urethral discharge is present in prepubertal boys. Urethral specimens are not recommended among asymptomatic boys. Only standard culture systems should be used. Expert opinion suggests nucleic acid amplification tests (NAATs) may be an alternative *only* if confirmation is available but culture systems for *C. trachomatis* are unavailable. Confirmation tests should consist of a second U.S. Food and Drug Administration–approved NAAT that targets a different molecule from the initial test.

[‡]Test abuser. Test victim at initial visit and at 12-week follow-up visit if there is no history of immunization.

Table 29-21. Implications of Commonly Encountered Sexually Transmitted Infections for Diagnosis and Reporting of Suspected Sexual Abuse of Infants and Prepubertal Children

Sexually Transmitted/ Associated Infection Confirmed	Evidence for Sexual Abuse	Suggested Action
Gonorrhea*	Diagnostic	Report[†]
Syphilis*	Diagnostic	Report[†]
Human immunodeficiency virus[‡]	Diagnostic	Report[†]
Chlamydia*	Diagnostic	Report[†]
Trichomonas vaginalis	Highly suspicious	Report[†]
Condylomata acuminata (anogenital warts)	Suspicious	Report[†]
Genital herpes	Suspicious	Report[†§]
Bacterial vaginosis	Inconclusive	Medical follow-up

Adapted from the American Academy of Pediatrics Committee on Child Abuse and Neglect Guidelines for the evaluation of sexual abuse of children. Pediatrics 1999;103:186-191. Correction published in Pediatrics 1999;103:1049.

*If not likely to be perinatally acquired.

[†]Reports should be made to the agency in the community mandated to receive reports of suspected child abuse or neglect.

[‡]If not likely to be perinatally or transfusion acquired.

[§]Unless there is a clear history of autoinoculation.

SYSTEMIC DISEASE

The STDs and their sequelae that are most often associated with systemic symptoms include HIV, syphilis, HSV, hepatitis B, PID, reactive arthritis, and disseminated gonorrhea infection. See later discussion for relevant disease presentations and management.

DIAGNOSTIC AND THERAPEUTIC CONSIDERATIONS

BACTERIAL VAGINOSIS

BV is a noninflammatory disturbance of the normal vaginal ecosystem and is one of the most common causes of vaginal discharge in adolescents. Although not considered to be an STD, BV occurs

Table 29-22. Postexposure Prophylaxis for Sexually Transmitted Diseases* after Sexual Assault in Adolescents

Ceftriaxone, 125 mg intramuscularly in a single dose
plus
Metronidazole, 2 g orally in a single dose
plus
Azithromycin, 1 g orally in a single dose *or* doxycycline, 100 mg orally twice daily for 7 days
Post-exposure hepatitis B virus immunization if no previous immunization; follow-up doses should be administered at 1-2 months and 4-6 months

Adapted from Centers for Disease Control and Prevention: Sexually transmitted diseases treatment guidelines 2002. MMWR Morb Mortal Wkly Rep 2002;51:1-80.

*Excluding human immunodeficiency virus infection.

Table 29-23. **Recommendations for Human Immunodeficiency Virus (HIV) Postexposure Assessment of Children and Adolescents within 72 Hours of Sexual Assault**

Review HIV/AIDS local epidemiology and assess risk of HIV infection in assailant

Evaluate circumstances of assault that may affect risk of HIV transmission

Consult with specialist in HIV treatment if postexposure prophylaxis is considered

If the victim appears to be at risk of HIV transmission from the assault, discuss antiretroviral prophylaxis, including toxicity, and unknown efficacy with patient (or guardian)

If the victim is (or if guardian chooses for the child) to receive antiretroviral postexposure prophylaxis, provide enough medication until the return visit at 3-7 days after initial assessment to reevaluate patient and to assess tolerance of medication; pediatric dosages should not exceed adult doses

HIV antibody test at original assessment, 6 weeks, 3 months, and 6 months

Adapted from Centers for Disease Control and Prevention: Sexually transmitted diseases treatment guidelines 2002. MMWR Morb Mortal Wkly Rep 2002;51:1-80.

AIDS, acquired immunodeficiency syndrome.

Table 29-25. **Treatment Regimens for Bacterial Vaginosis**

Nonpregnant Females

Metronidazole, 500 mg orally twice daily for 7 days

or

Metronidazole gel, 0.75%, one full applicator (5 g) intravaginally once a day for 5 days

or

Clindamycin cream, 2%, one full applicator (5 g) intravaginally once a day for 7 days

Pregnant Females

Metronidazole, 250 mg orally three times daily for 7 days

or

Clindamycin, 300 mg orally twice daily for 7 days

Adapted from Centers for Disease Control and Prevention: Sexually transmitted diseases treatment guidelines 2002. MMWR Morb Mortal Wkly Rep 2002;51:1-84.

more frequently among sexually active females. BV is thought to result from the replacement of the normal H_2O_2-producing vaginal flora with organisms such as *G. vaginalis, M. hominis, Mobiluncus* species, *Bacteroides* species, and other anaerobes. BV is asymptomatic in almost 50% of females diagnosed with this disorder. Usual symptoms include vaginal odor and vaginal discharge.

BV is diagnosed by the presence of a gray-white, malodorous (fishy), homogenous, nonviscous vaginal discharge. The clinical diagnosis of BV is made by the presence of at least three of the four criteria listed in Table 29-24 or by more sophisticated laboratory techniques listed in Table 29-16.

Treatment is recommended for all symptomatic patients. Options for treatment include oral and vaginal regimens (Table 29-25). Abstinence from alcohol during treatment with metronidazole and for 24 hours afterward should be stressed because of the disulfiram-like effect of that drug. No treatment of the sexual partner is indicated.

VULVOVAGINAL CANDIDIASIS

Candida species are common microbes that can be isolated from the vagina in 10% to 55% of asymptomatic, healthy women of reproductive age. It is probably a commensal organism that becomes an

Table 29-24. **Amsel Criteria for Diagnosis of Bacterial Vaginosis**

Vaginal discharge: thin, homogenous, white, uniformly adherent

Vaginal pH > 4.5

Positive result of whiff test: fishy odor after mixing discharge with 10% KOH

>20% clue cells on microscopic examination: bacteria-coated squamous epithelial cells, where both the periphery (cell membrane) and cytoplasm have a granular, irregular, "moth-eaten" appearance

KOH, potassium hydroxide.

invasive pathogen under certain circumstances. Increased rates of infection are noted in pregnant girls and women, especially during the third trimester; in some oral contraceptive users; in patients with poorly controlled diabetes mellitus; in patients with high-calorie, high-carbohydrate, and high-fiber diets; and in patients who are taking corticosteroids or broad-spectrum antibiotics. Most vaginal yeast infections (85% to 90%) are caused by *Candida albicans.* Other candidal species and *Torulopsis glabrata* infections are increasing in frequency.

Acute pruritus and vaginal discharge are the main complaints of symptomatic patients. The odorless discharge may be watery or thick and sometimes resembles cottage cheese. At times, the patient may also complain of vulvar burning sensation, vaginal soreness, external dysuria, or dyspareunia. On examination, the labia can be edematous and erythematous; pustulopapular lesions may exist peripherally. The vaginal mucosa may be erythematous, but the cervix is normal. Table 29-16 describes the diagnostic features of VVC.

VVC is easily treated with many topical azole antifungal preparations whose active agent is clotrimazole, miconazole, buto-conazole, terconazole, or tioconazole. Clinical and microbiologic cure rates are 80% to 90% for most regimens. Oral fluconazole, in a 150-mg single dose, is as effective as the topical treatments. A longer duration of treatment (10 to 14 days) may be needed for severe and recurrent infections.

TRICHOMONIASIS

T. vaginalis is a sexually transmitted, unicellular, flagellated, anaerobic protozoan that exists as an extracellular parasite in the human lower genitourinary tract (see Fig. 29-2). females appear to have more acute manifestations than do males. Many girls and women have no symptoms, but vaginal discharge, abnormal vaginal odor, vulvar pruritus, dyspareunia, dysuria, and lower abdominal discomfort are the usual findings. In males who are symptomatic, urethral discharge has been noted. Table 29-16 lists diagnostic techniques.

Trichomoniasis is easily treated in about 85% to 95% of infected patients with metronidazole in a 2-g single dose accompanied by concurrent partner treatment with the same regimen. Abstinence from alcohol for 24 hours should be stressed because of the disulfiram-like effect of metronidazole. Topical treatments are not effective. Nonresponders should be retreated with a 7-day course of 500 mg of metronidazole twice daily. If this regimen fails, a third alternative is 2 g of metronidazole daily for 3 to 5 days. However, a partner's nonadherence to treatment should be explored because this is a common cause of reinfection. A single 2-g dose of metronidazole is recommended during pregnancy.

CHLAMYDIA INFECTION

C. trachomatis is the most common reported pathogen among adolescents. Chlamydia is frequently asymptomatic in both sexes. Most sexually active adolescents are unaware of their risk for chlamydia infection. Although often asymptomatic, chlamydia can manifest as various STD syndromes, depending on the site of infection. Affected patients of both sexes may develop urethritis. Females may develop MPC.

Sequelae of uncomplicated chlamydia infection can be devastating for females. Infection can ascend into the pelvis, causing PID. Chlamydia screening and treatment of adolescent girls consequently reduces the incidence of PID. Females with a prior chlamydia infection are also at increased risk of infertility, ectopic pregnancy, and chronic pelvic pain.

Chlamydia sequelae are rare among males. The incidence of epididymitis among males is much lower than the incidence of PID among females. There is no evidence of a causal association between chlamydial and gonorrheal urethritis and male infertility.

Exudative STDs involving mucosal surfaces, such as chlamydia, can result in sequelae among patients of both sexes. Reactive arthritis, a postinfectious inflammatory arthritis, can follow a localized genitourinary chlamydia infection. Like other exudative STDs, chlamydia can facilitate both HIV transmission and acquisition.

Diagnostic options are presented in Table 29-13. The CDC's recommended treatment options are listed in Table 29-14 and Table 29-26. All sexual partners should be evaluated and treated. Abstinence should be recommended for at least 7 days after initiation of therapy for both infected patients and sex partners. A "test of cure" is not routinely recommended after treatment of adolescent chlamydia infection. However, providers should consider advising all with chlamydia infection to be rescreened 3 to 4 months after treatment. Some experts recommend testing adolescents for chlamydia every 6 months because the risk of repeat infection is high.

GONORRHEA INFECTION

Adolescent females aged 15-19 years have the highest reported rate of gonorrhea in the United States. In addition to age, other demographic risk factors for gonorrhea include African American race, lower socioeconomic status, early onset of sexual activity, single marital status, and prior gonorrhea infection. *N. gonorrhoeae* infections can manifest as various STD syndromes. Both males and females may develop urethritis, proctitis, or pharyngitis. Females

Table 29-26. Treatment for Pediatric* Uncomplicated Genital *Chlamydia trachomatis* and *Neisseria gonorrhoeae* Infections

Pathogen	Treatment
C. trachomatis	Erythromycin base or ethylsuccinate, 50 mg/kg/day orally divided into 4 doses daily for 14 days[†]
	or
	Azithromycin, 1 g orally in a single dose[‡]
N. gonorrhoeae[§]	Ceftriaxone, 125 mg intramuscularly in a single dose[§]

Adapted from Centers for Disease Control and Prevention: Sexually transmitted diseases treatment guidelines 2002. MMWR Morb Mortal Wkly Rep 2002;51:1-80.

*Younger than 8 years.

[†]For children weighing <45 kg.

[‡]For children weighing ≥45 kg.

[§]Children weighing ≥45 kg should be treated with a regimen recommended for adults.

may develop MPC. Sensitive NAATs have shown that gonorrhea infection can be asymptomatic in both sexes.

As in chlamydia infections, females may develop PID as a sequela and males in rare cases develop epididymitis. Both sexes are at risk of developing disseminated gonorrhea infection. Gonorrhea facilitates HIV transmission and acquisition.

Diagnostic options are presented in Table 29-12.

The CDC's recommended treatment options are listed in Tables 29-14 and 29-26. Some providers prescribe azithromycin for treatment of gonorrhea infection. However, a single 1-g azithromycin dose produces suboptimal gonorrhea cure rates. A single 2-g dose provides adequate therapy, but a high frequency of gastrointestinal side effects and its high cost prohibit its use. Cefixime is currently not available in the United States.

Fluoroquinolones have not been recommended for persons younger than 18 years because they damage articular cartilage in juvenile animal models. However, among children treated with fluoroquinolones, no joint damage attributable to therapy has been observed. Quinolones should not be used to treat gonorrhea infections acquired in Asia or the Pacific, including Hawaii and California, because of documented resistance in those areas.

GENITAL HERPES SIMPLEX VIRUS INFECTIONS

Genital herpes, caused by HSV-1 and HSV-2, is the most common cause of genital ulcers in the United States. An estimated 1.5% of all adolescents aged 12-19 years are infected with HSV-2. Demographic and behavioral risk factors include female gender, nonwhite race, and greater number of lifetime sex partners. Clinical disease develops with approximately a third of HSV-2 infections; a large proportion of genital herpes infections go unrecognized.

Although HSV-2 is responsible for most genital herpes infections, the frequency of HSV-1 genital infections is rising. A prior HSV-1 infection appears to be protective against development of symptoms with HSV-2 infection but not protective against infection with HSV-2 virus.

HSV-infected patients can present with a primary infection, which can be asymptomatic; a first clinical episode, which may not necessarily occur during the primary infection; or a recurrent episode. Usually first clinical episodes are more painful and prolonged than are subsequent ones. Recurrent episodes occur less frequently with a genital HSV-1 infection and with intervals between episodes becoming longer.

Symptomatic primary genital herpes infection is characterized by prolonged systemic and local symptoms. Systemic symptoms typically develop a week after exposure to infection and last for about a week. Systemic symptoms, more common among females, manifest as fever, headache, malaise, and myalgias. Local symptoms typically develop a week after exposure to infection, reach their maximum intensity 7 to 10 days after onset of symptoms, and gradually recede over the following week. Local symptoms include pain, itching, dysuria, vaginal or urethral discharge, and tender bilateral inguinal adenopathy. Painful lesions usually begin as papules or vesicles that rapidly spread over the genital area. Multiple small pustular lesions coalesce into large areas of ulcerations, eventually crusting over and reepithelializing. Crusting does not occur over mucosal surfaces. Lesions typically do not leave scars. New lesions commonly develop during the end of the first week of symptoms. Viral shedding usually continues for 2 weeks. An episode, from onset of lesions to complete resolution, can last up to 3 weeks.

Primary HSV infection can cause other conditions, including nongenital lesions, cervicitis, urethritis, cystitis, proctitis, and pharyngitis. Systemic complications such as hepatitis, pneumonia, thrombocytopenia, and monoarticular arthritis may occur.

Recurrent genital herpes imparts a less severe and shorter duration of local and systemic symptoms. Females usually develop more severe episodes than do males. Typically, patients develop prodromal symptoms, which can vary from mild tingling sensations to shooting pains in the buttocks or lower extremities, before the appearance of lesions. The lesions of recurrent infections are usually unilateral (80% to 95%) and involve a much smaller area. The average number of lesions is five in females and eight in males. Most patients experience pain for 4 to 6 days. Some patients may experience dysuria or tender adenopathy. The mean time to heal is 10 days, and the mean duration of viral shedding is 4 days. Considerable variability exists in the clinical manifestation and frequency of recurrent episodes. Therefore, herpes should be considered in the evaluation of all genital lesions.

Complications of genital herpes include central nervous system disease such as aseptic meningitis, autonomic dysfunction, and transverse myelitis; extragenital lesions, most commonly located in the buttocks, groin, or thigh area; disseminated infection; vertical transmission, resulting in neonatal herpes; and facilitation of HIV infection.

Asymptomatic viral shedding is common with genital HSV infection. Clinicians need to stress to infected patients that they may be contagious during the prodrome and during the symptom-free periods, and clinicians should offer strategies to decrease risk of transmission to sexual partners.

The clinical diagnosis of genital herpes should be confirmed by laboratory testing to distinguish between virus types. Because recurrences are usually less frequent after initial episodes of HSV-1 infection, knowledge of virus type helps determine the prognosis. HSV isolation by cell culture is the preferred virologic test for patients who present with open genital ulcers or other mucocutaneous lesions. HSV antigen detection tests do not distinguish between HSV-1 and HSV-2. Tzanck preparations and cervical Pap smears are insensitive and nonspecific for diagnosis of HSV infection.

For serologic testing of HSV, the serologic type-specific glycoprotein G (gG)–based assays should be specifically requested. A test using an assay for HSV antibodies must be based on the HSV-specific glycoprotein G2 for the diagnosis of HSV-2 infection and the glycoprotein G1 for diagnosis of HSV-1 infection. Older assays that do not accurately distinguish between HSV-1 and HSV-2 antibodies, despite claims, remain on the market. U.S. Food and Drug Administration–approved gG-based type-specific assays include POCkit HSV-2 Rapid Test (Diagnology, Belfast, Northern Ireland), and HerpeSelect-1 ELISA IgG, HerpeSelect-2 ELISA IgG, and HerpeSelect 1 and 2 Immunoblot IgG (Focus Technologies, Herndon, Virginia). The reported sensitivities range from 80% to 98%, and specificities are reported to be higher than 96% for detection of HSV-2 antibodies. False-negative results may occur early after infection, and false-positive results can occur in patients with a low likelihood of HSV infection.

HSV is a manageable but not curable chronic infection. Although systemic antiviral medication partially controls signs and symptoms of clinical episodes, it does not eradicate latent virus or affect the frequency or severity of recurrences after the drug is discontinued. Counseling regarding the natural history of genital herpes, sexual and perinatal transmission, and methods to reduce transmission, such as consistent condom use and abstinence during clinical episodes, is an important component of clinical management.

Table 29-27 lists CDC-recommended regimens for first clinical episodes of genital herpes. Most patients presenting with first episodes should receive antiviral therapy despite mild manifestations because therapy can prevent progression to severe and prolonged symptoms. Duration of treatment may be extended if healing is incomplete after 10 days of therapy.

Table 29-28 lists episodic therapy that can be used for recurrent HSV disease. Effective episodic treatment of recurrent herpes decreases the duration of symptoms and viral shedding by 1 to 2 days. The patient can be provided with a prescription for the medication and instructions to self-initiate treatment immediately when symptoms begin because effective episodic treatment requires initiation of therapy during the prodromal period or within 1 day of lesion onset.

Table 29-27. Treatment Regimens for First Clinical Genital Herpes Episode

Acyclovir, 400 mg orally three times a day for 7-10 days
or
Acyclovir, 200 mg orally five times a day for 7-10 days
or
Famciclovir, 250 mg orally three times a day for 7-10 days
or
Valacyclovir, 1.0 g orally twice a day for 7-10 days

Adapted from Centers for Disease Control and Prevention: Sexually transmitted diseases treatment guidelines 2002. MMWR Morb Mortal Wkly Rep 2002;51:1-80.

Table 29-29 lists CDC-recommended suppressive therapy for recurrent HSV disease. Suppressive therapy reduces the frequency of genital herpes recurrences by 70% to 80% among patients experiencing frequent recurrences (i.e., >6 episodes per year). Patients with less frequent recurrences may also benefit from suppressive therapy. Patients should understand that suppressive therapy reduces but does not eliminate subclinical viral shedding. Because the frequency of recurrent outbreaks typically diminishes over time, continuation of therapy should be periodically reassessed (e.g., once a year).

HUMAN IMMUNODEFICIENCY VIRUS INFECTION

HIV infection is increasing among adolescents in the United States, and sexual contact is the most common cause of new infections in adolescents. Over 50% of new adolescent cases occur in females, the majority from heterosexual infection. HIV transmission in adolescent males occurs most commonly via male-to-male sex. There is an increased prevalence of HIV infection among African American and Hispanic adolescents.

Most adolescents are asymptomatic, and thus HIV testing is necessary to identify infected patients. Indications for HIV testing are listed in Table 29-9. Adolescents need to be informed about the importance of testing. Diagnosis allows early initiation of therapy and decreases transmission to others. State laws regarding adolescent consent for HIV counseling and testing vary.

Adolescents with sexually acquired HIV infection frequently have additional STDs and high levels of sexual activity.

Acute retroviral syndrome, a mononucleosis-like illness, frequently develops within a few weeks of primary infection with HIV. Signs and symptoms may include fever, sweats, malaise, myalgias, anorexia, nausea, diarrhea, pharyngitis, truncal exanthem, and lymphadenopathy. Possible neurologic manifestations range from aseptic meningitis to Guillain-Barré syndrome or encephalitis. Acute opportunistic

Table 29-28. Treatment Regimens of Episodic Therapy for Recurrent Genital Herpes

Acyclovir, 400 mg orally three times a day for 5 days
or
Acyclovir, 200 mg orally five times a day for 5 days
or
Acyclovir, 800 mg orally twice a day for 5 days
or
Famciclovir, 125 mg orally twice a day for 5 days
or
Valacyclovir, 500 mg orally twice a day for 3-5 days
or
Valacyclovir, 1.0 g orally once a day for 5 days

Adapted from Centers for Disease Control and Prevention: Sexually transmitted diseases treatment guidelines 2002. MMWR Morb Mortal Wkly Rep 2002;51:1-80.

Table 29-29. Treatment Regimens of Suppressive Therapy for Recurrent Genital Herpes*

Acyclovir, 400 mg orally twice a day
or
Famciclovir, 250 mg orally twice a day
or
Valacyclovir, 500 mg orally once a day
or
Valacyclovir, 1.0 g orally once a day

Adapted from Centers for Disease Control and Prevention: Sexually transmitted diseases treatment guidelines 2002. MMWR Morb Mortal Wkly Rep 2002;51:1-80.

*Continuation of suppressive therapy should be periodically reassessed (e.g., once a year).

infections occasionally occur. Peripheral lymphocyte counts are low; transaminase elevation is common. If acute HIV infection is suspected, a serologic test for HIV should be performed, but the result is likely to be negative because antibodies are not yet present. An HIV polymerase chain reaction test is usually positive at this stage. Such patients should be referred to an HIV clinic for early antiretroviral therapy.

There is substantial variation in the rate of progression from HIV infection to acquired immunodeficiency syndrome (AIDS) in untreated patients. Because the median time to develop AIDS is about 10 years, most infected adolescents are asymptomatic at the time of diagnosis. Clinical manifestations of AIDS are protean and can affect virtually every organ system (Table 29-30).

Treatment of adolescents with HIV infection is best done at an HIV clinic or by a pediatric infectious disease specialist. High HIV plasma RNA (viral load) and a low CD4 T cell count are related predictors of disease progression and risk of opportunistic infections. Therapy includes antiretroviral medications and prophylaxis against

Table 29-30. Organ-Specific Manifestations of Acquired Immunodeficiency Syndrome

Immune
Lymphadenopathy
Hepatosplenomegaly
Lymphopenia
Opportunistic infections (bacterial sepsis, recurrent otitis media, *Mycobacterium avium* complex or *Mycobacterium kansasii, Mycobacterium tuberculosis,* histoplasmosis, cryptococcosis, *Salmonella* species, *Nocardia* species, coccidioidomycosis, CMV)

Constitutional
Fever
Weight loss, failure to thrive
Fatigue
Night sweats
Malaise

Muscle and Nervous Systems
Aseptic meningitis
Developmental delay or regression after reaching milestones
Encephalopathy
Progressive multifocal leukoencephalopathy
Dementia (cognitive impairment)
Peripheral neuropathy
Bell palsy
Ataxia
Myelopathy
Headache
Depression
Spasticity
Paresis
Lymphoma (primary CNS)
Seizures
Strokes
Polymyositis/pyomyositis
Opportunistic infections (toxoplasmosis)

Pulmonary
Lymphoid interstitial pneumonia
Opportunistic pneumonias (*Pneumocystis carinii,* CMV)

Cardiac
Cardiomyopathy
Opportunistic infections (myocarditis)

Gastrointestinal
Parotitis
Hairy leukoplakia
Gingivitis
Periodontitis
Oral ulceration
Oral and esophageal thrush
Esophagitis
Gastritis
Hepatitis
Cholecystitis
Cholangitis
Diarrhea (enterocolitis)
Pancreatitis
Opportunistic infections (HSV, *Candida* species, CMV, cryptosporidiosis, isosporiasis)

Ocular
Retinitis
Opportunistic infections (CMV)

Cutaneous
Seborrhea dermatitis
Psoriasis
Atopic dermatitis
Ichthyosis
Opportunistic infections (HSV, zoster, varicella, *Bartonella* species causing bacillary angiomatosis, Norwegian scabies)

Hematologic
Thrombocytopenia
Anemia
Leukopenia
Lymphopenia

Malignancies
Lymphomas
Leiomyosarcomas
Kaposi sarcoma
Cervical cancer

Renal
Nephropathy

CMV, cytomegalovirus; CNS, central nervous system; HSV, herpes simplex.

opportunistic infection. Identification and treatment of HIV-infected pregnant adolescents substantially decreases the risk of mother-to-child HIV transmission. Compliance with medical therapy is a major problem in adolescent patients, with unstable living situation the most significant risk factor for poor adherence.

HUMAN PAPILLOMAVIRUS ANOGENITAL INFECTIONS

Genital HPV infection is probably the most prevalent STD in the United States. Adolescent females have almost a 50% risk of acquiring an HPV infection. Most HPV infections are transient. Repeat HPV tests become negative in most female adolescents within 24 months. However, HIV-infected patients are more likely to have persistent HPV infection.

Genital warts and cervical squamous intraepithelial lesions are clinical manifestations of HPV that are important to diagnose. Genital warts have already been discussed in this chapter.

The majority of cervical cancer is caused by persistent HPV infection. HPV may cause cytologic abnormalities on Pap smear. However, most abnormal Pap smears in adolescents are not associated with high-grade cervical dysplasia. Cervical cancer screening among adolescents should begin 3 years after the onset of vaginal intercourse or by age 21 years.

SYPHILIS

Syphilis is caused by the spirochete *T. pallidum.* Syphilis prevalence rates among adolescents are much lower than those of other STDs. Adolescent prevalence rates are highest among African Americans. Syphilis is more common in the southern United States than any other U.S. region. The disease is most readily transmitted during sexual contact by organisms living in open lesions of the genital and anal skin or mucosa. Organisms can also be transmitted by oral contact. After inoculation of *T. pallidum,* the incubation period averages 21 days, with a range of 10 to 90 days.

Primary syphilis begins with a papule which progresses to an ulcer over 1 to 3 weeks. More than one lesion can be present. The typical ulcer (chancre) can range in size from 2 to 20 mm. Unless it is secondarily infected, it has a clean base with rounded borders that feel rubbery to palpation. The ulcer is usually painless but can be tender to palpation. The ulcer heals gradually within a few weeks. Almost 50% of patients have bilateral, usually nontender, nonsuppurative, regional lymphadenopathy that can persist for months.

Secondary syphilis represents disseminated infection and develops 6 to 24 weeks after inoculation, or about 3 to 6 weeks after the appearance of a chancre. Multiple organ systems can be involved, including the skin, lymphatics, gastrointestinal tract, bones, kidneys, eyes, and central nervous system. Most patients have symptoms of fever, malaise, anorexia, weight loss, pharyngitis, laryngitis, arthralgia, and lymphadenopathy. Epitrochlear nodes are suggestive of syphilis. Most patients have a rash that manifests as macular, maculopapular, papular, papulosquamous, or, in rare cases, pustular lesions. Vesicles are not present. The lesions occur on the trunk at first and may be pruritic. Different types of lesions can occur simultaneously. Two thirds of patients have lesions on their palms and soles. Occasional patients may have a temporary patchy alopecia or loss of eyebrow hair. These closed skin lesions are relatively noninfectious but may persist for months. If a squamous component of the rash is present, it may resemble pityriasis rosea, psoriasis, or lichen planus.

Other types of mucocutaneous lesions are highly infective because they contain large numbers of spirochetes. The plaques of condylomata lata occur in warm, moist intertriginous locations, such as the vulva, scrotum, anal verge, inner thighs, and axillary folds. Mucous patches may occur in the mouth, pharynx, vulva, vagina, cervix, glans penis, and anal canal.

Asymptomatic involvement of the central nervous system can occur in 8% to 40% of untreated patients; cerebrospinal fluid (CSF) samples demonstrate elevated protein levels and lymphocyte counts. Symptoms of aseptic meningitis develop in only 1% to 2% of untreated patients. Anterior uveitis is rare. Other rare manifestations of secondary syphilis include glomerulonephritis, nephrotic syndrome, hepatitis, arthritis, and periostitis.

Latent syphilis infection lacks clinical manifestations. A latent infection is detected by serologic testing. Latent syphilis acquired within the preceding year is referred to as *early latent* syphilis. All other cases of latent syphilis are considered *late latent* syphilis or latent syphilis *of unknown duration.*

Identifying the organism from exudate or tissue through darkfield examination or direct fluorescent antibody tests makes the definitive diagnosis of primary or secondary syphilis. These techniques are technically difficult, and consultation with an STD specialist or the health department is recommended.

A presumptive syphilis diagnosis can be made by using a nontreponemal test (i.e., Venereal Disease Research Laboratory [VDRL] or rapid plasma reagin) *and* confirming positive results with a treponemal test (i.e., fluorescent treponemal antibody absorbed and *T. pallidum* particle agglutination). Nontreponemal test antibody titers are usually correlated with disease activity; treponemal test antibody titers are not. A fourfold change in a nontreponemal test titer (e.g., from 1:16 to 1:4) is considered necessary to demonstrate a clinically significant difference between the same two serologic nontreponemal test results. Treponemal test antibody titers usually are poorly correlated with disease and should not be used to assess treatment response. Nontreponemal test results usually become nonreactive sometime after treatment, whereas most reactive treponemal tests remain reactive throughout the life of the patient. Although rapid plasma reagin and VDRL are equally valid assays, quantitative results from the two tests cannot be compared. Therefore, providers should consistently use the same nontreponemal test for an individual patient. Providers should consult with an STD specialist or the health department for evaluation of neurosyphilis and for interpreting syphilis test results for an HIV-infected patient.

All patients diagnosed with syphilis should be tested for HIV infection. Syphilis-infected patients who have symptoms or signs suggesting neurologic disease should have an evaluation that includes a CSF analysis. Consultation with an infectious diseases specialist or the health department is recommended.

Syphilis during pregnancy places the fetus at risk for congenital syphilis. All pregnant females should be screened for syphilis. Pregnant females in populations in which syphilis is known to be a public health problem should be screened again during the third trimester and at delivery. Consultation with the health department is recommended for management and follow-up of pregnant patients diagnosed with syphilis.

Children diagnosed with syphilis after the newborn period should have birth and maternal records reviewed to assess whether the child has congenital or acquired disease. Acquired disease should be reported to child-protection services. In addition, a CSF examination to detect asymptomatic neurosyphilis should be performed.

All cases of syphilis should be reported to the health department to assist with follow-up and partner notification.

The treatment of all stages of syphilis is best achieved with parenteral penicillin G. Preparation and dosage depends on the disease stage and clinical manifestations. Table 29-31 shows CDC-recommended syphilis treatment regimens. Providers should consult with an STD specialist or the health department for managing treatment and follow-up for patients with a diagnosis of neurosyphilis and for HIV-infected patients with a diagnosis of syphilis.

Patients should be followed up at 6 and 12 months after treatment for clinical and laboratory evaluation. Patients should be retested with the same nontreponemal test used at diagnosis. Patients with persistent or recurrent signs or symptoms and those with a sustained fourfold increase in the nontreponemal test titer should be re-treated

Table 29-31. Treatment Regimens for Syphilis

Primary and Secondary Syphilis

Adults	Benzathine penicillin G, 2.4 million U IM in a single dose
Children*	Benzathine penicillin G, 50,000 U/kg IM, up to 2.4 million U, in a single dose
Penicillin allergy†	Doxycycline, 100 mg orally twice daily for 14 days *or* Tetracycline, 500 mg four times daily for 14 days

Early Latent Syphilis

Adults	Benzathine penicillin G, 2.4 million U IM in a single dose
Children*	Benzathine penicillin G, 50,000 U/kg IM, up to 2.4 million units in a single dose

Late Latent Syphilis or Latent Syphilis of Unknown Duration

Adults	Benzathine penicillin G, 7.2 million U total, administered as 3 doses of 2.4 million U IM each at 1-week intervals
Children*	Benzathine penicillin G, 50,000 U/kg IM, up to 2.4 million U administered as 3 doses at 1-week intervals

Adapted from Centers for Disease Control and Prevention: Sexually transmitted diseases treatment guidelines 2002. MMWR Morb Mortal Wkly Rep 2002;51:1-80.

*Children beyond the neonatal period.

†Some specialists recommend ceftriaxone, 1 g IV or IM daily for 8-10 days or azithromycin, 2 g orally in a single dose.

IM, intramuscularly.

and reevaluated for HIV infection. A CSF analysis should be performed in suspected cases of treatment failure.

COMPLICATIONS OF SEXUALLY TRANSMITTED DISEASES

PELVIC INFLAMMATORY DISEASE

PID is an acute clinical syndrome caused by microorganisms ascending from the lower female genital tract through the endometrium to the level of the fallopian tubes. It may involve contiguous structures, including the ovaries, pelvic peritoneum, and pelvic cavity. It involves endometritis, salpingitis, tuboovarian abscess, and pelvic peritonitis. It has a broad clinical spectrum that includes the following manifestations: acute, silent, atypical, a residual or chronic syndrome, and postpartum or postabortal occurrence. Unless a diagnostic procedure such as laparoscopy or ultrasonography is performed, it is difficult to enhance clinical specificity.

Adolescence is the age group with the highest rates of PID. Short-term complications include perihepatitis (Fitz-Hugh-Curtis syndrome, inflammation of the liver capsule) and tuboovarian abscess. Long-term consequences from tubal scarring and occlusion include infertility, ectopic pregnancy, and chronic pelvic pain.

Table 29-32. Diagnostic Criteria for Pelvic Inflammatory Disease

Minimum Criteria

Uterine or adnexal tenderness (unilateral or bilateral)
or
Cervical motion tenderness

Additional Criteria to Increase Specificity of Minimum Criteria

Abnormal cervical or vaginal mucopurulent discharge
Presence of WBCs on saline microscopy of vaginal secretions
Oral temperature > 38.3° C (101° F)
Elevated erythrocyte sedimentation rate or C-reactive protein
Laboratory evidence of *Neisseria gonorrhoeae* or *Chlamydia trachomatis* at cervix

Adapted from Centers for Disease Control and Prevention: Sexually transmitted diseases treatment guidelines 2002. MMWR Morb Mortal Wkly Rep 2002;51:1-80.

WBC, white blood cell.

PID is a polymicrobial infection. Sexually transmitted organisms, particularly *C. trachomatis* and *N. gonorrhoeae*, are often implicated. The altered vaginal flora that occurs with BV can often be found in the upper genital tract of women diagnosed with PID, which implicates BV as an important cofactor in the development of PID. In many PID cases, no pathogen is identified.

The diagnostic criteria and differential diagnosis of PID are presented in Tables 29-32 and 29-33. Most girls and women with PID have mucopurulent cervical discharge or evidence of white blood cells on a microscopic evaluation of a vaginal fluid saline preparation. If the cervical discharge appears normal and if there are no white blood cells noted on the wet preparation, PID is unlikely to be the disease, and alternative causes of pain should be sought.

When the diagnosis is suspected, the following laboratory studies improve the specificity of the diagnosis: saline wet preparation of vaginal fluid for evidence of inflammation, complete blood cell count with differential, erythrocyte sedimentation rate or C-reactive protein measurement, urinalysis, urine culture, and diagnostic tests for *N. gonorrhoeae* and *C. trachomatis*. An HIV antibody test should be offered, and counseling should be performed after the patient has clinically improved. A sensitive pregnancy test should be performed routinely in patients with suspected PID. This excludes the diagnosis of ectopic pregnancy and guides antibiotic treatment. Ultrasonography may be helpful if the diagnosis is in question, if ectopic pregnancy is a strong consideration, or if a tuboovarian abscess is considered.

Table 29-33. Differential Diagnosis for Pelvic Inflammatory Disease

Ectopic pregnancy
Ovarian cyst (with or without torsion)
Acute appendicitis
Endometriosis
Pyelonephritis
Septic or incomplete abortion
Pelvic thrombophlebitis
Functional pain
Psoas-pelvic abscess
Mesenteric adenitis
Pelvic adhesions
Chronic intestinal disease (e.g., inflammatory bowel disease)

Antibiotic treatment regimens for PID are generally empirical and must be broad in spectrum. All regimens should be effective against *N. gonorrhoeae* and *C. trachomatis,* even when endocervical tests are negative. Providing coverage against anaerobes and other gram-negative organisms is also important. Treatment should be initiated as soon as a presumptive diagnosis is made. Table 29-34 lists CDC-recommended antibiotic treatment regimens for PID. Addition of metronidazole or clindamycin to the oral doxycycline regimen improves anaerobic coverage at the risk of decreasing compliance.

PID is often treated in the outpatient setting. Indications for hospitalization include a diagnostic suspicion of a surgical emergency such as ovarian torsion or appendicitis, severe illness, pregnancy, tuboovarian abscess, or inability to tolerate or failure to respond to outpatient therapy. Adolescents with a diagnosis of PID, who are treated as outpatients, must be monitored with a repeat visit within 48 to 72 hours to ascertain adequate clinical improvement versus need for hospitalization.

EPIDIDYMITIS

Epididymitis is an unusual complication of sexually transmitted urethritis. Ascent of *N. gonorrhoeae* or *C. trachomatis* to the epididymis occurs in fewer than 1% of patients. Urethritis, often asymptomatic, usually accompanies sexually transmitted epididymitis. Epididymitis presents with an abrupt onset of unilateral testicular pain and edema (see Chapter 28). A hydrocele and palpable swelling of the testicle usually are present. Testicular torsion should be considered, and an expert should be consulted if the diagnosis is in question.

Table 29-35 lists the evaluation for epididymitis. Table 29-36 lists CDC-recommended treatment regimens. Treatment must begin at the time of presentation. Hospitalization should be considered when severe pain suggests other diagnoses, such as testicular torsion, when patients are febrile, or if patients may not comply with treatment.

Table 29-34. Treatment Regimens for Pelvic Inflammatory Disease

Parenteral Regimens (One of the Following)

Cefotetan, 2g IV q12h, *or* cefoxitin, 2 g IV q6h, *plus* doxycycline, 100 mg IV or PO q12h OR

Clindamycin, 900 mg IV q8h, *plus* gentamicin, loading dose (2 mg/kg body weight) IV or IM, followed by a maintenance dose (1.5 mg/kg) q8h

Parenteral therapy may be discontinued 24 hr after clinical improvement and continue

    Doxycycline, 100 mg PO b.i.d., *or* clindamycin, 450 mg orally q.i.d. continued for 14 days of total therapy

      For tuboovarian abscess, addition of either metronidazole, 500 mg PO b.i.d., *or* clindamycin, 450 mg PO q.i.d., to oral doxycycline provides better coverage against anaerobes

Outpatient Regimens (One of the Following)

Ofloxacin, 400 mg PO b.i.d., *or* levofloxacin, 500 mg PO q.d. for 14 days, *with or without* metronidazole, 500 mg PO b.i.d. for 14 days OR

Ceftriaxone, 250 mg IM in a single dose, *or* cefoxitin, 2 g IM, with probenecid, 1 g PO in a single dose once, *or* other parenteral third-generation cephalosporin (e.g., ceftizoxime or cefotaxime) *plus* doxycycline, 100 mg PO b.i.d. for 14 days, *with or without* metronidazole, 500 mg PO b.i.d. for 14 days

Adapted from Centers for Disease Control and Prevention: Sexually transmitted diseases treatment guidelines 2002. MMWR Morb Mortal Wkly Rep 2002;51:1-80.

IM, intramuscularly; IV, intravenously; PO, per os (orally).

Table 29-35. Diagnostic Evaluation for Epididymitis

Gram-stained smear of urethral exudate or intraurethral swab specimen for diagnosis of urethritis and for presumptive diagnosis of gonococcal infection

Diagnostic test for urethral *Neisseria gonorrhoeae* and *Chlamydia trachomatis* infection

Examination of first-void urine for leukocytes if the urethral Gram stain is negative or not available; culture and Gram-stained smear of uncentrifuged urine should be obtained

Syphilis serologic profile and HIV counseling and testing

Adapted from Centers for Disease Control and Prevention: Sexually transmitted diseases treatment guidelines 2002. MMWR Morb Mortal Wkly Rep 2002;51:1-80.

HIV, human immunodeficiency virus.

Bed rest, scrotal elevation, and nonsteroidal antiinflammatory agents afford symptomatic relief.

Patients treated as outpatients should be reevaluated in 3 days. If significant clinical improvement has not occurred, hospitalization and referral to a urologist may be indicated. Patients who have persistent tenderness and swelling after treatment should be evaluated for tuberculosis, fungal epididymitis, and neoplasm.

PREVENTION

Although most pediatric health care providers are not specifically trained to deliver effective STD prevention, providers can deliver the following services that can affect individual risks and patient population prevalence rates.

1. Explain to *all* adolescent patients and their parents the concept of confidential preventive services.
2. Confidentially ask *all* adolescent patients whether they are sexually active.
3. Confidentially screen *all* sexually active adolescents for STDs.
4. For patients with positive results of tests for an STD, facilitate partner notification and treatment if possible.
5. Provide information on STD-preventive behaviors, such as abstinence and correct and consistent condom use.
6. Closely monitor sexually active adolescents with STD screening and risk reduction counseling (i.e., repeat visits every 4 to 6 months instead of annually).

Table 29-36. Treatment Regimens for Epididymitis

One of the following:

For epididymitis most likely caused by gonoccocal or chlamydial infection:

    Ceftriaxone, 250 mg IM in a single dose, *plus* doxycycline, 100 mg orally twice daily for 10 days

For epididymitis most likely caused by enteric organism, or for patients who are allergic to cephalosporins and/or tetracyclines:

    Ofloxacin, 300 mg orally twice daily for 10 days*

    Levofloxacin, 500 mg orally once daily for 10 days*

Adapted from Centers for Disease Control and Prevention: Sexually transmitted diseases treatment guidelines 2002. MMWR Morb Mortal Wkly Rep 2002;51:1-80.

*Fluoroquinolones have not been recommended for persons younger than 18 years because they damage articular cartilage in juvenile animal models. Among children treated with fluoroquinolones, no joint damage attributable to therapy has been observed. Quinolones should not be used to treat possible gonorrhea infections acquired in Asia or the Pacific, including Hawaii, or California.

IM, intramuscularly.

Table 29-37. Red Flags and Things Not to Miss

Diagnosis of More than One Sexually Transmitted Disease in the Same Patient

If patient is diagnosed with syphilis, gonorrhea, or human immunodeficiency virus

If patient reports engaging in unprotected sex with multiple partners

If patient is immunocompromised

If patient has a history of sexually transmitted diseases

Abdominal Pain in an Adolescent Girl

Pelvic inflammatory disease
Tuboovarian abscess
Ectopic pregnancy
Appendicitis
Ovarian cyst (rupture or torsion)

Fever, Rash, Malaise, Arthalgia

Disseminated goncoccemia
Reactive arthritis
Human immunodeficiency virus infection

Rape

Pregnancy

Treatment of Partners

Asymptotic Cervicitis or Urethritis

7. Remain informed on state and federal minor consent laws regarding STD care.

In a busy pediatric clinical setting, effective HIV and STD prevention counseling presents a challenge. The CDC promotes delivering one or two brief (15- to 20-minute) "client-centered" HIV prevention counseling sessions. Providers help patients (1) identify the specific behaviors putting them at risk of acquiring or transmitting HIV and (2) commit to steps to reduce their HIV risk.

The provider should focus on the adolescent's personal risk or circumstances. A personalized risk assessment encourages the patient to identify, understand, and acknowledge his or her own behaviors and circumstances that put him or her at increased risk of acquiring STDs and HIV. The session should include an exploration of previous attempts to reduce risk and identification of successes and challenges in previous risk-reduction efforts. This in-depth risk assessment allows the provider to help the adolescent consider ways to reduce personal risk and commit to a single, explicit step to reduce risk. In the follow-up session, the provider asks the patient to describe the risk-reduction step attempted, acknowledges positive steps made, and helps the patient identify and commit to additional behaviors. The provider should also offer appropriate referrals, such as for substance abuse. By using this prevention model, providers can effectively help reduce their adolescent patients' high-risk sexual behaviors and prevent infection with new STDs.

RED FLAGS

Red flags are presented in Table 29-37.

REFERENCES

Introduction

Centers for Disease Control and Prevention: Youth risk behavior surveillance— United States, 2001. MMWR Morb Mortal Wkly Rep 2002;51(SS-4): 13-15. Available at: http://www.cdc.gov/mmwr/PDF/SS/ SS5104.pdf (accessed November 14, 2003).

History, Physical Examination, and Laboratory Testing

American Medical Association: AMA Guidelines for Adolescent Preventive Services (GAPS): Recommendations and Rationale. Baltimore, Williams & Wilkins, 1994.

Centers for Disease Control and Prevention: Revised guidelines for HIV counseling, testing, and referral. MMWR Morb Mortal Wkly Rep 2001;50:1-57.

Woods ER, Neinstein LS: Office visit, interview techniques, and recommendations to parents. In Neinstein LS (ed): Adolescent Health Care, 4th ed. Philadelphia, Lippincott Williams & Wilkins, 2002, pp 59-78.

Genital Ulcer Disease and Herpes Simples Virus

Centers for Disease Control and Prevention: Sexually transmitted diseases treatment guidelines 2002. MMWR Morb Mortal Wkly Rep 2002; 51(No. RR-6):12-78.

Corey L, Handsfield HH: Genital herpes and public health. JAMA 2000; 228:791-794.

Corey L, Wald A: Genital herpes. In Holmes KK, Sparling PF, March PA, et al (eds): Sexually Transmitted Diseases, 3rd ed. New York, McGraw-Hill, 1999, pp 285-334.

Fleming DT, McQuillan GM, Johnson RE, et al: Herpes simplex virus type 2 in the United States, 1976 to 1994. N Engl J Med 1997;337:1105-1111.

Langenberg AGM, Corey L, Ashley RL, et al: A prospective study of new infections with herpes simplex virus type 1 and type 2. N Engl J Med 1999;341:1432-1438.

Wald A, Zeh J, Selke S, et al: Virologic characteristics of subclinical and symptomatic genital herpes infections. N Engl J Med 1995;333:770-775.

Wald A, Zeh J, Selke S, et al: Reactivation of genital herpes simplex virus type 2 infection in asymptomatic seropositive persons. N Engl J Med 2000;342:844-850.

Genital Warts and Human Papillomavirus

Cain JM, Howett MK: Preventing cervical cancer. Science 2000;288: 1753-1754.

Centers for Disease Control and Prevention: Sexually transmitted diseases treatment guidelines 2002. MMWR Morb Mortal Wkly Rep 2002;51: 53-59.

Ho GYF, Bierman R, Beardsley L, et al: Natural history of cervicovaginal papillomavirus infection in young women. N Engl J Med 1998;338: 423-428.

Koutsky LA, Kiviat NB: Genital human papillomavirus. In Holmes KK, Sparling PF, March PA, et al (eds): Sexually Transmitted Diseases, 3rd ed. New York, McGraw-Hill, 1999, pp 347-360.

Moscicki AB, Ellenberg JH, Vermund SH, et al: Prevalence of and risks for cervical human papillomavirus infection and squamous intraepithelial lesions in adolescent girls. Arch Pediatr Adolesc Med 2000;154:127-134.

Moscicki AB, Hills N, Shiboski S, et al: Risks for incident human papillomavirus infection and low-grade squamous intraepithelial lesion development in young females. JAMA 2001;285:2995-3002.

Saslaw D, Runowica CD, Solomom D, et al: American Cancer Society guidelines for the early detection of cervical neoplasia and cancer. CA Cancer J Clin 2002;52:342-362.

Sawaya GF, Brown AD, Washington AE, Garber AM: Current approaches to cervical-cancer screening. N Engl J Med 2001;344:1603-1607.

Cervicitis, Uethritis, Vaginitis, and Upper Genital Tract Diseases

Burstein GR, Romaplo AM: Chlamydia. In MB Goldman, MC Hatch (eds): Women and Health. San Diego, Calif, Academic Press, 1999, pp 273-284.

Burstein GR, Zenilman JM: Non-gonococcal urethritis—A new paradigm. Clin Infect Dis 1999;(Suppl 1):S66-S73.

Centers for Disease Control and Prevention: Sexually transmitted diseases treatment guidelines 2002. MMWR Morb Mortal Wkly Rep 2002;51:3053.

Centers for Disease Control and Prevention: Take action on HEDIS. Available at: *http://www.cdc.gov/nchstp/dstd/Reports_Publications/ HMOletter.pdf* (accessed September 15, 2003)

Chacko MR, Woods CR Jr: Gynecologic infections in childhood and adolescence. In Feigin RD, Cherry JD (eds): Textbook of Pediatric Infectious Diseases, vol 1, 4th ed. Philadelphia: WB Saunders, 1998, pp 509-548.

Holmes KK, Stamm WE: Lower genital tract infections in women. In Holmes KK, Sparling PF, March PA, et al (eds): Sexually Transmitted Diseases, 3rd ed. New York, McGraw-Hill, 1999, pp 761-782.

Hook EW III, Handsfield HH: Gonococcal infections in the adult. In Holmes KK, Sparling PF, March PA, et al (eds): Sexually Transmitted Diseases, 3rd ed. New York, McGraw-Hill, 1999, pp 451-466.

Kamb ML, Newman K, Peterman TA, et al: Most bacterial STDs are asymptomatic [abstract 022]. Oral presentation at Sexually Transmitted Infections at the Millennium Conference, Baltimore, May 2000.

Scholes D, Stergachis A, Heidrich FE, et al: Prevention of pelvic inflammatory disease by screening for cervical chlamydial infection. N Engl J Med 1996;334:1362-1366.

Westrom L, Eschenbach D: Pelvic inflammatory disease. In Holmes KK, Sparling PF, March PA, et al (eds): Sexually Transmitted Diseases, 3rd ed. New York, McGraw-Hill, 1999, pp 783-810.

Sexual Assault

American Academy of Pediatrics, Committee on Adolescence: Care of the adolescent sexual assault victim. Pediatrics 2001;107:1476-1479.

American Academy of Pediatrics, Committee on Child Abuse and Neglect: Guidelines for the evaluation of sexual abuse of children: Subject review (RE9819). Pediatrics 1999;103:186-191. Corection published in Pediatrics 1999;103:1049.

Centers for Disease Control and Prevention: Sexually transmitted diseases treatment guidelines 2002. MMWR Morb Mortal Wkly Rep 2002; 51(RR-6):69-74.

Hammerschlag MR: Use of nucleic acid amplification tests in investigating child sexual abuse. Sex Transm Infect 2001;77:153-154.

Human Immunodeficiency Virus and Prevention

American Academy of Pediatrics, Committee on Pediatric AIDS and Committee on Adolescence: Adolescents and human immunodeficiency virus infection: The role of the pediatrician in prevention and intervention. Pediatrics 2001;107:188-190.

Centers for Disease Control and Prevention: Revised guidelines for HIV counseling, testing, and referral. MMWR Morb Mortal Wkly Rep 2001; 50(RR-19):1-57.

30 Menstrual Problems and Vaginal Bleeding

Marjorie Greenfield

Abnormal vaginal bleeding (Table 30-1) is a common problem reported by adolescents. The severity can range from a minor inconvenience to a medical emergency. Ninety-five percent of abnormal bleeding in adolescents is dysfunctional uterine bleeding (DUB). The term *dysfunctional* denotes abnormal bleeding without discernible pelvic disease; such bleeding is usually caused by a hormonal abnormality. The history, physical examination, and possibly a few blood tests should rule out most other causes of bleeding and allow appropriate management of DUB.

THE OVULATORY MENSTRUAL CYCLE

HYPOTHALAMUS

Gonadotropin-releasing hormone (GnRH), a decapeptide secreted in pulses from the hypothalamus, is transported down a portal system to the pituitary gland. The pulsatile secretion of GnRH from the hypothalamus allows secretion of follicle-stimulating hormone (FSH) and luteinizing hormone (LH) but has only a permissive effect and is not involved in regulation of their blood levels. Factors that interfere with hypothalamic function can reduce production of FSH and LH.

PITUITARY

Pituitary gland production of FSH and LH responds to negative feedback of circulating estrogen. There is also a positive feedback mechanism that increases LH production when estrogen levels rise sharply in the midcycle, producing the "LH surge" (Fig. 30-1). In adolescents, the positive feedback mechanism and LH surge are the last parts of the system to mature.

OVARY

Follicular Phase

The ovary controls the menstrual cycle. When estrogen and progesterone levels decline and a menstrual period begins, the pituitary gland, released from negative feedback inhibition, secretes FSH, stimulating the development of new ovarian follicles. As the dominant follicle emerges, it produces large amounts of estrogen. This rapid rise in estrogen leads to the LH surge; the LH surge triggers ovulation. Estrogen levels do not rise to the level that triggers positive feedback until the follicle is ready for ovulation; the follicle itself controls the timing of ovulation.

Luteal Phase

After ovulation, the follicle becomes a corpus luteum, a factory for progesterone synthesis. After 14 days, if conception has not occurred, the corpus luteum ceases its function, estrogen and progesterone levels decline, and menstruation begins as a result of

withdrawal of hormonal support to the endometrial lining. If pregnancy were to occur, human chorionic gonadotropin (hCG) from the conceptus would stimulate the corpus luteum to continue producing progesterone.

ENDOMETRIUM

Histologic Changes through the Cycle

The sequence of hormonal changes during the menstrual cycle leads to a synchronous response of the endometrium. Estrogen, in the first half of the cycle, causes the *proliferative phase,* characterized by endometrial growth and thickening. Progesterone, in the second half of the cycle, causes the *secretory phase,* creating glandular differentiation in the estrogenized endometrium, readying it for implantation of a conceptus.

Normal Control of Menstrual Bleeding

Menstruation occurs when a sequence of hormonally determined events in the endometrium leads to an organized sloughing of the endometrial surface. As estrogen and progesterone levels decline, the spiral arterioles undergo spasms in rhythmic waves, and the surface of the endometrium becomes ischemic. As the surface weakens, it loses its integrity, allowing menstrual blood to escape. Thrombin and platelet plugs limit blood loss (see Chapter 50). The superficial endometrium collapses and is shed. Menstrual flow stops as a result of synchronized vasoconstriction, tissue collapse, vascular stasis (clotting of blood in exposed vessels), and estrogen-induced "healing." The self-limited character of menstrual bleeding depends on adequate clotting mechanisms and normal ovulatory hormonal events. This becomes important in the attempt to understand causes of abnormal menstrual bleeding.

UTERINE BLEEDING IN THE ADOLESCENT

NORMAL ADOLESCENT CYCLES

Normal adolescent menstrual cycles are not necessarily the same as normal ovulatory adult cycles (see Table 30-1). Among girls aged 13 to 16 who were evaluated by serial serum progesterone levels, only 33% of cycles were ovulatory in girls who had been menstruating for less than 1½ years. Even 5 years after menarche, only 80% of the cycles were ovulatory. This anovulatory state is believed to result from immaturity of the hypothalamic-pituitary-ovarian (HPO) axis; the positive feedback mechanism for the LH surge is not consistently functional. Anovulatory cycles are, therefore, the norm for young adolescents.

The normal cycle in a teenager is light to moderate bleeding lasting 2 to 8 days every 21 to 40 days. The best explanation for the cyclicity of bleeding in normal but anovulatory adolescents is that although the positive feedback mechanism of ovulation is not

Table 30-1. Normal and Abnormal Menses

Normal cycle (adolescent): bleeding every 21-45 days for 2-8 days

Normal cycle (adult, ovulatory): bleeding every 24-35 days for 3-7 days

Menorrhagia: prolonged or excessive regular periods

Menometrorrhagia: heavy, irregular periods

Oligomenorrhea: infrequent periods

Intermenstrual bleeding: bleeding between regular menstrual periods

Dysfunctional uterine bleeding: abnormal uterine bleeding not caused by local uterine pathology; cause usually hormonal

developed, there is negative feedback of estrogen on pituitary FSH. As estrogen levels rise, FSH decreases, causing the ovarian follicles to stop producing estrogen. The withdrawal of hormonal support causes the endometrium to slough, an "estrogen withdrawal bleed." As the inhibition on the pituitary gland is released, FSH increases and the ovarian production of estrogen resumes. This allows for regular "menses" in the anovulatory adolescent. The bleeding is not quite as controlled and consistent as the cycles of estrogen-progesterone withdrawal bleeding in an ovulatory woman, but the decline in estrogen levels is effective at decreasing the thickness of the uterine lining enough so that bleeding is not excessive. This pattern, interspersed with occasional ovulatory cycles, appears to control bleeding adequately in most teenage girls.

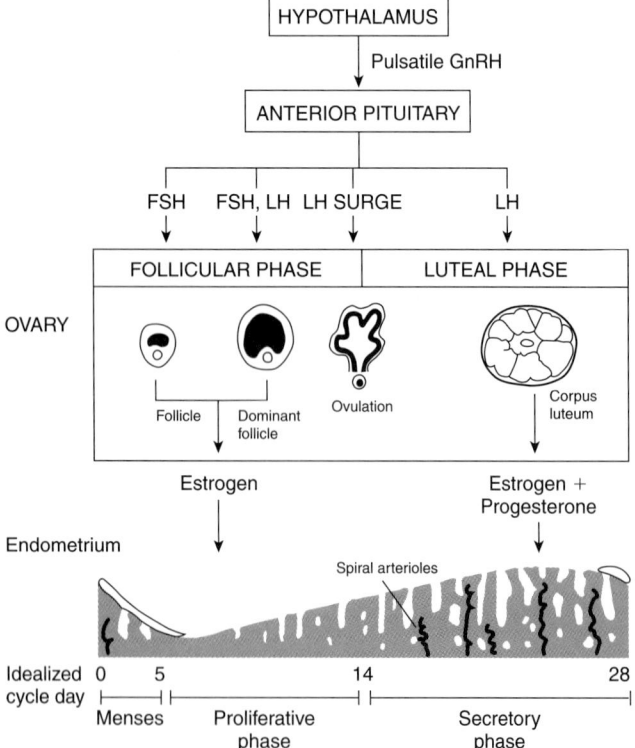

Figure 30-1. Hypothalamic-pituitary-ovarian endometrial axis: changes over time. FSH, follicle-stimulating hormone; GnRH, gonadotropin-releasing hormone; LH, luteinizing hormone. (Adapted from Nesse R: Managing abnormal vaginal bleeding. Postgrad Med 1991;89:207.)

ABNORMAL ADOLESCENT MENSTRUAL CYCLES: DYSFUNCTIONAL UTERINE BLEEDING

Problems develop when the *negative* feedback does not occur and estrogen levels stay constant. Because hormone levels do not decline to allow a withdrawal bleed, a normal cyclic menstrual pattern is not seen. Constant levels of circulating estrogen stimulate the uterine lining to become abnormally thick and unstable. As dyssynchronous breakdown in the endometrial structure occurs, bleeding can be heavy and unpredictable, lasting days to months and leading to hemodynamic instability and anemia. This classic description of severe DUB may or may not be superimposed on a pattern of oligomenorrhea or amenorrhea.

DEVELOPING A DIFFERENTIAL DIAGNOSIS

DUB, manifesting as heavy irregular menses, is the most common type of abnormal vaginal bleeding in teenagers. Other patterns of bleeding suggest other diagnoses (Table 30-2). Normal menses followed by intermenstrual bleeding may indicate a structural process, such as endometrial polyps or cervicitis, in which the hormonal environment does not control the bleeding. Normal menses with bleeding after intercourse can be from a vaginal or cervical lesion. Dark, possibly foul-smelling blood after the normal menstrual period suggests an obstructed uterine horn or hemivagina with slow leaking of sequestered blood through a fistulous tract. A detailed menstrual history can give clues to the diagnosis.

In addition to the menstrual history, a sexual history, a medical history, a review of systems, a pelvic examination with a Papanicolaou (Pap) smear, and a urine pregnancy test are necessary to identify the site and cause of bleeding (Figs. 30-2 to 30-5). Additional testing is determined by the emerging differential diagnosis (Table 30-3).

COMMON CAUSES OF ABNORMAL UTERINE BLEEDING

Anovulation

In contrast to the cyclical changes in estrogen levels seen with "normal" anovulatory cycles in teenagers, problematic bleeding is a result of chronic anovulation associated with a steady state of estrogen, FSH, and LH. Constant levels of estrogen provide constant stimulation of endometrial growth and can lead to hemorrhage, anemia, infertility, and endometrial cancer. As few as 50% of patients revert to regular cycles by 4 years after presentation.

Coagulopathy

Of nonpregnant adolescent girls admitted to the hospital for menorrhagia, as many as 19% have a coagulopathy. As the severity of the menorrhagia increases, coagulation problems are more likely to be present. Severe iron deficiency anemia, requirement for transfusion, and hemorrhage at first menses each confers an even greater chance of finding a coagulopathy.

Idiopathic thrombocytopenia purpura, von Willebrand disease, and, less often, thrombocytopenia caused by systemic disease, such as leukemia or systemic lupus erythematosus, can manifest with menorrhagia (see Chapter 50). Screening for coagulopathy with a platelet count, prothrombin time, and activated partial thromboplastin time, plus von Willebrand disease screening with ristocetin cofactor/von Willebrand factor activity test, von Willebrand factor antigen test, and factor VIII clotting activity assay, is usually adequate. If coagulopathy is still strongly suspected, consultation with a hematologist may be necessary to rule out the rare coagulopathies that are not detectable with these initial tests.

Table 30-2. Differential Diagnosis of Abnormal Vaginal Bleeding in Adolescents

	Bleeding Pattern			Evaluation	
	MR	*MMR*	*IB*	Suggestive Finding; *Diagnostic Finding*	Treatment
Source: Uterus				**Common Causes**	
Anovulation	+	+		No extrauterine source of bleeding seen on examination *Responds appropriately to treatment*	See Table 30-5
Coagulopathy	+			More commonly found in cases of severe bleeding especially if onset at menarche; family history, ROS suggestive of clotting disorder; ecchymoses, petechiae may be seen on examination *Abnormal PT, PTT, platelet count, bleeding time, or test for von Willebrand disease*	Treat coagulopathy; oral contraceptives may help with menorrhagia; complete menstrual suppression sometimes required See also Chapter 50
Complication of pregnancy		+		History of late period; pregnancy symptoms (nausea, breast tenderness) *Positive urine or blood pregnancy test*	See Figure 30-6
Source: Vagina				**Uncommon Causes**	
Injury			+	History *Visible laceration*	Surgical or topical hemostasis; suture or allow to heal by secondary intention
Foreign body (e.g., retained tampon or contraceptive sponge)			+	History, foul discharge *Visible foreign body*	Removal
Cancer			+ +	Lesion seen, ± abnormal cytologic findings *Biopsy*	Referral to specialist; therapy chosen per type and stage of tumor
Source: Cervix				**Less Common Causes**	
Neoplasia					
Dysplasia/carcinoma			+	Bleeding point on cervix; abnormal cytology *Colposcopy with directed biopsies*	LEEP, laser, cryotherapy, or cone biopsy
Cervical polyp			+	*Polyp seen*	Grasp with clamp or ring forceps and twirl off polyp in office; send specimen to pathologist
Hemangioma			+	Lesion seen	Conservative versus excision or ablation
Infection (cervicitis) (see Chapter 29)					
Herpes			+	Cervical vesicles ± ulceration, ± pelvic pain, tenderness; Pap smear sometimes shows multinucleated giant cells *Culture positive for herpes*	If primary infection, consider oral famcyclovir, 250 mg b.i.d. × 7-10 days
Human papillomavirus (HPV)			+	Flat or raised warts seen on cervix *Pap smear + colposcopy necessary to differentiate from dysplasia; HPV typing may determine risk of cancer*	Laser, LEEP, cryotherapy, trichloroacetic acid or 5-fluorouracil cream after Pap smear and colposcopy; treat for dysplasia or symptoms
Trichomonas			+	Friable inflamed cervix; yellow-green vaginal discharge, pH 7-8 *Saline preparation: motile flagellates*	Metronidazole, 2 g orally once each for patient and sexual partners
Source: Uterus				**Less Common Causes**	
Neoplasia					
Fibroid	±		±	± Enlarged uterus on examination; palpable fibroids *Abnormal findings on ultrasound, and/or hysteroscopy*	NSAID sometimes helpful for menorrhagia; myomectomy via hysteroscope, laparoscope, or laparotomy may be needed
Endometrial polyps			+	History of spotting superimposed on normal menstrual cycle *Hysteroscopy, saline sonogram, and/or D&C*	D&C or hysteroscopic excision
Malignant uterine tumor		±	±	Abnormal Pap smear, enlarged uterus, tissue at cervical os. *Biopsy*	Surgery determined by type of tumor and stage

Continued

Table 30-2. Differential Diagnosis of Abnormal Vaginal Bleeding in Adolescents—cont'd

	Bleeding Pattern			Evaluation	Treatment
	MR	*MMR*	*IB*	**Suggestive Finding;** *Diagnostic Finding*	**Treatment**
Source: Uterus				**Less Common Causes**	
Ovarian tumor producing estrogen (bleeding is uterine)		+		Adnexal mass on examination or ultrasonography *Surgical diagnosis and staging*	Surgery
Foreign body					
IUD	+		+	No other cause of bleeding (patient ovulatory, not pregnant, no PID) *IUD in uterus; responds to therapy*	NSAID sometimes useful for menorrhagia; removal if PID coexists or if necessary to control bleeding
Infection					
PID	+		+	Tender uterus and adnexae; purulent cervical discharge ± ↑ WBC count, ESR, or fever *Clinical diagnosis, tests often positive for gonorrhea, chlamydia*	CDC guidelines (see Chapter 29)
Postpartum or postabortal endometritis ± retained products of conception			+	± ↑ WBC count, ESR, fever *Recent pregnancy; tender uterus*	D&C if retained tissue seen on sonogram; broad-spectrum antibiotics, methergine
Congenital partially obstructed hemivagina or uterine horn			+	Foul, dark blood after menses *Abnormal pelvic examination and/or pelvic ultrasonography*	Refer for surgical treatment

CDC, Centers for Disease Control and Prevention; D&C, dilation and curettage; ESR, erythrocyte sedimentation rate; IB, intermenstrual bleeding, IUD, intrauterine device; LEEP, loop electroexcisional procedure; MMR, menometrorrhagia; MR, menorrhagia; NSAID, nonsteroidal anti-inflammatory drug; Pap, Papanicolaou; PID, pelvic inflammatory disease; PT, prothrombin time; PTT, partial thromboplastin time; ROS, review of systems; WBC, white blood cell.

Bleeding and Hormonal Contraceptives

Abnormal bleeding during the first few months of low-dose oral contraceptive use is common and can be managed with reassurance if pregnancy is not suspected. Bleeding usually normalizes within three to four cycles. Prolonged use of combination estrogen-progesterone oral contraceptives, skin patches, vaginal rings, progestin-only oral contraceptives (mini-pill), and injectable or implantable progestin contraceptives may lead to deciduation and atrophy of the endometrium. This thin uterine lining may bleed unpredictably. Endometrial atrophy is best treated with supplemental estrogen, which thickens and stabilizes the uterine lining. For girls with normal pelvic examination findings and a negative pregnancy test, conjugated equine estrogens (e.g., Premarin), 1.25 mg, or estradiol, 2 mg taken daily with the oral contraceptive for 7 days, should regulate bleeding for many cycles afterward. This regimen may need to be repeated if the problem recurs. Doubling up on the birth control pill or giving the next dose of injectable contraceptive early does not diminish the bleeding, because this provides a progestin-dominant stimulus to an already atrophic endometrium. If estrogen supplementation is not successful, other causes of bleeding should be considered. Many girls have some breakthrough bleeding if they are late in taking a pill, especially in long-term pill users. Reminding the patient of the need to take pills consistently can help to prevent breakthrough bleeding.

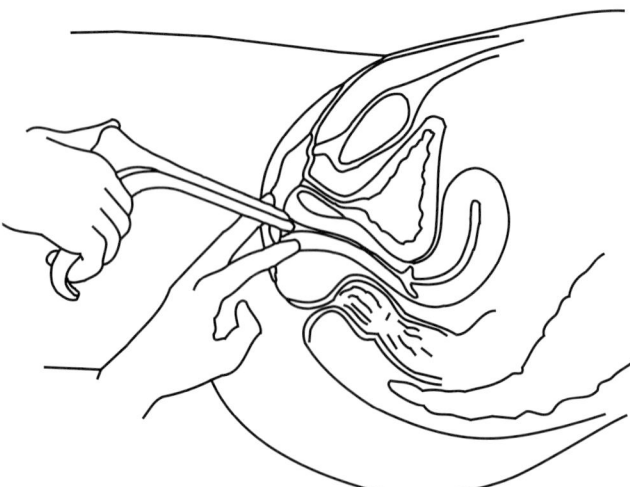

Figure 30-2. Sagittal section of the speculum examination. The Huffman (narrow Pederson) vaginal speculum is essential for examining adolescents. With blades 1.5 cm wide and 11 cm long, it is narrow enough to be tolerated by a virginal adolescent and also deep enough to reach the cervix. With one hand (usually the non-dominant hand), the examiner separates the patient's labia minora and visualizes the introitus. The speculum is then inserted at an oblique angle. (From Swartz MH: *Textbook of Physical Diagnosis: History and Examination,* 2nd ed. Philadelphia, WB Saunders, 1994, p 380.)

Illness and Medication

Medications and illnesses that cause abnormal uterine bleeding do so by their effects on coagulation or on the hormonal milieu (Table 30-4).

Chronic illnesses such as diabetes, cystic fibrosis, and sickle cell anemia can lead to anovulation. This chronic anovulation confers the short-term and long-term risks of unopposed estrogen exposure. If the patient's medical condition cannot be improved, cyclic progestins or oral contraceptives should be considered if there are no contraindications (Table 30-5).

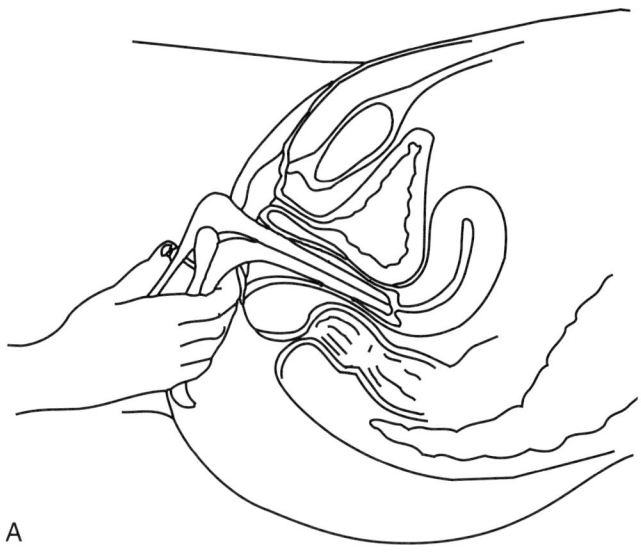

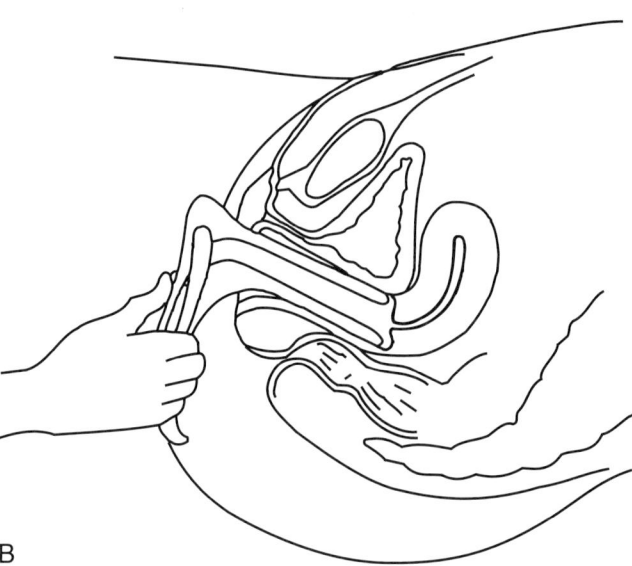

Figure 30-3. Sagittal-section illustrating the position of the speculum during inspection of the cervix. The examiner fully inserts the speculum before opening the blades. **A,** The angle of insertion is about 45 degrees to the examining table. As the blades are opened, the speculum is carefully maneuvered so that the cervix is fully seen. **B,** The thumb lever is then locked in place. (From Swartz MH: Textbook of Physical Diagnosis: History and Examination, 2nd ed. Philadelphia, WB Saunders, 1994, p 381.)

Pregnancy Complications

Pregnancy can manifest with abnormal bleeding that may or may not be preceded by an episode of amenorrhea. Particularly abnormal pregnancies, such as ectopic pregnancies or those about to end in miscarriage, may manifest with abnormal bleeding without a "missed period." The urinary hCG pregnancy tests in use today are positive in more than 98% of patients with ectopic pregnancies. Highly diluted urine may yield false-negative results. A negative serum hCG level essentially rules out the possibility that abnormal bleeding is caused by a complication of pregnancy (Fig. 30-6).

MANAGEMENT OF ABNORMAL BLEEDING
(see Table 30-5)

ACUTE MANAGEMENT

Treatment and evaluation of severe abnormal bleeding are usually begun simultaneously. The urine pregnancy test can be used to triage the patient; a negative blood hCG level effectively rules out pregnancy. Hemodynamic stability is assessed, and replacement of blood and fluids is used as needed. It is important to complete relevant blood work (complete blood cell count, prothrombin time, activated partial thromboplastin time, and, if possible, von Willebrand screening) before a blood transfusion is started. Most patients with bleeding severe enough to require hospitalization are anovulatory. Although both estrogens and progestins have been used to stop acute anovulatory bleeding, few studies are available to compare their effectiveness (Table 30-6). If the acute bleeding is caused by a coagulopathy, the underlying problem (see Chapter 50) should be addressed, although hormonal protocols for management of the vaginal bleeding can be employed simultaneously and are often successful.

LONG-TERM FOLLOW-UP AND PREVENTION OF RECURRENCE

Once the initial bleeding is controlled, or if the patient with moderate/severe bleeding is not actively bleeding at presentation, therapeutic goals include prophylaxis against recurrence, prevention of the long-term sequelae of unopposed estrogen stimulation to the endometrium, and treatment of anemia. Although the underlying cause of chronic anovulation may not be found, a basic workup should be performed (see section on amenorrhea).

To prevent recurrence of bleeding, cyclic progestins or oral contraceptives should be used for 3 to 6 months. They decrease the thickness of the uterine lining and allow for orderly estrogen-progestin withdrawal bleeds. Because the uterine lining is usually quite thick at the onset of treatment, the first progestin withdrawal period may be quite severe but should not last longer than 1 week. This must be explained to the patient so that the heaviness of the next period is not viewed as failure of treatment. As the endometrial height diminishes with each succeeding menstrual period, bleeding should become lighter.

For the teenager who does not need contraception, it is acceptable to discontinue treatment after 3 to 6 months and observe the patient for development of ovulatory cycles. Of girls who have severe DUB, 50% will have long-term problems with chronic anovulation and its associated risks of recurrent hemorrhage and uterine cancer. Therefore, a few months after treatment is stopped, the clinician should review the patient's menstrual calendar and document ovulation. Prospective documentation of premenstrual symptoms (breast tenderness), a luteal phase serum progesterone level, or a basal body temperature chart is adequate for documenting ovulation (Table 30-7). If the patient remains anovulatory, cyclic progestin or oral contraceptive treatment should be reinstituted to prevent recurrent abnormal bleeding and to diminish the long-term risk of endometrial carcinoma.

For the adolescent who needs contraception, it is best to continue oral contraceptives or equivalent treatment with skin patches or vaginal ring. There is no evidence that even long-term oral contraceptive use has any effect on the menstrual cycle within 1 year of discontinuance. Those who are anovulatory before using oral contraceptives, however, may continue to be anovulatory after the pills are stopped.

Failure of anovulatory bleeding to respond to hormonal treatment is an indication to reevaluate the patient.

AMENORRHEA

Amenorrhea or absence of menstrual periods is a symptom, not a diagnosis. Causes can be grouped into two categories: (1) end-organ

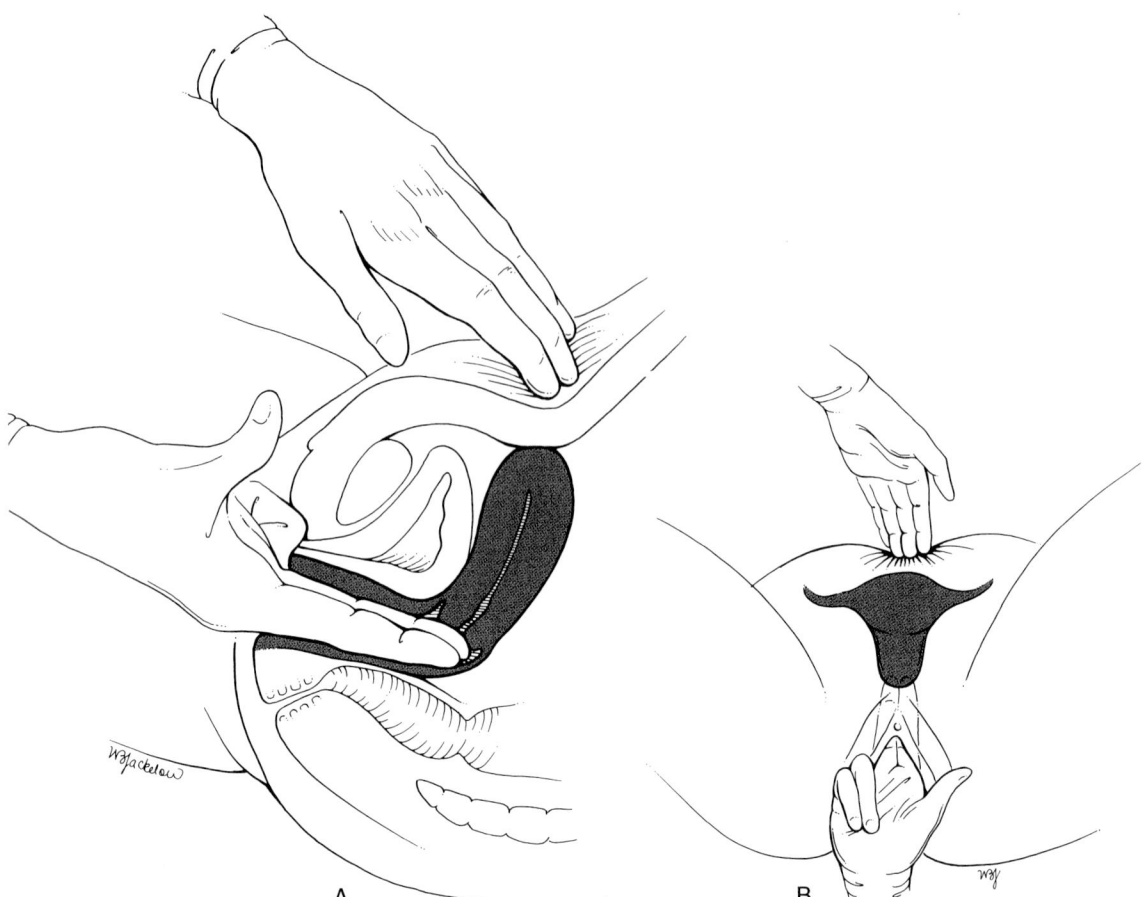

Figure 30-4. The bimanual examination. Palpation of the uterus is performed with one or two fingers of the examiner's dominant hand inside the patient's vagina and with the examiner's other hand on the patient's lower abdomen. As the uterus is trapped between the examining hands, pressure with the abdominal hand causes the cervix to move against the inside finger or fingers, giving the examiner an appreciation of the uterine size, shape, configuration, mobility, and tenderness. An empty bladder facilitates the examination. By pressing the vaginal examining finger or fingers into the lateral fornix anteriorly, superiorly, and laterally and pressing on the patient's abdomen so that the vaginal and abdominal fingers try to appose, the examiner can palpate the adnexal structures as they move between the examining hands. This provides an appreciation of adnexal size, shape, mobility, and tenderness. A rectoabdominal examination may also be used to assess the uterus or adnexa if a vaginal examination is not tolerated. **A,** Sagittal section through the pelvic organs. **B,** Position of the uterus between the examining hands. (From Swartz MH: Textbook of Physical Diagnosis: History and Examination, 2nd ed. Philadelphia, WB Saunders, 1994, p 385.)

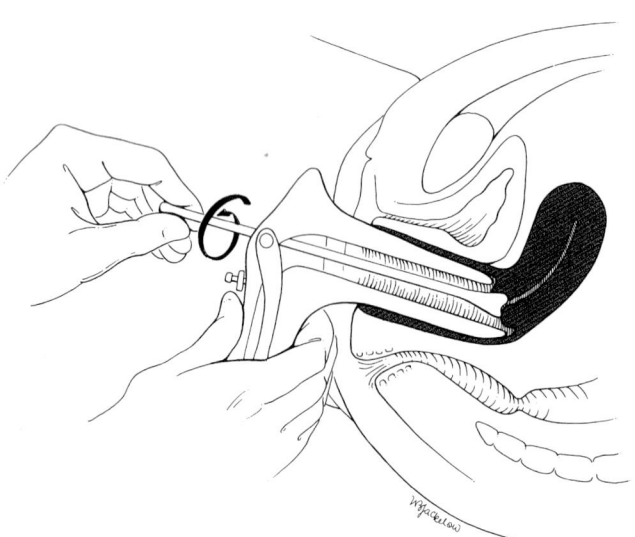

Figure 30-5. Obtaining smear for the Papanicolaou test. The endocervical brush and the longer end of the spatula are placed in the cervical os and rotated for cell collection. (From Swartz MH: Textbook of Physical Diagnosis: History and Examination, 2nd ed. Philadelphia, WB Saunders, 1994, p 383.)

or outflow tract anomalies and (2) inadequate hormonal stimulation to the endometrium.

Primary amenorrhea is traditionally defined as no menstrual period by age 16 years or no menses in the absence of breast development by age 13 years. Age 14.5 years is the 95th percentile for menarche. Secondary amenorrhea denotes 3 to 6 months without menstrual bleeding in a previously menstruating girl or woman, although shortly after menarche, 12 to 18 months without periods may be normal. The evaluation of amenorrhea is driven by the patient's needs and concerns, not necessarily by definitions. A 16-year-old with 8 weeks of amenorrhea may need a pregnancy test. A 10-year-old with stigmata of Turner syndrome need not wait until age 13 for an evaluation of amenorrhea.

Certain processes, such as imperforate hymen or müllerian agenesis (absence of the uterus and proximal vagina) can cause only primary amenorrhea. Other processes can cause amenorrhea at any time, depending on when the disease occurs. Anorexia nervosa, if it develops before menarche, can cause primary amenorrhea with or without pubertal delay. If anorexia develops later, it may cause secondary amenorrhea.

Congenital anatomic conditions that cause only primary amenorrhea are suspected from the initial history and physical examination findings. Once these few specific diagnoses are ruled out, primary and secondary amenorrhea are evaluated similarly.

Table 30-3. Diagnostic Approach to Abnormal Uterine Bleeding in Adolescence

Evaluation Method	Comments	When Needed
History		
Menstrual	Last menstrual period, pattern of cycles, recent change, molimina (i.e., premenstrual symptoms), dysmenorrhea	Always
Medical	Pelvic pain, fever, vaginal discharge, coagulopathy, endocrine problems, major illness	Always
Sexual	History of sexual intercourse (including most recent date), birth control used, history of abnormal Pap smear or sexually transmitted infection	Always
Social	Stress, eating disorder, exercise, drugs, alcohol abuse, domestic violence	Always
Medications	Anticoagulants, hormones, drugs with endocrine or coagulation effects	Always
Family history	Clotting disorders, endocrinopathies	Always
Physical Examination		
General	Weight Body habitus, hirsutism, Tanner stage Stigmata of endocrine or coagulation disorders Signs of trauma	Always
Pelvic	To assess source of bleeding and possible cause	Always
External genitalia, vagina, cervix	Cervix and vaginal walls can usually be visualized even with a Huffman (narrow Pederson) speculum, even in a young virginal adolescent	
Uterus, adnexa	By rectoabdominal examination if bimanual examination not tolerated	
Rectovaginal or rectoabdominal		
Tests		
Pregnancy test	If urine test results are negative and suspicion is high, check serum hCG	Always, if sexual contact is a possibility
Hemoglobin or hematocrit	With or without retic count, iron studies, ferritin	If bleeding is heavy or objective quantification is desired*
Clotting studies	Platelet count, PT, PTT, bleeding time, vWF testing	In menorrhagia at first period, severe bleeding, family history or personal history of coagulopathy and menorrhagia or failure to respond to treatment
Blood type and screen	Treat Rh-negative teenagers who miscarry with RhoGAM	If pregnant or hemodynamically compromised
Gonorrhea and chlamydial probes	Specimen can be obtained during examination; discarded if results rule out suspicion of infection	If any chance of sexually transmitted infection
Pelvic ultrasonography		If bimanual examination results are abnormal or if there is suspicion of congenital anomaly
Hysteroscopy/endometrial sampling		If bleeding is superimposed on normal ovulatory cycles *and* no extrauterine bleeding site is apparent; or if bleeding does not respond to hormonal therapy and coagulation studies and pregnancy test are negative
Heme in urine, heme in stool		If bleeding site is not apparent

*Patient's assessment of menstrual blood loss is notoriously inaccurate. Even pad counts can vary tremendously among women with similar blood loss, although six to eight pads or tampons per day is considered the upper limit of normal. Hematologic parameters can be objective measures of severity of bleeding.

hCG, human chorionic gonadotropin; Pap, Papanicolaou; PT, prothrombin time; PTT, partial thromboplastin time; vWF, von Willebrand factor.

OVERVIEW OF PROCESSES THAT LEAD TO AMENORRHEA

Causes of amenorrhea may be divided into compartments: end-organ, outflow tract, and three other compartments that lead to inadequate hormonal stimulation to the endometrium: the ovary, the pituitary, and the hypothalamus. The history, physical examination, and a few simple tests can usually identify which compartment has led to the problem. In teenagers, end-organ and outflow tract conditions are probably congenital, manifesting as primary amenorrhea with

Table 30-4. Medications that Can Cause Abnormal Uterine Bleeding

Hormonal Effects

Estrogens: oral estrogens, estrogen patch
Progestins: oral progestins, progestin-only "mini-pill," injectable or implantable progestin
Estrogen/progestin: combination oral contraceptives, skin patches, vaginal rings
Androgens: anabolic steroids, danazol
Prolactin: many drugs raise prolactin levels, including estrogens, phenothiazines, tricyclic antidepressants, benzodiazepines, metaclopromide, and other drugs that deplete dopamine levels or block dopamine receptors

Anticoagulant Effects

Warfarin, heparin
Aspirin, other nonsteroidal antiinflammatory drugs
Chemotherapeutic agents that result in thrombocytopenia

normal secondary sexual development. Once these are ruled out, the general evaluation for amenorrhea can begin.

CONGENITAL CAUSES OF PRIMARY AMENORRHEA IN ADOLESCENTS WITH NORMAL SECONDARY SEXUAL DEVELOPMENT (Table 30-8)

Obstruction to Menstrual Outflow

Congenital conditions, such as *imperforate hymen, transverse vaginal septum,* and (in rare cases) cervical anomalies, can obstruct menstrual outflow. The diagnosis is suspected when cyclic pain

Table 30-5. Management of Dysfunctional Uterine Bleeding

Mild (Hgb ≥ 11 mg/dL)

Reassurance
Instruction to keep a menstrual calendar
Iron supplementation
Periodic reevaluation: 2-3 months

Moderate (Hgb 9-11 mg/dL)

Actively bleeding: hormonal hemostasis—oral estrogen protocol,* then as for not actively bleeding
Not actively bleeding: iron supplementation, regulate cycles with cyclic progestins† or oral contraceptives‡ for 3-6 months, then reevaluate

Severe (Hgb ≤ 8 mg/dL or hemodynamically unstable)

Not actively bleeding: transfusion if necessary, then as for moderate DUB
Actively bleeding: transfusion/fluid replacement, hormonal hemostasis by IV or oral estrogen protocol, D&C if unable to stop bleeding with IV estrogen, then same as for moderate DUB

*See Table 30-6.

†Medroxyprogesterone acetate (Provera), 10 mg/day or equivalent for 12 days each month.

‡Any 30- to 35-μg estrogen ethinyl estrodiol pill.

D&C, dilation and curettage; DUB, dysfunctional uterine bleeding; Hgb, hemoglobin; IV, intravenous.

and abnormal anatomy are found. A mass (hematocolpos and/or hematometra) may be palpable.

Inability of the Endometrium to Respond to Hormonal Stimulation

Absence of the uterus or, in rare cases, absence or severe scarring of the endometrium can cause amenorrhea. The most common diagnosis in this category is *müllerian agenesis* (absence of the uterus and proximal vagina). A less common cause is *androgen insensitivity syndrome* (see Chapter 31). *Asherman syndrome,* or uterine scarring, is caused by prior dilation and curettage and/or severe uterine infection. The scarred endometrium does not respond to hormones, and menses are scanty or absent. This is extremely rare in teenagers.

Müllerian Agenesis

Müllerian agenesis, also known as *Mayer-Rokitansky-Kuster-Hauser* syndrome, is associated with urinary tract and skeletal anomalies. Affected girls and women have normal gonadal function and completely normal secondary sexual development. Cyclic abdominal pain, if present, is mittelschmerz (ovulation pain). The vagina is usually a dimple or small in-pouching for which a procedure is needed later in life to allow sexual intercourse. Usually the uterus is absent, but there may be a small uterine remnant, usually without endometrium. These individuals cannot become pregnant, but with assisted reproductive technology, they can provide eggs to be fertilized with the male partner's sperm and gestated in the uterus of a surrogate.

Androgen Insensitivity Syndrome

Androgen insensitivity syndrome, formerly known as *testicular feminization,* occurs in persons who are phenotypically female but are chromosomally XY and lack androgen receptors. In complete androgen insensitivity syndrome, the external genitalia appear female, and the vagina is very shallow. The müllerian and wolffian duct systems are absent. At puberty, breasts develop as a result of gonadal estrogens. Axillary and pubic hair is absent. Malignant transformation of intraabdominal testes can occur, usually after age 25 years. In complete androgen insensitivity syndrome, gonadectomy is delayed until after puberty, to allow smooth secondary sexual development and prevent the majority of tumors.

Explaining the Diagnosis

The diagnosis of müllerian agenesis or androgen insensitivity can be psychologically traumatic. Just as she is forming her identity as a woman, the patient discovers she is "not normal" and cannot achieve the milestone of menarche. At the same time, she learns of impediments to reproduction and to sexual intercourse. Explanation to the patient that her vagina did not form completely and that she needs a procedure to help deepen it can give her words for her condition that she can use when she chooses to tell others about it. A multidisciplinary approach with counseling and, if possible, group support or contact with an older girl who has been through treatment can be helpful.

CAUSES OF AMENORRHEA IN ADOLESCENTS WITH NORMAL ANATOMY

Inadequate hormonal stimulation to the endometrium is the most common cause of secondary amenorrhea and of pubertal delay. There are three general situations that fall under this description:

- chronic anovulation (which includes polycystic ovarian syndrome)
- hypogonadotropic hypogonadism (including the "athletic triad")
- ovarian failure (hypergonadotropic hypoestrogenism)

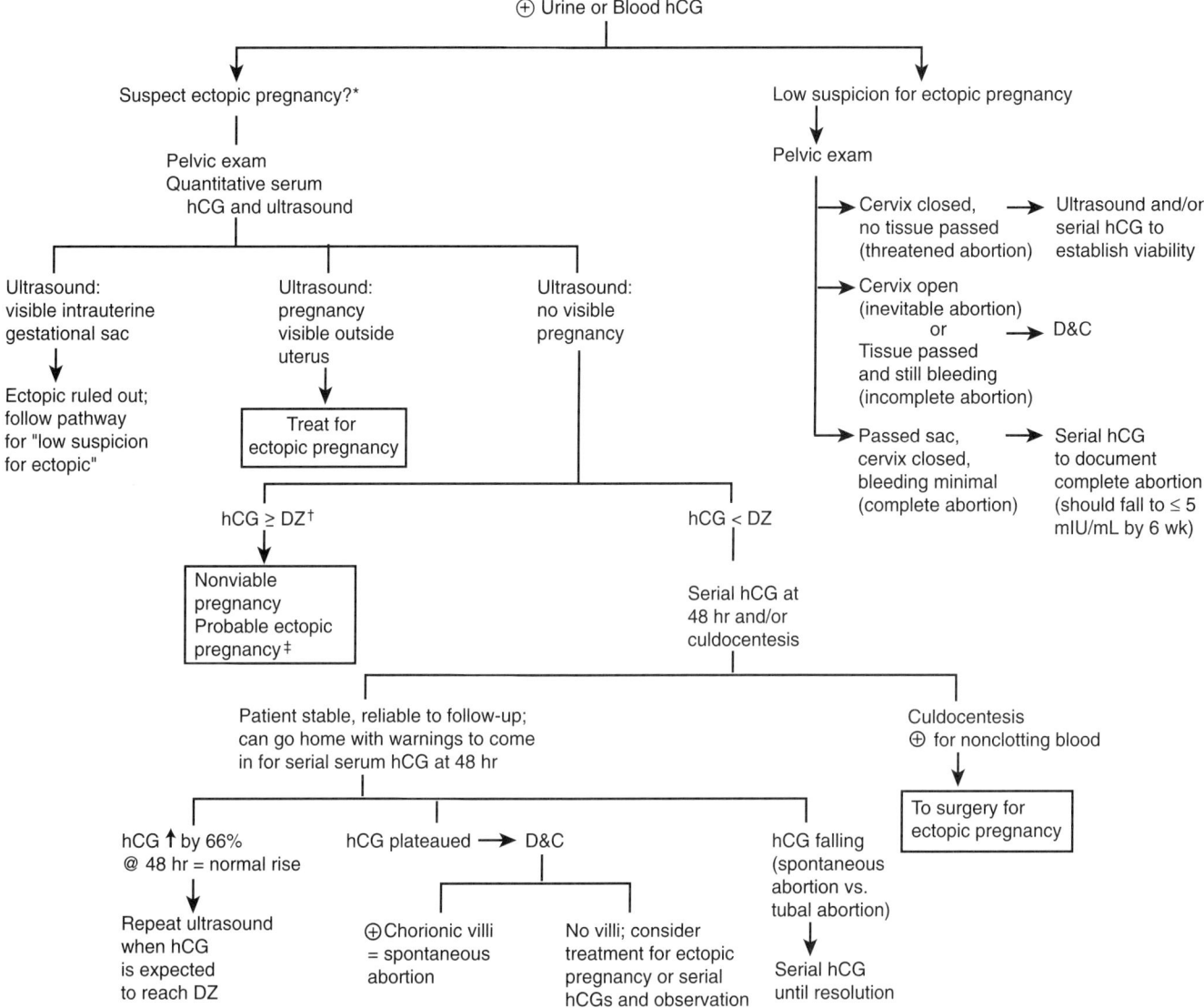

* Patient with pelvic/abdominal pain or risk factors (prior ectopic, prior tubal surgery, prior pelvic inflammatory disease, prior gonorrhea or chlamydia infection, chronic pelvic pain). If ruptured tubal pregnancy suspected (e.g., hemodynamic instability with pelvic pain), may take patient to surgery with only positive pregnancy test or positive culdocentesis.

† DZ (discriminatory zone) is the hCG value at which a normal pregnancy would be expected to be visible on the ultrasound. Transvaginal scanning, which visualizes a pregnancy a few days earlier than the abdominal scan, has a lower DZ. Each institution should assess its own DZ based on ultrasound technology and the type of hCG test used. According to the 2nd International Reference Preparation, the DZ for transvaginal ultrasound is usually ≤ 1500 mIU/mL; DZ for abdominal sonogram is about 6000 mIU/mL.

‡ Can treat for presumed ectopic in OR or as for plateaued hCG below.

Figure 30-6. Evaluation of abnormal bleeding in pregnancy. DZ, discriminatory zone; D&C, dilation and curettage; hCG, human chorionic gonadotropin.

Anovulation

In chronic anovulation, the ovary makes estrogen, but ovulation does not occur. Because there is no ovulation, there is no cyclic elevation of progestins and no progestin withdrawal bleeding. Obesity, stress, hypothyroidism, and hyperprolactinemia can all lead to chronic anovulation. Nonetheless, a cause is usually not found.

If hirsutism is present, it is evaluated with attention to ruling out the rare case of late-onset congenital adrenal hyperplasia, Cushing syndrome, and tumor of the ovary or adrenal gland (Fig. 30-7).

Polycystic ovarian syndrome (PCOS) can be a *result* of chronic anovulation. Patients with PCOS may have cystic ovaries, hirsutism, obesity, and amenorrhea or DUB. Insulin resistance and acanthosis nigricans are sometimes observed. PCOS is best considered an extreme at the end of the spectrum of manifestations of chronic anovulation. Patients with PCOS are usually treated as anovulatory (see later discussion), although insulin-sensitizing agents such as metformin are also effective.

Table 30-6. Medications to Stop Acute Anovulatory Bleeding

Medication	Dosage	Comments
Estrogens		Usually causes nausea
IV conjugated equine estrogens (Premarin)*	25 mg IV q4h Maximum 4 doses	One published study only; study showed effectiveness at stopping acute bleeding from many causes
Conjugated equine estrogens (Premarin)*	2.5 mg PO q6h × 5 days	
Combination Estrogens/ Progestins		May cause nausea, progestin side effects (see under "Progestins")
High-dose oral contraceptive pills*	50 µg ethinyl/estradiol pill q.i.d. × 5-7 days	Outpatient method that provides estrogen and progestin
Progestins		No comparison studies of progestins versus estrogen or oral contraceptives; theoretically less effective if bleeding has been prolonged and endometrial basalis layer is exposed, because progestins only "organize" an already estrogenized proliferative endometrium; side effects of progestins are similar to normal premenstrual symptoms: breast tenderness, depression, bloating, water retention
Medroxyprogesterone acetate (Provera)	10-40 mg per 24 hr PO × 12 days	
Norethindrone acetate (Aygestin)	5-10 mg per 24 hr PO × 12 days	
Megesterol	40-120 mg/day × 12 days	

*Must be immediately followed by 12-21 days of progestin-dominant therapy. Usually 30-50 µg estrogen daily oral contraceptives, although medroxyprogesterone acetate, 10 mg/day, can be used.

IV, intravenously; PO, per os (orally); q.i.d., four times per day.

Table 30-7. Differentiating Ovulatory from Anovulatory Menstrual Cycles

	Ovulatory	Anovulatory
Menses	There is regularity of interval, flow, and duration, usually 28 ± 7 days lasting 3-7 days	Variable flow, duration, and interval
Dysmenorrhea	Possibly cramps with bleeding*	No cramps or cramps only with passing clot
Molimina† (premenstrual symptoms)	Possibly breast tenderness,* fluid retention, abdominal bloating, mood disturbance	None
Mittelschmerz	Possible midcycle unilateral pelvic pain	None
Basal body temperature	Biphasic basal body temperature, taken each day, usually before rising in A.M.	Monophasic basal body temperature
Serum progesterone	High serum progesterone 1–2 days before menses (5 ng/mL)	Serum progesterone ≤1 ng/mL 1-12 days before bleeding

*Presence of these signs in a reliable historian strongly suggests ovulatory cycles.

†Best documented prospectively and/or correlated with basal body temperature.

Hypogonadism

Ovarian Failure

In patients with hypergonadotropic hypogonadism, FSH and LH levels are in the menopausal range because the ovaries do not make estrogen, which would otherwise provide negative feedback. Ovarian failure may be caused by gonadal dysgenesis, or the ovaries may appear normal. *Gonadal dysgenesis* is associated with Turner syndrome and other X chromosome deletions and mosaic conditions (see Chapter 31). Some persons with Turner syndrome are chromosomally XY/XO mosaic and require gonadectomy at the time of diagnosis to prevent malignant transformation of the intraabdominal streak testis. Because of this risk, the karyotype must be obtained for all adolescents with unexplained ovarian failure, to evaluate for the presence of Y chromosomal material. Other less common causes of ovarian failure include autoimmune oophoritis, galactosemia, and exposure to cytotoxic chemotherapy or radiation therapy. Some ovarian failure is idiopathic.

Hypothalamic Amenorrhea

Hypogonadotropic hypogonadism is another low-estrogen condition. The pituitary gland, hypothalamus, or both are not appropriately cycling to stimulate the ovary to produce estrogen. FSH and LH levels in these cases are low or normal. This is found in the adolescent athletic triad of amenorrhea, disordered eating, and osteoporosis. Low body weight, chronic illness, anorexia nervosa, intense exercise, hypothyroidism, and hyperprolactinemia can all cause hypothalamic amenorrhea. Intracranial tumors, such as craniopharyngioma and prolactinoma, can also lead to this type of amenorrhea.

Amenorrhea Related to Hormonal Contraceptives

Amenorrhea that occurs while a person is using birth control pills, patches, rings, or long-acting implantable or injectable contraceptives is caused by the progestin-dominant hormonal environment provided

Table 30-8. Congenital Anatomic Causes of Primary Amenorrhea with Normal Breast Development*

Diagnosis	Müllerian Agenesis	Androgen Insensitivity (AI)	Transverse Vaginal Septum	Imperforate Hymen
Patients with primary amenorrhea[†]	15%	1%	3%	1%
Patients with primary amenorrhea and apparent obstruction or absence of vagina[†]	75%	5%	15%	5%
Chromosomes[‡]	46,XX	46,XY	46,XX	46,XX
Gonads	Ovaries	Testes	Ovaries	Ovaries
Serum testosterone[‡]	Normal female level	Normal male level (high)	Normal female level	Normal female level
Vagina	Absent or shallow	Absent or shallow	Obstructed by septum which may be thick or thin, high or low	Obstructed by thin membrane, which may look blue from hematocolpos
Axillary/pubic hair	+	Absent unless AI is incomplete	+	+
Cyclic pain	±	−	+	+
Uterus	Absent or rudimentary	Absent	Present	Present
Mass	−	−	+ Can present with acute urinary retention as hematocolpos mass obstructs urethra	+ Can present with acute urinary retention
Introitus bulges with Valsalva maneuver	−	−	−	+
Associated anomalies	Urinary tract and skeletal	Inguinal hernias; gonadal malignancy in adulthood	Major urinary tract abnormalities in 15%	Possibly some increase in urinary tract abnormalities
Treatment	Vaginal dilation or surgical neovagina	Gonadectomy after age 16-18 Vaginal dilation or surgical neovagina	Surgical approach depends on extent and location of septum; may be extensive; should be done as soon as possible	Excision of hymen as soon as possible; diagnostic needle aspiration contraindicated because of risk of infection
Fertility	Advanced reproductive technology required; in vitro fertilization surrogate with uterus to gestate pregnancy	Not fertile	Variable, low septa have a better prognosis than do high septa	Usually fertile

*Cervix not visible on pelvic examination. Short vagina; may be absent or obstructed.

[†]Data from Reindollar RH, Byrd JR, McDonough PG: Delayed sexual development: A study of 252 patients. Am J Obstet Gynecol 1981;140:371.

[‡]Sometimes useful in differentiating müllerian agenesis from androgen insensitivity.

+, present; −, absent; ±, may be present or absent.

to the endometrium and by suppression of ovulation. As long as pregnancy has been ruled out, further workup is generally not necessary. The endometrium in these cases is decidualized and atrophic. Short-term additional estrogen taken with the combination birth control pills usually leads to resumption of menses. Conditions such as eating disorders and stress do not play a role in creating amenorrhea in a girl receiving hormone therapy because the hormonal environment provided to the endometrium is independent of her endogenous hormones.

Menstrual cycles are expected to revert to normal by 6 months after discontinuance of oral contraceptive pills and by 12 months after the last depot-medroxyprogesterone acetate (Depo-Provera) injection. For amenorrhea that continues after that point, evaluation is indicated.

EVALUATION OF THE AMENORRHEIC ADOLESCENT

The evaluation for amenorrhea (Table 30-9) is rarely performed on an emergency basis. An organized history and physical examination with cautious use of ancillary tests can usually identify the general category in which the patient's condition fits. Within that category, serious medical conditions can be ruled out before treatment is initiated. Even when there is an obvious predisposing factor, such as intense competitive exercise, the protocol should be followed to allow precise identification of the current hormone state and to rule out serious coinciding conditions.

History

The history should cover the patient's general health, including any immediate problems at the time of her birth, major illness, chronic illness, and exposure to chemotherapy or pelvic or central nervous system radiation therapy. Pubertal milestones are identified. Eating habits, emotional stress, exercise habits, sexual activity, birth control method, use of drugs and medications, and any change in weight must be addressed. Review of systems can identify sex hormonal abnormalities, including hirsutism, hot flashes, presence of cyclic abdominal pain, and/or premenstrual symptoms. Is there a breast discharge suggestive of a prolactinoma? Are there symptoms of any other hormonal syndrome, such as hypothyroidism? (See Chapter 49.) Are there any symptoms that might suggest an intracranial tumor, such as significant headaches or loss of peripheral vision?

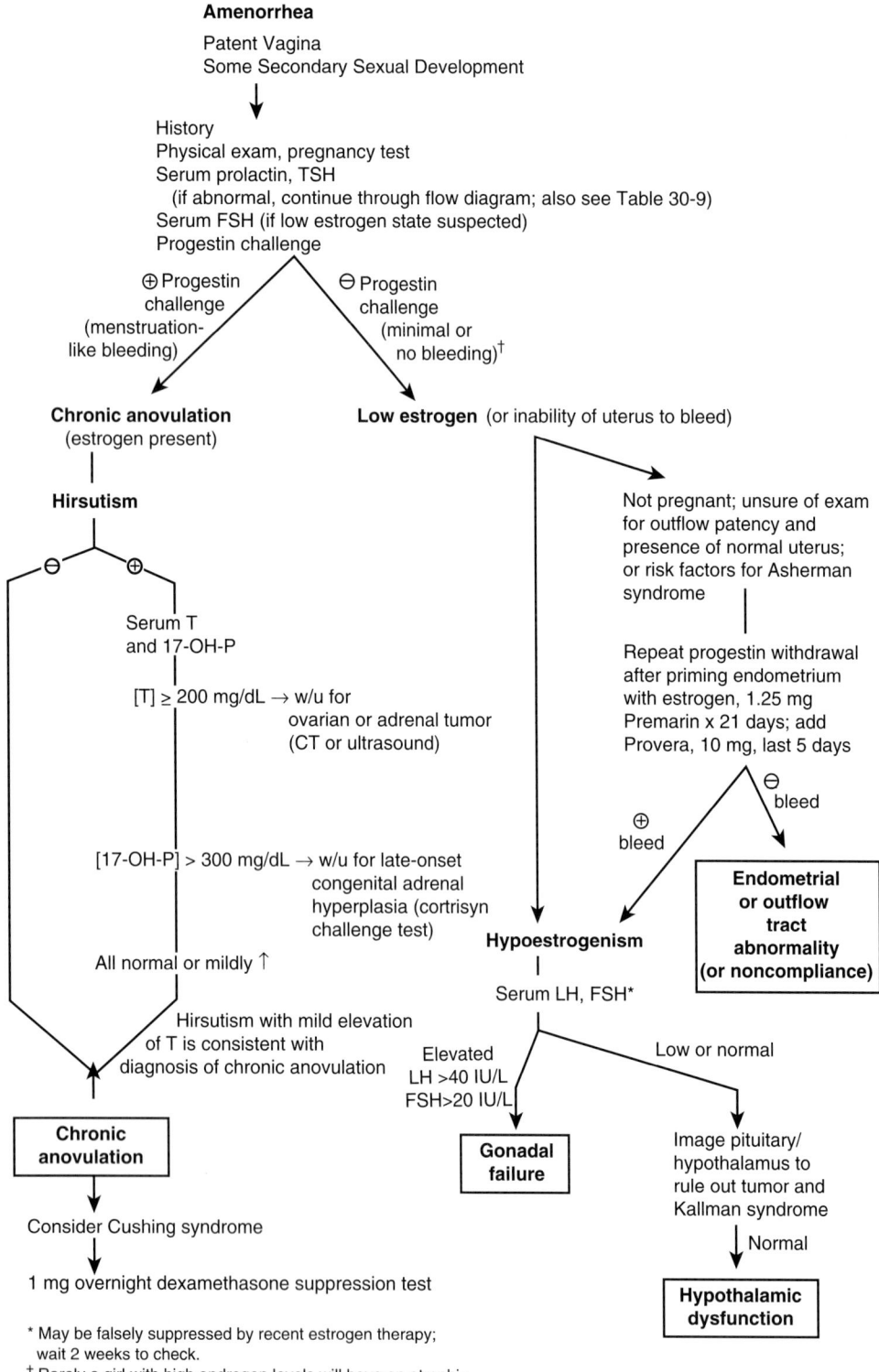

Figure 30-7. General workup for amenorrhea. CT, computed tomography; FSH, follicle-stimulating hormone; LH, luteinizing hormone; 17-OH-P, 17-hydroxyprogesterone; T, testosterone; TSH, thyroid-stimulating hormone.

Physical Examination

General appearance, pulse, and blood pressure should be noted. Vital signs may be depressed in anorexia nervosa and other starvation states. Weight and height should be plotted on a growth chart. Vision and fundi must be checked carefully. Secondary sexual characteristics may be undeveloped (delayed puberty), normal, or abnormal (hirsutism). Sexual maturation staging (see Chapter 59), observation

for evidence of hirsutism or virilization, nipple expression to check for galactorrhea, and palpation of the thyroid are performed. The abdomen should be examined to identify a pelvic mass, which may indicate hematocolpos or pregnancy.

On pelvic examination, external genitalia should be observed for estrogen effect. Are the tissues pink, moist, and full, or red, thin, and atrophic? Is the vagina patent? Is the cervix visible or at least palpable?

Table 30-9. General Workup for Amenorrhea in Girls with Normal Anatomy and Some Secondary Sexual Development

Visit 1

From History and Physical Examination

1. Some secondary sexual development (for pubertal delay, see Chapter 59)
2. Patent vagina
3. Cervix seen or palpated
4. Uterus palpated or visualized by ultrasonography

Suspect Inadequate Hormonal Stimulation to Endometrium

1. Assess estrogen status, prolactin, and thyroid function
   a. Serum PRL, thyroid-stimulating hormone (TSH)
   b. Serum follicle-stimulating hormone (FSH) if hypoestrogenic state is suspected
   c. For assessment of estrogen status, perform progestin challenge

Schedule Next Visit in 3-4 Weeks

Visit 2

Review Results of PRL and TSH

1. ↑ PRL (or any galactorrhea) requires evaluation for pituitary adenoma; CT with contrast or MRI is needed to check for pituitary tumor; many medications can lead to elevation of PRL (see table 30-4); any elevation of PRL can lead to ovulatory dysfunction
2. ↑ TSH necessitates assessment of free T$_4$; if hypothyroid, thyroid hormone replacement may completely resolve ovulatory dysfunction
3. Even if PRL or TSH levels are abnormal, continue workup to identify where the patient's condition falls in the spectrum of ovulatory dysfunction (see Fig. 30-7)

Review of Response to Progestin Challenge

1. Was there menstruation-like bleeding?
2. Follow flowsheet to identify hormonal state of the patient (see Fig. 30-7)
3. Remainder of care plan depends on the hormonal state (normal versus low estrogen) and on the compartment that has caused the problem

CT, computed tomography; MRI, magnetic resonance imaging; PRL, prolactin.

On bimanual examination (see Fig. 30-4), if the uterus is palpable, is it normal in size or prepubertal? Are the ovaries palpable? If the digital examination and speculum examination are not tolerated, the vagina can be probed with a saline-moistened swab to determine its length.

On rectovaginal or rectoabdominal examination, are there any masses consistent with hematometria or hematocolpos? If there is evidence of an obstructed or absent vagina, a rectoabdominal examination can be performed to check for a mass and to identify the uterus if present. Ultrasonography is helpful in corroborating the physical examination findings.

In girls without pubertal development, estrogen levels are always low. Visualization of the cervix in these cases is not as important as it is in the pubertal adolescent with delayed menarche, because abnormal anatomy is rarely found. The cause of the delay is almost always hypothalamic, pituitary, or ovarian. In the postpubertal girl, if the physical examination demonstrates normal female external genitalia and a patent vagina with visualization or palpation of the cervix, the workup can then progress to the general evaluation for amenorrhea. The cause is usually in the HPO axis.

Evaluation of the Hypothalamic-Pituitary-Ovarian Axis

Laboratory Studies and the Progestin Challenge (see Fig. 30-7)

After obtaining the history and physical examination results, the examiner should assess for hypothyroidism and prolactinoma with serum levels of thyroid-stimulating hormone (TSH) and prolactin. At the same time, an assessment of the estrogen status of the patient is performed. Because single blood estrogen levels are unreliable, physiologic testing is done by progestin challenge. Progestins cause bleeding only if the endometrium is in a proliferative state, primed by prior estrogen exposure. The progestin challenge test is positive if menstruation-like bleeding occurs within 2 weeks after treatment with 5 days of 5 to 10 mg of oral medroxyprogesterone acetate or any equivalent dose of a progestin.

Progestin Challenge Results

Bleeding that occurs after the progestin challenge proves that there is a functional uterus and outflow tract. The amount of bleeding is approximately proportional to the amount and duration of prior estrogen exposure. If bleeding is similar to a menstrual period, the patient's condition belongs to the category of chronic anovulation with an estrogenized endometrium.

Failure of the progestin challenge to lead to menstruation-like bleeding indicates a low-estrogen state or the inability of the uterus to demonstrate bleeding. If the patient may have been pregnant for a few days at the time of the progestin challenge, the pregnancy test should be repeated 2 weeks later. If the pelvic findings are entirely normal and the patient has no historical risk factors for Asherman syndrome, her condition belongs to the category of hypogonadism (hypoestrogenic amenorrhea). If there is any question of the ability of the uterus to bleed, progestin withdrawal should be repeated after priming the endometrium with estrogen.

Although the general rule is that failure to bleed after progestin withdrawal indicates a low estrogen state, there is one rare exception. A few girls with very high androgen levels, as may be seen in polycystic ovarian syndrome or late-onset congenital adrenal hyperplasia, may have an atrophic endometrium (and failure to have a withdrawal bleed after progestins) despite the presence of estrogen. Severe hirsutism is not usually seen with true low-estrogen states.

THINGS NOT TO MISS

The examiner must never forget that the most common cause of amenorrhea in the general population is pregnancy. The examiner needs to obtain a private history, earn the patient's confidence, and provide confidentiality if it is requested. When the diagnosis is in doubt, a pregnancy test should be conducted even if the patient does not admit to sexual activity. Commercially available urine pregnancy tests turn positive by the first missed period. In rare cases, women with abnormal pregnancies (ectopic and those about to miscarry) have hCG levels too low to detect in the urine. A blood hCG level is diagnostic.

TREATMENT OF AMENORRHEA

End-Organ and Outflow Tract Anomalies

In all cases of outflow obstruction, it is important to allow menstrual blood to escape, because failure to do so can lead to severe endometriosis and scarring of the reproductive organs. The procedure may be as simple as hymenotomy, or it may involve complicated vaginal and cervical reconstruction. All efforts should be made to preserve reproductive function.

If the uterus is absent, as in müllerian agenesis and androgen insensitivity syndrome, treatment is aimed at creating adequate vaginal depth for satisfactory sexual intercourse once that is desired. These procedures are best held off until the patient is mature and motivated, because they entail the patient's taking responsibility for ongoing dilation of her vagina. The presence of a Y chromosome, as in androgen insensitivity syndrome, necessitates surgical gonadectomy to prevent malignancy. Estrogen replacement therapy is then necessary.

Hormonal Causes of Amenorrhea

If the underlying cause is identified, such as hypothyroidism, obesity, or an eating disorder, treatment should be aimed at the specific problem. Often, however, a specific cause is not found or is not easily treated.

Regardless of cause, hormonal replacement is indicated in order to improve self-image and to prevent the sequelae of untreated sex hormone abnormalities (Table 30-10). In general, hypoestrogenic states necessitate estrogen-progestin hormone replacement therapy or oral contraceptives to complete pubertal development, to prevent vaginal atrophy, and to possibly help avert osteoporosis. Patients with chronic anovulation require cycling with 12 days of progestins at least every 2 or 3 months to bring about withdrawal bleeding. This helps prevent excessive bleeding, endometrial hyperplasia, and cancer. An alternative treatment is oral contraceptives, or equivalent treatment with the contraceptive patch or vaginal ring, which have the added benefit of suppressing ovarian androgens (thus ameliorating hirsutism) and providing contraception. The length of time to continue therapy depends on whether spontaneous cycles can be expected to resume. In the obese girl with PCOS, a modest weight loss of 20 to 30 pounds often leads to resumption of ovulatory cycles.

DYSMENORRHEA

Dysmenorrhea is defined as crampy lower abdominal or low back pain temporally associated with menstruation. It is a common problem that causes much suffering and interferes in some cases with school attendance. In one study, 60% of 12- to 17-year-old girls reported some dysmenorrhea; 14% frequently missed school.

Dysmenorrhea is categorized as either the very common *primary* dysmenorrhea, associated with no clinically detectable pelvic pathologic process, or the much less common *secondary* dysmenorrhea, caused by an underlying pelvic abnormality. Primary dysmenorrhea usually begins with the onset of menstrual flow and lasts from hours to a few days. The cramping may be accompanied by nausea, vomiting, diarrhea, and/or headache. Primary dysmenorrhea begins when the cycles become ovulatory, usually by the third postmenstrual year.

MECHANISM OF PRIMARY DYSMENORRHEA

Primary dysmenorrhea by definition is not associated with clinically discernible pelvic pathology. The pain results from uterine contractions caused by high levels of prostaglandins originating in the premenstrual secretory endometrium. Women with dysmenorrhea

Table 30-10. Hormone Replacement Options for Amenorrheic Conditions*

	Hormone Replacement	Benefits of Therapy	Risks of Therapy
Chronic anovulation (estrogen present)	Progestin therapy with medroxyprogesterone acetate, 5-10 mg/day PO or 5 mg norethindrone acetate 12 days/ month every 1-3 months	Diminishes risk of sudden menorrhagia and of endometrial hyperplasia/ cancer later in life; creates predictable normal menses	Some premenstrual symptoms may occur while the patient is taking progestin; does not provide contraception or address cause of amenorrhea; does not suppress androgens to treat hirsutism
	Low-dose oral contraceptive pills (20-35 μg of estrogen) or contraceptive patch	Same as for progestin therapy; provides contraception; improves hirsutism by suppressing ovarian androgens	Does not address cause of amenorrhea; some parents object to their daughters' taking oral contraceptives; side effects can include nausea, headache, and breakthrough bleeding
Hypogonadism (low-estrogen state)†	Oral medroxyprogesterone acetate 5-10 mg/day or 2.5-5 mg norethindrone acetate on days 1-12 of the month (by calendar) plus oral conjugated estrogens, 0.625 mg/day	Prevents osteoporosis,‡ heart disease, and atrophic vaginal changes; eliminates hot flashes if present	Does not address cause of amenorrhea; does not provide contraception (if ovulation is possible, given the diagnosis); premenstrual symptoms may occur while the patient is taking progestins; some adolescents prefer oral contraceptives to "medications"
	Low-dose oral contraceptive pills (20-35 μg of estrogen)	Same as HRT; provides contraception in case of spontaneous ovulation (if that is a possibility); many adolescents prefer taking oral contraceptives to taking "medications"	Same as risks of oral contraceptives for chronic anovulation

*These options may need modification according to the individual's response.

†See Chapter 59 for treatment of pubertal delay.

‡Estrogen therapy may not prevent bone loss in girls with amenorrhea and low body weight.

HRT, hormone replacement therapy.

have greater resting uterine tone during menses and more severe contractions than do asymptomatic controls. Treatment with non-steroidal antiinflammatory drugs (NSAIDs) diminishes these objective findings as well as the sensation of cramps. Systemic release of prostaglandins probably accounts for the other symptoms, such as nausea and diarrhea, often seen with primary dysmenorrhea.

Because progesterone from the postovulatory corpus luteum induces the change from a proliferative to a secretory endometrium, primary dysmenorrhea occurs only in ovulatory cycles. Anovulatory bleeding may cause cramping as a clot passes through the cervix, but as a rule it is not associated with pain.

SECONDARY DYSMENORRHEA

A small percentage of adolescents with menstrual pain have underlying pathologic processes. Table 30-11 presents the differential diagnosis of menstrual pain.

EVALUATION OF DYSMENORRHEA

History

Routine inquiry enables girls who are suffering from dysmenorrhea to get treatment. It is important to assess the timing of pain, the degree of disruption of daily routines, the associated symptoms, the response to over-the-counter medications, and the sexual history. The history helps to differentiate primary from secondary dysmenorrhea. Dysmenorrhea associated with one specific menstrual period in a sexually active adolescent suggests a pregnancy complication or pelvic inflammatory disease (PID). Menstrual pain beginning at menarche or at any other time during which the cycles are believed to be anovulatory suggests outflow tract obstruction, because anovulatory bleeding does not cause primary dysmenorrhea. Endometriosis may be difficult to diagnose because its manifestation may be similar to that of primary dysmenorrhea. However, endometriosis that is diagnosed in the adolescent is often associated with intermittent,

Table 30-11. Differential Diagnosis of Dysmenorrhea

	Description of Pain	Occurrence of Dysmenorrhea in Anovulatory Cycles	Diagnosis	Treatment
Primary	Crampy lower abdominal/low back pain ± radiation to upper thighs ± nausea, vomiting, diarrhea, headache; begins at time of menstrual flow; lasts 1-3 days	No	Normal abdominal and pelvic examination; internal pelvic examination can be reserved for sexually active girls and older teenagers; rectoabdominal examination assesses pelvic pathology	NSAIDs and/or oral contraceptives; see Table 30-12
Secondary				
Congenital partial outflow obstruction (e.g., rudimentary uterine horn, obstructed hemivagina)	Pain begins at or shortly after menarche and occurs with bleeding	Yes	Pelvic examination ± ultrasonography ± laparoscopy; found in 8% of adolescents who underwent laparoscopy for pain	Surgical relief of obstruction
Endometriosis	Increasingly severe dysmenorrhea ± chronic pelvic pain exacerbated during menses	No	Found in 16% to 70% of adolescents who underwent laparoscopy for pelvic pain; pelvic examination finding may be normal or there may be tenderness of the uterosacral ligaments/*cul-de-sac* and/or ovarian masses; although congenital obstruction of menstrual outflow increases chance of endometriosis, most teenagers with endometriosis have normal anatomy; diagnosis is by laparoscopy	Surgical and/or hormonal therapy; post-treatment prophylaxis with oral contraceptives
Atypical secondary dysmenorrhea				
Pelvic inflammatory disease	Pain during or immediately after menses	Yes	Pelvic examination: tender uterus and adnexa, ± cervicitis, ± ↑ WBC count, ± ↑ ESR, ± fever	Follow CDC recommendations (see Chapter 29)
Pregnancy complication	Pain and bleeding may coincide and may be interpreted by the patient as a painful menstrual period	N/A	UCG, or serum hCG	See Figure 30-6

CDC, Centers for Disease Control and Prevention; ESR, erythrocyte sedimentation rate; hCG, human chorionic gonadotropin, N/A, not applicable; NASIDs, nonsteriodal anti-inflammatory drugs; UCG, urinary chorionic gonadotropin; WBC, white blood cell.

non–menstrually related pelvic pain that worsens before and during menses.

Examination and Testing

In the evaluation of dysmenorrhea, an internal pelvic examination can be reserved for girls who are sexually active, for older adolescents, for girls who do not respond to standard treatment with NSAIDs or oral contraceptives, and for those with atypical manifestations. If necessary, a rectoabdominal examination or ultrasound study can diagnose a pelvic mass and may be better tolerated than vaginal examination in young virginal adolescents.

If the pain is associated with one particular period, pregnancy and PID should be ruled out. PID is a clinical diagnosis based on history, vital signs, abdominal and pelvic examination, and white blood cell count (see Chapter 29).

The goals of treatment of endometriosis in an adolescent with dysmenorrhea include alleviation of pain and, if possible, prevention of progression of the disease. If endometriosis is suspected on the basis of tenderness on pelvic examination or failure to respond to NSAIDs and oral contraceptives, the benefits of laparoscopy to make the diagnosis should be weighed against the risks. For adult patients in whom the history strongly suggests endometriosis, some experts recommend empirical treatment with GnRH analogues, rather than starting with laparoscopy. This may also be an efficacious and cost-effective approach for adolescents.

TREATMENT OF DYSMENORRHEA (Table 30-12)

NSAIDs work by decreasing production of prostaglandins in the endometrium. About 80% of women with primary dysmenorrhea obtain relief of pain and the associated gastrointestinal symptoms with most NSAIDs.

Oral contraceptives are successful in diminishing primary dysmenorrhea by inducing atrophy of the endometrium; the result is decreased production of prostaglandins. Because this effect may take 3 or 4 months to develop, NSAIDs should be offered concurrently for the first few treatment cycles. Low-dose oral contraceptives, if not contraindicated, are the treatment of choice for dysmenorrhea in sexually active adolescents requiring contraception.

Acupuncture, transcutaneous electrical nerve stimulation, supplemental ω-3 fatty acids, and calcium antagonists have also shown some promise in treating primary dysmenorrhea.

SUMMARY AND THINGS NOT TO BE MISSED

The examiner should not miss the opportunity to treat the adolescent with primary dysmenorrhea who is suffering in silence. The examiner also should not mistake acute pelvic pain with vaginal bleeding for dysmenorrhea but should consider pregnancy complications and PID in the differential diagnosis of sudden onset of "menstrual" pain.

The practitioner should consider endometriosis and/or congenital anomaly with partial menstrual outflow obstruction in cases of severe dysmenorrhea with abnormal pelvic findings, poor response to the usual therapies, or generalization of pelvic pain beyond the time of the menstrual flow.

VAGINAL BLEEDING IN THE PREPUBERTAL CHILD

Vaginal bleeding is abnormal in white girls younger than 8 and in girls of African descent younger than 7. It is always abnormal in the absence of secondary sexual characteristics. Although childhood vaginal bleeding is uncommon, it can be caused by serious problems such as intracranial tumors, vaginal malignancy, and sexual abuse. The source of bleeding in a young girl can be the lower genital tract or the uterus.

ETIOLOGY

In a child without signs of puberty, a vulvovaginal source of bleeding is most likely. Common causes within this category include vaginal foreign body, infectious vulvovaginitis, urethral prolapse, vulvar injury, and lichen sclerosus. There are also some common vulvovaginal conditions that only rarely manifest with bleeding. In condyloma acuminatum, mild vulvar trauma or secondary infection can lead to bleeding. During a pinworm infestation, scratching can result in bleeding excoriations.

Uncommon lower genital tract conditions, including vaginal or cervical malignancy, vaginal polyps, and hemangiomas of the vagina, vulva, or cervix, can manifest with vaginal bleeding. Although malignancy is rare, it was found in 12% to 21% of the patients in published series of cases of early childhood vaginal bleeding and must not be missed.

Except for a small amount of endometrial bleeding as the newborn withdraws from relatively high fetal levels of estrogen, *uterine bleeding* is always pathologic in childhood. Possible causes include

- precocious puberty
- isolated premature menarche
- autonomous estrogen secretion from either an ovarian or adrenal tumor
- exposure to exogenous estrogen

Table 30-12. Treatment of Primary Dysmenorrhea			
	Medication	**Regimen**	**Comments**
NSAID	Ibuprofen, 200 mg	2 tablets PO q4-6h	Over-the-counter
	Naproxen sodium, 275 mg	2 tablets to start, then 1 PO q6h	
	Naproxen sodium, 550 mg	1 tablet PO q12h	12-hr regimen is appealing to patients
	Mefenamic acid, 250 mg	2 tablets to start, then 1 PO q6h	Suggested in some studies as most effective drug
Oral contraceptives or contraceptive patch	Any low-dose pill (≤35 μg of estrogen) or ortho Evra	Cyclic	Particularly useful if birth control method is needed; a few cycles may be needed to reach maximum effectiveness

*Aspirin has not been shown to be better than placebo in the treatment of primary dysmenorrhea. NSAID treatment is effective if started at the onset of cramping and bleeding.
NSAID, nonsteroidal antiinflammatory drug; PO, per os (orally).

Vulvovaginal Sources of Bleeding
(Table 30-13 and Fig. 30-8)

Vaginal Foreign Body

Vaginal bleeding is more predictive of vaginal foreign body than is vaginal discharge. The chief complaint of vaginal bleeding without discharge results in the finding of vaginal foreign body in 50% of cases. In contrast, if the bleeding is associated with vaginal discharge, there may be less than a one-in-five chance of finding a foreign body. Usually the foreign body consists of a small wad of what appears to be toilet paper or other fibrous material. This is neither palpable on rectoabdominal examination nor visible on a sonogram or radiograph. Other items, such as small toys, pen tops, and safety pins have been reported. The child usually does not recall or admit to placing the foreign object in the vagina.

How did the foreign material get into the vagina? The prepubertal hymen is acutely and uncomfortably sensitive to touch, and normal masturbation in girls is thought to involve clitoral and labial manipulation, with less than 1% of girls engaging in vaginal or anal penetration. Among girls referred from a general outpatient pediatric practice to a child gynecology clinic who were subsequently found to have vaginal foreign bodies, most met criteria for confirmed sexual abuse. The approach to evaluation of the girl with a vaginal foreign body needs to include an assessment for the possibility of sexual molestation (see Chapter 36). A screening interview of the child alone with a trained professional and cultures for sexually transmitted infections are indicated.

Infectious Vulvovaginitis

Vulvovaginitis most commonly manifests with discharge or irritation, but vaginal bleeding is sometimes reported. Although most vulvovaginitis is caused by irritants or mixed bacteria, vaginal bleeding is most commonly seen in single-organism infections with group A streptococci, *Shigella* species, and, on occasion, gonococci. Diagnosis is made from visualization of vaginal discharge and from culture yielding a specific pathogen. The treatment for bacterial vulvovaginitis includes either culture-driven or broad-spectrum systemic antibiotic therapy and local hygiene measures, such as sitz baths, wiping from front to back after defecation, and appropriate hand washing.

Urethral Prolapse

Urethral prolapse is an eversion of the urethral mucous membrane through the meatus. Careful examination reveals red, friable, and sometimes necrotic tissue at the urethra, which is occasionally mistaken for cervical prolapse or a vaginal tumor. Many approaches to treatment have been reported. Local care with sitz baths is often all that is needed. Topical estrogen cream or antibiotics have been used. Surgical resection of the mucosa can be reserved for cases in which initial treatment fails or when bleeding or necrosis is severe.

Trauma

Vulvovaginal trauma in girls is usually caused by straddle injury. Other reported mechanisms of injury include vaginal penetration and tearing resulting from sudden forced stretching of the perineum from leg abduction. Evaluation of the child with vulvovaginal trauma requires a detailed history of how the injury occurred, with attention to the consistency and plausibility of the story. The hymen is lacerated only if the injury involved penetration into the vagina. A suspicion of sexual abuse requires a report to the proper authorities and evaluation of the ongoing safety of the child (see Chapter 36).

A vulvar laceration that is bleeding but that can be completely visualized is treated with ice packs, pressure, and suturing if necessary. Vulvar hematomas are common and usually self-limited

as tissue pressure controls continued expansion. Hematomas with overlying lacerations often develop bacterial cellulitis. A surgical approach with evacuation of the hematoma and ligation of bleeding vessels can be reserved for situations in which the hematoma is very large or continues to expand. If the bleeding points cannot be isolated, the hematoma cavity can be packed for 24 hours.

If the apex of the laceration cannot be seen, examination with the patient under sedation or general anesthesia is necessary to assess for trauma to the hymen or vagina. Hymenal laceration implies that the injury has penetrated the vagina. Because the vaginal wall is very thin, penetrating vaginal injuries often extend into adjacent structures. If the laceration extends to the vaginal apex, exploratory surgery is necessary to exclude extension into the peritoneal cavity. If hematuria is found, cystourethrography is recommended to evaluate the bladder and urethra. Urethral obstruction from a hematoma may necessitate suprapubic catheter placement. Home care after initial treatment of vulvar injury includes ice packs for 6 hours, followed by warm sitz baths two to three times a day to promote comfort and help prevent secondary infection.

Malignancy

Vaginal or cervical *botryoid sarcoma* (embryonal rhabdomyosarcoma) can manifest as a grapelike mass that is visible at the introitus. *Endodermal sinus tumor* has a similar appearance. The diagnosis of these malignancies is made from biopsy. Because these tumors grow below the epithelium of the vagina, superficial biopsy may not be diagnostic.

Vaginal clear cell adenocarcinoma is rare and should become even more so as the cohort of women exposed to diethylstilbestrol (DES) in utero continues to age. DES was taken off the market in 1972, and the youngest people exposed in utero are now in their 30s. Vaginal adenocarcinoma is occasionally seen in girls who were not DES-exposed.

Lichen Sclerosus

Lichen sclerosus is a hypotrophic dermatologic condition often found in the vulvar area. It appears as a thinning of the skin to a parchment-like appearance. The classic appearance is of an hourglass surrounding the introitus and anus. As a result of the thinness of the epidermis, minor trauma can lead to significant bleeding and subepithelial bruising. Lichen sclerosus has been misdiagnosed as fungal infection, hemangioma, sexual abuse, and severe vulvar trauma. The diagnosis is usually clinical, based on the characteristic appearance, but biopsy can confirm the diagnosis if necessary.

Uterine Sources of Vaginal Bleeding

If the external examination and vaginoscopy do not demonstrate a vulvovaginal source of bleeding, uterine bleeding should be suspected. Other indications that the source may be uterine include growth spurt, secondary sexual development, ovarian cyst, abdominal tumor, or risk factors for precocious puberty, such as previous cranial irradiation or stigmata of McCune-Albright syndrome.

Except for the occasional neonatal estrogen withdrawal bleeding, all uterine bleeding in children is pathologic, usually indicating estrogen effect on the endometrium. Serious underlying conditions, including brain tumor and malignant ovarian tumor, may yield no signs or symptoms other than vaginal bleeding at presentation. Causes of uterine bleeding in children are categorized in the following sections (Fig. 30-9) (see Chapter 59).

Precocious Menarche

Cyclic menses with no other secondary sexual characteristics has been termed *precocious menarche*. The cause is not known, but it is

Table 30-13. **Causes of Lower Genital Tract Bleeding in Girls**

	Diagnostic Features	Management
Common Causes		
Vaginal foreign body	Vaginal bleeding with or without discharge; usually a wad of toilet paper or other fibers; case reports of small toys, pen tops, safety pins; may be seen on unaided visual examination especially when patient is in the knee-chest position; vaginoscopy* is "gold standard" to make diagnosis and to rule out additional masses in vagina	Removal of foreign body usually resolves bleeding/discharge; persistent or recurrent bleeding is suggestive of additional foreign material; possibility of sexual abuse should be considered
Infectious vulvovaginitis	Vaginal discharge usually reported; may follow URI (group A streptococci) or diarrheal episode (*Shigella*); vulva may look reddened from primary infection or from irritating secretions; wet preparation shows white blood cells; vaginal culture may grow specific organism	If no response to local hygiene measures and specific antibiotics, consider EUA or vaginoscopy to look for another cause (e.g., foreign body)
Urethral prolapse	Careful examination demonstrates red edematous or necrotic mass encircling urethral meatus; vagina can be identified posterior to mass; sometimes occurs after hard Valsalva maneuver; age range: 5-9 yr	Sitz baths with or without estrogen cream or oral or topical antibiotics; usually effective within 2 weeks; urethral catheterization if patient cannot void; resection or cautery of mass with anesthesia if local care fails or if patient is symptomatic or tissue is necrotic
Lichen sclerosus	Vulvar ecchymoses and abrasions may be seen with minimal trauma; characteristic white parchment-like thin skin, often in hourglass symmetric pattern around introitus/anus; biopsy is diagnostic but unnecessary when lesion is characteristic; some cases improve at puberty	Recommend good hygiene, prevention of trauma (e.g., loose clothes, padded bicycle seat); no treatment needed in asymptomatic patients; topical corticosteroids can diminish irritation
Trauma	Evaluate for possibility of neglect or abuse to determine whether it is safe for patient to be discharged home Straddle injury: evaluate extent of lacerations/stability of hematoma Penetrating injury: evaluate extent of injuries and perform EUA; perform laparotomy or laparoscopy if wound extends to vaginal apex; evaluate bladder and rectum if laceration extends into vagina or if urine or stool test is positive for blood	EUA needed when injuries are more than minor; small vulvar hematoma; pressure, ice pack, rest, and evaluation of size stability; large or expanding hematoma: incision or evacuation of clots and ligation of visible vessels or pack; repair lacerations; careful evaluation for abuse or neglect necessary
Malignancy Sarcoma botryoides (embryonal rhabdomyosarcoma of vagina or cervix) or endodermal sinus tumor of vagina	Grapelike mass protruding from vagina; peak age, 2 yr (90% < 5 yr); biopsy is diagnostic, but tumor is below epithelium (can be missed); full staging required	Initial treatment is chemotherapy followed by surgery or radiation; exenteration is no longer standard first-line care
Adenocarcinoma of vagina or cervix	Vaginoscopy with biopsy; staging required; expect incidence in children to diminish because most adenocarcinomas of the vagina occurred in girls exposed to DES in utero and DES has been off the market for more than 30 years	Radical surgery
Uncommon Causes		
Human papillomavirus	Lesions can be single or multiple, 1 mm to large cauliflower-like masses, flesh-toned or pink or white; abrasion or secondary infection with ulceration can lead to vulvar bleeding	Evaluate for sexual abuse especially if diagnosed after age 2 years; for small vulvar condylomata, office podophyllin or TCA Large or resistant to treatment: laser ablation under general anesthesia; recurrence rate: 25% Cervical/vaginal lesions: laser in operating room with patient under general anesthesia; colposcopy with biopsy if indicated
Pinworms (*Enterobius vermicularis*)	Transparent tape (Scotch tape) test shows eggs; flashlight examination at night can show worms at vagina or anus	Mebendazole; evaluate family members, classmates, and playmates; clean and trim patient's fingernails
Hemangiomas of lower genital tract	Urethral, vulvar, vaginal, and cervical hemangiomas have been reported; appear purple or dark-red and soft; blanching occurs with pressure; overlying epithelium is usually intact, but bleeding occurs when trauma leads to ulceration; biopsy, if done, should be in hospital with blood replacement available	Treatment can be withheld if no symptoms; many spontaneous regressions; successful reported treatments include surgical excision, laser ablation, topical estrogen, and systemic corticosteroids

*Vaginoscopy: With the availability of fiberoptics, visualization of the full length of the vagina can be performed with only a 3- to 5-mm-diameter instrument. A hysteroscope or cystoscope with saline as the distending medium is ideal. In a cooperative child, fiberoptic vaginoscopy can be accomplished in the office. A nasal speculum can be substituted, if necessary, during examination of prepubertal girls under anesthesia.

DES, diethylstilbestrol; EUA, examination under anesthesia; TCA, trichloroacetic acid; URI, upper respiratory infection.

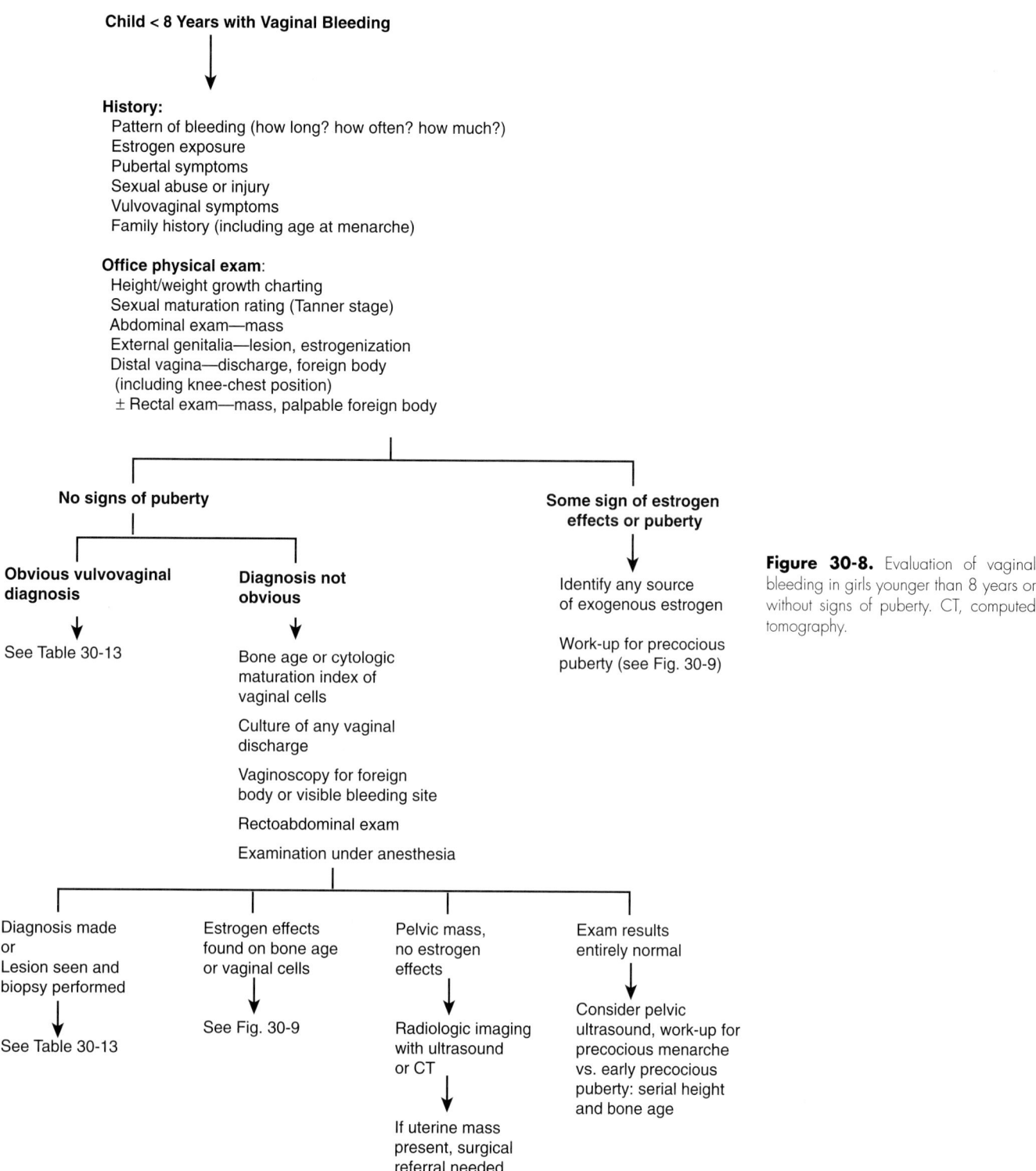

Figure 30-8. Evaluation of vaginal bleeding in girls younger than 8 years or without signs of puberty. CT, computed tomography.

considered a rare form of incomplete precocious puberty. In these children, there is a small increase in serum estrogen levels that does not lead to short stature. Gonadotropin levels are prepubertal. After other sources of vaginal bleeding are ruled out by examination with anesthesia and vaginoscopy, growth rate and/or bone age can be monitored over months to ensure that menstruation was not an early sign of precocious puberty. In precocious menarche, normal adult height and fertility are achieved.

Complete Precocious Puberty

In complete precocious puberty, more than one manifestation of puberty has occurred. Growth acceleration and breast development may precede uterine bleeding, but the sequence of pubertal events may be disordered, with uterine bleeding as the initial finding. Adrenarche may or may not coexist. The menstrual bleeding may be

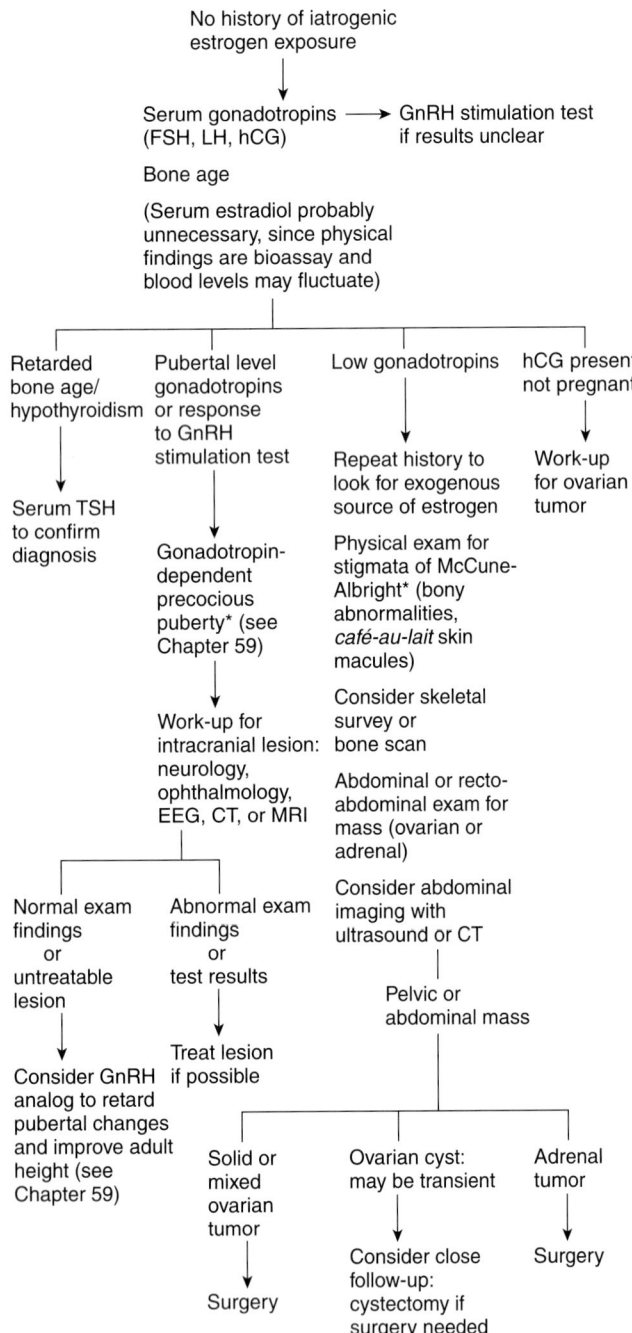

*Follicular cysts are often found with true precocious puberty and with McCune-Albright syndrome. Surgical treatment is not effective at ameliorating pubertal development in these syndromes.

Figure 30-9. Evaluation of uterine bleeding in a child with estrogen effects or other pubertal findings. CT, computed tomography; EEG, electroencephalography; FSH, follicle-stimulating hormone; GnRH, gonadotropin-releasing hormone; hCG, human chorionic gonadotropin; LH, luteinizing hormone; MRI, magnetic resonance imaging; TSH, thyroid-stimulating hormone.

anovulatory or ovulatory. Causes of complete precocious puberty (see Chapter 59) are as follows:

1. central or gonadotropin-dependent precocious puberty
2. peripheral or gonadotropin-independent pseudoprecocious puberty
   a. exogenous estrogen

b. estrogen-secreting tumors of the ovary or adrenal gland
   c. apparent autonomous function of the ovary (McCune-Albright syndrome, follicular cysts of the ovary)
3. gonadotropin and gonadotropin-like molecules (e.g., hCG) not derived from maturation of the HPO axis
4. mixed peripheral and central precocious puberty

Other Causes of Uterine Bleeding in Children

Uterine malignancy is extremely rare in children. Findings include no secondary sexual characteristics and irregular bleeding whose source is in the uterus. A preliminary diagnosis is made from abdominal or rectal examination, hysteroscopic examination with the patient under general anesthesia, or ultrasonography. Full staging and treatment are carried out according to oncology protocol.

EVALUATION (see Figs. 30-8 and 30-9)

History

The history is used to differentiate vulvovaginal from uterine causes of bleeding. The pattern of bleeding (how long, how often, how much), previous vulvovaginal symptoms or trauma, and any possibility of sexual abuse must be addressed. Evidence of estrogen effects, including growth spurt, known estrogen exposure, and family history of precocious puberty, should be sought.

Physical Examination

The general physical examination includes height, weight, sexual maturation rating (formerly known as Tanner staging) with particular attention to breast budding, and abdominal examination. External genitalia should be visualized in the frog-leg position, which can be done with the patient semisitting on an examination table, in stirrups, or in the parent's lap. Vulvar lesions are noted. Is there evidence of estrogen effect? Is there vaginal discharge of fluid, pus, or blood? The knee-chest position may allow better visualization of the vaginal walls. Specimens for culture, if indicated by signs of vaginitis, can be obtained by small calcium alginate swab (Calgiswab), by nonbacteriostatic saline lavage with an eyedropper, or by the catheter-within-a-catheter technique of Pokorny. Cotton swabs are abrasive as they pass through the hymen and should be avoided. The rectoabdominal examination can assess for a pelvic mass. Further examination and testing are determined by findings.

The genital examination can be frightening for children. Time spent developing rapport, engendering the child's trust, and assuring the child (truthfully) that she can stop the examination at any time pays off when the examination is completed. The examiner should give as much control as possible, such as letting the child choose who will be in the room and decide whether she wants to climb up to the table or be lifted by her parent. Sometimes an adequate result can be obtained with the girl herself separating the labia and keeping the examiner's hands off. Physicians need to reinforce for her that when it comes to her private parts, "no means no," even in the doctor's office. That said, distraction often works well. If the child is not able to allow an office examination, she can be examined under sedation or anesthesia, if necessary.

Summary and Things Not to Miss

In the list of causes of vulvovaginal bleeding, the most concerning possibilities include malignancy and sexual abuse. Both diagnoses require a high index of suspicion and may mandate persistence on the part of the evaluator.

When bleeding is uterine, the cause of the endometrial hormonal stimulation is most important. If the source of hormones cannot be eliminated, attention must be turned to ameliorating peripheral effects of early sex steroid exposure.

REFERENCES

Normal and Abnormal Menstrual Bleeding in the Adolescent

Gordon CM: Adolescent gynecology, part I—Common disorders: Menstrual disorders in adolescents: Excess androgens and polycystic ovary syndrome. Pediatr Clin North Am. 1999;46:519.

Kadir RA, Economides DL, Sabin CA, et al: Assessment of menstrual blood loss and gynaecological problems in patients with inherited bleeding disorders. Haemophilia. 1999;5:40.

Mitan LAP, Slap GB: Adolescent medicine: Adolescent menstrual disorders. Med Clinics North Am 2000;84:851.

Speroff L, Glass RH, Kase NG: Dysfunctional uterine bleeding. In: Clinical Gynecologic Endocrinology and Infertility, 6th ed. Baltimore, Lippincott Williams & Wilkins, 1999, p 575.

Speroff L, Glass RH, Kase NG: Oral contraception. In: Clinical Gynecologic Endocrinology and Infertility, 6th ed. Baltimore, Lippincott Williams & Wilkins, 1999, p 867.

Speroff L, Glass RH, Kase NG: Regulation of the menstrual cycle. In: Clinical Gynecologic Endocrinology and Infertility, 6th ed. Baltimore, Lippincott Williams & Wilkins, 1999, p 201.

Amenorrhea

Aiman J, Smentek C: Premature ovarian failure. Obstet Gynecol 1985;66:9.

Byrne J, Fears TR, Gail MH, et al: Early menopause in long-term survivors of cancer during adolescence. Am J Obstet Gynecol 1992;166:788.

Coney PJ: Effect of vaginal agenesis on the adolescent: Prognosis for normal sexual and psychological adjustment. Adolesc Pediatr Gynecol 1992;5:8.

Glueck CJ, Wang P, Fontaine R, et al: Metformin to restore normal menses in oligo-amenorrheic teenage girls with polycystic ovary syndrome (PCOS). J Adolesc Health 2001;29:160.

Neinstein LS, Castle G: Congenital absence of the vagina. Am J Dis Child 1983;137:669.

Reindollar RH, Byrd JR, McDonough PG: Delayed sexual development: A study of 252 patients. Am J Obstet Gynecol 1981;140:371.

Russell JB, Mitchell D, Musey PI, et al: The relationship of exercise to anovulatory cycles in female athletes: Hormonal and physical characteristics. Obstet Gynecol 1984;63:452.

Sabatini S: The female athlete triad. Am J Med Sci 2001;322:193.

Speroff L, Glass RH, Kase NG: Amenorrhea. In: Clinical Gynecologic Endocrinology and Infertility, 6th ed. Baltimore, Lippincott Williams & Wilkins, 1999, p 421.

Speroff L, Glass RH, Kase NG: Anovulation and the polycystic ovary. In: Clinical Gynecologic Endocrinology and Infertility, 6th ed. Baltimore, Lippincott Williams & Wilkins, 1999, p 487.

Dysmenorrhea

Bevan JA, Maloney KW, Hillery CA, et al: Bleeding disorders: A common cause of menorrhagia in adolescents. J Pediatr 2001;138:856.

Davis AR, Westhoff CL: Primary dysmenorrhea in adolescent girls and treatment with oral contraceptives. J Pediatr Adolesc Gynecol 2001;14:3.

Klein JR, Litt IF: Epidemiology of adolescent dysmenorrhea. Pediatrics 1981;68:661.

Laufer MR, Groitein L, Bush M, et al: Prevalence of endometriosis in adolescent girls with chronic pelvic pain not responding to conventional therapy. J Pediatr Adolesc Gynecol. 1997;10:199.

Ling FW: Randomized controlled trial of depot leuprolide in patients with chronic pelvic pain and clinically suspected endometriosis. Pelvic Pain Study Group. Obstet Gynecol 1999;93:51.

Proctor ML, Roberts H, Farquhar CM: Combined oral contraceptive pill (OCP) as treatment for primary dysmenorrhoea. Cochrane Database Syst Rev 2001;(4):CD002120.

Schroeder B, Sanfilippo, JS: Adolescent gynecology, part I—Common disorders: Dysmenorrhea and pelvic pain in adolescents. Pediatr Clin North Am 1999;46:555.

Smith RP: Pressure-velocity analysis of uterine muscle during spontaneous dysmenorrheic contractions in vivo. Am J Obstet Gynecol 1989;160:1400.

Speroff L, Glass RH, Kase NG: Menstrual disorders. In: Clinical Gynecologic Endocrinology and Infertility, 6th ed. Baltimore, Lippincott Williams & Wilkins, 1999, p 557.

Speroff L, Glass RH, Kase NG: Oral contraception. In: Clinical Gynecologic Endocrinology and Infertility, 6th ed. Baltimore, Lippincott Williams & Wilkins, 1999, p 867.

Zhang WY, Li Wan Po A: Efficacy of minor analgesics in primary dysmenorrhoea: A systematic review. Br J Obstet Gynaecol 1998;105:780.

Vaginal Bleeding in the Prepubertal Child

Eberlein WR, Bongiovanni AM, Jones IT, et al: Ovarian tumors and cysts associated with sexual precocity. Pediatrics 1960;57:484.

Friedrich WN, Grambsch P, Broughton D, et al: Normative sexual behavior in children. Pediatrics 1991;88:456.

Herman-Giddens ME: Vaginal foreign bodies and child sexual abuse. Arch Pediatr Adolesc Med 1994;148:195.

Hill NCW, Oppenheimer LW, Morton KE: The aetiology of vaginal bleeding in children: A 20-year review. Br J Obstet Gynaecol 1989;96:467.

Imai A, Horibe S, Tamaya T: Genital bleeding in premenarcheal children. Int J Gynaecol Obstet 1995;49:41.

Kellogg ND, Parra JM, Menard S: Children with anogenital symptoms and signs referred for sexual abuse evaluations. Arch Pediatr Adolesc Med 1998;152:634.

Lyon AJ, DeBruyn R, Grant DB: Transient sexual precocity and ovarian cysts. Arch Dis Child 1985;60:819.

Merritt DF: Evaluation of vaginal bleeding in the preadolescent child. Semin Pediatr Surg 1998;7:35.

Paradise JE, Willis ED: Probability of vaginal foreign body in girls with genital complaints. Am J Dis Child 1985;139:472.

Perlman SE: Management quandary. Premenarchal vaginal bleeding. J Pediatr Adolesc Gynecol 2001;14:135.

Pokorny SF: Prepubertal vulvovaginopathies. Obstet Gynecol Clin North Am 1992;19:39.

Richardson DA, Hajj SN, Herbst AL: Medical treatment of urethral prolapse in children. Obstet Gynecol 1982;59:69.

Root AW: Precocious puberty. Pediatr Rev 2000;21:10.

31 Ambiguous Genitalia

Jack S. Elder

The infant with ambiguous genitalia presents a challenge in diagnosis and management for the physician and parent. Questions of diagnosis and management have profound and lifelong implications for the patient and family. Advances in genetics, endocrinology, and surgical techniques have enabled earlier diagnosis as well as improved treatment.

EMBRYOLOGY

All embryos possess indifferent internal and external genital structures that will feminize unless they are acted on by a masculine influence. Sexual characteristics emerge from common bipotential precursors, and errors are possible at each stage of development.

Normal sexual differentiation is the result of a series of well-regulated steps (Figs. 31-1 to 31-3). Initially, the indifferent gonad forms on the genital ridges at 3 to 5 weeks' gestation. Chromosomal information dictates whether a gonad will differentiate into a testis or an ovary.

The sex-determining Y (SRY) gene, which codes for the *testis-determining factor,* is located on the short arm of the Y chromosome (see Fig. 31-3). The testis-determining factor causes the primordial germ cells to become organized into testicular cords starting in the sixth week of gestation. The SRY gene sequentially affects autosomal genes to induce Sertoli cell development in the bipotential primordial gonad. By the ninth week, Leydig cells are formed and testosterone production begins.

An ovary forms in the presence of two X chromosomes. Both X chromosomes appear to be active in the germ cell and oocyte from the onset of meiosis to ovulation. In the formation of an ovary, the primitive cords break up into cell clusters that give rise to the ovarian medulla, and in the seventh week of gestation, the surface epithelium gives rise to cortical cords, which eventually develop into follicular cells in the fourth month of gestation. In XX embryos, the medullary cords regress.

The fetal gonads dictate the development of the genital ducts (see Fig. 31-1). At the seventh week of gestation, the fetus has indifferent mesonephric (wolffian) and paramesonephric (müllerian) ducts. These structures complete their development during the third month. In the male embryo, testosterone secreted by the Leydig cells of the fetal testes diffuses into the target cells and binds to a cytoplasmic receptor. Under the influence of local testosterone, the wolffian duct becomes the epididymis, the vas deferens, the seminal vesicle, and the ejaculatory duct (see Fig. 31-1). The testosterone diffuses into the target cells and binds to a cytoplasmic receptor. This receptor-testosterone complex stimulates the differentiation of the wolffian duct structures. The Sertoli cells in the fetal testes secrete müllerian-inhibiting substance (MIS), also termed *antimüllerian hormone*. The remnants of the müllerian duct in the male fetus are the appendix testis (a short stalk-like structure on the upper pole of the testis) and the prostatic utricle (a tiny diverticulum in the prostatic urethra).

In the female embryo, the absence of MIS production allows the müllerian ducts to develop into the fallopian tubes, the uterus, and the upper third of the vagina (see Fig. 31-1). In the absence of testosterone, the vestigial wolffian duct structures remain as the Gartner duct and the epoophoron and paroophoron.

The external genitalia start developing via a common pathway from the cloacal folds in the third week of gestation, modifying into the urogenital sinus, the genital tubercle, the urethral folds, and the genital (labioscrotal) swellings (see Fig. 31-2). Dihydrotestosterone (DHT) is the active hormone that stimulates the development of the male external genitalia. Testosterone is converted into DHT by the 5α-reductase enzyme, which is present in cells in the urogenital sinus. Intracellular DHT binds to the androgen receptor, causing the genital tubercle and the urethral plate to elongate into the phallus. By the third month of gestation, the urethral folds fuse in the midline to form the urethra, and the genital swellings fuse to form the scrotum.

Female external genitalia differentiate in the absence of DHT. The genital tubercle forms the clitoris, the genital swellings become the labia majora, and the urethral folds become the labia minora (see Fig. 31-2). The vagina is formed from the urogenital sinus.

By the 15th week of gestation, differentiation of the external genitalia is complete. The male genitalia continue to enlarge throughout the second and third trimesters.

CLASSIFICATION OF INTERSEX DISORDERS

Sexual differentiation is a well-regulated sequence of events. Developmentally, chromosomal sex determines gonadal sex, which then determines phenotypic sex.

A straightforward organizational scheme for intersex disorders is based on the histologic features of the gonads (Table 31-1). The five possible classifications are female pseudohermaphroditism, male pseudohermaphroditism, mixed gonadal dysgenesis, true hermaphroditism, and gonadal dysgenesis (Table 31-2).

A patient with an intersex disorder may have ambiguous genitalia, normal-appearing external genitalia (female or male), or a minor abnormality such as hypospadias and an undescended testis.

EVALUATION

The child with ambiguous genitalia should be evaluated by a team consisting of a geneticist (dysmorphologist), pediatric endocrinologist, pediatric urologist, and ethicist (Fig. 31-4). Decisions regarding the evaluation, gender assignment, and long-term management need to be made jointly on the basis of the diagnosis and the future potential for successful sexual function.

HISTORY AND PHYSICAL EXAMINATION

A thorough history taking and physical examination must be performed, with full attention given to the history of the pregnancy, the family history, and the pedigree. Identically afflicted relatives should be identified, but more subtle signs must not be missed.

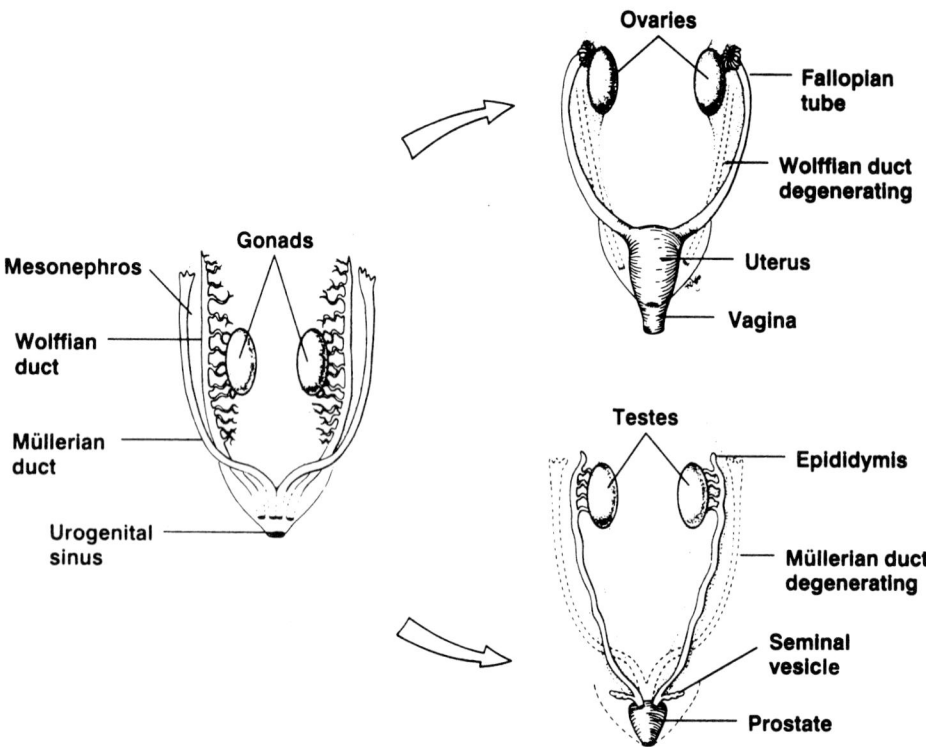

Figure 31-1. *Development of the internal genitalia from the indifferent stage. (From Rubenstein SC, Mandell J: The diagnostic approach to the newborn with ambiguous genitalia. Contemp Urol 1994;6:13. Reprinted with permission from Natalie Johnson.)*

Sudden infant death, infertility, amenorrhea, hirsutism, and variant forms of sexual development in any relative should be investigated. The mother should be questioned about any medication, especially hormones, taken during pregnancy.

On physical examination, the genitalia should be meticulously examined and documented; one important finding is a gonad located in the scrotum or the labioscrotal fold. Any phenotypically male infant with bilateral nonpalpable testes or subcoronal hypospadias and cryptorchidism should undergo full evaluation. Rectal examination may disclose a cervix. Other potential findings include hyperpigmentation of the areola and labioscrotal folds (congenital adrenal hyperplasia [CAH]), palpation of the uterus as a thickened structure, hypertension, signs of dehydration and failure to thrive, and associated congenital anomalies.

DIAGNOSTIC STUDIES

Laboratory analysis provides an important tool for the evaluation and treatment of these conditions. An initial study is a karyotype determination. Testing of multiple tissues (blood lymphocytes, skin fibroblasts) may be necessary if chromosomal mosaicism is suspected. The finding of Barr bodies in a buccal smear may be inaccurate in the newborn, and this evaluation is generally not obtained.

If the gonads are nonpalpable, the serum 17-hydroxyprogesterone level should be measured (Fig. 31-5). Serial serum electrolyte levels should also be determined because the most common cause of intersex disorder, CAH (from 21-hydroxylase deficiency), may result in life-threatening salt wasting (hyponatremia, hyperkalemia, acidosis). Steroid profiles, such as testosterone, androstenedione, adrenocorticotropic hormone (ACTH), plasma renin, and 11-deoxycortisol determinations, are necessary on occasion.

Voiding cystourethrography and retrograde genitography determine whether the uterus, cervix, and vagina are present. Abdominopelvic ultrasonography should be performed to study the pelvic organs for the presence of a uterus and the inguinal area for the presence of gonads (testes or ovotestes) and for the size and presence of the kidneys and adrenal glands. If the bladder is empty during the study,

it should be filled by means of a small feeding tube to allow visualization of the pelvic structures. Inability to discern the cervix or vagina by radiography does not exclude their existence. Endoscopy, cystourethroscopy, and vaginoscopy allow more complete examination of the genitalia, and if these tests are performed with contrast material under fluoroscopic control, the anatomy may be defined more accurately.

Exploratory laparotomy (or laparoscopy) and gonadal biopsy are used in selected cases to confirm the gonadal histologic and morphologic features of the wolffian and müllerian duct structures to aid in the assignment of sex. At the time of exploration, gonadal tissue at high risk for malignant degeneration may be removed if necessary. Laparotomy and biopsy are indicated if the results will affect the sex of rearing or if there is a risk of gonadal malignancy in the future.

FEMALE PSEUDOHERMAPHRODITISM

Female pseudohermaphroditism is the condition of a person with a 46,XX karyotype who is partially virilized; it is the most common intersex disorder. The ovaries and müllerian derivatives are normally developed, and sexual ambiguity is limited to the external genitalia. Because patients with this disorder have normal internal structures, they are potentially fertile. The timing of intrauterine exposure to androgen determines the severity of the masculinization. If the differentiating external genitalia are exposed to androgens, there may be complete labioscrotal fusion and possibly a phallic urethra. In contrast, androgen exposure primarily during the second and third trimesters causes only clitoral hypertrophy.

The most common cause of genital ambiguity in the newborn is one form of CAH, the frequency of which is estimated to be 1 in 14,000 births of white infants (Table 31-3). CAH results from a deficiency in the activity of one of the enzymes required for cortisol biosynthesis (Table 31-4; see also Fig. 31-5).

Cholesterol is the building block for adrenal hormone synthesis. Through a series of enzymatic reactions, cholesterol is converted to cortisol, aldosterone, and sex hormones (see Fig. 31-5). CAH is caused

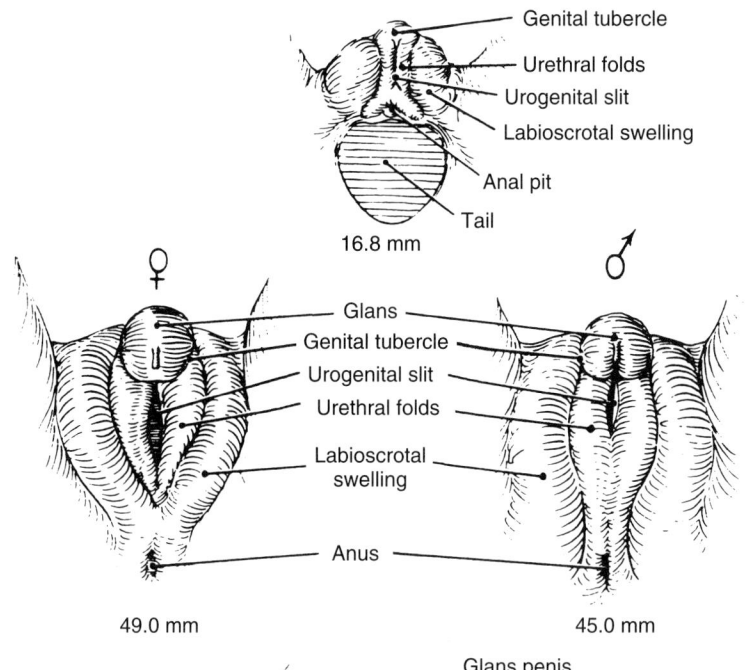

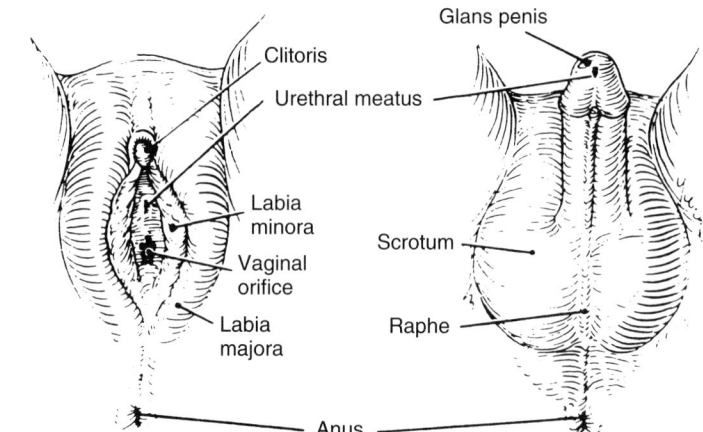

Figure 31-2. Differentiation of male and female external genitalia from indifferent primordia. (From Grumbach MM, Conte FA: Disorders of sex determination. In Wilson JD, Foster DW [eds]: Williams Textbook of Endocrinology. Philadelphia, WB Saunders 1998.)

by a deficiency of an enzyme in this pathway, resulting in decreased synthesis of the desired hormone and an elevated ACTH level, secondary to reduced cortisol feedback on the fetal hypothalamic-pituitary-adrenal axis. The elevated ACTH level causes an overproduction of the precursors of cortisol proximal to the enzyme deficiency, which are then transformed to various androgens, including dehydroepiandrosterone, androstenedione, and androstenediol.

CAH is an autosomal recessive disorder. Girls and boys are affected in equal frequencies. However, genital ambiguity occurs primarily in girls. The condition in boys is not discovered at birth unless the boys experience a salt-losing crisis, are identified by universal state-wide postnatal screening tests, are identified through prenatal screening performed because of the birth of an affected sibling, or have one of the less common enzyme defects. Precocious puberty develops in untreated boys with CAH.

CAH is the only intersex disorder that can be life-threatening if untreated. More than 90% of the cases are a result of a deficiency of the enzyme 21-hydroxylase, whereas deficiency of the 11β-hydroxylase enzyme accounts for another 5% of cases. Less common are deficiencies of the enzymes 3β-hydroxysteroid dehydrogenase, 17α-hydroxylase, and desmolase (see Table 31-3).

A 21-hydroxylase deficiency may be mild or severe. The severe or "salt-wasting" type of 21-hydroxylase deficiency is a life-threatening disease and manifests with impaired secretion of cortisol and aldosterone, resulting in anorexia, vomiting, hyponatremia, hyperkalemia,

acidosis, dehydration, and circulatory collapse. This usually occurs after the fifth day of life. The more severe the enzymatic defect, the more masculine the phenotype is (Figs. 31-6 and 31-7). There is also a "simple virilizing" type of CAH with normal aldosterone biosynthesis and a mild "nonclassic" form in which the infant is asymptomatic, but androgen excess develops during childhood or at puberty.

Other causes of *adrenal insufficiency* with or without intersex signs in infancy and childhood are noted in Table 31-5; manifestations are noted in Table 31-6.

The second most common cause of CAH, 11β-hydroxylase deficiency, results in decreased production of cortisol and corticosterone and increased production of desoxycorticosterone, a steroid with a salt-retaining effect. There is marked heterogeneity in the clinical and hormonal manifestations of this autosomal recessive disorder. Typically, affected girls present with ambiguous genitalia at birth and may become hypertensive either in infancy or later in childhood. Affected boys appear normal at birth, but hypertension and precocious puberty develop. There is no salt-wasting component to the classic form of this syndrome, but in rare cases, gene mutations result in a salt-wasting form of the condition.

Other enzyme deficiencies that lead to CAH include deficiencies of 3β-hydroxysteroid dehydrogenase, 17α-hydroxylase, and desmolase. These conditions do not cause female pseudohermaphroditism; girls with these conditions are not virilized.

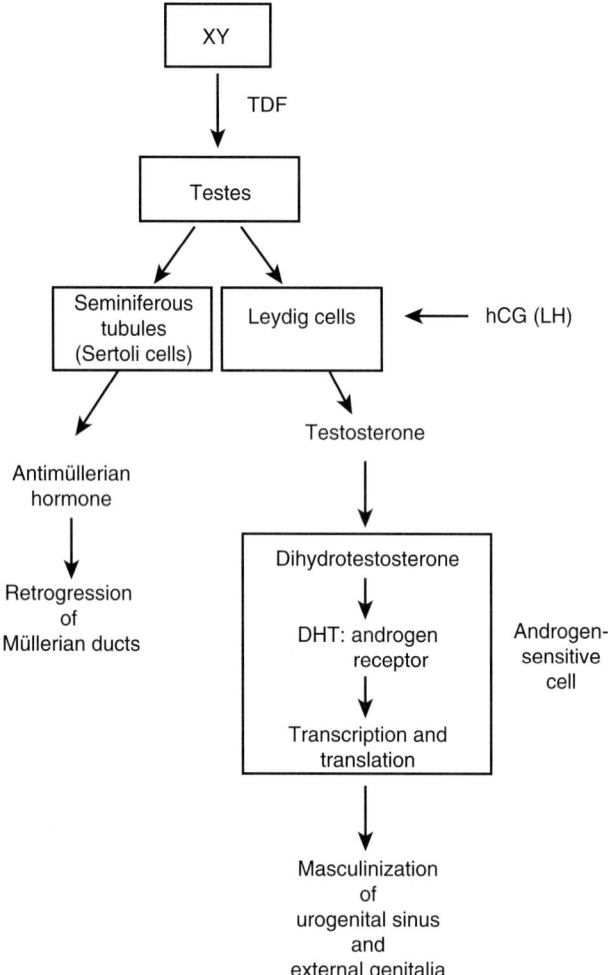

Figure 31-3. A diagrammatic scheme of male sex determination and differentiation. DHT, dihydrotestosterone; hCG, human chorionic gonadotropin; LH, luteinizing hormone; TDF, testis determining factor. (From Wilson JD, Foster DW [eds]: Williams Textbook of Endocrinology. 8th ed. Philadelphia, WB Saunders, 1992, p 918.)

Table 31-1. Classification of Intersex Disorders

Disorder	Gonads	Karyotype
Female pseudohermaphroditism	Ovaries only	46,XX
Male pseudohermaphroditism	Testicles only	46,XY
True hermaphroditism	Ovarian and testicular tissue Ovary and testis Ovotestis and testis Ovotestis and ovary Two ovotestes	46,XX; 46,XY; and mosaic
Mixed gonadal dysgenesis	Testis and streak gonad	45,XO/46,XY with mosaicism
Pure gonadal dysgenesis	Streak gonads only	46,XX or 46,XY or 45,XO

severity of the enzyme deficit. Any phenotypically male neonate with nonpalpable testes should be evaluated for CAH.

In full-term newborns with a 21-hydroxylase deficiency, serum levels of 17-hydroxyprogesterone are typically elevated, ranging from 3000 to 40,000 ng/dL (normal, 100 to 200 ng/dL); in those with mild forms, the level is at the upper limit of normal. In premature infants, 17-hydroxyprogesterone levels may be normally elevated (false positive). Measurement of urinary 17-ketosteroid and pregnanetriol level is not usually performed. Salt-losing patients often have hyponatremia and hyperkalemia on a regular or low-salt diet. In newborns with the 11-hydroxylase deficiency, plasma 11-deoxycortisol and 11-deoxycorticosterone levels are elevated. Radiologic evaluation includes a pelvic ultrasound study to try to identify a uterus and ovaries, an inguinal ultrasound study to try to identify gonads (testes, if present, indicate that the patient does not have CAH), and an adrenal ultrasound study, because 50% of neonates with CAH have adrenal glands that are enlarged or at the upper limit of normal in size.

TREATMENT

Initial management is directed at correcting or preventing hypoglycemia, hyponatremia, hyperkalemia, hypovolemia, and shock. In addition to saline infusion and correction of electrolyte abnormalities, hydrocortisone therapy is started. When the child is stabilized and receiving appropriate doses of glucocorticoids and mineralocorticoids, surgical management is considered. The procedure, termed *feminizing genitoplasty,* involves (1) clitoroplasty, in which the erectile tissue of the clitoris is removed, preserving normal clitoral sensation, and (2) vaginoplasty, in which the lower vagina is exteriorized (see Fig. 31-7).

PRENATAL SCREENING

The 21-hydroxylase deficiency is an autosomal recessive condition; consequently, there is a 25% risk that a sibling of an affected child will have CAH. The gene for CAH is linked with the human leukocyte antigen class I and class II genes. DNA probes for these genes can be used to define the sequences associated with CAH. If genetic material can be obtained from the embryo or fetus (by chorionic villus biopsy at 10 weeks' gestation) with an affected sibling before the external genitalia have completely developed, treatment may be

Another cause of female pseudohermaphroditism is excessive androgen production by the mother, which occurs with adrenal or ovarian tumors or human chorionic gonadotropin (hCG)–dependent luteoma of pregnancy.

EVALUATION

Patients with CAH and ambiguous genitalia are genetically female with normal ovaries (Table 31-7). The karyotype is 46,XX. Because there is no production of testosterone or MIS by the male gonads, the wolffian structures are absent, and the development of the fallopian tubes, the uterus, and the upper vagina is normal. Only the development of the external genitalia is affected in such patients. Examination of girls with the 21-hydroxylase or 11-hydroxylase enzyme deficiency reveals variable degrees of virilization. With the mildest forms, there is simply clitoral hypertrophy and a normally positioned vagina; in the most severe forms, there is complete labioscrotal fusion, a long phallus with a urethral opening at its tip, and a high insertion of the vagina on the urethra (see Figs. 31-6 and 31-7). The gonads are nonpalpable because the ovaries do not descend into the inguinal canal or labia unless an inguinal hernia is present. The severity of the virilization effect is directly proportional to the

Table 31-2. Etiologic Classification of Hermaphroditism

Female Pseudohermaphroditism

Androgen exposure
  Fetal source
    21-Hydroxylase (P450 c21) deficiency
    11β-Hydroxylase (P450 c11) deficiency
    3β-Hydroxysteroid dehydrogenase II (3β-HSD II)
      deficiency
    Aromatase (P450$_{arom}$) deficiency
  Maternal source
    Virilizing ovarian tumor
    Virilizing adrenal tumor
    Androgenic drugs
  Undetermined origin
    Associated with genitourinary and gastrointestinal tract
      defects

Male Pseudohermaphroditism

Defects in testicular differentiation
  Denys-Drash syndrome (mutation in WT1 gene)
  WAGR syndrome (*W*ilms tumor, *a*niridia, *g*enitourinary
    malformation, *r*etardation)
    Deletion of 11p13
  Camptomelic syndrome (autosomal gene at 17q24.3-q25.1)
    and SOX 9 mutation
  XY pure gonadal dysgenesis (Swyer syndrome)
    Mutation in SRY gene
    Unknown cause
  XY gonadal agenesis
Deficiency of testicular hormones
  Leydig cell aplasia
  Mutation in LH receptor
  Lipoid adrenal hyperplasia (P450 scc) deficiency; mutation
    in steroidogenic acute regulatory protein
  3β-HSDII deficiency
  17-Hydroxylase/17,20-lyase (p450 c17) deficiency
  Persistent müllerian duct syndrome
    Gene mutation, müllerian-inhibiting substance (MIS)
    Receptor defects for MIS
Defect in androgen action
  5α-Reductase II mutations
  Androgen receptor defects
    Complete androgen insensitivity syndrome
    Partial androgen insensitivity syndrome
    (Reinfenstein and other syndromes)
  Smith-Lemli-Opitz syndrome
    Defect in conversion of 7-dehydrocholesterol to
      cholesterol

True Hermaphroditism

XX
XY
XX/XY chimeras

From Rapaport R: Hermaphroditism (Intersexuality). In Behrman RE, Kliegman RM, Jenson HB (eds): Nelson Textbook of Pediatrics, 16th ed. Philadelphia, WB Saunders, 2000, p 1760.

given to prevent virilization of the genitalia. If dexamethasone is administered to the mother at 10 weeks' gestation, it will cross the placenta and suppress the overproduction of cortisol precursors. Amniotic fluid can also be assayed for 17-hydroxyprogesterone as a complementary study. The earlier the initiation of dexamethasone therapy, the less likely it is that significant virilization will occur in the fetus with CAH.

Postnatal screening is available in many states and measures 17-hydroxyprogesterone on routine heel stick samples examined for phenylketonuria and other metabolic disorders. This is used primarily to detect salt-losing conditions before affected persons develop an adrenal crisis.

MALE PSEUDOHERMAPHRODITISM

Male pseudohermaphroditism is the condition of a person who is chromosomally male (46,XY) and has normal testes who undergoes incomplete virilization (Table 31-8; see also Table 31-2). The abnormality includes a spectrum of conditions, including failure of target tissue response to testosterone or dihydrosterone, failure of conversion of testosterone to dihydrosterone, a defect in testicular differentiation, a disorder in testosterone synthesis, and a defect in production of MIS.

Some of these conditions do not result in obviously ambiguous genitalia; however, in all cases, sexual differentiation is abnormal.

ANDROGEN RESISTANCE (INSENSITIVITY)

Testicular feminization (complete androgen resistance or insensitivity syndrome) is an X-linked disorder of patients with a 46,XY karyotype who have an abnormality of the androgen receptor, either qualitatively abnormal or at undetectable low levels. During embryonic development, differentiation of the wolffian ducts and virilization of the external genitalia are inhibited, and secretion of MIS causes regression of the müllerian ducts. Consequently, affected individuals have bilateral testes; normal female external genitalia with a short, blind-ending vagina; and wolffian-derived internal duct structures. At puberty, breasts develop, but the patients do not menstruate or develop any pubic or axillary hair.

Diagnosis usually occurs at puberty after evaluation for amenorrhea (see Chapter 30). Androgen resistance results in increased luteinizing hormone secretion, which causes elevated levels of both testosterone and estradiol. The elevated level of estradiol is responsible for breast development. Markedly elevated serum luteinizing hormone and testosterone levels and a 46,XY karyotype establish the diagnosis. The assignment of female sexual identity should be reinforced. The diagnosis of testicular feminization may be made before puberty when a phenotypic girl undergoing hernia repair is found to have an inguinal or labial testis.

Treatment includes bilateral orchiectomy because there is a significant risk of gonadal cancer with age. Estrogen replacement then becomes necessary. If complete androgen resistance is diagnosed in a prepubertal girl, the decision of whether to perform bilateral gonadectomy at the time of diagnosis or delay the procedure until pubertal development has occurred is controversial. Because of the underdeveloped müllerian structures, patients are candidates for vaginoplasty, which is usually performed with a segment of large or small bowel.

There is spectrum of X-linked *incomplete* androgen resistance syndromes. Müllerian development does not occur, and wolffian duct derivatives usually are hypoplastic. In these syndromes (Reifenstein, Lubs, Gilbert-Dreyfus), development of the external genitalia is variable and ranges from genital ambiguity to severe hypospadias with chordee (ventral penile curvature). The testes are small and are often undescended. Biopsy of the testes reveals azoospermia. At puberty, there is usually poor virilization, absent or sparse axillary and pubic hair, and gynecomastia. Serum luteinizing hormone, testosterone, and estradiol levels are elevated. Gender assignment of these patients depends on their phenotype and gender identity. Some who have a phenotype of a mild virilized female with clitoromegaly choose not to have any reconstructive surgery. Phenotypic boys and men with severe hypospadias and chordee can undergo satisfactory urethral reconstruction and resemble normal boys and men.

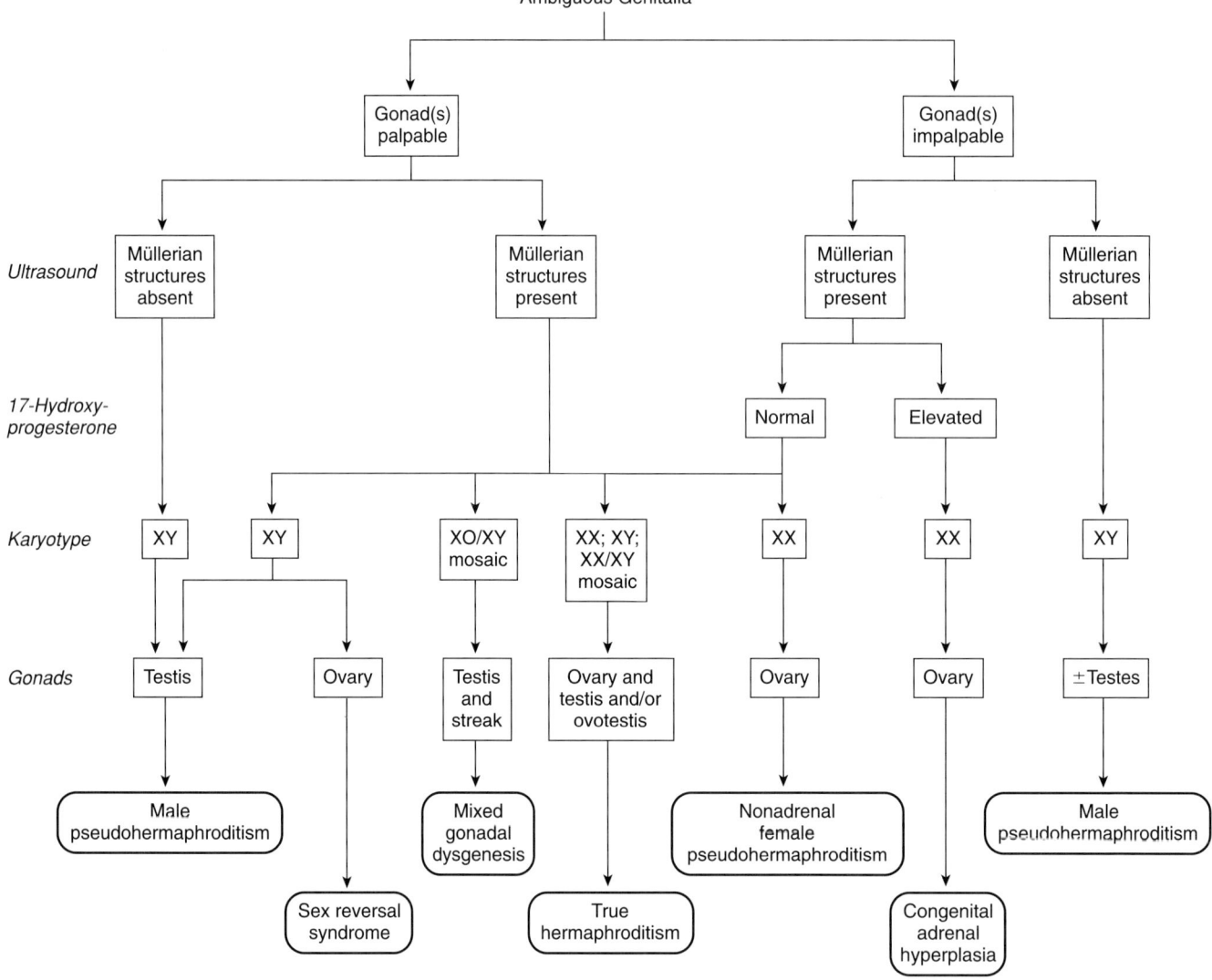

Figure 31-4. Algorithm portraying evaluation of an infant with ambiguous genitalia.

5α-REDUCTASE DEFICIENCY

External genital development in boys is stimulated by the 5α-reduced product of testosterone, DHT (see Fig. 31-3). Boys and men with a 5α-reductase deficiency have a small phallus or ambiguous genitalia with perineoscrotal hypospadias, a bifid scrotum, and inguinal or scrotal/labial testes. Because the testes produce MIS, there is a blind vaginal pouch that opens into the urogenital sinus or urethra. However, the wolffian duct derivatives are present. In untreated patients, at puberty the female phenotype transforms into a masculine phenotype with penile/phallic enlargement, scrotal rugation and pigmentation, enlargement and descent of the testes into the labioscrotal folds, and deepening of the voice. In addition, at puberty gender identity often changes from female to male in untreated individuals.

The diagnosis is suggested by a high testosterone-to-DHT ratio, either under basal conditions or after gonadal stimulation with hCG. Genitography shows wolffian duct structures. Early diagnosis of 5α-reductase deficiency is important for allowing appropriate gender identification.

In many cases, DHT therapy results in significant phallic enlargement, and hypospadias repair can then be performed, which results in a satisfactory male appearance. If the genitalia are clearly female, however, bilateral orchiectomy and estrogen replacement are indicated.

ABNORMAL TESTICULAR DIFFERENTIATION

If testicular differentiation is abnormal, genital development is also often abnormal.

In the *vanishing testis syndrome,* the testes form but involute during gestation. If testicular regression occurs before 8 weeks' gestation, the embryo has no testosterone or MIS, and female external genitalia and müllerian development result. Testicular regression also may occur late in gestation, usually from testicular torsion. In this instance, the individual has a normal phallus but bilateral impalpable testes, and müllerian derivatives are absent. In these patients, the karyotype is 46,XY. Usually, the baseline gonadotropin levels are high, and the testosterone level is low. After a series of hCG injections, the serum testosterone level should rise dramatically in normal boys and men with functioning testes but is unchanged in those with the vanishing testis syndrome.

Although the diagnosis of anorchia can be made by endocrine methods, confirmation with laparoscopy is recommended. Management includes treatment with exogenous testosterone at puberty. Patients with this disorder are sterile.

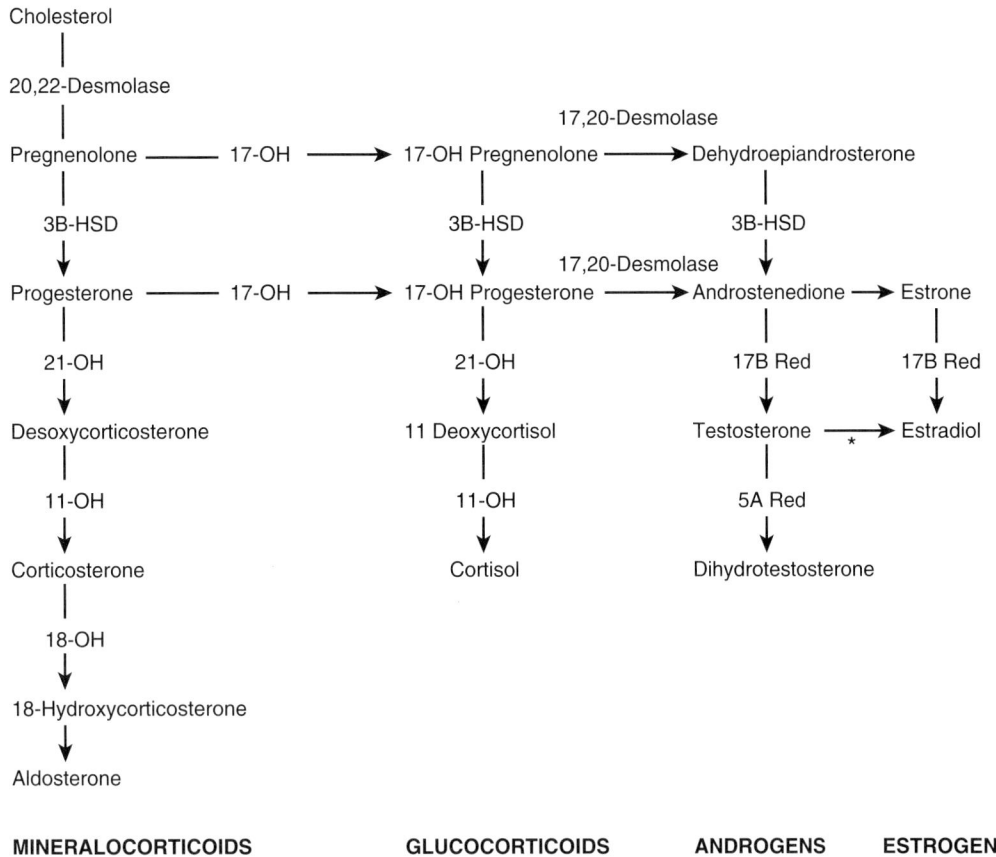

Figure 31-5. Scheme of adrenal steroid biosynthesis. 11-OH, 11β-hydroxylase; 17-OH, 17α-hydroxylase; 18-OH, 18-hydroxylase; 21-OH, 21-hydroxylase; 3B-HSD, 3β-hydroxysteroid dehydrogenase; 17B Red, 17β-reductase; 5A Red, 5α-reductase.

DISORDER OF TESTOSTERONE SYNTHESIS

Five enzymes are involved in the biosynthesis of testosterone: 20,22-desmolase, 3β-hydroxysteroid dehydrogenase, 17α-hydroxylase, 17,20-desmolase, and 17-ketosteroid reductase. The first three enzymes also are involved in the production of corticosteroids; thus, a deficiency of one of these enzymes also causes CAH (see Fig. 31-5).

A defect in *desmolase activity* causes severe adrenal and gonadal insufficiency. Because testosterone is not produced, most affected boys and men have female external genitalia with a blind vaginal pouch, undeveloped wolffian duct derivatives, and no müllerian structures. Sonography demonstrates large, lipid-laden adrenal glands, and the disorder has been termed *congenital lipoid adrenal hyperplasia.* Death from adrenal insufficiency often occurs in infancy. The diagnosis is made by demonstration of low levels of all steroids in urine and plasma and an absent adrenal response to ACTH.

A defect in 3β-hydroxysteroid dehydrogenase results in reduced testosterone production but increased dehydroepiandrosterone production, allowing some virilization of affected boys and men; the typical appearance is severe hypospadias with chordee. In its complete form, deficiencies of aldosterone, cortisol, estradiol, and testosterone occur. The usual presentation is adrenal crisis with severe salt loss, although milder forms have been described. The diagnosis is made by detection of the precursors of aldosterone and cortisol, pregnenolone, 17-hydroxypregnenolone, and dehydroepiandrosterone. Treatment is similar to that of patients with 21-hydroxylase deficiency, except for the need for gonadal steroids at puberty.

A defect in the *17α-hydroxylase enzyme* results in impaired synthesis of 17α-hydroxypregnenolone and 17α-hydroxyprogesterone, which in turn results in impaired synthesis of cortisol and sex steroid. Affected individuals may experience hypertension, hypokalemia, and alkalosis. Because of impaired testosterone synthesis, the external genitalia in affected boys and men show minimal or no virilization. The diagnosis is suspected in 46,XY persons with ambiguous or female genitalia, hypokalemic alkalosis, and hypertension. The diagnosis of 17α-hydroxylase deficiency is confirmed by demonstration of high levels of corticosterone, deoxycorticosterone, progesterone, and pregnenolone, as well as low levels of aldosterone and renin.

A defect in *17,20-desmolase activity* or *17β-hydroxysteroid dehydrogenase* activity causes reduced testosterone secretion and thus ambiguous genitalia in persons with the 46,XY karyotype. They have virilization of the wolffian duct derivatives, and müllerian structures are absent. Inguinal or intraabdominal testes are common. An unusual feature of 17β-hydroxysteroid dehydrogenase deficiency in boys and men is that at puberty significant virilization can occur, often in association with gynecomastia. Affected patients have elevated levels of androstenedione and estrone and low levels of testosterone and estradiol.

In most patients with the 46,XY karyotype and a disorder in testosterone synthesis, the genitalia are female or ambiguous in appearance. If the sex of rearing is decided to be male, early hypospadias repair and orchiopexy are recommended. If a female gender is assigned, however, gonadectomy and clitoroplasty should be performed, and vaginoplasty may be necessary at puberty.

Table 31-3. Diagnosis and Treatment of Congenital Adrenal Hyperplasia

Disorder	Signs and Symptoms	Laboratory	Therapeutic Measures
Lipoid congenital adrenal hyperplasia	Salt-wasting crisis Male pseudohermaphroditism	Low levels of all steroid hormones, with decreased or absent response to ACTH Decreased or absent response to hCG in male pseudohermaphroditism ↑ ACTH ↑ PRA	Glucocorticoid and mineralocorticoid administration Sodium chloride supplementation Gonadectomy of male pseudohermaphrodite Sex hormone replacement consonant with sex of rearing
3β-HSD deficiency	Classic form: Salt-wasting crisis Male and female pseudohermaphroditism Precocious puberty Disordered puberty	↑↑ Baseline and ACTH-stimulated Δ5 steroids (pregnenolone, 17-OH pregnenolone, DHEA, and their urinary metabolites) ↑ ACTH ↑ PRA Suppression of elevated adrenal steroids after glucocorticoid administration	Glucocorticoid and mineralocorticoid administration Sodium chloride supplementation Surgical correction of genitals and sex hormone replacement as necessary consonant with sex of rearing
3β-HSD deficiency	Nonclassic form: Precocious puberty, disordered puberty, menstrual irregularity, hirsutism, acne, infertility	↑ Baseline and ACTH-stimulated Δ5 steroids (pregnenolone, 17-OH pregnenolone, DHEA, and their urinary metabolites) ↑ Δ5/Δ4 serum and urinary steroids Suppression of elevated adrenal steroids after glucocorticoid administration	Glucocorticoid administration
21-OH deficiency	Classic form: Salt-wasting crisis Female pseudohermaphroditism Postnatal virilization	↑↑ Baseline and ACTH-stimulated 17-OH progesterone and pregnanetriol ↑↑ Serum androgens and urinary metabolites ↑ ACTH ↑ PRA Suppression of elevated adrenal steroids after glucocorticoid administration	Glucocorticoid and mineralocorticoid replacement Sodium chloride supplementation Vaginoplasty and clitoral recession in female pseudohermaphroditism
21-OH deficiency	Nonclassic form: Precocious puberty, disordered puberty, menstrual irregularity, hirsutism, acne, infertility	↑ Baseline and ACTH-stimulated 17-OH progesterone and pregnanetriol ↑ Serum androgens and urinary metabolites Suppression of elevated adrenal steroids after glucocorticoid administration	Glucorticoid administration
11β-Hydroxylase deficiency	Classic form: Female pseudohermaphroditism Postnatal virilization in boys and girls Hypertension	↑↑ Baseline and ACTH-stimulated compound S and DOC and their urinary metabolites ↑↑ Serum androgens and their urinary metabolites ↑ ACTH ↓ PRA Hypokalemia Suppression of elevated steroids after glucocorticoid administration	Glucocorticoid administration Vaginoplasty and clitoral recession in female pseudohermaphroditism
11β-Hydroxylase deficiency	Nonclassic form: Precocious puberty, disordered puberty, menstrual irregularity, hirsutism, acne, infertility	↑ Baseline and ACTH-stimulated compound S and DOC and their urinary metabolites ↑ Serum androgens and their urinary metabolites Suppression of elevated steroids after glucocorticoid administration	Glucocorticoid administration
17α-OH/17,20-lyase deficiency	Male pseudohermaphroditism Sexual infantilism Hypertension	↑↑ DOC, 18-OH DOC, corticosterone, 18-hydroxycorticosterone Low 17-α-hydroxylated steroids and poor response to ACTH Poor response to hCG in male pseudohermaphroditism ↓ PRA ↑ ACTH Hypokalemia Suppression of elevated adrenal steroids after glucocorticoid administration	Glucocorticoid administration Surgical correction of genitals and sex hormone replacement in male pseudohermaphroditism with sex of rearing Sex hormone replacement in female pseudohermaphroditism

Adapted from Miller WL, Levine LS: Molecular and clinical advances in congenital adrenal hyperplasia. J Pediatr 1987;111:1. From Behrman RE, Kliegman RM, Jenson HB (eds): Nelson Textbook of Pediatrics, 16th ed. Philadelphia, WB Saunders, 2000, p 1731.

ACTH, adrenocorticotropic hormone (corticotropin); DHEA, dehydroepiandrosterone; DOC, deoxycorticosterone; hCG, human chorionic gonadotropin; HSD, hydroxysteroid dehydrogenase; PRA, plasma renin activity.

↑, increased; ↑↑, greatly increased; ↓, decreased.

Table 31-4. Causes of Virilization in Girls	
Condition	Additional Features
P-450 C_{21} deficiency (21-hydroxylase)	Salt loss in some
3β-Hydroxysteroid dehydrogenase deficiency	Salt loss
P-450 C_{11} deficiency (11β-hydroxylase)	Salt retention/hypertension
Androgenic drug exposure (e.g., progestins)	Exposure by 12th wk of gestation
Mixed gonadal dysgenesis*	Karyotype: 45,X/46,XY
True hermaphrodite	Testicular and ovarian tissue present
Maternal virilizing adrenal or ovarian tumor	Rare; positive history
Idiopathic	Unknown cause

Adapted from Styne DM: Endocrine disorders. In Behrman RE, Kliegman RM (eds): Nelson Essentials of Pediatrics. 2nd ed. Philadelphia, WB Saunders, 1994, p 636.

*Or mosaic Turner syndrome.

PERSISTENT MÜLLERIAN DUCT SYNDROME

Also termed *hernia uteri inguinale,* persistent müllerian duct syndrome is an X-linked condition that results from a defect in the production of MIS, an abnormality in the secretion of MIS, or a lack of response by the müllerian duct to MIS. This form of male pseudohermaphroditism does not cause ambiguous genitalia. The typical presentation is an infant or child with an inguinal hernia and cryptorchidism in whom routine exploration discloses müllerian structures (fallopian tube and uterus) as well as an epididymis and vas. In many cases, transverse testicular ectopia is present.

Treatment includes removal of the müllerian structures; care must be taken not to injure the wolffian duct derivatives.

MIXED GONADAL DYSGENESIS

Mixed gonadal dysgenesis is the second most common cause of ambiguous genitalia in newborns. Most affected patients have chromosomal mosaicism with a 45,XO/46,XY karyotype. Nearly all have incomplete virilization (Fig. 31-8). Patients with a more feminine phenotype typically have genital ambiguity with phallic enlargement, a urogenital sinus, and varying degrees of labioscrotal fusion. Internal genitalia include a unilateral streak gonad; persistent müllerian duct structures (fallopian tube, uterus, and vagina) ipsilateral to the streak; a contralateral testis, which may or may not be undescended; and frequently a fallopian tube on the side of the testis. Individuals with a more feminine phenotype usually have an intraabdominal testis, whereas in those with a more masculine phenotype, the testis is usually inguinal or scrotal. Approximately 33% of patients have somatic stigmata of *Turner syndrome:* a shield-shaped chest, webbed neck, cubitus valgus, multiple pigmented nevi, and short stature. Approximately 60% are reared as girls because of the diminutive phallus, which is usually hypospadiac.

Histologically, the streak gonad is composed of fibrous connective tissue resembling ovarian stroma. The testis lacks germinal elements but at puberty has abundant Leydig and Sertoli cells. Thus, at puberty most patients with a retained testis undergo virilization, and the serum testosterone level is in the normal adult range. It is thought that the incomplete virilization at birth represents delayed development of the testis in utero.

Management depends on several factors. First, the testis lacks germinal elements. Second, most patients have significant hypospadias,

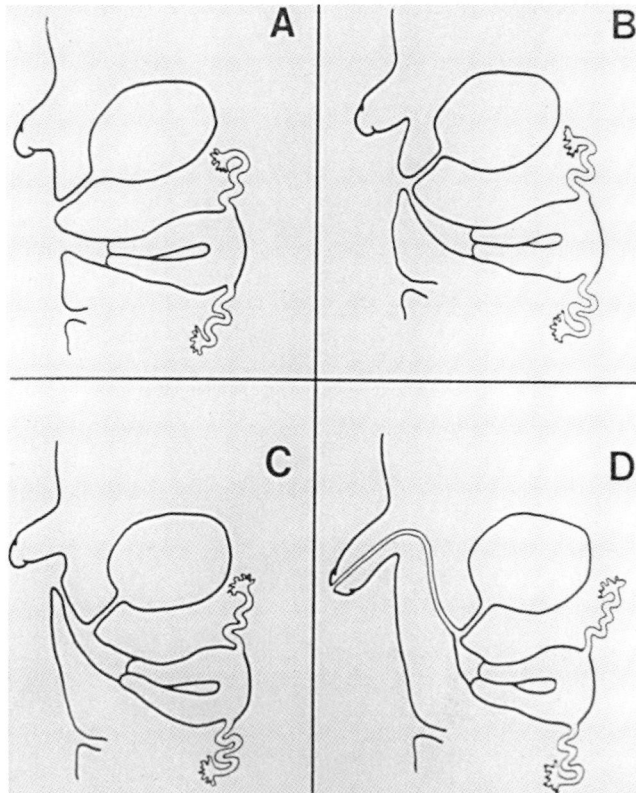

Figure 31-6. Spectrum of external virilization in congenital adrenal hyperplasia. **A,** Clitoromegaly. **B** and **C,** Progressive labioscrotal fusion. **D,** Complete virilization with penile urethra. (From Griffin JE, Wilson JD: Disorders of sexual differentiation. In Walsh PC, Retik AB, Stamey TA, Vaughan ED Jr [eds]. Campbell's Urology, 6th ed. Philadelphia: WB Saunders, 1992:1509.)

with a uterus and a vagina. Individuals with a male gender assignment must undergo reconstructive surgery, but usually the appearance of the penis can be relatively normal if the corporal bodies of the penis are sufficiently long. Third, gonadal tumors develop in 25% of patients and include seminoma, gonadoblastoma, dysgerminoma, and embryonal cell carcinoma. Tumors may develop in either the testis or the streak gonad. If a tumor develops in an intraabdominal testis, ipsilateral müllerian structures are always present. Tumors may develop in a scrotal streak gonad but not in a scrotal testis if it descended before birth. If a tumor is present in a streak gonad, it is also present in the contralateral intraabdominal testis. Approximately 50% of affected patients are less than 148 cm in height. For these reasons, most infants with mixed gonadal dysgenesis are reared as girls. If gender assignment is female, early exploratory laparotomy and prophylactic gonadectomy are advisable.

TRUE HERMAPHRODITISM

True hermaphroditism is the least common of the intersex disorders. In an individual with this condition, the gonads contain both ovarian and testicular tissue. Patients may have an ovotestis on one side and an ovary or testis on the other (unilateral), bilateral ovotestes (bilateral), or a testis on one side and an ovary on the other (lateral). The most common finding is an ovary on the left side and a testis on the right. Nearly all patients have a urogenital sinus, and most have a uterus. The ductal system usually follows from the ipsilateral gonad: a fallopian tube on the side of the ovary and an epididymis on the side of the testicle. If an ovotestis is present, the adjacent ducts

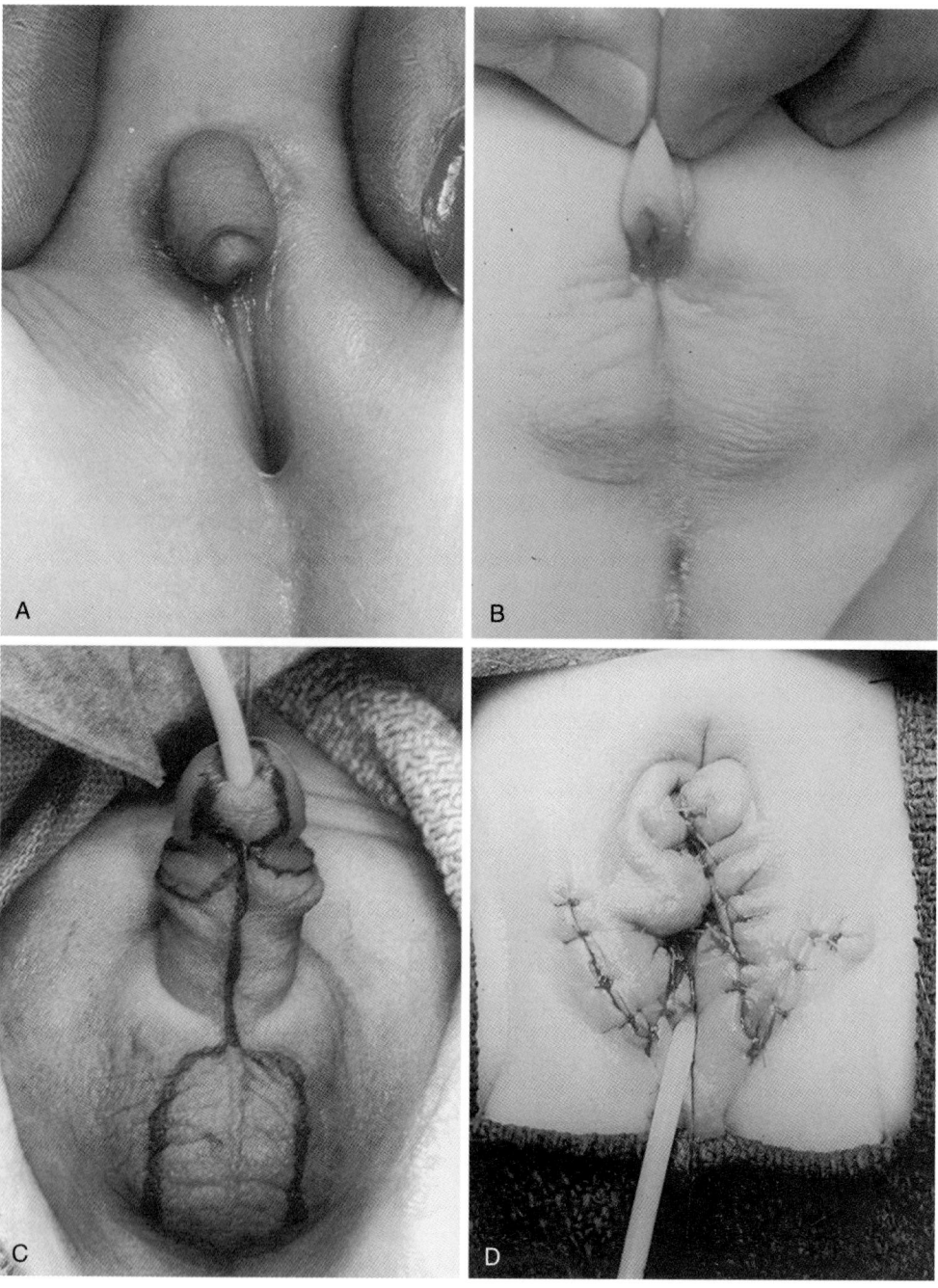

Figure 31-7. Spectrum of virilization of external genitalia in girls with congenital adrenal hyperplasia (CAH). **A,** Clitoromegaly without labioscrotal fusion. **B,** Mild clitoromegaly with labioscrotal fusion. **C,** Severe virilization in a girl with CAH. **D,** Same patient as in part C after feminizing genitoplasty.

may be wolffian, müllerian, or both. If an ovotestis is present, it may be anywhere along the course of normal testicular descent, and often it is associated with an inguinal hernia. The appearance of the external genitalia is variable. Nearly all affected persons have incomplete virilization; that is, they have hypospadias.

At puberty, 80% of affected patients develop gynecomastia, and 50% menstruate. Individuals reared as boys may show cyclic hematuria. Ovulation is more common than spermatogenesis, but both are uncommon.

Sixty percent of affected patients have a 46,XX karyotype, but the SRY gene has been detected in many. Twenty percent have a 46,XY karyotype; the remainder demonstrate mosaicism or chimerism. Gonadal neoplasms have been reported in patients with an XY cell line. Because most have a masculine phenotype, approximately 70% have been reared as boys.

The primary consideration in these patients is gender assignment. If the phallus is diminutive, the infant probably should be reared as a girl, irrespective of the internal genitalia, because the potential for phallic growth is minimal. If there are both a phallus and a vagina, the sex of rearing should be based on the findings at exploratory laparotomy. If a testis that can be placed in the scrotum is identified, the infant should be raised as a boy. If there are normal müllerian structures on one side that are associated with an ovary, strong consideration should be given to rearing the infant as a girl. After gender assignment, the contradictory gonadal tissue and internal ducts should be excised.

Table 31-5. Causes of Adrenal Insufficiency in Infancy and Childhood

Congenital Adrenal Hypoplasia
Secondary to ACTH deficiency
Autosomal recessive
X-linked

Adrenal Hemorrhage

Congenital Adrenal Hyperplasia
P-450$_{scc}$ (cholesterol side chain cleavage) deficiency
3β-Hydroxysteroid dehydrogenase deficiency
P-450 C$_{21}$ (21-hydroxylase) steroid dehydrogenase deficiency
P-450 C$_{11}$ (11β-hydroxylase) deficiency
P-450 C$_{17}$ (17-hydroxylase) deficiency

Isolated Deficiency of Aldosterone Synthesis
P-450$_{c11}$ (18-hydroxylase) deficiency
P-450$_{c11}$ (18-hydroxysteroid dehydrogenase) deficiency

Pseudohypoaldosteronism: End-Organ Unresponsiveness to Aldosterone

Congenital Adrenal Unresponsiveness to ACTH

Addison Disease
Autoimmune
Infections of the adrenal gland
  Tuberculosis
  Histoplasmosis
  Meningococcosis
Infiltration of the adrenal gland
  Sarcoidosis
  Hemochromatosis
  Amyloidosis
  Metastatic cancer
Adrenoleukodystrophy

Drugs (Suppress Adrenal Steroidogenesis)
Withdrawal of steroid therapy given for more than 7-10 days
Metyrapone
Ketoconazole

From Styne DM: Endocrine disorders. In Behrman RE, Kliegman RM (eds): Nelson Essentials of Pediatrics, 2nd ed. Philadelphia, WB Saunders, 1994, p 639.
ACTH, adrenocorticotropic hormone.

Table 31-6. Clinical Manifestations of Adrenal Insufficiency

Cortisol Deficiency
Hypoglycemia
Inability to withstand stress
Vasomotor collapse
Hyperpigmentation (primary adrenal insufficiency with ACTH excess)
Apneic spells
Hypoglycemic seizure
Muscle weakness, fatigue

Aldosterone Deficiency
Vomiting
Hyponatremia
Urinary sodium wasting
Salt craving
Hyperkalemia
Acidosis
Failure to thrive
Volume depletion
Hypotension
Dehydration
Shock
Diarrhea
Muscle weakness

Androgen Excess or Deficiency (Caused by Enzyme Defect)
Ambiguous genitalia

From Styne DM: Endocrine disorders. In Behrman RE, Kliegman RM (eds): Nelson Essentials of Pediatrics, 2nd ed. Philadelphia, WB Saunders, 1994, p 639.
ACTH, adrenocorticotropic hormone.

Table 31-7. Diagnostic Tests for Suspected Congenital Adrenal Hyperplasia

Test	Finding
Blood	
Karyotype	46,XX
17-Hydroxyprogesterone	Elevated
Testosterone	Elevated
11-Deoxycortisol	Elevated (with 11β-hydroxylase deficiency)
Androstenedione	Elevated
Serial electrolytes	↓ Na, ↑ K
Radiology	
Ultrasonography (pelvis, inguinal canal, adrenal glands)	
Genitogram	

K, potassium; Na, sodium.
↓, decreased; ↑ increased.

GONADAL DYSGENESIS

TURNER SYNDROME

Although patients with gonadal dysgenesis do not have ambiguous genitalia, the condition represents an important disorder of sexual differentiation. The karyotype is 45,XO, and this abnormality is found in 1 in 10,000 newborn girls. Typical features include short stature, sexual infantilism at puberty, and distinctive somatic abnormalities. At birth, loose skin folds on the neck are apparent, as is lymphedema of the extremities. Later, characteristic facial features become apparent, including prominent low-set ears, epicanthal folds, ptosis, low posterior hairline, and micrognathia. Affected patients have a shield-shaped chest and often a webbed neck. Associated anomalies may include renal abnormalities, coarctation of the aorta, cubitus valgus, puffy hands and feet, and short fourth metacarpals. Treatment includes estrogen replacement at puberty. All affected patients are sterile.

PURE GONADAL DYSGENESIS

Individuals with pure gonadal dysgenesis have normal female external genitalia, but the internal structures are similar to those in patients with Turner syndrome (bilateral streak gonads, müllerian

Table 31-8. Causes of Inadequate Masculinization in Boys

Condition	Additional Features
Testicular feminization syndrome (complete)*	Female external genitalia, absence of müllerian structures
Testicular feminization syndrome (partial)*	Same as for complete syndrome, with ambiguous external genitalia
Partial androgen insensitivity syndromes	Family history frequently positive
5α-Reductase deficiency	Autosomal recessive, virilization at puberty
Vanishing testis syndrome	Unknown or vascular event; may occur at >12 weeks' gestation
P-450$_{scc}$ deficiency	Salt loss
3β-Hydroxysteroid dehydrogenase deficiency	Salt loss
P-450$_{c17}$ deficiency	Salt retention/hypertension
17,20-Desmolase deficiency	Adrenal function normal
17β-hydroxysteroid oxidoreductase deficiency	Adrenal function normal
Dysgenetic testes	Possible abnormal karyotype
Leydig cell hypoplasia	Rare

Adapted from Styne DM: Endocrine disorders. In Behrman RE, Kliegman RM (eds): Nelson Essentials of Pediatrics, 2nd ed. Philadelphia, WB Saunders, 1994, p 636.

*Or androgen insensitivity.

duct development, and sexual infantilism). The patients are normal or tall in height, have few congenital anomalies, and have either a 46,XX or 46,XY karyotype. Those with the 46,XY form often have clitoromegaly. Gonadal tumors may arise in patients with a 46,XY karyotype, and prophylactic gonadectomy is recommended for these individuals. Patients may present with amenorrhea. Virilization indicates the presence of a tumor of one of the streak gonads.

Gonadal dysgenesis is characterized by abnormal testicular development, and in the 46,XY form, there is a variety of phenotypic differences, ranging from normal male to genital ambiguity, depending on the extent of testicular development. The condition may be sporadic or familial. Swyer syndrome consists of the female phenotype with female internal genitalia, normal or tall stature, and sexual infantilism with primary amenorrhea. These patients have streak gonads that do not secrete testosterone or antimüllerian substance, and therefore müllerian derivatives develop.

All of these patients are at risk for dysgerminoma, seminoma, and gonadoblastoma. Consequently, at laparotomy, gonadectomy (removal of the streak gonads) is recommended. Pubertal development should be initiated by estrogen replacement therapy in patients reared as girls.

AMBIGUOUS GENITALIA ASSOCIATED WITH DEGENERATIVE RENAL DISEASE

DENYS-DRASH SYNDROME

Denys-Drash syndrome is the clinical triad of genital abnormalities, nephropathy, and Wilms tumor. Most persons with this condition have a female phenotype or ambiguous genitalia and dysgenetic gonads. Although 46,XY is the most common karyotype, some patients with 46,XXY and 46,XX karyotypes and with hypoplastic

gonads or streak gonads have been reported. The nephropathy is progressive into end-stage renal disease and is caused by focal or diffuse mesangial sclerosis. In this syndrome, Wilms tumor typically develops before the age of 2 years and is frequently bilateral. Denys-Drash syndrome is an autosomal dominant disorder.

WAGR SYNDROME

"WAGR" syndrome refers to the association of *W*ilms tumor, *a*niridia, *g*enitourinary anomalies, including hemihypertrophy, and mental *r*etardation. Some of these patients have ambiguous genitalia, and some develop bilateral gonadoblastoma. The syndrome is secondary to a deletion at chromosome 11p13.

GENDER ASSIGNMENT AND MANAGEMENT

When a baby is born, the parents, the family, and their friends immediately want to know the baby's weight and its gender. If the neonate has ambiguous genitalia, the possible confusion among the medical team regarding gender assignment can have a profound effect on how the baby is viewed and treated by his or her family. Gender assignment in these patients is an emergency.

It is noteworthy that the issue of gender assignment or reassignment has become extremely controversial. Recommendations should be made by a multidisciplinary team. Important issues include (1) the presence of other congenital anomalies; (2) the size of the phallus; (3) the potential for providing a cosmetically and functional male or female genital appearance after reconstructive surgery; (4) the potential for gonadal malignancy; (5) the potential for fertility, including the use of artificial reproductive technology; (6) the potential for sex steroid production; (7) the neurologic status of the patient; and (8) parental preferences.

The initial discussion with the parents should include the fact that the genitalia of the child are incompletely formed and that more extensive testing must be performed before gender assignment. Until a definite sex has been assigned, the newborn should be referred to as "the baby," rather than "he," "she," or "it." The infant should never be alluded to as "half-boy and half-girl." For inquisitive family and friends, the parents may simply state that the baby is quite ill and will need to be hospitalized for several days; most of the time, no further questions regarding the baby's gender will follow. It sometimes takes several days to identify the cause of the ambiguous genitalia; only after the cause is determined can the gender assignment be made. In the unlikely event that an intersex condition is found for the first time in an older child, the assigned gender should not be changed except in very unusual circumstances.

When a neonate with ambiguous genitalia is assigned a male gender, current surgical techniques allow a remarkably normal genital appearance as long as the phallus is satisfactory in size. If the penis is diminutive, it may be necessary to give two or three monthly injections of testosterone enanthate to determine whether there is significant phallic growth potential. Nearly all of these infants have hypospadias, often with chordee. If there is significant chordee, the stretched penile length may be difficult to assess accurately and tends to be underestimated. In the absence of chordee, the stretched penile length is determined with a ruler pressed into the suprapubic fat pad above the symphysis pubis. The measurement includes the tip of the glans to the base (excluding redundant foreskin). The width is measured at midshaft during stretching. A micropenis has a stretched length or width below 2.5 standard deviations of the mean for age. At 40 weeks' gestation, this measurement (micropenis) is approximately 27 to 30 mm for length and 9 to 10 mm for diameter. Clitoral enlargement is present if the clitoris exceeds 6 mm in a full-term neonate. Gonadal (testis) size is considered small if the longest diameter is less than 0.8 cm. If a male gender assignment is made,

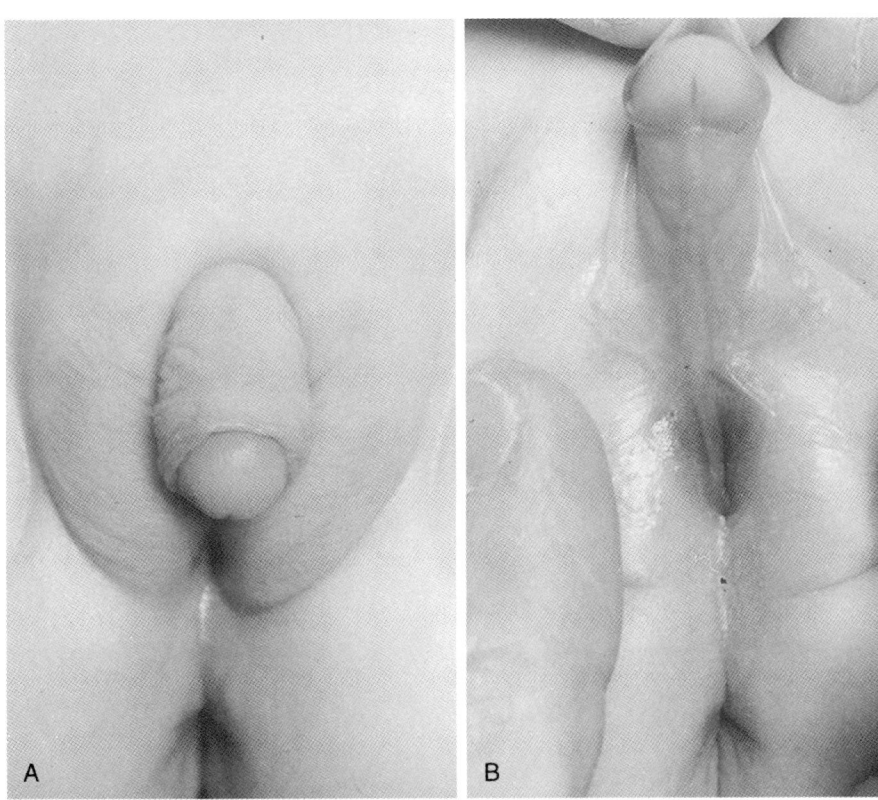

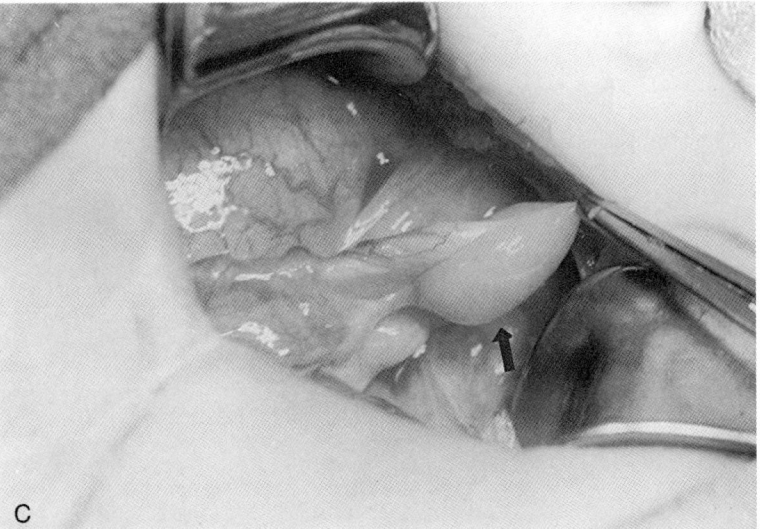

Figure 31-8. Patient with mixed gonadal dysgenesis. **A** and **B**, External genitalia shows normal-sized phallus and hypospadiac urethra. **C**, Laparotomy shows streak gonad (arrow).

the reconstructive procedure can be performed at 6 to 12 months of age, usually with one procedure.

If the patient is assigned a female gender, reconstructive surgery, termed *feminizing genitoplasty,* should be performed as soon as is feasible from a medical standpoint. This procedure involves both a clitoroplasty and a vaginoplasty. If only clitoromegaly is present, only a reduction clitoroplasty is necessary. Reconstructive surgical techniques have allowed this procedure to be performed in a way that allows an excellent cosmetic appearance and satisfactory sexual function. In this procedure, the corporal bodies of the clitoris are removed, and the glans (tip of the phallus) and the neurovascular bundle, which provides sensation, are preserved. In patients with mixed gonadal dysgenesis or true hermaphroditism, reduction clitoroplasty may be performed shortly after laparotomy and gonadal biopsy. In infants with CAH, genitoplasty needs to be deferred until the baby is stable from a medical standpoint. If the vagina opens onto

a urogenital sinus, a vaginoplasty must be performed in conjunction with reduction clitoroplasty. In patients born without a vagina, bowel vaginoplasty is usually deferred until puberty.

For infant girls with CAH, the sex of rearing nearly always should be female. With feminizing clitoroplasty, the cosmetic and functional anatomic result should be quite satisfactory. With proper hormonal regulation, these individuals can bear children, and the likelihood of tumor formation is no different from that in other women. If there is full masculine development with labioscrotal fusion (scrotum) and a phallus with a urethra at its tip, whether to assign a male or female gender is controversial, because some authorities think that the individual's brain may have already undergone sex steroid imprinting as male.

In a patient with male pseudohermaphroditism secondary to complete androgen resistance, a female gender assignment is most appropriate. The testes have a 6% to 30% risk of undergoing malignant degeneration in adulthood and therefore should be removed. Timing of gonadectomy is controversial, however: Some investigators recommend the procedure during childhood, whereas others advocate waiting until after puberty to allow feminization because of augmented estradiol secretion. If the testes are to be removed after puberty, the caregiver must be careful in explaining to the patient the reason for the procedure and should not refer to the gonads as testicles. After gonadectomy, estrogen support must be initiated.

Individuals with an incomplete form of androgen resistance have a variable phenotypic appearance. The müllerian structures are absent, and the wolffian structures are generally hypoplastic. In some cases, significant virilization occurs at puberty. In general, a male gender assignment should be made only if there is an excellent response with significant phallic growth after parenteral administration of testosterone.

In boys with a 5α-reductase deficiency, pseudovaginal perineoscrotal hypospadias is apparent. These boys have normal testes and wolffian duct derivatives, but external virilization is absent. Although some of these boys may be assigned a female gender, marked virilization occurs at puberty with penile enlargement, testicular descent, scrotal rugation, and deepening of the voice. Consequently, these patients are good candidates for a male gender assignment if they have an adequate response to parenteral androgens.

In children with a 46,XY karyotype and a disorder in testosterone synthesis, the genital appearance is variable, from female to hypospadiac male. However, the tissue response to testosterone stimulation should be normal. Some of these patients, such as those with a 17α-dehydrogenase defect, eventually restore their capacity for testosterone synthesis and show significant virilization at puberty. All have bilateral testes, which may be intraabdominal, inguinal, or labioscrotal. In these patients, the enzyme defect should be identified and androgen stimulation initiated to determine whether there is sufficient penile growth response to allow a male gender assignment.

Children with persistent müllerian duct syndrome have a normal penis and wolffian duct derivatives but internally have a fallopian tube or tubes and a uterus. The likelihood of gonadal malignancy is low. These patients are reared as boys, but the likelihood of fertility is reduced. Complete excision of the müllerian duct derivatives often results in injury to the vas deferens and is often unnecessary.

In neonates with mixed gonadal dysgenesis, the phenotypic appearance is variable, from predominantly masculine to predominantly feminine. After puberty, the testis contains no spermatogonia. Consequently, the patient is sterile, irrespective of gender assignment. Furthermore, in 25% of cases, a gonadal tumor develops, either in the streak or in the testis. If the patient has a female phenotype, a female gender assignment should be made. However, those with a normal-sized phallus and a scrotal testis can be reared as male. In such patients, the streak gonad should be promptly removed. If a child with mixed gonadal dysgenesis is reared as a boy, the short stature may be treated with growth hormone.

Patients with pure gonadal dysgenesis have bilateral streak gonads and a female phenotype without ambiguous genitalia. Because the risk of tumor development in the streak is 30%, prophylactic gonadectomy is necessary.

Patients with true hermaphroditism have variable karyotypes and phenotypes. Gender assignment in these patients can be a difficult decision. In general, ovarian tissue functions better than testicular tissue. For example, the ovary produces estrogen in a cyclic pattern that allows breast development and, in some cases, menses and ovulation. In fact, pregnancy in true hermaphrodites has been reported. In contrast, spermatogenesis in testicular tissue is uncommon, and testosterone production is often inadequate. Furthermore, testes have a 2% to 3% likelihood of undergoing malignant degeneration. Nevertheless, approximately 70% of affected patients are assigned a male gender. The most important criterion is the phallic size. If the penis is small, one way to test it is to measure the serum testosterone level and reassess stretched penile length after hCG stimulation, because a poor response to hCG is predictive of poor penile growth and masculinization at puberty. After a decision regarding assignment of gender, all discordant gonadal tissue must be removed. In addition, if a female gender assignment is made, feminizing genitoplasty should be performed before hospital discharge.

RED FLAGS

Danger signs include manifestations of adrenal insufficiency, in addition to a male phenotype without a palpable testis in the scrotum, hyperpigmentation (increased ACTH production), and hypertension. Although normal at birth, male patients with CAH experience an adrenal crisis once circulating placental-maternal steroid hormones are catabolized and excreted. This phenomenon often occurs between the 3rd and 10th days of life. The initial diagnosis in the boy with salt-losing CAH may be sepsis, pyloric stenosis, meningitis, or other more common neonatal conditions.

REFERENCES

Ahmed SF, Cheng A, Dovey L, et al: Phenotypic features, androgen receptor binding, and mutational analysis in 278 clinical cases reported as androgen insensitivity syndrome. J Clin Endocrinol Metab 2000;85:658.

American Academy of Pediatrics Section on Endocrinology and Committee on Genetics: Technical report: Congenital adrenal hyperplasia. Pediatrics 2000;106:1511.

Barthold JS, Kumasi-Rivers K, Uphadhyay J, et al: Testicular position in the androgen insensitivity syndrome: Implications for the role of androgens in testicular descent. J Urol 2000;164:497.

Baskin LS: Fetal genital anatomy reconstructive implications. J Urol 1999;162:527.

Berenbaum SA: Effects of early androgens on sex-typed activities and interests in adolescents with congenital adrenal hyperplasia. Horm Behav 1999;35:102.

Birnbacher R, Marberger M, Weissenbacher G, et al: Gender identity reversal in an adolescent with mixed gonadal dysgenesis. J Pediatr Endocrinol Metab 1999;12:687.

Borer JG, Nitti VW, Glassberg KI: Mixed gonadal dysgenesis and dysgenetic male pseudohermaphroditism. J Urol 1995;153:1267.

Cheikhelard A, Luton D, Philippe-Chomette P, et al: How accurate is prenatal diagnosis of abnormal genitalia? J Urol 2000;164:984.

Damiani D, Fellous M, McElreavey K, et al: True hermaphroditism: Clinical aspects and molecular studies in 16 cases. Eur J Endocrinol 1997; 136:201.

DeSautel MG, Stock J, Hanna MK: Müllerian duct remnants: Surgical management and fertility issues. J Urol 1999;162:1008.

Diamond M: Pediatric management of ambiguous and traumatized genitalia. J Urol 1999;162:1021.

Diamond M, Sigmundson HK: Sex reassignment at birth: Long term review and clinical implications. Arch Pediatr Adolesc Med 1997;151:298.

Farkas A, Chertin B, Hadas-Halpren I: 1-Stage feminizing genitoplasty: 8 years of experience with 49 cases. J Urol 2001;165:2341.

Forest MG: Prenatal diagnosis, treatment, and outcome in infants with congenital adrenal hyperplasia. Curr Opin Endocrinol Diabet 1997;4:209.

Forest MG: Diagnosis and treatment of disorders of sexual development. In DeGroot LJ, Jameson JL (eds): Endocrinology, 4th ed. Philadelphia, WB Saunders, 2001, p 1974.

Ganesan A, Smith GHH, Broome K, et al: Congenital adrenal hyperplasia: Preliminary observations of the urethra in 9 cases. J Urol 2002;167:275.

Grumbach MM, Conte FA: Disorders of sex differentiation. In Wilson JD, Foster DW, Kronenberg HM, Larsen PR (eds): Williams Textbook of Endocrinology, 9th ed. Philadelphia, WB Saunders, 1998, p 1303.

Hovatta O: Pregnancies in women with Turner's syndrome. Ann Med 1999;31:106.

Kaefer M, Diamond D, Hendren WH, et al: Incidence of intersexuality in children with cryptorchidism and hypospadias: Stratification based on gonadal palpability and meatal position. J Urol 1999;162:1003.

Kuhnle U, Bullinger M, Schwarz HP: The quality of life in adult female patients with congenital adrenal hyperplasia: A comprehensive study of the impact of genital malformations and chronic disease on female patients' life. Eur J Pediatr 1995;154:708.

Meyer-Bahlburg HFL: Variants of gender differentiation. In Steinhausen H-C, Verhulst FC (eds): Risks and Outcomes in Developmental Psychopathology. New York, Oxford University Press, 1999, p 298.

Meyer-Bahlburg HFL, Gruen RS, New MI, et al: Gender change from female to male in classical congenital adrenal hyperplasia. Horm Behav 1996; 30:319.

Miller WL: Dexamethasone treatment of congenital adrenal hyperplasia in utero: Experimental therapy of unproved safety. J Urol 1999;162:537.

Mueller RF: The Denys-Drash syndrome. J Med Genet 1994;31:471.

Reiner WG, Gearhart JP, Jeffs R: Psychosexual dysfunction in males with genital anomalies: Late adolescence, Tanner stages IV to VI. J Am Acad Child Adolesc Psychiatr 1999;38:865.

Schober JM: Long-term outcomes and changing attitudes to intersexuality. BJU Int 1999;83(Suppl 3):39.

Schober JM: Sexual behaviors, sexual orientation and gender identity in adult intersexuals: A pilot study. J Urol 2001;165:2350.

Shapiro E: Sonographic appearance of normal and abnormal fetal genitalia. J Urol 1999;162:530.

Slijper FME, Drip SLS, Molenaar JC, et al: Long-term psychological evaluation of intersex children. Arch Sex Behav 1998;27:125.

Sheldon CA, Gilbert AA, Lewis AG: Vaginal reconstruction: Critical technical principles. J Urol 1994;152:190.

Snyder HM, Retik AB, Bauer SB, et al: Feminizing genitoplasty: A synthesis. J Urol 1983;129:1024.

Speiser PW: Prenatal treatment of congenital adrenal hyperplasia. J Urol 1999;162:534.

Stratakis CA, Rennert OM: Congenital adrenal hyperplasia: Molecular genetics and alternative approaches to treatment. Crit Rev Clin Lab Sci 1999;36:329.

Zucker KJ, Bradley SJ, Oliver G, et al: Psychosexual development of women with congenital adrenal hyperplasia. Horm Behav 1996;30:300.

DEVELOPMENTAL/ PSYCHIATRIC DISORDERS

32 Mental Retardation and Developmental Disability

Gregory S. Liptak

DEFINITIONS

Mental retardation is defined as limitations in intelligence and adaptive skills that begin in childhood. The formal definition of mental retardation has been based on the intelligence quotient (IQ) derived from formal testing. Unfortunately, although the IQ score is an average of many abilities, it has been viewed as a single entity. In 1992, the American Association on Mental Retardation defined mental retardation as an IQ less than 70 or 75, with onset of limitations before age 18 years and with limitations in two or more adaptive skills (Table 32-1). Further characterization is noted in Table 32-2. The association recommends that once a child has received a diagnosis of mental retardation, the strengths and weaknesses in four domains should be described. These domains are intellectual functioning and adaptive skills, psychological and emotional considerations, physical health and etiologic considerations, and environmental considerations. This process can then be used to identify the social supports that the child would require to maximize his or her potential. For example, a child could be described as "a 4-year-old child who is mentally retarded with good social skills but who needs supports in self-direction and safety."

The term *developmental disability* is used to describe a broader array of conditions, including mental retardation. Developmental disabilities may be isolated, as in the child with impaired vision, or may be multiple, as in the child with delays in fine motor, gross motor, and social functioning. There may be considerable overlap in specific disorders in terms of the affected functions (Fig. 32-1).

EPIDEMIOLOGY

Developmental disabilities are common; about 5.5% of patients in a general practice may have cognitive and language disorders, and 4.0% may have motor abnormalities. These disabilities and their prevalence rates per 1000 children include (1) mental retardation (10.3), (2) cerebral palsy (CP) (2.0), (3) hearing impairment (1.0), and (4) visual impairment. Overall, chromosomal disorders (24%), syndromes (12%), perinatal-postnatal hypoxic-ischemia or infectious or traumatic injury (2.6%), intrauterine infection (7%), inborn errors of metabolism (5%), and undetermined factors (18%) account for most instances of severe mental retardation (Table 32-3).

Delayed development is more frequent in certain populations, such as those of low socioeconomic status, including the homeless. The prevalence of specific conditions that cause developmental delay varies with gender, age (especially inasmuch as many conditions, such as chromosomal anomalies, are associated with high mortality rates and are less frequent after infancy), and location. The distribution of etiologic factors in children with mental retardation also differs with the degree of delay. Chromosomal disorders, such as trisomy 21 (Down syndrome), are more common in moderately and severely retarded individuals, whereas environmental deprivation is more common in those with mild retardation. The percentage of children having retardation with an unknown cause is also greater in the mildly affected group. Genetic methods help identify the cause in adolescents with severe retardation and may determine a diagnosis in about 80% of cases in which the cause was previously undiagnosed. These diagnoses include fragile X syndrome, Rett syndrome, CATCH-22 (cardiac defects, abnormal face, thymic hypoplasia, cleft palate, hypocalcemia—defects on chromosome 22), subtelomeric deletion syndromes, and Angelman syndrome.

DIAGNOSIS

Pursuing a single cause for delayed development in a child is important for providing insight into prognosis, recurrence risk, therapies, counseling, and linkage with a supportive group. From a community perspective, having specific diagnoses helps in the development of prevention strategies. However, it is not sufficient. Identification of the child's functional abilities, strengths and weaknesses, overall physical health, and environmental factors is critical for optimizing the child's health, development, and functioning. In addition, the origin of developmental disability is not apparent in many children, or there may be multiple possible causal factors or multiple disabilities. For example, as many as 23% of children with developmental disabilities may have two disabilities; 6% may have three or more. Even if a specific diagnosis cannot be made, early identification of developmental delay can lead to a program of early intervention or remediation that will improve the child's ultimate functioning.

IDENTIFICATION

Identifying a child who is at increased risk for developmental delay requires a process of selection (screening). The screening process may be minimal, as with the child who has obvious multiple congenital anomalies or when the parents express concern about their child's development; or the screening may require a more formal test, as in the general screening of children who have no apparent risk factors. Once a child is identified as being at increased risk, a comprehensive evaluation needs to be performed.

The greater the number of biologic risk factors, the greater is the likelihood that the child will develop abnormally. For prenatal and perinatal risk factors, a combination of three or more factors was predictive of later developmental delay; in one study, 11% of mothers had three or more risk factors but accounted for 43% of the children with disabilities.

- *Biologic risks* include intracranial hemorrhage; intrauterine growth retardation; very low birth weight (usually <750 g); hypoxic-ischemic encephalopathy; brain anomalies documented on computed tomography (CT); symptomatic hypoglycemia; severe hyperbilirubinemia; microcephaly or macrocephaly; congenital infections; acquired central nervous system (CNS) infection; seizures; maternal drug use; exposure to toxins (lead); severe neonatal lung disease; failure to thrive; or congenital malformations such as holoprosencephaly, schizencephaly, or lissencephaly (which have been linked to specific genes that influence brain development).

Table 32-1. Definition of Mental Retardation

Assumptions
1. Assessments performed on the child are sensitive to differences in culture, language, communication, and behavior
2. The demands and constraints of the child's environment (home, neighborhood, school) must be considered
3. Even children with limitations have strengths that should be considered

Criteria
1. Intelligence quotient (IQ) equal to or below 70-75, *plus*
2. Limitations exist in two or more of the following adaptive skills:
   a. Communication
   b. Self-care
   c. Home living
   d. Social skills
   e. Community use
   f. Self-direction
   g. Health and safety
   h. Functional academics
   i. Leisure
   j. Work
3. Limitations manifest before age 18 yr

- *Sociocultural risks* include poverty; a lack of prenatal care or health insurance; adolescent or single-parent status of the mother; maternal mental illness; a history of child abuse, neglect, or family violence; poor parenting skills; homelessness; divorce; or disordered bonding and attachment.

Sociocultural risks have a profound effect on development and interact with biologic risk factors. Biologic risk factors that can lead to intellectual impairment do not always have the same magnitude of neurodevelopmental consequences for children from middle or upper socioeconomic backgrounds as they do for poor children. Except in children with catastrophic circumstances, child-rearing conditions that support and enrich early development may compensate for biologic deficits. Sociocultural conditions such as small family size, higher level of parental education, and fewer changes in residence have a more powerful effect than many biologic risks and seem to be important predictors of developmental functioning beyond infancy.

SCREENING FOR SPECIFIC ABNORMALITIES

Defects in vision, hearing, and language can have devastating effects on development; early intervention to ameliorate these problems can improve outcomes. All children should be screened on a regular basis for these conditions.

Visual Defects

Children at high risk for development of defects in vision (see Chapter 43) include those with strabismus (especially after 4 months of age), hydrocephalus, congenital infection, asphyxia, congenital anomaly of the central nervous system, prematurity with overexposure to oxygen, and family history of childhood onset of visual impairment. All neonates should routinely undergo an evaluation of their fundi for the presence of a red reflex, which can be obscured by cataract or tumor, as well as inspection of the globe, which may be affected by congenital glaucoma. Infants with nystagmus who do not follow visually by 3 months of age, who have dissociation between visual behavior and motor behavior, or whose parents express concern about their vision should undergo a formal ophthalmologic evaluation.

Preschool children should undergo periodic evaluations of extraocular movements to rule out strabismus and amblyopia; the evaluation should involve visual inspection of the child's eyes, the Hirschberg light test, and the cover-uncover test. As early in the child's development as possible, specific tests of monocular and binocular vision such as Allen cards (3 to 5 years), the Snellen chart (>5 years), or the Titmus tester (>4 years) should be performed.

Loss of Hearing

Early detection of hearing loss is critical for optimizing the language development of these children. Previous hearing screening strategies were based on identifying children at high risk for hearing loss. These strategies, however, missed a significant number of children. This has led to the implementation of universal hearing screening for newborns in some states. In areas where this has not been implemented, screening for hearing loss should begin in the neonatal period for newborns at high risk by using otoacoustic emissions or brainstem auditory evoked potentials. Criteria for classifying a child at high

Table 32-2. Severity of Mental Retardation and Adult Age Functioning

Level	Mental Age as Adult*	Adult Adaptation
Mild	9-11 yr	Reads at 4th-5th grade level; simple multiplication/division; writes simple letter, lists; completes job application; basic independent job skills (arrive on time, stay at task, interact with coworkers); uses public transportation, may qualify for driver's license; keeps house, cooks using recipes
Moderate	6-8 yr	Sight-word reading; copies information, e.g., address from card to job application; matches written number to number of items; recognizes time on clock; communicates; some independence in self-care; housekeeping with supervision or cue cards; meal preparation, can follow picture recipe cards; job skills learned with much repetition; uses public transportation with some supervision
Severe	3-5 yr	Needs continuous support and supervision; may communicate wants and needs, sometimes with augmentative communication techniques
Profound	<3 yr	Limitations of self-care, continence, communication, and mobility; may need complete custodial or nursing care

From Dr. Robert L. Schum, Grand Rounds Presentation at Children's Hospital of Wisconsin, 2003.
*International Statistical Classification of Diseases and Related Health Problems, 10th revision (World Health Organization).

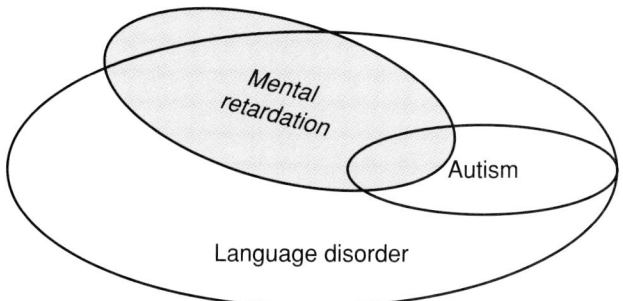

Figure 32-1. Relationship of autism, language disorders, and mental retardation. (Modified from Simms MD, Schum RL: Preschool children who have atypical patterns of development. Pediatr Rev 2000;21:147-158.)

risk include prematurity or low birth weight (usually <1500 g); hereditary hearing loss; use of potentially ototoxic drugs such as aminoglycoside antibiotics and furosemide; craniofacial anomaly (cleft palate); congenital infection, particularly rubella and cytomegalovirus; meningitis; hyperbilirubinemia necessitating an exchange transfusion; severe neonatal asphyxia; head trauma; persistent fetal circulation; and parental suspicion that the child does not hear. Newborns born weighing 1500 g or less or with gestations of 32 weeks or less, or both, may have an incidence of hearing loss of 15% (14% conductive or unspecified and 1% sensorineural). At 5 years of age, 2% of these neonates at high risk may have severe problems with communication.

For older children, parental concern about hearing loss has a sensitivity of approximately 44%. If parents express concern about their child's ability to hear and if the child has recurrent episodes of otitis media, mastoiditis, or one of the perinatal risk factors, a formal audiometric screening is performed. The value of routine screening of all preschool children with audiometry has been questioned.

Table 32-4 lists the latest acceptable age ("limit ages") for the appearance of abilities; absence of these milestones may indicate a disorder of hearing. Deaf infants may smile, coo, and babble; however, their vocalizations usually cease after 8 months of age.

Speech and Language Disorders

Disorders of speech and language development, prevalent in 3% to 20% of preschool children, are the most common reason for referral to early intervention programs and are correlated with subsequent learning problems. The most common cause of delayed language development is global mental retardation. Although the optimal age at which to intervene for a child with abnormal language development is uncertain, the consensus is that delayed diagnosis decreases the likelihood of successful treatment. A number of screening tests, such as the Language Development Survey (sensitivity of 0.87 and specificity of 0.86 in comparison to the Bayley Mental Developmental Index), the Clinical Linguistic and Auditory Milestone Scale (CLAMS) (sensitivity, 0.66; specificity, 0.79), and the Early Language Milestone Scale (sensitivity of 0.87 and specificity of 0.70 in comparison to the Sequenced Inventory of Communication Development), are available; none is completely practical for use in an office setting. A very brief sentence repetition screening test has a sensitivity of 0.76, a specificity of 0.92, a positive predictive value of 0.54, and a negative predictive value of 0.97 in comparison to a standard battery of tests.

Other Conditions

Newborn screening for inborn errors of metabolism, which can have profound effects on development, are routinely performed in all states. The specific diseases screened for vary by state and may include phenylketonuria, galactosemia, maple syrup urine disease, homocystinuria, biotinidase deficiency, and hypothyroidism. In most states, tandem mass spectroscopy identifies the common disorders such as inborn errors of fatty acid metabolism, phenylketonuria, and

Table 32-3. Prevalence of Select Conditions Associated with Developmental Delay

Condition	Prevalence per 100,000	Comments
Cerebral palsy	250-270	Represents many causes
Significant hearing loss	150	In neonatal period
Down syndrome	98-125	Prevalence at birth
Fragile X syndrome	117	Predominantly in boys
Meningomyelocele	60-100	Prevalence at birth
Klinefelter syndrome	100	15% have intelligence quotient (IQ) < 80
Fetal alcohol syndrome	60-800	Present at birth
Congenital HIV infection	5-50	Preventable with maternal and neonatal therapy
Blindness	41-88	At 10 yr of age
Infantile hydrocephalus	64	Prevalence at birth
Neurofibromatosis	33	5% have mental retardation
Trisomy 18	30	Prevalence at birth
Trisomy 13	20	Prevalence at birth
Turner syndrome	20	IQ may be normal
Prader-Willi syndrome	13-20	In childhood
Galactosemia	14	In infancy
Phenylketonuria	6-12	In infancy
Anophthalmia	6	Consider other anomalies
Rett syndrome	4-5	In girls 2 to 18 yr of age
Histidinemia	3	At birth
Acrocephalosyndactylia (Apert syndrome)	1-2	Present at birth

HIV, human immunodeficiency syndrome.

Table 32-4. Latest Acceptable Age for Skills Related to Hearing*

Age (mo)†	Activity
3	Not startling to loud sounds
6	Not smiling to voice; not vocalizing
9	Does not localize speech or other sounds
12	Not babbling multiple sounds and syllables
18	No words
24	<50% of speech understandable

Adapted from the Arizona Speech, Language, Hearing Association.

*A child who does not demonstrate the activity by the stated age should have formal audiometry performed.

†Corrected for gestational age.

Table 32-5. Items Used to Identify Neonates at Increased Risk for Developmental Delay

Item	Comment
Apgar scores	<3 at 5 min or <5 at 10 min, and HIE
Abnormal EEG	
Neonatal seizures	Hypoglycemia, hypoxia, intracranial hemorrhage, or infection confer high risk
Intracranial hemorrhage	Grade III or higher; PVL
Hydrocephalus	Especially with other anomalies, thin cortical mantle, or parenchymal lesions
Central nervous system anomalies	Seen on CT scan or ultrasonography
Prematurity	<32 wk
Small for gestational age	<3rd percentile (intrauterine growth retardation)
Dysmorphic features	Three or more minor or one or more major
Chromosomal anomaly	Trisomies, fragile X, XO
Ventilation required	Longer than 2 wk
Small head circumference	<3rd percentile
Meningitis/encephalitis	Bacterial (group B streptococci, *Escherichia coli*) Viral (herpes simplex)
Hypoglycemia	Symptomatic
Congenital infection	Cytomegalovirus, toxoplasmosis, syphilis, rubella, herpes simplex, varicella-zoster, HIV
Hyperbilirubinemia	Requiring exchange transfusions
Associated medical problems	Such as retinopathy of prematurity, heart disease, bronchopulmonary dysplasia, necrotizing enterocolitis

CT, computed tomography; EEG, electroencephalography; HIE, hypoxic-ischemic encephalopathy; HIV, human immunodeficiency virus; PVL, periventricular leukomalacia.

galactosemia, as well as more unusual metabolic diseases. Although most of these conditions are extremely rare, early treatment can lead to improved developmental outcomes.

Prenatal screening of α-fetoprotein with maternal serum is also common. Low levels have been associated with Down syndrome, whereas elevated levels have been associated with open neural tube defects and other anomalies, such as gastroschisis. Adding serum tests for estradiol and human chorionic gonadotropin is useful in screening for Down syndrome and several trisomies, including 13 and 18. This screening is typically followed by high-resolution ultrasonography and, if indicated, amniocentesis. A "biophysical profile," which includes amniotic fluid volume, fetal breathing movements, nonstress test, and fetal movements, can be helpful in evaluating the health of the fetus. Prenatal screening for other specific conditions, such as Tay-Sachs disease, is being performed in genetic populations at high risk for those conditions.

GENERAL SCREENING

All infants and children should be screened for developmental delays. The Denver II screening test is widely used, but it has modest sensitivity (0.56) and specificity (0.43). Parent report instruments, such as the Parents' Evaluation of Developmental Status, Ages and Stages Questionnaires, and Child Development Inventories, have excellent psychometric properties and require less time for the pediatrician than instruments that require direct examination. If the parents' report indicates a potential concern, the physician can perform an office screening test, such as the Hawaii Early Learning Profile (for children from birth to 3 years), or can refer the child directly to an early intervention program for evaluation.

Another strategy for screening children for developmental delay is to develop an inventory of items that leads to an index of risk (Table 32-5). Although these indices have been shown to have good concurrent sensitivity and specificity, they may not always predict future function because they do not account for environmental and other factors such as attention. For example, 7.6% of children in the United States repeat kindergarten or first grade. Factors associated with increased risk of grade retention include poverty, male gender, low maternal education, hearing loss, speech defects, low birth weight, enuresis, and exposure to household smoking. On the other hand, high maternal education and residence with both biologic parents at age 6 years were associated with a decreased risk of retention.

Inventories of risk can be coupled with other screening assessments of the child, the child's environment, or both. Table 32-6 gives the limit ages of motor milestones. In infants who both are premature and have delays in the achievement of these milestones, CP is more likely to be present. The sensitivities and specificities of these items range from 0.70 to 0.94. Similar criteria, based on motor skills, for screening children who have specific conditions, such as spina bifida, have been developed, although most have not undergone extensive psychometric evaluation. Any risk inventory should be administered jointly with evaluations of the environment, such as the Home Observation for Measurement of the Environment.

The most commonly used method of general screening is to rely on parental report, which may have a sensitivity of 80%, a specificity of 94%, a positive predictive value of 76%, and a negative predictive value of 95%. In a similar population, parental concerns regarding speech and language problems may have a sensitivity of 83%, specificity of 72%, positive predictive value of 72%, and negative predictive value of 83%. Although parental history is important, it should not be the only criterion used. A lack of parental worry about a child's development is no guarantee that the development is normal.

Many practitioners ask parents to fill out parent report measures, such as the Ages and Stages Questionnaire or the Infant/Child Monitoring Questionnaire. These questionnaires, which are specific for preschool-age children, can be administered before the pediatric visit and reviewed during the visit.

Table 32-6. Latest Acceptable Age for Skills Related to Motor Functioning

Milestone	Age (mo)*
Roll prone to supine	4.5
Roll supine to prone	6.0
Sit with arms supported	6.75
Sit without support	8.0
Creep	8.5
Come to sitting	9.5
Crawl	9.75
Pull to standing	10.25
Cruise	11.0
Walk independently	14.75

Adapted from Allen MC, Alexander GR: Motor milestones of very preterm infants at risk for cerebral palsy. Dev Med Child Neurol 1992;34: 226-232.

*Corrected for gestational age.

COMPREHENSIVE ASSESSMENT

History

Once a child is identified as being at risk for developmental delay, a primary care physician should obtain a comprehensive evaluation. Further evaluations by specialty physicians, therapists (physical, occupational, speech), and other experts may be indicated. Table 32-7 outlines some of the information that should be sought.

An assessment of the child's current level of functioning and previous developmental milestones should be obtained for all areas of development, including cognitive, fine motor, gross motor, speech and language, and socialization skills. A system for differentiating common categories of disorders is noted in Table 32-8.

Delays isolated to a single, specific area such as expressive language are more likely to be transient than are generalized delays. Because the guidelines of the DDST end at school age, many physicians are unaware of milestones that children achieve after 5 years of age. Guidelines are available, and school records can be used to help evaluate functioning.

If the child's development has deteriorated (regressed), a *progressive encephalopathy* is likely to be present. *Progressive* disorders are often a result of metabolic or storage diseases, whereas *static* encephalopathies are usually caused by structural abnormalities or are the result of a previous trauma (including hypoxia). Tables 32-9 and 32-10 list "extrinsic" and "intrinsic" causes of neurologic deterioration. More than 300 neurodegenerative disorders have been described; additional classifications based on progression and age are noted in Tables 32-11 and 32-12 and in Figures 32-2 to 32-5.

Neurodegenerative disorders are often categorized as involving white matter, gray matter, basal ganglia, or the entire central nervous system. White matter diseases (e.g., adrenoleukodystrophy) affect long tracts and manifest with loss of motor skills, spasticity, disturbed gait, areflexia (if peripheral nerve involvement), or ataxia, whereas gray matter diseases (e.g., ceroid lipofuscinoses) manifest with seizures and abnormalities of cognition, vision, and hearing. Many disorders classified as "white matter" or "gray matter" manifest with a mixed picture of signs and symptoms. Diseases that involve primarily the basal ganglia, such as Huntington disease, manifest with mental deterioration, behavioral changes, rigidity, ataxia, dysarthria, seizures, and incoordination. As these diseases progress, neurologic signs and symptoms become more widespread and less specific.

The history should include prenatal, perinatal, and neonatal events as well as serious acute illnesses, recurrent illnesses, and trauma. Details regarding nutrition and exposure to toxins should be sought.

A detailed family pedigree outlining the previous two generations can identify any familial conditions similar to the patient's problem and identify consanguinity.

An evaluation of the home, including family composition, resources, stresses, and social supports, should be sought. Information regarding a typical day can provide insights into the child's routine activities, nutritional status, and parent-child interactions (whether the parent spends time playing with the child or participates in stimulating activities). Because a child's temperament can affect the manifestations of developmental delay or even be mistaken for developmental delay or a psychiatric condition, a temperamental profile should be obtained.

In addition to developing rapport with the family, the act of taking the history can provide insights into the child's developmental status. While the interview is occurring, the child's interactions with the environment (light, sound) and with people should be observed. The child's general neurologic functioning can also be assessed; level of alertness, facial symmetry, extraocular movements, occurrence of tics, use and symmetry of extremities, locomotion, and posture should be noticed. Parental interactions with the child should also be noted.

Physical Examination

Any child suspected of having developmental delay should have a complete physical examination, which may reveal a recognizable pattern of malformation (Tables 32-13 and 32-14). In addition to a qualitative evaluation to obtain a comprehensive view of the child and to determine whether the child is ill, precise quantitative measurements include weight, length (or height), and head circumference; facial features, such as inner canthal distance, palpebral fissure length, and ear length; hand and foot measurements as well as dermatoglyphics; and measurement of male genitalia (penile length and testicular volume).

If a child has an unusual appearance, biologic family members should be examined either directly or from photographs to determine any resemblance. If the child does not resemble anyone in the family, a new genetic mutation or autosomal recessive condition may be responsible. Examination of the skin of family members may be helpful in conditions such as tuberous sclerosis and neurofibromatosis.

Although the presence of multiple minor physical anomalies has been associated with developmental delay (see Table 32-14), most children with minor anomalies develop normally.

A conscientious neurologic evaluation should be performed. In addition to general mentation and cerebellar signs, a careful motor examination, including evaluation of gait, muscle tone, deep tendon reflexes, and strength, is indicated. Infants should be evaluated for the presence of primitive reflexes, such as the asymmetrical tonic neck response, and postural responses (e.g., response to being tipped sideways while sitting up). Children who have normal motor milestones or who appear alert may nonetheless have significant developmental delay.

Laboratory Studies

Routine Blood and Urine Tests

Most children who present with possible developmental delay do not require routine laboratory studies. If a child demonstrates failure to thrive (see Chapter 13), developmental regression, vomiting (see Chapter 16), or lethargy, metabolic screening should be performed (Table 32-15).

The first step is to make certain that the child underwent a neonatal metabolic screening evaluation with normal findings. Because of some risk of false-negative results, a metabolic screen should be repeated. This includes evaluating levels of serum amino acids, urinary

Table 32-7. Information to Obtain about a Child with Suspected Developmental Disabilities

Item	Possible Significance
Parental Concerns	Parents are quite accurate in identifying developmental problems
Current Levels of Developmental Functioning	Used to monitor child's progress
Temperament	May interact with disability or be confused with developmental delay
Prenatal History	
Alcohol ingestion	Fetal alcohol syndrome; an index of caretaking risk
Illegal drug, toxin, medication exposure	Developmental toxin (e.g., phenytoin); may be an index of caretaking risk
Radiation exposure	Damage to CNS
Nutrition	Inadequate fetal nutrition
Prenatal care	Index of social situation
Injuries, hyperthermia	Damage to CNS
Smoking	Possible CNS damage
HIV exposure	Congenital HIV infection
Maternal PKU	Maternal PKU effect
Maternal illness	Toxoplasmosis, rubella, CMV, HIV, herpesvirus infections
Perinatal History	
Gestational age, birth weight	Biologic risk from prematurity and small for gestational age
Labor and delivery	Hypoxia or index of abnormal prenatal development
Apgar scores	Hypoxia, cardiovascular impairment
Specific perinatal adverse events; see Table 32-5	Increased risk for CNS damage
Neonatal History	
Illness: seizures, respiratory distress, hyperbilirubinemia, metabolic disorder; see also Table 32-5	Increased risk for CNS damage
Malformations	May represent syndrome associated with developmental delay
Family History	
Consanguinity	Autosomal recessive condition more likely
Mental functioning	Increased hereditary and environmental risks
Illnesses (e.g., metabolic disease)	Hereditary illness associated with developmental delay
Family member died young or unexpectedly	May suggest inborn error of metabolism or storage disease
Family member requires special education	Hereditary causes of developmental delay
Social History	
Resources available (e.g., financial, social support)	Necessary to maximize child's potential
Educational level of parents	Family may need help to provide stimulation
Mental health problems	May exacerbate child's conditions
High-risk behaviors (illicit drug use, sexual promiscuity)	Increased risk for HIV infection; index of caretaking risk
Other stressors (e.g., marital discord)	May exacerbate child's conditions or compromise care
Other History	
Gender of child	Important for X-linked conditions
Developmental milestones	Index of developmental delay; regression may indicate progressive condition
Head injury	Even moderate trauma may be associated with developmental delay or learning disabilities
Serious infections (e.g., meningitis)	May be associated with developmental delay
Toxic exposure (e.g., lead)	May be associated with developmental delay
Physical growth	May indicate malnutrition; obesity, short stature associated with some conditions
Recurrent otitis media	Associated with hearing loss and abnormal speech development
Visual and auditory functioning	Sensitive index of impairments in vision and hearing
Nutrition	Malnutrition during infancy may lead to delayed development
Chronic conditions such as renal disease or anemia	May be associated with delayed development

CMV, cytomegalovirus; CNS, central nervous system; HIV, human immunodeficiency virus; PKU, phenylketonuria.

organic acids, blood glucose, lactate and pyruvate, plasma ammonia, acyl carnitine, and lead and thyroid function tests. Serum electrolytes may indicate an anion gap, which is a nonspecific finding that can be seen with a variety of disorders. In most children with developmental disorders, their causes are not determined by metabolic testing.

Once suspicions have been narrowed to a group of conditions (on the basis of clinical presentation, neuroimaging, and laboratory screening tests), specific evaluations (such as microscopy or biochemical analyses) of blood, urine, and tissue samples (liver, muscle, skin) can be undertaken. On the other hand, some children have distinctive features (phenotypes), and specific tests can be obtained without prior screening. For example, 7-dehydrocholesterol can be evaluated in an infant who has the features of Smith-Lemli-Opitz syndrome, or very-long-chain fatty acids can be evaluated to

Table 32-8. Differential Diagnosis of Atypical Patterns of Development

	Mental Retardation	Developmental Language Disorder	Specific Language Impairment	Autism/Pervasive Developmental Disorder	Asperger Syndrome
Cognitive ability	Delayed	Normal/delayed	Normal	Normal/delayed	Normal
Language ability	Delayed	Disordered	Disordered	Disordered	Normal
Social ability	Normal	Normal	Normal	Abnormal	Abnormal
Family history	Negative	Speech/language	Speech/language	Affective disorder/social deficits	Social deficits

From Simms MD, Schum RL: Preschool children who have atypical patterns of development. Pediatr Rev 2000;21:147-158.

determine whether a child has a peroxisomal disorder such as Zellweger syndrome.

Genetic Evaluation

Standard cytogenetic analysis (karyotyping and banding) is used to detect abnormalities in the number of chromosomes (e.g., trisomy 21 in Down syndrome) and duplications or deletions of chromosomal material visible in the microscope (e.g., 5p– in cri-du-chat syndrome). Molecular cytogenetic techniques, such as fluorescent in situ hybridization (FISH), permit the detection of chromosomal rearrangements that are beyond the resolution of standard cytogenetic analysis. Conditions that can be diagnosed with FISH include Prader-Willi syndrome (deletion in 15q11 [paternal]) and Angelman syndrome (deletion in 15q11 [maternal]), which are contiguous gene syndromes. Other conditions that can be diagnosed using FISH are the CATCH-22 (cardiac abnormality, T-cell deficit, clefting, and hypocalcemia in association with the 22q11.2 deletion) syndrome (also known as DiGeorge and velocardiofacial syndromes, involving deletion in 22q11), Williams syndrome (deletion in 7q11), Miller-Dieker syndrome (deletion in 17p13), Smith-Magenis syndrome (deletion in 17p11), and Langer-Giedion syndromes (deletion in 8q24).

In addition, many children with mental retardation of unknown origin have subtelomeric deletions.

Direct mutation analysis is used to identify conditions wherein specific mutations within a gene responsible for the condition have been identified. The techniques used to detect these mutations include oligonucleotide hybridization analysis, Southern blot analysis,

Table 32-9. Select "Extrinsic" Conditions Associated with Developmental Regression

Neoplasms and their therapy
  Leukemia
  Tumors
  Histiocytosis
Increased intracranial pressure
  Hydrocephalus, including ventricular shunt malfunctions
  Subdural hematoma or effusion
  Tumors
Infections
  Encephalitis, including HIV infection
  Meningitis
Endocrine
  Hypothyroidism
  Adrenocortical insufficiency
Other
  Collagen-vascular disease (e.g., SLE)

HIV, human immunodeficiency virus; SLE, systemic lupus erythematosus.

polymerase chain reaction, and direct sequencing. Conditions that can be diagnosed with these direct mutation analysis techniques include fragile X syndrome (expansion of FMR1 on Xq27), Huntington disease or chorea (gene located at 4p16), and neurofibromatosis types 1 (17q11) and 2 (22q12). Other techniques such as denaturing high-performance liquid chromatography and direct sequencing can be used to identify the MECP2 coding region for mutations in Rett syndrome. Table 32-16 lists some common chromosomal defects that are associated with developmental delay. For all children who have severe developmental delay with multiple congenital abnormalities, cytogenetic analyses should be performed. If previous chromosomal analyses were performed more than 5 years previously, they should be repeated. For children with developmental delay and hypopigmentation not pathognomonic for a specific condition (e.g., neurofibromatosis), chromosome analysis of cells from peripheral blood may be helpful. If the results are normal, a skin biopsy should be performed for analysis of skin fibroblasts, because these may be abnormal, whereas lymphocytes appear normal.

Controversy exists regarding the routine screening for fragile X syndrome of all children with mental retardation who do not have features suggesting other chromosomal aberrations. Proponents argue that the knowledge potentially gained with regard to prognosis and familial issues (e.g., risks to future children) outweighs the cost. Others have argued that children should be screened and that only those at high risk should have chromosome analysis. Table 32-17 presents one screening method; a score of 5 or greater leads to a sensitivity of 0.88 and specificity of 0.98 in comparison to chromosome analysis. Once fragile X syndrome is identified in a family, molecular studies may be substituted for cytogenetic techniques in subsequent testing.

Whenever a clinician screens a child for a chromosomal anomaly, the physician should provide clinical information to the laboratory, including the child's differential diagnosis, so that the technicians can choose the proper techniques.

Neuroimaging

Ultrasonography. An ultrasound study of the head performed before the anterior fontanelle closes can provide a general anatomic picture of the brain, including a view of the posterior fossa. This technique is insensitive to lesions involving the subdural space, and its success depends more on the skill of the interpreter than that of other imaging studies. It does not expose the child to radiation, nor is sedation required in most instances. Its primary uses include identifying and monitoring intraventricular hemorrhage and hydrocephalus; these functions are useful, especially in the preterm infant.

Computed Tomography Scans. CT provides greater detail than does ultrasonography, including details of bone structures and the subdural space. It can be used with contrast material to further delineate structures, such as tumors, or to differentiate white from gray matter. However, CT exposes the child to radiation, and most young children require sedation to undergo this procedure.

Table 32-10. Select "Intrinsic" Conditions Associated with Developmental Regression

Age at Onset (Yr)	Conditions	Comments
<2, with hepatomegaly (see Chapter 18)	Fructose intolerance	Vomiting, hypoglycemia, poor feeding, failure to thrive (when given fructose)
	Galactosemia	Lethargy, hypotonia, icterus, cataract, hypoglycemia (when given lactose)
	Glycogenosis (glycogen storage disease) types I–IV	Hypoglycemia, cardiomegaly (type II)
	Mucopolysaccharidosis types I and II	Coarse facies, stiff joints
	Niemann-Pick disease, infantile type	Gray matter disease, failure to thrive
	Tay-Sachs disease	Seizures, cherry-red macula, edema, coarse facies
	Zellweger (cerebrohepatorenal) syndrome	Hypotonia, high forehead, flat facies
	Gaucher disease type II	Extensor posturing, irritability
	Carbohydrate-deficient glycoprotein syndromes	Dysmyelination, cerebellar hypoplasia
<2, without hepatomegaly	Krabbe disease	Irritability, extensor posturing, optic atrophy and blindness
	Rett syndrome	Girls with deceleration of head growth, loss of hand skills, hand wringing, impaired language skills, gait apraxia
	Maple syrup urine disease	Poor feeding, tremors, myoclonus, opisthotonos
	Phenylketonuria	Light pigmentation, eczema, seizures
	Menkes kinky hair disease	Hypertonia, irritability, seizures, abnormal hair
	Subacute necrotizing encephalopathy of Leigh	White matter disease
	Cerebrooculofacioskeletal syndrome (of Pena and Shokeir)	Reduced white matter, failure to thrive
	Canavan disease	White matter disease
	Pelizaeus-Merzbacher disease	White matter disease
2–5	Niemann-Pick disease types III and IV	Hepatosplenomegaly, gait difficulty
	Wilson disease	Liver disease, Kayser-Fleischer ring; deterioration of cognition is late
	Gangliosidosis type II	Gray matter disease
	Ceroid lipofuscinosis	Gray matter disease
	Mitochondrial encephalopathies(e.g., myoclonic epilepsy with ragged red fibers [MERRF])	Gray matter disease
	Ataxia-telangiectasia	Basal ganglia disease
	Huntington disease (chorea)	Basal ganglia disease
	Hallervorden-Spatz syndrome	Basal ganglia disease
	Metachromatic leukodystrophy	White matter disease
	Adrenoleukodystrophy	White matter disease, behavior problems, deteriorating school performance, quadriparesis
5–15	Adrenoleukodystrophy	Same as for adrenoleukodystrophy in 2- to 5-yr-olds
	Multiple sclerosis	White matter disease
	Neuronal ceroid lipofuscinosis, juvenile and adult (Spielmeyer-Vogt and Kufs disease)	Gray matter disease
	Schilder disease	White matter disease, focal neurologic symptoms
	Refsum disease	Peripheral neuropathy, ataxia, retinitis pigmentosa
	Sialidosis II, juvenile form	Cherry-red macula, myoclonus, ataxia, coarse facies
	Subacute sclerosing panencephalitis	Diffuse encephalopathy, myoclonus; may occur years after measles

Magnetic Resonance Imaging. Magnetic resonance imaging (MRI) provides the greatest detail of the nonbone aspects of the central nervous system. It cannot be used in patients who have ferromagnetic implants or metallic foreign bodies. The scanning time is longer than for CT, and most young children require sedation. The contrast material usually used, gadolinium, is generally safer than the contrast agents used for CT. MRI is superior to CT in the evaluation of the posterior fossa. MRI can also be used for imaging the spinal cord. MRI can differentiate abnormalities of gray and white matter, as well as deep and cortical gray matter lesions. Special techniques include magnetic resonance angiography, which can identify blood flow, and cerebrospinal fluid flow imaging, which can identify flow in conditions such as Chiari II malformation. Magnetic resonance spectroscopy can be used to identify metabolites in the brain such as lactate, *N*-acetylaspartate, and choline. Conditions such as phenylketonuria, maple syrup urine disease, and Canavan disease have distinctive patterns on spectroscopy.

Table 32-11. Progressive Encephalopathy: Onset Before Age 2 Years

Acquired Immunodeficiency Syndrome Encephalopathy

Aminoacidurias

1. Homocystinuria
2. Maple syrup urine disease
   a. Intermediate form
   b. Thiamine-responsive form
3. Phenylketonuria

Hypothyroidism

Lysosomal Enzyme Disorders

1. Glycoprotein degradation disorders
   a. Mannosidosis type I
   b. Fucosidosis types I and II
   c. Sialidosis type II (infantile form)
2. Mucolipidoses
   a. Type II (I-cell)
   b. Type IV
3. Mucopolysaccharidoses
   a. Type I (Hurler)
   b. Type II (Sanfilippo)
4. Sphingolipidoses
   a. Gaucher disease type II (glucosylceramide lipidosis)
   b. GM_1 gangliosidosis types I and II
   c. GM_2 gangliosidosis (Tay-Sachs, Sandhoff)
   d. Globoid cell leukodystrophy (Krabbe)
   e. Metachromatic leukodystrophy (sulfatide lipidoses)
   f. Multiple sulfatase deficiency
   g. Niemann-Pick type A (sphingomyelin lipidosis)

Mitochondrial Disorders

1. Mitochondrial myopathy, encephalopathy, lactic acidosis, stroke
2. Progressive infantile poliodystrophy (Alper)
3. Subacute necrotizing encephalomyelopathy (Leigh)
4. Trichopoliodystrophy (Menkes)

Neurocutaneous Syndromes

1. Chédiak-Higashi syndrome
2. Neurofibromatosis
3. Tuberous sclerosis

Other Genetic Disorders of Gray Matter

1. Infantile ceroid lipofuscinosis (Santavuori)
2. Infantile neuroaxonal dystrophy
3. Lesch-Nyhan syndrome
4. Rett syndrome

Other Genetic Disorders of White Matter

1. Alexander disease
2. Galactosemia: transferase deficiency
3. Neonatal adrenoleukodystrophy
4. Pelizaeus-Merzbacher disease
5. Spongy degeneration of infancy (Canavan–Van Bogaert)

Progressive Hydrocephalus

From Fenichel GM: Clinical Pediatric Neurology: A Signs and Symptoms Approach, 2nd ed. Philadelphia, WB Saunders, 1993, p 116.

Indications for Various Imaging Modalities. Many studies have identified abnormalities of the brains of children with developmental delay on MRI that were not evident on CT. These abnormalities include delayed myelination, focal lesions, and hypoplastic white matter. In approximately 33% of children with developmental delay, the MRI scan is abnormal. Abnormal results are more likely to be found if the child has microcephaly or associated neurologic findings, such as seizures or a focal motor deficit; the scan is less likely to be positive if the child has no associated symptoms or is autistic. In most cases, the findings are nonspecific and do not help make a definite diagnosis or alter therapy. Nonetheless, diagnosing a form of cerebral dysplasia is helpful to the family, especially if there is a recurrence risk. The MRI scan may help clarify the timing of a lesion. For example, if a child who has CP at term is found to have periventricular leukomalacia in the first weeks of life, an abnormality that typically occurs before 38 weeks' gestation, it is likely that a prenatal event rather than an event during labor and delivery led to the CP.

MRI is most useful for the following conditions:

- children who have developmental regression, in which the scan can differentiate white from gray matter involvement, can guide subsequent specific metabolic studies, and can identify extrinsic causes of regression, such as leukemia and human immunodeficiency virus (HIV) infection
- children with intractable seizures for whom surgical intervention may be of help
- children with focal neurologic findings
- children thought to have intracranial tumors or masses, including neurofibromatosis, Sturge-Weber syndrome, and tuberous sclerosis
- children who have evidence of brainstem or posterior fossa dysfunction, such as Möbius syndrome or Chiari malformation

CT should be performed if intracranial calcifications are suspected, as with prenatal infections (toxoplasmosis, cytomegalovirus); if abnormalities of the skull (such as a craniofacial anomaly) or subdural space are in question; and to identify major malformations, such as holoprosencephaly.

Plain skull roentgenograms are helpful in the diagnosis of craniosynostosis and other craniofacial anomalies, such as Apert syndrome. CT scanning with three-dimensional reconstruction provides more detail in these situations.

Other Tests

Most neurometabolic disorders can be identified through serum, plasma, and urine tests in conjunction with neuroradiologic investigations. However, other tests can be helpful for identifying specific diagnoses or categories of diseases. Analysis of cerebrospinal fluid for elevated protein levels may help in the diagnosis of a disease affecting white matter; the presence of measles antibody can help identify subacute sclerosing panencephalitis. On occasion, cerebrospinal fluid evaluation of lactate, pyruvate, and amino acids may be helpful. Peripheral nerve conduction tests and electromyography may help confirm that the condition is associated with a peripheral neuropathy. Diminished deep tendon reflexes and prolonged nerve conduction times are noted in Krabbe disease, Refsum disease, metachromatic leukodystrophy, and infantile neuroaxonal dystrophy (see Chapter 38). Skin and muscle biopsies may identify conditions in which abnormal material is stored in cells, such as neuronal ceroid lipofuscinosis. Brainstem auditory evoked response is useful as an evaluation of hearing in infants and can also be used to evaluate brainstem functioning. Visual evoked response can be useful in determining the integrity of the visual pathways; however, it cannot determine visual acuity.

Table 32-12. Progressive Encephalopathy: Onset After Age 2 Years

Infectious Diseases
1. Subacute sclerosing panencephalitis
2. HIV infection

Lysosomal Enzyme Disorders
1. Glycoprotein degradation disorders
   a. Aspartylglycosaminuria
   b. Mannosidosis type II
2. Mucopolysaccharidoses types II and VII
3. Sphingolipidoses
   a. Gaucher disease type III (glucosylceramide lipidosis)
   b. GM_2 gangliosidosis (juvenile Tay-Sachs)
   c. Globoid cell leukodystrophy (late-onset Krabbe)
   d. Metachromatic leukodystrophy (late-onset sulfatide lipidoses)
   e. Niemann-Pick type C (sphingomyelin lipidosis)

Other Genetic Disorders of Gray Matter
1. Ceroid lipofuscinosis
   a. Late infantile (Bielschowsky-Jansk ý)
   b. Juvenile
2. Heller syndrome
3. Huntington disease
4. Mitochondrial disorders
   a. Late-onset poliodystrophy
   b. Myoclonic epilepsy with ragged red fibers (MERRF)
5. Xeroderma pigmentosum

Other Genetic Disorders of White Matter
1. Adrenoleukodystrophy
2. Alexander disease
3. Cerebrotendinous xanthomatosis

Modified from Fenichel GM: Clinical Pediatric Neurology: A Signs and Symptoms Approach, 2nd ed. Philadelphia, WB Saunders, 1993, p 117.

HIV, human immunodeficiency virus.

FORMAL NEURODEVELOPMENTAL ASSESSMENTS

Standardized evaluations of development are usually indicated as part of the evaluation of a child with developmental delays. These include tests of general intelligence, such as the Stanford-Binet test; tests of language, such as the Peabody Picture Vocabulary Test; tests of fine motor skills, such as the Bruininks-Oseretsky Test of Motor Integration; and tests of social adaptation, such as the Vineland Adaptive Behaviour Scales. Tests of educational achievement such as the Wide Range Achievement Test, which is a test of school achievement, or the Woodcock-Johnson Psychoeducational Battery, which has both an achievement component and a cognitive component, can be useful to identify the child's functional status. Other tests, such as the Halstead-Reitan Neuropsychological Battery and the Bender Visual Motor Gestalt test, can provide more specific information on the child's sensory motor abilities (such as visual-spatial integration).

The selection of the test battery should be related to the child's condition. For example, if autism is suspected, tests such as the Autism Diagnostic Observation Score and the Autism Diagnostic Interview–Revised should be used. The testing should provide a profile of the child's strengths and weaknesses and not just a series of scores. These results can also serve as a baseline for subsequent monitoring of the child's progress. The tests, which should be administered by trained people, should be adapted for alternate sensory and response modes. The Leiter International Performance Scale has been constructed for use in children with hearing loss. After the functional assessment has been completed, the child's progress should be monitored in a systematic manner.

DIAGNOSTIC STRATEGY

Figure 32-6 illustrates a strategy to identify and assess individuals with developmental delay. All children should be screened routinely for vision, hearing, and language. Children with abnormal findings should be referred for definitive evaluation, such as to an early intervention program. Using developmental surveillance techniques such as evaluation of the family and home environment (obtained as part of a routine history or by using the Home Observation for Measurement of the Environment), a checklist of milestones (such as the Hawaii Early Learning Profile), risk inventories (see Table 32-5), and parental assessments of a child's development (obtained either informally as part of a routine history or formally by a questionnaire such as the Infant/Child Monitoring Questionnaire), the clinician can identify children who are at increased risk for delayed development.

For children identified as being at increased risk, a comprehensive history, physical examination, and evaluation of the environment should be obtained. If the child has developmental regression, the steps outlined in Figure 32-5 should be followed. If the child does not have a terminal condition, formal neurodevelopmental testing should be performed to identify the child's functional profile in order to tailor the intervention to maximize the child's development. Continuous monitoring of the child's development should follow the diagnosis.

Children with delayed development *without regression* can be categorized into four groups:

1. children with microcephaly, macrocephaly, multiple physical anomalies, and pigmentary changes, who should undergo MRI and genetic evaluation
2. children whose manifestations seem to fit a specific disorder, such as fragile X syndrome, who should undergo genetic evaluation, specific biochemical tests, or both
3. children with focal neurologic signs or focal or repeated seizures, who should undergo MRI
4. all other children with delayed development

All children with delayed development should be referred for formal neurodevelopmental assessments.

Because many conditions can cause developmental delay, identifying those in whom treatment may dramatically improve the course becomes essential (Table 32-18). Although these conditions account for only a small proportion of children with delayed development, early recognition is critical. Enzyme replacement therapy and transplantation of liver, bone marrow, and fetal tissue may constitute treatment for more conditions in the future.

In addition to the primary condition leading to developmental delay, many children experience behavioral or psychological problems. For instance, children who have Tourette syndrome often have attention-deficit/hyperactivity disorder and obsessive-compulsive disorder. Psychiatric illnesses common to children with mild or moderate retardation include adjustment disorders, organic brain disease, affective disorders, and attention-deficit/hyperactivity disorder (see Chapter 35). Children with severe delay may exhibit stereotypic or self-destructive behaviors. Clinicians evaluating these children must be aware that these psychiatric conditions can interfere with functioning as much as the primary condition.

SPECIFIC CONDITIONS

Human Immunodeficiency Virus Infection

Developmental regression before the age of 2 years can be caused by infection with HIV. It is estimated that 1500 to 2000 new cases of HIV infection occur annually in neonates in the United States.

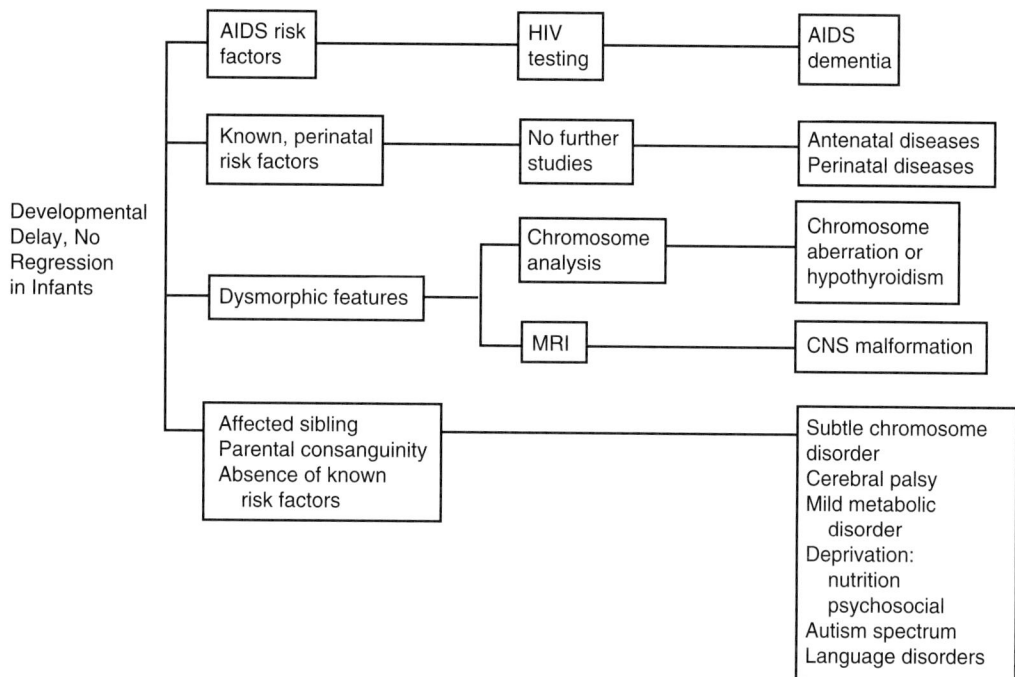

Figure 32-2. Evaluation of infants with developmental delay but no evidence of psychomotor regression. AIDS, acquired immunodeficiency syndrome; CNS, central nervous system; HIV, human immunodeficiency virus; MRI, magnetic resonance imaging. (Modified from Fenichel GM: Clinical Pediatric Neurology: A Signs and Symptoms Approach, 2nd ed. Philadelphia, WB Saunders, 1993, p 118.)

Approximately 20% of children infected with HIV prenatally or in the immediate perinatal period have signs and symptoms in the first year of life. The developmental regression or failure to progress (developmental plateau) is usually accompanied by other signs and symptoms, including failure to thrive, diarrhea, hepatosplenomegaly, lymphadenopathy, thrush, parotitis, and recurrent infections, including otitis media, bacteremia, pneumonia, and prolonged viral infections.

All children exhibiting developmental regression in the first 2 years of life should be screened for HIV, especially because current treatment can prolong life, prevent opportunistic infection, and improve developmental functioning. MRI scans of these children usually show cerebral atrophy with abnormalities of white matter; calcifications of the basal ganglia may be present as well. Children who exhibit symptoms early have a worse prognosis for survival than do those who do not develop symptoms until later.

A second group of children (80%) with congenital HIV infection presents later with a slower, less fulminant course. These children may demonstrate delays in speech and cognition, as well as hyperactivity and difficulties with attention, without any other signs or symptoms of HIV infection. If children who are at increased risk for HIV infection have nonspecific developmental delay, they should be screened for HIV infection. Treatment with antiretroviral agents such as zidovudine (AZT) has improved the IQ score and cognitive functioning of infected children.

Cerebral Palsy

CP refers to a group of conditions characterized by abnormalities of movement and posture after nonprogressive lesions of the immature brain. CP is not a single disorder or pathologic entity; rather, it is a heterogeneous collection of conditions. Although many cases of CP are "mixed," a classification scheme can be useful because rates of mental retardation and seizures vary with the different types (Table 32-19).

CP may be the result of prenatal factors such as congenital infections or malformations, perinatal factors such as hypoxia or intraventricular hemorrhage, or postnatal factors such as CNS infection, trauma, or hypoxia. CP is more common in preterm infants and in infants who are small for gestational age. The incidence of CP per 1000 births by birth weight is 90 among infants weighing less than 1500 g; 23 among infants small for gestational age weighing between 1500 and 2000 g; and 7 among infants of average size for gestational age weighing between 1500 and 2000 g.

Previously, it was believed that a difficult labor and delivery was a leading cause of CP. Although there are instances when asphyxia related to obstetric conditions such as cephalopelvic disproportion leads to CP, prenatal, often undetected events are more likely causes. Abnormalities of the CNS, such as cysts or ischemia, cause CP and may also lead to difficult labors and deliveries. Problems during pregnancy, such as amnionitis, and maternal clotting disorders have been associated with CP in these children.

Although the lesion in CP is static, the clinical picture of the child may change with maturation. For instance, the child who has a neonatal insult may be hypotonic for the first 6 months of life and then develop spasticity. Dyskinesia (dystonia and athetosis) and ataxia may not develop until the child is 18 months old. Earlier signs that should raise suspicion of CP include difficulty feeding because of abnormal oral motor patterns (tongue thrusting, tonic bite, oral hypersensitivity), irritability, difficulty with sleep, jittery or jumpy behavior, and delayed milestones, including head control. Exaggerated or persistent infantile reflexes, hyperreflexia, and asymmetry of extremity use may occur. The delay in reaching milestones; the presence of primitive or exaggerated reflexes, poor postural responses, abnormal posture, and spasticity; and abnormal results of a neurologic examination should suggest the diagnosis of CP. Repeated examination is necessary to exclude a degenerative condition; persistent subclinical seizures or adverse reaction to anticonvulsants may worsen the clinical condition of children with CP. In addition to seizures and mental retardation, children with CP have

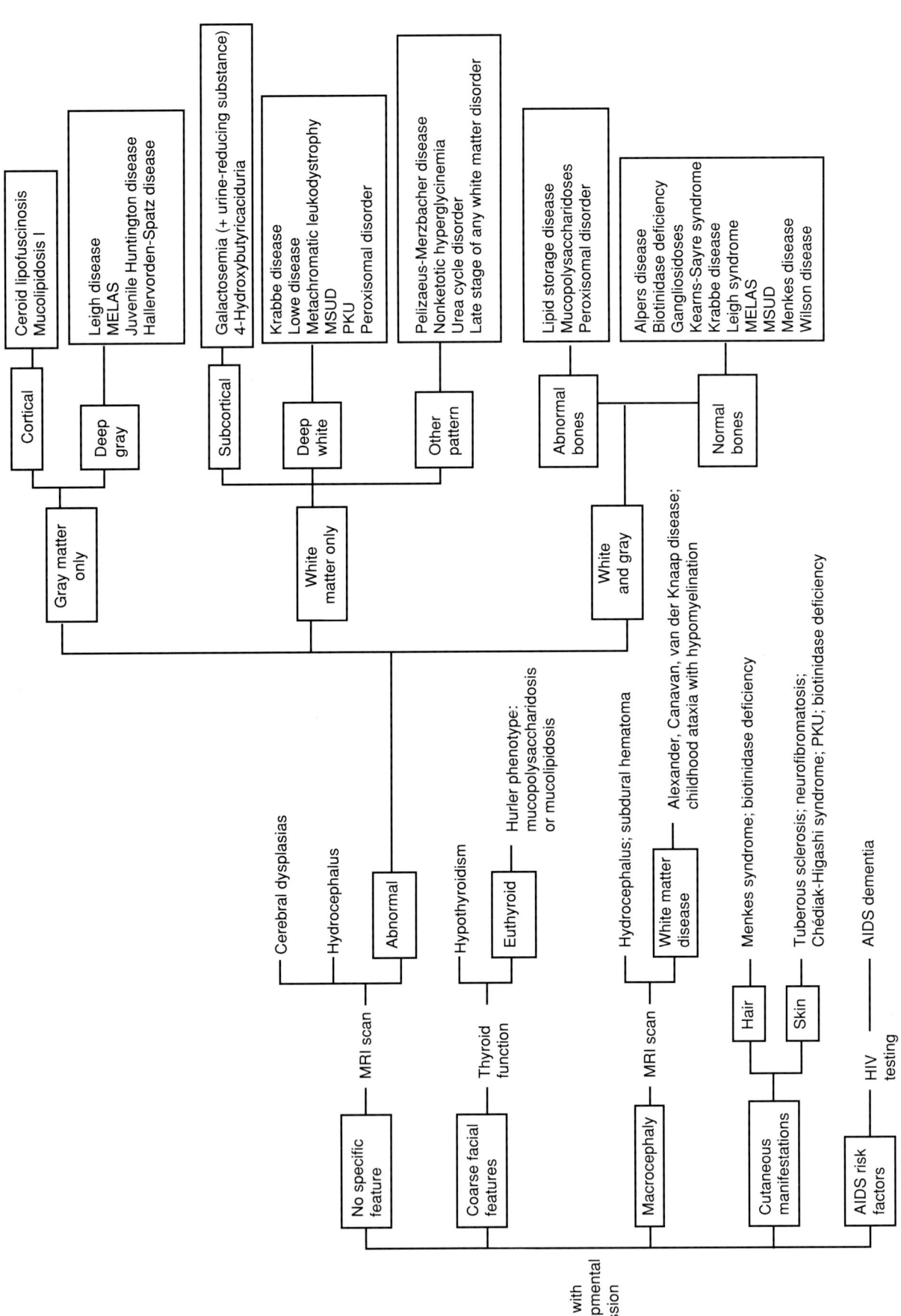

Figure 32-3. Evaluation of infants with progressive dementia. AIDS, acquired immunodeficiency syndrome; HIV, human immunodeficiency virus; MELAS, mitochondrial encephalomyopathy, lactic acidosis, and stroke-like symptoms; MRI, magnetic resonance imaging; MSUD, maple syrup urine disease; PKU, phenylketonuria. (Modified from Fenichel GM: Clinical Pediatric Neurology: A Signs and Symptoms Approach, 2nd ed. Philadelphia, VVB Saunders, 1993, p 121.)

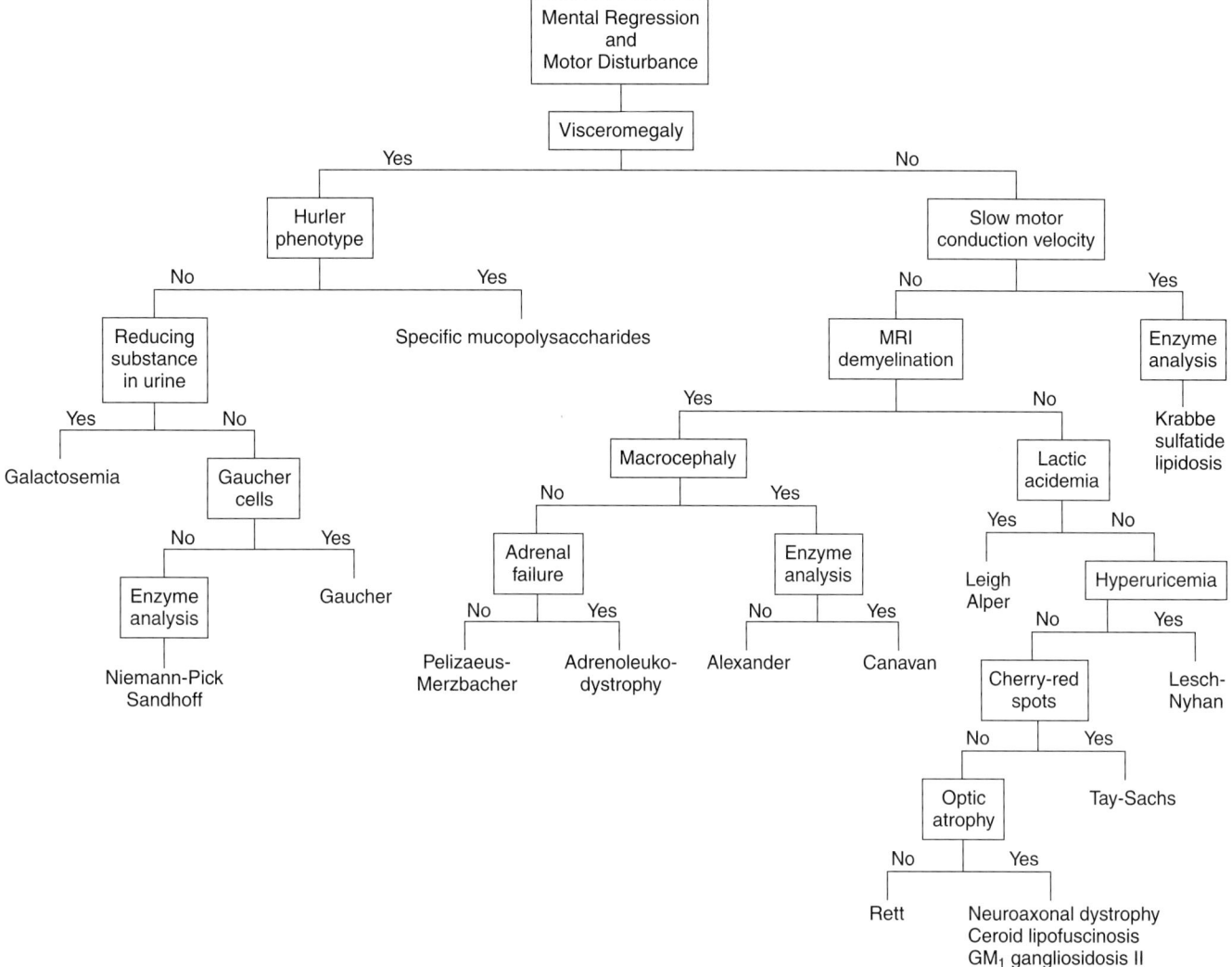

Figure 32-4. Evaluation of infants with progressive mental regression and motor disturbances. MRI, magnetic resonance imaging. (Modified from Fenichel GM: Clinical Pediatric Neurology: A Signs and Symptoms Approach, 2nd ed. Philadelphia, WB Saunders, 1993, p 131.)

an increased occurrence of visual problems, including strabismus, hearing loss, and growth failure. In older children with dyskinetic CP, symptomatic cervical spine degeneration may develop.

If a child with a diagnosis of dyskinetic CP has symptoms that worsen as the day progresses, *dopa-responsive dystonia* should be suspected. This rare but treatable form of dystonia may begin with toe-walking and difficulties with gait; it responds dramatically to the administration of levodopa. Other unusual inborn errors of metabolism, such as *arginase deficiency* and *glutaric aciduria,* may mimic CP. These conditions cause progressive deterioration, whereas CP does not.

Fragile X Syndrome

Fragile X syndrome is the most common genetic cause of mental retardation and is caused by an inheritable unstable DNA in the FMR1 gene of the X chromosome. A genetic sequence (C-C-G) is duplicated more than 200 times in affected individuals. Persons of both sexes with this unstable sequence who have fewer than 200 copies (premutation) are usually mildly affected or normal (are carriers). When transmitted by a women, this unstable sequence increases in size. Therefore, the daughters of male carriers who are clinically normal are carriers who are also generally clinically normal. Clinically normal female carriers may produce boys (the 50% that inherit

the abnormal X chromosome) who are abnormal. The greater the number of these abnormal sequences in the female carrier, the greater is the likelihood that she herself will have some developmental delay and will have abnormal sons. Girls and women who carry the full mutation are at high risk for having some manifestations of the condition.

The diagnosis of fragile X syndrome is difficult to make clinically, especially in young children. Physical features are neither constant nor specific and are less noticeable in those younger than 3 years. Table 32-17 lists some of the associated features. Others include macroorchidism in postpubertal boys, macrocephaly, flattened nasal bridge, and prominent epicanthal folds. Cognitive abilities vary from learning disabilities to severe impairment; seizures have been reported in about 20% of these individuals.

Children with fragile X syndrome often have autistic features, and 5% of boys with a diagnosis of autism have fragile X syndrome. However, 5% of severely retarded, nonautistic boys also have the fragile X gene. Therefore, this disorder per se is not a major cause of autism.

Autism

Developmental disorders are often revealed as disorders of language. The differential diagnosis of poor language development in the

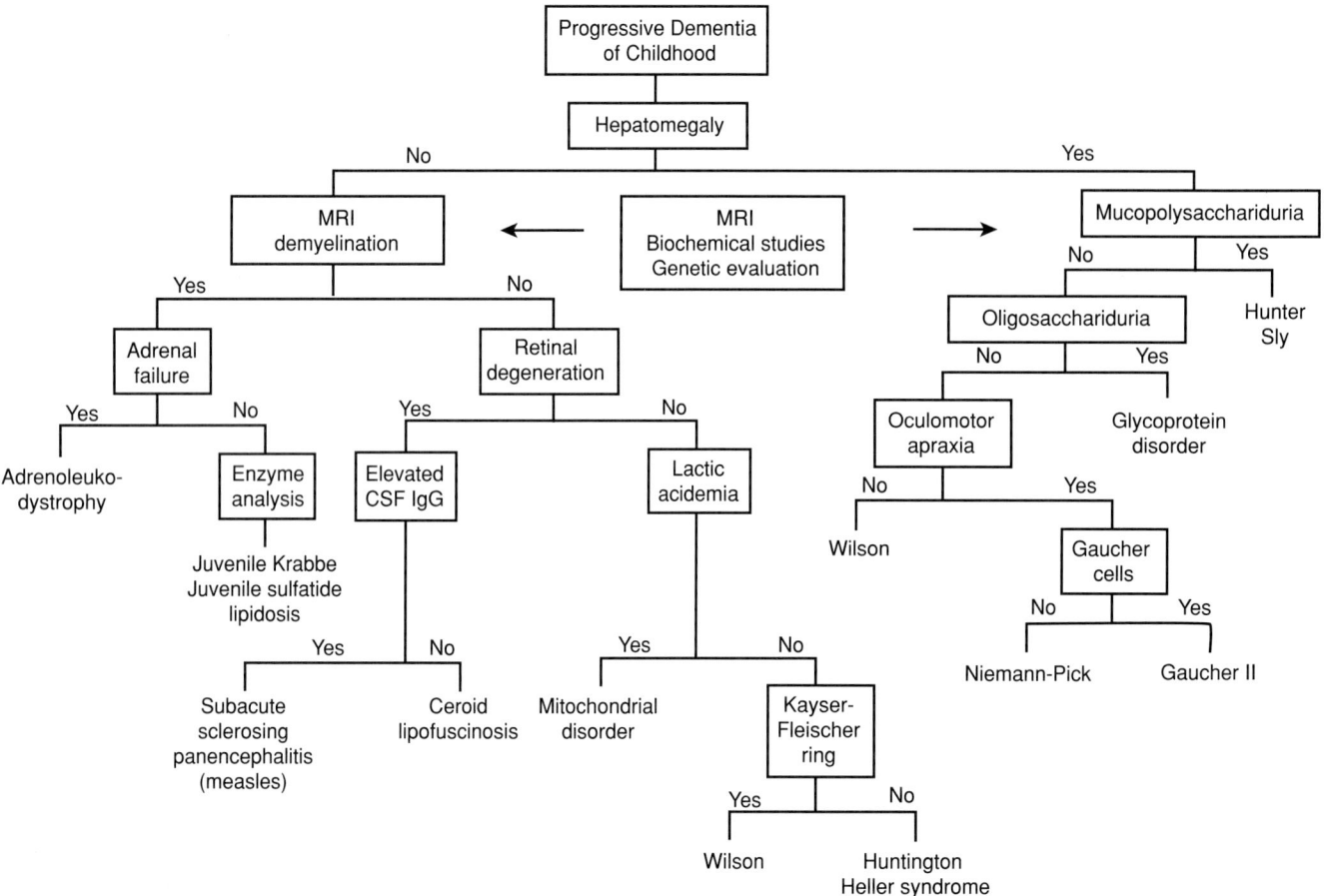

Figure 32-5. Evaluation of children with progressive dementia. CSF, cerebrospinal fluid; IgG, immunoglobulin G; MRI, magnetic resonance imaging. (Modified from Fenichel GM: Clinical Pediatric Neurology: A Signs and Symptoms Approach, 2nd ed. Philadelphia, WB Saunders, 1993, p 138.)

preschool child includes hearing impairment, mental retardation, expressive dysphasia, and autism. A single child may have features of more than one of these conditions. The diagnosis of autism is based on a constellation of clinical features and does not imply a single cause. The *Diagnostic and Statistical Manual of Mental Disorders, Fourth Edition* (*DSM-IV*) requires three criteria for the diagnosis: impaired reciprocal social interactions, abnormal verbal and nonverbal communication (eye-to-eye contact), and diminished repertoire of activities and interests, with onset during infancy or childhood.

Children with features of autism who do not meet all the criteria may still be considered to be part of the autistic spectrum disorder and may be designated as having pervasive developmental disorder, not otherwise specified (Table 32-20). Children with even less involvement may have Asperger syndrome.

Although certain diagnoses have been associated with autistic symptoms (untreated phenylketonuria, tuberous sclerosis, fragile X syndrome, Rett syndrome, Sotos syndrome, Angelman syndrome, hypomelanosis of Ito), most cases of autism have no known cause. Abnormalities of the cerebellum and limbic system have been hypothesized but not proved. Prenatal exposures to toxins, such as valproic acid, and conditions that affect the brain, such as Möbius and Joubert syndromes, have been linked to autism. Autism appears to result from abnormalities in many genes (polygenic). About 7% of siblings of autistic children have autism, and 30% have some autistic symptoms, such as delayed language.

Autism has a prevalence of about 40 to 60 in 100,000 and is more common in boys. During infancy, autistic children avoid eye contact, do not play with their parents or siblings, act deaf or visually impaired, and do not cuddle. They have delayed language skills and

may have echolalia. They tend to be irritable, have a strong need for routines in their daily lives, and often have stereotypic behaviors. They have what some people call "mind blindness," an inability to take another person's point of view as well as an inability to show empathy. Visual impairment, deafness, child abuse and neglect, and severe language disorders must be considered in children who present with autistic features. In general, the degree of aloofness (impaired social relatedness, such as solitary activities and poor social signals) in children with autism is much more severe than in children with the other disorders. Rett syndrome, which occurs in girls and is characterized by loss of hand function, ataxia, and characteristic hand wringing, also has autistic features.

Storage Diseases

Inborn errors of metabolism may manifest as an acute encephalopathy (often a result of an organic acidemia or hyperammonemia) or as a chronic progressive encephalopathy (cardiomyopathy, spasticity, hyperreflexia, liver dysfunction), often as a result of mitochondrial disorders or storage diseases (see Table 32-15).

- *Sphingolipidoses* (Tay-Sachs disease, Niemann-Pick disease, GM_1 gangliosidosis) are often associated with a cherry-red retinal spot, organomegaly, and mental retardation.
- *Glycoprotein degradation disorders* (e.g., mannosidosis, fucosidosis) may variably manifest with coarse facies, mental retardation, hepatosplenomegaly, and vacuolated lymphocytes.
- *Mucopolysaccharidoses* (e.g., the Hurler, Hunter, and Sanfilippo syndromes) may variably manifest with coarse facies, mental

Table 32-13. Physical Examination of a Child with Suspected Developmental Disabilities

Item	Possible Significance
General Appearance	May indicate significant delay in development or obvious syndrome
Stature	
Short stature	Williams syndrome, malnutrition, Turner syndrome; many children with severe retardation have short stature
Obesity	Prader-Willi syndrome
Large stature	Sotos syndrome
Head	
Macrocephaly	Alexander syndrome, Canavan disease, Sotos syndrome, gangliosidosis, hydrocephalus, mucopolysaccharidosis, subdural effusion
Microcephaly	Virtually any condition that can retard brain growth (e.g., malnutrition, Angelman syndrome, de Lange syndrome, fetal alcohol effects)
Face	
Coarse, triangular, round, or flat face; hypotelorism or hypertelorism, slanted or short palpebral fissure; unusual nose, maxilla, and mandible	Specific measurements may provide clues to inherited, metabolic, or other diseases such as fetal alcohol, cri du chat (5p– syndrome), or Williams syndrome
Eyes	
Prominent	Crouzon syndrome, Seckel syndrome, fragile X syndrome
Cataract	Galactosemia, Lowe syndrome, prenatal rubella, hypothyroidism
Cherry-red spot in macula	Gangliosidosis (GM_1), metachromatic leukodystrophy, mucolipidosis, Tay-Sachs disease, Niemann-Pick disease, Farber lipogranulomatosis, sialidosis type III
Chorioretinitis	Congenital infection with cytomegalovirus, toxoplasmosis, or rubella
Corneal cloudiness	Mucopolysaccharidosis types I and II, Lowe syndrome, congenital syphilis
Ears	
Low-set or malformed pinnae	Trisomies such as 18, Rubinstein-Taybi syndrome, Down syndrome, CHARGE association, cerebrooculofacioskeletal syndrome, fetal phenytoin effects
Hearing	Loss of acuity in mucopolysaccharidosis; hyperacusis in many encephalopathies
Heart	
Structural anomaly or hypertrophy	CHARGE association, CATCH-22, velocardiofacial syndrome, glycogenesis type II, fetal alcohol effects, mucopolysaccharidosis type I; chromosomal anomalies such as Down syndrome; maternal PKU; chronic cyanosis may impair cognitive development
Liver	
Hepatomegaly	Fructose intolerance, galactosemia, glycogenosis types I-IV, mucopolysaccharidosis types I and II, Niemann-Pick disease, Tay-Sachs disease, Zellweger syndrome, Gaucher disease, ceroid lipofuscinosis, gangliosidosis
Genitalia	
Macroorchidism	Fragile X syndrome
Hypogenitalism	Prader-Willi syndrome, Klinefelter syndrome, CHARGE association
Extremities	
Hands, feet, dermatoglyphics, and creases	May indicate specific entity like Rubinstein-Taybi syndrome or be associated with chromosomal anomaly
Joint contractures	Sign of muscle imbalance around joints: e.g., with meningomyelocele, cerebral palsy, arthrogryposis, muscular dystrophy; also occurs with cartilaginous problems such as mucopolysaccharidosis
Skin	
Café au lait spots	Neurofibromatosis, tuberous sclerosis, Bloom syndrome
Seborrheic or eczematoid rash	Phenylketonuria, histiocytosis
Hemangiomas and telangiectasia	Sturge-Weber syndrome, Bloom syndrome, ataxia-telangiectasia
Hypopigmented macules, streaks, adenoma sebaceum	Tuberous sclerosis, hypomelanosis of Ito
Hair	
Hirsutism	De Lange syndrome, mucopolysaccharidosis, fetal phenytoin effects, cerebrooculofacioskeletal syndrome, trisomy 18
Neurologic	
Asymmetry of strength and tone	Focal lesion, cerebral palsy
Hypotonia	Prader-Willi syndrome, Down syndrome, Angelman syndrome, gangliosidosis, early cerebral palsy
Hypertonia	Neurodegenerative conditions involving white matter, cerebral palsy, trisomy 18
Ataxia	Ataxia-telangiectasia, metachromatic leukodystrophy, Angelman syndrome

CHARGE, *c*oloboma, *h*eart defects, *a*tresia choanae, *r*etarded growth, *g*enital anomalies, *e*ar anomalies (deafness); CATCH-22, *c*ardiac defects, *a*bnormal face, *t*hymic hypoplasia, *c*left palate, *h*ypocalcemia—defects on chromosome 22; PKU, phenylketonuria.

Table 32-14. Examples of Minor Anomalies and Associated Syndromes*†

Head	Flat occiput: Down syndrome, Zellweger syndrome	**Teeth**	Anodontia: ectodermal dysplasia
	Prominent occiput: trisomy 18		Notched incisors: congenital syphilis
	Delayed closure of sutures: hypothyroidism, hydrocephalus		Late dental eruption: Hunter syndrome
	Craniosynostosis: Crouzon syndrome, Pfeiffer syndrome		Wide-spaced teeth: de Lange syndrome, Angelman syndrome
	Delayed fontanelle closure: hypothyroidism, Down syndrome, hydrocephalus	**Hair**	Hirsutism: Hurler syndrome
Face	Midface hypoplasia: fetal alcohol syndrome, Down syndrome		Low hairline: Klippel-Feil sequence, Turner syndrome
	Triangular facies: Russell-Silver syndrome, Turner syndrome		Sparse hair: Menkes, argininosuccinicacidemia
	Coarse facies: mucopolysaccharidoses, Sotos syndrome		Abnormal hair whorls/posterior whorl: Down syndrome
	Prominent nose and chin: fragile X syndrome		Abnormal eyebrow patterning: Waardenburg syndrome
	Flat facies: Apert syndrome, Stickler syndrome	**Neck**	Webbed neck/low posterior hair line: Turner syndrome
	Round facies: Prader-Willi syndrome	**Chest**	Shield-shaped chest: Turner syndrome
Eyes	Hypertelorism: fetal hydantoin syndrome, Waardenburg syndrome	**Genitalia**	Macroorchidism: fragile X syndrome
	Hypotelorism: holoprosencephaly sequence, maternal phenylketonuria effect		Hypogonadism: Prader-Willi syndrome
	Inner canthal folds/Brushfield spots: Down syndrome	**Extremities**	Short limbs: achondroplasia, rhizomelic chondrodysplasia
	Slanted palpebral fissures: trisomies		Small hands: Prader-Willi syndrome
	Prominent eyes: Apert syndrome, Beckwith-Wiedemann syndrome		Clinodactyly: trisomies, including Down syndrome
	Lisch nodules: neurofibromatosis		Polydactyly: trisomy 13
	Blue sclera: osteogenesis imperfecta, Turner syndrome		Broad thumb: Rubinstein-Taybi syndrome
Ears	Large pinnae/simple helices: fragile X syndrome		Syndactyly: de Lange syndrome
	Malformed pinnae/atretic canal: Treacher Collins syndrome, CHARGE association		Transverse palmar crease: Down syndrome
			Joint laxity: Down syndrome, fragile X syndrome
	Low-set ears: Treacher Collins syndrome, trisomies		Phocomelia: de Lange syndrome
Nose	Anteverted nares/synophrys: de Lange syndrome	**Spine**	Sacral dimple/hairy patch: spina bifida
	Broad nasal bridge: fetal drug effects, fragile X syndrome	**Skin**	Hypopigmented macules/adenoma sebaceum: tuberous sclerosis
	Low nasal bridge: achondroplasia, Down syndrome		Café au lait spots and neurofibromas: neurofibromatosis
	Prominent nose: Coffin-Lowry syndrome, Smith-Lemli-Opitz syndrome		Linear depigmented nevi: hypomelanosis of Ito
Mouth	Long filtrum/thin vermilion border: fetal alcohol effects		Facial port-wine hemangioma: Sturge-Weber syndrome
	Cleft lip and palate: isolated or part of syndrome		Nail hypoplasia or dysplasia: fetal alcohol syndrome, trisomies
	Micrognathia: Robin sequence, trisomies		
	Macroglossia: hypothyroidism, Beckwith-Wiedemann syndrome		

Modified from Levy SE, Hyman SL: Pediatric assessment of the child with developmental delay. Pediatr Clin North Am 1993;40:465-477.

*Increased incidence of minor anomalies have been reported in cerebral palsy, mental retardation, learning disabilities, and autism.

†The presence of three or more minor anomalies implies a greater chance that the child has a major anomaly and the diagnosis of a specific syndrome.

CHARGE, *C*oloboma, *h*eart defects, *a*tresia choanae, *r*etarded growth, *g*enital anomalies, *e*ar anomalies (deafness).

retardation, hepatosplenomegaly, dysostosis multiplex, and corneal clouding.

- *Neuronal ceroid lipofuscinosis* may manifest with mental retardation, vision loss, ataxia, and myoclonic seizures.
- *Peroxisomal disorders* (Zellweger syndrome, X-linked adrenoleukodystrophy, Refsum syndrome) variably manifest with mental retardation and encephalopathy, seizures, blindness, dysmorphic features, and deafness.

Congenital Infections

Bacteria, parasites, or viruses acquired before, during, or after birth may cause central nervous system infection and injury. The diagnosis is based on the clinical manifestations (Table 32-21) and culture or serologic evidence of infection (Table 32-22).

Postnatal Infections

CNS infection during infancy or childhood may cause encephalitis or meningoencephalitis with resultant mental retardation. Bacterial (pneumococcus, *Mycobacterium tuberculosis,* meningococcus) and viral (herpes simplex type 1 or 2, eastern or western equine encephalitis virus, West Nile virus, St. Louis encephalitis virus, HIV; in rare cases, mumps, enteroviruses, or California encephalitis virus) causes occur in infancy and early childhood and variably have neurodevelopmental sequelae. Secondary problems caused by the infection, such as hearing or visual loss, must also be considered. Late sequelae of prior viral infection such as measles or rubella panencephalitis may appear 10 to 20 years after the initial CNS disease and manifest as dementia, poor school performance, and progressive encephalopathy.

Table 32-15. Features Suggestive of Inherited Neurometabolic Disorders

Encephalopathy	Systemic Features
Mental retardation	Urinary odor
Developmental regression	Intrauterine growth
Cerebral palsy	retardation
Spastic diplegia	Failure to thrive
Spastic quadriplegia	Poor suck
Depressed sensorium	Vomiting repeatedly
Lethargy	Weak cry
Irritability	Cardiomyopathy
Stupor	Hepatomegaly
Coma	Fatty liver
Dementia	Fibrosis/cirrhosis
Hypotonia	
Seizures	**Hepatosplenomegaly**
Myoclonus	**Renal Tubular Acidosis**
Infantile spasms	**Susceptibility to Infections**
Extrapyramidal symptoms	**Bone Marrow Depression**
Dystonia	Neutropenia
Opisthotonos	Thrombocytopenia
Choreoathetosis	Pancytopenia
Cerebellar symptoms	**Seborrhea**
Ataxia	**Alopecia**
Hypoplasia	**Abnormal Hair**
Microcephaly	Pili torti
Macrocephaly	Trichorrhexis nodosa
Speech problems	
Eye-related problems	
Abnormal movements	
Apraxia	
Cherry-red spot	
Nystagmus	
Optic atrophy	
Tapetoretinal degeneration	

Modified from Chaves-Carballo E: Detection of inherited neurometabolic disorders. A practical clinical approach. Pediatr Clin North Am 1992;39:801–820.

DIAGNOSTIC HAZARDS

One of the risks in identifying children as developmentally delayed (or at risk of developmental delay) is that such identification can alter the perceptions of the child's family, making the child "vulnerable." This might lead to constraints on the child's experiences and diminished expectations of performance. When a child is born with a single risk factor, such as prematurity, and if the child has some difficulty during infancy, such as colic or slow weight gain, the parents may stop placing any demands on the child and treat the child as if he or she were retarded. The child, especially if he or she has a passive temperament, may respond to the environment by withdrawing and may indeed have delays in motor and other milestones. Identifying unusual physical characteristics (minor anomalies) may have the same negative effects.

Balanced against the risk of labeling is the need for parents to know their child's condition and to be responsible for informed decisions regarding care. Thus, as soon as the child's condition is fairly certain, this information should be shared with the family in a sensitive manner with an explanation of the margin of uncertainty. Positive as well as negative information about the child should be transmitted, and an effort should be made to identify the child's and parents' accomplishments during subsequent visits so that the visits are not viewed as entirely "fault finding."

When parents are informed that their child is not normal, they grieve for the "lost" normal child. This process of grieving involves stages that include denial, sadness, anger, and guilt. One parent may be experiencing persistent anger while another is still sad or depressed. This difference in stages may make communication between them exceedingly difficult. Grieving may occur at times other than the initial diagnosis: for example, on the first day of kindergarten.

These feelings may be expressed in nonfunctional ways, such as denial that leads to unending shopping for professionals who will "cure" the child or anger that is expressed at the clinician, thereby thwarting efforts at building a trusting relationship. However, many authorities believe that these emotions are essential steps that allow the parents to release the old dreams and secure new ones. The goal of the therapeutic clinician is not to prevent parents from expressing

Table 32-16. Chromosomal Abnormalities in Which Developmental Delay Is a Major Feature

Condition	Incidence	Comments
Trisomy 21	1/700	Down syndrome
Fragile X syndrome	1/800	Macroorchidism, hyperactivity, autistic-like behavior
47,XXY (Klinefelter syndrome)	1/1000	Small testes, problems in language skills
47,XXX	1/1000	Girls with learning and language problems; may have 48,XXXX
45,XO (Turner syndrome)	1/2000	Girls with short stature, broad neck, gonadal dysgenesis; visuospatial deficits common
Prader-Willi syndrome (abnormality of contiguous genes on chromosome 15; inherited from deletions of paternal chromosomes—monoparental disomy)	1/5000	Hypotonia in infancy, obesity, short stature, mild retardation
Angelman syndrome (chromosome anomaly similar to that in Prader-Willi syndrome; inherited from maternal deletion in chromosome 15—monoparental disomy)	Unknown	Ataxia, prognathism, absence of speech, severe retardation, inappropriate laughter
Trisomy 18	1/8000	Multiple congenital anomalies, severe developmental delay
Trisomy 13	1/20,000	Multiple congenital anomalies, severe developmental delay
5p– (cri du chat syndrome)	1/100,000	High-pitched cry, small stature, speech and language delays
4p– (Wolf-Hirschhorn syndrome)	1/100,000	Midline deficiencies, profound retardation, seizures
11p– (Wilms tumor, aniridia)	1/100,000	Ambiguous genitalia, aniridia, cataracts
17p– (Miller-Dieker syndrome)	1/100,000	Lissencephaly, microcephaly, seizures, cryptorchidism

Table 32-17. **Scoring System for Screening Individuals for Fragile X Syndrome***

Category	Score	Criteria
Family history	2	Retarded sibling, maternal uncle, aunt, nephew, niece, first cousin
	1	Any other affected relative
	0	No family history of retardation
Personality	2	Shyness, lack of eye contact followed by friendliness, verbosity, and echolalia
	1	Some of these characteristics
	0	No characteristic
Ears	2	Large and protruding
	1	Large, not protruding
	0	Other
Face	2	Long jaw, high and wide forehead
	1	Only one finding
	0	No findings
Body habitus	2	Slim, tall, rounded shoulders, hyperextensible fingers, lack of body hair, *or* obese with female fat distribution, striae, soft skin, lack of body hair (in boys and men)
	2	Slim *or* obese (girls and women)
	1	Only some features
	0	No features

*A score of 5 or greater has a sensitivity of 0.88 and specificity of 0.98 in comparison with chromosome analysis.

these feelings or hurrying them through the stages but to accept the parents at whatever stage they are in and to help them understand the normalcy of the stages.

Once a diagnosis has been established, the child's family can be given a prognosis for developmental outcome. Each child is unique; therefore, making a prognosis for an individual child on the basis of only statistical data is risky. Studies of children who have physical disability have shown that they are likely to walk if they have head control when seated by 9 months of age, if they sit by 24 months of age, and if they crawl by 30 months of age.

TREATMENT

The treatment of a child with developmental delay or mental retardation includes health maintenance, treatment of the underlying condition (if possible), treatment of associated conditions (such as hyperactivity, seizures, or drooling), relief of symptoms, anticipatory guidance to prevent secondary conditions, and environmental support. The overriding goal of these objectives is to optimize the functional status of the child.

Health maintenance should be the same as that provided for all children, including immunizations (except pertussis in undiagnosed progressive neurologic disorders and live vaccine for the child who has HIV infection), regular monitoring for physical growth and development, and screening for conditions such as anemia, tuberculosis, and lead poisoning. Specific growth charts are available for some conditions, including Down syndrome, Prader-Willi syndrome, and fragile X syndrome. Nutritional recommendations are available for children with CP. Affected children who are breast-fed appear to have better scholastic achievement scores.

Very few conditions (see Table 32-18) that lead to developmental delay can be "cured." Because many of these curable or treatable conditions are rare, medications that may be effective in their treatment could receive the support provided for "orphan drugs" under the Orphan Drugs Act.

Treatment of associated conditions depends on knowledge of the condition and the child, which argues for continuity of care. For example, the child with a behavioral or psychiatric problem may benefit from counseling, support, or psychopharmacologic medications. These medications can be used to reduce arousal symptoms and to improve affect, perceptual functioning, cognitive processing,

communication, and behavior (Table 32-23). Attention must be paid to the medication and condition. Valproic acid is more likely to cause hepatotoxicity in certain conditions, including GM_2 gangliosidosis, spinocerebellar degeneration, Friedreich ataxia, Lafora body disease, Alpers disease, and myoclonic epilepsy with ragged red fibers. Parents and capable children should be informed about the medication prescribed, including its side effects. Some written guidelines for parents and youth are available for psychopharmacologic medications. Many children who have developmental delay have epilepsy. Newer medications and modes of treatment such as stereotactic-guided surgery and vagal nerve stimulation are available to manage seizures.

Effective relief of symptoms also depends on knowledge of the child and the condition. Many children with CP have drooling and spasticity. Drooling has been controlled by the use of glycopyrrolate, scopolamine patch, or surgery to remove salivary glands. Spasticity has been treated with the injection of botulinum toxin, intrathecal or oral baclofen, tizanidine, and dorsal root rhizotomy.

Anticipatory guidance involves the same categories used in all children but may need to be modified because of the unique features of the child's condition. Prevention of secondary conditions requires specific anticipatory guidance. For example, in a child with CP, the following conditions necessitate prevention: aspiration pneumonia; malnutrition; falls; decubitus ulcers; deformities (contractures) of the foot, knee, and hip; kyphoscoliosis; osteoporosis; poor expressive communication; depression; and low self-esteem. Patients with CP may also need help in finding employment opportunities and recreation.

Although many different conditions can cause developmental delay, children with this problem and their families share many common characteristics, including chronicity of the condition (with no cure in most instances); inability to participate in peer activities; loss of the "ideal" child; increased expense; lost opportunities (such as the inability of a parent to return to work because he or she must care for the child at home); need for personal care (because the child cannot be left alone or with a sitter); confusing systems of health care, insurance coverage, and governmental agencies and rules; and social isolation.

Environmental support may be needed and may take the form of family therapy, financial counseling, and referral to a disease-oriented volunteer support group or enrollment in a school or preschool program or in a "Big Brothers/Big Sisters" program. Formal support includes early intervention for children from birth to 3 years

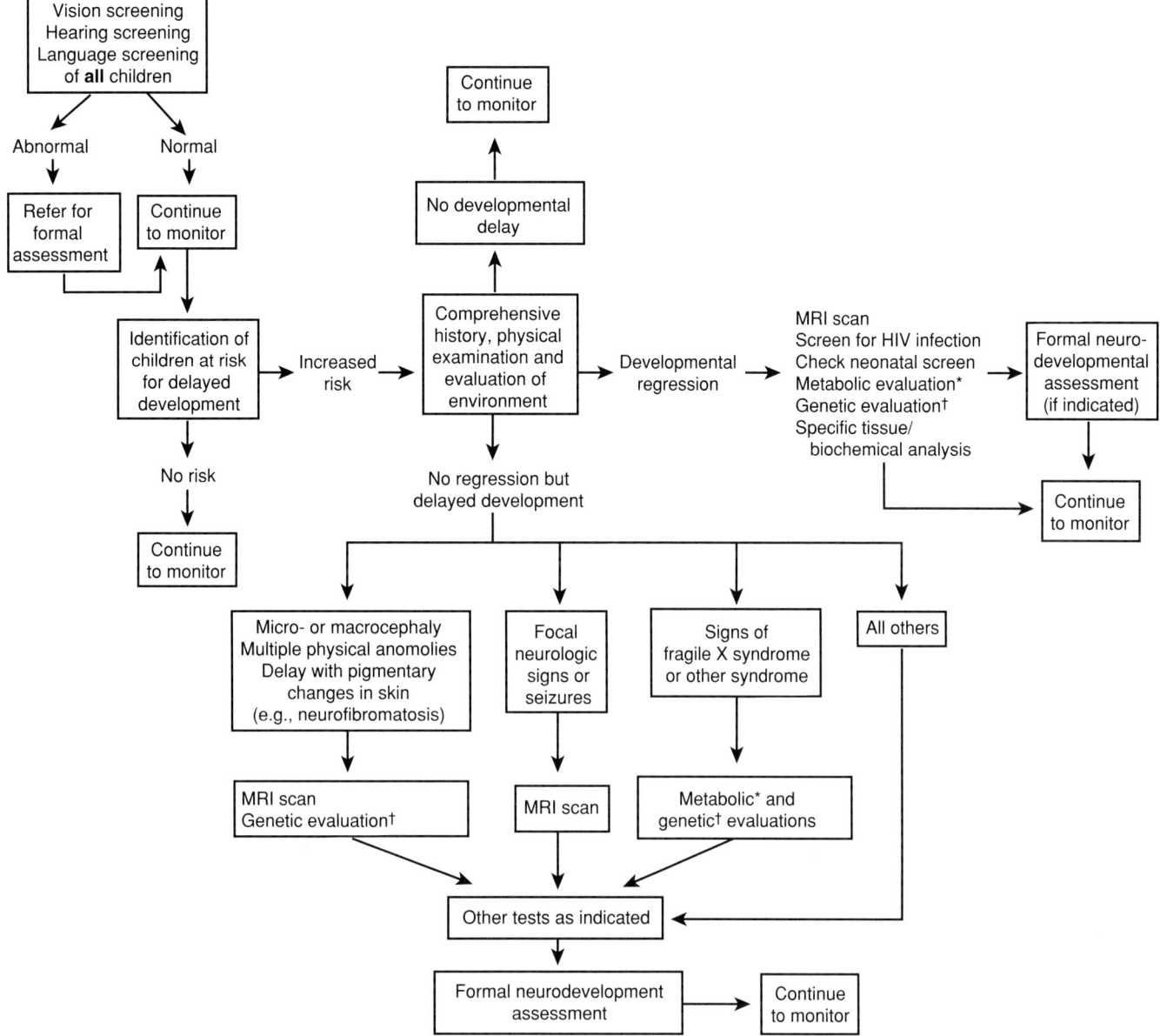

Figure 32-6. Diagnostic strategy for identifying and assessing individuals with developmental delay. *Metabolic evaluation includes serum amino acids, serum and urine organic acids, serum lactate, and ammonia. †Genetic evaluation includes karyotype, cytogenetics, specific gene probes, and dysmorphology consultation if indicated. HIV, human immunodeficiency virus; MRI, magnetic resonance imaging.

of age, preschool intervention through the school district for children from 3 to 5 years of age, and use of Individuals with Disabilities Education Act and Section 504 of the Rehabilitation Act for the school-age child. One time period during which supports have been limited is the transition of the adolescent to early adulthood. Although families should ideally be able to determine their children's needs and procure services, they may need assistance to do so. Care coordination (or case management) is one way of providing environmental support. This consists of determining the needs of the child and family, planning comprehensive care, facilitating and coordinating services, monitoring to ensure that the families have received the services they need, and empowering families to become increasingly independent in the care of their child.

Although treatment plans differ for different conditions, the mnemonic "MD'S DD BASICS" may help the clinician remember issues related to the care of children with developmental disabilities

(Table 32-24). Specific checklists that can be used to monitor the care of children with specific problems, such as Down syndrome, are also available (Table 32-25).

Because conventional medical care cannot cure many conditions associated with developmental delay, many complementary therapies have arisen. A number of them, such as patterning to learn motor skills, ingestion of megadoses of vitamins, and the indiscriminate injection of fetal tissue, have largely been discounted. Other treatments, such as the injection of secretin to improve functioning in autism and hyperbaric oxygen to help children with CP, have been the subjects of several published negative studies. Because it is difficult for families of a developmentally delayed child to abandon hope for a cure, and because traditional medicine is often ineffective in helping children with delayed development, the clinician should keep an open mind when discussing alternative therapies with families.

Table 32-18. Conditions in Which Early Treatment May Significantly Improve the Course of the Disease

Condition	Treatment
Galactosemia	Lactose-free diet
Fructosemia	Fructose-free diet
Hypoglycemia from any cause	Prevent hypoglycemia and/or provide glucose
Lead intoxication	Separate child from source of lead; chelation therapy (?)
Hypothyroidism	Thyroid replacement
Phenylketonuria	Phenylalanine-free diet
Maternal phenylketonuria	Phenylalanine-free diet during pregnancy
Maple syrup urine disease	Diet restricted in branched chain amino acids + dialysis or exchange transfusion
Recurrent otitis media	Antibiotic prophylaxis, pressure-equalizing tubes (?)
Malnutrition	Adequate nutrition
Increased intracranial pressure (e.g., hydro-cephalus, neoplasm)	Shunt ventricles or cystic structure
Congenital HIV infection	Prenatal/postnatal treatment with AZT (zidovudine)
Congenital toxoplasmosis	Prenatal treatment with spiramycin, pyrimethamine, and sulfonamide
Dopa-responsive dystonia	Responds to levodopa; may be misdiagnosed as cerebral palsy
Metachromatic leukodystrophy	Bone marrow transplantation
Niemann-Pick disease	Bone marrow transplantation, liver transplantation, implanted amniotic epithelial cells
Adrenoleukodystrophy	Bone marrow transplantation
Mucopolysaccharidosis type I	Bone marrow transplantation
Glycogen storage disease type IV	Liver transplantation
Menkes disease	Parenteral copper histidinate
Lesch-Nyhan syndrome	Allopurinol + bone marrow transplantation (?)
Krabbe disease	Bone marrow transplantation (?)

HIV, human immunodeficiency virus.

Table 32-19. Classification of Cerebral Palsy

Type	% of All CP	IQ < 50 (%)	Seizures (%)
Spastic diplegia	32	33	31
Spastic quadriplegia	24	64	56
Spastic hemiplegia	29	39	67
Dyskinetic	10	30	27
Ataxic	4	1	1

Table 32-20. Autistic Spectrum Disorders

Autistic Disorder (Classic Autism)
Severe qualitative deficits in social interaction and communication skills
Restricted and stereotyped patterns of behavior, interests, and activities
Onset before the age of 3 yr

Pervasive Developmental Disorder, Not Otherwise Specified (PDD-NOS)
Severe and pervasive deficits in social and communication skills *or*
Restricted and stereotyped patterns of behavior, interests, and activities, *but*
Symptoms do not meet the "threshold" for autistic disorder

Asperger Syndrome
Deficits in sociability and a narrow range of interests
No speech or language delays
Normal intellectual abilities
Motor clumsiness

Childhood Disintegrative Disorder
Previously completely normal children who undergo massive regression between 2 and 10 yr of age
Mental retardation

From Simms MD, Schum RL: Preschool children who have atypical patterns of development. Pediatr Rev 2000;21:147-158.

SUMMARY AND RED FLAGS

Developmental disabilities are common. Identifying children with developmental delay involves both specific attention to children with biologic and/or sociocultural risks and general screening practices, such as vision screening. The cause and diagnostic strategy depend on whether the child has delays in multiple or single domains and the pattern of onset (delayed acquisition of skills versus loss of milestones). A systematic diagnostic approach should be used with a thorough approach to the myriad diagnostic possibilities, with the recognition that some children do not have a single defined disease process (see Fig. 32-6). All children with developmental delay should be referred for a formal neurodiagnostic assessment and need meticulous monitoring to optimize their functional status.

Red flags include developmental regression (see Tables 32-9 and 32-10), developmental delay associated with vomiting or lethargy (see Table 32-15), and recognition of a treatable cause of delay (see Table 32-18).

Table 32-21. Distinguishing Features of Perinatal Congenital Infections

Agent	Maternal Epidemiology	Neonatal Features
Toxoplasma gondii	Heterophil-negative mononucleosis Exposure to cats or raw meat or immunosuppression High-risk exposure at 10-24 wk gestation	Hydrocephalus, abnormal spinal fluid, intracranial calcifications, chorioretinitis, jaundice, hepatosplenomegaly, fever, MR if symptomatic Many infants asymptomatic at birth *Treatment*: pyrimethamine plus sulfadiazine
Rubella virus	Unimmunized seronegative mother; fever ± rash Detectable defects with infection: 　　by 8 wk, 85% 　　9-12 wk, 50% 　　13-20 wk, 16% Virus may be present in infant throat for 1 yr *Prevention*: vaccine	Intrauterine growth retardation, microcephaly, microphthalmia, cataracts, glaucoma, "salt-and-pepper" chorioretinitis, hepatosplenomegaly, jaundice, PDA, deafness, blueberry muffin rash, anemia, thrombocytopenia, leukopenia, metaphyseal lucencies, B- and T-cell deficiency, MR if symptomatic Infant may be asymptomatic at birth
Cytomegalovirus (CMV)	Primary infection may be asymptomatic Heterophil-negative mononucleosis; infant may have viruria for 1-6 yr	Sepsis, intrauterine growth retardation, chorioretinitis, microcephaly, periventricular calcifications, blueberry muffin rash, anemia, thrombocytopenia, neutropenia, hepatosplenomegaly, jaundice, deafness, pneumonia Many asymptomatic at birth, MR if symptomatic *Prevention*: CMV-negative blood products
Herpes simplex type 2 virus	STD: primary genital infeciton may be asymptomatic; intrauterine infection rare, acquisition at time of birth more common	*Intrauterine infection*: chorioretinitis, skin lesions, microcephaly, MR *Postnatal infection*: encephalitis, localized or disseminated disease, skin vesicles, keratoconjunctivitis, MR if CNS infection *Treatment*: acyclovir
Varicella-zoster virus	Intrauterine infection with chickenpox during first trimester Infant develops severe neonatal varicella when maternal illness occurs 5 days before or 2 days after delivery	Microphthalmia, cataracts, chorioretinitis, cutaneous and bone aplasia/hypoplasia/atrophy, cutaneous scars, MR Zoster as in older child *Prevention of neonatal condition*: VZIG *Treatment of ill neonate*: acyclovir
Treponema pallidum (syphilis)	STD Maternal primary asymptomatic: painless "hidden" chancre Penicillin, not erythromycin, prevents fetal infection	*Presentation at birth* as nonimmune hydrops, prematurity, anemia, neutropenia, thrombocytopenia, pneumonia, heptosplenomegaly *Late neonatal presentation* as snuffles (rhinitis), rash, hepatosplenomegaly, condylomata lata, metaphysitis, cerebrospinal fluid pleocytosis, keratitis, periosteal new bone, lymphocytosis, hepatitis; MR possible *Late onset abnormalities* teeth, eye, bone, skin, CNS, ear *Treatment*: penicillin
Parvovirus B-19	Etiology of fifth disease; fever, rash, arthralgia in adults	Nonimmune hydrops, fetal anemia *Treatment:* in utero transfusion
Human immuno-deficiency virus (HIV)	AIDS: most mothers are asymptomatic and HIV-positive; high-risk history: prostitute, drug abuse, sexual partner of bisexual person, or hemophiliac	AIDS symptoms develop between 3 and 6 mo of age in 25%-40%; failure to thrive, recurrent infection, hepatosplenomegaly, neurologic abnormalities, MR *Management*: intravenous immunoglobulin, trimethoprim-sulfamethoxazole, antiretroviral therapy
Hepatitis B virus	Vertical transmission common; may result in cirrhosis, hepatocellular carcinoma	Acute neonatal hepatitis; many become asymptomatic carriers *Prevention:* HBIG, vaccine
Borrelia burgdorferi	Lyme disease, erythema chronicum migrans, meningitis, arthritis, carditis	Prematurity, rash, cortical blindness, fetal death?
Neisseria gonorrhoeae	STD, infant acquires at birth *Treatment:* cefotaxime, ceftriaxone	Gonococcal opthalmia, sepsis, meningitis *Prevention:* silver nitrate, erythromycin eye drops *Treatment:* intravenous ceftriaxone
Chlamydia trachomatis	STD, infant acquires at birth *Treatment:* oral erythromycin	Conjunctivitis, pneumonia *Prevention:* erythromycin eye drops *Treatment:* oral erythromycin
Mycobacterium tuberculosis	Positive PPD skin test, recent converter, positive chest roentgenogram, positive family member *Treatment:* INH and rifampin ± ethambutol	Congenital rare septic pneumonia; acquired primary pulmonary TB; MR if CNS symptoms; if asymptomatic, follow PPD *Prevention:* INH, bCG, separation *Treatment:* INH, rifampin, pyrazinamide
Trypanosoma cruzi (Chagas disease)	Central South American native, immigrant, travel Chronic disease in mother	Failure to thrive, heart failure, achalasia *Treatment:* nifurtimox

Modified from Kliegman RM: Fetal and neonatal medicine. In Behraman RE, Kliegman RM (eds): Nelson Essentials of Pediatrics, 2nd ed. Philadelphia, WB Saunders, 1994.

AIDS, acquired immunodeficiency syndrome; bCG, bacillus Calmette-Guérin; CNS, central nervous system; HBIG, hepatitis B immune globulin; INH, isoniazid; MR, mental retardation; PDA, patent ductus arteriosus; PPD, purified protein derivative; STD, sexually transmitted disease; TB, tuberculosis; VZIG, varicella-zoster immune globulin.

Table 32-22. Diagnosis of Congenital Infections

Serologic Findings

Syphilis: nontreponemal (VDRL) or treponemal (FTA-ABS)

Toxoplasmosis: ELISA, Sabin-Feldman dye test

Rubella: latex agglutination, enzyme immunoassay

Cytomegalovirus: ELISA

Herpes simplex viruses: several methods

Varicella-zoster virus: fluorescent antimembrane antibody

Lyme disease: ELISA

Human parvovirus B19: ELISA or RIA

Arboviruses: antibody capture ELISA (blood or CSF)

Serologic Studies Should Include

An acute sample from the infant for agent-specific IgM and IgG

A convalescent sample from the infant for agent-specific antibodies

A maternal sample for agent-specific IgG

Virologic Findings (Culture and PCR)

Cytomegalovirus: urine, saliva, blood leukocytes; occasionally, CSF

Rubella virus: urine, nasopharyngeal secretions

Herpes simplex viruses: skin lesions, throat, rectum, CSF

Varicella-zoster virus: skin lesions

Enteroviruses: CSF, throat, stool

Arboviruses: blood, CSF

When the agent is unknown, samples should include urine, throat washing, CSF, blood, rectal swab, and fluid from skin vesicles, if present.

From Bale JF, Murph JR. Congenital infections and the nervous system. Pediatr Clin North Am 1992;39:669-690.

CSF, cerebrospinal fluid; ELISA, enzyme-linked immunosorbent assay; FTA-ABS, fluorescent treponemal antibody absorption; IgM, immunoglobulin M; PCR, polymerase chain reaction; RIA, radioimmunoassay; VDRL, Venereal Disease Research Laboratory.

Table 32-23. Psychopharmacologic Agents that May be Useful in the Treatment of Children with Developmental Disabilities

Medication	Possible Indications
Carbamazepine	Mania, bipolar disorder, impulsivity, aggression, seizures, trigeminal neuralgia
Clomipramine	Obsessive-compulsion, depression
Clonazepam	Mania, bipolar disorder, seizure
Clonidine	Manic episodes, attention-deficit/hyperactivity disorder, aggression
Fenfluramine	Prader-Willi syndrome (to suppress appetite and control aggression)
Fluoxetine, other SSRIs	Obsessive-compulsion, depression
risperidone, olanzapine, aripiprazole	Aggressive, self-injurious behavior
Methylphenidate, dextroamphetamine, pemoline	Attention-deficit/hyperactivity disorder
Propranolol	Aggression, impulsivity
Valproic acid	Bipolar disorder, especially rapidly cycling

SSRI, selective serotonin reuptake inhibitors.

Table 32-24. Providing Primary Care to Children with Developmental Disabilities Using the Mnemonic "MD'S DD BASICS"

MD'S DD BASICS	Things to Check	Potential Consultant(s)
Motor	Ambulation, seating, position, spine	Orthopedist, physiatrist, PT, OT
Diet	Weight, fat stores, diet, feeding problems	Nutritionist/dietitian, speech pathologist, OT
Seizures	Seizure record; drug levels and side effects	Neurologist
Dermatology	Skin breakdown	Nursing, plastic surgeon
Dentistry	Teeth, gums	Dentist
Behavior	Aggression, self-injury, sleep, pica, interfering behavior	Psychologist, psychiatrist
Advocacy	Finances, family support, program aid	Social worker
Sensory	Vision, hearing	Ophthalmologist, audiologist
Infections	Immunizations, environment, lungs, urine	Infection control nurse
Constipation	Stools, gastroesophageal reflux	Gastroenterologist
Sexuality	Menses, sexual activity, masturbation, contraception, prevention of sexually transmitted diseases	Gynecologist, habilitation program

Adapted from Sulkes S: MD's DD BASICS: Identifying common problems and preventing secondary disabilities. Pediatr Ann 1995;24:245-254.

OT, occupational therapist; PT, physical therapist.

Table 32-25. **Medical Checklist for a Child with Down Syndrome**

Age	Condition	Monitoring
Birth to 2 mo	Etiology, recurrence risk	Chromosome analysis and genetic counseling
	Hypothyroidism	TSH, T_3, and T_4
	Congenital heart defect	Pediatric cardiology evaluation, including echocardiography
	Family stress	Referral to Down Syndrome Association
2-12 mo	Refractive errors, cataracts	Pediatric ophthalmologic evaluation
	Hearing loss; recurrent otitis media	Auditory brainstem evoked response
	Delayed development	Formal developmental evaluations
1-12 yr	Delayed development	Enrollment in early intervention program
	Hypothyroidism	Annual TSH
	Hearing loss	Auditory testing: annually between 1 and 3 yr and every 2 yr between 3 and 13 yr
	Refractive error	Opthalmologic examination every 2 yr
	Atlantoaxial instability	Cervical spine roentgenography at 2 and 12 yr
	Routine care	Dental examination at 2 yr, then every 6 mo (prophylaxis for subacute bacterial endocarditis, if indicated)
12-18 yr	Hypothyroidism	TSH annually
	Decreased hearing	Auditory testing every 2 yr
	Refractive error	Opthalmologic examination every 2 yr
	Mitral valve prolapse	Echocardiography

T_3, triiodothyronine; T_4, thyroxine; TSH, thyroid-stimulating hormone.

REFERENCES

Ad Hoc Committee on Terminology and Classification. Mental Retardation: Definition, Classification and Systems of Support. Washington, DC, American Association on Mental Retardation, 1992.

Allen MC, Alexander GR. Motor milestones of very preterm infants at risk for cerebral palsy. Dev Med Child Neurol 1992;34:226-232.

American Academy of Pediatrics, Committee on Genetics: Molecular genetic testing in pediatric practice: A subject review. Pediatrics 2000;106:1494-1497.

Barkovich JA: Pediatric Neuroimaging, 3rd ed. Philadelphia, Lippincott Williams & Wilkins, 2000.

Birch EE, Garfield S, Hoffman DR, et al: A randomized trial of early dietary supply of long-chain polyunsaturated fatty acids and mental development in term infants. Dev Med Child Neurol 2000;42:174-181.

Bradley RH, Caldwell BM, Brisby J, et al: The HOME inventory: A new scale for families of pre- and early adolescent children with disabilities. Res Dev Disabil 1992;13:313-333.

Burton BK: Inborn errors of metabolism in infancy: A guide to diagnosis. Pediatrics 1998;102:E69.

Byrd RS, Weitzman ML: Predictors of early grade retention among children in the United States. Pediatrics 1994;93:481-487.

Carey JC: Health supervision and anticipatory guidance for children with genetic disorders (including specific recommendations for trisomy 21, trisomy 18 and neurofibromatosis I). Pediatr Clin North Am 1992;39:25-53.

Chamberlin RW: Developmental assessment and early intervention programs for young children: Lessons learned from longitudinal research. Pediatr Rev 1987;8:237-247.

Chaves-Carballo E: Detection of inherited neurometabolic disorders: A practical clinical approach. Pediatr Neurol 1992;39:801-820.

Coplan J, Gleason JR: Quantifying language development from birth to 3 years using the Early Language Milestone Scale. Pediatrics 1990;86:963-971.

Einarsson-Backes LM, Stewart KB: Infant neuromotor assessments: A review and preview of selected instruments. Am J Occup Ther 1992;46:224-232.

Frankenburg WK, Dodds J, Archer P, et al: The Denver II: A major revision and restandardization of the Denver Developmental Screening Test. Pediatrics 1992;89:91-97.

Gabrielli O, Salvolini O, Coppa GV, et al: Magnetic resonance imaging in the malformative syndromes with mental retardation. Pediatr Radiol 1990;21:16-19.

Glascoe FP: Can clinical judgment detect children with speech-language problems? Pediatrics 1991;87:317-322.

Glascoe FP, Altemeier WA, MacLean WE: The importance of parents' concerns about their child's development. Am J Dis Child 1989;143:955-958.

Glascoe FP, Byrne KE, Ashford LG, et al: Accuracy of the Denver II in developmental screening. Pediatrics 1992;89:1221-1225.

Harbord MG, Finn JP, Hall-Craggs MA, et al: Myelination patterns on magnetic resonance of children with developmental delay. Dev Med Child Neurol 1990;32:295-303.

Harris SR: Early diagnosis of spastic diplegia, spastic hemiplegia, and quadriplegia. Am J Dis Child 1989;143:1356-1365.

Holm VA, Cassidy SB, Butler MG, et al: Prader-Willi syndrome: Consensus diagnostic criteria. Pediatrics 1993;91:398-402.

Holst K, Andersen E, Philip J, et al: Antenatal and perinatal conditions correlated to handicap among 4-year-old children. Am J Perinatol 1989;6:258-267.

Horwitz SM, Leaf PJ, Leventhal JM, et al: Identification and management of psychosocial and developmental problems in community-based, primary care pediatric practices. Pediatrics 1992;89:480-485.

Howlin P, Asgharian A: The diagnosis of autism and Asperger syndrome: Findings from a survey of 770 families. Dev Med Child Neurol 1999;41:834-839.

Iivanainen M, Kaakkola S: Dopa-responsive dystonia of childhood. Dev Med Child Neurol 1993;35:362-367.

Jankovic J: Tourette's syndrome. N Engl J Med 2001;345:1184-1192.

Kilmon CA, Barber N, Chapman K: Instruments for the screening of speech/language development in children. J Pediatr Health Care 1991;5:61-70.

Kirby RS, Swanson ME, Kelleher KJ, et al: Identifying at-risk children for early intervention services: Lessons from the Infant Health and Development Program. J Pediatr 1993;122:680-686.

Kopparthi R, McDermott C, Sheftel D, et al: The Minnesota Child Development Inventory: Validity and reliability for assessing development in infancy. J Dev Behav Pediatr 1991;12:217-222.

Labar D: Vagus nerve stimulation for intractable epilepsy in children. Dev Med Child Neurol 2000;42:496-499.

Laing S, Partington M, Robinson H, et al: Clinical screening score for fragile X (Martin Bell) syndrome. Am J Med Genet 1991;38:256-259.

Lovell RW, Reiss AL: Psychiatric disorders in developmental disabilities. Pediatr Clin North Am 1993;40:579-592.

Mazzocco M: Advances in research on the fragile X syndrome. Ment Retard Dev Disabil Res Rev 2000;6:96-106.

Morgan AW, Aldag JC: Early identification of cerebral palsy using a profile of abnormal motor patterns. Pediatrics 1996;98:692-697.

Najman JM, Bor W, Morrison J, et al: Child developmental delay and socio-economic disadvantage in Australia: A longitudinal study. Soc Sci Med 1992;34:829-835.

Nickel RE, Squires J: Developmental screening and surveillance. In Nickel RE, Desch LW (eds): The Physician's Guide to Caring for Children with Disabilities and Chronic Conditions. Baltimore, Paul H. Brookes, 2000, pp 15-30.

Palfrey JS, Frazer CH: Determining the etiology of developmental delay in very young children: What if we had a common internationally accepted protocol?! J Pediatr 2000:136:569-570.

Pellock JM: Managing pediatric epilepsy syndromes with new antiepileptic drugs. Pediatrics 1999;104:1106-1116.

Ramey CT, Ramey SL: Effective early intervention. Ment Retard 1992;30:337-345.

Rapin I: Hearing disorders. Pediatr Rev 1993;14:43-49.

Salt A, Gringras P, Dorling J, Hartley L: Developmental delay. In Moyer VA, Elliott EJ (eds): Evidence Based Pediatrics and Child Health. London, BMJ Books, 2000, pp 117-124.

Schaefer GB, Bodensteiner JB: Evaluation of the child with idiopathic mental retardation. Pediatr Neurol 1992;39:929-943.

Scheiner AP, Sexton ME: Prediction of developmental outcome using a perinatal risk inventory. Pediatrics 1991;88:1135-1143.

Shevell MI, Majnemer A, Rosenbaum P, et al: Etiologic yield of sub-specialists' evaluation of young children with global developmental delay. J Pediatr 2000;136:593-598.

Shonkoff JP, Hauser-Cram P, Krauss MW, Upshur CC: Development of infants with disabilities and their families: Implications for theory and service delivery [review]. Monogr Soc Res Child Dev 1992;57:v-vi, 1-153.

Shprintzen RJ: Velocardiofacial syndrome. Otolaryngol Clin North Am 2000;33:1217-1235.

Simms MD, Schum RL: Preschool children who have atypical patterns of development. Pediatr Rev 2000;21:147-158.

Snow BJ, Tsui JK, Bhatt MH, et al: Treatment of spasticity with botulinum toxin: A double-blind study. Ann Neurol 1990;28:512-515.

Stein LK: Factors influencing the efficacy of universal newborn hearing screening. Pediatr Clin North Am 1999;46:95-105.

Sturner RA, Kunze L, Funk SG, et al: Elicited imitation: Its effectiveness for speech and language screening. Dev Med Child Neurol 1993;35:715-726.

Sugimoto T, Yasuhara A, Nishida N, et al: MRI of the head in the evaluation of microcephaly. Neuropediatrics 1993;24:4-7.

Veen S, Sassen ML, Schreuder AM, et al: Hearing loss in very preterm and very low birthweight infants at the age of 5 years in a nationwide cohort. Int J Pediatr Otorhinolaryngol 1993;26:11-28.

Wasserman RC, Croft CA, Brotherton SE: Preschool vision screening in pediatric practice: A study from the Pediatric Research in Office Settings (PROS) Network, American Academy of Pediatrics. Pediatrics 1992;89:832-838.

Watkin PM, Baldwin M, Laoide S: Parental suspicion and identification of hearing impairment. Arch Dis Child 1990;65:846-850.

Yeargin-Allsopp M, Murphy CC, Oakley GP, et al: A multiple-source method for studying the prevalence of developmental disabilities in children: The Metropolitan Atlanta Developmental Disabilities Study. Pediatrics 1992;89:624-630.

Young Poussaint T, Barnes PD: Imaging of the developmentally delayed child. Magn Reson Imaging Clin North Am 2001;9:99-119.

33 Dysmorphology

R. Stephen S. Amato

Dysmorphology is the subset of clinical genetics that concerns structural abnormalities that alter appearance. Normal human morphology varies on a wide continuum; outside this range are discontinuous traits termed *birth defects* that generally have a significant and obvious effect on appearance. The clinical challenges are to identify and describe birth defects and to differentiate normal variable morphology (human variation in appearance) from the abnormal and place the totality of morphologic findings in the context of a specific diagnosis. Description, identification, and diagnosis provide insight into the nature of the condition, enable an estimate of recurrence risk, make possible a prediction for prognosis, and guide appropriate interventions. Common definitions of underlying mechanisms for dysmorphology are noted in Table 33-1; a glossary of terms used in dysmorphology is presented in Table 33-2.

Often the geneticist-morphologist is asked to view a child with the expectation that the total picture will lead to an instant identification of a syndrome or condition. Instant identification happens more frequently with the more common or better known conditions. Most often, however, a diagnosis is difficult with many complex disorders; knowledge, skill, attention to detail, the use of the current medical literature, and review of standard reference sources are required for diagnosis.

There is a wide array of possibilities for diagnoses when the examiner is confronted with a child with a medical problem or birth defect and unusual morphologic findings (Tables 33-3 and 33-4). Often, there is no obvious or easy answer. A detailed medical history needs to be collected, and a thorough physical examination should be conducted. First, all the data are assembled; next, what may be significant is culled from what is minor or just normal variation. There are many diagnostic tests, some based on molecular methods, and there are excellent types of imaging, but these tests are expensive, may only be performed in specialized labs, and may require genetic material from other family members. Even the "classical" chromosome analysis has numerous variations with specific fluorescent-labeled probes for various chromosomal sites. Testing must be used judiciously to confirm a diagnosis or to select among possibilities, but many tests are too specific to be of help when the condition is a total unknown. Before any laboratory or imaging testing is done, the examiner should address the question "Does the description correlate with a described condition or syndrome?" Often, the working diagnosis is the succinct and relevant description of the child, which amounts to a list of findings arranged in order of importance or significance from the perspective of the examiner.

Table 33-1. Mechanisms, Terminology, and Definitions of Dysmorphology

Terminology	Definition	Example
Malformation sequence	Single, local tissue morphogenesis abnormality that produces a chain of subsequent defects	DiGeorge sequence of primary fourth brachial arch and third and fourth pharyngeal pouch defects that lead to aplasia or hypoplasia of the thymus and parathyroid glands, aortic arch anomalies, and micrognathia
Deformation sequence	Mechanical (uterine) forces that alter structure of intrinsically normal tissue	Oligohydramnios produces deformations by in utero compression of limbs (dislocated hips, equinovarus foot deformity), crumpled ears, dislocated nose, or small thorax
Disruption sequence	In utero tissue destruction after a period of normal morphogenesis	Amnionic membrane rupture sequence, leading to amputation of fingers/toes, tissue fibrosis, and destructive tissue bands
Dysplasia sequence	Poor organization of cells into tissues or organs	Neurocutaneous melanosis sequence with poor migration of melanocyte precursor cells from the neural crest to the periphery, manifesting as melanocytic hamartosis of skin, meninges, and so forth
Malformation syndrome	Appearance of multiple malformations in unrelated tissues without an understandable unifying cause; with enhanced genetic investigation, a single etiology may become identified	Trisomy 21 Teratogens

Table 33-2. Glossary of Selected Terms Used in Dysmorphology

Terms Pertaining to the Face and Head

Brachycephaly: A condition in which head shape is shortened from front to back along the sagittal plane; the skull is rounder than normal

Canthus: The lateral or medial angle of the eye formed by the junction of the upper and lower lids

Columella: The fleshy tissue of the nose that separates the nostrils

Glabella: Bony midline prominence of the brows

Nasal alae: The lateral flaring of the nostrils

Nasolabial fold: Groove that extends from the margin of the nasal alae to the lateral aspects of the lips

Ocular hypertelorism: Increased distance between the pupils of the two eyes

Palpebral fissure: The shape of the eyes based on the outline of the eyelids

Philtrum: The vertical groove in the midline of the face between the nose and the upper lip

Plagiocephaly: A condition in which head shape is asymmetric in the sagittal or coronal planes; can result from asymmetry in suture closure or from asymmetry of brain growth

Scaphocephaly: A condition in which the head is elongated from front to back in the sagittal plane; most normal skulls are scaphocephalic

Synophrys: Eyebrows that meet in the midline

Telecanthus: A wide space between the medial canthi

Terms Pertaining to the Extremities

Brachydactyly: A condition of having short digits

Camptodactyly: A condition in which a digit is bent or fixed in the direction of flexion (a "trigger finger"–type appearance)

Clinodactyly: A condition in which a digit is crooked and curves toward or away from adjacent digits

Hypoplastic nail: An unusually small nail on a digit

Melia: A suffix meaning "limb"(e.g., amelia—missing limb; brachymelia—short limb)

Polydactyly: The condition of having six or more digits on an extremity

Syndactyly: The condition of having two or more digits at least partially fused (can involve any degree of fusion, from webbing of skin to full bony fusion of adjacent digit)

From Berhman RE, Kliegman RM: Nelson Essentials of Pediatrics, 4th ed. Philadelphia, WB Saunders, 2002, p 149.

Table 33-3. Causes of Congenital Malformations

Monogenic (7.5% of Serious Anomalies)
X-linked hydrocephalus
Achondroplasia
Ectodermal dysplasia
Apert disease
Treacher Collins syndrome

Chromosomal (6% of Serious Anomalies)
Trisomies 21, 18, 13
XO, XXY
Deletions 4p– 5p–, 7q–, 13q–, 18p–, 18q–, 22q–
Prader-Willi syndrome (50% have partial deletion of chromosome 15)

Maternal Infection (2% of Serious Anomalies)
Intrauterine infections (e.g., herpes simplex, CMV, varicella-zoster, rubella, and toxoplasmosis)

Maternal Illness (3.5% of Serious Anomalies)
Diabetes mellitus
Phenylketonuria
Hyperthermia

Uterine Environment (% Unknown)
Deformation
Uterine pressure, oligohydramnios: clubfoot, torticollis, congenital hip dislocation, pulmonary hypoplasia, seventh nerve palsy

Disruption
Amniotic bands, congenital amputations, gastroschisis, porencephaly, intestinal atresia

Twinning
Conjoined twins, intestinal atresia, porencephaly

Environmental Agents (% Unknown)
Polychlorinated biphenyls
Herbicides
Mercury
Alcohol

Medications (% Unknown)
Thalidomide
Diethylstilbestrol
Phenytoin
Warfarin
Cytotoxic drugs
Isotretinoin (vitamin A)
D-pencillamine
Valproic acid

Unknown Etiologies
Polygenetic
Anencephaly/spina bifida
Cleft lip/palate
Pyloric stenosis
Congenital heart disease

Imprinting of Genes
Prader-Willi syndrome
Beckwith-Wiedemann syndrome

Sporadic Syndrome Complexes (Anomalads)
CHARGE syndrome
VATER syndrome
Pierre Robin syndrome
Prune-belly syndrome

Nutritional
Low folic acid–neural tube defects

From Berhman RE, Kliegman RM: Nelson Essentials of Pediatrics, 4th ed. Philadelphia, WB Saunders, 2002, p 148.

CMV, cytomegalovirus; CHARGE, *c*oloboma, *h*eart defects, *a*tresia choanae, *r*etarded growth, *g*enital anomalies, *e*ar anomalies (deafness); VATER, *v*ertebral defects, *a*nal atresia, *t*racheoesophageal fistula with *e*sophageal atresia, and *r*adial and renal anomalies.

Table 33-4. Examples of Human Developmental Abnormalities According to Primary Cause

Condition	Clinical Findings	Genetics and Pathogenesis
Single Gene		
Aniridia	Reduced or absent iris, frequent retinal, lens, and/or corneal abnormalities	Autosomal semidominant loss-of-function mutations in the paired-like transcription factor *PAX6*; also observed along with Wilms tumor and genitourinary abnormalities as part of the 11p13 WAGR deletion syndrome (Wilms tumor, aniridia, ambiguous genitalia, mental retardation)
Rubenstein-Taybi syndrome	Mental retardation, broad thumbs and toes, down-slanting palpebral fissures, hypoplastic maxilla, prominent nose, congenital heart disease	Heterozygosity for loss-of-function mutations in the autosomal gene encoding CREB-binding protein (CBP), a transcriptional coactivator for many different target genes
Waardenburg syndrome	Deafness, white forelock, pale and/or asymmetric eye pigmentation; cases due to *PAX3* mutations have abnormally wide space between the inner eyelids and occasional upper-limb defects	Autosomal semidominant loss-of-function mutations in one of two different genes: *PAX3*, which encodes a paired-like transcription factor expressed in the neural tube and somites, or *MITF*, which encodes a bHLH transcription factor expressed in developing pigment cells
Synopolydactyly	Interphalangeal webbing and extra digits in hands and feet	Semidominant gain-of-function mutation in *HOXD13*
Holoprosencephaly	Defective morphogenesis and bilateral cleavage of the forebrain and midface causes manifestations ranging from mild (single central incisor) to severe (microcephaly, cyclopia)	Approximately 10% of cases caused by heterozygosity for loss-of-function mutations in *SHH*, which encodes a dosage-sensitive paracrine signaling molecule; other etiologies include single-gene loci, multifactorial causes, and chromosomal imbalance syndromes
de Lange syndrome	Growth and mental retardation, upper-limb deficiencies, synophrys, depressed nasal bridge, anteverted nares, thin upper lip	Usually sporadic and probably new dominant mutation of unknown gene; rare sibling recurrence may be germline mosaicism
Multifactorial and/or Teratogenic		
Cleft lip with or without cleft palate	Absence of midline tissue from the upper lip, may extend posteriorly to involve the hard and soft palate	Isolated occurrences usually polygenic and associated with recurrence risks of 3%–5%; less frequently, associated findings suggest syndromic cause
Fetal alcohol syndrome	Microcephaly, optic nerve hypoplasia, developmental delay, facial abnormalities, hyperactive behavior	Prenatal exposure to ethanol during critical periods of brain development directly causes death of developing neurons
Retinoic acid embryopathy	Microtia (small ears), conotruncal cardiac malformations, posterior fossa malformations, thymus and parathyroid abnormalities	Exposure to isotretinoin causes abnormalities of neural crest– and branchial arch–derived structures
Chromosomal Imbalance		
Trisomy 21	Growth and mental retardation, abnormal facial features, hypotonia, endocardial cushion defect, duodenal atresia	50% increase in dosage for 250 genes on chromosome 21
Velocardiofacial syndrome	Cleft palate, prominent pear-shaped nose, conotruncal heart malformations, learning disabilities	Heterozygous microdeletion in 22q11 that contains 20 genes; individual genes responsible for morphogenetic abnormalities not yet identified

From Nussbaum RL, McInnes RR, Willard HF: Thompson and Thompson Genetics in Medicine, 6th ed. Philadelphia. WB Saunders, 2001, p 338.

HUMAN VARIATION

Normal human variation is enormous. A common sense argument can be made for variation by pointing out the ability of people to recognize and differentiate thousands of individuals whom they have met; computer programs for human recognition are based on this premise. A more biologic argument can be made by noting the problem of finding tissue match donors for organ transplantation. Nonetheless, humans differ little from one another in their DNA; variation is currently estimated as about eight bases per 10,000. Subgroups of the population may share many alleles and superficially resemble one another but still differ appreciably at the molecular level. Because persons in the same family or same group may resemble one another, any attempt at identifying a condition as an abnormality should include inspection of close relatives for their appearance. Unusual morphologic findings in a child who resembles his or her parents do not exclude a dysmorphic condition, but they probably mean that the child has another clinical finding that is of concern, motivating the questions for evaluation. The finding may be an obvious birth defect, short or large stature, developmental delay, mental retardation, or another significant problem. Many children have phenotype variations or minor anomalies; the more minor anomalies that are present, the greater is the probability that an underlying syndrome or a major organ anomaly is present (Table 33-5).

THE MOLECULAR BIOLOGY OF SYNDROMES

The identification of syndromes and practice in the field of dysmorphology have been viewed as tedious assignments that are based on arcane classifications from encyclopedic data sources. Computer programs have been devised to assist with diagnosis, but accessibility of programs is limited, and their utility is not as great as was anticipated. Syndromes are still identified by searching standard sources for a matching set of findings; there is no shortcut to this process. The careful and complete description is the phenotype (the physical appearance or behavioral expression); DNA analysis when available may provide the genotype and confirm the diagnosis, but it cannot unerringly define the phenotype. For decades, it has been possible to identify an individual from a database of millions on the basis of his or her physical fingerprints. It is much easier to identify one individual out of millions than it is to classify an individual in a group according to an arbitrary constellation of findings superimposed on a genome that is unique for the individual. The advent of molecular and biochemical diagnostic methods for identifying genes and gene products has begun to ease the burden on the geneticist by providing diagnostic and confirmatory tests for syndrome identification (Table 33-6; see Table 33-4). A surprise of the Human Genome Project was the proposed relatively low number of genes (28,000 to 40,000). However, there is a complexity of gene products as exemplified by an average of three proteins per gene resulting from

---

Table 33-5. Minor Anomalies and Phenotype Variants

Craniofacial	**Hand**
Large fontanel	Simian creases
Flat or low nasal bridge	Bridged upper palmar creases
Saddle nose, upturned nose	Clinodactyly of fifth digit
Mild micrognathia	Hyperextensibility of thumbs
Cutis aplasia of scalp	Single flexion crease of fifth digit (hypoplasia of middle phalanx)
Eye	Partial cutaneous syndactyly
Inner epicanthal folds	Polydactyly
Telecanthus	Short, broad thumb
Slanting of palpebral fissures	Narrow, hyperconvex nails
Hypertelorism	Hypoplastic nails
Brushfield spots	Camptodactyly
Ear	Shortened fourth digit
Lack of helical fold	**Foot**
Posteriorly rotated pinna	Partial syndactyly of second and third toes
Preauricular with or without auricular skin tags	Asymmetric toe length
Small pinna	Clinodactyly of second toe
Auricular (preauricular) pit or sinus	Overlapping toes
Folding of helix	Nail hypoplasia
Darwinian tubercle	Wide gap between hallux and second toe
Crushed (crinkled) ear	Deep plantar crease between hallux and second toe
Asymmetric ear sizes	**Others**
Low-set ears	Mild calcaneovalgus
Skin	Hydrocele
Dimpling over bones	Shawl scrotum
Capillary hemangioma (face, posterior neck)	Hypospadias
Mongolian spots (African Americans, Asians)	Hypoplasia of labia majora
Sacral dimple	
Pigmented nevi	
Redundant skin	
Cutis marmorata	

Approximately 15% of newborns have one minor anomaly; 0.8% have two minor anomalies, and 0.5% have three. If two minor anomalies are present, the probability of an underlying syndrome or a major anomaly (congenital heart disease, renal, central nervous system, limbic) is fivefold that in the general population. If three minor anomalies are present, the probability that there is a major anomaly is 20%-30%.

Table 33-6. Some Chromosomal Deletion Syndromes for which There Is a Commercially Available DNA Probe for Fluorescent In Situ Hybridization (FISH) Analysis

Condition	Brief Description	Probe
Williams syndrome	Proportionate short stature, mild-moderate to severe mental retardation, cocktail party patter for conversation, stellate pattern of iris pigmentation, supravalvular aortic stenosis, recessed nasal bridge, and wide mouth with full lips	7q11
WAGR syndrome	Wilms tumor, aniridia, growth delay, mental retardation, and genitourinary anomalies	11p13
Prader-Willi syndrome Angelman syndrome	Distinct syndromes with common or overlapping areas of deletion; phenotype depends on gender of the parent of origin of the deletion *Prader-Willi syndrome:* hypotonia in infancy, short stature, obesity, mild-moderate and occasionally severe mental retardation, small hands and feet (caused by paternal deletion of 15q11-13 or maternal uniparental disomy for chromosome 15) *Angelman syndrome:* severe mental retardation, absence of speech, ataxia, tremulous movements, large mouth, frequent drooling (caused by maternal deletion of chromosome 15q11-13 or paternal uniparental disomy)	15q11
Smith-Magenis syndrome	Brachycephaly, prognathism, self-destructive behavior, wrist biting, pulling out nails, head banging, indifference to pain, severe mental retardation, hyperactivity, social behavior problems	17p11.2
Miller-Dieker syndrome	Microcephaly, narrow temples, hypotonia/hypertonia, abnormal posturing, seizures, severe to profound mental retardation, poor growth, lissencephaly and other brain abnormalities on CT or MRI	17p13
Velocardiofacial (VCF) syndrome (overlaps with DiGeorge syndrome)	*VCF:* cleft palate, congenital heart disease, learning and/or behavior problems, long face, prominent nose, limb hypotonia, slender hands with tapering fingers *DiGeorge syndrome:* T cell deficiency, immunoglobulin deficiency	22q11

CT, computed tomography; MRI, magnetic resonance imaging; WAGR, Wilms tumor, aniridia, genitourinary anomalies, and mental retardation.

alternative splicing of exons and use of coding sequences in introns. The functions of numerous identifiable but unique DNA sequences remain to be evaluated. Allelic mutations can result in different-appearing syndromes. Mutations in the fibroblast growth factor receptor 3 gene can cause achondroplasia (a significant reduction in long bone growth and other skeletal problems), hypochondroplasia (a milder reduction in long bone growth), isolated craniosynostosis (premature closure of skull sutures), Crouzon syndrome with acanthosis nigricans; and thanatophoric dysplasia (a lethal skeletal dysplasia with hypoplastic thorax). The result of the molecular diagnostic study becomes the criterion for the condition or syndrome, but the morphologic description defines the parameters of the gene expression in a specific person. It is important to note that the genotype in an asymptomatic individual does not necessarily predict the final appearance or expressivity of the condition (phenotype). The morphology becomes complementary to the genotype, rather than defining the condition. For many syndromes, there is no confirmatory test, but the availability of clear descriptions will enhance understanding of the underlying molecular mechanisms.

THE CHILD WITH MORPHOLOGIC ABNORMALITIES

The evaluation of a child, especially a neonate or even a fetus, with morphologic abnormalities or other birth defects must be conducted with sensitivity and compassion, as well as with crisp and objective observation. The clinician must recognize the need to describe abnormalities adequately to parents and in the medical record but must not depict the infant as an alien-like being with the selection of frightening words derived from animal likenesses (carp mouth, simian crease) or mythologic constructs (gargoyle, monster).

A detailed history is an integral part of any medical assessment; however, the clinician needs to be aware that detailed questions about pregnancy, maternal health and habits, environmental exposures, and family history can have the unintended consequence of placing blame on an individual or the paternal or maternal family (see Table 33-3). Most birth defects occur sporadically without a family history. Autosomal recessive disorders typically happen in one or more siblings without a family history; many autosomal dominant conditions occur as new mutations. Even sex-linked conditions may have no prior family occurrence or an occurrence identified in a "remote" relative such as the maternal grandmother's brother. These cautions being noted, the examiner must obtain a complete history to assess whether any patterns may exist in the family.

MEDICAL HISTORY

Many conditions have some expression in utero. Environmental agents can cause morphologic problems and alterations in growth and development of the embryo and fetus. Prenatal history is helpful even if findings are negative, but very specific questions must be formulated. For example, questions about maternal health, assisted reproductive methods, pregnancy diagnosis, prepregnancy vitamin supplements, maternal weight gain, detection of fetal movement, uterine bleeding, maternal serum α-fetoprotein screening, fetal ultrasound assessment, diagnostic studies such as chorionic villi sampling and amniocentesis, and gestational diabetes are all important to establish. Maternal intake of prescription and nonprescription medications, alcohol, and "recreational" drugs, maternal smoking, and mother's inhalation of organic solvents (called "huffing") are very common, and all can affect a fetus, lead to morphologic changes, and otherwise affect fetal growth and development. Viral illnesses and rashes are germane to note, as are times of exposure during the pregnancy.

Parvovirus B19, rubella virus, cytomegalovirus, *Toxoplasma* species, herpes simplex virus, varicella virus, and *Treponema pallidum* (syphilis) are microorganisms that can be teratogenic or affect organ function. Fetal exposure to these organisms at a vulnerable time can be critical; conversely, exposures after formation of an organ are not expected to have a morphologic effect on the organ. The fetal upper lip and palate form and fuse between 4.5 weeks and 10 weeks of gestation. Exposures at 12 weeks of gestation cannot affect the process of lip and palate formation that was already complete. Chronic exposure to alcohol or episodic "binge" drinking can have adverse effects at any time. If exposure occurs after organ formation, growth may be affected. On occasion, a discrepancy is discovered between an ultrasound report and a neonatal clinical finding: for example, a "normal" cerebellum reported at 17 weeks of gestation and absence of the cerebellum at term. Before concluding that some process happened between 17 and 40 weeks of gestation, it is important to review the actual studies done at 17 weeks. This type of investigation can help pinpoint the timing of in utero problems or can eliminate erroneous hypotheses if the study of the fetus at 17 weeks was actually incomplete or inconclusive.

Events at the time of labor and delivery should be examined. Perinatal anoxia is often blamed for infants' problems, but infants with a syndrome or genetic condition may be predisposed to perinatal problems, including fetal distress or neonatal adaptive difficulties.

For older children, a medical history that includes a complete problem list, prior interventions, and medications is necessary to delineate the problems.

DEVELOPMENTAL HISTORY

A developmental history establishes the pattern for acquisition of developmental milestones. A screening tool such as the Denver Developmental Assessment Test can assist in the evaluation of younger children. It is important to establish whether a child is making progress, remaining static, or showing signs of developmental regression by losing landmarks of development (see Chapter 32). The last possibility is the most ominous for prognosis and warrants aggressive evaluation for diagnosis and possible treatment.

FAMILY HISTORY

Most syndromes, birth defects, or "dysmorphic" conditions occur without a family history, but a positive finding is invaluable in identifying a specific condition. In most populations, about 5% of children have a biologic father who is not the mother's current partner. This fact needs to be considered but must be handled with absolute discretion.

In taking a family history, it is helpful to methodically identify each family member by name, age, sex, relationship, and current health. It is customary to start with the siblings of the patient (the proband), proceed to the parents and the parents' siblings and their children, and then consider the four grandparents and their siblings. This approach is more helpful than the generic question, "Does anyone in the family have anything like this?" Many parents may be unaware of neonatal deaths in older relatives (the proband's grandparents or uncles and aunts).

Most people are unfamiliar with the term *consanguinity,* but the examiner can ask whether there are ancestors in common or inquire about the place of origin and the size of the community from which the families derive. Maiden names of women should always be noted. Self-identified, remote ancestry may help identify a fruitful area to investigate because certain conditions may be more common in certain ethnic population groups. *Consanguinity* refers to couples who have ancestors in common within two or three generations, whereas group identity is not consanguinity.

PHYSICAL EXAMINATION AND ASSESSMENT FOR MORPHOLOGIC ABNORMALITIES

The examination of an individual for problems of morphology must include all elements of a complete physical examination. Care must be taken not to overlook complicating acute problems such as signs of airway obstruction, sepsis, seizures, congestive heart failure, or increased intracranial pressure. While assessing a child's morphology, no physician should miss the immediate, life-threatening signs indicative of the need for intervention.

INSPECTION

The general observation of a child is important. If a child has an unusual appearance and the differences do not seem to be familial variations as judged by observing parents, then it is necessary to describe how the child appears different. When the variation is a discontinuous variable—that is, a birth defect (e.g., there is an extra digit on the ulnar side of each hand; there is a cleft of the lip on the left that extends into the left nostril, and there is a notch in the gum

---

Table 33-7. Clinical Findings that May Be Present with Trisomy 21*

Stature smaller than that of peer age group	Lax joints, including laxity of the atlantoaxial articulation (the latter predisposing the patient to C1-C2 dislocation)
Developmental delays	Short, broad hands, feet, and digits; single palmar crease, clinodactyly
Congenital heart disease (e.g., endocardial cushion defect and ventricular septal defect)	Exaggerated space between 1st and 2nd toes
Structural abnormalities of the bowel (e.g., tracheoesophageal atresia, duodenal atresia, annular pancreas, duodenal web, and Hirschsprung disease)	Velvety, loosely adhering mottled skin (cutis marmorata) in infancy; coarse, dry skin in adolescence
Central hypotonia	Statistically increased risk for leukemia, Alzheimer disease, hypothyroidism
Brachycephaly	
Delayed closure of fontanels	
Small midface, hypoplastic frontal sinuses, myopia, and small (short) ears	

From Behrman RE, Kliegman RM: Nelson Essentials of Pediatrics, 4th ed. Philadelphia, WB Saunders, 2002, p 142.

*An individual may exhibit any combination of these findings. There is no correlation between the number of physical findings and eventual level of mental performance. The increased risk for leukemia is significant but probably no greater than 1% for any individual. Alzheimer disease is relatively common in persons with trisomy 21 who die in middle adult life, but its frequency in all adults with Down syndrome is not known.

Table 33-8. Ultrasonographic and Pathologic Findings of Trisomic Conditions

Abnormality	Trisomy 21	Trisomy 18	Trisomy 13
IUGR	+	++	++
CNS abnormalities	−	+	++
Holoprosencephaly	−	−	++
Mild ventricular dilatation	+	+	+
Agenesis of the corpus callosum	−	+	+
Dandy-Walker variant	−	++	+
Spina bifida, NTD	−	++	+
Face	−	+	++
Cyclopia	−	−	++
Cleft lip or palate	−	+	++
Microphthalmia	−	++	+
Duodenal atresia	++	−	−
Esophageal atresia	+	++	−
Cardiac defects	+	++	++
Echogenic intracardiac foci	+	−	++
Diaphragmatic hernia	−	++	+
Cystic hygroma	+	+	+
Hydrops	+	+	+
Omphalocele	−	+	+
Echogenic bowel	++	+	+
Short femur or humerus	+	++	−
Radial aplasia or limb reduction	−	++	+
Clenched hands or wrists	−	++	+
Polydactyly	−	−	++
Club feet or rocker-bottom feet	−	++	++
Renal abnormalities	+	+	++
Choroid plexus cysts	+?	++	−
Single umbilical artery	−	++	++

From Nyberg DA, Souter VL: Sonographic markers of fetal aneuploidy, Clin Perinatol 2002;27:762.

IUGR, intrauterine growth retardation; CNS, central nervous system; NTD, neural tube defect.

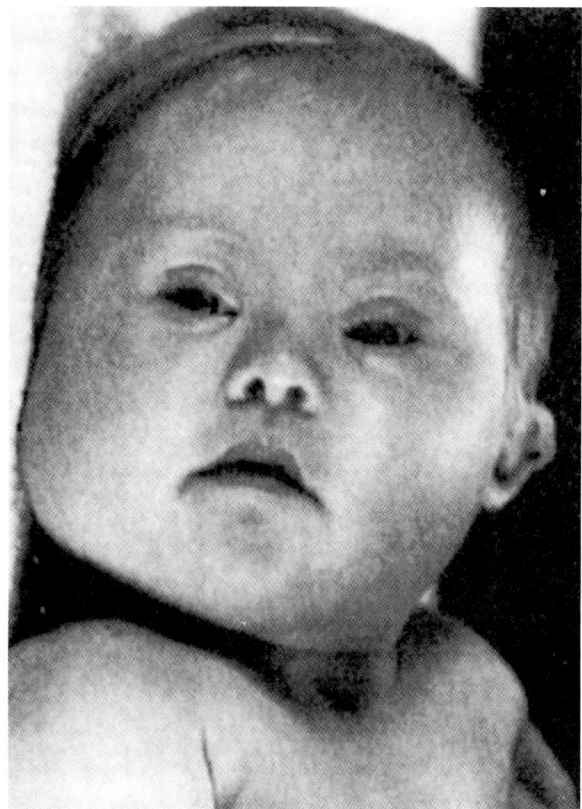

Figure 33-1. Facial appearance of a child with Down syndrome. (From Wiedemann HR, Kunze J, Dibbern H: Atlas of Clinical Syndromes: A Visual Guide to Diagnosis, 3rd ed. St. Louis, Mosby, 1989.)

glad for confirmatory tests. Most cases of trisomy 21 can be identified by inspection, but there is not the same degree of certainty about every dysmorphic patient.

Reference books on syndromology, human malformations, and deformations are excellent resources for assistance with diagnosis; however, most illustrations in texts focus on individuals with the most exaggerated findings to illustrate the condition. Birth defects are discrete (discontinuous) variables, but human features occur in a continuum. Diagnosis becomes a process of identifying the variables by a systematic evaluation of the entire individual.

ANTHROPOMETRICS

The Centers for Disease Control and Prevention published new growth curves for children and adolescents that were based upon a heterogeneous U.S. population more representative of various ethnic and ancestral groups than were previous charts. There are separate curves for height, weight, head circumference, and stature for boys and girls aged 0 to 36 months, and there are corresponding curves for boys and girls aged 2 to 18 years, in addition to curves for body mass index, but without curves for head circumference. There are also references for anthropometric measurements of various body parts from the fetus to adult age. If a child's measurements are discrepant from the norms—that is, over the 97th percentile or under the 3rd percentile—it is possible to transpose the actual measurement up or down to the 50th percentile on the same line to determine the height age or weight age equivalent. Height can be plotted versus weight on the stature curve to determine whether these parameters are proportional. Thus, a child can be identified as small or tall for age and

behind the cleft)—the task is easier. Such birth defects may be considered major abnormalities. The subtle malformations are often minor abnormalities, but both major and minor findings are relevant to diagnosis (see Table 33-5). Some conditions may be obvious on inspection alone, especially to an experienced observer. Typical manifestations of Down syndrome (Tables 33-7 and 33-8; Figs. 33-1 to 33-3), trisomy 13 or 18 (Table 33-9; Figs. 33-4 to 33-6), severe manifestations of de Lange syndrome, and those of Williams syndrome may represent a quick diagnosis; however, even these classical syndromes may manifest in atypical and subtle ways, and careful assessment is necessary to identify them. The expectation that, with enough experience, a physician, even a geneticist or a dysmorphologist, can unerringly identify every case of a common syndrome (even one so common and well known as trisomy 21) is not true. Human diversity is so great that even the most experienced clinicians are

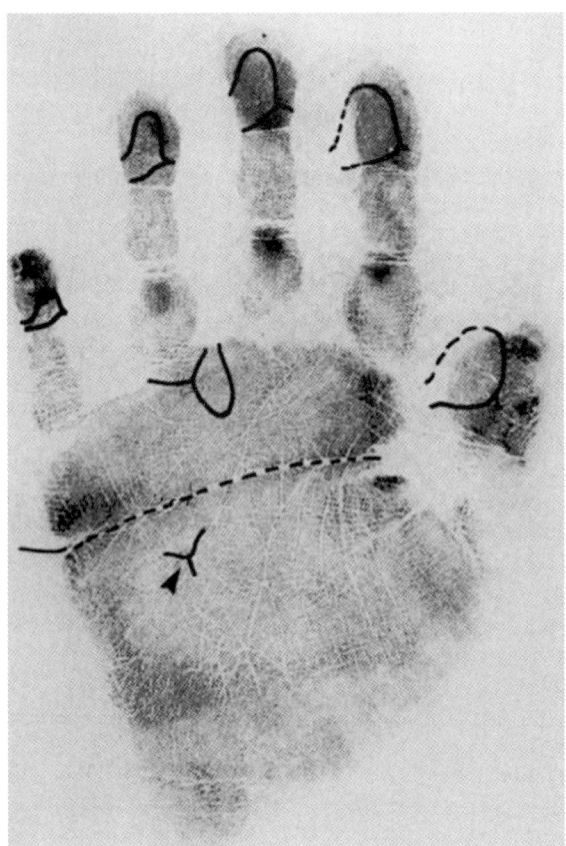

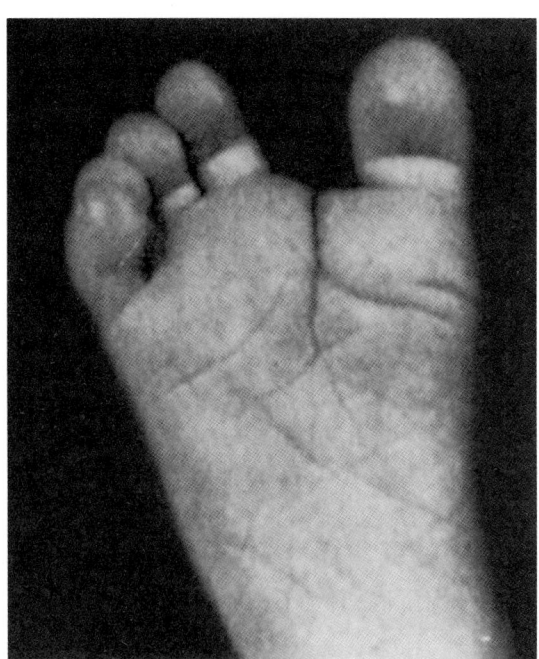

Figure 33-3. "Prehensile" foot in a 1-month-old child. (From Wiedemann HR, Kunze J, Dibbern H: Atlas of Clinical Syndromes: A Visual Guide to Diagnosis, 3rd ed. St. Louis, Mosby, 1989.)

Figure 33-2. Characteristic dermal patterns of the palm of a child with Down syndrome: a single flexion crease (simian crease), axial triradius (*arrowhead*) in distal position, a pattern area on the palm between the third and fourth digits, and ulnar loops on all 10 digits. (From Nussbaum RL, McInnes RR, Willard HF: Thompson & Thompson Genetics in Medicine, 6th ed. Philadelphia, WB Saunders, 2001, p 160.)

Table 33-9. Findings that May Be Present in Trisomy 13 and Trisomy 18

	Trisomy 13	Trisomy 18
Head and face	Scalp defects (e.g., cutis aplasia)	Small and premature appearance
	Microphthalmia, corneal abnormalities	Tight palpebral fissures
	Cleft lip and palate in 60%-80% of cases	Narrow nose and hypoplastic nasal alae
	Microcephaly	Narrow bifrontal diameter
	Microphthalmia	Prominent occiput
	Sloping forehead	Micrognathia
	Holoprosencephaly (arhinencephaly)	Cleft lip or palate
	Capillary hemangiomas	Microcephaly
	Deafness	
Chest	Congenital heart disease (e.g., VSD, PDA, and ASD) in 80% of cases	Congenital heart disease (e.g., VSD, PDA, and ASD)
	Thin posterior ribs (missing ribs)	Short sternum, small nipples
Extremities	Overlapping of fingers and toes (clinodactyly)	Limited hip abduction
	Polydactyly	Clinodactyly and overlapping fingers; index over 3rd, 5th over 4th; closed fist
	Hypoplastic nails, hyperconvex nails	Rocker-bottom feet
		Hypoplastic nails
General	Severe developmental delays and prenatal and postnatal growth retardation	Severe developmental delays and prenatal and postnatal growth retardation
	Renal abnormalities	Premature birth, polyhydramnios
	Nuclear projections in neutrophils	Inguinal or abdominal hernias
	Only 5% live longer than 6 mo	Only 5% live longer than 1 year

From Behrman RE, Kliegman RM: Nelson Essentials of Pediatrics, 4th ed. Philadelphia, WB Saunders, 2002, p 142.

ASD, atrial septal defect; PDA, patent ductus arteriosus; VSD, ventricular septal defect.

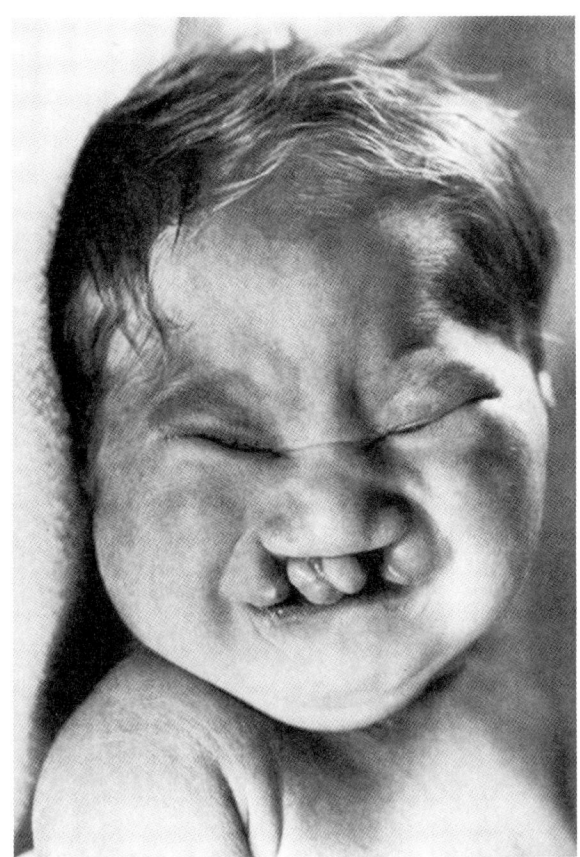

Figure 33-4. Facial appearance of a child with trisomy 13. (From Wiedemann HR, Kunze J, Dibbern H: Atlas of Clinical Syndromes: A Visual Guide to Diagnosis, 3rd ed, St. Louis, Mosby, 1989.)

appropriate or inappropriate in weight (either too heavy or too thin) for height (see Chapter 60). A child with short stature and proportionate weight has proportionate short stature. Head growth is an important factor in assessing brain growth as well as skull growth and suture closure. Abnormally small head size (microcephaly) and abnormally large head size (macrocephaly) are considered in proportion to stature with consideration for chronologic age. A child 7 years of age but with a height age of 4 and proportionate weight and head circumference does not truly have microcephaly, but proportionate short stature.

A helpful diagnostic assessment for children of discrepant size is the bone maturation or bone age, determined by radiograph: generally of the left hand and wrist, according to the standards of Gruleich and Pyle, but occasionally, for infants, by radiograph of the hemiskeleton (Sontag et al., 1939).

EXAMINATION

The details of morphology are documented in much more detail than is ordinarily the case in a general physical examination. Diagnosis is often based on the language used in the description. Even if a diagnosis is not clear, the description is the starting point of the evaluation. It is helpful to have an anatomic outline for assessing morphology in an orderly and systematic manner (Tables 33-10 to 33-14). Items usually included in a general medical examination are not generally included in this list.

ASSEMBLING THE DATA

After the history and examination are complete, the abnormal findings are listed. In general, the order is in a sequence ranked by perceived importance. In determining the order, the clinician may consider the magnitude of the deviation, but uniqueness is important in differentiating conditions. Subtleties can be significant; for example, inverted nipples (common in carbohydrate-deficient glycoprotein syndrome) or redundant umbilical skin (in company with abnormal anterior chamber of the eye and abnormally shaped teeth in Rieger syndrome) can be very helpful in identifying a condition.

The description of history and morphology becomes the working diagnosis. Even if the clinician cannot find a match in the standard

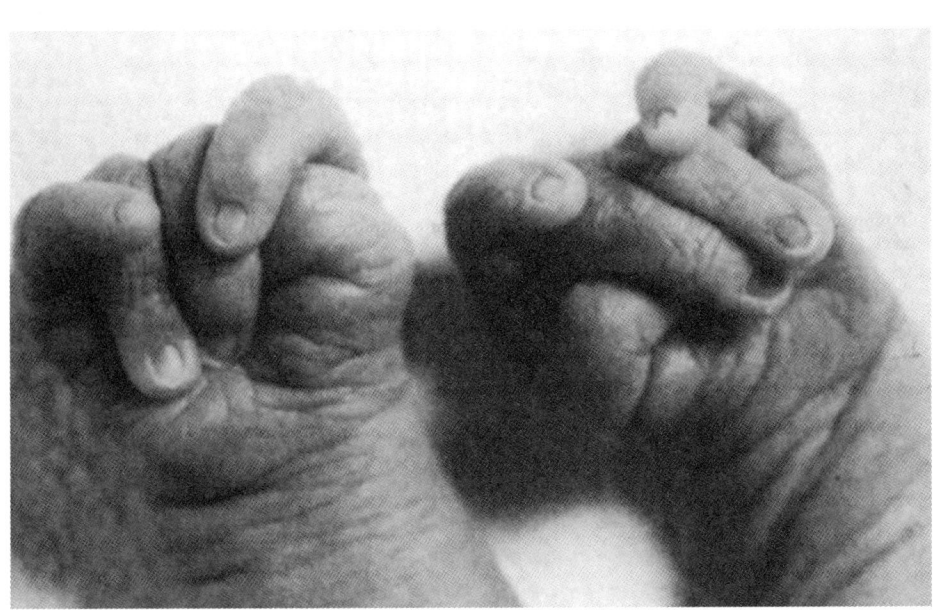

Figure 33-5. Trisomy 18: Overlapping finger and hypoplastic nails. (From Wiedemann HR, Kunze J, Dibbern H: Atlas of Clinical Syndromes: A Visual Guide to Diagnosis, 3rd ed. St. Louis, Mosby, 1989.)

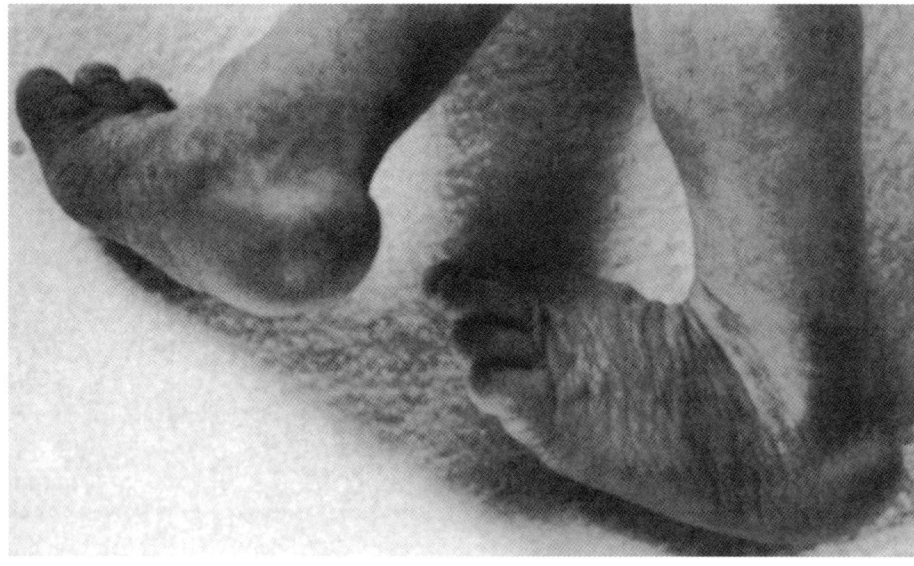

Figure 33-6. Trisomy 18: Rocker bottom feet (protruding calcanei). (From Wiedemann HR, Kunze J, Dibbern H: Atlas of Clinical Syndromes: A Visual Guide to Diagnosis, 3rd ed. St. Louis, Mosby, 1989.)

Table 33-10. Features of Congenital Syndromes Found on Physical Examination

Examination Site	Syndrome
Skin	
Cutis marmorata	Trisomy 21, hypothyroidism, de Lange syndrome
Café-au-lait spots	Neurofibromatosis
Ash-leaf hypopigmented macules	Tuberous sclerosis
Vesicular-linear pigmented macules	Incontinentia pigmentosa
Facial angioma	Sturge-Weber syndrome
Edema	Turner syndrome, Noonan syndrome, trisomy 21
Cutis aplasia	Trisomy 13
Sparse hair	Cartilage-hair hypoplasia, ectodermal dysplasias, oculodentodigital anomalies
Hypertrichosis	de Lange syndrome, fetal hydantoin syndrome, fetal alcohol syndrome, trisomy 18
Head	
Macrocephaly	Hydrocephalus, achondroplasia, Hallermann-Streiff syndrome, Hunter syndrome, Hurler syndrome, mucopolysaccharidosis type VII, Proteus syndrome, Robinson syndrome, Sotos syndrome, Weaver syndrome, Krabbe disease
Microcephaly	Cerebral dysgenesis, Aicardi syndrome, Angelman syndrome, Bloom syndrome, fetal alcohol syndrome, fetal rubella syndrome, maternal PKU, Seckel syndrome, Smith-Lemli-Opitz syndrome, Williams syndrome; trisomies 13 and 18; chromosome 3p, 4p, 5p, 11q, 13q, 18p deletions
Craniosynostosis	Apert syndrome, Carpenter syndrome, Crouzon syndrome, Pfeiffer syndrome, craniofrontonasal dysplasia, fetal hyperthyroidism, adrenal genital syndrome (Table 33-11)
Face	See Table 33-12
Neck	
Short	Klippel-Feil and Sprengel anomalies, Turner syndrome, Noonan syndrome, trisomy 21, Meckel-Gruber syndrome, Morquio syndrome, Scheie syndrome, CHARGE association, spondyloepiphyseal dysplasias
Redundant or webbed skin folds	Turner syndrome, Noonan syndrome, XXXX syndrome, trisomy 21, Klippel-Feil anomaly, Zellweger syndrome, Aarskog syndrome
Chest	
Thoracic hypoplasia	Thanatophoric dysplasia, Jeune asphyxiating thoracic dystrophy, achondroplasia, camptomelic, dysplasia, cleidocranial dysostosis, hypophosphatasia, short-rib–polydactyly syndrome
Pectus excavatum or carinatum	Marfan syndrome, Aarskog syndrome, Coffin-Lowry syndrome, homocystinuria, Morquio syndrome, mucopolysaccharidosis type VII, Noonan syndrome, osteogenesis imperfecta, Turner syndrome, XYY syndrome
Abdomen	See Table 33-13
Genitalia	See Chapter 31
Extremities	See Table 33-14

CHARGE, coloboma, heart disease, atresia choanae, retarded growth and development and/or central nervous system anomalies, genital hypoplasia, and ear anomalies and/or deafness; PKU, phenylketonuria.

Table 33-11. The Common Craniosynostoses Syndromes

Syndrome	Craniofacial Features	Additional Features	Prenatal Diagnosis
Apert syndrome	Irregular craniosynostosis, short AP diameter, full forehead and flat occiput, flat facies, hypertelorism, strabismus, down-slanting palpebral fissures, small nose, maxillary hypoplasia	Mental delay in more than half of the patients; agenesis of corpus callosum; ventriculomegaly; cleft palate; osseous or cutaneous syndactyly (mitten hands); fusion of C5-C6	Sonographic and molecular prenatal diagnosis were reported; because two mutations in *FGFR2* account for 98% of all mutations, mutation analysis in prenatally suspected sporadic cases is possible
Crouzon syndrome	Frontal bossing, ptosis, maxillar hypoplasia, parrot-like nose, short AP and wide lateral dimensions, hypertelorism	Mental delay, hydrocephaly, agenesis of corpus callosum, clefting, acanthosis nigricans, poor sight, hearing loss	Prenatal diagnosis in affected patients or with familial history was reported; molecular diagnosis was reported in familial case with known mutation
Pfeiffer syndrome	Brachycephaly, high forehead, hypertelorism, small nose with low nasal bridge, narrow maxilla; type 1—mild expression; type 2—severe malformations with cloverleaf skull; type 3— same type as type 2 without the cloverleaf skull deformity at birth	Broad distal phalanges of thumb and big toe, small middle phalanx of fingers, partial syndactyly	Sonographic diagnosis was reported on type 2; no molecular prenatal diagnosis has been reported; such diagnosis is feasible in suspected cases

From Dar P, Gross SJ: Craniofacial and neck anomalies. Clin Perinatol 2000;27:820.

AP, anteroposterior.

references concerning the syndrome identification, a descriptive diagnosis is invaluable for providing the constellation of findings that delineate the problems.

MINIMAL DIAGNOSTIC CRITERIA

The key phenotypic elements of a syndrome, which unquestionably identify it and differentiate it from all other similar conditions, have been termed the *minimal diagnostic criteria*. In the absence of a definitive laboratory test, establishing the diagnostic criteria is a logical and ideal goal for achieving uniformity of diagnosis. Unfortunately, minimal diagnostic criteria are difficult to decide upon and are enumerated for only a few conditions. Reasonably successful efforts at identifying diagnostic criteria for two relatively common conditions, neurofibromatosis type 1 (NF-1) (Table 33-15) and Marfan syndrome (Table 33-16), have been achieved through consensus conferences. The molecular abnormalities for each condition have been identified, but laboratory testing for each is not yet practical. Both conditions are inherited in an autosomal dominant pattern, but cases can arise from new mutations. It is instructive to view the criteria for these two conditions to appreciate the issues involved. The criteria for NF-1 were established first in 1988 (see Table 33-15) through a National Institutes of Health consensus conference. In NF-1, a family history that includes an affected parent is a major help (and major criterion) for diagnosis. When there is no positive family history, an index case is subjected to more criteria. The criteria are quite specific and include easily documented findings. However, criteria do not include learning disabilities, mental retardation, scoliosis, short stature, asymmetric limb growth, endocrine and neuroendocrine tumors, hypertension, or epilepsy, any of which may be present in NF-1. These conditions are germane, but not unique, to NF-1.

Diagnostic criteria for Marfan syndrome are given in Table 33-16. A family history that includes an affected parent is a major criterion and decreases the burden of diagnosis to finding a significant additional criterion and a minor finding. Often, the key criterion in the child of a parent with Marfan syndrome is a dilated aortic root. Many clinicians make a presumptive diagnosis and would prescribe prophylactic β blockers on these criteria alone. When there is an index case with a negative family history, the diagnosis is made by evaluating five body systems: cardiovascular, skeletal, ocular, cutaneous, and pulmonary. Criteria from two systems, with findings from a third, must be met. Although there can be debate about major and minor criteria, defining systems of relevance for diagnosis supplies a framework for making an analysis and leads to more uniformity.

The concept of minimal diagnostic criteria is laudable but difficult to achieve. When available, the minimal diagnostic criterion is the confirmatory laboratory test; however, the confirmatory laboratory test does not necessarily define the parameters of the phenotype of the syndrome.

DIAGNOSTIC TESTS

There is no universal test for establishing the nature of a birth defect or morphologic syndrome. Chromosome analysis with detailed banding detects trisomies, translocations, deletions, and duplications large enough to be resolved at the banding level achieved (Tables 33-17 and 33-18). Fluorescent-labeled DNA probes can identify submicroscopic deletions or rearrangements beyond the limit of banding resolution. It is not always practicable for a laboratory to screen for all known deletion syndromes, and so it is necessary to screen for deletions that may fit the morphology or phenotype of the patient.

Some examples of those syndromes for which there are commercially available probes are given in Table 33-6. Specific gene

Table 33-12.   Common Syndromes, Sequences, and Associations with Facial Anomalies

Facial Anomaly	Chromosomal Anomalies*	Single Gene Syndromes, Associations, and Sequences†‡	Teratogene Embryopathies
Frontal bossing	Trisomy 18	Achondroplasia, acromesomelic dysplasia, Apert syndrome, Beal syndrome, craniofrontonasal dysplasia, Crouzon syndrome, ectocermal dysplasia, Freeman-Sheldon syndrome, Jarcho-Levine syndrome, Killian syndrome, leprechaunism, Marshal-Smith syndrome, OPD types I and II, Pfeiffer syndrome, pyknosynostosis, Robinson syndrome, Rubinstein-Taybi syndrome, Russell-Silver syndrome, Schinzel-Giedion syndrome, Sotos syndrome	Fetal trimethadione syndrome, fetal valproate syndrome
Hypotelorism	Trisomy 13	Holoprosencephaly sequence, maternal PKU, Langer-Giedion syndrome, Meckel-Gruber syndrome, Williams syndrome	Fetal hydantoin syndrome
Hypertelorism	Cat-eye syndrome, triploidy, trisomies 13 and 8	Aarskog syndrome, acrodysostosis, Apert syndrome, CHARGE association, cleft lip sequence, craniofrontonasal dysplasia, Crouzon syndrome, Gorlin's syndrome, Holt-Oram syndrome, lethal Marshal syndrome, multiple pterygium syndrome, Noonan syndrome, Opitz syndrome, OPD types I and II, Pena-Shokeir syndrome, Pfeiffer syndrome, Robert syndrome, Robinow syndrome, SGBS, Sotos syndrome, Weaver syndrome	Fetal methotrexate syndrome, fetal hydantoin syndrome, retinoic acid embryopathy
Lateral displacement—inner canthi		Dubowitz syndrome, Freeman-Sheldon syndrome, frononasal dysplasia, Waardenburg syndrome, Pena-Shokeir syndrome, VCFS	Fetal valproate syndrome
Up-slanting palpebral fissures	Trisomies 13, 18, and 21	AR chondrodysplasia punctata, Jarcho-Levin syndrome, Miller-Dieker syndrome, Pfeiffer syndrome, Prader-Willi syndrome	Fetal hydantoin syndrome
Down-slanting palpebral fissures	Cat-eye syndrome	Aarskog syndrome, Apert syndrome, VCFS, lethal multiple pterygium syndrome, Miller syndrome, Nager syndrome, Noonan syndrome, OPD type II, Opitz syndrome, Robinow syndrome, Seckel syndrome, SGBS, Sotos syndrome, Treacher Collins syndrome, Weaver syndrome	
Prominent eyes		Anencephaly, Apert syndrome, Beckwith-Wiedemann syndrome, craniometaphyseal dysplasia, Crouzon syndrome, fibrochondrogenesis, Kniest dysplasia, Marshall syndrome, Pena-Shokeir syndrome, Robinow syndrome, Schinzel-Giedion syndrome, Seckel syndrome, Stickler syndrome	Fetal aminopterin/methotrexate syndrome
Microphthalmia		Aicardi syndrome, CHARGE association, frontonasal dysplasia sequence, Goltz syndrome, Meckel-Gruber syndrome, microphthalmia-linear skin, Proteus syndrome, Albright syndrome, Walker-Warburg syndrome	Fetal alcohol syndrome; fetal rubella syndrome, fetal warfarin syndrome
Small nose		Aarskog syndrome, acrodysostosis, acromesomelic dysplasia, achondrogenesis,	Fetal alcohol, hydantoin, trimethadione, valproate and warfarin syndromes

Anomaly	Chromosomal*	Single-gene syndromes†	Teratogen
Prominent nose	Trisomy 8 and 13	Apert syndrome, Bloom syndrome, de Lange syndrome, fibrochondrogenesis, Jarcho-Levin syndrome, Killian syndrome, Marshall syndrome, maternal PKU, Miller-Dieker syndrome, Optiz syndrome, OI type II, OPD type I, Pfeiffer syndrome, Robinow syndrome, SGBS, Stickler syndrome, Williams syndrome, Yunis-Varon syndrome, Zellweger syndrome	
Low-set ears	Cat-eye syndrome, trisomy 21, triploidy, trisomy 9, mosaic	Arteriohepatic dysplasia, floating harbor syndrome, Langer-Giedion syndrome, pyknodysostosis, Rubinstein-Taybi syndrome, Seckel syndrome, Smith-Lemli-Opitz syndrome, VCFS; Branchiooculofacial syndrome, Costello syndrome, de Lange syndrome, fibrochondrogenesis, Miller-Dieker syndrome, Noonan syndrome, OPD type II, Pena-Shokeir syndrome, Rubinstein-Taybi syndrome, Schinzel-Giedion syndrome, Seckel syndrome, short-rib polydactyly syndrome, Smith-Lemli-Opitz syndrome, Treacher Collins syndrome	Fetal aminopterin/methotrexate syndrome
Large protruding ears	Turner syndrome, 47,XYY	COFS, Cohen syndrome, fragile X syndrome, Langer-Giedion syndrome, leprechaunism syndrome, trichorhinophalangeal syndrome, Weaver syndrome	
Microtia	Trisomy 21	—	
Micrognathia	Cat-eye syndrome, trisomies 13 and 18, triploidy, Turner syndrome	Achondrogenesis type IA and IB, Bloom syndrome, campomelic dysplasia, COFS, Cohen syndrome, de Lange syndrome, Dubowitz syndrome, Hurler syndrome, Langer-Giedion syndrome, lethal multiple pterygium, Marshal-Smith syndrome, maternal PKU, Meckel-Gruber syndrome, Miller syndrome, Miller-Dieker syndrome, Möbius syndrome, Mohr syndrome, Nager syndrome, oculoauriculovertebral syndrome, Opitz syndrome, oral-facial-digital syndrome, OPD type I, Pallister Hall syndrome, Pena-Shokeir syndrome, pynodysostosis, Robert syndrome, Russell-Silver syndrome, Seckel syndrome, Smith-Lemli-Opitz syndrome, Stickler syndrome, Treacher Collins syndrome, VCFS, Weaver syndrome, Zellweger syndrome	Retinoic acid embryopathy
Prognathism		Acrodysostosis, Angelman syndrome, Beckwith-Wiedemann syndrome, fragile X syndrome, Sotos syndrome	
Macroglossia	Trisomy 21	Beckwith-Wiedemann syndrome, Robinow syndrome, SGBS	—

From Dar P, Gross SJ: Craniofacial and neck anomalies. Clin Perinatol 2000;27:814-815.

*Only common aneuploidies are listed. Rare chromosomal deletion and duplication syndromes diagnosed on routine karyotype were not included except for the common cat-eye syndrome (duplication of 22q11.2).

†Included are only single-gene syndromes, associations, or sequences previously diagnosed by prenatal sonography or that the authors believe will assist in future prenatal diagnosis.

‡Diagnosis of microdeletion syndromes available through fluorescence in situ hybridization.

AR, autosomal recessive; CHARGE, coloboma, heart disease, atresia choanae, retarded growth and development and/or central nervous system anomalies, genital hypoplasia, and ear anomalies and/or deafness; COFS, cerebrooculofacioskeletal syndrome; OI, osteogenesis imperfecta; OPD, otopalatodigital syndrome; PKU, phenylketonuria; SGBS, Simpson-Golabi-Behmel syndrome; VCFS, velocardiofacial syndrome.

Table 33-13. Characteristics of Anterior Abdominal Wall Anomalies

Anomaly	Structural Defects	Incidence	Karyotype	Prognosis
Body stalk anomaly	Short or absent umbilical cord, combined with any of the following: ventral wall defect or abnormality of the limbs, spine, face, or cranium	1 in 14,000	Normal	Usually lethal
Gastroschisis	A right paraumbilical defect of the abdominal wall allowing evisceration of the fetal intestines	0.3-2 in 10,000	Normal	73% survival
Pentalogy of Cantrell	Thoracoabdominal ectopia cordis, pericardial defect, cleft sternum, associated congenital heart defects, anterior diaphragmatic defects, and supraumbilical anterior abdominal wall defect	1 in 100,000	Trisomies 13, 18, and 21	Usually lethal
Cloacal exstrophy	Exstrophy of the bladder, omphalocele, imperforate anus, and spinal defects	1 in 200,000	Normal	Usually lethal, but if mild, amenable to surgical correction
Bladder exstrophy	Absence of anterior abdominal wall and anterior bladder wall	1 in 40,000	Normal	Amenable to surgical correction
Omphalocele	Abdominal contents, covered by peritoneum and amnion, herniated into the base of the umbilical cord	1-3 in 10,000	Associated chromosomal anomalies mainly trisomies 13 and 18, but also trisomy 21, and triploidy, Beckwith-Wiedemann syndrome	Prognosis dependent on presence or absence of associated aneuploidy Amenable to surgical correction

From Robinson JN, Abuhamad AZ: Abdominal wall and umbilical cord anomalies. Clin Perinatol 2000;27:952.

abnormalities and most triplet repeat expansions are not detected by analysis of the karyotype or fluorescent in situ hybridization studies.

Diagnostic imaging is invaluable in assessing central nervous system malformations. Computed tomographic scans of the brain are easier to obtain because they are quicker and show abnormalities containing calcifications, which are very difficult to see on magnetic resonance images (MRIs). MRIs are unequaled in providing detail about brain structures, including the cerebellum, patterns of myelination, and subtleties not visible on computed tomographic scan.

The presence of moderate to profound mental retardation and/or severe behavior problems warrants sophisticated chromosome analysis and brain imaging with MRIs (see Chapter 32). Bone age testing is indicated with short stature, growth delay, or large stature.

Specific laboratory tests involving molecular diagnostics or biochemical methods are often available. As with consideration for using fluorescent in situ hybridization probes for chromosomal deletion syndromes, specific laboratory tests are most useful for confirming or establishing a diagnosis that is strongly suspected, not for searching randomly. With a pattern of sex-linked mental retardation or with a boy who has a relatively normal appearance, mental delay, especially severe delays in expressive language, and perhaps prominent ears and/or macroorchidism, the clinician would request molecular diagnostic testing for fragile X syndrome (cytogenetic analysis for this entity is no longer appropriate.) The presence of short stature, microcephaly, developmental delay, ptosis, upturned nose, genital abnormalities, hand abnormalities (e.g., polydactyly, camptodactyly), and perhaps a cleft palate would suggest Smith-Lemli-Opitz syndrome, and the biochemical analysis for 7-dehydrocholesterol, if levels are elevated, confirms the diagnosis.

Table 33-14. **Conditions in Which Limb Defects Are a Prominent Feature**

Conditions	Limb Defects	Other Notable Features	Inheritance
Acromesomelic dysplasia	Short distal limbs, with brachydactyly	Low thoracic kyphosis, disproportionately large head	AR
Amniotic band syndrome	Asymmetric amputations, deformations	Facial deformities, oligohydramnios	Sporadic
de Lange syndrome	Micromelia, phocomelia, oligodactyly	Synophrys, initial hypertonicity, mental retardation	Mostly sporadic
Ectrodactyly–ectodermal dysplasia–clefting syndrome	Partial to complete ectrodactyly	Cleft lip and palate, ectrodermal defects, genitourinary anomalies	AD
Fanconi pancytopenia syndrome	Radial ray defect	Pancytopenia, hypopigmentation, genitourinary anomalies	AR
Femoral hypoplasia–unusual facies syndrome	Femoral hypoplasia	Cleft palate, short nose; associated with maternal diabetes	Mostly sporadic
Grebe syndrome	Marked distal limb reduction, polydactyly	Many stillbirths and neonatal deaths	AR
Holt-Oram syndrome	Variable upper limb defect	Cardiac anomaly	AD
Isolated polydactyly	Postaxial polydactyly	—	AD
Larsen syndrome	Dislocations of elbows, wrists, hips, and knees; talipes equinovalgus or varus; spine abnormalities	Flat face with depressed nasal bridge	? AD
Poland anomaly	Distal hypoplasia of upper extremities with syndactyly, oligodactyly, brachydactyly	Unilateral hypoplasia of anterior chest wall hypoplasia or absent nipple	Sporadic
Thrombocytopenia–absent radius syndrome	Bilateral absence of radius; abnormalities of ulna, humerus, and lower extremities	Thrombocytopenia, congenital heart defect	AR
Roberts syndrome	Tetraphocomelia, ectrodactyly	Microcephaly, mental retardation, severe growth deficiency, cleft lip or palate, ocular defects, high neonatal mortality	AR

From Dugoff L, Thieme G, Hobbins JC: Skeletal anomalies. Clin Perinatol 2000;27:997.

AD, autosomal dominant; AR, autosomal recessive.

Table 33-15. **Diagnostic Criteria for Neurofibromatosis Type 1***

I	Family history (an affected parent)
II	Six or more café-au-lait spots ≥0.5 cm in prepubertal children ≥1.5 cm in postpubertal individuals
III	One or more plexiform neurofibromas
IV	Two or more neurofibromas
V	Freckling of the armpits or in skin folds
VI	Two or more Lisch nodules of the iris
VII	Optic glioma
VIII	Osseous dysplasia of the sphenoid bone and/or long bone cortex

From National Institutes of Health Consensus Developmental Conference: Neurofibromatosis Conference Statement. Arch Neurol 1988;45:575.

*There must be positive findings in two or more categories.

SUMMARY AND RED FLAGS

Syndromes and isolated congenital malformations are of concern because of the possibility of acute life-threatening organ dysfunction (cyanotic heart disease, gastrointestinal obstruction, airway obstruction, intracranial hypertension) and the long-term prognosis and risk of serious chronic medical problems and disabilities. Red flags in the neonate reflect anatomic anomalies interfering with cardiopulmonary function, enteric feeding, or neurologic function. Long-term concerns include significant neurologic and cognitive developmental problems, especially seizures, developmental delay, and, most worrisome, developmental regression. Acute care in a neonatal intensive care unit with pediatric surgery coverage is indicated for all neonates with obvious anomalies of the head and face, airway, heart, abdominal wall, gastrointestinal tract, genitourinary tract, and spine.

Table 33-16.　Diagnostic Criteria for Marfan Syndrome*

I	Family history (an affected parent)	
II	Cardiovascular system	1. Dilatation of the aortic root[†] 2. Aortic aneurysm[†] 3. Mitral valve prolapse 4. Pulmonary artery dilatation
III	Skeletal system (In general, a combination of four criteria should be present.)	1. Positive wrist and thumb sign[†] 2. Upper and lower segment ratio ≥ 1 SD below the mean for age and/or arm span:height ratio ≥ 1.05[†] 3. Scoliosis >20 degrees or spondylolisthesis[†] 4. Pectus carinatum[†] 5. Severe pectus excavatum[†] 6. Elbow extension <170 degrees[†] 7. Pes planus caused by medial displacement of the medial malleolus[†] 8. Radiographic evidence of depression of the floor of the acetabulum[†] 9. Joint hypermobility 10. Dental crowding with high arched palate 11. Facial dysmorphology (dolichocephaly, malar hypoplasia, retrognathism, medial up-slanting palpebral fissures)
IV	Ocular system	1. Ectopia lentis[†] 2. Flat cornea (measured by keratometry) 3. Increased axial eye length (by ultrasonography) 4. Hypoplastic iris or ciliary muscle, causing decreased miosis
V	Pulmonary system	1. Spontaneous pneumothorax 2. Apical blebs (determined by CT scan)
VI	Cutaneous system and dura	1. Lumbosacral dural ectasia determined by MRI or CT imaging[†] 2. Stretch marks (independent of weight change, child bearing, or repetitive exercises) 3. Incisional hernia

Modified from DePape A, Devereaux RB, Dietz HC, et al: Revised diagnostic criteria for the Marfan syndrome and related conditions. Am J Med Genetics 1996;62:417-426.

*There must be positive findings in two systems and minimal findings in a third system.

[†]Major criterion that has high diagnostic specificity.

CT, computed tomographic; MRI, magnetic resonance imaging.

Table 33-17.　Common Deletions and Their Clinical Manifestations

Deletion	Clinical Abnormalities
4p–	Wolf-Hirschhorn syndrome: The main features are typical "Greek helmet" facies with ocular hypertelorism, prominent glabella and frontal bossing, microcephaly, dolichocephaly, hypoplasia of the eye socket, ptosis, strabismus, nystagmus, bilateral epicanthic folds, cleft lip and palate, beaked nose with prominent bridge, hypospadias, cardiac malformations, and mental retardation
5p–	Cri-du-chat syndrome: The main features are hypotonia, short stature, characteristic cry, microcephaly with protruding metopic suture, moonlike face, hypertelorism, bilateral epicanthic folds, high arched palate, wide and flat nasal bridge, and mental retardation
9p–	The main features are craniofacial dysmorphology with trigonocephaly, slanted palpebral fissures, discrete exophthalmos, arched eyebrows, flat and wide nasal bridge, short neck with pterygium colli, genital anomalies, long fingers and toes, cardiac malformations, and mental retardation
13q–	The main features are low birth weight, failure to thrive, and severe mental retardation; facial features include microcephaly, flat wide nasal bridge, hypertelorism, ptosis, micrognathia; ocular malformations are common; the hands have hypoplastic or absent thumbs and syndactyly
18p–	A few patients (15%) are severely affected and have cephalic and ocular malformations, cleft lip and palate, and varying degrees of mental retardation; most (80%) have only minor malformations and mild mental retardation
18q–	The main features are hypotonia with "froglike" position with the legs flexed, externally rotated, and in hyperabduction; the face is characteristic with depressed midface and apparent protrusion of the mandible, deep-set eyes, short upper lip, everted lower lip ("carplike" mouth); antihelix of the ears is very prominent; varying degrees of mental retardation and belligerent personality
21q–	The main features are hypertonia, microcephaly, downward-slanting palpebral fissures, high palate, prominent nasal bridge, large low-set ears, micrognathia, and varying degrees of mental retardation; they may have skeletal malformations

From Behrman RE, Kliegman RM, Jenson HB: Nelson Textbook of Pediatrics, 16th ed. Philadelphia, WB Saunders, 2000, p 328.

Table 33-18. Microdeletions and Their Clinical Manifestations

Deletion	Syndrome	Clinical Manifestations
7q23–	Williams	Round face with full cheeks and lips, stellate pattern in iris, strabismus, supravalvular aortic stenosis and other cardiac malformations, varying degrees of mental retardation, and a very friendly personality
8q24.1–	Langer-Giedion or trichorhinophalangeal, type II	Sparse hair, multiple cone-shaped epiphyses, multiple cartilaginous exostoses, bulbous nasal tip, thickened alar cartilage, upturned nares, prominent philtrum, large protruding ears, and mild mental retardation
11p13–	WAGR	Hypernephroma (Wilms tumor), aniridia, male genital hypoplasia of varying degrees, gonadoblastoma, long face, upward-slanting palpebral fissures, ptosis, beaked nose, low-set poorly formed auricles, and mental retardation
15q11–13 (pat)	Prader-Willi	Severe hypotonia at birth, obesity, short stature (responsive to growth hormone), small hands and feet, hypogonadism, and mental retardation
15q11–13 (mat)	Angelman	Hypotonia, fair hair, midface hypoplasia, prognathism, seizures, jerky ataxic movements, uncontrollable bouts of laughter, and severe mental retardation
16p13–	Rubinstein-Taybi	Microcephaly, ptosis, beaked nose with low-lying philtrum, broad thumbs and large toes, and mental retardation
17p11.2	Smith-Magenis	Brachycephaly, midfacial hypoplasia, prognathism, myopia, cleft palate, short stature, behavioral problems, and mental retardation
17p13.3–	Miller-Dieker	Microcephaly, lissencephaly, pachygyria, narrow forehead, hypoplastic male external genitals, growth retardation, seizures, and profound mental retardation
20p12–	Alagille	Bile duct paucity with cholestasis; heart defects, particularly pulmonary artery stenosis; ocular abnormalities (posterior embryotoxin); skeletal defects, such as butterfly vertebrae; long nose with broad midnose
22q11–	DiGeorge–velocardiofacial CATCH-22	Hypoplasia or agenesis of the thymus and parathyroid glands, hypoplasia of auricle and external auditory canal, conotruncal cardiac anomalies, cleft palate, short stature, behavioral problems

From Behrman RE, Kliegman RM, Jenson HB. Nelson Textbook of Pediatrics 16th ed. Philadelphia, WB Saunders, 2000, p 331.

CATCH-22, cardiac defects, abnormal facies, thymus hypoplasia, cleft palate, and hypocalcemia caused by chromosome 22 defects; WAGR, Wilms tumor, aniridia, genitourinary anomalies, and mental retardation.

REFERENCES

Bone Age and Physical Measurements

Greulich WW, Pyle SI: Radiographic Atlas of Skeletal Development of the Hand and Wrist, 2nd ed. Stanford, Calif, Stanford University Press, 1959.

Hall JG, Froster-Iskenius UG, Allanson JE: Handbook of Normal Physical Measurements. New York, Oxford University Press, 1989.

Keats TEE: Atlas of Roentgenographic Measurement. St. Louis, Mosby-Yearbook, 1990.

Sontag LW, Snell D, Anderson M: Skeletal maturation. Am J Dis Child 1939;58:949.

Syndrome References

Bonthron D, Fitzpatrick D, Porteous M, Trainor A: Clinical Genetics: A Case-Based Approach. Philadelphia, WB Saunders, 1998.

Bronstein RA, Cornstock CH: Central nervous system anomalies. Clin Perinatol 2000;27:791-812.

Bukowski R, Saade GR: Hydrops fetalis. Clin Perinatol 2000;27:1007-1032.

Dar P, Gross SJ: Craniofacial and neck anomalies. Clin Perinatol 2000;27:813-838.

Devine PC, Malone FD: Noncardiac thoracic anomalies. Clin Perinatol 2000;27:865-900.

Dugoff L, Thieme G, Hobbins JC: Skeletal anomalies. Clin Perinatol 2000;27:979-1006.

Gleason PF, Eddleman KA, Stone JL: Gastrointestinal disorders of the fetus. Clin Perinatol 2000;27:901-920.

Goodman RM, Gorlin RJ: The Malformed Infant and Child—An Illustrated Guide. New York, Oxford University Press, 1983.

Gorlin RJ, Cohen MM Jr, Hennekam RCM: Syndromes of the Head and Neck, 4th ed. New York, Oxford University Press, 2001.

Jacobs AM, Toudjarska I, Racine A, et al: A recurring FBN1 gene mutation in neonatal Marfan syndrome. Arch Pediatr Adolesc Med 2002;156:1081-1084.

Jones KL: Smith's Recognizable Patterns of Human Malformations, 5th ed. Philadelphia, WB Saunders, 1997.

Malone FD, D'Alton ME: Anomalies peculiar to multiple gestations. Clin Perinatol 2000;27:1033-1046.

McKusick VA: Mendelian Inheritance in Man, 12th ed. Baltimore, Johns Hopkins University Press, 1998. Available on line as: OMIM: Online Mendelian Inheritance in Man, *http://www3.ncbi.nim.nih.gov/OMIM/*

Nyberg DA, Souter VL: Sonographic markers of fetal aneuploidy. Clin Perinatol 2000;27:761-789.

Robinson JN, Abuhanad AZ: Abdominal wall and umbilical cord anomalies. Clin Perinatol 2000;27:947-978.

Roizen NJ, Patterson D: Down's syndrome. Lancet 2003;361:1281-1288.

Saphier CJ, Gaddipati S, Liat E, et al: Prenatal diagnosis and management of abnormalities in the urologic systems. Clin Perinatol 2000;27:921-946.

Simpson JL, Elias S: Genetics in Obstetrics and Gynecology, 3rd ed. Philadelphia, WB Saunders, 2003.

Simpson LL: Structural cardiac anomalies. Clin Perinatol 2000;27:839-864.

Stevenson RE, Hall JG, Goodman RM: Human Malformations and Related Anomalies, Vols. 1 and 2. New York, Oxford University Press, 1993.

34 The Irritable Infant

Emory M. Petrack

An irritable infant is a challenge to the parents and physician. Although most infants may be irritable at times, an irritable infant is defined here as a patient younger than 1 year of age who, according to the caregiver, cries excessively or is excessively fussy or cranky. There are many causes of infant irritability (Tables 34-1 and 34-2); most irritable infants do not have significant underlying pathologic processes. However, there are serious entities that must not be missed (Table 34-3).

DIAGNOSTIC APPROACH

The approach to the crying infant is directed toward a thorough history and physical examination, coupled with the judicious use of laboratory and roentgenographic studies. Patients without prior medical problems (e.g., sickle cell anemia) who cry for more than 2 hours and whose parents believe that this episode is longer than any previous episode represent approximately 0.2% of emergency department visits. The final diagnoses in these irritable infants underscore the importance of a thorough evaluation. The history provides important information in directing the evaluation in approximately 20% of cases. The final diagnosis is evident from the initial physical examination in 41%, from initial laboratory or roentgenographic studies in 20% (Table 34-4), and from subsequent follow-up evaluations in 39%.

In 61% of these irritable infants, the crying may result from a serious underlying cause, defined as a condition with the potential to cause harm if it is not promptly treated. In 75% of these seriously ill infants, the diagnosis can be made or accurately suspected by the end of the physical examination. Many seriously ill infants may continue to cry excessively after their evaluation; most infants without serious conditions stop crying. Abnormal physical findings or persistent crying beyond the initial assessment may be predictive of serious illness, with a sensitivity of 100% (95% confidence interval: 90% to 100%), a specificity of 77% (95% confidence interval: 54% to 91%), and a positive predictive value of 87% (95% confidence interval: 72% to 95%).

As with any potentially ill patient, initial attention is given to the evaluation and stabilization of the patient; the next step is to obtain a careful history and perform a physical examination (Fig. 34-1). Every component of the physical examination has the potential to uncover findings that may direct the clinician to a specific diagnosis (Table 34-5). Every part of the patient's body should be carefully examined after clothing is removed. This initial evaluation should be performed with the intent of specifically looking for serious conditions (see Table 34-3) and should include a fluorescein examination of the eye to detect a corneal abrasion and retinoscopy to detect retinal hemorrhages.

In patients with normal findings on physical examination, further evaluation is based on the ability to console the patient during the evaluation. In patients with normal examination results, very few consolable patients have a serious condition, whereas about 60% of inconsolable patients have a serious illness. In the consolable infant, the clinician should consider nonurgent causes of crying (Table 34-6).

However, these patients must be monitored closely (at 24-hour intervals or sooner) for the development of a serious condition.

In the persistently inconsolable infant, laboratory studies are needed to assist in the diagnostic process, and patients are best monitored in the hospital until a diagnosis can be established. Some ancillary tests to consider are

- a complete blood cell count, erythrocyte sedimentation rate, and/or C-reactive protein measurement (for infection or inflammation)
- analysis of cerebrospinal fluid (C-reactive protein) (for meningitis or encephalitis)
- hemoglobin electrophoresis (for signs of sickle cell disease)
- serum pH and electrolyte (for electrolyte abnormalities, metabolic diseases)
- urinalysis and culture (for urinary tract infection)
- stool guaiac (for intussusception, gastroenteritis, cow's milk allergy)

Other possible tests include a skeletal survey or bone scan (for trauma, abuse) and a computed tomographic (CT) scan of the head (for intracranial hemorrhage or hydrocephalus).

Despite the many possible causes of irritability, the most likely diagnosis in infants younger than 4 months of age is either above-average crying in a normal infant or infantile colic. The information that the physical examination is normal (coupled with assurances about conditions that have been ruled out) may reduce parental stress. Other issues concerning feeding (overfeeding or underfeeding), teething, and parental stress are all important to explore. Caregivers should be questioned about the options for increased support from family or friends during this stressful period. Of most importance, because a definitive diagnosis has not been established, infants should receive follow-up evaluation within 24 hours to ensure that a more serious illness was not missed.

SPECIFIC DIAGNOSES

INFANTILE COLIC (EXCESSIVE CRYING, PAROXYSMAL FUSSING, PERSISTENT CRYING)

Infantile colic is a controversial topic, and there is still marked disagreement regarding its cause and management. A uniform definition for infantile colic is lacking, and there exists an inability to incorporate double-blind strategies to assess some of the interventions for it and an overreliance on maternal recall for documenting length of crying. Furthermore, colic is a relatively self-limited condition that usually lasts less than 3 months. Because of these facts, there may not be enough time to adequately assess the success of a particular therapy. Nonetheless, colic is a common problem, occurring in 20% to 30% of infants.

Definition

Colic refers to unexplained paroxysms of irritability, fussing, or crying. Episodes occur more than three times per week, last longer than 3 hours per day, and usually are present for 3 weeks. Paroxysms

Table 34-1. Differential Diagnosis in the Irritable Infant

Central Nervous System Encephalitis Hydrocephalus Intracranial hemorrhage Meningitis Pseudotumor cerebri Tumor **Eyes** Corneal abrasion Foreign body Glaucoma **Ears** Otitis media, externa Foreign body **Nose** Foreign body **Mouth** Foreign body Herpangina Herpes stomatitis Teething **Respiratory System** Bronchiolitis Foreign body aspiration Pneumonia Reactive airways Upper airway obstruction **Cardiovascular System** Anomalous coronary artery Congestive heart failure Supraventricular tachycardia **Gastrointestinal System** Anal fissure Appendicitis Constipation Feeding problems Gastroenteritis Gastroesophageal reflux	Incarcerated inguinal hernia Intussusception Malrotation Volvulus **Genitourinary Tract System** Testicular torsion Tourniquet syndrome of the penis Urinary tract infection **Musculoskeletal System** Cellulitis Diskitis Fractures Osteomyelitis Physical abuse Septic arthritis Soft tissue injury Tourniquet syndrome of the digit **Skin** Dermatitis Insect bites **Miscellaneous** Colic Drug ingestion Electrolyte disorder Fever Hypoglycemia Hypoxia Inborn error of metabolism Lactose intolerance Neonatal drug withdrawal (from maternal use) Parenting difficulties Sepsis Sickle cell anemia crisis Vaccine reaction Viral syndrome

Table 34-2. Acute and Subacute Causes of Infant Irritability

Acute (<48-72 hours)	Subacute (>3-4 Days)

Infectious
 Encephalitis
 Herpangina
 Herpes stomatitis
 Meningitis
 Osteomyelitis
 Otitis media
 Sepsis
 Urinary tract infection
 Viral syndrome
Surgical
 Appendicitis
 Hernia*
 Intussusception
 Testicular torsion
 Volvulus
Cardiovascular
 Congestive heart failure
 Supraventricular tachycardia
Trauma
 Minor
 Intracranial hemorrhage
 Insect or spider bites, bee sting
 Physical abuse
Other
 Dermatitis
 Fever
 Vaccine reaction
 Drugs
 Corneal abrasion
 Anal fissure*
 Hair tourniquet
 Electrolyte disturbances*
 Hypoglycemia*
 Foreign body in ear, nose, eye, oropharynx
 Sickle cell anemia crisis
 Hypoxia
 Teething
 Abdominal pain
  Constipation
  Gastroenteritis
  Gastroesophageal reflux
 Colic*
	Colic*
	Feeding problems*
	Parenting difficulties
	Dermatitis
	Teething
	Abdominal pain
	 Constipation
	 Gastroenteritis
	 Gastroesophageal reflux
	 Anal fissure*
	Infectious
	 Diskitis
	 Encephalitis
	 Herpangina
	 Herpes stomatitis
	 Meningitis
	 Osteomyelitis
	 Otitis media
	 Urinary tract infection
	 Viral syndrome
	Trauma
	 Minor
	 Insect or spider bites
	 Physical abuse
	Other
	 Drugs
	 Foreign body in ear, nose, eye, oropharynx
	 Toxin exposure
	 Lactose intolerance
	 Inborn error of metabolism
	 Congenital lesions*
	  Heart disease
	  Glaucoma
	  Hydrocephalus
	  Central nervous system abnormality

*Most commonly seen in infants younger than 3 months.

generally occur in the evenings, usually start between 3 and 21 days of age, and subside by 3 to 4 months of age. In an infant with colic, no underlying disease is responsible for the crying. Crying and fussing are normal parts of early infant development. Normal crying gradually increases from birth until 2 months of age, when the child may cry for a total of 2.5 hours per day. The distinction between normal crying and colic is not clear. Colic may simply represent a point further along on a continuum of infant behavior.

Cause

The cause of colic is unclear. Colic may not represent a single entity but, rather, may be a common endpoint for various processes. Some of the proposed theories for the causes of colic are dietary antigens (milk proteins), abnormal peristalsis, excessive gas production, and infant temperament.

Some of the dietary antigens that have been implemented as a possible cause for colic are cow's milk proteins (whey or casein) and soy protein; maternal consumption of cow's milk has been associated with colic in purely breast-fed infants. Unfortunately, no specific laboratory test exists for diagnosing protein allergy in relation to infantile colic. In some infants, crying time may decrease with the elimination of soy or cow's milk protein. However, reexposure of a diet-treated group to soy or cow's milk antigen may not result in an increase in crying time. Despite the conflicting evidence, dietary protein may play some role in a subset of crying infants.

Another theory of the origin of colic implicates abnormal peristalsis or excessive intestinal gas. Colicky infants often exhibit intermittent episodes of crying that appear to be associated with pain. The infant seems to achieve relief after the passage of flatus. It is difficult to know whether these episodes of colic are a result of excess gas or whether the excess gas is a result of significant periods

Table 34-3. Diagnoses Not to Be Missed (Red Flags)

Acute surgical abdomen
Anomalous coronary artery
Congestive heart failure
Corneal abrasion
Electrolyte disturbances
Foreign body
Incarcerated hernia
Intussusception
Physical abuse
Serious infectious illness
Supraventricular tachycardia
Testicular torsion
Tourniquet syndromes

of crying with aerophagia. If there are excessive gas, watery diarrhea, and cramps, it is possible that lactose malabsorption is present. Lactose feeding with a hydrogen breath test confirms this diagnosis. Infants with lactose malabsorption should respond to a non–lactose-containing formula.

The role of abnormal peristalsis and infant crying is suggested by the reduction of infant crying with dicyclomine hydrochloride, which is an anticholinergic agent. Because of the severe side effects of this drug (including hypersensitivity reactions and apnea), it is no longer approved for use in infants younger than 6 months. Drugs that have been shown to have no effect in treating colic are simethicone, dimethicone, alcohol, and phenobarbital. In addition, several reports have been published of infants presenting with cyanosis and apnea who were treated for colic with the following medications: dimenhydrinate (Dramamine) plus phenobarbital, hyoscyamine sulfate, atropine sulfate, and scopolamine hydrobromide (Donnatal). The clinician must be aware that parental distress from prolonged, unexplained infant crying can lead to the use of inappropriate and even dangerous remedies.

Table 34-4. Utility of Ancillary Studies in Infants with Acute Excessive Crying

Diagnostic Study	No. of Patients in Whom Study Proved Useful (n = 11)	Final Diagnosis (n)
Skeletal radiography	2	Tibial fracture (1) Clavicular fracture (1)
Lumbar puncture/ cerebrospinal fluid analysis	2	Pseudotumor cerebri (1)* Encephalitis (1)
Electrocardiography	2	SVT
CT of the head	2	Pseudotumor cerebri (1)* Subdural hematoma (1)
Barium enema	1	Intussusception
Esophagraphy	1	GE reflux/esophagitis
Amino and organic acid studies	1	Glutaric aciduria
Urinalysis	1	Urinary tract infection

Adapted from Poole S: The infant with acute, unexplained, excessive crying. Pediatrics 1991;88:450-455.

*One patient, with pseudotumor cerebri, required lumbar puncture and head CT to establish the diagnosis.

CT, computed tomography; GE, gastroesophageal; SVT, supraventricular tachycardia.

Another theory relates to infant temperament. Some infants have an increased sensitivity to surrounding stimuli, leading to excessive crying. Parental anxiety concerning the crying infant may interact with the infant's native temperament to create an environment that exacerbates the problem. Some aspect of this infant-maternal relationship is frequently associated with a significant number of children with the diagnosis of colic (Fig. 34-2).

Clinical Features

The most prominent feature of the infant with colic is significant crying or irritability. It is important to carefully characterize the nature of the crying, including the duration, intensity, and time of day when it occurs. The crying is intense and often inconsolable. Episodes typically occur in the late afternoon or evening. The parent is often quite distressed about the inability to soothe the infant. At times of the day when the infant is not exhibiting this behavior, the activity level, amount of feeding, and general appearance are normal. In addition, there is no suggestion of any other pathophysiologic process.

In infantile colic, both the physical examination and laboratory results are normal. Even though the clinician may suspect infantile colic from the history alone, it is extremely important to perform a thorough physical examination to rule out other diagnoses (see Fig. 34-1 and Table 34-5). If the infant remains inconsolable during the evaluation, the clinician needs to perform a series of laboratory investigations to rule out other conditions (see Fig. 34-1 and Table 34-4). If the infant has normal physical findings, is consolable, and has a history consistent with infantile colic, laboratory tests are usually not required.

Treatment

Before a management plan is chosen, other serious illnesses must be ruled out (see Tables 34-1 and 34-2). In the initial presentation, colic can be confused with other, more significant disease processes necessitating immediate intervention.

The following approach to the infant with colic is recommended:

1. The level of distress and anxiety that the crying is causing the parents should be recognized and acknowledged with empathy. Severe colic can be associated with an intense level of frustration and anger for the entire family. It is not acceptable to acknowledge colic simply as a developmental phenomenon that the infant will soon outgrow.
2. The parents should be reassured that, according to a thorough history and physical examination, no specific problem exists regarding the infant's physical or emotional health. The clinician should acknowledge that the infant appears to be crying more than the average infant and that such crying can be quite stressful for the family.
3. Although still controversial, changing the infant's formula is probably helpful in only a subset of infants with colic. In addition, although some clinicians switch from lactose-based to soy-based formulas, soy protein may be as antigenic as cow's milk protein and can cause irritability. If an allergic cause is suspected, a formula change to a hydrolyzed casein formula (Nutramigen) may be considered. A change in formula may not be without undesirable behavioral consequences, including development of parental anxiety concerning the possibility of an intrinsic abnormality in their infant. Appropriate counseling should help to allay this fear.
4. Although increased carrying of young infants may reduce normal crying time, such a reduction has not been shown to occur in infants with colic. Parents might try to respond to excessive crying by feeding the baby, holding the baby, giving the baby a pacifier, or putting the infant to bed. It has also been suggested that perhaps some background noise or vibration, as occurs during an automobile ride, might be useful. The possibility of overstimulation as a

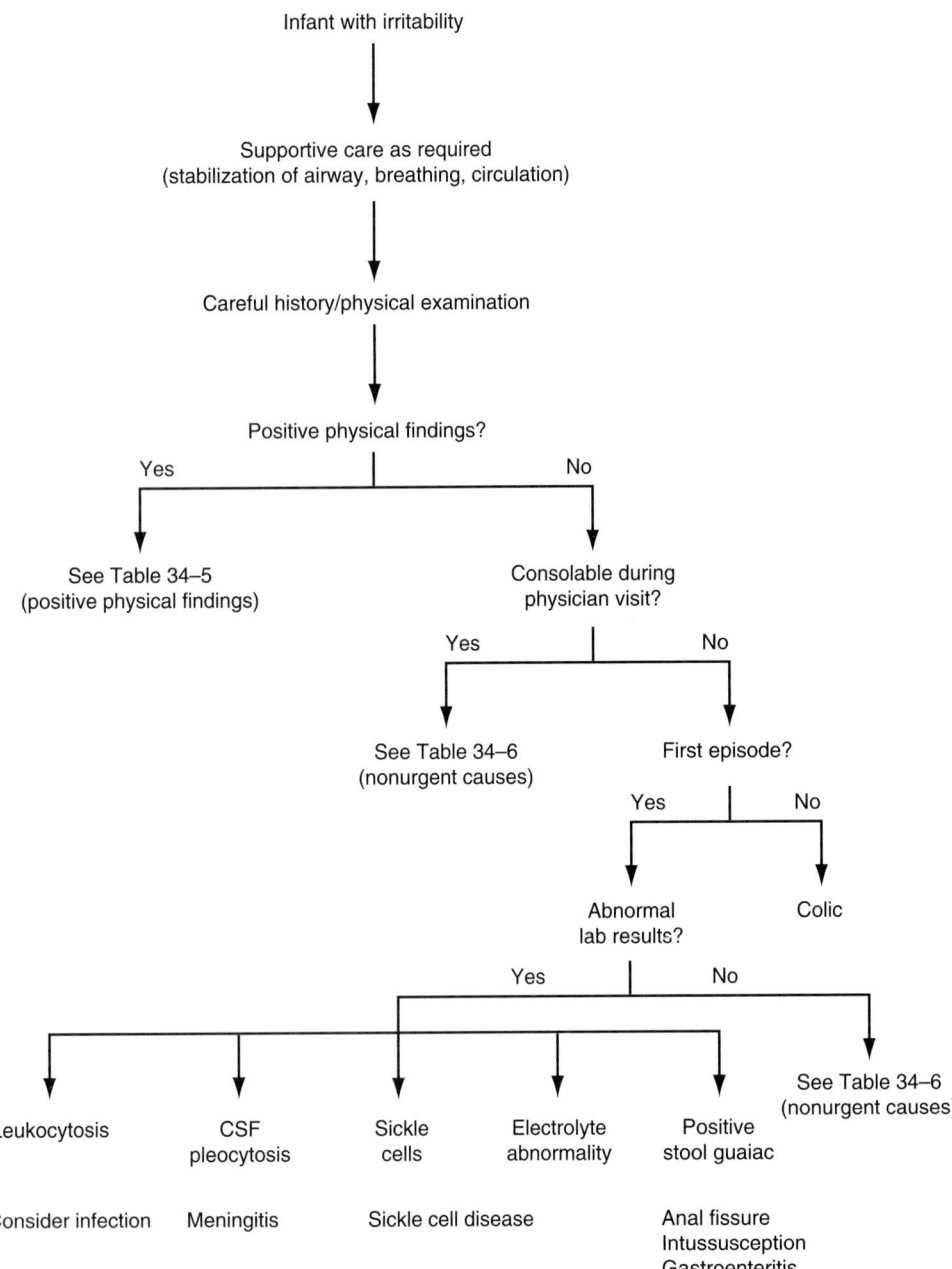

Figure 34-1. Approach to the irritable infant. CSF, cerebrospinal fluid.

cause of colic should also be entertained. If the infant remains inconsolable after 20 to 30 minutes of active intervention, it is probably worthwhile attempting to decrease stimulation by attempting to put the infant to bed in a quiet environment.

5. The use of various medications to reduce colic remains controversial. These medications also have potential serious and life-threatening side effects. No specific drug therapy can be recommended for the treatment of colic.

6. The clinician should give encouragement to the parents that altering the way they handle the crying and interact with the infant during colicky periods should reduce the amount of crying. While not minimizing the impact of colic on the family, the clinician should explain to the family the natural history of colic. The primary caregiver should be encouraged to seek support and periodic relief from the infant's care.

7. Close follow-up is important. This element is especially critical if the clinician has any doubt concerning the establishment of the correct diagnosis.

TOURNIQUET SYNDROMES

In tourniquet syndromes, a filamentous material, such as hair or a thread from clothing, becomes wrapped around an appendage, causing ischemia. Some of the reported appendages that can be affected by this syndrome are the fingers, the toes, the penis, and the uvula. Almost 2% of infants with prolonged crying may have a tourniquet syndrome. Hair that is initially moist can tighten as it dries after becoming wrapped around an affected appendage. With surrounding edema, the hair may become partially or completely obscured in the skin, which makes the diagnosis difficult to establish. This syndrome should be suspected in any irritable infant who has a well-demarcated line separating normal tissue from a distal dusky, edematous appendage.

With penile hair strangulation, the distal penis is noted to be swollen, edematous, and sometimes discolored. The hair is often deeply imbedded in a groove that is covered with edematous tissue. Because the hair is often not visible, an erroneous diagnosis of

Table 34-5. Positive Findings on Physical Examination

Physical Finding	Possible Diagnoses	Specific Tests to Consider
Skin	Dermatitis (eczema)	
	Abuse	Skeletal survey
	Vaccine reaction	
	Abrasion, cellulitis	
	Insect bite	
	Viral exanthem	
Fever with		
Inflamed eardrum	Otitis media	
CVA tenderness	Urinary tract infection	UA, urine/blood culture
Bone tenderness, erythema	Osteomyelitis, arthritis	CBC, ESR, blood culture, bone scan, arthrocentesis
Tachycardia	Supraventricular tachycardia	Electrocardiography
	Congestive heart failure	CXR
	Dehydration	Electrolyte levels
	Trauma	Hematocrit, UA, CT
	Blood loss, anemia	Hematocrit
Tachypnea	Hypoxia	Pulse oximetry, ABG, CXR
	Respiratory illness	Pulse oximetry, ABG, CXR
	Salicylate ingestion	ABG, salicylate level
	Acidosis	ABG
Ears	Otitis media	
	Foreign body	
Eyes	Corneal abrasion	Fluorescein stain
	Foreign body	Fluorescein stain
	Fundi (hemorrhage, papilledema)	CT
Nose	Foreign body	
Mouth	Herpangina	
	Stomatitis	
	Teething	
Respiratory findings		
Wheezing	Asthma, bronchiolitis, foreign body	Pulse oximetry, ABG, CXR
Crackles	Pneumonia, CHF	Pulse oximetry, ABG, CXR
Abdominal findings	Reflux esophagitis	pH probe, endoscopy
	Volvulus	Upper barium study
	Intussusception	Barium enema
	Appendicitis	Abdominal radiograph, CT scan
	Testicular torsion	Nuclear scan, Doppler scan
	Gastroenteritis	
	Hernia	
	Anal fissure	
Genitourinary findings	Testicular torsion	Nuclear scan, Doppler scan
	Sexual abuse	
	Hair tourniquet	
	Nephrolithiasis	CT scan
Extremity findings	Trauma	Radiographic study
	Hair tourniquet	
	Osteomyelitis-arthritis	Radiographic study, bone scan, arthrocentesis
Neurologic findings	Meningitis	LP
	Pseudotumor cerebri	Head CT, LP
	Cerebral palsy	

ABG, arterial blood gas; CBC, complete blood count; CHF, congestive heart failure; CT, computed tomography; CVA, costovertebral angle; CXR, chest x-ray study; ESR, erythrocyte sedimentation rate; LP, lumbar puncture; UA, urinalysis.

paraphimosis might be made. Failure to recognize penile strangulation can lead to numerous complications, including urethral fistula, gangrene, deformity of the glans, urethral stricture, or loss of part of the penis. Therefore, this diagnosis should be considered in all infants presenting with a swollen penis.

Management of tourniquet syndromes consists of the expeditious removal of the strand. The strand may be dissolved by a hair depilatory agent, removed with tweezers, or cut. Because of the edema obscuring the strand, the only recourse may be to cut the strand through a skin incision perpendicular to the demarcation line.

Almost 38% of patients require surgical intervention for penile strangulation. Because of the need to rapidly reestablish tissue perfusion, coupled with the difficulty in removing the strand from edematous tissue, it is important to request surgical consultation as soon as the diagnosis is established.

TEETHING

Many complaints, ranging from fever to irritability, have been ascribed to teething. Parents often attribute normal processes and

Table 34-6. Nonurgent Causes of Infant Irritability

Colic
Constipation
Feeding problems
Parenting difficulties
Teething
Vaccine reaction
Viral syndrome

events to teething. For example, teething infants often experience mild fever, drooling, crying, or feeding or sleeping difficulties. Even though teething may be associated with these symptoms, it may not be the cause.

From interviews with parents and pediatricians, the consensus is that teething is associated with irritability. A longitudinal survey of parental reports of primary tooth eruption supports this notion. Irritability was related to anterior (incisors) and posterior (cuspids and molars) tooth eruption in 69% and 97% of infants, respectively. In addition, of the 19 symptoms accompanying tooth eruption, irritability was the most frequently occurring symptom. Even though tooth eruption may be associated with irritability, teething should be considered as a diagnosis of exclusion. Just as in the evaluation of the infant with colic, more serious underlying causes must be considered (see Table 34-3).

Management consists of allowing the infant to bite on any appropriate hard object, such as a teething ring, biscuit, pretzel, bagel, or frozen washcloth.

Some infants might find rubbing of the erupting tooth by the parent's finger to be helpful. Additional relief might be obtained from the use of an analgesic, such as acetaminophen, or the application of a topical anesthetic agent.

DRUG REACTIONS

Although various therapeutic medications and illicit drugs have been said to be responsible for infant irritability, there is little information supporting such an association. In a series of reports, maternal oral decongestants have been associated with infant irritability through their transmission in breast milk. Cessation of maternal use led to a rapid improvement in infant behavior. If this effect is caused by maternal transmission, it seems reasonable to suggest that direct treatment of the infant with these agents may also lead to irritable behavior. Although still controversial, it has been suggested that illicit drugs, including cocaine, opiates, and marijuana, precipitate irritability through breast milk. In the neonate, irritability may also be a symptom of drug withdrawal, resulting from maternal addiction to drugs such as heroin, methadone, amphetamines, or barbiturates during pregnancy. Neonatal drug withdrawal usually occurs in the first week of life but may be delayed 2 to 3 weeks if the mother used methadone. Manifestations include crying, sneezing, emesis,

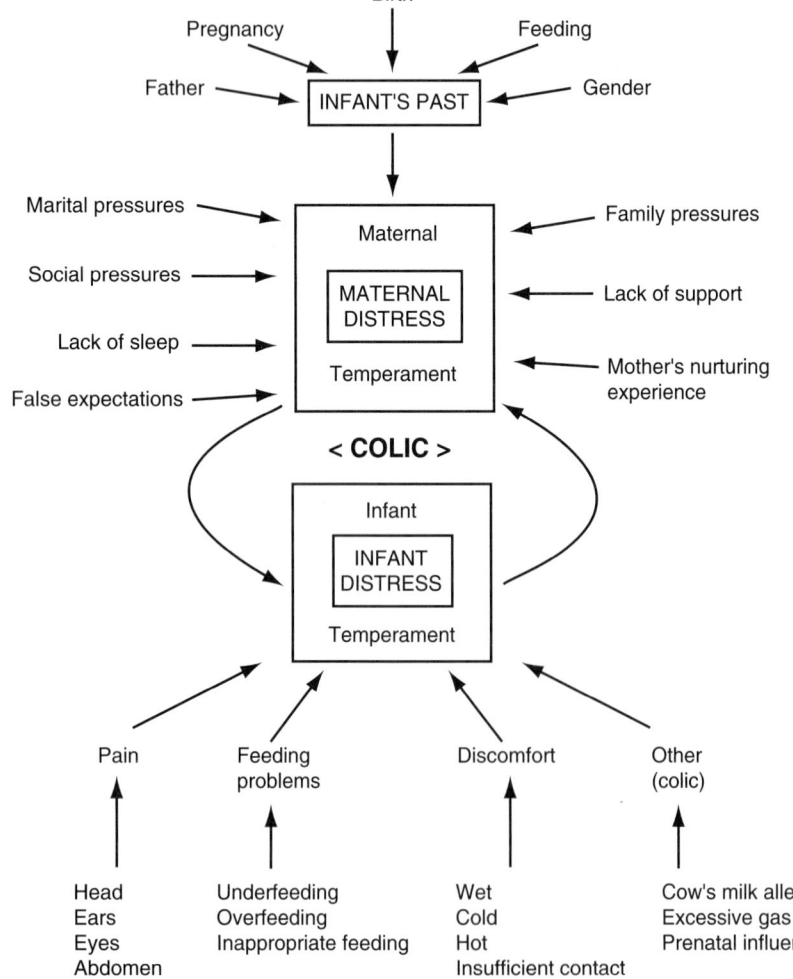

Figure 34-2. Interaction of stresses acting on mother and crying infant. (Adapted from Hewson P, Oberklaid F, Menahem S: Infant colic, distress, and crying. Clin Pediatr 1987;26:74.)

seizures, poor feeding, hiccups, diarrhea, sleeplessness, hyperactivity, and tremors.

Treatment of neonatal drug withdrawal includes replacing the opiate with paregoric or methadone or suppressing symptoms with phenobarbital. In the evaluation of the irritable neonate, a careful infant and maternal drug history are important to obtain along with urine drug toxicology profile if indicated.

IMMUNIZATION REACTIONS

Some infants may become irritable after administration of childhood immunizations. Irritability after administration of the diphtheria-tetanus-pertussis vaccine was common, with fretfulness in 70% of infants and irritability for more than 3 hours after 1% of doses. Fortunately, it appears that the current practice of using an acellular pertussis component results in irritability much less commonly, although quantitative data are not available. The irritability associated with immunizations may be attenuated by acetaminophen.

SUMMARY AND RED FLAGS

Although at times a simple diagnosis is easily established, the infant with excessive irritability often presents a significant challenge. Establishment of the likely diagnosis, combined with exclusion of significant pathophysiologic processes (see Table 34-3), is a prerequisite to the formulation of an appropriate management plan. Through a logical and stepwise approach, the clinician can usually establish the cause and develop a treatment plan (see Table 34-1). When the clinician cannot determine the underlying cause, close follow-up monitoring should result in optimal patient care.

Red flags include inconsolability; abnormal level of consciousness or abnormal vital signs; evidence of trauma or anemia (blood loss, sickle cell, leukemia); vomiting; diarrhea; hematochezia and abdominal tenderness or distention; signs of tourniquet syndrome; eye tearing, photophobia, or conjunctival irritation (corneal abrasion); abnormalities of growth, including head circumference; and signs of cardiorespiratory compromise.

REFERENCES

The Irritable Infant

Harkness M: Corneal abrasion in infancy as a cause of inconsolable crying. Pediatr Emerg Care 1989;5:242-244.

Ludwig S: Shaken baby syndrome: A review of 20 cases. Ann Emerg Med 1984;13:104-107.

Poole S: The infant with acute, unexplained, excessive crying. Pediatrics 1991;88:450-455.

Reijneveld SA, Brugman E, Hirasing RA: Excessive infant crying: The impact of varying definitions. Pediatrics 2001;108:893-897.

Trocinski D, Pearigen P: The crying infant. Emerg Med Clin North Am 1998;16:895-910.

Infantile Colic

Barr R, Kramer M, Pless I, et al: Feeding and temperament as determinants of early infant crying/fussing behavior. Pediatrics 1989;84:514-521.

Barr R, McMullan S, Spiess H, et al: Carrying as colic "therapy": A randomized controlled trial. Pediatrics 1991;87:623-630.

Carey W: The effectiveness of parent counseling in managing colic. Pediatrics 1994;94:37.

Danielsson B, Hwang C: Treatment of infantile colic with surface active substance (simethicone). Acta Paediatr Scand 1985;74:446-450.

Garrison M, Christakis D: A systematic review of treatments for infant colic. Pediatrics 2000;106:184-190.

Hardoin R, Henslee J, Christenson C: Colic medication and apparent life-threatening events. Clin Pediatr 1991;30:281-285.

Hill DJ, Heine RG, Cameron DJS, et al: Role of food protein intolerance in infants with persistent distress attributed to reflux esophagitis. J Pediatr 2000;136:641-647.

Hill D, Menahem S, Hudson I, et al: Charting infant distress: An aid to defining colic. J Pediatr 1992;121:755-758.

Hunziker U, Barr R: Increased carrying reduces infant crying: A randomized controlled trial. Pediatrics 1986;77:641-648.

Lothe L, Lindberg T: Cow's milk whey protein elicits symptoms of infantile colic in colicky formula-fed infants: A double-blind crossover study. Pediatrics 1989;83:262-266.

Lothe L, Lindberg T, Jakobsson I: Cow's milk formula as a cause of infantile colic: A double-blind study. Pediatrics 1982;70:7-10.

Lucassen PLBJ, Assendelft WJJ, Gubbels JW, et al: Effectiveness of treatments for infantile colic. BMJ 1998;316:1563-1569.

Miller A, Barr R: Infantile colic: Is it a gut issue? Pediatr Clin North Am 1991;38:1407-1423.

Parkin P, Schwartz C, Manuel B: Randomized controlled trial of three interventions in the management of persistent crying of infancy. Pediatrics 1993;92:197-201.

Singer J: A fatal case of colic. Pediatr Emerg Care 1992;8:171-172.

St James-Roberts I: Persistent infant crying. Arch Dis Child 1991;66:653-655.

St James-Roberts I: Managing infants who cry persistently. BMJ 1992;304:997-998.

Taubman B: Parental counseling compared with elimination of cow's milk or soy milk protein for the treatment of infant colic syndrome: A randomized trial. Pediatrics 1988;81:756-761.

Tourniquet Syndromes

Alpert J, Filler R, Glaser H: Strangulation of an appendage by hair wrapping. N Engl J Med 1965;273:866-867.

Curran J: Digital strangulation by hair wrapping. J Pediatr 1966;69:137-138.

Haddad F: Penile strangulation by human hair. Urol Int 1982;37:375-388.

McClure W, Gradinger G: Hair strangulation of the glans penis. Plast Reconstr Surg 1985;76:120-123.

McNeal R, Cruickshank J: Strangulation of the uvula by hair wrapping. Clin Pediatr 1987;26:599-600.

Teething

Macknin M, Piedmonte M, Jacobs J, et al: Symptoms associated with infant teething: A prospective study. Pediatrics 2000;105:747-752.

Seward M: Local disturbances attributed to eruption of the human primary dentition. Br Dent J 1971;130:72-77.

Seward M: General disturbances attributed to eruption of the human primary dentition. J Dent Child 1972;39:178-183.

Drug Reactions

Chasnoff I, Lewis D, Squires L: Cocaine intoxication in a breast-fed infant. Pediatrics 1987;80:836-838.

Mortimer E: Drug toxicity from breast milk? [letter]. Pediatrics 1977;60:780-781.

Rogers W: Fussy baby: A new cause [letter]. Pediatrics 1979;63:347-348.

Zuckerman B, Bresnahan K: Developmental and behavioral consequences of prenatal drug and alcohol exposure. Pediatr Clin North Am 1991;38:1387-1406.

Vaccine Reactions

Ipp M, Gold R, Greenberg S, et al: Acetaminophen prophylaxis of adverse reactions following vaccination of infants with diphtheria-pertussis-tetanus toxoids-polio vaccine. Pediatr Infect Dis J 1987;6:721-725.

Long S, Deforest A, Smith D, et al: Longitudinal study of adverse reactions following diphtheria-tetanus-pertussis vaccine in infancy. Pediatrics 1990;85:294-302.

Pickering L (ed): American Academy of Pediatrics 2000 Red Book: Report of the Committee on Infectious Diseases, 25th ed. Elk Grove Village, Ill, American Academy of Pediatrics, 2000.

35 Unusual Behaviors

William J. Swift   Hugh F. Johnston*

Unusual behaviors in children are common and consist of psychiatric conditions that range from variations in normal behavior to life-threatening suicide attempts. Almost 20% of children have a diagnosable psychiatric illness that can result in a high degree of stress in the family. These unusual behaviors may be grouped into the following chief complaints: suicidal thoughts and attempts, disruptive behaviors, hallucinations, unexplained physical complaints, and delayed development.

HISTORY

The history is the most important tool for identifying the psychiatric disorder (Table 35-1). The first step in conducting the history is to ensure the child's safety with regard to injury to the child either by the child (suicide attempt) or by someone else (physical or sexual abuse). After the child's safety is ensured, the history should focus on the stressors that may be precipitating the behavior and on the symptoms that may distinguish which disorder or disorders are causing the behavior.

Besides psychiatric illnesses, the clinician should also focus on possible medical causes of these behaviors, including medication side effects, substance abuse, and medical illnesses ranging from encephalopathies to endocrinopathies (e.g., hypothyroidism). Because comorbidity is common in children with psychiatric illnesses, the clinician should consider combinations of illnesses that may cause these symptoms. The clinician should obtain the information from multiple sources, interviewing the parents and the child separately, or interviewing other adults who have spent a significant amount of time with the child (e.g., a teacher). Interviewing the child separately provides a better chance of uncovering destructive behaviors (e.g., substance abuse or sexual activity) and of obtaining the child's perspective. Because of the strong genetic predisposition in some of these disorders, a detailed psychiatric family history should be obtained. Often these disorders are undiagnosed; hence, the family history should include both the presence of symptoms and diagnoses in family members.

Because many of these disorders have symptoms that occur in clusters, a diagnostic manual that classifies these symptom clusters into individual diagnoses has been developed. This manual, the *Diagnostic and Statistical Manual of Mental Disorders, Fourth Edition (DSM-IV)*, contains descriptive diagnostic criteria that are based on the presence or absence of various symptoms.

SUICIDAL THOUGHTS AND ATTEMPTS

Suicide is the third leading cause of death in adolescents. The thought of killing oneself as a solution to a problem is common among adolescents and young adults. Of children younger than 15 years,

9% have thought of suicide, 2% have seriously considered suicide, and 1% have attempted suicide. Among college students, there is a fivefold increase in suicide ideation, with 43% thinking of suicide at some point, 15% seriously considering suicide, and 5% attempting suicide. Because of this high prevalence of suicide ideation, the assessment for the risk of suicide is the first part of the evaluation of any child who presents with unusual behaviors. The approach in evaluating suicide ideation is based on whether the child is just thinking of suicide or is making suicide threats or attempts (Fig. 35-1).

SUICIDAL THOUGHTS

When suicidal ideation is present, most parents report that the child has previously thought of committing suicide. However, the office interview may be the first time that the child verbalizes this thought.

The clinician needs to determine the seriousness of these thoughts. To assess risk, the interviewer should focus on the risk factors for completed suicides. These risk factors are male sex, adolescence, conscious plan, available means (medications or firearms), depression, hopelessness, impulsiveness, low frustration tolerance, use of intoxicants, sexual identity conflicts, recent death of family member or friend, and previous suicide attempts. Although depression is an important risk factor for suicide, only half of adolescents who attempt suicide have clinically diagnosable depression. In the nondepressed group, the crucial characteristics for suicide are impulsivity and low frustration tolerance.

Other than for the most frivolous thoughts of suicide, any adolescent who is thinking of suicide should be persuaded to discuss this issue with a responsible adult and should be encouraged to seek counseling. If significant risk factors exist for suicide, the patient should be referred to a child psychiatrist or other mental health provider on an emergency basis.

SUICIDE THREATS AND ATTEMPTS

Once the patient's thoughts of suicide have escalated to suicide threats or attempts, the patient's life is in great danger. This is a medical emergency; the patient should be immediately referred to an experienced mental health professional. Because the child's problem-solving abilities and judgment are impaired, someone else must ensure the child's safety. This usually necessitates a psychiatric hospitalization.

Only after suicide risk is accurately assessed can outpatient management be considered. After a suicide gesture or attempt, the accuracy of this assessment depends on the patient's cooperating and having a clear consciousness. If the patient is uncooperative, stuporous, or confused, the evaluation results are unreliable, and the patient is assumed to be potentially suicidal. Once the patient is alert, he or she must be able to communicate a plausible theory that led to the suicidal behavior. Without such a theory, the patient has no insight into his or her actions, and hence the clinician cannot predict whether the suicide attempt will be repeated. Even with a plausible theory, the crucial factors that led to the act must be changed before the clinician can

*This chapter is an updated and edited version of the chapter by Theodore Reeves Warm and Robert L. Findling that appeared in the first edition.

Table 35-1. Essential Elements of the Patient's History

Assess suicide potential (ensure safety)
Interview child alone
Interview multiple sources
Obtain family history for symptoms and disorders
Rule out medical causes, including substance use
Consider comorbidities
Inquire about past mental health referrals

consider discharging the patient from the hospital. A highly agitated mental state may also suggest high suicide risk.

Finally, the patient must be sincerely glad to be alive. People who have attempted suicide frequently promise that they will not do it again. Because of the high incidence of repeat attempts, these promises are unreliable. The combination of not being remorseful, no plausible theory, and being unable to resolve or change the initiating factors warrants inpatient care and is a red flag. Because of the inherent difficulties in predicting suicidal acts, it is best for the clinician to err on the side of safety when in doubt.

DISRUPTIVE BEHAVIORS

Disruptive behaviors are the most common chief complaint of unusual behavior in a patient presenting to a health care provider's office. These behaviors may be associated with a wide variety of diagnoses, ranging from attention-deficit/hyperactivity disorder (ADHD) to schizophrenia. These conditions may be divided into those that are chronic (Fig. 35-2) and those that are episodic and recent in onset (Figs. 35-3 and 35-4). Disruptive behaviors may be further subdivided

into those treated by a primary health care provider and those that should be treated by a mental health specialist.

CHRONIC DISRUPTIVE BEHAVIOR

Chronic disruptive behaviors are usually brought to the attention of the health care provider because of an acute crisis (e.g., school failure, destruction of property). The precipitating event that leads to consultation may be an escalation in the severity of the behavior or a change in the family or school that makes such behaviors less tolerable. The *DSM-IV* lists three main diagnoses within the category of disruptive behavioral disorders: ADHD, oppositional defiant disorder (ODD), and conduct disorder. It is common for a child to present with combinations of these disorders.

Treatment by Primary Care Physician

Attention-Deficit/Hyperactivity Disorder

The cardinal features of this condition are hyperactivity (being fidgety, on the move), distractibility (short attention span), and impulsiveness (acting without forethought) (Table 35-2). The prevalence of this condition is four to nine times higher in boys than in girls. Difficulty in appropriately diagnosing this disorder is in differentiating age-appropriate hyperactivity/inattentiveness from pathologic behavior. The *DSM-IV* has divided this condition into three subtypes: ADHD—combined type; ADHD—predominantly inattentive type; and ADHD—predominantly hyperactive-impulsive type.

To diagnose these conditions, the examiner must note at least six of nine symptoms for inattention or six of nine symptoms for hyperactivity/impulsivity. Symptoms must be present for at least 6 months, be maladaptive, and be inconsistent with the child's developmental age.

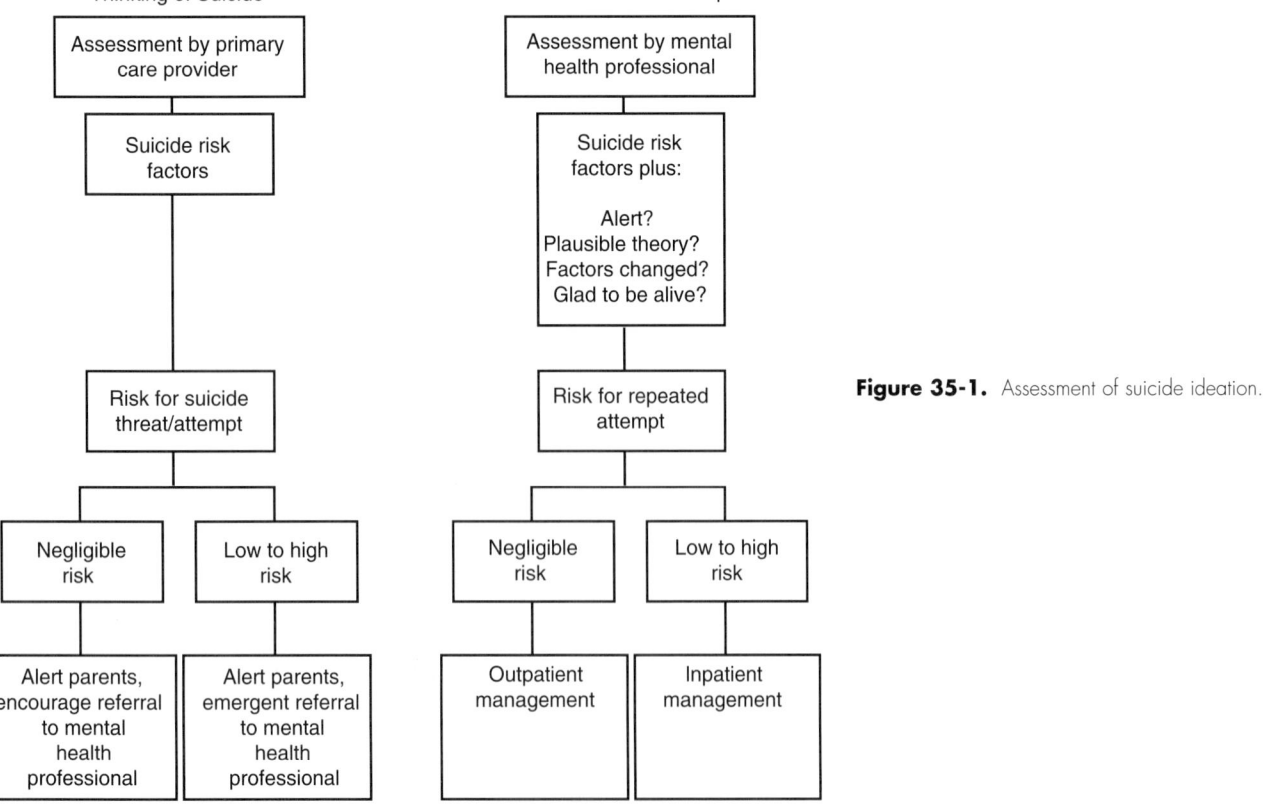

Figure 35-1. Assessment of suicide ideation.

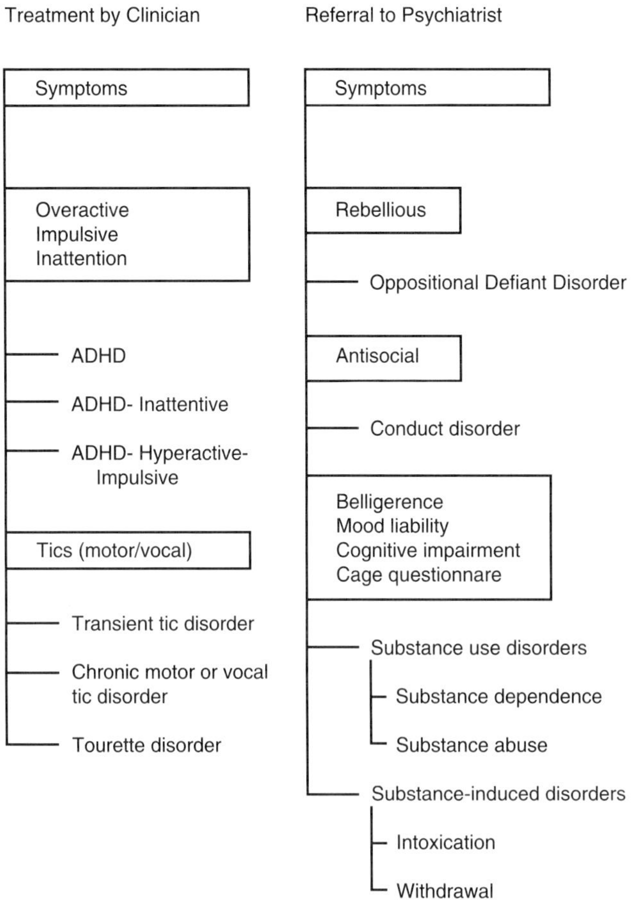

Treatment by Clinician

| Symptoms |

| Overactive
Impulsive
Inattention |

—— ADHD

—— ADHD- Inattentive

—— ADHD- Hyperactive-
Impulsive

| Tics (motor/vocal) |

—— Transient tic disorder

—— Chronic motor or vocal
tic disorder

—— Tourette disorder

Referral to Psychiatrist

| Symptoms |

| Rebellious |

—— Oppositional Defiant Disorder

| Antisocial |

—— Conduct disorder

| Belligerence
Mood liability
Cognitive impairment
Cage questionnare |

—— Substance use disorders

—— Substance dependence

—— Substance abuse

—— Substance-induced disorders

—— Intoxication

—— Withdrawal

Figure 35-2. Evaluation of chronic disruptive behaviors. ADHD, attention-deficit/hyperactivity disorder.

The nine symptoms of *inattention* are (1) careless schoolwork, (2) difficulty in sustaining attention, (3) inattentiveness (child does not listen), (4) failure to finish work, (5) disorganization, (6) avoidance of tasks that require sustained attention, (7) loss of objects necessary for tasks, (8) easy distractibility, and (9) forgetfulness. The nine symptoms of *hyperactivity/impulsivity* are (1) fidgeting or squirming in one's seat, (2) inappropriately getting out of one's seat, (3) inappropriately running or climbing on objects, (4) inability to play quietly, (5) often being on the go, (6) talking excessively, (7) stating answers before questions are completed, (8) difficulty in waiting one's turn, and (9) interrupting others.

For the diagnosis, some of these symptoms must be present before the child is 7 years of age, they must occur in at least two separate settings (home, school), and they must significantly impair the child's social or academic function.

The chronic hyperactivity of this syndrome may be subtle. Although children with ADHD tend to move around more than other children, the hyperactivity may be of concern only in certain situations. These circumstances are those in which the child is expected to be quiet (school, places of worship). Some children with ADHD can sit and be attentive in quiet and relaxed situations, whereas a noisy and active setting (unstructured classroom) precipitates inappropriate behavior. As these children become older, they also become less overtly hyperactive; an adolescent may only feel restless. This restlessness may also significantly contribute to academic underachievement. Despite intentions for diligent studying, the restlessness may cause the affected teenager to feel the need to walk around, which distracts him or her from studies.

Impulsivity significantly contributes to the child's morbidity. Just as impulsive children's activities change rapidly, so do their emotions. An impulsive child whose emotions quickly escalate is at risk for physically aggressive behaviors such as hitting or biting. In older children, the impulsive aggression is manifested as explosive behavior. Because of their explosive behavior, inability to wait their turn in a game, and then talking back to teachers, these children have great difficulty with both peer and teacher relations. Impulsivity can also be potentially life-threatening because the child may act before considering the consequences. This may manifest as risk-taking behaviors (sexual activity, substance use) or as actions such as running into the street after a ball without checking for oncoming traffic.

Hyperactivity and impulsivity in children are readily apparent to adults; however, the manifestations of inattention and distractibility are not as overtly visible. In young children, inattentive behavior consists of shifting from one activity to another and having difficulty finishing tasks. The parents may incorrectly consider these actions to represent a lack of motivation. In adolescents, inattentive behavior may result in poor school performance. These children may forget to do homework or may need excessively long periods to complete assignments because of their inability to focus on their work. Because the assumptions about an inattentive child's character are often inaccurate (lazy, behavior problem), the clinician should consider the diagnosis of attention-deficit disorder (with or without hyperactivity) in any child who is academically underachieving.

Potential problems in the diagnosis of ADHD are the duration of symptoms, the definition of abnormal age-specific symptoms, and the absence of symptoms in certain settings. Because ADHD is a chronic disorder, the diagnosis necessitates that symptoms be present for at least 6 months. Acute changes in a child's behavior are usually the result of a recent psychological stressor and should not be considered a part of ADHD.

The second problem is defining when a behavior is abnormal. Children normally become less active and impulsive as they get older. The classroom teacher represents an excellent resource who can determine whether the patient's level of activity and degree of impulsivity are abnormal. Standardized behavioral checklists (filled out by the parents and teachers) report the degree of patient's abnormal behaviors with regard to an age-specific reference population.

The final problem is the common misconception that hyperactive children demonstrate their inattentive, impulsive, and hyperactive behaviors in the examination room. Most children with ADHD are attentive and still during a brief outpatient visit. The clinician should not rely on observations performed in the office but should instead obtain information from multiple sources, including parents, teachers, day care workers, and even a direct classroom observation by a trained health care professional.

Before settling on a diagnosis of ADHD, the clinician must rule out the other psychiatric and medical causes for these symptoms. Some of the psychiatric conditions that may resemble this condition or occur with it are learning disorders, oppositional behavior, and other psychiatric illnesses that may better account for the symptoms (pervasive developmental disorders, mood disorders, anxiety disorders, substance abuse). Because of the high association of learning disorders with ADHD, each evaluation should include an assessment for learning problems. This assessment consists of individual testing by a psychometrician to assess the child's abilities and deficiencies.

Because of the genetic predisposition to ADHD, a psychiatric family history should also be obtained. In this family history, the parents may report feelings of restlessness or difficulties in completing tasks. In the medical evaluation for ADHD, further diagnostic testing should be directed by the results of a complete history and thorough physical examination. The preschool-aged child should be screened for lead poisoning and iron deficiency, whereas the older child should undergo further diagnostic tests, as directed by the results of history and physical examination, to rule out such conditions as hyperthyroidism, absence seizures, hearing loss, and substance abuse.

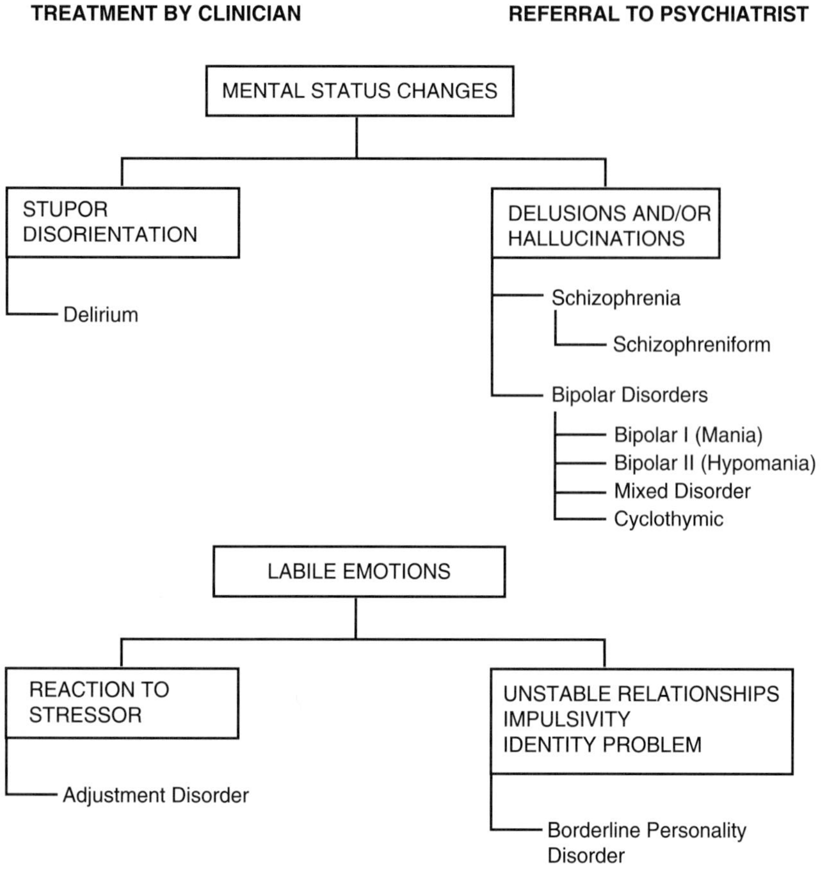

TREATMENT BY CLINICIAN   **REFERRAL TO PSYCHIATRIST**

```
              ┌─────────────────────────────┐
              │   MENTAL STATUS CHANGES      │
              └─────────────────────────────┘
       ┌──────────────┴─────────────────────────┐
┌──────────────────┐              ┌──────────────────────┐
│ STUPOR           │              │ DELUSIONS AND/OR     │
│ DISORIENTATION   │              │ HALLUCINATIONS       │
└──────────────────┘              └──────────────────────┘
   └── Delirium                      ├── Schizophrenia
                                     │     └── Schizophreniform
                                     │
                                     └── Bipolar Disorders
                                           ├── Bipolar I (Mania)
                                           ├── Bipolar II (Hypomania)
                                           ├── Mixed Disorder
                                           └── Cyclothymic
```

Figure 35-3. Evaluation of episodic disruptive behaviors.

```
              ┌─────────────────────────────┐
              │      LABILE EMOTIONS         │
              └─────────────────────────────┘
       ┌──────────────┴─────────────────────────┐
┌──────────────────┐              ┌──────────────────────────┐
│ REACTION TO      │              │ UNSTABLE RELATIONSHIPS   │
│ STRESSOR         │              │ IMPULSIVITY              │
└──────────────────┘              │ IDENTITY PROBLEM         │
   └── Adjustment Disorder        └──────────────────────────┘
                                     └── Borderline Personality
                                         Disorder
```

REFERRAL TO PSYCHIATRIST

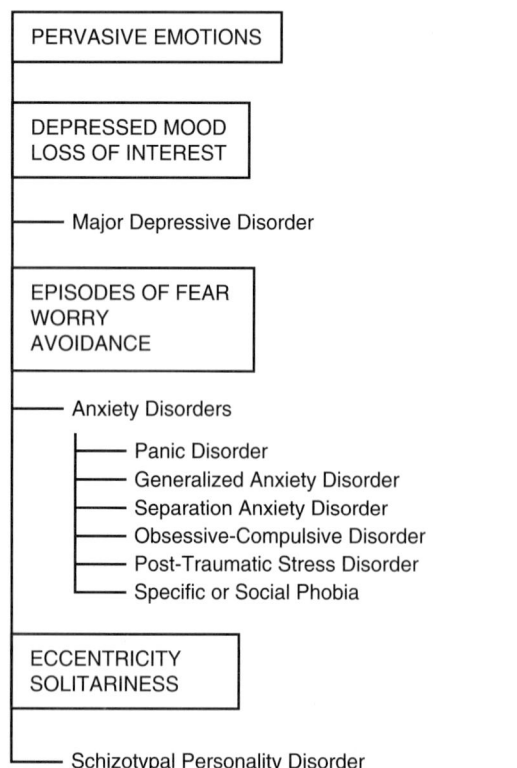

Figure 35-4. Evaluation of episodic disruptive behaviors with pervasive emotions.

ADHD, a chronic illness, may cause problems throughout the patient's lifetime. Psychotropic medications usually reduce some of the outward symptoms of this condition (e.g., hyperactivity); however, the patient can have significant morbidity unless the patient learns how to deal with the learning and behavior problems associated with this condition. Therefore, successful treatment requires a multidisciplinary approach consisting of family education, psychological counseling, academic remediation, behavior modification, and psychotropic medications.

Table 35-2. Challenges in Diagnosis and Treating Attention-Deficit/Hyperactivity Disorder (ADHD)

Problems in Diagnosing ADHD

No hyperactivity report may be present in teenagers; instead, the patient may have only restlessness

Differentiating inattention from lack of motivation is difficult

Differentiating age-appropriate from pathologic behavior (behavioral checklists, teacher's report) is difficult

Hyperactive children have normal behavior in quiet, structured settings

Sudden onset of hyperactivity is secondary to a stressor and not to ADHD

Comorbidities (learning disabilities, conduct disorder, oppositional defiant disorder) should be ruled out

Problems in Treating ADHD

Treatment must be multifactorial and not consist just of stimulants

Behavioral modification must have realistic goals, with consistent and frequent rewards

The first step in treating ADHD is to educate the family with regard to the causes, potential problems, chronicity, and treatment of this condition. Additional important resources are books from the lay press as well as support groups for parents who have children with ADHD.

The second step in treating ADHD is to initiate coping skills that can be used to enhance socially appropriate behavior (e.g., task completion, turn taking in games) at home and in school. These coping skills include establishing a predictable schedule for family activities (bedtime, mealtime routines), distracting the child to another activity when the child's excitement level accelerates, and instituting individually tailored, reward-based behavior modification techniques. For behavior modification to be successful, the following elements are essential:

1. identification of specific behaviors to work on
2. selection of tasks small enough to ensure the child some success
3. an attractive chart for recording success
4. reliable rewards with small items or privileges (preferably daily)
5. small punishments for failure to comply (loss of television or telephone for the evening)
6. consistent reward and punishment for the corresponding behavior

Some of the problems in successfully implementing behavioral techniques are unrealistic expectations, inconsistency, and delays in rewarding success. In the classroom, the child should be placed in the front to make classroom distractions less apparent to the child.

Many children with ADHD have significant trouble with their self-esteem because of poor school performance, difficulty in peer relations, and intrafamilial discord. To address the child's emotional issues and problems with self-image, the clinician may recommend psychotherapy.

Behavior modification programs, psychosocial interventions, psychological therapies, and parent education are all useful interventions in the management of ADHD. However, for most children, the efficacy of such interventions is relatively small in comparison to the typical response produced by stimulant medication. Furthermore, many failed behavior modification programs become successful after the child has been appropriately treated with medications. Methylphenidate preparations (Ritalin, Concerta, and others) and amphetamine preparations (Dexedrine, Adderall, and others) are the mainstay of stimulant treatment. Pemoline (Cylert) has fallen out of favor because of this drug's potential for causing liver toxicity. Three other classes of medications have demonstrated efficacy for ADHD: tricyclic antidepressant medications (e.g., imipramine, nortriptyline), bupropion (Wellbutrin), and antihypertensives belonging to the α_2-agonist class such as clonidine (Catapres) and guanfacine (Tenex). The therapeutic effect of these alternative medications is, on balance, much less than that of the stimulants. Atomoxine (Strahera) is a promising nonstimulant option for the treatment of ADHD. Atomoxine is valuable for patients who do not tolerate or respond to stimulant medications.

If stimulant therapy is initiated, the clinician needs to perform follow-up at regular intervals to assess efficacy (using such parameters as school performance, standardized behavioral checklists) and side effects (e.g., tics, tremors, hypertension, weight loss). Stimulants can cause weight loss by appetite suppression. Using the medication only on school days can minimize this effect.

Because ADHD is associated with long-term dysfunction, children with this disorder are at increased risk for continuing academic underachievement and reduced occupational status in adulthood.

Tic Disorders

Children with tic disorders usually present first to the primary care provider. According to the *DSM-IV*, tics are motor movements or vocalizations that are sudden, rapid, recurrent, nonrhythmic, and involuntary. Tics become worse during stress but may improve during activities requiring moderate (physical or mental) activity.

Muscle spasms differ from tics because they are slower and last longer.

Tics need to be differentiated from medication-induced movement disorders as well as from the abnormal movements associated with various neurologic conditions. Pathologic non-tic movements are chorea (dancing, random), athetosis (writhing, sinuous movements), dystonia (twisting, slow contractions), myoclonus (shocklike jerks), and hemiballismus (violent, unilateral motions). Simple motor tics may consist of eye blinking, neck jerking, or shoulder shrugging, whereas examples of complex motor tics are repetitive grooming behaviors, deep knee bends, and smelling of objects. Simple vocal tics may be throat clearing or grunting sounds, whereas complex vocal tics may consist of repeating inappropriate words or phrases (e.g., coprolalia—the repetitive, stereotyped vocalization of obscenities).

According to the *DSM-IV*, conditions that make up the tic disorders are

- transient tic disorder (motor or vocal tics of <1 year's duration)
- chronic motor or vocal tic disorder (motor or vocal tics > 1 year's duration)
- Tourette disorder (motor *and* vocal tics > 1 year's duration)

There is some evidence that group A β-hemolytic streptococcal infections are associated with pediatric autoimmune neuropsychiatric disorders (PANDAS) such as tics and obsessive-compulsive disorders (OCDs). The working criteria for a diagnosis of PANDAS are

- presence of OCD and/or tic disorder
- pediatric onset
- abrupt onset and episodic course
- association with group A β-hemolytic streptococcal infections
- association with neurologic abnormalities, such as motor hyperactivity, choreiform movements, or tics

In children who meet these criteria, PANDAS should be considered, because antibiotic therapy may eradicate the OCD or tic symptoms.

Tourette Disorder. Tourette disorder is a chronic illness consisting of multiple motor and vocal tics of at least 1 year's duration. The incidence of this condition is 4 to 5 per 10,000. In some families, this illness is inherited as an autosomal dominant condition, with 70% penetrance in female carriers and 99% penetrance in male carriers. Because of this difference in penetrance, Tourette disorder is 1.5 to 3 times more common in boys than in girls. The median age for presentation is 7 years, but some cases are reported as early as 2 years. Even though coprolalia is popularly thought to be associated with this illness, fewer than 10% of affected patients have this form of complex vocal tics. The *DSM-IV* criteria for Tourette disorder are

1. multiple motor and vocal tics lasting longer than 1 year with no tic-free intervals longer than 3 months
2. age of onset before 18 years
3. no medical causes (drugs, neurologic diseases) for the tics

Children with chronic tic disorders frequently have other psychological conditions, such as ADHD and OCD. In addition, the tics may cause the patient's peers to socially ostracize the patient. Because of the combination of ADHD and obsessive-compulsive behaviors with the tics, these children are not accepted by their peers and frequently frustrate their teachers and family members. This increase in stress can worsen the tics, which can further compound the problem. Because of these issues, the family may need counseling.

If the symptoms are not severe, the only necessary therapy may be psychological support. If the symptoms become problematic, the patient may need to be treated with low dosages of antipsychotic drugs, such as haloperidol (Haldol) or pimozide (Orap). Risperidone (Risperdal), an atypical antipsychotic agent, has some efficacy in the treatment of Tourette disorder. Because pimozide can cause the prolongation of the QT interval, an electrocardiogram should be obtained before therapy is initiated and at regular intervals. Because stimulant therapy can aggravate tics, children with both Tourette disorder and ADHD may be treated with clonidine. In patients with chronic tics and OCDs, both conditions may be treated with medications that potentiate serotonin activity (clomipramine or a selective serotonin reuptake inhibitor).

Treatment by Psychiatrist

When treating children severely affected by disruptive behavioral disorder symptoms (or any severe psychiatric disorder), the primary care provider is best advised to team up with the local mental health "system" in providing ongoing care (see Fig. 35-2). This system might include a social worker to provide counseling therapy and overall case coordination; a chemical dependency specialist if addictions are an issue; a psychologist to provide psychometric testing and to assist with school programming, and a child and adolescent psychiatrist if there are unusually complex medication and/or psychological issues.

Oppositional Defiant Disorder

Oppositional defiant disorder is a chronic condition in which the patient is stubbornly rebellious toward all authority. This behavior is more than just a reaction to a stressful situation or the normal show of independence during adolescence. According to the *DSM-IV,* affected patients exhibit a consistent pattern during a 6-month period of at least four or more of the following behaviors:

1. frequently losing temper
2. often arguing with authority figures
3. defying rules
4. deliberately annoying adults
5. blaming others for his or her actions
6. becoming easily annoyed by others
7. being angry
8. being vindictive

This diagnosis should not be made if the patient meets the *DSM-IV* criteria for conduct disorder or if the symptoms occur during the course of a mood, anxiety, or psychotic disorder. In mood and psychotic disorders, children exhibit oppositional behavior as a reaction to their illness and hence they should be classified under their primary mood or psychotic disorder.

The prevalence of ODD ranges from 2% to 16%, depending on the population. In prepubertal children, it occurs more frequently in boys; however, in adolescents, its incidence is equal in both sexes. Most children present before 8 years of age. Affected preschool-aged children sometimes exhibit increased motor activity and difficulty in being comforted, and they overreact to situations. Affected school-aged children have low self-esteem and a low tolerance for frustration.

Some of the theories on the causes of ODD are learned behavior (secondary gain from defiant behavior), fixation at a negative stage of behavior development (the "terrible twos"), and poor parenting skills. There may also be a genetic component because the disorder commonly occurs in families with mood or psychotic disorders (especially with maternal depression) and with chronic disruptive behaviors (ADHD, conduct disorder).

Children with ODD are at marked risk for other psychological disorders. Because of the association of ADHD with ODD, children with ODD should also be evaluated for ADHD. In addition, these patients may be at increased risk for conduct disorder, antisocial personality disorder (as adults), substance abuse, major depressive disorder, and suicide.

Because of the difficulty in treating ODD, mental health professionals are the ones who usually manage this condition. Therapy is directed toward treating comorbid disorders (ADHD, substance abuse, suicide ideation). In addition, various psychotherapeutic modalities (individual, group, family) are employed to improve the child's functioning. The role of the primary care provider is early recognition and referral to a mental health specialist. Success of therapy depends on early intervention before the dysfunctional patterns are firmly established. The clinician can enhance compliance with psychotherapy by being supportive and by explaining to the family that therapy often requires months of slow progress and demands active family participation.

Conduct Disorder

Children who chronically violate the rights of others may be diagnosed as having conduct disorder. According to the *DSM-IV,* a child has conduct disorder if he or she has repetitively violated the rights of others and of society. Children with this diagnosis have performed three or more of the following behaviors within the past year with at least one occurring in the previous 6 months:

1. aggression toward people or animals (intimidation, initiation of fights; use of weapons; cruelty to people; cruelty to animals; rape; confrontational theft ["mugging"])
2. destruction of property (arson, vandalism)
3. deceitfulness (nonconfrontational theft [house breaking, "conning"])
4. serious violation of rules (curfew violation, running away, truancy before age 13)

For running away to qualify as a symptom, it must occur twice (or once if it was lengthy) and must not be an attempt to escape sexual or physical abuse. Conduct disorder is subdivided into childhood onset (symptoms occur before 10 years of age) and adolescent onset (symptoms occur at or after 10 years of age). It is also subdivided by severity of the offense, such as mild (truancy), moderate (vandalism, nonconfrontational theft), and severe (rape, confrontational theft).

The prevalence of conduct disorders is higher among males than females. Children initially present with lying, initiating of fights, and truancy; as they get older, they progress to more violent acts. Boys are more likely to exhibit acts of violence (fighting and stealing) than are girls, who are more likely to exhibit truancy, runaway behavior, and sexual promiscuity. Of concern is that 50% of these children may develop antisocial personality disorder, which is a severe conduct disorder of adulthood that is usually associated with criminal activity; the earlier the onset of conduct disorder, the greater is the risk of developing antisocial personality disorder as an adult. These children have a high frequency of depression (suicide ideation), personality disorders, anxiety disorders, ADHD, and substance abuse.

Although the cause of conduct disorder is unknown, both genetic and psychosocial factors play a role. The psychosocial factors associated with conduct disorder are parental rejection, difficult infant temperament, physical or sexual abuse, early institutional living, and lack of appropriate discipline. A biochemical or genetic cause for this condition has been postulated because of the high prevalence of this condition in families with psychiatric disorders, ADHD, and conduct disorder.

Therapy is best managed by mental health professionals. The therapy consists of individual and/or family psychotherapy, judicious use of residential treatment centers, and treatment of comorbid conditions (substance abuse, ADHD, depression). The behavior in children with conduct disorders can markedly improve if their ADHD is treated with stimulants and their depression is treated with antidepressants. The success of therapy depends on early recognition and intervention before the destructive behaviors are firmly established. The role of the primary care provider is early recognition, referral, and enhancement of compliance with treatment.

Unfortunately, there is no compelling evidence to suggest that any treatment is effective for severe conduct disorder. As a result, behavioral containment and control to protect the individual and society may be the most feasible goals.

Substance Use

The presence of unusual disruptive behaviors can be the result of the intoxication or the withdrawal of a psychoactive agent. Some of these behaviors are belligerence, mood lability, and cognitive impairment. As many as 90% of high school seniors have tried psychoactive drugs (nicotine or ethanol), and almost 60% have tried illicit drugs. Almost 20% of high school seniors drink ethanol to the point of intoxication on a weekly basis. More than half of adolescents who drink do so in automobiles. Some of the illicit drugs used are tetrahydrocannabinol (THC, found in marijuana), central nervous system (CNS) depressants (benzodiazepine, phenobarbital), hallucinogens (lysergic acid diethylamide [LSD], methylene-dioxymethamphetamine [MDMA or "ecstasy"], phencyclidine piperidine [PCP]), opiates (heroin), stimulants (sympathomimetics, amphetamine, cocaine), and inhalants (toluene, Freon, nitrous oxide). The *DSM-IV* divides the diagnoses attributable to drugs into substance use (dependence and abuse) and substance-induced disorders (intoxication, withdrawal).

Substance dependence according to the *DSM-IV* consists of three or more symptoms occurring at the same time during a 12-month period:

1. tolerance (higher doses of the drug are needed to achieve the same effect)
2. withdrawal (the drug is needed to suppress symptoms)
3. drug use that entails taking larger amounts or use over a longer period than intended
4. desire or effort to cut down use
5. drug-seeking activity
6. social or occupational impairment
7. continued use despite physical or psychological complications

Substance abuse is considered present when any drug use leads to significant adverse consequences, such as repetitive absences from work or school, expulsion from school, driving while impaired, and arrests. The diagnosis of substance abuse does not require tolerance or withdrawal.

The role of the primary care provider is to identify the patients who are using or abusing drugs. This identification can be made by the patient history, the results of the physical examination, and urine toxicology testing. Because of the high prevalence of substance use, the clinician should have a high index of suspicion in any patient who presents with psychiatric symptoms, high-risk behaviors (runaway, delinquency), unexplained somatic complaints, and acute changes in behavior or mental status (Tables 35-3 and 35-4). The interview should begin without the presence of the parents and should be conducted in a manner that does not make the patient defensive. The interview may begin with the clinician asking whether the patient's friends have ever tried drugs and whether the patient has ever partied with these friends. One series of questions that may assist the clinician in determining whether a patient has a substance use disorder is the so-called CAGE questionnaire (Table 35-5). The CAGE questionnaire has a sensitivity of 90% and a specificity of 79% for detecting ethanol abuse. This questionnaire may also be used for other substances.

If there is suspicion of substance abuse, urine and blood toxicology testing should be performed. Some of the physical findings associated with drug use (see Tables 35-3 and 35-4) are

- red skin (anticholinergic drugs, jimson weed, LSD, THC, MDMA, alcohol withdrawal)
- dilated pupils (stimulants, hallucinogens, withdrawal syndromes)
- pinpoint pupils (opiates)
- ataxia (CNS depressants, MDMA)
- lateral nystagmus (CNS depressants)
- vertical nystagmus (PCP)

The general time after ingestion in which a drug may be detected in the urine depends on the drug, the amount ingested, and the chronicity of use. The following drugs are listed with the times after use in which the drugs may be detected:

- alcohol: 12 hours
- heroin: 24 hours
- cocaine: 4 to 6 days, as benzoylecgonine
- marijuana: single use, 5 days; long-term daily use, 30 days
- phenobarbital: 33 days
- PCP (overdose): 9 days

If a clinician identifies a patient as a substance user, the unusual behavior should not be attributed solely to the drug. Instead, the clinician must consider other psychiatric conditions associated with drug use: ADHD, ODD, conduct disorder, schizophrenia, and mood disorders. The clinician must also consider the complications associated with drug use: human immunodeficiency virus infection, hepatitis B infection, cerebrovascular accidents (resulting from stimulants), bacterial endocarditis (resulting from intravenous use), asthma (resulting from THC use), and injuries from violence, accidents, or suicide attempts.

If the clinician suspects substance use, the patient should be referred to a mental health specialist. The treatment of drug use or abuse consists of detoxification, treatment of comorbid conditions, and psychological intervention to help maintain sobriety. Detoxification involves the termination of use of the substance as well as the management of potential withdrawal symptoms (from opiates, amphetamines, barbiturates, and, less often, cocaine). Sobriety maintenance is attempted by addressing coexisting psychiatric disorders and implementing psychosocial interventions. Although pharmacologic treatment for abuse prevention is sometimes used in adults (such as disulfiram for alcohol abuse), this form of intervention is not often employed with adolescents.

Central Serotonin Syndrome

Central serotonin syndrome results from excessive serotonin activity in the CNS from dietary supplements (L-tryptophan) or use of drugs that enhance CNS serotonin levels (serotonin reuptake inhibitors [SRIs] or selective serotonin reuptake inhibitors [SSRIs]). Certain drugs increase synaptic serotonin release (amphetamine, cocaine, MDMA, fenfluramine, mescaline, psilocin, L-dopa); others are serotonin agonists (lithium, LSD) or inhibit serotonin degradation (monoamine oxidase inhibitors, MDMA). In addition to SRRIs and SRIs, other drugs that inhibit serotonin reuptake include tricyclic antidepressants, meperidine, dextromethorphan, and MDMA.

The triad of cognitive-behavioral, autonomic nervous system, and neuromuscular signs and symptoms are characteristic of the central serotonin syndrome. Patients frequently manifest behavior alterations that include confusion, disorientation, agitation, and irritability. Coma, anxiety, seizures, hallucinations, and hypomania are less common.

Autonomic features include hyperthermia, diaphoresis, and tachycardia; hypertension, mydriasis, and tachypnea are less common. Neuromuscular features include myoclonus, hyperreflexia, tremor, rigidity, restlessness, hyperactivity, and ataxia. Other toxic ingestions (salicylates, sympathomimetic agents, or anticholinergic drugs), other withdrawal symptoms, and neuroleptic malignant syndrome are included in the differential diagnosis (see Table 35-3).

Serum drug levels are usually normal if the patient has been prescribed an SSRI or SRI. Management includes stopping the drug and treating complications such as hyperthermia with cooling, benzodiazepines (clonazepam), and mechanical ventilation. Some physicians administer propranolol or cyproheptadine, a nonspecific postsynaptic 5-HT$_{1A}$ and 5-HT$_2$ inhibitor. The mortality rate is 10% to 15%; most patients recover within 24 hours of discontinuing the agent.

Table 35-3. **Immediate Effects of Substance Abuse**

Substance	Immediate Effects	Duration of Action	Toxicity	Signs and Symptoms of Withdrawal	Treatment of Overdose
Alcohol	Respiratory depression, central nervous system (CNS) depression, ataxia, slurred speech, hypoglycemia	Depends on amount ingested and adolescent's tolerance	Cirrhosis, gastrointestinal, hemorrhage, thiamine and folate deficiency, CNS depression, impaired motor performance and mental function, stupor, deep anesthesia, death	Insomnia, restlessness, anxiety, tremulousness, hypertension, tachycardia, diaphoresis; auditory or visual hallucinations or both, seizures, delirium tremors are rare in adolescents	Supportive ventilation if needed
Amphetamine, other stimulants	↑ Blood pressure (BP), activity, and alertness; tachycardia; insomnia, anorexia; ↓ fatigue, euphoria; excitation; aggression; hostility	2-8 hr	Agitation; ↑ heart rate, BP, and temperature; hallucinations; paranoia, psychosis; convulsions; death, arrhythmias	Apathy, hallucinations, irritability, excessive sleep, depression, psychosis, suicidal thoughts, sudden death	Paranoia with haloperidol; seizures with diazepam
Nicotine	↑ BP and heart rate; ↓ temperature; CNS stimulation, skeletal muscle relaxation	Minutes	CNS stimulation	Restlessness, anxiety, insomnia, agitation, nausea, headache, ↑ appetite, inability to concentrate	None
Cocaine, crack	↑ Alertness, exultation, euphoria, insomnia; ↓ appetite; ↑ BP and heart rate; aphrodisiac, local anesthesia	15-30 min	Agitation; ↑ temperature, pulse, and BP; tremors; convulsions, tachyarrhythmias; paranoia, psychosis; cerebral hemorrhage; myocardial infarction; death	Apathy, long periods of sleep, irritability, depression, suicidal thoughts, disorientation	Paranoia with haloperidol; seizures with diazepam; cooling for hyperthermia; nitroprusside, labetalol for hypertension
Inhalants (solvents, gasoline)	Respiratory depression, CNS depression, ataxia, slurred speech, bradycardia	5-30 min	Arrhythmias, hallucinations, seizures, encephalopathy, renal tubular acidosis, hepatitis, peripheral neuropathy, lead poisoning, sudden death	Rare: chills, hallucinations, headache, abdominal pain, muscle cramps, delirium tremens	Organ-specific therapies
LSD, other hallucinogens	Dysphoria; hallucinations; anxiety; paranoia; psychosis; ↑ BP, heart rate, and temperature; dilated pupils; incoordination; ↑ creativity	2-12 hr; can produce exhaustion lasting for days	Long intense "trips"; psychotic reactions not always reversible; flashbacks; suicide attempts; deaths with some drugs	None	Reassurance; haloperidol
Marijuana, hashish	Euphoria, ↓ reaction time, ↓ inhibitions, ↑ appetite	2-4 hr	Dysphoria, acute anxiety attacks, acute psychosis, fatigue, paranoia, lack of motivation	Insomnia, hyperactivity, ↓ appetite	Psychological support
PCP and PCP analogues	Ataxia, nystagmus, ↑ BP, slurred speech, dysphoria, hallucinations, aggression, paranoia, confusion, hyperthermia	Hours to days	Psychosis; convulsions, coma, seizures, ↑ or ↓ BP, muscle rigidity; paranoia; flashbacks; suicide attempts, accidents	None	Haloperidol, diazepam, cooling for hyperthermia

Continued

Table 35-3. Immediate Effects of Substance Abuse—cont'd

Substance	Immediate Effects	Duration of Action	Toxicity	Signs and Symptoms of Withdrawal	Treatment of Overdose
Opioids	Euphoria, ataxia, slurred speech, miosis, stupor, respiratory depression	Hours	Respiratory depression, hypothermia, hypotension, pulmonary edema, apnea, coma, death	Increased sympathetic nervous system activity, hunger, antisocial behavior gooseflesh, diaphoresis, rhinorrhea, diarrhea, yawning	Naloxone; ventilation
Sedative-hypnotics	Respiratory depression, coma, hypotension	Variable by drug type and class	Alcohol enhances toxicity of benzodiazepines	Irritability, anxiety, depression	Supportive ventilation; Flumazenil* for benzodiazepines
γ-Hydroxybutyrate (GHB)	Sedation, respiratory depression, "date rape drug"	1-2 hr	Death if taken with alcohol or other intoxicants	Uncertain	Supportive ventilation if needed
Flunitrazepam (Rohypnol) ("Roofies")	Potent sedative benzodiazepine; as per GHB	4-6 hr	Amnesia	Uncertain	Supportive ventilation if needed
MDMA ("Ecstasy")	Amphetamine-like effects (see those for amphetamines)	4-5 hr	↑ BP, ↑ temperature, seizures, hyponatremia, cerebral infarction, arrhythmias, hepatic or renal failure, behavioral effects, death	Uncertain	Treat hyperthermia by cooling, dantrolene

Data from Jones RL: Substance abuse. In Shearin RB (ed): Handbook of Adolescent Medicine. Kalamazoo, Mich: Upjohn Company, 1983, pp 133-152; Abramewicz M (ed): Treatment of acute drug abuse reaction. Med Lett 1987;29:83; Kreipe RE, McAnarney ER: Adolescent medicine. In Behrman RE, Kliegman RM (eds): Nelson Essentials of Pediatrics, 2nd ed. Philadelphia, WB Saunders, 1994, p 244.

*Flumazenil is a benzodiazepine antagonist that may produce vomiting, acute withdrawal symptoms, or seizures. It should be used cautiously after an airway is secured.

LSD, lysergic acid diethylamide; PCP, phencyclidine; MDMA, 3,4-methylenedioxymethamphetamine.

EPISODIC (RECENT) DISRUPTIVE BEHAVIORS

Episodic disruptive disorders may be either an acute presentation of an illness in a previously healthy individual or an episodic flare-up of a chronic disorder. These conditions may be subdivided according to the patient's mental status (confusion or delusion), emotional state (labile or pervasive), and the best expert to treat the condition (primary care provider or mental health specialist) (see Figs. 35-3 and 35-4).

Mental Status Changes

Delirium

Delirium is characterized by deficits in cognition and consciousness that develop over a short time (Table 35-6). According to the *DSM-IV,* the criteria for the diagnosis of delirium are

1. a disturbance of consciousness with reduced ability to focus or sustain attention
2. a change in cognition (drowsiness, disorientation) or perceptual disturbances (illusions, hallucinations)
3. an onset over a short period of time
4. a medical cause for the symptoms

The symptoms of delirium develop acutely and fluctuate throughout the course of the illness. Besides altered sensorium, the patient also has reversal of the sleep/wake cycle and may exhibit disruptive behaviors consisting of psychomotor agitation or retardation.

Delirium is caused by global cerebral dysfunction. Hence, any agent that can cause coma can also cause delirium. Some of these causes are represented by the mnemonic AEIOU-TIPS, which stands for *a*lcohol, *e*ncephalopathy (lead, Reye syndrome, inborn errors of metabolism, encephalitis), *i*nsulin (hypoglycemia or hyperglycemia), *o*piates, *u*remia, *t*rauma, *i*nfection, *p*oisonings, and *s*eizures. Because the aforementioned causes of delirium are potentially life-threatening, an expedient and comprehensive medical evaluation is needed.

Children with delirium present with perceptual disturbances consisting of misinterpretations (hearing a sound and thinking it represents something else), illusions (visual misinterpretations), and hallucinations (seeing something that is not actually there). The hallucinations of delirium are different from those of psychoses (e.g., schizophrenia) because they are usually visual and acute in onset, whereas those resulting from psychoses are usually auditory and subacute or chronic. The hallucinations occurring with psychoses may have a delusional component.

The treatment of delirium is directed toward the underlying medical problem. Some patients with delirium may be aggressive and assaultive. A psychiatric consultation may be helpful in differentiating the hallucinations into medical versus psychotic causes and in assisting in the pharmacologic and behavioral or environmental management of the agitated patient. Benzodiazepines, high-potency antipsychotic agents (haloperidol), or both may reduce the agitation; however, the dosages must be carefully titrated to prevent the side effects of these medications from contributing to the patient's altered sensorium. Because patients with delirium are frightened and confused, their agitated behavior may respond to frequent reassurances, implementation of expected routines, a consistent environment, and frequent reorientation.

Table 35-4. Long-Term Effects, Adulteration, and Methods of Administration of Substances that Adolescents Abuse

Substance	Long-Term Effects	Tolerance	Dependence		Adulteration or Substitution	Method of Administration
			Psychological	*Physical*		
Alcohol	Blackouts; behavioral changes; ↑ accidents; homicide; suicide; gastritis; peptic ulcer; alcoholic hepatitis; fatty liver; pancreatitis	Yes	Yes	Yes	Methanol	Ingested
Amphetamine, other stimulants (speed)	Weight loss, insomnia, anxiety, paranoia, hallucinations; skin abscesses and amphetamine psychosis after injections	Yes	High	Yes	More than 90% of speed is adulterated with caffeine, asthma medicatons, PCP, LSD, strychnine, sugars	Ingested, injected
Tobacco	↑ Risk of chronic bronchitis, heart disease, and cancer (oral cancer with smokeless tobacco)	Yes	Yes	Yes	No	Smoke inhaled, snuff dipping, chewed
Cocaine, crack	Nasal perforation with snorting, weight loss, insomnia, anxiety, paranoia, hallucinations, soft tissue abscesses with injections	Yes	High	Yes, especially after smoking or injection	Local anesthetics, sugars, PCP	Snorted, smoked, ingested, injected
Inhalants (solvents, gasoline, "white out," etc.)	Liver damage with toluene, trichloroethylene, gasoline; ancmia with tetraethyl lead; leukemia with benzene; kidney damage with trichloroethylene	Yes, especially with toluene	Yes	Yes	None	Sniffing rags soaked with the compound, inhaling fumes through the mouth
LSD, other hallucinogens	Flashbacks, pronounced personality changes, ↑ risk of chronic psychosis	Yes, cross-tolerance with mescaline, DMT, and psilocybin	Degree unknown	No	Sold as tablets, in liquids, in microdots in many colors; often adulterated with or substituted for other drugs	Ingested, injected, sniffed
Marijuana, hashish	Great variety involving several body systems; ↓ motivation	Yes	Degree unknown	No	With PCP	Smoke inhaled, ingested
PCP and PCP analogues	Personality disorders, flashbacks, catatonia, neuropsychological disturbances, increased risk of schizophrenia	Yes	High	Degree unknown	Often added to other drugs or advertised as other drugs	Ingested, injected, smoked
Opioids	↓ Motivation, antisocial behavior, crime to support habit, skin abscesses, endocarditis, osteomyelitis, nephritis, hepatitis, HIV, amenorrhea	Yes	Yes	Yes	Quinine, sugar	Ingested, injected subcutaneous (skin-popping), intravenous

Modified from Jones RLK: Substance abuse. In Shearin RB (ed): Handbook of Adolescent Medicine. Kalamazoo, Mich: Upjohn Company, 1983, pp 133-152; Kreipe RE, McAnarney ER: Adolescent medicine. In Behrman RE, Kliegman RM (eds): Nelson Essentials of Pediatrics, 2nd ed. Philadelphia, WB Saunders, 1994, p 245.

DMT, dimethyltryptamine; HIV, human immunodeficiency virus; LSD, lysergic acid diethylamide; PCP, phencyclidine.

If the underlying medical condition for delirium is promptly treated before irreversible CNS damage develops, the patient should make a full recovery. However, if damage has occurred, the patient may develop dementia. *Dementia* is a chronic, irreversible, and possibly progressive disease that includes memory impairment and

one of the following symptoms:

1. aphasia (inability to name an object)
2. apraxia (inability to carry out motor activities despite understanding the task and having intact motor abilities)
3. agnosia (inability to recognize objects)

Table 35-5. CAGE Questionnaire*

C: Have you ever tried to *C*ut down on drinking?
A: Have you ever been *A*nnoyed by criticism of your drinking?
G: Have you ever felt *G*uilty about your drinking?
E: Have you ever had a morning *E*ye-opener (a drink to prevent withdrawal symptoms)?

*CAGE questioning has a sensitivity of 90% and a specificity of 79% for detecting alcohol abuse.

4. problems with executive function (inability to engage in age-appropriate planning, organizing, sequencing, abstracting)

In children, dementia can also manifest as a loss of developmental milestones or deteriorating school performance.

Schizophrenia

Schizophrenia is a chronic disorder that may flare into an active phase of very disruptive behavior (Table 35-7). This disruptive behavior consists of delusions, hallucinations, disorganized speech, and catatonic behavior. According to the *DSM-IV*, the diagnostic criteria for schizophrenia are two or more of the following present for a 1-month period:

1. delusions
2. hallucinations
3. disorganized speech
4. catatonic behavior
5. negative symptoms, such as flat affect

These characteristic signs and symptoms must appear in the context of significant social and educational dysfunction. There must also be continuous indications of the disturbance for at least 6 months (prodrome, active phase, residual period). Medical causes and mood disorders need to be excluded. The diagnosis of schizophrenia is further subdivided by the primary symptom complex into the following types: paranoid, disorganized, catatonic, residual, and undifferentiated.

During the prodromal phase, the patient may develop increasing negative symptoms, such as social withdrawal, flattening of affect, alogia (speaking in brief sentences), and avolition (lack of desire to do anything). The flat affect may consist of a reduction in body language, lack of eye contact, and emotional unresponsiveness. During this period, the patient may also have unusual beliefs that are not of the magnitude of true delusions or hallucinations. The patient may have magical thinking or may perceive that someone is talking to him or her, but no words are hallucinated. This prodromal state must be present for 6 months before the diagnosis of schizophrenia can be made.

During the acute phase of schizophrenia, the patient has at least two characteristic symptoms (or one characteristic if the delusions are bizarre) for more than 1 month, unless the symptoms have been

Table 35-6. Approach and Red Flags for Delirium

1. Symptoms evolve in hours
2. Level of consciousness waxes and wanes
3. Urgent medical evaluation (AEIOU-TIPS) is required
4. All poisons and medications in the home should be reviewed
5. Hallucinations are usually visual or tactile

AEIOU-TIPS, alcohol, encephalopathy, insulin, opiates, uremia-trauma, infection, poisonings, seizures.

Table 35-7. Approach and Red Flags for Psychoses

General
Strong family history of symptoms or disorders
Delusions
Comorbidities should be ruled out
Increased suicide risk

Schizophrenia
Declining function unless treated
Duration of symptoms > 6 mo
Symptoms: hallucinations, disorganized speech, flat affect, disorganized/catatonic behavior

Bipolar Disorders*
Past episodes of mania or hypomania
Should be considered for any disruptive behavior that does not respond to treatment

Major Depressive Disorders*
Can manifest with behavioral problems and irritability instead of depressed mood
Should not be overattributed to a stressor
Risk for developing bipolar disorders

*Bipolar and some depressive disorders are classified as mood disorders, but in severe cases patients may show psychotic features.

shortened by treatment. The most common delusions (erroneous beliefs) in this disorder are persecutory (patient is being spied on) and referential (events or comments are directed toward the patient). Other less common delusions are somatic (internal organs are replaced by others), religious, and grandiose. The most common hallucinations are auditory, but they may emanate from any sensory modality.

For hallucinations to support the diagnosis of schizophrenia, the patient must have a clear sensorium. The disorganized speech may be incomprehensible, and the patient may be unable to organize a logical conversation. The behavior problems consist of inappropriate dress, disheveled appearance, unprovoked aggression, and catatonia (decreased response to the environment).

If symptoms have not been present for 6 months, the provisional diagnosis of schizophreniform disorder is used. Approximately two thirds of patients with schizophreniform disorder have symptoms that last longer than 6 months and hence are reclassified as having schizophrenia.

The prevalence of schizophrenia ranges from 0.5% to 1.0%. Even though some cases have been reported in children as young as 5 years of age, most cases of schizophrenia manifest between the late teens and early 30s.

Results of monozygotic twin studies support both an environmental cause and a biologic cause for schizophrenia. Among children who have a first-degree biologic relative with schizophrenia, there is a 10-fold increase in schizophrenia over the incidence in the general population. Neuroimaging studies have consistently noted increased ventricular size in the brains of schizophrenics in comparison with normal persons.

The differential diagnosis of schizophrenia consists of the same medical causes of delirium and dementia plus the mood disorders and pervasive developmental disorders. In addition, ingestions (e.g., amphetamines, cocaine, PCP, hallucinogens) may produce similar symptoms.

The prognosis of schizophrenia is guarded, with significant morbidity and mortality (suicide, especially early in the illness). This chronic disorder is associated with exacerbations and remissions. Even with optimal therapy, patients with schizophrenia have significant social deficits, poor initiative, and abnormal thought processes.

The treatment of schizophrenia consists of the use of atypical antipsychotic agents (risperidone, olanzapine, clozapine in treatment-resistant cases), psychotherapy, and educational interventions. The patient often benefits from socialization groups plus individual and/or group therapy. The families of patients with schizophrenia also need emotional support and guidance. Because of the abnormalities in the thinking process and the neuropsychological deficits, patients often need an individual educational program. This disease is difficult to treat, and therefore the therapy is managed best by a psychiatrist. The primary care provider may assist in the management by conducting the medical evaluation and by educating the family. Families often confuse schizophrenia with dissociative identity (or multiple personality) disorder; they are unrelated.

Bipolar Disorders

Bipolar disorder, formerly called manic-depressive disorder, is a mood disorder. The most common mood disorder is major depressive disorder. Bipolar disorder manifests acutely, with severe problems in thinking and behavior that lead to significant impairment in functioning (see Table 35-7). Disturbances in thinking associated with mania include racing thoughts (rapidly changes topics), distractibility, and delusions of grandeur. Problematic behaviors during a manic episode include recklessness (excessive participation in social activities, promiscuity, buying sprees), agitation, decreased sleep, and excessive talkativeness.

The bipolar disorders are divided into the following categories:

- bipolar I disorder (episodes of mania usually with episodes of depression)
- bipolar II disorder (major depression with only hypomanic episodes)
- mixed bipolar disorder (daily occurrence of both manic and depressive features)
- cyclothymic disorder

Cyclothymic disorder is a chronic, cyclic illness of hypomania and depressive symptoms (no major depressions). Approximately 15% to 50% of patients with cyclothymic disorder will eventually develop bipolar I or II disorder.

According to the *DSM-IV,* a manic episode consists of an abnormally elevated (euphoric), expansive, or irritable mood for at least 1 week unless treated. This mood disturbance is associated with at least three (four if patient is irritable) of the following symptoms:

1. grandiosity
2. decreased desire for sleep
3. talkativeness
4. racing thoughts
5. distractibility
6. excessive goal-directed activity (or psychomotor agitation)
7. reckless pursuit of pleasure

Hypomanic episodes consist of the same symptoms except that the symptoms are present for a shorter time (4 days), are not associated with any psychotic activity (delusions or hallucinations), and are not severe enough to cause major social or academic dysfunction. About 10% of patients with hypomania progress to mania.

The differential diagnosis of bipolar disorders includes the medical conditions that cause coma or delirium. Some specific medical conditions whose presenting symptoms resemble bipolar disease are thyroid disorders (hypothyroidism or hyperthyroidism), Cushing disease, and multiple sclerosis. Substance-induced mood disorders (e.g., cocaine, tricyclic and SSRI antidepressants) must also be considered. The clinician should obtain a detailed family history because of the high prevalence of these disorders in parents of children with bipolar disorders. Because the condition is often undiagnosed in parents, the questions should be directed toward the presence of the *symptoms* for bipolar disorders.

Some of the psychiatric disorders that frequently occur with bipolar disorders are eating disorders, ADHD, conduct disorders, panic disorders, social phobias, adjustment disorders, and substance-related disorders. These conditions may manifest with symptoms that imitate bipolar disorders (e.g., distractibility of ADHD instead of mania). The clinician must decide whether the symptoms are caused by a bipolar disorder or by some other psychiatric disorder. ADHD can be differentiated from mania because the hyperactive behavior of ADHD is more likely to manifest in childhood and progress to restlessness in the teenager, whereas teenagers with mania present acutely with excessive activity. Because patients with bipolar disorders can also present with hallucinations and delusions, schizophrenia must be ruled out. Likewise, patients with initial diagnoses of schizophrenia have been found after years of follow-up to have bipolar disorders.

The lifetime prevalence of bipolar I disorders is 0.4% to 1.6%, and that of bipolar II disorders is 0.5%. Approximately 15% of adolescents with recurrent major depression eventually develop bipolar illnesses. A 2- to 15-fold increase of bipolar disorders in children of affected parents supports a biologic determinant for this condition. Manic patients have biologic abnormalities in neuroendocrine function (increased cortisol production, absence of dexamethasone nonsuppression) and in neurotransmitter systems.

Although bipolar disorders can develop in childhood, the average age of onset is 20 years for men and women. The natural history of bipolar disorders is a chronic illness with episodes of mania, hypomania, and major depression; 15% of patients have four or more episodes per year. Risk factors for initiation of a manic episode are disruption of the normal sleep cycle (crossing multiple time zones), the postpartum period, and recent onset of major depression (about 70% of manic or hypomanic episodes are associated with recent major depression). With therapy, many patients recover fully between episodes; however, 30% of patients with bipolar I disorder and 15% of those with bipolar II disorder have persistent interpersonal and occupational disorders. Ten percent to 15% of patients with bipolar disorders eventually commit suicide.

Because of the severe morbidity and mortality with this disorder and the complexities of treatment, psychiatrists manage bipolar disorders. Treatment consists of medications and psychotherapy. Medications used to treat bipolar disorder include lithium carbonate, carbamazepine, valproic acid, benzodiazepines, and antipsychotic agents. Various forms of psychotherapy are often employed in conjunction with a close liaison with schools to promote scholastic success as well as to maximize the patient's well-being.

The role of the primary care provider in the management of bipolar disorders is early detection. Mixed (manic and depressed) states with marked dysphoric, agitated affect and explosive anger occur more frequently in youths than in adults. Guidelines that may lead to early diagnosis are as follows:

1. Know and recognize the symptoms for mania and hypomania.
2. Remember that depressed patients often have bipolar disorders.
3. Obtain a thorough family history to look for symptoms of mood disorders.
4. Consider bipolar illnesses in patients with any disruptive disorder that does not respond to treatment.
5. Assess for drug and/or alcohol use (may induce bipolar disorder and is frequently a comorbid condition).

Once the primary care provider suspects bipolar disorders, the patient should be referred to a psychiatrist. Because of the manic symptoms (elation, angry outbursts when thwarted, delusions of grandeur) that accompany this disorder, these patients may vigorously argue and refuse referral. Family members must often be enlisted to insist on referral.

Labile Emotions

Adjustment Disorder

Adjustment disorder (see Fig. 35-3) is an excessive or maladaptive response to stress. A recognizable stressor must be present in order to make this diagnosis. Some of the typical stressors for children and adolescents are separations, painful injuries, illness, treatment of an illness (hospitalization, surgery), parental divorce, change of residency, academic failure, and conflict with peers.

The *DSM-IV* criteria for adjustment disorder are as follows:

1. The symptoms develop within 3 months of the stressor.
2. Significant impairment (social, academic) results.
3. The symptoms do not meet criteria for mood or anxiety disorder.
4. The symptoms do not represent bereavement.
5. The symptoms abate 6 months after termination of the stressor.

This disorder is further subdivided by the patient's symptoms, such as depressed mood, anxiety, and/or conduct disorder.

The prevalence of adjustment disorder ranges from 10% to 30% in mental health clinics. Besides the morbidity secondary to the social and/or academic impairment, these patients may be at increased risk for suicide. If the stressor is an illness or treatment, the morbidity of the medical condition may increase as a secondary consequence of noncompliance. The differential diagnosis of adjustment disorder is mood or anxiety disorder, exacerbation of a personality disorder, or post-traumatic stress disorder. The primary care provider may intervene with advice, insight, reassurance, and, if necessary, a referral to a mental health professional for short-term counseling.

Borderline Personality Disorder

Borderline personality disorder (see Fig. 35-3) is a chronic personality disorder characterized by intense mood lability, impulsivity, and identity disturbances. Patients with this disorder also have unstable and intense interpersonal relationships. According to the *DSM-IV*, the diagnosis of this condition requires five or more of the following features:

1. frantic efforts to avoid abandonment
2. intense interpersonal relationships alternating between extreme idealization and devaluation
3. unstable self-image
4. impulsivity
5. recurrent suicide attempts and/or self-mutilating behaviors
6. marked mood reactivity (short periods of intense anxiety or dysphoria)
7. feelings of emptiness
8. difficulty in controlling anger
9. stress-related paranoia

The prevalence of borderline personality disorder in the general population is 2%, occurring predominantly in females. Risk factors for this illness include abuse, neglect, and early parental loss. A fivefold prevalence among children with affected parents, coupled with the social risk factors, suggests both a genetic and a psychosocial cause.

This disorder usually manifests during adolescence or early adulthood as a fulminant crisis around an unstable and intense relationship. These crises often involve a suicide attempt because of severe impulsivity and mood lability. Approximately 10% of affected patients commit suicide. The morbidity is compounded by the physical sequelae from these multiple attempts (scarring, mutilation, brain anoxia). In addition to their suicide attempts, these individuals commonly quit school, relationships, or work just before reaching a goal, even when success is imminent. Other comorbid conditions associated with borderline personality disorder are mood disorders, substance abuse, eating disorders (especially bulimia), ADHD, and post-traumatic stress disorder. The suicide attempts, the failed life opportunities, and the comorbid conditions all add to the overall morbidity of this condition.

Although borderline personality disorder may be diagnosed in patients younger than 18 years, most child and adolescent psychiatrists are reluctant to do so. There are two reasons for this diagnostic circumspection: (1) borderline personality disorder has decidedly negative connotations for many health care professionals, and these connotations can be so stigmatizing that they might interfere with the quality of care; and (2) the entire process of differential diagnosis is much more difficult in adolescence because the developmental shifts typical of this phase are dramatic enough to blur the boundaries between borderline personality disorder and its common comorbid conditions, particularly the mood disorders (unipolar and bipolar), psychotic disorder, and post-traumatic stress disorder. The presence of substance abuse and family turmoil, which are frequently associated with borderline personality disorder, adds other layers of complexity to the diagnostic picture. Nevertheless, the diagnosis is appropriate and valid for some adolescent patients who show a pervasive pattern of instability and impulsivity and have a history of significant maltreatment (physical, sexual) in childhood.

Borderline personality disorder is difficult to treat. Even though the patients are very reasonable and appealing between the crises, the primary care provider should refer them to a mental health specialist because of the serious mortality and morbidity associated with this chronic recurrent disorder.

Treatment consists of psychotherapy and the use of psychotropic agents to treat target symptoms. The course of treatment is often lengthy, with frequent exacerbations and remissions.

Pervasive Emotions

Major Depressive Disorder

Because of the associated risk of suicide and significant social and academic impairment, depression is a serious condition. Even though a child may be pervasively sad, he or she may also present with behavior problems and irritability (see Table 35-7). According to the *DSM-IV*, major depressive disorder consists of at least a 2-week period of a depressive mood (irritability in some children) or loss of interest in pleasurable activities that results in significant impairment. During this period, the patient has at least five of the following symptoms:

1. depressed mood (irritability in some children)
2. loss of interest/pleasure
3. loss of appetite or overeating
4. sleep disorders
5. fatigue
6. feeling of worthlessness or guilt (patient may be delusional)
7. poor concentration
8. suicidal ideation or thoughts of death

These symptoms should not be secondary to bereavement, medical conditions, substance abuse, or bipolar disorders. Patients may also present with somatic complaints, psychosis, or both. The psychotic symptoms are typically auditory hallucinations and delusions of guilt, medical illnesses, or deserving punishment.

The occurrence of major depressive disorders in adolescence from a community-screened population is 4% to 5%. There is also a threefold increase of major depression in children whose parents have the disorder. Other evidence suggesting a biologic component to the illness includes abnormalities on polysomnograms (reduced latency to onset of rapid eye movements in early sleep) and abnormal levels of neurotransmitters.

The differential diagnosis of major depression encompasses various medical disorders, including neurologic disorders (causes of coma or delirium), endocrine disorders (hypothyroidism, hyperparathyroidism), side effects from medications (H_2 blockers, isotretinoin [Accutane]), and substance abuse or use. The patient should be screened for thyroid or parathyroid disorders and for substance abuse. Numerous psychiatric conditions are comorbid with major depression. In children, these conditions are ODD, conduct disorder, ADHD, and anxiety disorders. In adolescents, these illnesses are ODD, conduct disorder, ADHD, anxiety disorders, eating disorders, and substance abuse or use.

Major depressive disorders can manifest at any age; however, the average age of presentation is the mid-20s. Children usually present with somatic complaints, social withdrawal, and irritability, whereas adolescents often present with psychomotor retardation, negative self-cognition of guilt and worthlessness, and excessive sleep. Approximately 10% to 15% of children with major depression eventually develop bipolar disorders. Fifty percent of children with major depression have multiple episodes, frequently associated with significant stressors. Approximately 25% of patients with certain chronic medical conditions (cancer, diabetes) develop major depressive disorder during the course of illness. Beyond the social and academic dysfunction caused by the major depression and its associated comorbid conditions (ADHD, behavior disorders), 15% of patients eventually commit suicide.

The main difficulty in diagnosing major depression is that the gravity of the depressive mood is often not apparent to the parents and the clinician. Unlike patients with bipolar disease, these patients do not present with disruptive behaviors. Instead, they present with irritability, sullenness, or meanness. The parents and/or clinician may attribute this behavior to normal adolescence ("just going through a phase"). These children do not appear sad and deny having any problems. The clinician should have a high index of suspicion of major depression in any child who presents with sullenness and irritability. Guidelines for evaluating such a patient are as follows:

1. Assess suicidal ideation and ensure the patient's safety.
2. Interview multiple sources (coaches, teachers) to determine the child's function and symptoms.
3. Obtain a thorough family history for symptoms and diagnoses of mood disorders.
4. Rule out bipolar disorders (mania and hypomania).
5. Investigate primary or comorbid conditions (e.g., substance abuse).
6. Consider the role of life stressors in relationship to the symptoms.

Emotional reaction to adverse stressors is a normal part of life. The clinician must decide whether the reaction to the stressor is normal, an adjustment disorder, or major depression.

Treatment of major depression is usually conducted by a psychiatrist and consists of psychotherapy and/or psychopharmacologic interventions. The SSRIs such as sertraline (Zoloft) and fluoxetine (Prozac) are the first-line medications for juvenile depression. When major depression causes significant impairment in function, a trial of antidepressants should be considered. Besides medications, psychotherapy (individual, group, and family) is beneficial in treating depressed children. Because major depression often interferes with academic performance, a close liaison with the school system is important.

The role of the primary care provider is early recognition and referral. Because children with major depression often do not present with problematic behavior, the family is reluctant to seek psychiatric care. The primary care provider is a trusted advisor who can encourage a referral to a mental health provider.

Anxiety Disorders

Anxiety disorders (see Fig. 35-4) are the most prevalent psychiatric disorders in children and adolescents. These disorders are characterized by intense episodes of distress, which consist of fear, worry, avoidance, or terror. The anxiety disorders are

- panic disorder
- separation anxiety disorder
- specific phobia
- social phobia
- OCD
- post-traumatic stress disorder
- acute stress disorder
- generalized anxiety disorder

Some of the medical conditions that manifest with anxiety symptoms and hence must be ruled out are metabolic disorders (hypoglycemia), endocrine disorders (thyroid or parathyroid), neurologic diseases, ingestion of stimulants (caffeine, psychostimulants), drug withdrawal, and catecholamine-producing tumors (pheochromocytoma, carcinoid).

The SSRIs have enhanced the treatment of childhood anxiety disorders; these medications include fluoxetine, sertraline, fluvoxamine (Luvox), and citalopram (Celexa). The SSRIs are very similar in most respects and are generally well tolerated. Some children become behaviorally activated in response to a SSRI. This activation/agitation side effect usually responds to a dosage adjustment or changing to a different SSRI medication. Another anxiolytic medication that is well tolerated and safe is buspirone (BuSpar); it is often not quite as effective as the SSRIs, but it is a useful alternative. Although the SSRIs were initially marketed as antidepressants, they have nonspecific antianxiety properties that are useful in treating all of the anxiety disorders.

Panic Disorder. According to the *DSM-IV*, panic disorders consist of recurrent unexpected panic attacks, during which one of the attacks is followed by a concern of having additional attacks, worry about the implications of the attack (loss of control), or a significant change in behavior (social avoidance). A panic attack consists of at least four of the following symptoms:

1. palpitations (tachycardia)
2. sweating
3. shaking
4. shortness of breath
5. sensation of choking
6. chest pain
7. nausea
8. dizziness
9. emotional detachment
10. paresthesia
11. chills
12. fear of dying
13. fear of "going crazy"

These symptoms may result in hyperventilation syndrome, which causes respiratory alkalosis, tetany, paresthesia, dizziness, or fainting. Panic attacks occur suddenly, peak within 10 minutes, and may occur with agoraphobia. Agoraphobia is an intense anxiety about having a panic attack in a place from which the person cannot escape or in which help may not be available. Because of this anxiety, the individual either avoids the situation (being outside the home alone) or endures the situation with marked distress.

The 1-year prevalence rate of panic disorders ranges from 1.5% to 3.5%. Thirty percent to 50% of individuals with panic disorder also have agoraphobia. The age of onset is bimodal, with the largest peak occurring in adolescence and a smaller one in the mid-30s. Panic disorder in prepubertal children occurs but is rare.

Patients with panic disorders have a high degree of comorbid conditions. Fifty percent to 65% of patients may have major depressive disorder. Patients with panic disorder are also at great risk for substance abuse because they often seek pharmacologic agents (THC, alcohol, benzodiazepines) to reduce their symptoms. There is a relatively high frequency of other anxiety disorders such as social phobia (in 15% to 30% of patients), OCDs (in 8% to 10%), and generalized anxiety disorders (in 25%) that occur with panic disorders. The physical complaints that accompany this disease often cause patients to miss work or school and seek medical care, which adds to the financial cost of the disorder.

Many adolescents with panic disorder can be treated in the primary care setting. SSRIs such as sertraline and citalopram are very effective in blocking panic attacks and are well tolerated. Patients with many comorbid conditions, severely impaired patients, and younger patients should be referred to a child psychiatrist.

Generalized Anxiety Disorder. In this condition, the child displays excessive worries and concerns over many issues. According to the *DSM-IV*, the diagnostic criteria for a generalized anxiety disorder are

1. anxiety and worry about various issues for more than 6 months
2. difficulty in controlling the worry
3. significant dysfunction

In addition, affected children have one of the following symptoms: fatigue, restlessness, irritability, sleep disturbances, poor concentration, and muscle tension. Patients may also have symptoms of depression or somatic complaints (abdominal pain, headaches).

The lifetime prevalence of generalized anxiety disorder is 5%; most cases develop during childhood and adolescence. The clinical course of this disorder is chronic and fluctuating and worsens with stress. It is also associated with mood disorders, other anxiety disorders, and substance abuse.

Once the condition is recognized, the treatment consists of reducing stress in the environment, psychotherapy, and medication. The psychotherapy focuses on helping the child obtain a sense of control over this emotional state. As an adjunct to psychotherapy, many children benefit from the use of SSRIs.

Separation Anxiety Disorder. In this condition, there is excessive anxiety at the separation from home or a loved one that is developmentally inappropriate. According to the *DSM-IV*, the symptoms are present for more than 4 weeks, occur before the age of 18 years, and consist of at least three of the following:

1. distress with separation (home, loved one)
2. worry about losing loved ones
3. worry about an event (kidnapping) causing separation
4. refusal to go to school
5. reluctance to be alone
6. refusal to fall asleep alone
7. repeated nightmares of separation
8. somatic complaints

These symptoms may worsen when the child anticipates a separation.

The prevalence of separation anxiety disorder is 4%; the onset is usually during early childhood. Affected patients are often demanding and intrusive, which leads to family conflict. Major depressive disorders and panic disorder with agoraphobia are common comorbid conditions.

For simple and uncomplicated cases, the primary care provider may institute simple behavioral techniques, such as initiation of brief separations so that the child may see that separation does not lead to catastrophic consequences. Parents, who are anxious and fearful about upsetting the child, often complicate the situation. For more complex and severe cases (family strife or comorbid condition present), the patient should be referred to a psychiatrist. The treatment includes behavioral and supportive psychotherapy. Many cases can be successfully treated without resorting to medications. If the psychosocial treatment stalls, a trial of an SSRI (e.g., sertraline, citalopram) may help.

Obsessive-Compulsive Disorder. This disorder consists of recurrent behaviors over which the patient has little control. According to the *DSM-IV*, obsessions are recurrent thoughts that are inappropriate and cause marked anxiety. Some common obsessions are

- contamination (acquiring an illness from someone or something)
- doubts (needing to check and recheck the stove many times to make sure it is off; even so the patient is riddled with doubt that it is actually off)
- order (distress with asymmetry)
- aggression
- sexual acts

Compulsions are repetitive and excessive acts designed to reduce anxiety (hand washing and checking behaviors are two common examples).

According to the *DSM-IV*, the obsessive-compulsive behaviors are time consuming (take >1 hour per day) or significantly interfere with the patient's function. The lifetime prevalence in a community-based sample for OCD is 2.5%. The origin of this condition is unknown; however, there is a higher predominance among children whose parents have either Tourette syndrome or OCD. There is some evidence that group A β-hemolytic streptococcal infections are associated with PANDAS such as tics and OCD. In younger children with sudden onset of OCD, this diagnosis should be considered, because antibiotic therapy may eradicate the symptoms of OCD.

The presentation usually occurs earlier in male patients (6 to 15 years of age) than in female patients (20 to 29 years of age). Children may present with anxiety, stress, poor concentration, or declining school performance. The differential diagnosis includes anxiety disorders, major depression, hypochondriasis, and tic disorders.

Conditions commonly comorbid with OCD include major depression, anxiety disorders, eating disorders, and Tourette disorder. In addition, the obsessions and compulsions may lead to social avoidance, frequent visits to the doctor, and substance abuse. In this chronic disorder, 80% of patients have waxing and waning symptoms with exacerbations secondary to stress, 15% have a progressive deterioration in function, and 5% have occasional episodes with minimal symptoms.

The treatment is usually directed by a psychiatrist and consists of cognitive-behavioral therapy and psychotropic medications. Cognitive-behavioral interventions are designed to provide patients with a sense of control over their thoughts and behaviors. Medications that potentiate serotonin activity (clomipramine, fluoxetine) may be successful in alleviating the symptoms. The response to treatment is quite variable: Some patients experience a complete remission, whereas others remain significantly disabled. OCD may manifest as a dermatitis that has resulted from excessive washing behaviors.

Post-traumatic Stress Disorder. In this condition, the patient has a severe reaction to an extremely threatening stressor. According to the *DSM-IV*, the characteristics of this syndrome may be summarized by the mnemonic TRAUMA, which stands for *t*raumatic event, *r*eexperience, *au*tonomic, symptoms of longer than 1 *m*onth's duration, and *a*voidance. The traumatic event must be very severe (e.g., life-threatening) and cause fear and horror in the victim. This event is then reexperienced as thoughts, dreams, or flashbacks (which occur when the patient is awake). The patient also experiences intense distress (psychological and/or physiologic) when exposed to a situation that resembles the traumatic event. The autonomic symptoms consist of sleep disturbances, irritability, poor concentration, or hyperventilation. The avoidance consists of either avoiding circumstances associated with the event (certain people, places, and activities) or withdrawal from relationships (emotional detachment, diminished interest, inability to love). Children's symptoms are similar to those of adults, except that their dreams are frankly nightmares, their fear is manifested in disorganized or agitated behavior, and their reenactment may consist of repetitive play (airplane crash reenacted as throwing a toy plane against the wall). In addition, children frequently complain of somatic complaints (e.g., headaches).

The lifetime prevalence of post-traumatic stress disorder in a community ranges from 1% to 14%; however, it is three to four times higher among those exposed to extreme stress (disaster victims). Patients with this condition have an increased risk for panic disorders, social phobia, substance abuse, OCD, somatization disorder, and major depressive disorders.

The differential diagnosis includes adjustment disorders, panic disorders, OCDs, and psychoses (flashbacks versus hallucinations). In adjustment disorders, the stressor must be recognizable, whereas in post-traumatic stress disorder, it must be extreme. In acute stress disorder, the symptoms can simulate post-traumatic stress disorder except that the symptoms occur soon after an event (<4 weeks) and rapidly resolve (<4 weeks). In post-traumatic stress disorder, the intrusive thoughts center on the stressor, whereas in OCD, they are unrelated.

Patients with post-traumatic stress disorder are usually treated by a mental health professional. Treatment generally consists of psychotherapy. In adults, psychotropic medications improve the symptoms; however, there has been little research on the use of this approach in children. Nevertheless, many psychiatrists would consider a trial of an antianxiety agent in children who are not responding to psychotherapy.

Specific and Social Phobias.

Fears are common throughout childhood; however, phobias are internal fears that cause severe anxiety and distress. According to the *DSM-IV,* diagnostic criteria of a specific phobia are as follows:

1. An intense fear is caused by a particular stimulus.
2. The presence or the thoughts of a stimulus cause anxiety.
3. Stimuli are avoided or endured with great distress.
4. Symptoms lead to significant dysfunction.

Some of the specific phobias involve animals, environmental situations (e.g., heights), blood or injection, and situational conditions (e.g., enclosed places).

Social phobias are similar to specific phobias except that the stimulus is either social or performance related. The lifetime prevalences of specific and social phobias from a community-based sample are 10% to 11% and 3% to 13%, respectively. The onset of specific phobias is bimodal, with the peaks occurring in childhood and in the mid-20s, whereas social phobias begin in adolescence. Boys are as likely as girls to have social phobias, but girls are more likely to have specific phobias. In both conditions, the anxiety in children is manifested as clinging, crying, tantrums, and "freezing" (not moving). In social phobias, the children refuse to participate in group play, stay close to familiar adults, and appear excessively timid in unfamiliar social functions.

Social phobias tend to be chronic, with fluctuations precipitated by stressors. Comorbid conditions associated with social phobias are other anxiety disorders (panic disorder with agoraphobia), mood disorders, and substance abuse. The comorbid conditions associated with specific phobias are other anxiety disorders. In both conditions, the phobias can place significant limitations (academic, work, social life) on a person's function in society. In children, social phobia often manifests as refusal to attend school. For instance, the child reports somatic complaints (headache, stomachache) in the morning before school that vanish when the child is allowed to remain home. Sensitive interviewing can often elicit the underlying fear of social scrutiny.

Primary care providers, using behavioral therapy, may manage uncomplicated phobias; however, complex cases should be referred to a psychiatrist. The primary treatment of phobias is behavior therapy with the use of desensitization with graded exposure to the feared item. For significant dysfunction that remains, pharmacotherapy with anxiolytics (SSRIs, benzodiazepines) has been reported to be effective.

Personality Disorders

Personality disorders consist of chronic maladaptive traits that lead to psychosocial dysfunction and distress. Even though the personality disorders can manifest with labile erratic emotions (borderline personality disorder, histrionic personality disorder) and anxiety (obsessive-compulsive personality disorder), schizotypal personality disorder can manifest with pervasive and eccentric behavior (see Fig. 35-4). Most child psychiatrists are slow to make a personality disorder diagnosis in a child or adolescent. This reluctance is because many aspects of a youngster's personality are changing and in flux throughout development, making the reliability and validity of such diagnoses suspect. According to *DSM-IV,* personality disorder categories may be applied to children or adolescents in the relatively unusual instances in which the individual's particular maladaptive personality traits appear to be pervasive, persistent, and unlikely to be limited to a particular developmental stage or an episode of an Axis I disorder.

Schizotypal Personality Disorder. This personality disorder consists of a long-standing pattern of marked difficulty in forming close relationships, coupled with eccentric behaviors. This condition occurs in about 3% of the population. Children and adolescents present with solitariness, poor peer relations, social anxiety, and peculiar thoughts; they appear odd and are often teased by their peers. The patients may seek treatment for the acute onset of anxiety or depression. Some of these patients may respond to a stressor with a transient psychosis.

According to the *DSM-IV,* this diagnosis can be made if the patient has five or more of the following symptoms:

1. ideas but not delusions of reference (incorrect interpretations of external events as having an unusual meaning specifically for the person)
2. superstitions
3. illusions
4. odd thinking
5. suspiciousness
6. rigid affect
7. peculiar behavior and/or appearance
8. lack of close friends
9. excessive social anxiety

The origin of this condition is unknown; however, there is a familial tendency for it. The differential diagnosis includes schizophrenia, mood disorders, and pervasive developmental disorders (Asperger syndrome, autistic disorder). Therapy is best directed by a psychiatrist and includes psychotherapy (to deal with the acute problem as well as the underlying personality disorder) and psychotropic agents to treat acute manifestations of anxiety, depression, or psychosis.

HALLUCINATIONS

The presence of hallucinations is of extreme concern to parents because it conjures up the image of an uncontrollable, mentally disturbed person. To the primary care provider, hallucinations are a warning that a serious medical or psychological condition may be present (Fig. 35-5). Because of these concerns, hallucinations necessitate a prompt and urgent evaluation. The first step is to assess the patient's mental status. If the abnormal mental status consists of confusion, the examiner should consider the medical causes of delirium. If delusions are present, schizophrenia and mood disorder must be ruled out. Most hallucinations associated with delirium are visual, whereas those observed in psychoses are typically auditory. Most children who present with hallucinations have a normal mental status.

Hallucinations occur in as many as 5% of normal children. Even though these hallucinations can be of any sensory modality, they are mostly auditory. The hallucinations may be perceived as chatter or as a voice that chastises the child. Hallucinating children may also have symptoms of anxiety or depression secondary to a recognizable stressor. Most hallucinations in children with a normal mental status can be managed by the primary care provider through reassurance to the parents. In more extreme cases, a consultation with a child psychiatrist may be necessary to rule out other conditions (acute phobic

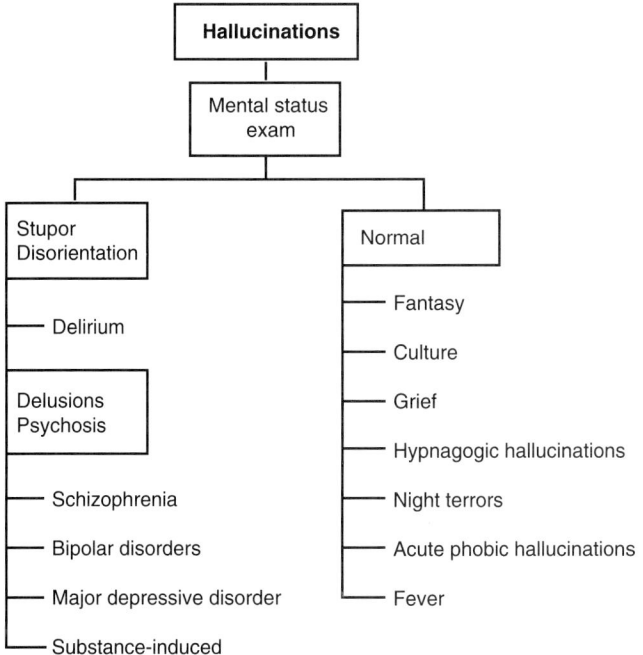

Figure 35-5. Evaluation of hallucinations.

hallucinations). The contexts in which children with a normal mental status may hallucinate include beliefs (fantasy, cultural), grief, sleep, acute phobic hallucinations, and fever.

FANTASY

The concept of hallucination is based on the assumption that a person can differentiate the real from the imaginary. Children under 3 years of age confuse reality with imagination. By 4 years of age, children understand the concept of "pretend," and by 7 years of age, they understand imagination but act as though the fantasy is still real (e.g., imaginary companion). By age 8 years, most children are reliably able to distinguish inner thoughts from voices. Some children are involved in more fantasy than are their classmates and may use it as entertainment or comfort. On occasion, they may get carried away by their fantasies and become quite fearful. Most of these children proceed to healthy psychological adjustment; however, the extremes may be an early manifestation of schizotypal personality disorder.

CULTURE

Hallucinations may be supported by cultural, religious, and parental beliefs. For example, seeing religious visions or hearing voices from God during excitable, fundamentalist religious services are accepted and even encouraged by the participants. Even more common are parental beliefs in supernatural spirits and ghosts. This becomes problematic when adults accept the child's report of a supernatural experience as reality. This acceptance may frighten both the child and the adult.

Treatment of these hallucinations consists of recognizing the context in which they occurred and reassuring the family that the child is normal. In addition, the child's reality testing would be helped and his or her fearfulness reduced if the family can reassure the child that the hallucination is just imagination and that there is nothing to fear. A problem arises when the family believes in supernatural events. To reduce confrontation, the clinician should first acknowledge that supernatural beliefs are common, determine the extent of the adult's belief in the supernatural, and assess the parent's level of certainty

that a supernatural event caused the child's experience. If the parent expresses some uncertainty, acknowledgment of that uncertainty would help the child. If the parents are adamant in their beliefs, they will not be able to reassure their frightened child. In place of the parents, the clinician may need to rely on a trusted family member who is less certain. If asked, the clinician may explain that doctors are scientists who seek explanations that are not supernatural. This approach may avoid a detrimental confrontation between the parents and the health care provider.

GRIEF

Hallucinations after the death of a loved one are easily recognized because they are usually visual and occur in the context of grief. These hallucinations can also be auditory, in which the deceased's voice is speaking to the child. The family's reaction and interpretation of these hallucinations are highly dependent on their cultural and religious beliefs. Some families may perceive these events as a supernatural or a religious experience. Although these hallucinations may be frightening to young children, many find them a reassuring reunion. If these experiences cause a problem, the treatment consists of reassurance from a parent or a recognized religious leader from the family's place of worship.

HYPNAGOGIC HALLUCINATION

Dreamlike hallucinations can occur as a person falls asleep (hypnagogic) or as a person is awakening (hypnopompic). These hallucinations can also occur as part of post-traumatic stress disorder (flashback) or narcolepsy (periods of irresistible sleep, cataplexy, and hypnopompic or hypnagogic hallucinations). When these hallucinations occur independently of these syndromes, treatment consists only of reassurance.

NIGHT TERRORS

Night terrors are frequently mistaken as hallucinations. This condition is one of the parasomnias, a category that includes sleepwalking and sleep talking. According to the *DSM-IV,* night terrors (sleep terror disorder) consist of episodes in which the child appears to arouse during the night and cries or screams inconsolably. During these episodes, there is intense fear and autonomic arousal (tachycardia, sweating). On awakening, the child has no memory of the event. Episodes of night terrors last from 1 to 10 minutes, during which the child may speak but does not make sense. Night terrors occur during stage 4 deep sleep and not during rapid eye movement sleep.

The prevalence of night terrors ranges from 1% to 6%. It usually begins during early childhood and resolves spontaneously during adolescence. The occurrence of night terrors is inconsistently associated with stressors. Seizure disorders, especially of the temporal and frontal lobes, can produce fear and complex behavior patterns resembling night terrors. Hence, a seizure disorder should be considered in patients with persistent and significant symptoms.

Treatment for night terrors consists of education and reassurance. If the night terrors occur in unusually long clusters, a brief course of low-dose benzodiazepine therapy or a tricyclic antidepressant administered at bedtime may interrupt the clusters.

ACUTE PHOBIC HALLUCINATIONS

Acute phobic hallucinations are relatively common, occur in preschool-aged children, and consist of episodes of hallucinations coupled with panic. These hallucinations last from 10 to 60 minutes and may occur any time of the day but are present mostly at night. A child may become very frightened during an episode. The child may state that bugs are crawling over him or her and attempt to remove them, cry, or hide. Because of the acute change in mental status, this condition must be differentiated from the medical and psychotic causes of hallucinations (delirium).

The actual cause of acute phobic hallucinations is unknown. The symptoms usually last 1 to 3 days and diminish over 1 to 2 weeks. If the condition does not quickly abate, it responds well to low dosages of benzodiazepines.

FEVER

Preschool-aged children may hallucinate during times of high fevers. These hallucinations are temporary and are not associated with future mental disorders. Management of fever-induced hallucinations consists of ruling out the medical causes of delirium and reassuring the family.

UNEXPLAINED PHYSICAL COMPLAINTS

Parents may present to the primary care provider with "unexplained physical complaints" on behalf of the child. These complaints may be inconsistent with the results of the physical examination or laboratory tests (severe abdominal pain in a smiling child) and may fail to respond to any medical therapy, or the symptoms may be changed if they are not producing the appropriate response. These unexplained complaints might be caused by overprotectiveness, excessive worry, underlying psychological conditions, or manipulation. Clinicians can easily become annoyed when they suspect that they are being manipulated (Table 35-8).

These unexplained physical complaints may be the manner in which a patient copes with a stressor. The patient may not be aware of the stressor, nor may the patient realize that these symptoms emanate from his or her effort to cope with the problem. The clinician should empathize with the patient, then state the conditions that the child does not have (with serious diseases ruled out), and state that the symptoms are real. The health care provider should address the issue that stress can cause or make symptoms worse and should recommend that the possibility of stress be evaluated while the clinician continues to monitor the patient for other medical illness.

The various conditions that contribute to unexplained physical complaints are organized on the basis of whether the parent or the child is the complainer (Fig. 35-6).

PARENTS' COMPLAINTS

Vulnerable Child Syndrome

Vulnerability begins when an apparently healthy child suddenly develops a life-threatening illness. Even though the child may recover completely from the illness, the parents fear that the condition will recur. After a life-threatening illness, parents universally and appropriately rethink the illness to determine whether any warnings were overlooked. After appraising the oversight and/or the absence of warnings, the family usually returns to normal activity except for some increased wariness.

Some parents are so traumatized by this life-threatening event that they live in constant dread of its recurrence. They may also manifest some of the features of post-traumatic stress disorder. These parents are fearfully attentive to every nuance of change in the child. The child may incorporate this fear and be reluctant to separate from the parent, which delays the development of independence and self-confidence. Because the parents live every day as if it is the child's last, they are reluctant to discipline the child. Consequently, the child does not learn self-control and consideration of others, which can lead to significant personality dysfunction.

During the course of a life-threatening illness, the primary care provider should anticipate the development of the vulnerable child syndrome, warn the parents of this syndrome, and reassure the family that the life-threatening illness is not likely to recur. If the syndrome has already developed, some parents may benefit by realizing that their fears are based on the past and, with reassurance, can relax.

Hypochondriasis by Proxy

Parents may worry excessively about the child's health because of a preceding life-threatening event (vulnerable child) or mistrust of the medical profession (missed diagnosis in a family member) or as an expression of their own fear of having a serious condition themselves (hypochondriasis by proxy). These parents do not invent the child's symptoms but instead experience an exaggerated worry about symptoms. The evaluation of a parent's excessive concern over the child's health may be further subdivided into specific concerns versus general medical worries.

The specific medical concerns for the child's health are those caused by a prior life-threatening event or by a misfortunate experience with the medical profession. Reassurance after an appropriate and thorough medical evaluation may reduce parental anxiety. When the parent reveals the past incident that led to distrust of the reassurances of doctors, the clinician may be able to reduce the parent's worry through open discussion on the differences between past and current events.

If the parent reports that he or she worries about everything, the clinician should determine whether this is a recent development or a long-term characteristic. Parents with acute onset of general medical worries about their children may suffer from a recent stressor or may have anxiety, depressive behavior, or OCD. Because these conditions cause enormous distress in the parent, they merit a referral to a psychiatrist.

Parents with long-term, generalized, and excessive concern about a child's health may have hypochondriasis. Hypochondriasis, according to the *DSM-IV,* is a preoccupation with fears of having a serious disease that are based on misinterpretation of one or more bodily signs or symptoms. In addition, these fears are chronic (>6 months in duration) and persist despite an appropriate medical evaluation. The prevalence of hypochondriasis in a general medical practice ranges from 4% to 9%. The onset can occur at any age but usually occurs in early adulthood. This condition may cause the deterioration of the parent-physician relationship as a result of frustration and anger. In addition, it compounds the morbidity by excessive and inappropriate medical testing. Even though hypochondriasis is characterized as a chronic condition that waxes and wanes, complete remission can occur. Factors that are favorable to a remission are acute onset, associated medical conditions, lack of secondary gain, and absence of personality disorder.

Simple reassurance does not address the chronic fear or worry expressed by parents with hypochondriasis. Reassurance may paradoxically cause the deterioration of the parent-physician

---

Table 35-8. Essential Elements of the Management of Unexplained Physical Complaints

Avoid feeling manipulated or angry
Avoid the following behaviors:
  Ordering more tests to prove the child is healthy
  Tricking the patient with a placebo
  Stating that the symptoms do not exist
Proper management consists of
  Addressing parents'/child's worries
  Conducting an appropriate medical evaluation
  Stating what medical conditions are ruled out
  Introducing stress as a possible cause of the symptoms
  Exploring stress while monitoring for other medical illnesses

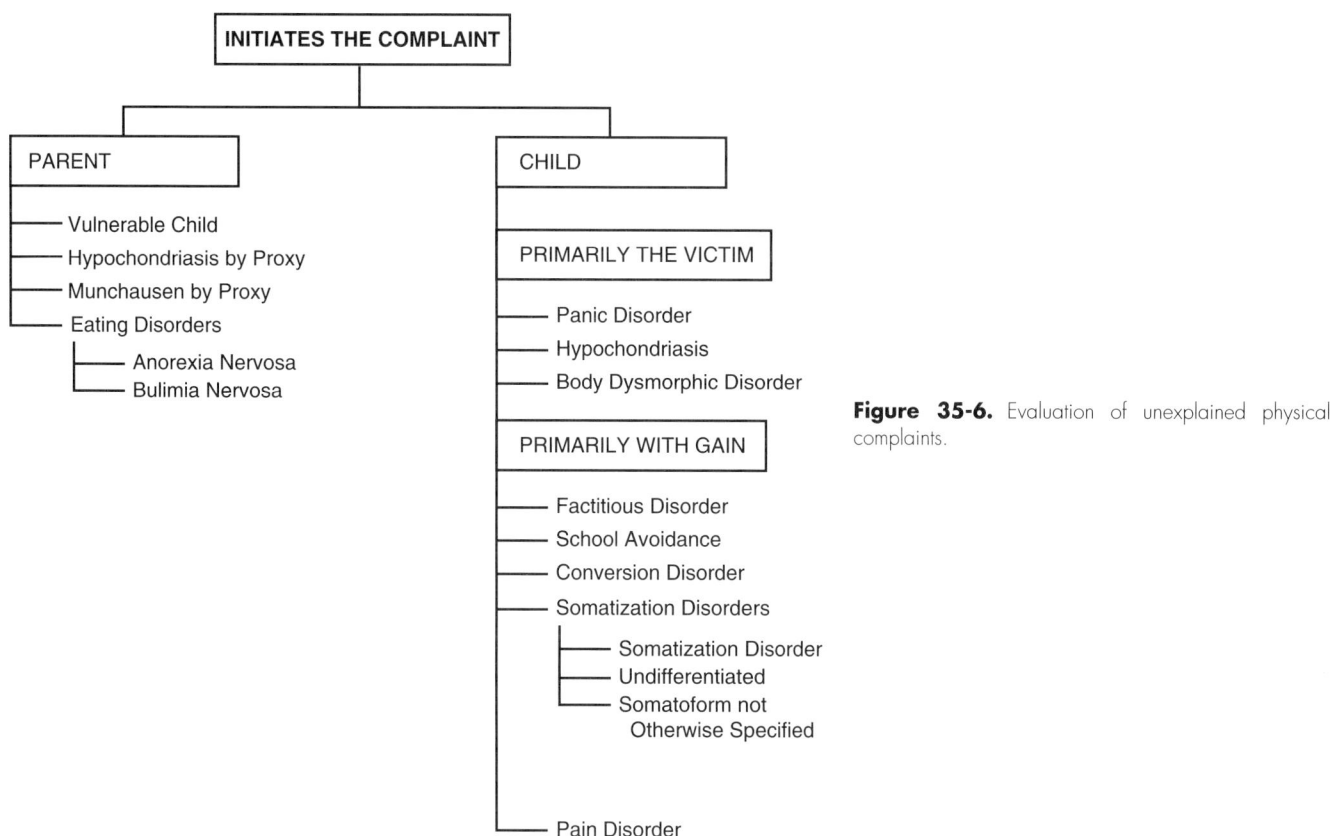

Figure 35-6. Evaluation of unexplained physical complaints.

relationship. This deterioration may lead to the referral (by parent or clinician) of the child to a subspecialist for further medical evaluation. Instead of simple reassurance, the treatment consists of empathy, education of the parents, reassurance about the child's medical health, and referral of the parents to the appropriate mental health professional.

Factitious Disorders (Munchausen Syndrome by Proxy)

According to *DSM-IV*, factitious disorder is defined as a condition in which the patient either feigns or produces symptoms and physical findings to fulfill an underlying need to assume the sick role and receive care. In addition, there is also no external reward for these symptoms, in contrast to malingering, in which the symptoms result in either economic gain or in avoidance of responsibilities. In Munchausen syndrome by proxy (see Chapter 36), a caregiver feigns or produces the symptoms in a child and then seeks medical care.

The perpetrator (or offender) in Munchausen syndrome by proxy is usually the mother. The offender may also have had a history of factitious disorder that is quiescent as long as the symptoms can be inflicted on someone else. The victim can be of any age but is usually a toddler. When the victim is an older child, he or she may collaborate with the offender. Usually, the offender focuses on one victim at a time; however, all siblings in the home are potentially at risk.

The most commonly induced or feigned symptoms in children are

- bleeding (stool or urine contaminated with parent's blood)
- diarrhea (laxative induced)
- vomiting (emetic induced)
- fever (induced by injection of bacteria)
- CNS depression (medication induced)
- seizures (hypoxia secondary to smothering or hypoglycemia from insulin injection)

- apnea (smothering)
- rashes (contact dermatitis)

Potential warning signs for this condition are unexplained and prolonged illnesses, incongruous symptoms and signs, ineffective medical treatments, prior episodes of sudden infant death syndrome, and widespread allergies.

The offending caregiver may not seem worried about the child's medical condition. Some caregiverss may form an unusually close relationship with the medical staff; however, there are many exceptions, in which the caregiver is instead neglectful, disruptive, and argumentative.

Besides the morbidity of the induced symptoms, the rate of mortality from this syndrome is as high as 9%. When a clinician suspects Munchausen syndrome by proxy, the first step is to ensure the child's safety, which usually means admission to a medical ward (Table 35-9). The next step is to develop a definitive investigative plan with a multidisciplinary team consisting of mental health professionals, physicians, social services, child abuse specialists, and the legal system. This plan may include

1. typing the blood in the specimen and comparing it with the child's blood
2. toxicology studies of stool (laxatives), vomitus (emetics), or urine (substance use)
3. species-specific insulin levels (pork/beef) for unexplained hypoglycemia
4. surveillance by covert video camera (with hospital legal advice and an approved protocol)

Events occurring only in the presence of the offender is circumstantial evidence and by itself will probably not lead to conviction in a court of law. In addition, referring the caregiver to a mental health provider is unfruitful and rarely results in the collection of any evidence.

With evidence in hand, the team should confront the perpetrator in a nonaccusatory manner. The offender may confess; however,

Table 35-9. Essential Elements of the Management of Munchausen Syndrome by Proxy

1. Maintain high index of suspicion
2. Ensure child's safety
3. Assemble multidisciplinary team
4. Collect evidence, including covert video surveillance, before confronting parent with the suspected diagnosis
5. Parental personality is a poor predictor
6. Realize that confrontation rarely results in a confession
7. Present evidence to legal system to determine
   a. Necessity of removal of child from home
   b. Institution of a close monitoring system

usually the caregiver denies his or her involvement, becomes angry, and threatens to take the child out of the hospital. During this time, the caregiver is also at great risk for depression and suicide. Psychotherapy for caregivers with Munchausen syndrome by proxy is rarely successful and cannot guarantee the child's safety. Instead, the multidisciplinary team, in conjunction with the legal system, needs to decide whether to remove the child from the caregiver's custody or institute a close surveillance program.

Eating Disorders

With eating disorders (Table 35-10), it is usually the concerned parent who initiates the visit to the health care provider. The eating disorders are anorexia nervosa (severe weight loss with or without induced purging) and bulimia nervosa (stable weight, uncontrolled binge eating, and induced purging). These disorders manifest with unexplained physical complaints, such as protracted diarrhea, persistent vomiting, weight loss, and/or amenorrhea. Adolescents who deliberately induce these symptoms to control caloric intake are very concerned about the weight and shape of their bodies. These patients go to great lengths to hide their intent and symptoms. Some of the ways of hiding these disorders are wearing baggy clothes, excessive and vigorous exercise to get into shape for sports or ballet, selection of healthy food because of low-fat or low-calorie content, complaints of allergies that ruin the taste and smell of food, and secret purging (induced vomiting and/or

diarrhea). Because of frequent concealment, the detection of these potentially lethal conditions is a diagnostic challenge.

Anorexia Nervosa

According to the *DSM-IV,* anorexia nervosa is defined as

1. refusal to maintain body weight at 85% of what is appropriate
2. intense fear of gaining weight
3. distorted perception of body size
4. in postpubertal girls, an absence of three consecutive menstrual cycles

The prevalence of anorexia nervosa ranges from 0.5% to 1%; almost 90% of cases occur in girls. Although this condition is associated with higher socioeconomic status, it can occur in persons from a variety of socioeconomic backgrounds and in all ethnic groups. The cause of anorexia nervosa is multifactorial and complex. It is associated with psychological (recent stressor), cultural (industrialized nations with abundance of food), environmental, and biogenetic influences.

Besides the weight loss, patients with anorexia nervosa may develop symptoms of depression or withdraw socially secondary to the physiology of semistarvation. Actual loss of appetite is rare in these patients; instead, they may develop obsessive-compulsive behavior regarding food (e.g., they may collect recipes or hoard food). These patients may also have inflexible thinking or feel the need to control their environment.

Anorexia nervosa may affect every organ system; presenting symptoms and signs are secondary to malnutrition and purging. The symptoms of malnutrition are fatigue, depression, and amenorrhea. The physical findings of malnutrition are bradycardia, hypothermia, hypotension, emaciation, hair loss, yellow skin (hypercarotenemia), and lanugo (fine body hair).

If the patient controls caloric intake by vomiting, he or she may present with hypertrophic salivary glands, dental erosions (secondary to gastric acid irritation), and abrasions and/or calluses on the dorsum of the hand (secondary to manual induction of vomiting). The metabolic abnormalities related to starvation and purging consist of leukopenia, anemia, hyperamylasemia (resulting from parotid gland irritation from gastric acid if the patient is binging and purging), metabolic alkalosis (resulting from vomiting), metabolic

Table 35-10. Characteristics of Anorexia Nervosa and Bulimia Nervosa

Characteristics	Anorexia Nervosa	Bulimia Nervosa
Intense preoccupation with food	Yes	Yes
Weight loss	Severe	Fluctuates
Female	90%-95%	90%-95%
Family history	+ for anorexia nervosa	+ for depression
Methods of weight control	Severe food restrictions, emesis, exercise	Restriction and binges with self-induced vomiting and diuretic and/or laxative abuse
Guilt/shame	None	Yes
Denial	Yes	None
Personality	Withdrawn/asexual	Outgoing/heterosexual
Onset (age)	Bimodal (13-14 yr and 17-18 yr)	17-25 yr
Endocrinopathy/metabolism	Amenorrhea, increased growth hormone, osteoporosis, hypercarotenemia, hypothermia	Menstrual irregularities, hypokalemia
Cardiovascular complications	Bradycardia, hypotension, arrhythmias	Ipecac toxicity, arrhythmias
Gastrointestinal	Constipation, elevated hepatic enzymes	Gastric dilation and rupture, Mallory-Weiss syndrome, esophagitis, parotid enlargement, dental enamel erosion
Psychiatric	Depression, suicide, obsessional fears, social phobia	Impulsive behaviors, alcohol-drug addictions, depression, suicide

From Tershakovec AM, Stallings VA: Pediatric nutrition and nutritional disorders. In Behrman RE, Kliegman RM (eds): Nelson Essentials of Pediatrics, 2nd ed. Philadelphia, WB Saunders, 1994, p 66.

acidosis (resulting from laxative abuse), decreased triiodothyronine level, hypomagnesemia, hypocalcemia, hypozincemia, and electrolyte abnormalities (resulting from diuretic abuse and dehydration).

These patients also have regression of the hypothalamic-pituitary-gonadal axis, which results in low estrogen levels in girls and low testosterone levels in boys.

In evaluating an adolescent with unexplained weight loss, the examiner must rule out the medical causes of cachexia such as malignancy, malabsorption, or inflammatory bowel disease. Interview data that support a diagnosis of anorexia nervosa are a restrictive dietary history, distorted perception of body shape, and rationalization of behavior (e.g., weight loss for ballet).

Once the medical causes for weight loss have been ruled out, the examiner must consider the psychiatric differential diagnosis for anorexia nervosa and its associated comorbid conditions. These conditions are major depressive disorder, schizophrenia, substance abuse (stimulants), OCD (multiple obsessions besides food), social phobia, body dysmorphic disorder, and bulimia nervosa. If the depression does not resolve with the correction of the malnutrition, the clinician should also consider the diagnosis of major depressive disorder. In addition, patients who try to control their caloric intake with pharmacologic agents are more likely to exhibit impulsive behavior (sexuality) and substance abuse (stimulants).

Anorexia nervosa is associated with both life-threatening psychological conditions (major depressive disorder, suicide) and medical conditions (electrolyte abnormalities, starvation). The lifelong rate of mortality secondary to anorexia nervosa in patients who require hospitalization is more than 10%. Some of the possible medical complications are osteoporosis (resulting from hypocalcemia with low serum estrogen levels), cardiomyopathy (resulting from ipecac abuse), anemia, sepsis (resulting from malnutrition-induced immunodeficiencies), arrhythmias (resulting from electrolyte abnormalities, prolonged corrected QT interval), and superior mesenteric artery syndrome. The superior mesenteric artery syndrome, which is characterized by postprandial vomiting and pain (mesenteric ischemia) secondary to intermittent gastric outlet obstruction, is more common in anorexic patients because of their emaciation.

The treatment of anorexia nervosa requires a multidisciplinary approach involving the primary care provider, a nutritionist, and a psychiatrist. Inpatient management may be necessary. The decision about where to admit the patient (medical versus psychiatric unit) is based on the medical stability of the patient and the patient's willingness to cooperate with a nutritionally sound refeeding program. For the medically stable but uncooperative patient, the patient should be admitted to the psychiatric unit, where the focus is behavioral, emphasizing slow weight restoration.

The nutritionist can assist in the management by developing a nutritionally sound diet that ensures a safe rate of weight gain. Too rapid a refeeding may result in steatorrhea.

The psychiatric treatment consists of behavior therapy to ensure compliance with the refeeding program as well as various forms of psychotherapies (individual, group, or family). The comorbid conditions that also may need to be addressed are depression (suicidal ideation), anxiety disorder (OCD, social phobia), body dysmorphic disorder, and substance use. Psychopharmacology is generally unsuccessful in treating anorexia nervosa unless the intent is to treat comorbidity (e.g., depression). Anorexia nervosa is a chronic condition that in many cases necessitates long-term psychosocial support and medical monitoring.

Bulimia Nervosa

This condition consists of binge eating and inappropriate means for maintaining weight (purging). According to the *DSM-IV,* the diagnostic criteria for bulimia nervosa are

1. lack of control in eating an excessive amount of food during a set period of time

2. inappropriate methods for controlling weight gain (purging)
3. binge eating and using inappropriate methods for controlling weight gain, occurring at least twice a week for 3 months
4. distorted perception of body shape
5. not meeting criteria for anorexia nervosa (weight not below 85% of age-appropriate ideal body weight)

Bulimia nervosa is twice as common as anorexia nervosa and has a later onset (late adolescence). Like anorexia nervosa, it is more common in girls (90%) and can occur in any socioeconomic background. Almost 90% of patients control their weight gain by purging. Other methods for controlling weight are excessive exercise and fasting before binge eating.

Comorbid psychological conditions are common in bulimia and include mood disorders (major depression, especially in those who purge), personality disorders, substance use, and anxiety disorders.

Approximately 30% of patients who use medications to control weight also have substance use disorders (alcohol, stimulants).

The comorbid medical conditions of bulimia nervosa are associated with vomiting or medication abuse. These conditions are esophagitis and gastritis, cardiomyopathy (from ipecac abuse), hypokalemia (from diuretic abuse), kidney stones (from diuretic abuse), metabolic alkalosis (from vomiting), metabolic acidosis (from laxative abuse), and increased amylase levels.

Some patients with diabetes mellitus develop a variant of bulimia nervosa. These patients may control their weight gain by reducing their intake of insulin.

Concealment of symptoms coupled with the lack of cachexia makes bulimia nervosa difficult to detect. Some patients may present to the clinician because of a parent's detection of binge eating and purging. Physical findings that suggest recurrent vomiting are dental erosion, parotid hypertrophy, callous abrasions on the dorsum of the hand (Russell sign), and pharyngeal irritation.

In contrast to anorexia nervosa, significant medical complications occur less commonly in bulimia nervosa. Most patients with bulimia nervosa can be treated in an outpatient setting. Treatment is orchestrated by a psychiatrist and is directed toward both the underlying condition and the comorbid conditions. Patients often respond to individual or group therapy. For other patients, antidepressant medications (e.g., sertraline, fluoxetine) may ameliorate some of the symptoms. For some patients, treatment may be very successful, with remission that persists for years. Unfortunately, for others, bulimia nervosa is a disorder of exacerbations, remissions, and chronic residual dysfunction that necessitates long-term management by a psychiatrist.

CHILD'S COMPLAINTS

One way in which the body responds to a psychological stressor is by the development of medical symptoms. Evidence that supports a stressor as a cause of the symptom is the potential gain from the symptom and the temporal relationship of the stressor and the symptom. For example, a child may develop chronic fatigue symptoms on the anniversary of his or her mother's death, or a patient's persistent abdominal pain from prior flare-ups of Crohn disease may prevent the patient from returning to school, despite medical evidence that the disease is in remission. These symptoms seem real to the child and cause a great deal of distress (see Fig. 35-6). Some of the extreme manifestations of these concerns or complaints are the anxiety disorders and the somatoform disorders.

The child's complaints may be further subdivided according to whether the child primarily suffers (is the victim) or gains (consciously or unconsciously) from the symptoms. Some patients in the victimized group may still receive secondary gain (more attention from parents). Patients with conditions that usually result in secondary gain may obtain relatively little gain in comparison with the suffering caused by the symptoms (see Fig. 35-6).

To address the psychological causes for the symptoms, the primary care provider must first rule out the possibility of any medical condition. Once that is accomplished, the child needs to be reassured of his or her health. The underlying psychological problem needs to be recognized and treated.

Primarily the Victim

Panic Disorder and Hypochondriasis

Panic disorder and hypochondriasis can manifest with medical symptoms (see Fig. 35-6). In panic disorder, the patient has recurrent and unexpected panic attacks that are not necessarily preceded by a recognizable stressor. The attacks are characterized by an autonomic discharge, resulting in flushing, sweating, palpitations, chest pain, hyperventilation, dizziness, paresthesias, and a fear of imminently dying. In hypochondriasis, the child either fears that he or she has a serious illness or focuses on minor discomforts with a worry that he or she may have a life-threatening illness. Hypochondriasis is often associated with other anxiety and depressive disorders; consequently, these young patients may appear sad, irritable, or fatigued. Treatment centers on an appropriate medical evaluation to reassure the patient, coupled with a referral to a mental health professional.

Body Dysmorphic Disorder

Almost all children and adolescents have some concern regarding their physical appearance that leads to some distress. These concerns may be focused on their complexion, their developing bodies, or the shape of their facial features. According to the *DSM-IV*, patients have body dysmorphic disorder when they are preoccupied with excessive concerns regarding their body's appearance; this preoccupation leads to significant social and academic dysfunction. Onset often occurs during adolescence. Patients with body dysmorphic disorder often seek medical treatment for their perceived disfigurement. Unfortunately, even a result that is cosmetically acceptable to someone else does not alleviate the patient's worry. Because of these concerns, the patient is at significant risk for major depressive disorder and suicide.

The differential diagnosis of body dysmorphic disorder includes normal concerns about appearance, eating disorders, delusional disorder, social phobia, major depressive disorder, and OCD (multiple obsessions besides body image). Because of the risk of major depression and suicide, patients with body dysmorphic disorder should be referred to a psychiatrist.

Primarily with Gain

Factitious Disorder

Factitious disorder consists of patients' inducing symptoms or signs to assume the sick role and receive care. There is no financial gain as is found with malingering. The onset of this disorder usually occurs in early adulthood; however, it can also occur in childhood. Patients are at risk for substance use disorders (using agents to induce symptoms) as well as for complications from associated diagnostic workups and unnecessary surgical procedures. When these individuals are older, they may induce symptoms in their own children (Munchausen syndrome by proxy). On confrontation, they may either change their symptoms or try to seek medical care elsewhere. Treatment for this chronic disorder is psychotherapy.

School Avoidance

School avoidance occurs when a child uses medical symptoms to avoid school unnecessarily. If these symptoms become severe enough (duration > 4 weeks, associated worries of separation, significant dysfunction), they may represent an early manifestation of separation anxiety disorder (see section on disruptive behaviors). The symptoms of school avoidance may involve any organ system but are usually abdominal pain, headaches, or both. These pains are worse in the morning (especially on Mondays). In more severe cases, the symptoms may develop on Sunday evenings. Anxiety about attending school and the pattern of gain are quickly apparent.

The cause of the anxiety may be a conflict with a teacher or classmates. In adolescents, the anxiety may be caused by a recurrent stressor, such as an embarrassing situation (e.g., gym class) or conflict with peers. Some factors that may contribute to the development of this disorder are fear of losing one's parents, reduction of fear when the patient stays at home, parental sharing of their emotional distress, recent family tragedy, and an increasing understanding of death (i.e., that it is universal, permanent, and unpredictable). Patients with school avoidance may also have an anxiety disorder (social phobia) or major depressive disorder. Establishing the differential diagnosis of school avoidance is often difficult and complex.

Treatment of simple school avoidance consists of correction of school-based fears (e.g., about a teacher or peers) by parental intervention with the school, reassurance, education of the parents regarding their inadvertent reinforcement of separation anxiety, and immediate return to school. The longer the absence, the harder it is for the child to return. To get the child back to school, the parent may have to either accompany the child to the classroom or institute a stepwise return to the classroom (e.g., beginning in the principal's office, then going to the library, and finally returning to the classroom). The child should be referred to a psychiatrist if there is an underlying psychiatric disorder (anxiety or depressive disorder); if a grade school–aged child does not return to school within approximately 1 week; or if a child in junior high/middle school does not return within a few days. If there is a significant anxiety or depressive component, the psychiatrist may prescribe a temporary course of benzodiazepines or SSRI antidepressants.

Conversion Disorders

According to the *DSM-IV*, the diagnostic criteria for conversion disorders are symptoms associated with voluntary motor or sensory function (not factitious symptoms or pain symptoms), preceded by a recent stressor, unexplained by a medical evaluation, and causing significant distress or prompting medical evaluation.

In children younger than 10 years, the typical presenting symptoms are either pseudoseizures or gait disturbances. Older individuals may present with such symptoms as paralysis of a limb, paresthesias, blindness, or aphonia. These symptoms are relatively easy to identify because they do not follow an anatomic nerve distribution, nor do the actions fit the symptoms (a "blind" person never bumping into anything). Pseudoseizures are more difficult to document and may require continuously videotaped electroencephalographic telemetry. The patient may react to the symptoms either with indifference (*la belle indifference*) or in a dramatic manner.

The prevalence of conversion disorder is 1 to 30 per 10,000 in the general population. The onset is usually in late adolescence to early adulthood. A typical episode is acute, follows a recent stressor, and is of relatively short duration (<4 weeks). The symptoms often appear to solve a psychological conflict (blindness prevents seeing something that should not be seen). Some common childhood stressors associated with conversion disorders are grief and incest.

Approximately 25% of the patients have a relapse within a year. Factors that are associated with a favorable prognosis are acute onset; identifiable stressor at time of onset; above-average intelligence; and symptoms of paralysis, aphonia, or blindness. Major depressive disorder and personality disorders are associated with conversion disorders.

Management is usually conducted by a mental health provider. Treatment consists of empathy, a face-saving explanation for the symptoms, explanation of the relationship of stressors to symptoms, reduction of stressors, reassurance that the symptoms will remit, introduction of techniques to reduce stress (relaxation imagery), and a stepwise rehabilitation program with physical therapy. Because of the high rate of comorbidity associated with this disease, patients need to be monitored for depressive symptoms and suicidal ideation. In some cases, patients benefit from dynamic psychotherapy; however, many adolescents with conversion disorders are not self-reflective as to the psychological basis of their symptoms and hence do not respond well to an exploratory psychotherapy.

Somatization Disorder

According to the *DSM-IV,* somatization disorder (Briquet syndrome) consists of a history of multiple physical complaints consisting of at least four pain symptoms, two gastrointestinal symptoms, one neurologic symptom, and one sexual symptom (impotency, menorrhagia). These multiple symptoms occur over years, are not produced factitiously or by a medical condition, begin before the age of 30 years, and cause significant dysfunction. Two milder manifestations of somatization disorder, which are more commonly seen in children, are undifferentiated somatoform disorder (one symptom > 6 months' duration) and somatoform disorder not otherwise specified (one symptom < 6 months' duration).

The prevalence of somatization disorder is 0.2% to 2% in girls and less than 0.2% in boys. Associated comorbid conditions are major depressive disorder, panic disorder, substance abuse, and personality disorders (borderline personality disorder and antisocial personality disorder). This is a chronic condition that rarely remits. The psychiatric differential diagnosis is extensive and includes mood disorders (major depression), schizophrenia with somatic delusions, panic disorders (symptoms occur only during an attack), generalized anxiety disorder, and factitious disorder.

Recognition is the major problem in the management of this condition. These patients are often referred to multiple medical subspecialists for reassurance purposes. If the underlying psychological problem is not addressed, reassurance is rarely successful. Proper management consists of an appropriate medical evaluation to rule out medical causes for the symptoms, recognition of this psychological disorder, and prompt referral to a mental health specialist.

Pain Disorder

Pain disorder is a somatoform disorder in which the patient has significant pain that leads to medical attention. According to the *DSM-IV,* this pain is related to stress and causes significant dysfunction. In addition, it is neither self-inflicted nor related solely to a medical condition. The symptoms may occur with or without a previous (but resolved) medical condition. Psychological factors and a medical condition, acting in concert, commonly play roles in the development of pain disorder.

The actual prevalence of pain disorder is unknown; however, it appears to be quite common. The comorbid conditions associated with pain disorders are substance abuse (to alleviate symptoms), mood disorders (usually with chronic pain), and anxiety disorders (usually with acute pain). Sometimes a parent or other relative has served as a "pain model" for the young person.

Two methods by which this syndrome may manifest are the "continuation" syndrome and the "let-down" syndrome. In the continuation syndrome, the symptoms from the medical disease persist even after the biologic abnormalities have completely resolved. The let-down syndrome occurs in highly successful and hard-working students who are under a lot of stress. These symptoms provide them with a legitimate excuse to escape the rigorous demands imposed by themselves or others. The patient's recognition of the conflict over ambition is important in the resolution of this condition.

Treatment of pain disorder consists of an appropriate medical evaluation and prompt referral to a mental health professional. The psychological treatment is similar to that for conversion disorder.

DELAYED DEVELOPMENT

Delayed development (see Chapter 32) is a broad category of illnesses that can cause specific or general delay. The causes of developmental delay encompass many conditions; in more than half the cases, a medical condition has caused the delay. These medical conditions include genetic disorders (5%); alterations of embryonic development (30%), perinatal or prenatal disorders (10%), and other medical illness of childhood (5%). Another 15% to 20% of cases are caused either by deprivation or by severe mental disorders (pervasive developmental disorders).

Specific developmental delays may be secondary to a medical condition such as cerebral palsy or to learning disorders (reading, mathematics, written expression disorders); to communication disorders (expressive and/or receptive); to developmental coordination disorder; or to psychiatric disorders (selective autism). This part of the chapter concentrates on the psychiatric causes of general and specific delay (Fig. 35-7).

PSYCHIATRIC CAUSES OF GENERAL DELAY

Pervasive Developmental Disorders

Pervasive developmental disorders cause severe impairment in social development, language development, and/or imaginative play. In addition, these disorders are often associated with severe to profound mental retardation (intelligence quotient < 50). The pervasive developmental disorders are

- autistic disorder
- Rett syndrome
- childhood disintegrative disorder
- Asperger syndrome

The diagnosis of pervasive developmental disorder not otherwise specified may be used if the patient does not fulfill the diagnostic criteria for the aforementioned disorders.

Autistic Disorder

According to the *DSM-IV,* the diagnosis of autism is made if the patient has six or more symptoms in the following three categories: social interaction (at least two symptoms), communication (at least one symptom), and repetitive, stereotypic behavior (at least one symptom). In addition, the symptoms need to occur before the patient is 3 years of age. The problems with social interactions are sparsity of nonverbal communication (body gestures), failure to develop peer relationships, lack of sharing or showing things to others, and lack of emotional reciprocity. In early infancy, parents may notice that these infants do not cuddle well. Affected infants fail to respond to voice to the point that the parent worries that the child is deaf. The language and symbolic impairments include a delay or a lack of any verbal communication, difficulties in sustaining a conversation, echolalia or nonsensical words, and lack of imaginative play.

The degree of language impairment and overall intelligence are two of the best predictors of prognosis. The stereotypic and repetitive behavior of these children includes intense preoccupation with an interest (mimicking an actor), inflexible adherence to routines (behavioral outbursts when the routines are not adhered to), repetitive motor movements (rocking), and preoccupation with parts of an object.

The prevalence of autistic disorder is 2 to 5 per 10,000; more than 75% of cases occur in boys. This disorder is biologically based

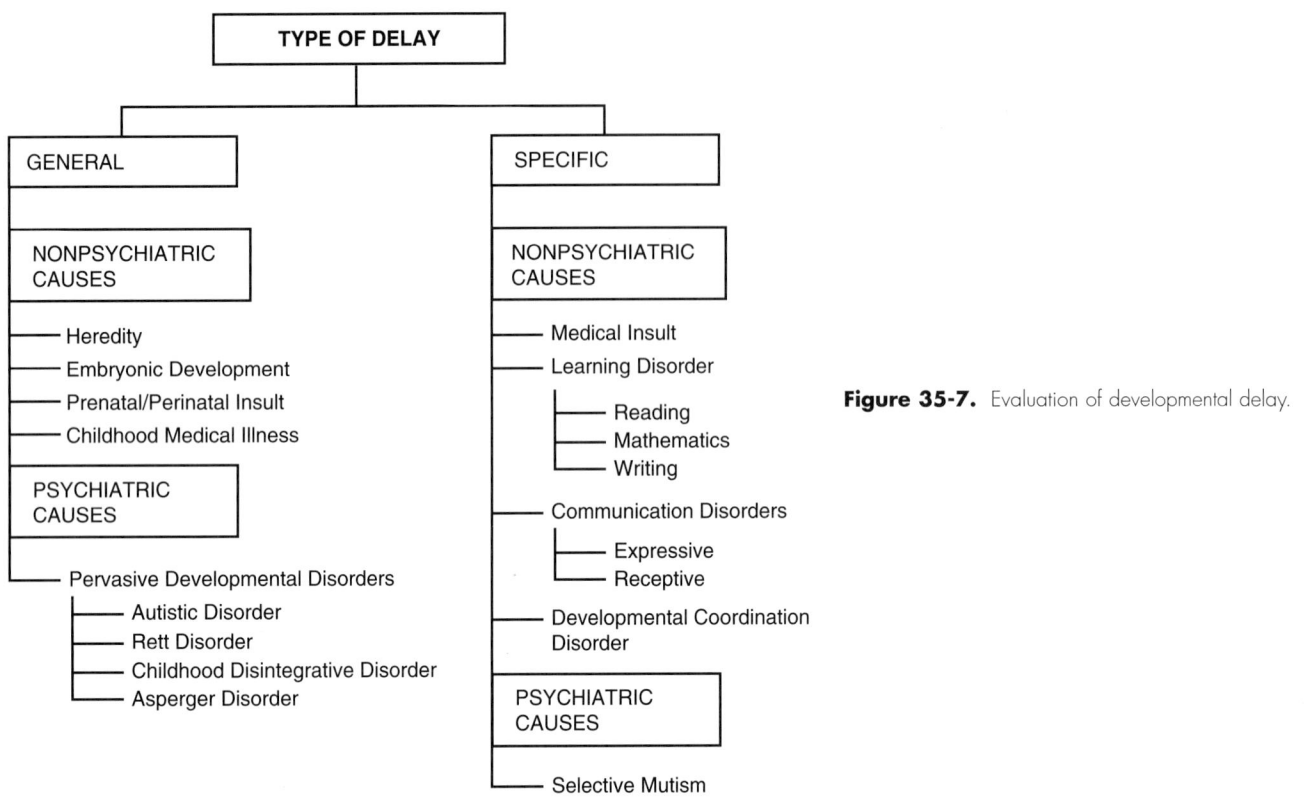

Figure 35-7. Evaluation of developmental delay.

because of the neurochemical and neuroanatomic abnormalities occurring in it, coupled with the increased risk of the disorder among siblings in affected families. Some of the medical conditions associated with autistic disorder are encephalitis, phenylketonuria, birth anoxia, and fragile X syndrome.

Children with autistic disorder may be hyperactive, impulsive, and aggressive and may engage in self-injurious activities. These children may also have unusual reactions to stimulation, such as an oversensitivity to touch or a high pain threshold. As these children become older, they may show some willingness to passively engage in social encounters. Older children may also have extraordinary long-term memory (e.g., for songs, baseball statistics) but use the information inappropriately. The comorbid conditions of autistic disorder are significant: 25% of affected patients have seizures, and 75% have moderate to profound mental retardation (intelligence quotient < 50). As adults, about 30% may have some degree of independent living. Because of the severity of the symptoms, depression is common in less cognitively impaired patients who have some insight into their condition.

The differential diagnosis of autistic disorder includes the other pervasive developmental disorders, communication disorders, schizophrenia, and mental retardation.

The cornerstone of treatment is to foster the patient's ability to communicate, to develop the patient's social skills, and to facilitate learning. These interventions are usually performed in special education settings. Pharmacologic interventions are sometimes used to address specific behavioral problems such as aggressiveness or sleep disruption. SSRIs are frequently prescribed to reduce the intensity of restrictive, repetitive behaviors and interests.

Rett Syndrome

Infants with Rett syndrome are normal until 5 months of age. Between 5 and 48 months of age, the toddler exhibits decelerated growth of the head circumference, loss of purposeful hand movements (hand wringing), poor gait or truncal movements, loss of social engagement, and severely impaired language development with psychomotor retardation. This condition is extremely rare and has been reported only in girls. The loss of skills is persistent and progressive, ending in severe and profound mental retardation. As the patients approach adolescence, there may be some improvement in social interests and developmental milestones. Seizure disorders frequently complicate this disorder, and many patients with Rett syndrome die prematurely.

Childhood Disintegrative Disorder

In this condition, the child is normal until at least 2 years of age. Between 2 and 10 years of age, the patient loses at least two of the following skills: language, social skills, motor skills, bowel or bladder control, and the ability to play. The child also has problems in two of the following areas: social interaction, communications, or repetitive behavior. Autistic disorder differs from childhood disintegrative disorder in that it occurs earlier (usually in infancy) and causes significant problems in all three areas. Childhood disintegrative disorder is a very rare condition.

The origin is unknown; however, occasionally, a disorder causing developmental regression (metachromatic leukodystrophy) may be associated with it. After the loss of skills, this condition plateaus, from which there may be a slight improvement. Childhood disintegrative disorder is also complicated by severe mental retardation and an increased frequency of seizure disorders.

Asperger Syndrome

The diagnostic features of Asperger syndrome consist of severe impairment in social interactions coupled with restrictive, repetitive behaviors. According to the *DSM-IV,* the diagnostic criteria for Asperger syndrome consist of at least two impairments of social interactions (poor nonverbal communication, failure to develop peer relationships, lack of sharing, lack of emotional reciprocity) coupled with one or more repetitive, stereotypic patterns of behavior (repetitious motor movements, preoccupation with parts, inflexible adherence to rituals, intense preoccupation with a topic). Asperger syndrome differs from autistic disorder in that there are no impairments in cognitive function, including language. In addition, patients with Asperger disorder are curious about the environment and develop appropriate self-help and adaptive (other than social) behaviors. Asperger syndrome and autistic disorder are almost certainly closely related, differing primarily in severity, with autism at the more severe end of the spectrum and Asperger syndrome at the milder end (although the social relatedness impairment remains significant).

The prevalence of Asperger syndrome is unknown. Affected preschool-aged children may have motor delay and clumsiness. As the patient gets older, difficulties with social interactions and empathy arise. The duration of this disorder is probably lifelong.

PSYCHIATRIC CAUSES OF SPECIFIC DELAY

Selective Mutism

The patient with selective mutism has a persistent failure to speak in certain situations (for instance, the classroom), even though the individual can speak in other situations (at home). These symptoms last for at least 1 month (but not limited to the first month of school). In addition, the symptoms are not caused by embarrassment from a speech problem (stuttering) or unfamiliarity with a language. Affected children are excessively shy and withdrawn and fear social embarrassment, whereas at home they may be controlling, seeking proximity to the parents, or completely normal.

The differential diagnosis includes communication disorders (not restricted to certain situations), pervasive developmental disorders (absence of language is in all settings), and social phobia. Patients with social phobia may present with selective mutism. Although patients with selective mutism do exhibit a specific and persistent delay in speaking in social, extrafamilial situations, many experts now consider selective mutism to be a childhood variant of social phobia, an anxiety disorder. Behavior therapy applied both at home and at school appears to be the most effective intervention. There is some suggestion that the addition of an SSRI (fluoxetine, sertralin, ritalopram) may augment the impact of behavioral interventions.

SUMMARY AND RED FLAGS

Unusual behaviors are common in children. The primary physician is charged with recognizing and treating the most common of these and with recognizing and referring those that are serious or unusual (see Table 35-1). Suicide is the third leading cause of death in adolescents. When thoughts of suicide have escalated to threats or attempts, the patient's life is in danger (see Fig. 35-1). Delirium and psychoses may be either an acute manifestation of a new illness or a recurrent episode in a chronic disorder (see Tables 35-6 and 35-7). Many psychiatric illnesses have comorbid psychiatric and medical conditions necessitating a diligent and collaborative approach to management (see Figs. 35-2 to 35-4). Red flags include risk-taking behavior, violence, poor school performance, poor attention to personal appearance and hygiene, deteriorating social interaction, suicide attempts without remorse, reduced appetite, weight loss, reduced or excessive sleeping, and hallucinations.

REFERENCES

General References

American Psychiatric Association: Diagnostic and Statistical Manual of Mental Disorders, 4th ed. Washington, DC: American Psychiatric Association, 1994.

Dulcan MK, Martini DR: Concise Guide to Child and Adolescent Psychiatry 2. Washington, DC: American Psychiatric Press, 1999.

Klykylo WM, Kay J, Rube D: Clinical Child Psychiatry. Philadelphia, WB Saunders, 1998.

Werry JS, Aman MG: Practitioner's Guide to Psychiatric Drugs for Children and Adolescents. New York: Plenum Press, 1999.

Suicide

Brent DA: Risk factors for adolescent suicide and suicidal behavior: Mental and substance abuse disorders, family environmental factors, and life stress. Suicide Life Threat Behav 1995;25:52-63.

De Wilde EJ, Kienhorst I, Diekster R, et al: The specificity of psychological characteristics of adolescent suicide attempters. J Am Acad Child Adolesc Psychiatry 1993;32:51-59.

Hergenroeder AC, Kastner L, Farrow J, et al: The pediatrician's role in adolescent suicide. Pediatr Ann 1986;15:787-798.

Pfeffer CR, Klerman G, Hurt S, et al: Suicidal children grow up: Rates and psychological risks of suicide attempts during follow-up. J Am Acad Child Adolesc Psychiatry 1993;32:106-113.

Pilowsky DJ, Wu Li-Tzy, Anthony JC: Panic attacks and suicide attempts in mid-adolescence. Am J Psychiatry 1999;156:1545-1549.

Chronic Disruptive Behaviors

American Academy of Pediatrics, Committee on Substance Abuse: Role of the pediatrician in prevention and management of substance abuse. Pediatrics 1993;91:1010-1013.

Burd L, Kerbeshian PJ, Barth A, et al: Long-term follow-up of an epidemiologically defined cohort of patients with Tourette syndrome. J Child Neurol 2001;16:421-437.

Cantwell DP: Attention deficit disorder: A review of the past 10 years. J Am Acad Child Adolesc Psychiatry 1996;35:978-987.

Garfinkel BD, Amrami KK: Assessment and differential diagnosis of attention deficit hyperactivity disorder. Child Adolesc Psychiatr Clin North Am 1992;1:311-324.

Herrerias CT, Perrin JM, Stein MT: The child with ADHD: Using the AAP clinical practice guidelines. Am Fam Physician 2001;63:1803-1810.

Kazdin AE, Bass D, Siegel T, et al: Cognitive-behavioral therapy and relationship therapy in the treatment of children referred for antisocial behavior. J Consult Clin Psychol 1989;57:522-535.

Leckman JF, Hardin MT, Riddle MA, et al: Clonidine treatment of Gilles de la Tourette's syndrome. Arch Gen Psychiatry 1991;48:324-328.

Leonard HL (ed): New research on atomoxetine for ADHA. Brown University Child and Adolescent Psychopharmacology Update 2003;5:1,5,6.

Loeber R, Burke JD, Lahey BB, et al: Oppositional defiant and conduct disorder: A review of the past 10 years, part I. J Am Acad Child Adolesc Psychiatry 2000;39:1468-1484.

Mannuzza S, Klein RG, Bessler A, et al: Adult outcome of hyperactive boys: Educational achievement, occupational rank, and psychiatric status. Arch Gen Psychiatry 1993;50:565-576.

Mayfield D, McLeod G, Hall P: The CAGE questionnaire: Validation of a new alcoholism screening instrument. Am J Psychiatry 1974;131: 1121-1123.

Moffitt TE: Adolescent-limited and life course persistent antisocial behavior: A developmental taxonomy. Psychol Rev 1993;100:674-701.

The MTA Cooperative Group: A 14-month randomized clinical trial of treatment strategies for attention deficit/hyperactivity disorder. Arch Gen Psychiatry 1999;56:1073-1086.

Smith HE, Margolis RD: Adolescent inpatient and outpatient chemical dependence treatment: An overview. Psychiatr Ann 1991;21:105-108.

Stokes A, Bawden HN, Camfield PR, et al: Peer problems in Tourette's disorder. Pediatrics 1991;87:936-942.

Episodic Disruptive Behaviors

Acute reactions to drugs of abuse. Med Lett 2002;44:21-24.

Arnold DH: The central serotonin syndrome: Paradigm for psychotherapeutic misadventure. Pediatr Rev 2002;23:427-432.

Bernstein GA, Borchardt CM, Perwin AR: Anxiety disorders of childhood and adolescence: A review of the past 10 years. J Am Acad Child Adolesc Psychiatry 1996;35:1110-1119.

Birmaher B, Ryan ND, Williamson DE, et al: Childhood and adolescent depression: A review of the past 10 years, part I. J Am Acad Child Adolesc Psychiatry 1996;35:1427-1439.

Birmaher B, Ryan ND, Williamson DE, et al: Childhood and adolescent depression: A review of the past 10 years, part II. J Am Acad Child Adolesc Psychiatry 1996;35:1575-1583.

Famularo R, Fenton T, Kinscherff R: Child maltreatment and the development of post traumatic stress disorder. Am J Dis Child 1993;147:755-760.

Geller B, Luby J: Child and adolescent bipolar disorder: A review of the past 10 years. J Am Acad Child Adolesc Psychiatry 1997;36:1168-1176.

March JS, Leonard HI: Obsessive-compulsive disorder in children and adolescents: A review of the past 10 years. J Am Acad Child Adolesc Psychiatry 1996;35:1265-1273.

Marenco S, Weinberger DR: The neurodevelopmental hypothesis of schizophrenia: Following a trail of evidence from cradle to grave. Dev Psychopathol 2000;12:501-527.

Moreau D, Weissman MM: Panic disorder in children and adolescents: A review. Am J Psychiatry 1992;149:1306-1314.

Murphy ML, Pichichero ME: Prospective identification and treatment of children with pediatric autoimmune neuropsychiatric disorder associated with group A streptococcal infection (PANDAS). Arch Pediatr Adolesc Med 2002;156:356-361.

Petti TA, Vela RM: Borderline disorders of childhood: An overview. J Am Acad Child Adolesc Psychiatry 1990;29:327-337.

Pfefferbaum B: Posttraumatic stress disorder in children: A review of the past 10 years. J Am Acad Child Adolesc Psychiatry 1997;36:1503-1511.

Snider LA, Seligman LD, Ketchen BR, et al: Tics and problem behaviors in schoolchildren: Prevalence, characterization and associations. Pediatrics 2002;110:331-336.

Volkmar FR: Childhood and adolescent psychosis: A review of the past 10 years. J Am Acad Child Adolesc Psychiatry 1996;35:843-851.

Wagner KD: Generalized anxiety disorder in children and adolescents. Psychiatr Clin North Am 2001;24:139-153.

Weller EB, Weller RA, Svadjian H: Mood disorders. In Lewis M (ed): Child and Adolescent Psychiatry: A Comprehensive Textbook, 2nd ed. Baltimore: Williams & Wilkins, 1996, pp 650-665.

Hallucinations

Nagera H: The imaginary companion. Psychoanal Study Child 1969;24:165-196.

Schreier HA, Libow JA: Acute phobic hallucinations in very young children. J Am Acad Child Adolesc Psychiatry 1986;25:574-578.

Unexplained Physical Complaints

American Psychiatric Association: Practice guidelines for eating disorders. Am J Psychiatry 1993;150:207-228.

Benjamin PY: Psychological problems following recovery from acute life-threatening illness. Am J Orthopsychiatry 1978;48:284-290.

Eminson DM, Postlewaite RJ: Factitious illness: Recognition and management. Arch Dis Child 1992;67:1510-1516.

Fluoxetine Bulimia Nervosa Collaborative Study Group: Fluoxetine in the treatment of bulimia nervosa: A multicenter, placebo controlled, double-blind trial. Arch Gen Psychiatry 1992;43:139-147.

Fritz GK, Fritsch S, Hagino O: Somatoform disorders in children and adolescents: A review of the past 10 years. J Am Acad Child Adolesc Psychiatry 1997;36:1329-1338.

Hill K, Maloney M: Anorexia nervosa and bulimia. In Klykylo WM, Kay J, Tube D (eds): Clinical Child Psychiatry. Philadelphia: WB Saunders, 1998, pp 279-288.

Lehmkuhl G, Blahz B, Lehmkuhl U, et al: Conversion disorder (DSM-III-R 300-1), symptomatology and course in childhood and adolescence. Eur Arch Psychiatry Neurol Sci 1989;238:155-160.

Levy JC: Vulnerable children: Parents' perspectives and the use of medical care. Pediatrics 1980;65:956-963.

Maisami M, Freeman JM: Conversion reaction in children as body language: A combined child psychology/neurology team approach to the management of functional neurological disorder in children. Pediatrics 1987;80:46-52.

Meadows R: Management of Munchausen's syndrome by proxy. Arch Dis Child 1985;60:385-393.

Rosenberg D: Web of deceit: A literature review of Munchausen's syndrome by proxy. Child Abuse Negl 1987;2:547-563.

Turgay A: Treatment outcome for children and adolescents with conversion disorder. Can J Psychiatry 1990;35:585-587.

Wachsmuth JR, Garfinkel PE: The treatment of anorexia nervosa in young adolescents. Child Adolesc Psychiatr Clin North Am 1993;2:145-160.

Wentz E, Gillberg I, Gillberg C, et al: Ten-year follow up of adolescent onset anorexia nervosa: Physical health and neurodevelopment. Dev Med Child Neurol 2000;42:328-333.

Delayed Development

Cook EH, Rowlett R, Jaselskis C, et al: Fluoxetine treatment of children and adolescents with autistic disorder and mental retardation. J Am Acad Child Adolesc Psychiatry 1992;31:739-745.

Klin A, Volkmar FR: The pervasive developmental disorders: Nosology and profiles of development. In Luthar SS, Burack JA, Cichetti D, Weisz JR (eds): Developmental Psychopathology: Perspectives on Adjustment, Risk and Disorder. New York: Cambridge University Press, 1997, pp 208-226.

Tanguay PE: Pervasive developmental disorders: A 10-year review. J Am Acad Child Adolesc Psychiatry 2000;39:1079-1095.

Volkmar FR: Childhood disintegrative disorder: Issues for DSM-IV. J Autism Dev Disord 1992;22:625-642.

Volkmar FR, Nelson DS: Seizure disorder in autism. J Am Acad Child Adolesc Psychiatry 1990;29:127-129.

36 Child Abuse

Robert M. Reece

DEFINITIONS

Local statutes define for local jurisdictions what should legally be considered child abuse. Public Law 93-247, the Child Abuse Prevention and Treatment Act of 1974, defines child abuse as "the physical or mental injury, sexual abuse, negligent treatment, or maltreatment of a child under the age of 18 years by a person who is responsible for the child's welfare under circumstances which indicate the child's health or welfare is harmed or threatened thereby."

Kempe (1978) succinctly defined child physical abuse as "non-accidental physical injuries as a result of acts or omissions on the part of the child's parents or guardians." Child care lapses in environmental control, repetitive accidental poisonings, and failure to provide food, shelter, clothing, medical care, emotional support, or education should all be included as manifestations of maltreatment.

Definitions of child sexual abuse depend on the context because there are legal, psychosocial, medical, and cultural situations within which it can be defined. Definitions are often omitted from descriptions of child sexual abuse, with the manifestations of the abuse serving to illustrate the phenomenon, thereby avoiding the task of drawing a line between abuse and other events. It is often left to observers, who must claim that they "know it when they see it." However, definitions do exist, and several are presented here to allow some delineation of this epidemic.

The National Center on Child Abuse and Neglect of the U.S. Department of Health and Human Services defines child sexual abuse as "contacts or interactions between a child and an adult for the sexual stimulation of the perpetrator or another person or [as] sexual contacts or interactions between a child and a significantly older child who has power or control over the [younger] child."

The definition of child sexual abuse proposed by Kempe (1978) is "the involvement of children and adolescents in sexual activities they do not understand, to which they cannot give informed consent or that violate social taboos."

Legal definitions describe "sexual activity" as being divided into two categories: (1) sexual conduct, or intercourse, and (2) sexual contact, or the touching of the erogenous zones of another person for the purpose of sexually arousing or gratifying either person. Local jurisdictions then define levels of severity attached to the sexual activities described, taking into account the act itself, the age of the victim, and his or her capacity to object or defend against the act.

PREVALENCE

In 1999, on the basis of data contained in "Child Maltreatment 1999: Reports from the States to the National Child Abuse and Neglect Data System," the Department of Health and Human Services estimated that there were 2,974,00 referrals of possible maltreatment and, after investigation, 826,000 cases of substantiated child maltreatment. This is a prevalence of 11.8 per 1000 children. The distribution of the forms of maltreatment was as follows: neglect,

58.4%; physical abuse, 21.3%; sexual abuse, 11.3%; and miscellaneous forms making up the balance. These figures represent a decline of 19.2% from 1993. However, not all states report these statistics, and the various states have widely variable procedures for screening in reports, investigating reports and substantiating cases. The figures from 1993 and 1999 were collected by different methods. Until uniform data collection systems are in place, the trends that are reported must be viewed with some skepticism.

SEXUAL ABUSE

DIAGNOSTIC STRATEGIES

A child who has been sexually abused may come to the attention of a physician by having told someone of the abuse or by exhibiting behavioral or physical signs and symptoms.

Historical information may be derived from several sources:

1. Witnessed events: The observation of sexual activity by an adult with a child may be seen by another child or adult. The details of this witnessed event should be clear as to time, the nature of the activity observed, and the positive identification of the individuals involved.
2. Admission by the perpetrator.
3. Disclosure by the victimized child: This disclosure may be proximate in time to the event or events, but it is often delayed, sometimes for months or even years after the last episode. It may be disclosed to an adult caretaker, a trusted friend, or an authority figure (police, child protection worker, teacher, physician, therapist, or other health care provider).
4. Previous medical encounters: In some cases, previous medical examinations will have been performed, and this information can provide important data.

Medical History

A complete medical history, including the prenatal history, obstetric and perinatal events, childhood illnesses and hospitalizations, surgical procedures, and other contact with medical professionals, should be detailed. A careful review of systems may reveal symptoms referable to the current complaint. This exercise helps to avoid the pitfalls of misattribution of medical conditions to sexual abuse, and it also demonstrates good medical diagnostic work if the case comes to trial, in which the strength of the legal case may rest on the medical evidence.

Family and Social History

It is the province of the examining physician to gather pertinent family and social history. This should include a description of the social and economic milieu. The marital status of the caretaking parent, the identity of the other members of the household, and the status of adult partners and friends who are occasional members of

611

the household should be learned in order to understand the ecology of the allegation. Inquiries into a history of abuse in the childhood of the adult caretaker or current domestic violence should be made. Is there exposure to high risks of violence, drugs or alcohol, nutritional problems, or diseases? Are there psychiatric disorders apparent in the caretaker or in those with him or her at the time of the visit? Is there a history of emotional disorder in the caretaker or the child? Has there been previous involvement with law enforcement or social service agencies?

The occurrence of allegations of sexual abuse within the context of divorce or custody disputes has brought this situation to the forefront in the public mind. Examination of peer-reviewed literature indicates a very low incidence of sexual abuse in all divorce and custody cases (2%) and a higher incidence of proven "malicious" false allegations (5% to 14%). Nonetheless, all allegations of sexual abuse must be taken seriously and warrant thorough investigations. The emotional landscape of divorce is such that there may also be an increased incidence of all types of abuse perpetrated against the children trapped in these struggles.

Behavioral Signs and Symptoms

Nonspecific signs and symptoms can occur in a child reacting to a wide range of stresses and conflicts (enuresis, encopresis, disturbed sleep or eating patterns, changes in school performance, mood swings, or just depression, irritability, temper outbursts). These can be present in sexually abused children but are not diagnostic for sexual abuse. Specific symptoms or signs of sexual abuse are the byproduct of inappropriate sexual exposure and are associated with sexual function in some way. Thus, unexpected knowledge in young children about sexual matters, unusual curiosity about sexual or excretory functions, asking others to engage in sexual acts, acting out sexually with toys or other children, or abnormal masturbatory activities are examples of behavioral symptoms suggestive of sexual abuse. Research has cast some doubt on the specificity of sexualized behaviors, and these behaviors must therefore be put into the context of the total information about each case.

Physical Signs and Symptoms

There are also specific and nonspecific physical manifestations and important legitimate reasons for certain presenting complaints that must be taken into account when a child is evaluated for possible sexual abuse. A child may have an innocent injury to private parts through play (straddle injury, penetrating injury); may have dysuria, abdominal pain, proctitis, vaginitis, or vulvitis from nonsexually acquired infections (streptococcal cellulitis, intravaginal foreign body); or may have a nonsexual dermatologic problem (lichen sclerosus et atrophicus, severe contact dermatitis secondary to poor hygiene, seborrheic dermatitis). The 4-year-old who has a foul-smelling vaginal discharge not caused by a foreign body, has vaginal bleeding, or demonstrates decreased anal tone with accompanying fecal soiling, however, has physical signs that suggest sexual abuse until careful evaluation proves otherwise.

The Medical Interview

Because of the nature of the information involved, the medical interview in a possible sexual abuse case may intimidate otherwise self-assured pediatricians. The examiner must derive information from the child about what may be confusing, painful, and frightening to him or her that may be perceived by the child in a completely different way than by adults. The objectives of the interview are to determine

- the elements of the abuse
- who was involved
- when and how often it occurred
- where it occurred

The initial goal is to make the child comfortable and unafraid. The child and the adult bringing the child for the session should be informed of what will happen during the visit. It is often helpful to address children's universal fear of pain by assuring them that they are not going to have "shots" or any painful procedure during the course of the examination. In girls, the caregiver should be told that the examination does not involve the type of gynecologic examination used for adults and that nothing is to be inserted into the child's vagina. The child can be reassured that the trusted adult with whom he or she came can be present during the examination. The caregiver should be interviewed separately from the child, and the interview with the child should be conducted after rapport has been established with him or her.

The first step in interviewing the child is to explain in simple terms that the examiner is a "kid's doctor" and that at first the examiner just wants to get to know the child. This can be done by "making friends" with the child in the form of "getting to know you" questions about his or her friends, pets, neighborhood, school, or interests (sports, television, music, or hobbies). Allowing the child to select a beverage or a treat before the interview can enhance this process. In some clinics, younger children are presented with a choice of small stuffed animals to take home with them, and the animal is used for demonstration of the elements of the examination. The stuffed animal can be used to familiarize the child with the colposcope, allowing the child to look at the toy through the colposcope and then to take a picture of the animal with the flash attachment. This engages the child with the instrument and serves to demystify the process.

The interview must not involve leading questions, must be open-ended, and must include various forms of projective techniques for eliciting information. Projective techniques can include drawing, playing with toys in the room, and using dollhouses and dolls. The use of anatomically detailed dolls is controversial. Many sexual abuse evaluation centers have turned to other means of conducting these interviews.

The interviewer should be supportive, unrushed, and friendly, and the interview should be conducted in a child-friendly environment. If more than one session is required, the same interviewer should conduct all sessions.

Eliciting information should start with general questions and proceed to more specific ones. Using an approach suggesting ignorance or puzzlement on the part of the examiner instills self-confidence in the child, and it allows the examiner to ask clarifying questions in the form of "I don't really understand what you said about..." or "I'm not really sure about one thing that you told me." Establishing the routines in the child's family environment can be a transition from the general discussion about the world outside of the home to the world within the home. It also allows a subtle transition to the more private areas of the child's life:

Where do you sleep?
Who puts you to bed?
Who helps you with your bath?

Once rapport has been established, greater focus can be brought to the issues of possible sexual abuse. The child may be asked whether he or she knows the reason for this visit and whether he or she could help make the examiner understand what might have happened. This can be augmented by a discussion of "good touch, bad touch" or by asking the child to identify body parts on a picture. The language used by the interviewer influences the success of eliciting accurate information. The interviewer should use developmentally sensitive language that includes short, single-clause questions; the active voice; the clear use of names over pronouns; single negatives; short, understandable words; simple verbs; and direct statements. The child should be praised for the effort in the interview but not for the content. The use of phrases such as "some children have told me that..." or indicating in some other way that this discussion does not necessarily relate to the child but to other people is of use by giving the topic at hand an impersonal, abstract cast.

These techniques may elicit the exposition of the events in graphic and lengthy detail or may cause shutdown. The posing of the questions that turn from nonthreatening to threatening requires a sense of timing that experienced interviewers acquire and use intuitively. Most children, if comfortable, will disclose a clear and credible description of their experience.

The Credibility of Children's Histories of Sexual Abuse

From medical, psychosocial, and legal perspectives, it is necessary to evaluate the credibility of a child's recounting of what happened to him or her if sexual abuse is a consideration. Because children are often eager to please and wish to provide the "right" answer, it is important that the examiner use clearly worded questions that encourage children to provide answers that will be viewed nonjudgmentally. The interviewer should not suggest correct answers or scenarios, because children are prone to suggestibility.

The issue of lying in childhood has been studied and may be classified according to the reasons for lying. Reasons for lying include avoidance of punishment; getting something that the child could not get otherwise; protection of friends from trouble; self-protection; winning the admiration or interest of others; avoidance of embarrassment; maintenance of privacy; and demonstration of the child's power over an authority. Children do not lie to get into trouble, and the disclosure of sexual abuse, especially because the perpetrator has often intimidated or threatened the child not to tell about "their secret," puts the child at distinct risk. Consequently, when a child discloses sexual abuse to someone who has gained his or her trust, it usually represents the child's desire to escape from further harm and should be accepted as a truthful representation of the events described. In rare instances, however, a child can be programmed to tell a lie about sexual abuse by an unscrupulous caretaker whose motive is other than the child's best interests. Skilled interviewers are able to detect such prevarication, and careful questioning leads to the exposure of this attempted deception.

The issue of children's competency in testifying to the events around a sexual abuse allegation becomes a legal question; persons performing the medical evaluation are responsible for gathering information in the most objective manner, using the best techniques available, and for delivering this information clearly and without bias at the time of legal proceedings. Disclosure information obtained during the conduct of a medical examination is admissible in court according to the "hearsay exception" rule.

The Physical Examination

Usually, permission for the performance of an evaluation for sexual abuse should be obtained from the legal guardian. If the legal guardian is suspected of being the perpetrator, is shielding the perpetrator, or is for some other reason obstructing the evaluation of the child, some legal consultants believe the authority to perform necessary evaluations is covered under the child abuse reporting statutes. It is advisable in questionable cases to obtain legal advice before proceeding.

The site of the examination and the time of the alleged event or events determine, to some extent, the approach to the physical examination. If the alleged sexual abuse is thought to have occurred within the past 72 hours and to have involved contact with the perpetrator's genitalia, the collection of forensic evidence should be considered as an adjunct to the examination (see Chapter 29). If more than 72 hours have elapsed since the alleged contact and the child is being seen in an emergency setting or where the examiners are inexperienced in conducting such evaluations, the child should be examined with attention given to treatable acute injury (bleeding, tissue damage necessitating surgical care) or to signs or symptoms of infection necessitating culture analysis and treatment. If these services are not present and the child is otherwise healthy and is in

no danger of being reexposed to the perpetrator, the child can be examined at a scheduled appointment by professionals familiar with sexual abuse evaluations. This approach avoids needless duplication of interviewing and examinations.

The goals of the physical examination are as follows:

1. "Primum non nocere": "First, do no harm."
2. Diagnose and treat, when necessary, injured tissue.
3. Diagnose and treat sexually transmitted diseases (STDs).
4. Diagnose and make decisions regarding pregnancies for patients in the childbearing years.
5. Thoroughly examine and document medical forensic evidence when indicated.
6. Make decisions about disposition and further diagnosis or therapy.
7. Document the findings with a consideration of both medical and legal aspects.

The elements of the physical examination should be explained again to the caregiver and to the child after the medical interview. This explanation can be made to the child in the presence of the caregiver so that reassurances can be made to the caregiver and interpretation by the caregiver to the child can enhance the compliance of the child. If photographic colposcopy is to be done, it should be explained to both the child and the caregiver that only numbers identify any pictures taken and that no one will be able to recognize who is in the pictures. The absence of painful procedures during the examination should be stressed, and the child should be assured that he or she has control over the procedure. Children should be told that the examiner is going to listen to their heart and lungs; look at their eyes, nose, and ears; check to see whether they have any lumps in their tummies; and look at their knees, toes, and "bottom" to "make sure they are OK." The examiner can also state that "if anytime during the examination you want me to stop, just tell me, and I'll stop, and we'll talk about what I'm doing."

It is important to tell children that this kind of examination should be done only by a doctor or nurse when their mother (or other trusted caregiver) is present. They should be told that no one else is allowed to perform this kind of examination. The child should be encouraged to ask questions about the examination before it is begun and anytime during the examination. Offering to let the child listen to his or her heart with the stethoscope is also helpful in establishing trust. If a colposcope is to be used, allowing children to look through the lens and to photograph a toy gains their interest in the instrument. Some colposcopes have been equipped with a long cable so that the child can actually trip the shutter when photographs are to be taken, and this focuses the child's attention on this activity.

A general physical examination should then proceed, with note of any medical findings relevant to the sexual abuse issue and to general medical conditions. During the examination, the child can be told what the examiner has seen or heard and what will be done next. Carrying on a conversation with children about subjects of interest to them builds rapport and makes the next phase of the examination easier.

Under no circumstances should the child be forced to undergo any part of the examination. If the child is unable to cooperate after several attempts, the examination can be rescheduled. If two attempts at an examination have failed, an examination with the child under anesthesia may be scheduled.

Equipment

The success of an anogenital examination depends on the availability of necessary equipment. Although the colposcope is increasingly used in these evaluations and has been successful in augmenting knowledge about normal and abnormal anogenital findings, its use is not mandatory. It is necessary, however, to have adequate examination tables, optimal lighting, some form of magnification (hand lens or otoscope), and a child-friendly environment for the examination.

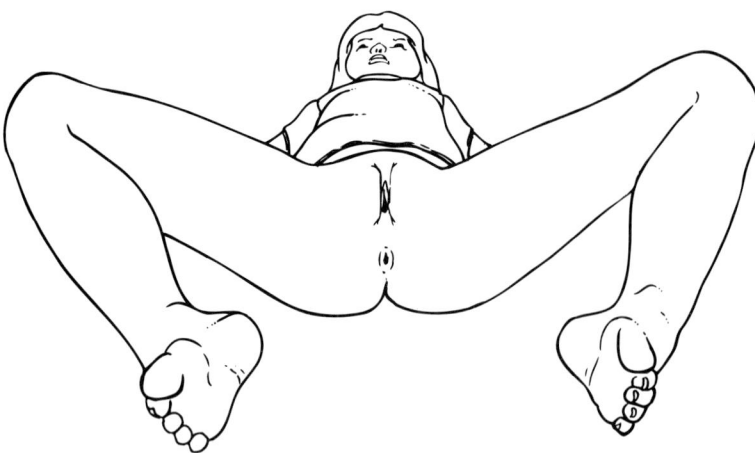

Figure 36-1. Supine frog-leg position for genital examination. (From Giardino AP, Finkel MA, Giardino ER, et al: A Practical Guide to the Evaluation of Sexual Abuse in the Prepubertal Child. Newbury Park, Calif, Sage Publications, 1992, p 69.)

It is also desirable to be able to provide the child with toys or distracting objects. In addition, the requisite laboratory materials for the collection, transport, culturing, and confirmation of specimens involved in diagnosing STDs; a microscope and wet mount materials; and experienced medical assistants with knowledge of the need to preserve the chain of evidence are essential. When forensic evidence is needed, a sex crimes kit is necessary, along with expertise in collecting and delivering such evidence so that the legal chain of evidence is maintained.

Positions for Examination

Most specialists in sexual abuse have children assume the supine frog-leg and the knee-chest positions, either alone or in combination, during examination. The frog-leg position is arguably more comfortable for the prepubertal child and more frequently employed (Fig. 36-1). The child can assume this position on a flat table surface with or without stirrups. As the child approaches adolescence, the use of stirrups makes the examination more acceptable because the adductor muscles of the thigh may be less pliant. The knee-chest position is less natural and comfortable; it is less stable when the examiner tries to focus for colposcopic photography (Fig. 36-2). However, some investigators maintain that without employing both positions, the posterior rim of the hymen may be incompletely evaluated.

In both the frog-leg and the knee-chest positions, separation and traction of the labia are necessary to visualize the introitus and the edges of the hymenal membrane. Simple lateral movement by the thumbs and forefingers of the examiner can accomplish this (Fig. 36-3). The labia majora should be drawn downward and outward (traction) (Fig. 36-4). Various movements during this traction enable the floor of the perineum to open, allowing good visualization. Examination of the anus can be done with the child in these same positions or in the left lateral decubitus position (Fig. 36-5).

The appearance of the normal anatomy of a prepubertal girl is shown in Figure 36-6. An example of penetrating sexual abuse is noted in Figure 36-7.

Types of Sexual Abuse

Sexual abuse occurs by way of a variety of sexual contacts. Fondling (passing the whole hand over the buttocks or genitalia) usually produces no physical findings, but when it progresses to digital contact and ultimately penetration, the resulting trauma can range from erythema to abrasion or laceration of the vaginal walls, depending on the amount of force, the penetrating object (finger,

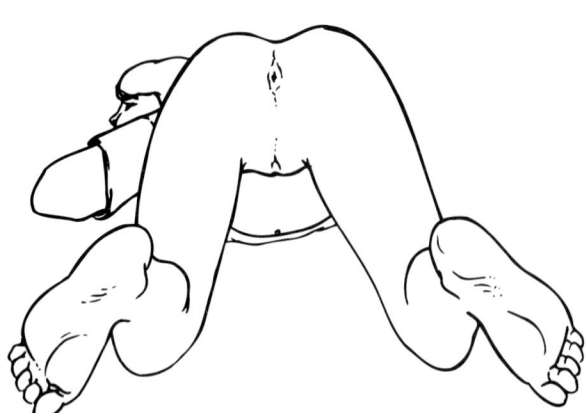

Figure 36-2. Knee-chest position for genital examination of the prepubertal child, to supplement examination in the supine frog-leg position. (From Giardino AP, Finkel MA, Giardino ER, et al: A Practical Guide to the Evaluation of Sexual Abuse in the Prepubertal Child. Newbury Park, Calif, Sage Publications, 1992, p 71.)

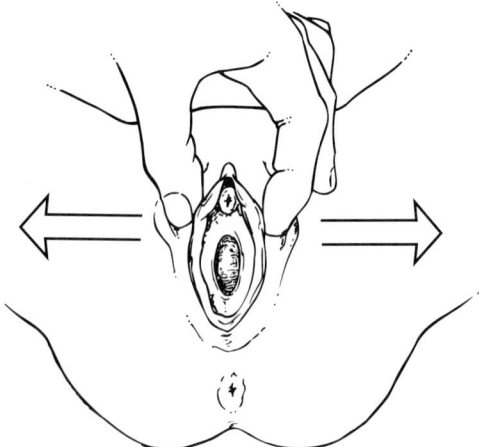

Figure 36-3. Examination of female external genitalia by simple lateral movement by the thumbs and forefingers of the examiner. (From Giardino AP, Finkel MA, Giardino ER, et al: A Practical Guide to the Evaluation of Sexual Abuse in the Prepubertal Child. Newbury Park, Calif, Sage Publications, 1992, p 73.)

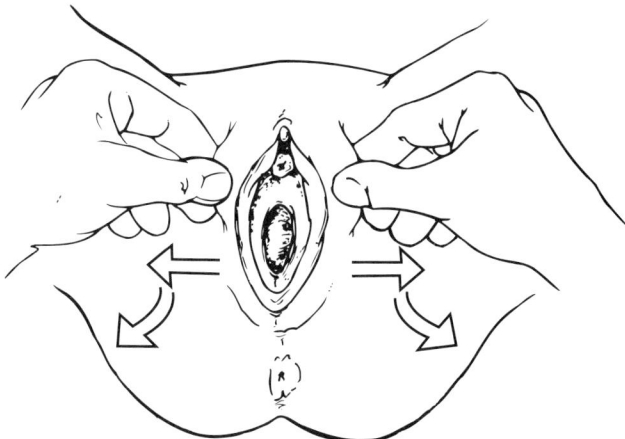

Figure 36-4. Examination of female external genitalia with the labia majora drawn downward and outward (traction). (From Giardino AP, Finkel MA, Giardino ER, et al: A Practical Guide to the Evaluation of Sexual Abuse in the Prepubertal Child. Newbury Park, Calif, Sage Publications, 1992, p 72.)

penis, instrument), and the degree of penetration involved. Chronic digital abuse can be manifested by changes in the hymenal contour, healed transections, or the attenuation of the hymenal membrane until it is barely visible. When acute penile contact occurs, it can produce erythema, edema, bruising of the vulvar and perivestibular tissue, hymenal distortion, transections, vaginal edema, erythema, or abrasions. In long-standing cases, the vaginal orifice may take on a distinctly dilated character (see Fig. 36-7).

Oral-genital contact by the perpetrator can cause petechiae, edema, bruising, and abrasions, but in most instances, no residual trauma is seen.

Anal findings are even more nonspecific because of the natural distensibility of the anal sphincter. Bruising, laxity of the anal sphincter, and immediate dilation of the anus during the examination (especially in the absence of stool in the rectum) are worrisome findings. Major forced trauma to the anus and perianal structures produces more significant injuries; findings of this magnitude are rare. The perpetrators of child sexual abuse generally intend not to produce discernible injuries, because they want continuing access to their victims.

Classification of Anogenital Findings in Children with Suspected Abuse

Most sexually abused children will have negative findings of medical examinations (range of positive findings, from 2% to 20%).

The determination of normal and abnormal in the examination of sexually abused prepubertal girls has been difficult. One classification of medical findings in child sexual abuse examinations includes the following (Table 36-1):

Class 1: Normal. Variations in the appearance of the hymen, perihymenal tissues, and perianal tissues are documented in more than 10% of the subjects in studies of nonabused children.

Class 2: Nonspecific. Findings may be the result of sexual abuse but may also be the result of other nonabusive causes.

Class 3: Suspect. Findings are rarely seen in nonabused children and have been noted in children with documented abuse but have not been clearly proven to occur only as a result of abuse.

Class 4: Suggestive of abuse or penetration. Findings, or a combination of findings, can be reasonably explained only by postulating that sexual abuse or penetrating injury has occurred. This type of finding mandates a report to law enforcement and a child protective service, even if the child is unable to give a clear history of molestation, under the assumption that there is no clear and consistent history of accidental penetrating injury.

Class 5: Clear evidence of penetrating injury. Findings can have no explanation other than penetrating trauma to the hymen or perianal tissues.

The assessment and likelihood of abuse are noted in Table 36-2.

Laboratory Evidence

Prepubertal children with STDs are considered the victims of sexual abuse (see Chapter 29). The most common STDs acquired through sexual abuse are gonorrhea, syphilis, and chlamydial infection (Table 36-3). Other STDs associated with sexual abuse are herpes simplex, condyloma acuminatum, trichomoniasis, human immunodeficiency virus (HIV) infection, and pediculosis pubis. Several studies have indicated low yields when cultures are obtained from all children who are having sexual abuse evaluations. Most investigators now obtain cultures from children when there is evidence of vaginal discharge, when there is known contact with the genitalia of an infected perpetrator, or when there is a history of vaginal discharge.

The Centers for Disease Control and Prevention recommend that the following be obtained from selected child sexual abuse victims at high risk:

- gonorrheal cultures from pharyngeal, anal, and urethral or vaginal sites
- chlamydial cultures from vaginal and anal sites in girls and from anal and urethral sites in boys
- serologic testing for syphilis, HIV, hepatitis B
- examination for anogenital warts or ulcerative lesions
- in girls, culture or wet mounts of vaginal secretions for microscopic examination for *Trichomonas* species and bacterial vaginosis

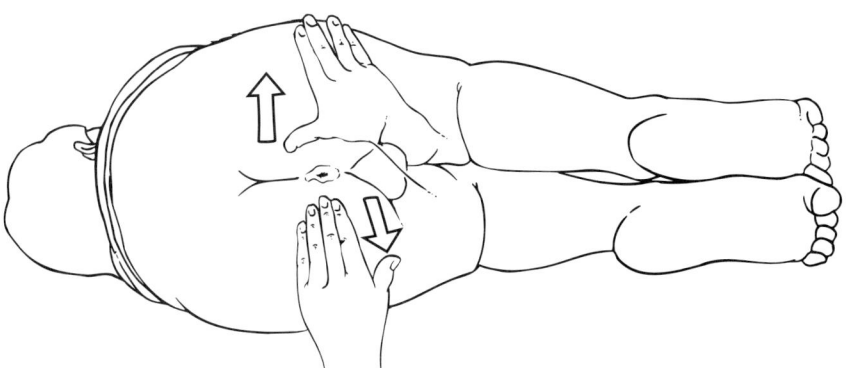

Figure 36-5. Hand placement for separation of the buttocks to view external anal tissues with the child in the left lateral decubitus position. (From Giardino AP, Finkel MA, Giardino ER, et al: A Practical Guide to the Evaluation of Sexual Abuse in the Prepubertal Child. Newbury Park, Calif, Sage Publications, 1992, p 74.)

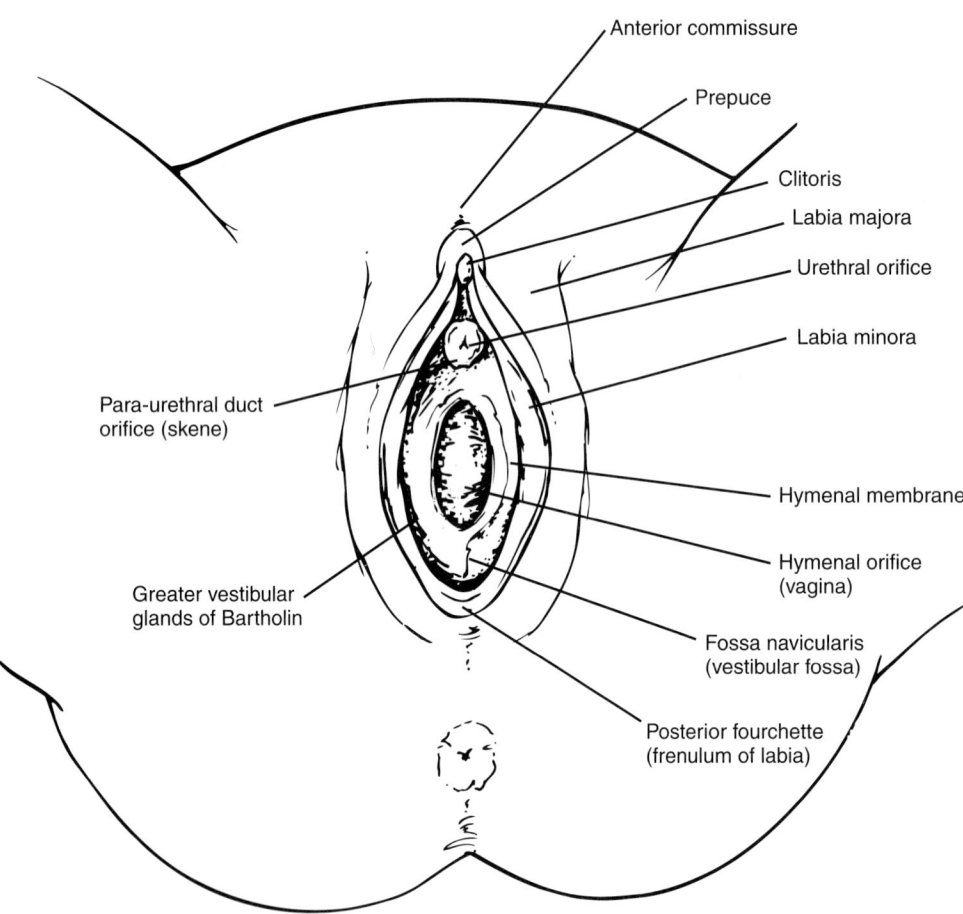

Figure 36-6. Normal anatomy of female external genitalia. (From Giardino AP, Finkel MA, Giardino ER, et al: A Practical Guide to the Evaluation of Sexual Abuse in the Prepubertal Child. Newbury Park, Calif, Sage Publications, 1992, p 32.)

- in adolescents, cultures for gonorrhea and chlamydia from all sites of penetration or attempted penetration, testing for *Trichomonas* species and bacterial vaginosis
- repeat serologic testing 2, 6, 12, and 24 weeks after the assault

Although histories from children, especially the young, cannot supply adequate information as to the type of contact, older children are often able to give quite accurate histories of the events of sexual contact. More selective testing can be based on the epidemiology of diseases in a given locale. The safest course of action is to adhere to strict guidelines, but clinical judgment based on the circumstances of each individual case should be applied.

For information on specific therapy for STDs, see Chapter 29.

Collection of Forensic Materials

Five conditions should be adhered to before the collection of specimens:

1. Specific details of collection, labeling, and packaging of specimens should be determined with the processing laboratory.
2. A specimen collection protocol should be used to ensure that all appropriate specimens are collected.
3. Collection kits should be standardized.
4. The procedures for collecting specimens should be explained in advance to the child and to his or her caretaker.
5. Proper consent should be obtained before performing the collection.

If forensic evidence is to be gathered, it should be done within 72 hours of the event, because material is rarely recoverable after that time (Table 36-4). The handling of collected specimens should be documented to maintain a chain of evidence and to prevent legal challenges about confusing specimens from different patients.

DIFFERENTIAL DIAGNOSIS

The correct diagnosis of sexual abuse in children can lead to intervention that is sometimes life-saving. In many cases, the recognition of abuse provides the opportunity for the child to enter a new, protected, and nourished life. The long-term outcome for some adults in whom the diagnosis was not made in childhood is a life of mistrust, maladjustment, and a multitude of psychogenic medical complaints. We do not know the outcome in children in whom a misdiagnosis of child sexual abuse has occurred. Such an error sets in motion a process that is, at the very least, disruptive and, in the worst case, tragic. It behooves the diagnostician to be aware of possible diagnoses that may be confused with sexual abuse (Table 36-5).

DIAGNOSTIC FORMULATION

Few cases of alleged sexual abuse follow a smooth course from the chief complaint to a firm and unassailable diagnosis. Individuals who provide clear and convincing disclosure information, exhibit behavioral signs and symptoms known to be induced by sexual abuse, and demonstrate definitive anatomic changes secondary to the trauma of sexual abuse may not have their cases supported by the protective and judicial systems. Children who provide disclosure information that is borderline or equivocal may nonetheless be the victims of abuse. The evaluators must be able to gather meaningful

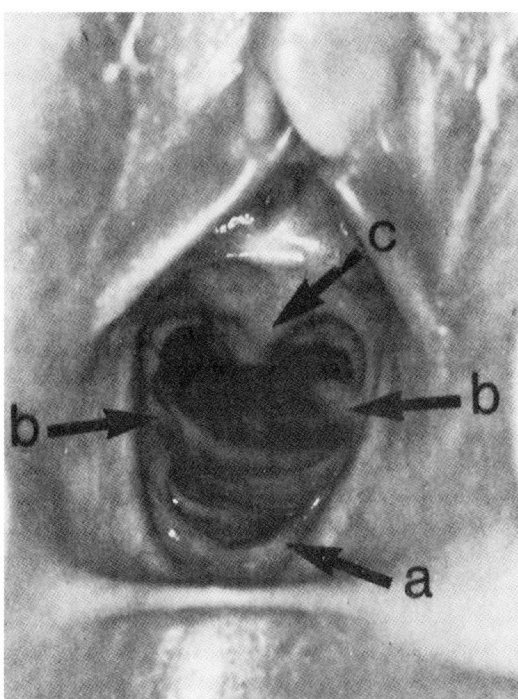

Figure 36-7. View of the genitalia of a 7-year-old girl sexually molested by her father and uncle; labial traction method. Narrow hymenal rim (*arrow a*) with exposed ridges (*arrows b*) at the 3- and 9-o'clock positions, anterior column (*arrow c*), and enlarged hymenal orifice. Colposcopic photographs (magnification, ×10). (From McCann J: Use of the colposcope in childhood sexual abuse examinations. Pediatr Clin North Am 1990;37:863-881.)

information and to analyze and synthesize it so that a balanced, accurate, and holistic appraisal of the case is accomplished.

The three critical components of diagnosis of child sexual abuse are

1. the disclosure information
2. the physical and behavioral signs and symptoms
3. the positive results of the medical examination

Foremost in importance are the quality and credibility of the child's description of the events and the techniques used in eliciting the information. A disclosure statement is theoretically possible in all cases if sexual abuse has occurred in a verbal child. This is the best and most reliable evidence. The diagnostic value of physical and behavioral signs depends on the specificity of those factors for sexual abuse. Such physical and behavioral signs/symptoms are variably present and can be legally challenged if it is possible to cast doubt about their origin. The finding of definitive diagnostic anatomic changes is of great value but occurs in a low proportion of cases (15% to 30%). Positive culture or serologic results for STDs have value in direct proportion to the STD involved, the detection method used, and the specificity of the STD for sexual abuse.

REPORTING CHILD ABUSE

In all 50 states, there exist uniform statutes mandating that physicians report to the child protective services bureau in their local jurisdiction all cases in which there exists a "reasonable" suspicion that child abuse has occurred. Absolute certainty is not required, and in many cases, more information needs to be elicited by the child protection agency to decide whether a case is founded. The person who reports is immune from legal action by caretakers, unless it can be proved that malicious intent was present; there are both civil and criminal penalties for failing to report when suspicion exists. Consultation is usually readily available from child protection agencies by telephone on a 24-hour basis if there is doubt about the need to report.

Table 36-1. Proposed Classification of Anogenital Findings in Children

Normal (Class 1)

Periurethral (or vestibular) bands
Longitudinal intravaginal ridges
Hymenal tags
Posterior (inferior) hymenal rim measuring at least
   1 mm wide
Estrogen changes (uniformly thickened, redundant hymen)
Hymenal clefts in the anterior (superior) half of the hymenal
   rim: on or above the 3- to 9-o'clock line, patient supine
Hymenal bumps or mounds
Diastasis ani (smooth area) at 6 or 12 o'clock position in the
   perianal area
Anal tag/thickened fold in midline
Increased perianal pigmentation

Nonspecific (Class 2)

Erythema of vestibule or perianal tissues
Increased vascularity of vestibule or hymen
Labial adhesions
Vaginal discharge
Lesions of condyloma acuminata in a child younger
   than 2 yr old
Anal fissures
Flattened anal folds
Anal dilation with stool present
Venous congestion of perianal tissues

Suspected for Abuse (Class 3)

Enlarged hymenal opening (>2 standard deviations
   above mean for age and position)
Immediate venous congestion of perianal tissues with
   edema and/or distorted anal folds
Anal dilation of at least 20 mm with stool not visible
   in rectal vault
Posterior hymenal rim less than 1 mm in all views
Condyloma acuminata in a child older than 2 yr of age
Acute abrasions or lacerations in the vestibule or on the labia
   (not involving the hymen)

Suggestive of Abuse/Penetration (Class 4)

Combination of two or more suspected anal findings or two
   or more suspected genital findings
Scar of fresh laceration of the posterior fourchette
Perianal scar

Clear Evidence of Penetrating Injury (Class 5)

Areas in the posterior (inferior) half of the hymenal rim
   with an absence of hymenal tissue, confirmed in knee-chest
   position
Obvious hymenal transections
Perianal lacerations extending beyond (deep to) the external
   anal sphincter
Recent hymenal-vaginal lacerations
Lacerations through the hymen and posterior fourchette or
   perineum

Table 36-2. Overall Assessment of the Likelihood of Sexual Abuse

Class 1: No Evidence of Sexual Abuse

1:1   Normal examination, no history, no behavioral changes, no witnessed abuse

1:2   Nonspecific findings with another known cause, and no history or behavioral changes

1:3   Child considered at risk for sexual abuse but gives no history and has nonspecific behavioral changes

1:4   Physical findings of injury consistent with accidental trauma with history given

Class 2: Possible Abuse

2:1   Class 1, 2, or 3 findings in combination with significant behavioral changes, especially sexualized behaviors, but child unable to give history of abuse

2:2   Presence of condyloma or herpes simplex type I (genital) in the absence of a history of abuse, with otherwise normal examination findings

2:3   Child has made a statement but given no detailed or consistent history

2:4   Class 3 findings with no disclosure of abuse

Class 3: Probable Abuse

3:1   Child gives a clear, consistent, detailed description of molestation, with or without other findings present

3:2   Class 4 or 5 findings in a child, with or without a history of abuse, in the absence of any convincing history of accidental penetrating injury

3:3   Culture-proven infection with *Chlamydia trachomatis* (child >2 yr of age) in a prepubertal child; also, culture-proven herpes simplex type 2 infection in a child or documented *Trichomonas* infection

Class 4: Definite Evidence of Abuse or Sexual Contact

4:1   The finding of sperm or seminal fluid in or on child's body

4:2   A witnessed episode of sexual molestation; this also applies to cases in which pornographic photographs or videotapes are acquired as evidence

4:3   Nonaccidental, blunt penetrating injury to the vaginal or anal orifice

4:4   Positive, confirmed cultures for *Neisseria gonorrhoeae* in a prepubertal child, or serologic confirmation of acquired syphilis

4:5   Pregnancy

Problems in diagnosis are noted in Table 36-6, and indications for consultation with other experts are noted in Table 36-7.

PHYSICAL ABUSE

Two separate domains exist in cases of suspected physical abuse. The first domain, which is a strictly medical one, requires a traditional medical or surgical approach to diagnosis and management. The second domain requires a decision as to whether the observed phenomenon is the result of inflicted injury, a medical disease process, or an accidental injury. Standard medical and surgical approaches are the central concerns in the first domain, with optimal management necessary to obtain the best short-term outcome. Within the second domain lies the challenge of securing the best comprehensive outcome for the child and family. This requires the skills and wisdom of the interdisciplinary team at both the hospital and the community levels.

ACCIDENT OR ABUSE?

An accident is defined as an event that occurs incidentally, casually, or by chance. It is presumed that such an event was at least consciously unintentional and that if such circumstances were under conscious control, an attempt would have been made to avert the anticipated event. An intentional event or action is one that occurs voluntarily and is under conscious, or perhaps even unconscious, control, reflecting an underlying conflict or impulse.

In possible child abuse cases, there is a continuum from what appears to be a volitional act to what appears to be a chance event. The distinction must be made, taking into account the setting of the event (social context, location of encounter), the biases of the observer and the reporter, the type of injury (likelihood of observed injury or injuries being caused by an accidental mechanism), and the future risk to the child, if it is at all predictable.

The approach both to the medical or surgical diagnosis and to the determination of the cause of the observed condition, however, is a traditional medical one: accurate and comprehensive historical investigation, thorough physical examination, and discerning selection of laboratory and imaging studies.

Several questions help to distinguish accidental from inflicted injury:

1. What is the age of the patient? Developmental stages of childhood determine what kinds of injuries are likely to be seen. The motor skills of the child determine what the child could have done to incur injury. What are the normal behaviors of a child at this particular age? What is this child developmentally capable of doing? Is the child "hyperactive" either in the eyes of his or her caretakers or in actuality? Is the child a "daredevil"? Is the child obstreperous, combative, or "annoying" and therefore more likely to be disciplined harshly?

2. Is the history plausible? Could this injury have been sustained in the manner described?

3. Does the history change with changing information supplied to the caretaker? Adjustments in the account of the injury may be made by caretakers to fit the evolving information, which indicates that the history is being tailored to fit the new information.

4. Does the history change when related in subsequent accounts by other family members?

5. Are there nonfamilial eyewitnesses to the injury?

6. Was the injury unwitnessed by the caretaker? The lack of information as to how a serious injury has occurred should raise the index of suspicion for an abusive origin.

7. Is the caretaker's demeanor defensive, belligerent, hostile, or passive and not in keeping with the seriousness of the patient's condition?

8. Is the social situation in which the injury occurred a high-risk environment? The presence of community or intrafamilial violence, substance abuse, chaotic living arrangements, poverty, social isolation, transient lifestyles, mental health problems, or discord among family members should serve as a red flag.

9. Can the described mechanism of injury account for the observed injury? The concept of the discrepant history is a central one in distinguishing between accidental and inflicted injury. Often the injury is explained by claims that it was caused by a fall. According to a large literature, falls from short distances are discounted as being responsible for serious injuries, but short falls down steps, off beds, off couches, off tables, and in baby walkers are often offered as the mechanisms of serious injuries in actual abuse cases. The role of torsion must be considered in fractured bones, and it should be remembered that for a torsion injury to exist, one end of a long bone is twisted in the opposite direction of the other by a large force. The issue of how much force is required to produce injuries is often raised. Information derived from the medical literature helps to answer this question.

Table 36-3. Incubation, Diagnosis, and Implications of Sexually Transmitted Diseases (STDs) in Prepubertal Children

STDs	Incubation	Diagnosis	Relationship to Sexual Abuse
Gonococcal infection	2-7 days	Culture confirmed by two or more confirmatory tests	Certain*
Syphilis	10-90 days	RPR or VDRL test confirmed by FTA-ABS or MHA-TP test	Certain*
Chlamydial infection	Variable	Culture only: rapid techniques lack adequate specificity	Probable*
Human papillomavirus	1-9 mo (? 20 mo)	Inspection, application of acetic acid, or biopsy and viral typing infection	Probable*
Trichomoniasis	4-20 days	Wet mount of discharge, culture more sensitive	Probable*
Herpes simplex virus type 2 infection	2-14 days	Culture with viral typing	Probable*
Herpes simplex virus type 1 infection	2-14 days	Culture with viral typing	Possible
Bacterial vaginosis	7-14 days?	"Clue cells" on wet mount and positive "whiff" test	Uncertain
Genital mycoplasma	2-3 wk?	Culture	Uncertain
HIV infection	6 wk–18 mo	ELISA confirmed by Western blot	Uncertain

From Finkel MA, De Jong AR: Medical findings in child sexual abuse. In Reece RM, Ludwig S (eds): Child Abuse: Medical Diagnosis and Management. Philadelphia, Lippincott Williams & Wilkins, 2001, pp 207-286.

*Except when perinatal transmission is documented.

ELISA, enzyme-linked immunosorbent assay; FTA-ABS, fluorescent treponemal antibody absorption; HIV, human immunodeficiency virus; MHA-TP, microhemagglutination-*Treponema pallidum;* RPR, rapid plasma reagin; VDRL, Venereal Disease Research Laboratory.

10. What else might produce the clinical picture? The development of a differential diagnosis is critical in investigating all possible causes for the clinical and radiographic findings.

HEAD INJURIES

More fatalities and long-term morbidity are due to abusive head injury than to any other form of maltreatment. The types of abusive head injuries range from asymptomatic tissue swelling to mild or moderate bruising to skull fracture to intracranial bleeding, diffuse axonal shearing injury, and brain swelling resulting in stupor, coma, and death. When a child younger than 3 years of age comes for medical care with a serious head injury without a readily apparent major trauma history (motor vehicle accident, fall from heights over 10 feet), the chances that this is an inflicted injury are quite high.

Data Collection

While a seriously head-injured child is being evaluated and treated medically, it is crucial for a detailed, analytic, but not challenging or accusatory history to be obtained from the caretakers. The person collecting the history should ideally be someone with experience in child abuse cases who does not have immediate responsibility for the medical treatment required by the child.

As a rule, abusing parents tell a misleading story about how the "accident" happened and are sometimes quite inventive in describing the event. Gentle probing, with inquiries and request for clarification about questionable portions of the history, often elucidates the mechanism of injury and shows discrepancies in the history. The interviewer should establish a timeline of events beginning with the last time the caretakers believed that the child was completely "normal." A thorough description of all events involving the child after that time up to and including the injury event, the caretakers' response to the event, and the solicitation of medical care should be sought. This helps to determine when the child became symptomatic and who had physical access to the child.

The history of the pregnancy, labor and delivery, and neonatal course and a family history of medical diseases are important, with particular attention to bleeding and clotting disorders, neurologic diseases, metabolic and bone diseases, or other genetic conditions of the family. This comprehensive evaluation eliminates the necessity of returning to the caretakers for missing data as the case progresses. The medical history of the child, including previous injuries and serious illnesses or hospitalizations, along with a review of systems, should be obtained. Exploration of the social milieu with attention to the living arrangements and the relationships of household members should be done.

Physical Examination

The physical examination of the child with a head injury involves the risk of ignoring less urgently compromised organ systems (see Chapter 40). Ignoring bleeding visceral organs is the most glaring and potentially disastrous omission, but overlooking cutaneous injuries can deprive the diagnostician of important clinical data because of the fleeting nature of these injuries. Likewise, inspection of the oral cavity for intraoral lesions is important, as is a search for scalp lesions hidden under the hair. The neck should be carefully inspected for signs of injury (strangulation, hand- or finger-inflicted bruising). The presence of bruises on the back or thighs or in the perineum should also be noted. Photodocumentation of such injuries is highly desirable. The use of digital cameras is becoming widespread. All forms of photodocumentation have been challenged legally, but if the images produced are said to represent what the examiner saw at the time of the examination, these legal maneuvers are answered.

The examination of the fundi is of utmost importance. This should ideally be carried out by pupillary dilatation and indirect ophthalmoscopic inspection or, in lieu of that capability, by direct ophthalmoscopy. Although retinal hemorrhages are the most common finding in child abuse, other lesions may also be seen. These include retinal detachment, optic nerve injury, and cupping of the optic nerve secondary to raised intracranial pressure. Although retinal hemorrhages are not pathognomonic for inflicted head trauma, they are present in a high percentage of abuse cases, are not present in most accidental head trauma cases, and are seldom seen in children who have undergone cardiopulmonary resuscitation. The presence of widespread, bilateral, multilayered retinal hemorrhages extending to the periphery of the retina are highly specific for inflicted head injury.

Table 36-4. **Collecting Forensic Specimens in Sexual Abuse Cases**

1. Obtain 2-3 swabbed specimens from each area of body assaulted (for sperm, acid phosphatase, P30, MHS-5 antigen, blood group antigen determinations). The number of swabs required depends on local laboratory. Most laboratories request air-dried specimens, which require drying for 60 min before they can be packaged.
2. Mouth: Swab under tongue and buccal pouch next to upper and lower molars. These areas are locations where seminal fluid is most likely to be persistent.
3. Vagina: Use dry or moistened swab or 2 mL saline wash. Remember that overdilution of secretions may produce false-negative results of tests for acid phosphatase. Secretions may also be collected with a pipette or eyedropper.
4. Rectum: Insert swab at least $\frac{1}{2}$ to 1 inch beyond anus.
5. Specimens should be taken from any other suspicious site on the body. Saline- or sterile water-moistened swabs may be used to lift any stains suspected to be dried seminal fluid or blood. An alternate method is to scrape off the dried stains with the back of a scalpel blade into a clean envelope or tube.
6. Make saline wet mount of specimens from all assaulted orifices and examine immediately for presence of motile and nonmotile sperm.
7. Some forensic laboratories request a dry smear of each secretion sample using clean glass microscope slides; others prefer to prepare their own slides from swab specimens.
8. Collect saliva specimen to determine the victim's antigen secretion status. Saliva may be collected using 3-4 sterile swabs or a 2×2 gauze pad that the victim placed in the mouth.
9. Obtain a venous blood sample from the victim for antigen secretor status. This sample from the victim will be used in the analysis of the identity of the perpetrator.
10. Save torn or bloody clothes or any clothing when semen staining is suspected, using Wood lamp. Semen may fluoresce with a blue or green color under the ultraviolet light of the Wood lamp, although fluorescence under UV light is nonspecific. Various skin infections; congenital or acquired skin pigmentary changes; and chemicals, including systemic and topical medications, cosmetics, soaps, and industrial chemicals, may fluoresce under UV light.
11. If the victim was wearing a tampon, pad, or diaper during the assault or if a fresh tampon, pad, or diaper was used after the abuse, save this for analysis; seminal fluid products may be found on these items. Plastic bags should be used only on dry specimens and only if so directed by the laboratory. Sealed plastic may promote the growth of *Candida* and other organisms that might destroy some of the evidence.
12. Save any foreign material found on removal of clothing. Fiber analysis or trace analysis may provide evidence that links the specimens to the perpetrator or the location of the abuse.
13. Collect samples of combed pubic hair or scalp hair and fingernail scrapings. These procedures are often considered optional. Pubic hair, scalp hair, or skin fragments from scratching may be used to help identify the perpetrator. Control samples of the victim's body or scalp hair are collected for comparison. Usually, it is recommended that the hairs be plucked rather than cut, although the additional trauma of plucking 10 to 20 hairs from a child may not be warranted unless foreign hair material is found on the child's body. Some protocols recommend considering cutting hairs or collecting plucked hairs at a later time if needed.
14. Specimens should also be taken to screen for sexually transmitted diseases. The recommended procedures are detailed in the text. Swabs should *not* be air dried because air drying kills the organisms and causes the cultures for these diseases to be falsely negative. Specimens for culture should be sent quickly to a microbiology laboratory for processing and not be included with the materials to be processed in the forensic laboratory.

From Finkel MA, De Jong AR: Medical findings in child sexual abuse. In Reece RM, Ludwig S (eds): Child Abuse: Medical Diagnosis and Management. Philadelphia, Lippincott Williams & Wilkins, 2001, p 268.

MHS-5, mouse antihuman semen-5; UV, ultraviolet.

Laboratory Studies

Children with head trauma severe enough to warrant admission to the hospital should also undergo laboratory studies to support diagnoses of associated trauma in other organ systems, to anticipate hematologic and biochemical alterations sometimes attendant to head trauma, and to document and monitor their neurologic status. These studies are listed in Table 36-8.

Imaging Studies

In most instances of moderate to severe head injury, the first imaging modality should be computed tomography (CT) scanning without contrast media, because it is readily available in most hospitals and can be performed safely with life support systems operating during the procedure (Figs. 36-8 and 36-9). Bone windows should be employed along with the standard scan. Plain radiographs of the skull usually show existing skull fractures better than do CT scans but are of no value in demonstrating intracranial bleeding or parenchymal brain injury. Magnetic resonance imaging (MRI) is

ordinarily used as a confirmatory test rather than as an initial one because of the longer scan times and need for life support, but MRI shows parenchymal changes and smaller subdural hematomas in superior detail (see Fig. 36-8). Some of the newer techniques in MRI are gaining acceptance, and in time MRI may supplant CT scanning as the imaging modality of choice.

CT scans of the abdominal viscera are valuable when there is elevation of liver and pancreatic enzymes or when there is reason to believe hepatic or pancreatic damage is present. If splenic or renal laceration is suspected, CT scans delineate these injuries.

Skeletal radiologic surveys are recommended for serious head trauma, because the diagnosis of abuse may be made or supported if unsuspected traumatic injuries are found in other parts of the skeleton. Such accompanying skeletal fractures are seen in some cases of abusive head injury. Posterior rib fractures and the classic metaphyseal lesions at the ends of long bones provide strong evidence in favor of an abusive origin. Subtle acute posterior rib fractures may be difficult to visualize on the initial skeletal survey but can be demonstrated with bone scan scintigraphy or with follow-up thoracic films in 10 to 14 days, which reveal callus formation at the fracture site (Fig. 36-10).

Table 36-5. **Conditions Confused with Child Sexual Abuse**

Dermatologic Conditions

Erythema and excoriations
Diaper rash
Poor hygiene
Candida infection
Pinworms
Allergy/irritants
Bruises
Hematologic disorders
Mongolian spots
Hypersensitivity vasculitis
Purpura fulminans
Coining and other folk practices
Phytodermatitis
Other
Lichen sclerosus
Seborrheic, atopic, and contact dermatitis
Lichen planus
Lichen simplex chronicus
Psoriasis

Congenital Conditions

Midline pits, fusion defects, shiny areas
Prominent median raphe
Midline tags
Linea vestibularis
Diastasis recti (depressed fan-shaped areas)
Genital hemangiomas

Injuries

Straddle injuries
Violent abduction of the legs
Motor vehicle accidents
Self-destructive behavior in retarded children
Female circumcision

Anal Conditions

Severe or chronic constipation and megacolon
Postmortem anal dilation
Neurogenic patulous anus (myotonic dystrophy)

Anal Conditions—cont'd

Fistula
Inflammatory bowel disease
Pinworms
Lichen sclerosus
Hemolytic-uremic syndrome
Rectal polyps or tumor
Eversion of the anal canal/rectal prolapse

Urethral Conditions

Prolapse
Caruncle
Hemangioma
Polyps
Papilloma
Cyst
Condyloma
Sarcoma botryoides
Prolapsed bladder or ureterocele

Infections

Vaginitis with organisms not sexually transmitted
Group A β-hemolytic streptococcus
Shigella species
Pinworms
Nonpathologic *Neisseria* species
Haemophilus species
Varicella
Molluscum
Perinatally acquired
  Chlamydia
  Syphilis
  Herpes simplex virus (HSV)
  Human papillomavirus (HPV) infection
Autoinoculation
  HSV type 1
  HPV (warts)
Infection with cyclic/idiopathic neutropenia
Non–sexually transmitted disease causes of genital ulcers

Adapted from Bays JA: Conditions mistaken for child sexual abuse. In Reece RM, Ludwig S (eds): Child Abuse: Medical Diagnosis and Management. Philadelphia, Lippincott Williams & Wilkins, 2001, pp 287-306.

The types of injuries in serious abusive head injury include skull fractures, subdural or subarachnoid bleeding (see Fig. 36-8), cerebral edema (see Fig. 36-9), diffuse axonal injury, parenchymal tears and contusions, and injuries to the cervical spinal cord. The shaken-baby syndrome/shaken-impact syndrome (SBS/SIS) occurs mainly in infants, usually younger than 1 year, but has been described in older children as well. In fact, there have been reports of shaken-adult syndrome, with the signs, symptoms, and clinical and radiographic findings identical to those seen in SBS. A key factor in these cases is the disparity in size between the perpetrator and the victim. Perpetrators are men in 75% of cases and women in 25%. Parents, baby sitters, other relatives, and unrelated adults have all been implicated. It is highly unlikely that children younger than 5 years could be perpetrators of SBS/SIS.

Shaking alone or shaking with impact by slamming the child against a hard or soft surface with resultant deceleration and hypoxia are the responsible factors producing the subdural hematoma, diffuse axonal injury, and consequent cerebral edema leading to raised intracranial pressure. Whether shaking alone or shaking plus impact is required to cause the damage is debated. The clinical picture is one of neurologic devastation, resulting in death in approximately 25% of the victims and long-term neurologic morbidity in the majority (57% to 65%) of the survivors. The most important consideration in SBS/SIS is that the lesions are injuries to the brain and that the attendant subdural and subarachnoid bleeding are only markers of the traumatic and hypoxic injuries. Retinal hemorrhages are seen in the majority of the cases, and the types of retinal hemorrhages—extensive, multiple, involving numerous layers of the retina—are almost never seen in any other condition and thus can be said to be diagnostic unless another major accidental injury can be demonstrated (e.g., major motor vehicle crash, falls from five stories).

ABDOMINAL AND THORACIC INJURIES

Abdominal and thoracic injuries are the second most common cause of death in child abuse (Table 36-9). They account for 6% to 8% of all injuries in physical abuse, and most of these are abdominal injuries. Reported fatality rates are between 40% and 50%.

Table 36-6. Pitfalls in Child Abuse Evaluation:
12 Costly Errors

1. A desire not to make the diagnosis
2. Failure to assemble past information on medical conditions and medical encounters
3. Too great a reliance on the information developed by others
4. Transference-countertransference with custodial parent (formation of alliances or development of hostilities)
5. Overinterpretation or underinterpretation of signs and symptoms
6. Overinterpretation or underinterpretation of physical findings
7. Failure to know about conditions mistaken for sexual abuse
8. Faulty laboratory techniques resulting in either false-positive or false-negative reports
9. Use of techniques easily challenged in court
10. Impatience about arriving at a diagnostic conclusion
11. Failure to understand normative data with regard to psychosexual development
12. Failure to prepare adequately for court appearances

The following features help distinguish abusive from accidental abdominal injuries:

1. Abusive injuries are more common in younger children (median age 2.6 years versus 7.8 years in accidental cases).
2. Vague histories often account for the abusive injuries. In contrast, accidental injuries are often witnessed or otherwise well documented: 70% of the injuries in the accidental group are caused by motor vehicle accidents and 20% by falls from great heights.

Table 36-7. When to Seek Consultation

1. If clinician is not prepared to work in an interdisciplinary group
2. If clinician is not prepared to see the case through from initial encounter through the investigation and ultimate legal resolution
3. If clinician's knowledge base about any of the components of the evaluation is too narrow
4. If there are areas of uncertainty about the diagnosis

Table 36-8. Laboratory Studies in Physical Abuse Cases

Complete blood cell count with morphology analysis; serial hematocrit levels
Serum electrolytes, blood urea nitrogen, creatinine, serum and urine osmolality
Urinalysis
Liver function studies (aspartate aminotransferase, alanine aminotransferase, bilirubin, alkaline phosphatase)
Serum amylase
Creatine phosphokinase
Cultures of blood, urine, cerebrospinal fluid (if safe to perform lumbar puncture)
Prothrombin time, partial thromboplastin time, platelet count
Stool for blood
Arterial blood gases

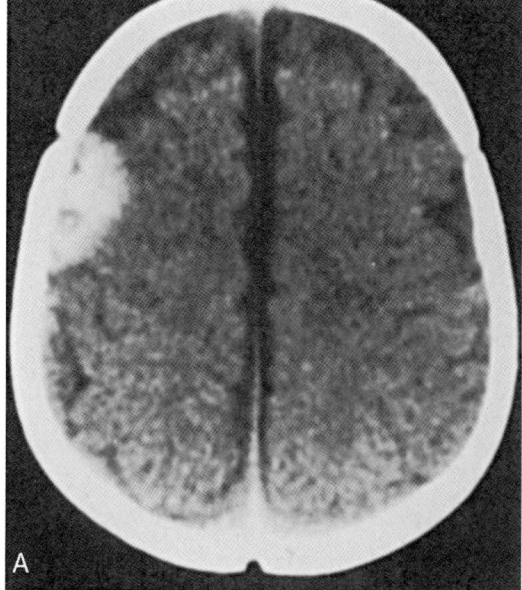
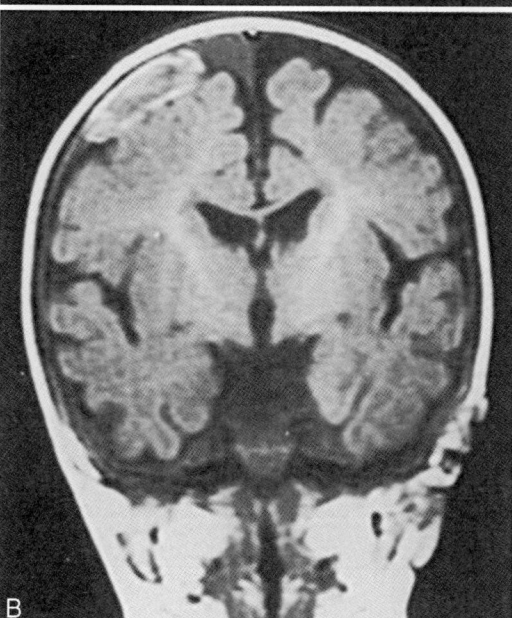

Figure 36-8. Images in a 6-month-old with seizures. **A,** Axial unenhanced computed tomographic image reveals a focal acute high-density hematoma over the right cerebral convexity. There is generalized enlargement of the extracerebral spaces, reflecting either chronic subdural hematoma or brain atrophy. **B,** Coronal T1-weighted magnetic resonance image shows the acute right convexity subdural hematoma as a mass with high signal intensity. A subacute subdural hematoma with lower signal intensity surrounds the acute lesion. There is also generalized brain atrophy with increased extracerebral space; the normal cerebrospinal fluid over the left cerebral convexity is of lower signal intensity than is the subacute hematoma over the right convexity. (From Merten DF, Carpenter BLM: Radiologic imaging of inflicted injury in the child abuse syndrome. Pediatr Clin North Am 1990;37:815-839.)

3. Delay in seeking medical care is seen in abusive injuries, in contrast to the accidental group, in which care is typically sought promptly.
4. Abusive injuries occur to hollow viscera most often, whereas a solid organ is more often injured in accidents.
5. The mortality rate from abuse is higher (>50%) than in accidental injuries (~20%).

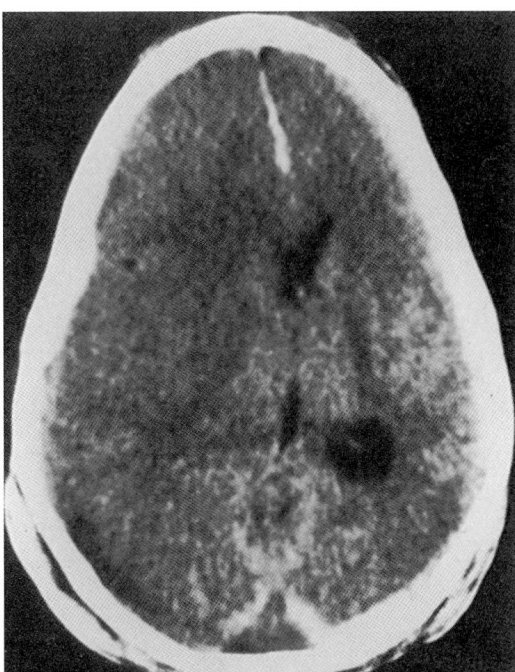

Figure 36-9. Unenhanced computed tomographic image in an abused 3-month-old infant reveals generalized right-sided decrease in brain density caused by diffuse cerebral edema. The right lateral ventricle is effaced, and there is a shift of midline structures to the left. Posterior and anterior subdural interhemispheric hemorrhages are also present. (From Merten DF, Carpenter BLM: Radiologic imaging of inflicted injury in the child abuse syndrome. Pediatr Clin North Am 1990;37:815-839.)

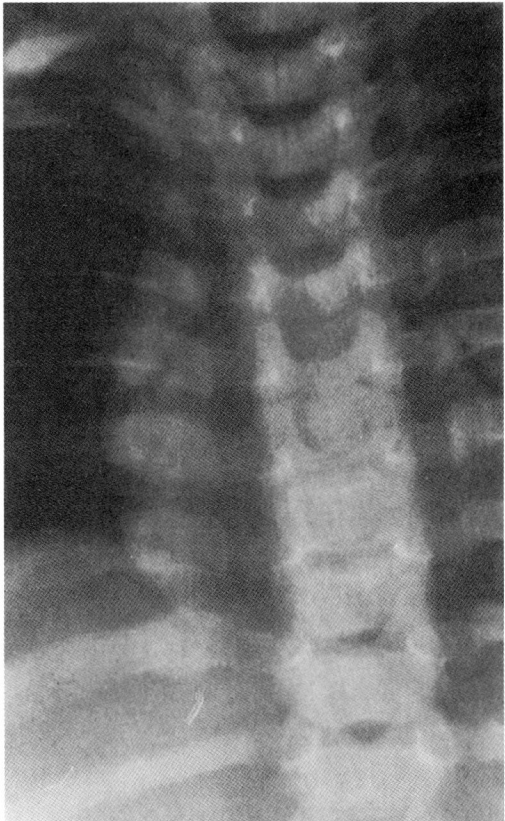

Figure 36-10. Chest radiograph in a 7-month-old infant with an "accidental" skull fracture also reveals multiple healing fractures of the right sixth through ninth ribs adjacent to the costovertebral junctions. (From Merten DF, Carpenter BLM: Radiologic imaging of inflicted injury in the child abuse syndrome. Pediatr Clin North Am 1990;37:815-839).

There is a hierarchy of injury to the abdominal organs, with hollow viscera being the most commonly affected. Ninety percent of hollow visceral injuries are seen in the duodenum or jejunum; the remainder are in the terminal ileum. The second most common organ for abusive injury is the liver, particularly the more midline portion, and the third most common is the pancreas.

Clinical Manifestations

The manifestations of abdominal injury can be quite striking, with distention, exquisite tenderness, vomiting, shock, or unconsciousness. However, most children with abdominal injuries, either inflicted or accidental, have no obvious abdominal wall cutaneous injuries. Some children have only minimal signs and symptoms; florid symptoms develop only after several hours. Often there are injuries to other parts of the body, making attention to the abdomen less of a perceived priority. Rapid deterioration can occur if blood loss is not identified and treated.

Laboratory Studies

The pertinent laboratory studies are listed in Table 36-8.

Imaging Studies

The initial imaging study to diagnose abdominal or thoracic injury is plain radiography. Two frontal views of the abdomen, one with the patient supine and one with the patient erect, are recommended. If the child is too ill for an erect view to be obtained, a horizontal beam cross-table lateral view can be used. This technique usually identifies obstruction, perforation (pneumoperitoneum), hemoperitoneum, or ascites. If there is obstruction, contrast media can be used to localize the lesion. Barium is the preferred contrast medium unless perforation is suspected, in which case a water-soluble contrast medium should be used. A frontal view of the chest is recommended for possible thoracic injuries, including rib fractures. A skeletal survey should also be obtained at the earliest possible opportunity, especially in severely injured children, because future opportunities may not occur and important forensic evidence may be lost. Contrast studies of the genitourinary tract have been rarely indicated since the advent of CT scanning, but voiding cystourethrography may be needed if lower urinary tract rupture needs delineation.

The CT scan is the most useful imaging technique for evaluation of solid organ injuries. Contrast studies are better for showing hollow organ lesions; the contrast CT scan may demonstrate extravasation or a leakage of contrast material, which is usually an indication for surgical exploration. Most intramural hematomas without perforation do not necessitate intervention but resolve with supportive care unless there are bleeding complications. Abdominal ultrasonography also helps identify solid organ trauma and hematoma formation (liver, spleen, pancreas, kidney).

Clues to thoracic and abdominal trauma are noted in Table 36-9.

SKELETAL INJURIES

The actual incidence of skeletal injuries in child abuse is unknown, although an estimate of fractures in abused children younger than 1 year of age is as high as 70%. Nearly 50% of these fractures are clinically unsuspected, and almost 50% involve more than one bone.

Table 36-9. Types of Abdominal and Thoracic Injuries

Organ	Injury	Signs/Symptoms/Diagnostic Findings
Hypopharynx	Traumatic perforation	Feeding difficulty, drooling, palatal abrasion, sloughing lesion pharynx
Esophagus	Traumatic perforation	Coughing, blood-tinged sputum
		Interstitial emphysema, emesis, mediastinitis, rib fractures on radiographic study
Stomach	Traumatic perforation	Shock and collapse
		Distended abdomen
		Free peritoneal air on plain radiographic study
Duodenum	Blunt abdominal trauma	High intestinal obstruction
		Gastric dilatation
		Vomiting
Jejunum, ileum	Blunt trauma	Possible peritonitis secondary to perforation
		Obstruction
Colon, rectum	Blunt trauma	Lower abdominal pain
	Anal penetration	Pain, constipation
Genitourinary tract	Sexual abuse	Bruising, abrasions, tears of external genitalia
	Sadistic abuse	Rupture of bladder
Liver	Blunt trauma	Abdominal distention
		Shock, collapse
		Elevated aspartate aminotransferase, alanine aminotransferase, bilirubin
		CT or ultrasound evidence of injury
Spleen	Blunt trauma	Peritoneal irritation, left shoulder pain
		Blood loss, shock
		Associated rib fractures
		CT or ultrasound evidence of injury
Pancreas	Deep epigastric blunt trauma	Abdominal distention, tenderness
		Elevated amylase
		CT or ultrasound evidence of injury

CT, computed tomography.

Most abuse fractures (80%) are seen in children younger than 18 months, and only 2% of all fractures in this age group are of accidental origin.

The skeletal survey, especially in children with head and visceral injuries, is extremely important in suspected abuse of children younger than 2 years because of the high likelihood that it will reveal unsuspected fractures.

The differential diagnosis of skeletal trauma is noted in Table 36-10.

Types of Fractures

Extremity Fractures

These are the most common abusive fractures; certain types of extremity fractures are more specific for abuse. The "classic metaphyseal lesion" of the long bones has long been identified as the most specific for inflicted injury and is considered pathognomonic for abuse (Fig. 36-11). This so-called corner fracture, bucket-handle fracture, metaphyseal flag, or metaphyseal fragmentation fracture is a planar fracture through the primary spongiosa region of the end of the long bones, producing a disk-like fragment at this site. The fractured portion of the bone, depending on the projection of the x-ray beam, appears as a fragment (corner fracture) or a semilunar loop (bucket-handle fracture). The torsional forces necessary to produce these lesions are those associated with SBS or the application of rotational vectors to the long bones.

The most common long bone fracture in child abuse involves the diaphysis, occurring four times more frequently than metaphyseal fractures. The femur, humerus, and tibia are the long bones most often affected by transverse or oblique/spiral fractures. There are no specific types or locations for abusive fractures, which emphasizes the need for careful history taking, attention to the age of the child, and use of the skeletal survey for children younger than 2 years. Toddler fractures or oblique fractures of the tibia in children aged 9 months to 3 years are common accidental injuries that can occur without the knowledge of caretakers. They produce symptoms of limp, disinclination to bear weight on the affected leg, or pain on standing.

Fractures resulting from abuse may also involve the forearms and, rarely, the clavicle. Fractures of the hands and feet, scapulae, and pelvis are unusual in child abuse.

Rib Fractures

Often unsuspected clinically and discovered through skeletal surveys, rib fractures nevertheless constitute 25% of fractures seen in abuse (see Fig. 36-10). Most of these are posterior fractures, occurring near the costovertebral articulation. They result when the rib arcs rotate poteriorly across the vertebral transverse process, producing a levering effect on the rib. The second most common location for rib fractures is in the midaxillary line. The fracture line in posterior fractures is usually on the anterior (visceral) surface of the rib, whereas the fracture line in the midaxillary fracture is on the outer surface of the rib. Because these fractures are produced by compressions of the thorax while the child is being held during shaking or when the child is forcefully picked up in anger by a caretaker, they are often multiple and bilateral. Overlying bruises of the thoracic wall may be observed but are often absent. Unless the fractures have been present long enough to produce callus, they

Table 36-10. Differential Diagnosis of Skeletal Trauma

Obstetric trauma
Prematurity
Nutritional-metabolic defects
Scurvy
Rickets
Secondary hyperparathyroidism (renal osteodystrophy)
Menkes syndrome
Mucolipidosis type II (I-cell disease)
Methotrexate osteodystrophy
Prostaglandin therapy
Hypervitaminosis A
Congenital syphilis
Osteomyelitis
Congenital insensitivity to pain
Cerebral palsy-myelodysplasia
Skeletal dysplasias
Osteogenesis imperfecta
Infantile cortical hyperostosis (Caffey disease)
Leukemia
Metastatic neuroblastoma
Histiocytosis X
Toddler fracture
Normal variant
Physiologic periosteal new bone

Adapted from Brill PW, Winchester P, Lachman PS, et al: Differential diagnosis of child abuse. In Kleinman PK: Diagnostic Imaging of Child Abuse. St. Louis, Mosby, 1998, pp 178-236; and Radkowski MA: The battered child syndrome: Pitfalls in radiological diagnosis. Pediatr Ann 1983;12:894.

may not be discernible on plain radiography; in these cases, bone scintigraphy is most useful.

Vertebral Body Fractures

These fractures are being diagnosed more frequently and may be common. They are anterior vertebral body compression fractures and are thought to be caused from hyperflexion during shaking or other violent handling.

Skull Fractures

Skull fractures are classified as simple and complex. Simple fractures are linear and do not cross suture lines; complex fractures are multiple, cross suture lines, are displaced, are comminuted, are diastatic, or are depressed. Complex fractures do not result from trivial trauma, and although they can be the result of accidental trauma, such trauma nearly always has a consistent history. Complex skull fractures alleged to have been acquired by falls from short heights or in unwitnessed falls are highly suspect for abuse.

Imaging Techniques

The skeletal survey is the preferred diagnostic technique for fractures in suspected child abuse. Although radionuclide scintigraphy has certain useful applications (acute subtle fractures, rib fractures), it is not without inherent technical shortcomings and is dependent on the level of competence of the radiologist interpreting it. Table 36-11 details the views recommended for the skeletal survey.

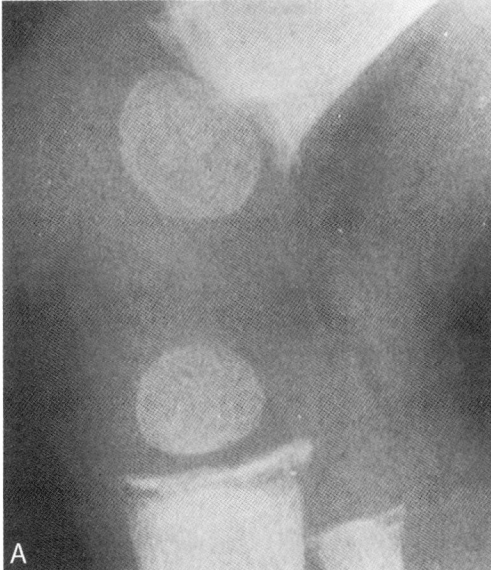
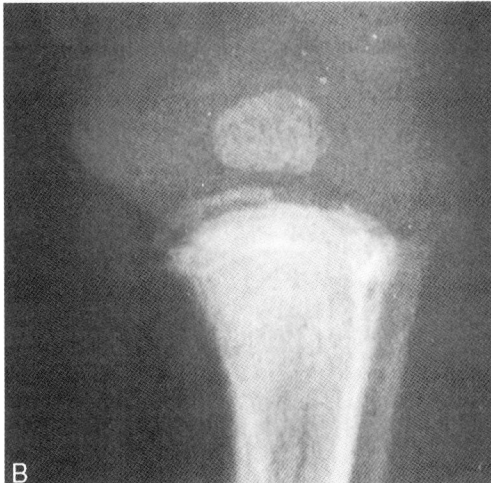

Figure 36-11. Metaphyseal fracture. **A,** Lateral view of the knee in a 5-month-old infant reveals a complete metaphyseal fracture of the tibia and an incomplete fracture of the fibula. There are corner fractures of the femur. **B,** Bucket-handle fracture of the tibia in a 3-month-old infant. (From Merten DF, Carpenter BLM: Radiologic imaging of inflicted injury in the child abuse syndrome. Pediatr Clin North Am 1990;37:815-839.)

Table 36-11. Elements of the Skeletal Survey

Skull: Frontal and lateral (lateral to include the cervical spine)
Spine: Frontal and lateral thoracolumbar spine (lateral to include the sternum)
Chest: Frontal (for rib and spinal detail)
Extremities
  Upper: Frontal (to include shoulder and hands*)
  Lower: Frontal (to include lower lumbar spine, pelvis, and feet†)

From Cooperman D, Merten DF: Skeletal manifestations of child abuse. In Reece RM, Ludwig S (eds): Child Abuse: Medical Diagnosis and Management. Philadelphia, Lippincott Williams & Wilkins, 2001, p 125.

*Separate views of the hands and feet in larger infants and children.

†At least two views of each fracture should be obtained.

Dating of Fractures

Physicians are often asked to pinpoint the time of injury in child abuse cases. The ability to narrow the time frame is limited, but there are some precepts of value (Table 36-12).

CUTANEOUS INJURIES

The most common manifestations of child abuse are cutaneous injuries. These types of lesions include bruises, abrasions, lacerations, petechiae, ecchymoses, and burns (Figs. 36-12 and 36-13). The characteristics of skin lesions important for distinguishing inflicted injuries from accidental ones are the location (Table 36-13), pattern, presence of multiple lesions of different ages, and failure of new lesions to appear during hospitalization or after removal of the child from the caretaker.

The inflicting instrument may be discerned from the shape of the skin lesion (Fig. 36-14). The typical lesion left by a looped electric cord used for whipping may appear elliptic; a belt, buckle, or wire coat hanger leaves a bruise conforming to its shape; the human hand may leave parallel linear stress petechiae, representing the spaces between the fingers, or scalloping lesions conforming to the metacarpal-phalangeal junction; adult human bites leave characteristic lesions, which can be measured and compared with the dentition of the alleged perpetrator; gags leave down-turned lesions at the corners of the mouth; lesions around the neck suggest ligatures applied in that location; ligatures applied to wrists and ankles to restrain the child leave rope burns or pressure lines to those structures; bruises of the upper arms or in the rib cage suggest encirclement bruises resulting from hard pressure applied during shaking or violent handling.

Dating of bruises is imperfect because of the variability of skin color, location of the bruise, healing characteristics, and varying age groups of the children involved in abuse.

Color photography of bruises, with clear identification of the patient, color card, and the date the photograph is taken, can be of great value for documenting bruises.

BURNS

Between 12% and 30% of burns in children are nonaccidental, and burns represent approximately 10% of all abuse cases; 87% of inflicted burns are scald burns, and 13% are flame injuries. The peak age of burn victims is 13 to 24 months. The classic lesion is the immersion burn involving the buttocks and ankles, sustained when a child is held down in extremely hot water. There is often a doughnut lesion of the buttocks, sparing the portion of the buttocks

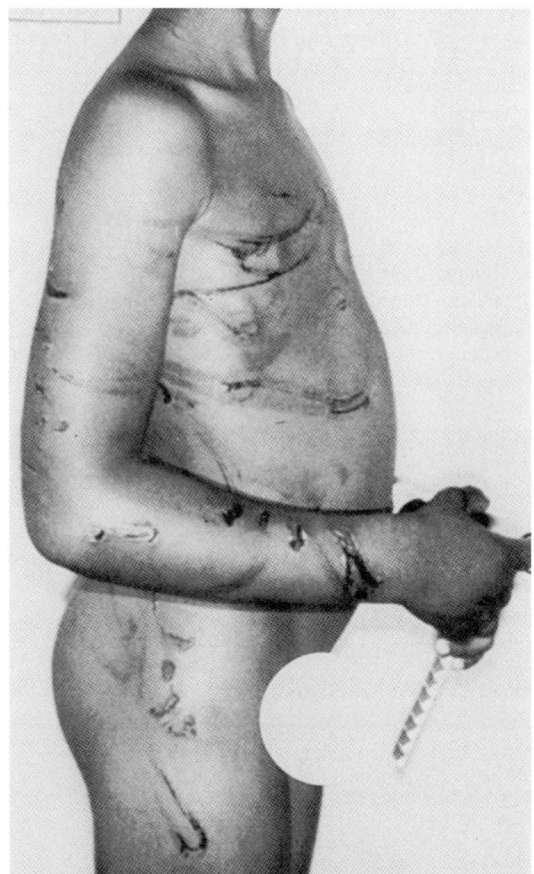

Figure 36-12. Lash marks from an electric cord. Such marks are distinctive. The deep lacerations, which are looped if the cord is looped, result in deep tissue damage, and there is a potential for keloid formation on healing. (From Johnson CF: Inflicted injury versus accidental injury. Pediatr Clin North Am 1990;37:791-815.)

hot plate	light bulb	curling iron	car cigarette lighter	steam iron
knife	grid	cigarette	forks	immersion

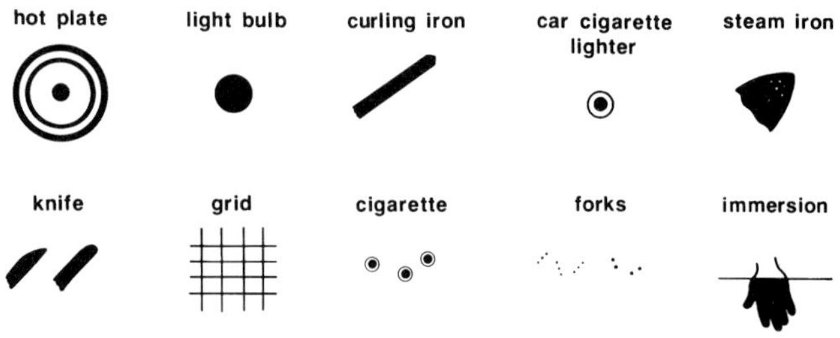

Figure 36-13. Marks from burns. (From Johnson CF: Inflicted injury versus accidental injury. Pediatr Clin North Am 1990;37:791-815.)

Table 36-12. Dating Fractures

Category	Early (Days)	Peak (Days)	Late (Days)
1. Resolution of soft tissues	2-5	4-10	10-21
2. Periosteal new bone	4-10	10-14	14-21
3. Loss of fracture line definition	10-14	14-21	
4. Soft callus	10-14	14-21	
5. Hard callus	14-21	21-42	42-90
6. Remodeling	3 months	1 yr	2 yr to epiphyseal closure

From O'Connor JF, Cohen J: Dating fractures. In Kleinman PK (ed): Diagnostic Imaging in Child Abuse. St. Louis, Mosby, 1998, p 176.

Table 36-13. Location of Cutaneous Injuries

Inflicted	Accidental
Upper arms	Shins
Trunk	Hips (iliac crest)
Upper anterior legs	Lower arms
Side of face	Prominences of spine
Ears and neck	Forehead
Genitalia	Under chin

Adapted from Pascoe JM, Hildebrandt HM, Tarrier A, Murphy M: Patterns of skin injury in nonaccidental and accidental injury. Pediatrics 1979;64:245.

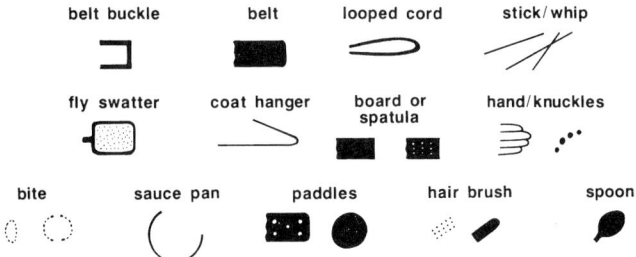

Figure 36-14. Marks from objects. (From Johnson CF. Inflicted injury versus accidental injury. Pediatr Clin North Am 1990;37:791-815.)

resting against the relatively cooler porcelain of the tub. Sharp demarcation lines are typically seen at the borders of burned and spared skin. These lesions, plus the stocking-glove immersion burns, represent easy diagnoses, because they are so obviously caused by restraint of the child. Likewise, burns of the palms and soles are diagnostic for inflicted injury unless the caretaker has an unusually convincing history of a mechanism of injury. Table 36-14 summarizes the distinguishing characteristics of inflicted versus accidental burns.

Nonaccidental burns also seem to carry a higher correlation with social pathologic disorders than do other forms of child abuse. In most inflicted burn cases, the children either are known to the state's protective service agencies or have been previously admitted to the hospital with a variety of diagnoses, including failure to thrive, poisoning, lead intoxication, fractures, head injuries, and previous burns.

POISONING

Although reports of intentional poisoning of children are small in number, the true incidence is difficult to determine. Repetitive accidental poisoning in childhood may have no relationship to home safety but is intimately associated with parental psychopathologic disorders and disturbed family relationships. The clinical indicators of abuse by poisoning are noted in Table 36-15.

Poisonous substances may include household agents (salt, pepper, talc, water, caustic agents, air freshener, laxatives), drugs of misuse (cocaine, ethanol or isopropyl alcohol, opiates, barbiturates, lysergic acid diethylamide [LSD], phencyclidine [PCP], marijuana), prescription drugs (barbiturates, anticonvulsants, insulin, imipramine, opiates, phenothiazines), or others (arsenic, ipecac, acetaminophen, aspirin, mineral oil, Epsom salt, ethylene glycol) (see Chapter 40).

MUNCHAUSEN SYNDROME BY PROXY

Munchausen syndrome by proxy (MSBP) is a bizarre form of child abuse in which the child is the victim of a form of mental illness of the mother, the psychodynamics of which are poorly understood. The condition is defined as a circumstance in which

1. Illness is simulated or produced by a parent (almost invariably the mother) or someone who is in a caretaker role.
2. The child is brought persistently for medical assessment and care, which results in multiple medical and sometimes surgical procedures.
3. The perpetrator denies knowledge about the cause of the child's illness.
4. Acute symptoms and signs in the child abate when the child is separated from the perpetrator (see Chapter 35).

The goal of the diagnostic process is to gather evidence that the illness is simulated or faked (Table 36-16). The strategy of this process is to gather the team of caregivers in the hospital setting and discuss the evolving information on a regular basis. It is wise to alert the child protection agency, law enforcement, and prosecuting

Table 36-14. Inflicted versus Accidental Burns

	Inflicted	Accidental
History	Burns attributed to sibling	Compatible with observed injury
	Unrelated adult seeks medical care	
	Differing accounts of injury	
	Treatment delay >24 hr	
	Prior "accidents"	
	No parental concern	
	Lesion incompatible with history	
Location	Buttocks, perineum, genitalia	Front of body
	Ankles, wrists	Random and injury-specific
	Palms, soles	
Pattern	Sharply demarcated edges	Associated irregular splash burns
	Stocking-glove distribution	
	Full thickness	Partial thickness
	Symmetrical	Asymmetrical
	Burns older than history indicates	
	Burn neglected, infected	
	Numerous lesions of varying ages	One traumatic event
	Pattern of burn consistent with instrument	
	Large area of uniform, dry contact burn	

Table 36-15. Clinical Indicators of Abuse by Poisoning

Age
<1 yr or between 5 and 10 yr

History
Nonexistent, discrepant, or changing
Does not fit child's development
Previous poisoning in this child
Previous poisoning in siblings
Does not fit circumstances or scene
Third party, often a sibling, is blamed
Delay in seeking medical care

Toxin
Multiple toxins
Substances of abuse
Bizarre substances

Presentation
Unexplained seizures
Life-threatening events
Apparent sudden infant death syndrome
Death without obvious cause
Chronic unexplained symptoms that resolve when the child is protected
Other evidence of abuse or neglect

From Bays JA: Clinical indicators of abuse by poisoning. Personal communication.

Table 36-16. Munchausen Syndrome by Proxy (MSBP): Methods of Fabrication and Corresponding Diagnostic Strategies

Presentation	Method of Simulation and/or Production	Method of Diagnosis
Bleeding	1. Warfarin poisoning 2. Phenolphthalein poisoning 3. Exogenous blood applied 4. Exsanguination of child 5. Addition of other substances (paint, cocoa, dyes)	1. Toxicology screen 2. Diapers positive 3. Blood group typing (major and minor) ^{51}Cr labeling of erythrocytes 4. Mother caught in the act 5. Testing, washing
Seizures	1. Lying by offender 2. Poisoning Phenothiazines Hydrocarbons Salt Imipramine 3. Suffocation/carotid sinus pressure	1. Other MSBP features/retrospective 2. Analysis of blood, urine, IV fluid, milk 3. Witnessed Forensic photos of pressure points
Central nervous system depression	1. Drugs Lomotil Insulin Chloral hydrate Barbiturates Aspirin Diphenhydramine Tricyclic antidepressants Acetaminophen Hydrocarbons 2. Suffocation	1. Assays of blood, gastric contents, urine IV fluid; analysis of insulin type 2. See apnea and seizures
Apnea	1. Manual suffocation 2. Poisoning Imipramine Hydrocarbon 3. Lying by offender	1. Patient with pinch marks on nose Video camera (hidden) Mother caught Diagnosis of exclusion 2. Toxicology (gastric/blood) Chromatography of IV fluid 3. Diagnostic process of elimination
Diarrhea	1. Phenolphthalein/other laxative poisoning 2. Salt poisoning	1. Stool-diaper positive 2. Assay of formula/gastric contents
Vomiting	1. Emetic poisoning 2. Lying by offender	1. Assay for drug 2. Admit to hospital
Fever	1. Falsifying temperature 2. Falsifying chart	1. Careful charting, rechecking, urine temperature 2. Careful charting, rechecking Duplicating temperature chart in nursing station, urine temperature
Rash	1. Drug poisoning 2. Scratching 3. Caustics applied/painting skin	1. Assay 2. Diagnosis of exclusion 3. Assay/wash off

Modified from Rosenberg PA: Munchausen syndrome by proxy. In Reece RM (ed): Child Abuse: Medical Diagnosis and Management. Malvern, Pa, Lea & Febiger, 1994, pp 266-279.

attorney's office that such a case is being investigated and sometimes to involve them at the outset of the investigation. A child psychiatrist and child psychologist should be added to the team, and the hospital legal counsel, if not a member of the child protection team, should also attend the meetings.

Covert video surveillance is sometimes employed in these cases and should be done with the full understanding of the ward team, the hospital administration, and the legal department. There are arguments about the use of covert video surveillance, but those who favor its use argue that the goals of the hospital should be to render a diagnosis and to protect children; there are sometimes no options for collecting data except in this manner.

Extremely careful notes in the chart (or alternative record) are essential because the details are the most important ingredients in the formulation of the diagnosis. When the case comes to court, it is essential that all involved with the proceeding are prepared to present their information and are sure of their facts. The ultimate outcome of the child's well-being rests on this. Seldom does an opportunity occur to diagnose MSBP on a subsequent admission of the same child.

In studies examining the long-term outcome of MSBP, the victims of this form of child abuse almost uniformly fare poorly unless the diagnosis is made promptly and the child is removed from the custody and care of the perpetrator.

REFERENCES

General

Reece RM, Ludwig S (eds): Child Abuse: Medical Diagnosis and Management. Philadelphia. Lippincott Williams & Wilkins, 2001.
Visual Diagnosis of Child Abuse [CD-ROM]. Elk Grove Village, Ill, American Academy of Pediatrics, 2001.

Sexual Abuse

Adams JA: Classification of anogenital injuries: An evolving process. APSAC Advisor 1993;6:11-13.
Bays JA: Conditions mistaken for child sexual abuse. In Reece RM, Ludwig S (eds): Child Abuse: Medical Diagnosis and Management. Philadelphia, Lippincott Williams & Wilkins, 2001.
Committee on Child Abuse and Neglect: Shaken baby syndrome: Rotational cranial injuries—Technical report. Pediatrics 2001;108:206-210.
Ekman MAM: Kids' testimony in court: The sexual abuse crisis. In Edman P (ed): Why Kids Lie. New York: Scribner's, 1989.
Finkel MA, DeJong AR: Medical findings in child sexual abuse. In Reece RM, Ludwig S (eds): Child Abuse: Medical Diagnosis and Management. Philadelphia, Lippincott Williams & Wilkins, 2001.
Giardino AP, Finkel MA, Giardino ER, et al: A Practical Guide to the Evaluation of Sexual Abuse in the Prepubertal Child. Thousand Oaks, Calif, Sage Publications, 1992.
Heger A, Emans SJ: Evaluation of the Sexually Abused Child. New York, Oxford University Press, 2000.

Physical Abuse

DiScala C, Sege R, Li G, et al: Child abuse and unintentional injuries. Arch Pediatr Adolesc Med 2000;154:16-22.
Duhaime AC, Alario A, Lewander W, et al: Head injury in very young children: Mechanisms, injury types and ophthalmologic findings in 100 hospitalized patients younger than 2 years of age. Pediatrics 1992;90: 179-185.
Duhaime AC, Christian CU, Rorke LB, et al: Non-accidental head injury in children—The "shaken baby syndrome." N Engl J Med 1998;338: 1822-1829.
Hight DW, Bakalar H, Lloyd J: Inflicted burns in children. JAMA 1979;242:517-520.
Jenny C, Hymel KP, Ritzen A, et al: Analysis of missed cases of abusive head trauma. JAMA 1999;281:621-626.
Kempe CH: Sexual abuse, another hidden epidemic. Pediatrics 1978; 62:382-386.
Kleinman PK: Diagnostic Imaging of Child Abuse. St. Louis, Mosby, 1998.
Kleinman PK, Marks S, Blackbourne B: The metaphyseal lesion in abused infants: A radiologic and histopathologic study. AJR Am J Roentgenol 1986;146:895-905.
Ledbetter DJ, Hatch E, Feldman K, et al: Diagnostic and surgical implications of child abuse. Arch Surg 1988;123:1101-1105.
Levin AV: Retinal hemorrhages and child abuse. In David TJ (ed): Recent Advances in Pediatrics, vol 18. New York, Blakiston, 2000.
Merten DF, Radkowski M, Leonidas J: The abused child: A radiological reappraisal. Radiology 1983;146:377-383.
O'Connor JF, Cohen J: Dating fractures. In Kleinman PK (ed): Diagnostic Imaging of Child Abuse. St. Louis, Mosby, 1998.
Pascoe JM, Hildebrandt M, Tarrier A, Murphy M: Patterns of skin injury in nonaccidental and accidental injury. Pediatrics 1979;64:245-247.
Reece RM, Sege R: Childhood head injuries: Accidental or inflicted? Arch Pediatr Adolesc Med 2000;13:3-10.
Taylor D: Child abuse and the eye. Eye 1999;13:3-10.
Worlock T, Stower M, Barbor P: Patterns of fractures in accidental and non-accidental injury in children. A comparative study. BMJ 1986;293: 100-105.

NEUROSENSORY DISORDERS

37 Headaches in Childhood

Ajay Gupta   Bruce H. Cohen

Headaches are a common reason why children make a special visit to their physician's office or an emergency department. The term *headache* refers to a nonspecific symptom that consists of any pain or discomfort in the skull, face, facial structures, and pharynx. The pain from headaches affects the quality of life and is an important cause of lost time from school. A classification of headaches is noted in Table 37-1. A headache may also be the initial manifesting symptom of a serious medical condition (Tables 37-2 to 37-4).

PATHOPHYSIOLOGY

A headache is a result of referred pain from parts of the head and neck other than the brain, because no pain receptors exist in the brain. Intracranial structures that mediate pain include the dura, large arteries, and venous structures (venous sinuses). Extracranial structures that may mediate pain include the periosteum, pharynx, orbit, sinus, middle ear, teeth, and muscles of the neck, face, and head. The cranial structures are innervated by the fifth, ninth, and tenth cranial nerves. The upper cervical spinal cord roots innervate the structures of the posterior scalp and neck. Pain results from traction or inflammation of vessels or dura, dilatation of vessels, or sustained contraction of the scalp or neck muscles. Diseases of the extracranial structures (e.g., sinusitis) can cause headaches by referred pain.

DIAGNOSTIC APPROACH

Primary headaches (e.g., migraine headaches) do not have an identifiable cause. *Secondary headaches* are caused by intracranial or extracranial pathologic processes. The first step in evaluating a child with headache is to rule out a secondary headache, using a thorough history and physical examination combined with selective use of neuroimaging and laboratory tests. The second step, for the child with a primary headache, is to determine the specific primary headache syndrome (migraine, tension, or cluster headache) and the degree of headache-related disability.

HISTORY

An accurate history guides the physician toward the diagnosis. Because the description of aura and pain from classic migraine headaches is so typical, the physician can be confident of the diagnosis if the physical examination findings are normal (Table 37-5). Older children usually provide accurate details; parents need to assist younger children in providing the history.

The history should begin with a general medical history, which includes information about current illnesses, chronic medical problems, and past and current medications (Table 37-6). The next step is to define the headache pattern and the pain profile (Table 37-7; see Table 37-6). In most cases, a single phenotypic headache is present. If the patient has more than one type of headache, the physician must obtain a specific history for each type (Table 37-8). Patients should be questioned about the onset, the frequency, and the duration of the pain, as well as any changing patterns of headache frequency. The temporal pattern of headaches is useful in creating a differential diagnosis (Table 37-9). The severity of pain may be constant or may escalate through the duration of the headache. Special note should be made if the pain awakens the patient from sleep or if the headache is present when the patient wakes up in the morning, which may indicate increased intracranial pressure (ICP). Once the headache pattern has been defined, the physician should have a precise sense of the temporal pattern of the headaches.

The patient should be asked to describe the location of the pain (Figs. 37-1 to 37-3). If the pain is unilateral, it should be noted whether the pain is always on one side or on either side at different times (Table 37-10). The patient may be able to characterize the quality of the pain and to report whether the pain is sharp or dull and constant or throbbing.

It is important to determine the intensity of the discomfort; however, the clinician must be careful in determining how the intensity is ascertained. Pain is a subjective symptom with a significant emotional component that may be subject to the influences of age, culture, duration, and previous encounters with physicians. The intensity of the headache is not necessarily correlated with the seriousness of the disease. A patient may unintentionally exaggerate the description of the pain for attention. Likewise, the clinician should never dismiss the patient with a mild chronic headache as not having a serious medical problem. Headaches caused by brain tumors may initially be mild but persistent, whereas pain caused by muscle contraction headaches can be quite severe.

A common method for assessing the severity of pain is the "1-to-10 scale," in which the patient ranks the pain between 1 (mildest) and 10 (worst). This scale is most helpful for evaluating chronic headaches or for trying to determine the efficacy of treatment. In older patients, descriptive phrases, such as *mild, moderate, severe,* and *excruciating,* may suffice. In children who may have difficulty verbalizing the pain, the nine-face interval scale or the linear analog scale is more reliable (Fig. 37-4).

The family history is important because of the genetic component in some headaches, such as migraines and aneurysms (see Table 37-6). The patient should recall events around the onset of headaches, such as trauma, intake of particular foods or food additives (Table 37-11), physical activities (exertional headache), or presence of an aura (migraine). The clinician should note any symptoms that suggest neurologic dysfunction, such as hemiparesis, visual loss, ataxia, confusion, diplopia, scotomas, vertigo, and hemisensory phenomena. Response to medication can be helpful information, and the physician should ask about both over-the-counter medication and prescription medication, including medication that has not been prescribed for the patient. A response to medication may occur with primary or secondary causes of headache; a response is not diagnostic. For example, relief of an acute headache by a triptan (e.g., sumatriptan) is not diagnostic of migraine; triptans may be effective for other causes of headache. In patients with recurring headaches, a headache diary helps with the diagnosis and with the assessment of the efficacy of a particular therapy (see Table 37-8). Overuse of

Table 37-1. 1988 International Headache Society Classification

Migraine without Aura

1. At least five attacks fulfilling 2 to 4
2. Attacks last 2 to 72 hours
3. At least two of the following:
   Unilateral
   Pulsating
   Moderate to severe intensity
   Aggravated by routine physical activity
4. During headache at least one of the following:
   Nausea or vomiting
   Photophobia and phonophobia

Migraine with Aura

1. At least two attacks fulfilling 2
2. At least three or more of the following:
   One or more reversible symptoms indicating focal cerebral cortical or brainstem dysfunction
   At least one aura symptom develops gradually over 4 or more minutes, or two or more symptoms occur in succession
   No aura lasts more than 60 minutes
   Headache follows aura with a free interval of <1 hour
3. Typical auras include
   Homonymous visual disturbance
   Unilateral paresthesias
   Unilateral weakness
   Aphasia or other speech difficulty

Episodic Tension

1. At least 10 episodes fulfilling 2 to 4
2. Headache lasting 30 minutes to 7 days
3. Two or more of the following:
   Pressing/tightening quality
   Mild to moderate intensity
   Bilateral
   Not aggravated by routine activity
4. Both of the following:
   No nausea or vomiting
   Phonophobia or photophobia is absent

Chronic Tension Type

1. Average headache frequency >15 days/month for >6 months fulfilling 3 and 4 listed above for episodic tension

Headache Associated with Trauma

Headache Associated with Disorder of Sinuses or Other Facial or Cranial Structures

From Headache Classification Committee of the International Headache Society: Proposed classification and diagnostic criteria for headache disorders, cranial neuralgias, and facial pain. Cephalalgia 1988;8(Suppl 7):9-96.

Table 37-2. Differential Diagnosis of Headache

1. Vascular headache of migraine type
   a. Classic migraine
   b. Common migraine
   c. Cluster headache
   d. Hemiplegic and ophthalmoplegic migraine
   e. "Lower half" headache
2. Muscle-contraction (tension) headache
3. Combined headache: vascular and muscle-contraction
4. Headache of nasal vasomotor reaction
5. Headache of delusional, conversion or hypochondriacal states
6. Nonmigrainous vascular headaches
   a. Systemic infections
   b. Miscellaneous: hypoxic states, carbon monoxide poisoning, chemical vasodilator effects (e.g., nitrates), caffeine withdrawal, cerebral ischemia, postconcussion or postconvulsive states, "hangovers," hypoglycemia, hypercapnia, hypertensive states, pheochromocytoma
7. Traction headache
   a. Primary or metastatic tumors: meninges, brain, or vasculature
   b. Hematomas: epidural, subdural, parenchymal
   c. Abscesses: epidural, subdural, parenchymal
   d. Post–lumbar puncture headache
   e. Pseudotumor cerebri
8. Headache due to overt cranial inflammation
   a. Intracranial: meningitis, subarachnoid hemorrhage, iatrogenic (postoperative, postpneumoencephalogram, etc.), arteritis, phlebitis
   b. Extracranial: vasculitis, cellulitis
9. Ocular headache
   Increased intraocular pressure, ocular muscle contraction, trauma, tumor, inflammation
10. Aural headache
    Trauma, inflammation, infection, tumor of the ear
11. Nasal/sinus headache
    Allergic, infectious, inflammatory, traumatic, tumor of the nose and/or paranasal sinuses
12. Dental headache
    Infection, trauma, tumor, inflammation, iatrogenic
    Temporomandibular joint syndrome
13. Cranial/neck headache
    Disorders of cervical spine, cervical nerve roots, scalp/neck muscles, tendons, ligaments
14. Cranial neuritides
    Traction, trauma, inflammation, infection, tumor
15. Cranial neuralgia
    Trigeminal
    Glossopharyngeal

Chronic post-traumatic headache is often multifactorial, usually related to 1b, 2, and/or 13 above.

Adapted from the Ad Hoc Committee on Classification of headache, National Institute of Neurological Diseases and Blindness: Classification of headache. JAMA 1962;179:717-719.

analgesic medications by patients with a history of headaches can create a headache syndrome. All classes of headache medications can paradoxically cause headaches that may be worse on waking and exacerbated by activity. Stopping the medication improves the situation.

PHYSICAL EXAMINATION

Children with headache should have a thorough physical examination (Table 37-12). Many causes of headache, including some serious diseases early in their course, do not cause abnormal findings on physical examination (see Table 37-7). When the results of the neurologic examination are abnormal (Table 37-13), a structural brain lesion is possibly present, and a neuroimaging study is warranted.

NEUROIMAGING AND LABORATORY INVESTIGATIONS

There are various indications for ordering neuroimaging studies (Table 37-14). Magnetic resonance imaging (MRI) of the brain is the preferred study, although noncontrast computed tomographic (CT) scanning of the brain is useful in an emergency situation or when MRI is contraindicated. Routine blood work is not indicated in

Table 37-3. Systemic Infection in which Headache May Be a Prominent Symptom

Common Illness	Uncommon Illness	Uncommon, but Most Serious
Viremia	Typhoid fever	Meningitis (bacterial, viral)
Influenza	Tularemia	Brain abscess
Pharyngitis	Toxoplasmosis	Retropharyngeal abscess
Otitis media	Cytomegalovirus infection	Orbital cellulitis
Sinusitis	Mumps	Cervical osteomyelitis
Mononucleosis	Measles	Suppurative intracranial thrombophlebitis
Pneumococcal pneumonia	Poliomyelitis	Subdural empyema
Mycoplasma pneumonia	Psittacosis	Encephalitis
	Dengue	Septicemia
	Trichinosis	Endocarditis
	Q fever	Rocky Mountain spotted fever
	Legionnaires disease	Malaria
	Leptospirosis	
	Typhus	

Adapted from Reilly BM: Practical Strategies in Outpatient Medicine, 2nd ed. Philadelphia, WB Saunders, 1991, p 90.

patients with a history suggestive of a primary headache syndrome and normal findings in physical and neurologic examination. In some instances, findings in the history, physical examination, or neuroimaging dictate laboratory evaluation (Table 37-15).

SUDDEN SEVERE HEADACHE

A sudden and severe headache is alarming and usually prompts a visit to the physician. The diagnostic approach (see Fig. 37-5) is different than for the patient with recurrent headaches. The physician must note that every patient with migraines (and other non–life-threatening headaches) has a first severe headache. This headache may even be associated with an abnormal neurologic state, fever, or other worrisome features. Neuroimaging (see Table 37-14) and laboratory tests (see Table 37-15) may be indicated in the evaluation of an acute, severe headache. Additional indications for neuroimaging include an abnormal finding in a neurologic examination; reduced visual acuity; poor growth; neuroendocrine manifestations (galactorrhea, secondary amenorrhea); behavioral changes; seizures; increased headache frequency; and increased pain with awakening, coughing, straining, or position changes.

Table 37-4. Secondary Headache: Systemic and Metabolic Causes

Common	Uncommon
Hyperthyroidism	Carbon monoxide poisoning
Hypothyroidism	Toxic hemoglobinopathies
Anemia	Pheochromocytoma
Polycythemia	Parathyroid disease
Hypoxemia	Cushing disease
Hypercarbia	Addison disease
Hypoglycemia	Vitamin A intoxication
Hypertension	Lead poisoning
Uremia	Cranial neoplasm
Hyponatremia	Chronic leukemia-lymphoma
Pseudotumor cerebri	Subarachnoid
	hemorrhage–aneurysm
	Glaucoma
	Uveitis (iritis)

Adapted from Reilly BM: Practical Strategies in Outpatient Medicine, 2nd ed. Philadelphia, WB Saunders, 1991, p 111.

SPECIFIC HEADACHE DISORDERS

MUSCLE CONTRACTION (TENSION) HEADACHES

Most children and adolescents experience an occasional muscle contraction headache, usually in response to stress, exhaustion, or hunger (see Table 37-5 and Fig. 37-1). Frequent muscle contraction headaches, also called *tension headaches,* occur in about 15% of older children. Younger children may also have muscle contraction headaches; however, muscle contraction headaches do not cause persistent headaches in this age group. These headaches can be annoying, painful, and disabling. A muscle contraction headache often accompanies other headache disorders or is the end result of a migraine. In addition, structural cervical or cranial musculoskeletal abnormalities may cause muscle contraction (tension) headaches.

Clinical Features

These headaches have a typical pattern and are usually chronic and nonprogressing. Patients awaken feeling well, with the pain beginning gradually and escalating throughout the day. The pain is constant, squeezing, nonpulsatile, and located in a band extending from the front of the head, across the temples, and toward the occiput or neck (see Fig. 37-1). Nausea and photophobia may accompany these headaches but are not a constant feature. In patients with long-standing pain, the headaches can assume characteristics of migraines.

Chronic muscle contraction headaches are defined as headaches occurring at least 15 days a month for at least 6 months. Often, the child or adolescent has daily headaches. A detailed psychosocial history is important because it may uncover the cause for the headache. Adjustment disorders and depression may be either the primary cause or a secondary reaction to chronic pain. Sleep disturbances, school absences, and chronic analgesic use are common in this group. A negative psychosocial history can also occur in patients with chronic muscle contraction headaches. In some highly motivated and successful children, the headaches may be a reaction to the stress associated with achievement. In this instance, school attendance is usually perfect and the patient continues to achieve in all realms.

Patients with muscle contraction headaches have normal neurologic and physical findings except for tenderness along the affected muscles. These muscles often feel tight, and palpation can trigger the pain. There are no laboratory tests to diagnose these headaches.

Table 37-5. Clinical Features of Most Common Chronic Headache Syndrome

Feature	Classic Migraine	Common Migraine	Muscle Contraction
Prodrome	Visual or neurologic	None (or vague)	None
Quality	Throbbing, pulsatile	Throbbing	Tight, squeezing Sometimes throbbing
Location	Unilateral	Usually unilateral	Usually bilateral
Associated symptoms	Nausea, vomiting, photophobia	Usually nausea; anorexia	Depression
Usual duration	Several hours	Several hours	Highly variable
Usual frequency	Several per year	1–2 per month	Daily or several per week
Patient's typical response	Hibernates in dark room	"Sick"	Rarely interrupts usual activities
	Tries to sleep	Can't work	"I can live with it"
	Frightened by prodrome		

Modified from Reilly BM: Practical Strategies in Outpatient Medicine, 2nd ed. Philadelphia, WB Saunders, 1991, p 101.

Treatment

Patients usually do not seek the advice of a physician for the occasional muscle contraction headache because rest and over-the-counter analgesics (acetaminophen or ibuprofen) usually alleviate the pain. In contrast, patients with chronic, frequent headaches may require a multidisciplinary approach to their management. Some may benefit from physical therapy through the use of progressive range-of-motion exercises aimed at strengthening the neck muscles. Other patients may benefit from the assistance of a psychologist. Besides addressing underlying adjustment disorders, the psychologist can assist by teaching the patient stress management (relaxation techniques, biofeedback). It is important for the patient to realize that certain types of stress are normal. The patient needs to know that stress is not going to be eliminated and that he or she must learn to cope. To reduce stress, the daily schedule should be regulated, with a focus on exercise, proper diet, and sleep. Because caffeine, nicotine, and alcohol may contribute to the headaches, the patient should avoid using these drugs. If the headaches are affecting the activities of normal childhood and adolescence, individual therapy, family therapy, or both are warranted.

Over-the-counter analgesics are the most appropriate treatments for the occasional severe headache. Aspirin is contraindicated in children and teens because of the risk of Reye syndrome (see Chapter 40). Other medications (low-dose tricyclic antidepressants) for treating chronic headaches exist; however, the clinician must be careful to ensure that these medications are used properly and are not abused. Treating only the symptom and not the cause (stress) may actually prolong the patient's condition and expose the patient to the potential side effects of the medications. Benzodiazepines, narcotics, and barbiturates should be avoided because of their addictive potential, although these agents can be used rationally and successfully in

Table 37-6. Headache History

General Medical History

Presence of other acute medical problems or symptoms
Chronic medical problems
Current medication use or overuse
Previous medication used for headaches
Previous long-term medication use or overuse
Intake of caffeine, vitamin A, alcohol, cocaine

Pattern

When did the headaches begin?
Frequency and change in frequency
Duration of headaches
Pattern to the time of day
Presence of headaches on weekends, weekdays
Are headaches preceded by a warning?

Description of Pain

Location
Quality
Intensity
Effects of position, Valsalva maneuver, and movement

Associated Factors

Trauma
Are headaches associated with other activity?
Does any medication make the headache better?
Do the following occur before, during, or immediately after the headache: visual disturbance, vertigo, weakness, paresthesias, nausea, vomiting, changes in sensorium?

Family History

Migraines
Aneurysm (autosomal dominant polycystic kidney disease, inherited disorders of collagen synthesis)

Table 37-7. Headache Disorders with No Neurologic Signs

Headache Disorder	Pain Profile
Muscle contraction	CN, AI
Common migraine	AI, CN
Cluster	AI
Hypertension, uncomplicated	AI, CN
Fever	AS
Ice cream headache	AS
Anoxia	AS
Medication overuse	CN
Caffeine withdrawal	AS, AI
Coital headache	AS, AI
Early hydrocephalus or brain mass	CP
Cough headache, uncomplicated	AI
Meningitis, uncomplicated	AS
Sinusitis, dental or pharyngeal abscess	AI
Temporomandibular joint syndrome	CN
Postconcussive syndrome	CN
Conversion disorder	CN

AI, acute intermittent; AS, acute, singular (occurs only with the causative condition); CN, chronic nonprogressive; CP, chronic progressive.

Table 37-8. The Headache Diary for Recurring Headaches*

Date
Time of onset
Time of resolution
Maximum level of pain (mild, moderate, or severe, *or* 1-10)
Associated phenomena:
  Sleep
  Food
  Position, Valsalva maneuver
  Medication use or overuse

*If more than one type of headache exists, the types should be defined and labeled, and separate data should be recorded for each type.

the responsible patient who has infrequent and severe muscle contraction headaches. Ergot alkaloids should also be avoided because of their addictive properties and the high incidence of side effects in children. The calcium channel blockers and β blockers are helpful only if there is a significant migrainous component to the headache.

Some patients may benefit from prophylactic therapy. In these patients, a single, daily standard dose of ibuprofen, naproxen, or amitriptyline may prevent headaches. Amitriptyline given at dosages far below what is effective in the treatment of depression can have an excellent effect in preventing muscle contraction headaches.

Table 37-9. Differential Diagnosis of Headaches Based on the Time Course

New Acute Severe Headache

Viral syndrome
Acute sinusitis, pharyngitis
Migraine
Migraine variant
Meningoencephalitis
Intracranial hemorrhage
Head trauma
Brain tumor
Substance abuse (e.g., cocaine)
Medications
Carbon monoxide poisoning
Ventriculoperitoneal shunt malfunction
Hypertensive encephalopathy
Intracranial venous sinus thrombosis

Recurrent Acute Headaches

Migraine and migraine variants
Tension-type headache
Substance abuse
Medications
Postepileptic event
Cluster headaches
Intermittent raised intracranial pressure
  (e.g., from colloid cyst in the third ventricle)

Chronic Progressive Headaches

Hydrocephalus
Brain tumor
Intracranial infections (e.g., brain abscess, infection of the
  ventriculoperitoneal shunt, tuberculosis, cryptococcal
  meningitis)
Chronic subdural hematoma
Pseudotumor cerebri (benign intracranial hypertension)
Primary or secondary central nervous system vasculitis

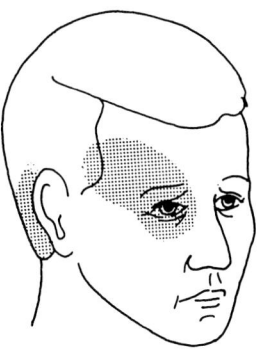
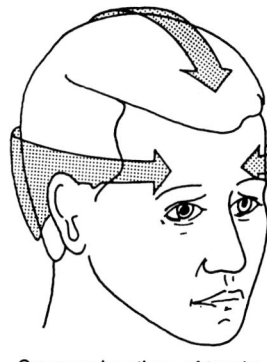

Common locations of migraine headache—tension headache may also be unilateral

Common locations of tension headache—migraine may occur in the same location

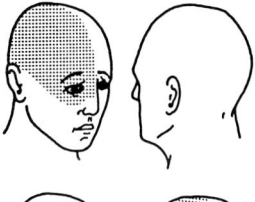
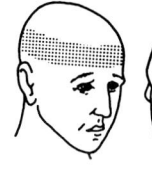
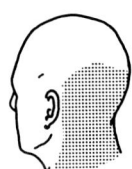

"Hatband" distribution

Occipital distribution

A **B**

Figure 37-1. Common location of migraine (**A**) and tension (**B**) headaches. (From Reilly BM: Practical Strategies in Outpatient Medicine, 2nd ed. Philadelphia, WB Saunders, 1991.)

Because amitriptyline can cause sleepiness, it is usually given as a single bedtime dose, ranging from 10 to 75 mg (adolescent age dose).

In patients with chronic headaches, overuse of analgesic medications may paradoxically produce headaches. These headaches are often difficult to distinguish from tension headaches but may be

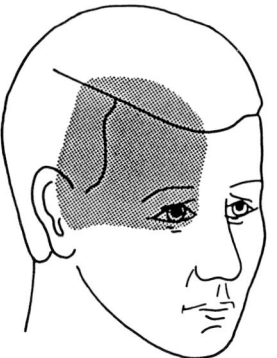
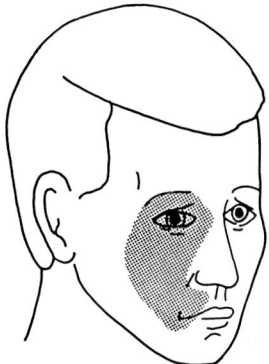

Ocular disease?
Frontal sinusitis?
Temporomandibular syndrome?
Temporal arteritis?
Tension headache?
Migraine?
Cluster?

Ocular disease?
Maxillary sinusitis?
Dental infection?
Allergic/vasomotor rhinitis?
Nasopharyngeal tumor?
Trigeminal neuralgia?
Migraine?
Cluster?

Figure 37-2. Periorbital headache. (From Reilly BM: Practical Strategies in Outpatient Medicine, 2nd ed. Philadelphia, WB Saunders, 1991.)

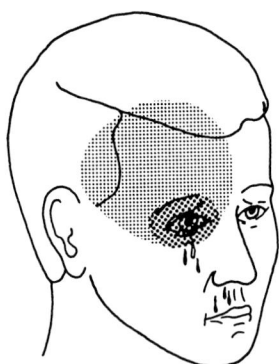

Periorbital or
frontotemporal
location is
usual

Tears and
nasal stuffiness,
often unilateral,
accompany the
headache

Duration is
usually brief
(1 hour)

Figure 37-3. Cluster headache. (From Reilly BM: Practical Strategies in Outpatient Medicine, 2nd ed. Philadelphia, WB Saunders, 1991.)

present on awakening or increase with physical activity. The treatment is to stop the medication.

MIGRAINE HEADACHES

Types of Migraines

Common and Classic Migraines

By 15 years of age, at least 5% to 10% of children have had a migraine headache (see Fig. 37-1 and Tables 37-1, 37-5, and 37-10). Migraine and migraine variants also occur in early childhood but at an unknown prevalence. The general description of this headache type usually makes the diagnosis straightforward. A family history of migraines and a history of motion (car) sickness are common in patients with migraines.

With a few exceptions, childhood migraines are very similar to those in adults. During childhood, migraines affect more boys than girls, which is contrary to the adult experience. In children, the headaches are less frequent, are shorter in duration, and respond better to treatment. Vomiting and abdominal pain are also more common in children than in adults. Of adults, 18% of women and 6% of men have migraines.

The pattern of migraines is highly variable. Migraines may be sporadic; however, they can also occur at almost any interval. Without prophylactic treatment, most patients have between 1 to 4 migraines a month. There is often no temporal pattern, although in some patients the headaches may cluster around a certain event. In postpubertal women, migraines may cluster around particular phases of the menstrual cycle. Unless the migraines tend to cluster, patients rarely have pure migraines more than twice a week. Mild or moderate headaches often occur between the more severe migraine attacks.

In the *classic migraine,* the headache is preceded by an aura, which is caused by vasoconstriction and diminished blood flow to the affected region of the brain. The aura associated with the classic migraine is visual and may consist of blurred vision, spreading scintillating scotomas, flashing lights, zigzag lines, and hemianopsia. These features should last less than 60 minutes. Sensory auras are less common than visual auras and consist of numbness or tingling, which may be followed by weakness. Transient hemiparesis (hemiplegic migraine), aphasia, and alteration of consciousness (confusional migraine) are rare auras. With *common migraines,* there is no specific aura; however, the patient may feel fatigued or ill immediately before the headache.

The onset of the pain is gradual and develops over minutes to an hour. Some patients, however, have a sudden onset of severe pain. Less severe migraines consist of a dull, constant pain. As the severity increases, the pain becomes throbbing. The headache is often unilateral but may be bilateral. The pain may be frontal or facial, instead of the more typical temporal location. As the headache proceeds, the pain can generalize to the entire cranium. In children with basilar artery migraines, the pain is occipital. Intense nausea and, less often, vomiting often accompany migraines. Skin pallor is also a common finding. Nasal congestion and tearing may occasionally be present.

Table 37-10. **Differential Diagnosis of Commonly Confused Chronic Unilateral Headache Syndromes**

Feature	Common Migraine	Cluster	Trigeminal Neuralgia	Temporomandibular Joint Syndrome	Tension*
Prodrome	None	None	None	None	None
Quality	Throbbing	Ache, severe	Sharp, "electric" jabs	Dull ache	Dull ache
Location	Hemicranial Periorbital	Periorbital	Cheek, jaw, lower lip	Preauricular, jaw spreading to temple, eye, and neck	Temple, occiput and neck
Associated symptoms	Nausea	Tearing; rhinorrhea	None	Limited jaw motion or "clicking"	Depression; muscle tightness
Usual duration	3-8 hours	½-2 hours	10-60 seconds, repetitively over 1-3 hrs	Several hours, or constant	Hours-days, constant
Usual frequency	1-2 per month	1-4 per day, during cluster†	Daily‡ but episodic	Daily‡	Daily‡
Patient's typical response	"Sick" Quiet	Paces the floor, agitated	Avoids trigger points	Depression Teeth grinding	Depression, coping

Modified from Reilly BM: Practical Strategies in Outpatient Medicine, 2nd ed. Philadelphia, WB Saunders, 1991, p 102.

*Tension headache is usually bilateral but may be confused with these syndromes when unilateral.

†A typical cluster will last several weeks.

‡Frequency of these syndromes is highly variable, but daily occurrence is common.

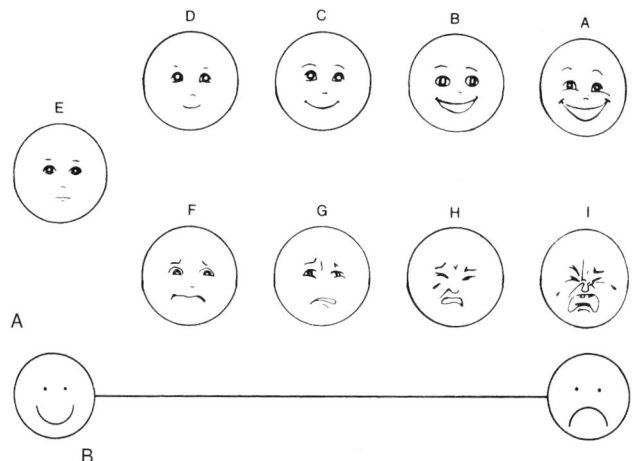

Figure 37-4. Assessing pain in young children. **A,** Nine-face interval scale. Faces A through D represent varying magnitudes of positive affect; faces F through I represent varying magnitudes of negative affect. **B,** Linear analog scale. The child places an X on the line to identify the relative severity of headache. (Adapted from Beyer JE, Wells N: The assessment of pain in children. Pediatr Clin North Am 1989;36:846.)

Because most patients are sensitive to motion, light, and noise during a migraine attack, they search for a dark and quiet place to sleep. The patient usually awakens within 2 to 12 hours feeling fatigued but usually pain free.

Certain factors are known to trigger migraine attacks in susceptible patients. Patients need to be questioned about the temporal association of their migraines with these factors because eliminating the precipitant may prevent some or all of the migraines. The most common identified precipitants to migraines are specific foods and food additives, such as chocolate, hard cheeses, onions, yeast, and beans (see Table 37-11). Because caffeine withdrawal can precipitate

Table 37-11. Possible Dietary Precipitants of Migraine

Ripened cheeses (cheddar, Emmentaler, Stilton, Brie, Camembert, brick, blue, Swiss, Gouda, Roquefort, mozzarella, Parmesan, provolone, Romano)	Fermented sausage and aged, canned, cured, or processed meats (bologna, salami, pepperoni, summer sausage, hot dogs), bacon
Pickled herring	Canned soups with monosodium glutamate
Chocolate	Pizza
Anything fermented, pickled, or marinated	Hot fresh yeast breads, coffee cake, doughnuts, sourdough bread
Olives, pickles	Chicken livers
Sour cream, yogurt, buttermilk, chocolate milk	Brewer's yeast, meat tenderizers, seasoned salt
Sauerkraut, onions	Citrus foods
Sunflower seeds	Tea, coffee, cola
Nuts, peanut butter	Banana
Beans, except string beans	Foods containing large amounts of monosodium glutamate (Chinese foods)
Avocados, figs, raisins, papaya, passion fruit, red plums	Corn
Alcoholic beverages	Egg

Data from Diamond S, et al., Modern Medicine, July 1986, pp 76-86; and Mansfield LE: Food allergy and headache. Whom to evaluate and how to treat. Postgrad Med 1988;83:46. Reprinted from Reilly BM: Practical Strategies in Outpatient Medicine, 2nd ed. Philadelphia, WB Saunders, 1991, p 116.

Table 37-12. Important Components of the Physical Examination in the Child with Headaches

General Examination

Airway, breathing, circulation, and blood pressure
Growth, including head circumference
Mental status, behavior profile
Head, neck, eye, ear, nose, and throat examination for swelling, tenderness, trauma, or infection
Dental examination
Skin examination for rashes, neurocutaneous lesions, pallor
Evidence of external trauma
External bleeding, petechia

Neurologic Examination

Meningeal signs
Fundus, eye movements, and pupillary reaction
Facial asymmetry
Motor strength in all extremities
Deep tendon reflexes
Gait
Romberg sign
Cerebellar signs (e.g., finger-to-nose test, rapid alternating movements, and action tremors)
Palpation of shunt track if ventriculoperitoneal shunt present

a migraine attack, all caffeinated beverages should be avoided. Some of the food additives that may trigger a migraine are sulfites, nitrites, and monosodium glutamate (MSG). MSG is found in Chinese-style foods, canned and dehydrated soups, proprietary spices (seasoned salts), salad bars, and many packaged foods. Because food additives are commonly used in the food industry, susceptible patients are advised to read all labels. Aside from foods, other precipitants include menstruation, hunger, estrogen (oral contraceptives), lack of sleep, stress, heat, and exertion.

Some patients with migraines are extremely sensitive to exertion, especially on hot days. Their headaches may be precipitated by strenuous activities, such as summer practice sessions for varsity sports or a marching band. The headaches may be prevented by proper dress and prophylactic indomethacin therapy.

Complicated Migraine

Patients with a complicated migraine have neurologic deficits that persist during and after the headache. These deficits include hemisensory symptoms, hemiparesis, aphasia, visual loss, and alteration in consciousness. In most cases, the neurologic deficit precedes the headache. These symptoms usually last about as long as the headache but can last for days. Permanent neurologic deficits are rare but can occur if the vasoconstriction is severe and causes infarction.

Complicated migraines begin in childhood and evolve into the more typical migraine pattern as the patient gets older. In some children with this disorder, their attacks are precipitated by mild head trauma, such as striking the head against a wall or using the head to hit a soccer ball.

Two genetic disorders may mimic complicated migraine. Autosomal dominant familial hemiplegic migraine and episodic ataxia type 2 are caused by mutations of a neuronal calcium channel. Patients may present with hemiplegic migraine, episodic ataxia, or both. Acetazolamide is effective in treating this disorder. MELAS (mitochondrial encephalopathy, lactic acidosis, and strokelike attacks) is a mitochondrially inherited disorder, with a high frequency of hemiplegic migraine-like attacks. Recovery from attacks is variable. This diagnosis must be considered in children with coexisting epilepsy, mental retardation or regression, and myopathy. A DNA

Table 37-13. Headache Disorders Associated with Neurologic Signs

Headache Disorder	Pain Profile	Neurologic Sign
Complicated migraine	AI	Hemiparesis, aphasia, paresthesia, hemianopsia
Basilar artery migraine	AI	Ataxia, visual disturbance, vertigo, tinnitus, paresthesia
Acute confusional migraine	AI	Alteration in sensorium, stupor, agitation, fugue state
Ophthalmoplegic migraine	AI	Paresis of eye movement, dilated pupil, ptosis
Vasculitis	CP, AI	Seizure, changes in sensorium
Brain neoplasm or mass	CP	Papilledema, focal deficit
Hydrocephalus	CP, AI	Papilledema, bilateral sixth nerve palsies, increased motor tone, impaired upward gaze and Parinaud syndrome
Pseudotumor cerebri	CP	Papilledema, constricted visual fields, enlarged blind spot
Subarachnoid hemorrhage, ruptured aneurysm	AS	Changes in sensorium, focal neurologic signs, meningismus
Subdural or epidural hemorrhage	CP	Focal neurologic signs, papilledema, changes in sensorium
Sagittal sinus thrombosis	AS	Papilledema, focal neurologic deficits, changes in sensorium, seizures
Meningitis; encephalitis	AS	Papilledema, focal neurologic deficits, changes in sensorium, seizures
Optic neuritis	AS	Papillitis, decreased visual acuity, afferent pupillary defect

AI, acute intermittent; AS, acute, singular (occurs only with the causative condition); CP, chronic progressive.

test for the most common mitochondrial mutation is available. Migraines are also common in a variety of other mitochondrial disorders.

Basilar Artery Migraine

The basilar artery is more prone to involvement in childhood migraines, which leads to brainstem or occipital lobe dysfunction. The headache is usually occipital and may be intense. Neurologic abnormalities include ataxia, nausea, and vomiting. In some patients, the headache may be a minor component of the syndrome. Visual changes can also occur and can include vivid visual images. Vertigo, tinnitus, and paresthesia are less common symptoms that accompany a basilar artery migraine.

Table 37-14. Role of Neuroimaging Studies

When to Order a Neuroimaging Study

The "thunderclap headache" or "worst headache of my life"
The first severe headache
Abnormal neurologic findings
Chronic or progressive headaches
Unilateral headaches that never alternate sides
Headache associated, even briefly, with alteration of sensorium
Presence of papilledema
Meningeal signs without fever
Recent worsening

Advantages of Magnetic Resonance Imaging (MRI)

Most vascular malformations are detected
Accurate detection of tumors in temporal lobes and posterior fossa, and small tumors that obstruct CSF flow (quadrigeminal plate and third ventricular)
Paranasal sinuses usually included in the examination without special request
More sensitive for detecting transependymal CSF in cases of borderline hydrocephalus
Diagnostic for Chiari malformations
Magnetic resonance angiography can detect many aneurysms
Magnetic resonance venography can detect cortical vein and dural sinus thrombosis

Advantages of Computed Tomography

Less expensive and easier access than MRI
Shorter imaging time, important in evaluating ill patients
May be used in patients with pacemakers, metal implants (surgical clips), and cosmetic tattoos (MRI may turn off pacemakers and dislodge the clips; tattoos distort the image)

CSF, cerebrospinal fluid.

Table 37-15. Potentially Useful Laboratory Tests in Children with Headaches

Laboratory Test	Possible Cause of Headache
Complete blood count	Infection (elevated white blood cell count); bleeding diathesis (thrombocytopenia); anemia
CSF examination	Infection, vasculitis, pseudotumor cerebri, subarachnoid hemorrhage after CT is normal
Toxicology screen	Substance abuse
Hypercoagulation panel	Unexplained venous sinus thrombosis
ESR, ANA, ANCA	Vasculitis
Genetic tests	Familial hemiplegic migraine, MELAS
EEG	Seizure disorder
VP shunt radiographic series	Malfunctioning VP shunt

ANA, antinuclear antibody; ANCA, antineutrophil cytoplasmic antibodies; CSF, cerebrospinal fluid; CT, computed tomography; EEG, electroencephalogram; ESR, erythrocyte sedimentation rate; MELAS, mitochondrial encephalomyopathy, lactic acidosis, and strokelike symptoms; VP, ventriculoperitoneal.

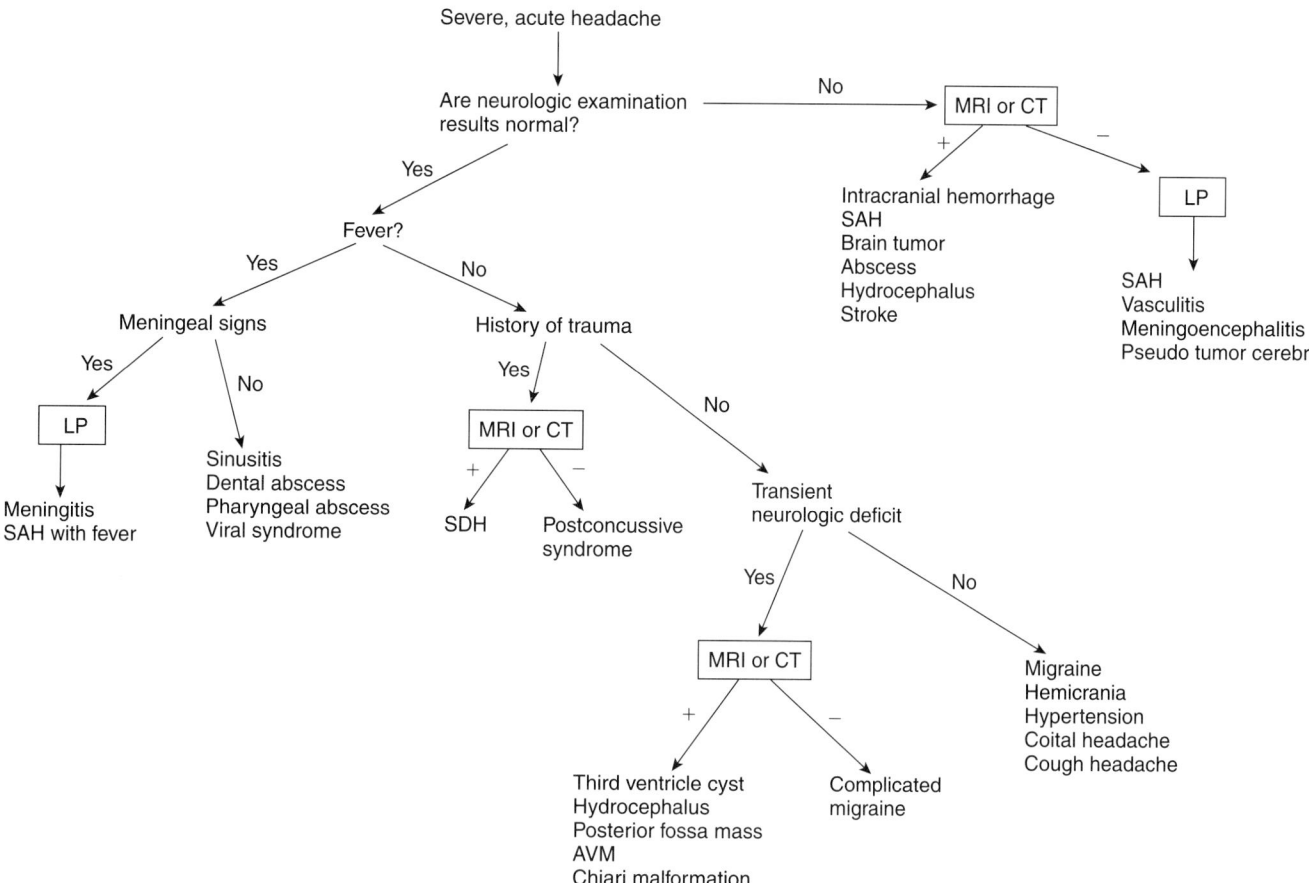

Figure 37-5. Evaluation of an acute, severe headache. *Boxes* indicate tests. AVM, arteriovenous malformation; CT, computed tomography; LP, lumbar puncture; MRI, magnetic resonance imaging; SAH, subarachnoid hemorrhage; SDH, subdural hematoma.

Acute Confusional Migraine

This disorder begins after 5 years of age and usually converts to typical migraine as the patient gets older. Acute confusional migraine begins with an alteration in consciousness, which can include varying degrees of lethargy, agitation, and stupor. A fugue-like state has also been described with these migraines. Attacks last a few hours, with the child eventually falling asleep. The child awakens without memory of the incident.

Ophthalmoplegic Migraine

Cranial nerve palsies, usually of the third cranial nerve, may accompany this type of a migraine. Physical findings usually include pupillary dilatation and ptosis. Other cranial nerves involved during these headaches are the fourth cranial nerve (causing loss of downward and medial eye movement) and the sixth cranial nerve (causing loss of lateral eye movement). The ophthalmoplegia may persist for a few weeks after the headache. In younger children, a headache may not be associated with this disorder. An MRI study is warranted because ophthalmoplegia, even if transient, is associated with serious conditions, such as aneurysms and tumors.

Amaurosis fugax (ophthalmic transient ischemia) manifests as monocular visual loss lasting minutes; in childhood, it is often caused by migraines.

Migraine Status

Most migraines last 6 to 12 hours; however, some patients are susceptible to prolonged headaches. A prolonged headache may last for days and is usually associated with protracted vomiting and dehydration. Diagnosis is based on a propensity for previous prolonged migraine attacks.

Treatment of Migraines

Treatment can help most patients with migraine headaches. If precipitating factors can be identified, they should be avoided. If medication is necessary, the physician and patient must decide whether the goal is to prevent the migraines (prophylactic management) or to stop or lessen the headache once it starts (abortive management). The choice of treatment depends on the age of the patient and the frequency and severity of the headaches.

Abortive Management

Abortive management is most effective when medication is taken as soon as possible. Children may need to be able to take the medication at school. If abortive therapy is used, the medication should be taken at the first symptom, whether it is the aura or the headache. The characteristics of the headache dictate the therapeutic decision making: Patients with less severe symptoms may respond to non-steroidal antiinflammatory drugs (NSAIDs). In contrast, patients with more severe symptoms do not need to "fail" a trial of NSAIDs before taking more effective medications. This only prolongs patient suffering and school absences, increases dissatisfaction with the physician, and leads to poor utilization of resources, with frequent emergency room and office visits. Patients with significant nausea or emesis may not tolerate an oral agent.

Table 37-16 outlines a general approach for the acute treatment of childhood migraine. NSAIDs, such as ibuprofen or naproxen sodium, are useful for mild to moderate migraine. There are two principal benefits of adding a dopamine antagonist such as metoclopramide. First, it reduces nausea and emesis. Second, its prokinetic action improves the rate of absorption of concurrent medication, leading to faster headache relief. Metoclopramide may cause drowsiness and extrapyramidal symptoms, which are mostly transient and reversible with benzodiazepines or diphenhydramine. Other agents that combat nausea in migraine include prochlorperazine, diphenhydramine, and trimethobenzamide. The rectal form of trimethobenzamide is useful in children with intractable emesis during a migraine. If possible, patients should rest and try to fall asleep. Sleep relieves symptoms, and many patients awaken free of pain.

The combination of isometheptene mucate, dichloralphenazone, and acetaminophen (Midrin), may be used in moderate migraine. The combination of aspirin, the barbiturate butalbital, and caffeine (Fiorinal) is another treatment option.

The triptans are selective agonists of the serotonin (5-HT) receptors, mainly receptor subtypes 5-HT_{1B} and 5-HT_{1D}. Triptans are highly effective for the treatment of migraine. A wide variety of preparations are available, with different pharmacologic properties (Table 37-17). The subcutaneous (SC) form of sumatriptan is ideal for rapid-onset migraine that is associated with nausea and emesis, which precludes oral medication. Oral sumatriptan has a slower onset of action than the SC form; the onset of action of the intranasal spray is intermediate between those of the oral and SC forms. Sumatriptan also relieves migraine-associated symptoms such as nausea, emesis, photophobia, and sonophobia.

Adverse effects of sumatriptan are uncommon in children. Atypical sensations such as tingling and numbness over body parts; anxious feeling; sensations of heaviness or tightness of the chest and throat; and feeling of warmth, burning, cold, or pressure are symptoms reported by patients after taking triptans and are therefore referred to as "triptan symptoms." The symptoms are generally mild and always transient, with resolution within 1 to 2 hours. They are more common and intense with sumatriptan than with newer triptans. The reported incidences in adults are 42% with SC sumatriptan

and 8% with oral sumatriptan. The incidence in children appears to be lower. Minor pain, erythema, or tingling is also common at the injection site after SC sumatriptan. Some children may report a bad taste after intranasal sumatriptan. Cardiovascular adverse effects are rare; the incidence of coronary vasospasm and cardiac ischemia appears to be about one per million doses. Nevertheless, caution should be exercised in children with underlying heart disease, and the presence of coronary insufficiency is a contraindication. Other conditions that are contraindications to the use of 5-HT_1 agonists are hypertension, peripheral vascular disease, and pregnancy. Neurologic vascular events have been reported only rarely in adults and are caused mostly by treatment of a misdiagnosed stroke in evolution. Some patient with complicated migraines may be at increased risk of developing cerebrovascular events, and therefore it is imperative that proper diagnosis of the migraine syndrome is made before 5-HT_1 agonists are considered. Triptans and other vasoconstrictive agents are generally contraindicated in complicated migraine episodes such as hemiplegic migraine, basilar migraine, ophthalmoplegic migraine, and migraine attacks associated with other neurologic abnormalities. The second-generation triptans rizatriptan and zolmitriptan have several potential advantages over sumatriptan: They have better oral bioavailability, more rapid onset of action after an oral dose, increased central nervous system penetration, a longer duration of action with a lower rate of headache recurrence, and a decreased incidence and severity of "triptan symptoms."

Dihydroergotamine (DHE) is a nonselective 5-HT_1 agonist, with affinity for 5-HT_1, 5-HT_2, 5-HT_3, adrenergic, and dopaminergic receptors. Common adverse effects of DHE are nausea, emesis, abdominal pain, diarrhea, and leg cramps. DHE is available in intravenous, intramuscular, and intranasal preparations. The intravenous form is recommended for use in severe prolonged migraine and is the treatment of choice for status migrainosus. Metoclopramide or prochlorperazine can be used with intravenous DHE to ameliorate nausea and emesis. Intranasal DHE is an effective alternative to triptans for treatment of acute migraine. DHE is contraindicated in children with peripheral vascular disease and heart disease with coronary insufficiency; it should not be used concurrently with triptans or other vasoconstrictor agents.

Table 37-16. Stratification of Acute Childhood Migraine into Four Treatment Groups*

Mild/Moderate Attack with No or Mild Nausea	Moderate Attack with Nausea, with or without Vomiting	Severe Attack with Debilitating Symptoms	Severe Intractable Attack >72 Hours (Status Migrainosus)
Oral NSAID Oral metoclopramide	Children >12 years Oral isometheptene mucate–dichloralphenazone–acetaminophen (Midrin) Oral/intranasal sumatriptan Oral/MLT rizatriptan Oral zolmitriptan Intranasal DHE Rectal or oral antiemetics Children <12 years NSAID Rectal or oral antiemetics	Children >12 years SC sumatriptan Intranasal/oral sumatriptan MLT/oral rizatriptan Intranasal DHE Rectal or oral antiemetics May add naproxen (Naprosyn) for longer attack Children <12 years IV metoclopramide IV diphenhydramine or rectal prochlorperazine IV/oral NSAID IV hydration	Children >6 years IV DHE IV metoclopramide IV ketorolac IV diphenhydramine IV prochlorperazine (>50 kg) IV hydration Children <6 years IV DHE May use drugs similar to severe attack Other options IV steroids IV valproate IV magnesium sulfate (no pediatric experience for valproate or magnesium)

Modified from Gupta A, Rothner AD: Treatment of childhood headaches. Curr Neurol Neurosci Rep 2001;1:144-155.

*One or a combination (preferably with different mechanisms of action) of drugs may be chosen from one treatment group depending on the clinical circumstances. Only one 5-HT agonist or vasoconstrictor agent should be used during an episode.

DHE, dihydroergotamine; IV, intravenous; MLT, orally disintegrating tablets; NSAID, nonsteroidal antiinflammatory drug.

Table 37-17. Selective 5-HT Agonists in Childhood Migraine

Drug	Route	Onset of Action (min)	T½ (hr)	Bio-availability (%)	Dose for 30-50 kg (age, approx. 12-17 yr)		Dose for >50 kg		Comments
					Initial	*Max/24 hr*	*Initial*	*Max/24 hr*	
Sumatriptan	Oral	30	2-3	15	25 mg	50 mg	50 mg	100 mg	Watch for "triptan
	Nasal	15	2-3	20	5-10 mg	10-20 mg	20 mg	40 mg	symptoms"
	SC	10	2-3	90	0.1 mg/kg	Repeat × 1	6 mg	12 mg	especially with SC form. Nasal is 5 and 20 mg/spray
Rizatriptan	Oral	30	3	50	5 mg	10 mg	5-10 mg	10-20 mg	
	MLT	30	3	50	5 mg	10 mg	5-10 mg	10-20 mg	MLT form dissolves in mouth
Zolmitriptan	Oral	45	3	40	2.5 mg	5 mg	2.5-5 mg	10 mg	

Modified from Gupta A, Rothner AD: Treatment of childhood headaches. Curr Neurol Neurosci Rep 2001;1:144-155.

The physician must be aware that drug-dependent states can develop, even with nonnarcotic medications. Therefore, medication use must be monitored carefully. If a patient is using analgesics more than 1 day a week, abortive management should be considered unsuccessful and should be abandoned.

Prophylactic Management

For children with frequent migraines (every 1 to 2 weeks), daily medication is a more appropriate choice (Table 37-18). The most commonly used prophylactic medications are β blockers, amitriptyline, and cyproheptadine. The goal is to prevent as many headaches as possible at a dose that has tolerable side effects. Medication should be started at a low dose to minimize sedation and other adverse effects. The dose should be increased every 1 to 2 weeks if the headaches are not controlled. If intolerable side effects develop, the medication should be tapered and another begun in its place.

In the younger patient, cyproheptadine (an antihistamine with serotonin antagonist properties) should be the first choice because it is very well tolerated. The major side effects are excessive appetite and weight gain; this drug may not be acceptable to teenagers. Dose escalation is usually in 1- to 2-mg increments every 1 to 2 weeks.

β Blockers (e.g., propranolol) are second-line medications and are generally well tolerated. The major dose-limiting effects include fatigue, weight gain, and cardiovascular β blockade. Because of these effects, this medication can interfere with the lifestyle of active teenagers and athletes. This group of medications is an excellent choice if the headaches are controlled at a dose below that which causes β blockade. Dose escalation of propranolol is usually in weekly increments of 10 to 20 mg. Long-acting (sustained-release) preparations are available once the headaches are controlled.

Amitriptyline, a tricyclic antidepressant with serotonin antagonist properties, is usually a good choice for teenagers with migraines. In addition to controlling migraines, amitriptyline is also effective against mixed migraine–tension headache disorders. Because of the sedative properties of amitriptyline, a single daily bedtime dose is usually administered. The starting dose is 10 mg at bedtime, with dose escalation of 10 mg every 1 to 2 weeks until adequate control is achieved. Dose-limiting side effects include dry mouth, weight gain, fatigue, and constipation. Most older patients cannot tolerate more than 75 mg a day. A pretreatment electrocardiogram should be obtained because tricyclic antidepressants prolong the QT interval. This medication should not be prescribed if a prolonged QT interval is found because it may precipitate severe ventricular arrhythmias (torsades de pointes) that are refractory to treatment.

CLUSTER HEADACHES

Cluster headaches rarely occur before adolescence but are common in young adults and are more common in men than in women (see Fig. 37-3). Episodes of pain are intermittent, with long periods of remission; hence the name "cluster." Cluster pain is localized to the eyes and temples but can spread to other parts of the head. The pain begins suddenly and rapidly increases to an excruciating level; patients may think they are dying and plead for relief at any cost. Patients find it impossible to rest, and they become agitated and restless during an attack. They may yell, scream, pace around, or bang their head against the wall. This is in sharp contrast to a migraine attack where the patient is quiet and withdraws to a dark cool room for sleep. Most cluster headaches last 30 minutes to 2 hours. The headaches occur in bouts lasting from 4 to 8 weeks, with one or two bouts occurring a year. During these periods, alcohol should be avoided because it can precipitate a headache. Cluster headaches are more common in smokers. Lacrimation, rhinorrhea, sweating, and nasal stuffiness usually accompany the headache. These headaches usually occur at a particular time of day, most occurring at night.

The management of cluster headaches is directed at both the prophylaxis of headaches during clusters and the treatment of acute headache. The acute headache responds to oxygen inhalation, subcutaneous sumatriptan, or parenteral DHE. A short course of steroids may help induce a prompt remission. Prophylactic agents include verapamil, lithium, prednisone, and methysergide.

VASCULITIS HEADACHES

Vasculitis is an important cause of headaches in adults, although in children it rarely manifests as headaches. Instead, the headaches may be part of the constellation of symptoms associated with this illness. Because of the increased risk of systemic hypertension in patients with vasculitis, it is important to include a blood pressure measurement as part of the complete history and physical examination. When systemic lupus erythematosus and mixed connective tissue disorders affect the central nervous system, children often have seizures and mental status changes. These changes can occur with or without headaches.

HYPERTENSION-RELATED HEADACHES

Systemic hypertension, both acute and chronic, may be associated with headaches. The pain is probably caused by alterations in the regulation of cerebral blood flow. Acute hypertension typically

Table 37-18. Medications for Migraine Prophylaxis in Children

Class	Medication	Efficacy/Side Effects*	Dose	Contraindications (C/I) and Common Side Effects (SE)	Comments/Precautions
β Blockers	Propranolol	4+/2+	<35 kg: 10-20 mg t.i.d. >35 kg: 20-40 mg t.i.d. Max: 160-240 mg/day	C/I: asthma, heart failure, and heart block SE: depression, decreased athletic performance, hypotension	Do not stop abruptly Sustained-release preparation
Tricyclic antidepressants	Amitriptyline	4+/2+	Start 5-10 mg q.h.s., increase to 5 mg/kg/day Max dose, 100-150 mg/day	C/I: glaucoma, seizures, cardiac disorders SE: sedation, anticholinergic symptoms, arrhythmias	May obtain ECG before starting treatment; do not stop abruptly, especially when on high doses for long time Monitor ECG, heart rate, and blood pressure
	Nortriptyline	4+/2+	Start 10 mg q.h.s. Max dose, 50-75 mg/day	Similar to those for amitriptyline Less sedating	Similar to those for amitriptyline
Calcium channel blockers	Verapamil	2+/1+	4-10 mg/kg/day in 3 divided doses Max adult dose, 480 mg/day	C/I: heart failure, heart block SE: constipation, hypotension	Sustained-release preparation available
Antiepileptic drugs	Valproate	4+/2+	10-30 mg/kg/day in 2 or 3 divided doses Higher doses may be needed	C/I: hepatic disease SE: liver toxicity, thrombocytopenia, pancreatitis, nausea, sedation, alopecia, weight gain	Monitor LFT and CBC at start and periodically
Antiserotonin	Cyproheptadine	2+/1+	Start 2 mg q.h.s. Max doses, 2-6 yr: 12 mg/day in 3 divided doses 7-16 yr: 20 mg/day in 3 divided doses	C/I: asthma, glaucoma, gastrointestinal or genitourinary obstruction SE: increased appetite and weight gain	Morning doses may cause school-time sedation
NSAIDs	Naproxen (Naprosyn)	2+/2+	5-20 mg/kg/dose q8-12h Max dose, 1250 mg/day for 2-4 weeks	C/I: Gastrointestinal bleeding, ulcer disease SE: platelet dysfunction, tinnitus	For prompt relief while other agent is being introduced
Vitamins	Riboflavin	2+/−	100-400 mg/day	SE: Hypersensitivity, yellow discoloration of urine	Administer with food

Modified from Gupta A, Rothner AD: Treatment of childhood headaches. Curr Neurol Neurosci Rep 2001;1:144-155.

*Efficacy and potential for side effects of medications are rated on a scale of 1+ to 5+. − is no side effect.

CBC, complete blood cell count; ECG, electrocardiogram; LFT, liver function tests; NSAID, nonsteroidal antiinflammatory drug.

occurs in a child with post-streptococcal glomerulonephritis, renal failure, or collagen-vascular disease. Although hypertension is an uncommon cause of headaches in children, the diagnosis of hypertension is straightforward, and treatment of the hypertension alleviates the headaches (see Chapter 12). Many patients with hypertension have no headaches.

Headaches can be part of malignant hypertension syndrome, in which case retinal exudates and microscopic hematuria are usually present. Severe hypertension can also cause an intracerebral hemorrhage. Use of cocaine causes headaches through various mechanisms, including hypertension, vasoconstriction, hypersensitivity vasculitis, and subarachnoid hemorrhage.

FEVER-RELATED HEADACHES

Headaches are common in febrile patients, regardless of the source of the fever (see Table 37-3). The pain is usually bifrontal and bitemporal but may also involve the occiput and neck. The pain may be throbbing and may increase with neck flexion. Any abnormalities seen during the neurologic examination (nuchal rigidity, altered mental status) suggest that factors other than fever may be the source of the headache and must be evaluated.

ICE CREAM HEADACHES

This common headache affects about 33% of children and 90% of patients with migraines. This disorder occurs more in the summer. Within 30 seconds of quickly ingesting a cold drink or ice cream, a severe, boring pain develops deep inside the head. The pain lasts for only several seconds to a minute. Once this condition is recognized as such, no further evaluation or treatment is necessary.

CHRONIC PAROXYSMAL HEMICRANIA

Chronic paroxysmal hemicrania consists of frequent and intense unilateral headaches (see Table 37-9). This disorder is much more common in women than in men. Although it usually begins in adulthood, chronic paroxysmal hemicrania can affect older children and adolescents. The average headache lasts about 10 minutes (range, a few minutes to 45 minutes). Patients can have as many as 10 to 20 attacks a day, and the pain can awaken the patient from sleep. Sudden head movement can also precipitate an attack.

This headache responds dramatically to indomethacin therapy. Relief of symptoms occurs within a few days of beginning the medication. Other NSAIDs are of no benefit. Because the symptoms of chronic paroxysmal hemicrania are similar to those of vascular malformations of the brain, a neuroimaging study should be performed to rule out these malformations before the diagnosis of chronic paroxysmal hemicrania is made.

ANOXIA AND CARBON MONOXIDE HEADACHES

Anoxia, hypoxia, and carbon monoxide poisoning may produce headaches through dilatation of cerebral arteries, which in turn causes an increase in cerebral blood flow. In children with illnesses that predispose them to hypoxia (chronic lung disease, obstructive sleep apnea), treatment should be directed at alleviating the source of the hypoxia. High altitudes can also lead to an acute hypoxic state, in which case symptoms can be treated with altitude descent, acetazolamide, and dexamethasone.

Low-level carbon monoxide poisoning should be suspected in any child with chronic headaches. The diagnosis is difficult to confirm with an arterial hemoglobin carbon monoxide (HgCO) level because the half-life of HgCO in room air is only 4 hours. Hence, the level may be normal only a few hours after exposure. One way of diagnosing and treating this condition is removing the cause of the exposure. Some sources of carbon monoxide exposure are heavy urban traffic in which the patient is a car passenger; methylene dichloride paint strippers; kerosene space heaters; a gasoline engine running in an attached garage; cigarette smoking; and faulty home furnaces. In severe carbon monoxide poisoning, the patient is treated with 100% oxygen (carboxyhemoglobin half-life, 50 minutes) or hyperbaric oxygen (2 to 3 atm; carboxyhemoglobin half-life, 30 minutes) until the HgCO level is less than 15% and both the metabolic acidosis and mental status changes have resolved.

CAFFEINE WITHDRAWAL HEADACHES

The threshold for withdrawal for each person is variable, but when caffeine is ingested in sufficient quantities for prolonged periods, sudden withdrawal can lead to vascular headaches. In the most common scenario, consumption occurs on weekdays, and because of schedule differences, the caffeinated beverage is not consumed on the weekend. This syndrome is easily diagnosed by history or by use of a headache diary. Treatment is removal of all sources of caffeine from the diet, such as tea, coffee, caffeinated soft drinks, "pep" pills, and diet pills.

EXERTIONAL HEADACHES

Coughing, running, swimming, competitive sports, or sexual activity may precipitate exertional headaches. The headaches usually begin during or after the activity and may be associated with nausea and occasional vomiting. They are generalized or localized to one side and last from 30 minutes to 12 hours. History and examination findings are usually normal. The headaches may interfere in performance of the youngster preparing for competitive sports. Indomethacin is the treatment of choice and can be used as needed before the activity or for daily treatment, if circumstances so dictate. More than 85% of patients show excellent response to indomethacin. Monitoring of side effects is important if daily long-term treatment is used.

TRACTION HEADACHES

One of the greatest concerns in the evaluation of a child with headaches is whether the headache is caused by increased ICP.

Increased ICP causes headaches by generating traction on the dura and vessels at the base of the brain. Some processes (brain tumors, pseudotumor cerebri) result in constant headaches because ICP is continuously increased. Other conditions (colloid cyst of the third ventricle) may cause intermittent headaches through transient increases in ICP.

Persistently Increased Intracranial Pressure

Neoplasms and Hydrocephalus

In children with headaches, a concern about a brain tumor is probably the key reason why patients request, and physicians order, an imaging study. The mechanism of brain tumors that causes headaches may be either increased ICP or direct traction on the dural or vascular structures. Headaches caused by hydrocephalus can develop rapidly, whereas traction from tumor growth causes a slow and progressive headache. However, at the time of presentation, most patients with headaches caused by tumors or hydrocephalus have chronic and progressive headaches, in which the frequency and severity of pain escalate over time. Tumors may produce hydrocephalus by obstructing cerebrospinal fluid (CSF) flow.

With or without a brain tumor, hydrocephalus usually causes a generalized headache. Slowly developing hydrocephalus initially causes mild pain, whereas rapidly developing hydrocephalus causes severe pain. Most patients with hydrocephalus have morning headaches that lessen after they arise. Those who do not follow this pattern have constant pain.

When the headache is solely a result of tumor without accompanying hydrocephalus, the location of the headache may or may not be related to the tumor site. Patients with posterior fossa tumors usually have occipital pain, but if hydrocephalus is also present, the pain may be generalized. It is important to note that many patients with brain tumors have no particular pattern to their headaches. Initially, their pain may be mild, and over-the-counter analgesics provide adequate pain relief. If the pain pattern is typical, the severity and frequency of pain increase slowly. Patients with brain tumors near the optic chiasm may have visual disturbances and endocrine deficiencies or galactorrhea. Diplopia may be present if the third or sixth cranial nerve is compressed (nonlocalizing signs); ptosis may also be present.

The examination often reveals abnormal findings, including papilledema and neurologic deficits. Common focal neurologic findings include eye movement abnormalities, facial weakness, swallowing difficulties, hemiparesis, and ataxia. Nonlateralizing signs include increased motor tone and bilateral sixth nerve palsies. Increased motor tone may not be a constant finding and may manifest as transient shivering. Tenderness or rigidity of the neck is a sign of increased ICP. Macrocephaly is present in young children with unfused cranial sutures and in those with long-standing hydrocephalus. Other signs of hydrocephalus are a bulging fontanelle and widened cranial sutures. The head growth chart is especially important in the evaluation of children with hydrocephalus. Head growth is abnormal if the plot of sequential head circumferences crosses percentile lines. Papilledema is usually absent in children with an open fontanelle and may also be absent in children with posterior fossa tumors (with or without hydrocephalus).

The *Parinaud syndrome* is the triad of upward-gaze paresis, poor pupillary reaction to light, and retraction nystagmus on convergence. This constellation of physical findings is seen in patients with hydrocephalus or tumors in the pineal region. The presence of Parinaud syndrome always warrants neuroimaging.

Increased ICP that is caused by hydrocephalus and/or brain tumors should be suspected in any child with chronic progressive headaches, abnormal neurologic examination results, nuchal rigidity, or abnormal head growth. Patients with these signs and symptoms should undergo a neuroimaging study (see Table 37-14).

Nonneoplastic Masses

Nonneoplastic masses, such as hemorrhage, cysts, and abscesses, can also cause headaches. Intracranial hemorrhage should be suspected in any child with a concussion causing amnesia or loss of consciousness or with a head injury resulting in abnormal neurologic examination results (e.g., altered mental status, focal findings). Most intracranial hemorrhages are detected by the initial neuroimaging study performed immediately after the injury; however, some subdural and a few epidural hematomas may take weeks to develop after the trauma.

Cysts are classified as arachnoid, epidermoid, and dermoid. Slow-growing cysts often produce headache patterns similar to those of neoplasms. Epidermoid and dermoid cysts can have sinus tracts that communicate with the skin. If these cysts become infected, their clinical manifestation resembles a brain abscess.

A brain abscess should be considered in any child with a right-to-left cardiac shunt, chronic mucosal surface infections (sinus, otitis, dental), and a recent onset of persistent, chronic headaches. Patients with a brain abscess may present with progressive neurologic dysfunction and may deteriorate quickly.

Aneurysmal Rupture

Arterial aneurysms may be congenital (berry) or caused by an infectious process (mycotic). Rupture of an arterial aneurysm is rare in children. The rupture produces an excruciating headache, known as a *thunderclap headache.* Patients state that this is "the worst headache of my life." The pain is acute in onset and associated with nuchal rigidity, emesis, and changes in sensorium. The neurologic examination findings may be nonfocal. CT scans reveal blood in the cisterns and meninges in 85% of cases. If the CT scan shows no pathologic process, a lumbar puncture is necessary in all patients thought to have a ruptured aneurysm. The spinal fluid in a ruptured aneurysm is bloody, xanthochromic, or both. In half the cases, patients report having previous headaches before having the headache associated with the rupture. These earlier headaches may be caused by leakage of blood from the aneurysm. If the clinician suspects a leaking or ruptured aneurysm, rapid neurologic and neurosurgical care is mandatory. Arteriovenous malformations may produce similar manifestations.

Pseudotumor Cerebri

Even though pseudotumor cerebri is also known as benign intracranial hypertension, it is associated with significant morbidity. The headache in pseudotumor cerebri can be intermittent or constant and may resemble a migraine. Papilledema is usually present at the time of presentation. In severe cases, the retinal blind spot may enlarge, and the visual fields may become constricted. This syndrome is more common in older children and adolescents, girls and women, and obese individuals. The characteristic findings are chronic progressive or nonprogressive headaches, papilledema, normal neuroimaging, and raised ICP.

Pseudotumor cerebri may be either idiopathic or secondary to a variety of medical conditions (Table 37-19). Because papilledema is a common finding in this syndrome, a neuroimaging study must be performed before the lumbar puncture to rule out other causes of papilledema (tumor, hydrocephalus) (see Table 37-14). The opening pressure from the lumbar puncture (in the lateral position) in pseudotumor cerebri is elevated (range, 240 to 600 mm H_2O). The results of the physical examination (except papilledema, visual field changes, and occasional sixth nerve palsy), neuroimaging studies, and CSF studies are usually normal.

In the evaluation of a patient with pseudotumor cerebri, a detailed history and physical examination are needed to rule out the many secondary causes of this syndrome (see Table 37-19). Specifically in young children, obstruction of the intracranial venous sinuses by

---

Table 37-19. Conditions Associated with Pseudotumor Cerebri

Intracranial Venous Drainage Obstruction
Mastoiditis and lateral (sigmoid) sinus obstruction
Extracerebral mass lesions
Congenital atresia or stenosis of venous sinuses
Head trauma
Cryofibrinogenemia
Polycythemia vera
Paranasal sinus and pharyngeal infections

Cervical or Thoracic Venous Drainage Obstruction
Intrathoracic mass lesions and postoperative obstruction of
venous return

Endocrine Dysfunction
Pregnancy
Menarche
Marked menstrual irregularities
Oral contraceptives
Obesity
Withdrawal of corticosteroid therapy
Addison disease
Hypoparathyroidism
"Catch-up" growth after deprivation, treatment of cystic
fibrosis, correction of heart anomaly
Initiation of thyroxine treatment for hypothyroidism
Adrenal hyperplasia
Adrenal adenoma

Hematologic Disorders
Acute iron deficiency anemia
Pernicious anemia
Thrombocytopenia
Wiskott-Aldrich syndrome

Vitamin Metabolism
Chronic hypervitaminosis A
Acute hypervitaminosis A
Hypovitaminosis A
Cystic fibrosis and hypovitaminosis A
Vitamin D–deficiency rickets

Drug Reaction
Tetracyclines
Perhexiline maleate
Nalidixic acid
Sulfamethoxazole
L-Asparaginase
Indomethacin
Penicillin

Prophylactic Antisera

Miscellaneous
Galactosemia
Galactokinase deficiency
Lyme disease
Sydenham chorea
Sarcoidosis
Roseola
Hypophosphatasia
Paget disease
Maple syrup urine disease
Turner syndrome

Adapted from Burg FD, Ingelfinger JR, Wald ER (eds): Gellis and Kagan's Current Pediatric Therapy, 14th ed. Philadelphia, WB Saunders, 1993, p 67.

infection or dehydration and thrombosis, trauma, and chronic middle ear or mastoid infection should be considered, and magnetic resonance venogram and special views may be necessary to visualize the mastoid air cells.

The goal of treatment is to lower the ICP and alleviate the headaches. Lumbar puncture is a fast, reliable, but temporary method for achieving both goals. Most patients require multiple lumbar punctures before their symptoms resolve. If the visual fields are affected, the treatment must be aggressive, with serial lumbar punctures, until the fields return to normal. If symptoms persist despite serial lumbar punctures, a lumbar-to-peritoneal drain or optic sheath decompression may be necessary to provide long-term drainage for the spinal fluid. The primary cause should be addressed when possible. In obese patients, weight loss may also be helpful. Corticosteroids provide quick relief from the headache and associated visual impairment. Because steroids can cause rapid weight gain, their use should be avoided if at all possible. Ocular findings should be monitored closely because patients may develop permanent visual impairment.

Transient Increased Intracranial Pressure

Cough headaches are intermittent headaches caused by transient increases in ICP that result from activities that elevate intrathoracic pressure (exertion, coughing, bending). The pain is maximum and severe at the onset of the activity and then resolves in seconds. Patients are usually asymptomatic between events. Cough headaches, which are much shorter than are exercise-induced vascular headaches, may be caused by both benign and life-threatening conditions. Structural causes of cough headache include brain tumors and Chiari malformations. The results of the physical examination are usually normal, even when structural lesions cause this syndrome. To rule out these structural lesions, patients with cough headaches should undergo MRI.

Colloid cyst of the third ventricle is another life-threatening condition that causes cough headaches. With changes in position, this cyst functions as a ball valve and intermittently impedes the flow of CSF. This obstruction causes transient increases in ICP. Sometimes, the patient may be asymptomatic during these episodes of increased ICP. At other times, the patient may experience severe intermittent headaches, increased muscle tone (posturing) that resembles shivering, coma, and death. The ICP returns to normal when position is changed or when the increased CSF pressure overcomes the obstruction. Physical findings are normal between events. The diagnosis is made by neuroimaging studies (MRI). Treatment consists of CSF diversion or removal of the cyst.

Decreased Intracranial Pressure

Abnormally low ICP causes headaches by the same mechanism as that of increased ICP: traction on the dura and vessels at the base of the brain. The most common cause of a headache from decreased ICP is leaking CSF after a lumbar puncture. This headache can occur after any lumbar puncture but is more commonly associated with older children, use of large-bore spinal needles, and multiple attempts at obtaining CSF. Patients describe a severe headache within seconds after assuming an upright position. The headache disappears soon after the patient lies down.

Treatment consists of bed rest until the leak seals. A blood patch is used when the leak fails to seal during bed rest. This procedure consists of injecting the patient's own blood into the epidural space, thus "patching" the dural leak. Other causes of low-pressure headaches include CSF leaks from fractures or tumors at the base of the skull.

HEADACHES CAUSED BY INFLAMMATION

Any inflammatory process involving the head or neck can cause headaches. The pain may be from direct inflammation of the brain

---

Table 37-20. Chronic Facial Pain: Differential Diagnosis

Orbital Pain	**Nasal/Cheek Pain**
Ocular disease	Sinusitis
Migraine	Facial cellulitis
Cluster	Neoplasm (nasopharynx, sinus)
Sinusitis	Vasomotor rhinitis
Orbital cellulitis	Allergic rhinitis
Tolosa-Hunt syndrome	Trigeminal neuralgia
Intracranial aneurysm	Midline granuloma
Cavernous sinus disease	Wegener granulomatosis
Giant cell arteritis	TMJ syndrome
Neoplasm	Dental disease
Graves disease	Postherpetic neuralgia
Neoplasm, frontal lobe	Atypical odontalgia
Trigeminal neuralgia	Cluster
Postherpetic neuralgia	
Zoster	**Poorly Localized/Vague**
	Sinus disease
Ear/Periauricular Pain	TMJ syndrome
Chronic external otitis	Depression
Relapsing polychondritis	Conversion reaction
Cholesteatoma	Neoplasm
TMJ syndrome	Muscle contraction
Migraine	
Carotidynia	**Dental/Jaw Pain**
Glossopharyngeal neuralgia	Toothache
Thyroiditis	TMJ syndrome
Muscle contraction	Sinusitis
Carotid aneurysm	Neoplasm
Cervical spine disease	Trigeminal neuralgia
Neoplasm	Parotid disease
Zoster	Atypical odontalgia
	Postherpetic neuralgia

Adapted from Reilly BM: Practical Strategies in Outpatient Medicine, 2nd ed. Philadelphia, WB Saunders, 1991, p 106.

TMJ, temporomandibular joint.

---

and dura (meningitis), or it may be referred from extracranial inflammation (sinusitis, dental abscesses) (Table 37-20).

Intracranial Inflammation

With meningitis and meningoencephalitis, the headache is acute in onset and generalized. Fever, nuchal rigidity, alteration in sensorium, and abnormal neurologic findings usually accompany an inflammatory process of the meninges (see Chapter 52).

Extracranial Inflammation

The headache associated with sinusitis can be acute or chronic. The headache is frontal or ocular when the frontal or maxillary sinuses are involved. When the ethmoid or sphenoid sinuses are infected, the headache can be frontal or occipital. Some of the symptoms and signs associated with sinusitis are purulent rhinorrhea, halitosis, cough (worse at night), tenderness to palpation over the sinuses or teeth, and fever. In addition, these patients may have a medical history of allergic rhinitis or previous sinusitis. If a radiographic study is needed to confirm the diagnosis, a sinus CT scan is preferred over routine sinus roentgenograms because CT scanning is more sensitive in diagnosing sinusitis and costs the same.

The headaches from dental abscesses may be aching or knifelike. Dental abscesses can be a complication of dental caries, tooth extractions, and root canal procedures. The examination results may be normal, or the examination may reveal gingival swelling, redness, or pain.

Inflammation of the eye and orbit usually causes localized pain (see Table 37-20). The signs and symptoms of periorbital cellulitis are periorbital redness and tenderness, whereas in orbital cellulitis, the patient may have chemosis, proptosis, ophthalmoplegia, and visual loss. A corneal abrasion should always be suspected in the irritable infant and in the patient with excruciating eye pain. Diagnosis is made by fluorescein examination of the cornea (see Chapter 43).

Optic neuritis (inflammation of the optic nerve) often causes ipsilateral retroorbital pain. Optic neuritis may occur as a single entity, or it can be part of the manifestation of multiple sclerosis. This disorder is rare in children but common in adolescents. The ophthalmologic examination reveals papillitis (resembling papilledema), afferent pupillary defect, and decreased visual acuity. Often, the findings may be normal except for decreased visual acuity. A neuroimaging study should be performed because of the ocular findings and to rule out multiple sclerosis. Optic neuritis is treated with intravenous corticosteroids.

TEMPOROMANDIBULAR JOINT SYNDROME

Malocclusion of the temporomandibular joint (TMJ) can cause chronic headaches. The pain is localized to the side of the affected joint. Some patients report constant pain, whereas others have pain only with jaw movement. An identifying "click" occurs when the patient opens the mouth. Not every person with a click has TMJ syndrome, and not everyone with TMJ syndrome has headaches. Gum chewing may exacerbate the pain associated with TMJ syndrome. In patients without TMJ syndrome, gum chewing may cause headaches through overuse of the temporalis muscles. Patients with symptomatic TMJ syndrome often find relief with the use of a bite plate worn during sleep.

POSTCONCUSSIVE SYNDROME

Chronic headaches can occur as part of the postconcussive or post-traumatic syndrome. The headache is generally constant and may have qualities of both chronic muscle contraction and migraine headaches. For example, some patients may have nausea, vomiting, and visual auras. Other features of this syndrome are fatigue, dizziness, vertigo, poor memory, decreased reaction times, and inability to concentrate. The neurologic findings are usually normal. Symptoms begin soon after the head injury (within 1 to 7 days) and can persist for years. About 70% of patients recover within a year, but 15% are still symptomatic after 3 years. The pathophysiologic mechanism of this syndrome is unknown.

Even though postconcussive syndrome is more common in persons with a history of psychologic or psychosomatic illness, it is not an imaginary phenomenon. A neuroimaging study may be necessary to rule out the presence of a chronic subdural hematoma, which is rare. Patient education is the most important element of treatment. Some patients may also benefit from psychotherapy. NSAIDs, amitriptyline, and propranolol may be helpful, but narcotics should be avoided because of their addictive potential in the treatment of chronic headaches.

OCCIPITAL NEURALGIA

The greater occipital nerve is a continuation of the C2 nerve root, which innervates the posterior scalp. Irritation or inflammation of this nerve can produce occipital pain that may be intermittent or persistent. The pain is described as ranging from "pins and needles" to lancinating. On physical examination, affected patients have decreased sensation over the C2 dermatome, limitation of cervical movements, and tenderness to palpation over the posterior scalp. Whiplash injury, atlantoaxial subluxation, weight lifting, wrestling, and arthritis are associated with this syndrome. Most patients respond to some combination of cervical collar, muscle relaxants, NSAIDs, and physical therapy. In severe cases, repeated nerve blocks with steroids and a local anesthetic provide relief.

CONVERSION DISORDER

Headaches associated with conversion disorders are very difficult to diagnose and treat accurately. The frequency and severity of these headaches increase without lasting relief from any pharmacologic or physical therapy. Some patients appear as if they are in pain, whereas others look perfectly normal despite claiming to be in considerable pain. Secondary muscle contraction pain can occur, which further complicates the diagnosis. The neurologic findings in conversion disorders are normal. As patient and family anxiety grows, the physician's anxiety also increases, resulting in the ordering of many blood tests and neuroimaging studies.

The two problems in treating conversion disorder headaches are (1) to convince the family that there is no physical cause for these headaches, and (2) to uncover the origin of the conversion disorder. The physician with a preestablished rapport with the family is clearly at an advantage in convincing the family that no physical cause exists for the headaches. The origins of a conversion disorder are difficult to uncover and require the finesse of an experienced therapist. Psychologic intervention is mandatory, not only to identify the source of the problem but also to offer appropriate consoling.

SUMMARY AND RED FLAGS

Headaches are a common cause of morbidity in children. Although muscle contraction and migraine headaches are the most common causes of headaches in children, the clinician must rule out life-threatening conditions in the evaluation of each patient with a headache. A thorough history and physical examination are the best diagnostic tools aiding the clinician in determining which patients have a serious and life-threatening cause for their headaches. The red flags from this evaluation are thunderclap headache, cough headache, the first severe headache, chronic or progressive headaches, persistently unilateral headaches, any persistently abnormal neurologic findings (>1 hour), meningeal signs, papilledema, and alterations of sensorium. A new headache in a patient with a chronic medical condition, particularly an immunosuppressed patient, and headaches associated with activities are other red flags. Patients with these red flags need a complete emergency evaluation that includes neuroimaging studies (see Table 37-14).

REFERENCES

Annequin D, Tourniaire B, Massiou H: Migraine and headache in childhood and adolescence. Pediatr Clin North Am 2000;47:617-631.

Appleton R, Farrell K, Buncic JR, et al: Amaurosis fugax in teenagers. Am J Dis Child 1988;142:331-333.

Becker WJ: Evidence based migraine prophylactic drug therapy. Can J Neurol Sci 1999;26:S27-S32.

Caruso JM, Ferri R, Exil G, et al: The efficacy of divalproex sodium in the prophylactic treatment of children with migraine. Ann Neurol 1998;44:567.

Dahlof CGH, Hargreaves RJ: Pathophysiology and pharmacology of migraine. Is there a place for antiemetics in future treatment strategies? Cephalalgia 1998;18:593-604.

Dalessio DJ: Relief of cluster headache and cranial neuralgias. Promising prophylactic and symptomatic treatments. Postgrad Med 2001;109:69-72.

Digre KB: Not so benign intracranial hypertension. BMJ 2003;326:613-614.

Dodick DW, Rozen TD, Goadsby PJ, et al: Cluster headache. Cephalalgia 2000;20:787-803.

Green MW: A spectrum of exertional headaches. Med Clin North Am 1085;85:1085-1092.

Guidetti V, Galli F: Recent development in paediatric headache. Curr Opin Neurol 2001;14:335-340.

Gupta A, Rothner AD: Treatment of childhood headaches. Curr Neurol Neurosci Rep 2001;1:144-154.

Headache Classification Committee of the International Headache Society: Classification and diagnostic criteria for headache disorders, cranial neuralgias and facial pain. Cephalalgia 1988;8:1-96.

Jensen VK, Rothner AD: Chronic nonprogressive headaches in children and adolescents. Semin Pediatr Neurol 1995;2:151-154.

Jones JS, Nevai J, Freeman MP, et al: Emergency department presentation of idiopathic intracranial hypertension. Am J Emerg Med 1999;17:517-521.

Joutel A, Bousser MG, Biousse V, et al: A gene for familial hemiplegic migraine maps to chromosome 19. Nat Genet 1993;5:40-45.

Kaniecki R: Headache assessment and management. JAMA 2003;289:1430-1433.

Kosmorsky G: Pseudotumor cerebri. Neurosurg Clin North Am 2001;12:775-797.

Lessell S: Pediatric pseudotumor cerebri (idiopathic intracranial hypertension). Surv Ophthalmol 1992;37:155-166.

Lewis DW: Headaches in children and adolescents. Am Fam Physician 2002;65:625-632.

Lewis DW, Ashwal S, Dahl G, et al: Practice parameter: Evaluation of children and adolescents with recurrent headaches: Report of the Quality Standards Subcommittee of the American Academy of Neurology and the Practice Committee of the Child Neurology Society. Neurology 2002;59:490-498.

Linder SL: Treatment of childhood headache with dihydroergotamine mesylate. Headache 1994;34:578-580.

Linder SL, Winner P: Pediatric headache. Med Clin North Am 2001;85:1037-1053.

Lipton RB, Stewart WF, Stone AM, et al: Stratified care vs step care strategies for migraine. The Disability in Strategies of Care (DISC) study: A randomized trial. JAMA 2000;284:2599-2605.

Lipton RB, Stewart WF, Von Korff M: Burden of migraine: Societal costs and therapeutic opportunities. Neurology 1997;48:S4-S9.

Mark AS, Casselman J, Brown D, et al: Ophthalmoplegic migraine; reversible enhancement and thickening of the cisternal segment of the oculomotor nerve on contrast-enhanced MR images. Am J Neuroradiol 1998;19:1887-1891.

Maytal J, Lipton RB, Solomon S, et al: Childhood onset cluster headaches. Headache 1992;32:275-279.

Practice parameter: The utility of neuroimaging in the evaluation of headache in patients with normal neurologic examinations (summary statement). Report of the Quality Standard Subcommittee of the American Academy of Neurology. Neurology 1994;44:1353-1354.

Rothner AD: Headaches in children and adolescents. Child Adolesc Psychiatr Clin North Am 1999;8:727-745.

Rothner AD: Evaluation of headache. In Winner P, Rothner AD (eds): Headache in Children and Adolescents. Hamilton, Ontario, BC Decker, 2001.

Senior K: New understanding into the mechanics of migraine. Lancet 2002;359:500.

Soler D, Cox T, Bullock P, et al: Diagnosis and management of benign intracranial hypertension. Arch Dis Child 1998;78:89-94.

Steiner TJ, Fontebasso M: Headache. BMJ 2002;325:881-886.

Tronvik E, Stivner LJ, Helde G, et al: Prophylactic treatment of migraine with an angiotensin II receptor blocker. JAMA 2003;289:65-69.

Winner P: Triptans in childhood and adolescence. Sem Pediatr Neurol 2001;8:22-26.

38 Hypotonia and Weakness

Saleem I. Malik   Michael J. Painter*

IDENTIFICATION OF MUSCLE WEAKNESS AND HYPOTONIA

Hypotonia (abnormally diminished muscle tone) may be acute or chronic, progressive or static, isolated or part of a complex clinical situation; it affects children of all ages (Table 38-1). It may or may not be associated with weakness (Tables 38-2 to 38-5). The evaluation of children with hypotonia can be simplified by a thoughtful, analytic approach to the differential clues that are useful in identifying an underlying cause (Tables 38-6 and 38-7; Figs. 38-1 to 38-3).

Hypotonia is usually defined functionally as diminished resistance to movement as a limb is passively moved through a range of motion about a joint. The assessment of muscle tone can also be made by several observations, including

- evaluation of spontaneous posture
- extent of mobility of joints
- response to flapping of distal extremities
- response to postural changes

The method of evaluating muscle tone and strength depends on the age of the patient.

Muscle tone is defined as the resistance experienced by the examiner to movement of limbs about joints. Muscle tone is divided into postural and phasic. Postural tone is that experienced by the steady flexion or extension of a joint and is caused by the resultant uniform resistance of muscle to passive movement. Antigravity posture of muscle is caused by postural tone. Phasic tone is the catch experienced when an extremity is rapidly flexed or extended. The anatomic structures responsible for muscle tone are contained in a closed circuit formed by the muscle spindle, which is connected to the spinal cord by sensory afferent pathways. The sensory afferent fibers synapse directly or indirectly with anterior horn α and γ motor neurons. The α motor neurons end at the neuromuscular junction, and the γ motor neurons end at the muscle spindle, completing the closed circuit. It is the level of activity of γ motor neuron and its influence on the muscle spindle that sets the level of resting muscle tone. This lower motor neuron pathway is closely monitored and influenced by descending pathways from the cerebral cortex, basal ganglia, brainstem, and cerebellum. These descending pathways constitute a portion of the upper motor neuron.

The maintenance of normal muscle tone requires the integrity of the entire central and peripheral nervous systems, from the cerebral cortex, cortical white matter pathways, basal ganglia, cerebellum, brainstem, spinal cord, peripheral nerve, neuromuscular junction, and muscle (see Table 38-6). Diseases that affect the function of the nervous system at any level may result in abnormal muscle tone (see Tables 38-6 and 38-7). Many neonates and infants with hypotonia have disorders of the brain. Most older children and adolescents with hypotonia have a disorder of the motor unit (anterior horn cell, peripheral nerve, neuromuscular junction, and muscle) (Fig. 38-4).

---

*This chapter is an updated and edited version of the chapter by Warren Cohen that appeared in the first edition.

THE HYPOTONIC INFANT

CLINICAL EVALUATION

In an infant, historical information must include a complete obstetric history as well as accurate data about perinatal events, diet, toxic exposure, and family diseases.

Muscle Strength

Muscle strength cannot be measured directly in infants (Table 38-8), but numerous clinical clues allow the careful observer to identify weakness. The most important of these is the spontaneous posture. The weak infant has diminished or no spontaneous movement, often in striking contrast to the usual vigorous and plentiful movements of the infant with normal strength (Fig. 38-5). The lower extremities are abducted, and the lateral surfaces of the thighs lie against the examination table, whereas the upper extremities lie extended alongside the body or flexed in a flaccid position beside the head. With marked weakness, there are no movements that overcome the pull of gravity. The immobility of the weak infant results in flattening of the occipital bone, which is often associated with occipital hair loss. When placed in a sitting posture, the infant droops forward, the shoulders droop, the head falls forward, and the arms hang limply.

Passive Tone

Passive tone can be assessed by evaluating the resistance to movement of the limbs through a range of motion at the joints. Evaluation of the shoulders, elbows, wrists, hips, knees, and ankles is especially helpful. The examiner senses a "looseness" of the limbs as the limbs are moved.

In addition, grasping the midportion of the infant's limb and passively flapping the extremity allow the examiner to evaluate the degree of limpness of the distal extremity. In the hypotonic infant, the hands and feet wave limply; in the normal infant, the ankle and wrist are maintained fairly rigidly in line with the rest of the extremity.

Even in normal infants, there is a wide variation of muscle tone. Passive muscle tone varies and is particularly diminished after feeding and before sleep. There is profound hypotonia in all infants during sleep. Tone can also be affected by the position of the head. The child whose head is turned to one side may be manifesting an asymmetric tonic neck response, with increased extensor tone on the side of the body to which the head is turned and increased flexor tone on the contralateral side. This asymmetry of tone may be elicited even in the child who does not exhibit the typical "fencer's" posture. Therefore, examination of an infant should always be conducted while the infant's head is in the midline; the same is true for eliciting muscle stretch reflexes. Hypotonia can also be associated with heart failure, sepsis, acidosis, failure to thrive, and other systemic-generalized serious conditions affecting the baby's general health (see Table 38-1).

Table 38-1. Causes of Hypotonia and Weakness in Infancy and Childhood

Systemic	Connective Tissue	Cerebral	Spinal Cord	Anterior Horn Cell	Peripheral Nerve	Neuromuscular Junction	Muscle
Common							
Sepsis	Stickler syndrome	Hypoxic-ischemic brain injury	Myelodysplasia	Spinal muscular atrophies	Postinfectious polyneuropathy (Guillain-Barré syndrome)	Botulism	Duchenne muscular dystrophy
Heart failure	Marfan syndrome	Brain malformation	Spinal cord tumor		Toxic neuropathies	Infantile myasthenia	Becker muscular dystrophy
Acidosis	Achondroplasia	Intrauterine infection	Epidural abscess		Isoniazid	Transient neonatal myasthenia	Myotonic dystrophy
Failure to thrive		Postnatal brain injury	Transverse myelitis		Vincristine		Inflammatory muscle disease (dermatomyositis-myositis)
Hypoxia			Trauma (transection or compression)		Nitrofurantoin		
Renal failure					Zidovudine		
Hypoglycemia							
Down syndrome							
Prader-Willi syndrome							
Noonan syndrome							
Fragile X syndrome							
Uncommon							
Amino acid disorders	Ehlers-Danlos syndrome	Progressive encephalopathies	Neonatal spinal cord transection	Möbius syndrome	Chronic inflammatory demyelinating polyneuropathy	Toxic organophosphate poisoning	
Organic acid disorders	Osteogenesis imperfecta	Mitochondrial disease	Hypoxic-ischemic myelopathy		Hereditary motor and sensory neuropathy (Charcot-Marie-Tooth disease)	Postneuromuscular blocking agents (vecuronium)	
Urea cycle disorders	Velocardiofacial syndrome		Arteriovenous malformation		Dejerine-Sottas disease		
Scurvy					Familial dysautonomia		
Rickets							
Sotos syndrome							
Angelman syndrome							
Rett syndrome							
Smith-Lemli-Opitz syndrome							
Rare							
Lowe syndrome		Miller-Dieker syndrome	Arthrogryposis	Poliomyelitis	Refsum disease		Other muscular dystrophies
Zellweger syndrome		Walker-Warburg syndrome		Incontinentia pigmenti	Giant axonal neuropathy		Congenital myopathies
Neonatal adrenal leukodystrophy				Fazio-Londe disease	Metachromatic leukodystrophy		Metabolic myopathies
Mucolipidosis type IV				Infantile neuroaxonal dystrophy	Krabbe disease		Mitochondrial myopathies
Tay-Sachs disease				GM_2 gangliosidosis			Arthrogryposis
Gangliosidosis				Anterior spinal artery occlusion			
Mannosidosis				Arthrogryposis			

Table 38-2. **Nonparalytic Conditions: Hypotonia without Significant Weakness**

1. **Disorders of the Central Nervous System**
   a. Nonspecific mental deficiency
   b. Birth trauma, intracranial hemorrhage, intrapartum asphyxia, and hypoxia
   c. Hypotonic cerebral palsy
   d. Metabolic disorders: lipidoses (leukodystrophies); mucopolysaccharidoses; aminoacidurias; congenital disorders of glycosylation*; Leigh and Zellweger syndromes
   e. Chromosomal abnormalities
      Down syndrome

2. **Connective Tissue Disorders**
   Congenital laxity of ligaments
   Ehlers-Danlos and Marfan syndromes
   Osteogenesis imperfecta; arachnodactyly

3. **Prader-Willi Syndrome**

4. **Metabolic; Nutritional; Endocrine**
   Organic acidemias; hypercalcemia; rickets; celiac disease; hypothyroidism; renal tubular acidosis

Modified from Dubowitz V: Muscle Disorders in Childhood, 2nd ed. London, WB Saunders, 1995, p 459.

*Carbohydrate-deficient glycoproteins.

Table 38-3. **Acute Generalized Weakness**

Infectious Disorders
1. Acute infectious myositis
2. Acute inflammatory polyradiculoneuropathy (Guillain-Barré syndrome)
3. Enterovirus and West Nile virus infections

Metabolic Disorders
1. Acute intermittent porphyria
2. Hereditary tyrosinemia

Neuromuscular Blockade
1. Botulism
2. Tick paralysis

Periodic Paralysis
1. Familial hyperkalemic
2. Familial hypokalemic
3. Familial normokalemic

Poisoning
1. Opiates
2. Barbiturates
3. Other sedatives
4. Magnesium

Modified from Fenichel GM: Clinical Pediatric Neurology: A Signs and Symptoms Approach. Philadelphia, WB Saunders, 1993, p 187.

Joint Extensibility

The extent to which the joints may be extensible provides an indirect clue to the presence of hypotonia. Examination of mobility at the elbows, wrists, hips, and knees is helpful. The hypotonic infant may assume unusual postures in the presence of joint hyperextensibility. The "scarf sign" is a particularly useful sign of hyperextensibility in the young infant. With the infant in a semireclining position, the hand

Table 38-4. **Progressive Proximal Weakness**

Spinal Cord Disorders
Juvenile Spinal Muscular Atrophies
1. Autosomal recessive
2. Autosomal dominant
3. GM$_2$ gangliosidosis (hexosaminidase A deficiency)

Myasthenic Syndromes
1. Familial limb-girdle
2. Myasthenia gravis
3. Slow channel syndrome

Myopathies
1. Muscular dystrophies
   a. Duchenne and Becker dystrophies
   b. Facioscapulohumeral syndrome
   c. Limb-girdle dystrophy
2. Inflammatory myopathies
   a. Dermatomyositis
   b. Polymyositis
   c. Inclusion body myositis
3. Metabolic myopathies
   a. Acid maltase deficiency
   b. Carnitine deficiency
   c. Debrancher enzyme deficiency
   d. Lipid storage myopathies
   e. Mitochondrial myopathies
   f. Myophosphorylase deficiency
4. Endocrine myopathies
   a. Adrenal cortex
   b. Parathyroid
   c. Thyroid

Modified from Fenichel GM: Clinical Pediatric Neurology: A Signs and Symptoms Approach. Philadelphia, WB Saunders, 1993, p 171.

is pulled across the chest toward the opposite shoulder and the position of the elbow is noted. The presence of joint hyperextensibility is confirmed if the elbow passes the midline; this is suggestive of hypotonia.

Postural Reflexes

Traction Response

The traction response is the most useful and most sensitive of the postural reflexes in infants. With the infant lying supine, the infant's hands are grasped, and the infant is pulled up to a sitting position (Fig. 38-6). Once the sitting posture is attained, the head is held erect in the midline. During the maneuver, the examiner notes the infant's attempt to counter the traction by flexion of the arms.

In an infant younger than 3 months, the plantar grasp should also be evident. In addition, there should be flexion at the elbow, knee, and ankle in response to the maneuver. The degree to which the head and neck pull up along with the trunk depends on the child's age (see Fig. 38-6).

In infants younger than 33 weeks' gestation, there is no traction response. From 33 weeks to term, the infant has head lag but responds to the traction maneuver by flexing the neck flexors in an attempt to lift the head. The full-term infant exhibits a traction response with minimal head lag, and when the sitting posture is attained, the head may be held erect momentarily and then fall forward.

By age 3 months, there should be no head lag, and the head should be aligned with the plane of the back as the child is pulled to sitting. The absence of flexion of the limbs in response to the examiner's pull and the presence of head lag inappropriate for age suggests hypotonia.

Table 38-5. Progressive Distal Weakness

Spinal Cord Disorders

Motor Neuron Diseases
1. Juvenile amyotrophic lateral sclerosis
2. Spinal muscular atrophies
   a. Genetic forms
   b. Nonfamilial Asian

Neuropathies
1. Hereditary motor sensory neuropathies (HMSN)
   a. HMSN I: Charcot-Marie-Tooth
   b. HMSN II: neuronal Charcot-Marie-Tooth
   c. HMSN III: Dejerine-Sottas
   d. HMSN IV: Refsum
2. Other genetic neuropathies
   a. Familial amyloid neuropathy
   b. Giant axonal neuropathy
   c. Pyruvate dehydrogenase deficiency
   d. Sulfatide lipidoses: metachromatic leukodystrophy
   e. Other leukodystrophies
3. Neuropathies with systemic diseases
   a. Drug induced
   b. Systemic vasculitis
   c. Toxins
   d. Uremia
4. Idiopathic neuropathy
   a. Chronic axonal neuropathy
   b. Chronic demyelinating neuropathy

Myopathies
1. Hereditary distal myopathies
2. Myotonic dystrophy

Scapulo(humeral)peroneal Syndrome
1. Bethlem myopathy
2. Emery-Dreifuss syndrome
3. Scapulohumeral syndrome with dementia
4. Scapuloperoneal neuronopathy

Modified from Fenichel GM: Clinical Pediatric Neurology: A Signs and Symptoms Approach, 2nd ed. Philadelphia, WB Saunders, 1993, p 181.

Axillary Suspension

The response to axillary suspension allows assessment of generalized and shoulder girdle tone. The infant is held under the arms, lifted, and suspended from the axillae without the thorax's being grasped. In infants with normal tone and strength, the shoulder girdle muscles exert enough strength to allow the infant to be suspended without slipping through the examiner's grasp. In addition, the infant's head is held midline and the legs are held with some flexion at the hips, knees, and ankles. The hypotonic infant droops with legs extended and head falling forward, and the absence of resistance of the muscles of the shoulder girdle allows the infant to slip through the grasp of the examiner as the baby's arms fling upward.

Ventral Suspension

The response to ventral suspension allows assessment of tone of the trunk, neck, and extremities (see Fig. 38-6). The examiner holds the infant, who is lying prone. The infant is supported only by the examiner's hand on the abdomen. A normal infant holds the head erect and the back straight and holds the extremities with some flexion at the elbows, hips, knees, and ankles. A full-term neonate makes intermittent attempts to hold the head straight, maintains the back

straight, and can flex the limbs. The hypotonic infant droops in the examiner's palm, as if in the shape of an inverted U, with the head and legs dangling limply.

DIAGNOSTIC APPROACH

A careful perinatal history is obtained to identify possible features suggestive of perinatal hypoxic-ischemic brain injury. The infant who has a neurologic dysfunction attributable to perinatal asphyxia should have demonstrated evidence of an acute encephalopathy during the neonatal period (disturbance of consciousness, poor feeding, seizures, autonomic dysfunction).

A computed tomographic study or magnetic resonance imaging (MRI) of the head is helpful to identify evidence of brain malformation, intrauterine infection, hypoxic brain injury, intracranial hemorrhage, or hydrocephalus. If the history suggests seizures, an electroencephalogram should be obtained.

An ophthalmologic evaluation may detect evidence of ocular malformation (cataracts, microphthalmia, optic hypoplasia), evidence of intrauterine infection (chorioretinitis), or retinal/macular abnormality (retinitis pigmentosa, cherry-red spot) (see Chapter 43).

In some cases, requesting a hearing evaluation or brainstem auditory evoked response may be appropriate. A lumbar puncture is necessary only if acute or chronic (intrauterine) meningitis is suspected.

Figure 38-1 summarizes the approach to the hypotonic newborn. After a thorough history and careful physical examination, it should be determined whether the infant has signs of encephalopathy. A computed tomographic scan or MRI of the head is obtained to detect any anatomic abnormalities. If the scan does not reveal an abnormality and if the neonate exhibits increased reflexes and tone over time, a diagnosis of *static encephalopathy* can be made. If hypotonia persists, anterior horn cell disease, congenital myopathy, or neuromuscular junction disease should be considered (see Table 38-1, Table 38-6, and Fig. 38-4).

If the baby is not encephalopathic, the practitioner should determine whether a systemic disease (Prader-Willi syndrome or Down syndrome) is present. Is the motor-sensory level consistent with myelodysplasia or spinal cord injury? In addition, causes of arthrogryposis multiplex congenita must be considered (Table 38-9).

If the baby is markedly weak, the examiner should check to see whether the mother is also weak or whether she displays myotonia. If either is true, then transplacental-derived transient neonatal myasthenia gravis or myotonic dystrophy, respectively, is a possibility (Table 38-10). If neither is the case, then myopathy (Table 38-11), congenital myasthenia, infant botulism (Table 38-12), or anterior horn cell disease must be considered (see Tables 38-4 and 38-5).

Common Disorders

Hypoxic-Ischemic Encephalopathy

Hypoxic-ischemic encephalopathy is a general term that describes a child with sustained hypoxic and ischemic injury (most commonly in the perinatal period) that results in varying degrees of mental and motor developmental impairment. The typical child with severe hypoxic-ischemic encephalopathy is markedly hypotonic during the neonatal period and demonstrates other manifestations of encephalopathy (seizures, poor suck, poor feeding, impaired alertness, hypotonia, or hypertonia). Seizures are present in 50% of the patients with moderate to severe encephalopathy. Neonates with hypoxic-ischemic injury may also be jittery. Over the course of weeks to several months, signs of hyperreflexia and hypertonia begin to evolve, generally in a rostral-caudal progression. In some infants, hypotonia persists and is the prominent motor sign. The term *hypotonic cerebral palsy* is often used to describe this group. In most of

Table 38-6. Distinguishing Features in Motor Weakness

	Upper Motor Unit		Lower Motor Unit			
	Brain	Spinal Cord	Anterior Horn Cell	Peripheral Nerve	Neuromuscular Junction	Muscle
Deep tendon reflexes	Normal to ↑	↓ Acutely; ↑	↓ To absent	↓ To absent (lost early)	Normal	Normal to ↓
Strength	Normal	↓	↓	↓	↓	↓
Tone	↑ (Spasticity)	↓ Acutely; ↑	↓ (Flaccid)	↓	↓	↓
Level of consciousness	↓	Normal	Normal	Normal	Normal	Normal
Fasciculations	Absent	Absent	Present	Rare	Absent	Absent
Primitive reflexes, including Babinski	Present	±	Absent	Absent	Absent	Absent
Atrophy	Less prominent	Less prominent	Present	Present	Absent	Present; pseudohypertrophy
Sensation	Normal	Absent below lesion	Normal	±	Normal	Normal
Location	Generalized; may be hemiplegic	Below lesion	Symmetric for SMA; asymmetric for poliomyelitis	Symmetric for GBS; asymmetric for mononeuritis; usually distal	Symmetric	Symmetric; usually proximal
Creatine phosphokinase	Normal	Normal	Normal	May be elevated	Normal	↑
Other	Seizures Focal lesions Regression Developmental delay	Back pain Bowel or bladder dysfunction	Facial involvement late	Abnormal nerve conduction velocity Nerve biopsy	Response to tensilon (myasthenia) Constipation, dilated pupils (botulism)	Tender muscles (myositis) Gower sign (dystrophies)

GBS, Guillain-Barré syndrome; SMA, spinal muscular atrophy; ± present or absent.

Table 38-7. Common Causes of Hypotonia and Weakness

	Hypoxic Ischemic Encephalopathy	Brain Malformation	Spinal Cord Transection	Transverse Myelitis	Spinal Cord Tumor	Spinal Muscular Atrophy	Polio-myelitis	Guillain-Barré	Myasthenia Gravis	Botulism	Myopathy
Dysmorphism, malformation		✓									
Seizures, MR, lethargy	✓	✓									
Motor/sensory level			✓	✓	✓						
Hypotonia	✓	✓	✓	✓	✓	✓	✓	✓	✓	✓	✓
Hypertonia	✓	✓	✓	✓	✓						
Reflexes increased	✓	✓	✓	✓	✓						
Reflexes decreased	✓	✓	✓	✓	✓	✓	✓	✓		✓	Decreased or normal
Proximal weakness						✓			✓		✓
Distal weakness							✓	✓			
Abnormal CT/MRI	✓	✓	✓	✓	✓						
Abnormal NCV			✓	✓	✓		✓	✓	✓	✓	
Abnormal EMG	✓	✓	✓		✓	✓	✓	✓	✓	✓	✓
Acute onset weakness	Initially		✓	✓			✓	✓		✓	Inflammatory, metabolic myopathies
Chronic progressive weakness					✓	✓			✓		✓

CT, computed tomography; EMG, electromyography; MRI, magnetic resonance imaging; MR, mental retardation; NCV, nerve conduction velocity.

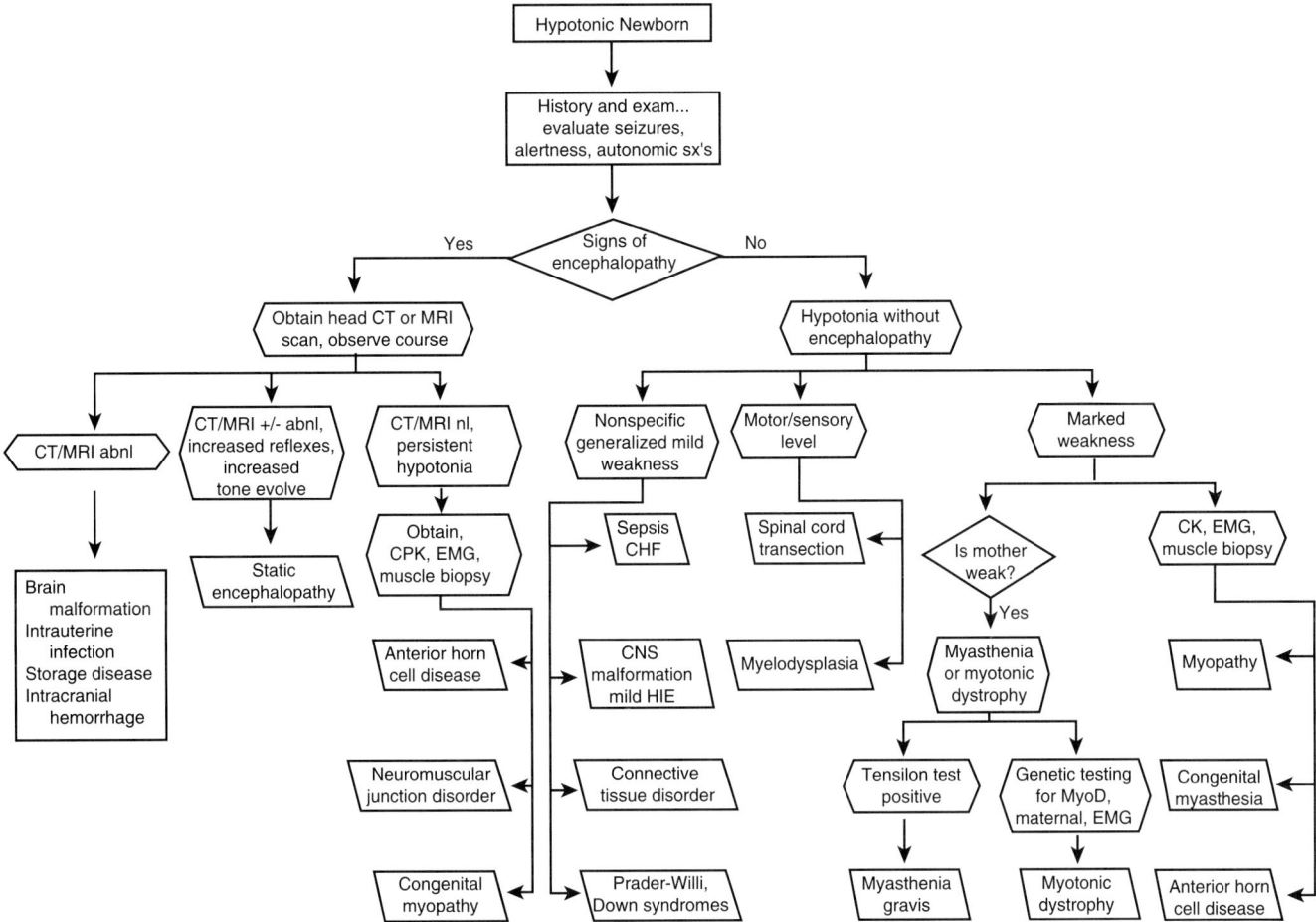

Figure 38-1. Approach to the hypotonic newborn. abnl, abnormal; CHF, congestive heart failure; CNS, central nervous system; CPK (CK), creatine phosphokinase; CT, computed tomography; EMG, electromyography; HIE, hypoxic-ischemic encephalopathy; MRI, magnetic resonance imaging; MyoD, myotonic dystrophy; nl, normal; sx, signs.

the infants, however, signs of spasticity or dyskinetic movements develop, and these children represent the more common cases of spastic cerebral palsy and dyskinetic cerebral palsy.

The diagnosis is established by a nonprogressive but often evolving clinical course, with supportive evidence provided by the perinatal history, fetal heart rate monitoring, acid-base status of the fetus, Apgar scores, and pathologic conditions of placenta. Important intervention issues include physical therapy, referral for early services, special education, nutritional counseling, prevention of contractures, and adaptive equipment.

Brain Malformations

Brain malformation can arise as a result of a chromosomal disorder, as a component of a multiple malformation syndrome, or as an isolated abnormality. When associated with chromosomal disorder or multiple malformation syndromes, the other associated features are the primary clues to diagnosis. In isolated brain malformation, the primary features are microcephaly (in most cases) and cognitive and motor developmental impairment. The MRI scan can detect abnormalities of development of the hemispheric structures (agenesis of the corpus callosum, holoprosencephaly), abnormalities of cortical cellular migration (lissencephaly, pachygyria), and cerebral heterotopias as well as brainstem and cerebellar malformations.

Uncommon Disorders

Progressive Encephalopathies of Infancy

Progressive encephalopathies of infancy account for a small number of children with persistent hypotonia (see Chapter 32). These disorders are recognizable by a progressive deterioration of neurologic function and by diagnostically specific clues. The infant's development is normal for some time and then plateaus; this is followed by developmental regression, with loss of previously acquired skills (see Chapter 32). Hypotonia is a feature of many of these disorders, at least at some point during the course of the illness (Tay-Sachs disease), and some disorders feature hypotonia as the result of the combination of central nervous system injury and an associated polyneuropathy (Krabbe and metachromatic leukodystrophies). Progressive disorders that may be associated with hypotonia include neonatal adrenoleukodystrophy, mannosidosis, fucosidosis, Gaucher disease types 2 and 3, GM_1 gangliosidosis, infantile neuroaxonal dystrophy, infantile Refsum disease, Krabbe leukodystrophy, metachromatic leukodystrophy, mucolipidosis type IV, and Tay-Sachs disease. The diagnosis of these disorders is based on recognition of clinically suggestive clues and on results of specialized biochemical and molecular genetic testing (see Chapter 32). If such a disorder is suspected, the infant should be referred to appropriate genetic and neurologic specialists.

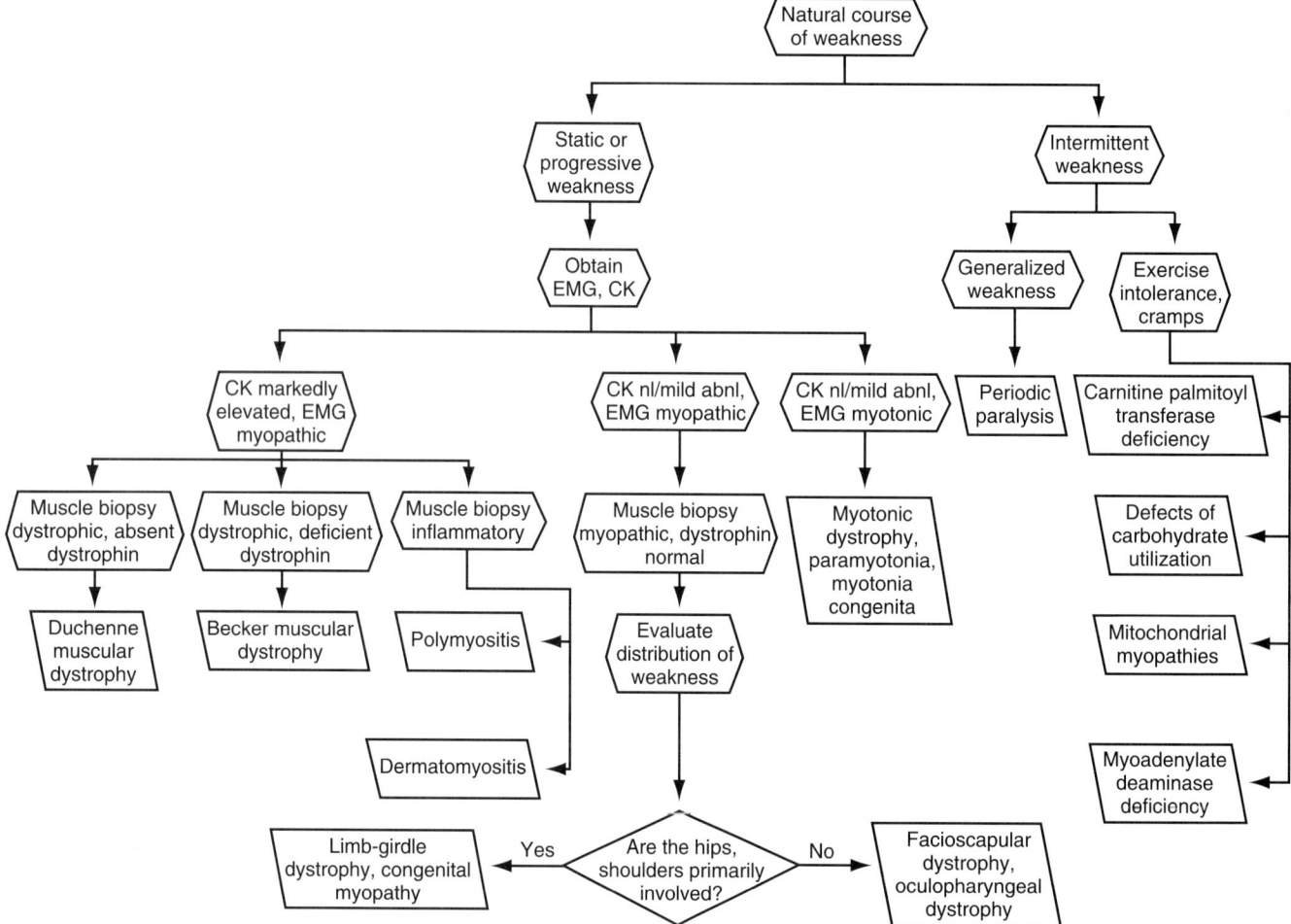

Figure 38-2. Diagnostic approach to the child with muscle disease. abnl, abnormal; CK, creatine kinase; EMG, electromyography; nl, normal.

Mitochondrial Diseases

Mitochondrial diseases often affect both the brain and muscle and clinically manifest hypotonia, probably as a combination of both cerebral dysfunction and myopathy (Tables 38-13 and 38-14). The diagnosis is based on recognition of clinical symptoms, presence of lactic acidosis, presence of ragged red fibers on muscle histologic examination, and mitochondrial abnormalities identifiable on a muscle electron microscopic examination. The diagnosis of many mitochondrial diseases is possible by specific mitochondrial DNA testing. Other inborn errors of metabolism may produce hypotonia by central mechanisms (organic acidurias, hyperammonemia) or by interfering with muscle metabolism (Table 38-15).

Brain Malformation Syndromes

Miller-Dieker Syndrome.   A cortical malformation, lissencephaly, produces severe developmental impairment and hypotonia early in life, and hypertonia develops later. The facial changes include bitemporal hollowing, up-turned nares, thin vermilion boarder, and small jaw. Visible deletion of chromosome band 17p13.3 is seen in about half the affected patients.

Walker-Warburg Syndrome.   The combination of brain malformation (polymicrogyria, cerebellar malformation) and an associated congenital muscular dystrophy produces marked hypotonia in infancy.

THE HYPOTONIC OLDER CHILD

CLINICAL EVALUATION

Posture and Strength

Observation of the child's spontaneous posture may suggest the presence of weakness. Muscle strength can be observed as the child performs functional tasks, including pulling to sit spontaneously from a prone position, arising to stand from a sitting or lying position (Gower sign) (Fig. 38-7), standing on one leg independently, hopping, walking, running, and climbing stairs. The wheelbarrow maneuver can be used to functionally assess strength in the upper extremities. In the child older than 5 years, manual muscle testing can be performed if the child is cooperative (see Table 38-8). The examiner evaluates each muscle group independently, comparing the child's muscle strength in resistance to the examiner's. The child with muscle weakness has difficulty performing motor tasks and may exhibit unusual postures (lordosis) or might manifest the Gower maneuver (see Fig. 38-7) or toe-walking and, on manual muscle testing, may be easily overcome by the examiner's strength.

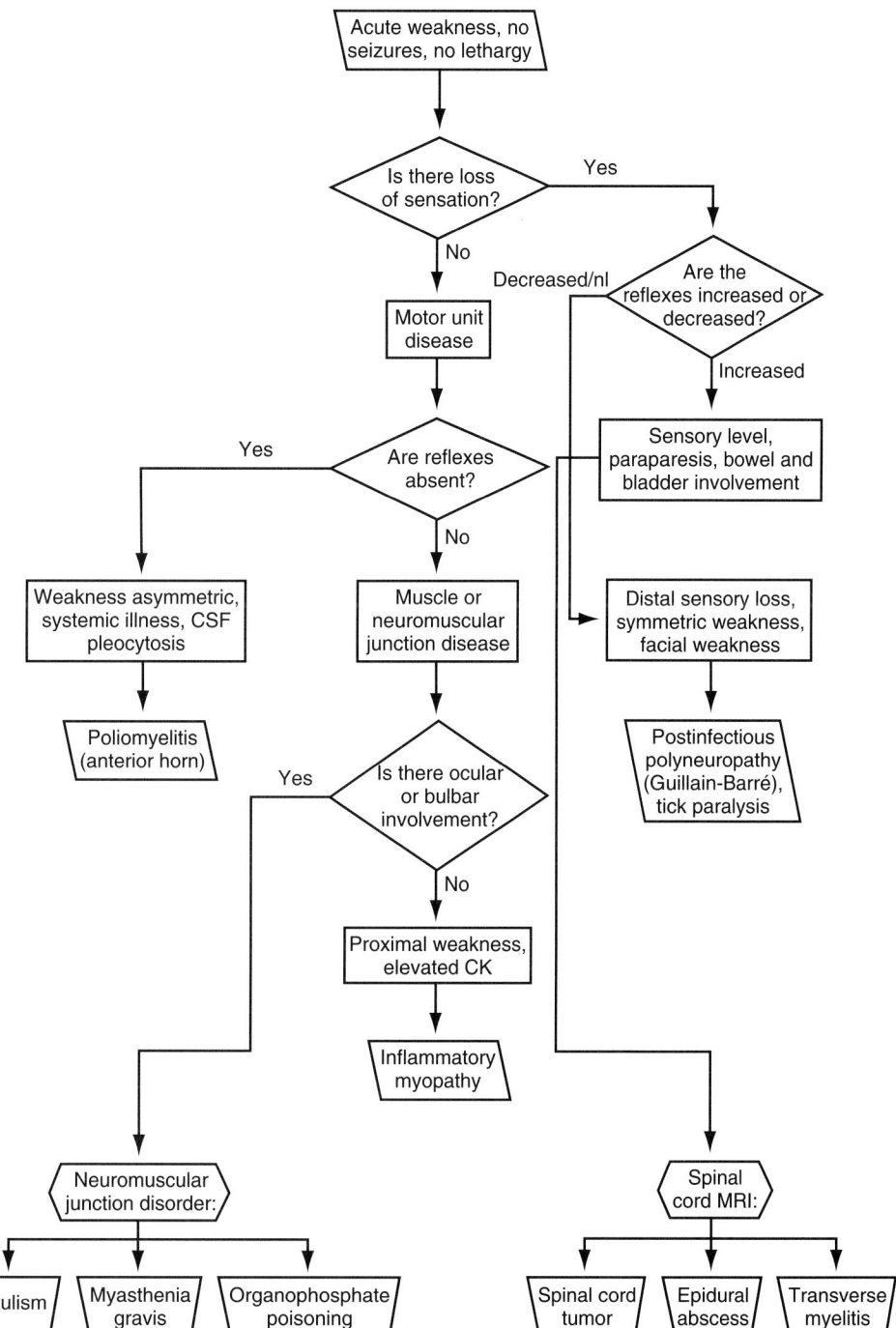

Figure 38-3. Diagnostic approach to the child with acute weakness. CSF, cerebrospinal fluid; CK, creatine phosphokinase; MRI, magnetic resonance imaging; nl, normal.

Passive Tone

Passive muscle tone is more consistent during the waking hours in the child than in the infant. The major joints should be moved through a range of motion and the extent of resistance noted. Flapping the distal extremities provides a useful clue. Lifting the lower extremity briskly at the knee while the patient lies supine is a useful test of muscle tone. In the normal child, the foot briefly drags along the examination table, then rises with the leg. In the hypertonic child, the leg remains extended stiffly at the knee. In the hypotonic child, the lower leg hangs limply and the foot drags as the knee is raised.

Joint Extensibility

The hypotonic child demonstrates hyperextensibility of joints, especially at the elbows, wrists, knees, and ankles. Examination of the small muscles of the fingers may also be helpful.

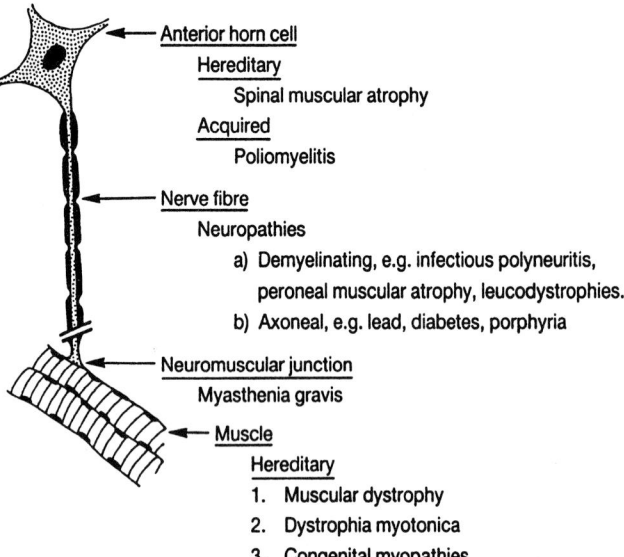

Figure 38-4. Disorders of the lower motor neuron: anatomical approach. (From Dubowitz V: Muscle Disorders in Childhood, 2nd ed. London, WB Saunders, 1995, p 2.)

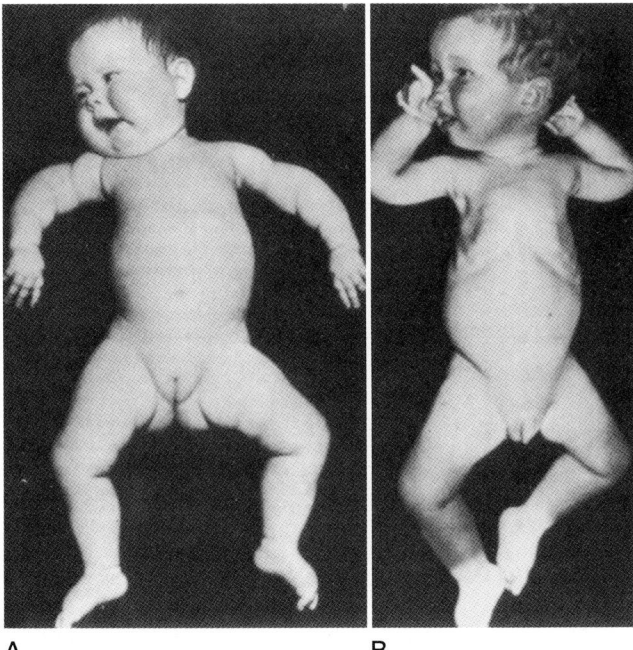

A   B

Figure 38-5. Werdnig-Hoffmann disease: characteristic postures. Six-week-old **(A)** and 1-year-old **(B)** infants with severe weakness and hypotonia from birth. Note the frog-leg posture of the lower limbs and internal rotation ("jug-handle") **(A)** or external rotation **(B)** at shoulders. Intercostal recession is especially evident in B, and facial expressions are normal. (From Volpe JJ [ed]: Neurology of the Newborn, 3rd ed. Philadelphia, WB Saunders, 1995, p 609.)

DIAGNOSTIC APPROACH

The diagnosis of a particular neurologic disorder depends on the location of the lesion (i.e., which part of the nervous system is impaired or abnormal), the patient's age, and whether the condition is progressive or static (see Tables 38-1 and 38-6). Figure 38-2 outlines an algorithm for determining the cause of muscle weakness in a child (see also Tables 38-2 to 38-5).

ANATOMIC LOCALIZATION

The initial approach is to identify the location of dysfunction along the axis of the nervous system. Disorders of the cerebral cortex commonly cause hypotonia in infants and children. Some progressive neurologic disorders affect both the brain and peripheral nerves (metachromatic leukodystrophy, a lipid storage disorder and some mitochondrial disorders). Other progressive disorders may affect both brain and muscle (Walker-Warburg syndrome, neonatal myotonic dystrophy, and some mitochondrial disorders).

Sometimes disturbance of function at one site conveys a predilection for injury to another site in the nervous system. Children with

Table 38-8. Grading Muscle Strength
0: No contraction
1: Minimal contraction only
2: Moves in horizontal plane but not against gravity
3: Moves against gravity but not against resistance
4: Moves against gravity and minimal resistance
5: Moves against gravity and full resistance

congenital muscle weakness (congenital myopathy) are likely to have had severe respiratory impairment at birth that resulted in secondary anoxic injury to the brain. Because hypotonia is nonspecific with regard to localizing the site of nervous system dysfunction, the evaluation of the child with hypotonia must begin with a search for other clues that might identify the location of the abnormality.

IS THE PROBLEM A SYSTEMIC DISORDER?

Systemic disorders (see Table 38-1) are a common cause of generalized hypotonia in infants and even in toddlers and children. Hypotonia is commonly seen in association with sepsis and other infections, heart failure, failure to thrive, hypercalcemia, renal failure, hypothyroidism, acidosis, hypoxia, hyperammonemia, hypoglycemia, rickets, scurvy, amino and organic acid disorders, severe malnutrition, and other chronic disorders. This observation warrants a careful search for a systemic or metabolic abnormality in children with hypotonia, particularly (but not exclusively) when the onset of hypotonia is acute (see Table 38-3 and Fig. 38-3). Most of these disorders cause hypotonia by causing a disturbance of cerebral cortex function.

Frequently overlooked causes of hypotonia are those that are not traditionally considered neurologic disorders. Connective tissue disorders often produce a clinical picture similar to those of neurologic causes of hypotonia in infancy and early childhood, with associated delay of developmental milestones (velocardiofacial syndrome, achondroplasia, Marfan syndrome, Ehlers-Danlos syndrome). In several congenital disorders, hypotonia is a regular feature as a result of a combination of abnormalities of neurologic, muscle, and connective tissue function, including Sotos syndrome, Prader-Willi syndrome, Angelman syndrome, Noonan syndrome, Rett syndrome, and Smith-Lemli-Opitz syndrome.

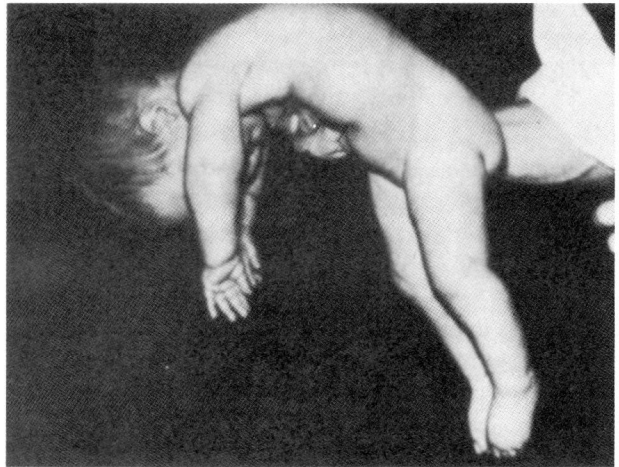

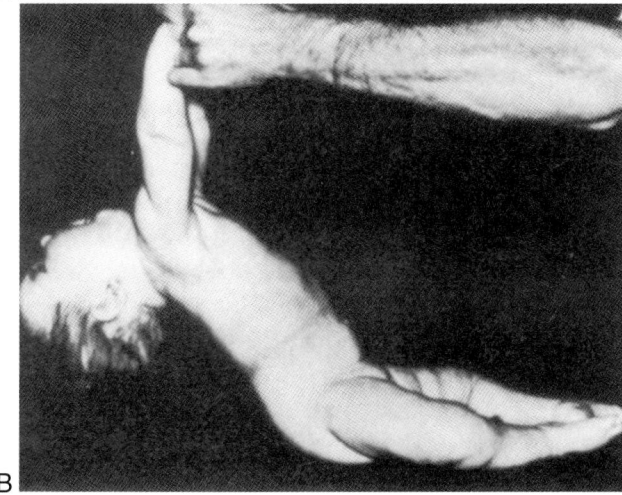

Figure 38-6. Werdnig-Hoffmann disease: clinical manifestations of weakness of limb and axial musculature in a 6-week-old infant with severe weakness and hypotonia from birth. Note the marked weakness of the limbs and trunk on ventral suspension **(A)** and of the neck **(B)** on pull to sit. (From Volpe JJ [ed]: Neurology of the Newborn, 3rd ed. Philadelphia, WB Saunders, 1995, p 609.)

Table 38-9. Major Causes of Arthrogryposis Multiplex Congenita

Site of Major Pathologic Findings	Disorder
Cerebrum	Microcephaly; migrational disorders: lissencephaly-pachygyria (e.g., Zellweger syndrome), polymicrogyria, agenesis of corpus callosum; fetal alcohol syndrome; cytomegalovirus infection; leptomeningeal angiomatosis; encephaloclastic processes: porencephalies, hydranencephaly, multicystic encephalomalacia; hydrocephalus
Anterior horn cell	Developmental agenesis/hypoplasia/dysgenesis (amyoplasia congenita); Werdnig-Hoffmann disease; X-linked spinal muscle atrophy; Möbius syndrome; cervical spinal atrophy; lumbar spinal atrophy; lumbosacral meningomyelocele; sacral agenesis; other
Peripheral nerve or root	Hypomyelinative polyneuropathy; axonal (?) polyneuropathy; neurofibromatosis
Neuromuscular junction	Infant of myasthenic mother; congenital myasthenia; infant of mother with multiple sclerosis(?)
Muscle	Congenital muscular dystrophy; congenital myotonic dystrophy; myotubular myopathy; central core disease; nemaline myopathy; congenital polymyositis, congenital fiber type disproportion; glycogen storage myopathy (muscle phosphorylase deficiency, phosphofructokinase deficiency)
Primary disorder of joint and/or connective tissue	Marfan syndrome; other disorders of connective tissue; intrauterine periarticular inflammation
Intrauterine mechanical obstruction	Uterine abnormality; amniotic bands; oligohydramnios; twin pregnancy; extrauterine pregnancy

From Volpe JJ (ed): Neurology of the Newborn, 3rd ed. Philadelphia, WB Saunders, 1995, p 600.

Diagnostic Considerations

Any child with hypotonia and weakness should be evaluated for a systemic disorder. Laboratory evaluation, such as electrolyte measurements, renal function tests, thyroid function tests, and acid-base balance assessment, should be considered for common metabolic disorders. Laboratory evaluation should also be considered for uncommon metabolic disorders in children with chronic hypotonia, especially those with other neurologic findings and those with recurrent bouts of lethargy, pronounced hypotonia, vomiting, or acidosis. Appropriate metabolic screening tests include plasma and urine amino acid quantification, urine organic acid quantification, and measurements of blood ammonia, blood lactate, and pyruvate.

Cytogenic studies should be done for any hypotonic child who additionally demonstrates microcephaly, growth retardation, congenital malformations, dysmorphism, global developmental delay, or features of specific disorders (Down or Prader-Willi syndrome).

Connective tissue disorders should be considered, especially if joint hyperextensibility and hypotonia are disproportionate to the extent of weakness and in the absence of other neurologic abnormalities or microcephaly (see Table 38-2). The diagnosis of these disorders is generally based on clinical criteria, but molecular genetic testing is becoming increasingly available.

If unusual neurologic or dysmorphic features are present, specific disorders, such as Rett syndrome, Angelman syndrome, Prader-Willi syndrome, Noonan syndrome, Sotos syndrome, and fragile X syndrome, must be considered.

Common Disorders

Down Syndrome

The child with Down syndrome generally has recognizable features, including microcephaly, up-slanted palpebral fissures, epicanthal folds, a flat nasal bridge, a protuberant tongue, excess posterior

Table 38-10. Clinical Features of Congenital Myotonic Dystrophy

Clinical Feature	% of Cases Exhibiting Feature
Reduced fetal movements	68
Polyhydramnios	80
Premature birth (<36 wk)	52
Facial diplegia	100
Feeding difficulties	92
Hypotonia	100
Atrophy	100
Hyporeflexia or areflexia	87
Respiratory distress	88
Arthrogryposis	82
Edema	54
Elevated right hemidiaphragm	49
Transmission via mother	100
Neonatal mortality	41
Infant death in siblings	28
Mental retardation in survivors	100

From Volpe JJ (ed): Neurology of the Newborn, 3rd ed. Philadelphia, WB Saunders, 1995, p 635.

nuchal skin, and simian palmar creases (see Chapter 33). Hypotonia and associated weakness are almost constant findings. As the child grows, the muscle strength generally improves, but the hypotonia persists.

The diagnosis is established by chromosome analysis. Important intervention issues include genetic counseling, referral for early intervention therapeutic services, special education, and monitoring for medical complications, including hypothyroidism, hearing loss, and atlantoaxial dislocation.

Prader-Willi Syndrome

Prader-Willi syndrome manifests in early infancy with marked hypotonia and virtually no other identifiable symptoms. As the child grows, the phenotypic features become more apparent, including microbrachycephaly, almond-shaped palpebrae, short stature, and small hands and feet. At age 3 to 6 years, the child has a disorder of appetite that results in ravenous food-seeking behaviors, impaired satiety, and eventual marked obesity. Weakness associated with the disorder is most prominent in the neonate and older infant and gradually lessens, whereas the hypotonia persists.

The molecular diagnosis can be obtained by chromosome analysis in many of the children and by fluorescent in situ hybridization study. Seventy percent to 75% of affected children have deletion of

chromosome 15q11-q13 of paternal origin, and 20% to 25% have maternal disomy. Because the clinical findings are nonspecific during the early months, such testing should be performed in any neonate or infant with hypotonia of unknown cause. Important intervention issues include genetic counseling, referral for early services, special education, nutritional counseling, behavior management, and monitoring for medical complications of the disorder, including glucose intolerance and complications of morbid obesity.

Uncommon Disorders

Metabolic Disorders

Metabolic disorders that are associated with hypotonia include the following (see Tables 38-1, 38-14, and 38-15):

* amino acid and organic acid disorders
* Lowe syndrome
* peroxisomal disorders (infantile Refsum syndrome, infantile adrenoleukodystrophy, Zellweger syndrome)
* acyl coenzyme A dehydrogenase deficiencies
* storage disorders (mannosidosis, Krabbe disease, sialuria, mucolipidosis type IV, Tay-Sachs disease)

Neurologic Disorders

Neurologic disorders associated with hypotonia are often recognizable by unusual neurologic features:

* Angelman syndrome: awkward gait, inappropriate laughter, seizures (fluorescent in situ hybridization testing reveals that 65% to 75% have deletion of 15q11-q13 chromosome of maternal origin—same chromosome as that affected in Prader-Willi syndrome)
* Rett syndrome: autism, loss of hand use, characteristic wringing hand movements

Congenital Malformation Syndromes

Congenital malformation syndromes are recognizable by their characteristic features:

* Sotos syndrome: macrocephaly, macrosomia, down-slanted palpebrae, mild ventriculomegaly
* Noonan syndrome: short stature, down-slanted palpebrae, ear abnormalities, congenital heart disease, wide-spaced nipples and shield chest, pectus deformities
* Lowe syndrome: cataracts, aminoaciduria, hypotonia

Connective Tissue Disorders

Connective tissue disorders associated with hypotonia, and particularly with joint hyperextensibility, can also generally be recognized

Table 38-11. Specific Congenital Myopathies: Distinguishing Clinical Features

	Neonatal Hypotonia and Weakness	Severe Form with Neonatal Death	Facial Weakness*	Ptosis*	Extraocular Muscular Weakness*
Central core disease	+	0	0	0	0
Nemaline myopathy	+	+	+	0	0
Myotubular myopathy	+	+	+	+	+
Congenital fiber type disproportion	+	0	+	0	0

From Volpe JJ (ed): Neurology of the Newborn, 3rd ed. Philadelphia, WB Saunders, 1995, p 649.

*+, often a prominent feature.

Table 38-12. Infantile Botulism versus "Congenital Myasthenia"

	Infantile Botulism	"Congenital Myasthenia"
Generalized hypotonia and weakness	+	+/−
Facial weakness, ptosis	+	+
Pupillary abnormality	+	−
Constipation	+	−
Response to anticholinesterase	−	+
Electromyography	Incremental response	Decremental response

Modified from Volpe JJ (ed): Neurology of the Newborn, 3rd ed. Philadelphia, WB Saunders, 1995, p 628.

by their associated symptoms:

- Stickler syndrome: micrognathia, Pierre Robin cleft palate
- velocardiofacial syndrome: congenital heart disease, micrognathia, hypocalcemia, T cell disorders, cleft palate
- achondroplasia: disproportionate short stature, risk of brain stem compression
- Ehlers-Danlos syndrome: skin bruising and scarring, skin hyperelasticity
- Marfan syndrome: tall stature, long, thin arms and fingers, ectopic lens, blue sclera, aortic dissection, mitral valve prolapse
- osteogenesis imperfecta: fractures

Table 38-13. Clinical Features of Mitochondrial Disease

Nervous System
1. Ataxia
2. Central apnea
3. Deafness
4. Dementia
5. Hypotonia
6. Mental retardation
7. Neuropathy
8. Ophthalmoplegia
9. Optic atrophy
10. Retinitis pigmentosa
11. Stroke
12. Peripheral neuropathy

Heart
1. Cardiomyopathy
2. Conduction defects

Kidney
1. Aminoaciduria
2. Hyperphosphaturia

Skeletal Muscle
1. Exercise intolerance
2. Myopathy

Other
1. Anemia
2. Lactic acidosis
3. Recurrent bowel obstruction (pseudoobstruction)
4. Myoclonic epilepsy

From Fenichel GM: Clinical Pediatric Neurology: A Signs and Symptoms Approach, 2nd ed. Philadelphia, WB Saunders, 1993, p 205.

Table 38-14. Mitochondrial Disorders

Complex I (NADH–Coenzyme Q Reductase)
1. Congenital lactic acidosis, hypotonia, seizures, and apnea
2. Exercise intolerance and myalgia
3. Kearns-Sayre syndrome
4. Metabolic encephalopathy, lactic acidosis, and stroke (MELAS)
5. Progressive infantile poliodystrophy
6. Subacute necrotizing encephalomyelopathy

Complex II (Succinate–Coenzyme Q Reductase)
1. Encephalomyopathy (?)

Complex III (Coenzyme QH$_2$–Cytochrome-*c* Reductase)
1. Cardiomyopathy
2. Kearns-Sayre syndrome
3. Myopathy and exercise intolerance with or without progressive external ophthalmoplegia

Complex IV (Cytochrome-*c* Oxidase)
1. Fatal neonatal hypotonia
2. Menkes syndrome
3. Myoclonus epilepsy and ragged red fibers (MERRF)
4. Progressive infantile poliodystrophy
5. Subacute necrotizing encephalomyelopathy
6. Transitory neonatal hypotonia

Complex V (Adenosine Triphosphate Synthase)
1. Congenital myopathy
2. Neuropathy, retinopathy, ataxia, and dementia
3. Retinitis pigmentosa, ataxia, neuropathy, and dementia

Modified from Fenichel GM: Clinical Pediatric Neurology: A Signs and Symptoms Approach, 2nd ed. Philadelphia, WB Saunders, 1993, p 206.

IS THE PROBLEM IN THE CEREBRUM OR CEREBELLUM?

Several clues suggest that hypotonia is caused by abnormality of cerebral function. The presence of associated symptoms attributable to dysfunction of the cerebral cortex is the most useful:

- acute impairment of consciousness
- acute or chronic impairment of cognitive abilities (mental status examination or poor school grades, respectively)
- seizures

Delayed language and social development are typical of chronic problems. The presence of microcephaly or macrocephaly is also an important clue. The presence of brisk reflexes, clonus, an asymmetric tonic neck response, and the Babinski sign suggests possible cerebral cortical dysfunction (upper motor neuron disorder). The presence of dysmorphism or of congenital malformations suggests the possibility of a cerebral malformation. Congenital ocular malformations (e.g., microphthalmia or optic hypoplasia) are frequently associated with congenital brain malformation.

The presence of hypertonia mixed with signs of hypotonia strongly suggests a cerebral origin. This may seem paradoxical, but it is often overlooked that many children with cerebral causes of hypotonia have signs of hypertonia as well. This may occur as an evolutionary phenomenon in the development of spasticity; cerebral palsy is often characterized by hypotonia in infancy with later development of spasticity. In some children with cerebral dysfunction, the coexistence of hypotonia and hypertonia is persistent. Thus, an infant with hypotonia of the neck and trunk musculature who also exhibits scissoring of the lower extremities or persistent fisting of the hands (typical signs of hypertonia) can be presumed to have a cerebral dysfunction.

Table 38-15. Glycogenoses that Affect Muscle

Type	Enzyme Deficiency	Eponymous or Other Names	Subunit; Isozyme	Clinical Features	Other Tissues/ Systems Affected
II	α-1,4-Glucosidase (acid maltase)	Pompe disease	—	Severe form: generalized, resembles infantile spinal muscular atrophy	Heart, nervous system, leukocytes, liver, kidneys
				Mild form: resembles limb-girdle dystrophy	?Heart
III	Amylo-1,6-glucosidase ("debranching enzyme")	Limit dextrinosis Forbes disease Cori disease	—	Infantile hypotonia Mild weakness	Hepatic Hypoglycemia Ketosis Leukocytes Cardiac
IV	α-1,4-Glucan: α-1,4-glucan 6-glycosyl transferase ("branching enzyme"; amylo [1,4 → 1,6] transglucosidase)	Amylopectinosis	—	Usually no muscle symptoms In some, wasting or weakness	Hepatomegaly Cirrhosis Liver failure Cardiac
V	Muscle phosphorylase	McArdle disease	M	Exercise intolerance Muscle cramps Fatigue Myoglobinuria	None
VII	Phosphofructokinase	Tarui disease	M	Exercise intolerance Muscle cramps Fatigue Myoglobinuria	Hemolytic anemia
VIII	Phosphorylase *b* kinase		α β	Exercise intolerance Muscle stiffness Weakness	Liver Cardiac
IX	Phosphoglycerate kinase		A	Exercise intolerance Muscle cramps Fatigue Myoglobinuria	Hemolytic anemia Central nervous system
X	Phosphoglycerate kinase		M	Exercise intolerance Muscle cramps Fatigue Myoglobinuria	Hemolytic anemia Seizures Mental retardation
XI	Lactate dehydrogenase		M	Exercise intolerance Muslce cramps Fatigue Myoglobinuria	Acroerythema

Modified from Dubowitz V: Muscle Disorders in Childhood, 2nd ed. London, WB Saunders, 1995, p 178.

Signs of cerebellar dysfunction (ataxia, titubation, dysmetria, and impairment of coordination) are often useful diagnostic clues (see Chapter 42). The cerebellum helps maintain normal muscle tone, and diseases of the cerebellum typically are associated with some degree of hypotonia.

IS THE PROBLEM IN THE SPINAL CORD?

Classically, spinal cord dysfunction produces spastic weakness of all four extremities or paraparesis of the lower extremities (Tables 38-16 to 38-18). However, particularly after acute injury to the spinal cord and in some chronic disorders of the spinal cord, hypotonia may be the prominent motor sign. The typical associated findings of hyperreflexia, clonus, Babinski signs, and sensory loss (with a sensory level) are important clues, as is the disparity between the weakness and sensory impairment of the extremities in contrast to the normal strength and function of the head and neck.

Spinal cord injury resulting from birth trauma is frequently overlooked as a cause of hypotonia in the newborn. A history of a lengthy or difficult (breech or vertex) delivery should suggest spinal cord injury, and care should be taken not to falsely attribute motor dysfunction in these infants to anoxic brain injury. The bones of the cervical spine are normal, but MRI demonstrates the cord lesion. This diagnosis should *never* be missed, because neurosurgical intervention is often required. To make matters more confusing, many spinal cord–injured neonates also have anoxic encephalopathy because of the traumatic nature of the delivery.

Finally, the extent to which the hypotonia of neonatal hypoxic-ischemic injury is caused by hypoxic injury to the spinal cord has not yet been fully evaluated. Any child with suspected spinal cord injury should undergo MRI.

If spinal cord injury is suspected, the clinician should accomplish the following:

1. Immobilize the patient's head and neck.

Table 38-19. Typical Electrophysiologic Features of Neuropathies and Myopathies

	Nerve Conduction Velocity	F response	H reflex	Electromyography
Inflammatory myopathy or dystrophy	Normal	Normal	Normal	Fibrillations; positive sharp waves; small motor units
Metabolic myopathy	Normal	Normal	Normal	Small motor units
Axonal neuropathy	Normal	Normal	Normal	Fibrillations; positive sharp waves; fasciculations; large motor units with distal predominance
Demyelinating neuropathy	Slowed diffusely	Delayed or absent diffusely	Delayed or absent	Normal motor units
Radiculopathy	Normal	Delayed or absent in damaged root	Delayed or absent if S1 is involved	Fibrillations; positive sharp waves; fasciculations; large motor units if chronic
Motoneuron disease	Normal	Normal	Normal	Fibrillations; positive sharp waves; fasciculations; large motor units diffusely

From Wyngaarden JB, Smith LH Jr, Bennett JC (eds): Cecil Textbook of Medicine, 19th ed, vol 2. Philadelphia, WB Saunders, 1988, p 2038.

(Table 38-19). The electromyogram (EMG) may demonstrate fibrillations and large motor unit potentials that are reduced in number.

Diagnostic Considerations

The patient is examined for distribution of weakness, reflexes, and the presence of tongue fasciculations. Creatine kinase levels and an EMG are obtained, and a lumbar puncture is performed when acute poliomyelitis is suspected.

Common Disorders

Anterior Horn Cell Disease

Spinal muscular atrophy represents a group of heterogeneous genetic disorders characterized by degeneration of anterior horn cells in the spinal cord (Table 38-20). *Werdnig-Hoffmann disease* is the prototype for the spinal muscular atrophies and is inherited as an autosomal recessive trait. Manifestations begin early in life and even occasionally in the prenatal period (e.g., decreased fetal movements, congenital contractures, polyhydramnios caused by poor swallowing, poor respiratory effort at birth). Neonates and young infants experience progressive weakness and hypotonia, which result in poor head and body control and a flaccid, motionless, extended posture with alert facies (see Figs. 38-5 and 38-6). Fasciculations may be noted in the tongue, over muscles with little subcutaneous fat, and as a fine tremor of the outstretched fingers. Bilateral paralysis of the diaphragm may be present before loss of deep tendon reflexes or detection of muscle weakness.

The diagnosis is by blood DNA analysis for mutation in either survival motor neuron gene or neuronal apoptosis inhibitor protein gene on chromosome 5q13. If genetic test results are positive, no further evaluation is necessary. If mutation tests are negative, a more traditional evaluation, including serum enzyme levels, electromyographic nerve conduction studies, and muscle biopsy, is pursued.

Neuropathies

Neuropathies are characterized by hypotonia, weakness, and diminished or absent reflexes (Tables 38-21 and 38-22; see Fig. 38-3). Neuropathies may be primarily motor or sensory, and the child's symptoms may be either acute or chronic weakness or discomfort caused by paresthesias and dysesthesias. In chronic sensory neuropathies, the child may sustain injuries (e.g., burns or even fractures) that are unnoticed. Autonomic symptoms associated with some neuropathies include orthostatic hypotension, gastrointestinal dysmotility, and abnormalities of sweating. In general, the reflexes in neuropathies are diminished disproportionately to the extent of muscle weakness; that is, the reflexes may be markedly reduced or absent, whereas the muscle strength is only mildly diminished. Nerve conduction studies and EMGs demonstrate slowing of nerve conduction velocities and features that suggest either primary axonal involvement (fibrillations, normal or mildly slow nerve conduction velocity) or demyelination (marked slowing of nerve conduction velocity) (see Table 38-19).

Guillain-Barré syndrome is an acute demyelinating polyneuropathy that frequently follows an upper respiratory tract infection or *Campylobacter*-associated diarrhea. The disorder is characterized by ascending motor weakness and areflexia. The weakness is usually symmetric, ascends and progresses over various periods (usually 1 to 2 weeks), and may cause serious respiratory compromise by producing weakness of the respiratory muscles. Therefore, all patients must

Table 38-20. Spinal Muscular Atrophy: Clinical Classification

Type	Disease	Onset	Course	Age at Death
1. Severe	Werdnig-Hoffman	Birth to 6 months	Never sit	Usually <2 years
2. Intermediate	—	<18 months	Never stand	>2 years
3. Mild	Kugelberg-Welander	>18 months	Stand alone	Adult

From Munsat TL: Workshop Report: International SMA [Spinal Muscular Atrophy] Collaboration. Neuromuscul Disord 1991;1:81. Reprinted in Dubowitz V: Muscle Disorders in Childhood, 2nd ed. London, WB Saunders, 1995, p 327.

Table 38-21. Mnemonic for Peripheral Neuropathy: CHANCE-IT

Collagen Vascular Diseases	Hereditary	Autoimmune	Nutrition	Cancer	Endocrine	Infectious	Toxin or Trauma
Periarteritis nodosa	HMSN	GBS	Vitamin deficiencies (B_1, B_6, B_{12}, E)	Eaton-Lambert	Diabetes mellitus	*Campylobacter* (GBS)	Tick-toxin
	HSAN	Immunizations			Hyperthyroidism	Diphtheria	INH
	HSN				Hypothyroidism	Lyme (cranial)	DDI
SLE	Metabolic (porphyria)	Chronic inflammatory polyneuropathy			Acromegaly	Leprosy	DDC
Vasculitis	Refsum disease				(entrapment)	HIV	Organophosphates
Angiitis	Leukodystrophies (e.g., Krabbe, metachromatic)					Herpes-zoster	Lead
						Rabies	Mercury
							Thallium
							Arsenic
Granulomatous (sarcoidosis)							Vincristine
							Uremia
Wegener granulomatosis	Amyloid (familial)						Chloramphenicol
Henoch-Schönlein purpura	Congenital abetalipoproteinemia						Nitrofurantoin
Mononeuritis multiplex	Fabry disease						Acrylamide
	Tangier disease						Cyanide
							N-Hexane
							Glue sniffing
							Buckthorn toxin
							Carbon monoxide
							Entrapment
							Obstetric trauma

DDC, dideoxycytidine; DDI, dideoxyinosine; GBS, Guillain-Barré syndrome; HIV, human immunodeficiency virus; HMSN, hereditary motor-sensory neuropathy–Charcot-Marie-Tooth syndrome; HSAN, hereditary sensory-autonomic neuropathy–Riley-Day syndrome (dysautonomia); HSN, hereditary sensory neuropathy; INH, isoniazid; SLE, systemic lupus erythematous.

Table 38-22. Polyneuropathies with Possible Onset in Infancy

Axonal

1. Familial dysautonomia
2. Hereditary motor-sensory neuropathy type II
3. Idiopathic with encephalopathy
4. Infantile neuronal degeneration
5. Subacute necrotizing encephalopathy

Demyelinating

1. Acute inflammatory demyelinating polyneuropathy (Guillain-Barré syndrome)
2. Chronic inflammatory demyelinating polyneuropathy
3. Congenital hypomyelinating neuropathy
4. Globoid cell leukodystrophy
5. Hereditary motor-sensory neuropathy type I
6. Hereditary motor-sensory neuropathy type III
7. Metachromatic leukodystrophy

Modified from Fenichel GM: Clinical Pediatric Neurology: A Signs and Symptoms Approach, 2nd ed. Philadelphia, WB Saunders, 1993, p 158.

be tested for respiratory function (negative inspiratory forces and vital capacity). There may also be paresthesias. A Miller-Fisher variant involves ophthalmoplegia and ataxia, whereas autonomic nervous system involvement may produce hypotension or hypertension and bradyarrhythmias or tachyarrhythmias. In addition to an abnormal nerve conduction velocity, the cerebrospinal fluid protein level is usually elevated after the first week of illness.

Treatment includes careful monitoring of respiratory status, autonomic dysfunction, and strength. Intravenous immunoglobulin and plasmapheresis are two treatment options for progressive disease. Intravenous immunoglobulin, when given during the first week, is as effective as plasmapheresis and may be of greater efficacy and associated with fewer side effects.

Congenital hypomyelinating neuropathy also manifests as infantile hypotonia. Nerve biopsy shows axons without evidence of myelination. Molecular genetic analysis may show a point mutation in the myelin protein zero gene.

Muscle and Neuromuscular Junction Disorders

Neuromuscular junction disorders must be differentiated from *muscle diseases*. Both are characterized by hypotonia, weakness, and normal to diminished reflexes (see Tables 38-5 and 38-6). The degree of muscle weakness is usually more pronounced than the extent of loss of reflexes, just the reverse of the case observed in neuropathies. Disorders of the neuromuscular junction are identifiable by electromyographic response to repetitive stimulation and by response to edrophonium chloride (Tensilon) intravenously (Fig. 38-8; see Tables 38-6 and 38-19). In most muscle disorders, weakness is most prominent in the proximal muscles, and the sensory examination findings are normal. The creatine kinase level is elevated in many but not all muscle disorders. The nerve conduction velocities are normal, and the EMG demonstrates small, short, abundant potentials. The muscular dystrophies (Table 38-23) and other myopathies (see Table 38-4) are typical of muscle disorders and usually produce progressive proximal muscle weakness (see Table 38-4).

Myopathies

Muscular dystrophy, both Duchenne and Becker, are X-linked recessive disorders caused by mutations on the short arm of the X chromosome in the XP21 region. This mutation results in absent or decreased muscle intracellular protein dystrophin. Most young infants are not obviously symptomatic. Poor head control may be noted, but early motor milestones are achieved on time (sitting, walking). Nonetheless, the walking child may assume a hyperlordotic posture by 1½ to 2 years of age; the Gower sign, demonstrating proximal leg weakness, is often present by age 3 years (see Fig. 38-7). The typical waddling antalgic Trendelenburg gait is often noted by 5 to 6 years of age. Eventually, there is muscle atrophy; the calves may be enlarged (pseudohypertrophy) because of proliferation of fat and collagen with possibly some muscle hypertrophy.

With time, proximal muscle weakness makes ambulation difficult, and the patient requires a wheelchair. Respiratory muscle failure eventually develops; pulmonary insufficiency is aggravated by thoracic kyphoscoliosis. Additional complications include myocardiopathy, mental retardation (20% to 30%), contractures, scoliosis, and malignant hyperthermia on exposure to various anesthetic agents.

The diagnosis of Duchenne muscular dystrophy is suspected from the history (including the family history), physical examination

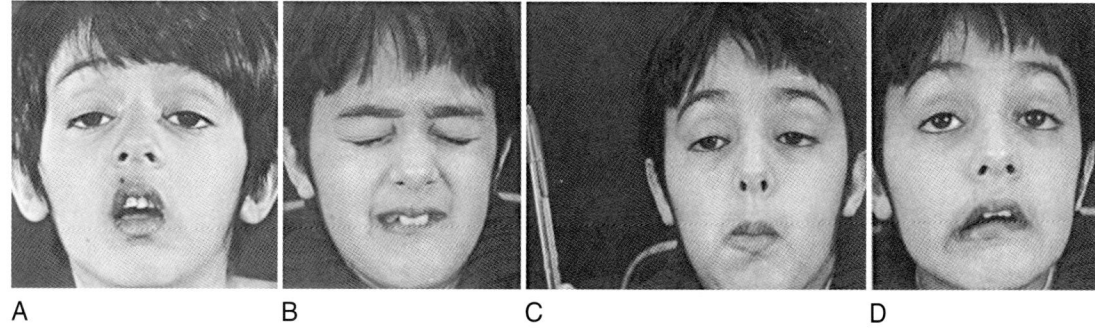

A   B   C   D

Figure 38-8. Congenital myasthenia. This child was referred at 4 years of age with a history of swallowing difficulty. By 2 years, his walking had not progressed further, and he was unable to run or climb stairs. His parents had also noted some ptosis in the first year. On examination he had obvious ptosis, limited ocular movement, associated weakness of facial movement, an expressionless face, open mouth and an inability to close the eyes tightly (**A**). There was general hypotonia with joint laxity. The child got up from the floor with a Gower sign and could not stand on one leg or run. A diagnosis of myasthenia was confirmed by demonstrating response decrement to repeated ulnar nerve stimulation. A definite improvement in the ptosis and his ability to get up from the floor was noted after intravenous edrophonium chloride (Tensilon). He was treated with pyridostigmine and showed a definite improvement, but with time, he needed an increased dosage and frequency. His performance improved after each dose and tended to wane as the next dose became due. He still had a Gower sign on rising from the floor, marked ptosis, external ophthalmoplegia, and facial weakness (**B** to **D**). His parents are first cousins, and so this is probably a case of autosomal recessive infantile (congenital) myasthenia. (From Dubowitz V: Muscle Disorders in Childhood, 2nd ed. London, WB Saunders, 1995, p 414.)

Table 38-23. Muscular Dystrophies

	Genetic Type	Age at Onset (yr)	Age at Disabililty (yr)	Pattern of Weakness
Duchenne	X-linked	0-5	10-15	Proximal
Becker	X-linked	5-15	15-25	Proximal
Limb-girdle	Autosomal recessive	10-30	20-40	Proximal
Facioscapulohumeral	Autosomal dominant	10-30	30-50	Proximal arm, face
Myotonic	Autosomal dominant	10-30	30-50	Distal limbs, face
Scapuloperoneal	Autosomal dominant	20-30	30-50	Proximal arm, distal leg
Emery-Dreifuss	X-linked	5-15	25-50	Proximal arm, distal leg

From Fenichel GM; Clinical Pediatric Neurology: A Signs and Symptoms Approach, 2nd ed. Philadelphia, WB Saunders, 1993, p 174.

findings, and an elevated serum creatinine phosphokinase (often 10,000 to 30,000 IU/L). Muscle biopsy or genetic testing confirms the diagnosis. Treatment is supportive and includes exercise, physical therapy, bracing, seating, special education, and emotional support. Most affected patients die by age 20 to 25 years.

Myotonic dystrophy is a common muscle disorder of childhood that is distinct in that it causes primarily a distal distribution of muscle weakness and is associated with myotonia, a phenomenon characterized by persistent muscular contraction with apparent delay in relaxation of muscles. A child with myotonia has difficulty releasing a ball after gripping it tightly or letting go of a doorknob.

In *congenital myotonic dystrophy,* the newborn infant appears with severe generalized hypotonia and weakness, often with swallowing and sucking difficulty, facial diplegia, and congenital joint contractures (talipes equinovarus, arthrogryposis). In *childhood-onset myotonic dystrophy,* the phenomenon of myotonia is often the first symptom and is usually described by the child as "stiffness," which is often exacerbated by exposure to cold. Myotonia usually is present by age 10 years, but significant distal muscle weakness is not usually evident until the end of the second decade. This is a slowly progressive disorder with multisystemic involvement, including the development of cataracts, premature male-pattern baldness, facial muscle atrophy resulting in "hatchet face" appearance, cervical kyphosis, cardiac arrhythmias, and testicular atrophy. Useful diagnostic tests include EMG (which reveals a characteristic electrical pattern of myotonia), and muscle biopsy. Myotonic dystrophy is a trinucleotide repeat expansion disorder at chromosome region 19q13.3. Genetic testing establishes the diagnosis.

Dermatomyositis

See Chapter 44.

Neuromuscular Junction Disorders

Myasthenia gravis is caused by the presence of antiacetylcholine receptor antibodies, which produce neuromuscular blockade at the level of the neuromuscular junction. Antibodies may be acquired by the transplacental route (transient neonatal myasthenia gravis) in infants born to mothers with this disease. These patients usually demonstrate generalized hypotonia and difficulty feeding a few hours after birth. Otherwise, they are alert, and pupils are reactive. Complete recovery in 4 to 6 weeks is the rule. Congenital infantile myasthenia gravis is less common and is caused by several genetic defects causing either defective release of acetylcholine (presynaptic) or abnormal receptor response (postsynaptic). Clinically, all congenital myasthenic syndromes are seronegative for acetylcholine receptor antibodies and can manifest either as prominent ocular findings or with respiratory or feeding difficulties. Congenital infantile

myasthenia gravis is less common than that acquired in older childhood. In all types, the cranial nerves are most often affected, producing ptosis (see Table 38-12 and Fig. 38-8) and diplopia, followed by facial weakness and dysphagia. The pupillary light response is intact. Although the deep tendon reflexes may be reduced, these reflexes are never completely lost. Generalized motor weakness ensues. The disease is characterized by rapid fatigue of muscles; patients are more symptomatic as the day progresses.

The diagnosis is suspected from the history of fatigability of extraocular muscles and is confirmed by the presence of antiacetylcholine receptor antibodies and a positive result of the edrophonium test. This short-acting cholinesterase inhibitor acutely elevates the level of acetylcholine in the neuromuscular junction, thus overcoming the receptor blockade. Ptosis, ophthalmoplegia, and fatigability are rapidly corrected (in seconds) but return to baseline levels within 1 to 2 minutes.

Therapy includes long-acting cholinesterase inhibitors (neostigmine, pyridostigmine) and atropine if the cholinesterase inhibitors produce untoward muscarinic effects (e.g., increased secretions.) Prednisone is useful because of the autoimmune nature of the disease. Thymectomy in noncongenital or nonfamilial cases or plasmapheresis may also be of value. Hashimoto thyroiditis with resultant hypothyroidism may complicate myasthenia gravis. Neonatal myasthenia gravis is transient, and anticholinesterase therapy is needed for a few days to a few weeks after birth.

Infantile botulism is caused by the germination of *Clostridium botulinum* organisms in the infant's gastrointestinal tract with local endogenous toxin production. Toxin is absorbed into the circulation and eventually inhibits the release of neuronal acetylcholine in the peripheral nervous system.

Infantile botulism is common between the ages of 2 and 6 months of life; many affected infants are breast-fed and may have a prior history of constipation. The sources of *C. botulinum* include honey, corn syrup, soil, and dust. Manifestations include lack of fever, poor feeding (poor sucking and swallowing), constipation, a weak cry and smile, hypotonia, ptosis (see Table 38-12), mydriasis, ileus, bladder atony, and hypotonia. Respiratory arrest and inappropriate antidiuretic hormone secretion may ensue. There is a descending paralysis, as symptoms are usually first noted in the cranial nerves.

Food-borne botulism is manifested after ingestion of preformed toxin in poorly canned foods. Affected children have nausea and vomiting with dilated pupils, diplopia, dysphagia, dysarthria, dry mouth, and hypotonia.

The diagnosis of infant botulism is confirmed by recovery of the organism or the toxin from stool, blood, or food. Treatment is supportive, with careful attention to respiratory function and nutrition. No antitoxin or antibiotics are needed. Aminoglycoside antibiotics may exacerbate weakness, because they have neuromuscular blocking effects. In food-borne botulism, antitoxin and penicillin therapy are indicated.

SUMMARY AND RED FLAGS

In the neonate and older infant, hypotonia is more commonly associated with systemic diseases that indirectly affect the central nervous system. However, various disorders are related to the nervous system and necessitate immediate attention. Meningomyelocele is usually discovered by prenatal fetal ultrasonography or at birth. Like an encephalopathic infant, any child with an acute neurologic process needs thorough investigation. Hypotonia and weakness can arise from dysfunction at many potential sites of the nervous system. An accurate diagnosis requires careful anatomic localization (see Table 38-6).

Acute weakness, paralysis, or loss of function also warrants immediate attention and follow-up (see Fig. 38-3). Ascending motor weakness with absence of deep tendon reflexes that develops over a few days suggests Gillian-Barré syndrome and is a medical emergency. In addition, spine pain, a motor-sensory level, bowel and bladder dysfunction, and upper motor neuron signs strongly suggest a lesion in the spinal cord and constitute a medical *and* possibly a surgical emergency.

REFERENCES

Central Nervous System

Knebusch M: Acute transverse myelitis in childhood: Nine cases and review of the literature. Develop Med Child Neurol 1998;40:631-639.
Knoll JHM, Lalande M: Cytogenetic and molecular studies in Prader-Willi and Angelman syndrome. Am J Med Genet 1993;46:2.
Malki J, Sheth P: Mapping of acute (I) spinal muscular atrophy to chromosome 5q12-q14. Lancet 1990;336:271-273.

Muscle Disorders

Buist NRM, Powell BR: Approaches to the evaluation of muscle diseases. Int Pediatr 1992;7:320-326.
Bushby KMD: Recent advances in understanding muscular dystrophy. Arch Dis Child 1992;67:1310-1312.
Darras B: Molecular genetics of Duchenne and Becker muscular dystrophy. J Pediatr 1990;117:1-15.
Darras BT, Friedman NR: Metabolic myopathies: A clinical approach; part I. Pediatr Neurol 2000;22:87-97.
Darras BT, Friedman NR: Metabolic myopathies: A clinical approach; part II. Pediatr Neurol 2000;22:171-181.
Emery AEH: The muscular dystrophies. Lancet 2002;359:687-695.
Mendell JR: Congenital muscular dystrophy searching for definition after 98 years. Neurology 2001;56:993-994.
Miller G, Wessel HB: Diagnosis of dystrophinopathies: Review for the clinician. Pediatr Neurol 1993;9:3-9.
Pizzuti A, Fu YH: An unstable triplet repeat in a gene related to myotonic muscular dystrophy. Science 1992;255:1256.
Ptacek LJ, Johnson KJ, Griggs RC: Genetics and physiology of the myotonic muscle disorders. N Engl J Med 1993;328:482-488.
Reardon W, Newcombe R, Fenton I, et al: The natural history of congenital dystrophy: Mortality and long-term clinical aspects. Arch Dis Child 1993;68:177-181.

Peripheral Neuropathy

Abd-Allah SA, Jansen PW, Ashwal S: Intravenous immunoglobulin as therapy for pediatric Guillain-Barré syndrome. J Child Neurol 1997;12:376.

Acute flaccid paralysis syndrome associated with West Nile virus infection—Mississippi and Louisiana, July-August 2002. MMWR Morbid Mortal Wkly Rep 2002;51:825-828.
De Jonghe B, Sharshar T, Lefaucheur JP, et al: Paresis acquired in the intensive care unit. JAMA 2002;288:2859-2867.
Dematteis M, Pepin JL, Jeanmart M, et al: Charcot-Marie-Tooth disease and sleep apnoea syndrome: A family study. Lancet 2001;357:267-272.
Dyck PJ, Dyck PJB: Atypical varieties of chronic inflammatory demyelinating neuropathies. Lancet 2000;355:1293-1294.
Epstein MA, Sladky JT: The role of plasmapheresis in childhood Guillain-Barré syndrome. Ann Neurol 1990;28:65-69.
Gruenewald R, Ropper AH, Lior H, et al: Serologic evidence of *Campylobacter jejuni/coli* enteritis in patients with Guillain-Barré syndrome. Arch Neurol 1991;48:1080-1082.
Hughes RAC: Peripheral neuropathy. BMJ 2002;324:466-469.
Hughes RAC: Sensory form of Guillain-Barré syndrome. Lancet 2001;357:1465-1466.
Hund EF, Borel CO, Cornblath DR, et al: Intensive management and treatment of severe Guillain-Barré syndrome. Crit Care Med 1993;21:433-446.
Jansen PW, Perkin RM, Ashwal S: Guillain-Barré syndrome in childhood: Natural course and efficacy of plasmapheresis. Pediatr Neurol 1992;9:16-20.
Lupski JR: Charcot-Marie-Tooth polyneuropathy: Duplication, gene dosage, and genetic heterogeneity. Pediatr Res 1999;45:159-165.
Lupski JR, Chance PF, Garcia CA: Inherited primary peripheral neuropathies: Molecular genetics and clinical implications of CMT1A and HNPP. JAMA 1993;270:2326-2330.
Moore PM, Cupps TR: Neurological complications of vasculitis. Ann Neurol 1983;14:155-167.
Nguyen DK, Agenarioti-Belanger S, Vanasse M: Pain and the Guillain-Barré syndrome in children under 6 years old. J Pediatr 1999;134:773-776.
Rantala H, Uhari M, Niemel M: Occurrence, clinical manifestations, and prognosis of Guillain-Barré syndrome. Arch Dis Child 1991;66:706-709.
Ropper AH: The Guillain-Barré syndrome. N Engl J Med 1992;326:1130-1136.
Said G: Value of nerve biopsy? Lancet 2001;357:1220-1221.
Shahar E, Shorer Z: Immune globulins are effective in treatment of severe Guillain-Barré syndrome. Pediatr Neurol 1997;16:32.
Shaw PJ: Motor neurone disease. BMJ 1999;318:1118-1121.
Tabarki B, Coffinieres A, Van den Bergh P: Critical illness neuromuscular disease: Clinical, electrophysiological, and prognostic aspects. Arch Dis Child 2002;86:103-107.
Vedanarayanan VV, Evans OB, Subramony SH: Tick paralysis in children: Electrophysiology and possibility of misdiagnosis. Neurology 2002;59:1088-1090.
Winer J: Guillain-Barré syndrome revisited. BMJ 1992;304:65-66.

Neuromuscular Junction

Drachman DB: Myasthenia gravis. N Engl J Med 1994;330:1797-1810.
Havard CWH, Fonseca V: The natural course of myasthenia gravis. BMJ 1990;1409-1410.
Horslen SP, Clayton PT, Harding BN, et al: Olivopontocerebellar atrophy of neonatal onset and disialotransferrin developmental deficiency syndrome. Arch Dis Child 1991;66:1027-1032.
Spinal muscular atrophies [editorial]. Lancet 1990;336:280-282.
Vincent A, Palace J, Hilton-Jones D: Myasthenia gravis. Lancet 2001;357:2122-2128.

39 Paroxysmal Disorders

Andrew Bleasel   Elaine Wyllie

DEFINITIONS

An *epileptic seizure* is a paroxysmal alteration in behavior, motor function, or autonomic function or a combination of these, occurring in association with excessive synchronous neuronal activity in the central nervous system (CNS).

A *convulsion* is a generalized tonic-clonic ("grand mal") seizure in which bilateral tonic or tonic-clonic motor involvement of the upper and lower limbs occurs in association with loss of consciousness.

Acute symptomatic seizures are seizures occurring in association with a transient acute structural or metabolic CNS insult.

Epilepsy is a disorder in which there are *recurrent* unprovoked epileptic seizures.

Nonepileptic paroxysmal disorders comprise a variety of episodic behavioral and motor phenomena that cause people to seek medical advice. These episodes may result from physiologic processes, intercurrent organic illness, or psychiatric illness.

The adjective *ictal* refers to the events or phenomena occurring during an epileptic seizure.

The adjective *interictal* describes behavior or clinical observations between epileptic seizures, most often used in reference to findings on electroencephalogram (EEG).

EPIDEMIOLOGY AND CAUSES OF SEIZURES AND EPILEPSY

Approximately 1% of children have at least one afebrile seizure before the age of 14 years; most seizures occur before the age of 3 years. If febrile seizures are included, approximately 3.5% of children experience some kind of seizure by the age of 15 years. Of children experiencing seizures, the majority (>50%) have febrile convulsions; 13% have acute symptomatic seizures other than febrile convulsions; 8% have single, unprovoked seizures of unknown cause; and 25% have chronic epilepsy. The incidence of acute symptomatic seizures is highest in the first year of life; the most common causes of these predominantly neonatal seizures are infection and metabolic insults. After age 4 years, head injury is the most common cause of acute symptomatic seizures, and infection is the next most common.

The incidence of recurrent unprovoked seizures among children younger than 15 years has been estimated to be between 45 to 85 per 100,000 in developed countries. It is highest in younger children; in those younger than 1 year, it is about 100 per 100,000. The *prevalence* of active epilepsy—patients taking antiepileptic drugs (AED)—is between 4.3 and 9.3 per 1000, or about 0.5% to 1% of the population.

Between 60% and 80% of children with epilepsy have no identifiable etiologic factors for the disease. Population-based studies report the following presumed causes for 23% of children with symptomatic epilepsy: developmental (epilepsy in association with neurologic abnormalities present since birth) in 13%; infection in

5%; head trauma in 3%; and miscellaneous causes in 2%. Other identifiable causes include tumors, malformations of cortical development, vascular malformations, and cerebral infarction.

SEIZURE CLASSIFICATION

Table 39-1 outlines the clinical and EEG classification of epileptic seizures.

PARTIAL SEIZURES

Partial seizures are seizures in which the first clinical and EEG changes indicate initial activation of a system of neurons limited to part of one cerebral hemisphere. *Simple partial seizures* do not involve loss or impairment of consciousness. The clinical symptoms and signs of simple partial seizures reflect the functional anatomy of the region of the brain undergoing the abnormal neuronal discharge. In all cortical areas, there may be spread of a focal seizure beyond the region of onset; this may be reflected in a march of motor or sensory symptoms in contralateral body parts if the seizure activity spreads to primary motor or sensory cortex. Certain cortical areas do not produce symptoms when involved; seizures beginning in a so-called silent cerebral area may produce symptoms and signs only on spread to eloquent cortex.

Focal motor seizures produce clonic movements of the limb or limbs contralateral to the primary motor cortex involved. Other focal motor seizures include version of the head and eyes, vocalization, and speech arrest. Involvement of primary *somatosensory* or *special sensory* cortex produces crude somatosensory experiences such as paresthesia or numbness, often with a dysesthetic quality, and visual, auditory, olfactory, or gustatory phenomena. Symptoms arising from special sensory cortex seizures vary in complexity according to the extent of involvement of the association cortex surrounding the primary special sensory cortex (e.g., flashes of uncolored light in comparison with structured visual hallucinations). Focal seizures involving the limbic system produce *psychic symptoms,* such as distorted memory experiences; sensations of unreality or detachment; distorted time sense; fearfulness, depression, or a sense of well-being; distorted perceptions of surroundings, objects, or self; and structured hallucinations.

When consciousness is impaired, the seizure is classified as a *complex partial seizure.* Impairment of consciousness is defined as an alteration in awareness of external stimuli; this may be combined with a loss or impairment of responsiveness to external stimuli. Assessment of consciousness during seizures is often difficult. It is possible to be unresponsive because of an aphasia, an apraxia, paralysis, or even distraction without being unaware or unconscious of one's surroundings. At the same time, it is possible to be responsive to external stimuli but to have altered awareness, often demonstrated by complete amnesia for peri-ictal events, which implies that memory was not acquired during the seizure because of neuronal dysfunction.

Table 39-1. **Classification of Seizures**

Partial Seizures

Simple partial seizures
  With motor signs
  With somatosensory or special sensory symptoms
  With autonomic symptoms or signs
  With psychic symptoms
Complex partial seizures
  Simple partial onset followed by impairment of
    consciousness, with or without automatisms
  With impairment of consciousness at the onset, with or
    without automatisms
Partial seizures, secondarily generalized seizures
  Simple partial, complex partial, or simple to complex
    partial before generalizing; the evolution may be to
    generalized tonic-clonic, tonic, or clonic seizures

Generalized Seizures

Absence seizures
  Simple, complicated, atypical
Myoclonic seizures
Clonic seizures
Tonic-clonic seizures
Tonic seizures
Atonic seizures

Unclassified Epileptic Seizures

From: Commission on Classification and Terminology of the International League Against Epilepsy: Proposal for Revised and Clinical Electroencephalographic Classification of Epileptic Seizures. Epilepsia 1981;22:489-501.

An *aura* is the portion of a seizure that is experienced before loss of consciousness. The aura that precedes a complex partial seizure is itself a simple partial seizure. An aura may be suspected if there is a change in behavior before seizures, such as interrupting an activity to seek out parents or complaining of an epigastric discomfort.

Automatisms are semipurposeful movements that usually occur with impairment of consciousness either during or after an epileptic seizure. They may be a perseveration of an activity in progress at ictal onset or novel semipurposeful movements arising during the seizure. They are most often a mixture of masticatory, oral, and lingual movements and simple fragmentary limb movements, such as fidgeting with a held object or pulling at clothing. In infants, oroalimentary automatisms are more likely than gestural automatisms and must be distinguished from the normal behavior of infants.

GENERALIZED SEIZURES

Generalized seizures are defined as seizures in which the first clinical changes indicate initial involvement of both hemispheres. Motor involvement, if present, is bilateral, as are the initial EEG changes. Consciousness is impaired in most generalized seizures but not in all; for instance, brief myoclonic seizures and some atonic seizures may not be associated with any impairment of consciousness.

Absence seizures ("petit mal") begin with sudden interruption of activity and with staring; they are usually brief and end abruptly without postictal confusion. *Simple absence seizures* consist of only motionlessness and a blank stare. Absence seizures are more typically accompanied by added motor features and may be referred to as *complicated absence seizures*. Clonic motor activity may occur, most often involving only the eyelids and facial muscles, but it may be manifested as generalized myoclonic jerks of the trunk and limbs. Changes in muscle tone are common; increased tone is usually maximal in the axial musculature and may be predominantly flexor or extensor, symmetric or asymmetric. Alternatively, there may be a

loss of muscle tone associated with the seizure, so that the head droops, objects are dropped, or the person slumps; falling is unusual. Automatisms may be seen in 40% to 50% of absence seizures and are more common in absence seizures of long duration. Lip smacking, swallowing, fumbling or searching hand movements, or ambulation can appear during the seizure, or preictal activities may be continued in a slow, automatic manner. Paroxysmal alterations in autonomic function may also accompany absence seizures, including pupillary dilation, pallor, flushing, sweating, salivation, piloerection, or a combination of these. *Atypical absence seizures* are described as absence seizures with a less abrupt beginning and end, with more pronounced changes in muscle tone, and of longer duration. Table 39-2 is a comparison of the clinical features of absence seizures, complex partial seizures, and episodic daydreaming.

Tonic-clonic seizures are perhaps the most dramatic of the epileptic seizures. The tonic phase begins with sudden sustained contraction of facial, axial, and limb muscle groups, and there may be an initial involuntary stridorous cry or a moan secondary to contraction of the diaphragm and chest muscles against a partially closed glottis. The tonic contraction is maintained for seconds to tens of seconds, during which time the child falls if standing, is apneic and may become cyanotic, may bite the tongue, and may pass urine. The clonic phase of the seizure begins when the tonic contraction is repeatedly interrupted by momentary relaxation of the muscular contraction. This gives the appearance of generalized jerking as the contraction resumes after each relaxation. At the end of the clonic phase, the body relaxes and the patient is unconscious with deep respiration. If roused, the patient is confused, may complain of muscle soreness, and usually wishes to sleep. The tonic-clonic sequence and the unconscious postictal state are very important historical points in the differential diagnosis of psychogenic convulsive events and epileptic tonic-clonic seizures.

Myoclonic jerks are sudden, brief, shocklike contractions of muscles. They may involve the whole body or a portion of the axial musculature such as face and trunk, or they may be limited to the limbs. They can be isolated or repetitive, irregular or rhythmic. Myoclonus may arise from cortical, brainstem, and spinal cord neuronal groups. Some forms of myoclonus of brainstem or spinal origin occurring without other seizure types are not regarded as epileptic myoclonus but thought of as movement disorders.

Generalized clonic seizures may occur without a preceding tonic phase, and the postictal phase is usually shorter than for tonic-clonic seizures.

Generalized tonic seizures begin in the same way as tonic-clonic seizures. The tonic contraction subsides without the intervening relaxation-recontraction clonic phase. The extent of muscle involvement may vary from patient to patient and from seizure to seizure in a single patient. A massive generalized contraction produces facial grimacing, neck and trunk flexion or extension, abduction of the arms, and flexion of the hips. Subtle tonic seizures may produce only facial grimacing and slight neck and trunk flexion. Tonic seizures may be accompanied by pronounced autonomic activity with diaphoresis, flushing, pallor, and tachycardia even when the muscular contraction is slight.

Atonic seizures are characterized by a sudden decrease or loss of postural muscle tone. The extent of muscle involvement may vary; an atonic seizure may be limited to a sudden head drop with slack jaw or may result in a fall because of loss of axial and limb muscle tone. The falls are referred to as "drop attacks," and because they are unprotected, they often result in injury.

Status epilepticus exists when epileptic seizures are prolonged or are frequently repeated without recovery between the seizures. The time most often defined is 30 minutes or longer, but seizures continuing for more than 5 to 10 minutes warrant immediate attention. Status epilepticus is most commonly characterized as convulsive or nonconvulsive status epilepticus. Convulsive status epilepticus may involve repetitive or prolonged generalized tonic-clonic, myoclonic, or tonic seizures. Nonconvulsive status epilepticus may involve

Table 39-2. **Differential Diagnosis of Episodic Unresponsiveness without Convulsions**

Clinical	Absence Seizures	Complex Partial Seizures	Staring, Inattention
Frequency	Multiple daily	Rarely more than 1-2 per day	Daily, situation dependent: e.g., may occur only at school
Duration	Often <10 s, rarely >30 s	Average duration >60 s, rarely <10 s	Seconds to minutes
Aura	Not present	May be present	Not present
Abrupt interruption of child's activity	Yes: e.g., speech arrest midsentence, pause while eating, playing or fighting	Yes	Activities such as play or eating are not abruptly interrupted, no sudden onset
Eyelid flutter	Common, often with upward eye movement	Uncommon but may be present	No
Myoclonic jerks	Common	Uncommon	Not present
Automatisms	Occur in longer absences, usually mild	Frequent and often prominent	No
Responsiveness	Unresponsive	Unresponsive	Responds to touch
Postictal impairment	None	Postictal confusion and malaise is typical; drowsiness may also occur	No
EEG	Generalized 3-Hz spike-and-wave complexes	Regional epileptic discharges (most often frontal or temporal)	Normal
MRI	Normal	Focal structural lesions not uncommon (e.g., tumor)	Normal
First-line medication	Valproate, ethosuximide	Carbamazepine, phenytoin, valproate	None

EEG, electroencephalogram; MRI, magnetic resonance imaging.

repeated or continuous absence seizures or complex partial seizures with an altered state of consciousness lasting hours or even days. Status epilepticus has a significant acute mortality rate only partly because of the underlying cause of the seizures (encephalitis, anoxia).

HISTORY AND PHYSICAL EXAMINATION

The assessment of children presenting with unexplained episodes of disturbed consciousness or abnormal movements depends almost entirely on the history, because there are rarely any abnormal physical signs. By their very nature, paroxysmal disorders are not present most of the time. Witnesses to the episodes are the most informative sources, and it is imperative that witnesses are sought and interviewed. A description of the events from the patient should be obtained whenever possible. Even young children can describe potentially diagnostic symptoms, and parents may sometimes unwittingly misrepresent symptoms. It is valuable to have parents and witnesses mimic the behavior or events witnessed to clarify the nature of ictal motor activity.

In the history taking, the clinician should always attempt to confirm the diagnosis of seizures. This is especially important with first seizure presentations, when alarm and concern about the consequences may obscure a more benign diagnosis. The clinician should determine whether the "first seizure" really is the first seizure. Have there been previous unrecognized subtle partial seizures or remote generalized tonic-clonic seizures? Were there provocative factors such as sleep deprivation, intercurrent illness, or fever? Are there associated disturbances in motor function, cognitive function, or development (Fig. 39-1)? The history and physical examination must also be explored for possible underlying causes, such as perinatal hypoxia-asphyxia, metabolic or degenerative disease, cerebral tumors, or neurocutaneous disease (Table 39-3). A thorough family history is valuable; the presence of consanguinity, migraine, sleep disorders, neonatal seizures, febrile seizures, epilepsy, and mental

retardation should be noted. Single-gene epilepsy syndromes account for a small percentage of all epilepsy, but distinct genetic disorders can be identified clinically (Table 39-4). Additional genetic epilepsy syndromes include familial benign rolandic epilepsy, juvenile myoclonic epilepsy, autosomal dominant temporal lobe epilepsy with auditory symptoms, familial partial epilepsy with variable foci, familial febrile seizures, and childhood absence seizures.

DIAGNOSTIC EVALUATION OF A SEIZURE DISORDER

ELECTROENCEPHALOGRAPHIC STUDIES

After a detailed history and physical examination, the EEG is the next step in the evaluation. The incidence of EEG epileptiform activity in normal children without a history of seizures is very low (<2%); many positive records show benign focal epileptiform discharges of childhood. The incidence of epileptic seizures in patients with focal spikes is 83%, whereas for generalized spikes, it is probably much lower. In a child with suspected seizures, the finding of focal or generalized epileptiform activity on the EEG supports a diagnosis of epilepsy, whereas repeatedly negative EEG studies argue against such a diagnosis and should prompt the physician to consider alternative diagnoses and to attempt to record the episodes.

An EEG should include at least 20 to 30 minutes of recording and should include hyperventilation, photic stimulation, and sleep, all of which potentially activate epileptiform discharges, increasing the diagnostic yield. Hyperventilation produces absence seizures in about 80% of children with childhood absence epilepsy. Intermittent photic stimulation produces generalized epileptic discharges in a number of the generalized epileptic syndromes. Recording during wakefulness and sleep performed after sleep deprivation probably has the highest yield. Recording of the EEG during light non–rapid eye movement sleep can easily be achieved by administration of sedative agents such as chloral hydrate. If benign focal epilepsy of

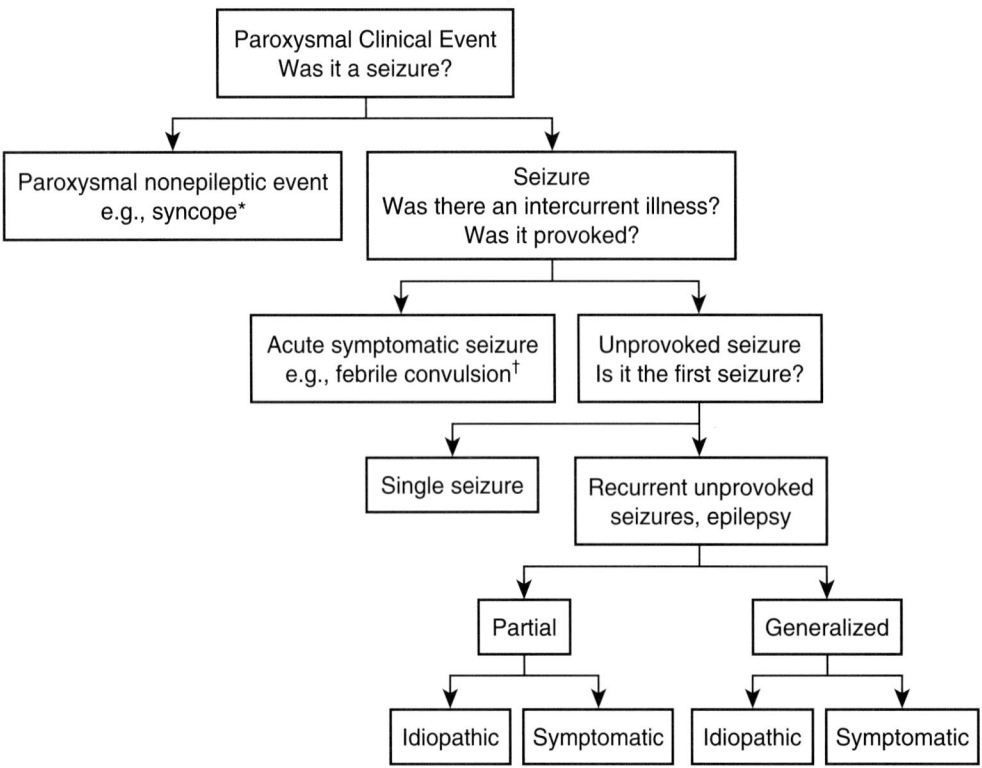

Figure 39-1. Steps for confirming the diagnosis and type of seizures.

* See Tables 39-13, 39-18, 39-19, and Chapter 42
† See Tables 39-12 and 39-14

childhood is suspected, a period of recording in sleep is essential; a negative EEG study performed during wakefulness and sleep argues against the diagnosis. In juvenile myoclonic epilepsy, discharges may appear only in the mornings on awakening. It is often impractical to monitor overnight, but it may be possible to use ambulatory EEG monitoring if diurnal EEG with sleep and wakefulness has been unhelpful and the diagnosis is still in question.

Repeated outpatient EEGs after earlier negative studies may provide positive studies by increasing the total sampling time. In patients not responding to treatment, repeated studies may reveal previously unrecorded focal or generalized discharges that would support a modification of AED therapy. Overnight recording in the hospital provides for prolonged sampling of the interictal EEG in wakefulness and spontaneous sleep. For any patient with refractory seizures or an uncertain diagnosis, the use of video and EEG monitoring is usually helpful in clarifying the diagnosis. Defining the exact seizure type may lead to modification of drug treatment or consideration of epilepsy surgery, or a nonepileptic paroxysmal disorder may be discovered.

NEUROIMAGING STUDIES

Magnetic resonance imaging (MRI) is superior to computed tomography for the evaluation of epilepsy. Any patient with focal epilepsy should have MRI of the brain unless the syndrome is clearly that of benign focal epilepsy of childhood with centrotemporal spikes. MRI should also be performed in the other benign focal epilepsies of childhood, because these syndromes are less clearly defined and may be mimicked by structural lesions. MRI may also reveal an abnormality in patients with symptomatic generalized epilepsy. Structural neuroimaging is important in the assessment of candidates for surgical resection in patients with intractable seizures.

EVALUATION OF THE FIRST SEIZURE

There is no clinical sign or diagnostic investigation that determines with certainty whether a child presenting with a first seizure has epilepsy or has had an isolated seizure. The assessment of patients with a first seizure must include a search for etiologic agents and features that may indicate the risk of recurrence. Factors to be considered include the circumstances of the seizure, the health of the child in the time before the seizure, the recent sleep patterns, the possibility of abuse or trauma, and the chance of ingestion of prescription or street drugs.

A number of prospective studies have addressed the recurrence risk after a first unprovoked seizure, usually defined as a seizure or flurry of seizures within 24 hours in patients older than 1 month. In a pediatric population, the recurrence rate is probably 40% to 50%.

The most important predictor of recurrence appears to be the existence of an underlying neurologic disorder. The existence of mental retardation or cerebral palsy is a common antecedent to epilepsy, as is a history of significant head injury. An EEG with generalized or focal epileptiform discharges or with focal or generalized slowing is also predictive of recurrence. Partial seizures are more likely to be associated with recurrence, although patients with such seizures are also more likely to have an existing neurologic deficit or an abnormal EEG. The duration of the first seizure or a presentation in status epilepticus does not seem to be associated with a higher incidence of recurrence. A family history of epilepsy is not a predictor of recurrence. Earlier age at onset, particularly before the age of 12 months, has been associated with a higher risk of recurrent seizures.

Treatment with AEDs lowers the recurrence rate by about 50%. However, most authorities believe that the majority of patients with a first seizure should not be treated. In adults or adolescents, the issues of driving and employment are paramount and may influence

Table 39-3. Neurocutaneous Syndromes

Clinical Syndromes and Findings	Investigations
Sturge-Weber Syndrome	
Facial hemangioma, "port-wine stain" upper face, division of cranial nerve V; bilateral in 30%, absent in 5%, associated truncal and limb hemangiomas in 45%	CT scan; calcification, MRI scan with gadolinium
Intracranial leptomeningeal angiomatosis	EEG; attenuation of background rhythms, epileptiform discharges
Epilepsy in 70%-90%, usually before 2 yr and before hemiparesis, intractable in 35%	
Mental retardation in 50-60%	
Hemiparesis in 30%, often with hemisensory deficit and hemianopia	
Tuberous Sclerosis	
Diagnostic criteria	
Any one of the following:	
Facial angiofibroma (adenoma sebaceum, nasolabial folds, and nose: become more prominent with age) or periungual fibromas	Physical examination
Cortical tubers, subependymal nodule, giant cell astrocytoma	MRI examination, T_1 and T_2 sequences, with gadolinium
Multiple retinal hamartomas (usually asymptomatic) or multiple renal angiomyolipomas (usually asymptomatic, may manifest as hematuria, hypertension, or renal failure)	Funduscopic examination and renal ultrasonography, abdominal CT scan
Or any two of the following:	
Infantile spasms (seizures in 90%, most commonly generalized; infantile spasms and myoclonus)	History and physical, EEG; focal or generalized abnormalities
Hypomelanotic papules (ash leaf spots; in 80%-90%, 1-2 cm oval or leaf-shaped)	Wood lamp examination in darkened room
Single retinal hamartoma	Funduscopic examination
Subependymal or cortical calcification on CT scan	CT scan of the brain
Single renal angiomyolipomas or cysts	Renal ultrasonography or abdominal CT scan
Cardiac rhabdomyomas (single or multiple, may obstruct outflow, cause arrhythmias or conduction defects)	Echocardiography, ECG
First-degree relative with tuberous sclerosis (autosomal dominant disorder, 80% of cases represent new mutations)	Examination of parents; echocardiography, MRI scans
Also associated:	
Mental retardation in 50%-66%	
Shagreen patches; hamartomatous skin lesion in lumbosacral region in 20%	
Pulmonary involvement, fibrosis	Chest radiograph
Skeletal abnormalities	Hand, feet (cystic), long bone (sclerotic) radiographic changes
Epidermal Nevus Syndrome	
Hamartomatous lesions; subclassified according to most predominant histologic and clinical features (e.g., linear nevus sebaceus, see below)	Careful examination of scalp, skin folds, and conjunctiva; funduscopic examination
Sporadic, affects both sexes equally; CNS abnormalities are common with epidermal nevus syndrome, including seizures (25% of patients), mental retardation, and neoplasia; also, skeletal abnormalities, including kyphoscoliosis and hemiatrophy	Spine and limb radiographs as appropriate
Linear nevus sebaceus; hairless verrucous yellow-orange or hyperpigmented plaques on the face and scalp	
Epilepsy in 76%	
Mental retardation in 60%	
Associated neuronal migration disorders	MRI scan of the brain
Malignant transformation of the skin lesion	
Other Neurocutaneous Syndromes Associated with Seizures	
Neurofibromatosis; cutaneous lesions include café au lait spots, axillary freckling, neural tumors; seizure type includes generalized tonic-clonic, partial complex, and partial simple-motor	MRI scan of the brain
Incontinentia pigmenti; involvement includes linear papular-vesicular cutaneous lesions at birth, later pigmentation, ocular and dental anomalies; female-to-male ratio > 20:1 (boys may die in utero); seizure type includes neonatal-onset and later generalized tonic-clonic	Skin biopsy; ophthalmology examination
Hypomelanosis of Ito (incontinentia pigmenti achromians)	

CNS, central nervous system; CT, computed tomography; ECG, electrocardiogram; EEG, electroencephalogram; MRI, magnetic resonance imaging.

Table 39-4. Monogenetic epileptic channelopathies

Type of Channelopathy/Specific Disease	Gene Map Locus on Chromosome	Gene Mutation
Voltage-gated channelopathies		
Sodium channelopathies		
Familial generalized epilepsy with febrile seizures plus	2q24	*SCN1A*
	19q13.1	*SCN1B*
	2q23-q24.3	*SCN1A*
Benign familial neonatal-infantile convulsions	2q24	*SCN2A*
Severe myoclonic epilepsy of infancy	2q24	*SCN1A*
Intractable childhood epilepsy with generalized tonic-clonic seizures	2q24	*SCN1A*
Potassium channelopathies		
Benign familial epilepsy or neonatal convulsions	20q13.3	*KCNQ2*
	8q24	*KCNQ3*
Ligand-gated channelopathies		
ACh receptor channelopathies		
Autosomal dominant frontal nocturnal epilepsy	20q13.2	*CHRNA4*
	1p21	*CHRNB2*
	15q24	*ENFL2*
GABA$_A$ receptors channelophathies		
Familial generalized epilepsy with febrile seizures plus	5q31.1-q33.1	*GABRG2*

From Celesia GG: Are the epilepsies disorders of ion channels? Lancet 2003;361:1238.

ACh, acetylcholine; GABA, γ-aminobutyric acid.

the decision to treat a first seizure. In children, there is almost no indication for chronic AED treatment in response to a single seizure, and the implications of a second seizure are less pronounced. Nonetheless, activities such as bathing and swimming must be carefully supervised. If there is a second seizure, the risk of further seizures increases significantly. The decision to begin AED therapy is usually made after a patient has had two or more seizures in a short interval of time (6 to 12 months).

STATUS EPILEPTICUS

Convulsive status epilepticus is a medical emergency. Studies of adults and children presenting with status epilepticus show that 33% have no history of epilepsy, another third have a history of chronic epilepsy, and an acute illness or insult has caused status epilepticus in another third. Status epilepticus is more likely to develop in patients with symptomatic localization-related and generalized epilepsies than in those with idiopathic epilepsy; however, one of the most common precipitants of status epilepticus, cessation or disruption of a regular AED, affects both groups. Other important causes of status epilepticus include systemic febrile illnesses, intracranial infections (meningitis, encephalitis), poisoning, acute metabolic disorders, and head injury.

The goals of the emergency management of status epilepticus are as follows:

1. Maintain normal cardiorespiratory function and cerebral oxygenation.
2. Stop clinical and electrical seizure activity, and prevent its recurrence.
3. Identify precipitating factors.
4. Correct any metabolic disturbances (hypoglycemia, hyponatremia) and prevent systemic complications such as cardiovascular collapse, cardiac arrhythmia, pneumonia, and renal failure.

Table 39-5 sets out a plan of initial assessment and management of convulsive status epilepticus. Lorazepam and diazepam offer a rapid anticonvulsant action when given intravenously but must be combined with a primary AED. Side effects include sedation, depressed respiration, decreased ability to protect the airway, and hypotension. Either phenytoin (or intramuscular fosphenytoin in the absence of intravenous access) or phenobarbital could be used in conjunction with the benzodiazepines; fosphenytoin is less sedating than phenobarbital. If the status epilepticus consists of frequent, repeated generalized seizures with return of consciousness between episodes, fosphenytoin or phenobarbital loading is more appropriate than bolus doses of benzodiazepines, because benzodiazepines alter the level of consciousness, which complicates the assessment. Valproate can be given intravenously and may be the appropriate therapy for patients with known idiopathic and symptomatic generalized epilepsies when they are stable or instead of fosphenytoin or phenobarbital.

Nonconvulsive status epilepticus may arise when frequent complex partial seizures or absence seizures occur. In both of these settings, discrete seizures may not be identifiable; instead, the child may present with confusion, clouded consciousness, and partial responsiveness or a stuporous state, all of which can last hours or even days. This clinical picture is more typical of absence status epilepticus. In complex partial status epilepticus, which is probably a less common phenomenon, it is more likely that obvious fluctuations in the level of responsiveness with automatisms occur; this suggests repeated seizures and intervening postictal confusion. This form of status epilepticus is not a medical emergency because cardiorespiratory function is not endangered. However, delay in therapy is not advisable, especially if complex partial status is suspected, in which case treatment should follow that outlined for convulsive status epilepticus.

In absence status epilepticus, intravenous benzodiazepines are usually effective but should be used in conjunction with intravenous valproate, ethosuximide, or clonazepam.

CLASSIFICATION OF EPILEPSIES AND EPILEPTIC SYNDROMES

The classification of epilepsies and epileptic syndromes has two broad divisions: generalized seizures and partial seizures (Table 39-6).

Table 39-5. Management of Convulsive Status Epilepticus

Priority	Examination and Laboratory Investigations	Management
On arrival	Airway patency and respiratory rate, inspect pharynx, chest auscultation, BP, pulse, temperature; Level of consciousness; response to command, pain; Serum Na, K, glucose, creatinine, Ca, Mg; CBC, liver function studies, AED levels; Serum and urine toxins screen; Arterial blood gases, chest radiograph	Airway protection; suction pharynx and give supplemental oxygen Rectal antipyretic to lower temperature if elevated IV access and administer: 25% glucose IV, 2-4 mL/kg, and* lorazepam IV, 0.1 mg/kg (to a maximum 8 mg) as bolus and fosphenytoin IV, 20 mg/kg at 150 mg/min with ECG monitoring and collection of serum level after loading dose If immediate IV access is not possible, give diazepam, 0.3-0.5 mg/kg rectally, and fosphenytoin IM and arrange for central line or intraosseous access
After initial treatment	Neck stiffness, funduscopy, signs of trauma, rashes, symmetry of motor function and reflexes	If patient is febrile: appropriate cultures, other studies depending on age and other symptoms If any suspicion of head injury: obtain urgent CT scan
If seizures continue	Patient's level of consciousness becomes depressed with lorazepam and PB, and an EEG is necessary to assess adequacy of therapy	Arrange ICU bed and consider intubation; give further bolus of lorazepam, 0.05-0.1 mg/kg, and push PHT serum level above 30 mg/L with further loading dose (~10 mg/kg) In ICU setting, if seizures continue with PHT levels of 30-40 mg/L, then add PB, 20 mg/kg IV loading over 15-30 mins Continued clinical or electrical seizures may necessitate induction of pentobarbital therapy: loading dose of 5-15 mg/kg, followed by IV infusion of 1-3 mg/kg/hr, titrated by EEG monitoring to achieve burst suppression pattern; maintain for 24-48 hr and review Elective intubation and ventilation, arterial line, BP monitoring
After stabilization or in tandem with escalating therapy	Lumbar puncture; if acute febrile illness with papilledema or focal neurologic signs, then CT/MRI first	If LP is delayed and intracranial infection is suspected, then cover with antibiotic and antiviral therapy

*Give lorazepam if actively convulsing; this may not be required in patients with serial seizures who can be quickly loaded with fosphenytoin.

AED, antiepileptic drug; Ca, calcium; CBC, complete blood count; BP, blood pressure; ECG, electrocardiogram; ICU, intensive care unit; IM, intramuscularly; IV, intravenously; K, potassium; LP, lumbar puncture; Na, sodium; Mg, magnesium; PB, phenobarbital; PHT, phenytoin.

These two categories are divided into symptomatic or cryptogenic epilepsy and idiopathic epilepsy. *Symptomatic epilepsies* have a known cause, whereas *idiopathic epilepsies* have no identifiable cause but are not the result of an underlying brain disorder. Idiopathic epilepsy syndromes are thought to have a genetic origin. *Cryptogenic epilepsy* is thought to be symptomatic but without an identifiable cause; there is often evidence of underlying brain dysfunction such as mild mental retardation, focal neurologic signs, or specific learning disorders. Most epileptic syndromes are first manifested in childhood.

Classification of the epilepsies into specific syndromes provides a powerful framework for accurate communication, appropriate investigations, treatment strategies, and prognosis. At diagnosis, the clinician should attempt to determine whether the seizure disorder is focal or generalized and then whether there is evidence of underlying brain dysfunction. Both the partial and generalized idiopathic epilepsies most often respond favorably to treatment, and there is a good chance of long-term remission. The symptomatic and cryptogenic epilepsies respond less predictably to treatment, and the chance of remission is less certain. Identification of one of the epileptic encephalopathies of infancy and childhood has grave prognostic significance (Table 39-7). These epilepsies vary in the seizure types and EEG features but have certain features in common: specific age at onset and expression, intractable seizures, cognitive dysfunction, arrest in development, conspicuous interictal epileptic discharges in the EEG, and a poor response to treatment.

NEONATAL PERIOD

The paroxysmal disorders seen in the neonatal period (birth to 8 weeks) are given in Table 39-8.

Paroxysmal Nonepileptic Disorders

Jitteriness

Jitteriness or tremulousness is a common movement disorder of neonates. It can be confused with seizures, especially if superimposed on normal tonic postural reflexes. Jitteriness, characterized by rhythmic alternating movements of all extremities with equal velocity in flexion and extension, only occasionally has a clonic appearance. Jitteriness is not accompanied by eye deviation or staring, is stimulus sensitive, and can usually be stopped by gentle passive flexion of the moving limb.

Common associations of jitteriness in the newborn are hypoxic-ischemic encephalopathy, hypoglycemia, hypocalcemia, and drug withdrawal. Jittery neonates may be more likely to have seizures and epileptiform EEG abnormalities than are unaffected neonates. However, jitteriness may also appear in otherwise healthy infants. In this case, there are no associated insults or identifiable etiologic factors, and the children develop normally. Jitteriness then seems to behave as a benign movement disorder, resolving by 10 to 14 months but often earlier.

Table 39-6. Classification of Epilepsies and Epileptic Syndromes

Localization-Related (Focal, Partial) Epilepsies

Idiopathic
  Benign childhood epilepsy with centrotemporal spikes
  Childhood epilepsy with occipital paroxysms
Symptomatic
  The subclassification is determined by the anatomic location suggested by the clinical history, predominant seizure type, interictal and ictal EEG, and imaging studies; thus, SPS, CPS, or secondarily generalized seizures arising from frontal lobes, parietal, temporal, occipital, multiple lobes or an unknown focus
Localization related but uncertain symptomatic or idiopathic

Generalized Epilepsies

Idiopathic
  Benign neonatal familial convulsions
  Benign neonatal convulsions
  Benign myoclonic epilepsy in infancy
  Childhood absence epilepsy (pyknoepilepsy)
  Juvenile absence epilepsy
  Juvenile myoclonic epilepsy (impulsive petit mal)
  Epilepsy with grand mal seizures upon awakening
  Other generalized idiopathic epilepsies that do not conform exactly to the syndromes just described
Cryptogenic or symptomatic generalized
  West syndrome (infantile spasms)
  Lennox-Gastaut syndrome
  Epilepsy with myoclonic astatic seizures
  Epilepsy with myoclonic absences
  Symptomatic
  Nonspecific cause
    Early myoclonic encephalopathy
  Specific disease states manifesting with seizures

Epilepsies and Syndromes in which It Is Undetermined whether They Are Focal or Generalized

With both generalized and focal seizures
  Neonatal seizures
  Severe myoclonic epilepsy in infancy
  Epilepsy with continuous spike-and-wave patterns during slow-wave sleep
  Acquired epileptic aphasia (Landau-Kleffner syndrome)
  Without unequivocal generalized or focal features
  All cases with GTCS in which the EEG findings do not allow classification as definitely generalized or localization-related: e.g., sleep GTCS

Special Syndromes

Situation-related seizures
  Febrile convulsions
  Isolated seizures or isolated status epilepticus
Acute symptomatic seizures: e.g., alcohol withdrawal seizures, eclampsia, uremia

From Commission on Classification and Terminology of the International League Against Epilepsy: Proposal for Revised Classification of Epilepsies and Epileptic Syndromes. Epilepsia 1989;20:389-399.

CPS, complex partial seizures; EEG, electroencephalogram; GTCS, generalized tonic-clonic seizures; SPS, simple partial seizures.

Table 39-7. Cryptogenic and Symptomatic Epileptic Encephalopathies

Neonates and Infants

Early epileptic encephalopathy
Early infantile myoclonic epilepsy
Migratory partial seizures of infancy
West syndrome (infantile spasms)
Severe myoclonic epilepsy of infants
Epilepsy in association with inherited disorders of metabolism (see Table 39-10)
Lysosomal storage disorders
Urea cycle disorders
Aminoacidurias

Children and Adolescents

Lennox-Gastaut syndrome
Myoclonic-astatic epilepsy
Atypical benign partial epilepsy
Acquired epileptic aphasia (Landau-Kleffner syndrome)
Continuous spike-and-wave patterns in slow-wave sleep
Epilepsy in association with inherited disorders of metabolism (see Table 39-16)
Mitochondrial encephalomyopathies
Progressive myoclonus epilepsies
Epilepsy in association with systemic disorders involving the central nervous system
Systemic lupus erythematosus, other vasculitides

Another rare disorder, *familial trembling chin syndrome,* may appear in the neonatal-infancy period and cause concern. This unusual condition may have some relationship to familial essential tremor.

Benign Neonatal Sleep Myoclonus

Myoclonic jerks may appear during sleep in some healthy neonates. It has been reported within hours of birth and may disappear over

Table 39-8. Paroxysmal Disorders of the Neonatal Period

Paroxysmal Nonepileptiform Disorders

Jitteriness
Benign neonatal sleep myoclonus

Acute Symptomatic Seizures and Occasional Seizures*

Hypoxic-ischemic encephalopathy
Intraventricular hemorrhage
Acute metabolic disorders†
Sepsis-meningitis

Epileptic Syndromes

Benign idiopathic neonatal convulsions
Familial
Nonfamilial
Symptomatic focal epilepsy
Brain tumor
Malformations of cortical development
Inherited metabolic disease; mitochondrial disorders
Early-onset generalized epileptic syndromes with encephalopathy
Early myoclonic encephalopathy
Early infantile encephalopathic epilepsy

*See Table 39-10.

†Hypoglycemia, hypocalcemia, hypomagnesemia, hyponatremia, hypernatremia.

the next few months or persist into childhood. The jerks can be bilateral and synchronous or asymmetric; they may migrate between muscle groups during an episode. They are repetitive but do not disturb sleep. These jerks have been described in all stages of sleep but are most prominent in quiet sleep; they are not confined to sleep onset.

Features distinguishing this phenomenon from epilepsy are lack of associated seizures, presence exclusively during sleep with disappearance on awakening, normal EEGs, and normal psychomotor development.

Acute Symptomatic Seizures and Occasional Seizures

Classification

Most neonatal seizures are acute symptomatic seizures. The number of children who continue to have seizures after the neonatal period is relatively small. Neonatal seizures have been classified according to the clinical features of the ictus as subtle, tonic, clonic, and myoclonic. However, not all of these clinical seizure types have consistent ictal EEG patterns. The classification of neonatal seizures reflects the variable, poorly organized, and often subtle clinical expression of epileptic seizures at this age. Typical generalized tonic-clonic or absence seizures are not seen at this age, perhaps because of the limited capacity of the neonatal brain for interhemispheric synchrony. Patterns include the following:

- *Clinical seizures consistently associated with an EEG seizure pattern:* Clonic seizures with focal or multifocal jerking of the face or extremities fit this category, as do focal tonic seizures with focal tonic posturing of a limb or asymmetric posturing of the axial musculature.
- *Clinical seizures sometimes associated with an EEG seizure pattern:* Myoclonic seizures consist of single or multiple flexor jerks of the upper or lower limbs. An ictal EEG pattern is not always seen in this group. Fragmentary (multifocal) myoclonus is not always associated with an ictal EEG.
- *Clinical seizures not consistently associated with an EEG seizure pattern:* These include motor automatisms characterized by a diversity of signs, including any of the following: wide-eyed staring, rapid blinking, eyelid fluttering, drooling, sucking, repetitive limb movements such as "rowing" or "swimming" with the arms or "pedaling" with the legs, apnea, hyperpnea, and vasomotor skin color changes. This group may be subtle seizures and includes tonic eye deviation.

Generalized tonic seizures are manifested as tonic extension of the limbs or flexion of the upper limbs and extension of the lower limbs, sometimes mimicking decerebrate or decorticate posturing. The question has arisen whether abnormal posturing or automatisms without an ictal EEG pattern are epileptic seizures at all. Instead of an EEG seizure pattern, infants with subtle seizures typically have suppressed background rhythms. Generalized tonic seizures and focal and multifocal myoclonus are also often not associated with ictal EEG patterns, and when seen in stuporous or comatose children, the jerks may not be epileptic.

Some simple clinical observations should guide the assessment of neonates with episodic abnormal behaviors. Epileptic behaviors are typically repetitive and stereotyped but are not provoked by stimulation of the child or increased with increasing intensity of a stimulus. Nonepileptic movements may disappear with repositioning of a limb or the child. Gentle restraint of a limb should be able to suppress or abort nonepileptic motor activity, whereas epileptic movements are still palpable. Apneas, tachyarrhythmias, or bradyarrhythmias suggesting autonomic activation are not typical of nonepileptic phenomena. The association of abnormal eye movements with unusual behavior or limb movements suggests a seizure rather than nonepileptic behavior.

Diagnostic Investigations

EEG monitoring can be useful in the evaluation of suspicious fluctuations in vital signs in neonates who are paralyzed and intubated or comatose or in neonates with subtle but repetitive episodes of unusual behavior.

Proper treatment must include a thorough search for the cause of the seizures, because many conditions necessitate specific treatment. The possible etiologic factors are numerous and diverse (Tables 39-9 and 39-10). The most common cause is hypoxic-ischemic

---

Table 39-9. Causes of Neonatal Seizures

Ages 1-4 Days

Hypoxic-ischemic encephalopathy
Drug withdrawal, maternal drug use of narcotic or barbiturates
Drug toxicity: lidocaine, penicillin
Intraventricular hemorrhage
Acute metabolic disorders
  Hypocalcemia
    Perinatal asphyxia, small for gestational age
    Sepsis
    Maternal diabetes, hyperthyroidism, or hypoparathyroidism
  Hypoglycemia
    Perinatal insults, prematurity, small for gestational age
    Maternal diabetes
    Hyperinsulinemic hypoglycemia
    Sepsis
  Hypomagnesemia
  Hyponatremia or hypernatremia
    Iatrogenic or inappropriate antidiuretic hormone secretion
Inborn errors of metabolism
  Galactosemia
  Hyperglycinemia
  Urea cycle disorders
Pyridoxine deficiency (must be considered at any age)

Ages 4-14 Days

Infection
  Meningitis (bacterial), encephalitis (enteroviral, herpes simplex)
Metabolic disorders
  Hypocalcemia
    Diet, milk formula
  Hypoglycemia, persistent
    Inherited disorders of metabolism: galactosemia, fructosemia, leucine sensitivity
    Hyperinsulinemic hypoglycemia
    Anterior pituitary hypoplasia, pancreatic islet cell tumor
    Beckwith syndrome
Drug withdrawal, maternal drug use of narcotic or barbiturates
Benign neonatal convulsions, familial and nonfamilial
Kernicterus, hyperbilirubinemia

Ages 2-8 Weeks

Infection
  Herpes simplex or enteroviral encephalitis, bacterial meningitis
Head injury
  Subdural hematoma, child abuse
Inherited disorders of metabolism
  Aminoacidurias, urea cycle defects, organic acidurias
  Neonatal adrenoleukodystrophy
Malformations of cortical development
  Lissencephaly
  Focal cortical dysplasia
Tuberous sclerosis
Sturge-Weber syndrome

Table 39-10. Inherited Disorders of Metabolism and Neurodegenerative Diseases Associated with Seizures in Infants

Disorder	Clinical Features and Laboratory Findings	Investigations
Neonates		
These disorders are rare. The clinical features are nonspecific and usually do not distinguish between the inherited disorders of metabolism; however, they may suggest that a search for these conditions is warranted: 　Metabolic or degenerative disorder in another sibling 　Normal immediately after birth with symptoms and signs developing in the first days to weeks of life 　Food intolerance; vomiting, diarrhea, not settling after feedings 　Lethargy, may become stuporous after feeding 　Hypotonia 　Seizures; tonic, clonic, subtle neonatal seizures; myoclonus in some disorders 　Late signs: weight loss, failure to thrive, psychomotor retardation	Initial investigations in neonatal seizures: 　Urinalysis, ketones, glucose, 2,4-DNPH screen 　Serum Na^+, K^+, Ca^{2+}, Mg^{2+}, glucose, blood urea nitrogen, creatinine 　Serum ammonia, lactate, and pyruvate 　Liver function tests, complete blood cell count, arterial blood gas measurements 　Lumbar puncture and CSF analysis 　EEG 　CT or MRI scan may be indicated
Aminoacidurias		
Maple syrup urine disease	An unusual maple syrup odor of urine may be detected; severe metabolic acidosis and increased anion gap; urine positive for ketones; boiled urine reacts with 2,4-DNPH to give yellow precipitate	Serum and urine amino acid analysis; Elevated serum leucine, isoleucine and valine
Organic acidurias 　Propionic acid 　Methylmalonic acid 　Isovaleric acid 　Glutaric acid	Hyperammonemia, metabolic acidosis and increased anion gap, ketosis, low blood urea nitrogen; secondary elevation of lactate and hypoglycemia may be present and secondary carnitine deficiency may occur; glycine level may be elevated in these disorders Thrombocytopenia, neutropenia, and anemia Characteristic body odor in some of these disorders	Serum and urine organic acid analysis Serum carnitine measurement
Urea cycle disorders	Hyperammonemia without ketoacidosis or hematologic abnormalities	Urine orotic acid and serum ammonia and citrulline measurements
Nonketotic hyperglycinemia 　D-glycericacidemia	Intractable seizures and severe encephalopathy, often with coma, within the first weeks of life; may have the clinical syndrome of early myoclonic encephalopathy; myoclonic seizures, burst suppression on EEG, severe psychomotor retardation	Elevated urine and plasma glycine levels, normal organic acid pattern and ammonia level
Pyridoxine dependency	No specific clinical features; must be suspected in all neonatal seizures without alternative cause and especially those not responding to simple measures	Therapeutic trial of pyridoxine; high dosage must be given for a period of weeks
Peroxisomal diseases 　Zellweger syndrome 　Adrenoleukodystrophy 　Refsum disease	Characteristic facies Neonatal form Infantile form	Serum very-long-chain fatty acid analysis
Infants		
Pyruvate dehydrogenase deficiency Pyruvate carboxylase deficiency	Metabolic acidosis and increased anion gap, lactic acidosis, with normal lactate-to-pyruvate ratio (10:20); hyperammonemia may be seen; normoglycemic; serum, urine, and CSF alanine levels may be elevated Lactate-to-pyruvate ratio is normal or elevated The clinical features are nonspecific: encephalopathy, hypotonia, and seizures; intermittent hyperventilation may be present Both these disorders can manifest later in childhood with developmental delay and episodic symptoms such as ataxia and vomiting	Serum lactate and pyruvate measurement Serum, urine, and CSF amino acids measurement
Biotinidase deficiency	Refractory seizures, rash, alopecia; lactic and organic acidosis	
Aminoacidurias 　Phenylketonuria	Onset in infancy with developmental delay and seizures; seizures occur in about 25%, and the infant may have severe epilepsy with West syndrome; deficiency of phenylalanine hydroxylase causes the accumulation of phenylalanine and phenylacetic acid	Detection and quantification of urinary and plasma amino acids

Table 39-10. Inherited Disorders of Metabolism and Neurodegenerative Diseases Associated with Seizures in Infants—cont'd

Disorder	Clinical Features and Laboratory Findings	Investigations
Infants—cont'd		
Phenylketonuria variant with biopterins deficiency	Hypotonia and seizures develop at or after 6 months of age; generalized motor seizures, erratic myoclonus, and oculogyric seizures	Detection and quantification of urinary and plasma amino acids
Tay-Sachs disease GM$_2$ gangliosidosis	Abnormalities appear in the first weeks to months of life with irritability and acoustic startle or myoclonus, not seizures, in the first months; developmental delay and cherry-red macular spots are present; seizures develop in the 2nd year of life; erratic myoclonus, partial seizures, and slowing of background rhythms on EEG	Blood sample and skin biopsy; hexosaminidase A deficiency detectable in blood lymphocytes and cultured fibroblasts
Sandhoff disease	Similar in phenotype to Tay-Sachs disease	Hexosaminidase A and B deficiency detectable in blood lymphocytes, cultured fibroblasts
GM$_1$ gangliosidosis Pseudo-Hurler disease	Dysmorphic features; developmental delay appears with decreased responsiveness in the first weeks of life, then arrest of development after 3-6 months of age; seizures are frequent without specific characteristics; cherry-red spots at maculae; in the other mucopolysaccharidoses—Hunter, Hurler, and Sanfilippo—seizures are not often a prominent feature	Skin biopsy, blood β-galactosidase deficiency found in blood lymphocytes and cultured fibroblasts
Leigh disease (subacute necrotizing encephalopathy)	A clinical syndrome resulting from various enzyme disorders Usually manifesting in infancy with regression of motor skills, hypotonia, lethargy, respiratory disorders (typically hyperventilation and apnea), and seizures; other features are nuclear and supranuclear oculomotor paralysis, brainstem dysfunction, choreoathetosis, cerebellar ataxia, and pyramidal signs	CSF lactate measurement; MRI of the brain (may show midbrain periaquaductal signal abnormalities) Muscle biopsy for oxidative metabolism analysis and DNA studies
Menkes disease	Sex-linked inheritance on long arm of X chromosome; hypotonia, failure to thrive, abnormal temperature regulation, hypothermia or hyperthermia, fragile wiry hair, poor pigmentation, generalized seizures, often infantile spasms	Deficiency of serum copper and ceruloplasmin
Krabbe disease	Appears before 3-6 months of age; rigidity develops in an irritable, crying infant; opisthotonic posturing of the neck and trunk; generalized motor seizures may occur but must be distinguished from tonic spasms; affected children become blind with optic atrophy	Skin biopsy and blood Galactocerebrosidase deficiency
Angelman syndrome	Developmental delay from birth, characteristic facies, ataxia with jerky limb movements, inappropriate laughter ("happy puppet"), seizures in 86% of patients	Chromosome 15 abnormality on fluorescent in situ hybridization analysis
Early infantile type of ceroid-lipofuscinosis	Massive myoclonus at 3-18 months; hypotonia, ataxia, impaired vision, dementia; vanishing EEG; no enzymatic defect identified; diagnosis must be based on clinical features and skin biopsy showing ceroid	Skin biopsy, rectal biopsy; genetic testing available
Other Rare Metabolic Disorders with Encephalopathy Seizures in Infancy		
Glutaric aciduria type II, multiple acyl-CoA dehydrogenase deficiency		Dicarboxylicaciduria
Medium-chain acyl–CoA dehydrogenase deficiency		Increased urinary *N*-acetylaspartic acid
Canavan–van Bogaert disease		

CoA, coenzyme A; CSF, cerebrospinal fluid; CT, computed tomography; DNPH, dinitrophenylhydrazine; EEG, electroencephalogram; MRI, magnetic resonance imaging.

encephalopathy (60% to 65%); however, it is important to make a positive diagnosis of this historically and to exclude conditions such as local anesthetic toxicity, pyridoxine-dependent seizures, and metabolic encephalopathies that may masquerade as perinatal asphyxia.

Prognosis

The prognosis for normal development after neonatal seizures depends on the cause of the seizures. Approximately 50% of neonates with seizures develop normally, 30% have neurologic sequelae, and 15% to 20% die. The likelihood of recurrent seizures is 15% to 30% overall. Generalized myoclonic jerks may be the harbinger of infantile spasms in later months. Fifty percent of neonates with hypoxic-ischemic encephalopathy–related seizures develop normally, but fewer than 10% of neonates with seizures and intraventricular hemorrhage develop normally. Neonates with seizures caused by CNS infection, hypoglycemia, structural brain malformations, and birth trauma do poorly, whereas those with seizures caused by hypocalcemia (in the absence of asphyxia), drug withdrawal (from maternal drug use), and stroke usually do well.

The EEG may add prognostic information; children with a normal background are unlikely to have any neurologic deficits, but severe abnormalities of the background rhythms, such as burst-suppression patterns, suppression of background rhythms, and electrocerebral silence, are associated with a 90% chance of a poor outcome, including death. Moderate abnormalities of the EEG in the form of amplitude asymmetries and patterns immature for the patient's conceptional age are associated with intermediate outcomes and are of less value in isolation from other clinical data.

Treatment

The primary treatment of neonatal seizures is the treatment of the underlying cause. Some neonates also require treatment with an AED, most commonly phenobarbital. At an intravenous loading dose of 18 to 20 mg/kg, phenobarbital should produce a serum level of approximately 18 to 20 mg/L (Table 39-11). A daily maintenance dose of 3 to 5 mg/kg keeps serum levels in this range. The serum level can be increased to 40 to 60 mg/L with further loading doses before consideration of a second drug for persistent seizures. Frequent estimations of serum levels are needed, and some free levels should be determined during the course of treatment with high total levels, because protein binding is lower in neonates than in older children. All neonates with seizures should have a trial of pyridoxine and folinic acid treatment if the cause is not identified and seizures persist.

If a self-limited or correctable short-term insult is the cause, the clinician may administer a loading dose with phenobarbital and give no maintenance therapy, simply observing for recurrent seizures. Alternative management would be to administer a loading dose of phenobarbital and give maintenance doses throughout an illness or to treat for a maximum of 3 months if the time during which the child is at risk for seizures is uncertain.

In the setting of refractory seizures with adequate serum levels of phenobarbital and no treatable exacerbating factors, phenytoin is most commonly chosen as a second drug. Fosphenytoin, the phosphate-ester pro-drug of phenytoin, has several advantages over phenytoin, including the intramuscular route of administration and a

lower risk of bradycardia. An intravenous loading dose of 15 to 20 mg/kg can be used. The half-life of phenytoin in neonates may vary between 6 and 140 hours, with a mean of 30 hours. The maintenance dosage may be difficult to predict; thus, frequent assessments of serum levels are indicated. Protein binding is lower than in older children (see Table 39-11).

Epileptic Syndromes

Benign Idiopathic Neonatal Convulsions, Familial and Nonfamilial

Some neonatal seizures occur in otherwise healthy neonates without perinatal risk factors or identifiable causes that remit spontaneously and are not followed by developmental delay; these include benign idiopathic neonatal convulsions and benign familial neonatal convulsions.

Benign idiopathic neonatal convulsions are common and may account for 2% to 7% of neonatal seizures. The disorder is sometimes referred to as "fifth-day fits," although the seizures may begin between 1 and 7 days of age. The seizures are typically focal and multifocal clonic seizures that may in rare cases develop into status epilepticus. The seizures remit within hours or days. Although normal at the onset of seizures, affected neonates may become drowsy and hypotonic during the seizures and for a few days after the seizures remit. The distinctive interictal EEG pattern is referred to as *theta pointu alternant*: intermittent θ rhythms in the rolandic area, often asynchronous between the hemispheres and associated with sharp waves. This pattern may occur in 60% of neonates with benign idiopathic neonatal convulsions but is not specific for the disorder, being seen in other neonatal encephalopathies. Normal interictal EEGs have also been reported. Long-term follow-up data are not yet complete, but the majority of affected children appear to have normal psychomotor development and no increased risk for the development of epilepsy. Currently, this diagnosis may be made only after exclusion of other causes of neonatal seizures, and the diagnostic workup must include a lumbar puncture and a computed tomographic scan or MRI to exclude neonatal stroke (see Chapter 41).

Benign familial neonatal convulsions are less common. There is a distinctive family history of transient neonatal seizures that shows autosomal dominant inheritance. The onset of seizures is usually between 2 and 4 days after birth, but in some cases, onset may occur at 1 to 3 months of age. The neonates are otherwise healthy without risk factors for seizures. The seizures are usually brief clonic seizures, but some neonates have tonic seizures. This group differs from the nonfamilial cases in that the seizures may persist longer, the interictal EEG is generally nonspecific (theta pointu alternant is reported in very few cases), and later seizures occur more frequently, in approximately 10% to 15% of children. Abnormalities in two

Table 39-11. Neonatal Antiepileptic Medication: Pharmacokinetic Parameters

Antiepileptic	Routes of Administration	% Protein Bound	Loading Dose	Half-life (Hours)	Maintenance Dosage (mg/kg/day)	Therapeutic Range (mg/L)
Phenobarbital	IV, PR, PO	24	20 mg/kg	40-200	3-5	10-30
PHT	IV, PO	85-90	15-20 mg/kg	6.9-140*	IV: 8-10 PO: 18-20	5-20
Fosphenytoin	IV, IM	70, displaces PHT	15-20 mg/kg†	Fosphenytoin > PHT, 8-15 min	18-20	5-20
Diazepam	IV, PR	84	0.1-0.3 mg/kg/dose‡	31-75	3	0.3-0.7
Lorazepam	IV	85	0.05 mg/kg/dose§	18-73	NA	NA

*Great variation, shorter if exposed to enzyme-inducing drugs (e.g., phenobarbital) and within first 2-3 week of life.

†Dosage is in PHT equivalents per kilogram.

‡Can be given every 15 minutes to a maximum of 2 mg.

§Up to two doses only.

IM, intramuscularly; IV, intravenously; PHT, phenytoin; PO, per os (orally); PR, per rectum.

potassium channel genes, *KCNQ2* on chromosome 20 and *KCNQ3* on chromosome 8, have been found in some kindreds (see Table 39-4).

Pyridoxine-Dependent Seizures

This is a rare autosomal recessive disorder in which seizures usually appear within the first 3 months of life, often within hours of birth but, in rare cases, as late as 2 to 5 years of age. The EEG may show focal, multifocal and generalized epileptiform activity. The seizures, myoclonic, generalized tonic-clonic and partial, and EEG discharges disappear over hours in response to intravenous 50 to 100 mg of pyridoxine. The children require long-term pyridoxine, 50 to 100 mg/day. The outcome may nonetheless be poor, with developmental delay despite early treatment.

Symptomatic Focal Epilepsy

Malformations of Cortical Development. Disorders of cell migration within the CNS may result in profound anatomic abnormalities and dysfunction or a spectrum of lesser abnormalities, ranging from focal areas of cortical dysgenesis and clinical deficits to subcortical collections of neurons (heterotopia) seen only under the microscope. Migrational abnormalities are rare but are commonly associated with seizures.

Lissencephaly, or agyria, is a profound abnormality characterized by a smooth brain without development of the normal gyral pattern and sulci; there are often large heterotopia in the white matter, and neuroimaging studies may reveal the appearance of a "double cortex."

Hemimegalencephaly is characterized by gross enlargement of one hemisphere with no normal cortical development within that hemisphere and by often recognizable MRI scan abnormalities in the normal-sized hemisphere. More restricted abnormalities may occur in the form of a limited area of gyral enlargement and distortion called *pachygyria.*

Schizencephaly refers to unilateral or bilateral clefts in the cerebral hemispheres, usually with abnormal arrangement (polymicrogyria) of the cortical gray matter lining the clefts.

Porencephaly refers to fluid-filled cavities within the brain. Porencephalic cysts communicate with both the subarachnoid space and the ventricular system and are lined not by cortical gray matter but rather by gliotic tissue, because they result from loss of tissue as a consequence of insults, typically infarction, during development.

Early-Onset Generalized Epileptic Syndromes with Encephalopathy

Early myoclonic encephalopathy appears in neonates before 2 to 3 months of age, usually within the first 2 weeks of life. Myoclonus appears at the onset but may be fragmentary. Partial motor seizures, massive myoclonus, or infantile spasms may also occur. The EEG does not show hypsarrhythmia; rather, it shows a suppression-burst pattern that may later evolve into a hypsarrhythmic pattern. There is a failure or arrest of psychomotor development and a high rate of mortality before 12 months of age. A number of patients have had nonketotic hyperglycemia or congenital malformations of the nervous system. Familial cases with an identifiable inborn error of metabolism (glycine encephalopathy, D-glycericacidemia, propionic acidemia, methylmalonic acidemia) have also been reported.

Early epileptic encephalopathic with suppression-burst EEG pattern (Ohtahara syndrome) has an onset during the same period. The affected child experiences intractable tonic seizures or epileptic spasms, and the EEG shows a suppression-burst pattern. Affected children have a severe encephalopathy, and the prognosis for remission from seizures or for normal development is very poor. Many of these patients have malformations of cortical development.

There appear to be neonates in whom the EEG features and clinical course of these two syndromes overlap; these syndromes may evolve into West syndrome and the Lennox-Gastaut syndrome.

INFANCY

The paroxysmal disorders of infancy (8 weeks to 2 years) are shown in Table 39-12.

Paroxysmal Nonepileptic Disorders

Infantile Syncope

Cyanotic Infant Syncope (Breath-Holding Spells). Cyanotic infant syncope consists of episodes of loss of consciousness followed by tonic stiffening in crying infants (see Chapter 6). These episodes have also been called *breath-holding spells, anoxic*

Table 39-12. Paroxysmal Disorders in Infants

Nonepileptiform Disorders
Infantile syncope*
  Cyanotic breath-holding spells
  Pallid syncope
Shivering attacks
Paroxysmal torticollis
Extrapyramidal drug reactions, dystonia
Gastroesophageal reflux with dystonia†
Rumination†
Stereotypic movements, autism, Rett syndrome, coexisting
  deafness and blindness†
Withholding, constipation†
Masturbation
Spasmus nutans
Opsoclonus
Benign paroxysmal vertigo
Myoclonus
  Nonepileptic; anxiety, excitement, acute metabolic
    encephalopathy
  Benign myoclonus of early infancy
Hyperexplexia†
Alternating hemiplegia of childhood
Sleep disorders*
  Jactatio capitis, head banging

Acute Symptomatic Seizures, Occasional Seizures
Febrile convulsions*
Meningitis, encephalitis*
Head injury, child abuse
Poisoning
Intercurrent medical illness, renal, liver disease, cardiac
  left-to-right shunt and embolism
Metabolic disease, rickets

Epileptic Syndromes
Symptomatic focal epilepsy†
West syndrome
Early myoclonic encephalopathy‡
Early infantile encephalopathic epilepsy‡
Malformations of cortical development‡
Neurocutaneous disorders (see Tables 39-1 and 39-3)
  Tuberous sclerosis
  Sturge-Weber syndrome
  Incontinentia pigmenti
  Epidermal nevus syndrome
Severe myoclonic epilepsy in infancy

*Common.
†See childhood section for discussion.
‡See neonatal section for discussion.

seizures, and *convulsive syncope,* but *cyanotic infant syncope* may be a better term because the loss of consciousness appears to be the result of transient impairment of cerebral perfusion. The subsequent tonic posturing in the typical attack is not epileptic but is thought to have the same brainstem origin as decerebrate or decorticate posturing. In rare cases, typical infant syncope may evolve into a true but short generalized tonic-clonic seizure or, in rare cases, status epilepticus, presumably triggered by the anoxia.

Cyanotic infant syncope is common, seen in 4.6% of a large cohort of children monitored from birth, and can be mistaken for tonic-clonic seizures. A thorough history is usually sufficient for diagnosing this condition. The peak incidence is between 6 and 18 months of age, but it may occur in neonates or in children as old as 6 years of age. The typical clinical picture is an infant who is frightened, frustrated, or surprised; begins to cry vigorously; and then becomes apneic and cyanotic before becoming unconscious, stiff, or limp. The crucial diagnostic point is the history of an external event precipitating the episode. The striking features that are so easily confused with an epileptic seizure are the tonic posture or the clonic movements that may occur after the child has lost consciousness. The child regains consciousness rapidly, after being positioned horizontally, without a prolonged postictal state, although there may be a tendency to sleep. The differential diagnosis is noted in Table 39-13.

Although the spells appear to be unpleasant for the child, they do not result in late sequelae and do not necessitate intensive investigation. The child should be evaluated for anemia; treatment of iron deficiency anemia reduces the frequency of syncopal events. Treatment with carbamazepine, phenytoin, or valproate may decrease the frequency or severity of postsyncopal convulsions in the rare child with epileptic seizures triggered by the anoxic event.

Pallid Infant Syncope. Pallid infant syncope occurs in response to transient cardiac asystole in children with a hypersensitive cardioinhibitory reflex. This form is less common but more alarming. There is minimal crying, perhaps only a gasp, and no obvious apnea before the loss of consciousness. Again, there is a precipitating event; the child appears to lose consciousness after minimal injury or fright, collapses limply, and then may have posturing and clonic movements before regaining consciousness (see Table 39-13).

Pallid infant syncope, if frequent and troublesome or if followed by prolonged generalized tonic-clonic convulsions, can be treated with atropine, which blocks the vagus nerve–mediated asystole. Most affected children require no medical treatment.

Sleep Disorders

Also referred to as head banging or rocking, jactatio capitis nocturna consists of rhythmic to-and-fro movements of the head or rocking of the body. It occurs typically at the transition from wakefulness to sleep, early in the evening or after arousal during the night. This behavior is quite common, occurring in up to 15% of children; it begins in infancy or early childhood but may persist up to 10 years of age. The child is not awake during the episode and does not remember the events, which usually last less than 15 minutes.

Clonazepam at bedtime may be helpful if the episodes are prolonged, threaten to injure the child, or appear to be interfering with normal sleep patterns. In most cases, it is sufficient to ensure that the bed area is padded to prevent injury.

Table 39-13. Differential Diagnosis of Infantile Syncope

Clinical	Infantile Syncope	Pallid Syncope	Tonic-Clonic Seizures	Infantile Spasms
Age range	1-6 yr; peak, 6-18 mo	1-6 yr	All ages	4-12 mo
Precipitating factors	Present (e.g., minor trauma, frustration, fright)	Present (e.g., minor trauma, frustration, fright)	Usually none	None
Occurrence in sleep	Never	Never	Common	At transition from awake to sleep and sleep to awake
Sequence of events	Crying → exhale; apnea → cyanosis, loss of consciousness; opisthotonos → relaxation, resumption of breathing	Upset, usually not crying → sudden pallor → limp fall with fainting → tonic posture, or clonic jerks may occur	Sudden loss of consciousness → increased tone, followed by synchronous jerking of body and limbs → unconsciousness; duration, 1-2 min	Sudden sustained flexion or extension of proximal limbs and trunk; duration, 2-20 s; seizures usually occur multiple times daily
Postictal symptoms	Usually minimal; infant may be lethargic and irritable	Usually minimal; quick return to normal	Usually marked; unconsciousness initially, then confusion and lethargy	Rapid return to preictal state
Interictal EEG	Normal	Normal	Frequently abnormal with epileptiform discharges	Abnormal background and epileptiform discharges
Ictal EEG	Reflects global cerebral hypoxia, diffuse rhythmic slowing → suppression → slowing with return of consciousness	Reflects global cerebral hypoxia; diffuse, rhythmic slowing → suppression → slowing with return of consciousness	EEG seizure patterns; postictal diffuse suppression, then slowing	High-amplitude slow transient waves → diffuse suppression
Pathophysiology	Respiratory arrest without asystole	Vagal bradycardia or temporary asystole	Primary CNS event	Primary CNS event, age-related epileptic seizure

CNS, central nervous system; EEG, electroencephalogram.

Shivering Attacks

Shivering or shuddering attacks are brief episodes characterized by sudden flexion of the head and trunk associated with a rapid tremulous contraction of the musculature. The appearance is exactly that of a sudden brief shudder experienced normally when exposed to cold. In this condition, however, the shuddering occurs repeatedly. Some infants experience more than 100 brief shudders per day. There may be clustering, with intervals of several weeks free of the episodes. The child may assume a characteristic posture with flexion of head, trunk, and elbows and adduction of elbows and knees.

The attacks have been described in children between the ages of 4 months and 10 years, although most often the onset seems to occur in infancy and early childhood. The phenomenon is nonepileptic and benign, eventually disappearing. Some children and their relatives have been reported to have an essential tremor. The shuddering is faster and of lower amplitude than myoclonus and is paroxysmal, not sustained, as occurs with a tremor.

Paroxysmal Torticollis

Torticollis is an abnormal posturing of the head and neck, with the head flexed toward the shoulder and the neck rotated with the chin turned toward the opposite shoulder. The posturing is paroxysmal, although variable in duration, lasting minutes or days, and there is no loss of consciousness. Some children have associated pallor, agitation, and vomiting, and the disorder has been suspected to result from labyrinthine dysfunction, like benign paroxysmal vertigo of childhood. The disorder is self-limited and remits in early childhood. There is an association with migraine in patients later in life and among their relatives.

There are various causes of torticollis (see Chapter 52). In older children, torticollis may occur as a focal dystonia persisting to adulthood. Familial cases have been described, and in some, the torticollis may be the earliest manifestation of a more generalized dystonia. Sustained abnormal posturing should prompt appropriate radiologic investigations to exclude inflammatory or neoplastic disorders of the upper cervical spinal cord, posterior fossa, cervical spine, or soft tissues of the neck. In very rare cases, gastroesophageal reflux manifests with dystonic posturing of the neck and upper trunk. Adverse extrapyramidal reactions to phenothiazines and related drugs may produce dystonic posturing of the neck and trunk.

Masturbation

Episodes of genital self-stimulation may occur in young children. Infant girls may assume stereotyped posturing with tightening of the thighs or applied pressure to the suprapubic or pubic area, not associated with manual stimulation of the vulva or rhythmic movements. The episodes vary in duration from minutes to hours and are often accompanied by irregular breathing, facial flushing, and diaphoresis.

Spasmus Nutans

Spasmus nutans is a rare disorder of unknown origin characterized by nystagmoid eye movements, head nodding, and torticollis. Head nodding may develop before the nystagmus and can be horizontal, vertical, or mixed. Both the head movements and the nystagmus may be paroxysmal, allowing confusion with seizures. There is no loss of consciousness during an episode. Small-amplitude rapid eye movements are typical; they tend to be asymmetric between the eyes and may even be monocular. The eye movements vary in prominence with different directions of gaze (see Chapter 43).

This is a self-limited disorder with onset between 4 and 18 months of age and not persisting after age 3 years, although nystagmus alone may persist in some children. Investigations should include imaging of the brain, optic nerves and chiasma, because some cases have been associated with CNS tumors.

Benign Paroxysmal Vertigo

Benign paroxysmal vertigo may be confused with seizures, because attacks develop suddenly, are accompanied by ataxia, and may cause the infant to fall. There is pallor, distress, and assumption of a motionless, often supine, position but no loss of consciousness; older children can recall the event. There may be vomiting; nystagmus should be visible during the episode. Attacks last seconds to minutes and vary in frequency, sometimes occurring daily. Older children can identify symptoms of nausea and vertigo and are less likely to be thought to be experiencing seizures. The children are normal between attacks. The condition is closely related to migraine, with many shared symptoms and the later development of more typical migrainous headache. Treatment for repeated attacks may include dimenhydrinate.

Benign Myoclonus of Early Infancy

This uncommon syndrome may resemble the cryptogenic form of infantile spasms at onset, with bilateral myoclonic jerks developing in a previously normal infant. However, this is a benign, probably nonepileptic condition occurring in infants 3 to 8 months of age and disappearing after a period of weeks or months. The pattern of myoclonus may differentiate it from infantile spasms, including predominant involvement of the head, neck, and upper limbs with adversive head movements or tremors without involving the lower limbs.

The EEG is normal. Myoclonic movements are not accompanied by an EEG seizure pattern. These abnormal movements may necessitate monitoring to establish the nonepileptic diagnosis. There is no arrest of normal development or regression as is seen in West syndrome. Most important, the myoclonus remits, not persisting after 2 years of age, and there is increased risk for other seizure patterns after its cessation.

Alternating Hemiplegia of Childhood

Alternating hemiplegia of childhood is a rare syndrome of episodic hemiplegia that usually manifests in infancy with the following diagnostic criteria:

1. onset before age 18 months, often before age 6 months
2. recurrent episodes of fluctuating hemiparesis or hemiplegia, affecting both sides of the body and disappearing during sleep
3. other paroxysmal phenomena: tonic seizures, dystonic posturing, choreoathetosis, nystagmus and other paroxysmal oculomotor disturbances, and autonomic dysfunction, occurring during or between hemiplegic episodes
4. progressive cognitive and neurologic deficits

The pathophysiologic mechanism remains unknown, although there are reports of mitochondrial dysfunction in some cases and an autosomal dominant pattern of inheritance in others. The differential diagnosis includes paroxysmal choreoathetosis and dystonia syndromes, familial hemiplegic migraine, transient ischemic attacks associated with cerebral vascular abnormalities such as moyamoya disease or cardiac emboli, mitochondrial disorders, hyperviscosity, sickle cell anemia crises, inherited disorders of metabolism (pyruvate dehydrogenase deficiency and Leigh disease), and epileptic seizures with postictal paralysis (see Chapter 41). Symptomatic treatment is available with flunarizine, a calcium channel blocker.

Acute Symptomatic Seizures and Occasional Seizures

Febrile Convulsions

Febrile convulsions are common and are defined as seizures occurring between the ages of 6 months and 5 years in association with a fever in the absence of intracranial infection or other identifiable cause. Patients with a history of previous afebrile seizures are not included in the affected population. The temperature elevation is variable. The highest incidence of febrile convulsions occurs between 1 and 2 years of age, and 85% of febrile convulsions occur before the age of 4 years. The incidence is between 2% and 5%; it is slightly more common in boys.

The seizures are usually brief with bilateral clonic or tonic-clonic motor involvement without any postictal paralysis or a prolonged postictal state of confusion or drowsiness. The seizures generally occur well within the first 24 hours of a febrile illness, not necessarily when the fever is highest; they may be the first indication of illness. Complicated or severe febrile convulsions are defined as those lasting longer than 15 minutes, recurring during a single febrile illness, having unilateral or focal features, or followed by postictal paralysis. Seizures occurring late in a febrile illness should raise suspicions of encephalitis, brain abscess, or meningitis. Abnormal behavior associated with a febrile delirium and even violent shivering may be mistaken for seizure activity.

Evaluation. The initial investigation must include a search for the cause of the febrile illness. For this diagnosis, it is essential that primary CNS infection be ruled out as the cause of both the fever and the seizures. It is suggested that children younger than 12 months of age should routinely have a lumbar puncture when presenting with a febrile seizure; many clinicians would not perform a lumbar puncture in an otherwise healthy child with an uncomplicated febrile seizure over the age of 2 years. A lumbar puncture must be performed if there is any suspicion of intracranial infection and when features of the seizure or postictal state suggest a focal or lateralized seizure (see Chapter 52). In a child with focal seizures, fever, and signs of encephalitis, herpes simplex must be suspected. Computed tomography or MRI and EEG may be part of the workup if an underlying CNS infection is suspected or a preexisting neurologic deficit has been revealed by the history.

Treatment. Treatment of a child still in convulsion on arrival at the hospital should include prompt attention to protection of the airway and circulation. Giving acetaminophen rectally should lower the fever. If the convulsion does not cease promptly with lowering of the fever, rectal diazepam should be administered. Some children may require hospital admission. The family should be advised that future fevers with temperatures above 38° C (100.4° F) be treated with regular acetaminophen or ibuprofen.

There is no increased rate of mortality from febrile convulsions, and the mental and neurologic development can be expected to be normal after a simple febrile convulsion. However, approximately 30% of febrile convulsions recur in future febrile illness, and the parents should be warned of this. Recurrence is most likely in the first 6 to 12 months after the initial febrile convulsion. Other factors that increase the chance of recurrence are onset at a young age, preexisting neurologic abnormalities, and family history of epilepsy or febrile convulsions.

Most authorities would advise no treatment for almost all children with febrile convulsions. Rare exceptions include children presenting with prolonged (>15 minutes) seizures and children younger than 12 months old with multiple recurrences. For prolonged seizures, rectal diazepam could be considered as an abortive therapy. For children with frequent recurrences, one option is rectal or oral diazepam during febrile illnesses. If these intermittent therapies are ineffective or impractical, chronic phenobarbital or valproate could be considered for the rare child with prolonged or very frequent febrile convulsions.

Informing and reassuring parents of the benign nature and usual course of febrile convulsions are very important and may be of greater value than any medication.

Prognosis. There appears to be an increased risk of epilepsy among children with febrile convulsions. Overall, the risk is approximately 3%. Risk factors increasing the likelihood of future epilepsy include existence of a prior neurologic abnormality, prolonged convulsions (>30 minutes), focal or lateralized features of the seizure, and repeated convulsions within 24 hours. The incidence of epilepsy increases from 4% of those without risk factors to 49% of those with three risk factors. Risk factors for epilepsy with generalized seizures are more than three febrile seizures and epilepsy in a first-degree relative, which suggests that febrile convulsions in these individuals may be a manifestation of an increased predisposition to epilepsy. For epilepsy with partial seizures, the risk factors are prolonged convulsions, focal features of the seizure, and repeated seizures within 24 hours, which suggest either a causative role for febrile convulsions in partial epilepsy or a preexisting brain lesion. The number of recurrences of febrile seizures has not been shown to be a risk factor for later epilepsy. There is no evidence that AED treatment of febrile seizures affects the risk for later development of afebrile seizures.

Epileptic Syndromes

West Syndrome

West syndrome, or severe encephalopathic epilepsy in infants, is characterized by infantile spasms, the hypsarrhythmic EEG pattern, and developmental delay. It is a severe form of epilepsy, usually with evidence of diffuse cerebral dysfunction and a poor prognosis in most cases. The incidence is about 1 per 4000 to 6000 infants, with onset between 3 and 12 months of age; peak onset is 4 to 8 months.

The spasm is a brief bilateral tonic contraction of muscles of the trunk, neck, and limbs, usually symmetric. The extent of muscle involvement varies from a powerful contraction that "jackknifes" the body to minimal contraction of truncal muscles that causes only stiffening. The classic spasm, "salaam attack," begins with a jerklike contraction of trunk and limb musculature, which is maintained for a few seconds. Spasms may involve truncal flexion, extension, or both. Eye movements are commonly associated with the spasm either as deviation or as repetitive nystagmoid jerks. Apnea is common but tachypnea is uncommon. Children may cry or even appear to giggle at the end of the spasm. The seizures occur daily, frequently with hundreds being recorded per 24-hour period, often clustered together. Seizures may increase during the transitions from sleep to wakefulness and wakefulness to sleep.

Electroencephalographic Features. The hypsarrhythmic EEG pattern is a high-amplitude, chaotic slowing of generalized distribution without interhemispheric synchronization and with multifocal sharp waves throughout. Hypsarrhythmia is more frequent in younger infants and early in the course of the disorder, and it is more common to find some modified variant of it.

Differential Diagnosis. Differential diagnosis for the seizures themselves can include colic, exaggerated Moro reflexes, or normal myoclonic jerks on falling asleep or waking. Two myoclonic syndromes occur in this age group and must be distinguished from infantile spasms: (1) benign myoclonus of early infancy (see preceding "Infancy" section) and (2) benign myoclonic epilepsy.

Benign myoclonic epilepsy is a rare syndrome described in previously normal infants with onset between 4 months and 3 years. The infant has brief repetitive myoclonic jerks that involve the head and upper limbs and rarely the lower limbs; they occur daily in drowsiness and wakefulness. The ictal EEG shows 3-Hz spike-and-wave or polyspike activity during the events. The background EEG rhythms are normal. There are no other seizure types, and the infant does not have behavioral or cognitive disturbances. The long-term prognosis is favorable for development and remission of seizures after response to treatment with an AED. Some affected patients have had tonic-clonic seizures in adolescence.

An EEG pattern of suppression-burst activity heralds a poor prognosis, and some groups have proposed that infants with a consistent EEG pattern of this nature and a much earlier onset of seizures may have distinct epileptic syndromes separable from the majority of patients with West syndrome. These related syndromes, *early infantile epileptic encephalopathy* and *early myoclonic encephalopathy,* are discussed in the preceding "Infancy" section.

Evaluation. Investigation of patients with infantile spasms is directed at determining the cause and then classifying the condition into cryptogenic and symptomatic groups. The most common etiologic factor found is perinatal hypoxic-ischemic insult. Other important associations include intrauterine infection, prematurity, intracranial hemorrhage, malformations of cortical development, tuberous sclerosis, head injury, CNS infection, and inborn errors of metabolism. Approximately 10% to 15% of patients have no identifiable underlying cause and a history of normal development before the onset of their illness; this subset is referred to as *cryptogenic,* or *idiopathic, West syndrome.* This subset of patients is likely to have a much better long-term outcome: 38% are normal or mildly impaired, in comparison with only 5% in the symptomatic patients.

About 50% of infants go on to have other seizure types when spasms cease. Persistence of the epilepsy in most of the patients is associated with loss of the spasms and development of other seizure types, such as tonic seizures, simple partial seizures, and tonic-clonic seizures.

Treatment. Treatment with corticosteroids aborts the spasms in a significant number of infants. Regimens vary, including initial doses of adrenocorticotropic hormone or prednisone. The spasms should cease and the EEG patterns improve if the child has responded. After 1 to 2 weeks at maximum dosages, the corticosteroid is gradually decreased until it is discontinued altogether after 2 to 3 months.

Vigabatrin may be effective for infantile spasms, and it has been shown to be particularly effective in the treatment of infantile spasms with tuberous sclerosis. Topiramate and lamotrigine are being evaluated for possible efficacy. Valproate, nitrazepam, and clonazepam may also be helpful. The combination of valproate and lamotrigine is often more efficacious than either medication used alone.

Severe Myoclonic Epilepsy in Infancy

Severe myoclonic epilepsy in infancy is a rare cryptogenic generalized epilepsy appearing in the first year of life. The syndrome differs from the myoclonic syndromes already described (early myoclonic encephalopathy and early infantile encephalopathic epilepsy) by its later onset and the EEG findings. A mutation of a voltage-gated sodium channel gene is seen in 30% of cases (see Table 39-4).

The child may present with febrile or afebrile seizures, usually with normal psychomotor development preceding the onset of seizures, and often with a family history of epilepsy. The seizures are generalized or unilateral clonic seizures; myoclonic seizures appear later (and may not be a major feature of the disorder despite the name), between 8 months and 4 years of age; and partial seizures and atypical absences may occur. The interictal EEG may be normal initially and only later show fast, generalized spike-and-wave epileptiform discharges and focal abnormalities.

The seizures are usually refractory to AEDs, and psychomotor development eventually becomes retarded. Ataxia and signs of pyramidal tract dysfunction may become apparent.

CHILDHOOD

The paroxysmal disorders of childhood (2 to 12 years) are given in Table 39-14.

Table 39-14. Paroxysmal Disorders of Childhood

Nonepileptiform Disorders
Breath-holding spells*†
Syncope‡
Migraine and migraine equivalents, recurrent abdominal pain, cyclic vomiting*
Tic*
Spasmodic torticollis†
Drug reactions, dystonia
Paroxysmal choreoathetosis
Gastroesophageal reflux
Benign paroxysmal vertigo†
Myoclonus, nonepileptic; anxiety, excitement, acute metabolic encephalopathy†
Hyperexplexia
Masturbation†
Withholding, constipation*
Daydreaming, staring spells*
Stereotypic movements, autism, coexistent deafness and blindness
Munchausen syndrome by proxy
Hyperventilation‡
Psychogenic seizures‡
Transient global amnesia‡
Sleep*
  Head banging, jactatio capitis†
  Pavor nocturnus
  Somnambulism, somniloquy

Acute Symptomatic Seizures, Occasional Seizures
Febrile convulsions*
Brain tumor
Meningitis, encephalitis
Head injury, child abuse
Poisoning
Intercurrent medical illness, renal, liver disease, cardiac right-to-left shunt, and embolism
Metabolic disease, rickets

Epileptic Syndromes
Benign partial epilepsies*
Symptomatic focal epilepsy*
Epilepsia partialis continua
Rasmussen encephalitis
Hemiconvulsion hemiplegia syndrome
Childhood absence epilepsy*
Epilepsy with myoclonic absences
Lennox-Gastaut syndrome
Myoclonic astatic epilepsy
Landau-Kleffner syndrome
Epilepsy with continuous spike-and-wave patterns during slow-wave sleep

*Common.
†See infant section for discussion.
‡See adolescent section for discussion.

Paroxysmal Nonepileptic Disorders

Migraine and Migraine Equivalents

Migraine is a common disorder, and some episodes may be confused with seizures because of their paroxysmal nature and association with neurologic deficits or altered consciousness (see Chapter 37).

In *cyclic vomiting,* recurrent attacks of nausea, vomiting, and abdominal pain occur on a daily or weekly basis. There is no clouding of consciousness. Typically, there are symptom-free intervals lasting weeks to months. Migraine may develop later, or there may be a strong family history of migraine, and there appears to be some overlap of the cyclic vomiting with migraine.

Tic Disorders

Tics are common. They are sudden, brief, purposeless involuntary movements or utterances that occur repetitively (see Chapter 35). Tics may be thought to be myoclonic seizures, and, indeed, some tics may have a rapid myoclonic character. Myoclonus cannot be suppressed by the patient, may have an ictal EEG correlate, and may be associated with other seizure types.

Table 39-15 outlines some of the clinical features of episodic abnormal movements that may appear in children.

Sleep Disorders

Night Terrors and Confusional Arousals. *Night terrors* are a common phenomenon in children and are most frequent in boys aged 5 to 7 years. Up to 15% of children younger than 7 years have experienced some form of these episodes. The attacks are characterized by sudden arousal from sleep, often screaming in terror, and then crying with agitation and tachycardia. There may be vigorous and potentially injurious motor activity in older children, such as running

or hitting the bed or wall. The striking feature of these episodes is that the child is inconsolable but seemingly awake. The episodes arise out of slow-wave non–rapid eye movement sleep, usually occurring 1 to 2 hours after bedtime, and are not responses to dream imagery (i.e., not nightmares). Episodes last several minutes. Prior sleep deprivation, febrile illness, emotional stress, and some medications (sedatives/hypnotics, neuroleptics, stimulants, antihistamines) may be precipitants. In contrast to the experience of nightmares, children are amnestic for the events and their distress in night terrors.

Confusional arousals are less dramatic attacks with similar origin from slow-wave sleep and are more typical in younger children. The affected child stirs and begins crying and whimpering inconsolably. These arousals may be prolonged in infants, lasting up to 30 to 40 minutes.

There is no specific treatment for these events; parents should be educated about the nature of these arousals and reassured that they are self-limited. Although efforts to calm the child may seem to prolong the attacks, it is probably best if a parent sits with the child, if only to prevent injury. Frequent disruptive attacks or those with potentially injurious motor activity may be decreased by short-term treatment with low-dose tricyclic antidepressants or benzodiazepines.

Somnambulism. Somnambulism, or sleepwalking, is common in childhood: Approximately 15% of children have walked in their sleep, especially in the 2- to 3-year-old age group, and 2.5% are habitual

---

Table 39-15. Abnormal Involuntary Movements

Movement	Characteristics	Associations
Tics	Brief involuntary movements (motor tics) or sounds (phonic or vocal tics), occurring against a background of normal motor activity Tics may be simple, sudden brief movements such as shrugging a shoulder, blinking, or grimacing; or complex, more coordinated movement that might appear purposeful, such as hitting or touching Snorting, sniffing, or throat clearing are examples of simple phonic tics and short utterances, echolalia, or coprolalia are complex phonic tics	Idiopathic tic disorders Tourette syndrome
Tremor	Movements caused by rhythmically alternating contractions of a muscle group and its antagonists The movements may involve proximal and axial muscles Classified as resting, postural, or action tremors according to the response to these maneuvers	Physiologic tremor, essential tremor
Chorea	Random brief limb movements of variable duration, these can be incorporated into voluntary movements by the patient	SLE Wilson disease Postinfectious
Athetosis	Slow writhing movements of the extremities, often distal extremities The movements are random Often involuntary movements of this type have some features of chorea and are termed *choreoathetoid*	Kernicterus
Dystonia	Sustained muscle co-contraction of agonist and antagonist muscle groups, frequently causing twisting and repetitive movements or abnormal postures The velocity of the movements varies, usually being sustained at the height of the involuntary contraction for a second or longer The duration also varies in different syndromes; in spasmodic torticollis, there may be rhythmic jerks or spasms into the abnormal posture Subclassified by extent (focal, segmental, multifocal and generalized) and relationship to movement (action and rest)	Idiopathic (inherited) syndromes Postlesional syndromes
Myoclonus	Rapid brief muscle jerks with an irregular or occasionally rhythmic quality Can be epileptic or nonepileptic in origin	Encephalopathies Idiopathic and symptomatic epilepsies
Ballismus	Wild, large-amplitude, irregular limb movements	Postlesional
Asterixis	Repetitive movements caused by sudden, brief, irregular lapses in posture of an extremity.	Metabolic encephalopathies
Dyskinesia	Sometimes used as a general term to describe abnormal involuntary movements	

SLE, systemic lupus erythematosus.

sleepwalkers, having episodes at least once a month. The age at onset peaks between 4 and 10 and between 8 and 15 years. There is a family history of sleepwalking and other parasomnias for 60% to 80% of patients. These episodes of apparent unresponsiveness and "automatisms" could be mistaken for complex partial seizures or a postictal state.

Hyperekplexia

A startle response is normally seen in children and adults in response to sudden, unexpected stimuli. The typical response consists of a facial grimace, eye blink and brief head nod, shoulder elevation, abduction of the arms with elbow flexion, truncal flexion, and knee flexion. Startle is exaggerated with anxiety, fatigue, and sleep deprivation. Hyperekplexia is characterized by an excessive startle response interfering with daily living, usually causing patients to fall stiffly in the posture of the startle response and sustaining injury, with preserved consciousness. A history of infantile stiffness of the trunk and limbs and nocturnal myoclonus is present in many affected patients. There appears to be an infantile expression of the disorder, with severe hypertonia occurring with handling; the hypertonia may be so severe as to cause apnea, bradycardia, and even sudden death.

Generalized seizures have been reported in some cases; mental retardation and delayed motor development appear to be common. The background EEG is usually normal. There may be some improvement with clonazepam or valproate therapy. Linkage analysis has mapped a gene for this condition to chromosome 5q33-35, and mutations in the *GLRA1* gene, encoding the α1 subunit of the glycine receptor, have been found in families with an autosomal dominant or recessive inheritance pattern.

In some epileptic syndromes, such as the Lennox-Gastaut syndrome, generalized seizures may be precipitated by sudden unexpected stimuli. This phenomenon has been termed *startle-induced epileptic seizures* or *startle epilepsy.* Startle-induced seizures can normally be differentiated from nonepileptic startle responses by the presence of other seizure types and EEG abnormalities.

Self-Stimulatory Behavior

Repetitive purposeless movements may be performed by physically and intellectually handicapped children and by autistic children. Combined with unresponsiveness, these behaviors may be mistaken for automatisms in complex partial seizures. The important features that distinguish such behavior from epileptic activity are the setting in which it occurs, the variable content and duration of the "attacks," and the complete failure of the episodes to interrupt more stimulating activities. However, it may be very difficult to determine the nature of the episodes by interview; video and EEG monitoring may be required.

Factitious Disorder (Munchausen Syndrome) by Proxy

Factitious disorder is a consistent simulation of illness that leads to unnecessary investigations and treatments. When parents pursue such deception and cause their children to be investigated and treated, the situation is referred to as factitious disorder (or Munchausen syndrome) by proxy. Presentations with a history of paroxysmal loss of consciousness or seizures are common. The syndrome is described in children under 6 years of age; the mother is often the perpetrator (see Chapters 35 and 36).

Seizures refractory to carefully prescribed AEDs must always prompt a review of the diagnosis, and the clinician must also be careful to consider fabricated presentations.

Acute Symptomatic Seizures and Occasional Seizures

Febrile convulsions remain one of the most common causes of occasional seizures in early childhood. Head injury is more common in childhood than in infancy, but the list of other potential causes of seizures, including brain tumor, intracranial infection, and poisoning, is very similar. In addition, some metabolic and neurodegenerative disorders manifest in childhood, not in infancy (Table 39-16).

Epileptic Syndromes

Benign Partial Epilepsies of Childhood

Partial seizures and focal EEG discharges usually suggest the presence of a localized cerebral lesion. There is a group of idiopathic partial epilepsies beginning in children without abnormalities on neurologic examination or neuroimaging studies and frequently with a family history for epilepsy. The benign partial epilepsies of childhood (BPECs) are characterized by partial seizures and focal epileptiform discharges, both with age-dependent spontaneous recovery, in the absence of anatomic lesions.

Clinically, the seizures begin between 18 months and 12 years of age, most often at 8 to 10 years; there is no neurologic deficit or developmental delay. The seizures are brief and stereotyped in an individual, although they vary among patients. The seizures do not have a prolonged postictal deficit, are usually infrequent, and respond well to AED treatment. The focal epileptiform discharges occur with normal background rhythms. The sharp waves or spikes have a characteristic structure and are often very frequent, increasing during sleep. Rare generalized epileptiform discharges may occur, but if they are prominent, the diagnosis of BPEC should be questioned.

The most well-defined form of BPEC is *benign epilepsy with centrotemporal spikes and seizures,* often referred to as *benign rolandic epilepsy.* Brief hemifacial motor seizures with anarthria and drooling are typical. Consciousness is typically preserved, although this may not be true with longer seizures. A somatosensory aura involving the tongue, cheek, or gums may precede the motor seizure. Many seizures occur at night as tonic-clonic seizures, presumably secondary generalized with unwitnessed partial onset. Onset is between 3 and 13 years, with a peak onset at 9 to 10 years; there is a male-to-female predominance of approximately 3:2.

Management depends on seizure frequency; if the typical EEG discharges have been found in a child without seizures or after a first seizure, there is usually no indication to treat with AEDs. If seizures are infrequent and nocturnal, the option of no treatment should be discussed. AED treatment should be considered for patients experiencing more frequent seizures, troublesome seizures during the day, or seizures associated with any morbidity such as postictal headaches or lethargy. The seizures are usually controlled easily with a variety of AEDs, including carbamazepine or gabapentin.

The seizures of BPEC resolve spontaneously before 16 years of age, and so all treated patients should have AEDs withdrawn at least by that time. The EEG may be helpful in deciding when to withdraw treatment. Patients older than 14 years who are seizure-free for 1 to 2 years with normal EEGs should withdraw from treatment; the clinician should strongly consider a trial of withdrawal in patients 10 to 14 years old who are seizure-free and have a normal EEG. Younger patients with active EEGs are likely to have recurrence of seizures with AED withdrawal.

Benign childhood epilepsy with occipital paroxysms forms a subset of idiopathic partial epilepsies of childhood. There are two types of this subset: one with early onset (peak onset at 3 to 5 years), nocturnal seizures with tonic eye deviation, and vomiting and another with later onset (peak onset at 7 to 9 years) characterized by seizures beginning with visual symptoms, which is consistent with an occipital origin. Hemiclonic seizures or the automatisms of temporal lobe complex seizures often follow, according to whether the seizure spreads to suprasylvian or infrasylvian regions. A severe headache may follow the visual auras and a diagnosis of childhood migraine is often considered. The EEG typically shows high-amplitude sharp waves or spike-and-wave complexes recurring at

Table 39-16. Inherited Disorders of Metabolism and Neurodegenerative Diseases Associated with Seizures in Childhood and Adolescence

Name	Clinical Features and Laboratory Findings	Investigations
Syndrome of Progressive Myoclonus Epilepsy		
Multiple specific disorders cause the clinical syndrome of PME Prominent myoclonus; irregular repetitive, spontaneous or with action, stimulus sensitive Associated seizures types; usually tonic-clonic but also tonic, absence, and partial seizures Progressive neurologic deterioration, with prominent ataxia and other motor signs developing later Progressive dementia, varying in degree between the specific disorders		
Most cases are caused by the following five disorders:		
Unverricht-Lundborg	Onset, ages 8-15 years; myoclonus and GTC seizures, cerebellar ataxia, slowly progressive but mild cognitive decline; patients have long survival in comparison to other disorders in this group	Chromosome 21q22; cystatin B mutations Clinical diagnosis, must exclude other causes of PME syndrome
Myoclonus epilepsy and ragged red fibers (MERRF)	Onset, ages 5-12 years (range, 3-62 years); myoclonus, GTC seizures, progressive ataxia, dementia Other features include deafness, optic atrophy, neuropathy, myopathy, pyramidal signs, dysarthria and nystagmus There may be clinical overlap with other mitochondrial encephalomyopathies: mitochondrial encephalomyopathy with lactic acidosis and strokelike episodes (MELAS) and Kearns-Sayre syndrome	Serum and CSF lactate and pyruvate measurements Muscle biopsy; light microscopy, electron microscopy (EM), biochemical analysis of oxidative metabolism, and DNA studies
Lafora body disease	Onset, ages 10-19 years; generalized clonic, GTC seizures and partial seizures with visual auras; myoclonus develops later and becomes very disabling; severe dementia; death within 5 years of disease onset Lafora bodies (intracellular amyloid inclusions) are found in skin, muscle, neurons, and hepatocytes	Biopsy of skin must include eccrine sweat glands (i.e., axilla) to exclude Lafora bodies Chromosome 6q24; gene *EPM2A* produces laforin
Neuronal ceroid lipofuscinosis		
Late infantile form (Jansky-Bielschowsky)	Onset, ages 2-4 years; severe epilepsy, myoclonic, GTC, atonic, atypical absence seizures (not tonic, vs. Lennox-Gastaut syndrome), progressive severe dementia, ataxia, pyramidal and extrapyramidal signs, visual loss later, usually death in adolescence Ophthalmologic examination necessary; EEG; marked photic sensitivity to 1-Hz stimulation, electroretinogram (ERG) and visual evoked potential (VEP) abnormalities	Skin, conjunctival, or rectal mucosal biopsy; skin biopsy is the most practical and least morbid Lipopigment accumulation in lysosomes, best seen in eccrine secretory cells; the inclusions have a characteristic structure on EM that differs between the different subtypes of neuronal ceroid lipofuscinosis EEG, ERG, and VEP testing
Juvenile form (Batten-Spielmeyer-Vogt)	Onset, ages 4-10 years; usually manifests with decreased visual acuity secondary to retinal degeneration, psychomotor delay, cerebellar and extrapyramidal signs, later onset of seizures, and GTC and myoclonus Progressive severe dementia accompanies the other neurological signs Death in early adulthood ERG and VEP abnormalities	Same as for late infantile form
Adult onset (Kufs)	Onset, ages 11-50 years; dementia, psychiatric symptoms, cerebellar signs, and extrapyramidal signs are most prominent; seizures often tonic; visual disturbances are less common; fundi are normal; on EEG, marked photic sensitivity to 1-Hz stimulation	
Sialidosis		
Type 1	Onset, ages 8-20 years; decreased visual acuity and macular cherry-red spot; action- and stimulus-induced myoclonus; cerebellar ataxia; no dementia or decreased length of survival A peripheral neuropathy may be present	Urine specimen, blood sample for cultured leukocytes, and skin biopsy to obtain cultured fibroblasts for enzyme analysis
Type 2	Onset, ages 10-30 years; described in Japanese patients	Same as for type 1

Table 39-16. Inherited Disorders of Metabolism and Neurodegenerative Diseases Associated with Seizures in Childhood and Adolescence—cont'd

Name	Clinical Features and Laboratory Findings	Investigations
	Dysmorphic features and PME syndrome Elevated excretion of urinary sialylated oligosaccharides, enzyme analysis shows deficiency of α-*N*-acetylneuraminidase (type 1), additional deficiency of β-galactosidase (type 2)	
Less common causes of PME syndrome in this age group:		
Juvenile neuronopathic Gaucher disease; PME, supranuclear palsy, and splenomegaly; no dementia; pancytopenia on CBC, leukocytes show low β-glucocerebrosidase activity		CBC, leukocytes for enzyme analysis
Dentatorubral-pallidoluysian atrophy, seen in Japanese patients; PME is one manifestation		Clinical diagnosis in life
Neuroaxonal dystrophy; may appear as PME; also, chorea, lower motor neuron signs; axon steroids in neurons, may be seen in autonomic nerve endings around eccrine secretory coils		Peripheral nerve biopsy, skin biopsy
Late-onset GM₂ gangliosidosis; sensitivity to acoustic stimulus; myoclonus, severe dementia, dystonia, pyramidal signs; cherry-red spot may be seen at macula		Hexosaminidase A activity
Hallervorden-Spatz disease		Clinical diagnosis in life
Action myoclonus–renal failure syndrome, described in French-Canadians; tremor, PME, and, later, proteinuria and renal failure; no dementia		Clinical diagnosis, renal function
Other Rare Disorders with Seizures in Childhood and Adolescence		
Juvenile Huntington disease	Onset, age >3 years; developmental delay; dystonia; GTC, atypical absence, myoclonic seizures; parkinsonian features may be present	
Alpers syndrome	Progressive neurologic degeneration of childhood A clinical syndrome; now suspected to be a mitochondrial encephalopathy Normal at birth, then failure to thrive with developmental delay, myoclonic jerks, seizures, episodes of status epilepticus, hypotonia, and visual loss followed by spastic quadriparesis Epilepsy partialis continua may be present The spectrum of clinical features includes deafness, ataxia, chorea and liver disease	Muscle biopsy
Rett syndrome	Onset, ages 1-2 years; in girls only; delay or regression in motor development, loss of language, ataxia, "hand-ringing" mannerism Seizures occur later; myoclonic, partial, and generalized tonic-clonic Episodes of apnea, ataxic breathing, and hyperventilation; pyramidal signs	Muscle biopsy for mitochondrial enzyme analysis and histologic study, although cause is unknown, genetic testing
Maple syrup urine disease	Less severe forms may manifest late, even in adulthood, with episodic symptoms of encephalopathy and ataxia and possibly seizures	Urine and serum amino acids
Porphyria	Onset, late adolescence, after puberty; 15% of affected patients have seizures during an acute attack of porphyria	Urinary porphyrins

CBC, complete blood cell count; CSF, cerebrospinal fluid; EEG, electroencephalogram; GTC, generalized tonic-clonic; PME, progressive myoclonus epilepsy.

1 to 0.5 Hz posteriorly, usually maximal in the occipital regions. The discharges are present when the eyes are closed and should disappear with eye opening. There is some controversy about the specificity of the electroclinical features and whether these cases are true variants of benign childhood epilepsy. The conditions are relatively uncommon, and the same EEG pattern may be seen with symptomatic occipital epilepsy.

Acquired Epileptic Aphasia and Continuous Spike-and-Wave Patterns in Slow-Wave Sleep

These two conditions are age-related epileptic encephalopathies with disturbances in language and cognition occurring in association with persistent focal or bilaterally synchronous epileptiform activity and

seizures without an underlying structural lesion. In each, the epileptiform activity is thought to disturb synaptogenesis and connectivity in the maturing brain. Although they are rare, some authorities consider them part of the spectrum of benign childhood epilepsy. Epileptic aphasia, or the *Landau-Kleffner syndrome,* begins in a previously normal child (peak age at onset, 5 to 7 years) with the regression of language. There is a severe auditory agnosia, speech may disappear, the child often appears to be deaf, and there is usually a marked deterioration in behavior. Childhood psychosis and the autistic spectrum disorders are often considered in the differential diagnosis. Seizures occur but are not frequent and cannot explain the language deficits. The EEG in sleep shows almost continuous bilateral epileptiform discharges maximal over the temporal regions. The seizures are partial and easily controlled with medication, but the language regression and the EEG discharges do not remit with conventional AEDs. Treatment with corticosteroids does improve the condition in many children, but more than half have persistent language and learning deficits despite the eventual disappearance of the EEG abnormalities. In *continuous spike-and-wave patterns in slow sleep,* there is a more diffuse cognitive dysfunction, and more than 85% of the sleep EEG record is occupied by bilaterally synchronous epileptiform discharges. The disorder typically manifests at 5 to 7 years of age, and there is a broader spectrum of seizure types, including absences, atonic seizures, and complex partial seizures, which may be frequent in some patients.

Symptomatic Focal (Localization-Related) Epilepsy

The most common seizure type in symptomatic focal epilepsy in children is the complex partial seizure. Complex partial seizures may arise from temporal, frontal, parietal, or occipital lobes but most often from the temporal lobe. The causes of focal epilepsy in childhood are diverse and include birth asphyxia, later anoxic episodes, head injury, neoplasms, infection, malformations of cortical development, the cerebral lesions of neurocutaneous syndromes, vascular malformations, and cerebral infarction. Mesial temporal sclerosis is the most common finding in temporal lobes resected to treat refractory focal epilepsy in adults. The incidence of mesial temporal sclerosis in childhood nonidiopathic focal epilepsy has not yet been determined. MRI is a crucial diagnostic procedure and can reveal a variety of structural abnormalities.

Symptomatic focal epilepsy commonly evolves as a medically refractory disorder; however, in some patients, it can be amenable to surgical resection. The investigation of children for epilepsy surgery is a highly specialized process that follows documentation of medical intractability. Concordant evidence of a single epileptogenic region within the brain must be found with ictal video and EEG monitoring, both structural neuroimaging (MRI) and functional neuroimaging (single photon emission computed tomography and positron emission tomography) and neuropsychologic evaluation. If a focus can be demonstrated, it must be shown that resection of that area will not cause loss of sensorimotor or cognitive function. In the case of temporal foci, the risk of postoperative memory dysfunction must be addressed. In seizures with foci from extratemporal sites, it may be necessary to map cortical sensorimotor and language function by cortical stimulation to determine the limits of a surgical resection.

Childhood Absence Epilepsy

Childhood absence epilepsy is an idiopathic generalized epilepsy beginning in previously normal children between 3 and 12 years of age, with peak incidence at 6 to 7 years of age; girls are more frequently affected. It accounts for only about 8% to 10% of school-aged children with epilepsy. There is a family history of epilepsy in approximately 15% to 25% of patients. The absence seizures are simple or, more often, complicated with mild automatisms or other motor features. Absence seizures are very frequent, occurring daily, but they respond well to therapy. The EEG is normal apart from runs of 3-Hz spike-and-wave complexes; clinical seizures are associated with discharges lasting more than 2 to 3 seconds. The discharges and clinical seizures can be produced by hyperventilation. Prognosis is generally favorable, with remission in approximately 80% of cases by late adolescence. Generalized tonic-clonic seizures occur in 40% to 50% of patients with childhood absence epilepsy. They typically develop years after the onset of absences and may appear after remission from the absence seizures. Usually, the tonic-clonic seizures are infrequent and medically controllable.

Treatment with ethosuximide or valproate controls absence seizures in most patients. However, ethosuximide offers no protection against tonic-clonic seizures, whereas valproate is also effective against tonic-clonic seizures. Therefore, valproate is the drug of choice if both seizure types are present. If either ethosuximide or valproate proves ineffective after an adequate trial at maximum tolerated doses, a trial of the other should be commenced. Combination ethosuximide and valproate therapy has been effective in some patients with absence seizures not controlled by either drug alone. Clonazepam may also be effective, but it is associated with sedative and behavioral side effects. Alternatives may include lamotrigine, topiramate, or zonisamide, although few data about their efficacy in this setting are available.

Epilepsia Partialis Continua and Rasmussen Encephalitis

Epilepsia partialis continua describes continuous partial motor seizures usually manifesting as repetitive clonic jerks of the face, upper limb, lower limb, or larger portion of one half of the body that continue in this localized manner for hours to days or months. These focal seizures, with occasional secondary generalization, are caused by circumscribed rolandic or perirolandic cortical processes that include vascular lesions, focal cortical dysplasia, neoplasms, and unidentified focal areas of atrophy.

The focal seizures in this condition are generally impossible to control with AEDs, and surgical management with a limited cortical resection may be necessary. The risk of motor and sensory deficits limits possible resections, and careful mapping of the site of seizure onset and its relationship to functional cortex is required. Mitochondrial encephalomyopathies (mitochondrial encephalomyopathy with lactic acidosis and strokelike episodes) and an inherited disorder of metabolism (nonketotic hyperglycinemia) have also been reported to cause epilepsia partialis continua.

Rasmussen encephalitis is a clinically defined syndrome of predominantly lateralized cerebral dysfunction, with onset of seizures between 2 and 10 years of age. A variety of seizure types can occur, including focal motor seizures and complex partial seizures with secondary generalization, myoclonus, and epilepsia partialis continua; they are refractory to management with AEDs. The disorder is characterized by a progressive hemiparesis, language disturbances if the dominant hemisphere is affected, and intellectual decline. Progressive hemispheric atrophy, maximal in the central, temporal, and frontal regions, can be documented with neuroimaging studies. Pathologic specimens show nonspecific changes suggestive of encephalitis, although no etiologic agent has been identified. Worsening of the neurologic deficits can be expected over time, although the seizures may lessen and even "burn out."

Functional hemispherectomy, performed early in the course of the disease before complete hemiparesis, should control seizures, arrest the motor deterioration, and in most cases lead to stabilization or even improvement in language and intellectual function. However, significant morbidity and mortality rates are associated with the surgery, and the child is left with a paretic upper limb, although he or she can walk unaided.

Lennox-Gastaut Syndrome

The Lennox-Gastaut syndrome is characterized by generalized seizures and epileptiform discharges with delayed mental development and behavioral problems beginning between the ages of 1 and 8 years. The patients have a mixed seizure disorder with multiple seizure types; the typical seizures are axial tonic seizures, atypical absences, and atonic seizures, although patients may also have tonic-clonic, myoclonic, and complex partial seizures. The seizures are not easily controlled and are usually frequent, often several occurring per day. Episodes of status epilepticus are common, and nonconvulsive stupor with continuous spike-and-wave discharges or a stuporous state with repeated tonic seizures is typical. The waking EEG has abnormally slow background activity, and the EEG correlates of sleep may also be poorly organized. The epileptiform abnormalities consist of slow (<3 Hz) spike-and-wave discharges, multifocal spikes, or sharp waves and paroxysmal fast activity (>10 Hz) in sleep.

AEDs are always indicated but rarely able to control seizures completely. More often, some reduction in frequency and severity of seizures may be obtained. Monotherapy should be attempted with substitution of another agent if the initial drug proves ineffective. However, because of multiple seizure types, patients commonly need combinations of AEDs. Valproate should be used as a first-line agent for patients with atonic, tonic, and myoclonic seizures and may be helpful with tonic-clonic seizures. Patients with refractory tonic-clonic seizures or partial seizures as well as generalized seizures may benefit from the addition of lamotrigine. Combinations of AEDs must be monitored carefully for drug toxicity and unwanted interactions. Carbamazepine has been reported to exacerbate atypical absence seizures in some patients. Phenytoin can be an effective drug in controlling generalized tonic-clonic and tonic seizures. Barbiturates may be effective, although they are often poorly tolerated, and drug-related drowsiness may exacerbate tonic seizures in some patients. Other alternatives include clonazepam, topiramate, and levetiracetam. Felbamate has been reported to improve control of the debilitating tonic or atonic "drop attacks" in patients with this syndrome.

An issue perhaps peculiar to this notoriously refractory seizure disorder is the need to consider what level of seizure activity can be tolerated. For instance, the best control achieved may be infrequent daytime tonic seizures in the setting of daily absence seizures and frequent nocturnal tonic seizures. AED toxicity may be particularly noxious in these patients, leading to increased numbers of falls, worsening behavior, lethargy, and exacerbation of seizures.

A major source of morbidity and an important management issue is repeated falls associated with tonic and atonic seizures. Appropriate restriction in daily activities and the wearing of helmets with face protection are often required. Division of the anterior portion of the corpus callosum has been successful in controlling the falls associated with tonic or atonic seizures, but not all patients benefit, and seizure control is not complete.

Myoclonic Astatic Epilepsy

Although sometimes seen as a variant of the Lennox-Gastaut syndrome, myoclonic astatic epilepsy has been described as a distinct entity. Patients have a mixed seizure disorder with myoclonus, atypical absences, and tonic-clonic seizures but not tonic seizures. The term *astatic* refers to loss of station or posture with abrupt falling during myoclonic seizures. The peak age at onset is between 2 and 5 years, and the range is from 7 months to 6 years. Approximately one third of patients have a family history of epilepsy.

In comparison with the interictal EEG in Lennox-Gastaut syndrome, that in myoclonic astatic epilepsy shows faster generalized spike-and-wave and polyspike-and-wave epileptiform discharges. The absence of tonic and partial seizures and the EEG findings distinguish this syndrome from Lennox-Gastaut syndrome.

The course is variable, but a proportion of patients have a favorable one. A certain small group of children with an apparently unfavorable, even catastrophic-looking initial clinical presentation may respond well to valproate therapy and have spontaneous remission of seizures.

Panayiotopoulos Syndrome

This common and benign syndrome affects children between 3 and 6 years of age. The seizures may be prolonged and mimic nonepileptic conditions. The seizures have an autonomic component and often manifest with associated emesis, pallor, hypersalivation, and flaccidity. The EEG demonstrates occipital or extraoccipital spikes. Seizures occur during nocturnal sleep or daytime naps. Children may appear confused and may develop focal or generalized motor seizures. The outcome is good, with remission occurring in 2 years. Treatment with AEDs is not always needed.

ADOLESCENCE

The paroxysmal disorders of adolescence (12 to 18 years) are shown in Table 39-17.

Paroxysmal Nonepileptiform Disorders

Syncope

Loss of consciousness with falling is the salient feature of syncope (see Chapter 42 and Table 39-18).

Psychogenic Seizures

Nonepileptic paroxysmal abnormal behaviors (psychogenic seizures) may be a manifestation of psychiatric illness or emotionally based. Psychiatric disease, particularly panic attacks, may be mistaken for epilepsy.

Table 39-17. Paroxysmal Disorders of Adolescence

Nonepileptiform Disorders
More Common
Syncope
Migraine
Psychogenic seizures
   Dissociative states, conversion disorders
   Panic attacks, hyperventilation
Daydreaming
Sleep
   Nocturnal myoclonus, hypnic jerks
   Narcolepsy
   Somnambulism
   Somniloquy

Less Common
Episodic rage
Malingering
Paroxysmal choreoathetosis
Tremor
Tic
Drug reactions, dystonia
Transient global amnesia

Acute Symptomatic Seizures, Occasional Seizures
More Common
Drug abuse
Head injury
Meningitis and encephalitis

Less Common
Brain tumor
Intercurrent medical illness, endocrine disorder, systemic
   neoplasia

Epileptic Syndromes
More Common
Symptomatic localization-related epilepsy
Juvenile myoclonic epilepsy

Less Common
Juvenile absence epilepsy
Epilepsy with generalized tonic clonic seizures on awakening
Epilepsia partialis continua (Kojewnikow syndrome)
Rasmussen encephalitis
Progressive myoclonic epilepsy (see Table 39-16)

Table 39-18. Differential Diagnosis of Syncope

Clinical	Syncope	Tonic-Clonic Seizures
Precipitating factors	Almost always: patient is standing; environment is warm; fright; pain	Usually none, although sleep deprivation or awakening may be contributory
Prodrome	Lightheaded, dizzy, queasy; vision dims; loss of color, "grey out"; sweating May be averted by head down or recumbency	Aura or sense of déjà vu or jamais vu may be present
Occurrence in sleep	Never	Common
Evolution	Limp faint → fall → motionless unconsciousness, often with pallor, clammy skin; there may be a tonic phase with generalized stiffening	Sudden loss of consciousness → increased tone and massive truncal flexion or extension, followed by synchronous jerking of body and limbs with rubor or cyanosis and sweating → unconsciousness
Skin	Pale and cool	Flushed, cyanosed, warm
Incontinence	Rare	Occasional
Self-injury	Rare	Common (biting tongue)
Degree of postictal confusion	Minimal	Marked
Family history	Often positive for syncope	May be positive for seizures
Interictal EEG	Usually normal	Frequently abnormal, epileptiform discharges

Panic attacks may begin without the patient's being able to identify an external precipitant, and then the sense of dread or fear may be mistaken for a psychic aura. Many of the symptoms experienced, including palpitations, paresthesia, formication, lightheadedness, and carpopedal spasm, result from hyperventilation and tachycardia. There may be some apparent disturbance of consciousness. Historically, the sequence of events is important, especially the hyperventilation and associated symptoms. The patient may be asked to hyperventilate in the office to see whether symptoms are reproduced; hyperventilation must continue for 3 to 5 minutes with good effort for a negative result to be useful.

Rage attacks may occur and be confused with epileptic seizures. Often seen in intellectually impaired patients, they represent intense frustration in the presence of an inability to vent the frustration in other ways or to communicate it. Rage attacks may also occur in children with normal intelligence or in those taking anabolic steroids.

Psychogenic seizures are common. Among adults, 20% of patients referred with refractory seizures are found to have psychogenic seizures; in children, the number is smaller. Psychogenic seizures may appear as a manifestation of a conversion disorder. Psychogenic seizures or hysterical seizures probably occur in a dissociative state. Typically, they are characterized by marked motor activity such as pelvic thrusting, arching of the back, thrashing of the limbs, and even self-injury. The episodes may have a gradual onset with build-up of motor activity, and they usually last longer than epileptic seizures (Table 39-19). Other forms that the psychogenic seizure may take include a gradual slump to a motionless supine position with unresponsiveness and eyes closed, often with some flickering of the eyelids, referred to by some people as a "swoon."

Deliberate simulation of an epileptic attack may occur in some patients with epilepsy in an effort to manipulate their environment or circumstances, and in this case the differential diagnosis may include school refusal.

Evaluation. The interictal EEG is repeatedly normal in patients with psychogenic seizures. For definitive diagnosis, it may be necessary to record a clinical episode with continuous video and EEG monitoring.

Serum prolactin or creatinine kinase levels may also be helpful in the differential diagnosis of psychogenic seizures and epilepsy. Elevation of serum prolactin level can be seen within 30 minutes after a tonic-clonic or a temporal or frontal complex partial seizure but not after a psychogenic seizure. The test specimen must be compared with a baseline serum prolactin level collected at the same time of day, not within 24 hours of one of the episodes. Marked elevation of serum creatinine kinase level can be seen for 2 to 3 days after a tonic-clonic convulsion but generally not after a psychogenic seizure. However, elevation of creatinine kinase level reflects muscle damage, and a vigorous psychogenic episode with injury is also followed by elevation of creatinine kinase level.

Treatment. Treatment of psychogenic seizures must include an identification of underlying psychosocial and psychiatric problems by psychiatric personnel. Major mood disorders and severe environmental stress, especially sexual abuse, are common among children and adolescents with psychogenic seizures and should be considered in every case.

Presentation of the nonepileptic diagnosis to the patient after monitoring of a typical spell must be positive ("These attacks are not epileptic and will not necessitate chronic medication or further neurologic investigation") and truthful ("We don't know exactly what is causing them, but emotional factors are clearly playing a major role").

The prognosis of psychogenic seizures in the pediatric population is much better than in adults, with 80% of patients seizure-free at 3-year follow-up.

Acute Symptomatic Seizures and Occasional Seizures

The causes of acute symptomatic seizures in adolescence include those described in the preceding neonatal and childhood sections except for febrile convulsions. Head injury may be more common among adolescents, because participation in contact sports and motor vehicle accidents occur in the middle to late teen years. Street drug abuse can be associated with seizures.

Epileptic Syndromes

Juvenile Myoclonic Epilepsy

Juvenile myoclonic epilepsy has an onset between 12 and 18 years of age. The hallmark of the disorder is early-morning myoclonus involving axial and upper limb muscles, usually with sparing of

Table 39-19. Differential Diagnosis of Psychogenic Seizures

Clinical Factors	Psychogenic Seizures	Epileptic Seizures
Age at onset	Usually older than 8-10 years Predominates in girls; 15%-30% of patients are boys	Any gender, no sex predominance
Duration of seizures	May be very prolonged	Usually seconds to minutes
Evolution	May have a very gradual onset and ending	Usually more abrupt onset
Quality of convulsive movements	Thrashing, asynchronous limb movements, often with partial responsiveness	Usually rhythmical and synchronous with loss of consciousness
Stereotypical attacks	Typically variable	Typically stereotyped
Examination during the seizure	May resist examination, combative	Usually unresponsive and amnestic for ictal events
Self-injury	Rare	Common in GTC seizures
Incontinence	Rare	Common in GTC seizures
During sleep	No; may occur nocturnally but while patient is awake	Common
Changes in seizure frequency with medication	Rare	Usual
Interictal EEG	Repeatedly normal	Often abnormal
Ictal EEG	No EEG seizure patterns; normal rhythms while patient is unresponsive	EEG seizure patterns
Pitfalls in diagnosis	1. Psychological factors may not be immediately apparent 2. Misleading information may be given by parents (as in Munchausen syndrome by proxy)	1. Asynchronous vigorous automatisms are found in frontal lobe seizures 2. Bilateral limb movements and posturing without loss of consciousness occurs in supplementary motor seizures 3. EEG seizure patterns may be absent during some seizures (e.g., auras, SMA)

EEG, electroencephalogram; GTC, generalized tonic clonic; SMA, supplementary motor area.

facial muscles. Episodes typically occur on awakening. Tonic-clonic seizures occur in the majority of patients. The history of early-morning myoclonic jerks may not be volunteered and should be asked of all patients presenting with generalized tonic-clonic seizures. The patients may not have identified the myoclonus and instead describe nervousness, shakiness, or clumsiness for the first 1 to 2 hours of a morning. Fatigue, sleep deprivation, stress, and alcohol exacerbate the seizures. The tonic-clonic seizures typically begin with a clustering of repeated myoclonic jerks. Absence seizures occur in 15% to 40% of patients. Neurologic examination findings and IQ are normal. The interictal EEG shows spike-and-wave complexes at 3.5 to 6 Hz. Linkage analysis of patients and their family members has suggested that the disorder is linked to chromosome 21.

Valproate is the preferred AED. Lamotrigine is an effective agent and is often used because of concern about the possible side effects of valproate (weight gain and potential hormonal disturbance). Alternatives may include topiramate and zonisamide, although extensive data concerning their efficacy in this setting are not available. The seizures are well controlled in 80% to 90% of patients, but lifelong treatment is required, because relapse is common even after prolonged seizure-free intervals. It is estimated that more than 90% of patients suffer relapse within the first 6 to 12 months after cessation of AEDs.

Juvenile Absence Epilepsy

In comparison with childhood absence epilepsy, juvenile absence epilepsy has a later onset, at about the time of puberty, and the seizures are less frequent (less than daily). Neurologic examination findings and IQ are normal. The EEG shows generalized spike-and-wave discharges, usually at rates faster than 3 Hz. Tonic-clonic seizures may occur, usually on awakening, more frequently than in childhood absence epilepsy.

The treatment is the same as that for childhood absence epilepsy, but the prognosis for complete remission on therapy is less favorable.

Epilepsy with Generalized Tonic-Clonic Seizures on Awakening

This idiopathic generalized epilepsy involves generalized tonic-clonic seizures occurring more than 90% of the time within 2 hours of awakening or in an early-evening period of relaxation. Sleep deprivation and disruption are often potent precipitants of seizures. The age at onset of the seizures is usually between 10 and 20 years; a family history of epilepsy occurs in approximately 10% to 13% of cases. Myoclonic and absence seizures may also be present, and the distinction between juvenile myoclonic epilepsy and juvenile absence epilepsy is not clear. The EEG may show generalized spike-and-wave complexes or polyspikes.

Treatment starts with valproate, although barbiturates may be very effective. Lamotrigine is also used because of concern about the side effects of valproate. Topiramate and zonisamide may also be helpful. The prognosis for complete control of seizures on therapy is very good: 65% to 79% of patients have experienced remission with therapy. Avoidance of precipitating factors that disrupt sleep patterns is important. The relapse rate if AEDs are stopped is high (83%).

PRINCIPLES OF ANTIEPILEPTIC DRUG USE

The goal of AED therapy is to use a single agent in adequate dosages to completely control seizures. If seizures recur, the dosage of an AED should be gradually increased to achieve the maximum tolerated dose for the patient without causing symptoms of drug toxicity. Therapeutic ranges are derived from population studies in which the serum levels of patients with seizures controlled by an AED were compared with those of patients experiencing side effects. The therapeutic levels should be used as a guide. They should not be interpreted as the "normal" levels; the "therapeutic" level is that which controls the individual's seizures without causing symptoms of toxicity.

If one agent does not control the seizures, another AED should be substituted and tried as monotherapy. An adequate trial of therapy entails the maximum tolerated dose of an AED for a period of time in which several of the patient's seizures (or clusters of seizures) would usually occur or for at least 2 months, whichever is longer. This interval may be shortened in infants and children with very frequent seizures. Changes in AED dosages and regimens should be made gradually, and due regard must be given to time taken to reach steady-state serum concentrations on the new regimen (Tables 39-20 and 39-21).

If the child with epilepsy fails to achieve complete control of seizures on monotherapy with one of the first-line drugs, an alternative first-line drug should be substituted and, if unsuccessful, followed by a trial of monotherapy with one of the more recent AEDs. Drug changes can be made gradually on an outpatient basis; the existing AED can be reduced by 20%, and the new AED commenced at the usual starting dosage (see Table 39-20). Each week, the dosage of the new AED can be increased with a corresponding reduction in the previous AED until the new drug is at the desired maintenance dosage and the previous AED has been discontinued. The physician

Table 39-20. Antiepileptic Medication: Clinical Usage

Antiepileptic	Indication	Introduction of Medication	Maintenance Dosage (mg/kg/day)	Side Effects	Monitoring of Serum Levels
First-Line Drugs					
Carbamazepine	Partial seizures and secondarily GTCS	No loading dose	10-30 as t.i.d. For controlled-release preparations, 20% increase in dosage as b.i.d.	Drowsiness, vertigo, diplopia, hyponatremia (SIADH), dose-dependent neutropenia, rash in 4%-10% Rare: serious blood dyscrasia, hypersensitivity reaction	Yes
Ethosuximide	Absence seizures, symptomatic generalized epilepsy with falls, negative myoclonus	Add 33% of maintenance dosage every 7 days	10-40 as t.i.d., with meals	Nausea, gastrointestinal discomfort, headache Rare: aplastic anemia	No
Lamotrigine	Partial seizures, primary generalized tonic-clonic seizures, absence seizures, myoclonus and as adjunct in Lennox-Gastaut syndrome	0.5 mg/kg/day; increase by 1 mg/kg/day weekly, increase 2nd wk during concomitant use of valproate	5-15 as b.i.d. or t.i.d. as monotherapy; 1-5 q.d. or b.i.d. with concomitant use of valproate	Rash, insomnia, headache, ataxia, drowsiness, diplopia Marked changes in half-life are dependent on co-medication Rare: Stevens-Johnson syndrome	May be useful with polytherapy
Phenytoin	Partial seizures and secondarily GTC seizures	Loading 10-20 mg/kg PO	5-10 as b.i.d.	Ataxia, diplopia, gingival hyperplasia, coarsening of facial features Chronic use: cerebellar atrophy Rare: hypersensitivity reaction	Yes
Valproic acid	Primary GTC seizures, myoclonus and absence seizures, partial seizures	Loading dose only for status epilepticus: 20 mg/kg	15-60 as b.i.d. or t.i.d.	Weight gain, hair loss, tremor at high dosage, ovarian cysts, hyperandrogenemia Rare: hepatotoxicity, pancreatitis, encephalopathy	Yes
Second-Line Drugs					
Clobazam	Partial seizures Adjunct in Lennox-Gastaut syndrome	Begin at night with 33% of maintenance dosage	0.5-1 as b.i.d.	Sedation	No
Phenobarbital	Partial seizures and GTC seizures	6-8 mg/kg PO for 2 days, then maintenance dosage	3-4 as b.i.d.	Drowsiness, behavioral changes, hyperactivity	Yes
Primidone	Partial seizures and secondarily GTC seizures	Begin with phenobarbital, increasing over 3 days, then add primidone	5-20 as b.i.d. or t.i.d.	Acute reaction: nausea, vomiting, vertigo Sedation	Yes
Third-Line Drugs					
Acetazolamide	Absence seizures May use as trial in refractory generalized epilepsy	33% of maintenance dosage for 1 week, then gradual increase over next weeks	10-20 as b.i.d. or t.i.d.	Altered taste, parasthesia, initial drowsiness, cross-reactivity with sulfonamide allergy Rare: renal calculi, precipitation of hepatic coma in liver failure	No

Table 39-20. Antiepileptic Medication: Clinical Usage—cont'd

Antiepileptic	Indication	Introduction of Medication	Maintenance Dosage (mg/kg/day)	Side Effects	Monitoring of Serum Levels
Clonazepam	Infantile spasms, myoclonus, reflex epilepsy; Second-line therapy for absence seizures and partial seizures	0.01-0.03 mg/kg/day for 1 week, then increase by 0.25-0.5 mg/day each week	0.03-0.1 as b.i.d. or t.i.d.	Sedation, drooling; behavioral change: irritable, aggressive, hostile	No
Chlorazepate	Adjunct for partial and secondarily GTC seizures	0.3 mg/kg/day for 1 week, then increase by 0.4-3 mg/day each week	7.5-15 as b.i.d.	Sedation, ataxia, drooling	No

Drugs for Special Circumstances

Diazepam	Prophylactic rectal use for febrile convulsions Status epilepticus	0.5-0.7 q8h when fever >38.5° C (see Table 39-5)		Sedation, ataxia, vertigo IV use: respiratory depression and apnea, hypotension	No
Lorazepam	Status epilepticus	0.03-0.22 mg/kg, IV bolus (see Table 39-5)		IV use: respiratory depression and apnea, hypotension	No
Midazolam	Status epilepticus	Can be given via buccal or intranasal route, also as infusion for status epilepticus: 0.15-0.2 mg/kg IV bolus, 1 μg/kg/min to start, then variable infusion, usually ≤18 μg/kg/min		IV use: sedation, respiratory depression, apnea, hypotension	No

More Recent Drugs

Felbamate	Partial seizures, adjunct for symptomatic generalized epilepsy	Add 25% of maintenance dosage every 4 days	45 as t.i.d.	Headache, insomnia, anorexia, nausea, and vomiting Rare: aplastic anemia, hepatitis	No
Gabapentin	Adjunct for refractory partial seizures	Add 25% of maintenance dosage every 2 days	30-60 as t.i.d. or q.i.d.	Drowsiness, fatigue, ataxia, nonspecific dizziness	No
Levetiracetam	Partial seizures	Add 25% of maintenance dosage every week	20-60 as b.i.d. in adults	Drowsiness, lethargy, headache	No
Nitrazepam	Infantile spasms Myoclonic seizures, reflex epilepsy Adjunct symptomatic generalized epilepsy	Add 25% of maintenance dosage every week	0.25-1 as b.i.d.	Sedation, impaired swallowing, drooling, ataxia	No
Oxcarbazepine	Partial seizures	Add 25% of maintenance dosage every week	20-50 as b.i.d. or t.i.d.	Rash less common and hyponatremia more common than with carbamazepine	Yes
Tiagabine	Partial seizures	0.1 mg/kg/day; increase by 0.1 mg/kg/day every 1-2 weeks	0.4-1.25 as b.i.d. to q.i.d.	Drowsiness, poor concentration, irritability, tremor Gradual introduction lessens cognitive side effects	No
Topiramate	Partial seizures GTC seizures, absences, myoclonus, epileptic spasms. Lennox-Gastaut syndrome	1 mg/kg/day, increase by 1 mg/kg/day every 1-2 weeks	5-10 as b.i.d.	Paresthesia, anorexia, drowsiness, poor concentration, word finding difficulties Gradual introduction lessens cognitive side effects Rare: renal calculi	No
Vigabatrin	Partial seizures Tuberous sclerosis and West or Lennox-Gastaut syndromes	Add 25% of maintenance dosage every week	10-50 as b.i.d. or q.d. Higher doses for infantile spasms, up to 100-150	Drowsiness, fatigue, gastrointestinal upset, weight gain, peripheral visual field defects Depression and psychosis reported in adults	No
Zonisamide	Partial seizures GTC seizures, myoclonus, epileptic spasms	2-4 mg/kg/day; increase by 2 mg/kg/day to maintenance dose	4-18 as q.d. or b.i.d.	Drowsiness, anorexia, nausea, headache, poor concentration, renal stones	Yes

b.i.d., twice a day; GTC, generalized tonic-clonic; IV, intravenous; q.d., every day; q.i.d., four times a day; SIADH, syndrome of inappropriate antidiuretic hormone; t.i.d., three times a day.

Table 39-21. Antiepileptic Medication: Pharmacokinetic Parameters

Antiepileptic	% Protein Bound	Metabolism/Elimination	Half-life (Hours)	Therapeutic Range (mg/L)[1]
First-Line Drugs				
Carbamazepine	75	Hepatic metabolism	5-20[2]	9-12
Ethosuximide	<10	Hepatic metabolism	30-60[3]	40-100
Lamotrigine	55	Hepatic metabolism	12-48[4]	5-20[5]
Phenytoin	90	Hepatic metabolism	10-60	10-20
Valproic acid	70-93	Hepatic metabolism	5-15	50-100
Second-Line Drugs				
Clobazam[6]	>90	Hepatic metabolism	10-30	NA[7]
Phenobarbital	40-50	Hepatic metabolism	35-125	15-40
Primidone	<20	Hepatic metabolism	3-20	6-12
Third-Line Drugs				
Acetazolamide	90-95	Hepatic metabolism	10-15[8]	10-14
Clonazepam	85	Hepatic metabolism	20-30	20-75
Clorazepate[9]	95-98	Hepatic metabolism	55-100	NA[7]
Drugs for Special Circumstances				
Diazepam	95-97	Hepatic metabolism	6-23	0.3-0.7
Lorazepam	90	Hepatic metabolism	8-25	NA[7]
Midazolam	95	50% Renal excretion	2-6	NA[7]
More Recent Drugs				
Felbamate	25-35	Hepatic metabolism	14-20	20-80
Gabapentin	0	Renal excretion	5-9	2.0-3.0
Levetiracetam	0	Renal excretion	6-8	NA[7]
Nitrazepam	85	Hepatic metabolism	20-30	0.1-0.2
Oxcarbazepine[10]	45	Hepatic metabolism	10-15	8-20
Tiagabine	96	Hepatic metabolism	7-9, enzyme inducers 4-7	NA[7]
Topiramate	10-15	60% renal excretion	18-30	NA[7]
Vigabatrin[11]	0	Renal excretion	5-8	NA[7]
Zonisamide	50	Hepatic metabolism	50-70, enzyme inducers 25-40	20-30

[1]To convert to μmol/L: 1000/molecular weight × concentration (mg/L) = μmol/L. Therapeutic levels are guidelines; the dose should control seizures without serious side effects.

[2]Carbamazepine causes autoinduction of hepatic metabolism over first 2-6 weeks of therapy; clearance increases, half-life shortens, and serum level can be expected to drop despite compliance with original dosage.

[3]Ethosuximide half-life is shorter in infants and younger children.

[4]Used as monotherapy, lamotrigine has a half-life of about 24 hr; with phenobarbital, phenytoin, or carbamazepine (hepatic enzyme inducers), the half-life is reduced to 12 hr, and with valproate (hepatic enzyme inhibition), it is increased to 48 hr.

[5]Higher serum levels are tolerated, especially with concomitant administration of valproate.

[6]*N*-desmethylclobazam is the major active metabolite, and its much longer half-life (mean, 42 hr; range, 30-100 hr) must be considered.

[7]There is no established target level for monitoring.

[8]Acetazolamide is bound to carbonic anhydrase; this complex dissociates very slowly, and so the biologic half-life is several days.

[9]Chlorazepate acts as a pro-drug and is converted to *N*-desmethyldiazepam, the active form of clorazepate; the data for protein binding and half-life are for *N*-desmethyldiazepam. There is no established target level for monitoring.

[10]Oxcarbazepine (10,11-dihydro-10-oxycarbamazepine) has a half-life of 1-2.5 hr. It is converted to an active metabolite, 10,11-dihydro-10-hydroxycarbamazepine; the data for protein binding, half-life, and serum levels are for the 10-hydroxy compound.

[11]The biologic half-life is approximately 5 days as a result of the irreversible inhibition of γ-aminobutyric acid transaminase by vigabatrin.

must warn the parents and child that AED toxicity or an increase in the seizure frequency may occur during the change-over period. More rapid medication changes, especially if barbiturates are to be stopped, often require that the patient be admitted to the hospital during the change-over period.

Only about 10% of patients achieve better control with the addition of a second drug to the first, and there is very little evidence that more than two drugs benefit patients. In rare instances, patients with specific syndromes may benefit from the use of multiple AEDs. Carbamazepine and phenytoin have often been given in combination to patients with poorly controlled epilepsy. This combination can be very effective in some patients. However, it is usually very difficult to achieve adequate serum levels of both drugs because of their hepatic enzyme–inducing properties, and any adverse effects may be additive. As a general rule, the combination is best avoided. The process of monotherapy trials should be efficient, with close follow-up of patients experiencing persistent seizures and with careful attention to possible causes of refractory seizures (Table 39-22). Failure to respond to two to three AEDs in monotherapy at maximum tolerated doses should prompt a referral for assessment in a specialty epilepsy program. In some patients, resistance to AED may be genetically determined by mutations affecting drug transport or in metabolizing proteins such as the multidrug resistance–associated family of drug transporters.

It is important to design dosage schedules that are realistic. Dosing more often than three times a day results in a high incidence

Table 39-22. Management of Seizures Refractory to Medical Therapy

Incorrect Diagnosis

Review seizure type

Complex partial seizures may be mistaken for absence seizures

Reflex epilepsy with uncontrolled precipitating factors, photosensitivity, reading epilepsy

Repeat EEG with hyperventilation, photic stimulation, and sleep recording

If results are negative, consider nonepileptic paroxysmal disorders

Psychogenic seizures (see Table 39-19)

Migraine

Porphyria, hypoglycemia, hypocalcemia

Continuing seizures: admit for video/EEG monitoring to record the event

Inappropriate Medication

Review anticonvulsant levels

A second AED may have caused a drop in the serum level of a first-line drug

Review seizure type

Phenobarbital and carbamazepine may exacerbate atypical absence seizures

Drowsiness caused by phenobarbital and benzodiazepine may exacerbate tonic seizures

Phenytoin often worsens the function of patients with progressive myoclonus epilepsy syndromes

Noncompliance with Medication or Medical Advice

Check AED levels; ask patient to record medication doses taken

Check sleep habits, drug use; arrange review by social worker, psychiatrist

Inability to cope with epilepsy and avoidance of precipitating factors (adolescence, low intelligence, dysfunctional home situation)

Review all patient's prescribed and over-the-counter medication; urine drug screen for drug abuse

Exacerbation by other medication or toxins

Intercurrent Illness or Metabolic Complication of Another Medication

Serum Na^+, K^+, glucose, Ca^{2+}, Mg^{2+}, creatinine, liver function studies, complete blood cell count, pregnancy test

Intractable Epilepsies

Up to one third of cases of symptomatic focal epilepsy are refractory to current medical therapy

After adequate attempt with two first-line medications and available new AEDs, refer for epilepsy surgery assessment

Symptomatic generalized epilepsies such as West syndrome and Lennox-Gastaut syndrome are often refractory

Need to reassess goals of therapy

Refer for surgical assessment if there are recurrent falls caused by tonic or atonic seizures in older child

Epilepsy with progressive neurologic deterioration: e.g., brain tumor, inherited disorders of metabolism, degenerative neurological disease, progressive myoclonus epilepsy, phakomatosis, systemic or cerebral vasculitis

Review history, family history, and physical examination; repeat neuroimaging; repeat EEG studies (see Tables 39-10 and 39-16)

AED, antiepileptic drug; CBC, complete blood count; EEG, electroencephalogram.

of poor compliance. Parents must be advised to be careful with other prescribed and over-the-counter medications. Many medications may interfere with the AED metabolism. Table 39-23 outlines indications for monitoring AED serum levels.

CHOICE OF ANTIEPILEPTIC DRUGS

Focal Epilepsies

Partial Seizures and Secondary Generalized Tonic-Clonic Seizures

Among the traditional AEDs, phenytoin, carbamazepine, phenobarbital, and primidone are equally effective in controlling partial and secondary generalized tonic-clonic seizures in adults. In the symptomatic focal epilepsies, only approximately 35% to 50% of patients become seizure free with AED monotherapy; another 20% to 30% experience more than a 75% reduction in seizure frequency. First-line treatment in this group of seizures is usually with carbamazepine or oxcarbazepine. Although the barbiturates and the benzodiazepines have been shown to be effective, the sedative and cognitive side effects prevent them from being drugs of first choice; they are generally reserved for patients in whom first-line drugs are not effective or tolerated. Valproate is also effective against partial seizures in children, although large comparative studies are not available.

Other drugs, including lamotrigine, vigabatrin, gabapentin, topiramate, zonisamide, and levetiracetam (see Table 39-20), have also been shown to be efficacious in treating refractory partial seizures. Their place in the order of management is not yet defined, but some are increasingly being used soon after failure with carbamazepine monotherapy.

Idiopathic Generalized Epilepsy

Primary Generalized Tonic-Clonic Seizures

It is widely thought that valproate should be the first-choice drug for primary generalized tonic-clonic seizures, especially if they occur in association with absence seizures or myoclonic seizures. Lamotrigine, topiramate, and zonisamide have also been shown to be effective for this seizure type. Phenytoin, carbamazepine, and valproate are equally effective in controlling primary generalized tonic-clonic seizures in adults, and between 60% and 70% of patients can become seizure free. Phenytoin does not control any associated absence seizures, and carbamazepine may exacerbate absence seizures. Phenobarbital and primidone are not the drugs of first choice because of potential adverse sedative and cognitive effects.

Absence Seizures

Ethosuximide and valproate are the two drugs of first choice for absence seizures. Monotherapy with valproate controls absence seizures in more than 90% of children with childhood absence epilepsy. Ethosuximide and valproate have been successfully

Table 39-23. Indications for Anticonvulsant Serum Level Monitoring

Introduction and stabilization of a patient on phenytoin

Alteration in seizure pattern or frequency

A change in the dosage of an anticonvulsant

Commencement or withdrawal of other medications that interfere with anticonvulsants

Symptoms of toxicity

To check patient compliance

combined in patients with refractory absence seizures. Clonazepam is also effective but has the disadvantages of sedation and development of tolerance with chronic treatment. Lamotrigine, topiramate, and zonisamide have been effective for absence seizures, but experience is limited.

Myoclonic Seizures

Specific myoclonic syndromes associated with absence seizures and tonic-clonic seizures, such as juvenile myoclonic epilepsy, are usually treated with valproate. Approximately 80% of patients with this epilepsy can become seizure free, although lifelong treatment is required with juvenile myoclonic epilepsy. Clonazepam is also useful in myoclonic syndromes, although sedation occurs, and it does not tend to be useful in the long term because of tolerance; there are even some reports of exacerbation of seizures with long-term high-dose clonazepam. Exacerbation of seizures is particularly frequent with this drug when abrupt withdrawal is attempted. Clonazepam must be withdrawn very gradually, and the daily dose is reduced by only 0.25 mg every 3 weeks. Lamotrigine, topiramate, and zonisamide have a role in the treatment of myoclonus. Lamotrigine is an effective agent for juvenile myoclonic epilepsy and may become an alternative monotherapy option of this syndrome in young women. Valproate is associated with the development of ovarian cysts and weight gain.

Symptomatic Generalized Epilepsies

Tonic, Atonic, and Atypical Absence Seizures

Drugs useful in the treatment of these seizures include valproate and benzodiazepines such as clonazepam and clobazam. Valproate monotherapy should be introduced first, although complete control of seizures is likely to occur in only 10% to 30% of patients. Carbamazepine and phenytoin are often not effective, and carbamazepine may exacerbate absence seizures in the Lennox-Gastaut syndrome. Primidone and phenobarbital often have unacceptable side effects of drowsiness or worsening intellectual handicap at the dosages needed to control seizures; sedation may increase the frequency of tonic seizures.

Because of the refractory nature of these seizures, patients often end up on a combination of drugs, and AED toxicity can be a great problem, exacerbating a patient's tendency to fall. A benzodiazepine, such as clonazepam or clobazam, in combination with valproate is often used. Felbamate has been shown to be a useful drug as adjunctive treatment of tonic and atonic seizures in the Lennox-Gastaut syndrome, but the risk of serious toxicity limits its use. Lamotrigine, topiramate, and zonisamide have efficacy against the spectrum of seizures in the symptomatic generalized epilepsies, and their use is being explored. The combination of valproate and lamotrigine has been shown to be very effective in the control of intractable generalized seizure disorders.

The *ketogenic diet* is a high-fat, low-carbohydrate, low-protein diet designed to induce a state of chronic ketosis and is an effective treatment option in children with intractable generalized seizures. The diet is most often used as second-line treatment of intractable symptomatic/cryptogenic generalized epilepsies, especially those with myoclonus. The efficacy varies among studies, but approximately 50% of children achieve a clinically significant reduction in seizures. The diet requires a tremendous effort on the part of the parents and is successful only with proper education and close support by experienced dietitians. Affected children are at risk for osteopenia, growth retardation, and renal calculi with long-term use of the diet. Although the diet cannot be used in some children with inborn errors of metabolism, it is the treatment of choice for epilepsy caused by pyruvate dehydrogenase deficiency and glucose transporter protein deficiency.

Palliative epilepsy surgery is available for patients with intractable tonic or atonic seizures causing "drop attacks" and falls. Surgical division of the corpus callosum can modify the intensity of these seizures so that the patient does not fall. Hemispherectomy may be indicated in Rasmussen syndrome. Local resection of areas of mesial temporal sclerosis in patients with refractory temporal lobe seizures is a highly successful therapy. Vagal nerve stimulation, through surgical placement of stimulating electrode on the left vagus nerve in the neck, is a technique developed to treat intractable partial seizures resistant to medication. It has also been used effectively in the symptomatic generalized epilepsies.

STOPPING ANTIEPILEPTIC DRUGS

Most children (60% to 75% of patients) remain seizure free when AEDs are withdrawn after a seizure-free interval on medication for more than 2 years. If relapse occurs, it is generally in the first few months after cessation of medication, and 60% to 80% of the relapses occur before 12 months after cessation. Patients with underlying neurologic disorders and deficits and those with multiple seizure types are more likely to suffer relapse. A long duration of epilepsy before remission carries a slightly higher risk of relapse. The EEG is a strong predictor in idiopathic epilepsy; among patients with frequent epileptic discharges that are recorded in generalized epilepsy, the rate of relapse is higher. The EEG is less useful as a predictor of relapse in focal epilepsy. For most children with epilepsy, it is recommended that children who have been seizure free for 2 years undergo a trial of AED withdrawal.

LIFESTYLE

Parents should be encouraged to let their children lead a normal lifestyle, although some activities are inherently more dangerous for people with epilepsy. In general, climbing to significant heights, bathing, and swimming alone are not safe for children with active epilepsy. The clinician must stress the importance of avoiding overprotection of the child. Participation in sports and other school activities should be encouraged within the limits of avoiding dangerous activities such as rock climbing and scuba diving, in which even a brief loss of awareness could result in serious injury or death. If seizures are well controlled, minimal restrictions apply. In children with active seizures characterized by loss of consciousness, the physician has to make judgments on the basis of an individual assessment, considering the nature of the seizures, their frequency, and the degree of supervision during the activity in question. Driving restrictions vary from state to state; however, it is advisable that an adolescent be seizure free for at least 2 years before applying for a driver's permit. In general, heavy-impact contact sports such as football are best avoided by children with active epilepsy but are not contraindicated for children in remission. In adolescents, some advice regarding birth control may be necessary because many adolescents are unaware of the interaction of AEDs and oral contraceptives.

RED FLAGS

Red flags include signs of increased intracranial pressure, focal seizures, signs suggestive of syndromes, developmental delay or regression, trauma, drug exposure, and multiple organ system dysfunction. Status epilepticus is a medical emergency, necessitating prompt treatment and investigations to identify precipitating factors (see Table 39-5).

REFERENCES

General

Berg AT, Shinnar S, Levy SR, et al: How well can epilepsy syndromes be identified at diagnosis? A reassessment 2 years after initial diagnosis. Epilepsia 2000;41:1269-1275.

Brown TR, Holmes GL: Epilepsy. N Engl J Med 2001;344:1145-1151.

Bye AM, Kok DJ, Ferenchild FT, et al: Paroxysmal non-epileptic events in children: A retrospective study over a period of 10 years. J Paediatr Child Health 2000;36:244-248.

Commission on Classification and Terminology of the International League Against Epilepsy: Proposal for revised classification of epilepsies and epileptic syndromes. Epilepsia 1989;30:389-399.

Dreifuss FE, Nordli DR: Classification of epilepsies in childhood. In Pellock J, Dodson WE, Bourgeois BFD (eds): Pediatric Epilepsy: Diagnosis and Therapy, 2nd ed. New York, Demos, 2001, pp 69-80.

Kotagal P, Lüders HO (eds): The Epilepsies: Etiologies and Prevention. San Diego, Calif, Academic Press, 1999.

Kramer U, Nevo Y, Neufeld MY, et al: Epidemiology of epilepsy in childhood: A cohort of 440 consecutive patients. Pediatr Neurol 1998;18:46-50.

Lerche H, Jurkat-Rott K, Lehmann-Horn F: Ion channels and epilepsy. Am J Med Genet 2001;106:146-159.

Wyllie E (ed): The Treatment of Epilepsy: Principles and Practice, 3rd ed. Philadelphia, Lippincott Williams & Wilkins, 2001.

Neonatal Period

Daoust-Roy J, Seshia SS: Benign neonatal sleep myoclonus: A differential diagnosis of neonatal seizures. Am J Dis Child 1992;146:681.

Parker S, Zuckerman B, Bauchner H, et al: Jitteriness in full-term neonates: Prevalence and correlates. Pediatrics 1990;85:17-23.

Shuper A, Zalzberg J, Weitz R, et al: Jitteriness beyond the neonatal period: A benign pattern of movement in infancy. J Child Neurol 1991;6:243-245.

Acute Symptomatic Seizures and Occasional Seizures

Mizrahi EM: Neonatal seizures and neonatal epileptic syndromes. Neurol Clin 2001;19:427-463.

Painter MJ, Scher MS, Stein AD, et al: Phenobarbital compared with phenytoin for the treatment of neonatal seizures. N Engl J Med 1999;341:485-489.

Epileptic Syndromes

Mizrahi EM, Clancy RR: Neonatal seizures: early-onset seizure syndromes and their consequences for development. Ment Retard Dev Disabil Res Rev 2000;6:229-241.

Plouin P: Benign familial neonatal convulsions and benign idiopathic neonatal convulsions. In Engel JP, Pedley TA (eds): Epilepsy: A Comprehensive Textbook. Philadelphia, Lippincott-Raven, 1997, pp 2247-2255.

Watanabe K, Miura K, Natsume J, et al: Epilepsies of neonatal onset: Seizure type and evolution. Dev Med Child Neurol 1999;41:318-322.

Early-Onset Generalized Epileptic Syndromes with Encephalopathy

Dulac O: Epileptic encephalopathy. Epilepsia 2001;42(Suppl 3):23-26.

Lombroso C: Early myoclonic encephalopathy, early infantile epileptic encephalopathy, and benign and severe infantile myoclonic epilepsies: A critical review and personal contributions. J Clin Neurophysiol 1990;7:380-408.

Wang PJ, Lee WT, Hwu WL, et al: The controversy regarding diagnostic criteria for early myoclonic encephalopathy. Brain Dev 1998;20:530-535.

Infancy

Cyanotic and Pallid Infant Syncope

DiMario FJ: Prospective study of children with cyanotic and pallid breath-holding spells. Pediatrics 2001;107:265-269.

Kelly AM, Porter CJ, McGoon MD, et al: Breath-holding spells associated with significant bradycardia: Successful treatment with permanent pacemaker implantation. Pediatrics 2001;108:698-702.

Mocan H, Yildiran A, Orhan F, et al: Breath holding spells in 91 children and response to treatment with iron. Arch Dis Child 1999;81:261-262.

Sleep Disorders

Dyken ME, Lin-Dyken DC, Yamada T: Diagnosing rhythmic movement disorder with video-polysomnography. Pediatr Neurol 1997;16:37-41.

Shivering Attacks

Kanazawa O: Shuddering attacks—Report of four children. Pediatr Neurol 2000;23:421-424.

Paroxysmal Torticollis

Chaves-Carballo E: Paroxysmal torticollis. Semin Pediatr Neurol 1996;3:255-256.

Drigo P, Carli G, Laverda AM: Benign paroxysmal torticollis of infancy. Brain Dev 2000;22:169-172.

Masturbation

Finklestein E, Amichai B, Jaworowski S, et al: Masturbation in prepubescent children: A case report and review of the literature Child Care Health Dev 1996;22:323-326.

Spasmus Nutans

Shaw FS, Kriss A, Russel-Eggitt I, et al: Diagnosing children presenting with asymmetric pendular nystagmus. Dev Med Child Neurol 2001;43:622-627.

Benign Paroxysmal Vertigo

Herraiz C, Calvin FJ, Tapia MC, et al: The migraine: Benign paroxysmal vertigo of childhood complex. Int Tinnitus J 1999;5:50-52.

Russell G, Abu-Arafeh I: Paroxysmal vertigo in children—An epidemiological study. Int J Pediatr Otorhinolaryngol 1999;49(Suppl 1):S105-S107.

Benign Myoclonus of Early Infancy

Maydell BV, Berenson F, Rothner AD, et al: Benign myoclonus of early infancy: An imitator of West's syndrome. J Child Neurol 2001;16:109-112.

Pachatz C, Fusco L, Vigevano F: Benign myoclonus of early infancy. Epileptic Disord 1999;1:57-61.

Alternating Hemiplegia of Childhood

Chaves-Vischer V, Picard F, Andermann E, et al: Benign nocturnal alternating hemiplegia of childhood: Six patients and long-term follow-up. Neurology 2001;57:1491-1493.

Ducros A, Denier C, Joutel A, et al: The clinical spectrum of familial hemiplegic migraine associated with mutations in a neuronal calcium channel. N Engl J Med 2001;345:17-24.

Mikati MA, Kramer U, Zupanc ML, et al: Alternating hemiplegia of childhood: Clinical manifestations and long-term outcome. Pediatr Neurol 2000;23:134-141.

Acute Symptomatic Seizures and Occasional Seizures

Baumann RJ, Duffner PK: Treatment of children with simple febrile seizures: The AAP practice parameter. American Academy of Pediatrics. Pediatr Neurol 2000;23:11-17.

Knudsen FU: Febrile seizures: Treatment and prognosis. Epilepsia 2000;41:2-9.

Shinnar S, Pellock JM, Berg AT, et al: Short-term outcomes of children with febrile status epilepticus. Epilepsia 2001;42:47-53.

Epileptic Syndromes

Dulac O, Plouin P, Schlumberger E: Infantile spasms. In Wyllie E (ed): The Treatment of Epilepsy: Principles and Practice, 3rd ed. Philadelphia, Lippincott Williams & Wilkins, 2001, pp 415-452.

Wong M, Trevathan E: Infantile spasms. Pediatr Neurol 2001;24:89-98.

Severe Myoclonic Epilepsy in Infancy

Scheffer IE, Wallace R, Mulley JC, et al: Clinical and molecular genetics of myoclonic-astatic epilepsy and severe myoclonic epilepsy in infancy (Dravet syndrome). Brain Dev 2001;23:732-735.

Childhood

Paroxysmal Nonepileptic Disorders

Rand DC, Feldman MD: Misdiagnosis of Munchausen syndrome by proxy: A literature review and four new cases. Harv Rev Psychiatry 1999;7: 94-101.

Rosenow F, Wyllie E, Kotagal P, et al: Staring spells in children: Descriptive features distinguishing epileptic and nonepileptic events. J Pediatr 1998;133:660-663.

Wyllie E, Glazer J, Benbadis S, et al: Psychiatric features of children and adolescents with pseudoseizures. Arch Pediatr Adolesc Med 1999; 153:244-248.

Tic Disorders

Jankovic J: Tourette's syndrome. N Engl J Med 2001;345:1184-1192.

Marcus D, Kurlan R: Tics and its disorders. Neurol Clin 2001;19:735-758.

Sleep Disorders

Guilleminault C, Pelayo R: Narcolepsy in children: A practical guide to its diagnosis, treatment and follow-up. Paediatr Drugs 2000;2:1-9.

Laberge L, Tremblay RE, Vitaro F, et al: Development of parasomnias from childhood to early adolescence. Pediatrics 2000;106:67-74.

Ohayon MM, Guilleminault C, Priest RG: Night terrors, sleepwalking, and confusional arousals in the general population: Their frequency and relationship to other sleep and mental disorders. J Clin Psychiatry 1999;60:268-276.

Stores G: Children's sleep disorders: Modern approaches, developmental effects, and children at special risk. Dev Med Child Neurol 1999;41: 568-573.

Hyperekplexia

Vergouwe MN, Tijssen MA, Peters AC, et al: Hyperekplexia phenotype due to compound heterozygosity for GLRA1 gene mutations. Ann Neurol 1999;46:634-638.

Self-Stimulatory Behavior

Tan A, Salgado M, Fahn S: The characterization and outcome of stereotypic movements in non-autistic children. Mov Disord 1997;12:47-52.

Epileptic Syndromes

Andermann F, Zifkin B: The benign occipital epilepsies of childhood: An overview of the idiopathic syndromes and of the relationship to migraine. Epilepsia 1998;39(Suppl 4):S9-S23.

Baglietto MG, Battaglia FM, Nobili L, et al: Neuropsychological disorders related to interictal epileptic discharges during sleep in benign epilepsy of childhood with centrotemporal or rolandic spikes. Dev Med Child Neurol 2001;43:407-412.

Holmes GL: Clinical spectrum of benign focal epilepsies of childhood. Epilepsia 2000;41:1051-1052.

Koutroumanidis M: Panayiotopoulos syndrome. BMJ 2002;324:1228-1229.

Robinson R, Gardiner M: Genetics of childhood epilepsy. Arch Dis Child. 2000;82:121-125.

Symptomatic Focal (Localization-Related) Epilepsy

Berg AT, Shinnar S, Levy SR, et al: Early development of intractable epilepsy in children: A prospective study. Neurology 2001;56:1445-1452.

Canafoglia L, Franceschetti S, Antozzi C, et al: Epileptic phenotypes associated with mitochondrial disorders. Neurology 2001;56:1340-1346.

Shields WD: Catastrophic epilepsy in childhood. Epilepsia 2000;41 (Suppl 2):S2-S6.

Childhood Absence Epilepsy

Panayiotopoulos CP: Absence epilepsies. In Engel JP, Pedley TA (eds): Epilepsy: A Comprehensive Textbook. Philadelphia, Lippincott-Raven, 1997, pp 2327-2346.

Wirrell E, Camfield C, Camfield P, et al: Prognostic significance of failure of the initial antiepileptic drug in children with absence epilepsy. Epilepsia 2001;42:760-763.

Epilepsia Partialis Continua and Rasmussen Encephalitis

Hart Y, Andermann F: Rasmussen's syndrome. In Lüders HO, Comair YG (eds): Epilepsy Surgery, 2nd ed. Philadelphia, Lippincott Williams & Wilkins, 2001, pp 145-156.

Lennox-Gastaut Syndrome

Farrell K: Symptomatic generalized epilepsy and the Lennox-Gastaut syndrome. In Wyllie E (ed): The Treatment of Epilepsy: Principles and Practice, 3rd ed. Philadelphia, Lippincott Williams & Wilkins, 2001, pp 525-536.

Myoclonic Astatic Epilepsy

Oguni H, Fukuyama Y, Tanaka T, et al: Myoclonic-astatic epilepsy of early childhood—Clinical and EEG analysis of myoclonic-astatic seizures, and discussions on the nosology of the syndrome. Brain Dev 2001;23: 757-764.

Singh R, Andermann E, Whitehouse WP, et al: Severe myoclonic epilepsy of infancy: Extended spectrum of GEFS+? Epilepsia 2001;42:837-844.

Adolescence

Andriola MR, Ettinger AB: Pseudoseizures and other nonepileptic paroxysmal disorders in children and adolescents. Neurology 1999; 53(5, Suppl 2):S89-S95.

Epileptic Syndromes

Genton P, Gelisse P: Juvenile myoclonic epilepsy. Arch Neurol 2001; 58:1487-1490.

Janz D: The idiopathic generalized epilepsies of adolescence with childhood and juvenile age of onset. Epilepsia 1997;38:4-11.

Scheffer IE: Autosomal dominant nocturnal frontal lobe epilepsy. Epilepsia 2000;41:1059-1060.

Diagnostic Evaluation of a Seizure Disorder

Duchowny M: Recent advances in candidate selection for pediatric epilepsy surgery. Semin Pediatr Neurol 2000;7:178-186.

Kuzniecky RI, Barkovich AJ: Malformations of cortical development and epilepsy. Brain Dev 2001;23:2-11.

Liamsuwan S, Grattan-Smith P, Fagan E, et al: The value of partial sleep deprivation as a routine measure in pediatric electroencephalography. J Child Neurol 2000;15:26-29.

Raybaud C, Guye M, Mancini J, Girard N: Neuroimaging of epilepsy in children. Magn Reson Imaging Clin North Am 2001;9:121-147.

Strain JD, Kushner DC, Babcock DS, et al: Imaging of the pediatric patient with seizures. American College of Radiology. ACR Appropriateness Criteria. Radiology 2000;215(Suppl):787-800.

Antiepileptic Drugs

Bourgeois BFD: New antiepileptic drugs in children: Which ones for which seizures. Clin Neurpharmacol 2000; 23:119-132.

Diaz-Arrastia R, Agostini MA, Van Ness PC:. Evolving treatment strategies for epilepsy. JAMA 2002;287:2917-2920.

Gericke CA, Picard F, de Saint-Martin A, et al: Efficacy of lamotrigine in idiopathic generalized epilepsy syndromes: A video–EEG-controlled, open study. Epileptic Disord 1999;1:159-165.

Panayiotopoulos CP: Treatment of typical absence seizures and related epileptic syndromes. Paediatr Drugs 2001;3:379-403.

Pedley TA, Hirano M: Is refractory epilepsy due to genetically determined resistance to antiepileptic drugs? N Engl J Med 2003;15:1480-1482.

Wallace SJ: Myoclonus and epilepsy in childhood: A review of treatment with valproate, ethosuximide, lamotrigine and zonisamide. Epilepsy Res 1998;29:147-154.

Wallace SJ: Newer antiepileptic drugs: Advantages and disadvantages. Brain Dev 2001;23:277-283.

40 Delirium and Coma

Larry A. Greenbaum*

Coma, delirium, or any alteration of consciousness is considered serious brain dysfunction and necessitates a rapid, methodical approach to evaluation and treatment. The causes of coma are numerous, diverse, and, in many cases, life-threatening.

DEFINITIONS

Consciousness is the state of awareness of self and environment. Coma is lack of any awareness of self or environment, even in the presence of painful or other external stimulation. Many terms have been used to describe the levels of consciousness between full awareness and coma. Table 40-1 presents a practical approach to defining levels of impaired consciousness. *Delirium* is an abnormal mental state characterized by irritability, agitation, lack of contact with the environment, and confusion. Periods of lucidity may alternate with the delirious state, and the patient is often very frightened by this change in mental status. Patients may proceed rapidly from delirium or lethargy to coma. Any alteration in the level of consciousness, be it defined as delirium, lethargy, obtundation, stupor, or coma, must be managed as a life-threatening emergency until proven otherwise.

Terms such as *lethargy, obtundation, stupor,* and *coma* are qualitative descriptions that do not precisely define an individual's level of consciousness. Many rating scales have been developed to objectively evaluate the level of awareness in a patient; this allows different observers to follow the progression of the patient's mental status over time. The scales can be used to direct the level of intervention necessary to treat the patient and may provide prognostic information. The most widely used grading system is the Glasgow Coma Scale (Table 40-2).

The Glasgow Coma Scale is a 15-point scale that evaluates three areas of central nervous system (CNS) function. A score of 15 indicates full function, whereas a score of 3 indicates no function. The first area of assessment is *eye opening,* in which the arousability and alertness of the patient are evaluated. Spontaneous eye opening indicates intact arousal mechanisms but does not imply awareness. Eye opening in response to speech may be a response to any verbal stimulation; it does not imply a response to a command to open the eyes. Eye opening in response to pain is tested by application of a painful stimulus to the extremities, not to the face. Facial pain may elicit a grimace, preventing opening of the eyes. Patients with facial injuries and periorbital edema may not be capable of opening their eyes, which prevents evaluation with this part of the scale.

Verbal responses require a high degree of integration within the CNS. Oriented responses indicate awareness of person, place, and time. Patients should know why they are in the hospital, as well as the day, month, and year. Confused speech implies that the patient can respond to questions and engage in conversation but that the

responses are disoriented or inappropriate. Inappropriate words imply that the patient can make intelligible utterances but that speech is used only in an exclamatory or random way, often through shouting and swearing. Nonspecific sounds are moans, groans, and other utterances containing no recognizable words. Lack of verbal response may be caused by conditions other than a depressed level of consciousness. Tracheal intubation, aphasia, and language barriers are examples of situations or conditions that may prevent evaluation

---

Table 40-1. States of Altered Consciousness or Unresponsiveness

Coma: A state of unarousable unresponsiveness; even strong exteroceptive stimuli fail to elicit recognizable psychological responses; unresponsive to pain

Stupor: Spontaneous unarousability interruptible only by vigorous, direct external stimulation; responsive only to pain

Hypersomnia, pathologic drowsiness, obtundation: Terms applied to an increase above the patient's normal sleep/wake ratio, often accompanied during wakefulness by reduced attention and interest in the environment; responsive to pain and other stimuli

Delirium: An acute or subacute reduction in awareness, attention, orientation, and perception ("clouding of consciousness"), usually fluctuating and accompanied by abnormal sleep/wake patterns and often psychomotor disturbances

Syncope: Brief loss of consciousness caused by global failure of cerebrovascular perfusion

Dementia: A sustained or permanent multidimensional or global decline in cognitive functions

Vegetative state: A sustained, complete loss of cognition, with sleep/wake cycles and other autonomic functions remaining relatively intact; can either follow acute, severe bilateral cerebral damage or develop gradually as the end stage of a progressive dementia

Locked-in state: Preservation of intellectual activity accompanied by severe or total incapacity to express voluntary responses as a result of damage to or dysfunction of descending motor pathways in the brain or peripheral motor nerves; most, but not all, such patients can use vertical eye movements to signal by code

Adapted from Plum F: Neurology/disturbances of consciousness and arousal. In Wyngaarden JB, Smith LH, Bennett JC (eds): Cecil Textbook of Medicine, 19th ed. Philadelphia, WB Saunders, 1992, p 2049.

---

*This chapter is an updated and edited version of the chapter by James B. Besunder and John F. Pope that appeared in the first edition.

Table 40-2. Glasgow Coma Scale

Activity	Best Response	Score
Eye opening	Spontaneous	4
	To speech	3
	To pain	2
	None	1
Verbal	Oriented	5
	Confused	4
	Inappropriate words	3
	Nonspecific sounds	2
	None	1
Motor	Follows commands	6
	Localizes pain	5
	Withdraws in response to pain	4
	Flexion in response to pain	3
	Extension in response to pain	2
	None	1
Total score		3-15

Adapted from Teasdale G, Jennet B: Assessment of coma and impaired consciousness. Lancet 1974;2:81.

of the verbal area of the Glasgow Coma Scale. In the intubated patient, this area of the scale is often assigned the letter "T," indicating tracheal intubation and the inability to rate verbal responses.

Motor functioning reflects mentation as well as the integrity of the major CNS pathways. A score of 6 is given if the patient follows commands. If the patient does not follow commands, a painful stimulus is applied via pressure to the nail bed of a finger. The response to this stimulus may be flexion, withdrawal, extension, or no response. If the response is withdrawal, another painful stimulus must be applied to the trunk, head, or neck to determine whether there is localization. A localizing response indicates that stimuli at more than one area cause the patient to purposefully move the extremity to remove the irritant. Withdrawal of the upper extremity consists of abduction of the shoulder and flexion of the elbow. Withdrawal is typically a rapid movement. The flexion response, or _decorticate posturing,_ is a slow adduction of the shoulder, flexion of the arm, wrist, and fingers along with extension, internal rotation, and vigorous plantar flexion of the lower extremity. The extensor response, or _decerebrate posturing,_ involves the adduction and internal rotation of the shoulder and pronation of the forearm.

For purposes of gauging global brain function, the best motor response from any limb is taken as the score. Variation in response from one side of the body to the other is indicative of an asymmetrical brain lesion. If the patient has a right hemiparesis, there may be a withdrawal response of the left arm and no response to painful stimulation of the right arm. With an asymmetrical brainstem injury, the patient may demonstrate decorticate posturing on one side and decerebrate posturing on the opposite side. In these instances, it is important to describe the patient's response in addition to assigning a score. Spinal cord lesions resulting in paralysis or significant orthopedic injuries to the extremities prevent evaluation of the motor portion of the Glasgow Coma Scale.

The Glasgow Coma Scale is not intended to take the place of a complete neurologic evaluation (Table 40-3); the score is like a vital sign in a patient with mental status changes. The scale is an objective measure of improvement or worsening of the patient's level of consciousness over time. Interventions are often based on the score.

Most patients with traumatic brain injury should undergo endotracheal intubation if their score is 8 or less. Deterioration of a patient's score by 2 or more points indicates a need for quick reevaluation of the patient and the possible need for interventions such as endotracheal intubation and diagnostic studies such as a brain computed tomography (CT) scan. The score has been used to assign a prognosis to patients with brain injury, particularly with traumatic brain injury; about 36% of children who suffer a traumatic brain injury and have scores of 3 to 5 die, in comparison with 1.7% of patients with scores of 6 or higher. It may take days to weeks for patients with initial scores of 3 to 5 to become conscious, as opposed to a few days in patients with scores of 6 or higher.

The Glasgow Coma Scale score has also been used as a prognostic indicator in nontraumatic coma. Children presenting after near-drowning with an initial score of 6 or higher have a good outcome. Patients presenting with a score of 5 or less have a high probability of mortality or profound neurologic sequelae, although a patient with a score of 4 or 5 may survive with minimal impairment. A score of 3 on transfer to an intensive care unit after near-drowning has been associated with a nearly 100% rate of poor outcome.

The Glasgow Coma Scale was designed and validated in adult patients, and the normal verbal and motor responses in this scale are not achievable during the first few years of life. Many groups have developed modified coma scales for children. The modifications are based on a child's age-appropriate developmental abilities. The Pediatric Glasgow Coma Scale appears to be a reliable scale for use in children 5 years of age or younger (Table 40-4).

Other scales have been developed to measure the level of consciousness in specific disease states, such as poisonings, Reye syndrome, and hepatic failure. The Reed classification of coma has been used in the setting of poisoning or intoxication (Table 40-5) and is used to evaluate increasing depths of coma encountered with CNS-depressant drugs. The cardiovascular system is included in this classification because toxic ingestions may depress myocardial contractility or cause vasodilation.

A staging system used in Reye syndrome is presented in Table 40-6. The Reye syndrome scale is similar to the Glasgow Coma Scale but has the additional feature of evaluation of brainstem function by observation of pupillary and oculocephalic reflexes. The Glasgow Coma Scale and Reye syndrome staging scale are based on the central syndrome of rostral-caudal deterioration. The _central syndrome_ describes the constellation of clinical findings in patients as brainstem function becomes impaired at progressively lower levels by compression from above (Fig. 40-1). Neurologic function in a patient with hepatic encephalopathy is graded according to the scoring system in Table 40-7. This scale focuses more on cortical functioning and less on evolution of the central syndrome. Patients with grade IV hepatic encephalopathy have cerebral edema from liver failure and may show signs of the central syndrome. The cerebral edema in Reye syndrome is a direct effect of the disease process, distinct from hepatic failure. This distinction explains the differences in the Reye and hepatic encephalopathy scales.

DIFFERENTIAL DIAGNOSIS

The differential diagnosis of delirium and coma in the child is extensive. The causes of coma in children without head injuries commonly include intracranial infections (meningitis, encephalitis), ischemia, epilepsy, metabolic encephalopathies, child abuse, poisoning, and cerebral vascular accidents. Approximately 25% of children from a large series of comatose patients have traumatic brain injuries. Table 40-8 presents causes of mental status changes in children. As can be seen, some diagnoses (subdural hematoma, hydrocephalus, cerebral edema) apply to more than one category. The age of the patient can help the clinician differentiate the

Table 40-3. The Neurologic Examination in Coma

1. Guarantee vital functions.
2. Feel the scalp for hematomas (overlying fracture lines); be sure the neck is not fractured; test *gently* for stiff neck.
3. Test language. Test arousability by words, loud sounds, noxious stimuli. If vocalizations occur, check quickly for appropriate phrases, actual words, and presence or absence of aphasia.
4. Perform a neuroophthalmologic examination.
   Funduscopy (if difficult, can be deferred until patient is stabilized).
      Papilledema (increased intracranial or venous sinus pressure)
      Hemorrhages (subarachnoid hemorrhage; hypertensive encephalopathy; hypoxic-hypercarbic encephalopathy)
   Pupils
      Light reaction: Use bright flashlight and, if necessary, a magnifying glass to be certain of findings. Absence means potentially fatally deep sedative poisoning or acute or chronic structural brainstem damage.
      Equality: 15% of normal patients have mild anisocoria, but new or >2 mm dilation means parasympathetic (third nerve) palsy.
      Extraocular movements: Absence acutely means deep drug poisoning, severe brainstem damage, polyneuropathy, or botulism.
      Dysconjugate deviation: At rest, this means an acute third, fourth, or sixth nerve palsy or internuclear ophthalmoplegia. Tonic conjugate deviation toward a paralytic arm and leg means forebrain seizures or a contralateral pontine destructive lesion; such deviation away from the paralytic arm and leg means forebrain gaze paralysis.
      Spontaneous eye movements: In comatose patients, nystagmus, bobbing, and independently moving eyes all mean brainstem damage.
      Oculocephalic (away from direction of head turning) or oculovestibular (toward cold caloric irrigation) responses: Absence of responses means drug overdose or severe brainstem disease; dysconjugate responses with equal pupils mean internuclear ophthalmoplegia; responses with unequal pupils mean third nerve disease.
5. Examine the motor systems.
   Strength
      Unilateral weakness or motionlessness of arm and leg means contralateral supraspinal upper motor neuron lesion, most often cerebral; if of arm, leg, and face, contralateral cerebral lesion. Occasionally. arm and leg weakness reflects contralateral brainstem lesion.
      Weakness or motionlessness of all four extremities implies metabolic disease; less likely is brainstem disease (tone and reflexes increased) or peripheral disease (tone and reflexes decreased).
   Attempt to elicit reflex posturing
      Arm flexed, leg extended: contralateral deep cerebral-thalamic lesion
      Arm and leg extended: thalamic or mesencephalic lesion
      Arms extended and legs flexed or flaccid: pontine lesion
      Legs flexed, arms flaccid: pontomedullary or spinal lesion
   Compare side-to-side reflexes and examine plantar responses.
6. Seek seizure activity or abnormal movements: (1) generalized, (2) focal, (3) multifocal, and (4) myoclonic.
   Control 1 immediately, 2 and 3 deliberately; if 4 is present, treat underlying disease.
   Acute tremor, asterixis, multifocal myoclonus: seek metabolic cause.
7. Inspect breathing.
   Regular hyperpnea: metabolic acidosis; pulmonary infarction; congestive failure or alveolar infiltration; sepsis; salicylism; hepatic coma
   Cyclically irregular (Cheyne-Stokes): low cardiac output plus bilateral cerebral or upper brainstem dysfunction
   Irregularly irregular gasping, slow or weak: lower. brainstem dysfunction (including hypoglycemia, drug effects); less often, peripheral ventilatory paralysis
8. Proceed with laboratory tests and emergency management as described in text.

Adapted from Plum F: Neurology/sustained impairments of consciousness. In Wyngaarden JB, Smith LH, Bennett JC (eds): Cecil Textbook of Medicine, 19th ed. Philadelphia, WB Saunders, 1992, p 2057.

likely causes of coma, although there is considerable overlap (Table 40-9).

MANAGEMENT APPROACH

The approach to the child with an alteration of consciousness can be divided into four parts: (1) stabilization, (2) rapid neurologic assessment, (3) reversal of immediately treatable toxic or metabolic causes, and (4) determination of level of CNS function and of the cause of the coma (Fig. 40-2).

STABILIZATION

ABCs

The initial step is a rapid but meticulous evaluation of the patient's *a*irway, *b*reathing, and *c*irculation (ABCs), including determination of vital signs. Obtunded, stuporous, or comatose patients usually require intubation unless their mental status is improving or can be readily reversed. Intubation may be necessary not only to secure an airway but also to treat hypoventilation, to protect the airway if a gag reflex is not present, and to facilitate hyperventilation therapy in a child with suspected intracranial hypertension. Manipulation of the neck, particularly extension, should be *avoided* when an airway is being stabilized or secured, unless a cervical spine injury can be ruled out.

Attention is next directed toward an assessment of the circulation; this mandates evaluation of vital signs, presence and volume of peripheral pulses, and adequacy of end-organ perfusion. Blood pressure must be high enough to support perfusion of vital organs. Patients may be in shock with a normal blood pressure and may manifest tachycardia and, often, tachypnea. In early shock, except for septic shock, peripheral pulses are diminished in comparison with central pulses. As shock progresses and stroke volume decreases, the pulse pressure narrows, and the peripheral pulses become weak or "thready" and finally nonpalpable. Early septic

Table 40-4. Pediatric Glasgow Coma Scale

Activity	Best Response	Score
Eye opening	Spontaneously	4
	To speech	3
	To pain	2
	None	1
Verbal	Oriented	5
	Words	4
	Vocal sounds	3
	Cries	2
	None	1
Motor	Obeys commands	5
	Localizes pain	4
	Flexion to pain	3
	Extension to pain	2
	None	1

Normal Total Score Based on Age

Birth-6 months	9
7-12 months	11
1-2 years	12
2-5 years	13
>5 years	14

Adapted from Simpson D, Reilly P: Pediatric coma scale. Lancet 1982;2:450.

Table 40-5. Reed Classification of Coma

Grade 0*	Asleep
	Can be aroused
	Will answer questions
Grade 1*	Comatose
	Withdraws from painful stimuli
	Intact reflexes
Grade 2*	Comatose
	Does not withdraw from painful stimuli
	No respiratory, circulatory depression
	Intact reflexes
Grade 3†	Comatose
	Reflexes absent
	No respiratory, circulatory depression
Grade 4†	Comatose
	Reflexes absent
	Respiratory or circulatory problems

Adapted from Ellenhorn MJ, Barceloux DE: Medical Toxicology, Diagnosis and Treatment of Human Poisoning. New York, Elsevier Science, 1988, p 17.

*Good prognosis.

†Very serious, may need measures to enhance elimination.

Table 40-6. Staging of Reye Syndrome

Stage I	Lethargy, follows verbal commands, normal posture, purposeful response to pain, brisk pupillary light reflex, and normal oculocephalic reflex
Stage II	Combative or stuporous, inappropriate verbalizing, normal posture, purposeful or nonpurposeful response to pain, sluggish pupillary reaction, conjugate deviation on doll's eye maneuver
Stage III	Comatose, decorticate posture, decorticate response to pain, sluggish pupillary reaction, conjugate deviation on doll's eye maneuver
Stage IV	Comatose, decerebrate posture and decerebrate response to pain, sluggish pupillary reflexes, and inconsistent or absent oculocephalic reflex
Stage V	Comatose, flaccid, no response to pain, no pupillary response, no oculocephalic reflex

From Tasker RC, Dean JM, Rogers MC: Reye syndrome and metabolic encephalopathies. In Rogers MC (ed): Rogers Textbook of Pediatric Intensive Care, 2nd ed. Baltimore, Williams & Wilkins, 1992, p 792.

typically lethargic or confused. Lethargy alternating with combativeness is often seen. Infants older than 1 to 2 months of age should normally focus on their parents' faces. Failure to recognize parents is a sign of poor perfusion. Infants may also be irritable and have a weak cry. As shock progresses, changes in level of consciousness become more profound. The child may progress from responding to voice to responding to pain only and may subsequently become unresponsive.

History

During stabilization, a history of the patient must be obtained by another physician or nurse if available. Pertinent questions should focus on the recent history preceding the change in mental status, the medical history, and a family history, particularly of seizures or encephalopathy. Did the child sustain any traumatic injuries in the previous few days? Has the child been febrile, or are there other signs or symptoms of infection or systemic disease? A dietary history in infants presenting with a depressed level of consciousness is paramount and may raise suspicion of hypoglycemia (fasting or emesis) or hyponatremia (ingestion of free water). Exposure to drugs or toxins should be suspected in any patient with a sudden onset of unexplained symptoms (coma, seizures) or a gradual onset of symptoms preceded by a period of confusion or delirium. The caregivers should be asked directly about possible access to medications, illicit drugs, and environmental toxins.

RAPID NEUROLOGIC ASSESSMENT

After stabilization, the next phase in management is a rapid neurologic assessment (see Table 40-3), which should take no more than a few minutes. The primary goal is to determine whether there is a potentially rapidly progressive intracranial process that may be life-threatening, such as an expanding mass lesion (subdural or epidural hematoma), and whether patients are rapidly deteriorating. A secondary objective is to provide prognostic and triage information to other personnel who may be involved with the child in the future. This information permits comparisons of sequential examinations and is important in the patient who receives medications

shock or "warm" shock is often characterized by a widened pulse pressure and bounding pulses.

End-organ perfusion is best evaluated in the skin, kidneys, and brain. The skin should be checked for temperature, color, and capillary refill. Cool extremities, pallor, mottling, peripheral cyanosis, and capillary refill of more than 2 seconds indicate poor perfusion. As perfusion worsens, the coolness of the extremities extends proximally. Urine output may not be helpful in the initial evaluation of a patient, but it becomes an important marker to monitor during therapy. As renal perfusion improves, urine flow rate increases. The patient's alteration in consciousness may be a consequence of shock. In early stages of shock, the patient is

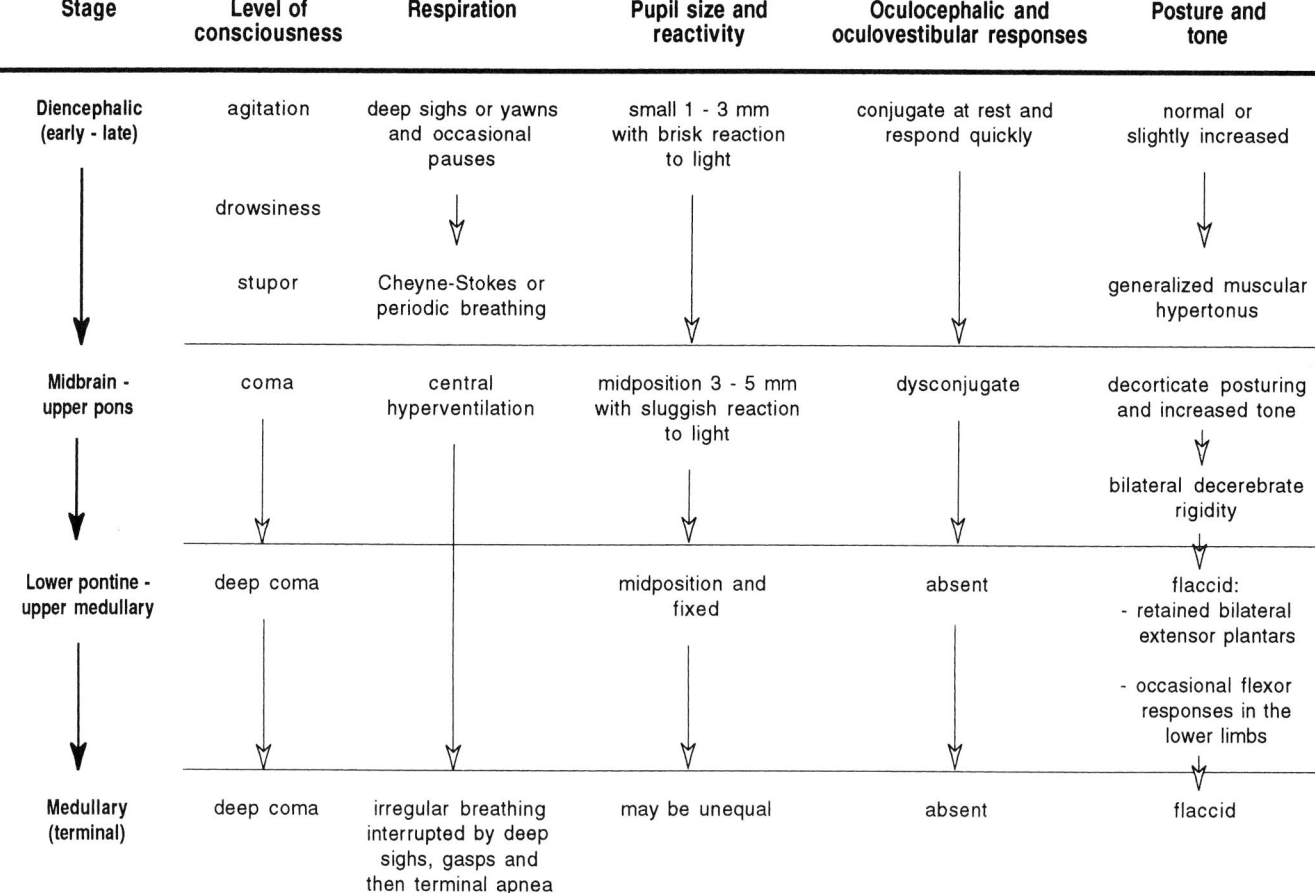

Stage	Level of consciousness	Respiration	Pupil size and reactivity	Oculocephalic and oculovestibular responses	Posture and tone
Diencephalic (early - late)	agitation	deep sighs or yawns and occasional pauses	small 1 - 3 mm with brisk reaction to light	conjugate at rest and respond quickly	normal or slightly increased
	drowsiness				
	stupor	Cheyne-Stokes or periodic breathing			generalized muscular hypertonus
Midbrain - upper pons	coma	central hyperventilation	midposition 3 - 5 mm with sluggish reaction to light	dysconjugate	decorticate posturing and increased tone
					bilateral decerebrate rigidity
Lower pontine - upper medullary	deep coma		midposition and fixed	absent	flaccid: - retained bilateral extensor plantars - occasional flexor responses in the lower limbs
Medullary (terminal)	deep coma	irregular breathing interrupted by deep sighs, gasps and then terminal apnea	may be unequal	absent	flaccid

Figure 40-1. Rostral-caudal deterioration in coma. (From Tasker RC, Dean JM, Rosen MC: Reye syndrome and metabolic encephalopathies. In Rogers MC [ed]: Textbook of Pediatric Intensive Care, 2nd ed. Baltimore, Williams & Wilkins, 1992, p 778.)

(neuromuscular blockers, CNS depressants) in the emergency department that may obscure subsequent neurologic findings. The rapid assessment includes an evaluation for traumatic injuries, focal neurologic findings, brainstem dysfunction, and clinically significant intracranial hypertension.

Traumatic Injuries

Traumatic injuries can result in life-threatening illnesses at any age, including newborns. The head and neck should be carefully inspected and the skull palpated for evidence of trauma (Table 40-10).

Table 40-7. Classification of Hepatic Encephalopathy

Grade 0	Normal
Grade I	Altered spatial orientation, sleep patterns, and affect
Grade II	Drowsy but arousable, slurred speech, confusion, and asterixis
Grade III	Stuporous but responsive to painful stimuli
Grade IV	Unresponsive, with decorticate or decerebrate posturing possible

From Rogers EL, Perman JA: Gastrointestinal and hepatic failure. In Rogers MC (ed): Textbook of Pediatric Intensive Care, 2nd ed. Baltimore, Williams & Wilkins, 1992, p 1151.

In infants, a bulging fontanelle represents raised intracranial pressure, which may have various causes. In the absence of a febrile illness, trauma, including that caused by shaken-baby syndrome (child abuse), should be suspected in any infant with a bulging fontanelle. Retinal hemorrhages are often present on funduscopic examination in children with the shaken-baby syndrome (see Chapter 36).

Focal Neurologic Findings

The presence of focal findings is determined by examination of a child's pupils for asymmetry in size or reactivity and examination of the motor system for asymmetrical movement of the extremities or face. The motor response is part of the Glasgow Coma Scale.

Brainstem Dysfunction

Brainstem function is evaluated by observing the child's respiratory pattern, assessing corneal reflexes, and testing oculocephalic (doll's eye) or oculovestibular (cold caloric) reflexes. The oculocephalic reflex should *not* be checked unless a cervical spine injury has been ruled out. Significant brainstem dysfunction is rarely associated with a normal breathing pattern (Fig. 40-3). Cheyne-Stokes respiration is a pattern of breathing in which periods of hyperpnea alternate with shorter apneic phases, observed in the presence of bilateral hemispheric or diencephalic dysfunction. It may also precede transtentorial herniation. The hyperpneic periods have a characteristic smooth, crescendo-decrescendo pattern.

Table 40-8. Etiologic Classification of Altered Mental Status in Children

Infectious	Metabolic/Systemic	Toxic*	Traumatic*	Anatomic	Hypoxic-Ischemic	Epileptic	Vascular	Psychological
Viral Aseptic meningitis* Encephalitis* ? Reye syndrome ? Hemorrhagic shock and encephalopathy syndrome Postinfectious encephalomyelitis Systemic infection with shock Bacterial Meningitis* Brain abscess Epidural empyema Subdural empyema Systemic infection with shock Toxic shock syndrome Fungal Fungal meningitis Fungal brain abscess Protozoan Meningitis Abscess Postimmunization encephalopathy	Hypoglycemia* Inborn errors of metabolism* Hyperammonemia Hepatic failure Renal diseases Uremic encephalopathy Hypertensive encephalopathy Dialysis encephalopathy (dysequilibrium syndrome) Hyperosmolar states Hypernatremia Hyperglycemia–diabetes mellitus* Hypoosmolar states Hyponatremia* Rapid decrease in osmolality in hyperosmolar states Endocrine disorders Adrenal insufficiency Hyperthyroidism and hypothyroidism Hyperparathyroidism and hypoparathyroidism Mineral abnormalities Hypercalcemia Hypocalcemia Hypermagnesemia Hypomagnesemia Hypophosphatemia Hypercapnia Hypoxia* Shock* Vitamin deficiency and dependency states Nicotinic acid Pantothenic acid Pyridoxine Thiamine Vitamin B_{12} Intussusception encephalopathy Methemoglobinemia Acidosis Alkalosis Porphyria Reye syndrome ? Hemorrhagic shock and encephalopathy syndrome Mitochondrial encephalopathies	Sympathomimetics Anticholinergics Phenothiazines PCP LSD Marijuana Cocaine Heavy metals (lead) Salicylates Organophosphates and carbamates Antihistamines Industrial solvents (inhaled) Alcohols Narcotics Sedative-hypnotics Barbiturates Carbon monoxide Tricyclic antidepressants Carbamazepine Cyanide Methaqualone	Concussion* Cerebral contusion Epidural hematoma Subdural hematoma Brainstem Epidural contusion Diffuse axonal shear injury Cerebral edema* Intraparenchymal hemorrhage Intraventricular hemorrhage (neonate)* Obstructive hydrocephalus Posttraumatic seizure Fat embolism	Tumor Hydrocephalus Hydrocephalus with shunt malfunction Subdural hematoma Epidural hematoma Brain abscess Subdural empyema Epidural empyema Cerebral edema Intracranial hemorrhage Cerebrovascular accident	Cardiac arrest Cardiac arrhythmia Severe shock Near-drowning Neonatal asphyxia* Hypoxemic respiratory failure Carbon monoxide poisoning Cyanide toxicity Anaphylaxis Asthma	Postictal state* Status epilepticus* Absence status Complex partial seizure	Embolism Spontaneous intraparenchymal hemorrhage Subarachnoid hemorrhage Vasculitis Lupus erythematosus Hypertensive encephalopathy Acute confusional migraine*	Conversion disorders* Catatonic schizophrenia

*Common.

LSD, lysergic acid diethylamide; PCP, phenylcyclohexyl piperidine (phenylcyclidine HCl); ?, unknown etiology.

Table 40-9. Common Causes of Altered Mental Status by Age

Neonate	Infant	Child	Adolescent
Hypoglycemia	Meningitis	Meningitis	Meningitis
Birth asphyxia	Bacterial	Bacterial	Bacterial
Congenital anomalies of the	Viral	Viral	Viral
central nervous system	Trauma	Encephalitis	Encephalitis
Systemic infection with shock	Abuse/shaken-baby syndrome	Trauma	Intentional ingestion
Cardiogenic shock	Asphyxia	Ingestion	Recreational drug/alcohol use
Congenital infection	Apparent life-threatening event	Reye syndrome	Suicide gesture or attempt
Bacterial meningitis	Intentional suffocation	Systemic infection with shock	Often involves multiple agents
Inborn errors of metabolism	Systemic infection with shock	Seizure	Trauma
Hypocalcemia	Ingestion	Near-drowning	Seizures
Intraventricular hemorrhage	Inborn errors of metabolism	Hypoglycemia	Diabetic ketoacidosis
Seizures	Hypoglycemia	Intussusception	Systemic infection with shock
Birth trauma	Hyponatremia	encephalopathy	Toxic shock syndrome
	Hypernatremia	Diabetic ketoacidosis	Reye syndrome
	Hypocalcemia		Spontaneous intracranial
	Encephalitis		hemorrhage
	Postimmunization		Psychological
	encephalopathy		
	Hemorrhagic shock and		
	encephalopathy syndrome		
	Intussusception encephalopathy		
	Seizures		

Central neurogenic hyperventilation is encountered with midbrain dysfunction; patients with this problem are tachypneic and hyperpneic. Apneustic breathing is associated with damage in the middle to lower pontine region. This pattern is characterized by a prolonged pause at full inspiration. Clusters of breaths separated by periods of apnea may be observed in patients with low pontine to upper medullary lesions, whereas medullary lesions result in ataxic or irregular breathing, slow regular breathing, or agonal respiration.

Absent or asymmetrical corneal reflexes or abnormal oculocephalic or oculovestibular reflexes also suggest serious brainstem involvement.

Intracranial Hypertension

Indications of clinically significant intracranial hypertension are usually apparent during an assessment of pupillary responses, vital signs, and motor responses (Tables 40-11 and 40-12). A unilaterally fixed and dilated pupil in a patient who is not awake represents uncal herniation precipitated by an increase in intracranial pressure in the supratentorial space. Impending central herniation from increased pressure on the caudal brainstem may be preceded by the *Cushing triad* of hypertension, bradycardia, and irregularities of respiration. The three components are not necessarily all present together, however. Decerebrate or opisthotonic posturing should also be considered a sign of raised intracranial pressure in an unresponsive patient. A lateral rectus palsy (cranial nerve VI) may also be an early sign of intracranial hypertension. A history of headaches, persistent vomiting, or ataxia may also suggest raised intracranial pressure.

A child with focal neurologic findings or brainstem dysfunction is considered to have a rapidly progressive intracranial lesion until proven otherwise. These children require an emergency head CT scan and an assessment for other life-threatening injuries if trauma is suspected. Vital signs should be monitored frequently. Intubation is performed before the CT scan if the Glasgow Coma Scale score is 8 or less or if signs of increased intracranial pressure are present. If raised intracranial pressure is suspected, the child should be hyperventilated and given mannitol before the CT scan. Children with altered mental status and a suspected head injury but without focal findings or brainstem dysfunction should also undergo emergency CT scanning. If their Glasgow Coma Scale score is 8 or less, an airway should be secured before the scan.

The absence of a history of trauma or physical findings suggestive of a rapidly progressive intracranial process does not preclude a traumatic or an anatomic cause of coma. A child may have a subarachnoid hemorrhage (ruptured aneurysm, arteriovenous malformation) or hydrocephalus without any of the aforementioned signs or symptoms of raised intracranial pressure.

REVERSAL OF IMMEDIATELY TREATABLE TOXIC OR METABOLIC CAUSES

Hypoglycemia and narcotic intoxication are two rapidly reversible causes of coma. Hypoglycemia is a medical emergency that must be reversed because sustained hypoglycemia may result in permanent neurologic damage (see Chapter 61). When vascular access is achieved, blood can be obtained for laboratory studies, including a blood glucose level determination. However, once an intravenous catheter has been placed, all unresponsive children should receive 0.5 to 1.0 g/kg (2 to 4 mL/kg) of 25% dextrose unless a diagnosis other than hypoglycemia is apparent. If the child's mental status improves or if there is laboratory confirmation of hypoglycemia, the dextrose bolus should be followed by a continuous infusion of glucose and electrolytes to prevent rebound hypoglycemia. Naloxone (0.1 mg/kg, maximum 2 mg; may repeat every 2 to 3 minutes if no response) is also administered to all children who have marked depression of consciousness without an obvious cause, particularly if hypoventilation is observed. Miosis is not a necessary finding because ingestion of multiple agents, including narcotics, may not result in small, constricted pupils. Large ingestions of narcotics may necessitate larger single doses of naloxone because of the competitive nature of its antagonistic effect, or they may necessitate multiple doses because its half-life is shorter than that of the narcotic ingested.

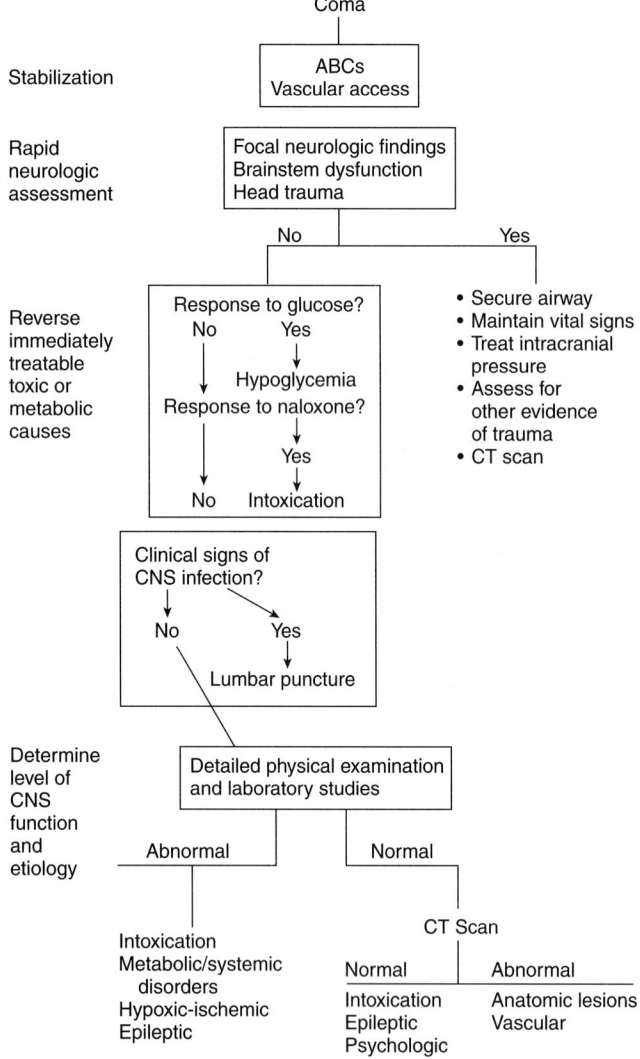

Stabilization — Coma → ABCs, Vascular access

Rapid neurologic assessment — Focal neurologic findings, Brainstem dysfunction, Head trauma

No → Reverse immediately treatable toxic or metabolic causes

Response to glucose?
No / Yes
Hypoglycemia
Response to naloxone?
No / Yes
Intoxication

Yes →
• Secure airway
• Maintain vital signs
• Treat intracranial pressure
• Assess for other evidence of trauma
• CT scan

Clinical signs of CNS infection?
No / Yes
Lumbar puncture

Determine level of CNS function and etiology — Detailed physical examination and laboratory studies

Abnormal
Intoxication
Metabolic/systemic disorders
Hypoxic-ischemic
Epileptic

Normal → CT Scan
Normal — Intoxication, Epileptic, Psychologic
Abnormal — Anatomic lesions, Vascular

Figure 40-2. Management approach to coma. ABCs, airway, breathing, and circulation; CNS, central nervous system; CT, computed tomography.

Table 40-10. Signs of Head Trauma Possibly Associated with Intracranial Disease

General	Signs of Basilar Skull Fracture
Lacerations	Hemotympanum
Hematomas	CSF rhinorrhea
Ecchymosis	CSF otorrhea
Swelling	"Raccoon eyes"
Palpable crepitations	Battle sign
Step-off of skull	

CSF, cerebrospinal fluid.

Another reversible cause of coma is a benzodiazepine ingestion. Flumazenil, a specific competitive antagonist of benzodiazepines, should not be routinely administered to unresponsive children in the emergency department. There are no compelling data suggesting that flumazenil reverses respiratory depression. Administration of flumazenil to a patient who has ingested multiple agents can precipitate seizures, particularly if the concomitant ingestion can cause seizures (e.g., tricyclic antidepressants).

The next question to be answered is whether there are clinical signs or symptoms of meningitis or encephalitis. Specifically, the child should be assessed for the presence of a bulging fontanelle, nuchal rigidity, and Kernig or Brudzinski signs (see Chapter 52). Prior administration of antibiotics does not affect meningeal irritation. Most (85%) children with meningitis have an alteration in mental status (53% lethargic, 22% stuporous, 10% comatose). Focal neurologic findings or seizures may be seen in children with meningitis.

If meningitis is suspected, a lumbar puncture, including measurement of the opening pressure, should be performed unless the procedure is contraindicated (Table 40-13). If a contraindication exists, the child should be stabilized, receive empirical antimicrobial therapy, and undergo head CT scanning. The patient should undergo lumbar puncture as soon as it is no longer contraindicated. If a patient presents with sudden nuchal rigidity not preceded by a prodromal illness, a subarachnoid hemorrhage should be suspected and a CT scan performed before the lumbar puncture.

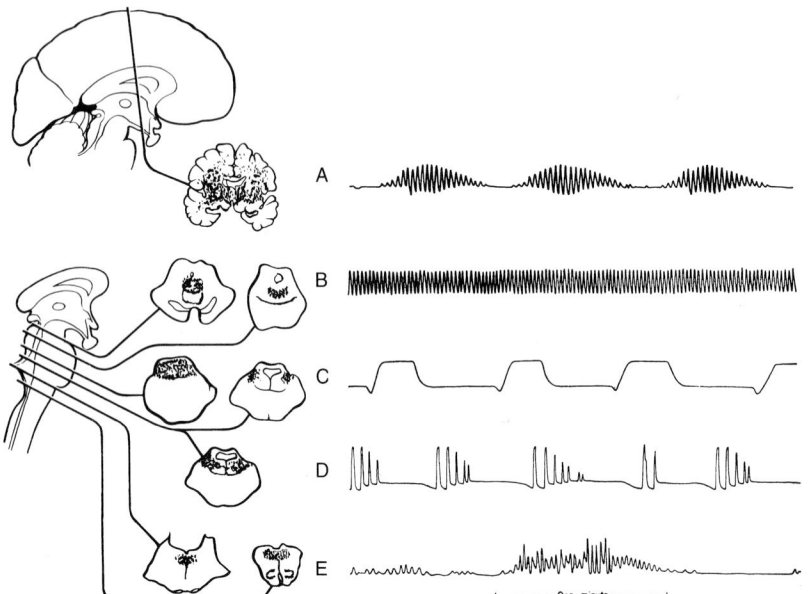

Figure 40-3. Abnormal respiratory patterns associated with pathologic lesions *(shaded areas)* at various levels of the brain. Tracings by chest-abdomen pneumography; inspiration reads up. **A,** Cheyne-Stokes respiration. **B,** Central neurogenic hyperventilation. **C,** Apneusis. **D,** Cluster breathing. **E,** Ataxic breathing. (Adapted from Plum F, Posner JB [eds]: The Diagnosis of Stupor and Coma, 3rd ed. Philadelphia, FA Davis, 1982, p 34.)

One minute

Table 40-11. Signs of Incipient Downward Herniation

	Central	Uncal
Arousal	Impaired early, before other signs	Impaired late, usually with other signs
Breathing	Sighs, yawns, sometimes Cheyne-Stokes respirations	No early change
Pupils	First, small reactive (hypothalamus); then one or both approach midposition	Ipsilateral pupil dilates, followed by somatic third nerve paralysis
Oculocephalic responses	Initially sluggish, later tonic conjugate	Unilateral third nerve paralysis
Motor signs	Early hemiparesis opposite to hemispheric lesion followed late by ipsilateral motor paresis and extensor plantar response	Motor signs late, sometimes ipsilateral to lesion

From Plum F: Neurology/sustained impairments of consciousness. In Wyngaarden JB, Smith LH, Bennett JC (eds): Cecil Textbook of Medicine, 19th ed. Philadelphia, WB Saunders, 1992, p 2050.

LEVEL OF CENTRAL NERVOUS SYSTEM FUNCTION AND CAUSE

The coma can be initially considered stable if (1) focal neurologic findings are not present, (2) there is no evidence of significant brainstem dysfunction, (3) intracranial pressure is not raised, (4) there is no evidence of head trauma or CNS infection, and (5) the child does not have a rapidly reversible toxic or metabolic cause. A detailed physical examination and laboratory evaluation can then be undertaken to determine the level of CNS function and the cause of the coma.

Physical Examination

Coma can be thought of as resulting from hemispheric or brainstem (including reticular activating formation) dysfunction. Dysfunction in either location may be produced by anatomic or nonstructural causes (referred to as *metabolic causes* in this discussion). The origin of coma (hemispheric versus brainstem) and its cause (metabolic versus structural) can be elucidated by evaluation of pupillary size and reactivity, eye movements, respiratory pattern, and motor responses. Pupillary light reflexes are generally preserved in metabolic encephalopathy, whereas their absence strongly suggests a structural lesion. The only exception to the latter is drug effect, particularly with potent anticholinergic compounds, such as glutethimide, atropine, or scopolamine, which produce fixed and dilated pupils. The balance between sympathetic and parasympathetic stimulation, which result in pupillary dilation and constriction, respectively, normally determines pupillary size and reactivity. A unilaterally dilated and fixed pupil is a sign of uncal herniation with entrapment of the oculomotor nerve. Parasympathetic fibers innervating the eye accompany the oculomotor nerve. Sympathetic fibers originate from at least four hypothalamic nuclei so that diencephalic dysfunction results in small, reactive pupils. Hypothalamic damage often results in ipsilateral miosis associated with *Horner syndrome* (miosis, ptosis, and anhidrosis).

Anhidrosis, in contrast to that observed with cervical lesions, involves the entire ipsilateral half of the body. This is an important clinical finding in that it may portend imminent transtentorial herniation. Injury to nuclei located in the midbrain disrupts both sympathetic and parasympathetic pathways, resulting in midsized, fixed pupils. Damage to the midbrain tectal regions also produces midposition or slightly large, fixed pupils. In contrast to nuclear damage, however, accommodation may be intact, so that pupillary size fluctuates spontaneously. Pontine lesions, principally hemorrhage, interfere with descending sympathetic fibers, causing symmetrically small pupils for which a magnifying glass may be needed to detect a light reflex. Lateral medullary lesions may also produce Horner syndrome, whereas central herniation results in fixed, dilated pupils. Figure 40-4 summarizes pupillary findings in comatose patients.

Evaluation of eye movements is helpful in differentiating hemispheric from brainstem causes of coma. Frontal regions of the cerebral hemispheres are responsible for voluntary eye movements, the quick phase of nystagmus, and control over brainstem reflexes that determine eye movements. Bilateral hemispheric depression may result in roving eye movements if brainstem function is intact. Because stimulation of a frontal gaze center causes conjugate deviation of the eyes to the opposite side, tonic lateral deviation of the eyes implies a seizure emanating from the contralateral hemisphere. Eye deviation may also result from an ipsilateral hemispheric injury with unopposed stimulation from the undamaged hemisphere or from a contralateral pontine lesion. The degree of eye deviation is usually more dramatic with hemispheric damage than with brainstem damage.

Table 40-12. Characteristics of Supratentorial Lesions Leading to Coma

Initiating symptoms usually cerebral-focal: aphasia; focal seizures; contralateral hemiparesis, sensory change, or neglect; frontal lobe behavioral changes; headache

Dysfunction moves rostral to caudal: e.g., focal motor → bilateral motor → altered level of arousal

Abnormal signs usually confined to a single or adjacent anatomic level (not diffuse)

Brainstem functions spared unless herniation develops

From Plum F: Neurology/sustained impairments of consciousness. In Wyngaarden JB, Smith LH, Bennett JC (eds): Cecil Textbook of Medicine, 19th ed. Philadelphia, WB Saunders, 1992, p 2050.

Table 40-13. Contraindications to Lumbar Puncture

Clinically important cardiorespiratory compromise in a neonate or young infant

Signs of raised intracranial pressure (pupillary changes, ptosis, hypertension, bradycardia, posturing, cranial nerve VI palsy, retinal changes)

Skin or soft tissue infection overlying area where lumbar puncture is to be performed

Focal neurologic findings

Suspected brain abscess (illness duration longer than expected for meningitis; focality)

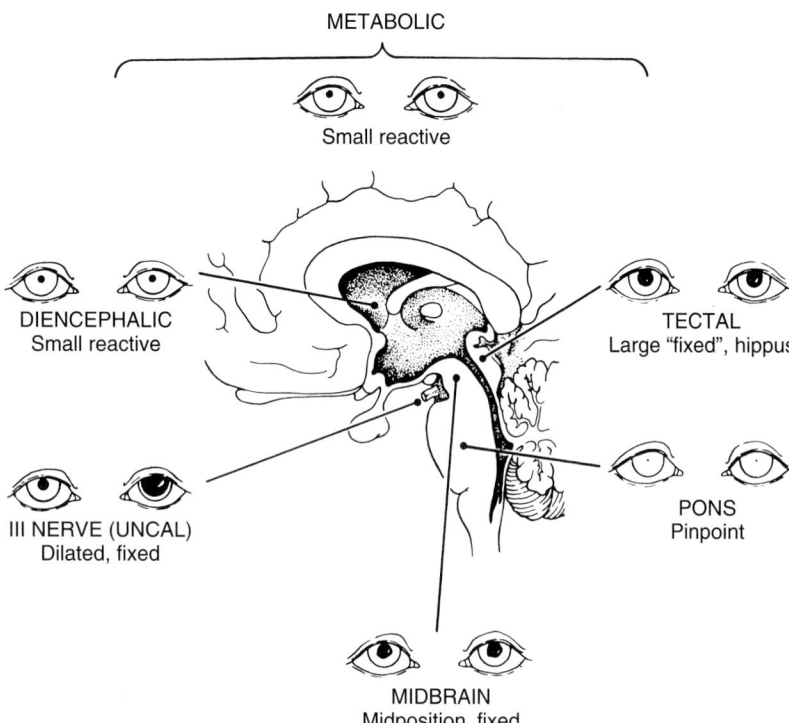

Figure 40-4. Pupils in comatose patients. (Adapted from Plum F, Posner JB [eds]: The Diagnosis of Stupor and Coma, 3rd ed. Philadelphia, FA Davis, 1982, p 46.)

If the patient's eyes are not moving, then reflex eye movements are tested by the oculocephalic and oculovestibular responses (Fig. 40-5). These maneuvers involve the same major neuronal pathways. Afferent fibers from the labyrinth, cerebellum, and cervical muscles reach the vestibular nuclei (cranial nerve VIII) in the medulla. Fibers from the vestibular nuclei then course to the ipsilateral abducens nuclei (cranial nerve VI). Fibers from the abducens nuclei then decussate in the midpons and ascend in the medial longitudinal fasciculus to reach the contralateral oculomotor nuclei (cranial nerve III). Positive reflexes indicate the absence of cortical input on an intact brainstem.

The oculocephalic reflex is elicited by rotating the child's head from side to side and observing the eye movements. If brainstem function is intact, the eyes deviate in a direction opposite to the head movement. Both left and right lateral rotation should be tested. This reflex should then be tested in a vertical plane by rapidly flexing and extending the neck. A positive response is upward gaze when the neck is flexed and downward deviation when the head is extended. Such maneuvers are contraindicated if cervical spine injury is suspected.

The oculovestibular reflex is tested by instilling ice water into the ear canal. The ear canal must be visualized to ensure that there is no obstruction and that the tympanic membrane is intact. The head is then placed at a 30-degree angle from the horizontal so that the semicircular canal is vertical, and up to 120 mL of ice water is then injected slowly into the external ear canal over a few minutes through an angiocatheter. After a minimum of 5 minutes, the other ear may be tested; this interval allows time for the oculovestibular system to reequilibrate. A positive response in an awake patient is nystagmus with the slow component toward the irrigated ear and the fast component away from the stimulus. With bilateral hemispheric depression, the fast phase of nystagmus dissipates, and the eyes are tonically deviated toward the irrigated ear. Both the oculocephalic and oculovestibular reflexes are absent in patients with low brainstem lesions because neurotransmission between the vestibular and abducens nuclei is interrupted. In patients with damage to the medial longitudinal fasciculus, the ipsilateral eye fails to adduct on irrigation of the contralateral ear canal. However, the opposite eye abducts normally. For example, with a lesion in the left medial longitudinal fasciculus, the right eye abducts, but the left eye does not, in response to irrigating the right ear canal. This reaction is caused by disruption of fibers between the abducens and the contralateral oculomotor nuclei (see Fig. 40-5).

In addition to assessing ocular motility, the examiner should test the corneal reflex and determine the presence or absence of a blink. The absence of a blink in response to a loud noise or bright light implies dysfunction of the pontine reticular formation secondary to either metabolic or structural causes. Unilateral absence of a blink implies a facial nerve lesion. The afferent limb of the corneal reflex is carried by the trigeminal nerve (cranial nerve V). The normal effector response involves both upward deviation of the eye (oculomotor nerve) and closure of the eyelid (facial nerve). A normal reflex suggests that the integrity of pathways between the midbrain and the pons has not been violated.

Examination of the motor system includes observation of body position, spontaneous movements, and response to noxious stimuli (Fig. 40-6). A normal body position usually denotes an intact brainstem, as do spontaneous, nonposturing movements. Hemiparesis or hemiplegia implies a structural lesion in the contralateral hemisphere or subcortical region or an ipsilateral spinal cord injury. The presence of hypertonia or hyperreflexia suggests previous corticospinal tract disease or an acute brainstem injury at the midbrain-pontine level. It can also be observed in patients with severe metabolic derangements, such as hepatic coma, hypoglycemia, anoxia, and uremia. Hypotonia implies bilateral hemispheric dysfunction or a medullary or spinal cord lesion. In patients with severe depression of brain function, motor function can be assessed only after the application of a noxious stimulus, such as a sternal rub or increasing subungual pressure to the fingernails or toenails. Ascending sensory pathways to the cerebral hemispheres are intact, and descending motor pathways are functioning to some degree if the response to a noxious stimulus includes verbalization or eye opening or a normal

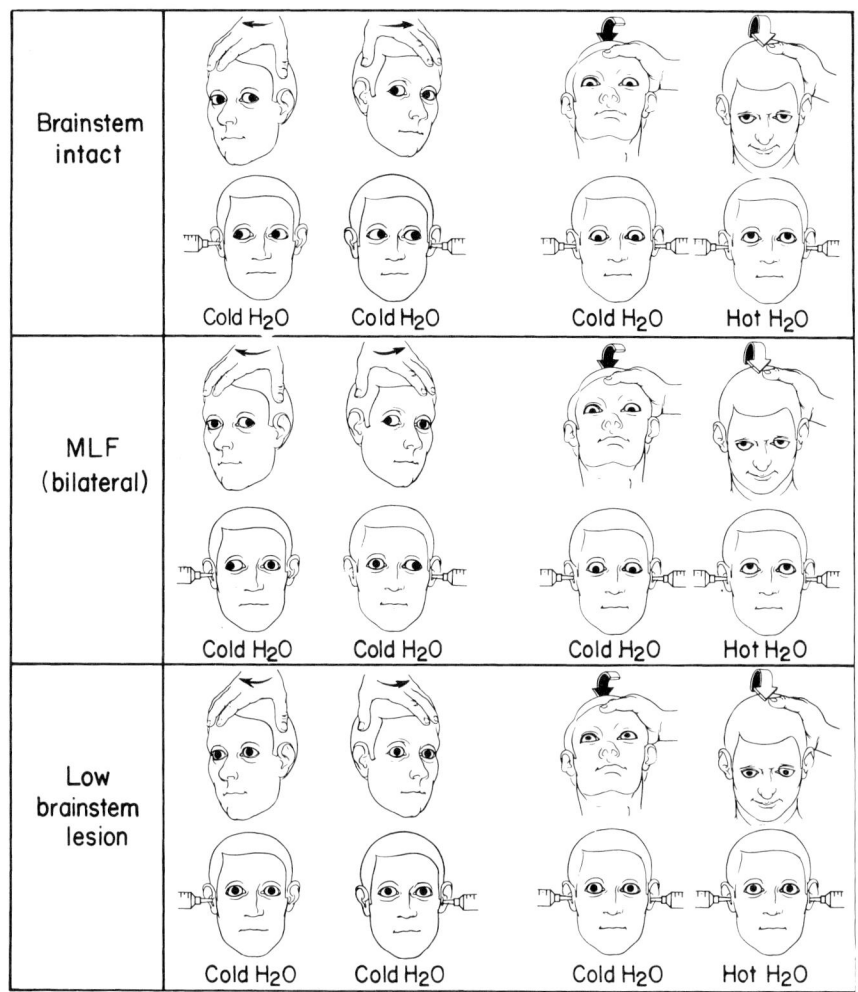

Figure 40-5. Ocular reflexes in unconscious patients. The *upper section* illustrates the oculocephalic (*upper row*) and oculovestibular (*lower row*) reflexes in an unconscious patient whose brainstem ocular pathways are intact. In the *middle section* of the drawing, the effects of bilateral medial longitudinal fasciculus (MLF) lesions on oculocephalic and oculovestibular reflexes are shown. The *left portion* of the drawings illustrates that oculocephalic and oculovestibular stimulation deviates the appropriate eye laterally and brings the eye, which would normally deviate medially, only to the midline, because the medial longitudinal fasciculus, with its connections between the abducens and oculomotor nuclei, is interrupted. The *right portion* is normal with MLF lesions. The *lowest section* of the drawing illustrates the effects of a low brainstem lesion. On the *left*, neither oculovestibular nor oculocephalic movements cause lateral deviation of the eyes, because the pathways are interrupted between the vestibular nucleus and the abducens area. Likewise, in the *right portion* of the drawings, neither oculovestibular nor oculocephalic stimulation causes vertical deviation of the eyes. (Adapted from Plum F, Posner JB [eds]: The Diagnosis of Stupor and Coma, 3rd ed. Philadelphia, FA Davis, 1982, p 55.)

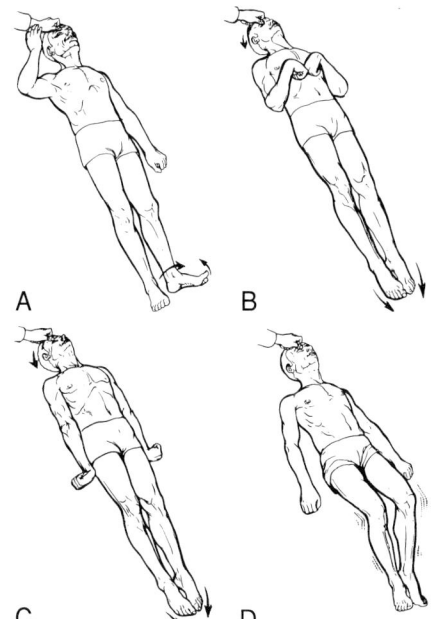

Figure 40-6. Motor responses to noxious stimuli. **A,** Localization of pain as patient attempts to remove stimulus. **B,** Decorticate posturing. **C,** Decerebrate posturing. **D,** Flaccid patient with no response. (Adapted from Plum F, Posner JB [eds]: The Diagnosis of Stupor and Coma, 3rd ed. Philadelphia, FA Davis, 1982, p 66.)

motor response, such as localization of the stimulus, withdrawal of the limb, or movement away from the stimulus.

Decorticate posturing implies hemispheric dysfunction with an intact brainstem (see Fig. 40-6). Decerebrate posturing is more ominous (see Fig. 40-6). Opisthotonos with clenched teeth is a severe form of decerebration. This response usually suggests brainstem compression or a severe structural injury to the midbrain-pontine region. It can also occur in association with severe metabolic diseases, such as hepatic coma, anoxia, and hypoglycemia. Less commonly, decerebrate posture may represent delayed cortical demyelination after a hypoxic-ischemic injury. Pontomedullary or spinal cord damage is associated with a flaccid response to noxious stimulation.

A patient's breathing pattern is also helpful in localizing the area of CNS dysfunction. Hyperventilation can be observed not only in midbrain structural lesions but also in toxic-metabolic encephalopathies as a primary response to stimulation of the respiratory center (salicylate, theophylline, hepatic coma) or as a compensatory response to a metabolic acidosis. This pattern is also seen with raised intracranial hypertension, as may occur in a child with meningitis. Hypoventilation with a normal rhythm, particularly if associated with a symmetrically depressed motor examination, usually implies global CNS depression secondary to drug ingestion.

A detailed physical examination should be performed next and may provide further clues to the cause of the coma (Table 40-14). Several laboratory or ancillary studies should be obtained in all patients, whereas ordering of other studies depends on clinical

Table 40-14. Physical Examination and Diagnosis of Coma

System	Sign	Disorder
Skin	Dry	Dehydration, myxedema, adrenal insufficiency, anticholinergic poisoning
	Moist	Syncope
	Pigment	Addison disease
	Nevi	Tuberous sclerosis with seizures
	Petechiae	Bacteremia, subacute bacterial endocarditis, idiopathic thrombocytopenic purpura
	Cyanosis	Hypoxia, congenital heart disease with cerebral embolism, methemoglobinemia
	Erythema	Carbon monoxide, atropine, or mercury intoxication
	Butterfly rash	Lupus erythematosus, tuberous sclerosis
	Desquamation	Vitamin A intoxication, scarlatina
	Nail changes	Splinter hemorrhage–endocarditis
		Mycotic infection and hypoparathyroidism
		Periungual fibroma (tuberous sclerosis)
Breath odor	Fruity	Diabetic ketoacidosis; amyl nitrate, alcohol, isopropyl alcohol poisonings
	Feculent	Hepatic encephalopathy
	Garlic	Selenium toxicity, arsenic poisoning, organophosphate poisoning
	Almonds	Cyanide poisoning
	Wintergreen	Methyl salicylate poisoning
	Ammoniacal	Uremia
	Acrid (pearlike)	Paraldehyde, chloral hydrate poisoning
Scalp	Contusions	Trauma
	Vasodilation	Sagittal sinus thrombosis
Eyes	Chemosis	Cavernous sinus thrombosis
	Periorbital ecchymosis	Blow-out orbital fracture
	Subhyaloid hemorrhage	Subarachnoid hemorrhage
	Vasospasm (retina)	Hypertensive encephalopathy
Ears	Hemorrhage	Basilar skull fracture
	Otitis media	Brain abscess, lateral sinus thrombosis
Nose	Cerebrospinal fluid rhinorrhea	Basilar skull fracture
Mouth	Scarred tongue	Seizure disorder
	Pigmentation	Addison disease
	Lead lines	Plumbism (lead intoxication)
Neck	Rigid	Meningitis, pneumonia, subarachnoid hemorrhage, encephalitis
Thyroid	Enlarged	Myxedema, thyrotoxicosis
Heart	Murmur	Subacute endocarditis, brain abscess
Abdomen	Hepatomegaly	Leukemia, hepatic failure, heart failure
Extremities	Fracture	Trauma, fat embolism
	Ecchymosis	Trauma, hemorrhagic diathesis

Adapted from Tait VF, Dean JM, Hanley DF: Evaluation of the comatose child. In Rogers MC (ed): Textbook of Pediatric Intensive Care, 2nd ed. Baltimore, Williams & Wilkins, 1992, p 741.

suspicions formulated from the history and physical examination (Table 40-15). Patients with suspected anatomic causes of coma should undergo emergency head CT scanning, whereas those with a suspected CNS infection should undergo lumbar puncture. Other studies to consider are electrocardiography to rule out conduction abnormalities, seen with many drugs; liver function studies; blood ammonia determination; measurement of calcium, magnesium, and phosphorus; and serum osmolality measurement. An *osmolal gap* as well as an anion gap should be calculated. The osmolal gap is the difference between the measured and calculated serum osmolality (normal is <5 to 10 mOsm/kg H_2O). Table 40-16 summarizes the differential diagnoses of an elevated anion or osmolal gap. Toxicology screens may be of value with suspected ingestions; however, the results must be interpreted cautiously. Because toxicology screens are not standardized, a "negative" result does not rule out an undetermined ingestion. Screening for certain agents, such as methanol and ethylene glycol, needs to be requested specifically, whereas tests for other compounds may yield false-negative results.

If physical examination and laboratory studies do not yield a diagnosis, a head CT scan should be obtained to rule out anatomic or vascular causes. If these results are normal, the most likely causes of coma are intoxication, psychological factors, or related to seizure. An electroencephalogram is indicated if encephalitis, encephalopathy, or seizure disorder is suspected. Magnetic resonance imaging may reveal subtle signs of edema, ischemia, or demyelination before these signs are visible on CT scan.

Table 40-25. Diagnostic Criteria for Hemorrhagic Shock and Encephalopathy Syndrome

Clinical	Laboratory	Exclusion Criteria
Shock	Falling hemoglobin level (>3 g/dL	Known infectious and
Coma and seizures	below admission level)	metabolic disorders
Bleeding	Falling platelet count (<150 × 10⁶/L)	Reye syndrome
Diarrhea	Prolonged PT and PTT	Toxin-mediated shock syndromes
Oliguria	Low fibrinogen level	
	Elevated fibrin degradation products	
	Elevated blood urea nitrogen concentration	
	Elevated plasma creatinine concentration	
	Elevated aspartate aminotransferase and	
	alanine aminotransferase levels	
	Metabolic acidosis	

Adapted from Levin M, Pincott JR, Hjelm M, et al: Hemorrhagic shock and encephalopathy: Clinical, pathologic, and biochemical features. J Pediatr 1989;144:195.

PT, prothrombin time; PTT, partial thromboplastin time.

encephalopathy, which has been reported in patients aged 17 days to 15 years. The median age at onset is 5 months; 87% of cases occur before 1 year of age. There is no seasonal or geographic variation. The clinical course is usually fulminant, with profound disseminated intravascular coagulation and bleeding from all venipuncture sites. The shock state is severe, resulting in extreme metabolic acidosis. Renal failure and hepatic failure develop, and the patients often die of cerebral edema with subsequent herniation. The mortality rate is 60% to 70%, and most survivors have a poor neurologic outcome.

The cause is unknown. A viral cause has been postulated, but no pathogens have been isolated. The occurrence of high fever in most patients has raised the question of thermal stress as a trigger of this syndrome in susceptible hosts. The high temperatures may also indicate a relationship to myopathic processes, such as malignant hyperthermia or neuroleptic malignant syndrome.

METABOLIC DISORDERS

Inborn errors of metabolism are complex and encompass many conditions. Table 40-26 is a partial list of inborn errors of metabolism that may manifest in the neonate with lethargy, seizures, and coma. The clinical manifestations of metabolic disease in the neonate can be nonspecific (Table 40-27). The infants are often thought to have sepsis and are evaluated and treated for presumptive infection. The presence of a documented infection does not preclude metabolic disease because some of these infants are prone to infection (e.g., galactosemia and *Escherichia coli* sepsis). A family history of a previous infant dying from an unexplained illness or other children in the family with neurologic disorders may provide clues to a metabolic cause. Laboratory abnormalities that may be seen in metabolic disease are listed in Table 40-28.

Infants with *urea cycle defects* often manifest altered mental status, coma (recurrent), and emesis. They cannot metabolize ammonia to urea; this leads to accumulation of ammonia in the blood. These disorders are inherited as autosomal recessive traits, except for ornithine transcarbamoylase deficiency, which is X-linked. Carbamyl phosphate and ornithine cannot be metabolized to citrulline in the absence of the enzyme ornithine transcarbamoylase. In this defect, carbamyl phosphate is shunted to produce orotic acid, which is detected in the urine, and plasma citrulline levels are low or absent.

The keys to the diagnosis of inborn errors of metabolism in the neonate are a high degree of suspicion, the appropriate screening studies (see Table 40-28), and, if the results are positive, a more detailed laboratory evaluation under the guidance of a specialist in metabolic diseases (Table 40-29).

Metabolic encephalopathy resulting from inborn errors of metabolism (partial, incomplete, stress, or fasting exacerbated) or from renal, hepatic, or toxic causes may also manifest in older children or adolescents. There may or may not be a family history or personal history of recurrent lethargy, emesis, repeated hospitalizations, or personality changes. Encephalopathy in older patients that results from endogenous substances (ammonia, organic acids, hypoglycemia, urea) or exogenous substances (opiates, barbiturates) may manifest within a wide range of symptoms (Table 40-30). The electroencephalograph may be of value in addition to the screening and specific tests noted in Table 40-15, Table 40-28, and Figure 40-7.

REYE SYNDROME

Reye syndrome is classically seen within 2 weeks after a prodromal viral infection, such as varicella, influenza B, or influenza A. There is a strong association between aspirin use and Reye syndrome, which led to the warning against the use of aspirin in children and adolescents. Reye syndrome can be seen in children of any age and has a peak incidence between ages 5 and 15 years. This syndrome is usually heralded by the abrupt onset of repeated vomiting, followed by combativeness and mental status changes, which can range from delirium to coma. Cerebral edema and increased intracranial pressure can develop. The mortality rate is high; death is usually secondary to cerebral herniation or myocardial depression from drugs used to treat intracranial hypertension.

Laboratory studies reveal an elevated serum ammonia concentration and elevated hepatic enzyme levels. The serum ammonia level may be initially normal, particularly during stage I (see Table 40-6). Affected patients may also be hypoglycemic and have a metabolic acidosis. They have microvesicular fatty metamorphosis of the liver, with swelling and disruption of hepatic mitochondria.

The incidence of Reye syndrome has decreased dramatically, and it is now an uncommon diagnosis. Reye syndrome should be thought of as a syndrome and not as a specific disease. A distinct etiologic factor has not been discovered, but the syndrome may represent a response to several different insults in susceptible hosts. Many genetic metabolic diseases may manifest with a picture similar to that of Reye syndrome. Although inborn errors of metabolism usually manifest in infancy, some may manifest later. Findings of

Table 40-26. Inborn Errors of Metabolism Manifesting with Seizures, Lethargy, and Coma in the Neonatal Period

Disorders of Carbohydrate Metabolism	Disorders of Amino Acid Metabolism	Organic Acidemias	Urea Cycle Defects	Lysosomal Storage Disorders	Other
Fructose-1,6-biphosphatase deficiency	Maple syrup urine disease	Methylmalonicacidemia	Carbamyl phosphate synthetase deficiency	Farber disease	Congenital adrenal hyperplasia
Galactosemia	Hypervalinemia	Propionicacidemia (ketotic hyperglycinemia)	Ornithine transcarbamylase deficiency	Fucosidosis	Hypophosphatasia
Hereditary fructose intolerance	Periodic hyperlysinemia	Isovalericacidemia	Citrullinemia		Menkes kinky hair syndrome
Glycogen storage disease, types I and III	Hyper-β-alaninemia	3-Methylcrotonyl CoA carboxylase deficiency	Argininosuccinicaciduria		Hereditary oroticaciduria
Pyruvate carboxylase deficiency	Nonketonic hyperglycinemia	Multiple carboxylase deficiency			Fatty acyl–CoA dehydrogenase deficiencies
Phosphoenolpyruvate carboxykinase deficiency	Pyroglutamic aciduria	Multiple acyl–CoA dehydrogenase deficiencies			Primary systemic carnitine deficiency
	Hyperornithemia-hyperammonemia-homocitrullinuria (HHH) syndrome	Hydroxymethylglutaryl (HMG)–CoA lyase deficiency			Zellweger syndrome
	Lysinuric protein intolerance	2-Methyl-3-hydroxybutyricacidemia			Neonatal adrenoleukodystrophy
	Methylenetetrahydrofolate reductase deficiency	D-Glycericacidemia			
	Sulfite oxidase deficiency				

Adapted from Burton BK. Inborn errors of metabolism: The clinical diagnosis in early infancy. Pediatrics 1987;79:359.

CoA, coenzyme A.

Table 40-27. Clinical Manifestations of Inborn Errors of Metabolism in the Neonatal Period

Lethargy
Coma
Seizures
Increased or decreased muscle tone
Poor suck and feeding
Vomiting
Diarrhea
Tachypnea and/or hyperpnea
Respiratory failure
Jaundice
Unusual odors
Cardiomegaly
Hepatomegaly

Table 40-29. Laboratory Evaluation of Suspected Metabolic Disease

Plasma ammonia
Arterial blood gas
Plasma amino acids
Plasma carnitine
Plasma pyruvate and lactate
Urinary amino acids
Urinary organic acids

Table 40-28. Laboratory Evidence of Metabolic Disease

Acidosis,* alkalosis
Hypoglycemia
Hyperammonemia
Elevated liver enzyme levels
Direct hyperbilirubinemia
Urine-reducing substance
Urine ketones

*High anion gap if increased organic acids (ketoacids, lactic acid) are produced. Normal anion gap if associated renal tubular acidosis (type I glycogen storage disease, galactosemia) is present.

Table 40-30. Characteristics of Metabolic Encephalopathy

Confusion, lethargy, delirium often precede or replace coma
Motor signs, if present, usually symmetrical
Bilateral asterixis, myoclonus appear
Pupillary reactions usually preserved; tonic calorics often present
Sensory abnormalities usually absent
Hypothermia common
Abnormal signs reflect incomplete brain dysfunction at multiple anatomical levels

From Plum F: Neurology/sustained impairments of consciousness. In Wyngaarden JB, Smith LH, Bennet JC (eds): Cecil Textbook of Medicine, 19th ed. Philadelphia, WB Saunders, 1992, p 2052.

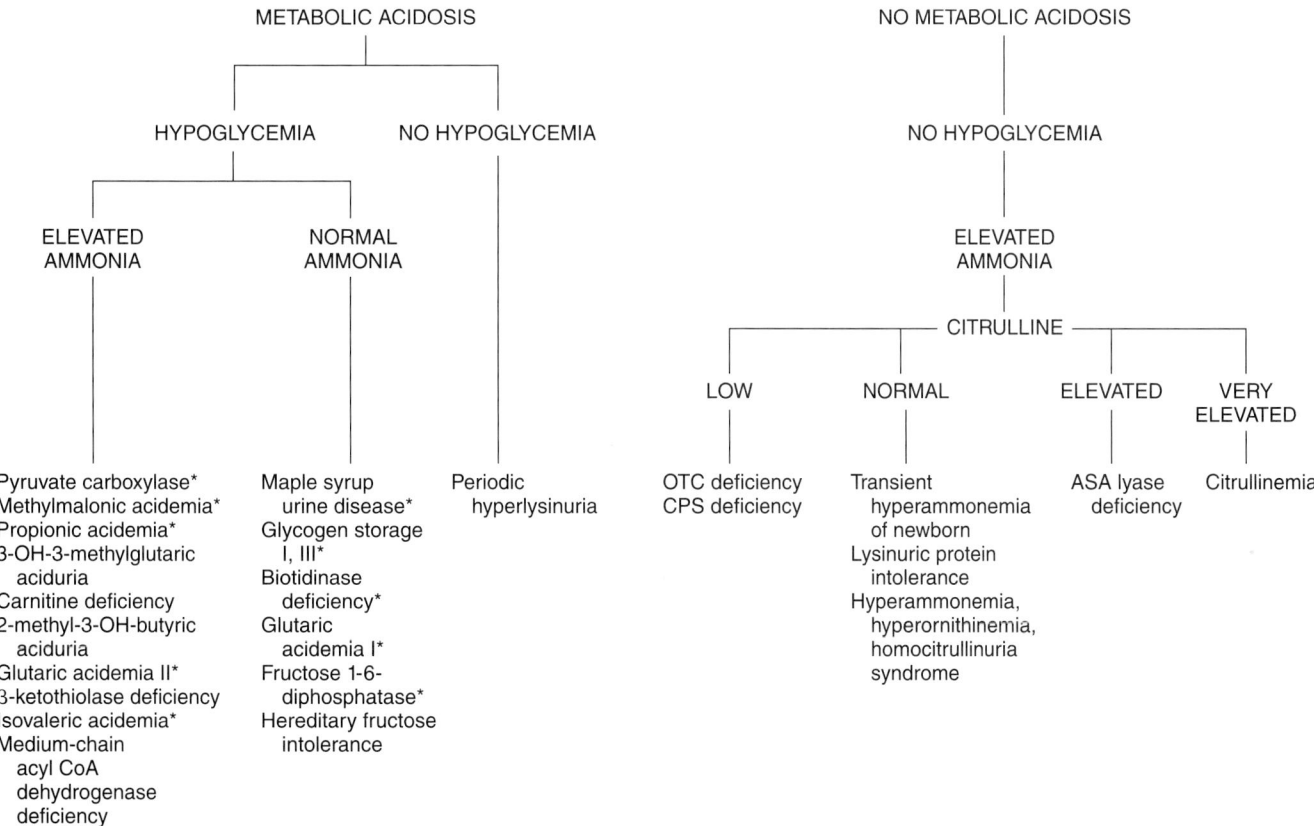

*Ketonuria.

Figure 40-7. An approach to evaluation of metabolic disorders in which symptoms are similar to those of Reye syndrome. In disorders with metabolic acidosis, the most useful diagnostic test is evaluation of organic acids. In the second group, plasma amino acids are most helpful. ASA, argininosuccinic acid; CoA, coenzyme A; CPS, carbamoyl phosphate synthetase; OTC, ornithine transcarbamoylase. (Adapted from Greene CL, Blitzer MG, Shapira E: Inborn errors of metabolism and Reye syndrome: Differential diagnosis. J Pediatr 1988;113:156.)

Table 40-31. Criteria for Diagnosis of Brain Death

Nature and Duration of Coma Must Be Known

Known structural disease or irreversible systemic metabolic cause

No chance of drug intoxication or hypothermia; no paralyzing or potentially anesthetizing drugs recently given for treatment

Body temperature must be above 34°C

Hypotension excluded

Six-hr observation of no brain function is sufficient in cases of known structural cause when no drug or alcohol is involved in causation or treatment; otherwise, 12 hr plus negative drug screen required (24 hr with anoxic injury); observation period may be shortened with the use of a confirmatory test (EEG, cerebral perfusion scan)

Absence of Cerebral and Brain Stem Function

No behavioral or reflex response to noxious stimuli above foramen magnum level, including absence of corneal, gag, and cough reflexes

Midposition or fully dilated, fixed pupils

No oculovestibular response to 50 mL ice water calories

Apneic off ventilator with oxygenation for 10 min with arterial $PCO_2 \geq 60$ mm Hg

Systemic circulation may be intact

Purely spinal reflexes may be retained

Supplementary (Optional) Criteria

EEG isoelectric for 30 min at maximal gain

Brainstem-evoked responses reflect absent function in vital brainstem structures

No cerebral circulation present on angiographic examination or cerebral perfusion scan

Modified from Plum F: Neurology/brain death. In Wyngaarden JB, Smith LH, Bennett JC (eds): Cecil Textbook of Medicine, 19th ed. Philadelphia, WB Saunders, 1992, p 2059.

EEG, electroencephalography; PCO_2, partial pressure of carbon dioxide.

hypoglycemia, acidosis, or hyperammonemia in any patient with altered mental status should lead the clinician to consider a metabolic origin. Figure 40-7 outlines an approach to the patient who presents with mental status changes, vomiting, and a Reye syndrome–like illness. Additional causes of hyperammonemia are valproic acid–induced hyperammonemia and the rare syndrome of elevated ammonia level seen after high-dose chemotherapy for malignancy.

SUMMARY AND RED FLAGS

Delirium and coma are common and potentially serious manifestations of a diverse group of life-threatening but potentially reversible disorders. Common causes vary by age, but toxic ingestion, trauma, seizures (postictal), infections, and metabolic disturbances, including inborn errors of metabolism, must be considered. Red flags include family or personal histories compatible with these disorders, signs of increased intracranial pressure, and rapidly progressive rostral-caudal deterioration (Table 40-31).

REFERENCES

Coma Scales

Durham SR, Clancy RR, Leuthardt E, et al: CHOP Infant Coma Scale ("Infant Face Scale"): A novel coma scale for children less than two years of age. J Neurotrauma 2000;17:729-737.

Fenichel GM: Altered states of consciousness. In Clinical Pediatric Neurology: A Signs and Symptoms Approach, 4th ed. Philadelphia: WB Saunders, 2001, p 47.

Lieh-Lai MW, Theodorou AA, Sarnaik AP, et al: Limitations of the Glasgow Coma Scale in predicting outcome in children with traumatic brain injury. J Pediatr 1992;120:195.

Simpson D, Reilly P: Pediatric coma scale. Lancet 1982;2:450.

Tatman A, Warren A, Williams A, et al: Development of a modified paediatric coma scale in intensive care clinical practice. Arch Dis Child 1997;77:519-521.

Wang MY, Griffith P, Sterling J, et al: A prospective population-based study of pediatric trauma patients with mild alterations in consciousness (Glasgow Coma Scale score of 13-14). Neurosurgery 2000;46:1093-1099.

Diagnosis and Management of Coma

Graham CA: Management of unexplained coma in children. Eur J Emerg Med 2000;7:241-244.

Kirkham FJ: Non-traumatic coma in children. Arch Dis Child 2001;85:303-312.

Liao YJ, So YT: An approach to critically ill patients in coma. West J Med 2002;176:184-187.

Wong CP, Forsyth RJ, Kelly TP, et al: Incidence, aetiology, and outcome of non-traumatic coma: A population based study. Arch Dis Child 2001;84:193-199.

Prognosis

Cheliout-Heraut F, Rubinsztajn R, Ioos C, et al: Prognostic value of evoked potentials and sleep recordings in the prolonged comatose state of children. Preliminary data. Neurophysiol Clin 2001;31:283-292.

Christophe C, Fonteyne C, Ziereisen F, et al: Value of MR imaging of the brain in children with hypoxic coma. AJNR Am J Neuroradiol 2002;23:716-723.

Forsyth RJ, Wong CP, Kelly TP, et al: Cognitive and adaptive outcomes and age at insult effects after non-traumatic coma. Arch Dis Child 2001;84:200-204.

Mandel R, Martinot A, Delepoulle F, et al: Prediction of outcome after hypoxic-ischemic encephalopathy: A prospective clinical and electrophysiologic study. J Pediatr 2002;141:45-50.

Robinson LR, Micklesen PJ, Tirschwell DL, et al: Predictive value of somatosensory evoked potentials for awakening from coma. Crit Care Med 2003;31:960-967.

Wohlrab G, Boltshauser E, Schmitt B: Neurological outcome in comatose children with bilateral loss of cortical somatosensory evoked potentials. Neuropediatrics 2001;32:271-274.

Toxicology

Abbruzzi G, Stork CM: Pediatric toxicologic concerns. Emerg Med Clin North Am 2002;20:223-247.

Bryant S, Singer J: Management of toxic exposure in children. Emerg Med Clin North Am 2003;21:101-119.

Hoffman RJ, Nelson L: Rational use of toxicology testing in children. Curr Opin Pediatr 2001;13:183-188.

Jones A: Recent advances in the management of poisoning. Ther Drug Monit 2002;24:150-155.

Liebelt EL, DeAngelis CD: Evolving trends and treatment advances in pediatric poisoning. JAMA 1999;282:1113-1115.

McGuigan ME: Poisoning potpourri. Pediatr Rev 2001;22:295-302.

Mokhlesi B, Leiken JB, Murray P, et al: Adult toxicology in critical care: Part I: General approach to the intoxicated patient. Chest 2003;123:577-592.

Powers KS: Diagnosis and management of common toxic ingestions and inhalations. Pediatr Ann 2000;29:330-342.

Trauma

American Academy of Pediatrics: Committee on Child Abuse and Neglect: Shaken baby syndrome: Rotational cranial injuries—Technical report. Pediatrics 2001;108:206-210.

Duhaime AC, Christian CW, Rorke LB, et al: Nonaccidental head injury in infants—The "shaken-baby syndrome." N Engl J Med 1998;338: 1822-1829.

Gedeit R: Head injury. Pediatr Rev 2001;22:118-124.

Hackbarth RM, Rzeszutko KM, Sturm G, et al: Survival and functional outcome in pediatric traumatic brain injury: A retrospective review and analysis of predictive factors. Crit Care Med 2002;30:1630-1635.

Ng SM, Toh EM, Sherrington CA: Clinical predictors of abnormal computed tomography scans in paediatric head injury. J Paediatr Child Health 2002; 38:388-392.

Prasad MR, Ewing-Cobbs L, Swank PR, et al: Predictors of outcome following traumatic brain injury in young children. Pediatr Neurosurg 2002;36:64-74.

White JR, Farukhi Z, Bull C, et al: Predictors of outcome in severely head-injured children. Crit Care Med 2001;29:534-540.

Hemorrhagic Shock and Encephalopathy

Chaves-Carballo E, Bouchama A: Fever, heatstroke, and hemorrhagic shock and encephalopathy. J Child Neurol 1998;13:286-287.

Ince E, Kuloglu Z, Akinci Z: Hemorrhagic shock and encephalopathy syndrome: Neurologic features. Pediatr Emerg Care 2000;16:260-264.

Jardine DS, Winters WD, Shaw DW: CT scan abnormalities in a series of patients with hemorrhagic shock and encephalopathy syndrome. Pediatr Radiol 1997;27:540-544.

Inborn Errors of Metabolism

Burton BK: Inborn errors of metabolism in infancy: A guide to diagnosis. Pediatrics 1998;102:E69.

Ellaway CJ, Wilcken B, Christodoulou J: Clinical approach to inborn errors of metabolism presenting in the newborn period. J Paediatr Child Health 2002;38:511-517.

Reye Syndrome

Belay ED, Bresee JS, Holman RC, et al: Reye's syndrome in the United States from 1981 through 1997. N Engl J Med 1999;340:1377-1382.

Casteels-Van Daele M, Van Geet C, Wouters C, et al: Reye syndrome revisited: A descriptive term covering a group of heterogeneous disorders. Eur J Pediatr 2000;159:641-648.

41 Stroke in Childhood

Michael J. Rivkin

Most cases of acute lateralized body weakness result from abnormalities of the blood supply to a portion of the central nervous system (CNS). *Stroke* serves as a term to denote the sudden onset of symptoms attributable to such an interruption of cerebral or spinal perfusion.

Childhood stroke has been reported in all racial and ethnic groups and occurs with an incidence of 2.5 cases per 100,000 population per year. The sequelae are not trivial. In addition to lasting lateralized weakness, learning disabilities, disturbances of language, visual deficits, and seizures may persist.

Brain damage resulting from stroke occurs in one of two general forms:

1. *Ischemia* consists of inadequate brain or spinal cord perfusion with consequent dearth of oxygen or other blood-delivered substances necessary for normal metabolic function.
2. *Hemorrhage* occurs when blood is released into the extravascular cranial space. In this circumstance, focal injury of brain or spinal tissue occurs as a result of pressure exerted by the space-occupying mass of blood.

Ischemic injury of brain occurs as a result of one of three mechanisms: embolism, thrombosis, or diminished systemic perfusion.

Embolic damage to brain occurs when material formed at a site in the vascular system proximal to the brain lodges in a blood vessel, thus blocking cerebral perfusion. Emboli originate most commonly from the heart, arising from a thrombus on cardiac chamber walls or from vegetations on valve leaflets. Artery-to-artery emboli are composed of clot or platelet aggregates that originate in vessels proximal to the brain but ultimately come to rest and occlude flow in vessels critical for cerebral perfusion. Systemic vein-to-cerebral artery emboli (paradoxical emboli) are possible in the presence of right-to-left shunts with cyanotic congenital heart disease or a patent foramen ovale.

Thrombosis denotes vascular occlusion caused by a localized process within a blood vessel or vessels. Although atherosclerosis underlies most thrombotic processes affecting adults, it is not common in children. Localized luminal clot formation occurs in polycythemia or in a hypercoagulable state. Alternatively, anatomic abnormalities may lead to clot formation or mechanical obstruction as is found in fibromuscular dysplasia, arteritis (vasculitis), or arterial dissection.

If *systemic pressure declines* enough to compromise cerebral perfusion, the CNS may sustain injury as a result of diminished perfusion. Cardiac pump failure (resulting from congenital heart disease or its surgical repair) and systemic hypotension resulting from hypovolemia represent common causes of hypotensive cerebral ischemic injury. With diminished cerebral perfusion, brain injury is more diffuse than the more focal injuries characteristic of thrombotic and embolic cerebral events.

Intracranial *hemorrhage* arises in one of two neuropathologic patterns:

1. *Subarachnoid* hemorrhage (SAH) occurs when blood flows from the intracranial vascular bed and onto the surface of the brain to mix with cerebrospinal fluid in the subarachnoid space. The most common source of such intracranial bleeding in early childhood is an arteriovenous malformation. Ruptured intracranial aneurysms also cause subarachnoid hemorrhage, especially in older children.
2. *Intracerebral* hemorrhage (ICH) denotes bleeding into the parenchyma of the brain. Severity and region of deficits caused by intraparenchymal hemorrhage are determined by the extent and location of bleeding in the brain.

The location, or focality, of the resultant deficit after a stroke depends on whether the event occurred in cortex, subcortical areas, brainstem, or cerebellum. Although alterations of blood flow result in permanent deficits, some cause only temporary ones. *Transient ischemic attacks* (TIAs) are brief episodes of focal, nonconvulsive neurologic deficit attributable to interruption of cerebral perfusion. As in stroke, the onset is abrupt. However, the episode must last less than 24 hours, and recovery must be complete. Progression of symptoms characterizes stroke when the underlying process, either ischemia or hemorrhage, widens its CNS domain with resultant expansion of symptoms and signs.

Whether short-lived or permanent, deficits are commonly motor. Loss of strength may occur as a lateralized weakness involving one half of the body (*hemiparesis*) or as complete loss of strength (*hemiplegia*). *Diparesis,* or *diplegia,* involves weakness of the legs and is found primarily in premature infants who have suffered bilateral hypoxic-ischemic brain injury, in full-term neonates after intracranial hemorrhage that has led to posthemorrhagic hydrocephalus, and in children suffering spinal cord injury below the neck. Involvement of the cerebellum often manifests as gait ataxia or impairment of fine motor coordination. Stroke occurring in the brainstem is reflected by cranial nerve dysfunction in the distribution of the vascular event. If long sensory or motor tracts running between brain and spinal cord are involved, dysfunction of these systems may be involved.

Distinction among the three processes underlying stroke—embolism, thrombosis, and hemorrhage—is possible according to clinical features (Table 41-1). Thrombotic strokes are often heralded by TIAs. The stroke frequently bears a stepwise tempo, and neurologic symptoms may appear haltingly. The cerebrospinal profile is normal. Embolic strokes are infrequently preceded by TIAs. Onset of the episode is abrupt, and neurologic symptoms are manifested immediately. A mild to moderate headache may accompany neurologic symptoms. Lumbar puncture yields normal cerebrospinal fluid. Intracerebral hemorrhage is frequently marked by headache. Severe headache of sudden onset marks SAH, in particular. Prodromal symptoms generally do not occur. However, previous seizures may suggest the existence of an arteriovenous malformation, whereas previous episodes of headache may be attributable to leaks from intracranial aneurysms. Consciousness is often lost, although it may be regained after a short while. Cerebrospinal fluid is bloody if SAH has occurred or if intraparenchymal bleeding reaches the ventricular system.

The signs of stroke found on physical examination often reflect interruption of the motor pathways extending from cortical upper motor neurons to the spinal cord lower motor neuron, the anterior horn cell. Upper motor neuron motor deficits seen in stroke patients

Table 41-1. **Stroke in children: Characteristics of Stroke by Mechanism**

Mechanism	Onset	Pace of Deficit Onset	Location	TIAs	Neck Pain	Headache	Impaired Consciousness
Embolism	Sudden	Abrupt	Remote site of origin	Rare	None	Common	Seldom found unless infarction is large
Thrombosis	During sleep or in the setting of hypotension	Stepwise	In situ	Yes	None*	Rare	Unusual
Hemorrhage	Rapid	Abrupt or rapid in progression	In subarachnoid space or in brain parenchyma	None	Yes	Yes	Frequent in subarachnoid hemorrhage and in large parenchymal hemorrhages

*Except in dissecting intimal tear of carotid artery.

TIAs, transient ischemic attacks.

may result from events occurring at any of several levels in the CNS: cerebral cortex, subcortical white matter, brainstem, or spinal cord. Despite the vast neurologic terrain in which stroke may occur, characteristics common to its occurrence at each of these locations can be found. A group of muscles is always involved. Never are individual muscles affected in isolation. The group of muscles affected may initially be flaccid and powerless, but the paralysis is rarely permanently complete.

Spasticity serves as the chronic functional manifestation of upper motor neuron injury caused by stroke. The *antigravity muscles,* consisting of arm flexors and leg extensors, are most commonly affected. As a result, the arms assume a position of flexion and pronation, whereas legs become extended and adducted. If the involved extremity is rapidly moved so that the affected muscles are quickly stretched, a short interval of free movement occurs until an abrupt catch is encountered, which eventually gives way to progressively easier passive movement (*clasp-knife rigidity*). Enhancement of deep tendon reflex response has been attributed to the interruption of descending inhibitory pathways as well as to increased activity of the γ neuron reflex loop.

Clonus, repetitive muscle contraction in response to tendon percussion or stretch, further reflects the enhanced response of tendon reflexes resulting from upper motor neuron injury in stroke. Reflex elicitation at one point, such as at the biceps muscle, may provoke reflex responses in adjacent muscle groups, such as brachioradialis or finger reflexes. Such *spread* of reflex responsiveness is commonly seen in patients whose upper motor neuron pathways have been injured by stroke. Features of upper motor neuron injury are compared with those of lower motor neuron injury in Chapter 38.

The causes of stroke in children differ from those in adults. Stroke in adults is associated largely with hypertension or atherosclerosis and their respective hemorrhagic and ischemic consequences. Stroke in children is more commonly caused by or related to congenital heart disease, infection, metabolic disorders, hematologic and coagulation diatheses, and collagen-vascular disease (Table 41-2). Nonetheless, despite the most thorough evaluation, the cause escapes detection in 25% to 33% of pediatric patients.

THE SETTINGS OF STROKE IN CHILDREN

The neonatal (Table 41-3) and adolescent age groups each carry risks for stroke not shared equally by the large number of children whose ages lie between 1 and 13 years. The clinical presentations and causes of stroke are best considered with respect to each of three pediatric age groups: neonates, children between 1 and 13 years of age, and adolescents.

NEONATES

Hypoxic-Ischemic Encephalopathy

Brain injury resulting from asphyxia, hypoxia, or ischemia is an important cause of neonatal neurologic morbidity. Tissue oxygen deficiency is presumed to underlie the neurologic injury caused by hypoxic-ischemic insults. An oxygen deficit may be incurred by either *hypoxemia* or *ischemia.* Hypoxemia is defined as a diminished oxygen content of blood. Ischemia is characterized by reduced blood perfusion in a particular tissue bed. Hypoxemia and ischemia often occur simultaneously or in sequence. Ischemia is likely to be the more important of these two insults.

Asphyxia denotes an impairment in gas exchange, which results not only in a deficit of oxygen in blood but also in an excess of carbon dioxide and thereby acidosis. Furthermore, sustained asphyxia usually results in hypotension and ischemia, which is consistent with the likely predominant importance of ischemia as the final common pathway to brain injury. Asphyxia is the most common clinical insult resulting in brain injury during the perinatal period.

Evidence of hypoxic-ischemic injury to the neonatal nervous system is reflected by a constellation of signs noticed early after birth (hypoxic-ischemic encephalopathy [HIE]). The asphyxiating event or events may occur at any point in the antepartum, intrapartum, or postpartum periods. On the basis of admittedly imprecise historical data, it has been concluded that insults sustained by the fetus during the antepartum period account for approximately 20% of cases of HIE. Maternal cardiac arrest or hemorrhage leading to transplacental and fetal hypotension represents such prenatal insults. Intrapartum events, such as abruptio placentae, uterine rupture, and traumatic delivery, may account for 35% of cases of HIE. In an additional 35% of infants displaying signs of HIE, markers of intrapartum fetal distress and antepartum risk, such as maternal diabetes, intrauterine growth retardation, or maternal infection, are found. Postpartum difficulties, such as cardiovascular compromise, persistent fetal circulation, and recurrent apnea, account for approximately 10% of HIE cases. Postpartum difficulties are found more commonly in premature than in full-term infants. Therefore, for at least 65% of cases of neonatal HIE, difficulties of the intrapartum period alone do not explain the encephalopathy.

Recognition of neonatal HIE requires careful observation and examination of the newborn in the context of a detailed history of pregnancy, labor, and delivery. Newborns who have sustained hypoxic-ischemic insults severe enough to cause permanent neurologic injury usually demonstrate abnormalities on neurologic examination. Indeed, a combination of low Apgar scores, fetal acidosis or distress, and an abnormal neurologic examination finding help define HIE. Nonetheless, if the hypoxic-ischemic damage has occurred well in advance of parturition, it may be asymptomatic in the neonate.

Table-41-2. Causes of Stroke in Children

Cardiovascular Disease

Congenital
 Aortic stenosis
 Mitral stenosis
 Ventricular septal defects
 Patent ductus arteriosus
 Cyanotic congenital heart disease involving right-to-left shunt
 PHACE syndrome
Acquired
 Endocarditis
 Kawasaki disease
 Cardiomyopathy
 Atrial myxoma
 Arrhythmia
 Paradoxical emboli through patent foramen ovale
 Rheumatic fever
 Prosthetic heart valve

Hematologic Abnormalities

Hemoglobinopathies
 Sickle (SS) disease
 Sickle (SC) disease
Polycythemia
Leukemia/lymphoma
Thrombocytopenias (e.g., ITP, TTP, HUS)
Disorders of coagulation
 Protein C deficiency
 Protein S deficiency
 Factor V (Leiden) resistance to activated protein C
 Antithrombin III deficiency
 Lupus anticoagulant
 Oral contraceptive pill
 Pregnancy and the postpartum state
 Disseminated intravascular coagulation
 Paroxysmal nocturnal hemoglobinuria
 Inflammatory bowel disease (thrombosis)
 L-asparaginase
 Prothrombin mutations

Inflammatory Disorders

Meningitis
 Viral
 Bacterial
 Tuberculosis
Systemic infection
 Viremia
 Bacteremia
 Local head and neck infections
 Postvaricella
Drug-induced inflammation/vasoconstriction
 Amphetamine
 Cocaine
 Ergots
Autoimmune disease
 Systemic lupus erythematosus
 Juvenile rheumatoid arthritis
 Takayasu arteritis
 Mixed connective tissue disease
 Polyarteritis nodosum
 Primary CNS vasculitis

Metabolic Disease Associated with Stroke

Homocystinuria/elevated homocysteine levels
Pseudoxanthoma elasticum
Fabry disease
Sulfite oxidase deficiency
Mitochondrial disorders
 MELAS
 Leigh syndrome

Intracerebral Vascular Processes

Ruptured aneurysm
Arteriovenous malformation
Fibromuscular dysplasia
Moyamoya disease
Migraine headache
Postsubarachnoid hemorrhage vasospasm
Hereditary hemorrhagic telangiectasia
Sturge-Weber syndrome
Carotid artery dissection

Trauma and Other External Causes

Child abuse
Head trauma/neck trauma
Oral trauma
Placental embolism
ECMO therapy
Lollypop stroke (pharyngeal trauma)

CNS, central nervous system; ECMO, extracorporeal membrane oxygenation; HUS, hemolytic uremic syndrome; ITP, idiopathic (immune) thrombocytopenia purpura; MELAS, mitochondrial encephalomyopathy, lactic acidosis, and stroke; PHACE, posterior fossa brain malformations, facial hemangiomas, arterial anomalies (cerebrovascular hypoplasia, aneurysms, stenosis, aberrancy), coarctation of the aorta, cardiac and eye defects; TTP, thrombotic thrombocytopenic purpura.

Mild HIE (stage 1) may be characterized by hyperalertness or by mild depression of the level of consciousness, which may be accompanied by uninhibited Moro and brisk deep tendon reflexes, signs of sympathetic activity (dilated pupils), and a normal or only slightly abnormal EEG. Typically, these symptoms last less than 24 hours. Moderate encephalopathy (stage 2) may be marked by obtundation, hypotonia, diminished number of spontaneous movements, and seizures. Infants with severe HIE (stage 3) are ill for more than 24 hours and are comatose. In addition, they are markedly hypotonic and display bulbar and autonomic dysfunction. The EEG is abnormal and may demonstrate a burst-suppression pattern or seizures, or it may be isoelectric.

Neonates with moderate or severe HIE may show variation in level of consciousness during the first days after birth. Initially, depression of level of alertness may appear to improve after the first 12 to 24 hours after birth. However, specific signs of improving alertness such as visual fixation or following are lacking. In addition, other persistent or progressive neurologic deficits, as well as functional deterioration of other extraneural systems, are inconsistent with a true improvement in neurologic state. Coma may persist, supervene, or even progress to brain death by 72 hours of life. If the infant survives 72 hours without losing all cerebral function, a variable amount of improvement may be observed.

Table 41-3. Causes of Stroke in Neonates

Hypoxic-ischemic encephalopathy
Cerebral venous thrombosis
Congenital coagulopathies, including hypercoagulable states
Thrombocytopenia (alloimmune or maternal idiopathic
  thrombocytopenic purpura)
Intracranial hemorrhage
Intraventricular hemorrhage
Polycythemia
Familial porencephaly
Organic acidemias
Methylmalonic acidemia
Propionic acidemia
Isovaleric acidemia
Unknown presumed emboli (placental, patent ductus
  arteriosus) of in utero onset

Diffuse hypotonia accompanied by a dearth of movement constitutes the most frequently observed motor deficit found early in the course of neonatal HIE. By the end of the first day, patterns of weakness that reflect the distribution of cerebral injury from a generalized hypoxic-ischemic insult may emerge. Affected full-term infants may demonstrate quadriparesis with predominant proximal limb weakness. This pattern of weakness derives from ischemia in the watershed or parasagittal region of the brain, which correspond to the border zones of circulation between the anterior and the middle cerebral arteries and the middle and the posterior cerebral arteries. Affected premature infants may have weakness primarily in the lower extremities because of perinatal ischemic injury of motor fibers subserving the legs. These fibers lie dorsal and lateral to the external angles of the lateral ventricles. Focal injury resulting from focal ischemia (stroke) may result in focal deficits reflective of the vascular territory in which the injury has occurred. These patterns are relatively subtle. As many as 70% of infants with moderate or severe HIE experience seizures by the end of the first day after birth.

Focal and multifocal ischemic brain injury may occur during the perinatal period. Such injury, most often infarction, occurs in a vascular distribution. Prenatal cerebral infarctions have been identified by intrauterine ultrasonography. In one autopsy study of neonates, 32 of 592 (5%) infants had had cerebral infarctions. Among neonates surviving only a few hours after birth, several had infarctions with subacute or chronic histologic characteristics, indicating that the ischemic insult occurred before parturition. Focal seizures are the heralding sign of neonatal stroke. Although clinical signs corresponding to the area of infarction are expected, they may be absent. Neonatal strokes may follow uneventful deliveries and may occur in otherwise normal-appearing infants. Stroke may also accompany asphyxia, coagulopathy, polycythemia, and sepsis. A predilection for these ischemic lesions to occur in the territory of the middle cerebral artery, especially the left, has been noted and remains unexplained.

A direct relationship between motor and cognitive deficits at 1 year of age and the severity of acidosis observed at birth in asphyxiated and symptomatic neonates has been described. The extent of these sequelae is dependent not only on the occurrence of asphyxia but also on its duration. The three stages of HIE also correlate with outcome at 1 year of age. Those neonates with mild (stage 1) HIE or those who demonstrate moderate (stage 2) HIE for less than 5 days usually develop normally. Persistence of moderate encephalopathy or appearance of severe (stage 3) HIE is associated with seizures and motor and cognitive delay during follow-up. Children with mild HIE as neonates tend to be free of handicap in motor, cognitive, and school performance. Greater impairment of performance in each of these developmental spheres is found among children who exhibited moderate or severe neonatal HIE.

The likelihood of long-term neurologic sequelae after HIE is increased by the presence of neonatal seizures. The EEG may provide valuable prognostic information after the occurrence of seizure. Interictal background abnormalities, such as a burst-suppression pattern, persistently low voltage, and electrocerebral inactivity, are highly correlated with poor outcome. Conversely, infants with normal EEGs or those revealing only maturational delay have much more favorable prognoses.

Neuroimaging is useful in determination of prognosis. Head ultrasonography has shown that severe periventricular intraparenchymal echodensities followed by evidence of tissue injury (cyst formation) are correlated with later motor and cognitive deficits in premature infants. Magnetic resonance imaging (MRI) performed early in the neonatal course of hypoxic-ischemic brain injury provides useful prognostic information. Most infants with MRI evidence of basal ganglia "hemorrhage," periventricular leukomalacia, or multicystic encephalomalacia after asphyxia ultimately demonstrate neurodevelopmental abnormalities. Diffusion-weighted imaging (DWI) reveals evidence of neonatal brain injury earlier than can T1- and T2-weighted pulse sequences. Indeed, DWI reveals focal injury when standard MRI and computed tomography (CT) are normal. Such early identification of brain injury serves as an important prerequisite for institution of effective therapy when it becomes available.

Idiopathic Cerebral Infarction in the Full-Term Neonate

Focal seizures have been identified as the most common clinical feature indicating the presence of stroke in the full-term nonasphyxiated infant. Even though lateralized findings on neurologic examination may be found, they need not be present as hallmarks of cerebral infarction. Furthermore, diminished movement of extremities on the side of the focal seizure may represent a postictal Todd paralysis rather than paresis from upper motor neuron injury caused by cerebral infarction. The recognition of focal seizure as a manifestation of cerebral infarction is important, because this may serve as the only sign of the cerebrovascular event. Initially, other neurologic signs may be absent. However, as the child grows, motor or cognitive impairment may become progressively more apparent during the first 1 to 3 years of life.

The cause of the cerebral infarction frequently escapes detection among neonates who have not been subjected to prenatal asphyxia. Indeed, in 37 of 51 reported cases of neonatal stroke, a cause could not always be identified. Causes of neonatal stroke that have been identified include those of embolic and thrombotic origins. Interestingly, a left hemispheric location has been noted to be the most common area involved; the reason for this neuroanatomic predilection has not been discovered. Emboli from placenta may lodge in cerebral vessels and result in stroke. In addition, congenital heart defects involving right-to-left shunts through septal defects or through a patent ductus arteriosus serve as settings for embolic stroke in neonates. Coagulopathies caused by congenital defects of coagulation (factor VIII, protein C or S, or antithrombin III deficiency and others) or by sepsis-induced disseminated intravascular coagulation may underlie neonatal embolic stroke. Fetal head trauma during labor and delivery that results in endothelial damage to cerebral vessels occasionally leads to thrombosis and resultant focal ischemia of the brain. Polycythemia and hypotension can each lead to intravascular stasis and rheologic abnormalities, resulting in cerebrovascular thrombosis in neonates. Meningitis and encephalitis cause diffuse or localized thrombosis as a result of vascular inflammation, leading to hemostasis and thrombosis.

Evidence of localized dysfunction of brain found on EEG consists of focal, persistent voltage reduction or of marked focal slowing and sharp wave activity. In some instances, EEG evidence of clinically observed seizures may be found. Each of these findings may exist while the EEG remains relatively normal over other regions of brain. The areas of electrical abnormality should correspond to the affected areas of brain revealed by neuroimaging. Cranial CT demonstrates a low-density region that eventually evolves into atrophy. Visualization of the involved area should not require contrast enhancement. MRI demonstrates low or isointense signal intensity on T1-weighted images and high signal intensity on T2-weighted images as a result of increased water content in the infarcted region of brain. DWI reveals the local area of edema before any other neuroimaging procedure and must be performed if the CT and MRI are normal.

Treatment is both supportive and symptomatic. Anticonvulsant treatment is given if seizures have occurred (see Chapter 39). Phenobarbital is often used and is administered in a loading dose of 20 mg/kg. Maintenance therapy of 3 to 5 mg/kg/day is sufficient. Alternatively, phenytoin may be beneficial because it does not reduce the level of consciousness. Short-acting benzodiazepines are helpful in the acute situation. Attention should be given to hydration status, acid-base balance, and hematocrit.

Estimation of developmental outcome is difficult. The periods of follow-up reported in neonatal stroke series have been highly variable. Although seizures frequently abate, chronic motor deficits often become apparent. MRI evidence of cerebral infarction may be helpful. Most infants with evidence of marked white matter damage or cystic/multicystic encephalomalacia have proved to have neurodevelopmental abnormalities on short-term follow-up. Nonetheless, neonates with no signs of HIE who present with focal seizures may develop with minimal sequelae.

Polycythemia

Neonates are much more commonly polycythemic (central venous hematocrit >65%) than are older children. Polycythemia has been estimated to be present in 1.5% of newborns. It is most commonly encountered in neonates who are born at high altitude, those who are small for gestational age, infants of diabetic mothers, or recipients in twin-twin transfusion syndrome; it may also be seen in neonatal hyperthyroidism or adrenogenital syndrome. Clinical signs of the elevated hematocrit are present in some but not all affected infants and include plethora, acrocyanosis, impaired renal function, poor feeding, apnea, tachypnea, hypoglycemia, and indirect hyperbilirubinemia. Neurologic symptoms include jitteriness, irritability, lethargy, seizures, and focal motor deficits.

Most cases of polycythemia are idiopathic or secondary to acquired abnormalities of fetal oxygen delivery. Nonetheless, other polycythemias bearing autosomal dominant or recessive inheritance patterns have been described. These familial polycythemias are associated with mutant hemoglobins that create abnormalities of oxygen delivery.

Polycythemia and its resultant hyperviscosity may contribute to stroke in neonates. Inadequate cerebral perfusion and cerebrovascular thrombosis cause cerebral ischemia. Although most of the systemic complications of polycythemia resolve with adequate treatment, neurologic signs frequently do not. Cerebral infarction resulting from polycythemia-related ischemia causes deficits that resolve either slowly or not at all. Neurologic sequelae may be present in up to 35% of neonates with symptomatic polycythemia.

If signs of polycythemia are found in a neonate, further evaluation should be undertaken. Venous or arterial hematocrit, rather than capillary hematocrit, should be measured. If the family history and physical examination findings suggest a hereditary polycythemia, hemoglobin electrophoresis should be undertaken. Routine hemoglobin electrophoresis does not elucidate high oxygen-affinity hemoglobinopathies in all cases. If clinical suspicion is high, the heat instability test for unstable hemoglobins and oxygen dissociation assays can be utilized. Neuroimaging should be used to assess for cerebral infarction.

Treatment of symptomatic patients consists of hematocrit reduction by a partial exchange transfusion until the hematocrit is reduced to 50% to 55%. The equation to calculate the amount of blood removed and the amount of normal saline infused is

$$\text{volume (milliliters)} = (\text{current hematocrit} - 50) \times \text{weight in kilograms} \times 90 \text{ mL/current hematocrit}$$

Neonatal Cerebral Venous Thrombosis

Thrombosis may occur in cerebral veins that conduct deoxygenated blood from the parenchyma to the dural sinus system. These sinuses—the sagittal, straight, transverse, cavernous, and petrous—then convey the blood to the jugular veins. Occlusion of flow anywhere in these venous conduits leads to ischemia, infarction, and even hemorrhage. Infection, dehydration, polycythemia, congenital heart disease, extracorporeal membrane oxygenation, and protein C deficiency and other hypercoagulable states such as factor V Leiden and methyltetrahydrofolate reductase mutations have all been implicated as causes of cerebral venous thrombosis in neonates. However, often no cause is found for this occlusion of the cerebral venous system in neonates. Most affected patients are full-term infants. Adjacent areas of brain parenchyma reveal neuropathologic changes typical of infarction.

The only signs may be lethargy and focal seizures. The features of slowly developing focal motor deficits, headache, and cranial nerve dysfunction found in older children and adults with cerebral venous thrombosis is seldom observed.

Neuroimaging reveals the venous stasis best if magnetic resonance phase imaging, which detects blood flow, or magnetic resonance venography is performed, as well as conventional T1- and T2-weighted imaging. Treatment of underlying infection, metabolic disorder, or coagulopathy is necessary. However, if the cerebral venous thrombosis appears to be idiopathic, no anticoagulation is necessary. Follow-up information has been limited, but the neurologic prognosis appears good in the idiopathic cases.

Intracranial Hemorrhage in the Neonate

Intracranial hemorrhage occurs in neonates in one of four different neuroanatomic distributions: subdural (SDH), subarachnoid (SAH), intraparenchymal (IPH), or intraventricular (IVH).

Whereas SDH occurs more commonly in full-term infants, the other three types of hemorrhage are more common in premature infants.

Subdural Hemorrhage

SDH in neonates usually results from head trauma during birth. Thus, factors of labor and delivery promoting the application of increased force on the fetal head are liable to promote SDH. Cephalopelvic disproportion, rigidity of the bony pelvis, prolonged duration of labor, unusual presentations, or the need for prolonged manipulation or forceps application may each generate increased forces on the fetal head and cause SDH. As a result, shearing forces may create tears in the vein of Galen or tears of superficial cerebral veins. If forces are extreme, tears at the junction of falx and tentorium can generate large subdural blood collections in the relatively small posterior fossa, culminating in compression of the brainstem and cerebellar tonsillar herniation. The incidence of SDH has steadily declined recently as a result of improved obstetric practice.

Clinical features of SDH depend on the location and size of the hemorrhage. Tentorial laceration (Fig. 41-1) can cause stupor or even coma. Pupillary and extraocular movement abnormalities are common. Dystonic postures such as retrocollis or opisthotonos are seen. Finally, abnormalities of respiratory pattern regulation such as apneustic or ataxic respirations are seen and signify imminent

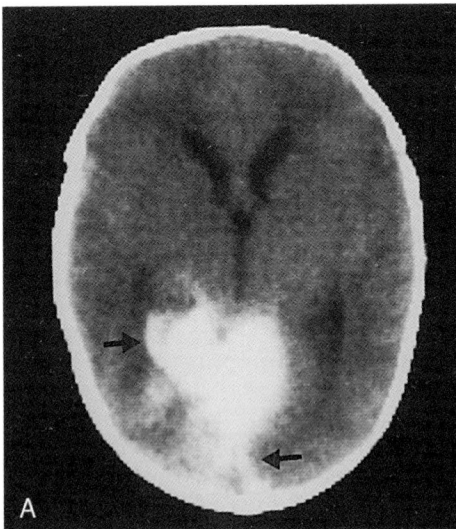 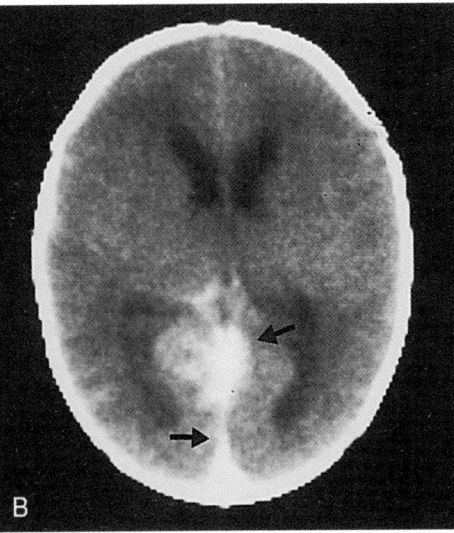

Figure 41-1. A and B, Generalized tonic seizures, lethargy progressing to coma, and irregular respiratory pattern were observed in a 1-day-old full-term infant. Cranial computed tomographic scan demonstrates a hyperdense region emanating from the falx and tentorium (*arrows*) caused by traumatic tear of tentorium, which resulted in hemorrhage from the straight sinus.

respiratory arrest. Less severe SDHs in the posterior fossa evolve more slowly and cause less severe brainstem dysfunction. Subdural collections of blood over the cerebral surfaces that result from tears of superficial cerebral veins may be asymptomatic. Minimal manifestation consists of irritability. With time the blood may liquefy and draw water into the area by osmotic forces, thus expanding the size of the lesion. If the collection is sufficiently large, seizures occur. Greater pressure may cause oculomotor dysfunction, accompanied by pupillary dilation and ablated pupillary light responses.

SDH may escape diagnosis in the first few weeks of life and appear later as a chronic subdural effusion; in this situation, the clinician must suspect child abuse (see Chapter 36). Such an occurrence is marked by a rapidly enlarging head circumference and increased transillumination of the skull. There may also be a combination of acute and chronic SDH in cases of child abuse. Symptomatic SDH is often treated with subdural taps (through the anterior fontanel) to remove the blood and relieve the pressure.

Subarachnoid Hemorrhage

Blood can occupy the subarachnoid space in one of two ways. First, blood may reach the subarachnoid space after hemorrhage has occurred in the cerebral parenchyma or in the periventricular region. Second, SAH may result from disruption of the superficial leptomeningeal arteries or of the fragile vessels bridging the subarachnoid space; disruption of either vascular structure leads to direct bleeding into the subarachnoid space, so-called primary SAH. Primary SAH commonly occurs after hypoxic-ischemic brain insults and after fetal head trauma.

Mild SAH is clinically the most common type, occurring as an occult phenomenon with few if any manifestations. Greater amounts of blood collecting over the convexities may result in focal motor deficits and often benign seizures. Large SAH accumulating over the convexities has been associated not only with seizures but with infarction of underlying cerebral cortex. The presence of accompanying infarction is indicated by the occurrence of focal seizures. A history of difficult labor and delivery may be associated with large SAH. Cerebral infarction in the setting of SAH has been observed more commonly in full-term infants than in premature infants.

When SAH is mild, the neurologic outcome can be good. Even in cases of SAH accompanied by an infrequent seizure or cerebral infarction, the prognosis is often favorable. Adverse consequences appear to be more dependent on the severity of any underlying intrapartum trauma or hypoxic-ischemic brain injury.

Intraparenchymal and Intraventricular Hemorrhage

IPH of the brain occurs in both full-term and preterm infants. Cerebral hemorrhage in the absence of IVH occurs most commonly in full-term infants. Hemorrhage into the parenchyma of the cerebral hemispheres can be caused by head trauma, vascular malformation, coagulopathy, thrombocytopenia, tumor, or infarction. A common cause of prenatal, intrapartum, and postnatal hemorrhage is alloimmune thrombocytopenia, caused by acquired antiplatelet antibodies when a mother becomes sensitized to paternal antigens on fetal platelets. Maternal immune thrombocytopenia may also affect the fetus, producing thrombocytopenia in utero. However, the incidence of neonatal cerebral hemorrhage is much lower in immune thrombocytopenia than in alloimmune thrombocytopenia. Vitamin K deficiency should be considered for breast-fed full-term neonates who present with intracranial hemorrhage. In the absence of recognized coagulation or anatomic abnormalities, cerebral hemispheric IPH has been attributed to hemorrhagic infarction. In premature infants, parenchymal hemorrhage most often occurs in conjunction with severe IVH. Hemorrhage from the friable, unsupported germinal matrix leads to accumulation of intraventricular blood and, often, ventricular distention. These events, in turn, cause impairment of blood flow in the medullary veins located in the periventricular white matter, preventing blood drainage into the greater cerebral venous system. Eventually, the periventricular venous congestion leads to ischemia and a resultant venous infarction.

Developmental outcome in full-term infants with IPH depends on the location and extent of the underlying cause. The occurrence of posthemorrhagic hydrocephalus or of moderate to severe asphyxia is predictive of abnormal outcomes, including motor impairment or cognitive delay. In premature infants, the simultaneous occurrence of IVH with IPH carries high risk for major motor deficits and marked cognitive impairment.

Evaluation of Stroke in Infants

Head ultrasonography detects areas of increased echogenicity in the cerebral cortex. In especially severe cases of ischemia, increased echogenicity of injured subcortical structures such as the thalamus and basal ganglia can be appreciated. Ischemic cortical injury involving the territory of the middle cerebral artery (frontal and parietal lobe regions surrounding the central sulcus) is better revealed by ultrasonography than are other vascular territories. The principal advantages of cranial ultrasonography are its easy portability to the patient's bedside and its lack of radiation exposure to the infant.

CT of the brain is useful, particularly for evaluation of full-term infants after a suspected cerebral insult. Diffuse injury appears as abnormal generalized attenuation throughout the cerebral parenchyma with loss of the distinction between gray and white matter; this abnormality may represent cerebral edema. Focal and multifocal brain injury is readily detected by cranial CT.

MRI scans obtained within the first 4 days of life in full-term infants with signs of severe HIE reveal white matter abnormalities and indistinct gray matter–white matter junctions on T2-weighted images. DWI can identify areas of recent infarct even earlier than conventional T1- and T2-weighted images. Subsequent images can show chronic changes such as cerebral atrophy, paucity of white matter, delayed myelination, and ventriculomegaly. MRI has proved useful in documenting delay of myelination, a sequel to perinatal ischemic white matter injury not readily discerned with CT. This additional capability has provided a potential explanation for subtle motor deficits found in children who have ischemic brain injury in the perinatal period. As observed in MRI studies of adults, neonatal focal cerebral ischemic injuries may be identified early in their course. MRI also detects neonatal hypoxic-ischemic injuries of basal ganglia not well detected by either head ultrasonography or CT. Moreover, MRI with venography is the procedure of choice in the neonatal period for identification of venous thrombosis.

Laboratory testing for the wide variety of etiologic factors underlying stroke should be conducted. The causes include infection, liver dysfunction, coagulopathy, prothrombotic states, organic and amino acid inborn errors of metabolism, urea cycle disorders, and mitochondrial abnormalities.

CHILDREN AGED 1 TO 13 YEARS

When stroke occurs in children, focal symptoms are reported and corresponding localized deficits are noted on the neurologic examination, which correlate neuroanatomically with the involved region of the CNS. In older children able to cooperate, findings elicited are helpful in localizing the site of the cerebrovascular event. Lateralized weakness often signifies injury to the contralateral hemisphere, including the regions governing movement. Such motor impairment accompanied by cranial nerve dysfunction on the side of the head *opposite* to the side of extremity weakness suggests brainstem infarction at a location above the pyramidal decussation. Findings of the sensory examination also may be helpful. Preservation of primary sensory modalities provides assessment of spinothalamic axis (pain and temperature) and posterior column (proprioception) integrity. Loss of pain and temperature sensation on one side of the body, combined with motor weakness, and the presence of proprioceptive deficits on the other side indicate that the cerebrovascular event is in the spinal cord. If the same distribution of motor and sensory disturbances occurs but is accompanied by cranial nerve dysfunction, a brainstem site of injury is likely. Finally, impairment of cortically based sensations such as graphesthesia and stereognosis on one side of the body implies a *contralateral* hemispheric cause of the observed cortical sensory deficit.

Analysis of language function in the older child may provide help in localizing the region of the cerebrovascular event. Unilateral lesions of the dominant hemisphere involving the frontal lobe immediately anterior to the motor strip supplying the face results in a characteristic speech disturbance. *Broca (nonfluent) aphasia* consists of the patient's inability to utter or to write the words or phrases that he or she wishes to express. Although the patient knows the thoughts that he or she wishes to express, the volitional motor function for written or oral expression cannot be mustered. Infarction in the more posterior superior temporal lobe results in an aphasia of a different type: *Wernicke aphasia,* characterized by marked impairment of auditory comprehension. Comprehension of written matter may be impaired as well. Although the patient remains fluent in speech, language is peppered with unintelligible utterances that are meaningless

(neologisms) or are similar but incorrect versions of the intended word (paraphasias). The larger the injury to this region, the more severe is the impairment of language. Speech in most right-handed people and in 50% of left-handed people is governed by the left hemisphere (so-called left hemispheric dominance). The remaining minority share right hemispheric dominance.

The causes of stroke in 1- to 13-year-old children may be considered in two general groups: (1) ischemic stroke and (2) intracranial hemorrhage. The ischemic category comprises embolic, thrombotic, and hypotensive causes of stroke. The category of intracranial hemorrhage includes both IPH and SAH.

Ischemic Stroke in Children

Congenital Heart Disease

Congenital heart disease remains the most common diagnosable cause of stroke in childhood. Children with cyanotic congenital heart disease (right-to-left shunts or mixing lesions) face the greatest risk (see Chapter 10). An embolic stroke constitutes the most common cerebrovascular event. Cardiac defects involving right-to-left shunts allow emboli originating in peripheral venous circulation to bypass their filtration and removal by the pulmonary vascular bed. Thus, emboli entering the heart via venous return may be shunted to the peripheral arterial circulation, only to lodge in the cerebrovascular tree (Fig. 41-2).

Patent foramen ovale contributes significantly to the occurrence of stroke in children and young adults. Echocardiographic evaluation of young patients who have had stroke reveals patent foramen ovale or evidence of right-to-left shunting in many. Transesophageal echocardiography conducted with Valsalva bubble studies for evidence of direct right-to-left flow is the most useful diagnostic test.

Valvular defects can cause stroke. Mitral valve prolapse may contribute to the occurrence of embolic stroke in the young. Small emboli are dislodged from the abnormal valve leaflets. Mitral valve prolapse has been estimated to underlie 20% to 30% of strokes in patients younger than 30 years. Echocardiography in both

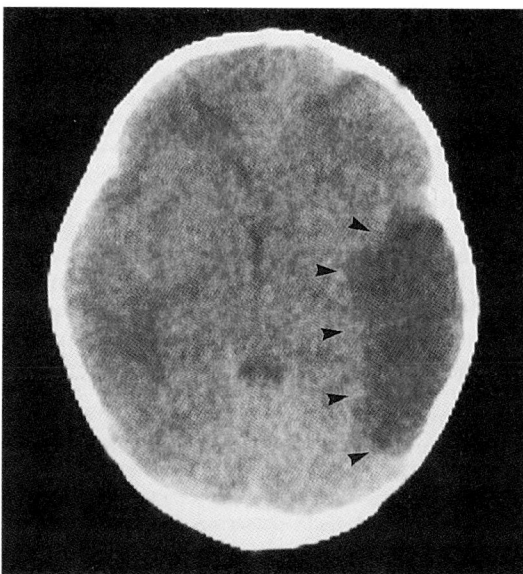

Figure 41-2. Cranial computed tomographic scan of a 3-month-old boy with trisomy 21 and tetralogy of Fallot who, after cardiac catheterization, had focal seizures involving the right side of the face and right arm. Region of hypodensity in left hemisphere (*arrowheads*) reflects infarction of the left middle cerebral artery territory, most likely caused by embolic occlusion of that vessel.

two-dimensional and M modes proves most helpful in discerning the cardiac valvular abnormality. Rheumatic valvular disease (mitral, aortic), once a common cause of embolic stroke, has become an infrequent cause of childhood stroke. Infected valves in bacterial endocarditis pose considerable risk for the occurrence of embolic stroke (native, prosthetic, rheumatic, or congenitally abnormal valve). Infective mitral and aortic valvular vegetations may dislodge and travel distally to occlude cerebral arteries. The most common organisms found are streptococci and staphylococci (see Chapter 11). Even after vegetations have been successfully sterilized, they may embolize and cause stroke. Emboli from infected valvular vegetations may embolize, travel to the cerebral vasculature, and seed the adventitia of the cerebral vessel. The resultant infection and inflammation results in weakening of the vessel and development of a *mycotic aneurysm.* Aneurysms may lie dormant for some time before their rupture leads to SAH or IPH and resultant neurologic signs.

Procoagulopathies

Several disorders of coagulation can lead to embolic or thrombotic stroke. Adverse consequences of antiphospholipid antibodies have been identified in all age groups. Children, adolescents, and young adults experience the cerebrovascular consequences of these antibodies most often. Antiphospholipid antibodies, including the lupus anticoagulant (LAC), are polyclonal antibodies found in serum that are able to bind to both neutral and negatively charged phospholipids (see Chapter 50). LAC and anticardiolipin antibodies were first associated with thrombotic or embolic cerebrovascular events in patients with systemic lupus erythematosus (SLE). Subsequently, patients suffering stroke with no evidence of underlying immune-mediated illness other than the LAC or anticardiolipin antibody were found. The antibody prolongs the partial thromboplastin time (PTT) in vitro but acts as a procoagulant in vivo. A common finding associated with coagulation testing among children with arterial ischemic stroke is the presence of anticardiolipin antibody. The presence of these antibodies in a patient who concurrently smokes cigarettes, has findings positive for antinuclear antibodies, or suffers from hyperlipidemia may impart a higher risk for stroke than if the patient carries the antibody alone. The antibody's presence is indicated by a prolonged PTT and a falsely positive serum Venereal Disease Research Laboratory result. The antibody's presence can be conclusively demonstrated functionally and immunologically. Although cerebral infarction and TIAs constitute the most frequently observed neurologic manifestations related to the presence of these antibodies, migraine headache, seizures, and monocular visual disturbances are also associated. Therapy for patients with antiphospholipid antibodies who have suffered stroke has not been fully substantiated by randomized prospective study. Nonetheless, low-dose anticoagulation has been advocated.

Absence of specific serum proteins that act as inhibitors of coagulation may lead to stroke in children. Two of these proteins, protein S and protein C, have been associated with thrombotic or embolic cerebrovascular disease in the young. Protein C and its cofactor protein S act as anticoagulants and synergistically attenuate coagulation by deactivating the activated forms of factors V and VIII. Absence of (or resistance to) either of these proteins disrupts the balance of coagulation toward increased spontaneous clotting and can result in stroke. In addition, antithrombin III opposes the action of the activated forms of factors II, IX, X, XI, and XII through the irreversible formation of inactivating complexes with these factors. Deficiencies of proteins S and C as well as of antithrombin III may cause arterial thrombotic or embolic stroke or venous infarction. Although their deficiencies are often congenital, they may be acquired through liver disease or nephrotic syndrome. Factor V Leiden, prothrombin 20210A, and lipoprotein A are all important factors that may contribute to the pathogenesis of arterial ischemic stroke in children. Elevated lipoprotein A, protein C deficiency, and sickle cell anemia

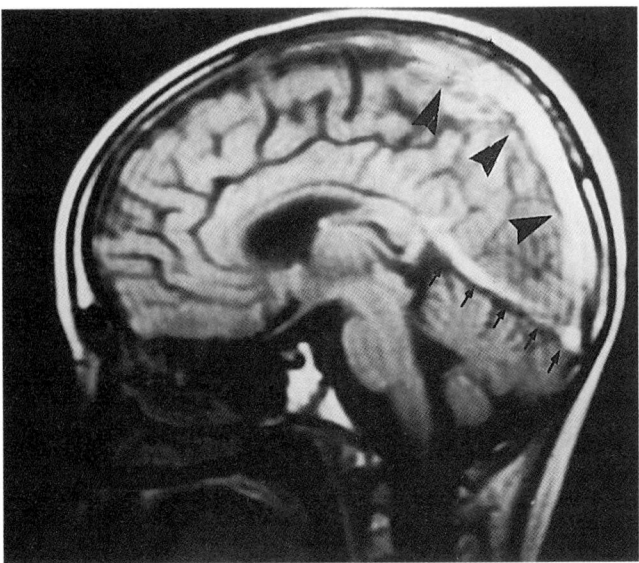

Figure 41-3. Cranial T1-weighted magnetic resonance imaging scan of a 9-year-old boy treated with L-asparaginase for acute lymphoblastic leukemia, who experienced new headache, seizures, and lethargy. Bright signal in superior sagittal sinus (*arrowheads*) and in straight sinus (*arrows*) denotes L-asparaginase–induced cerebral venous thrombosis.

increase the risk of recurrent strokes. A screening battery of tests, including prothrombin time, PTT, and specific immunologic and functional testing for the proteins suspected of being deficient is essential for diagnosis. Treatment with anticoagulation therapy after stroke has been recommended.

Cancer and its treatment may predispose children to cerebrovascular ischemic events. Promyelocytic leukemia and its treatment have been observed to provoke disseminated intravascular coagulation, leading to stroke. Lymphoreticular cancers more than solid tumors have been linked to thrombotic and embolic strokes. In addition, dural sinus and cerebral venous thrombosis have been found after therapy with L-asparaginase (Fig. 41-3). TIAs occurring after induction chemotherapy for acute lymphoblastic leukemia have been observed. Cranial radiation therapy may induce an occlusive vasculopathy, leading to focal cerebral ischemia.

Autoimmune Disorders

Autoimmune disorders may cause neurologic disturbance and cerebrovascular involvement (Table 41-4). Symptoms of abrupt onset with accompanying deficits referable to the CNS have long been associated with SLE. A CNS vasculitis had been presumed to underlie the CNS manifestations of SLE; however, autopsy study of patients suffering from SLE revealed a virtual absence of cerebrovascular inflammation. Rather, small areas of infarction relate to proliferative changes in cerebral arterioles that lead to luminal occlusion. Large areas of infarction are more probably related to LAC-derived thromboembolism or to embolism from the sterile cardiac valve leaflet vegetations associated with SLE (Libman-Sacks endocarditis). Additional causes of CNS illness include thrombocytopenic hemorrhage, steroid-induced pseudotumor or psychosis, and CNS infection.

True cerebral arterial vasculitis may be an isolated disease or seen in association with recognizable systemic autoimmune disorders. Isolated angiitis of the CNS may affect small, medium-sized, or large vessels. Multiple regions of infarction are often found on MRI. Neuropathologic evidence of polymorphonuclear leukocyte or monocyte infiltration leading to intimal proliferation and vessel wall necrosis is found. The inflammation affects blood flow and predisposes to thrombosis.

Table 41-4. Autoimmune Disorders Associated with Central Nervous System (CNS) Involvement

Disorder	CNS Manifestations
Systemic lupus erythematosus	Migraine headache, seizures, stroke, cerebellar dysfunction, transverse myelopathy, aseptic meningitis, psychosis
Mixed connective tissue disease	Seizures, stroke, cerebellar dysfunction, trigeminal neuropathy
Polyarteritis nodosum	Migraine headache, stroke, subarachnoid hemorrhage, seizures
Wegener granulomatosis	Migraine headache, subarachnoid hemorrhage, stroke
Takayasu arteritis	Seizure, stroke
Henoch-Schönlein purpura	Headache, stroke, seizures, chorea
Primary CNS vasculitis	Headache, stroke, seizure

Table 41-5. Genetic Causes of Stroke

Thrombotic/Embolic Stroke
Homocystinuria or elevated homocysteine levels
Fabry disease
Fibromuscular dysplasia
Procoagulopathies*
Sickle cell anemia

Hemorrhage
Factor VIII deficiency
Factor IX deficiency
Factor XI deficiency
Familial intracranial aneurysm
Sickle cell disease
Familial cavernous angioma
Glanzmann thrombasthenia
X-linked thrombocytopenia

Unknown Mechanism
Familial porencephaly
Organic acidemia
Mitochondrial disorders

Rare Monogenic Disorders
APP, CST3, BRI genes (autosomal dominant amyloid angiopathies)
NOTCH3 gene (cerebral autosomal dominant arteriopathy with subcortical infarcts and leukoencephalopathy [CADASIL])
KRIT1 gene (cavernous angiomas)

*Protein C, protein S, and antithrombin III deficiencies and factor V Leiden or prothrombin 20210A mutations.

Stroke may occur in the course of *polyarteritis nodosa.* Involvement of the CNS is found in 20% to 40% of such patients.

Wegener granulomatosus, a necrotizing vasculitis of the upper pulmonary system, rarely affects the CNS; stroke is uncommon. When the CNS is affected, extension of sinus or nasal inflammation into the basilar skull frequently has occurred.

Mixed connective tissue disease, which clinically overlaps with polymyositis, SLE, and progressive systemic sclerosis, can involve the CNS. Cranial neuropathy, most commonly trigeminal nerve dysfunction, has been the most frequently cited deficit. Stroke manifesting as sudden-onset hemiparesis and aphasia has been reported in children afflicted with mixed connective tissue disease.

Takayasu arteritis, involving the aorta and its principal branches, has been associated with thrombotic stroke. Inflammation-induced luminal constriction leading to thrombosis is thought to cause cerebral ischemia in children. Angiographic improvement of vessels in the carotid tree is observed with immunosuppressive treatment. Necrotizing arteritis with inflammatory infiltrate has been found in both meningeal and cerebral vessels of children suffering from *Henoch-Schönlein purpura.* Both fixed and transient deficits may occur in this disorder.

Treatment with steroids or other immunosuppressive agents proves most helpful in these disorders. Long-term anticoagulation has not been studied but should be considered with appropriate caution in acute situations.

Inflammation of cerebral vessels may also occur in the course of *bacterial meningitis.* The subarachnoid arteries become immersed in exudate. The vessel wall is affected by the inflammatory process. If this condition allowed to proceed long enough, thrombophlebitis ensues. Vascular occlusion results, with consequent features of stroke. Antibiotics combined with steroids early in the course of treatment form the cornerstone of therapy.

Metabolic Disorders Causing Stroke

Homocystinuria, a disorder of homocysteine metabolism, can cause thrombotic stroke in children. Abnormal homocysteine metabolism results from one of three inheritable enzymatic defects. The most striking phenotype results from deficiency of cystathionine synthetase, the enzyme that facilitates the catabolism of homocysteine to cystathionine. Accumulation of not only homocysteine but also methionine results. Children affected by this autosomal recessive disorder (Table 41-5) have marfanoid habitus, global developmental delay, lens dislocation, and thromboembolism. Thromboemboli may travel to cerebrovascular beds, causing stroke. Serum hyperhomocystinuria injures the vascular endothelium. The denuded vessel wall then becomes a site for thrombosis. The resulting thrombus may remain at its site of origin or it may embolize to a distal locus. Therefore, stroke may have thrombotic or embolic characteristics. Both arterial and venous infarctions may result. Treatment is dietary and aimed at reducing levels of homocysteine in serum. Pyridoxine administration and methionine restriction are effective in 30% to 40% of treated patients. Some patients without homocystinuria but with elevated homocysteine levels may be at risk for vascular morbid conditions, including stroke.

Sulfite oxidase deficiency, another autosomal recessive disorder, results in the accumulation of serum sulfite. The associated phenotype may result from deficiency of either the enzyme or its associated and essential pterin-containing molybdenum cofactor. Mental retardation, seizures, lens displacement, and acute hemiplegia result. The mechanism of the strokelike episodes has not been fully elucidated. It is possible that ischemic mechanisms are not involved and that direct metabolic neurotoxicity accounts for the sudden onset of deficits resembling those of stroke. Sulfites and *S*-sulfocysteine accumulate in urine. Dietary attempts to reduce sulfite accumulation have been unsuccessful.

Fabry disease, a lipid storage disease attributable to ceramide trihexosidase deficiency, results in accumulation of the sphingolipid trihexoside in the kidneys, vascular endothelium, and corneas. Symptoms become apparent in childhood or adolescence. Angiokeratomas and painful paresthesia often constitute the first symptoms. Renal failure follows. However, because of endothelial accumulation of sphingolipid in vessel walls, cerebrovascular occlusion results in stroke. Recurrent stroke is common in this rare X-linked disorder. Supportive care, as well as recombinant enzyme therapy, and treatment designed to improve renal function and minimize pain are instituted.

The manifestations of *mitochondrial disorders* include recurrent and sometimes catastrophic stroke. The syndrome of mitochondrial encephalomyopathy, lactic acidosis, and strokelike episodes (MELAS) manifests in childhood and results from a mutation of mitochondrial DNA. The most common biochemical finding is a deficiency of complex I of the electron transport chain. An elevated serum or cerebrospinal fluid lactate level serves as its chemical signature, and molecular confirmation of the diagnosis can be secured from blood. Although some features of MELAS are shared by other mitochondrial syndromes, hemiparesis of abrupt onset is fairly specific for this syndrome. Excruciating headache resembling migraine may precede the strokelike episodes. Seizures and sensorineural hearing loss are almost always present at some point in the course of the illness. Neuropathologic study of brains from patients with MELAS has shown cystic cavities and necrosis of cortex with relative sparing of white matter.

Other metabolic disorders have been associated with stroke in childhood. Urea cycle defects, especially ornithine transcarbamoylase deficiency manifesting in girls, can cause stroke. Deficiency of arginase, another important enzyme of the urea cycle, has been observed in association with hemiparesis and diparesis of subacute onset. Finally, familial lipoprotein disorders, especially those featuring a dearth of high-density lipoprotein or an abundance of triglycerides, have been associated with stroke in children. In most cases, a family history of hyperlipidemia is found.

Moyamoya Disease

Moyamoya disease commonly affects children younger than 15 years and manifests with TIAs or sudden-onset fixed motor deficits. Progressive narrowing and occlusion of the intracranial portion of the internal carotid arteries are characteristic. Endothelial proliferation, fibrosis, and intimal thickening characterize the vascular disease. Resultant proliferation of collateral vessels from the basilar skull circulation creates an intricate latticework of compensatory blood flow. The appearance on angiography is characteristic and consists of a fine vascular network located at the base of the brain. *Moyamoya* means "hazy" or "puff of smoke" (Fig. 41-4).

Children usually present with acute hemiplegia as a result of uncompensated occlusion of the internal carotid artery. Because the anatomic abnormality is often bilateral, the hemiplegia may alternate. Disturbance of fine motor function has been observed. Chorea has been reported in association with moyamoya syndrome. Although the vascular abnormality may be congenital, moyamoya syndrome can occur as a sequel to a primary disorder causing internal carotid artery occlusion. It has been found in children with sickle cell disease, neurofibromatosis, tuberculous meningitis, and fibromuscular dysplasia. Evidence suggesting a hereditary origin in some cases has been reported in Japan.

Optimal treatment has not been determined. Evidence of inflammation has not been found. Calcium channel blockers have been reported to increase collateral vessel diameter, improve perfusion, and ameliorate neurologic symptoms. Several surgical procedures (extracranial-intracranial or dural-intracranial bypass) designed to reestablish effective perfusion of endangered brain have been performed.

Sickle Cell Disease

Acute hemiplegia may be found in children with sickle cell disease (see Chapter 48). Cerebral infarction occurs in approximately 6% of patients. It may be an isolated event, or it may occur in the setting of a sickle crisis. Neurologic signs include hemiparesis, aphasia, and visual disturbances. Cerebral infarction may also be clinically silent. Neuroimaging studies, particularly MRI, reveal that stroke occurs in watershed distributions between two cerebrovascular territories, affecting both the gray and white matter of the cortex. The proposed pathophysiologic mechanisms encompass both sickling in large vessels, leading to thrombotic hypoperfusion, and diminished flow in small cerebral vessels as a result of the decreased compliance of sickled erythrocytes. Cerebral vessels reveal endothelial proliferation, disruption of the elastic lamina, and stenosis. Cerebral hyperemia

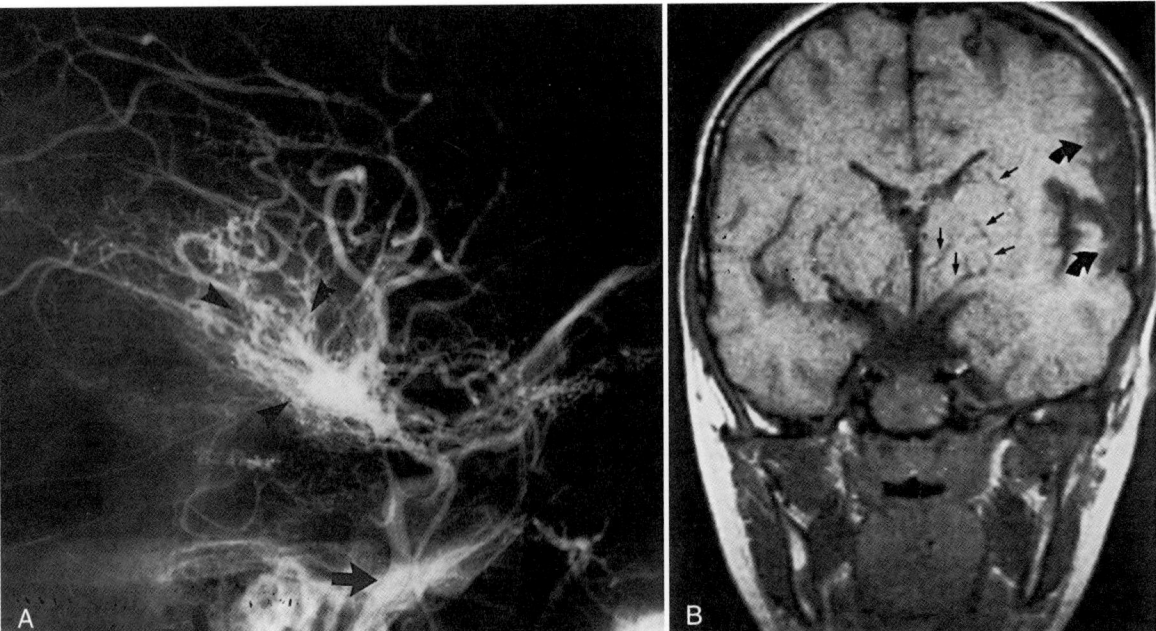

Figure 41-4. Sudden onset of right hemiparesis in a 6-year-old boy. **A,** Cerebral angiogram shows left internal carotid artery (*arrows*) leading to a highly arborized, telangiectatic network of vessels (*arrowheads*) typical of moyamoya disease. The typical middle cerebral artery vascular tree is absent. **B,** Cranial coronal magnetic resonance imaging scan of the same patient shows region of low signal in the middle cerebral artery territory and denotes infarction (*curved arrows*). Flow voids in the basal ganglia (*straight arrows*) are radiographic manifestations of the basilar collateral circulation typical of this vascular anomaly.

thought to be caused by vasodilation has been suggested as a mechanism contributing to the occurrence of watershed infarctions in sickle cell patients. Recurrences are common. Exchange transfusion diminishes the observed hyperemia and reduces the occurrence of stroke in these patients. Children who have suffered large strokes demonstrate correspondingly multifaceted deficits of cognitive function. Those in whom focal strokes have occurred show more subtle neuropsychologic deficits. Children with sickle cell disease who have silent infarctions may demonstrate school dysfunction as the only manifestation of neurologic involvement of the disease. These children can demonstrate twice the rate of school difficulties found in children with sickle cell disease without infarctions.

SAH also occurs among children with sickle cell disease. The frequency of SAH is less than that of infarction, occurring in fewer than 2%. Whereas ruptured cerebral aneurysm is frequently found in adults with sickle cell disease who have SAH, it is absent in affected children with SAH. The clinical findings of SAH differ from those of infarction in patients with sickle cell disease. Severe headache, vomiting, and alteration in mental state characterize SAH in children with sickle cell disease. Meningeal signs and focal neurologic deficits may be found on examination. Angiography should be performed on all patients to detect any surgically correctable vascular lesion underlying the hemorrhage. Medical therapy consisting of transfusion therapy has been suggested.

Intracranial Hemorrhage

Coagulopathies

Although some coagulation disturbances may predispose a patient to ischemic stroke (hypercoagulable states), others may promote intracranial bleeding (see Chapter 50). The hemophilias (A and B) are X-linked disorders that may result in intracranial bleeding. Bleeding may occur in either intraparenchymal or subarachnoid locations. Hemophilia A arises from factor VIII deficiency. Patients with this disorder may experience intracranial bleeding in association with head trauma. Unfortunately, spontaneous intracranial bleeding not associated with head trauma also occurs. The risk of spontaneous bleeding rises with the severity of factor VIII deficiency.

Hemophilia B derives from a deficiency of factor IX. Intracranial bleeding is seen less frequently among these patients than among patients with hemophilia A. Hemophilia B is encountered much less frequently than hemophilia A, and this difference may account for the less frequent observation of intracranial bleeding.

Clinical symptoms depend on the intracranial location of the hemorrhage. If the bleeding occurs in the subarachnoid space, symptoms of severe headache, nuchal rigidity, and meningismus are found. Mental status is frequently altered. If bleeding occurs within brain parenchyma, focal features, including hemiparesis, may be found.

Thrombocytopenia

Severe thrombocytopenia rarely leads to cerebral hemorrhage, especially if the cause is idiopathic (immune) thrombocytopenic purpura. Thrombocytopenia caused by bone marrow failure (drug-induced suppression, aplastic anemia, malignancy) may pose a greater risk. Significant risk of intracranial hemorrhage is thought not to occur until the platelet count is less than $20,000/mm^3$. Small petechial hemorrhages into white matter are thought to be more common than are large parenchymal hemorrhages.

Causes of thrombocytopenia include idiopathic immune thrombocytopenic purpura, thrombotic thrombocytopenic purpura, hemolytic uremic syndrome, infection, and malignancy (replacement of bone marrow or drug-induced suppression). The features of these underlying causes dominate the clinical picture (see Chapter 50).

Vascular Malformations

Arteriovenous malformation (AVM) of the brain is the most common cause of intracranial hemorrhage in preadolescent children. The malformation represents a developmental anomaly that manifests with hemorrhage much more frequently in children than in adults. The AVM consists of dilated vascular channels, some of which reveal the highly muscularized walls of arterioles. Gliotic neural tissue resides in and among the vascular branches of the malformation. It is more common in boys. The most frequent presenting events associated with AVM in children are seizures and hemorrhage. Most AVMs reside in the cerebral hemispheres; 10% arise in the posterior fossa.

The clinical features of AVM hemorrhage consist of those found in IPH. Focal features depend on the area of brain in which the bleeding has occurred. A higher mortality rate has been observed in children than in adults harboring hemorrhagic AVMs. The risk of hemorrhage from an unruptured AVM is approximately 3% per year.

Initially, treatment of AVMs consisted of anticonvulsant therapy for secondary seizures. Surgery was reserved for AVMs that bled at presentation. The introduction of MRI has led to better localization of the malformation (Fig. 41-5). In addition, percutaneous selective

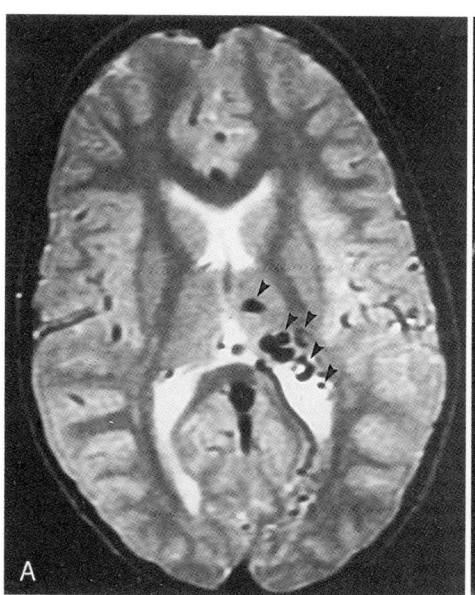
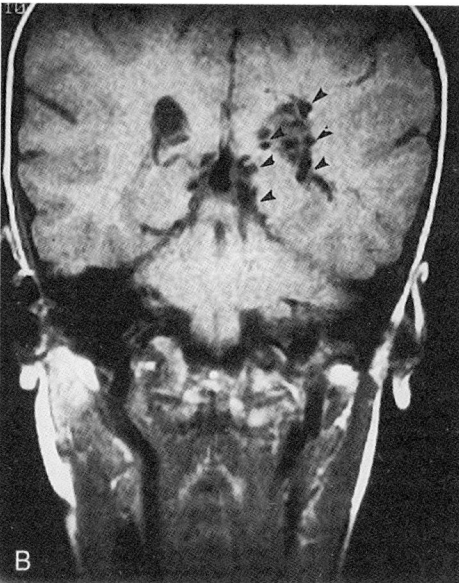

Figure 41-5. Cranial magnetic resonance imaging scan of a 6-year-old girl with recurrent headache. **A,** Axial view demonstrates flow voids deep in the left hemisphere near the lateral ventricle (*arrowheads*), consistent with arteriovenous malformation. **B,** Coronal view through parietal lobes also demonstrates numerous flow voids (*arrowheads*) indicative of arteriovenous malformation.

embolization of portions of the AVM or of the entire AVM has permitted the resection of AVMs thought previously to be inoperable. AVMs residing in critical regions of the CNS not amenable to surgery have been treated with stereotactic radiosurgery. Promising results have been obtained. Radiation damage to the CNS has complicated the recovery of approximately 3% of patients receiving this therapy.

Intracranial aneurysms constitute the most common cause of intracranial bleeding in all patients younger than 20 years and are more frequent in boys. In contrast to aneurysms in adults, the most common site of aneurysmal bleeding in children is along the intracranial portion of the internal carotid artery. The vertebral and basilar arteries are other common sites of intracranial aneurysm in children. In addition, intracranial aneurysms discovered in children tend to be larger than those found in adults. Although most aneurysms constitute vascular developmental anomalies, other causes exist, including mycotic aneurysms associated with bacterial endocarditis (Fig. 41-6). Acquired cerebral artery aneurysms have

been reported in children infected with the human immunodeficiency virus. Intracranial aneurysms are found with increased frequency among patients suffering from polycystic renal disease, those with aortic coarctation, and those with Ehlers-Danlos syndrome, in comparison with the general pediatric population. Intracranial aneurysms have been noted to exist in close association with AVMs in some pediatric cases.

All affected patients should be studied with angiography after aneurysmal bleeding. Patients should be closely observed for development of hydrocephalus and increased intracranial pressure. Aneurysmal bleeding resulting in significant SAH can precipitate cerebral vasospasm. Vasospasm, in turn, can cause a secondary cerebral infarction. Vasospasm occurs most commonly 7 to 10 days after the aneurysmal bleeding. Prophylaxis is the most effective treatment for vasospasm. Maintenance of blood pressure through intravascular volume expansion has been shown to reduce the incidence of posthemorrhagic vasospasm. Early enthusiasm for treatment with calcium channel blockers has attenuated.

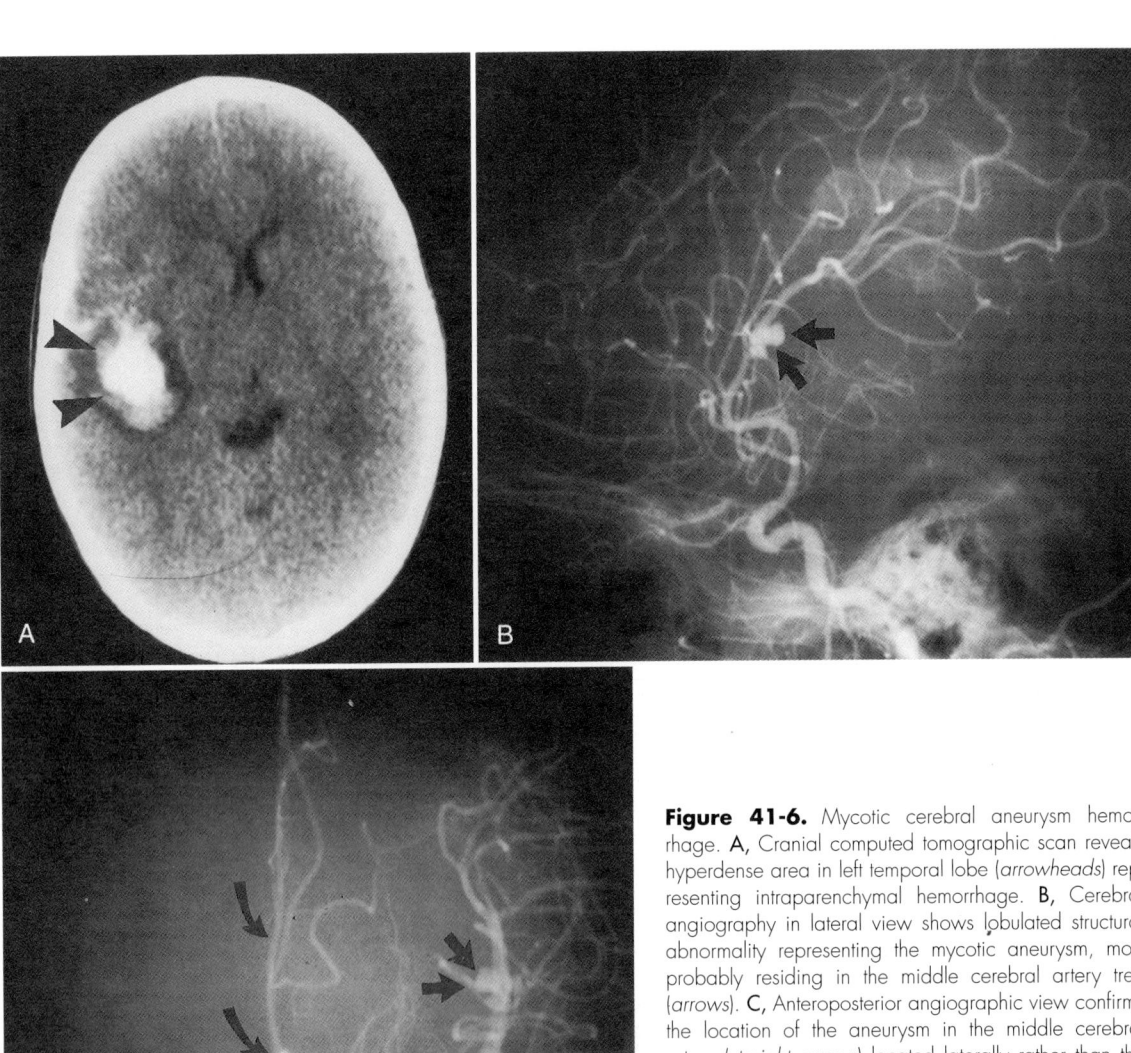

Figure 41-6. Mycotic cerebral aneurysm hemorrhage. **A,** Cranial computed tomographic scan reveals hyperdense area in left temporal lobe (*arrowheads*) representing intraparenchymal hemorrhage. **B,** Cerebral angiography in lateral view shows lobulated structural abnormality representing the mycotic aneurysm, most probably residing in the middle cerebral artery tree (*arrows*). **C,** Anteroposterior angiographic view confirms the location of the aneurysm in the middle cerebral artery (*straight arrows*) located laterally rather than the more medial anterior cerebral artery (*curved arrows*). The internal carotid artery (*open arrows*) gives rise to both the anterior and the middle cerebral arteries.

The syndrome of posterior fossa brain malformations, facial hemangiomas, arterial anomalies, coarctation of the aorta, and cardiac and eye defects (PHACE) is a constellation of disorders (see Table 41-2). CNS malformations affect the posterior fossa and include Dandy-Walker malformation, arachnoid cysts, cerebellar hypoplasia, and enlarged cisterna magna. Vascular anomalies include brachiocephalic artery and aortic arch anomalies (coarctation of aorta), cerebrovascular arterial hypoplasia, aneurysms, stenosis and aberrancies, and progressive occlusive arterial disease leading to stroke.

Evaluation of Stroke in Children

Neuroimaging provides the foundation of evaluation. Intracranial blood is rapidly seen with CT. The early stages of ischemic stroke, however, are detected with difficulty. MRI provides evidence of ischemia in the early stages of stroke. Magnetic resonance angiography has provided reliable information about the blood flow in and the structure of large intracranial vessels. Small intracranial vessels are poorly seen on magnetic resonance angiography, however, and invasive contrast angiography remains the neuroradiologic procedure of choice for full elucidation of the cerebral vasculature. Laboratory studies helpful in the evaluation of the child who has suffered stroke are determined by the patient's clinical features. Table 41-6 provides a synopsis of the tests most commonly employed.

ADOLESCENTS

The causes of adolescent stroke include those discussed for preadolescent children. Determination of stroke mechanism—embolic, thrombotic, or hemorrhagic—remains important. Nonetheless, stroke among adolescents may also be caused by other entities not commonly found in neonates or preadolescent children.

Fibromuscular Dysplasia

Fibromuscular dysplasia involves arteries throughout the body. First described in renal arteries, the pathologic features of fibromuscular dysplasia have been found in carotid, vertebral, and intracranial arteries. Fibromuscular dysplasia involves irregularly spaced focal zones of fibrous and muscular hyperplasia of the media, disruption of the elastic lamina, and eventration of the media. The constricted regions of vascular fibrosis alternate with regions of luminal dilation to create the characteristic beaded appearance on angiography. Fibromuscular dysplasia is more common in young girls and has been found in adolescents; with carotid involvement, a bruit may be auscultated in the neck. If renal arteries are affected, hypertension may be present. Neurologic symptoms signifying cerebrovascular involvement most commonly consist of TIAs and mild strokes. A thrombotic mechanism is presumed but has never been proven.

No treatment for symptomatic patients is established, although arterial dilation with metal dilators or transluminal angioplasty has been recommended.

Sexual Activity, Oral Contraception, and the Puerperium

Sexual intercourse generates marked increases in systemic blood pressure. Sustained hypertension elevates the risk of hypertensive intracranial hemorrhage. The risk for such a hemorrhage is heightened by the existence of an intracranial aneurysm or arteriovenous hemorrhage.

Oral contraceptives have been associated with stroke in young women. In some series, the combination of migraine headache and concurrent oral contraceptive use has been cited as a risk factor for stroke.

Table 41-6. Neuroradiologic, Laboratory, and Cardiovascular Assessment of Stroke in Children

Neuroradiologic Assessment
Rapid detection of intracranial blood
 Cranial CT
 Cranial MRI (also detects extravascular blood but is not as rapidly obtained as cranial CT images)
Detection of brain parenchymal changes related to stroke
 Cranial MRI, including diffusion weighted imaging
 Cranial CT (reveals changes later in course than MRI)
Detection of abnormal vascular structure
 Percutaneous cerebral angiogram (provides the most complete and accurate demonstration of extracranial and intracranial vasculature)
 Cranial MRA

Laboratory Assessment
Disturbance of RBC, WBC, or platelet number
 Hematocrit
 Platelet count
 WBC count with differential
Disturbance of coagulation
 PT, PTT
 Antithrombin III level
 Protein C level, protein S level; resistance to protein C assay
 Lupus anticoagulant detection, anticardiolipin antibody, antiphospholipid antibody
Metabolic disturbances
 Serum electrolytes, glucose
 Serum amino acids
 Urine organic acids
 Serum/CSF lactate and pyruvate
 Urine toxic screen
Disturbance of hemoglobin
 Hemoglobin concentration
 Hemoglobin electrophoresis
Inflammatory disturbances
 ESR
 ANA, RF
 CSF studies: glucose, protein, cell counts, special stains, cultures
Lipid and lipoprotein disturbances
 Serum triglycerides
 Serum cholesterol; if high, obtain fasting HDL

Cardiovascular Assessment
ECG
Standard and transesophageal echocardiogram

ANA, antinuclear antibodies; CSF, cerebrospinal fluid; CT, computed tomography; ECG, electrocardiography; ESR, erythrocyte sedimentation rate; HDL, high-density lipoproteins; MRA, magnetic resonance angiography; MRI, magnetic resonance imaging; PT, prothrombin time; PTT, partial thromboplastin time; RBC, red blood cell; RF, rheumatoid factor; WBC, white blood cell.

Pregnancy and the postpartum state have been considered periods of hypercoagulability. In addition, venous stasis increases. These two factors are believed to promote the occurrence of cerebral venous thrombosis and resultant cerebral venous infarction in pregnant patients and in patients immediately after parturition. Frequently, the initial manifestation is headache. Seizures, either focal or generalized, are common. Acute hemiparesis is the most common focal feature on neurologic examination. Papilledema can appear as intracranial pressure rises caused by resultant venous outflow obstruction in the head. The appearance of these signs or symptoms in a gravid or postpartum adolescent should raise suspicion about the existence of underlying cerebral venous thrombosis.

Diagnosis is made with cranial neuroimaging; MRI provides the best noninvasive assessment. If seizures occur, anticonvulsant treatment should be initiated. Once the diagnosis is confirmed, anticoagulants should be administered.

Cocaine Use

SAH can result from cocaine use. The probability of this occurrence is higher in cocaine users with occult intracranial aneurysms or arteriovenous malformations. Irrespective of the method of cocaine administration, SAH may occur. Cocaine produces tachycardia, hypertension, and vasoconstriction. The resultant sudden rise in systemic blood pressure is thought to precipitate SAH. Ischemic lesions have also been found. Nonetheless, intracranial hemorrhage appears to occur more commonly than ischemic infarction.

Treatment is supportive, with reduction of hypertension, hyperthermia, and tachycardia.

CAUSES OF STROKE UNRELATED TO AGE

Pharyngeal Infection

Pharyngeal infections have been associated with stroke caused by thrombotic occlusion of the carotid arteries in their cervical course. In childhood, stroke resulting from carotid occlusion more commonly occurs in the intracranial segment of the carotid artery. Infections of the cervical region such as tonsillitis, pharyngitis, cervical lymphadenitis, and necrotizing fasciitis have been found in children experiencing acute hemiplegia. In these instances, angiography has shown occlusion of the internal carotid artery located in its cervical segment. Neuroimaging has demonstrated ischemic infarction of the cortical region served by the middle cerebral artery, which arises from the carotid circulation. It is speculated that the soft tissue infection leads to an inflammatory arteritis. Vessel wall inflammation and direct pressure on the artery then lead to intravascular thrombosis and occlusion. Neurologic symptoms are noted in a patient with evidence of infection: fever, lethargy, sore throat or neck, difficulty swallowing, or cervical lymphadenopathy.

In these cases, prompt and aggressive antibiotic treatment constitutes the cornerstone of care. In some cases, surgical débridement of the infected area is necessary. Thrombolytic agents have been used to recanalize the occluded carotid artery. However, standardized, controlled trials of such treatment have not been performed.

Head and Neck Trauma

Head and neck trauma is an important cause of stroke in children. Neurologic symptoms may be delayed more than 24 hours in their appearance in relation to the time of inciting trauma. Stroke caused by carotid artery injury has been well documented. Most often, these cerebrovascular events occur after head and neck trauma sustained in motor vehicle accidents, bicycle accidents, fights, or falls. Hemiparesis is a common symptom at presentation if the cause resides in the carotid artery. Carotid angiography reveals internal carotid artery occlusion. The site of occlusion most often exists at the level of the carotid bifurcation. Pathologically, an intimal tear is found with attendant thrombus blocking the arterial lumen. In some cases, arterial dissection is found.

Vertebral artery injury from trauma may cause stroke in children. Traction injuries of the neck appear to cause vertebral artery injury. The vertebral artery is most vulnerable to traumatic injury at its atlantoaxial portion. The resultant strokes occur in the vertebrobasilar portion of the cerebral circulation. Symptoms are referable to the structures receiving blood from this system: brainstem, cerebellum, occipital lobes, and temporal lobes. Clinical symptoms of vertebrobasilar stroke include difficulty swallowing, ataxia, facial weakness, tinnitus, vertigo, anisocoria, extraocular movement palsies, dysmetria, cortical blindness, and mental status changes. Because both the long sensory and the motor tracts course through the brainstem, symptoms of general sensorimotor impairment may be found. Vertebral artery injury in children has been reported in the setting of athletic endeavor or automobile accidents. The resultant vertebrobasilar strokes are caused by thrombosis or vertebral artery dissection. Anticoagulation with antiplatelet agents has been proposed as therapy.

Migraine Headache

Stroke may occur in the setting of migraine headache. The occurrence of focal motor deficits during a migraine headache denotes *complicated migraine* (see Chapter 37). Acute hemiparesis has been well documented during these episodes and is believed to reflect the involvement of the cerebral circulation derived from the carotid artery. Symptoms such as ataxia, cortical blindness, and cranial nerve dysfunction are correlated with vertebrobasilar circulation involvement. Focal symptoms may be fixed or may occur as TIAs.

Initially, an association between migrainous stroke and discharged emboli from mitral valve prolapse was hypothesized, but studies have not supported the association. Although oral contraceptives confer hypercoagulability thought to predispose to stroke, the postulated additive risk for stroke with migraine headaches and oral contraceptives has been challenged. Angiographic studies on patients with focal deficits consistent with stroke in the setting of migraine headache reveal vasoconstriction of vessels in either the vertebrobasilar or the carotid circulations. The neuroanatomic position of the constricted vessels correlated with the location of the observed deficits. Ischemia provoked by vasoconstriction during prolonged migraine has been hypothesized as the mechanism of stroke in these patients.

Calcium channel blockers have been used for treatment, but definitive studies of their efficacy are awaited.

SUMMARY AND RED FLAGS

Acute hemiplegia most frequently represents stroke. Critical to the diagnosis of stroke are a history and physical examination findings that are consistent with the occurrence of stroke. Because stroke occurs most often in children as a consequence of an underlying process, circumspect consideration of the child's condition to determine whether such a predisposing condition exists will help determine the diagnosis with much greater accuracy.

Red flags in children with stroke include manifestations of underlying primary processes (e.g., trauma, medications, inborn errors, malignancy, coagulopathy), depressed level of consciousness, a positive family history of early-onset stroke (younger than 30 years), signs of increased intracranial pressure (see Chapter 40), a carotid bruit, hypertension, and the presence of prior TIAs.

Not all hemiplegia or all other focal deficits represent acute cerebrovascular events. Hemiparetic seizures, with their most striking features of acute lateralized weakness and preserved mental state, have been described as a form of partial epilepsy. In addition, seizures can be followed by a postictal (Todd) paralysis that may mimic the motor deficit of stroke. A search for a history of previous seizures is essential. A postictal paralysis is short-lived and is not associated with neuroradiologic characteristics of recent stroke. Preservation of consciousness, which is not a feature of generalized seizures, may help differentiate between epilepsy and cerebrovascular events. The EEG can be helpful in establishing the occurrence of seizure, but the diagnosis remains a clinical one.

Metabolic disturbances may cause focal motor deficits resembling stroke. Hypoglycemia and hyponatremia may each mimic stroke. Similarly, transient hemiparesis not associated with radiologic changes typical of stroke have been observed in juvenile diabetes mellitus. A survey for the existence of conditions that include these metabolic disturbances is important. Serum electrolyte and glucose levels should be measured. Similarly, severe anemia causing reduced oxygen delivery to the brain may result in evanescent focal motor deficits; evaluation of hematocrit is essential in any patient suspected of having suffered stroke.

Alternating hemiplegia of childhood may mimic stroke in children. This disorder appears to be sporadic in its occurrence. Early in its course, oculomotor and extrapyramidal features predominate, but eventually acute episodes of lateralized weakness supervene. The first symptoms of this disorder appear before the age of 18 months. Repeated episodes of lateralized hemiplegia are prominent. However, bilateral hemiplegia may occur. Extrapyramidal symptoms, oculomotor dysfunction, and dysautonomic features may also be present. Symptoms disappear during sleep. Developmental delay or mental retardation is present in all cases. Flunarizine, a calcium channel blocker, has shown some promise as a treatment in its apparent ability to reduce the frequency and duration of hemiplegic attacks, but experience with this drug is limited. Further study of this and other potential therapies are necessary.

Finally, multiple sclerosis may manifest in childhood with visual or motor disturbances suggestive of ischemic stroke; lesions change in space and time, and their effects are not often compatible with lesions at a neuroanatomic site distal to an arterial supply. MRI reveals demyelination in multiple sclerosis and other demyelinating processes.

REFERENCES

General

Fullerton HJ, Wu YW, Zhao S, et al: Risk of stroke in children: Ethnic and gender disparities. Neurology 2003;61:189.

Ganesan V, Chong WK, Cox TC, et al: Posterior circulation stroke in childhood. Neurology 2002;59:1552.

Kerr LM, Anderson DM, Thompson JA, et al: Ischemic stroke in the young. J Child Neurol 1993;8:266.

Riela A, Roach S: Etiology of stroke in children. J Child Neurol 1993;8:201.

Tournier-Lasserve E: New players in the genetics of stroke. N Engl J Med 2002;347:1711.

The Settings of Stroke in Children

Hypoxic-Ischemic Encephalopathy

Huppi PS, Inder TE: Magnetic resonance techniques in the evaluation of the perinatal brain: Recent advances and future directions. Semin Neonatol. 2001;6:195.

Rivkin M: Hypoxic ischemic brain injury in the term newborn: Neuropathology, clinical aspects, and neuroimaging. Clin Perinatol 1997;24:607.

Robertson,R, Ben-Sira L, Robson CD, et al: Magnetic resonance line scan diffusion imaging of term neonates with hypoxic-ischemic brain injury. AJNR Am J Neuroradiol 20;1999:1658.

Idiopathic Cerebral Infarction in the Full-Term Neonate

Butler I: Cerebrovascular disorders of childhood. J Child Neurol 1993;8:197.

Coker S, Beltran R, Myers T, et al: Neonatal stroke: Description of patients and investigation into pathogenesis. Pediatr Neurol 1988;4:219.

Lanska M, Lanska D, Horwitz S, et al: Presentation, clinical course and outcome of childhood stroke. Pediatr Neurol 1991;7:333.

McKinstry RC, Miller JH, Snyder AZ, et al: A prospective, longitudinal diffusion tensor imaging study of brain injury in newborns. Neurology 2002;59:824-833.

Polycythemia

Barron T, Gusnard D, Zimmerman R, et al: Cerebral venous thrombosis in neonates and children. Pediatr Neurol 1992;8:112.

Black V, Lubchenco L, Koops B, et al: Neonatal hyperviscosity: Randomized study of effect of partial plasma exchange transfusion on long-term outcome. Pediatrics 1985;75:1048.

Neonatal Cerebral Venous Thrombosis

Rivkin M, Anderson M, Kaye E: Neonatal idiopathic cerebral thrombosis: An unrecognized cause of transient seizures or lethargy. Ann Neurol 1992;32:51.

Wu YW, Miller SP, Chin K, et al: Multiple risk factors in neonatal sinovenous thrombosis. Neurology 2002;59:438.

Intracranial Hemorrhage in the Neonate

Bergman I, Bauer R, Barmada M, et al: Intracerebral hemorrhage in the full-term infant. Pediatrics 1985;75:488.

Children Aged 1 to 13 Years

Congenital Heart Disease

Bogousslavsky J, Regli F: Ischemic stroke in adults younger than 30 years of age. Arch Neurol 1987;44:479.

Jones H, Shekert R, Geraci J: Neurologic manifestations of bacterial endocarditis. Ann Intern Med 1969;71:21.

Lechat P, Mas J, Lascault G, et al: Prevalence of patent foramen ovale in patients with stroke. N Engl J Med 1988;318:1148.

Procoagulopathies

Golomb MR, MacGregor DL, Domi T, et al: Presumed pre- or perinatal arterial ischemic stroke: Risk factors and outcomes. Ann Neurol. 2001;50:163.

Levine S, Deegan M, Futrell N, et al: Cerebrovascular and neurologic disease associated with antiphospholipid antibodies: 48 cases. Neurology 1990;40:1181.

Nestoridi E, Buonanno FS, Jones RM, et al: Arterial ischemic stroke in childhood: The role of plasma-phase risk factors. Curr Opin Neurol 2002;15:139.

Pihko H, Tyni T, Virkola K, et al: Transient ischemic cerebral lesions during induction chemotherapy for acute lymphoblastic leukemia. J Pediatr 1993;123:18.

Strater R, Becker S, von Eckardstein A, et al: Prospective assessment of risk factors for recurrent stroke during childhood—A 5-year follow-up study. Lancet 2002;360:1540.

Autoimmune Disorders

Belman A, Leicher C, Moshe S, et al: Neurologic manifestations of Shoenlein-Henoch purpura. Pediatrics 1985;75:687.

Devinsky O, Petito C, Alonso D: Clinical and neuropathological findings in systemic lupus erythematosus: The role of vasculitis, heart emboli and thrombotic thrombocytopenic purpura. Ann Neurol 1988;23:380.

Graf W, Milstein J, Sherry D: Stroke and mixed connective tissue disease. J Child Neurol 1993;8:256.

Kohrman M, Huttenlocher P: Takayasu arteritis: A treatable cause of stroke in infancy. Pediatr Neurol 1986;2:154.

Lanthier S, Lortie A, Michaud J, et al: Isolated angiitis of the CNS in children. Neurology 2001;56:837.

Sigal L: The neurologic presentation of vasculitic and rheumatologic syndromes. Medicine 1987;66:157.

Metabolic Disorders Causing Stroke

Christodoulou J, Qureshi I, McInnes R, et al: Ornithine transcarbamoylase deficiency presenting with strokelike episodes. J Pediatr 1993;122:423.

Goto Y, Horai S, Matsuoda T, et al: Mitochondrial myopathy, encephalopathy, lactic acidosis, and stroke-like episodes (MELAS): A correlative study of the clinical features and mitochondrial DNA mutation. Neurology 1992;42:545.

Scheuerle A, McVie R, Beaudet A, et al: Arginase deficiency presenting as cerebral palsy. Pediatrics 1993;92:995.

Tulinius M, Holme E, Kristiamsson B, et al: Mitochondrial encephalomyopathies in childhood, I and II. J Pediatr 1991;119:242.

Moyamoya Disease

Karasawa J, Touho H, Ohnishi H, et al: Long-term follow-up after extracranial-intracranial bypass surgery for anterior circulation ischemia in childhood moyamoya disease. J Neurosurg 1992;77:84.

McLean M, Gebarski S, Van der Spek A, et al: Response of moyamoya disease to verapamil. Lancet 1985;1:163.

Rooney C, Kaye E, Scott R, et al: Modified encephaloduroarteriosynangiosis as surgical treatment of childhood moyamoya disease: Report of 5 cases. J Child Neurol 1991;6:24.

Sickle Cell Disease

Craft S, Schatz J, Glauser T, et al: Neuropsychologic effects of stroke in children with sickle cell anemia. J Pediatr 1993;123:712.

Pavlakis S, Bello J, Prohovnik I, et al: Brain infarction in sickle cell anemia: Magnetic resonance imaging correlates. Ann Neurol 1988;23:125.

Scahtz J, Brown RT, Pascual JM, et al: Poor school and cognitive functioning with silent cerebral infarcts and sickle cell disease. Neurology 2001;56:1109.

Steen RG, Xiong X, Langston JW, et al: Brain injury in children with sickle cell disease: Prevalence and etiology. Ann Neurol 2003;54:564.

Wang W, Kovnar E, Tonkin I, et al: High risk of recurrent stroke after discontinuance of five to twelve years of transfusion therapy in patients with sickle cell disease. J Pediatr 1991;118:377.

Thrombocytopenia

Woerner S, Abildgaard C, French M: Intracranial hemorrhage in children with idiopathic thrombocytopenic purpura. Pediatrics 1981;67:453.

Vascular Malformations

Broechler J, Thron A: Intracranial arterial aneurysms in children. Neurosurg Rev 1990;13:309.

Brown Y, Wiebers K, Forbes G: Unruptured intracranial aneurysms and arteriovenous malformations: Frequency of intracranial haemorrhage and relationship of lesions. J Neurosurg 1990;73:859.

Ito M, Yishuhara M, Wachi A, et al: Cerebral aneurysms in children. Brain Dev 1992;14:263.

Konsiolka D, Humphreys R, Hoffman H, et al: Arteriovenous malformations of the brain in children: A forty year experience. Can J Neurol Sci 1992;19:40.

Adolescents

Fibromuscular Dysplasia

Smith D, Smith L, Hasso A: Fibromuscular dysplasia of the internal carotid artery treated by operative transluminal balloon angioplasty. Radiology 1985;155:645.

Sexual Activity, Oral Contraception, and the Puerperium

Adams H, Butler M, Biller J, et al: Nonhemorrhagic cerebral infarction in young adults. Arch Neurol 1987;43:713.

Bousser M, Chiras J, Bories J, et al: Cerebral venous thrombosis—A review of 38 cases. Stroke 1985;16:199.

Cocaine Use and Stroke

Cregler L, Mark H: Medical complications of cocaine abuse. N Engl J Med 1986;315:1495.

Klonoff D, Andrews B, Obana W: Stroke associated with cocaine use. Arch Neurol 1989;46:989.

Toffol G, Biller J, Adams H: Nontraumatic intracerebral hemorrhage in young adults. Arch Neurol 1987;44:479.

Causes of Stroke Unrelated to Age

Pharyngeal Infection

Bush J, Givner L, Whitaker S, et al: Necrotizing fasciitis of the parapharyngeal space with carotid artery occlusion and acute hemiplegia. Pediatrics 1984;73:343.

Shillito J: Carotid arteritis: A cause of hemiplegia in childhood. J Neurosurg 1964;21:540.

Tagawa T, Mimaki T, Yabuuchi H, et al: Bilateral occlusions in the cervical portion of the internal carotid arteries in a child. Stroke 1985;16:896.

Head and Neck Trauma

Garg B, Ottinger C, Smith R, et al: Strokes in children due to vertebral artery trauma. Neurology 1993;43:2555.

Hope E, Bodensteiner J, Barnes P: Cerebral infarction related to neck position in an adolescent. Pediatrics 1983;72:335.

Lewis D, Berman P: Vertebral artery dissections and alternating hemiparesis in an adolescent. Pediatrics 1986;78:610.

Migraine Headache

Bogousslavsky J, Regli F, Van Melle G, et al: Migraine stroke. Neurology 1988;38:223.

Caplan L: Migraine and vertebrobasilar ischemia. Neurology 1991;41:55.

Conditions Resembling Stroke

Bourgeois M, Aicardi J, Goutieres F: Alternating hemiplegia of childhood. J Pediatr 1993;122:673.

Casaer P: Flunarizine in alternating hemiplegia in childhood. Neuropediatrics 1987;18:191.

Hanson P, Chodos R: Hemiparetic seizures. Neurology 1978;28:920.

Yarnell P: Todd's paralysis: A cerebrovascular phenomenon. Stroke 1975;6:301.

42 Syncope and Dizziness

David A. Lewis*

Dizziness is a common but very nonspecific chief complaint about which some elaboration by the patient is generally required for the physician to understand exactly what the patient is feeling. The description of the sensation is critical in distinguishing whether it is caused by vertigo, disequilibrium, lightheadedness, presyncope, or even ataxia (Table 42-1). Although the differential diagnoses of these entities may overlap, there are conditions that are most specific to each. All of the entities just named are conditions that may affect children at any age, but older children are more capable of articulating the abnormal sensation they feel. Children younger than 6 years of age may present with nausea, vomiting, ataxia, or frank syncope.

Syncope is the transient loss of consciousness and postural tone that results from inadequate cerebral perfusion. Syncope is a common phenomenon in children and adolescents that is usually benign. Fifteen percent to 20% of all young adults have had one episode of syncope in the past. It is critical to distinguish between syncope that is associated with exertion or activity versus syncope "at rest" (see later discussion). The history of the event, obtained from the patient or witnesses, is critical in establishing the differential diagnosis.

Presyncope is the feeling that the person is "about to pass out." The patient feels as if he or she is going to lose consciousness but does not. Presyncope may or may not reflect the same pathophysiologic process as true syncope. The diagnostic approach to presyncope, however, is essentially the same as for syncope.

Dizziness must be considered a change in mental status. It may potentially herald serious underlying central nervous system dysfunction. Dizziness must be better defined to distinguish *vertigo* from *lightheadedness*. The principal distinction with dizziness is the description of motion; swaying, whirling, or spinning is characteristic of vertigo. Lightheadedness often accompanies hyperventilation and is therefore frequently associated with psychologic stress, including anxiety, depression, and panic attacks. The history surrounding episodes of lightheadedness is vital for formulating the differential diagnosis.

The last of the "dizzy" feelings is disequilibrium. *Disequilibrium* refers to "balance problems" without vertigo. The characteristic historical feature is difficulty ambulating. A fairly rare complaint among children, disequilibrium in the young is most often caused by vestibular or cerebellar dysfunction and manifests as ataxia.

Ataxia is an impairment of coordination of movement and balance; this impairment is generally associated with dysfunction of the cerebellum or of the sensory and/or motor pathways connecting to the cerebellum. There are transient forms and progressive degenerative conditions. The trick is distinguishing between the poor coordination and true ataxia.

The common trait among all the "dizzy" feelings is primary or secondary central nervous system dysfunction. Dizziness should be considered a potential alteration in the patient's level of consciousness and must be taken seriously.

SYNCOPE

Syncope is a common phenomenon among children and adolescents. As many as 15% of children experience a syncopal event between the ages of 8 and 18 years. Before age 6 years, syncope is very unusual except in the setting of seizure disorders, breath-holding spells, and primary cardiac dysrhythmias. Syncope in children provokes great anxiety in parents, teachers, and other children who observe a syncopal episode. Fainting episodes cause a large number of health care visits and a surprising number of admissions to hospitals. The differential diagnosis of syncope is noted in Table 42-2.

The pathophysiologic mechanism of syncope seems to follow a common pathway with many inciting stimuli. Cerebral perfusion is compromised by a transient decrease in cardiac output as a result of vasomotor changes, decreasing venous return, primary dysrhythmia, or impairment of cerebral vascular tone. Adolescents subjected to a head-up tilt-table test report blurred vision and constriction of visual fields before losing consciousness, as well as nausea, pallor, sweating, and dizziness, which are accompanied by hypotension (systolic blood pressure < 60 mm Hg) and by bradycardia (heart rate < 40 beats/minute) with an occasional junctional rhythm and even asystole (Fig. 42-1). Symptoms are relieved by returning to the supine position.

Several situational factors can exacerbate this response, including

- warm temperature
- a confined space, such as being in a crowded room
- anxiety or fear
- sudden surprise
- the sight of blood
- pain, such as from needlesticks or shots

Other situational factors include urination, swallowing, coughing, defecation, and hair combing.

The response is caused by imbalance of parasympathetic and sympathetic tone, which results in peripheral vasodilatation, including venodilatation, but in no augmentation of venous return, because there is no accompanying increase in large skeletal muscle activity to augment systemic venous return and maintain cardiac filling. Subsequent vagal output results in inappropriate bradycardia and further compromises cardiac output. The child faints and becomes supine, which restores systemic venous return to the right side of the heart. At the same time, awakening is accompanied by increased sympathetic output, which restores the heart rate. The episode tends to be brief but may recur if the patient is "helped up" too quickly. One scenario in which this combination of events may be most dangerous is a hot, closed telephone booth, in which a patient cannot become supine and restore cardiac output. The magnitude of this vagal response should not be underestimated. In studies utilizing isoproterenol, despite the powerful β-adrenergic stimulation, susceptible patients become profoundly bradycardic and experience junctional rhythm or even asystole.

In obtaining the history of a syncopal episode, attention should be paid to the time of day, time of last meal, activities leading up to the

*Deceased.

743

Table 42-1. Syncope and Dizziness

	Vertigo	Presyncope	Disequilibrium	Lightheadedness
Patient complaint	"My head is spinning" "The room is whirling"	"I feel I might pass out" "I feel faint"	"I feel unsteady" "My balance is off"	"I feel dizzy" "I feel disconnected, drugged"
Associated features	Motion, swaying, spinning, nystagmus	Syncope: loss of postural tone, brief loss of consciousness Situational	Poor balance No vertigo or ataxia	Anxiety, hyperventilation, paresthesias, respiratory alkalosis, panic attacks
Usual cause	Vestibular disorders	Impaired cerebral perfusion	Sensory and/or central neurologic dysfunction	Anxiety and/or depressive disorders
Key differential diagnoses	Peripheral (labyrinthine-cochlear) vs. Central neurologic disorder	Neurocardiogenic (vagal) vs. Cardiac syncope vs. Neuropsychiatric syncope	Sensory deficit vs. Central neurologic disease	Anxiety/depression vs. Hyperventilation vs. Medication effects

event, and associated symptoms (palpitations, racing heart beat, chest pain, headache, shortness of breath, nausea, diaphoresis, visual changes, and hearing changes). Details, such as the patient's position (syncope while supine suggests a cardiac arrhythmia) when symptoms appeared, duration of the episode, and characterization of the patient's appearance during and immediately after the episode are also important. Almost without exception, by the time the patient presents to the office or emergency room, the physical examination findings in children and adolescents are normal. Therefore, the history becomes the most important piece of information for developing the differential diagnosis, diagnostic evaluation, and management plan.

NEUROCARDIOGENIC SYNCOPE

Neurocardiogenic syncope is a type of autonomic dysfunction that is also referred to as *vasodepressor syncope, vasovagal syncope,* and *reflex syncope.* Three mechanisms appear to exist:

1. The first response is primary bradycardia, sometimes to the extreme of sinus arrest and asystole, with subsequent hypotension (see Fig. 42-1). This is known as the *cardioinhibitory response.*
2. The second is a primary vasodepressor response that is characterized by hypotension, the heart rate being relatively preserved.
3. The third is a mixed and the most common response that features simultaneous hypotension and bradycardia.

The common pathway resulting in central nervous system dysfunction is cerebral hypotension and is also known as the *Bezold-Jarisch reflex* (Fig. 42-2). For most children and adolescents, prodromal warning signs herald the impending episode and can, after the first episode, allow the child enough time to prevent fainting by sitting with the head between the knees or by lying supine. The physiologic mechanisms of neurocardiogenic syncope have been demonstrated with head-up tilt-table testing. Tilt-table testing can be performed with or without invasive blood pressure monitoring. The goal is to reproduce the patient's symptoms under close monitoring. Various tilt angles and durations have been described, as has the use of isoproterenol as a provocative stimulus. There are data for normal adolescents, but there are minimal or no data regarding the reproducibility of tilt-table testing.

If the history suggests the diagnosis of neurocardiogenic syncope with normal physical examination findings and a normal electrocardiogram (ECG), treatment may be empirically started without tilt-table testing (Table 42-3). The first line of treatment is the use of salt supplementation (1 g/day orally) with the mineralocorticoid fludrocortisone acetate (Florinef) (0.1 mg/day orally). The average patient gains about 1 kg of water weight into the circulating volume over 2 to 3 weeks, and the increased volume allows blood pressure

to be maintained even in the presence of vasodilation. A tilt-table test is advisable if the patient does not respond to empirical volume-expansion therapy.

A second therapeutic choice is usually β-adrenergic receptor blockade, typically with atenolol or metoprolol. A second tilt-table test may be performed to confirm therapeutic success, but adolescent patients in particular have limited enthusiasm for a repeated tilt-table test. Alternative therapies may include theophylline or pseudoephedrine, disopyramide, or combinations of the drugs named earlier.

There are several causes of autonomic or neurocardiogenic syncope. Excessive vagal tone may be primary or secondary to breath holding, cough, swallowing (deglutition syncope), micturition or defecation, carotid sinus pressure sensitivity, and orthostasis. Of these, *breath-holding episodes* are among the most common and frightening, representing a frequent mechanism of syncope in children under age 6 years. Onset of breath holding is rare before the age of 6 months; the incidence peaks at age 2 years and resolves by ages 5 to 7 years. The incidence of breath-holding spells is approximately 5% of 1- to 5-year-olds. The family history is positive for more than 30%; this may suggest an autosomal dominant disorder with incomplete penetrance. Both sexes are equally affected. Typically, the child is startled or agitated, and a period of crying terminates with a prolonged noiseless expiration, visible cyanosis, and collapse. The episode is totally involuntary. Provocations include pain, anger, fear, or frustration. These episodes result in a great deal of parental anxiety. That anxiety is magnified when monitoring illustrates that the episode is accompanied by reflex increase in vagal tone, often accompanied by asystole for 15 to 30 seconds. Fifteen percent of patients have a brief (seconds) anoxic convulsion after syncope. After the episode, many children sleep. Most affected children "outgrow" these episodes, which rarely affect future central nervous function, such as cognition. Fifteen percent to 20% have vasovagal syncope as older children or young adults. Pallid breath-holding spells occur in fewer than 25% of episodes. Stereotypically, pallid spells begin with a sudden fright or pain, the patient quiets, then develops pallor, apnea, and bradycardia or brief asystole. Fifty percent of these patients reproduce this sequence with brief (<10-second) bilateral ocular pressure (oculocardiac reflex). Rare "malignant breath-holding" spells have been treated with placement of permanent cardiac pacemakers, with less than convincing results in affecting mortality. There may be some role for preventing the potential cerebral injury associated with profound hypotension during prolonged or repeated episodes of asystole. Nonetheless, most patients and families are treated expectantly with reassurance about the benign nature of the usual breath-holding spells. Oral iron therapy has been shown to decrease the frequency of breath-holding spells even in the absence of iron deficiency anemia.

Table 42-2. Syncope and Dizziness: Cause

Diagnosis	History	Symptoms	Description	Heart Rate/Blood Pressure	Duration	Postsyncope	Recurrence
Neurocardiogenic (Vasodepressor)	At rest	Pallor, nausea, visual changes	Brief ± convulsion	↓/↓	<1 min	Residual pallor, sweaty, hot; recurs if child stands too quickly	Common
Neuropathic postural tachycardia syndrome (also known as postural orthostatic tachycardia syndrome [POTS])	Chronic orthostatic intolerance	Lightheaded, dimming of vision, confusion; Blue-red color of legs	Brief; high catecholamine levels: a form of dysautonomia	↑/−	<1 min	Same as for neurocardiogenic	Common
Other Vagal							
Vasovagal	Needlestick	Pallor, nausea	Brief; convulsions rare	↓/↓	<1 min	Residual pallor; may recur if child stands	Situational
Micturition	Postvoiding	Pallor, nausea	Brief ± convulsion	↓/↓	<1 min	Same as above	(+)
Cough (deglutition)	Paroxysmal cough	Cough	Abrupt onset	May not change	<5 min	Fatigue or baseline	(+)
Carotid sinus	Tight collar, turned head	Vague, visual changes	Sudden onset, pallor	Usually ↓/↓	<5 min	Fatigue or baseline	(+)
Hypoglycemia	Fasting, insulin use	Gradual hunger, weakness, sweating	Pallor, sweating; loss of consciousness or seizures	No change or mild tachycardia	Variable	Relieved only by eating	(+)
Neuropsychiatric							
Hyperventilation	Anxiety	SOB, fear, claustrophobia	Agitated, hyperpneic ± Pallor	Mild ↓/↓	<5 min	Fatigue or baseline	(+)
Syncopal vertebrobasilar migraine	Headache	Aura, migraine, nausea		No change	<10 min	Headache, often occipital	(+)
Seizure (atonic) disorder	Anytime	± Aura	Convulsion or loss of tone ± incontinence	No change or mild tachycardia	Any duration	Postictal lethargy + confusion	(+)
Hysterical	Always an "audience" present	Psychologic distress	Gentle, graceful swoon	No change	Any duration	Normal baseline	(+)
Cerebral	At rest	Loss of consciousness	Brief; due to cerebral vasoconstriction	No change in HR or BP	<1 min	May have few	(+)
Benign paroxysmal vertigo	Sudden fall	Dizzy, nystagmus, nausea, sweating	Pallor, no loss of consciousness	↑/−	Any duration	Frightened	+
Cataplexy	Sudden sleep	Loss of tone	Sleep	−/−	Any duration	Daytime sleepiness	+
Breath-holding (hypoxic)	Agitation or injury	Crying	Cyanosis or pallor ± convulsion	↓/↓ Frequent asystole	<10 min	Fatigue, residual pallor	(+)
Cardiac Syncope							
LVOT obstruction	Exercise; Family history	± Chest pain, SOB	Abrupt during or after exertion, pallor	↑/↓	Any duration	Fatigue, residual pallor, sweating	(+)
Pulmonary hypertension	Anytime, especially exercise	SOB	Cyanosis and pallor	↑/↓	Any duration	Fatigue, residual cyanosis	(+)
Myocarditis	Postviral; Exercise	SOB, chest pain, palpitations	Pallor	↑/↓	Any duration	Fatigue	(+)
Tumor or mass	Recumbent, paroxysmal	SOB ± chest pain	Pallor	↑/↓	Any duration	Baseline	(+)
Coronary artery	Exercise; Family history	SOB ± chest pain	Pallor	↑/↓	Any duration	Fatigue, chest pain	(+)
Dysrhythmia	Anytime; Family history	Palpitations ± chest pain	Pallor	↑ or ↓/↓	Usually <10 min	Fatigue or baseline	(+)

BP, blood pressure; HR, heart rate; LVOT, left ventricular outflow obstruction; SOB, shortness of breath; −, no effect; ±, with or without; +, recurrence likely; (+), recurrence possible.

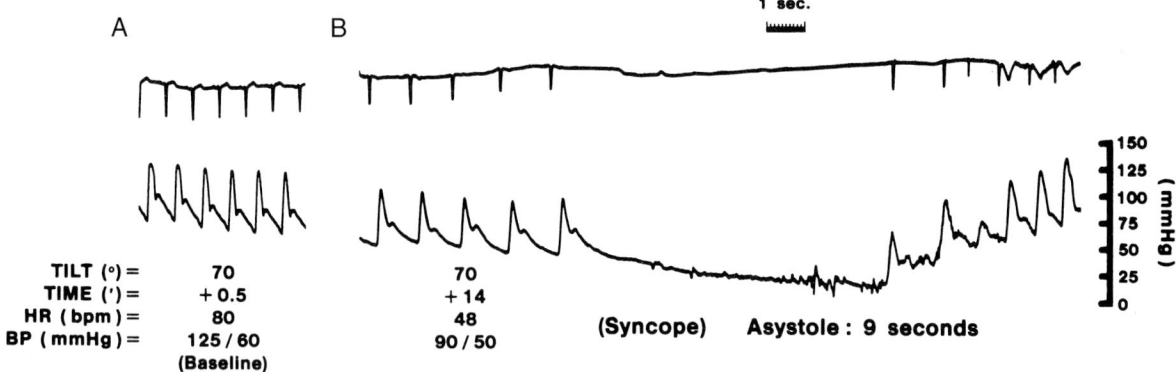

Figure 42-1. A, Baseline heart rate (HR) in beats per minute (bpm), blood pressure (BP), and rhythm 0.5 minutes after tilt to 70 degrees. B, Bradycardia and hypotension progressing rapidly to asystole with prompt recovery on returning to the supine position. This is an example of the cardioinhibitory response to orthostatic stress. (From Sra JS, Murthy VS, Jazayeri MR, et al: Use of intravenous esmolol to predict efficacy of oral beta-adrenergic blocker therapy in patients with neurocardiogenic syncope. J Am Coll Cardiol 1992;19:402-408, with permission from the American College of Cardiology Foundation.)

Reflex vagal bradycardia has been described in association with hair brushing, swallowing, stretching, orthodontic maneuvers, anomalies of the cervical spine, and dental trauma. Many of these episodes may actually be forms of carotid sinus sensitivity. Cough syncope probably is related to prolongation of high intrathoracic pressure that results in decreased venous return and subsequent decreased cardiac output.

The prodromal history is very important in evaluating neurocardiogenic or autonomic syncope. Syncope without warning, while the patient is supine, or during exercise implies a primary cardiac cause and is associated with greater morbidity and potential mortality.

CARDIAC SYNCOPE

A variety of cardiac conditions can result in hypotension and syncope. Table 42-2 lists several potential cardiac causes of syncope, both structural and arrhythmogenic. Diseases that produce hypotension (orthostatic or supine) frequently produce syncope or presyncope. Cardiac function and structure are usually normal before the episode; during the predisposing illness, cardiac filling pressures are often reduced because of reduced venous return from hypovolemia or decreased peripheral vascular resistance (peripheral pooling of blood). Dehydration from diarrhea and vomiting, hyperthermia, hyperpyrexia, heat exhaustion, polyuria (diabetes mellitus), or poor

intake from anorexia, together with the systemic effects of the primary illness, may produce orthostatic or true hypotension and syncope. In these conditions, dizziness, hypotension, or syncope occurs rapidly when the patient assumes an upright position (seconds). Toxins, as in *toxic shock syndrome,* may also contribute to orthostatic or true hypotension. Prolonged bed rest, combined with poor fluid intake during an illness, may also result in syncope or presyncope when the child arises to leave the bed. In most of these situations, intravenous fluid administration (normal saline, lactated Ringer solution) is sufficient to restore intravascular volume and venous return to alleviate postural or supine hypotension. Refractory hypotension suggests more serious pathologic processes, such as anaphylaxis, toxic shock syndrome, myocardial disease, or septic shock.

Dysrhythmias are common and are usually silent between episodes (see Chapter 7) (Table 42-4). Supraventricular tachycardia, ventricular tachycardia, and heart block are the most common types of dysrhythmia and may be primary or may result from medications or illicit drugs. Any form of acquired heart block carries a high mortality rate. One of the more common causes of acquired heart block is Lyme disease. Heart block may necessitate temporary or permanent electronic pacing to maintain cardiac output.

Primary cardiac conduction abnormalities that may result in syncope include Wolff-Parkinson-White syndrome, long QT syndrome, and catecholamine-sensitive ventricular tachycardia (see Table 42-4). Wolfe-Parkinson-White syndrome is characterized by a short PR interval, preexcitation seen as a widened QRS duration, and a delta wave on the proximal portion of the QRS. The delta wave represents the presence of accessory electrical tissue from atria to ventricle, with rapid antegrade conduction causing excitation of ventricular tissue before atrioventricular node–His bundle stimulation. If that pathway can conduct in the retrograde manner, a reentrant circuit is created, causing a narrow QRS complex tachycardia. This greatly shortens the diastolic ventricular filling time and results in diminished left ventricular end-diastolic volume, with subsequent decreased stroke volume and decreased cardiac output. Although the tachycardia is rarely sufficiently fast to result in syncope, some children have profound hypotension and rapid loss of consciousness. In adults, a similar mechanism results from atrial flutter or fibrillation if the ventricular response rate is fast.

Long QT syndromes are inherited abnormalities in the electrical recovery (repolarization) of the heart. Prolongation of the repolarization phase results in the risk of simultaneous depolarization, the "R-on-T" phenomenon, which causes disorganized ventricular electrical stimulation characterized by torsades de

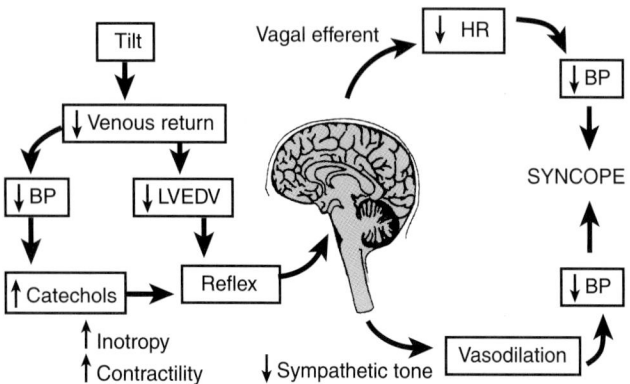

Figure 42-2. Tilt-table testing: the Bezold-Jarisch reflex. BP, blood pressure; HR, heart rate; LVEDV, left ventricular end-diastolic volume.

Table 42-3. Medications for Neurally Mediated Syncope

Medication	Principal Effects	Dosage	Adverse Effects
Fludrocortisone	Increases sodium, water retention Increases vascular sensitivity to NE	Start 0.1 mg PO q.d.-b.i.d. Rarely require >0.4 mg/day Maximum 1.0 mg/day	HTN, hypomagnesemia, hypokalemia, depression, edema, worsening migraine HA or acne
Midodrine	Direct α agonist: increases PVR and decreases venous capacitance	2.5-10 mg PO t.i.d. Maximum 40 mg/day	HTN, nausea
Methylphenidate	α agonist	5-10 mg PO t.i.d. Last dose before 6 p.m.	HTN, HA, CNS stimulation
Atenolol Metoprolol Pindolol	β blockers: reduces cardiac inotropy and mechanoreceptor activation, blocks vascular β_2 receptor (↑ PVR), central serotonin blockade	1-2 mg/kg/day as q.d. or b.i.d. 1-2 mg/kg/day as q.d. or b.i.d. 2.5-5 mg PO b.i.d.-t.i.d	Fatigue, bronchospasm, hypotension, bradycardia,* depression
Fluoxetine	SSRI: downregulates postsynaptic 5-HT receptors → reduces 5-HT effect on sympathetic activity	5-20 mg PO q.d.	CNS stimulation,† anorexia, nausea, diarrhea, fatigue, scalp pruritus
Nefazadone	SSRI	75-150 mg PO b.i.d.	
Sertraline	SSRI	25-100 mg PO q.d.	
Disopyramide	Negative inotrope Vagolytic Direct peripheral vasoconstriction	6-15 mg/kg/day Adult (typical): 200 mg CR b.i.d.	Anticholinergic effects, torsades de pointes

From Johnsrude CL: Current Approach to Pediatric Syncope. Pediatr Cardiol 2000;21:522-531.

*Less with pindolol.

†Less with newer SSRI.

b.i.d., twice per day; CNS, central nervous system; CR, continuous release form; HA, headache; Hct, hematocrit; 5-HT, serotonin; HTN, hypertension; NE, norepinephrine; PO, per os (orally); PVR, peripheral vascular resistance; q.d., every day; SSRI, selective serotonin reuptake inhibitor; t.i.d., three times per day.

Table 42-4. Syncopal Arrhythmogenic Disorders

Disorder	Arrhythmia	Comments
Long QT syndrome	Physical or emotional stress Induced VT or torsades de pointes (polymorphic VT)	$QTc = \dfrac{QT}{\sqrt{R\text{-}R}} > 450$ ms
Romano-Ward syndrome		AD: $LQT_{1, 2 \text{ and } 5}$ is mutated K⁺ channel; LQT_3 is mutated Na⁺ channel and is most lethal
Jervell and Lange-Nielsen syndrome		AR: $KVLQT_1$ gene; associated with sensorineural deafness
Acquired		Drugs: cisapride, certain antihistamines, erythromycin, tricyclic antidepressants, certain antiarrhythmic agents
Heart block	Bradycardia	Age-specific rates
Congenital		Associated with maternal SLE; less often with congenital heart disease Incidence 1 per 20,000 births
Acquired		Endocarditis, myocarditis, Lyme disease, tumor, rheumatic fever, drugs, Mt-myopathies, diphtheria, Rocky Mountain spotted fever, surgery
Wolfe-Parkinson-White syndrome	Delta wave, short PR interval, supraventricular tachycardias	Present at birth Must be seen when in sinus rhythm 0.1%-0.3% of population
Brugada syndrome	VT VF	Right bundle branch block with persistent ST elevation
Commotio cordis	VF, asystole	Initiated by blunt precordial chest trauma
Catecholamine-induced VT	VT (polymorphic)	AR or AD: Exercise- or catecholamine-induced VT once heart rate > 110; onset, >7 yr of age
Short coupled variant of torsades de pointes	VT	Rare
Idiopathic VF	VF	Rare; myocarditis must be ruled out

AD, autosomal dominant; AR, autosomal recessive; K⁺, potassium; Mt, mitochondrial DNA mutation; Na⁺, sodium; SLE, systemic lupus erythematosus; VF, ventricular fibrillation; VT, ventricular tachycardia.

pointes (coarse ventricular tachycardia), a potentially lethal dysrhythmia. There may be a family history of sudden cardiac death. Family studies with the same mutation have demonstrated that affected patients may not always have a long QT interval as defined for the syndrome. Some authorities have theorized that long QT syndromes may be responsible for some of the incidents of sudden infant death syndrome and drowning. Acquired prolongation of the QT interval may also be seen in electrolyte abnormalities (hyperkalemia) and with a variety of medications, including primary antiarrhythmic drugs (procainamide, quinidine, disopyramide, amiodarone), phenothiazines, antibiotics (erythromycin), antihistamines (e.g., astemizole [Hismanal]), and tricyclic antidepressants (imipramine [Tofranil], desipramine), which are used commonly in children with attention-deficit/hyperactivity disorder. For this reason, a toxicology screen may be warranted if there is any question of QT prolongation.

Patients who have undergone corrective or palliative surgery for congenital cardiac disease are at risk for some dysrhythmias that might result in syncope. Sinus node disease (in patients undergoing atrial surgery) may result in tachycardia-bradycardia episodes that can be associated with hypotension. Ventricular dysrhythmias are particularly common after repair of tetralogy of Fallot, double-outlet right ventricle, truncus arteriosus, and pulmonary atresia involving right ventriculotomy with subsequent ventricular scar formation.

Uncorrected structural heart disease is a relatively rare cause of a sudden decrease in cardiac output. However, hypertrophic cardiomyopathies, particularly idiopathic hypertrophic subaortic stenosis, can result in obstruction of left ventricular outflow with resultant high transmural pressure and secondary cardiac ischemia, which can be fatal (see Chapter 8). This type of obstruction is exacerbated by high sympathetic tone, which causes increased contractility and is a frequent mechanism of syncope associated with exercise in competitive athletics. The presence of an outflow tract murmur in the setting of syncope, especially if there is a positive family history, warrants evaluation with both electrocardiography and echocardiography. Any condition that impedes left ventricular outflow (valvar aortic stenosis, subaortic stenosis), left ventricular inflow or filling (mitral stenosis, pericardial tamponade), or blood flow through the pulmonary vasculature (primary or secondary pulmonary hypertension) may also result in syncope. In almost all cases, characteristic physical findings lead the clinician to the diagnosis. Pulmonary hypertension may be associated with cyanosis, as in *Eisenmenger syndrome*, in which case there is cerebral hypoxia resulting from right-to-left shunting, as well as decreased left ventricular output resulting from poor transpulmonary flow and decreased left ventricular filling (see Chapter 10).

Other rare causes of cardiac syncope are thoracic masses and intracardiac tumors or masses, coronary artery abnormalities, and inflammatory cardiac diseases (myocarditis). Masses or tumors, such as myxomas, fibromas, and rhabdomyomas, tend to produce paroxysmal symptoms, which are often associated with position changes, especially from the recumbent position. Coronary artery anomalies are usually not accompanied by signs of ischemia. Rather, the most common (Fig. 42-3) manifestation is syncope or sudden cardiac death from compression of the anomalous left main coronary artery as it courses between the pulmonary outflow and the aortic root. This usually occurs in a competitive athlete whose hypertrophied heart responds to catecholamine stimulation during activity and inadvertently compresses the anomalous coronary artery. Inflammatory conditions, such as heart block associated with Lyme disease and ventricular tachycardia associated with myocarditis or pericarditis, predispose to dysrhythmias.

Cardiac syncopal episodes can be accompanied by brief tonic-clonic seizure activity known as *Stokes-Adams syndrome*. The seizure activity appears 10 to 20 seconds after the onset of asystole and is usually of short duration with no subsequent postictal phase. This may explain why so many children with cardiac syncope frequently see a neurologist.

NEUROPSYCHIATRIC SYNCOPE

Primary neurologic causes of syncope are much more unusual in otherwise healthy children and adolescents than in adults. Convulsive disorders must be considered if there is a history of an aural prodrome, focal or generalized tonic-clonic activity, and a prolonged postictal phase of lethargy or confusion. This is especially true in children younger than 6 years. Prolonged postevent lethargy is unusual with more common causes of syncope if the vital signs have returned to normal. Seizures are the most likely cause of syncope in the recumbent patient. Absence or atonic seizures may appear without the aura, motor activity, and postictal confusion of generalized tonic-clonic seizures and must be distinguished from narcolepsy and temporal lobe seizures, which may occur with variable motor activity that sometimes appears purposeful but with more gradual loss of consciousness (see Chapter 39). Seizures are often accompanied by tachycardia and normal or elevated blood pressure. Hypertension with bradycardia and apnea should suggest increased intracranial pressure.

A premonitory aura may herald vertebrobasilar vascular spasm, which appears to occur in syncope associated with migraines.

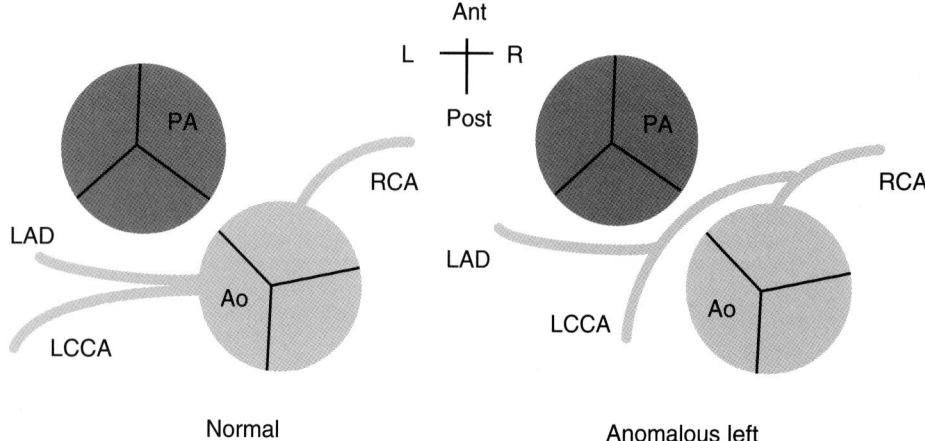

Figure 42-3. Coronary artery anomalies associated with sudden cardiac death. Ant, anterior; Ao, aorta; L, left; LAD, left anterior descending coronary artery; LCCA, left circumflex coronary artery; PA, pulmonary artery; Post, posterior; R, right; RCA, right coronary artery.

There may be a history of unilateral visual changes (poor vision), and the loss of consciousness usually has a somewhat longer onset and duration. Hemodynamic status remains stable throughout the episode. The patient frequently complains of headache after regaining consciousness. Vestibular migraine or migraine affecting the vertebrobasilar circulation can cause dizziness, vertigo, ataxia, confusion, and headache. There is often a positive family history of migraines.

Patients with a history of panic attacks or histrionic personalities may become syncopal secondary to hyperventilation. The mechanism is not completely understood but may involve the reaction of cerebral blood flow in response to hypocapnia and respiratory alkalosis. Tetany or paresthesias may be present in some patients. The history of the episode is, again, critical, and witnesses are especially helpful. The patient frequently relates a feeling of suffocation, smothering, shortness of breath, or chest tightness. In retrospect, the patient may also admit to numbness and tingling of the extremities and visual changes (Table 42-5). Hyperventilation and hypocapnia may be detected during the tilt-table test by measuring end-tidal CO_2.

Hypoglycemia should always be included as a cause of syncope, but it is exceedingly rare in children and adolescents. Certainly in the patient with insulin-dependent diabetes, hypoglycemia remains an important concern. As the blood glucose level drops, the patient feels weak, hungry, sweaty, agitated, and confused and eventually experiences altered mental status. Onset is gradual, and the patient remains hemodynamically stable, although tachycardia may be evident (see Chapter 61). Ingestion of oral hypoglycemic agents may exceed the body's normal gluconeogenesis capability, resulting in hypoglycemia.

Benign positional vertigo may begin before 6 years of age and manifests as a sudden fall, dizziness, and nystagmus with no loss of consciousness. Cataplexy, the sudden intrusion of rapid-eye-movement sleep in a previously awake patient, is a rare cause of loss of tone in children. If it is associated with narcolepsy, the patient may experience daytime sleepiness.

Cerebral syncope has been reported to occur as a loss of consciousness without hypotension or bradycardia. Local cerebral hemodynamic alterations (vasoconstriction) reduce cerebral blood flow, producing cerebral hypoxia. This is an uncommon condition.

Hysterical syncope is a diagnosis of exclusion. The patient is usually an adolescent and always has episodes in the presence of an audience. The patient is unusually calm in describing the episodes and relates details that may indicate no loss of consciousness. During the episode, there are no associated hemodynamic changes and no pallor, sweating, or respiratory changes. Typically, the patient falls gracefully and gently without injury. The key is to define what secondary gain the patient attains through the syncopal charade.

EVALUATION OF THE SYNCOPAL CHILD

History

Most children and adolescents who have a syncopal episode can be evaluated by their pediatrician. The history of the event is the critical information for most patients. A detailed account of what the patient felt immediately before losing consciousness, what the patient was doing, what the posture or position was, how the patient looked, how long the episode lasted, and associated signs or symptoms direct the diagnostic workup. A thorough and detailed family history is necessary to discover risk for sudden death, dysrhythmia, congenital heart disease, seizures, and metabolic disorders. The medication history, including nonprescribed, prescribed, and illicit drugs, as well as any accessible medication of other family members, should be gathered.

Physical Examination

Any person who has a syncopal episode should undergo a thorough physical examination, with special attention to the cardiovascular and neurologic systems. The examination should include obtaining vital signs with the patient supine and after standing for 5 to 10 minutes. On careful auscultation, the presence of an outflow tract murmur radiating to the neck, an abnormally loud second heart sound, or the presence of a long decrescendo diastolic murmur at the apex leads to more involved diagnostic testing. In most cases, patients with a history of syncope have normal physical findings at the time of the examination.

Diagnostic Tests

The history and physical examination findings guide the practitioner in determining the diagnostic tests. Because the child or adolescent who has had a syncopal episode is often evaluated hours or days after the episode, testing serum glucose and electrolytes or urine toxicology screening is usually of no value. All patients presenting with syncope need an ECG. The ECG should be inspected for the rhythm, with special attention to nonsinus rhythms and bradycardia. Measurements of the intervals should be performed manually regardless of any preprogrammed measurements printed on the ECG. Abnormalities of the PR, QRS, or QT/corrected QT (QTc) interval imply an underlying conduction abnormality. The P wave, QRS, and T wave amplitudes may indicate chamber enlargement or hypertrophy, each of which carries an increased risk for dysrhythmia. In the patient with a history of palpitations associated with syncope, 24-hour (ECG) Holter monitoring, with or without a subsequent patient-activated cardiac event recorder monitor, may help

---

Table 42-5. Symptoms Associated with Hyperventilation	
General	**Neurologic**
Fatigue	Dizziness
Diffuse weakness	Paresthesias (especially
Insomnia	distal)
Nightmares	Unsteadiness
Headache	Impaired memory and/or
"Feel cold"	concentration
Sweats	Slurred speech
	Blurred vision
Cardiovascular	
Palpitations	**Gastrointestinal**
Tachycardia	Globus hystericus
Precordial pain	Mouth dryness
Raynaud phenomenon	Dysphagia
	Bloating
Respiratory	Belching/flatulence
Shortness of breath	Abdominal pain
Chest pain	
Sighing respirations	**Psychic**
Yawning	Tension
"Can't get deep breath"	Anxiety
Paroxysmal nocturnal	Depression
dyspnea	Apprehension
Unexplained cough	
Dry mouth	
Musculoskeletal	
Muscle spasm	
Tremors	
Twitching	
Tetany	

From Reilly BM: Practical Strategies in Outpatient Medicine, 2nd ed. Philadelphia; WB Saunders, 1991, p 208.

capture the cardiac rhythm when the patient is symptomatic. If a heart murmur is appreciated, if there is a family history of sudden death or cardiomyopathy, or if the ECG is at all questionable, a cardiology consultation should be obtained, and two-dimensional, Doppler, and color-flow echocardiography should be performed. If the syncopal event is associated with exercise, echocardiography is critical; if the results are normal, a graded treadmill exercise stress test should be performed with full ECG and blood pressure monitoring. Patients with primary dysrhythmias may require cardiac catheterization and electrophysiologic testing with invasive monitoring (see Chapter 7). Patients with positional syncope with autonomic symptoms should undergo tilt-table testing with autonomic function testing that includes assessment of rhythmic breathing, carotid massage, Valsalva maneuver, and diving reflex elicited with ice to the face.

Patients exhibiting prolonged loss of consciousness, seizure activity, and a postictal phase of lethargy or confusion should be referred for neurologic consultation and electroencephalography. Without this history, the reported positive yield of electroencephalography is less than 1 in 300 studies. Likewise, neuroimaging studies generally have an exceptionally low yield in the absence of abnormality on physical examination.

SUMMARY AND RED FLAGS

The evaluation of the syncopal child or adolescent relies heavily on the ability to obtain a thorough, detailed history and to perform a physical examination. Hypotension, both supine and orthostatic, is a major red flag, as are associated palpitations or chest pain. Exertional syncope is a major red flag, and participation in gym class or sports must be restricted until a complete diagnostic workup is completed. Additional red flags include syncope while supine, a positive family history, prolonged loss of consciousness, prolonged seizures, prolonged postevent neurologic signs, and abrupt onset with no prodrome. Laboratory tests, except for the ECG, which is mandatory, are generally of limited value unless guided by pertinent positive or negative findings in the history and physical examination. The ECG allows screening for red flags (dysrhythmias), such as Wolfe-Parkinson-White syndrome, heart block, and long QT syndrome, as well as hypertrophic cardiomyopathies and myocarditis. The most common identifiable etiologic factor in otherwise healthy children and adolescents is neurocardiogenic or vasodepressor syncope, a usually benign and transient condition.

VERTIGO

The characteristic description of vertigo is the illusion of motion, usually described as spinning or whirling (see Table 42-1). The perception of motion may be internal ("My head is [or eyes are] spinning") or external ("The room is spinning or moving"). The sensation is usually rotatory, but it can be linear ("It feels like the swaying of a boat"). The patient's description is critical although potentially vague; further questioning may lead to the rather discrete differential diagnosis of vertigo.

The presence of associated symptoms may help if the patient's description leaves doubt about the type of dizziness. Nausea and vomiting frequently accompany vertigo, as do auditory changes, such as tinnitus, sensation of ear fullness, and unilateral deafness. This is especially important in small children who are unable to articulate the feeling of vertigo. Because middle ear infection can cause peripheral vertigo, some children seen with otitis media and vomiting may in fact have peripheral vertigo and secondary vomiting. If the dizziness usually occurs with abrupt changes in the position of the head, vertigo should be suspected. All vertigo reflects dysfunction of the vestibular-cochlear system.

The vestibular-cochlear apparatus with its associated reflex pathways is very complex. Dysfunction of the vestibular-cochlear apparatus is usually *central* (brainstem and eighth cranial nerve) or *peripheral* (distal or peripheral to the eighth cranial nerve).

Central vestibular disease refers to disorders of the brainstem, especially at the level of the vestibular nuclei or oculomotor nuclei or cerebellum (Table 42-6). Underlying causes of central vestibular dysfunction include

- acute vascular ischemic or thromboembolic events
- acute demyelinating diseases
- pharmacologic vertigo (alcohol, barbiturates, benzodiazepines)
- more indolent causes, including tumors of the brainstem or cerebellum and chronic demyelinating diseases
- trauma

Peripheral vertigo is generally unilateral and results in stimulation of the autonomic nervous system with resultant intense nausea, vomiting, pallor, and diaphoresis (Table 42-7; see Table 42-6). Peripheral vertigo can be caused by the following:

- middle ear infections
- paroxysmal positional vertigo

Table 42-6. Differences Between Peripheral and Central Vestibular Dysfunctions

Symptom/Sign	Peripheral	Central
Severity of vertigo	Marked	Often mild
	Nausea and vomiting common	
Nystagmus	Bilateral	Bilateral or unilateral
	Unidirectional	Bidirectional or unidirectional
	Rotatory/horizontal	May be vertical
	Never vertical	Usually no change with visual fixation
	Fast phase usually opposite to side of lesion	
	Improves with visual fixation	
	Begins within 2-10	Begins immediately
	Fatigues with time	Persistent
	Habituates	Reproducibly repetitive
Direction of environmental spin	Toward fast phase of nystagmus	Variable
Direction of past pointing	Toward slow phase of nystagmus	Variable
Tinnitus/deafness	Often present	Usually absent
Examples	Labyrinthitis	Multiple sclerosis
	Ménière disease	Vertebrobasilar ischemia (see Table 42-8)
	Positional vertigo (see Table 42-7)	

Modified from Reilly BM: Practical Strategies in Outpatient Medicine, 2nd ed. Philadelphia; WB Saunders, 1991, p 191.

Table 42-7. Peripheral Vestibulopathy

Syndrome	Usual Presentation	Typical Course	Hearing Loss?	Diagnosis	Treatment
(Benign) paroxysmal positional vertigo	Paroxysmal, brief, purely positional vertigo	Often polyphasic illness with gradual improvement but intermittent brief recurrences for weeks/months Does not cause ongoing severe vertigo	No	History Nylen-Bárány maneuvers	Wait
Vestibular neuronitis	Acute onset, severe vertigo, sometimes after viral respiratory infection	Severe ongoing vertigo for many hours or a few days Monophasic illness Resolves spontaneously No hearing loss	No	Clinical history Normal hearing Peripheral nystagmus Rapid (hours–days) resolution without recurrence	Wait
Infectious labyrinthitis	Usually mild vertigo accompanying obvious sinusitis, otitis media, or serous otitis	Resolves over several days with resolution of otitis/sinusitis Very rarely: severe purulent labyrinthitis, mastoiditis, meningitis	No, unless conductive loss due to otitis associated	ENT examination: otitis media? serous otitis? sinusitis?	Treat otitis, sinusitis; decongestants
Toxic vestibulopathy	Vertigo and/or hearing loss associated with use of toxic drugs	Usually dose related and reversible after withdrawal or dose reduction of offending drug	Depends on drug, but sensorineural deafness is common with aminoglycosides, aspirin, loop diuretics, platinum; hearing is usually normal with alcohol and quinidine	Peripheral vertigo with or without hearing loss while/after patient takes vestibulotoxic drugs; most are reversible with discontinuation of drug	Discontinue or adjust dose of drugs
Ménière disease	Episodic attacks of severe vertigo, usually with associated ear fullness sensation and/or hearing loss	Duration of attack, usually several hours; patient is well before and after attacks unless hearing loss progresses and persists	Usually sensorineural (90% unilateral) audiometry	Typical history with recurrences	Low-sodium diet Diuretics Surgery?
Cervicogenic vestibulopathy	Brief positional vertigo, associated with head and neck movements	Usually recurrent, brief, nondebilitating vertigo in patients with cervical spondylosis or other craniovertebral disease (rheumatoid arthritis, Klippel-Feil deformity)	No (but unrelated presbycusis common in this age group)	Typical history Nylen-Bárány maneuvers not consistent with benign positional vertigo Exclude: Vertebrobasilar ischemia Carotid sinus hypersensitivity	Vestibular exercises
Cholesteatoma	Indolent progression of symptoms	Indolent progression of symptoms	Conductive	Usually visible (at superior border of tympanic membrane) on otoscope examination of ear	Surgery
Otosclerosis	Progressive hearing loss, sometimes with intermittent vertigo	Indolent progressive hearing loss	Conductive	Family history Audiometry	Surgery
Labyrinthine hemorrhage	Sudden severe vertigo, usually in a patient on systemic anticoagulants (warfarin)	Gradual resolution over a few days	Variable	Syndrome similar to vestibular neuronitis, but history of anticoagulation is key	Wait Adjust and/or discontinue anticoagulants

Continued

Table 42-7. Peripheral Vestibulopathy—cont'd

Syndrome	Usual Presentation	Typical Course	Hearing Loss?	Diagnosis	Treatment
Post-traumatic					
Basilar (temporal bone) fracture	Severe vertigo, often with profound hearing loss immediately after head trauma	Gradual (days-weeks) resolution of vertigo; hearing loss, facial nerve injury often permanent	Often: sensorineural	Radiograph: fracture Hemotympanum? CSF otorrhea? Facial paresis?	Depends on extent of injury
Postconcussive	Ongoing, often mild/chronic vertigo after concussion, without fracture	Gradual resolution but often delayed for months-years	No	Persistent/chronic symptoms without evidence of other post-traumatic syndromes	Wait
Cupulolithiasis	Classic benign positional vertigo, but after head trauma	Same as for benign positional vertigo	No	Clinical history Nylen-Bárány maneuvers Exclude fistulas	Wait
Perilymphatic fistula	Trauma may be remote or indirect (swimming, diving injuries, for example) Usually, positional vertigo, recurrent; or mild persistent vertigo	Post-traumatic vertigo that does not improve over time	Often: mixed or sensorineural	Clinical history Positive fistula test Valsalva maneuver: symptoms worsen? Exclude fistulas	Surgery
Whiplash	Positional vertigo, worse with neck extension or turning, after deceleration neck injury	Gradual but slow improvement with resolution of neck symptoms	Usually none	Clinical history Exclude fractures and fistulas	Wait Physical therapy
Ossicular disruption	Hearing loss, acute vertigo, following head/facial trauma	Gradual (days) resolution of vertigo; hearing loss persists	Conductive	Clinical history Audiometry Exclude fistula	Surgery

Modified from Reilly BM: Practical Strategies in Outpatient Medicine, 2nd ed. Philadelphia; WB Saunders, 1991, pp 196-197.
CSF, cerebrospinal fluid; ENT, ear-nose-throat; TM, tympanic membrane.

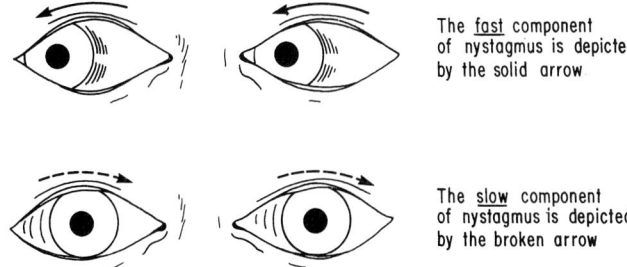

Figure 42-4. Fast nystagmus to the right. The appearance of the eyes is that of "frantic," jerky eye movements to the right: the direction of the fast component. (From Reilly BM: Practical Strategies in Outpatient Medicine, 2nd ed. Philadelphia, WB Saunders, 1991, p 192.)

- labyrinthitis
- vestibular neuronitis
- Ménière disease
- trauma

Patients suffering from acute ongoing peripheral vertigo appear very ill and very uncomfortable.

Acute ongoing vertigo is always accompanied by nystagmus. The rapidity of onset and the severity determine the degree of the nystagmus. Patients who complain of intermittent vertigo frequently do not have nystagmus between episodes. Figures 42-4 to 42-6 illustrate the appearance of central and peripheral vertigo-related nystagmus. Nystagmus in children with peripheral vestibular dysfunction is usually suppressed by visual fixation. Using an ophthalmoscope, the physician covers and uncovers the contralateral eye, inhibiting and permitting fixation. Peripheral nystagmus is frequently bilateral, unidirectional (slow and fast components in the same direction), and rotatory or horizontal (clockwise or counterclockwise). Therefore, nystagmus that is bidirectional, vertical, or unilateral should be considered central in origin.

Peripheral vestibular dysfunction has characteristic findings that can be elicited on physical examination. Deviation from these findings should imply central dysfunction and should direct the diagnostic workup to the central nervous system. Central vestibular dysfunction is much less common than peripheral vertigo and has a more serious underlying cause and higher rates of morbidity and mortality (Table 42-8).

The patient with peripheral vertigo typically falls toward or past points (Fig. 42-7) to the side of the lesion. The patient's surroundings appear to spin in the opposite direction, away from the lesion and in the same direction as the fast component of the nystagmus. The relationship of the direction that the patient falls, the direction the patient perceives the environment spinning, and the direction of the nystagmus is important in localizing the lesion. Such patients have abnormal neurologic examination findings, and all of the abnormalities are explainable on the basis of vestibular or cochlear dysfunction.

Patients with acute ongoing peripheral vestibular dysfunction frequently cannot walk and often have abnormal Romberg test findings (Fig. 42-8). They may complain of double vision and fine motor discoordination. Associated symptoms, such as dysarthria,

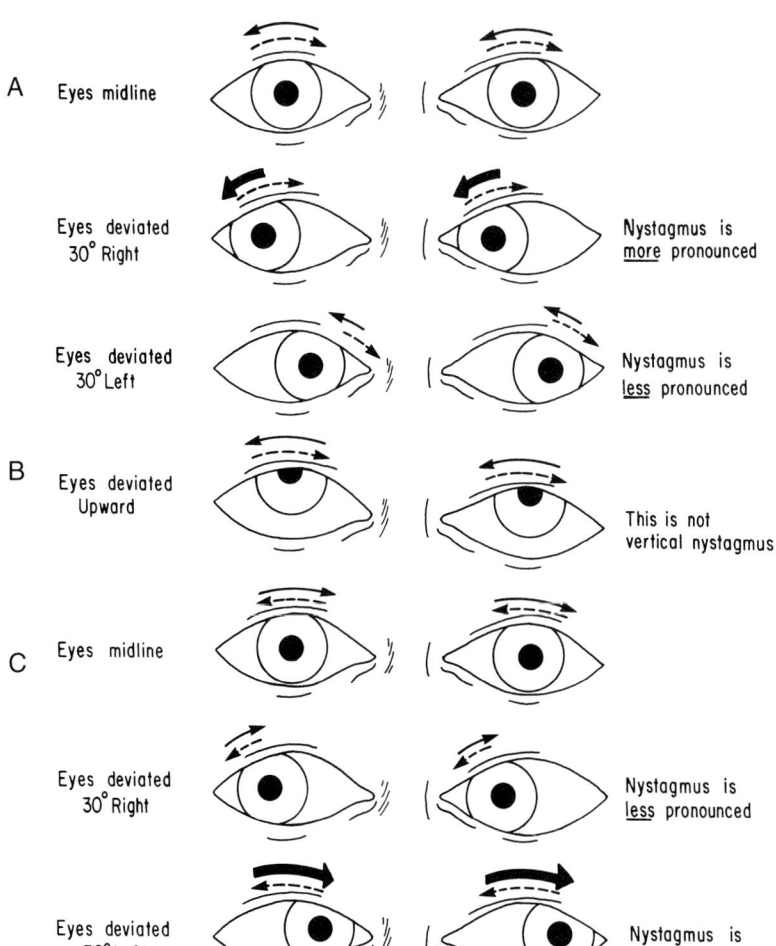

Figure 42-5. Peripheral nystagmus. **A,** In this case, nystagmus (fast right) affects each eye equally (bilateral), is unidirectional (the direction of fast and slow components stays the same in all gaze directions), and is horizontal and rotatory (i.e., the eyes move in the horizontal plane and in a counterclockwise direction during nystagmus). **B,** *Horizontal/rotatory* nystagmus, which occurs on vertical gaze, is *not* vertical nystagmus. **C,** In this instance, nystagmus (fast left) is horizontal/rotatory, unidirectional (fast component is always to the left), and bilateral. (From Reilly BM: Practical Strategies in Outpatient Medicine, 2nd ed. Philadelphia, WB Saunders, 1991, p 192.)

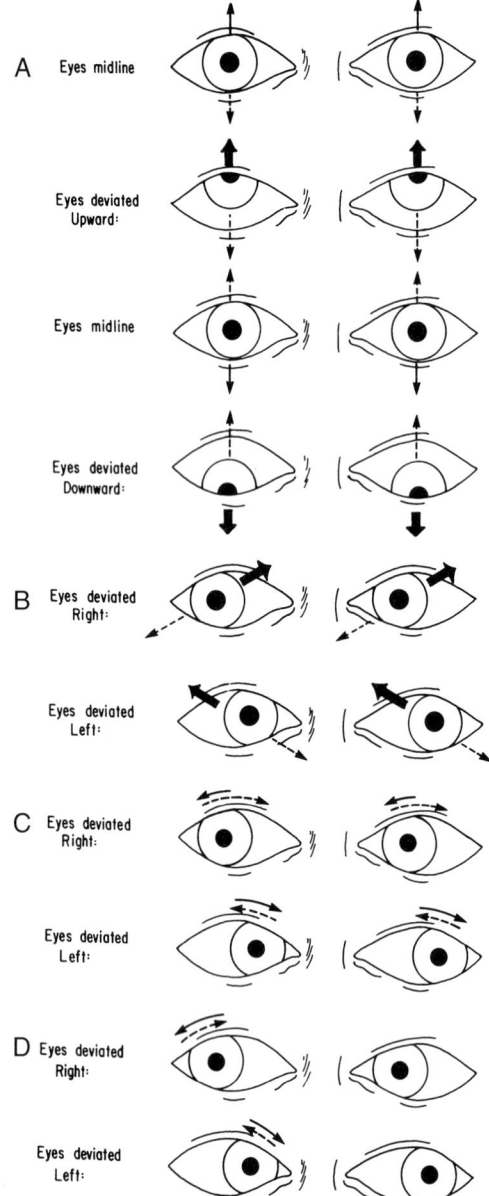

Figure 42-6. *Central nystagmus.* **A,** *Vertical nystagmus. Upper two panels: The fast (upward) component of vertical nystagmus is more prominent on upward gaze. Lower two panels: The fast component of vertical nystagmus is "down beating" and is even more prominent on downward gaze.* **B,** *Vertical nystagmus may persist on horizontal eye movements as well; this is still vertical nystagmus.* **C,** *Bidirectional nystagmus. The fast and slow components in this case change direction in different gaze directions.* **D,** *Unilateral nystagmus. Nystagmus in this instance affects only the right eye (and also changes direction; it is bidirectional as well). (From Reilly BM: Practical Strategies in Outpatient Medicine, 2nd ed. Philadelphia, WB Saunders, 1991, p 194.)*

dysesthesias, weakness, blindness, true diplopia, or hemiplegia, strongly imply a central mechanism, frequently of vascular origin. These are ominous findings, especially in a child with hemophilia, sickle cell disease, a history of congenital heart disease, or dysrhythmia. Likewise, the simultaneous presence of dysphagia, aphasia, pathologic reflexes, or unilateral cerebellar dysfunction (dysmetria, dysdiadochokinesia) with vestibular dysfunction is of central origin.

To make the diagnosis of acute ongoing peripheral vestibular dysfunction, the following must be demonstrated:

1. Vertigo must be a symptom.
2. Nystagmus must be carefully evaluated and must be of the peripheral type (bilateral, unidirectional, rotatory/horizontal).
3. There can be no neurologic signs or symptoms that cannot be explained by peripheral vestibular dysfunction.

Most patients do not have ongoing vertigo but give an episodic history. Provocational maneuvers of the head, such as the Nylen-Bárány maneuver, are utilized to elicit their symptoms (Fig. 42-9). Table 42-7 demonstrates the various types of peripheral vestibulopathy. Parainfectious (otitis media, upper respiratory tract) and post-traumatic causes are common in children and adolescents. Table 42-8 similarly demonstrates the characteristics of central vertigo; Table 42-6 illustrates differentiating features of positional nystagmus for peripheral versus central vertigo.

To treat persistent peripheral vertigo, the patient is asked to remain still in a dark room with the eyes closed. If symptoms of peripheral vertigo remain distressing to the patient, symptomatic treatment, including sedating (promethazine) or less sedating (meclizine) antivertiginous agents or transcutaneous scopolamine patches, may be indicated. Specific therapy may be needed for suppurative infections (labyrinthitis, otitis media, mastoiditis) and for central nervous system lesions that produce central vertigo.

Paroxysmal positional vertigo is common in adolescents and is characterized by brief (<30 seconds) episodes of disturbing vertigo when the patient turns over in bed, looks up or over the shoulder, or tosses the head to move hair away from the face. Between occurrences, there may be anxiety and apprehension about recurrence. The paroxysms can occur at any time of day, but they tend to cluster in the morning. Physical findings, including hearing, cranial nerves, and cerebellar function, are normal. The Nylen-Bárány maneuver (see Fig. 42-9) elicits a characteristic response, and the patient's symptoms, very reliably. Generally a benign but annoying condition, positional vertigo has a variable duration. Although it is usually transient, it can recur over a period of years. Most patients learn to avoid the positional maneuvers that provoke their episodes. Canalith repositioning maneuvers attempt to move the irritating free moving particles (canalithiasis) to a nonirritating position.

EVALUATION OF THE PATIENT WITH VERTIGO

History

The history is critical to the diagnosis of the vertiginous patient. A careful, detailed description of the prodrome and the actual symptoms, including timing, duration, direction of the spinning, associated symptoms, preceding infections (especially of the upper respiratory tract, such as otitis media or sinusitis), medications, and a history of trauma, such as occurs in swimming and diving, must be documented. A history of vertigo or any other neurologic condition is important.

Physical Examination

Special attention must be paid to the head, ears, eyes, nose, and throat examination. Good visualization of the tympanic membranes and of their mobility is necessary, along with testing both air and bony conduction with a tuning fork (Figs. 42-10 and 42-11). Visualization of the fundi is important. Palpation and percussion of the paranasal sinuses may be helpful in older children but is rarely useful in patients younger than 6 to 8 years. Testing of all the cranial nerves, including the olfactory nerve, should be done in an organized manner.

The neurologic examination must include evaluation of the gait, a Romberg test, and assessment of the visual fields and visual acuity. If nystagmus is not apparent, the Nylen-Bárány maneuver

Table 42-8. Central Vertigo

Cause	Usual Age at Onset	Clinical Clues	Diagnosis	Treatment
Vertebrobasilar ischemia	Young: migrainous	Known (suspected) vascular disease: hypertensive, diabetic Almost always accompanied by brainstem symptoms and signs: diplopia, dysarthria, dysesthesias, motor weakness	TIA: clinical history Stroke: neurologic examination CT scan may be unreliable MRI more sensitive Angiography?	TIA: aspirin; rarely, surgery Stroke: observe; rarely, anticoagulant
Cerebellar hemorrhage	Middle-aged	Hypertensive, anticoagulated, post-traumatic Sudden headache: diplopia, ataxia usually more prominent than vertigo	CT scan	Small hemorrhage: watch for worsening Large hemorrhage: surgical evacuation
Cerebellopontine angle tumors (Most: acoustic neuroma)	Middle-aged Young: neurofibromatosis type II	Hearing loss, tinnitus much more prominent than vertigo Mild disequilibrium Early: normal neurologic examination, except sensorineural hearing loss Later: Cranial nerves V and VII abnormal; papilledema?	Audiometry: retrocochlear, sensorineural hearing loss CT scan, MRI Internal audiometry canal tomography ENG, ABER	Surgery
Multiple sclerosis	Young (average age, 30)	Optic neuritis Internuclear ophthalmoplegia Spastic paraparesis/incontinence Vertigo first isolated symptom in only 10% of cases	Multiplicity of symptoms and signs dissociated in time and space MRI scanning CSF: oligoclonal bands	Steroids Long-term management
Drug toxicity	Any age	Alcohol, sedatives, tranquilizers, opiates, anticonvulsants	Discontinue drug	Discontinue drug
Basilar migraine	Young	Vertigo part of headache syndrome Usually positive family history	Clinical history	See Chapter 37
Vertiginous (temporal lobe) epilepsy	Young	Vertigo as aura to loss of consciousness Very rare	Clinical history Exclude other diagnoses EEG	Anticonvulsants
Cranial neuropathy	Variable	Many types, all uncommon: 　Herpes zoster: external ear/palate skin lesions and cranial nerve VIII symptoms 　Postinfectious: after viral syndromes: polyneuritis and/or cerebellitis and/or encephalitis 　Chronic meningitis: syphilis, tuberculosis, sarcoid, carcinomatous 　Vasculitis: Cogan syndrome, Wegener granulomatosus, temporal arteritis, syphilis 　Head and neck carcinoma 　Vascular compression syndromes		

Others: Heredofamilial disorders
　　　　(Friedreich ataxia, spinocere-
　　　　bellar degeneration, olivoponto-
　　　　cerebellar degeneration)
　　　Cerebellar degeneration (alcohol,
　　　　cancer)
　　　Tumor of brainstem, cerebellum
　　　Syrinx cervical cord
　　　Post-traumatic concussion

Modified from Reilly BM: Practical Strategies in Outpatient Medicine, 2nd ed. Philadelphia; WB Saunders, 1991, p 200.

ABER, auditory brainstem-evoked response; CT, computed tomography; CSF, cerebrospinal fluid; EEG, electroencephalogram; ENG, electronystagmography; MRI, magnetic resonance imaging; TIA, transient ischemic attack.

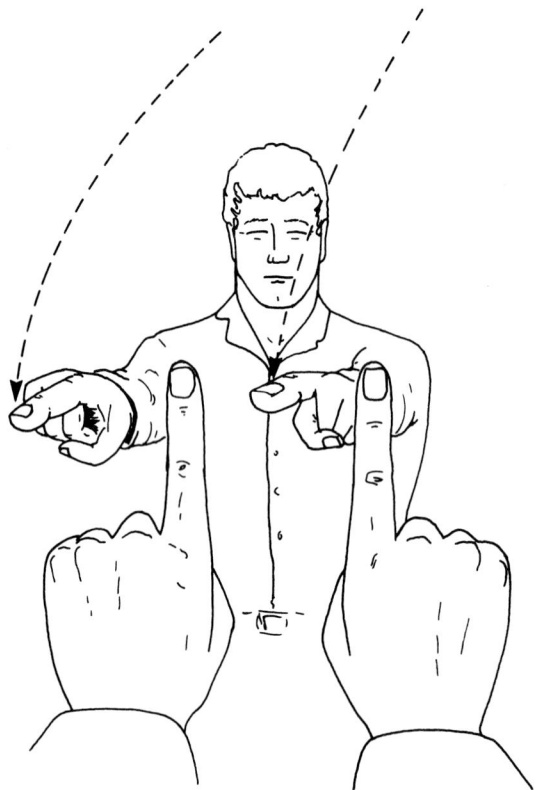

Figure 42-7. Past pointing. The patient is asked to raise the hands over the head and then, with the eyes closed, touch the examiner's fingers. This figure illustrates abnormal past pointing to the right; past pointing often points toward the side of the vestibular lesion. (From Reilly BM: Practical Strategies in Outpatient Medicine, 2nd ed. Philadelphia, WB Saunders, 1991, p 195.)

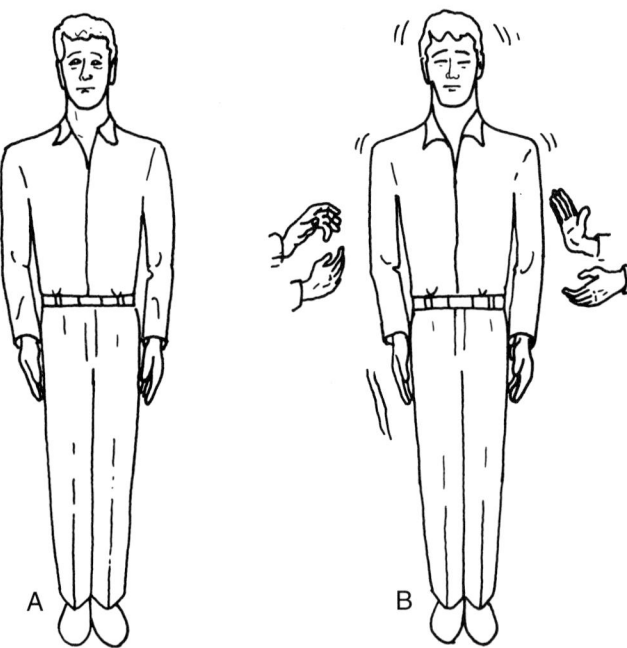

Figure 42-8. The Romberg test. The patient stands upright, feet together, arms at sides. The examiner should stand next to the patient. The test is performed in two stages: with the patient's eyes open and then with the eyes closed. Even a normal person may experience mild subjective disequilibrium and may "waver" with eyes closed. Thus, the Romberg test can sometimes simulate the feeling of disequilibrium. **A,** With eyes open, the patient can stand unsupported without difficulty. **B,** With eyes closed, the patient loses his or her balance. This test result suggests peripheral neuropathy or vestibular dysfunction or both. Cerebellar disease more often results in inability to maintain this posture with the eyes either open or closed. (From Reilly BM: Practical Strategies in Outpatient Medicine, 2nd ed. Philadelphia, WB Saunders, 1991, p 168.)

(see Fig. 42-9) should be performed and the presence or absence of nystagmus noted carefully. In most children and adolescents, the physical examination results are normal with only subtle findings when the symptoms are provoked.

Diagnostic Tests

The history and physical examination results direct the diagnostic workup and indicate which tests need to be performed. Imaging studies important in the workup of the vertiginous patient include computed tomography and magnetic resonance imaging. Both techniques allow visualization of the inner ear and the labyrinthine apparatus, as well as the brainstem and cerebellum. If an infectious cause is suspected, it may be useful to perform a lumbar puncture as long as increased intracranial pressure is not suspected. In the setting of trauma, the simple use of the pneumatic otoscope may allow the examiner to perform a "fistula test," reproducing or worsening the patient's symptoms because of an abnormal communication to the labyrinthine system. If hearing loss is a feature, audiometry and evoked response testing should be considered. A summary of diagnostic tests and their outcomes (diagnoses) is noted in Table 42-9.

SUMMARY AND RED FLAGS

Vertigo is characterized by the perception of movement, particularly rotational movement, and can be a most distressing and incapacitating

phenomenon. The history and physical examination findings, especially those of the head, ears, eyes, nose, and throat examination and neurologic examination, usually lead to the diagnosis, with laboratory tests and imaging studies generally having a confirmatory role. The history and examination should allow the examiner to distinguish between peripheral and central vestibular dysfunction.

In children and adolescents, peripheral vertigo is far more common than central vertigo. However, in certain at-risk populations, such as children with sickle cell disease, hemophilia, or congenital heart disease (especially children with right-to-left shunts or mixing lesions) and children receiving warfarin (Coumadin), the central causes resulting from hemorrhagic and thromboembolic phenomena must be remembered. Chronicity, persistence, vertical nystagmus, and signs of increased intracranial pressure are red flags. Because the diagnosis of vertigo requires that the patient be able to articulate the perception of movement, it is difficult to make this diagnosis in small children, and the condition must be carefully distinguished from other movement impairments, especially disequilibrium.

DISEQUILIBRIUM

When a "dizzy" patient describes feeling unsteady on his or her feet, off balance, or uncoordinated, the patient is describing a disturbance in the body's equilibrium system. The fundamental complaint is difficulty in walking, not from weakness but from a feeling of lack of control.

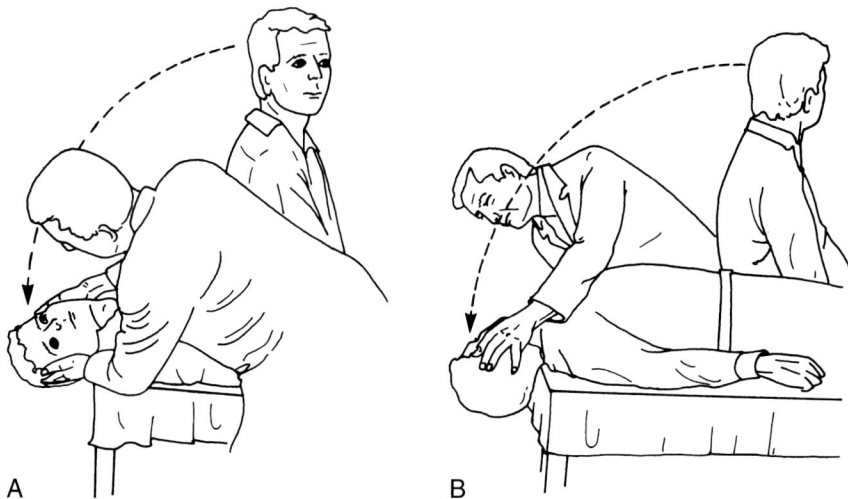

Figure 42-9. A and B, Patients are first observed, seated, with the eyes straight ahead. Any spontaneous nystagmus at rest, on horizontal gaze (no more than 30 degrees from the midline), or on vertical gaze is noted and analyzed. Extraocular movements are tested. Patients turn their head 30 to 45 degrees to one side and are then lowered quickly backward to the supine position, so that the head is extended down over the end of the examining table to about a 30-degree subhorizontal angle (A). The patient is now lying down, head turned to one side, and inclined backward, one ear facing the floor, with the examiner supporting the patient's head and neck. This position is maintained for 30 seconds. The patient's eyes are observed while in the midline and while they are looking down toward the floor. Induction of nystagmus is often accompanied by the onset of vertigo and a frantic urge to get up (especially when peripheral vestibular disease is the problem). The patient is then brought back to the upright position, the eyes are observed for 30 to 60 seconds (nystagmus may then occur again), and the maneuver is repeated, with the head now turned down to the opposite side (B). During the Nylen-Bárány maneuver, *positional* nystagmus should be observed for (1) the direction of slow/fast components; (2) the head position that elicits nystagmus; (3) the latency of onset of nystagmus (the time between assumption of the head position and the onset of nystagmus); (4) the persistence or fatigue of nystagmus (does nystagmus wane as the head position is maintained, or does it continue unabated?); (5) the intensity of vertigo induced; and (6) the presence or absence of habituation (does repeating the test in the vulnerable position cause a lesser or absent nystagmus response—habituation—or not?). (From Reilly BM: Practical Strategies in Outpatient Medicine, 2nd ed. Philadelphia, WB Saunders, 1991, p 204.)

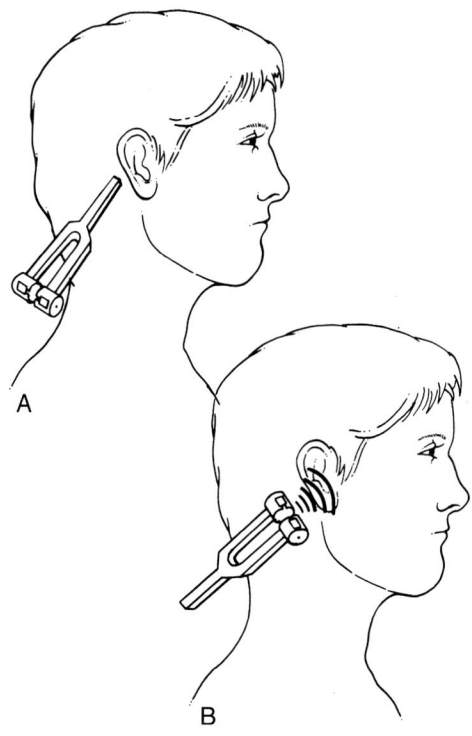

Figure 42-10. The Rinne test. The tuning fork is first placed on the mastoid process (A). When the sound can no longer be heard, the tuning fork is placed in front of the external auditory meatus (B). Normally, air conduction is better than bone conduction. (From Swartz MH: Textbook of Physical Diagnosis: History and Examination. Philadelphia, WB Saunders, 1989, p 175.)

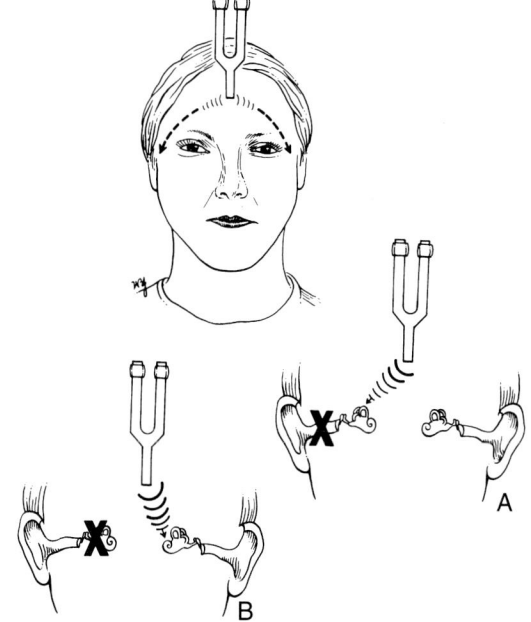

Figure 42-11. The Weber test. When a vibrating tuning fork is placed on the center of the forehead, the sound is normally heard in the center without lateralization to either side (**top**). A, In the presence of a conductive hearing loss, the sound is heard on the side of the conductive loss. B, In the presence of a sensorineural loss, the sound is better heard on the opposite (unaffected) side. (From Swartz MH: Textbook of Physical Diagnosis: History and Examination. Philadelphia, WB Saunders, 1989, p 176.)

Table 42-9. Approach to Diagnosis of Dizziness in Children

Presenting Complaint	Clinical and Laboratory Findings	Likely Diagnosis
Acute onset with hearing loss (all ages)	Fever +, infection +, toxin +, vomiting +	Labyrinthitis
	Fever −, tinnitus +, ear pressure +, vomiting +	Ménière syndrome
	Head trauma +, barotrauma +, exertion +	Perilymphatic fistula, concussion
	Fever −, head trauma −, infection −	Vascular occlusion
Recurrent paroxysmal vertigo with no hearing loss	As above	As above
Patient 16 months to 4 or 5 years	Nystagmus +, EEG normal, Eng ±	Benign paroxysmal vertigo
	Torticollis +, GE reflux +, EEG normal, ENG ±	Paroxysmal torticollis
Teen or older patient	Postinfection +, vomiting +, EEG normal, ENG + PPN	Vestibular neuronitis
All ages	Positional vertigo only, vomiting +, EEG normal, ENG + PPN	Paroxysmal positional vertigo
	Headache +, vomiting +, EEG normal, ENG ±	Migraine
Recurrent paroxysmal vertigo with no hearing loss but with loss of consciousness ± (all ages)	Headache +, vomiting +, EEG post. slow, ENG +	Migraine
	Headache −, vomiting −, EEG +, ENG +	Seizures
	Headache −, vomiting −, EEG normal, ENG normal	Hyperventilation
Chronic unremitting vertigo	Neurologic signs +, hearing loss +, cranial nerve deficits +, CT scan of brain +, MR image of brain +	Cerebellopontine angle tumor, cholesteatoma, cerebellar tumor, ependymoma
	Neurologic signs absent, metabolic workup normal, CT scan brain −, MR image brain −	Panic attacks, conversion reaction, depression
	Neurologic signs absent, metabolic workup abnormal	Metabolic disorder

From Eviatar L: Dizziness in children. Otolaryngol Clin North Am 1994;27:565.

CT, computed tomography; EEG, electroencephalogram; ENG, electronystagmography; GE, gastroesophageal; MR, magnetic resonance; PPN, paroxysmal positional nystagmus; +, positive, present; −, negative, absent; ±, positive or negative, present or absent.

Walking is a very complex activity. The constant integration of visual, vestibular, and proprioceptive afferent information regarding the changing spatial orientation is performed by using all levels of the central nervous system: the cerebral cortex, cerebellum, brainstem, spinal cord, and peripheral neuromuscular system. These spatial data are then utilized by the efferent system, producing both

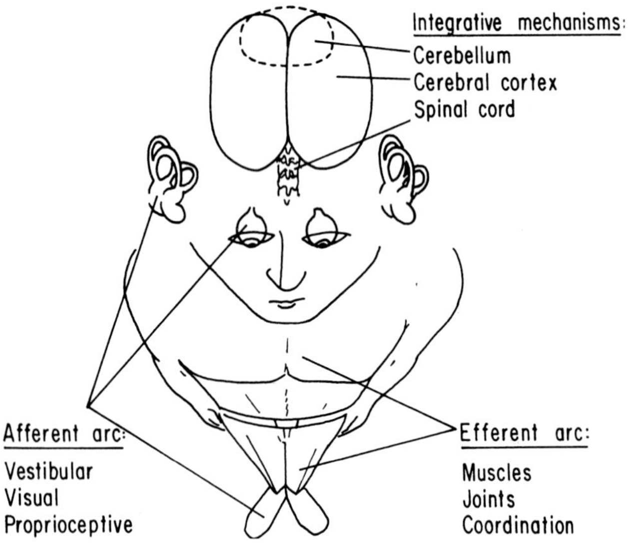

Figure 42-12. The afferent, integrative, and efferent components of the equilibrium system. (From Reilly BM: Practical Strategies in Outpatient Medicine, 2nd ed. Philadelphia, WB Saunders, 1991, p 166.)

Integrative mechanisms:
Cerebellum
Cerebral cortex
Spinal cord

Afferent arc:
Vestibular
Visual
Proprioceptive

Efferent arc:
Muscles
Joints
Coordination

voluntary and involuntary movements and spatial adjustments (Fig. 42-12). Disturbances in any of these pathways can result in difficulty with locomotion.

Disequilibrium, therefore, may result from any perceptual distortion of spatial orientation. The most common is visual impairment, to which any child who has played "Pin the Tail on the Donkey" or "Blind Man's Bluff" can attest. Humans depend a great deal on visual perception to orient themselves in space. Vestibulocochlear dysfunction can also severely impair a person's ability to ambulate. Peripheral neuropathies affecting proprioceptive function impair the ability of the central nervous system to accurately perceive the position of the limbs with regard to one another and to either the ground or the body. Disorders causing diffuse damage to the integrative mechanism or cortical or cerebellar diseases can impair proprioception as well. Likewise, efferent motor disability produces impairment of locomotion by producing weakness or apraxias (Table 42-10).

The diagnosis of the origin of disequilibrium, therefore, requires a well-organized, thorough history and physical examination, especially the neurologic examination. A single cause of disequilibrium is sometimes found; however, it is more common for the impairment to result from effects on multiple pathways: afferent, integrative, and efferent.

The history is critical for patients complaining of dizziness or difficulty ambulating. For children, this includes a detailed developmental history, because the differential diagnosis varies significantly for children who were walking and then stop and for those who do not achieve that milestone. For younger children, it may be very difficult to determine whether refusal or reluctance to walk is related to imbalance, pain (see Chapters 44 and 45), or weakness (see Chapter 38). Nausea and vomiting are usually associated with vertigo but tend to be rare with disequilibrium. Nausea and vomiting may accompany a viral illness that results in an acute cerebellar

Table 42-10. Disequilibrium

Cause	Clues	Gait/Romberg Test Result	Treatment
Most Common			
Multiple sensory deficits	Visual impairment? Hearing/vestibular dysfunction? Neuropathy? Spondylosis/degenerative joint disease? Neuropathy? Weakness?	Timid: slow, short stepped, apprehensive Remarkably improved with sensory assist (cane, companion) Romberg: normal or sensory	Sensory assist Correct/improve any/some of sensory deficits
Hyperventilation/ anxiety disorders	Young, healthy, anxious patient with *episodic "spells"* of disequilibrium; or Constant, chronic, elusive disequilibrium with or without obvious medical/psychosocial stress	Usually normal gait Romberg: normal or "Nonphysiologic"	Psychologic treatment; antianxiety medications
Vestibular disorders	*Chronic* unilateral vestibulopathy may cause ongoing disequilibrium: Ménière disease, cholesteatoma, fistula, acoustic neuroma, drug-induced vestibulopathy	Usually normal gait May veer to side of vestibular lesion Romberg: sensory	
Drug-induced	Central nervous system agents: tranquilizers, barbiturates, sedatives, alcohol, H_2 blockers, β blockers, calcium agents, indomethacin Vestibulotoxic agents: aspirin, loop diuretics, aminoglycosides, quinidine	Timid and/or ataxic gait Romberg: normal or cerebellar Romberg: sensory or normal	Discontinue or adjust dose of offending drug
Alcoholic	Heavy alcohol abuse may cause cerebellar and/or sensory degeneration Nystagmus uncommon	Ataxic gait Romberg: cerebellar or sensory	Often some (but incomplete) recovery from neuropathy with alcohol abstinence, vitamin therapy, physical therapy, nutritional therapy Cerebellar dysfunction often permanent, but abstinence, vitamins, nutrition may help
Painful ambulation	Arthritis? Claudication? Pain is limiting factor!	Limiping? Waddling? Normal gait? Romberg: usually normal	Find cause
Fear of falling	Normal examination No apraxia or ataxia Rarely, phobic	Timid gait Romberg: often cerebellar but fluctuates, inorganic	Reassure Rarely, phobic desensitization
Less Common			
Hypothyroidism	Weight gain or poor growth, cold intolerance, hoarseness, fatigue	Usually normal gait Severe: ataxic gait	Thyroid hormone
Hypoglycemia	Episodic; usually postprandial	Romberg: usually normal	Find cause (drug-induced, postprandial, insulinoma, etc.)
Apraxia	Usually diffuse cortical dysfunction or frontal lobe disease Usually apraxic in execution of other skilled movements (e.g., combing hair, brushing teeth)	Apraxic gait Romberg: normal	Find cause: CNS tumor subdural hematoma, normal-pressure hydrocephalus, multi-infarct state
Peripheral disease	Diabetes, alcoholism, pernicious anemia Only very severe (proprioceptive) neuropathy causes gait disorder	Sensory gait: footdrop and/or circus clown Romberg: sensory	Find cause: often irreversible
Cerebellar disease (nonalcoholic)	See Table 42-11	Ataxic gait Romberg: cerebellar	Find cause (see Table 42-11)

Continued

Table 42-10. Disequilibrium—cont'd

Cause	Clues	Gait/Romberg Test Result	Treatment
Less Common—cont'd			
Spasticity	Multiple sclerosis, spinal cord tumor/trauma Legs: weak, hyperreflexic, clonus Often bowel/bladder dysfuction	Spastic, scissors gait Romberg: often normal	Find cause: cord lesion, demyelinating disease, myelitis, etc.
Normal-pressure hydrocephalus	Urinary incontinence Cognitive impairment Gait disturbance	Ataxic/apraxic	CSF shunt
Hemiplegia	Prior cerebrovascular accident Hemiparesis on neurologic examination	Hemiplegic gait Romberg: often normal (if able to perform at all)	Find cause
Proximal myopathy	Severe bilateral proximal leg weakness: hip disease, muscular dystrophy, myositis, etc.	Waddling gait Romberg: normal	Find cause
Hysterical	Unpredictable, intermittent or bizarre "Secondary gain"	Gait varies: sometimes normal, timid, limping, apraxic Romberg: often cerebellar, but fluctuates, inorganic	Exclude organic causes Ongoing medical psychiatric treatment

Modified from Reilly BM: Practical Strategies in Outpatient Medicine, 2nd ed. Philadelphia; WB Saunders, 1991, pp 172-173.

CNS, central nervous system; CSF, cerebrospinal fluid.

ataxia and thus may precede the onset of disequilibrium. If nausea is simultaneous with the disequilibrium, drug or alcohol intoxication must be considered. Morning nausea or vomiting can be seen with increased intracranial pressure, as in hydrocephalus and posterior

Table 42-11. Cerebellar Ataxia

"Midline" (Ataxia, Nystagmus)	"Lateralizing" (Ataxia, Limb Incoordination, Dysarthria)
Acute	
Drug/alcohol intoxication-ingestion*	Ischemia/stroke: embolic, vasculitis
Post-traumatic	Hemorrhage: cerebellar, subdural
Cerebellar hemorrhage	Post-traumatic
Migraine	Abscess
Viral cerebellitis (varicella, enteroviruses, influenza, etc.*)	Viral cerebellitis (varicella, enteroviruses, influenza, etc.)*
Subacute	
Normal-pressure hydrocephalus	Primary neoplasm
Hypothyroidism	Metastatic neoplasm
Demyelinating disease	Demyelinating disease
Remote cancer effect	
Midline cerebellar tumor*	
Chronic	
Heredofamilial	Primary neoplasm
Cervical spondylosis	Arnold-Chiari malformation
Metabolic disease (rare)†	Familial spinocerebellar degeneration
	Metabolic diease†

Adapted from Dreyfus PM, Oshtory M, Gardner ED, et al: Cerebellar ataxia: Anatomical, physiological, and clinical implications. West J Med 1978;128:499-511 and from Reilly BM: Practical Strategies in Outpatient Medicine, 2nd ed. Philadelphia; WB Saunders, 1991, p 168.

*Common.

†Ataxia-telangiectasia, Hartnup disease, Refsum disease, abetalipoproteinemia, etc.

fossa tumors. Any history of head trauma, especially in toddlers, and any history of congenital heart disease with the potential for paradoxical embolization, including septic emboli resulting in brain abscess, must be taken seriously.

It is important to distinguish acute intermittent ataxia from more chronic or progressive forms (Tables 42-11 to 42-13). Drugs and postviral cerebellitis are common causes of acute sudden-onset ataxia. Varicella-associated postinfectious acute cerebellar ataxia usually comes after the infection, but in rare instances, it may occur before or during chickenpox. Its nature is benign. Metabolic hereditary disorders may cause intermittent symptoms provoked by fever, as in maple syrup urine disease, ataxia-telangiectasia, Hartnup disease, Refsum disease, pyruvate decarboxylase deficiency, abetalipoproteinemia, biotinidase deficiency, and some enzyme deficiencies. These must be distinguished from hypothyroidism, demyelinating disorders, muscular dystrophies, and neoplasms of the posterior fossa, brainstem, and spinal cord. Paraneoplastic effects of neuroblastoma produce ataxia, opsoclonus, and myoclonus. The Miller-Fisher variant of Guillain-Barré syndrome produces ataxia, ophthalmoplegia, and areflexia.

Progressive ataxias have a poorer prognosis. Age at onset can be used to distinguish some causes: Posterior fossa tumors and neuroblastoma generally occur within the first decade, Friedreich ataxia and Duchenne muscular dystrophy during the late first to second decades, and multiple sclerosis and diabetic peripheral neuropathy in the second decade.

Observation of the child's gait is an important component of the physical examination. Enough room should be found to allow the child to initiate walking, to proceed in a straight line for 10 to 20 paces, and to turn and return. The normal child, older than 2 to 3 years, initiates walking without hesitation and steps smoothly with a consistent stride length and height and a narrow base. The arms should swing freely and rhythmically, alternating with the feet, and there should be little sway in the trunk. When the child stops, there should be no hesitation again and no wavering or compensation. The observer should practice watching children walk normally to develop a sense for each part of the complex motion.

One of the most common gait abnormalities in children is the *wide-based gait*. Again, careful observation of toddlers at various stages of development familiarizes the observer with the transition from the wide-based, lurching steps of a 12-month-old

Table 42-12. Congenital Causes of Chronic Ataxia

Disorder	Age of Presentation	Clinical Manifestations	Mechanism of Ataxia, Diagnoses, and Treatment
Cerebellar hypoplasia	Early infancy (occasionally delayed)	Developmental delay, hypotonia, athetosis, chorea, delayed walking, ataxic gait	Absent cerebellar granular cells; CT shows small cerebellum
Vermal aplasia Dandy-Walker malformation	Early infancy	Macrocephaly, enlarged occipital region; ataxia	Hydrocephalus and cystic dilation of the fourth ventricle; treatment is by shunting of hydrocephalus and/or the posterior fossa cyst
Joubert syndrome	Early infancy	Neonatal episodic hyperpnea and apnea; hypotonia, nystagmus	MRI and CT demonstrate agenesis of the superior cerebellar vermis
Arnold-Chiari malformation	Variable	Headache, neck pain, lower cranial nerve dysfunction, nystagmus, ataxia; this variety does not have associated myelomeningocele	MRI and CT demonstrate caudal fourth ventricle; distortion of the brainstem; treatment is by posterior fossa decompression
Hydrocephalus	Variable	Macrocephaly, vomiting, ataxia	CT and MRI demonstrate enlarged lateral ventricles; in aqueductal stenosis, the third ventricle is particularly large, whereas the fourth ventricle is normal or small

From Behrman RE, Kliegman RM: Nelson Essentials of Pediatrics, 2nd ed. Philadelphia; WB Saunders, 1994, p 688.

CT, computed tomography; MRI, magnetic resonance imaging.

to the smooth, sure, rhythmic stride of children older than 2 to 3 years. Excessive trunk sway is typical of cerebellar ataxia. Waddling tends to be caused by proximal muscle weakness with a forward leaning, stiff appearance. It is important to distinguish an unsteady gait with irregular steps from a limp or a sensory deficit resulting in a high step with a slapping foot plant (see Chapter 45).

In a toddler, passive and active range of motion exercises should be performed to assure the observer that there is no joint or muscle pain. Reflexes, including the Babinski sign, should be carefully tested. Testing the sensory system in a toddler, especially proprioception, vibration, and two-point discrimination, can be a challenge. The Romberg test may also be difficult for younger children.

The Romberg test helps distinguish between cerebellar disequilibrium and sensory input impairment (see Fig. 42-8). To be reliable, the Romberg test requires some cooperation from the patient. Patients who can hold their position with only a minimal waver with their eyes closed have intact cerebellar and proprioceptive pathways. If the Romberg test result is "positive," the observer must distinguish between midline and lateralizing cerebellar disease. Ataxia with nystagmus is characteristic of midline cerebellar disease. Older children can also be asked to perform a heel-to-toe Romberg test. Lateralizing cerebellar diseases usually manifest dysmetria on finger-to-nose testing or the heel-shin maneuver; they may also show signs of dysdiadochokinesia with impairment of rapid, fine, alternating movements, such as sequential opposition of the thumbs and each fingertip or repetitive pronation-supination patting the hands on the knees, palm, and back. To perform these maneuvers, the patient must be old enough to cooperate and follow directions. Table 42-11 briefly demonstrates midline versus lateralizing cerebellar ataxias.

EVALUATION OF THE PATIENT WITH DISEQUILIBRIUM

History

A detailed developmental history, especially for a younger child, is obtained. The family history should also be complete. The examiner

should check for prodromal illnesses, especially viral (varicella) in nature:

- Is there any history of trauma?
- What is the character of the disability?
- Does the child feel unsteady standing, starting to walk, stopping, or turning?
- How do the parents characterize the child's gait?
- Are there associated symptoms, such as nausea, vomiting, pain, or vertigo?
- Does the child take or have access to any medications or alcohol?
- Is the disequilibrium intermittent or constant?
- Are there any other medical conditions of note?

Physical Examination

A thorough general physical examination should precede a very detailed neuromuscular examination. Presence of a goiter, cutaneous lesions of neurofibromatosis, or tuberous sclerosis may point to a diagnosis immediately. The neuromuscular examination should proceed from head to toe in an organized and systematic manner. Muscle tone, bulk, and symmetry of the face, trunk, and extremities are important. Cranial nerves should be examined, as should the sensory system (dermatome by dermatome). During the motor examination, the physician should isolate muscle groups and joints by observing the gait more than once, before assessing overall function. The Romberg test should be performed in all patients old enough to cooperate, as should the lateralizing cerebellar tests, such as the finger-to-nose and rapid, alternating movements. Attention to detail in the history and physical examination findings usually yields a diagnosis.

Diagnostic Tests

Other than for drug ingestion, obvious peripheral neuropathies or myopathies, focal extremity infections, or varicella-associated cerebellar ataxia, magnetic resonance imaging is the principal diagnostic test for children and adolescents with disequilibrium. Metabolic tests and thyroid function tests are indicated by either history or physical findings. Especially in younger children, imaging is necessary to rule

Table 42-13. Hereditary Causes of Ataxia

Disorder	Usual Age at Onset	Hereditary Pattern	Clinical Characteristics	Cause and Treatment
Friedreich ataxia	2-16 yr	Recessive	Ataxia, scoliosis, pes cavus, posterior column sensory loss, areflexia, cardiomyopathy	Supportive
Ataxia-telangiectasia	Early infancy (1-2 yr)	Recessive	Ataxia, oculomotor apraxia, sinopulmonary infections, telangiectasia of conjuctiva and skin	B and T cell dysfunction; cellular immunity is impaired; supportive
Machado-Joseph disease	12-15 yr	Dominant	Cerebellar, pyramidal, extrapyramidal degeneration; anterior horn cell disease; Portuguese ancestry	Supportive
Metachromatic leukodystrophy	1-2 yr	Recessive	Ataxia, peripheral neuropathy, spasticity, optic atrophy, dementia	Supportive
Refsum disease	4-7 yr	Recessive	Ataxia, neuropathy, retinitis pigmentosa, ichthyosis	Phytanic acid hydroxylase deficiency; phytol-free diet
Leigh disease	Infancy to adolescence	Recessive	Ataxia, lactic acidosis hypotonia, abnormalities of respiration	Some Leigh disorders of pyruvate metabolism; supportive
Wilson disease	Infancy to adulthood	Recessive	Hepatic disease, tremor, dystonia, athetosis, chorea	Ceruloplasmin deficiency; penicillamine
Abetalipoproteinemia	5-15 yr	Recessive	Ataxia, dysmetria, fat malabsorption, acanthocytosis, retinitis pigmentosa, sensory loss	Low-fat diet; vitamin E and A supplementation
Juvenile gangliosidosis	3-5 yr	Recessive GM_1 or GM_2 forms	Ataxia, spasticity, rigidity, dementia	None available
Ramsay Hunt syndrome	7-10 yr	Sporadic	Ataxia, tremor, myoclonus, dementia	Supportive
Marinesco-Sjögren syndrome	Infancy to 5 yr	Recessive	Cataracts, ataxia, growth failure, mental retardation	Supportive
Juveline sulfate lipidosis (juvenile MLD)	Infancy to 5 yr	Recessive	Dementia, ataxia, spasticity, aryl sulfidase A deficiency	Supportive

Modified from Behrman RE, Kliegman RM: Nelson Essentials of Pediatrics, 2nd ed. Philadelphia; WB Saunders, 1994, p 689.

MLD, metachromatic leukodystrophy.

out the posterior fossa tumors and demyelinating diseases. The lumbar puncture and analysis of the cerebrospinal fluid may also be indicated in cases preceded by a viral or infectious prodrome. When weakness is associated with the disequilibrium, there may be a place for electromyography and nerve conduction studies (see Chapter 38).

SUMMARY AND RED FLAGS

Because disequilibrium involves impairment of ambulation, it is seen only in toddlers and older children. Ataxia, however, can be seen in children before they are walking, and it may portend serious pathologic processes, including posterior fossa tumors, leukodystrophies, metabolic disorders, and familial-hereditary disorders. The history must be obtained carefully, with attention to developmental milestones, family history, and specifics of prodromal illnesses (chickenpox), associated symptoms, and a description of the gait. The physical examination must also be detailed and methodical, with special emphasis on the neuromuscular examination. Imaging studies of the central nervous system are usually required, especially in younger children, in whom the possibility of neoplasms is greatest.

LIGHTHEADEDNESS

Lightheadedness is the most difficult to characterize without using the term "dizzy." The lightheaded patient's description is vague and nonspecific. Terms such as "woozy," "spaced-out," "dreamy," "giddy," or "drugged" are frequently used. The key for the clinician is to elicit an adequate description from the patient to rule out vertigo, disequilibrium, and presyncope. The differential diagnosis for lightheadedness is then rather short in comparison with the other "dizziness" conditions (Fig. 42-13). Because of this, dizziness simulation tests are useful to distinguish the patient's complaint from atypical descriptions of vertigo, disequilibrium, and presyncope. The distinction between lightheadedness and presyncope is the most difficult to establish.

Besides the Nylen-Bárány maneuver (see Fig. 42-9), dizziness simulation tests include voluntary hyperventilation for 3 minutes, voluntary Valsalva maneuver, caloric testing of the ears, carotid massage, and tilt-table testing. All these may be used to distinguish lightheadedness from vertigo, disequilibrium, and presyncope. In the

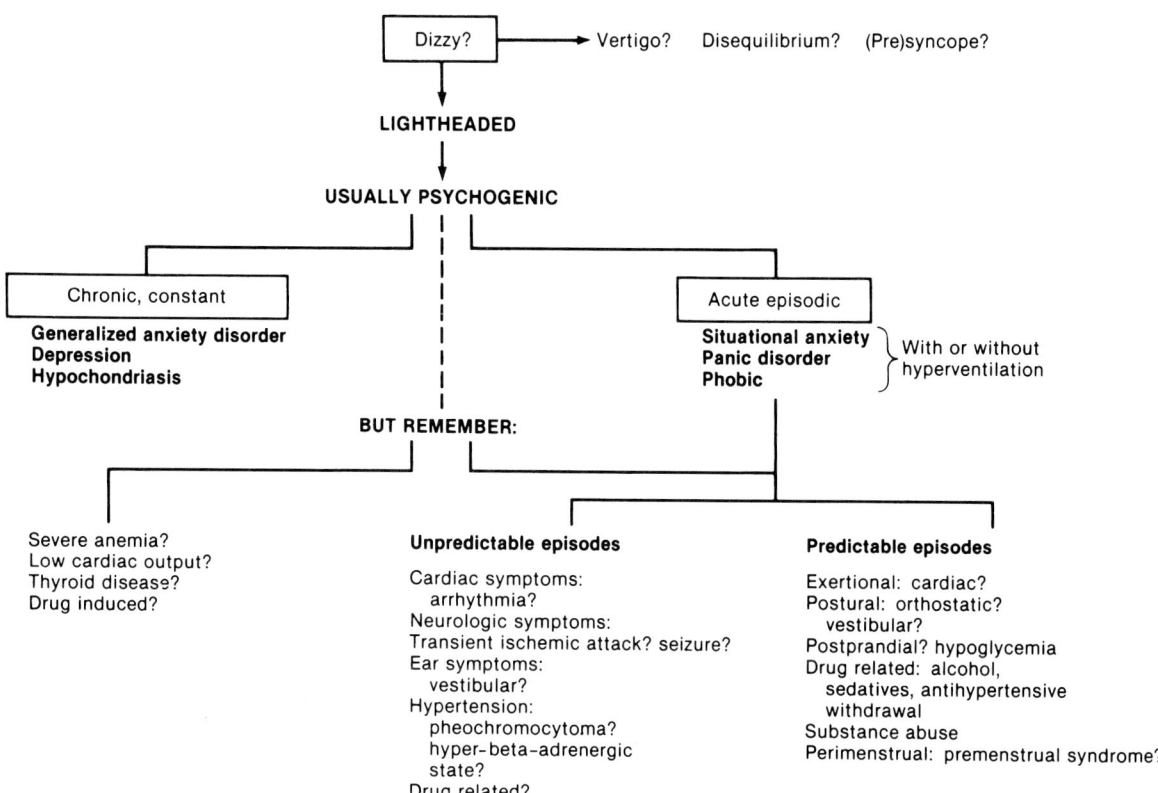

Figure 42-13. Evaluation for lightheadedness. (From Reilly BM: *Practical Strategies in Outpatient Medicine,* 2nd ed. Philadelphia, WB Saunders, 1991, p 206.)

patient who complains of lightheadedness, voluntary hyperventilation usually reproduces his or her symptoms. Voluntary hyperventilation in normal subjects produces a variety of symptoms (see Table 42-5). This test is predictive only if the patient's symptoms are precisely reproduced and all other investigation results are negative.

Lightheadedness that is episodic frequently follows a pattern related to the underlying psychogenic disorder: phobic disorders, post-traumatic stress syndrome, panic attacks, and anxiety disorders. Such situational anxieties, phobias, or panic attacks may occur with or without hyperventilation. Careful history taking is the key to recognizing the pattern. If the history is that of constant lightheadedness ("always there"), the origin is almost always psychogenic. This is a somatization generally of anxiety disorder or, on occasion, depression. The clinician must nonetheless remain cautious with predictable episodes, because postural episodes, drug-related episodes, and perimenstrual episodes can follow a pattern and represent physiologic abnormalities that predispose to lightheadedness.

Especially if the episodes of lightheadedness are unpredictable, the clinician is advised to consider a broader differential diagnosis. Severe anemia, low cardiac output, thyroid disease, and some medications may produce occasional lightheadedness. Of greater concern are episodes of lightheadedness associated with other symptoms, especially chest pain, seizures, confusion, and visual or auditory changes. Likewise, exertional lightheadedness must be pursued to definitively rule out a cardiac dysrhythmia.

If hyperventilation reproduces the patient's symptoms, it is not the diagnosis in and of itself. Hyperventilation is a feature of many psychogenic syndromes and may be acute or chronic. Part of the performance of the hyperventilation should be educating the patient to the feelings and to the scenario leading to the hyperventilation reaction. Even rather young children can then be trained to regulate their breathing to avoid the symptoms. However, this does not address the underlying cause of the hyperventilation reaction; that

requires patient, nonjudgmental, longer term counseling and careful categorization of the underlying disorder according to the *Diagnostic and Statistical Manual of Mental Disorders,* Fourth Edition, criteria (see Chapter 35). The clinician should not hesitate to consult a psychiatrist to facilitate this process as well as treatment of the definitive psychogenic disorder.

EVALUATION OF THE PATIENT WITH LIGHTHEADEDNESS

History

The patient is encouraged to describe symptoms without using the word "dizzy." The examiner should listen for descriptions suggesting vertigo, disequilibrium, or presyncope and should establish whether there is any pattern to the occurrence of the feeling of lightheadedness. The child, parents, or siblings are asked about associated symptoms, such as diaphoresis, hyperpnea, pallor or flushing, headache, and chest pain. It is probably best not to pursue psychiatric questioning at the very beginning of a relationship, so as not to give the impression that somatic symptoms are being minimized. However, after the more serious physiologic disorders are ruled out by history, physical examination, or diagnostic testing, the psychogenic disorders should be pursued.

Physical Examination

After a thorough general physical examination, including examination of the fundi, a full, detailed neurologic examination should be performed. In addition to allowing primary cardiac, endocrine, or neurologic disorders to be ruled out, the examination allows the clinician to gain the confidence of the patient and demonstrates the physician's concern about the patient's complaints. Dizziness simulation maneuvers, especially the Nylen-Bárány maneuver and voluntary hyperventilation, should be performed. Along the way, the patient should be given feedback, reassurance, and information about the purpose of various maneuvers in the physical examination.

Diagnostic Tests

In general, diagnostic testing is again directed by the history and physical examination findings. In the setting of lightheadedness, tests are generally done to rule out potentially serious cardiovascular and neurologic conditions. The dizziness simulation tests are very important and should be performed in precisely the same manner in every patient with this complaint, to maximize their reliability.

SUMMARY AND RED FLAGS

Lightheadedness must be distinguished from vertigo, disequilibrium, and presyncope. Frequently, the patient's description of the sensation is vague and uncertain. A pattern of the appearance of the symptoms may suggest an underlying cause. The coexistence of any other symptoms must be carefully sought. Physical findings are generally normal, including the neurologic examination; specific attention is given to cerebellar, vestibular, and sensory function. Voluntary hyperventilation in the supine position frequently reproduces the patient's lightheadedness. Hyperventilation may be acute or chronic and is a symptom itself, rarely a diagnosis.

Treatment must address the underlying psychogenic cause in order to be successful. Signs of depression as well as suicidal ideation must be determined.

REFERENCES

General

Alboni P, Brignole M, Menozzi C, et al: Diagnostic value of history in patients with syncope with or without heart disease. J Am Coll Cardiol 2001;37:1921-1928.

Johnsrude CL: Current approach to pediatric syncope. Pediatr Cardiol 2000;21:522-531.

Narchi H: The child who passes out. Pediatr Rev 2000;21:384-388.

Tanel RE: Putting the bite into the pediatric syncope evaluation. Pediatr Case Rev 2001;1:3-18.

Willis J: Syncope. Pediatr Rev 2000;21:201-204.

Syncope

Berger S, Dhala A, Friedberg D: Sudden cardiac death in infants, children, and adolescents. Pediatr Cardiol 1999;46:221-234.

Bradley T, Dixon J, Easthope R: Unexplained fainting, near drowning and unusual seizures in childhood: Screening for long QT syndrome in New Zealand families. N Z Med J 1999;112:299-302.

DiMario FJ Jr: Prospective study of children with cyanotic and pallid breath-holding spells. Pediatrics 2001;107:265-269.

Eirís-Pual J, Rodríguez-Nunez A, Fernandez-Martínez N, et al: Usefulness of the head-upright tilt test for distinguishing syncope and epilepsy in children. Epilepsia 2001;42:709-713.

Jacob G, Costa F, Shannon JR, et al: The neuropathic postural tachycardia syndrome. N Engl J Med 2000;343:1008-1014.

Kouakam C, Vaksmann G, Pachy E, et al: Long-term follow up of children and adolescents with syncope. Eur Heart J 2001;22:1618-1625.

Lahat H, Eldar M, Levy-Nissenbaum E, et al: Autosomal recessive catecholamine- or exercise-induced polymorphic ventricular tachycardia. Circulation 2001;103:2822-2827.

Pfammatter JP, Paul T: Idiopathic ventricular tachycardia in infancy and childhood. J Am Coll Cardiol 1999;33:2067-2072.

Priori SG, Napolitano C, Gioedano U, et al: Brugada syndrome and sudden cardiac death in children. Lancet 2000;355:808-809.

Ritter S, Tani LY, Etheridge SP, et al: What is the yield of screening echocardiography in pediatric syncope? Pediatrics 2000;105:E58.

Rodríguez-Nunez A, Fernandez-Cebrian S, Perez-Munuzuri A, et al: Cerebral syncope in children. J Pediatr 2000;136:542-544.

Salim MA, Ware LE, Barnard M, et al: Syncope recurrence in children: Relation to tilt-test results. Pediatrics 1998;102:924-926.

Shalev Y, Gal R, Tchou PJ, et al: Echocardiographic demonstration of decreased left ventricular dimensions and vigorous myocardial contraction during syncope induced by head-up tilt test. J Am Coll Cardiol 1991;18:746-751.

Thilenius OG, Quinones JA, Husanyi TS, Novak J: Tilt test for diagnosis of unexplained syncope in pediatric patients. Pediatrics 1991;87:334-338.

Vertigo

Dunn DW, Snyder H: Benign positional vertigo of childhood. Am J Dis Child 1976;176:1099.

Froehling DA, Bowen JM, Mohr DN, et al: The canalith repositioning procedure for the treatment of benign paroxysmal positional vertigo: A randomized trial. Mayo Clin Proc 2000;75:695-700.

Hotson JR: Clinical detection of acute vestibulocerebellar disorders. West J Med 1984;140:910-913.

Katsarkas A, Kirkham TH: Paroxysmal positional vertigo: A study of 255 cases. J Otolaryngol 1978;7:320-330.

Weisleder P, Fife TD: Dizziness and headache: A common association in children and adolescents. J Child Neurol 2001;16:727-730.

Disequilibrium

DeAngelis C: Ataxia. Pediatr Rev 1995;16:114-115.

Dinolfo EA, Adam HM: Evaluation of ataxia. Pediatr Rev 2001;22:177-178.

Dreyfus PM, Oshtory M, Gardner ED, et al: Cerebellar ataxia: Anatomical, physiological and clinical implications. West J Med 1978;128:499-511.

Kinast M, Levin HS, Rothner AD, et al: Cerebellar ataxia, opsoclonus and occult neural crest tumor. Am J Dis Child 1980;134:1057-1059.

Lightheadedness

Magarian GJ: Hyperventilation syndromes: Infrequently recognized common expressions of anxiety and stress. Medicine 1982;61:219-236.

Naschitz JE, Hardoff D, Bystritzki I, et al: The role of the capnography head-up tilt test in the diagnosis of syncope in children and adolescent. Pediatrics 1998;101:E6.

Tiwari S, Bakris GL: Psychogenic vertigo: A review. Postgrad Med 1981;70:69-77.

43 Eye Disorders

Mark S. Ruttum*

Some eye disorders in children can be diagnosed and successfully treated by the pediatrician; others should be referred to an ophthalmologist or other specialist for management. An example of the former is conjunctivitis or a corneal abrasion; strabismus and retinoblastoma are examples of the latter. The recognition and understanding of ocular symptoms and signs of a systemic disease or syndrome may be important in the context of a child's overall medical management.

EYE AND VISUAL SYSTEM ANATOMY

The anatomies of the eye and visual system are shown in Figures 43-1 and 43-2.

The optic nerves, made up of the converging nerve fiber layer of the retina, have intraorbital, intracanalicular, and intracranial portions. Partial decussation of the optic nerve fibers occurs in the chiasm (approximately 47% of fibers cross and 53% remain uncrossed), which gives binocular visual input to each side of the brain. The fibers of the optic nerves first synapse in the lateral geniculate bodies, where the visual input from each eye is separated into six distinct layers that originate from one eye or the other. From the lateral geniculate bodies, nerve fibers travel as the optic radiations to the visual cortex, where they again synapse and course out into various layers of primary and secondary visual cortex. It is in the visual cortex that the conscious process of "seeing" occurs.

DEVELOPMENT OF THE EYE AND VISUAL SYSTEM

The eyes and vision of a newborn are immature and require several years to reach adult proportions and functional status. By the ninth month of gestation, the retinal vessels have reached the periphery of the retina (an important factor in the pathogenesis of retinopathy of prematurity [ROP]), the optic nerve has completed myelination, and the pupillary membrane has disappeared. Postnatal relocation of cells in the macular region of the retina and reorganization of neuron-to-neuron connections in the visual cortex improve the poor visual acuity and other visual processes, which are not fully developed at birth but become so during the first year of life.

The visual acuity of the newborn has been estimated to be 20/200 to 20/400 and reaches the normal 20/20 level as early as 6 to 12 months of age, as tested with visually evoked cortical potential techniques. Visual acuity as measured with conventional letter or symbol recognition methods does not reach 20/20 until several years of age because of cognitive factors, not because of immaturity of the primary visual system. Binocular vision, including establishment of normal ocular alignment and depth perception, and improved facility of accommodation also develop rapidly in the first year of life.

The rapid maturation of visual function in the first year of life accounts for the extreme sensitivity of the visual system to abnormal visual input from strabismus or cataracts.

The majority of newborns are moderately hyperopic, but as many as 25% are myopic. Refractive error tends toward emmetropia through coordinated changes in the power of the refractive elements of the eye (the cornea and lens) and increase in the length of the eye. Heredity probably plays the major role in the refractive status of the eyes; the role played by the environment and visual experience is unknown. The developing visual system is less sensitive to refractive abnormalities than to visual deprivation from media opacities or strabismus, although significant and persistent refractive problems at this age can give rise to amblyopia.

AMBLYOPIA AND VISION SCREENING

Amblyopia is defined as a unilateral or, less commonly, bilateral reduction in visual acuity that cannot be immediately corrected with glasses or be attributed to a structural or organic abnormality of the eye or visual system. In children in whom visual acuity can be accurately measured, a practical definition of amblyopia is a two-line or greater difference between the best-corrected visual acuity of the eyes. For preverbal children, differences between the eyes in fixation and following behavior or fixation preference are used to diagnose amblyopia. Amblyopia results from abnormal visual experience early in life during the "sensitive" period for visual development. The sensitive period for amblyopia starts in early infancy and continues to at least the age of 6 years. The child's sensitivity is greatest early on, which means that the period of abnormal visual experience necessary to cause amblyopia is shorter than that in older children. The prevalence of amblyopia in the North American population is 2% to 4%.

Unilateral amblyopia results from three types of abnormal visual experience: strabismus, anisometropia (unequal refractive errors), and monocular visual deprivation (e.g., cataract, corneal opacity, severe ptosis). Bilateral amblyopia results from bilateral media opacities or significant bilateral refractive errors (ametropia).

Nearly all amblyopia is reversible if discovered at an early age and treated appropriately. Detection strategies for amblyopia can involve early recognition of factors that give rise to amblyopia or actual measurement of reduced visual acuity that may be caused by amblyopia. Most amblyogenic factors can be detected through routine pediatric screening such as red reflex evaluation and examination for strabismus. Screening for amblyogenic factors may be possible with photoscreening instruments. The theoretical advantages of a photoscreener are that an amblyogenic factor may be detected at an earlier age than with traditional examination techniques and that photoscreening can be done by less experienced medical personnel. Screening for anisometropia and regular refractive errors can also be accomplished more easily with photoscreening. Because photoscreening is an emerging technology, no system has proved to improve upon current amblyopia detection programs.

*This chapter is an updated and edited version of the chapter by Dennis M. Super that appeared in the first edition.

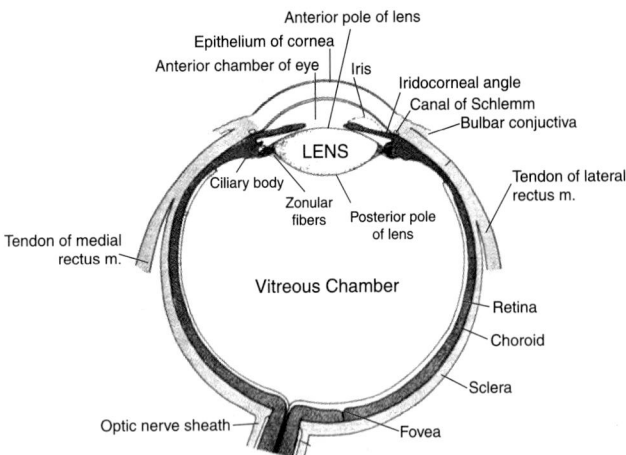

Figure 43-1. Anatomy of the eye, as seen in cross-section. (Modified from Reilly BM: *Practical Strategies in Outpatient Medicine*, 2nd ed. Philadelphia, WB Saunders, 1991, p 36.)

Currently recommended screening guidelines and referral criteria for amblyopia or amblyogenic factor detection in preschool children (aged 36 to 59 months) are presented in Table 43-1. The use of the Allen figures and other types of isolated symbols or letters is discouraged. Whenever possible, a line of symbols or isolated symbols with surrounding crowding bars is recommended (Fig. 43-3). Isolated symbols can lead to overestimates of the visual acuity of an eye with amblyopia and, thus, to the failure to detect this condition.

The treatment of amblyopia involves eliminating amblyogenic factors, providing a focused retinal image with appropriate optical correction, and forcing use of the amblyopic eye through occlusion of the sound eye or blurring the image it receives. For patients with visual deprivation amblyopia, the depriving factor must be removed by such means as ptosis surgery, treatment of an ocular or periorbital hemangioma, cataract surgery, corneal transplantation, or removal of blood in the vitreous humor. Optical correction is required for patients who have had cataract surgery and can be provided by spectacles, contact lenses, or intraocular lens implants. For patients with anisometropic amblyopia, optical correction usually involves spectacles or, less commonly, contact lenses.

An adhesive patch worn over the sound eye most commonly achieves enforced use of the amblyopic eye. Occlusive devices can be attached to glasses but may be less reliable if the child does not comply with spectacle wear. The use of the potent cycloplegic agent atropine sulfate is a commonly used method for encouraging use of the amblyopic eye. A drop of atropine is applied to the sound eye each day; this temporarily impairs its accommodative ability and, in the presence of sufficient hyperopia, prevents that eye from obtaining a

clear retinal image. Atropine "penalization" for amblyopia works best in hyperopic patients with mild to moderate amblyopia (visual acuity of 20/100 or better). Close follow-up of patients being treated for amblyopia is important for monitoring compliance with treatment and for preventing the development of iatrogenic amblyopia in the sound eye from excessive occlusion or penalization. Treatment is best accomplished before strabismus surgery is performed in patients with strabismic amblyopia. Parents must be instructed that strabismus surgery does not correct amblyopia and, conversely, occlusion or other forms of amblyopia treatment do not lead to resolution of strabismus.

STRABISMUS

Strabismus is defined as a lack of parallelism of the visual axes of the eyes. Less formally, it implies misalignment of the eyes in such a way that they are not simultaneously viewing the same object. Terms to describe eye alignment are noted in Table 43-2. Strabismus can be constant or intermittent and can be the same in all directions of gaze (comitant) or greater in one direction of gaze than in others (incomitant). Furthermore, it can be categorized as congenital or acquired, monocular or alternating. The direction of misalignment can be vertical or horizontal. Vertical strabismus is referred to as a hypertropia of the higher eye. Horizontal strabismus can be convergent (esotropia) or divergent (exotropia). The importance of strabismus detection derives primarily from the fact that it is the leading cause of amblyopia. Other reasons for detecting strabismus are the possibility of being able to restore normal binocular use of the eyes, improving depth perception, and minimizing the social and economic drawbacks to strabismus in society.

Strabismus detection can be simple, as in patients with a large angle of deviation (Fig. 43-4), or difficult, as in patients with more subtle deviations or no deviation at all (pseudostrabismus) (Fig. 43-5). In the case of a large manifest strabismus, inspection of the eyes is sufficient to confirm its presence. In most other instances, specific examination techniques must be relied upon. Evaluation of the symmetry of the corneal light reflexes from a penlight directed at the eyes can reliably detect many cases (see Fig. 43-4). With smaller angles of strabismus or when the results of the corneal light reflex are in doubt, the cover test should be performed (Fig. 43-6). The importance of providing attractive fixation targets for the child to view during the test cannot be overestimated. The examiner should adhere to the "one toy, one look" rule and have an array of age-appropriate fixation devices to maintain the child's interest. The penlight is not a good fixation target for performing the cover test; it does not present any detail requiring appropriate accommodation to see, and many children consider its brightness to be annoying and uncomfortable to watch.

Congenital esotropia is defined as convergent strabismus with onset in the first 6 months of life (see Fig. 43-4). Transient crossing

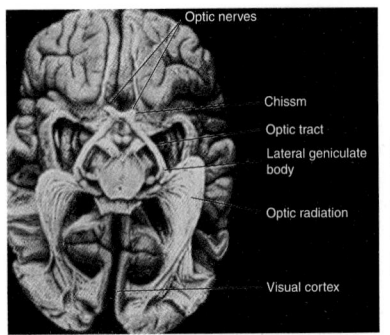

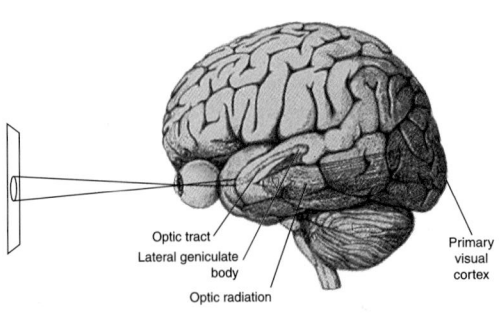

Figure 43-2. **A,** Dissection showing the visual pathways from the optic nerves to the visual cortex as viewed from the ventral aspect of the brain. **B,** Side view of the visual pathway from the eye to the visual cortex. (**A,** From Gluhbegovic N, Williams TH: *The Human Brain.* Hagerstown: Md, Harper & Row, 1980; **B,** From Hubel DH: *Eye, Brain, and Vision.* New York, WH Freeman, 1988.)

Table 43-1. Vision Screening Guidelines For Preschool Children

Function to Be Evaluated	Type of Test	Specific Test	Recommended Testing Procedures	Passing Criteria
Monocular distance acuity	Linear acuity	HOTV Lea symbols Tumbling E	Test distance = 10 ft (3 m)	Child must identify or match 4 out of 5 optotypes on the critical line with each eye tested monocularly.
	Isolated optotypes with surround bars *Note:* Isolated optotypes without surround bars should not be used; they overestimate acuity in individuals with amblyopia.	HOTV cards with surround bars	Pretest (performed binocularly): Test child's ability to perform test by having child identify or match each of the 4 optotypes on a line that is expected to be suprathreshold (20/100 or greater). Child must successfully identify each of the 4 optotypes.	
			Test procedure (performed monocularly): Test child's ability to identify or match optotypes on the line used in the retest. To proceed, child must identify or match 4 out of 5 optotypes on the pretest line. Then test child's ability to identify or match optotypes on the critical line. Repeat test procedure with the other eye.	Critical lines: 20/40 at 36-48 months 20/30 at 48-59 months
Stereopsis	Random dot stereogram	Random dot E	Test distance = 40 cm (630 arc sec) All testing, including pretesting, should be done binocularly with the polarized glasses on. Pretest: Test child's ability to perform test by having child identify the location of the 3-dimensional E on 4 out of 5 trials (E on left or right; above or below). Test procedure: Test child's ability to identify the location of the stereo E. Tester should use 5 presentations, varying location in a nonsystematic manner.	Child must locate stereo E on 4 out of 5 presentations.*

From Hartmann EE, et al: Preschool vision screening; Summary of a task force report. Pediatrics 2000;106:1105.

From a statistical perspective, it would be ideal to require that a child pass 5 out of 5 trials, because the probability of achieving this criterion by simply guessing is less than 5%. In reality, many children will have difficulty attending consistently for 5 trials. Therefore, the 4 out of 5 correct passing criterion is considered acceptable, even though the probability of passing by chance is 16.5%.

or divergence of the eyes is common in newborns and is probably not significant unless it persists beyond 3 months of age. In the classic form of congenital esotropia, there is a large-angle, constant deviation. Amblyopia occurs frequently. The cause of congenital esotropia is not known, but hereditary factors play a definite role. The incidence of congenital esotropia is less than 1% among neurologically normal infants but much higher in children with neurologic impairment.

Early correction of congenital esotropia may result in full or nearly full restoration of normal binocular function, a result not believed to be obtainable with correction of misalignment at older ages. Six months is considered the earliest age at which to perform strabismus surgery, but some authors have reported patients undergoing operation as early as 13 weeks of age who had binocular sensory outcomes (presence of stereopsis) superior to those who underwent operation later. Early detection and prompt referral of infants with suspected esotropia are indicated.

A second category of esotropia occurs in children whose eyes are initially straight but start to cross, at first intermittently, at 1 to 3 years of age. These children have excessive hyperopia and an abnormal relationship between accommodation and convergence. This type of esotropia is called *accommodative esotropia*. Amblyopia frequently develops. Treatment generally consists of correcting amblyopia and providing spectacles to correct hyperopia, thereby modulating the amount of accommodation required by the child (see Fig. 43-7). Bifocal spectacles may also be necessary for some forms of accommodative esotropia. Some ophthalmologists use the parasympathomimetic agent phospholine iodide in lieu of glasses for the management of accommodative esotropia or to facilitate "weaning" the child from glasses.

Esotropia caused by paralysis of a lateral rectus muscle, a sixth cranial nerve palsy, is not rare in children (Fig. 43-8). The onset may be sudden and associated with head trauma or a recent viral illness.

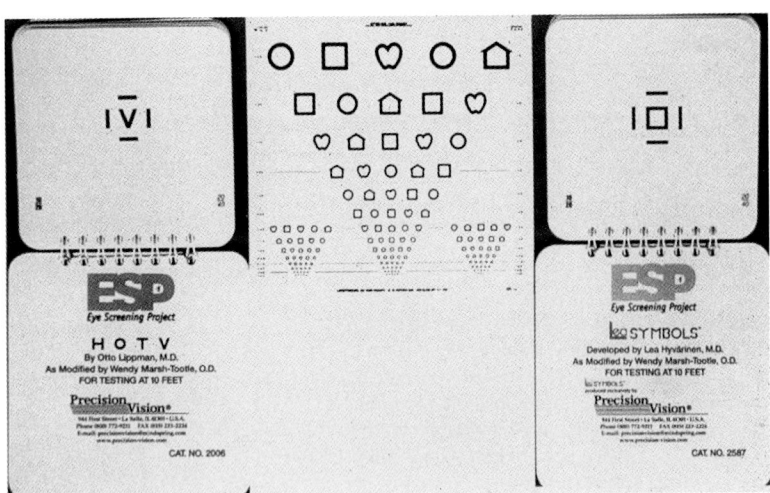

Figure 43-3. The Lea symbols in chart format (**middle**) and the Lea symbols and HOTV tests with crowding bars (**right** and **left**). All tests should be administered at a distance of 10 feet.

An older child may present with a face turn or closure of one eye to avoid diplopia, whereas a younger child may present with only the esotropia because of rapid development of suppression to eliminate diplopia. Neurologic investigation is indicated if the paralysis does not spontaneously abate in a few weeks (a so-called benign sixth nerve palsy believed to be postviral in origin) or if the child demonstrates other neurologic impairment or has papilledema.

Congenital exotropia is much less common than congenital esotropia. The presence of constant exotropia in the first year of life is a red flag because of its frequent association with coexisting ocular or systemic disease. The most common type of exotropia, however, called *intermittent exotropia,* manifests by 5 years of age; often parents notice it before a child is 2 years of age. This form of strabismus is manifest only part of the time, particularly when the child is tired or ill. Because the child maintains the ability to keep the eyes aligned part of the time, amblyopia is uncommon. Diplopia is prevented by active cortical suppression of input from the portion of the retina of the deviated eye that overlaps the central view of the fixating eye. When the eyes are straight, the child generally maintains normal binocular function, including stereopsis. Intermittent exotropia remains stable over long periods in most children; spontaneous resolution is rare. Treatment with part-time alternating occlusion or with minus-power spectacles as though the child were myopic is occasionally tried but seldom alters the natural history of the disorder. Vision therapy has not been shown to be effective. Eye muscle surgery is the only definitive treatment, although it has not been compared with other forms of treatment in a randomized clinical study. The optimum timing of surgery is controversial; some ophthalmologists advocate surgery soon after the diagnosis is made, regardless of the patient's age, and others recommend delaying surgery until the patient is at least 4 years of age, when initial surgical overcorrections, which are frequent, desirable, and usually temporary, can be managed more effectively.

Primary vertical strabismus is far less common than horizontal strabismus. A small vertical deviation in association with a larger amount of horizontal strabismus, however, is common, and is managed in conjunction with the horizontal deviation. One of the more common causes of hypertropia in children is congenital paralysis of the superior oblique muscle, a fourth cranial nerve paralysis. In some children, the "paralysis" is actually caused by an anatomic abnormality of the superior oblique tendon. Children with a superior oblique paralysis of any cause frequently present with a head tilt and face turned toward the side opposite the paralyzed superior oblique muscle. Superior oblique paralysis is one of the more common causes of ocular torticollis. An eye muscle disorder needs to be ruled out in any child with a chronic abnormality of head position. The anomalous head position and hypertropia caused by a superior oblique paralysis can be improved by eye muscle surgery in most instances.

An approach to the evaluation of strabismus is noted in Figure 43-9; other less common types of strabismus are listed in Table 43-3.

Table 43-2. Description of Alignment and Movement

Normal Ocular Alignment: Orthophoria

Latency

-phoria: development of abnormality only during certain conditions (fatigue, illness, cover test)

-tropia: abnormality present during normal conditions; deviation may be constant or intermittent

Direction of Deviation

Eso-: inward, horizontal deviation ("crossing")

Exo-: outward, horizontal deviation ("wall-eye")

Hyper-: upward, vertical deviation

Hypo-: downward, vertical deviation

Incyclo-: nasal torsional deviation of the superior pole of the cornea

Excyclo-: temporal torsional deviation of the superior pole of the cornea

Equality of Deviation

Concomitant: misalignment is equal in all positions of gaze

Noncomitant: misalignment varies significantly in different positions of gaze

Neuromuscular Dysfunction

Paralytic: misalignment secondary to a cranial nerve palsy, muscle weakness, or mechanical restriction (usually noncomitant)

Nonparalytic: no underlying neuromuscular dysfunction; usually concomitant but can be noncomitant

Tandem Movements of Both Eyes

-version: both eyes move in same direction (conjugate); direction of movement: leve- (left); dextro- (right); supra- (up); infra- (down)

-vergence: eyes move in opposite directions (disconjugate); convergence (inward movement), divergence (outward movement)

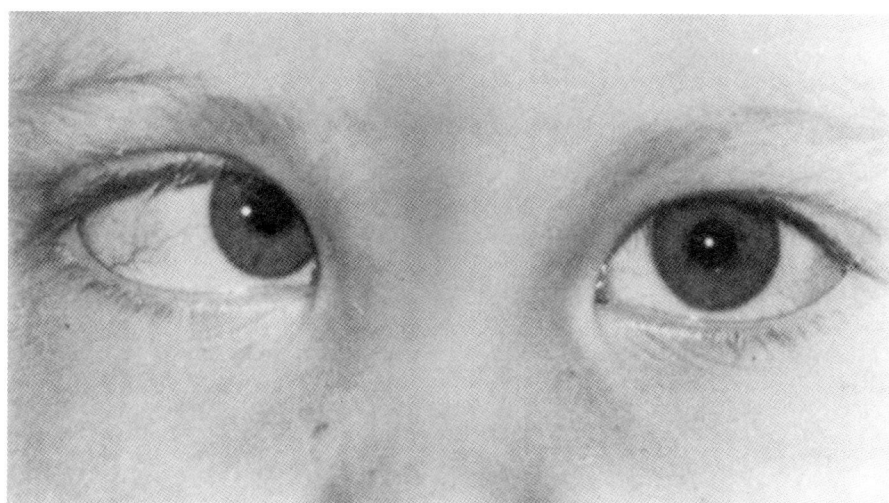

Figure 43-4. Corneal light reflex test reveals an asymmetrically placed reflex that is laterally displaced in the right eye. This indicates an inward deviation of the eye (esotropia). (From Lavrich JB, Nelson LB: Diagnosis and treatment of strabismus disorders. Pediatr Clin North Am 1993;40:739.)

REFRACTIVE ERRORS

Refractive errors include myopia (nearsightedness), hyperopia (farsightedness), and astigmatism. Refractive errors may be similar (isometropia) or different (anisometropia) between the two eyes.

MYOPIA

In patients with myopia, the parallel rays of light in the resting (nonaccommodating) eye are focused in front of the retina. The symptoms of myopia are squinting, viewing an object more closely than normal, and complaining of blurred far vision. Myopia is relatively common during childhood.

The incidence and degree of myopia increase with age, especially during growth spurts, as in adolescence. Because some forms of myopia are hereditary, children of myopic parents should be screened for myopia at an early age. Myopia may be associated with other ocular abnormalities, such as keratoconus (central conical protrusion of the cornea), cataracts, ectopia lentis (dislocated lens), spherophakia (overly spherical lens), glaucoma, and medullated (myelinated) nerve fibers. There is an increased prevalence of myopia in premature infants, especially with ROP, and in many genetic conditions (Marfan and Stickler syndromes).

Although myopia is usually the simple (physiologic) form with a healthy globe, some children have pathologic myopia that is associated with thinning of the sclera, choroid, and retina. Pathologic myopia is often associated with some degree of uncorrectable vision impairment. Because myopic patients are at a greater risk for retinal detachment, they should also take appropriate safety precautions, such as wearing polycarbonate spectacles, molded polycarbonate goggles, and appropriate headgear for sports. More than half of children with high degrees of myopia may have an underlying systemic association, such as Marfan, Stickler, Noonan, and Down syndromes, or a history of prematurity and developmental delay.

If myopia is sufficient to produce visual symptoms, concave (minus) lenses in the form of spectacles or contact lenses are prescribed to correct the refractive error. Prescription changes may be needed every 1 to 2 years (more frequently during growth spurts).

HYPEROPIA

In patients with hyperopia (farsightedness), parallel rays of light in the nonaccommodating eye would, if possible, be focused behind the retina. The process of accommodation (focusing), which alters the shape of the lens, can compensate for some degrees of hyperopia. Because children have a tremendous range of accommodation, moderately hyperopic children can see clearly without any visual

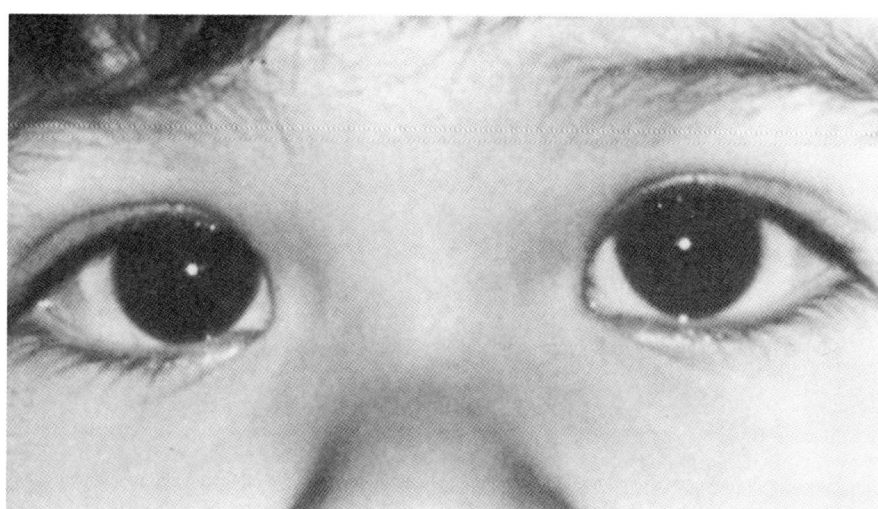

Figure 43-5. A child with pseudoesotropia. Note that the wide nasal bridge and prominent epicanthal folds create the illusion of an esotropia. The corneal light reflexes are centered in each eye; therefore, the eyes are straight. (From Lavrich JB, Nelson LB: Diagnosis and treatment of strabismus disorders. Pediatr Clin North Am 1993; 40:741.)

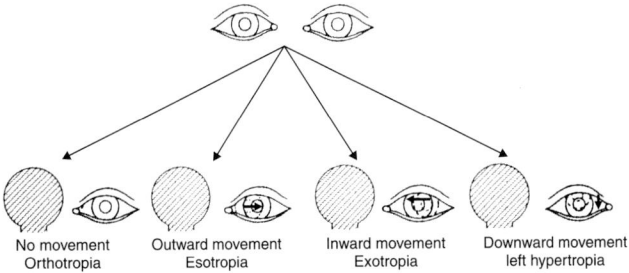

Figure 43-6. The cover test. In each instance, the occluder is placed over the right eye while the patient is viewing a fixation target and the examiner is watching for movement of the patient's left eye. If the left eye is not aligned, it will need to move to look at the fixation target. If there is no movement of the left eye, the test needs to be repeated by occluding the left eye and watching for movement of the right eye.

symptoms. Severely hyperopic children may be unable to fully compensate through accommodation. The greater accommodative effort may lead to symptoms of "eyestrain," which consist of headaches, fatigue, or eye rubbing. These symptoms may lead to a lack of interest in reading or in prolonged close work. Some children may also develop accommodative esotropia. If hyperopia is severe enough to produce symptoms or cause esotropia, convex (plus) lenses, usually in the form of glasses, are prescribed to correct the refractive error.

ASTIGMATISM

In the patient with astigmatism, the refractive power differs in various meridians of the eye. In most cases, astigmatism is caused by

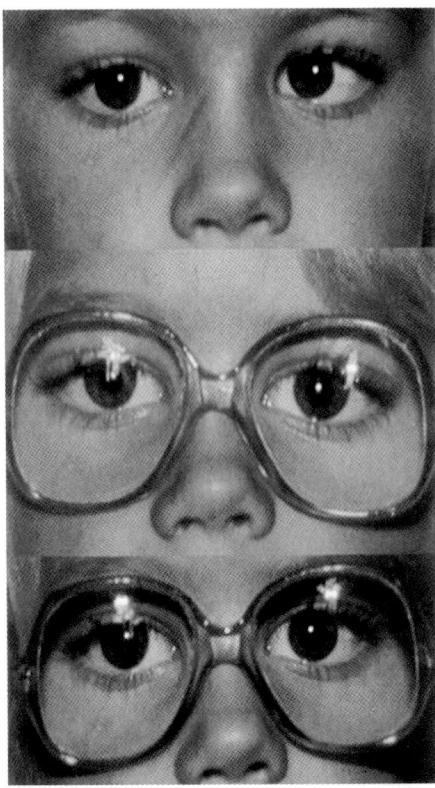

Figure 43-7. Accommodative esotropia (**top**). The deviation is completely controlled with glasses at both distant (**middle**) and near (**bottom**) fixation distances.

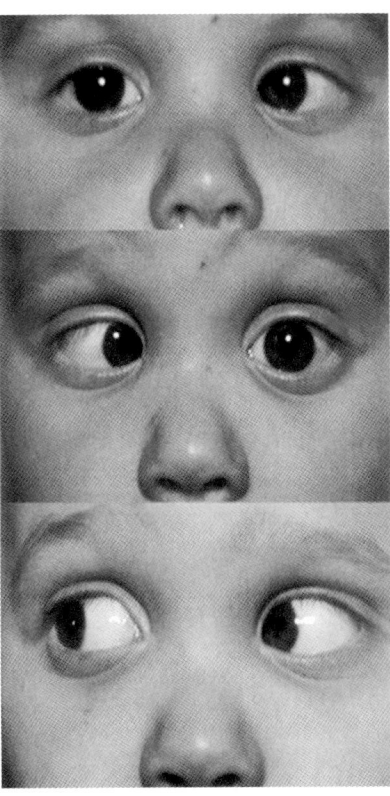

Figure 43-8. Left sixth cranial nerve palsy in a 4-year-old. A large manifest esotropia is present when the child looks straight ahead (**top**). The left eye does not abduct beyond the midline in gaze to the left (**middle**). Gaze to the right is normal (**bottom**).

abnormal curvature of the cornea; in rare cases, lens abnormalities may cause astigmatism. Infants and children with corneal distortion secondary to scarring (trauma or infection) or to external compression (ptosis or hemangioma of eyelid) are at an increased risk for astigmatism. Moderate levels of astigmatism may produce blurring of vision (far and near), leading to squinting, fatigue, headaches, and lack of interest in close-up work. High degrees of astigmatism can lead to amblyopia. Cylindric or spherocylindric lenses (usually glasses) are used to improve vision and comfort.

ANISOMETROPIA

In patients with anisometropia, the refractive error of one eye differs significantly from that of the other eye. The difference in refraction can be spheric (hyperopia or myopia) or cylindric (unequal amounts of astigmatism). Mild degrees of anisometropia usually cause no visual symptoms and do not lead to amblyopia. Amblyopia develops with higher degrees of anisometropia because the child uses the less ametropic eye and suppresses vision in the other. Strabismus frequently coexists with anisometropia, and both conditions may be involved in the pathophysiologic mechanisms of amblyopia. Anisometropia may initially be detected by comparison of the red reflex between the two eyes (Brückner test). The affected eye has the duller red reflex. Early detection and treatment of anisometropia are essential for the development of optimal visual function.

VISION IMPAIRMENT IN CHILDREN

Vision impairment is formally defined as best-corrected visual acuity of 20/70 or worse in both eyes. Impairment of vision exists as a continuum from 20/70 to no light perception. Legal blindness is said

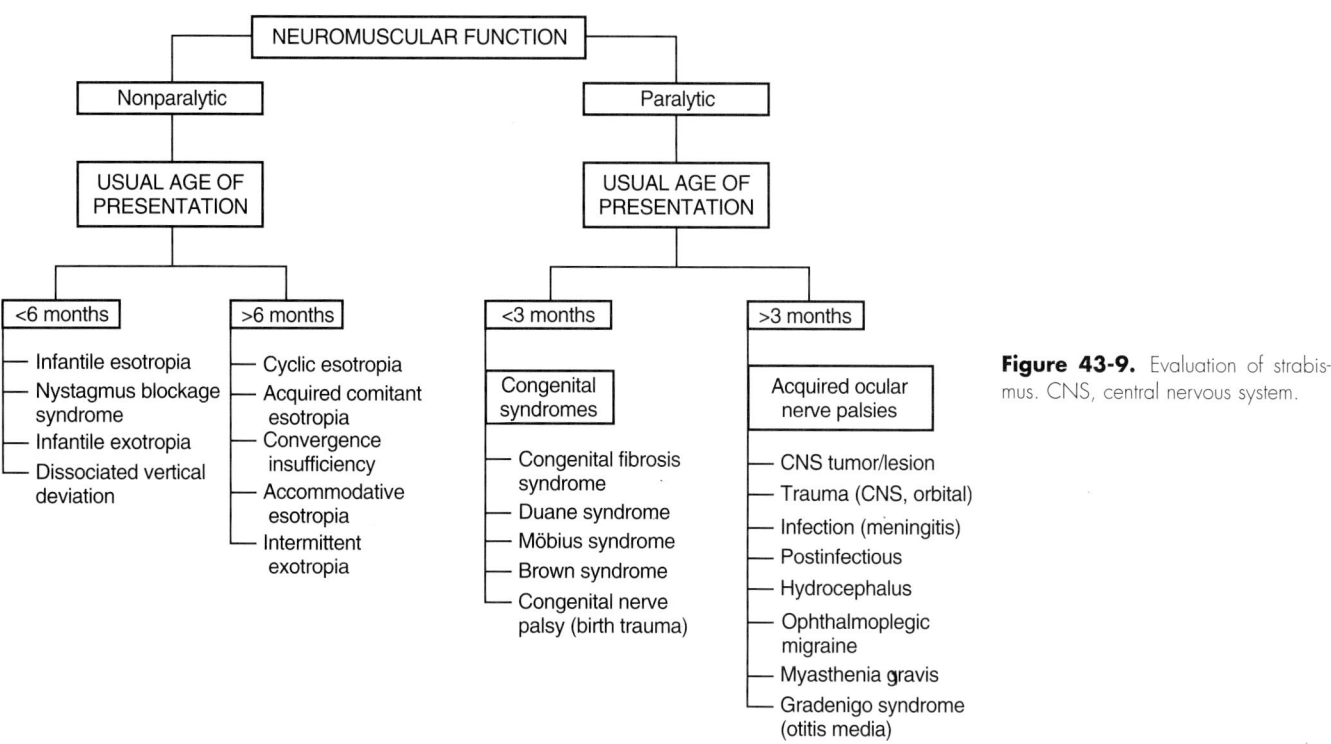

Figure 43-9. Evaluation of strabismus. CNS, central nervous system.

Table 43-3. Less Common Forms of Strabismus

Type of Strabismus	Presenting Symptoms and Signs	Cause	Treatment
Duane syndrome	Esotropia with deficient abduction or exotropia with deficient adduction of one eye; head turn	Absence of sixth nerve nucleus and aberrant innervation of lateral rectus muscle from third cranial nerve	Strabismus surgery for correction of large deviations or abnormal head position
Dissociated vertical deviation	One eye turns up intermittently, especially with fatigue	Eye movement abnormality related most commonly to congenital esotropia	Eye muscle surgery on superior rectus and inferior oblique muscles
Brown syndrome	Head tilt; inability to elevate eye in adduction	Restriction of free passage of superior oblique tendon through trochlea	Observation if not severe; superior oblique tendon surgery if severe
Möbius syndrome	Masklike facies; inability to abduct both eyes; difficulty closing eyes	Bilateral sixth and seventh nerve palsies	Protect corneas from exposure; strabismus surgery
Congenital fibrosis syndrome	Chin-up head position; inability to elevate eyes; ptosis	Autosomal dominant gene on chromosome 16 in some patients; absence of superior division of third nerve in others	Surgical release of tight extraocular muscles
Third nerve palsy	Exotropia and hypertropia; ptosis; dilated, nonreactive pupil	Congenital absence of third nerve; trauma; or tumor	Ptosis and strabismus surgery
Doubler elevator palsy	Chin-up head posture; inability to elevate one eye	Paresis of superior rectus muscle	Transposition strabismus surgery
Orbital floor fracture	Vertical diplopia; chin-up head position	Entrapment of orbital tissues in fracture	Repair of floor fracture; release of inferior rectus muscle restriction
Myasthenia gravis	Variable ptosis and eye movement abnormalities	Blockage of acetylcholine receptor sites by immune complexes	Treatment of systemic myasthenia; strabismus surgery if patient is stable

to be present when best-corrected visual acuity is 20/200 or less in each eye. Constricted visual fields may also play a role in the diagnosis of vision impairment or legal blindness. An infant or child whose visual acuity and visual field cannot be quantitated may be judged visually impaired on the basis of inability to fixate on and follow movement of the examiner's face or other objects or even, in severe instances, inability to perceive light. Milder vision impairment may be suspected on the basis of associated eye signs but can be difficult to confirm in a preverbal child because of compensatory behavior (holding objects close, a face turn) that allows the child to have relatively normal overall function and development. Observation of the child's behavior in the examination room (Table 43-4) and a detailed history (Table 43-5) taken from the parents about the child's visual behavior at home can be important in establishing the degree of impairment. Many visually impaired infants and children have nystagmus (Table 43-6), and the pupillary light reflex may be sluggish.

Visual inattentiveness in an infant deserves special attention because of the possibility that the child has a treatable but not obvious form of vision impairment such as bilateral congenital cataracts. Even if the cause of impairment is not remediable, early diagnosis is important for referral of the infant to an appropriate infant stimulation program and may be important for genetic counseling to the parents.

Vision impairment (monocular or binocular) acquired after infancy obligates the physician to search for a cause, because some causes are treatable (Tables 43-7 to 43-9).

RETINOPATHY OF PREMATURITY

Premature infants are at risk for the development of ROP because the retinal vessels have not yet grown out to the periphery of the retina and are susceptible to a variety of postnatal influences that can adversely affect their maturation. In more advanced stages of ROP, retinal neovascularization occurs. This pathologic process may stop or even reverse, but if it progresses, fibroglial proliferation may lead to traction on the retina and vitreous humor and result in a retinal detachment.

The international classification system for the acute stages of ROP describes the location, extent, and stage of the disease according to the position of the advancing wave of retinal vessels (Fig. 43-10). The retina is divided into zones I, II, and III. Zone I is centered on the optic nerve, from which the retinal arterioles emerge, and zone III exists as a crescent of retina mostly on the temporal side; zone II occupies the midportion of the retina in all four quadrants. The extent of disease describes the number of "clock hours" of retina involved with disease. The severity is indicated by stages 1 to 5.

ROP is rare in infants with a birth weight greater than 2000 g; the risk of ROP increases as birth weight and gestational age decrease. The prevalence of severe ROP is approximately 37% for infants weighing less than 750 g, 22% for those weighing between 750 and 999 g, and 8.5% for those weighing between 1000 and 1250 g. Supplemental oxygen administration also plays a definite but not isolated role in the pathogenesis of ROP. The amount of time that supplemental oxygen is given is a stronger correlate than is the level of oxygenation. Other correlates of ROP are multiple births, transfer to a hospital with a neonatal intensive care unit, white race, and complications of prematurity such as sepsis and intraventricular hemorrhage.

The management of ROP begins with a systematic program of eye examinations at well-defined times in infants judged to be at risk for developing ROP. Infants with a birth weight of less than 1500 g are first examined 5 to 6 weeks after birth. Follow-up examinations are performed every 2 weeks until the retina is fully vascularized.

Table 43-4. Red Flags in Inspection and Direct Ophthalmoscopy in Evaluating Visual Impairment

Physical Finding	Possible Pathologic Process
Inspection	
Globe	
Small	High hyperopia, persistent hyperplastic primary vitreous, phthisis bulbi (shrinkage related to deteriorating eye disease)
Large	Glaucoma, high myopia
Red eye	Inflammatory disease (infection, uveitis), trauma, tumor, glaucoma
Protrusion	Retrobulbar or orbital infection/tumor, hyperthyroidism
Sunken	Orbital fracture, Horner syndrome, atrophy, microphthalmia
Misalignment	Impairment of extraocular muscles: congenital weakness, muscle entrapment (tumor/trauma), cranial nerve palsy (infection, tumor, stroke, congenital)
Ophthalmoscopy	
Cloudy cornea	Anterior segment dysgenesis (Peter anomaly), glaucoma, trauma, infection, metabolic storage diseases (mucopolysaccharidoses)
Lens	
Cloudy	Cataracts (congenital versus systemic diseases)
Dislocated	Homocystinuria, Marfan syndrome
Cloudy vitreous	Retinoblastoma, detached retina, endophthalmitis, uveitis, hemorrhage
Optic disk	
Pale	Optic atrophy (congenital, trauma, tumor, hydrocephalus, degenerative neurologic disease)
Swollen	Increased intracranial pressure, optic neuritis
Hemorrhage	Optic neuritis, increased intracranial pressure
Retina/choroid	
Abnormal color	Retinitis pigmentosa (spicule pattern), chorioretinitis (atrophy with hyperpigmentation), Tay-Sachs disease (cherry-red macula)
Exudates	Diabetes mellitus, Coats disease, increased intracranial pressure
Hemorrhage	Hypertension, diabetes mellitus, increased intracranial pressure, trauma, blood disorders
Phakomata	Tuberous sclerosis (yellow plaques, nodules), von Hippel–Lindau disease (reddish globular mass), Sturge-Weber syndrome (choroidal hemangioma), neurofibromatosis (yellow plaques)
Blood vessels	
Constricted	Hypertension
Microaneurysm	Diabetes mellitus

LEUKOCORIA AND RETINOBLASTOMA

The term *leukocoria* means "white pupil." Leukocoria is a sign, not a specific disease. The causes of leukocoria are listed in Table 43-10. True leukocoria is never an insignificant finding; it mandates prompt

Table 43-5. Red Flags in History for Visual Impairment

Manifestation	Possible Pathologic Process
Child's Complaint	
Generalized blurred vision	
Far vision only	Myopia
Near vision only	Hyperopia, disorder of accommodation
Both far and near	Astigmatism or defect of visual pathways
Focal blurred vision (veil, shadow)	
Unilateral	Ipsilateral retinal or optic nerve
Bilateral	Chiasmal, postchiasmal, or bilateral prechiasmal lesion
Ghost/double vision	
With binocular vision	Cranial nerve or extraocular muscle
With monocular vision	Ocular media or macular disease
Changes in special visions	
Poorer color vision	Retinal or optic nerve disease
Poorer night vision	Retinal disease (retinitis pigmentosa)
Visual sensations	
Floaters, spots	Uveitis, retinal detachment, or hemorrhage
Shimmering lines or scotoma	Migraines
Visual hallucinations	Cerebral lesion, psychogenic
Parent's Observations	
Age-appropriate infant does not track	Severe ocular (myopia, cataracts) or systemic (meningitis) pathologic process
Objects viewed too closely	Decreased visual acuity related to refractive error; ocular or neurologic disorder
Squinting	Decreased visual acuity related to refractive error; ocular or neurologic disorder
Roving or wandering eyes	Nystagmus or strabismus; rule out ocular or neurologic disorder
Head tilting	Compensatory posturing for nystagmus, strabismus, astigmatism, or visual field defect
Bumping into objects	Visual field defect, decreased visual acuity
Reading problems	Visual impairment, visual processing disorder

referral to an ophthalmologist. The causes threaten either vision or life.

Retinoblastoma is the most feared cause of leukocoria because of its potential to metastasize and cause death. It is the most common malignant ocular tumor of childhood, with an incidence of about 1 per 15,000. Leukocoria, the most common presenting sign, is caused by light reflection from the tumor's white surface (Fig. 43-11). Some affected children may present with strabismus or, less commonly, with periocular inflammation, glaucoma, and proptosis. Retinoblastoma may occur bilaterally or multifocally in one eye in familial cases (germ cell mutation). It also occurs sporadically (usually a somatic cell mutation) when one eye is involved with a single tumor focus. Referral of a patient with suspected retinoblastoma to an ophthalmologist experienced in its diagnosis and management is critical. A child with bilateral retinoblastoma is also at risk for *trilateral retinoblastoma,* which includes a primary pineal gland tumor, a pinealoblastoma; cranial magnetic resonance imaging is indicated to rule out this entity. Examination of family members is routinely recommended in order to provide genetic counseling. The parents of a child with retinoblastoma should be informed about the risk for retinoblastoma in subsequent children, and those children should be examined as soon as practical. Genetic testing is also available.

CHILDHOOD CATARACTS

Congenital cataracts are a common cause of unilateral or bilateral vision loss in children, usually resulting from irreversible amblyopia in one or both eyes and occasionally from other accompanying structural ocular abnormalities (Table 43-11). Not all infants with cataracts have leukocoria, but all visually significant cataracts can be detected by careful evaluation of the red reflex (Fig. 43-12). Infants with bilateral, visually significant cataracts may present with visual inattentiveness or nystagmus, signs that significant impairment of vision has already occurred.

Most cases of unilateral cataract are idiopathic in origin or associated with other ocular anomalies (persistent hyperplastic primary vitreous, anterior segment dysgenesis). Bilateral cataracts are hereditary (usually autosomal dominant) in about one third of cases, associated with systemic or metabolic abnormalities in another third, and of unknown origin in the remaining third (see Table 43-11). Evaluation for a systemic cause should include a pediatric physical examination; ophthalmologic examination of the infant and family members; urine for reducing substances after lactose-containing milk feeding; and titers for toxoplasmosis, other infections, rubella, cytomegalovirus infection, and herpes simplex (TORCH). Other metabolic studies, chromosomal evaluation, and genetic consultation may be indicated. A workup to determine a systemic cause for a unilateral cataract is seldom fruitful.

Cataracts in older children may be newly acquired in some cases or a delayed manifestation of progressive congenital cataracts. Occasional unilateral cataracts are caused by an underlying congenital lens defect, which develops into a full-blown cataract at a later age. Trauma is also a common cause of an acquired unilateral cataract.

Ideally, unilateral cataracts must be removed and amblyopia treatment begun in the first month or two of life. Bilateral cataracts judged to be visually significant must be treated in the first several months of life to facilitate an optimal outcome.

Aphakic correction in infants younger than 6 to 12 months with bilateral cataracts is generally provided with extended-wear contact lenses or spectacles. Unilateral aphakia in this age group is best managed with a contact lens. A posterior chamber intraocular lens is an ideal way to correct unilateral aphakia in a child with a traumatic cataract. Intraocular lenses are also used with increasing frequency and at earlier ages in infants with unilateral or bilateral cataracts.

Table 43-6. Causes of Nystagmus and Poor Vision From Birth

Opacities of the Media
Bilateral corneal opacities
Bilateral cataracts

Retinal Disorders

Ophthalmoscopically visible

Optic nerve
  Optic atrophy
  Developmental anomalies
    Hypoplasia
    Coloboma
Macular disease
  Infections: "coloboma"
  Developmental
    Hypoplasia
    Traction
Rare bilateral association
  (e.g., retinal dysplasia, posterior PHPV)

Ophthalmoscopically variable

Achromatopsia (rod monochromatism)
Leber congenital amaurosis
Congenital stationary night blindness X-linked with myopia

Systemic Diseases
Neurologic disorders (e.g., hydrocephalus)
Metabolic disorders (e.g., Lowe syndrome)
Chromosomal abnormalities (e.g., Down syndrome)
Somatic malfunctions (e.g., de Lange syndrome)

Disturbances of Higher Centers, Cause Unknown
Congenital nystagmus
Spasmus nutans
Latent nystagmus
Occlusion nystagmus

Modified from Nelson LB, Calhoun JH, Harley RD: Pediatric Ophthalmology, 3rd ed. Philadelphia, WB Saunders, 1991, p 84.

PHPV, persistent hyperplastic primary vitreous (this is often unilateral).

There is accumulating evidence that an intraocular lens skillfully placed in the capsular bag (exactly what would be done for a cataract in an adult) is a safe, effective, and convenient way to manage aphakia in children. Management of aphakia with contact lenses or spectacles, however, still remains within the standard of care for many infants and children.

The management of a cataract is not finished after cataract surgery, as it would be in an adult. Amblyopia must be treated with occlusion of the sound eye, often for several years, until stable visual acuity can be demonstrated. Children who have had cataract surgery must be monitored indefinitely to evaluate for delayed complications such as glaucoma and retinal detachment.

GLAUCOMA IN CHILDHOOD

Glaucoma in childhood is divided into primary congenital glaucoma, primary developmental glaucoma that is related to other systemic or ocular abnormalities, and secondary glaucoma, which is caused by ocular trauma, inflammation, or previous surgery (Table 43-12).

Primary congenital glaucoma is defined as glaucoma that occurs in the first year of life and is unrelated to other ocular abnormalities. Only about 25% of affected infants have signs of glaucoma at birth;

in the remainder, signs develop during the first year. The incidence of congenital glaucoma is about 1 per 10,000, somewhat higher than retinoblastoma. There is a strong hereditary tendency. The incidence is much higher in societies with parental consanguinity. A recessively inherited form has been associated with a gene defect on the short arm of chromosome 2 and a dominantly inherited form on the long arm of chromosome 1. In the absence of a family history of congenital glaucoma, an affected parent has about a 5% chance of having an affected child.

The pathophysiologic mechanism of primary congenital glaucoma is unknown but is believed to be related to trabecular meshwork abnormalities in the drainage angle of the eye. This abnormality is posited to stem from a developmental arrest of the neural crest–derived anterior chamber tissue. The natural history of untreated congenital glaucoma is blindness resulting from progressive corneal opacification and optic nerve damage. As the entire eye enlarges from unrelenting elevated intraocular pressure, a condition of pseudoproptosis and "ox eye" appearance known as buphthalmos may result.

The classic triad of presentation of an infant with congenital glaucoma is epiphora, photophobia, and blepharospasm (Fig. 43-13). These symptoms appear to derive from the related corneal abnormalities, including enlargement, tears in the Descemet membrane, and edema. The differential diagnosis of congenital glaucoma includes conditions that demonstrate corneal opacities (Table 43-13) or an enlarged cornea (Table 43-14). Epiphora occurs also with conjunctivitis, corneal trauma, and nasolacrimal duct obstruction. Photophobia is observed in infants with corneal trauma or inflammation and with uveitis. Corneal opacification from chronic edema, an additional finding in congenital glaucoma, can also be found in infants with corneal dystrophies, metabolic storage diseases such as mucopolysaccharidoses, and forceps-related obstetric trauma (see Table 43-13).

The diagnosis of congenital glaucoma is confirmed by performing an examination with the patient under anesthesia. The diagnosis rests on a constellation of abnormal findings, including elevated intraocular pressure, corneal enlargement, anomalies of the drainage angle, and signs of damage to the optic nerve.

Topical and systemic medications (β blockers, carbonic anhydrase inhibitors) to lower intraocular pressure are frequently employed before the examination is performed, but surgery is the mainstay of treatment. Intraocular pressure can be controlled in about 80% of infants with angle surgery. Blindness results in up to 15% of affected eyes, and visual acuity is less than 20/50 in the majority of affected eyes. Amblyopia therapy with glasses and occlusion is generally necessary to obtain optimal visual acuity.

Primary developmental glaucoma and secondary glaucoma occur in infants and children with other ocular and systemic abnormalities (see Table 43-12). The management of these types of glaucoma is similar to that of primary congenital glaucoma but has a lower success rate, usually requires multiple operations, and may necessitate chronic administration of topical glaucoma medication.

CHILDHOOD UVEITIS

Uveitis is defined as inflammation of the uveal tissue of the eye, which includes the iris, ciliary body, and choroid. Inflammation can involve any or all of these structures, and terms such as *iritis, iridocyclitis, choroiditis,* and *chorioretinitis* are used to designate which portion of the uveal tissue is involved. Most cases of uveitis in childhood occur in the anterior part of the eye and are referred to as *iridocyclitis.*

A child with uveitis may have no symptoms or signs, as is common in the uveitis associated with juvenile rheumatoid arthritis (JRA), or can present with a "red eye" and complain of pain, photophobia, and blurred vision. There may be injection of the perilimbal

---

Table 43-7. Childhood Amaurosis (Blindness): Principal Neurologic Considerations

Congenital Malformations

Optic nerve hypoplasia
Congenital hydrocephalus
Hydranencephaly
Porencephaly
Micrencephaly
Encephalocele, particulary occipital type

Phakomatoses

Tuberous sclerosis
Neurofibromatosis (special association with
  optic glioma)
Sturge-Weber syndrome
von Hippel–Lindau disease

Tumors

Retinoblastoma
Optic glioma
Perioptic meningioma
Craniopharyngioma
Cerebral glioma
Posterior and intraventricular tumors when
  complicated by hydrocephalus

Neurodegenerative Diseases

Cerebral storage disease
  Gangliosidoses, particularly Tay-Sachs disease
    (infantile amaurotic familial idiocy), Sandhoff
    variant, generalized gangliosidosis
Other lipidoses and ceroid lipofuscinoses,
  particularly the late-onset amaurotic familial
  idiocies such as those of Janský-Bielschowsky
  and of Batten-Mayou-Spielmeyer-Vogt
Mucopolysaccharidoses, particularly Hurler
  syndrome and Hunter syndrome

Leukodystrophies (dysmyelination disorders),
  particularly metachromatic leukodystrophy and
  Canavan disease
Demyelinating sclerosis (myelinoclastic diseases),
  especially Schilder disease and Devic neuromyelitis
  optica
Special types: Dawson disease, Leigh disease,
  Bassen-Kornzweig syndrome, Refsum disease
Retinal degenerations: "retinitis pigmentosa" and its
  variants, and Leber congenital type
Optic atrophies: congenital autosomal recessive type,
  infantile and congenital autosomal dominant types,
Leber disease, and atrophies associated with hereditary
  ataxias: the types of Behr, of Marie, and of
  Sanger-Brown

Infectious Processes

Encephalitis, especially in the prenatal infection
  syndromes due to *Toxoplasma gondii*,
  cytomegalovirus, rubella virus, *Treponema pallidum*
Meningitis; arachnoiditis
Optic neuritis
Chorioretinitis

Hematologic Disorders

Leukemia with CNS involvement

Vascular and Circulatory Disorders

Collagen-vascular diseases
Arteriovenous malformations: intracerebral
  hemorrhage, subarachnoid hemorrhage

Trauma

Contusion or avulsion of optic nerves or chiasm
Cerebral contusion or laceration
Intracerebral, subarachnoid, or subdural hemorrhage

Drugs and Toxins

Modified from Harley RD: Pediatric Ophthalmology, 2nd ed. Philadelphia, WB Saunders, 1983, p 777.

CNS, central nervous system.

---

tissue (ciliary flush), and in advanced cases, the cornea may lose its luster from edema or deposition of calcium (band keratopathy) (Fig. 43-14). The pupil may have an irregular shape as a result of adhesions to the underlying lens (posterior synechiae). A cataract and glaucoma may result. Vision may be lost because of opacification of the ocular media, retinal edema, and amblyopia in a young child.

The diagnosis of uveitis can be made from an eye examination. Evaluation of the cause of the uveitis requires a thorough pediatric physical examination as well as supplementary radiologic and laboratory testing (Table 43-15). A chest radiograph may demonstrate tuberculosis and sarcoidosis. Serologic evaluation may include tests for syphilis, sarcoidosis, JRA, Lyme disease, and toxoplasmosis. In boys, haplotype testing for human leukocyte antigen B27 may be indicated because of the association between iritis and pauciarticular arthritis that may later evolve into ankylosing spondylitis.

The iritis in children with JRA is usually asymptomatic and chronic (see Chapter 44). The link between JRA and iritis is strongest in the pauciarticular form, when the onset occurs before the age of 7 years, and when the antinuclear antibody blood test is positive. Girls may be at higher risk than boys. JRA-associated uveitis may lead to blindness if not identified and treated aggressively.

The management of iritis in children is the elimination of intraocular inflammation with topical corticosteroid drops. Mydriatic drops are used to prevent the formation of posterior synechiae. Periocular injections of depot corticosteroid preparations and oral corticosteroids may be required for severe cases, but long-term use should be avoided. Nonsteroidal antiinflammatory drugs (NSAIDs) may allow a reduction in the corticosteroids necessary to treat chronic iritis. Systemic immunosuppressive medications, most commonly methotrexate, are reserved for children who have severe, persistent inflammation despite aggressive treatment with corticosteroids and NSAIDs.

Toxoplasmosis is the most common cause of posterior uveitis in children. Most ocular toxoplasmosis in the pediatric age group is probably acquired from the mother during pregnancy. In some instances, the infection is inactive at birth and goes unrecognized until inflammation occurs. Toxoplasmosis that is active at birth may result in widespread fetal tissue damage or may be associated with chorioretinitis, encephalomyelitis, and visceral disease. The diagnosis of toxoplasmosis is based on clinical findings, intracranial calcification in some children, and laboratory tests for specific immunoglobulin G and immunoglobulin M antibodies. Treatment of toxoplasmosis consists of combination therapy with pyrimethamine and sulfadiazine.

Toxocariasis is a rare cause of inflammation of the posterior segment of the eye. Caused by ingesting ova from dirt contaminated

Table 43-8. Causes of Monocular Visual Loss

Disorder	Timing	Pattern of Loss	Other Clues	Fundus Appearance	Pupil
Refractive error	Gradual*	Varies	Improves with pinhole	Normal	Normal
Cataract	Very gradual	Tunnel?	Opacity visible	Normal	Normal, but red reflex decreased
Corneal disease	Acute or chronic	Murky	Opacity visible or positive fluorescein uptake	Normal	Normal, but red reflex decreased
Iritis	Acute or chronic	Murky	Pain Ciliary flush	Normal	Small Disfigured?
Open-angle glaucoma	Gradual	Varies	Elevated pressures	Normal	Normal
Angle-closure glaucoma	Acute	Varies	Pain Steamy cornea Patient ill	Normal	Dilated Fixed
Central retinal occlusion	Acute	Varies	Painless Abrupt	Pale with cherry-red macula	Normal
Retinal detachment	Acute	Varies	Painless Floaters	Unremarkable or diagnostic	Afferent pupillary defect if extensive
Vitreous hemorrhage	Acute	"Dark"	Cannot see in the eye	Obscured	Normal, but red reflex decreased
Amaurosis fugax	Acute Transient	5-10 min	Carotid or heart disease, migraine	Normal	Normal
Migraine	Acute Transient	5-30 min	Headache History Scintillations	Normal	Normal
Optic neuropathy	Gradual or acute	Central scotoma	Toxins? Multiple sclerosis? Pituitary tumor? Virus?	Normal Pale optic disk?	Afferent defect?
Diffuse retinopathy	Gradual	Varies	Genetic? AIDS?	Retinal lesions	Afferent defect?
Papilledema (chronic)	Late	Varies	CNS tumor? Pseudotumor cerebri Hypertensive crisis?	Diagnostic	Normal
Endophthalmitis	Varies	Varies	Corneal infection? Penetrating injury? Systemic infection? Hypopyon?	Varies Often obscured	Varies

Modified from Reilly BM: Practical Strategies in Outpatient Medicine, 2nd ed. Philadelphia, WB Saunders, 1991, p 60.

*Refractive error may be more acute when caused by diabetes mellitus.

AIDS, acquired immunodeficiency syndrome; CNS, central nervous system.

with the canine parasite *Toxocara canis,* toxocariasis usually occurs in children aged 7 to 9 years old. Children typically present with a chronic, unilateral uveitis that can cause leukocoria and blurred vision. Diagnosis is based on an enzyme-linked immunosorbent assay for *Toxocara.* Treatment consists of management of intraocular inflammation with corticosteroids.

Several other entities can simulate uveitis in children and must be considered. These entities include retinoblastoma, leukemia, lymphoma, juvenile xanthogranuloma, and an intraocular foreign body.

NASOLACRIMAL PROBLEMS IN CHILDHOOD

The nasolacrimal system consists of tear-secreting glands and a drainage system. The lacrimal gland, located in the supertemporal orbit, is the primary producer of tears; accessory lacrimal glands in the upper eyelid supplement its output. The lacrimal drainage apparatus begins with puncta on the nasal aspect of the upper and lower eyelid margins. The puncta continue as canaliculi that course nasally to empty into the lacrimal sac. The lacrimal sac in turn drains inferiorly through the nasolacrimal duct just under the inferior turbinate (Fig. 43-15).

Developmental anomalies of the nasolacrimal drainage system are common and include atresia of the puncta or canaliculi (causing tearing but not infection), lacrimal-cutaneous fistula (causing tears to drain to the skin surface), and, by far the most common, failure of the distal nasolacrimal duct to achieve full patency (causing tearing and dacryocystitis).

Nasolacrimal duct obstruction occurs in about 5% of infants. A thin mucosal membrane at the distal end of the duct is the most common cause. Typically, the infant lacrimates and has a mucopurulent discharge that causes matting of the eyelids beginning at about 1 month of age. Pressure applied to the lacrimal sac with a finger or cotton swab often results in reflux of cloudy fluid from the puncta. The infection is usually polymicrobial, but a bacteriologic diagnosis is not necessary for clinical management. Nasolacrimal duct obstruction must be differentiated from the previously mentioned developmental anomalies—conjunctivitis, especially gonococcal or

Table 43-9. Organic Causes of Vision Loss in Infancy

Condition	Physical Findings	Comments
Corneal Disease		
Corneal forceps injury	Cloudy cornea	May lead to astigmatism and amblyopia; associated with intraocular hemorrhage, retinal detachment, or glaucoma
Sclerocornea	Opaque cornea	Scleralization of cornea; familial or sporadic; early keratoplasty possibly needed to provide vision
Anterior microphthalmia	Small cornea	Familial inheritance; associated with congenital cataracts, glaucoma, and/or colobomata
Anterior Chamber Diseases		
Peter anomaly	Corneal opacity with iridocorneal/lenticulocorneal adhesions	Maldevelopment of anterior segment of eye; associated with glaucoma and lens abnormalities
Persistent pupillary membrane	Bands or membranes obscuring pupil	Rupture of vessels in membranes may lead to hyphema; membrane may need to be removed to restore vision
Glaucoma	Tearing, enlarged eye, photophobia, cloudy cornea, pale optic disk	Increased intraocular pressure leading to blindness (optic nerve damage) Causes: anomalies of anterior segment, intraocular hemorrhage, ocular inflammatory disease, intraocular tumors Treatment: surgery
Iris and Lens Disorders		
Aniridia	Large, irregular, unreactive pupil	Hypoplasia of iris—type I: dominant or recessive (ataxia, mental retardation); type II: deletion of chromosome 11, associated with mental retardation, genitourinary anomalies, and Wilms tumor
Cataracts	Lens opacity	Multiple causes, ranging from familial inheritance to drugs
Anterior PHPV	Leukocoria (white pupillary reflex), lens opacity, cloudy cornea, small lens and eye	Persistence of fetal hyaloid vascular system, resulting in fibrovascular plaque on back of lens; as plaque contracts, ciliary process and lens become distorted Complications: glaucoma, cataract, intraocular hemorrhage, rupture of posterior capsule. Treatment: removal of membrane, lens aspiration. Prognosis: poor visual outcome
Retinal and Optic Nerve Disorders		
Posterior PHPV	Fibroglial veils around disk/macula, vitreous opacities (membrane, vessels)	Persistence of posterior fetal hyaloid vascular system; remnants of vascular system may cause traction detachment of retina
Chorioretinitis	Diffuse or local retinal atrophy demarcated by hyperpigmentation	Inflammation of posterior uveal with retinal involvement Causes: toxoplasmosis, histoplasmosis, herpes simplex, cytomegalic inclusion virus, syphilis, tuberculosis, and toxocariasis Other complications: glaucoma, detached retina
Retinoblastoma	Leukocoria	Neoplastic tumor with locus on chromosome 13; high incidence of secondary malignancy; poor prognosis with extraorbital metastasis
Retinopathy of prematurity	Leukocoria, cloudy vitreous; retinal white lines and ridges	Insult (hyperoxia) to vascularization of retina; associated with myopia and retinal detachment
Leber congenital retinal amaurosis	Normal findings to degeneration of retina	Failure of both rods and cones in retina; reduced or absent response to electroretinography; autosomal recessive
Achromatopsia	Color cannot be detected, photophobia	Failure of cone system in retina; autosomal recessive or X-linked; diagnosed with ERG
Congenital stationary night blindness	Disk anomalies, poor night vision	Defect in rod system of retina; autosomal recessive, dominant, or X-linked recessive
Optic nerve hypoplasia	Pale, small optic disk; peripapillary halo of pigmentation	Secondary to failure in differentiation or degeneration of retinal ganglion cell axons Some causes: septooptic dysplasia (hypopituitary, midline CNS defects), chromosomal defects (trisomy 13), albinism, fetal drug exposure (phenytoin, ethanol), infant of diabetic mother, CNS defects (hydrocephalus, anencephaly, encephalocele)
Optic nerve aplasia	Absence of retinal vessels and optic disk	Maldevelopment of optic nerve; associated with severe eye and CNS anomalies

Continued

Table 43-9. Organic Causes of Vision Loss in Infancy—cont'd

Condition	Physical Findings	Comments
Retinal and Optic Nerve Disorders—cont'd		
Morning glory disk anomaly	Enlarged, funnel-shaped disk	Associated with retinal detachments and midline defects (cleft palate, encephalocele, agenesis of corpus callosum)
Coloboma	White, wedge-shaped retinal defect; visual field loss	Malclosure of embryonic fissure that leaves a gap in the retina, hence exposing sclera; defect may extend to lens; associated with many congenital syndromes
Aicardi syndrome	Retinal lacunae, coloboma of optic disk	Occurs mostly in girls and women; associated with agenesis of corpus callosum, seizures, mental retardation, and vertebral anomalies
Albinism	Photophobia; blue-gray to yellow-brown iris; macular hypoplasia	Defect in formation of melanin, resulting in lack of pigment in eyes and sometimes skin; increased risk of skin cancer with hypopigmented skin

CNS, central nervous system; ERG, electroretinogram; PHPV, persistent hyperplastic primary vitreous.

chlamydial; herpes simplex keratitis; and congenital glaucoma—in which chronic tearing can be a prominent feature.

The initial management of nasolacrimal duct obstruction consists of administration of a topical antibiotic ointment or drop several times per day. A broad spectrum of bacterial coverage is desirable. A several-day course of topical antibiotic administration is usually sufficient to lessen the purulence; chronic administration of the antibiotic most probably leads to selection of resistant organisms and reduced effectiveness. Lacrimal sac massage should be combined with antibiotic treatment. The massage decompresses the lacrimal sac and, ideally, ruptures the membrane occluding the distal nasolacrimal duct by increased hydrostatic pressure. The conventional technique of massage is to place the index finger above the medial canthus and to stroke downward with firm pressure. Reflux of material through the puncta confirms that the sac is being properly massaged. In at least half of affected infants, the nasolacrimal duct obstruction resolves by 6 months of age. The proportion of those with obstruction remaining at 6 months that resolves by the age of 1 year is substantially smaller.

Surgical management of persistent nasolacrimal duct obstruction is indicated for children who continue to have tearing and eyelid crusting at 6 to 12 months of age. A probing of the nasolacrimal duct results in a cure in more than 90% of children younger than about 15 months.

A dacryocystocele is a variation of congenital nasolacrimal duct obstruction that occurs in newborns. These infants present with a bluish mass in the nasoorbital region; this mass is a dilated lacrimal sac that has both distal obstruction from a membrane and proximal obstruction from a one-way valve effect from an incompetent valve

of Rosenmüller (Fig. 43-16). The possibility that the bluish mass is a hemangioma, dermoid cyst, or an encephalocele must be considered. On occasion, the dilated sac is accompanied by bulging of the nasal mucosa at the distal end of the nasolacrimal duct. The nasal mass can compromise the infant's breathing. If the dacryocystocele fails to resolve with topical antibiotics and massage, or if cellulitis develops, systemic antibiotics and surgical decompression must be considered. Decompression is accomplished by relieving the distal obstruction by probing the nasolacrimal duct.

THE RED EYE

The term *red eye* usually refers to inflammation of the conjunctiva that causes the eye to appear red. Causes of red eye include infection

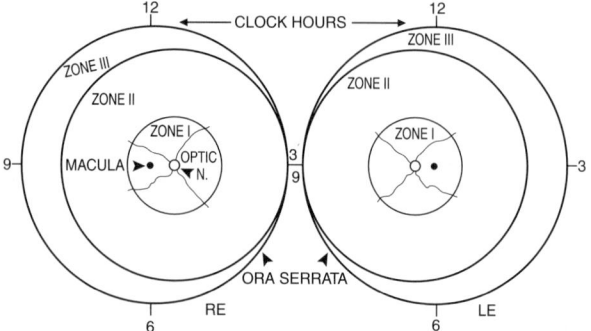

Figure 43-10. The international classification of retinopathy of prematurity (ROP). The stage of ROP is determined by the location, extent, and stage of disease according to the position of the advancing waves of retinal vessels.

Table 43-10. Differential Diagnosis of Leukocoria (White Pupillary Reflex)

Common Causes
Cataracts
Cicatricial retinopathy of prematurity
Exudative retinopathy
Fundus coloboma
Larval granulomatosus (toxocariasis)
Persistent hyperplastic primary vitreous
Retinoblastoma

Other Causes
Atrophic chorioretinal scars
Endophthalmitis
Glioneuroma
Hemangioma
Hamartoma
Leukemic ophthalmopathy
Incontinentia pigmenti
Medullated nerve fibers
Medulloepithelioma
Morning glory disk anomaly
Norrie disease
Organized vitreous hemorrhage
Phakomatoses
Retinal gliosis
Retinal dysplasia
Retinoschisis

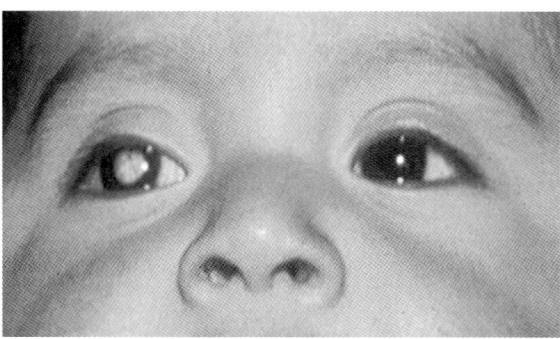

Figure 43-11. Infant with leukocoria of right eye caused by retinoblastoma.

of the ocular surface (cornea, conjunctiva, and sclera), allergy, intraocular inflammation, glaucoma, and trauma. Evaluation must be directed toward discerning whether a child's red eye is caused by a benign condition that can easily be treated with topical medication (bacterial conjunctivitis, allergic conjunctivitis) or whether the cause is potentially vision threatening (iritis, corneal ulceration, glaucoma) and requires ophthalmologic evaluation (Table 43-16).

In taking the history, the examiner should inquire about the mode of onset, associated illnesses, contact with other children with "pink eye," the presence of pain or itching, the characteristics of any discharge (watery, mucoid, purulent), and blurring of vision. The examination of the child should start with as precise a measurement of visual acuity as possible. The presence and type of discharge should be noted. Inspection of the surface of the eye with a penlight should determine whether the inflammation is diffuse or focal (e.g., perilimbal only) and whether the cornea has its normal luster. Foreign bodies must be looked for in cases associated with trauma. Fluorescein staining of the cornea to assess for a corneal abrasion should be considered. The red reflex should be checked.

The most common cause of a red eye in a child is infectious conjunctivitis (Table 43-17). *Streptococcus pneumoniae* is the most frequent bacterial pathogen, followed by *Haemophilus influenzae* and *Staphylococcus aureus*. *S. pneumoniae* and *H. influenzae* tend to cause acute conjunctivitis with morning crusting and difficulty opening the eyes. Subconjunctival hemorrhages may occur. *S. aureus* is more likely to cause chronic conjunctivitis with associated corneal involvement. A bacterial culture is not necessary in mild cases of suspected bacterial conjunctivitis because the infection tends to be self-limiting. Treatment with a broad-spectrum topical antibiotic ointment (bacitracin-polymyxin) or drop (trimethoprim-polymyxin) may relieve symptoms and shorten the course of infection, allowing the child to return to school or day care. Sulfacetamide preparations are inexpensive but have a narrower range of effectiveness and cause a great deal of stinging. Topical aminoglycosides and fluoroquinolones are reserved for more serious infections (corneal ulcers). Steroid-antibiotic combinations should be avoided because of the risk of worsening a bacterial corneal ulcer or an unsuspected herpes simplex infection.

Viral conjunctivitis tends to be associated with a watery or mucoid discharge. Follicles may be visible with low magnification on the palpebral conjunctiva, and a preauricular lymph node can often be palpated. Adenovirus types 3, 8, 11, and 19 are common pathogens; epidemic outbreaks are frequent. In children as old as 2 years, adenovirus can manifest with severe periorbital edema and erythema that mimics bacterial preseptal or orbital cellulitis; a conjunctival pseudomembrane is common in this setting.

Treatment is directed at symptoms and includes artificial tears and cool compresses. In older children, conjunctival and even corneal signs and symptoms predominate. A culture is not necessary and seldom helps guide therapy in acute cases. Treatment can be

with a topical antibiotic if a bacterial cause is suspected. Otherwise, treatment is largely supportive, with cool compresses providing symptomatic relief. Enteroviruses produce conjunctivitis, which may be hemorrhagic. Less frequent causes of viral conjunctivitis are herpes simplex and varicella. Both of these are usually associated with vesicular involvement of the eyelid and face. Treatment with specific antiviral medications is generally reserved for corneal involvement or an immunocompromised state. Topical corticosteroid medication is contraindicated because of the potential for worsening the infection.

The DNA poxvirus *Molluscum contagiosum* can cause a chronic conjunctivitis when lesions are located on the eyelid margin (Fig. 43-17). The conjunctivitis is caused by release of poxvirus particles into the tear film. Additional waxy, umbilicated lesions are oftentimes found elsewhere on the face. Treatment of the conjunctivitis requires excision or cryotherapy of lesions located on the eyelid margin.

Allergic conjunctivitis manifests with a bilateral watery or mucoid discharge and must always be considered in the differential diagnosis of bilateral red eyes. The child may rub the eyes because of pruritus; nasal allergic symptoms may also be present.

Systemic syndromes must also be considered in a child with a red eye. In the Stevens-Johnson syndrome, conjunctival inflammation is associated with other mucous membrane or cutaneous involvement. This disease can have severe ophthalmic consequences from conjunctival scarring and dry eye syndrome. Kawasaki syndrome is a febrile illness of young children who frequently manifest bilateral nonpurulent conjunctival injection and, in rare cases, iritis. Ophthalmic consultation may be indicated to assist in the diagnosis and management of children with Stevens-Johnson and Kawasaki syndromes.

EYELID AND ORBITAL PROBLEMS

Congenital abnormalities of the eyelids are relatively uncommon; they consist of entropion (inward turning of the eyelid margin), ectropion (eversion of the eyelid margin), epiblepharon (in which a horizontal fold of skin in the lower eyelid causes the lashes to rub against the cornea), and distichiasis (in which an accessory row of eyelashes more posterior than the normal ones rub against the cornea). All these may resolve spontaneously or, if necessary, can be corrected with eyelid surgery. Epicanthus consists of a crescent-shaped fold of skin, usually most prominent in the upper eyelid, that can make the child appear esotropic by obscuring the underlying sclera. Congenital ptosis (Fig. 43-18), defined as droopiness of the upper eyelid, is usually caused by abnormal development of the levator muscle. Other causes in children are congenital third nerve palsy and congenital Horner syndrome. Acute ptosis is a sign of increased intracranial pressure. Treatment of ptosis is usually delayed until the child is several years old unless it is causing amblyopia or, in bilateral cases, a severe chin-up head posture to allow the child to see. Surgical correction consists of resection of the levator muscle or suspension of the upper eyelid to the frontalis muscle with autogenous or cadaveric fascia lata.

Common causes of a mass in a child's eyelid or anterior orbit are tumors (capillary hemangioma), choristomas (dermoid cyst), or infections (chalazion). A hemangioma (Fig. 43-19) is the most common benign eyelid tumor of infancy and frequently extends into the orbit. The overlying skin frequently has a raised, red, and dimpled appearance, hence the name *strawberry hemangioma*. The lesion may increase in size when the infant cries. Similar skin lesions elsewhere on the body are common. Capillary hemangiomas often grow significantly in the first several months of life and may cause visual problems by occluding the visual axis, causing astigmatism from pressure against the eye or strabismus by physical displacement of the eye. The threat or actual development of amblyopia is an

Table 43-11. Differential Diagnosis of Cataracts

Developmental Variants

Prematurity (Y suture vacuoles) with or without retinopathy of prematurity

Genetic Disorders

Simple Mendelian Inheritance

Autosomal dominant (most common)
Autosomal recessive
X-linked

Major Chromosomal Defects

Trisomy disorders (13, 18, 21)
Turner syndrome (45X)
Deletion syndromes (11p13, 18p, 18q)
Duplication syndromes (3q, 20q, 10q)

Multisystem Genetic Disorders

Alport syndrome (hearing loss, renal disease)
Alström disease (nerve deafness, diabetes mellitus)
Apert syndrome (craniosynostosis, syndactyly)
Cockayne syndrome (premature senility, skin photosensitivity)
Conradi syndrome (chondrodysplasia punctata)
Crouzon syndrome (dysostosis craniofacialis)
Hallermann-Streiff syndrome (microphthalmia, small pinched nose, skin atrophy, and hypotrichosis)
Hypohidrotic ectodermal dysplasia (anomalous dentition, hypohidrosis, hypotrichosis)
Ichthyosis (keratinizing disorder with thick, scaly skin)
Incontinentia pigmenti (dental anomalies, mental retardation, cutaneous lesions)
Lowe syndrome (oculocerebrorenal syndrome: hypotonia, renal disease)
Marfan syndrome
Meckel-Gruber syndrome (renal dysplasia, encephalocele)
Myotonic dystrophy
Nail-patella syndrome (renal dysfunction, dysplastic nails, hypoplastic patella)
Marinesco-Sjögren syndrome (cerebellar ataxia, hypotonia)
Nevoid basal cell carcinoma syndrome (autosomal dominant, basal cell carcinoma erupts in childhood)
Peter anomaly (corneal opacifications with iris-corneal dysgenesis)
Reiger syndrome (iris dysplasia, myotonic dystrophy)
Rothmund-Thomson (poikiloderma: skin atrophy)
Rubinstein-Taybi syndrome (broad great toe, mental retardation)
Smith-Lemli-Opitz syndrome (toe syndactyly, hypospadias, mental retardation)
Sotos syndrome (cerebral gigantism)
Spondyloepiphyseal dysplasia (dwarfism, short trunk)
Werner syndrome (premature aging in 2nd decade of life)

Inborn Errors of Metabolism

Abetalipoproteinemia (absent chylomicrons, retinal degeneration)
Fabry disease (α-galactosidase A deficiency)
Galactokinase deficiency
Galactosemia (galactose 1-phosphate uridyltransferase deficiency)
Homocystinemia (subluxation of lens, mental retardation)
Mannosidosis (acid α-mannosidase deficiency)
Niemann-Pick (sphingomyelinase deficiency)
Refsum syndrome (phytanic acid α-hydrolase deficiency)
Wilson disease (accumulation of copper leads to cirrhosis and neurologic symptoms)

Endocrinopathies

Hypocalcemia (hypoparathyroidism)
Hypoglycemia
Diabetes mellitus

Congenital Infections

Toxoplasmosis
Cytomegalovirus infection
Syphilis
Rubella
Perinatal herpes simplex infection
Measles (rubeola)
Poliomyelitis
Influenza
Varicella-zoster

Ocular Anomalies

Microphthalmia
Coloboma
Aniridia
Mesodermal dysgenesis
Persistent pupillary membrane
Posterior lenticonus
Persistent hyperplastic primary vitreous
Primitive hyaloid vascular system

Miscellaneous Disorders

Atopic dermatitis
Drugs (corticosteroids)
Radiation
Trauma

Idiopathic

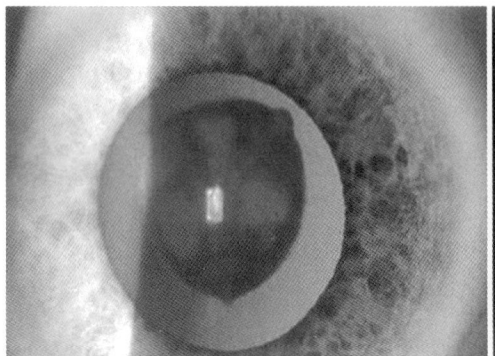 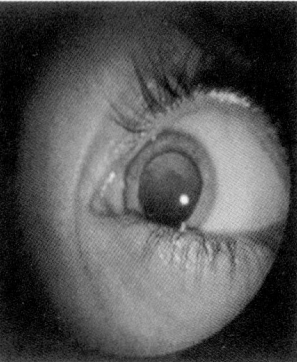

Figure 43-12. Left, Fundus reflex of an eye with a visually significant congenital cataract. The lens opacity is seen as black against the lighter fundus reflex. **Right,** Fundus reflex of a small, visually insignificant cataract. Nonetheless, this child requires referral for ophthalmologic evaluation.

Table 43-12. Childhood Glaucomas

I. Primary Genetically Determined Glaucoma
 	
A. Congenital open-angle glaucoma
B. Juvenile glaucoma
C. Primary angle-closure glaucoma
D. Primary glaucomas associated with systemic or ocular abnormalities
  1. Associated with *systemic* abnormalities
    a. Sturge-Weber syndrome
    b. Neurofibromatosis
    c. Pierre Robin anomalad
    d. Oculocerebrorenal syndrome (Lowe syndrome)
    e. Rieger syndrome
    f. Hepatocerebrorenal syndrome
    g. Marfan syndrome
    h. Rubinstein-Taybi syndrome
    i. Infantile glaucoma associated with mental retardation and paralysis
    j. Oculodental-digital syndrome
    k. Syndrome of microcornea, absent frontal sinuses, and open-angle glaucoma
    l. Mucopolysaccharidosis
    m. Trisomy 13
    n. Hurler disease
    o. Cutis marmorata telangiectasia
  2. Associated with *ocular* abnormalities
    a. Aniridia
    b. Congenital ocular melanosis
    c. Sclerocornea
    d. Familial hypoplasia of iris
    e. Anterior chamber cleavage syndrome
    f. Iridotrabecular dysgenesis and ectropion uveae
    g. Posterior polymorphous dystrophy
	II. Secondary Glaucoma
	
	A. Traumatic glaucoma
	  1. Acute
	    a. Angle concussion
	    b. Hyphema
	  2. Late onset with angle recession
	  3. Atriovenous fistula
	B. Intraocular neoplasm
	  1. Melanoma
	  2. Melanocytoma
	  3. Juvenile xanthogranuloma
	  4. Retinoblastoma
	  5. Leukemia
	C. Uveitis
	  1. Open-angle
	  2. Angle blockage
	    a. Synechial angle-closure
	    b. Iris bombé with pupillary block
	D. Lens-induced glaucoma
	  1. Subluxation-dislocation and pupillary block
	  2. Spherophakia and pupillary block
	  3. Phacolytic glaucoma
	E. Glaucoma after surgery for congenital cataract
	  1. Lens material blockage of trabecular meshwork
	  2. Pupillary block
	  3. Chronic open-angle glaucoma
	F. Steroid glaucoma
	G. Glaucoma secondary to rubeosis
	  1. Retinoblastoma
	  2. Coats disease
	  3. Medulloepithelioma
	H. Secondary angle-closure glaucoma
	  1. Retinopathy of prematurity
	  2. Microphthalmos
	  3. Nanophthalmos
	  4. Congenital iris-lens membrane
	I. Glaucoma associated with increased venous pressure
	  1. Idiopathic
	  2. Orbital disease
	J. Congenital rubella syndrome

From Nelson LB, Calhoun JH, Harley RD: Pediatric Ophthalmology, 3rd ed. Philadelphia, WB Saunders, 1991, p 259.

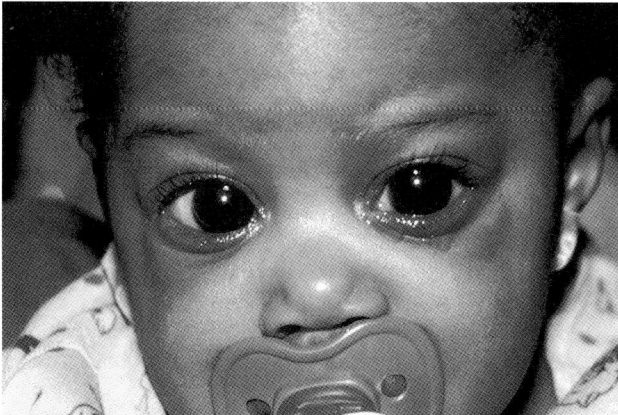

Figure 43-13. Bilateral congenital glaucoma in a 4-month-old infant. Note the large corneas and epiphora.

indication for treatment. Hemangiomas are generally sensitive to corticosteroids and shrink sufficiently to obviate the threat of amblyopia. Corticosteroids can be administered orally or intralesionally. Surgical excision of the hemangioma is rarely recommended. Hemangiomas that are not causing amblyopia but are cosmetically disfiguring are usually observed because the natural history of the lesion is to gradually involute over a period of several years, often leaving only mild atrophic skin changes.

A dermoid cyst is an encapsulated lesion composed of epidermal and dermal elements that develops along the sutural connections between orbital bones. The most common site is at the zygomatic-frontal suture in the superotemporal brow region; the next most common location is just inside the supernasal orbital rim along the frontal-nasal suture. On occasion, there is extension of the lesion into the orbit. Most dermoid cysts are about 1 to 2 cm in length and slightly mobile. They may grow slowly during childhood. Surgical excision is indicated to prevent severe inflammation that can accompany traumatic rupture of the cyst. In rare cases, a dermoid cyst causes astigmatism by pressing against the globe.

Rhabdomyosarcoma is the most common primary orbital malignancy in children. About 10% of all rhabdomyosarcomas originate in

Table 43-13. STUMPED: Differential Diagnosis of Neonatal Corneal Opacities

Diagnosis	Laterality	Opacity	Ocular Pressure	Other Ocular Abnormalities	Natural History	Inheritance
S—Sclerocornea	Unilateral or bilateral	Vascularized, blends with sclera, clearer centrally	Normal (or elevated)	Cornea plana	Nonprogressive	Sporadic
T—Tears in endothelium and Descemet membrane						
Birth trauma	Unilateral	Diffuse edema	Normal	Possible hyphema, periorbital ecchymoses	Spontaneous improvement in 1 month	Sporadic
Infantile glaucoma	Bilateral	Diffuse edema	Elevated	Megalocornea, photophobia and tearing, abnormal angle	Progressive unless treated	Autosomal recessive
U—Ulcers						
Herpes simplex keratitis	Unilateral	Diffuse with geographic epithelial defect	Normal	None	Progressive	Sporadic
Congenital rubella	Bilateral	Disciform or diffuse edema, no frank ulceration	Normal or elevated	Microphthalmos, cataract, pigment epithelial mottling	Stable, may clear	Sporadic
Neurotrophic—exposure	Unilateral or bilateral	Central ulcer	Normal	Lid anomalies, congenital sensory neuropathy	Progressive	Sporadic
M—Metabolic (rarely present at birth) (mucopolysaccharidoses IH, IS; mucolipidoses type IV)*	Bilateral	Diffuse haze, denser peripherally	Normal	Few	Progressive	Autosomal dominant
P—Posterior corneal defect	Unilateral or bilateral	Central, diffuse haze or vascularized leukoma	Normal or elevated	Anterior chamber cleavage syndrome	Stable; sometimes early clearing or vascularization	Sporadic, autosomal recessive
E—Endothelial dystrophy						
Congenital hereditary endothelial dystrophy	Bilateral	Diffuse corneal edema, marked corneal thickening	Normal	None	Stable	Autosomal dominant or recessive
Posterior polymorphous dystrophy	Bilateral	Diffuse haze, normal corneal thickness	Normal	Occasional peripheral anterior synechiae	Slowly progressive	Autosomal dominant
Congenital hereditary stromal dystrophy	Bilateral	Flaky, feathery stromal opacities; normal corneal thickness	Normal	None	Stable	Autosomal dominant
D—Dermoid	Unilateral or bilateral	White vascularized mass, hair, lipid arc	Normal	None	Stable	Sporadic

From Nelson LB, Calhoun JH, Harley RD: Pediatric Ophthalmology, 3rd ed. Philadelphia, WB Saunders, 1991, p 210.

*Mucopolysaccharidosis IH, Hurler syndrome; mucopolysaccharidosis IS, Scheie syndrome.

the orbit. The average age at onset is 5 to 7 years. Proptosis is the most common presenting sign and can develop rapidly over a period of days. Ptosis and strabismus are other presenting signs. A biopsy is required for confirmation of the diagnosis.

Neuroblastoma is the most common metastatic orbital tumor of childhood; 20% of all patients with neuroblastoma have ocular involvement. Ocular involvement can occur without orbital metastasis. An acquired Horner syndrome can occur with neuroblastoma located in the upper chest and involving the cervical sympathetic ganglions, and opsoclonus (rapid, multidirectional eye movements)

is a nonspecific presenting sign in some children. Metastatic neuroblastoma produces proptosis associated with periorbital ecchymosis. In about 50% of cases, there is bilateral orbital involvement. The average age at onset of neuroblastoma metastatic to the orbit is 2 years, much younger than that for rhabdomyosarcoma.

Other, less common orbital tumors in childhood are Ewing sarcoma, Wilms tumor, leukemia, and histiocytosis X. Ewing sarcoma is the second most common solid tumor metastatic to the orbit (after neuroblastoma). Orbital involvement occurs in 1% to 2% of children with leukemia.

Table 43-14. Differential Diagnosis of Enlarged Cornea

	Simple Megalocornea	Anterior Megalophthalmos	Primary Infantile Glaucoma with Buphthalmos
Inheritance	Autosomal dominant (?)	X-linked recessive (male preponderance)	Sporadic
Time of appearance	Congenital	Congenital	First year of life
Bilaterality	Bilateral Symmetrical	Bilateral Symmetrical	Unilateral or bilateral Asymmetrical
Natural history	Nonprogressive	Nonprogressive	Progressive
Symptoms	None	None	Photophobia, epiphora
Corneal clarity	Clear	Clear or mosaic dystrophy	Diffuse edema, tears in Descemet membrane
Intraocular pressure	Normal	Elevated in some adults	Elevated
Corneal diameter	13-18 mm	13-18 mm	13-18 mm
Corneal thickness	Normal	Normal	Thick
Keratometry	Normal	Normal; ↑ astigmatism	Flat
Gonioscopy	Normal	Excessive mesenchymal tissue	Excessive mesenchymal tissue
Globe diameter (A scan)	23-26 mm	23-26 mm	27-30 mm
Major ocular complications	None	Lens dislocation; cataract, <40 years; secondary glaucoma	Optic disk damage, late corneal edema
Associated systemic disorders	None	Occasionally Marfan and other skeletal abnormalities	None consistent

From Nelson LB, Calhoun JH, Harley RD: Pediatric Ophthalmology, 3rd ed. Philadelphia, WB Saunders, 1991, p 201.

OCULAR MANIFESTATIONS OF SYSTEMIC DISEASE

NEUROLOGIC DISEASE

Ocular abnormalities frequently accompany neurologic disease, and their detection can help in the localization and diagnosis of a specific condition. An afferent pupillary defect is an important finding that signifies diffuse unilateral retinal disease or, more commonly, unilateral optic nerve disease from conditions intrinsic to the optic nerve (a glioma in neurofibromatosis type 1) or extrinsic but applying

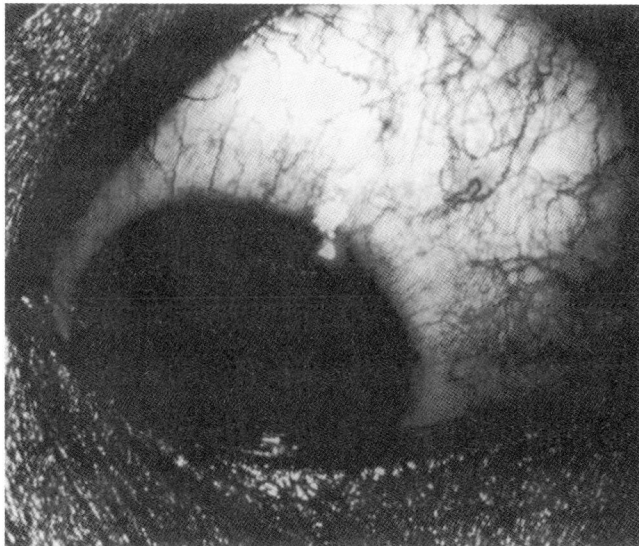

Figure 43-14. Ciliary flush associated with iritis. Note the straight, radially oriented vessels extending out from the iris. (From Reilly BM: Practical Strategies in Outpatient Medicine, 2nd ed. Philadelphia, WB Saunders, 1991, p 41.)

Table 43-15. Uveitis in Childhood

Anterior Uveitis
Juvenile rheumatoid arthritis (pauciarticular)
Sarcoidosis
Trauma
Tuberculosis
Kawasaki disease
Ulcerative colitis
Reactive arthritis
Spirochetal (syphilis, leptospiral)
Heterochromic iridocyclitis (Fuchs)
Viral (herpes simplex, herpes zoster)
Ankylosing spondylitis
Stevens-Johnson syndrome
Idiopathic
Drugs

Posterior Uveitis (Choroiditis: May Involve Retina)
Toxoplasmosis
Parasites (toxocariasis)
Sarcoidosis
Tuberculosis
Viral (rubella, herpes simplex, human immunodeficiency virus, cytomegalovirus)
Subacute sclerosing panencephalitis
Idiopathic

Anterior and/or Posterior Uveitis
Sympathetic opthalmia (trauma to other eye)
Vogt-Koyanagi-Harada syndrome (uveootocutaneous syndrome: poliosis, vitiligo, deafness, tinnitus, uveitis, aseptic meningitis, retinitis)
Behçet disease
Lyme disease

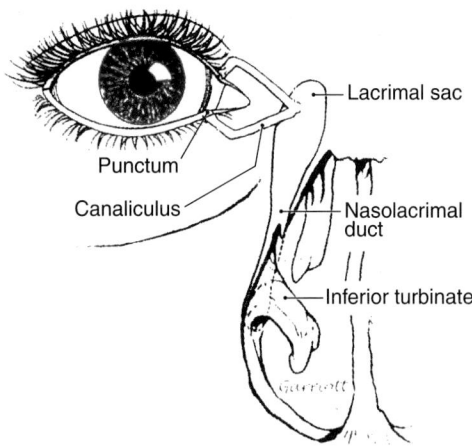

Figure 43-15. Anatomy of the nasolacrimal drainage system. (Modified from Rev Ophthalmol 2001;8:122. Reprinted with permission from Jobson Publishing, New York.)

Labels: Lacrimal sac; Punctum; Canaliculus; Nasolacrimal duct; Inferior turbinate

pressure on the nerve (an orbital tumor). The visual acuity of the affected eye is usually reduced in comparison with that of the normal eye. The presence of an afferent pupillary defect necessitates a comprehensive eye examination and imaging studies of the orbit and brain.

The seemingly acute onset of strabismus in a child may actually be the delayed recognition of intermittent, comitant strabismus related to significant hyperopia or a strong family history of strabismus. Strabismus of truly acute onset is most often incomitant and caused by paralysis of extraocular muscles innervated by the third or sixth cranial nerves. Cranial trauma and brain tumors are the most common causes of acute, incomitant strabismus in children. A sixth nerve palsy is of less localizing value than a third nerve palsy because of the more tortuous intracranial course of the sixth nerve. This nerve can be affected by direct pressure from a mass and indirectly by conditions that cause increased intracranial pressure. A patient with an acute sixth nerve paralysis typically has esotropia that increases when he or she gazes toward the affected side (see Fig. 43-8). The patient may have a compensatory face turn toward the side of the lesion to allow fusion and prevent diplopia. A third nerve paralysis usually causes exotropia and hypotropia of the involved eye (Fig. 43-20). There may also be ipsilateral ptosis and a dilated, nonreactive pupil.

Papilledema (Fig. 43-21) is a worrisome sign because of its association with conditions that cause increased intracranial pressure.

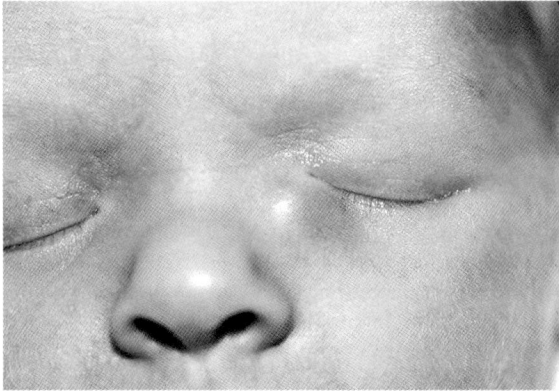

Figure 43-16. Dacryocystocele of the left lacrimal sac in a 2-week-old infant. The dacryocystocele resolved with a probing of the left tear duct.

The elevation of the optic nerve and blurring of the disk margins must be differentiated from papillitis or optic nerve drusen, which can have similar clinical appearances. Papillitis is more commonly unilateral (although it can manifest bilaterally) and is associated with reduced visual acuity and the presence of an afferent pupillary defect. Papilledema is almost always bilateral. Visual acuity is generally normal, although reduced visual acuity from optic atrophy can occur with chronic papilledema.

Visual field defects in children are uncommon despite parental concern about a child who seems to bump into objects frequently. Unilateral retinal or optic nerve disease can produce unilateral visual field defects, but these are almost always associated with reduced visual acuity in the involved eye. Bilateral visual field defects, particularly if symmetrical (homonymous), indicate disease of the optic radiations or visual cortex. Visual acuity may be entirely normal. Causes of bilateral visual field defects in children would be cerebrovascular accidents, pituitary or hypothalamic tumors, or congenital central nervous system abnormalities. Quantitative testing of the visual field of most children is difficult before the age of 10 years. Confrontation field tests can be performed to detect gross abnormalities of the visual field (hemianopsias). The technique of double simultaneous confrontation may be useful in younger children and is illustrated in Figure 43-22.

The phakomatoses (neurocutaneous syndromes) are a group of inherited disorders featuring multiple, discrete lesions of two or more organ systems, most commonly the skin and brain. Ocular involvement is common and may be a site of comorbidity or may serve as a marker for the overall condition (Lisch nodules of the iris in neurofibromatosis type 1).

Neurofibromatosis type 1 (NF-1) is by far the most common of the phakomatoses, with an estimated prevalence of 1 per 3000 to 5000. Lisch nodules of the iris, which can be diagnosed only by slit-lamp biomicroscopy because of their small size, are a cardinal feature of NF-1. Lisch nodules are tan, smooth-surfaced lesions on the iris surface that look like tapioca granules. They are usually not present until 5 years or older so their absence in a younger child does not exclude the diagnosis of NF-1. They have no particular malignant potential. Other ocular features of NF-1 are plexiform neurofibromas of the eyelid that give the eyelid margin a sigmoid shape and cause a variable amount of ptosis. Optic gliomas are the most significant ocular feature of NF-1 because of the possibility of vision loss. The gliomas can involve one or both optic nerves as well as the optic chiasm. The majority of optic gliomas in NF-1 are indolent. They are estimated to occur in 15% of patients with NF-1, but in only 1% to 5% of patients do symptoms develop (vision loss or proptosis). Treatment of optic gliomas is reserved for lesions that are documented to be growing and causing visual morbidity. In most affected children, this happens before age 10 years.

Neurofibromatosis type 2 is much less common than NF-1 and involves primarily the acoustic nerves. Ocular involvement can consist of posterior lens opacities that are generally not visually significant and hamartomas of the retina. Treatment of the eye conditions associated with neurofibromatosis type 2 is usually not necessary.

Tuberous sclerosis is an autosomal dominant disorder localized to chromosome 9. In children with tuberous sclerosis, angiofibromas of the eyelids and retinal lesions known as astrocytic hamartomas can occur but rarely cause significant problems with vision. The retinal lesions are not pathognomonic of tuberous sclerosis, inasmuch as similar lesions have been reported in NF-1 and in unaffected individuals.

In *von Hippel–Lindau disease*, retinal angiomas frequently develop and become ophthalmoscopically visible after 10 years of age. These angiomas have a propensity to leak, so that lipid can accumulate in the retina and the retina can become detached. The angiomas are more effectively treated with cryotherapy or laser when they are small, so children known to have von Hippel–Lindau disease should have regular eye examinations beginning at age 5 years.

Table 43-16. The Red Eye

Condition	Cause	Signs/Symptoms	Treatment
Bacterial conjunctivitis	*Haemophilus influenzae, H. influenzae aegyptius, Streptococcus pneumoniae, Neisseria gonorrhoeae, Staphylococcus aureus, Yersinia* species, cat-scratch bacillus less common	Mucopurulent unilateral or bilateral discharge, normal vision, photophobia usually absent Conjunctival injection and edema (chemosis); gritty sensation	Topical antibiotics: systemic ceftriaxone for *Gonococcus, H. influenzae*
Viral conjunctivitis	Adenovirus, ECHO virus, coxsackievirus	As above; may be hemorrhagic, unilateral enlarged preauricular lymph nodes	Self-limited
Neonatal conjunctivitis	*Chlamydia trachomatis, Gonococcus* species, chemical (silver nitrate), *S. aureus*	Palpebral conjunctival follicle or papillae; as above	Ceftriaxone for *Gonococcus* and oral erythromycin for *C. trachomatis*
Allergic conjunctivitis	Seasonal pollens or allergen exposure	Itching, incidence of bilateral chemosis (edema) greater than that of erythema, tarsal papillae	Antihistamines, steroids, cromolyn
Keratitis	Herpes simplex, adenovirus, *S. pneumoniae, S. aureus, Pseudomonas* species, *Acanthamoeba* species, chemicals	Severe pain, corneal swelling, clouding, limbus erythema, hypopyon, cataracts; contact lens history with amebic infection	Specific antibiotics for bacterial/fungal infections; keratoplasty, acyclovir for herpes
Endophthalmitis	*S. aureus, S. pneumoniae, Candida albicans,* associated surgery or trauma	Acute onset, pain, loss of vision, swelling, chemosis, redness; hypopyon and vitreous haze	Antibiotics
Anterior uveitis (iridocyclitis)	JRA, reactive arthritis, sarcoidosis, Behçet disease, Kawasaki disease, inflammatory bowel disease	Unilateral/bilateral; erythema, ciliary flush (in circumcorneal area), irregular pupil, iris adhesions; pain, marked photophobia, small pupil, poor vision, no discharge	Topical steroids, plus therapy for primary disease
Posterior uveitis (choroiditis)	Toxoplasmosis, histoplasmosis, *Toxocara canis*	No signs of erythema, decreased vision, no discharge	Specific therapy for pathogen
Episcleritis/scleritis	Idiopathic autoimmune disease (e.g., SLE, Henoch-Schönlein purpura)	Localized pain, intense erythema, unilateral; blood vessels bigger than in conjunctivitis; scleritis may cause globe perforation, no discharge	Episcleritis is self-limiting; topical steroids for fast relief
Foreign body	Occupational exposure	Unilateral, red, gritty feeling; visible or microscopic size	Irrigation, removal; check for ulceration
Blepharitis	*S. aureus, Staphylococcus epidermidis,* seborrheic, blocked lacrimal duct: rarely, molluscum contagiosum, *Phthirus pubis, Pediculus capitis*	Bilateral, irritation, itching, hyperemia, crusting, affecting lid margins	Topical antibiotics, warm compresses
Dacryocystitis	Obstructed lacrimal sac: *S. aureus, H. influenzae, Pneumococcus* species	Pain, tenderness, erythema and exudate in area of lacrimal sac (inferomedial to inner canthus); tearing (epiphora); possible orbital cellulitis	Systemic, topical antibiotics; surgical drainage
Dacryoadenitis	*S. aureus, Streptococcus* species, CMV, measles, EBV, enteroviruses, trauma, sarcoidosis, leukemia	Pain, tenderness, edema, erythema over gland area (upper temporal lid); fever, leukocytosis	Systemic antibiotics; drainage of orbital abscesses
Orbital cellulitis (postseptal cellulitis)	Paranasal sinusitis: *H. influenzae, S. aureus, S. pneumoniae,* other *Streptococcus* species	Rhinorrhea, chemosis, vision loss, painful extraocular motion, proptosis, opthalmoplegia, fever, lid edema, leukocytosis	Systemic antibiotics, drainage of orbital abscesses

Continued

Table 43-16. The Red Eye—cont'd

Condition	Cause	Signs/Symptoms	Treatment
Orbital cellulitis—cont'd	Trauma: *S. aureus* Fungi: *Aspergillus, Mucor* species if immunodeficient		
Periorbital cellulitis (preseptal cellulitis)	Trauma: *S. aureus,* *Streptococcus* species Bacteremia: *H. influenzae,* pneumococci, *Streptococcus pyogenes*	Cutaneous erythema, warmth, normal vision, minimal involvement of orbit, fever, leukocytosis, toxic appearance	Systemic antibiotics

Data from Rosenbaum JT, Nozik RA: Uveitis: Many diseases, one diagnosis. Am J Med 1985;79:545-547; Elkington AR, Khaw PT: The red eye. BMJ 1988;296:1720–1724; Wilhemus KR: The red eye. Infectious conjunctivitis, keratitis, endophthalmitis, and periocular cellulitis. Infect Dis Clin North Am 1988;2:99-116; Forrester JV: Uveitis: Pathogenesis. Lancet 1991;338:1498-1501; and Giolitti F: Acute conjunctivitis of childhood. Pediatr Ann 1993;22:353-356.

Modified from Behrman RE, Kliegman RM: Nelson Essentials of Pediatrics, 2nd ed. Philadelphia, WB Saunders, 1994, p 357–358.

CMV, cytomegalovirus; EBV, Epstein-Barr virus; ECHO, enteric cytopathogenic human orphan; JRA, juvenile rheumatoid arthritis; SLE, systemic lupus erythematosus.

Ocular involvement in *Sturge-Weber syndrome* is common. Abnormalities of the ocular circulation can occur when the eyelids are affected. These abnormalities range from increased conjunctival vascularity to angiomas of the choroid. Choroidal angiomas usually remain asymptomatic in childhood but can thicken in adolescence and cause degeneration of the overlying retina. Glaucoma is the most serious ocular complication and occurs in one third to one half of affected patients. Regular eye examinations in infancy may be necessary to rule out glaucoma. Treatment of glaucoma associated with Sturge-Weber syndrome may be more difficult and less effective than for other types of childhood glaucoma.

In the *ataxia-telangiectasia syndrome,* ocular features may be among the first recognizable signs. An ocular motor abnormality similar to congenital ocular motor apraxia may occur in which the child has difficulty initiating quick eye movements and has poor vestibuloocular reflexes. Telangiectasia develops in the conjunctiva in virtually all affected children beginning between the ages of 3 and 5 years.

Retinal vascular abnormalities can occur in both the *Wyburn-Mason syndrome* and in the *incontinentia pigmenti syndrome.* In the latter condition, the changes can mimic ROP with incomplete peripheral retinal vascularization. Retinal detachment can occur, and

Table 43-17. Conjunctivitis: Differential Diagnosis

	Clinical Findings				
Cause	*Unilateral or Bilateral*	*Discharge*	*Lids*	*Onset/Course*	Treatment
Viral* (usually adenovirus)	Bilateral	Thin, mucoid	Follicular	Gradual Upper respiratory tract infection? Preauricular adenopathy	Compresses
Herpes simplex	Unilateral	Thin, mucoid	Follicular	Gradual Keratitis Dendritic ulcer	Acyclovir
Bacterial	Unilateral or bilateral	Purulent	Papillary, purulent	Gradual	Topical antibiotics
Gonococcal	Unilateral	Purulent	Edema, inflamed	Hyperacute	Systemic antibiotics
Chlamydial	Unilateral or bilateral	Thin, mucoid	Follicular	Indolent Persistent Neonatal period Sexually active	Oral erythromycin any age or tetracycline (>10 years of age)
Allergic	Bilateral	Watery	Papillary	Gradual Seasonal Pruritic	Topical vasoconstrictors Systemic antihistamine Topical steroids
Vernal	Bilateral	Watery	Giant papillary	Adolescence Seasonal	Cromolyn?
Contact lens irritation	Bilateral	Watery	Giant papillary	Lenses	Adjust lens Change solution
Chemical	Unilateral or bilateral	Watery	Variable	Acute	Irrigate Remove irritant

Modified from Reilly BM: Practical Strategies in Outpatient Medicine, 2nd ed. Philadelphia, WB Saunders, 1991, p 46.

*Undifferentiated viral conjunctivitis, not caused by herpesvirus infection.

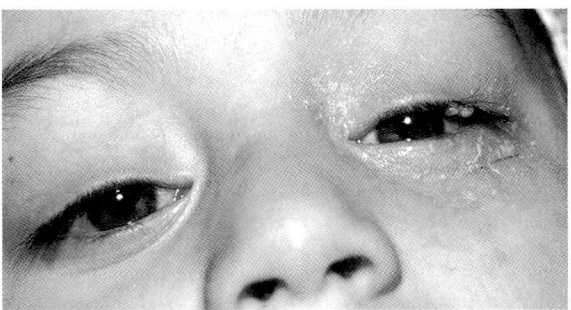

Figure 43-17. Chronic eczematoid and follicular conjunctivitis in only the left eye, caused by *Molluscum contagiosum*, in a 5-year-old. Note the elevated lesions on the lateral aspect of the left upper eyelid.

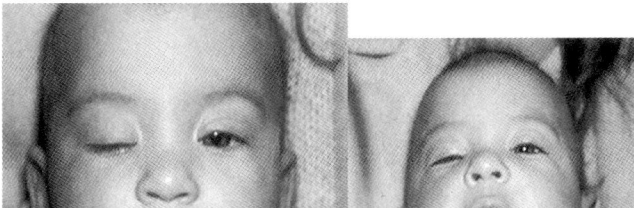

Figure 43-18. Congenital ptosis of the right upper eyelid. The child adopted a compensatory chin-up head posture to allow use of both eyes together and did not have amblyopia.

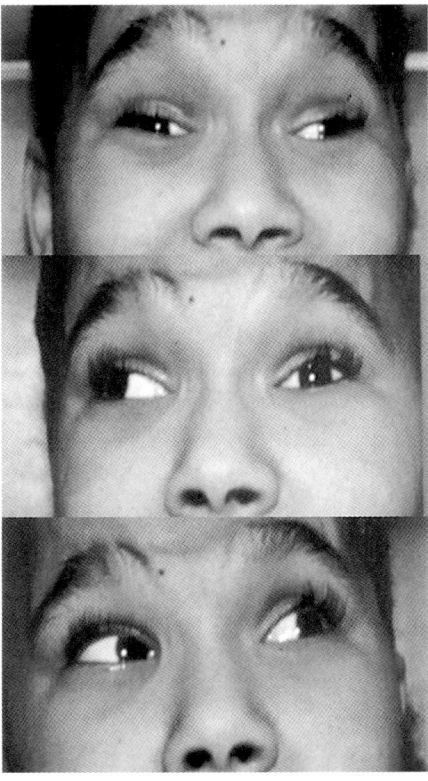

Figure 43-20. Left third cranial nerve palsy. The boy has exotropia (**top**), limitation of adduction of his left eye (**middle**), and normal gaze to his left (**bottom**).

the best mode of treatment is controversial. In Wyburn-Mason syndrome, a racemose angioma can develop in the retina with shunting of blood directly from arteries to veins. Vision can be normal or markedly reduced, depending on the location of the lesion. Treatment is not indicated for primary lesions.

DERMATOLOGIC DISEASE

Stevens-Johnson syndrome is characterized by bullous skin lesions, erosive involvement of mucous membranes, and systemic toxicity. Drugs, particularly sulfonamide medications, are common precipitating factors. Microbial agents, especially *Mycoplasma pneumoniae*, have also been implicated in this condition. Ocular involvement consists of eyelid edema and ulceration, conjunctival injection with vesicle formation in severe cases, and conjunctival scar formation that may result in adhesions between the palpebral and bulbar conjunctiva (symblepharons). The severity of late ocular complications depends primarily on the extent of conjunctival involvement. Malposition of the eyelids with corneal irritation from inward-turned eyelashes (trichiasis) can occur from severe conjunctival scarring. The most serious complication is dry eye syndrome, caused by

damage to the ducts of the lacrimal glands and obliteration of conjunctival mucus-forming cells (goblet cells). Eyelid surgery may be required, and the child with a dry eye may face a lifetime of needing ocular lubrication from artificial tears and ointments. Local treatment during the acute phase of the disease is recommended to prevent bacterial superinfections but may not have much influence on the eventual ocular outcome. *Toxic epidermal necrolysis* is associated with conjunctival inflammation that is usually less severe than the ocular involvement in Stevens-Johnson syndrome.

Hyperkeratotic disorders such as *lamellar ichthyosis* can cause deformity of the eyelids as well as changes in the conjunctiva and cornea. Although eyelid surgery may be required, the mainstay of treatment is ocular lubrication with artificial tears and ointments.

Ehlers-Danlos syndrome and *pseudoxanthoma elasticum*, disorders of skin elasticity, are associated with particular ocular abnormalities. Some patients with Ehlers-Danlos syndrome have myopic retinal

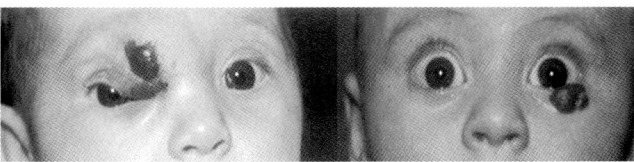

Figure 43-19. **Left,** A capillary hemangioma of the right upper eyelid and anterior orbit. This lesion necessitated treatment because it was causing amblyopia from astigmatism as a result of pressure against the globe and by occlusion of the visual axis. **Right,** This capillary hemangioma of the left lower eyelid is not causing amblyopia and does not necessitate treatment unless it grows substantially.

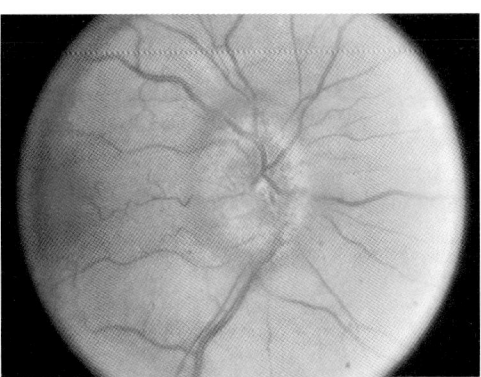

Figure 43-21. Papilledema of the right optic nerve.

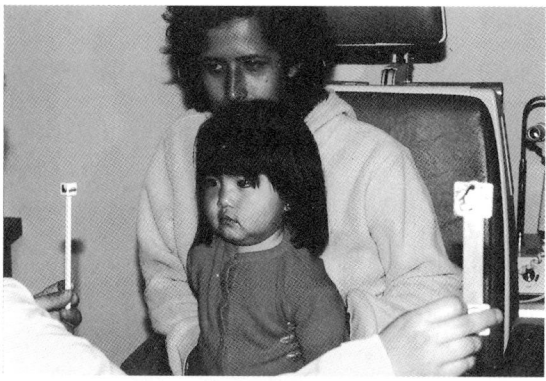

A

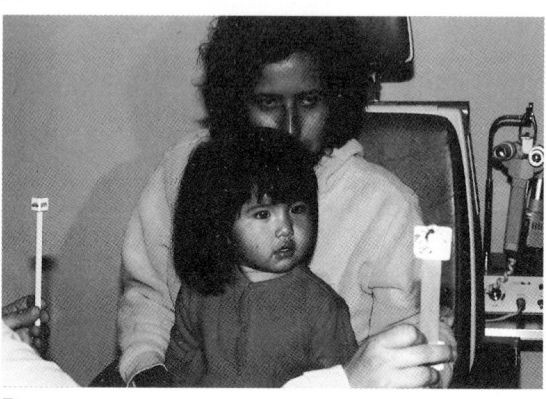

B

Figure 43-22. Visual field testing by the method of double simultaneous confrontation. A, The child's attention is directed toward the object held in the examiner's left hand. The picture in the examiner's right hand is slowly brought toward the midline. The child's attention switches to the latter object at about 45 degrees to the left of central fixation B, thus confirming the intactness of her visual field in the left periphery.

degeneration and retinal detachment. Cracks in the Bruch membrane of the retina, known as angioid streaks, can occur with both Ehlers-Danlos syndrome and pseudoxanthoma elasticum. Angioid streaks rarely occur before the second decade of life but can go on to cause macular degeneration of the retina.

Skin disorders causing neoplasia such as *juvenile xanthogranuloma* can affect the eye, sometimes even in the absence of typical skin lesions. Ocular complications from juvenile xanthogranuloma occur most commonly in infants and consist of nodular tumors of the iris and ciliary body. The iris lesions have thin-walled vessels that are prone to bleeding and to causing a hyphema. Glaucoma and iridocyclitis can also occur. The iris lesions may respond to topical corticosteroids.

HEMATOLOGIC DISORDERS

The *hemoglobinopathies* can have direct ocular consequences but seldom do so in the pediatric population. Patients with hemoglobin SC or S thalassemia are more prone to retinal vascular occlusive disease because of a higher hematocrit and greater blood viscosity than are patients with hemoglobin SS, but these retinal complications are frequently delayed until adolescence or early adulthood. Of greater concern in children with sickle cell disease are the complications that can ensue from sickled erythrocytes in general anesthesia or from ocular trauma that causes a hyphema.

Leukemia can cause ocular problems in children, although it does so less frequently than in adults. The choroid is most frequently affected in childhood leukemia, but choroidal involvement is usually not clinically apparent. Flame-shaped retinal hemorrhages are common and can be associated with other complications of leukemia such as anemia, thrombocytopenia, or coagulation disorders. Some retinal hemorrhages have white centers similar to those seen in bacterial endocarditis. Optic nerve involvement in leukemia results in edema and peripapillary hemorrhage that can severely affect visual acuity. Papilledema and loss of vision in leukemia represent an emergency, and such patients should receive radiation therapy promptly. Leukemic infiltrates in the anterior segment of the eye can produce iris lesions similar to those in juvenile xanthogranuloma. Leukemic cells can collect in the anterior chamber (hypopyon) and cause acute glaucoma. An anterior chamber tap may be required for cytologic confirmation. Leukemic involvement of the orbit is seen mainly with acute myelogenous leukemia and can be confused with orbital infection. There is a high correlation between leukemic involvement of the eye and that of the central nervous system, and, as such, it represents a poor prognostic feature.

CONGENITAL HEART DISEASE

Eye disease can be related to congenital heart disease by association, which is not surprising because there is a temporal relationship between the embryogenesis of the heart and that of the eyes; an embryopathic insult may result in malformations of both systems (Table 43-18). Congenital heart disease also can be a cause of eye disease as a direct effect of complications such as cyanosis or systemic hypertension.

In cyanotic congenital heart disease, hypoxemia and polycythemia can result in retinopathy and optic neuropathy. These changes are generally reversible on correction of the hypoxemia and polycythemia. In coarctation of the aorta, the retinal arteries can become diffusely tortuous, presumably as a result of the widened pulse pressure.

Table 43-18. Syndromes Associated with Ocular Abnormalities and Congenital Heart Disease

Syndrome	Primary Feature	Ocular Abnormality
CHARGE association	*C*oloboma, *h*eart disease, choanal *a*tresia, *r*etarded growth and development, *g*enital anomalies, *e*ar anomalies	Iris and chorioretinal colobomata
Marfan syndrome	Arachnodactyly, hyperextensibility, aortic dilatation	Lens dislocation, myopia, retinal detachment
Noonan syndrome	Webbed neck, pectus excavatum, cryptorchidism, pulmonic stenosis	Epicanthal folds, ptosis myopia, keratoconus, strabismus
Williams syndrome	Mental retardation, unusual facies, supravalvar aortic stenosis, hypercalcemia	Blue iris, stellate pattern of iris
Turner syndrome (XO)	Short stature, ovarian dysgenesis, webbed neck, broad chest, congenital lymphedema	Ptosis, strabismus, blue sclera, cataract

GASTROINTESTINAL DISORDERS

Ocular manifestations of inherited metabolic abnormalities of the gastrointestinal system occur primarily in the cornea and retina. Wilson disease is an autosomal recessive disorder of copper metabolism. Liver damage results at a young age, and damage to the basal ganglia can cause neurologic and psychiatric disorders. The distinctive ocular feature of *Wilson disease* is the Kayser-Fleischer ring, which represents copper deposition in the Descemet membrane of the peripheral cornea. An eye examination, including slit-lamp biomicroscopy of the cornea, is indicated in any child with hepatic or neurologic disease of unknown cause.

Alagille syndrome, an autosomal dominant condition with intrahepatic bile duct hypoplasia, is associated with a peripheral corneal finding known as posterior embryotoxon. This finding consists of thickening and anterior displacement of the Schwalbe line, which is the peripheral extent of the Descemet membrane of the cornea. It can best be seen with a slit-lamp biomicroscope. Posterior embryotoxon occurs in more than 90% of patients with Alagille syndrome, but because it also occurs in 15% of normal individuals, it is not pathognomonic for this syndrome.

Cataracts are a prominent feature of *galactosemia* associated with deficiency of the enzyme galactose-1-phosphate uridyltransferase. Newborns with hepatosplenomegaly, vomiting, diarrhea, and failure to thrive should be examined for cataracts in addition to assessment for galactosuria. Galactosemic cataracts are potentially reversible if lactose is eliminated from the diet promptly.

Pigmentary retinopathy is a prominent finding in *Zellweger cerebrohepatorenal syndrome,* characterized by deficient biogenesis of peroxisomes. Other reported ocular findings are epicanthal folds, corneal edema, posterior embryotoxon, optic atrophy, and nystagmus. Pigmentary retinopathy has also been reported in abetalipoproteinemia. This retinopathy is potentially reversible by vitamin E supplementation.

Inflammatory bowel disease also can be associated with ocular disease. Anterior uveitis occurs in both Crohn disease and ulcerative colitis. In turn, untreated chronic uveitis can lead to cataracts, glaucoma, and retinal edema. Conjunctivitis, keratitis, and retinal vasculitis are less frequent complications of these diseases.

GENITOURINARY DISEASE

Oculorenal syndromes may result from chromosomal abnormality syndromes or from inherited metabolic or developmental defects. The *WAGR syndrome* consists of *W*ilms tumor, sporadic *a*niridia, *g*enitourinary malformations, and mental *r*etardation. This association arises from deletion of the p13 region of chromosome 11, which leads to failure of a Wilms tumor suppressor gene. Any child with nonfamilial aniridia is at risk for Wilms tumor and needs appropriate genetic evaluation.

The *Bardet-Biedl syndrome* is an autosomal recessive disorder combining retinal dystrophy, polydactyly, obesity, and hypogenitalism. An electroretinogram may be the earliest means of detecting the cone-rod dystrophy in suspected cases. Visual acuity and the funduscopic appearance may be normal in the first decade of life, but both tend to worsen in the second decade.

Cystinosis is also an autosomal recessive disorder of cystine transport from lysosomes that leads to intracellular accumulation of cystine in many tissues, including the eyes and kidneys. Cystine crystals accumulate in the anterior layer of the cornea beginning in the first year of life. This can cause photophobia. Retinal deposits of cystine can lead to focal degeneration of the retinal pigment epithelium. Frequent topical administration of cysteamine drops can clear the cornea of cystine crystals and relieve ocular discomfort.

Alport syndrome is an X-linked syndrome characterized by nephritis, hearing loss, and ocular signs, particularly of the lens. An "oil droplet" appearance can be seen in the pupil with an ophthalmoscope. Perimacular flecks are frequently present in the retina but do not tend to reduce visual acuity.

The *Lowe oculocerebrorenal syndrome* is also an X-linked disorder comprising congenital cataracts, mental retardation, and renal tubular dysfunction. Glaucoma develops in a high proportion of affected boys and men. The carrier state can frequently be detected in girls and women by the appearance of numerous punctate opacities of the lens.

ENDOCRINE DISEASE

Thyroid ophthalmopathy related to *Graves disease* occurs in children much less frequently than in adults. It can be a cause of proptosis in children but is much less likely to cause optic neuropathy, corneal exposure, or severe extraocular muscle involvement.

Diabetes mellitus results in retinopathy at some point in nearly all persons with insulin-dependent type I diabetes. The prevalence of retinopathy is directly proportional to the duration of disease after puberty. It rarely occurs within 3 years of diagnosis, occurs in about 50% of patients at 7 years after diagnosis, and is seen in 90% at 15 years after diagnosis. Funduscopic signs of diabetic retinopathy are microaneurysms, retinal hemorrhages, cotton wool spots, and hard exudates. Proliferative diabetic retinopathy with development of new blood vessels is uncommon in children. Diabetic cataracts caused by sorbitol accumulation in the lens and lipemia retinalis are also rare complications of diabetes mellitus in children. There is accumulating evidence that good control of diabetes mellitus (as monitored by hemoglobin A_{1c}) may delay the onset and severity of retinal complications.

INFECTIOUS DISEASES

Intrauterine *rubella* infection has become a rarity in the United States because of immunization with the measles-mumps-rubella vaccine. A fetus infected transplacentally in the first trimester of pregnancy is prone to multiple congenital defects, including heart disease, microcephaly with mental retardation, and deafness. Ocular sequelae include cataracts, glaucoma, and chorioretinitis. Permanent visual impairment despite cataract surgery is common in these children.

A small percentage of infants with neonatal *herpes simplex* infection develop conjunctivitis, keratitis, chorioretinitis, and cataracts. Infants with disseminated herpes simplex infection, including retinal infection, are generally treated with acyclovir. Primary herpes simplex infection of the eye acquired after the perinatal period usually entails a vesicular eruption on the eyelids with subsequent conjunctival inflammation (Fig. 43-23). The cornea and intraocular structures are only infrequently involved, and treatment is directed toward the prevention of bacterial superinfection. Keratitis is an indication for topical antiviral therapy.

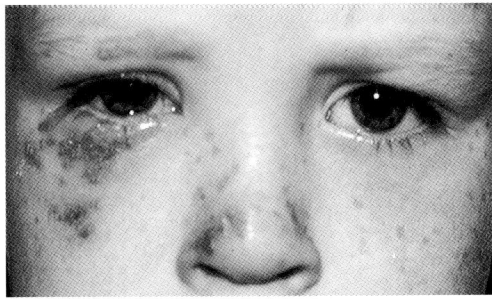

Figure 43-23. Vesicular eruptions of the right lower eyelid and the right side of the nose, caused by primary herpes simplex infection. The cornea was not involved.

Ophthalmia neonatorum is defined as conjunctival infection or inflammation occurring in the first month of life. Conjunctival irritation from silver nitrate solution administered as Crede prophylaxis was historically the most common cause, but this has become less common since the advent of therapy with topical tetracycline or erythromycin ointment as a substitute for silver nitrate. Almost any bacterial pathogen can cause conjunctivitis in a newborn, but infection with *Neisseria gonorrhoeae* is of particular concern because it produces a hyperacute, profusely purulent conjunctivitis that can lead to corneal perforation. Chlamydiae are a common cause of neonatal conjunctivitis and are acquired from an infected cervix during delivery. Because this organism can also cause pneumonia, systemic treatment with oral erythromycin is indicated. Unlike the majority of cases of conjunctivitis in older children, which is self-limiting and unlikely to cause ocular or systemic complications, neonatal conjunctivitis can have significant consequences. Evaluation with Gram and Giemsa stains and bacterial cultures are indicated. Chlamydiae can be diagnosed by culture or by fluorescent antibody-staining techniques or polymerase chain reaction techniques in certain laboratories.

Congenital toxoplasmosis is the form of this infection most likely to have ocular consequences in children. The infectious agent, *Toxoplasma gondii*, is acquired transplacentally and has particular affinity for the central nervous system, including the retina. Chorioretinitis is found in 80% of severely affected infants and can cause lesions in the macula that impair central vision. Ocular treatment is usually reserved for foci of infection in the retina that appear active and threaten vision.

Cytomegalovirus is also a transplacentally acquired infection. Retinal infection occurs in about 15% of infants with symptomatic systemic infection and, if severe and progressive, may necessitate treatment with systemic antiviral agents such as ganciclovir.

Varicella commonly causes lesions of the eyelids and, less commonly, of the conjunctiva. Keratitis and internal ophthalmoplegia with iritis are less common. Topical antibiotics may prevent bacterial superinfection. Systemic acyclovir is usually reserved for immunocompromised children.

Preseptal cellulitis (defined as infection confined to the eyelid tissues anterior to the orbital septum) is a common infection in children and needs to be distinguished from infection involving the orbit (Fig. 43-24). Preseptal infections may result from trauma and insect bites involving the eyelids or a primary bacteremia, or they

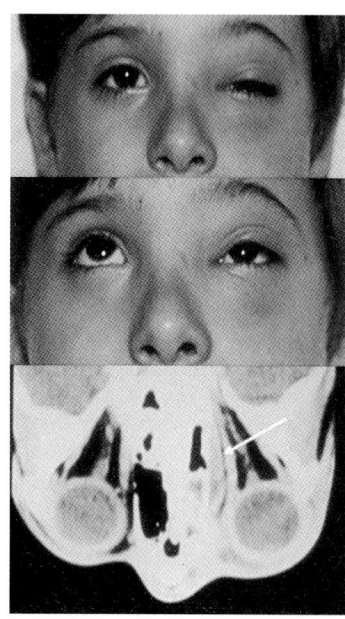

Figure 43-25. A subperiosteal abscess of the left orbit. Note the limitation of upward movement of the left eye (**middle**). The computed tomographic scan shows ethmoid sinusitis and a subperiosteal abscess bowing the left medial rectus muscle laterally (*arrow*).

may spread to the eyelids from the paranasal sinuses. The affected eyelids are swollen and red, and the infection can spread further into the eyebrow, forehead, and cheek. Proptosis and limitation of eye movements do not occur in preseptal cellulitis, but confirmation of this can be problematic because of the difficulty of opening the eye. *S. aureus,* group A streptococcus, and *S. pneumoniae* are the most common pathogens. Patients with signs and symptoms of systemic toxicity should be hospitalized for intravenous antibiotics; milder cases of preseptal cellulitis may be managed with oral antibiotics as long as appropriate follow-up is ensured.

Orbital cellulitis is an infection of the orbit, most frequently caused by spread of infection from the adjacent paranasal sinuses. Frequently, orbital cellulitis begins as a subperiosteal abscess that forms in the potential space between the periorbita (analogous to the periosteum of long bones) and the orbital bones (Fig. 43-25). Left untreated, this space-occupying mass can apply pressure to the optic nerve and cause permanent damage to vision. It can also spread into the intracranial space and result in cavernous sinus thrombosis or a subdural empyema or cerebral abscess. Systemic toxicity is quite common and severe with orbital cellulitis. Ocular signs include eyelid edema and erythema, proptosis, and inferior and lateral displacement of the globe with limited eye movements. Ocular movement is painful; visual activity may be reduced. If orbital cellulitis is suspected, computed tomography of the orbit and sinuses is indicated. Most children younger than 9 years who have small to medium-sized subperiosteal abscesses can be treated successfully with broad-spectrum intravenous antibiotics (ceftriaxone and vancomycin, ampicillin/sulbactam, or piperacillin/tazobactam). Close observation with periodic checks of vision and pupillary function is important in the first 24 to 48 hours of treatment. Older children, those with large subperiosteal abscesses, and children who fail to respond to intravenous antibiotics within 48 hours may require surgical drainage of the abscess.

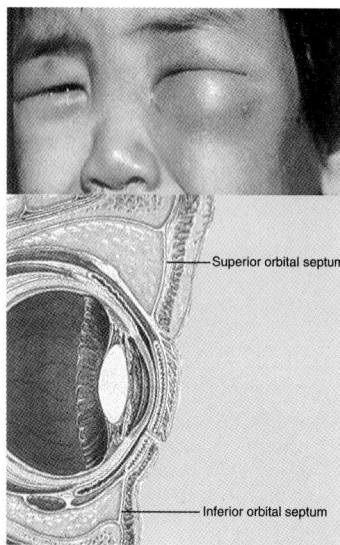

Superior orbital septum

Inferior orbital septum

Figure 43-24. Preseptal cellulitis in a young girl. The infection is confined to the space anterior to the superior and inferior orbital septa and does not involve the orbit.

OCULAR ALLERGY

Ocular allergy is common in children and often occurs in the context of other atopic diseases. The hallmarks of ocular allergy are itching and bilateral conjunctival inflammation, often occurring on a seasonal basis. The most common form of ocular allergy is seasonal allergic conjunctivitis, a type I hypersensitivity reaction that results in itching, mild conjunctival injection and edema, and a watery or thin mucoid discharge. Numerous follicles are present in the palpebral conjunctiva, and conjunctival scraping reveals eosinophils. Pharmacologic treatment includes oral antihistamines and H_1-receptor antagonists (chlorpheniramine, terfenadine, loratadine). Topical therapy consists of antihistamines, H_1 antagonists, and mast cell stabilizers (cromolyn sodium). Topical NSAIDs (ketorolac) may also be effective in the treatment of allergic conjunctivitis. Vernal keratoconjunctivitis and atopic keratoconjunctivitis are more severe forms of ocular allergy that result in hypertrophy of conjunctival and subconjunctival tissue and have the potential to harm vision by damaging the cornea. An ophthalmologist should treat these disorders.

ALBINISM

Albinism is a heterogeneous group of genetic disorders resulting from deficiencies in pigmentation. Clinically, albinism is divided into ocular and oculocutaneous forms. At least seven different gene defects can cause a reduction in melanin synthesis. Oculocutaneous albinism results from mutations in the tyrosinase gene or the P gene. Ocular albinism, an autosomal recessive or X-linked condition, mainly affects pigmentation in the visual system; it may be a mild form of oculocutaneous albinism or may involve other gene defects.

The most common ocular finding in albinism is iris transillumination, which may be observable in a darkened room by placing a penlight against the lower eyelid and noting the passage of light from both the pupil and the iris. Other frequent ocular findings are nystagmus, light fundus pigmentation (blonde fundus), and foveal hypoplasia. Visual acuity ranges from 20/40 to 20/200, the latter being considered legal blindness.

The Chédiak-Higashi and Hermansky-Pudlak syndromes can manifest features of albinism. If either of these conditions is suspected, hematologic consultation is recommended because of the lethal nature of these forms of albinism.

PSYCHOGENIC VISION DISORDERS

The clinician must determine whether visual symptoms are of organic or psychogenic origin. Some of the psychological conditions that may manifest with visual symptoms are factitious disorders, school avoidance, and conversion disorders (see Chapter 35). The incidence of psychogenic cause of vision loss is highest in older school-aged children (8 to 15 years); girls are affected more commonly than are boys.

Besides complaining of vision loss or blurring, the children with a psychogenic cause of the visual symptoms may also complain of abnormal visual sensations (spots, lines, or patterns, often in color), diplopia, polyopia, and a visual field defect. In addition to visual symptoms, the spectrum of psychogenic ophthalmic manifestations in these children may also include ocular discomfort ("eyestrain," asthenopia, or painful eye), headaches, exaggerated sensitivity to light, disorders of accommodation and convergence, blinking, and lid tics. Some children may even exhibit self-destructive behavior, such as gouging their eyes or pulling out their eyelashes.

RED FLAGS FOR PSYCHOGENIC VISION DISORDERS

The *red flags* that should alert the clinician to the possibility of a psychogenic vision problem are inconsistency, suggestibility, and the child's affect during the examination.

Inconsistency

If the cause of vision loss is organic, the symptoms are consistent across a variety of situations. If the vision is so poor as to interfere with schoolwork, it should also interfere with the child's performance in sports and in video games.

Suggestibility

Leading the patient to believe that the vision will be clearer as the examiner has the patient look through lenses of negligible power often yields a dramatic improvement in acuity. Similarly, a patient's visual field may expand to normal after the examiner suggests to the patient that the pupils will be "opened" after the administration of dilating drops.

Affect and Behavior during Testing

Some children are indifferent despite the purported severity of the disability, whereas others may appear annoyed, resentful, or belligerent. On reading the visual acuity chart, the child may stop abruptly and refuse to cooperate with the examiner. In addition, many youngsters may exhibit exaggerated grimacing, elaborate contortions, and frequent sighs during testing.

ETIOLOGY

Whether the symptoms are of conscious or unconscious origin, a precipitating factor often can be identified. The symptoms may be a response to problems at home (illness, divorce, abuse) or in school (peer relationships, school failure, trying to maintain a high level of achievement). Some children willfully feign a vision problem because they want glasses or attention. In each case, it is the physician's responsibility to perform a thorough examination to rule out any organic causes of visual loss, to demonstrate that the patient is capable of normal visual function, and to begin to address the psychogenic nature of the problem.

EVALUATION

For an assessment of visual symptoms, the child's response should be physiologically sound. For an assessment of visual acuity, the measurement of acuity should be identical regardless of the chart used (letter E, Snellen, or picture chart), the distance at which the child stands from the chart (adjusted for the shorter distance), and the use of a "zero power" lens despite suggestions from the examiner to the contrary. In a child who is blind in one or both eyes, the affected eye should be unable to fixate on an object (e.g., the patient's image on a tilted mirror), and there should not be any optokinetic nystagmus in response to a moving target in front of the patient.

In the assessment of a constricted visual field, the field constriction of psychogenic origin does not change proportionately when the test distance or object size is adjusted (the "tubular" field). In addition, the patient may involuntarily glance toward an object suddenly brought into view from the periphery.

Ophthalmologists have additional techniques that may be effective for accurate assessment of visual function:

- high-power lenses to surreptitiously blur the vision of one eye while having the patient read with both eyes open
- polarizing lenses and vectograph charts
- red-green goggles and colored charts to demonstrate intact vision in one or both eyes
- prisms to elicit diplopia or tell-tale refixation movements as the patient views the chart with both eyes open
- the Worth four-dot test to assess whether the patient sees with both eyes or has diplopia

Table 43-19. Specific Patterns of Nystagmus

Pattern	Description	Associated Conditions
Latent nystagmus	Conjugate jerk nystagmus toward viewing eye	Congenital vision defects, occurs with occlusion of eye
Manifest latent nystagmus	Fast jerk to viewing eye	Strabismus, congenital idiopathic nystagmus
Periodic alternating	Cycles of horizontal or horizontal-rotary movements that change direction	Caused by both visual and neurologic conditions
Seesaw nystagmus	One eye rises and intorts as other eye falls and extorts	Usually associated with optic chiasm defects
Nystagmus retractorius	Eyes jerk back into orbit or toward each other	Caused by pressure on mesencephalic tegmentum (Parinaud syndrome)
Gaze-evoked nystagmus	Jerk nystagmus in direction of gaze	Caused by medications, brainstem lesion, or labyrinthine dysfunction
Gaze-paretic nystagmus	Eyes jerk back to maintain eccentric gaze	Cerebellar disease
Downbeat nystagmus	Fast-phase beating downward	Posterior fossa disease, drugs
Upbeat nystagmus	Fast-phase beating upward	Brainstem and cerebellar disease, and some visual conditions
Vestibular nystagmus	Horizontal-torsional or horizontal jerks	Vestibular system dysfunction
Asymmetrical or monocular nystagmus	Pendular vertical nystagmus	Disease of retina and visual pathways
Spasmus nutans	Fine, rapid, pendular nystagmus	Torticollis, head nodding; idiopathic or gliomas of visual pathways

When all else fails, quietly hinting that a few eye drops might "clear things up" is often sufficient to get a child to read the 20/20 line.

TREATMENT

The approach to management should be supportive and nonpunitive. The clinician should never embarrass the child, accuse the patient of "faking," show anger, or subject the child to punishment. Glasses or medication that reinforces the concept of organic disease should be avoided. Reassurance and positive suggestion usually are sufficient to ease the child's symptoms. If symptoms persist or recur, the child should be referred to a psychologist or psychiatrist for further evaluation and management.

NYSTAGMUS

Nystagmus is defined as a rhythmic, to-and-fro movement of the eyes. Horizontal nystagmus is the most common form of nystagmus, but vertical nystagmus and torsional nystagmus also occur (Table 43-19). Nystagmus may be congenital or acquired. *Congenital nystagmus* is somewhat of a misnomer because the abnormal eye movements are generally not noted until an infant is 1 or 2 months of age, when the fixation reflex becomes established. Non-nystagmus eye movements are noted in Table 43-20.

Congenital nystagmus is often idiopathic; in this case, visual acuity is only moderately impaired, and the fundus examination findings and the electroretinogram are normal. A family history of nystagmus can frequently be ascertained. Congenital sensory defect nystagmus occurs with diseases that impair normal image formation (bilateral congenital cataracts) or image processing in both eyes (a retinal dystrophy or bilateral optic nerve atrophy or hypoplasia). Visual acuity is often more severely impaired than in idiopathic congenital nystagmus (20/200 or less), and visual loss may be progressive in some instances. The evaluation of a child with congenital nystagmus entails a thorough health and family history, a general physical examination, and an eye examination by an ophthalmologist with expertise in pediatric eye disorders (Figs. 43-26 and 43-27). A cranial magnetic resonance imaging scan is often indicated, and electroretinography and other electrophysiologic (electrooculography) or psychophysical tests (dark adaptation, color vision testing) may be useful in establishing a specific diagnosis. Fluorescein angiography may also help confirm a retinal dystrophy. Some children with congenital nystagmus adopt anomalous head positions to minimize the intensity of the nystagmus and improve visual acuity. Eye muscle surgery may be helpful in improving the abnormal head position.

Table 43-20. Specific Patterns of Non-nystagmus Eye Movements

Pattern	Description	Associated Conditions
Opsoclonus	Multidirectional conjugate movements of varying rate and amplitude	Hydrocephalus, diseases of brainstem and cerebellum, neuroblastoma
Ocular dysmetria	Overshoot of eyes on rapid fixation	Cerebellar dysfunction
Ocular flutter	Horizontal oscillations with forward gaze and sometimes with blinking	Cerebellar disease, hydrocephalus, or central nervous system neoplasm
Ocular bobbing	Downward jerk of eyes from primary gaze; eyes remain for a few seconds, then drift back	Pontine disease
Ocular myoclonus	Rhythmic to-and-fro pendular oscillations of the eyes, with synchronous nonocular muscle movement	Damage to red nucleus, inferior olivary nucleus, and ipsilateral dentate nucleus

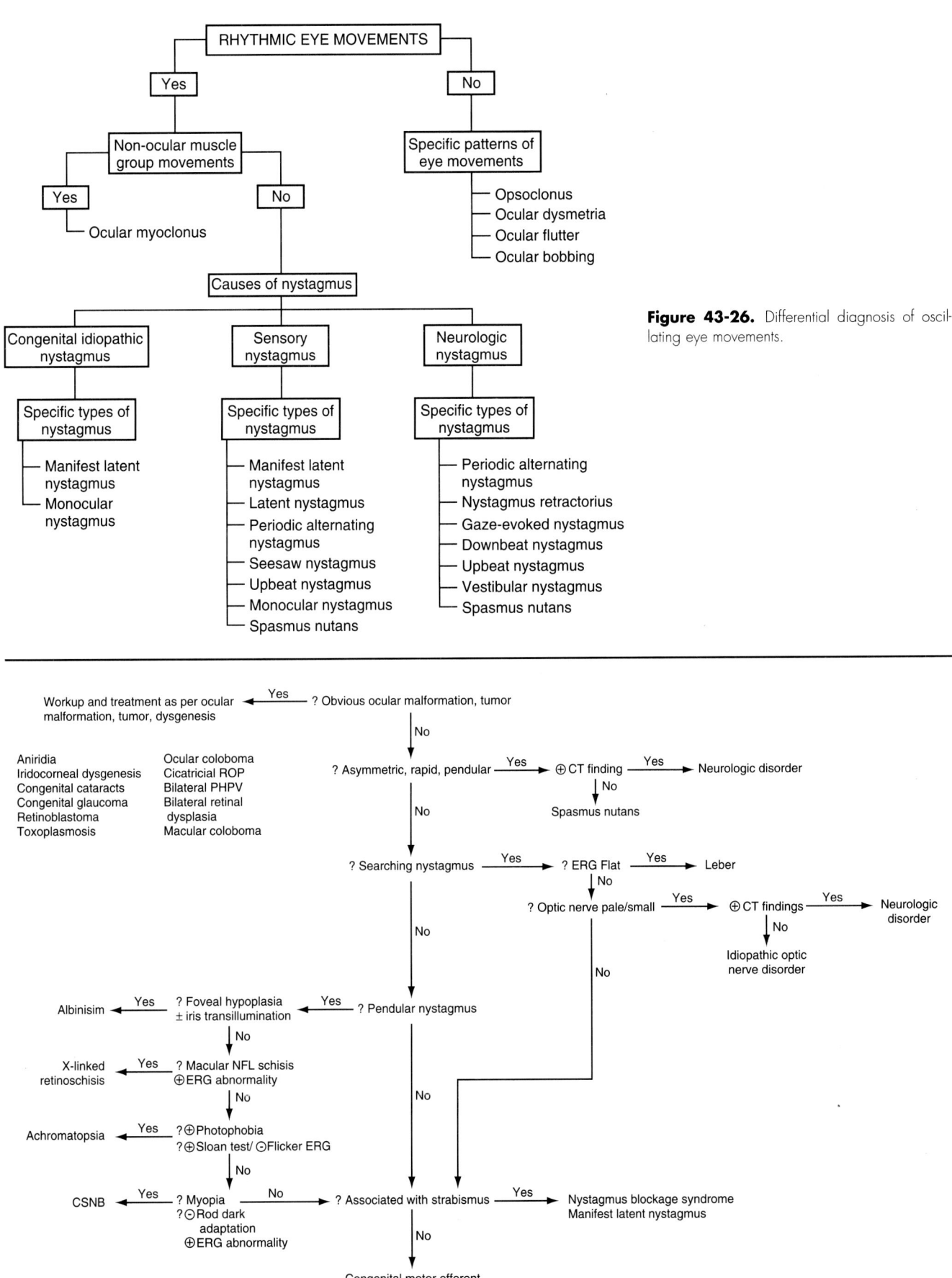

Figure 43-26. Differential diagnosis of oscillating eye movements.

Figure 43-27. Algorithm for the workup of an infant with nystagmus. CSNB, congenital stationary night blindness; CT, computed tomography; ERG, electroretinogram; NFL, nerve fiber layer; PHPV, persistent hyperplastic primary vitreous; ROP, retinopathy of prematurity. ⊕, positive; ⊖, negative. (From Nelson LB, Calhoun JH, Harley RD: Pediatric Ophthalmology, 3rd ed. Philadelphia, WB Saunders, 1991, p 493.)

Acquired nystagmus is less common than congenital nystagmus. Nystagmus that is truly acquired beyond the first few months of life is of concern and may represent a significant neurologic abnormality. It may be caused by central nervous system disorders, particularly of the cerebellum, brainstem, or suprasellar region. In children, the most common tumor causing acquired nystagmus is a craniopharyngioma. Vertically oriented nystagmus is also of great concern; it may be associated with the Arnold-Chiari malformation or drug intoxication.

Spasmus nutans is a special form of acquired nystagmus with onset between 3 and 15 months of age. The usual triad of findings consists of nystagmus (often a shimmering type of nystagmus that is frequently asymmetrical or even monocular), head nodding, and torticollis. This form of nystagmus is generally benign, but affected patients who were subsequently found to have chiasmal or suprachiasmal tumors have been reported. Neuroradiologic investigation may be indicated in uncertain cases. The diagnosis of spasmus nutans is confirmed if the nystagmus disappears by 3 to 4 years of age.

Opsoclonus is a special form of eye movement abnormality that is not truly nystagmus in that the bizarre, seemingly random oscillations of the eyes are not rhythmic and are frequently multivectorial. The most common cause of opsoclonus in children is acute cerebellar ataxia. The child presents with "dancing eyes and dancing feet." Opsoclonus can occur also with occult neuroblastoma, viral encephalitis, and hydrocephalus.

OCULAR TRAUMA

Trauma is a major cause of acquired visual loss in children (Fig. 43-28). Much of it is preventable, particularly that from sports injuries. Legislation has reduced the incidence of eye injuries from ice hockey to almost zero since the institution of mandatory face masks in children playing organized hockey. Legislation concerning the use of fireworks and BB guns could also reduce the number of cases of severe eye trauma in children. Child abuse is a frequent cause of eye injuries in young children and is theoretically avoidable through education of caregivers, but it has been frustratingly resistant to eradication.

Obtaining a history of the circumstances of an eye injury in children is important for ascertaining the potential seriousness of the injury. Assessment of visual acuity in the injured eye is also important for medical and legal reasons. The pediatrician should document whether the affected eye can perceive light, follow an object such as a small toy, or, in appropriate cases, read letters from an eye chart. All of these assessments are done with careful attention to occluding the sound or uninjured eye.

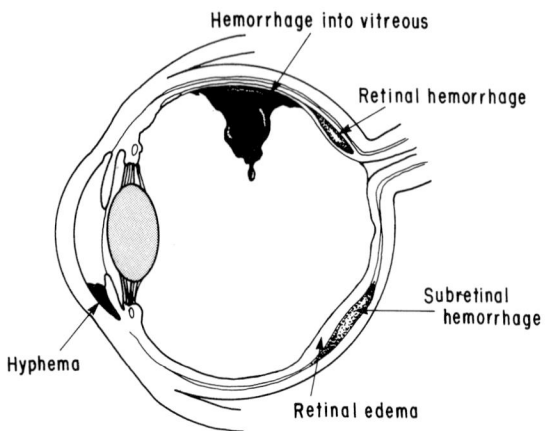

Figure 43-28. Various types of ocular hemorrhage after blunt trauma to the globe. (From Reilly BM: *Practical Strategies in Outpatient Medicine,* 2nd ed. Philadelphia, WB Saunders, 1991, p 68.)

The extent of the eye examination is determined by the child's level of cooperation. If the circumstances of the injury suggest a high likelihood of a perforating injury (from a sharp object that could go through the cornea or sclera), the eye should not be forced open but, rather, should be covered with a protective shield to prevent further injury until the child can be seen by an ophthalmologist. If a perforating injury is considered unlikely (a blunt or scratching type of injury), a sterile, topical ophthalmic anesthetic agent can be applied to the eye to reduce surface pain, which is a major cause of the child's reluctance to open the eye.

CORNEAL ABRASION AND CORNEAL FOREIGN BODY

A corneal abrasion should be suspected in any child with acute onset of ocular pain and conjunctival injection, regardless of whether the examiner can obtain a history of trauma. It is important to try to rule out a more severe eye injury if the history suggests the possibility of contact with a sharp or pointed object or severe blunt trauma. A child with a corneal abrasion usually presents with eye pain and photophobia. Examination may be difficult if the child does not voluntarily open his or her eyes. A drop of a topical anesthetic agent may eliminate the pain and cause the patient to suddenly become much more cooperative. If the topical anesthetic does eliminate eye pain, a diagnosis of corneal abrasion is more likely. The diagnosis can be confirmed by positive fluorescein staining of the cornea with a fluorescein paper strip moistened with normal saline or the topical anesthetic. Fluorescence occurs in the presence of blue light. Fluorescein adheres to areas of denuded corneal epithelium and persists through a blink, whereas areas of fluorescein pooling change with each blink.

The management of a corneal abrasion entails relief of pain, prevention of infection, and promotion of healing of the corneal epithelium. Ibuprofen or similar analgesics are usually sufficient for pain relief. A drop of a cycloplegic agent (cyclopentolate) may provide comfort by relieving ciliary spasm. Application of a topical antibiotic ointment such as erythromycin helps prevent infection and provides lubrication to the ocular surface to allow the new epithelium to slide in and adhere to the basement membrane of the cornea. There is a trend away from patching the eye in corneal abrasion because studies have not demonstrated a beneficial effect. Children generally do not like having their eyes patched. If a patch is applied, it should be placed snugly so that the eyelids cannot open and close. Follow-up 24 hours after treatment is indicated to make sure that the cornea is healing and not infected (corneal ulcer). Most abrasions heal completely within 24 to 48 hours.

The possibility of a foreign body embedded in the cornea, in the lower fornix, or, on occasion, on the tarsal conjunctiva of the upper eyelid must be considered. The pediatrician should evert the upper eyelid to inspect for a foreign body in the tarsal conjunctiva. Linear corneal epithelial defects with vertical orientation are a clue to a foreign body under the upper eyelid. A conjunctival foreign body can be irrigated out or swept out with a sterile applicator after a drop of topical anesthesia is applied. A corneal foreign body can be irrigated out, but attempting to sweep it out with an applicator is discouraged because the applicator may embed the foreign body deeper in the cornea. With appropriate magnification and lighting from a slit-lamp biomicroscope or loupes and a penlight, the foreign body may be gently removed from the cornea with a fine, blunt instrument (a corneal spud is an instrument designed for this). A needle can be used to remove the foreign body with caution in a cooperative child, but this should be done only with the magnification and illumination of a slit-lamp biomicroscope.

HYPHEMA

Any child with blunt ocular trauma causing a "black eye" should be evaluated for blood in the anterior chamber of the eye (hyphema)

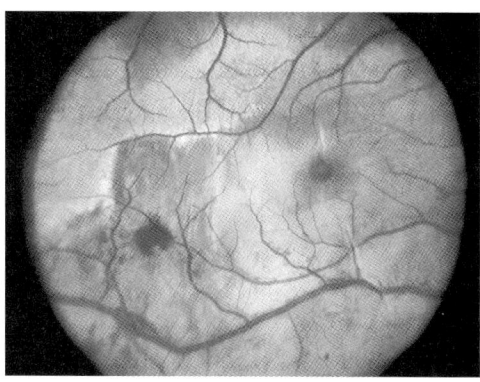

Figure 43-29. Hemorrhage and edema of the retina from blunt ocular trauma (commotio retinae).

(see Fig. 43-28). The visual acuity of the injured eye should be measured, if possible. The anterior segment and pupillary function can be examined with a penlight. Funduscopy should be attempted to look for associated retinal hemorrhage or edema (Fig. 43-29). The examining physician should be amenable to recommending ophthalmologic consultation, because a small hyphema or traumatic iritis may be detectable only with a slit-lamp biomicroscope. The primary goal of management of a hyphema is to allow the blood to slowly clear from the eye and to avoid recurrent bleeding, which greatly increases the risk of developing glaucoma, corneal blood staining, and amblyopia in a young child.

Eye Injuries in Child Abuse

In about 5% of cases of child abuse, the presenting sign involves the eye, and ocular injuries are detected in the course of examining many other child abuse injuries. Blunt injuries to the eyelids and anterior segment of the eye from fingers, fists, or belts may cause eyelid ecchymosis, subconjunctival hemorrhage, hyphema, cataract, and lens dislocation. The finding of such an injury should alert the physician to the possibility of child abuse.

The shaken-baby syndrome is a unique form of child abuse that is seen primarily in infants who have been violently shaken (see Chapter 36). Victims of shaken-baby syndrome are virtually always younger than 3 years and usually younger than 12 months old. Intracranial injury caused by shaking usually includes subdural hemorrhage. Retinal hemorrhages in all layers of the retina are the ocular hallmark of shaken-baby syndrome. In some instances, only scattered hemorrhages are seen, and in more severe injuries, retinal details cannot be seen because of vitreous blood or diffuse retinal hemorrhages (Fig. 43-30). Some shaken infants suffer permanent retinal damage that precludes the return of normal vision. Other shaken infants have

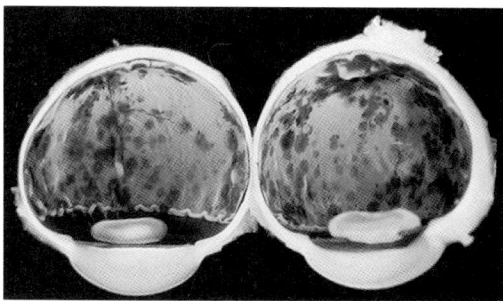

Figure 43-30. Gross pathologic specimen from an infant who died of shaken-baby syndrome. Note the diffuse retinal hemorrhages.

vision loss primarily as a result of injury to the visual pathways in the brain (cortical visual impairment). The severity of the damage to vision is strongly correlated with the overall neurologic damage.

VISUAL COMPLAINTS FROM CHILDREN

Frequently, a child is brought to the pediatrician because of a subjective visual complaint from the child rather than because of an abnormality observed by a parent. Symptoms associated with reading are common and include seeing blurred print, words "swimming" together, and skipping words or lines. Other children complain primarily of blurred distance vision. Uncommon visual phenomena may include seeing colored lights, objects appearing larger or smaller, seeing spots, and double vision. Eye pain localized to one or both eyes is also common. Frequent blinking is an exception to child-based complaints because the parent observes it. There are physiologic explanations for each of the complaints, and the child is usually interested in an explanation of the reason proposed for his or her complaint. A careful history of the exact nature of the complaint and any associated concerns should be sought and a screening eye examination performed. Specifically, distance and near visual acuity should be measured in each eye. A cover test or stereopsis test rules out manifest strabismus. An external eye examination may reveal a reason for eye pain or blinking (conjunctival injection, tearing, corneal abrasion, foreign body). Pupillary reactions should be assessed. Funduscopy should be done to evaluate optic nerve and retinal status. A color vision test may be helpful. Having the child read an age-appropriate passage may reveal information about the child's reading ability and the severity of the reading complaint. If the examination is normal, simple reassurance may ease the concerns of the child and parent, particularly if combined

Table 43-21. Symptoms and Signs that Should Raise Red Flags

Symptom or Sign	Most Worrisome or Urgent Cause
Leukocoria	Retinoblastoma
Acute onset of strabismus	Cranial nerve palsy from brain tumor, ↑ ICP*
Acute vision loss	Compression or infiltration of optic nerve by an orbital or intracranial lesion
Proptosis	Rhabdomyosarcoma
Sudden onset of ptosis	Third nerve palsy from tumor, ↑ ICP*
Severe headaches	↑ ICP*
Black eye	Trauma with associated hyphema
Light sensitivity	Uveitis
Head tilt or turn	Cranial nerve palsy causing strabismus, ↑ ICP*
Loss of corneal luster	Corneal edema from glaucoma or uveitis
Purulent conjunctivitis in a newborn	Gonococcal infection
Acquired anisocoria	Horner syndrome caused by neuroblastoma, ↑ ICP*
Bilateral cataracts in a newborn	Galactosemia
Retinal hemorrhages in an infant or toddler	Shaken-baby syndrome
Onset of nystagmus after early infancy	Brainstem or posterior fossa tumor

*↑ ICP, increased intracranial pressure.

with an offer to follow up on the complaint if it persists or if the parent notes objective changes in the child's eyes. If the complaint does persist or if the examination yields abnormal findings, referral to an ophthalmologist should be considered.

SUMMARY AND RED FLAGS

Ocular manifestations of vision loss, strabismus, and nystagmus may be caused by local ocular pathologic processes or by significant neurologic disease. Impaired visual function resulting from strabismus, cataracts, or other conditions may produce amblyopia and blindness. It is important to detect amblyopia because in nearly all cases, amblyopia is reversible if discovered early and treated appropriately. Symptoms and signs that suggest potentially life- or vision-threatening diseases are listed in Table 43-21.

REFERENCES

Anatomy and Neurophysiology of the Visual System

Livingstone MS: Art, illusion and the visual system. Sci Am 1988;258:78.

Wiesel TN, Hubel DH: Single-cell responses in striate cortex of kittens deprived of vision in one eye. J Neurophysiol 1963;26:1003.

Development of the Eye and Visual System

Tripathi BJ, Tripathi RC: Development of the human eye. In Bron AJ, Tripathi RC, Tripathi BJ (eds): Wolff's Anatomy of the Eye and Orbit, 8th ed. London, Chapman & Hall, 1997.

Amblyopia and Vision Screening

Donahue SP, Johnson TM, Leonard-Martin TC: Screening for amblyogenic factors using a lay network and the MTI photo-screener. Initial results from 15,000 preschool children in a statewide effort. Ophthalmology 2000;107:1637.

Kiorpes L, McKee SP: Neural mechanisms underlying amblyopia. Curr Opin Neurobiol 1999;9:480.

LaRoche GR: Detection, prevention, and rehabilitation of amblyopia. Curr Opin Ophthalmol 2000;11:306.

Tong PY, Bassin RE, Enke-Miyazaki E, et al: Screening for amblyopia in preverbal children with photoscreening photographs: II. Sensitivity and specificity of the MTI photoscreener. Ophthalmology 2000;107:1623.

Von Noorden GK: Amblyopia: A multidisciplinary approach. Proctor Lecture. Invest Ophthalmol Vis Sci 1985;26:1704.

Strabismus

Helveston EM, Neely DF, Stidham DB, et al: Results of early alignment of congenital esotropia. Ophthalmology 1999;106:1716.

Ing MR: The timing of surgical alignment for congenital (infantile) esotropia. J Pediatr Ophthalmol Strabismus 1999;36:61.

Von Noorden GK: A reassessment of infantile esotropia. XLIV Edward Jackson Memorial Lecture. Am J Ophthalmol 1988;105:1.

Vision Impairment in Children

Lambert SR, Taylor D, Kriss A: The infant with nystagmus, normal appearing fundi, but an abnormal ERG. Surv Ophthalmol 1989;34:173.

Mervis CA, Yeargin-Allsopp M, Winter S, et al: Aetiology of childhood vision impairment, metropolitan Atlanta, 1991-93. Paediatr Perinat Epidemiol 2000;14:70.

Retinopathy of Prematurity

Lee SK, Normand C, McMillan D, et al: Evidence for changing guidelines for routine screening for retinopathy of prematurity. Arch Pediatr Adolesc Med 2001;155:387.

O'Keefe M, Kafil-Hussain N, Flitcroft L, et al: Ocular significance of intraventricular haemorrhage in premature infants. Br J Ophthalmol 2001;85:357.

Paysse EA, Lindsey JL, Coats DK, et al: Therapeutic outcomes of cryotherapy versus transpupillary diode laser photocoagulation for threshold retinopathy of prematurity. J Am Assoc Pediatr Ophthalmol Strabismus 1999;3:234.

Reddy VM, Capone A Jr, Drack AV: The role of light toxicity in retinopathy of prematurity and congenital cataract. Am J Ophthalmol 1994;117:262.

Nasolacrimal Problems in Childhood

Paysse EA, Coats DK, Bernstein JM, et al: Management and complications of congenital dacryocele with concurrent intranasal mucocele. J AAPOS 2000;4:46.

Stager D, Baker JD, Frey T, et al: Office probing of congenital nasolacrimal duct obstruction. Ophthalmic Surg 1992;23:482.

The Red Eye

Fisher MC: Conjunctivitis in children. Pediatr Clin North Am 1987;34:1447.

Matoba A: Ocular viral infections. Pediatr Infect Dis 1984;3:358.

Ruttum MS, Ogawa G: Adenovirus conjunctivitis mimics preseptal and orbital cellulitis in young children. Pediatr Infect Dis J 1996;15:266.

Leukocoria and Retinoblastoma

Abramson DH, Frank CM, Susman M, et al: Presenting signs of retinoblastoma. J Pediatr 1998;132:505.

Mafee MF, Goldberg MF, Cohen SB, et al: Magnetic resonance imaging versus computed tomography of leukocoric eyes and use of in vitro proton magnetic resonance spectroscopy of retinoblastoma. Ophthalmology 1989;96:965.

Smith BJ, O'Brien JM: The genetics of retinoblastoma and current diagnostic testing. J Pediatr Ophthalmol Strabismus 1996;33:120.

Usalito M, Wheeler S, O'Brien J: New approaches in the clinical management of retinoblastoma. Ophthalmol Clin North Am 1999;12:255.

Childhood Cataracts

Birch EE, Stager DR: The critical period for surgical treatment of dense congenital unilateral cataract. Invest Ophthalmol Vis Sci 1996;37:1532.

Crouch ER Jr, Pressman SH, Crouch ER: Posterior chamber intraocular lenses: Long-term results in pediatric cataract patients. J Pediatr Ophthalmol Strabismus 1995;32:210.

Francis PJ, Berry V, Bhattacharya SS, et al: The genetics of childhood cataract. J Med Genet 2000;37:481.

Seaber JH, Buckley EG: Functional outcome of monocular and bilateral congenital cataract. Part 1: Visual acuity. Am Orthopt J 1997;47:29.

Glaucoma in Childhood

Talbot AW, Russell-Eggitt I: Pharmaceutical management of the childhood glaucomas. Expert Opin Pharmacother 2000;1:697

Wagner RS: Glaucoma in children. Pediatr Clin North Am 1993;40:855.

Childhood Uveitis

American Academy of Pediatrics Section on Rheumatology and Section on Ophthalmology: Guidelines for ophthalmologic examinations in children with juvenile rheumatoid arthritis. Pediatrics 1993;92:295.

Ceisler EJ, Foster CS: Juvenile rheumatoid arthritis and uveitis: Minimizing the blinding complications. Int Ophthalmol Clin 1996;36:91.

Mets MB, Holfels E, Boyer KM, et al: Eye manifestations of congenital toxoplasmosis. Am J Ophthalmol 1997;122:309

Tugal-Tutkun I, Havrlikova K, Powers WJ, et al: Changing patterns of uveitis in childhood. Ophthalmology 1996;103:375.

Eyelid and Orbital Problems

Castillo M, Mukherji SK, Wagle NS: Imaging of the pediatric orbit. Neuroimaging Clin North Am 2000;10:95.

Korn E: Oculoplastic update. Pediatr Ann 1990;19:316.

Volpe NJ, Jakobiec FA: Pediatric orbital tumors. Int Ophthalmol Clin 1992;32:201.

Weiss AH: The swollen and droopy eyelid. Signs of systemic disease. Pediatr Clin North Am 1993;40:789.

Ocular Manifestations of Systemic Disease

Bielory L, Wagner RS: Allergic and immunologic pediatric disorders of the eye. J Invest Allergol Clin Immunol 1995;5:309.

Brodsky MC, Baker RS, Hamed LM: Pediatric Neuro-ophthalmology. New York, Springer-Verlag, 1996.

Gottlob I: Nystagmus. Curr Opin Ophthalmol 2000;11:330.

Hamshere M, Cross S, Daniels M, et al: A transcript map of a 10-Mb region of chromosome 19: A source of genes for human disorders, including candidates for genes involved in asthma, heart defects, and eye. Genomics 2000;63:425.

Kerrison JB: Neuro-ophthalmology of the phacomatoses. Curr Opin Ophthalmol 2000;11:413.

Liu G, Keane-Meyers A, Miyazaki D, et al: Molecular and cellular aspects of allergic conjunctivitis. Chem Immunol 1999;73:39.

Oetting WS: Albinism. Curr Opin Pediatr 1999;11:565.

O'Hara MA: Ophthalmia neonatorum. Pediatr Clin North Am 1993; 40:715.

Ocular Trauma in Childhood

Kivlin JD, Simons KB, Lazoritz S, et al: Shaken baby syndrome. Ophthalmology 2000;107:1246.

Mills M: Funduscopic lesions associated with mortality in shaken baby syndrome. J AAPOS 1998;2:67.

ORTHOPEDIC DISORDERS

44 Arthritis

James J. Nocton*

A pediatrician must always consider the entire spectrum of complaints involving the musculoskeletal system (e.g., arthralgias, myalgias, joint swelling, poorly localized extremity pain, limping) and the possible associated illnesses. Patients rarely arrive in the clinic with a complaint of "arthritis." Instead, they have symptoms such as leg pain, knee swelling, or limitations of activity and function. These children may have arthritis, but many have alternative explanations. Gait disturbances, with an emphasis on orthopedic evaluation, are discussed in Chapter 45.

The differential diagnosis of extremity pain is extensive (Table 44-1). For many diagnoses, the history and physical examination are all that are necessary; for others, specific laboratory tests confirm a suspected diagnosis. Musculoskeletal symptoms may indicate pathologic processes localized and restricted to a single extremity or joint; or symptoms may be one component of a systemic illness.

Arthritis is a specific sign, indicating inflammation of the joint, and can be defined as (1) swelling of the joint or (2) limitation of motion combined with pain on motion, with tenderness, and/or with warmth. Arthritis should be distinguished from arthralgia (Table 44-2), bone pain, myalgia, and neuralgia. If arthritis is present, the diagnostic possibilities represent some specific diseases (Fig. 44-1). Arthritis is not a diagnosis; there are infectious, reactive or postinfectious, hematologic, traumatic, metabolic, oncologic, rheumatologic, and idiopathic causes of arthritis. The specific characteristics of the arthritis (number and location of joints involved, severity, degree of disability, chronicity), as well as the pattern of associated systemic signs and symptoms, lead to appropriate diagnosis and therapy.

HISTORY

Although the parents and child are usually the principal historians, it is often helpful to determine whether other adults have seen symptoms. Have day care providers reported problems to the parents? Has the school staff, coach, or physical education teacher noticed any problems similar to those seen at home? Obtaining consistent information from several observers in different settings determines the frequency of the symptoms, how disabling the symptoms have been, and the reliability of the history. If there are inconsistencies, it becomes difficult to formulate a diagnosis. Adolescents have a tendency to underreport their symptoms.

PAIN LOCATION

The pain must be localized as much as possible. There are several possible sources of extremity pain (Fig. 44-2). Pain directly over a joint or joints may indicate synovial inflammation, arthralgias secondary to viral infection, or mechanical joint problems such as ligament trauma, meniscal tears, or hypermobility. Pain near a joint could represent muscle, bone, tendon, enthesis (tendon insertion sites), or bursa disease, or it may be referred from a nearby joint. Pain could involve a whole limb or limbs, or a region of a limb, where it may reflect a neuropathy, myalgia, or a regional pain syndrome. On occasion, children complain of pain "all over," which suggests diffuse myalgias related to a systemic infection or, if chronic, fibromyalgia or a related chronic pain syndrome. Pain localized to a single small area is seen with infection, trauma, or tumor. Migrating joint pain or inflammation is more suggestive of some specific diagnoses such as acute rheumatic fever or immune complex–mediated diseases and is less consistent with trauma, septic arthritis (except gonococcus), osteomyelitis, or tumors.

PAIN CHARACTER

Arthritis is an aching discomfort and usually not severe enough to cause crying or screaming. Very severe pain should increase the suspicion of bone disease (osteomyelitis, leukemia, metastatic neuroblastoma, or bone tumors). Episodes of sporadic extreme pain are seen with pain syndromes such as "growing pains," fibromyalgia, and reflex sympathetic dystrophy or in situations in which psychogenic and behavioral factors contribute to the pain. With pain syndromes, children rate their pain as 10 on a scale of 1 to 10 and state that the pain is "constant." There may be an incongruity between their affect and their complaint (la belle indifference); for example, they may be smiling or laughing while they are describing the presence of excruciating discomfort. Pain that is sharp, radiating ("shooting"), or throbbing is unusual for arthritis and suggests an alternative explanation such as neuropathic pain, trauma, or psychogenic pain.

TIMING OF PAIN

Arthritis usually causes consistent patterns of discomfort. Symptoms are present daily, although often with day-to-day variability. Discomfort from pain and/or stiffness occurs on awakening or after other periods of inactivity, such as prolonged sitting in class or taking a long car ride. The morning stiffness may last for hours, but it generally improves with activity during the day. Some forms of arthritis, such as Lyme arthritis or spondyloarthropathies, may be more episodic. Lyme arthritis classically causes symptoms for days to weeks, usually in a single knee, interspersed with periods of improvement. Spondyloarthropathies can cause sudden increases in swelling and discomfort of one or more joints for several weeks at a time, followed by gradual spontaneous improvement.

Discomfort that occurs with activities and improves with rest is more suggestive of mechanical pain such as that associated with patellofemoral syndrome, hypermobility, tendonitis, or muscle strain. Affected children do not have symptoms in the morning or after naps, and these conditions are generally not associated with signs and symptoms of significant inflammation such as warmth, swelling, or limited range of motion.

Pain at night that wakes children from sleep may be seen in potentially serious conditions such as leukemia, bone tumors

* This chapter is an updated and edited version of the chapter by Arthur J. Newman that appeared in the first edition.

Table 44-1. **Conditions Causing Arthritis or Extremity Pain**

Rheumatic and Inflammatory Diseases

Juvenile rheumatoid arthritis
Systemic lupus erythematosus
Juvenile dermatomyositis
Polymyositis
Polyarteritis
Vasculitis
Scleroderma
Sjögren syndrome
Behçet disease
Overlap syndromes
Wegener granulomatosis
Sarcoidosis
Kawasaki syndrome
Henoch-Schönlein purpura
Chronic recurrent multifocal osteomyelitis

Seronegative Spondyloarthropathies

Juvenile ankylosing spondylitis
Inflammatory bowel disease
Psoriatic arthritis
Reactive arthritis associated with urethritis, iridocyclitis, and
mucocutaneous lesions

Infectious Illnesses

Bacterial arthritis (e.g., septic arthritis, *Staphylococcus
aureus,* pneumococcus, gonococcus, *H. influenzae*)
Lyme disease
Viral illness (parvovirus, rubella, mumps, Epstein-Barr virus,
hepatitis B)
Fungal arthritis
Mycobacterial infection
Spirochetal infection

Reactive Arthritis

Acute rheumatic fever
Reactive arthritis (post-infectious from *Shigella, Salmonella,
Yersinia, Chlamydia,* or meningococcus)
Serum sickness
Toxic synovitis of the hip
Postimmunization

Immunodeficiencies

Hypogammaglobulinemia
Immunoglobulin A deficiency
Human immunodeficiency virus

Congenital and Metabolic Disorders

Gout
Pseudogout
Mucopolysaccharidoses
Thyroid disease (hypothyroidism, hyperthyroidism)

Hyperparathyroidism
Vitamin C deficiency (scurvy)
Hereditary connective tissue disease (Marfan syndrome,
Ehlers-Danlos syndrome)
Fabry disease
Farber disease
Amyloidosis (familial Mediterranean fever)

Bone and Cartilage Disorders

Trauma
Patellofemoral syndrome
Hypermobility syndrome
Osteochondritis dissecans
Avascular necrosis (including Legg-Calvé-Perthes disease)
Hypertrophic osteoarthropathy
Slipped capital femoral epiphysis
Osteolysis
Benign bone tumors (including osteoid osteoma)
Histiocytosis
Rickets

Neuropathic Disorders

Peripheral neuropathies
Carpal tunnel syndrome
Charcot joints

Neoplastic Disorders

Leukemia
Neuroblastoma
Lymphoma
Bone tumors (osteosarcoma, Ewing sarcoma)
Histiocytic syndromes
Synovial tumors

Hematologic Disorders

Hemophilia
Hemoglobinopathies (including sickle cell disease)

Miscellaneous Disorders

Pigmented villonodular synovitis
Plant-thorn synovitis (foreign body arthritis)
Myositis ossificans
Eosinophilic fasciitis
Tendonitis (overuse injury)
Raynaud phenomenon

Pain Syndromes

Fibromyalgia
Growing pains
Depression (with somatization)
Reflex sympathetic dystrophy
Regional myofascial pain syndromes

(including benign tumors such as osteoid osteoma), or infections, but it also occurs with benign conditions such as "growing pains," muscle cramps, or "behavioral" pain. Those with the more dangerous illnesses usually have additional symptoms to suggest the diagnosis, while children with benign pains lack systemic symptoms, are well during the day, and have normal physical examination findings.

ACUITY

In most cases of chronic arthritis, children have symptoms for weeks to months, with a somewhat insidious onset before they seek medical attention. If the onset is more sudden and severe, the initial

evaluation focuses on possible diagnoses that necessitate more urgent treatment, such as trauma (including fractures), septic arthritis, or osteomyelitis. Acute rheumatic fever and other types of reactive arthritis, such as postinfectious arthritis, as well as arthritis or myositis associated with acute viral illnesses, may also manifest suddenly.

Affected children may state that they have had extremity pains "for years" or "all my life." These children often have either mechanical causes of their discomfort, such as hypermobility syndrome or patellofemoral syndrome; psychogenic or behavioral causes of pain; or other relatively benign conditions such as "growing pains." It is rare for such children to have an unrecognized arthritis.

Table 44-2. Distinguishing Characteristics of Arthritis and Arthralgia

Arthritis	Arthralgia
Prominent swelling	Minimal or no swelling
Morning stiffness	No morning stiffness
Symptoms improve with activity	Symptoms are exacerbated by activity
Stiffness follows rest	Pain improves with rest
Limited range of motion	Normal or excessive range of motion
Warmth of joint	No warmth
Symptoms usually daily, consistent	Symptoms usually intermittent

SIGNS OF INFLAMMATION

In most joints affected by arthritis, swelling and warmth are apparent. Exceptions include the shoulder and hip, in which the joints are too deep for these signs to be visible, and the joints of the spine, the temporomandibular joints, and the sacroiliac joints, in which the articular surface is small in relation to the surrounding soft tissues. In these areas, the physical examination is more helpful in detecting arthritis, because tenderness or pain with motion and limitation of motion should be elicited in patients who have arthritis.

DISABILITIES

The chief complaint is often a disability such as limping, trouble climbing stairs, or difficulty with writing. Some affected children have associated pain and signs of inflammation, whereas others have little or no discomfort.

If the chief complaint is the disability, begin by localizing the source of the disability. Is it a problem in the joint, the bones, the muscles, or the nerves? Muscle or nerve disease manifests primarily as weakness, although some children with myositis (particularly acute viral myositis) and sensory neuropathies also have pain. The rheumatic diseases associated primarily with myositis (dermatomyositis and polymyositis) cause proximal, symmetric weakness in the upper and lower extremities. The characteristic symptoms are difficulties climbing stairs, rising from the floor, taking the big step

HISTORY AND PHYSICAL EXAMINATION

ARTHRITIS
Common
  Rheumatic disease
  Infectious illness
  Reactive arthritis
  Spondyloarthropathy
Uncommon
  Trauma
  Malignancy
  Metabolic disease
  Hemophilia
  Immunodeficiency

NO ARTHRITIS
Common
  Orthopedic disorder
  Pain syndrome
  Viral illness
  Trauma
Uncommon
  Malignancy
    (primary or metastatic)
  Benign bone tumor
  Metabolic disease

Figure 44-1. Algorithm for determining possible causes of extremity pain, on the basis of the presence or absence of arthritis.

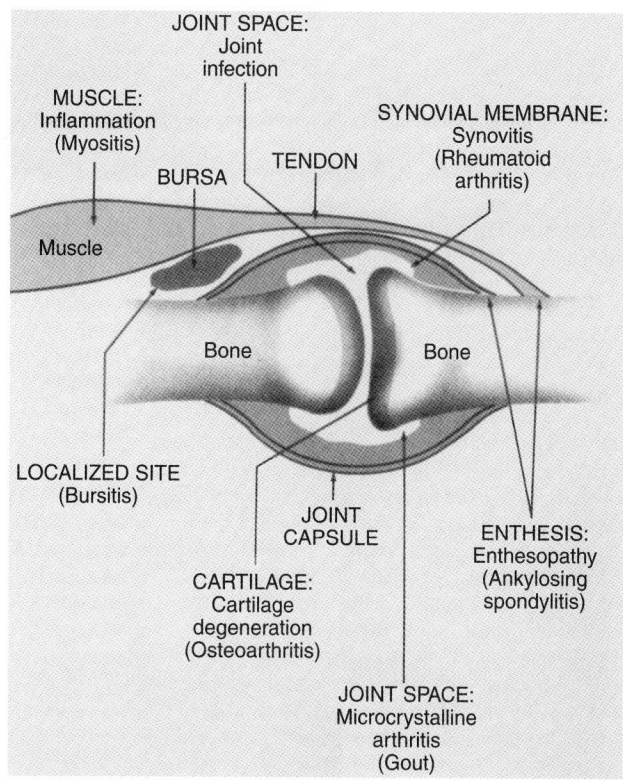

Figure 44-2. Location of musculoskeletal disease processes. The illustration depicts the site, pathophysiologic process, and typical disease (in parentheses). (From Fries JF: Approach to the patient with musculoskeletal disease. In Wyngaarden JB, Smith LH, Bennett JC [eds]: Cecil Textbook of Medicine, 19th ed. Philadelphia, WB Saunders, 1992, p 1488.)

onto a bus or into the family minivan, and washing or combing the hair, as well as fatigue and poor endurance. Isolated lower extremity or asymmetric weakness should increase suspicion of a neurologic disease.

Disabilities from arthritis are caused by the limited range of motion or pain of the joint rather than weakness. Limping, particularly in the mornings, walking on the toes (because of inability to extend the knee or Achilles tendon), and difficulty running and jumping are seen with lower extremity arthritis. The child with hand or wrist arthritis has difficulties opening bottles, turning doorknobs, manipulating buttons or snaps on clothing, and gripping pencils or eating utensils.

MEDICAL HISTORY

Various conditions are associated with arthritis, bone disease, or other rheumatic diseases. For example, there are numerous genetic syndromes and metabolic diseases associated with arthropathies (see Table 44-1). Endocrine disorders such as diabetes, hyperparathyroidism, and hypothyroidism are associated with arthropathy, periosteal inflammation, and muscle weakness, respectively. Arthritis is more frequent in patients with psoriasis and inflammatory bowel disease. Bone pain is common in hemoglobinopathies such as sickle cell disease. Cystic fibrosis and other chronic pulmonary diseases increase the likelihood of hypertrophic osteoarthropathy, which can cause pain. Arthritis or joint pain may occur after viral diseases or immunizations, presumably secondary to immune complex deposition in the joint, particularly with immunization against rubella and hepatitis B.

MEDICATIONS

Medications may cause the patient's symptoms (serum sickness reactions or swelling related to anaphylaxis). It is helpful to determine which medicines have improved symptoms. An adequate dose of antiinflammatory medication at least partially improves the discomfort of arthritis in most children. In rheumatic fever, antiinflammatory medications often result in dramatic improvement in symptoms. Conversely, the patient who continues to have severe pain despite adequate doses of antiinflammatory and analgesic medication is more likely to have an infection, a fracture, a tumor, or psychogenic pain.

FAMILY HISTORY

For some diseases, a positive family history increases the likelihood that other individuals in the family have that disease, but the genetics of the rheumatic diseases are complex, and none of the genetic associations are strong enough to confirm or eliminate a diagnosis solely on the basis of the family history. The family history is most helpful when either a spondyloarthropathy or lupus is considered as a diagnostic possibility. Ankylosing spondylitis, psoriasis, reactive arthritis, or inflammatory bowel disease in the family increases the likelihood that the child's arthritis is related to one of these entities. The presence of the human leukocyte (HLA) B27 antigen in these family members further increases the probability of a spondyloarthropathy in the child. Approximately 30% of patients with lupus have an affected first-degree relative. Less common familial illnesses that may cause rheumatic complaints include familial Mediterranean fever (recurrent fever, abdominal pain, joint pain), mucopolysaccharidoses, hemophilia, and muscular dystrophies. A family history of adults with "arthritis" is generally not helpful. In most instances, the family is referring to osteoarthritis rather than rheumatoid arthritis; even in families in which rheumatoid arthritis is present, there is usually a poor relationship between adult-type rheumatoid arthritis and the arthritis that occurs during childhood.

SOCIAL HISTORY

Determining the extent to which the problem has limited usual activities helps to gauge the severity of the problem. Has the child missed school because of pain? Has the child been able to participate in physical education, organized sports, or other physical activities such as dancing, swimming, and gymnastics? Is the older child participating in social activities with friends? In some instances, the limitations are directly related to pain or disability from arthritis, but school absences and the discontinuation of sports and social activities can be secondary to depression or psychogenic pain. It is helpful to ask the parents whether the child's mood or personality has changed recently and whether there have been any recent known psychosocial stressors such as problems at school or with friends or discord within the family. Fibromyalgia and other chronic pain syndromes in children are frequently associated with a history of psychosocial stress as well as depression.

The travel history is important in considering Lyme disease because the causative agent, the spirochete *Borrelia burgdorferi,* is transmitted by the bite of a deer tick that has a restricted geographical distribution. Lyme arthritis characteristically causes episodic joint effusions in one or a few large joints, most commonly the knee. A small percentage of patients develop chronic arthritis. The northeast (Connecticut, Rhode Island, Massachusetts), mid-Atlantic (Long Island, New York City suburbs, New Jersey, Southeastern Pennsylvania, Delaware, Maryland) and the upper Midwest (parts of Minnesota and Wisconsin) regions are the endemic regions in the United States. A child who has not traveled to these areas is unlikely to have Lyme disease. The arthritis may not appear until up to 2 years after the tick bite; a history of the classic rash (erythema migrans) is helpful.

REVIEW OF SYSTEMS

Some rheumatic diseases, including several forms of childhood arthritis, are systemic illnesses and cause fevers, poor appetite, weight loss, and fatigue. The absence of these symptoms helps eliminate specific illnesses as diagnostic possibilities. In the assessment of the presence of fever, the *pattern* of fever can be very helpful. Systemic-onset juvenile rheumatoid arthritis (JRA) typically produces one or two high temperature spikes each day, with many hours without fever in between (Fig. 44-3). Such a pattern is less likely to appear in other illnesses that cause more persistent fevers, such as infections or Kawasaki disease. A periodic fever pattern, in which fevers occur for several days, followed by weeks without fever, is seen in familial Mediterranean fever, cyclic neutropenia, the syndrome of fever, aphthous stomatitis, pharyngitis, and adenopathy (FAPA) (see Chapter 1), and other periodic fever syndromes. Systemic lupus erythematosus (SLE), vasculitis, rheumatic fever, serum sickness, inflammatory bowel disease, sarcoidosis, leukemia, and neuroblastoma may cause fevers associated with arthritis or extremity pains. These illnesses do not cause specific patterns of fever.

A decline in appetite is common and is more significant when associated with documented weight loss. Although most children with JRA do not have significant appetite changes, those with systemic JRA may have substantial appetite and growth disturbances. Severe polyarticular JRA may cause some appetite changes and mild weight loss. Children with Crohn disease or ulcerative colitis, both of which are often accompanied by abdominal pain and diarrhea, may demonstrate only poor appetite and a failure to thrive. SLE, vasculitis, scleroderma, chronic infections such as tuberculosis, and malignancies are additional causes of significant weight loss. An *increase* in weight should raise the suspicion of hypothyroidism or fluid retention.

Fatigue is common with any systemic illness, and it may be present in systemic-onset JRA, SLE, hypothyroidism, rheumatic fever, and fibromyalgia. The clinician should attempt to distinguish between generalized fatigue and specific muscle weakness. The presence of proximal muscle weakness, often associated with fatigue and poor endurance, is characteristic of polymyositis and dermatomyositis.

Systemic-onset JRA is nearly always accompanied by evanescent, pink, or salmon-colored macules, often a few centimeters in diameter or smaller but sometimes coalescing to form larger patches (Fig. 44-4). These may be generalized or localized on the trunk or extremities. The macules are usually not pruritic, appear with the fever spikes, and may resolve completely when the fever is absent.

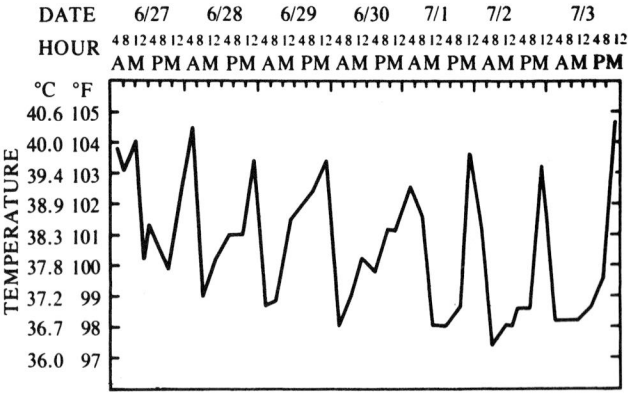

Figure 44-3. Graph of high, intermittent fever of a 3-year-old girl with systemic onset of juvenile rheumatoid arthritis. Most of the febrile spikes occurred in the late evening to early morning hours and were accompanied by a rheumatoid rash. (From Cassidy JT: Juvenile rheumatoid arthritis. In Kelley WN, Harris ED, Ruddy S, et al [eds]: Textbook of Rheumatology, 4th ed, vol 2. Philadelphia, WB Saunders, 1993, p 1193.)

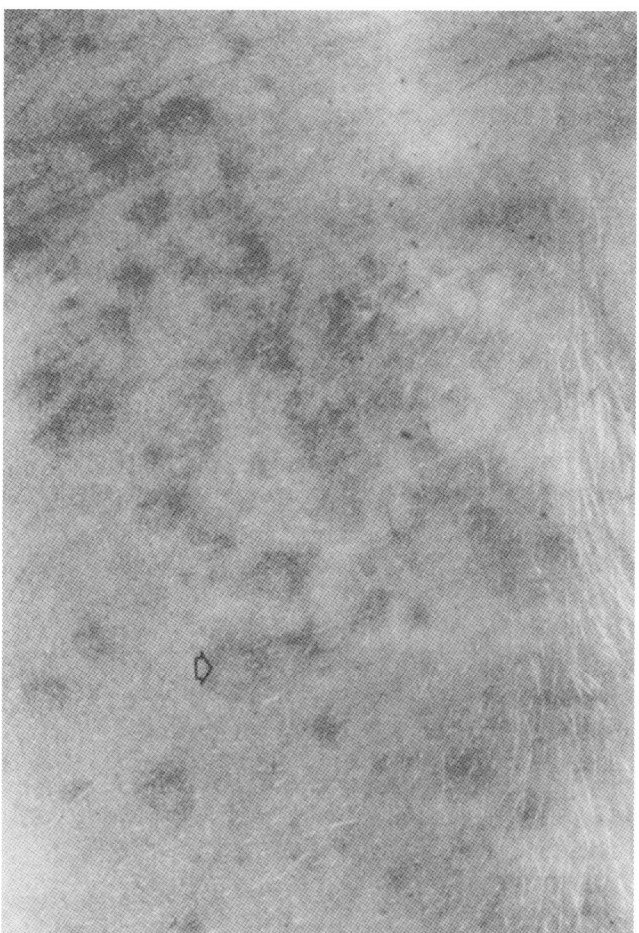

Figure 44-4. Rheumatoid rash. This was a faintly erythematous (salmon-colored), macular rash that was most prominent over the back but also involved the extremities and face. The individual lesions were transient, appeared in crops, and generally conformed to a linear distribution. Some of the lesions had central clearing (*arrow*). (From Cassidy JT: Juvenile rheumatoid arthritis. In Kelley WN, Harris ED, Ruddy S, et al [eds]: Textbook of Rheumatology, 4th ed, vol 2. Philadelphia, WB Saunders, 1993, p 1193.)

Sometimes parents do not notice the rash because of this fleeting nature. Acute rheumatic fever is associated with a specific rash, *erythema marginatum*, in only approximately 5% of cases. Erythema marginatum is also a fleeting rash, changing in distribution over time, and consists of erythematous patches with serpiginous borders that tend to migrate, usually over the trunk and proximal extremities. Because of their changes in distribution, families often confuse both of these rashes with "hives." The malar rash of SLE is a fixed, erythematous, nonblanching patch over the cheeks and nasal bridge that tends to spare the nasolabial folds. SLE may also cause vasculitic rashes, as well as nonspecific erythematous macular or papular lesions. Vasculitic rashes consist of palpable purpura and can sometimes be ulcerative. The characteristic skin lesions in dermatomyositis are essentially diagnostic: (1) A heliotrope rash is a purpuric discoloration of the upper eyelid, often accompanied by edema. (2) *Gottron rash* or *Gottron papules* are erythematous plaques or papules that appear on the extensor surface of the metacarpophalangeal and proximal interphalangeal joints of the hands. These are sometimes scaly and can be confused with psoriasis or eczema, were it not for the typical distribution. (3) Lesions similar to the Gottron lesions, occasionally erythema with some scaling, also appear on the

extensor surfaces of the elbows and knees and over the medial malleoli at the ankle. In addition, erythematous patches may appear on the shoulders, chest, or face, where the appearance can cause confusion with the malar rash of SLE.

Erythema migrans occurs in 60% to 80% of cases of Lyme disease, days to weeks after the tick bite. The lesion is expanding, beginning as a small papule and then forming a large erythematous, circular patch, usually at least 5 cm in diameter and often with some clearing in the center to produce a "target-like" appearance (Fig. 44-5). If untreated, the lesion usually lasts for several weeks and then gradually resolves. If dissemination occurs, some individuals develop multiple secondary lesions that appear similar to the primary lesion.

The history of other types of rashes or skin lesions may suggest other diagnoses. Measles and parvovirus infections, for example, have characteristic rashes. Petechiae may be seen with SLE, vasculitis, immune thrombocytopenia, or leukemia. Pallor or cyanosis of the digits, hands, and feet in association with cold temperature suggests Raynaud phenomenon, which may be associated with several rheumatic diseases, most notably SLE and scleroderma. Scleroderma causes tightening, thickening, and the development of a waxy texture to the skin, and it frequently begins on the hands, feet, and face. A history of photosensitivity is suggestive of SLE.

Questioning the parents about cognitive difficulties, including declining school performance or memory loss, helps screen for the possibility of subtle central nervous system involvement as part of SLE or vasculitis. Seizures or frank psychosis may also occur in these illnesses. Chronic neurologic Lyme disease typically causes short-term memory loss and mood disturbances, which may be subtle. Alopecia is frequently seen with SLE and may also occur with hypothyroidism. Ocular symptoms, such as pain or redness of the eye, occur with uveitis. Acute anterior uveitis (involving the iris and/or ciliary body) can be seen with reactive arthritis and other spondyloarthropathies. Chronic anterior uveitis is most common with pauciarticular JRA. Sarcoidosis in children is usually associated with posterior uveitis, although anterior uveitis also occurs. Ulcerations of the nose or hard palate may be present with SLE. Aphthous ulcerations can be seen with inflammatory bowel disease and Behçet disease. Frequent sinusitis is often a manifestation of Wegener granulomatosis.

The presence of chest pain might reflect pericarditis, in which case the symptoms are worse when the patient lies supine and improve with sitting up and leaning forward. Pericardial inflammation may be a component of systemic JRA and SLE. Similarly, pleuritic chest pain occurs with these illnesses. The presence of dysphagia suggests esophageal dysmotility, which may occur with inflammatory myopathies and scleroderma. Asking whether the child needs to cut the food into small pieces, needs to drink an unusual amount of fluid with meals, or takes a long time to complete a meal are helpful ways of assessing dysphagia. Abdominal pain, vomiting, and diarrhea are nonspecific but, if severe or if associated with melena or hematochezia, suggest Henoch-Schönlein purpura, inflammatory bowel disease, or vasculitis of the intestine. Testicular pain is seen with vasculitis, particularly polyarteritis nodosa. A history of recurrent genital and oral ulcerations is highly suggestive of Behçet disease. Peripheral edema, sacral edema, or periorbital edema may be present with illnesses causing glomerulonephritis, such as SLE and some of the vasculitides.

PHYSICAL EXAMINATION

Observing the child ambulate and explore the examination room provides a sense of the severity of the illness and the degree of disability. Particularly with young, fearful children, this period of observation may give a better sense of the range of motion of the joints or the degree of discomfort in the joints than the formal examination, when the child may be uncooperative.

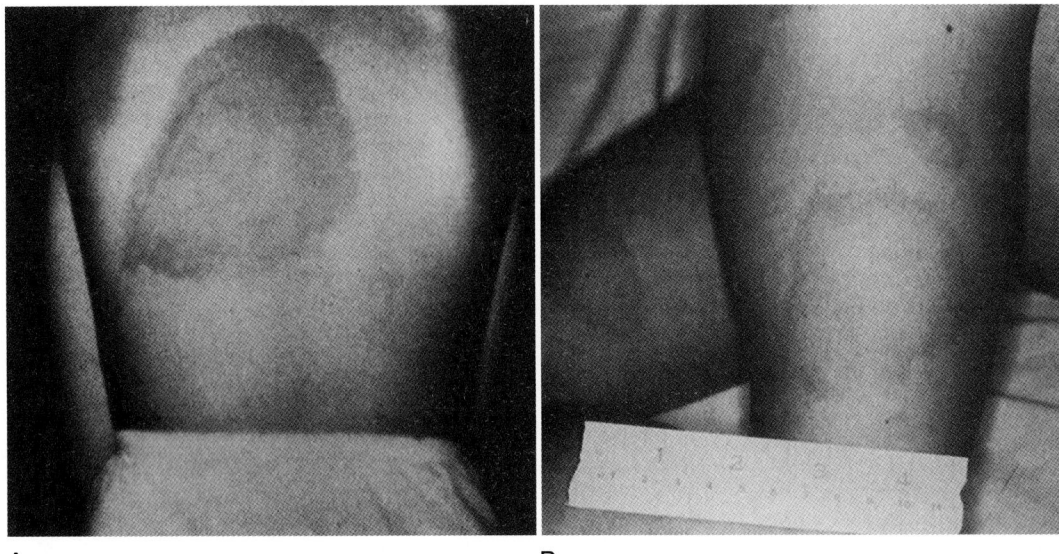

A   B

Figure 44-5. Erythema migrans (**A**) and secondary annular lesions (**B**), in different patients. The lesions began as red macules that expanded to form large rings. In **A**, the outer border is an intense red, the middle shows partial clearing, and the center is indurated. In **B**, the outer rims are red, and centers show nearly complete clearing. (From Steere AC, Malawista SE, Hardin JA, et al: Erythema chronicum migrans and Lyme arthritis: The enlarging clinical spectrum. Ann Intern Med 1977;86:685-698.)

The examination begins by reviewing the vital signs. Noting the presence of fever is critical, especially in the child with arthritis or localized extremity pain, because it may suggest an infectious process. Tachycardia may be caused by fever, anxiety, pericarditis, or myocarditis. Tachypnea suggests the presence of cardiac or pulmonary disease. Hypertension increases the suspicion of renal disease.

In any child with joint complaints, it is important to examine *all* of the joints because arthritis may be detected in joints that have not had symptoms. The neck and the joints of the upper extremities are examined with the child in a sitting position. Children with inflammation in the joints of the cervical spine usually have limitations in extension, lateral flexion, and rotation. This is tested by asking the child to look up at the ceiling, touch each ear to the ipsilateral shoulder, and touch the chin to each shoulder.

Arthritis of the temporomandibular joint is common with polyarticular JRA and can be overlooked. Children with chronic arthritis of these joints develop micrognathia as a result of delayed mandibular growth. The oral opening is often decreased, and there may be pain with opening and closing of the jaw, and tenderness to palpation directly over the joint.

Shoulder arthritis is identified by detecting limited range of motion and pain with motion. With the upper arm abducted to 90 degrees and the elbow flexed to 90 degrees, the clinician can then rotate the upper arm superiorly and inferiorly (external and internal rotation of the humerus, respectively), noting any limitation or pain. Alternatively, the patient can be asked to abduct and extend the arm, reaching behind the head to touch the contralateral scapula, and then to adduct and extend the arm, reaching behind the back and upward, again touching the contralateral scapula. The acromioclavicular joints and the sternoclavicular joints are occasionally affected by arthritis and should be palpated, noting any swelling or tenderness.

In the elbow, arthritis often produces detectable swelling and warmth. Elbow extension and flexion should also be tested, along with supination of the forearm and hand. Many children can normally hyperextend their elbows; therefore, it is helpful to compare the range of motion of the elbows.

The wrists are inspected for swelling and palpated for warmth and tenderness. Many children with wrist arthritis develop cysts of synovial fluid on the dorsal aspect of the wrist that may be fairly large but are usually nontender. Limitation in extension more than

flexion is common with wrist arthritis, as is limitation in radial deviation of the wrist. Children with arthritis frequently complain of pain or withdraw their arm with maneuvers to test flexion and extension in the wrist.

The metacarpophalangeal (MCP) joint and the proximal and distal interphalangeal (PIP and DIP) joints should be individually palpated, and any swelling, tenderness, or warmth should be noted. The examiner should flex and extend MCP joints, looking for limitations. To test the range of motion of the PIP and DIP joints, the child should try to supinate the hand and flex all of the digits, attempting to touch the fingertips to the palm. To examine the first MCP and thumb interphalangeal joint, the child should try to touch the tip of the thumb to the base of the fifth finger. Grip strength is determined by having the child tightly squeeze two of the clinician's fingers. Arthritis of the wrist or any of the small joints of the hand decreases grip strength.

The child should next lie in a supine position, either in the parent's lap or on the examination table so that the lower extremities can be examined. Each hip is taken through its range of motion, beginning with flexion by trying to bring the knee as close to the chest as possible, and any pain or limitation is noted. With the hip and knee each flexed to 90 degrees, internal and external rotation are tested by keeping the knee in a fixed position and turning the lower leg laterally and medially, thereby rotating the femur. The hip and knee are extended back to neutral supine position and abduction tested. With the child in the prone position, the examiner evaluates hip extension by placing one hand on the child's ipsilateral iliac crest and lifting the child's thigh posteriorly with the knee extended. Hip arthritis most often causes limitations with internal rotation and extension, usually in association with pain in the inguinal area.

The knee is inspected for effusions and other obvious deformities. Palpation of the knee reveals warmth, a common finding in knee arthritis, and synovial swelling or an effusion. Applying pressure in the suprapatellar area with one hand while palpating on either side of the patella with the other allows the detection of effusions more readily, as this forces excessive joint fluid that has accumulated in the suprapatellar area into the synovial space. Small effusions may be detected by eliciting a *bulge sign*. This is done by milking the medial and lateral depressions around the patella superiorly in an effort to push the fluid into the suprapatellar space and then gently pushing either medially or laterally just superior to the patella. This releases the fluid back into the synovial space, causing the area medial to the patella to bulge out. The popliteal fossa should be palpated, because fluid tends to track posteriorly as more accumulates, producing fullness in the popliteal fossa and sometimes a frank cyst, identical to the *Baker cysts* seen in adults with rheumatoid arthritis.

Palpating around the edges of the patella causes pain in many adolescents with patellofemoral syndrome (also known as chondromalacia patellae), a common cause of knee pain in active adolescents. In another maneuver that elicits pain in this syndrome, the patient relaxes the quadriceps muscles while the examiner pushes the patella inferiorly. While the examiner maintains pressure on the patella, the patient contracts the quadriceps. In addition to pain, a grinding sensation is often felt with this maneuver in patients with patellofemoral syndrome. The tibial tubercle and patellar tendon should be inspected and palpated for swelling and tenderness associated with Osgood-Schlatter disease and patellar tendonitis.

Flexing and extending the knee test the knee's range of motion. Most young children can touch their heel to their buttocks, and, as with the elbow, the ability to hyperextend the knee in childhood is common. The examiner can detect subtle limitations in extension by standing at the foot of the table and lifting the heels of the child off the table as the child holds his or her legs fully extended. If one knee is limited, the patella on that side is slightly more elevated.

Swelling in the ankles is often best seen when inspecting and palpating the posterior aspect of the ankle, where fullness on either side of the Achilles tendon may be appreciated, between the tendon and the malleoli. Warmth is common with ankle arthritis. Range-of-motion testing of the ankle should include both the ankle joint itself (tibiotalar) and the subtalar (talocalcaneal) joint. Cupping the child's heel with one hand and using the other hand to grasp the child's forefoot allows the examiner to move the forefoot superiorly (dorsiflexion) and inferiorly (plantar flexion). The hand cupping the heel is rocked laterally and medially to check inversion and eversion associated with motion at the subtalar joint. Holding the heel firmly with the cupped hand and gently rotating the forefoot with the other hand test the joints of the midfoot. Each of the metatarsophalangeal joints is palpated along with each of the toes. The toes are inspected for the presence of swelling. The plantar fascia and the Achilles tendon are palpated, and any tenderness or swelling is noted.

The child should stand so that the examiner can evaluate the back. The sacroiliac joints are palpated, any tenderness is noted, and the child is asked to keep the knees extended and bend forward, touching the hands to the ground if possible. The lumbar spine should curve forward normally without flattening. The Schober measurement, which reveals whether the lumbar spine flexes normally, is done by marking the lumbar spine at a point where a horizontal line connecting the iliac crests intersects the spine. Then the examiner measures 10 cm above and 5 cm below that spot while the child is standing. When the child bends forward, the distance between the top and bottom marks should increase to at least 21 cm as the vertebral bodies separate during flexion. A shorter distance suggests arthritis within the facet joints of the spine. Scoliosis is detected by noting any asymmetric elevation of the shoulder and upper back while the child bends forward.

Although the examiner is looking primarily for limitation of motion during the joint examination, the presence of hyperextensible joints may be significant. This is a common cause of pain associated with sports and other activities; it tends to improve with rest. Hypermobility, patellofemoral syndrome, frequent ankle sprains, and pes planus are frequently seen together. The hypermobile child or adolescent can hyperextend the knees and elbows, appose the thumb to the forearm while flexing the wrist, hyperextend the MCP joints so that the digits are parallel to the forearm when the wrist is extended, and easily put the palms flat on the floor while bending forward from a standing position with the knees locked. Extreme hypermobility is seen in individuals with Ehlers-Danlos syndrome or Marfan syndrome.

The presence of "trigger" points is consistent with fibromyalgia. These are exquisitely tender, well-localized points at the occiput, trapezius muscles, medial borders of the scapula; at the upper outer quadrant of the buttocks; at the second cervical space anteriorly; at the second costochondral space, just distal to the lateral epicondyle on the forearm; over the greater trochanter in the proximal leg; and over the medial aspect of the knees. Their presence in the older child with diffuse pain, fatigue, and difficulty sleeping is highly suggestive of fibromyalgia.

Proximal muscle strength testing should be performed in any patient complaining of weakness or fatigue. The deltoids, biceps, triceps, psoas, quadriceps, and hamstrings are tested. Neck flexor weakness is common in dermatomyositis and polymyositis, and it is tested by having the child lie supine and lift only his or her head. Most children are able to lift and keep the head elevated, even if asked to resist pressure with the examiner's hand against the forehead. To test muscle strength, the child performs a sit-up, although young, healthy children may have difficulty performing a sit-up. To test proximal leg strength, the child rises from a sitting position on the floor. In addition to strength testing, inspecting for muscular atrophy is useful. Chronic knee arthritis or hip disease leads to atrophy of the ipsilateral quadriceps. Similarly, ankle arthritis causes the gastrocnemius to atrophy; wrist arthritis leads to wasting of the forearm muscles; and elbow contractures cause atrophy of the triceps muscle. The atrophy is easily overlooked, and it is sometimes helpful to measure the circumference of the thigh, calf, or upper arm to detect asymmetry.

The skin and mucous membranes should be examined carefully, as there may be clues to the presence of systemic disease (Table 44-3).

Table 44-3. Skin Manifestations of Rheumatic Disease

Physical Finding	Possible Disease
Petechiae, purpura	Vasculitis (if palpable)
	Leukemia
	Meningococcemia
	Other infections
	SLE
Erythema nodosum	Inflammatory bowel disease
	Streptococcal infection
	Sarcoidosis
	Drugs
	Tuberculosis
	Fungal infection
Gottron papules	Dermatomyositis
Alopecia	SLE, hypothyroidism
Calcification	Dermatomyositis, CREST syndrome
Subcutaneous nodules	Polyarticular JRA, rheumatic fever
Oral ulcers	SLE, Behçet disease, inflammatory bowel disease, reactive arthritis
Genital ulcers	Behçet disease
Digital ulcers	Vasculitis, SLE, scleroderma
Tight, thickened skin	Scleroderma
Livedo reticularis	Antiphospholipid syndrome, SLE
Nail dystrophy or pits	Psoriasis
Edema	SLE, vasculitis, scleroderma, eosinophilic fasciitis, serum sickness
Desquamation	Kawasaki disease, scarlet fever
Cyanosis	Raynaud phenomenon, hypertrophic osteoarthropathy

CREST, calcinosis, Raynaud phenomenon, esophageal dysmotility, sclerodactyly, and telangiectasias; JRA, juvenile rheumatoid arthritis; SLE, systemic lupus erythematosus.

Systemic JRA, SLE, acute rheumatic fever, and dermatomyositis are associated with characteristic rashes. Petechiae or palpable purpura suggests vasculitis. Nodules are seen with acute rheumatic fever and some forms of JRA. Thickening and tightening of the skin, particularly over the distal extremities and face, are often present in scleroderma. Nasal or palatal ulcers suggest SLE, whereas aphthous ulceration may be seen with inflammatory bowel disease or Behçet disease. Alopecia, either well localized or diffuse, may be detected by the examiner without being recognized by the patient. The presence of peripheral or periorbital edema increases the suspicion of glomerulonephritis.

LABORATORY STUDIES

Laboratory testing should be considered when the diagnosis is unclear or when there is a suspicion of serious, life-threatening disease such as leukemia, septic arthritis, or osteomyelitis. JRA is not a diagnosis made by laboratory testing. Tests frequently seen in "arthritis panels" such as those for antinuclear antibody (ANA), rheumatoid factor (RF), and the erythrocyte sedimentation rate (ESR) are not specific for arthritis. If arthritis is detected on physical examination, laboratory testing aids in classifying the specific type of arthritis that is present.

A complete blood cell (CBC) count with differential is useful as a means of decreasing the suspicion of an acute infection or leukemia, which sometimes manifests with bone or joint pain or even frank arthritis. A normal CBC count is reassuring, but it is also helpful to compare the platelet count to the ESR. Because platelets are an acute phase reactant, their number should increase as the ESR increases. A normal or only slightly low platelet count in a child with a markedly elevated ESR increases the suspicion of leukemia.

An elevated white blood cell (WBC) count is often present with septic arthritis or osteomyelitis, but it is neither sensitive nor specific enough to change the diagnostic impression formulated after the history and physical examination. In systemic JRA, the WBC count may be markedly elevated, at 20,000 WBCs/mm³ or greater; the hemoglobin may be very low, at 6 or 7 mg/dL; and the platelet count is typically elevated. For many of the other inflammatory diseases that are associated with arthritis or extremity pain, a mild to moderate anemia as well as a mild thrombocytosis is common. SLE may demonstrate anemia, leukopenia, and thrombocytopenia.

The ESR is helpful in the rare instances when the physical examination is inconclusive regarding the presence or absence of an inflammatory condition. In uncooperative or obese children, it may be difficult to detect small effusions or subtle limitation in the range of motion. In these instances, an elevated ESR increases the suspicion of arthritis. In children who clearly have rheumatic disease or infection, the ESR is not diagnostically useful, but it may be used to monitor the disease.

A urinalysis is an excellent screen for glomerulonephritis, often present in patients with vasculitis or SLE. Proteinuria or red blood cell casts suggest renal involvement. The creatinine level is elevated with renal insufficiency. Severe proteinuria leads to hypoalbuminemia, which may also be seen without proteinuria in systemic JRA. Kawasaki disease is associated with sterile pyuria. Liver transaminases are elevated in patients with hepatitis and occasionally in patients with SLE. In those with myositis, elevated transaminases are frequently associated with increased creatine kinase, lactate dehydrogenase, and aldolase levels.

The ANA test is a sensitive screening test for SLE because it is positive in more than 95% of patients, who also usually have high ANA titers, typically values of 1:640 or higher. Lower ANA titers, usually in the range of 1:40 to 1:160, are seen in children with JRA, healthy children, or those with other illnesses. The ANA positivity varies in the different forms of JRA (see later discussion); those with a positive test result and younger than 7 years are at the greatest risk of developing uveitis and therefore should be evaluated more frequently by an ophthalmologist. The pattern of the ANA is rarely helpful. Homogeneous and speckled patterns are most common and are not specific for any illness. A peripheral or "rim" pattern is usually associated with anti–double-stranded DNA (anti-dsDNA) antibodies and is more specific for SLE. A nucleolar pattern suggests the presence of anti–SCL 70 antibodies, which may be seen in patients with scleroderma.

The ANA test is not specific and should not be used unless there is a strong suspicion of SLE or another rheumatic disease. A positive ANA finding is present in some asymptomatic healthy children; in children with viral illnesses, other infections, and other rheumatic diseases such as dermatomyositis; and in relatives of those with autoimmune illnesses such as SLE or hypothyroidism.

The RF test is not diagnostic. It is also not very sensitive. Only 5% of children with JRA have a positive RF result, and this usually occurs in teenagers with adult-like polyarticular disease. RF is an immunoglobulin M antibody directed against immunoglobulin G. In children with polyarthritis, the presence of RF is a poor prognostic factor; these children have a high likelihood of developing chronic, erosive arthritis. A positive test result for RF can be seen with other illnesses associated with the formation of immune complexes, including rheumatic diseases such as SLE or vasculitis, and with infectious diseases such as bacterial endocarditis and infectious mononucleosis. The RF test is not helpful diagnostically; it is useful for determining the prognosis of patients with chronic polyarticular arthritis.

If the history and physical examination findings are suggestive of SLE, additional autoantibody testing is helpful (Table 44-4). Anti-dsDNA antibodies and anti-Smith antibodies are highly specific for SLE. Antiribonucleoprotein antibodies may be seen in patients with SLE and, when present in isolation (without anti-dsDNA and anti-Smith antibodies), suggest *mixed connective tissue disease,* which has features of SLE, dermatomyositis, and scleroderma. Anti–Sjögren syndrome type A (anti-SSA [also known as anti-Ro]) and anti–Sjögren syndrome type B (anti-SSB [also known as anti-La]) antibodies are occasionally seen in patients with SLE but are not specific. They are seen in *Sjögren syndrome,* an illness producing chronic inflammation of the salivary and lacrimal glands and resulting in xerostomia and xerophthalmia.

Anticardiolipin antibodies, one of several antiphospholipid antibodies, may be present in SLE, but they are also seen in asymptomatic individuals and the *antiphospholipid antibody syndrome,* in which clinical manifestations are restricted to the complications of the hypercoagulable state associated with these antibodies. These complications include venous and arterial thromboses and recurrent spontaneous abortions. Many patients with SLE have a false-positive Venereal Disease Research Laboratory result because this measure is also a test for antiphospholipid antibodies. A positive direct Coombs test result, indicative of an autoimmune hemolytic anemia, is common in patients with SLE, although rarely is the hemolysis clinically significant. The complement proteins C3 and C4 are often depressed in patients with active SLE, which indicates consumption of C3 and C4 secondary to the formation of numerous immune complexes. Some patients with hereditary complement deficiencies develop SLE. Low levels of complement can be seen occasionally with the vasculitides and in other illnesses with immune complexes, such as bacterial endocarditis. The CH_{50} is a functional assay that measures the activity of the entire complement cascade. If any single complement protein is depressed, this may cause a decrease in the CH_{50}. The CH_{50} is less sensitive and less specific than testing for the individual complement components.

Wegener granulomatosis is the only vasculitis that can be diagnosed with confidence on the basis of serologic testing. Anti–proteinase 3 antibodies, previously identified as a cytoplasmic-staining antineutrophil cytoplasmic antibody, are 95% sensitive and specific for this disease. The antimyeloperoxidase antibody is much less specific; it is present with other vasculitides and a variety of infectious and inflammatory illnesses.

Table 44-4. Autoantibodies in Children

Test	Characteristics
Antinuclear antibody (ANA)	99% sensitive in SLE; very nonspecific
Anti–double-stranded DNA (dsDNA)	70%-80% sensitive for SLE; highly specific (nearly 100%)
Anti–single-stranded DNA (ssDNA)	Like ANA, sensitive for SLE but very nonspecific
Anti-Smith (Sm)	20%-35% sensitive in SLE; nearly 100% specific
Anti-SSA (Anti-Ro)	50% sensitive in SLE; seen in asymptomatic children and in Sjögren syndrome, scleroderma
Anti-SSB (Anti-La)	15% sensitive in SLE; seen in similar conditions as anti-SSA
Antiribonucleoprotein (RNP)	15%-40% sensitive in SLE; also seen in mixed connective tissue disease
Antihistone	Drug-induced SLE-like syndromes
Anti-IgG (RF)	30% of SLE patients; 5% of JRA; also seen in infections
Antineutrophil cytoplasmic (ANCA)	
Antiproteinase 3 (C-ANCA)	90%-95% sensitive and specific for Wegener granulomatosis
Antimyeloperoxidase (P-ANCA)	Very nonspecific; seen in other vasculitides, inflammatory bowel disease, other inflammatory diseases
Anti-RBC membrane (Coombs positive)	10%-50% sensitive in SLE; nonspecific, seen also in Evan syndrome, isolated hemolytic anemia
Anticardiolipin	Seen in SLE; nonspecific, seen in asymptomatic children and in those with antiphospholipid syndrome

IgG, immunoglobulin G; JRA, juvenile rheumatoid arthritis; RBC, red blood cell; RF, rheumatoid factor; SLE, systemic lupus erythematosus; SSA and SSB, Sjögren syndrome type A and type B.

Viral infections such as human parvovirus B19, Epstein-Barr virus, and rubella may be associated with arthralgias or arthritis, and testing for antibodies to these viruses may be helpful in some clinical situations. For diagnosing Lyme disease, the enzyme-linked immunosorbent assay (ELISA) is a very sensitive, but not specific, screening test. A positive ELISA is confirmed by Western blot (Table 44-5).

DIAGNOSTIC IMAGING

RADIOGRAPHS

Plain radiographs of the limbs are helpful as a means of excluding infections, trauma, leukemia, and solid bone tumors. Osteomyelitis usually causes periosteal elevation, which may be seen after approximately 1 week of illness. Chronic osteomyelitis causes abscesses that may be visualized on plain radiographs. Fractures, including stress fractures and small avulsion fractures, are occasionally detected even when the clinical information is not strongly suggestive. Leukemia can cause lucency within the metaphysis of

the long bones. Solid tumors, including *osteosarcomas, Ewing sarcoma,* and the benign *osteoid osteoma,* may all be identified on plain radiographs. Because knee pain may reflect referred pain from the hip, any child with unexplained knee or thigh pain should have pelvis and hip radiographs, including a "frog-leg" view. The young, limping child may have *Legg-Calvé-Perthes disease,* an avascular necrosis of the femoral head. A *slipped capital femoral epiphysis* is classically seen in an overweight patient in his or her early teens (see Chapter 45).

In the child with arthritis, soft tissue swelling or effusions within the joint may be identified on plain radiographs. Chronic arthritis may demonstrate bone erosions and juxtaarticular osteopenia. Radiographs are most useful in monitoring the course of the disease and can sometimes help guide management.

In children with suspected SLE, a chest radiograph may reveal an enlarged cardiac silhouette, suggestive of a pericardial effusion or the presence of pleural effusions. If Wegener granulomatosis is a consideration, a chest radiograph may reveal bilateral cavitating pulmonary nodules. Pulmonary hemorrhage, with bilateral alveolar infiltrates, can be seen with Wegener granulomatosis, as well as SLE and other vasculitides.

MAGNETIC RESONANCE IMAGING

Magnetic resonance imaging (MRI) is useful when plain radiographs either are unrevealing or have identified a poorly defined abnormality. The MRI, a sensitive test for osteomyelitis and avascular necrosis, can reveal small joint effusions that are not apparent on physical examination. MRI helps distinguish hemarthrosis from other forms of joint swelling and detects ligamentous and meniscal tears. The MRI provides better visualization and characterization of tumors than do plain radiographs. If myositis is suspected, MRI may reveal increased signal within the muscle as a result of inflammation and can help determine a potential biopsy site.

BONE SCAN

A bone scan is useful when plain radiographs are unremarkable and when the source of pain cannot be adequately localized. It is a sensitive test for inflammation in the bones and joints, and it can help

Table 44-5. Criteria for Diagnosing Lyme Disease

Characteristic clinical presentation
Exposure in an endemic area*
Positive Lyme ELISA, confirmed by positive Western blot
Western blots are considered positive if the following are present:
  For IgM, two of the following three bands must be present:
    23, 39, 41 kd
  For IgG, five of the following 10 bands must be present:
    18, 21, 28, 30, 39, 41, 45, 58, 66, 93 kd

*Mid-Atlantic and Southern New England coastal regions, northwestern Wisconsin, and eastern Minnesota are considered the most endemic regions in North America. Even within these regions, incidence of infection can vary widely.

ELISA, enzyme-linked immunosorbent assay.

Table 44-6. Affected Joint Distribution in Adults and Children with Nongonococcal Bacterial Arthritis

	Percentage of Cases	
Joint	*Adults*	*Children*
Knee	55	40
Hip	11	28
Ankle	8	14
Shoulder	8	4
Wrist	7	3
Elbow	6	11
Others	5	3
More than one joint, usually two	12	7

From Goldenberg DL: Bacterial arthritis. In Kelley WN, Harris ED, Ruddy S, et al (eds): Textbook of Rheumatology, 4th ed, vol. 2. Philadelphia, WB Saunders, 1993, p 1450.

distinguish arthritis from osteomyelitis, fractures, and tumors. Bone scans, like plain radiographs, are not as sensitive for osteomyelitis if obtained very early in the disease process, and a second scan should be considered if the initial study is negative. A bone scan may detect osteoid osteomas that are not apparent on plain radiographs. Reflex sympathic dystrophy usually demonstrates asymmetric increased uptake on the affected side.

OTHER IMAGING STUDIES

Ultrasonography helps evaluate the hip for transient synovitis. In a young child, it may be difficult to examine the painful hip; an ultrasonogram may identify an effusion. Ultrasonography is rarely helpful with other joints because effusions are more readily apparent on physical examination. *Echocardiography* is useful when acute rheumatic fever is a consideration. "Silent" valvulitis with resulting insufficiency is detected only by echocardiography. The echocardiogram can detect pericardial effusions in patients with SLE and coronary artery aneurysms in patients with Kawasaki disease.

Angiography is useful for the diagnosis of medium- or large-vessel vasculitis such as polyarteritis nodosa or Takayasu arteritis. *Computed tomography* of the chest is helpful in patients with Wegener granulomatosis (pulmonary nodules) and in those with scleroderma, in whom basilar lung fibrosis may be detected.

JOINT FLUID ASPIRATION

There are few indications for aspirating joint fluid diagnostically in the child with arthritis. The analysis of joint fluid in childhood is helpful for confirming or excluding three possible problems: (1) infectious arthritis, (2) hemarthrosis (either secondary to trauma or a coagulopathy), and (3) crystal diseases (gout, pseudogout). A fourth condition, the rare entity of *pigmented villonodular synovitis*, is suggested by the aspiration of a "chocolate-brown" synovial fluid from the knee.

Among these possibilities, only infection is a common consideration in childhood; infection can usually be excluded on the basis of the history and physical examination findings. The child with septic arthritis is typically febrile and has developed joint pain, swelling, warmth, and occasionally erythema, usually in a single joint (Table 44-6), within a short period of time (hours to a few days). When septic arthritis is suspected, the joint fluid is sent for cell count, protein analysis, glucose measurement, Gram stain, and culture (Tables 44-7 and 44-8). Some infectious arthritides develop more indolently, such as gonococcal arthritis, tuberculous arthritis, and opportunistic infections in immunocompromised hosts. Management is noted in Table 44-9. Teenagers with monarticular arthritis (Table 44-10) should undergo joint aspiration, regardless of other symptoms, if they have risk factors for gonococcal disease. Likewise, if there has been exposure to tuberculosis, or if a child is immunocompromised, joint fluid aspiration should be strongly considered.

If the child has sustained trauma and it is unclear from the history and physical examination whether a joint effusion is inflammatory or hemorrhagic, joint fluid analysis may be helpful. Similarly, if there is history of a bleeding disorder in the family or in the child, joint aspiration should be considered (Table 44-11; see Table 44-7).

Gout and pseudogout are unusual in childhood. Conditions that result in elevated serum uric acid levels predispose a child to gout, and if children with these conditions develop arthritis, the joint fluid should be analyzed for crystals. These conditions include leukemias, tumor lysis syndrome, renal failure, Down syndrome, Lesch-Nyhan syndrome, and type I glycogen storage disease.

ADDITIONAL TESTS

If weakness is present, an electromyogram (EMG) and a nerve conduction study help distinguish myopathies and myositis from neuropathies. Children with inflammatory myositis have a characteristic, albeit nondiagnostic, abnormal EMG. Peripheral neuropathies

Table 44-7. Classification of Synovial Effusions

Gross Examination	Normal	"Noninflammatory"	Inflammatory	Septic
Volume (knee)	<1 mL	Often >1 mL	Often >1 mL	Often >1 mL
Viscosity	High	High	Low	Variable
Color	Colorless to straw	Straw to yellow	Yellow	Variable
Clarity	Transparent	Transparent	Translucent	Opaque
WBCs/mm³†	<200	200-2000	2000-75,000	Often >100,000
PMNs†	<25%	<25%	Often >50%	>85%
Culture	Negative	Negative	Negative	Often positive
Mucin clot	Firm	Firm	Friable	Friable
Glucose	Nearly equal to blood	Nearly equal to blood	<50 mg/dL lower than blood	>50 mg/dL lower than blood

From Schumacher HR: Synovial fluid analysis and synovial biopsy. In Kelley WN, Harris ED, Ruddy S, et al (eds): Textbook of Rheumatology, 4th ed, vol 1. Philadelphia, WB Saunders, 1993, p 562.

†WBC count and PMN percentage are less if organism is less virulent or partially treated.

PMN, polymorphonuclear neutrophil; WBC, white blood cell.

Table 44-8. Synovial Fluid Examination in the Diagnosis of Bacterial Arthritis

Procedure	Important Technical Aspects	Diagnostic Yield
Culture	Plate immediately or inoculate in blood culture bottles	Nearly 100% positive in nongonococcal bacterial arthritis but only 25%-50% positive in gonococcal arthritis
Gram stain smear	Best yield if centrifuge fluid False-positive gram-positive from precipitated mucin	75% positive with gram-positive cocci, 50% with gram-negative bacilli, less than 25% in gonococcal arthritis
Leukocyte count and differential leukocyte count	Generally greater than 50,000 cells/mm^3 and greater than 80% PMNs	Significant overlap with noninfectious arthritis (RA, crystal-induced)
Glucose	Less than 50% of fasting, simultaneous blood glucose	Helpful but often not present and may be seen in RA
Detection of bacterial cell wall antigens	Counterimmunoelectrophoresis or similar immune test	Generally not useful, except in *Haemophilus influenzae* and *Streptococcus pneumoniae* arthritis

Modified from Goldenberg DL: Bacterial arthritis. In Kelley WN, Harris ED, Ruddy S, et al (eds): Textbook of Rheumatology, 4th ed, vol 2. Philadelphia, WB Saunders, 1993, p 1451.

PMN, polymorphonuclear neutrophil; RA, rheumatoid arthritis.

confirmed by nerve conduction studies may suggest the presence of a vasculitis or SLE.

Biopsies are most helpful in confirming the presence of vasculitis (Table 44-12) and to determine the extent of renal disease in a child with SLE. Wegener granulomatosis, Kawasaki disease, Takayasu arteritis, polyarteritis, and Henoch-Schönlein purpura are types of vasculitis that may be diagnosed on the basis of either clinical criteria alone (Kawasaki disease, Henoch-Schönlein purpura), a combination of clinical criteria and arteriography (Takayasu arteritis, polyarteritis), or clinical criteria and serologic profiles (anti–proteinase 3 antibodies in Wegener granulomatosis). Biopsies of affected tissue are often necessary to confirm a diagnosis. The most accessible affected tissue is acquired for biopsy first. In many children with vasculitis, this tissue is the skin. If there is no rash, muscle and nerve samples are taken for biopsy when EMG and nerve conduction studies reveal the presence of myositis or neuropathy. If neither of these sites is affected, then the risks and benefits of biopsy of affected organs are evaluated.

Synovial biopsy is rarely useful in the evaluation of arthritis. Biopsy is necessary to distinguish sarcoid arthropathy from JRA; sarcoid arthropathy is suspected when the young child has erythema nodosum, uveitis, and arthritis, as well as particularly "boggy" synovial effusions. In rare cases, synovial tumors, chronic indolent infections, or foreign bodies are detected by biopsy as well.

SPECIFIC DISEASES

JUVENILE RHEUMATOID ARTHRITIS

There are specific criteria for diagnosing JRA in a child (Table 44-13). There are at least five forms of JRA, each with a slightly different pattern of joint involvement, epidemiologic characteristics, associated features, and prognosis (Table 44-14). In Europe, the terms *juvenile chronic arthritis, juvenile arthritis,* and *juvenile idiopathic arthritis* have been used to describe the same group of illnesses. The old term *Still disease* is rarely used.

Pauciarticular Juvenile Rheumatoid Arthritis

This is the most common form of JRA, affecting half of all children with JRA. There are two subtypes of pauciarticular JRA. Pauciarticular type I, the more frequent subtype, most commonly manifests as monarticular arthritis of the knee. Most affected children have morning stiffness, mild discomfort, swelling, and warmth of the affected joint or joints, but they usually remain fairly functional. Most such children have a positive ANA test result, which places them at the highest risk for associated chronic anterior uveitis.

Pauciarticular JRA type II is referred to as a spondyloarthropathy because of the similarity in pattern and associated features to the seronegative spondyloarthropathies such as psoriatic arthritis, ankylosing spondylitis, and the arthritis of inflammatory bowel disease. The arthritis is more episodic and recurrent than other forms of

Table 44-9. Treatment of Bacterial Arthritis

1. Aspirate any possible infected joint immediately. Remove as much fluid as possible and perform synovial fluid culture, Gram stain, leukocytes count and differential leukocyte count, glucose with simultaneous blood glucose determinations, and crystal analysis.
2. If the fluid is purulent or if organisms are seen on the Gram stain smear, start antibiotics immediately:
    a. Organisms identified on Gram stain: If gram-positive cocci, start nafcillin or (if in hospital with methicillin-resistant *Staphylococcus aureus*) vancomycin. If gram-negative cocci, start ceftriaxone. If gram-negative bacilli, start an aminoglycoside and third-generation cephalosporin.
    b. Negative Gram stain: In children younger than 2 years, cover for penicillin-resistant *Haemophilus influenzae*, staphylococci, and gram-negative bacilli. In compromised hosts and intravenous drug users, cover for methicillin-resistent *S. aureus* and gram-negative bacilli.
3. When the specific bacterium is identified, adjust antibiotics if necessary. Administer antibiotics parenterally and in doses used to treat bacteremia.
4. Drain all purulent fluid with closed-needle aspiration, arthroscopy, or arthrotomy.
5. Reassess adequacy of treatment clinically and with serial synovial fluid analysis. If inadequate therapeutic response, obtain serum and synovial fluid bactericidal concentrations, and evaluate the efficacy of drainage.
6. Treat 4-8 wk for *S. aureus,* 2 wk for gonococcus. Treat intravenously until improvement occurs and then by mouth if organism is isolated and if serum levels on oral antibiotics are equal to those with intravenous therapy.

Modified from Goldenberg DL: Bacterial arthritis. In Kelley WN, Harris ED, Ruddy S, et al (eds): Textbook of Rheumatology, 4th ed, vol 2. Philadelphia, WB Saunders, 1993, p 1458.

Table 44-10. Differential Diagnosis of Monarticular Arthritis

Usually Monarticular	Often Polyarticular
Common	
Septic arthritis	Rheumatoid arthritis
Bacterial	Psoriatic arthritis
Tuberculous	Reactive arthritis
Fungal	Chronic articular
Lyme disease	hemorrhage
Avascular necrosis	Most JRA and juvenile
Hemarthrosis	spondylitis
Coagulopathy	Erythema nodosum/
Warfarin (Coumadin)	sarcoidosis
Trauma/overuse	Serum sickness
Pauciarticular JRA	Acute hepatitis B
Congenital hip dysplasia	Rubella
Osteochondritis dissecans	Henoch-Schönlein purpura
Reflex sympathetic dystrophy	Systemic lupus
Hemoglobinopathies	erythematosus
Stress fracture	Lyme disease
Osteomyelitis	Parvovirus
Metastatic tumor	Dialysis arthropathy
(neuroblastoma, leukemia)	Crystal-induced arthropathies
Synovial	Immune complex
osteochondromatosis	postbacteremia
Hypermobility	(meningococcus,
	Haemophilus influenzae)
Rare	
Pigmented villonodular	Undifferentiated connective
synovitis	tissue disease
Plant-thorn synovitis	Relapsing polychondritis
Familial Mediterranean fever	Enteropathic disease
Synovioma	Ulcerative colitis
Synovial metastasis	Regional enteritis
Intermittent hydrarthrosis	Whipple disease
Pancreatic fat necrosis	Chronic sarcoidosis
Gaucher disease	Hyperlipidemias types II
Behçet disease	and IV
Regional migratory	Still disease
osteoporosis	Pyoderma gangenosum
Sea urchin spine	Pulmonary hypertrophic
Amyloidosis (myeloma)	osteoarthropathy
Uric acid arthropathy	Chrondrocalcinosis-like
	syndromes caused by
	ochronosis, hemochro-
	matosis, Wilson disease
	Rheumatic fever
	Paraneoplastic syndromes

Modified from McCune WJ: Monarticular arthritis. In Kelley WN, Harris ED, Ruddy S, et al (eds): Textbook of Rheumatology, 4th ed, vol 1. Philadelphia, WB Saunders, 1993, p 369.

JRA, juvenile rheumatoid arthritis

Table 44-11. Hemarthroses

Trauma with or without fractures
Pigmented villonodular synovitis
Tumors
Hemangioma
Hemophilia or other bleeding disorders
von Willebrand disease
Anticoagulant therapy
Myeloproliferative disease
Thrombocytopenia
Scurvy
Ruptured aneurysm
Arteriovenous fistula
Idiopathic
Intense inflammatory disease

Modified from Schumacher HR: Synovial fluid analysis and synovial biopsy. In Kelley WN, Harris ED, Ruddy S, et al: (eds): Textbook of Rheumatology, 4th ed., vol 1. Philadephia, WB Saunders, 1993, p 563.

a family history of psoriasis, inflammatory bowel disease, or ankylosing spondylitis. Some children with this form of peripheral arthritis develop ankylosing spondylitis.

Polyarticular Juvenile Rheumatoid Arthritis

There are two subtypes of polyarticular JRA: RF-positive, and RF-negative. Patients with RF-positive disease tend to have more aggressive, destructive arthritis and more associated constitutional symptoms such as fatigue and poor appetite. The arthritis in these subtypes is symmetric and affects both small and large joints, and involvement of the small joints of the hands and feet, as well as the wrists, is very common. Chronic anterior uveitis may occur; it is

Table 44-12. Classification of Vasculitis

Arteritis Group
Kawasaki disease*
Polyarteritis nodosa
Cutaneous polyarteritis
Microscopic polyangiitis
Cogan syndrome

Leukocytoclastic Vasculitis
Henoch-Schönlein purpura*
Hypersensitivity vasculitis*
Hypocomplementemic urticarial vasculitis
Cryoglobulinemia

Granulomatous Vasculitis
Wegener granulomatosis*
Churg-Strauss syndrome
Lymphomatoid granulomatosis
Isolated central nervous system vasculitis

Giant Cell Vasculitis
Temporal arteritis/giant cell arteritis
Takayasu arteritis*

*Those labeled are the most common in childhood within each group. Others are rare in childhood.

Modified from Cassidy JT, Petty RE: Textbook of Pediatric Rheumatology, 4th ed. Philadelphia, WB Saunders, 2001, p 566.

chronic arthritis in childhood. Certain joints, such as the sacroiliac joints and the first metatarsophalangeal joint, are more commonly affected in children with spondyloarthropathies. Enthesitis, inflammation and pain at tendon insertion sites (e.g., Achilles tendon), tendon sheath swelling, and plantar fasciitis are common associated features; these children are at risk for acute uveitis. Arthritis may be the first manifestation of psoriatic arthritis or inflammatory bowel disease, preceding the other manifestations of these illnesses by years. Many affected children have HLA-B27 antigen; there may be

Table 44-13. Diagnostic Criteria for the Classification of Juvenile Rheumatoid Arthritis

Age at onset <16 years
Arthritis, defined as:
  Joint swelling or joint effusion
       Or
  The presence of at least two of the following:
    Limited range of motion
    Tenderness, or pain with motion
    Warmth or heat over the joint
Duration of arthritis at least 6 weeks
Onset-type classified at 6 months after onset as:
  Pauciarticular (or oligoarticular): four or fewer joints with arthritis
  Polyarticular: five or more joints with arthritis
  Systemic: any number of joints with arthritis associated with fever, other systemic symptoms and signs
Exclusion of other causes of childhood arthritis

Modified from Cassidy JT, Levinson JE, Bass JG, et al: A study of classification criteria for a diagnosis of juvenile rheumatoid arthritis. Arthritis Rheum 1986;29:274.

more common in younger patients, especially if their ANA test results are positive.

Systemic Juvenile Rheumatoid Arthritis

Any number of joints may be affected, but polyarticular involvement is most often eventually seen. Children with systemic JRA initially have a characteristic fever pattern of one or two high fever spikes each day, and an evanescent, pink, macular rash appears with the fever and may resolve completely as the child's fever abates (see Figs. 44-3 and 44-4). Initially, such children may be thought to have a fever of unknown origin (see Chapter 54). Constitutional symptoms such as fatigue, poor appetite, and weight loss are common. Generalized lymphadenopathy and hepatosplenomegaly are also common; pericarditis or pleural effusions may be seen. These children feel and appear ill during the fever spikes, but they may appear much improved once the fever abates. Very high peripheral WBC counts (20,000 WBCs/high-power field or greater), anemia and subsequent pallor, and thrombocytosis are characteristic laboratory findings. ANA and RF test results are usually negative, and uveitis is very rare.

Diagnosis

The diagnosis of JRA is based on clinical features. The differential diagnosis includes the diseases listed in Table 44-1 and in Tables 44-15 and 44-16. Lyme disease should always be considered (Table 44-17). Laboratory tests and imaging studies are used when necessary to exclude other illnesses. The ANA and RF tests are used to classify the subtype of JRA and to determine the risk of uveitis, but they are not diagnostic tests.

Treatment

The treatment of JRA is multidisciplinary. Medical treatment begins with nonsteroidal antiinflammatory drugs (NSAIDs). Naproxen is often used first because it is available as a liquid, can be given twice a day, and is approved for use in children. Physical therapy and occupational therapy (PT/OT) are a helpful adjunct to medication, as they promote range of motion of the stiff joint and the strengthening of muscles that may have become atrophic. Families are instructed about range-of-motion exercises and help the child perform these at

Table 44-14. Characteristics of Subtypes of Juvenile Rheumatoid Arthritis (JRA)
Pauciarticular Type I 35% of all cases of JRA Mostly girls (gender ratio, 4-8:1) Very young children (average age, 2 yr) Affects large joints; knee most common Chronic anterior uveitis more common (~15%-20%) No systemic symptoms ANA common (40%-90%); RF negative Prognosis favorable (most remissions occur within 5 years) **Pauciarticular Type II** 15% of all cases of JRA Mostly boys (gender ratio, 7:1) Preteens and adolescents Affects large joints, lower extremities, sacroiliac joints Acute anterior uveitis (~10%) Inflammatory bowel disease may develop ANA, RF negative Prognosis guarded; remission may occur, but patient at risk for spondylitis as adult **Polyarticular Rheumatoid Factor Positive** 5% of all cases of JRA Mostly girls Onset nearly always in teenagers Affects large and small joints Anterior uveitis less common Mild to moderate weight loss, fatigue ANA in 75%; RF in 100% Prognosis poor; remission unusual **Polyarticular Rheumatoid Factor Negative** 25% of all cases of JRA Mostly girls Any age Affects large and small joints Anterior uveitis in younger patients Minimal systemic symptoms ANA in 25%; RF negative Prognosis guarded; remission in some patients **Systemic Onset** 20% of all cases of JRA Boys and girls have same incidence Any age Any joint or number of joints Anterior uveitis very rare Fever, rash, poor growth, anemia ANA, RF negative Prognosis variable, worse in younger patients and in those with persistent systemic symptoms

ANA, antinuclear antibodies; RF, rheumatoid factor.

home. Ophthalmologic evaluations are necessary at specific intervals to screen for anterior uveitis. For patients at highest risk—children younger than 7 years of age with a positive ANA test result and pauciarticular or polyarticular JRA—ophthalmologic evaluations should be performed every 3 to 4 months for at least 4 years after diagnosis, every 6 months for 3 years after that, and then annually. Those with systemic JRA should have annual examinations since their risk is low. All others should have evaluations at 6-month intervals for the first 4 years after diagnosis, and annually thereafter.

Table 44-15. Differential Diagnosis: Rheumatic Disease

	Rheumatic Fever	Juvenile Rheumatoid Arthritis	Systemic Lupus Erythematosus	Kawasaki Disease	Dermatomyositis
Sex predilection	None	Dependent on subgroup	Girls > boys	None	Girls 3:2
Age at onset	3 yr or older	1 yr or older	Usually >8 yr	4 yr or younger	2 yr or older
Joint manifestations	Transient migratory arthritis: large joints	Pauciarticular or polyarticular Chronic (6 wk or more)	Arthralgia Transient arthritis Chronic arthritis	Pain and swelling of hands and feet Arthritis occasionally	Joint contractures; arthritis occasionally
Extraarticular manifestations	Fever Cardiac disease Chorea Rash, nodules	Dependent on subgroup: Systemic juvenile rheumatoid arthritis: fever, rash, etc. Pauciarticular: iridocyclitis	Occasionally multisystem disease, including nephritis	Fever Eye, oral, cutaneous lesions Lymphadenopathy Coronary vasculitis	Rash Muscle weakness, pain Gastrointestinal and respiratory system
Laboratory	Prior streptococcal infection Echo or ECG evidence of carditis	May have antinuclear antibodies, rheumatoid factor	Antinuclear antibodies Autoantibodies Low complement DNA antibody	Abnormal coronary vessels on Echo	Abnormal muscle enzymes, electromyogram, muslce biopsy
Pathogenesis	Post-streptococcal	Unknown	Immune complex disease	Unknown	Unknown
Diagnosis	Clinical (Jones criteria)	Clinical (juvenile rheumatoid arthritis criteria)	Clinical plus laboratory (systemic lupus erythematosus criteria)	Clinical (Kawasaki criteria)	Clinical Rash plus myositis Muscle biopsy
Natural history	Arthritis—transient: carditis may cause permanent damage	Chronic: arthritis may be destructive	Chronic or recurrent, may be fatal	Self-limited (often) Coronary vasculitis May be fatal	Chronic May be fatal
Therapy	Anti-inflammatory, group A streptococci prophylaxis to prevent recurrence	Anti-inflammatory Physical therapy	Antiinflammatory Corticosteroid Cytotoxic agents	Intravenous globulin Aspirin	Corticosteroid Cytotoxic agents

From Behrman RE (ed). Nelson Textbook of Pediatrics, 14th ed. Philadelphia, WB Saunders, 1992, p 620.
ECG, electrocardiogram; Echo, echocardiography.

Children with pauciarticular JRA usually require only treatment with an NSAID and PT/OT. The prognosis is generally favorable, with eventual remission likely for most children. If there is poor response or intolerance of NSAIDs, these children may benefit from steroid injections into the affected joint or joints. The response to steroid injections is variable, but many children experience complete resolution of arthritis for variable periods; on occasion, this resolution is permanent. Sulfasalazine is a second-line agent that has been most helpful for those with spondyloarthropathies, but it may also have benefit for younger children with pauciarticular JRA type I. It is usually combined with an NSAID in children who have not adequately responded to the NSAID alone.

Many children with polyarticular JRA require only the combination of NSAIDs and PT/OT. For those failing to respond, second-line agents such as sulfasalazine and hydroxychloroquine are considered if the arthritis is relatively mild and the child is functional. Hydroxychloroquine, an antimalarial with antiinflammatory properties, is generally well tolerated. The major risk from hydroxychloroquine is retinal toxicity. This is rare, especially when the dosage is

kept lower than 6.5 mg/kg/day, but children receiving this medication should have ophthalmologic evaluations every 6 months to screen for retinal toxicity. Those with more severe arthritis and/or disability may be treated with methotrexate. Methotrexate is very effective in reducing inflammation and disability in many children and adults with arthritis who have not responded to other medications. Subcutaneous administration is preferred because gut absorption is variable. Methotrexate is usually well tolerated, but there are concerns regarding hepatic toxicity, bone marrow suppression, and the potential over the long term for secondary malignancies. It is teratogenic and therefore should not be used during pregnancy. Children receiving methotrexate should have a CBC and liver transaminase measurements every 6 to 8 weeks. If elevated transaminase levels are detected and persist after either the drug is withheld for a short while or the dosage is reduced, the methotrexate should be discontinued. Methotrexate is most often used in combination with NSAIDs. On occasion, it is also used in combination with sulfasalazine and/or hydroxychloroquine in patients who fail to respond to these agents individually. Biologic agents should be considered in children who

Table 44-16. Differential Diagnosis: Nonrheumatic Conditions

	Septic Arthritis	Lyme Disease	Osteomyelitis	Viral Arthritis	Childhood Malignancy	Structural, Genetic	Growing Pains, Psychogenic
Sex predilection	Both	Both	Both	Girls > boys	Both	Either, depending on condition	Growing pains: boys > girls Psychogenic: girls > boys
Age at onset	<4 yr: *Haemophilus influenzae* Adolescence: Gonococcus Any age: *Staphylococcus aureus*	>2 yr	Any	More common in older children and adults	Any	Any	Growing pains: 2-8 yr Psychogenic: 6 yr or older
Joint manifestations	85% monarticular; joints swollen, hot, painful	Pauciarticular; episodic, recurrent	Sterile joint effusion adjacent to the area of bone infection	Transient arthritis: often polyarticular	Severe bone/joint pain, night pain	Local bone/joint pain or dysfunction	None or bizarre Features of reflex sympathetic dystrophy
Extraarticular manifestations	Fever, signs of sepsis, signs of gonococcal disease	Flulike illness, erythema migrans, neurologic, cardiac	Fever, signs of sepsis, bone pain	Those of underlying virus or vaccine	Those of underlying malignancy; no high fever, rash, or morning stiffness	Those of underlying conditions, dysmorphic features, structural abnormalities	Growing pains: none Psychogenic: bizarre
Laboratory	Cultures: joint fluid, blood, genital	Serologic: antibody to *Borrelia burgdorferi*	Culture: blood; bone: bone scan	Viral culture Serologic: rise in antibody titers	Hematologic abnormalities, abnormal radiograph or scan	Demonstration of abnormal structure or metabolic abnormality	Normal
Pathogenesis	Direct bacteremic synovial infection; occasional immune complex mechanism in gonococcal and meningococcal arthritis	*B. burgdorferi*: synovial and systemic infection	Direct bacteremic infection of bone, sympathetic joint effusion, or septic arthritis	Direct viral synovial infection, immune complex in some	Direct primary bone tumor or periarticular or bony infiltrate of malignant cells	Idiopathic or genetic	No organic disease
Diagnosis	Demonstration of organisms in joint fluid	Serologic	Demonstration of organisms: blood, bone; bone scan (early), radiograph (late)	Clinical, serologic, or viral culture	Bone marrow, tissue biopsy	Recognition of condition or syndrome	Clinical
Natural history	Joint destruction if untreated	Easily treated: may cause long-term CNS, skin, ocular disease	Bone/joint destruction if untreated	Arthritis transient	Joint manifestations may wax/wane	Chronic	Growing pains: benign Psychogenic: may become chronic and disabling
Therapy	Specific antibiotic	Specific antibiotic	Specific antibiotic	Symptomatic	That of underlying malignancy	That of underlying conditions	Recognition, reassurance, psychosocial attention

Modified from Behrman RE (ed): Nelson Textbook of Pediatrics, 14th ed. Philadelphia, WB Saunders, 1992, p 619.
CNS, central nervous system.

Table 44-17. **Manifestations of Lyme Disease by Stage***

| System† | Early Infection | | Late Infection |
	Localized Stage I	*Disseminated Stage 2*	*Persistent Stage 3*
Skin	Erythema migrans	Secondary annular lesions Malar rash Diffuse erythema or urticaria Evanescent lesions Lymphocytoma	Acrodermatitis chronica atrophicans Localized scleroderma-like lesions

Musculoskeletal		Migratory pain in joints, tendons, bursae,
		    muscle, bone
		Brief arthritis attacks
		Myositis‡
		Osteomyelitis‡
		Panniculitis‡
			Prolonged arthritis attacks
			Chronic arthritis
			Peripheral enthesopathy
			Periostitis or joint subluxations below
			    acrodermatitis

Neurologic		Meningitis Cranial neuritis, Bell palsy Motor or sensory radiculoneuritis Subtle encephalitis Mononeuritis multiplex Myelitis‡ Chorea‡ Cerebellar ataxia‡	Subtle mental disorders Axonal polyneuropathy Leukoencephalitis Encephalomyelitis Spastic parapareses Ataxic gait Dementia‡
Lymphatic	Regional lymphadenopathy	Regional or generalized lymphadenopathy Splenomegaly	
Heart		AV nodal block Myopericarditis Pancarditis	Cardiomyopathy
Eyes		Conjunctivitis Iritis‡ Choroiditis‡ Retinal hemorrhage or detachment‡ Panophthalmitis‡	Keratitis
Liver Respiratory		Mild or recurrent hepatitis Nonexudative sore throat Nonproductive cough Adult respiratory distress syndrome‡	
Kidney		Microscopic hematuria or proteinuria	
Genitourinary		Orchitis‡	
Constitutional symptoms	Minor	Severe malaise and fatigue	Fatigue

From Steere AC: Lyme disease. N Engl J Med 1989;321:586. Reproduced by permission of *The New England Journal of Medicine.*

*The staging system provides a guideline for the expected timing of the different manifestations of the illness, but this may vary in an individual case.

†The systems are listed from the most to the least commonly affected.

‡Because the inclusion of these manifestations is based on one or a few cases, they should be considered possible but not proven manifestations of Lyme disease.

AV, atrioventricular.

fail to respond to the medications just mentioned. Etanercept is a combination of soluble tumor necrosis factor receptor conjugated to the crystallized fragment portion of an immunoglobulin G molecule. Tumor necrosis factor is one of the main proinflammatory cytokines (along with interleukin-1) found in the joints of children with JRA, and this biologic agent binds strongly to tumor necrosis factor, thereby inhibiting its effect. Etanercept is effective, sometimes dramatically, in children with severe polyarticular JRA who failed to respond to methotrexate. It is administered subcutaneously twice a week. In the short term, it appears to be well tolerated; localized, mild injection site reactions are the most common adverse events.

The approach to children with systemic JRA is similar to that with polyarticular JRA. The usual sequence of treatment is NSAIDs initially, followed by methotrexate when necessary. Children with systemic JRA are at particular risk for severe adverse drug reactions; caution must always be used when the regimen is changed. Certain substances, such as gold and sulfasalazine, pose a greater risk for these children and should be avoided. Children with systemic JRA are most likely to require prednisone in order to control the systemic features of fever, poor appetite, and fatigue and to allow sufficient relief of joint discomfort. On occasion, those with severe pain and disability from polyarticular JRA may also require a brief course of prednisone. The use of prednisone in systemic or polyarticular JRA should be viewed as temporary, and dosages should be minimized, tapered, and discontinued when possible. When prednisone is added, methotrexate or other second-line agents should be considered, the plan being to taper and discontinue the prednisone once the other medications appear to be effective. Prednisone may also be indicated for potentially life-threatening conditions such as pericarditis. The long-term toxicity of prednisone is potentially more harmful than the disease. One method of avoiding some of the toxicity of long-term oral prednisone is to use intermittent intravenous administration of methylprednisolone. Children may start with weekly or twice-weekly doses, with the interval between doses gradually increased as the child improves. As with pauciarticular JRA, localized injections of steroids into one or more joints can be useful as an adjunctive treatment, particularly if a few joints are problematic.

SYSTEMIC LUPUS ERYTHEMATOSUS

In SLE there is B cell proliferation and increased production of immunoglobulins and specific autoantibodies, with subsequent immune-complex formation and deposition throughout the body. The cause is unknown, but it is more common in girls and women, African Americans, and persons with a first-degree relative with SLE. In childhood the peak onset is during the early teen years; it rarely occurs in children younger than 5 years. The potential clinical manifestations of SLE are numerous, and the illness demonstrates significant interindividual variability. Children with SLE have more severe disease, with a greater incidence of renal involvement and other serious manifestations, than do adults.

Diagnosis

SLE is suggested by the common manifestations of fever, rashes (specifically a malar rash), and arthritis in a school-aged child. The arthritis is most often symmetric, polyarticular, and frequently involves small joints of the hands and feet. Criteria were developed for the purpose of research studies and clinical application (Table 44-18). The presence of four or more of these 11 criteria is more than 90% sensitive and specific for SLE. Other clinical manifestations are listed in Table 44-19.

The ANA test is extremely sensitive, positive in more than 95% of children with SLE, usually in a high titer. However, it is not specific; testing for anti-dsDNA antibodies, anti-Smith antibodies, antiribonucleoprotein antibodies, anti-SSA, and anti-SSB antibodies should be performed in all children suspected of having SLE (see Table 44-4). Anti-dsDNA antibodies and anti-Smith antibodies are highly specific for SLE. Leukopenia, lymphopenia, thrombocytopenia, and an autoimmune hemolytic anemia, frequently with a positive result of a direct Coombs test, are common. Urinalysis is mandatory to screen for nephritis; proteinuria indicates disease. The anticardiolipin antibody test identifies antiphospholipid antibodies, a common finding in SLE that results in a hypercoagulable state, placing the patient at risk for thrombotic events. The complement proteins C3 and C4 are low in children with active SLE. Monitoring proteins C3 and C4 helps guide therapy; the levels should increase to normal as the illness is better controlled.

Treatment

Mild SLE is less common in childhood; patients with only cutaneous and joint manifestations may be managed with NSAIDs and/or hydroxychloroquine. These children are evaluated frequently and screened for the development of more serious complications. Those with organ involvement or severe constitutional symptoms require prednisone. Treatment is usually begun with a dosage of 1 to 2 mg/kg/day, with divided doses for those with more serious disease. Life-threatening manifestations are treated with intravenous "pulse" steroids, usually 30 mg/kg/day of methylprednisolone daily for 3 days, followed by daily oral prednisone. Once the clinical and laboratory manifestations improve, prednisone is carefully and slowly tapered, with close attention to the possibility of a flare of the disease, demonstrated either clinically or with decreasing complement levels and rising anti-dsDNA antibody titers.

Patients with severe renal disease or other organ manifestations that fail to respond to prednisone or methylprednisolone are candidates for more aggressive immunosuppressive therapy with cyclophosphamide and other agents. Cyclophosphamide is usually administered in monthly intravenous doses and is effective in treating severe lupus nephritis. Azathioprine, mycophenolate mofetil, cyclosporine, and methotrexate have also been used for various manifestations of SLE. Intravenous immune globulin can be beneficial for severe thrombocytopenia and hemolytic anemia.

Diet and exercise are important adjuncts. Limiting salt and fat is important for patients receiving prednisone or with renal disease, and supplements of calcium and vitamin D may help minimize the osteopenia associated with steroid use. Sun exposure should be limited and sun block used as necessary, because many children with SLE are photosensitive, and excessive exposure may lead to exacerbations. Psychological support is often necessary for teens affected with SLE, to aid in coping with an illness expected to be lifelong.

DERMATOMYOSITIS

In dermatomyositis, there is perivascular inflammation in muscles and skin, occasionally with gut and other organ involvement. It is more common in girls and can occur at any age; the average age at onset is 8 years. Weakness of proximal muscle—specifically the neck flexors, deltoids, biceps, triceps, quadriceps, psoas, and hamstrings—occasionally with accompanying mild muscle pain, fatigue, poor endurance, and a characteristic rash are the main manifestations. The skin manifestations include the heliotrope rash, a violaceous discoloration of the upper eyelids that is often accompanied by mild edema. Gottron rash consists of scaly, erythematous plaques or papules that appear over the MCP and PIP joints on the hands. Similar lesions are seen on the extensor surface of the elbows and knees and over the medial malleoli. The periungual capillaries may become grossly dilated and may develop thromboses that can be visualized either with the naked eye or with mild magnification. Some children develop more extensive erythroderma that may appear over the shoulders ("shawl sign") or in a V-neck distribution on the chest. The weakness may be subtle and not recognized for long periods. Frequent early symptoms include difficulties rising from the floor, climbing stairs, climbing in and out of a minivan, and combing the hair. The distribution of the rash, which may be misdiagnosed as eczema or psoriasis, is an early clue to the diagnosis.

Diagnosis

The diagnosis is suggested by the rash and proximal muscle weakness detected on physical examination (Table 44-20). Muscle enzymes are elevated in most, but not all, children with dermatomyositis. There may be elevations in only one or a few enzymes and therefore testing for aspartate aminotransferase, alanine aminotransferase, lactate dehydrogenase, creatine kinase, and aldolase should be performed. The child with a characteristic rash, clear proximal muscle weakness, and elevated muscle enzyme levels may not require additional testing for diagnosis. If weakness is questionable, or if the rash is not characteristic, an EMG can confirm the presence of muscle inflammation. MRI is a sensitive test for muscle inflammation and may be a less invasive method of evaluating the muscle. If there is any doubt regarding the diagnosis, a muscle biopsy is performed. The site for biopsy is determined by weakness on physical examination, or localization by EMG or MRI. The quadriceps or the deltoids are the easiest, most commonly used areas for biopsy. Involvement of the muscle may be spotty, and a normal finding on muscle biopsy does not exclude dermatomyositis. Typical findings

Table 44-18. 1982 Revised Criteria for Diagnosis of Systemic Lupus Erythematosus*

Criterion	Definition
Malar rash	Fixed erythema, flat or raised, over the malar eminences, tending to spare the nasolabial folds
Diskoid rash	Erythematous raised patches with adherent keratotic scaling and follicular plugging; atrophic scarring may occur in older lesions
Photosensitivity	Rash as a result of unusual reaction to sunlight (elicited by patient history or physician observation)
Oral ulcers	Oral or nasopharyngeal ulceration, usually painless, observed by a physician
Arthritis	Nonerosive arthritis involving two or more peripheral joints, characterized by tenderness, swelling, or effusion
Serositis	Pleuritis: convincing history of pleuritic pain or rub heard by a physician or evidence of pleural effusion *or* Pericarditis: documented by ECG or rub or evidence of pericardial effusion
Renal disorder	Persistent proteinuria greater than 0.5 g/day or greater than 3+ if quantitation not performed *or* Cellular casts: may be red blood cell, hemoglobin, granular, tubular, or mixed
Neurologic disorder	Seizures: in the absence of offending drugs or known metabolic derangements (e.g., uremia, ketoacidosis, or electrolyte imbalance) *or* Psychosis: in the absence of offending drugs or known metabolic derangements (e.g., uremia, ketoacidosis, or electrolyte imbalance)
Hematologic disorder	Hemolytic anemia: with reticulocytosis *or* Leukopenia: less than 4000/mm^3 total on two or more occasions *or* Lymphopenia: less than 1500/mm^3 on two or more occasions *or* Thrombocytopenia: less than 100,000/mm^3
Immunologic disorder	Positive LE cell preparation *or* Anti-DNA antibody to native DNA in abnormal titer *or* Anti-Sm: presence of antibody to Sm nuclear antigen *or* False-positive serologic test result for syphilis known to be positive for at least 6 mo and confirmed by negative *Treponema pallidum* immobilization or fluorescent treponemal antibody absorption test
Antinuclear antibody	An abnormal titer of antinuclear antibody by immunofluorescence or an equivalent assay at any time and in the absence of drugs known to be associated with "drug-induced lupus syndrome"

From Tan EM, Cohen AS, Fries JF, et al: The 1982 revised criteria for the classification of systemic lupus erythematosus. Arthritis Rheum 1982;25:1271.

*The proposed classification is based on 11 criteria. For the purpose of identifying patients in clinical studies, a person shall be said to have systemic lupus erythematosus if any four or more of the 11 criteria are present, serially or simultaneously, during any interval of observation.

ECG, electrocardiogram; LE, lupus erythematosus; Sm, Smith.

on biopsy include perivascular inflammation and perifascicular atrophy. The biopsy can help to exclude other potential myopathies such as muscular dystrophies and metabolic myopathies.

Treatment

Prednisone, 2 mg/kg/day, is the usual treatment for childhood dermatomyositis. Initial intravenous "pulses" of methylprednisolone, 30 mg/kg/day for 3 days, may be used for severe disease or in an attempt to limit the eventual total prednisone dose. Improvement is slow, and the prednisone dose is tapered gradually over a 1- to 2-year period. Attempts at rapid tapering often lead to flares of the disease and the need for higher doses of steroids. Some children do not respond adequately to prednisone, either with or without intravenous methylprednisolone. Methotrexate often helps to control the disease and allows tapering of the steroid. Cyclosporine, intravenous immune globulin, azathioprine, and mycophenolate mofetil are also used in place of or in addition to methotrexate for selected patients.

SCLERODERMA

Scleroderma is subclassified into systemic sclerosis and localized scleroderma (Table 44-21). Localized scleroderma (morphea or linear scleroderma), which is limited to the skin and subcutaneous tissues, is much more common in childhood and rarely progresses to involve internal organs. Systemic sclerosis is much more life-threatening because it has the potential to involve internal organs and cause more severe and widespread skin disease.

Morphea

Morphea is a patch of hardened skin that appears spontaneously on any part of the body. The skin becomes firm, stiff, atrophic, and discolored. There is absence of hair. Initially, the lesion appears violaceous, but then it fades to a yellowish-brown or dusky appearance in most individuals. The patches are nontender, and children are asymptomatic. Over years, the lesions tend to gradually fade and soften after an initial period of expansion. Biopsy reveals excessive

Table 44-19. Additional Manifestations of Systemic Lupus Erythematosus

Systemic	**Gastrointestinal**
Fever	Pancreatitis
Malaise	Mesenteric arteritis
Weight loss	Serositis
Fatigue	Hepatomegaly
Musculoskeletal	Hepatitis (chronic-lupoid)
Myositis, myalgia	Splenomegaly
Arthralgia	**Renal**
Cutaneous	Nephritis
Raynaud phenomenon	Nephrosis
Alopecia	Uremia
Urticaria	Hypertension
Panniculitis	**Reproduction**
Livedo reticularis	Infertility
Neuropsychiatric	Repeated abortions
Personality disorders	Neonatal lupus
Stroke	Congenital heart block
Peripheral neuropathy	**Hematologic**
Chorea	Anticoagulants (factors
Transverse myelitis	VIII, IX, XII, others
Migraine headaches	causing hemorrhage)
Mononeuritis multiplex	Antiphospholipid
Cardiopulmonary	antibodies (lupus
Endocarditis	anticoagulant causing
Myocarditis	thrombosis)
Pneumonitis	**Treatment-Induced**
Pulmonary hemorrhage	Steroid toxicity
Ocular	Immunosuprresion
Episcleritis	Opportunistic infections
Sicca syndrome	
Retinal cytoid bodies	

Modified from Kredich DW: Rheumatic diseases of childhood. In Behrman RE, Kliegman RM (eds): Nelson Essentials of Pediatrics, 2nd ed. Philadelphia, WB Saunders, 1992, p 289.

Table 44-20. Diagnostic Criteria for Polymyositis/Dermatomyositis

Progressive, symmetric weakness of proximal muscles and anterior neck flexors

Characteristic rash, including heliotrope (purple discoloration of eyelids, often with edema), Gottron sign (scaly erythema over the metacarpophalangeal and proximal interphalangeal joints), scaly erythematous patches over extensor surface of elbows and knees, and over the medial malleoli

Elevation of serum muscle enzymes (CK, SGOT, SGPT, LDH, aldolase)

EMG revealing short, small polyphasic motor units; insertional irritability, fibrillations; and high-frequency discharges

Abnormal muscle biopsy, revealing perivascular mononuclear cell infiltrate, perifascicular atrophy, and necrosis of muscle fibers

Modified from Bohan A, Peter JB: Polymyositis and dermatomyositis (first of two parts). N Engl J Med 1975;292:344.

CK, creatine kinase; EMG, electromyogram; LDH, lactate dehydrogenase; SGOT, serum glutamic-oxaloacetic transaminase; SGPT, serum glutamic-pyruvic transaminase.

Table 44-21. Classification of Scleroderma

Systemic Sclerosis

Diffuse: Systemic fibrosis, including widespread skin involvement (face, trunk, and both proximal and distal extremities) and internal organ involvement (lungs, kidneys, gastrointestinal tract, heart)

Limited (CREST syndrome): Skin fibrosis limited to distal extremities, face, and neck; internal organ involvement occurs late if at all, with pulmonary hypertension often being the most significant development

Localized Scleroderma

Morphea: single, discrete patch of fibrotic skin; no organ involvement

Generalized morphea: multiple, discrete patches of fibrotic skin; no organ involvement

Linear scleroderma: band of fibrosis on face (coup de sabre) or along an extremity, sometimes extending entire length; no organ involvement

CREST, calcinosis, Raynaud phenomenon, esophageal dysmotility, sclerodactyly, and telangiectasias.

amounts of collagen in the dermis, with diminished vascular structures and absence of hair follicles. There is no universally accepted treatment, which is considered only for cosmetic reasons. Topical and intralesional steroids have been used with varying success.

Linear Scleroderma

Linear scleroderma is similar to morphea, but rather than a patch, the area of hardened skin typically is a narrow band that may extend through an entire limb, part of the limb, or across the scalp and face ("coup de sabre" lesion). Cosmetically and functionally, linear scleroderma is much more severe than morphea, because the potential for limitation of limb use is greater or because of facial involvement. Growth of the limb may be affected, and involvement of the digits can cause significant functional difficulty. Children should receive physical and occupational therapy. There is no effective medical treatment, and, as with morphea, the skin tends to soften with time. Topical steroids, intralesional steroids, oral steroids, and methotrexate have been used with occasional success.

Systemic Sclerosis

Systemic sclerosis typically begins with severe Raynaud phenomenon, followed by thickening and tightening of the skin over the digits and hands and then the face, and then by varying degrees of progressive skin changes over the extremities and trunk. Difficulty opening the mouth and decreased facial expression are signs of facial involvement. As the skin over the hands tightens and hardens, pigment changes may occur, and flexion contractures of the small joints may develop. Renal disease, pulmonary fibrosis, pulmonary hypertension, esophageal and gut dysmotility, and cardiac disease may all occur. Anti–SCL-70 antibodies (anti-topoisomerase I) are present in approximately 30% to 40% of patients with systemic sclerosis and are very specific. There are no other helpful serologic tests. High-resolution computed tomography of the chest, esophagography, and echocardiography should be performed to screen for organ involvement and repeated at periodic intervals. Although there is no effective general treatment, intravenous cyclophosphamide and steroids have been shown to limit progression of pulmonary disease, angiotensin-converting enzyme inhibitors can limit renal disease, and prokinetic agents are helpful for patients with gastrointestinal involvement. The course of systemic sclerosis is variable; patients with rapid progression tend to have a less favorable outcome. A limited variant of scleroderma is known as the CREST syndrome (calcinosis, Raynaud phenomenon, esophageal dysmotility, sclerodactyly, and telangiectasias). Although less severe than systemic sclerosis, these patients can develop life-threatening pulmonary hypertension. The CREST syndrome is associated with anticentromere antibodies.

RHEUMATIC FEVER

Acute rheumatic fever is a post-streptococcal illness, resulting from a cross-reactive immune response to group A streptococcal pharyngitis (see Chapters 1 and 8). It is most common in children older than 5 years and occurs more often after infection with certain serotypes of group A streptococcus. There may be genetic reasons that predispose some children and adults to the illness. Signs and symptoms of rheumatic fever typically develop 1 to 3 weeks after streptococcal pharyngitis. Clinical manifestations have been grouped according to the Jones criteria, which separate major from minor criteria (Table 44-22).

The arthritis of rheumatic fever is usually very painful, disproportionate to the degree of swelling on physical examination. It is usually a migratory arthritis of the large joints; it rarely affects the fingers, spine, or toes. It tends to last in one joint for several days and then migrates to a different joint. The duration of joint symptoms is rarely longer than 3 to 4 weeks in untreated patients. If patients are treated with NSAIDs, the arthritis usually responds dramatically within 1 to 2 days. When rheumatic fever is a consideration and the diagnosis is unclear, it is helpful to avoid NSAID use early in the course, to avoid diagnostic confusion.

In the absence of carditis, rheumatic fever may be difficult to distinguish from early systemic JRA, Kawasaki disease, and viral illnesses causing fever, rash, and joint pain. The diagnosis is a clinical one, inasmuch as there is no diagnostic laboratory test. The Jones criteria were developed as a diagnostic aid, and the presence of two of the major criteria or of one major and two minor criteria *plus* evidence of recent streptococcal infection is considered diagnostic. Either a positive throat culture or elevations of the antistreptococcal antibodies (antistreptolysin O, anti-DNase B, antihyaluronidase) are the standard signs of recent streptococcal infection. Fulfilling the criteria is not necessarily specific, especially when the evidence of

recent streptococcal infection is based on mildly elevated serologic test results. Conversely, there are children with isolated chorea or classic rheumatic carditis who have rheumatic fever without necessarily fulfilling the Jones criteria. When a diagnosis of rheumatic fever is considered in a child with joint symptoms, it is important to distinguish arthritis from arthralgia and to evaluate the nature of the arthritis when present. If the arthritis is nonmigratory and not exquisitely tender, or if it involves unusual joints such as those in the hands, feet, and spine or lasts longer than 1 week in a single joint, then alternative diagnoses should be strongly considered.

Careful consideration of the diagnosis is especially important because of future implications regarding prognosis and treatment. Children with rheumatic fever may develop carditis with future episodes of streptococcal pharyngitis; each episode of carditis can produce additional heart valve damage. Therefore, prophylactic antibiotic treatment is recommended to minimize streptococcal infections, even for patients who do not have carditis with the initial attack. For those without carditis, most authorities recommend prophylaxis until age 18 years or for 5 years, whichever is longer. For patients with carditis, this recommendation is extended to age 25 years or for 10 years, again whichever is longer. Prophylaxis is usually either daily oral penicillin or monthly intramuscular injections of long-acting penicillin.

MYALGIA

Muscle pain needs to be distinguished from joint pain, bone pain, and the less common neuropathic pain in the child with extremity pain. If the complaint is localized to the muscles, the differential diagnosis is narrowed considerably. Intermittent benign bilateral myalgias of the calves or thighs are common in young children. These occur in a normally active child who has normal physical examination findings without weakness or systemic symptoms. The pains typically occur at night or at bedtime and resolve with massage or mild analgesia such as acetaminophen or ibuprofen, usually within 30 to 60 minutes. They can occur at varying frequencies and, in some children, may escalate periodically. Additional evaluation or treatment is unnecessary in most children, and eventually the pains resolve completely.

Myalgia may accompany polymyositis and dermatomyositis, and therefore every child complaining of muscle pain should undergo careful muscle strength testing. Myalgias may also be seen with vasculitis and systemic JRA. Many children with the acute onset of diffuse myalgia have a transient viral illness, and the myalgias resolve, usually within several days. Infection with influenza can cause an exquisitely painful myositis of the gastrocnemius muscles with resultant difficulty ambulating. The creatine kinase level may be very elevated. This condition is usually distinguished easily from a chronic inflammatory muscle disease by the sudden onset and localization to these specific muscles. Myoglobinuria may ensue and potentially affect renal function; therefore, these children should have a urinalysis, which yields positive results for heme in the presence of myoglobin but has no erythrocytes on microscopic examination. The myositis resolves within several days, and treatment is based on symptoms.

RADIAL HEAD SUBLUXATION

Radial head subluxation, or "nursemaid's elbow," is a traumatic process that occurs most frequently in young children—almost all younger than 4 years—as a result of a narrower radial head. The annular ligament encircles the proximal radius immediately distal to the radial head. If the radius is pulled distally with the elbow extended, as occurs when a young child is tugged by the arm, this ligament may slip over the radial head and become entrapped between the head of the radius and the humerus, producing the "nursemaid's elbow." When this occurs, the child typically holds the

---

Table 44-22. Jones Criteria for Diagnosis of Rheumatic Fever*

Major Criteria
Polyarthritis
Carditis
Erythema marginatum
Subcutaneous nodules
Chorea

Minor Criteria
Fever
Arthralgia
Elevated acute phase reactants (ESR or CRP)
Prolonged PR interval

Modified from Dajani AS, Ayoub EM, Bierman FZ, et al: Guidelines for the diagnosis of rheumatic fever: Jones Criteria, updated 1992. JAMA 1992;87:302-307.

*The presence of two major criteria or one major and two minor criteria plus evidence of preceding group A streptococcal infection (positive culture or rapid test, elevated antibodies) fulfills the criteria. The diagnosis may also be made in some instances of isolated chorea or isolated carditis alone, when other causes have been excluded.

CRP, C-reactive protein; ESR, erythrocyte sedimentation rate.

arm limply, elbow extended with hand pronated, and refuses any motion of the elbow. If the history suggests that the child experienced this type of trauma, and if observation and palpation of the arm does not disclose point tenderness, swelling, or discoloration suggestive of a fracture, an attempt may be made to reduce the subluxation without a need for radiographs. This is done by rotating the hand and forearm to a supine position and applying gentle traction on the radial head. As this is done, the annular ligament slips back around the head of the radius into position, and the child regains immediate use of the arm without pain. No additional treatment is necessary except for educating family and caregivers.

REFLEX SYMPATHETIC DYSTROPHY

Reflex sympathetic dystrophy is a regional pain syndrome that is rare in childhood and not well understood. After a seemingly minor injury, children develop intense pain in an extremity or part of the extremity, accompanied by intermittent autonomic changes such as discoloration, coolness, and localized excessive sweating. The pain leads to progressive disability of the extremity, occasionally leading to a fixed posturing of a hand, foot, or limb. Severely affected children become disabled, are unable to ambulate at times, and are often unable to attend school. There are frequently associated psychosocial stressors that need to be addressed. The treatment is analgesia, intense PT/OT, education, and psychological counseling. Some children improve dramatically within a few days of instituting therapy, whereas in others, treatment is difficult and the process lasts indefinitely. In some instances, sympathetic nerve blockade is helpful.

RED FLAGS

The differential diagnosis of arthritis is extensive. A thorough history and physical examination, especially over time, are helpful in making a diagnosis and initiating therapy in most patients. Potential pitfalls in diagnosis are noted in Table 44-23.

Red flags include manifestations suggestive of septic arthritis (fever, single joint, erythema, extreme tenderness, leukocytosis), malignancy (polyarthritis, night and nonarticular bone pain, absence of high fever, absence of obvious swelling or stiffness, positive

radiographic changes, and abnormal CBC count), Lyme disease, Kawasaki disease, and other treatable disorders. Multiorgan system involvement may be primary (as in SLE and rheumatic fever) or secondary to therapy and must be considered in order to avoid ongoing extraarticular involvement, which may be more life-threatening than the articular process.

In addition, the child with a history of injury and the acute onset of extremity pain may have a fracture or traumatic hemarthrosis and requires prompt evaluation. Trauma often precedes the development of osteomyelitis.

Any child with extremity pain, including arthritis, may have leukemia or neuroblastoma. Systemic symptoms, such as fatigue and poor appetite with weight loss, may accompany the pain and increase suspicion of malignancy. Deep bone pain caused by marrow invasion may not reveal any obvious physical findings. A normal or slightly low platelet count with an elevated ESR increases the suspicion of malignancy. If malignancy is suspected, a CBC count should be obtained, and then a bone aspiration should be performed. This is particularly important if treatment with steroids or other immunosuppressive medications is being considered. Steroids may alleviate a rheumatologic condition but may also place a child with leukemia at risk for relapse with steroid-resistant disease.

REFERENCES

General

Cassidy JT, Petty RE: Textbook of Pediatric Rheumatology, 4th ed. Philadelphia, WB Saunders, 2001.
Jacobs JC: Pediatric Rheumatology for the Practitioner, 2nd ed. New York, Springer-Verlag, 1993.
Klippel JH, Dieppe PA: Rheumatology, 2nd ed. London, Mosby, 1998.
Ruddy S, Harris ED, Sledge CB: Textbook of Rheumatology, 6th ed. Philadelphia, WB Saunders, 2001.

Juvenile Rheumatoid Arthritis

Giannini EH, Brewer EJ, Kuamina N, et al: Methotrexate in resistant juvenile rheumatoid arthritis. N Engl J Med 1992;326;1043-1049.
Glass DN, Giannini EH: Juvenile rheumatoid arthritis as a complex genetic trait. Arthritis Rheum 1999;42:2261-2268.
Hadchouel M, Prieur A-M, Griscelli C: Acute hemorrhagic, hepatic, and neurologic manifestations in juvenile rheumatoid arthritis: Possible relationship to drugs or infection. J Pediatr 1985;106:561-566.
Lovell DJ, Giannini EH, Reiff A, et al: Etanercept in children with polyarticular juvenile rheumatoid arthritis. N Engl J Med, 2000;342: 763-769.
Miller ML: Juvenile rheumatoid arthritis. Curr Probl Pediatr 1994;24: 190-198.
Ostrov BE, Goldsmith DP, Athreya BH: Differentiation of systemic juvenile rheumatoid arthritis from acute leukemia near the onset of disease. J Pediatr 1993;122:595-598.
Schaller JG: Juvenile rheumatoid arthritis. Pediatr Rev 1997;18:337-349.
Section on Rheumatology and Section on Ophthalmology: Guidelines for ophthalmologic examinations in children with juvenile rheumatoid arthritis. Pediatrics 1993;92:295-296.

Systemic Lupus Erythematosus

Boumpas DT, Austin HA, Fessler BJ, et al: Systemic lupus erythematosus: Emerging concepts. Part 1: Renal, neuropsychiatric, cardiovascular, pulmonary, and hematologic disease. Ann Intern Med 1995;122: 940-950.
Boumpas DT, Fessler BJ, Austin HA, et al: Systemic lupus erythematosus: Emerging concepts. Part 2: Dermatologic and joint disease, the antiphospholipid antibody syndrome, pregnancy and hormonal therapy, morbidity and mortality, and pathogenesis. Ann Intern Med 1995;123:42-53.
Cevera R, Khamashta MA, Font J, et al: Systemic lupus erythematosus: Clinical and immunologic patterns of disease expression in a cohort of 1,000 patients. Medicine 1993;72:113-124.
Lahita RG: Systemic Lupus Erythematosus, 2nd ed. New York, Churchill Livingstone, 1992.

Table 44-23. Potential Pitfalls in Diagnosis

DOs
1. Examine all joints.
2. Order radiographs of both affected and contralateral joints.
3. Ask parents to photograph swelling and rashes.
4. Insist on regular slit-lamp examinations even if arthritis is inactive.
5. Treat suspected septic arthritis or osteomyelitis even if the diagnosis is uncertain.
6. Encourage patient independence.

DON'Ts
1. Rule out organic disease if laboratory findings are negative.
2. Rule out organic disease if physical findings are normal at the patient's first visit.
3. Be worried about high fevers in children with systemic-onset juvenile arthritis.
4. Expect total compliance with the prescribed regimen.
5. Accept laboratory results at odds with your experience; repeat tests if necessary.
6. Be afraid to say, "I don't know."

Lang BA, Silverman ED: A clinical overview of systemic lupus erythematosus in childhood. Pediatr Rev 1993;14:194-201.

Mills JA: Systemic lupus erythematosus. N Engl J Med 1994;330:1871-1878.

Molta C, Meyer O, Dosquet C, et al: Childhood-onset systemic lupus erythematosus: Antiphospholipid antibodies in 37 patients and their first-degree relatives. Pediatrics 1993;92:849-853.

Ruiz-Irastorza G, Khamashta MA, Castellino G, Hughes GR: Systemic lupus erythematosus. Lancet 2001;357:1027-1032.

Waltuck J, Buyon JP: Autoantibody-associated congenital heart block: Outcome in mothers and children. Ann Intern Med 1994;120:544-551.

Yang L-Y, Chen W-P, Lin C-Y: Lupus nephritis in children: A review of 167 patients. Pediatrics 1994;94:335-340.

Infectious Arthritis

Baker DG, Schumacher HR: Acute monoarthritis. N Engl J Med 1993; 329:1013-1020.

Jackson MA, Burry VF, Olson LC: Pyogenic arthritis associated with adjacent osteomyelitis: Identification of the sequela-prone child. Pediatr Infect Dis J 1992;11:9-13.

Rose CD, Eppes SC: Infection-related arthritis. Rheum Dis Clin North Am 1997;23:677-695.

Sonnen GM, Henry NK: Pediatric bone and joint infections. Diagnosis and antimicrobial management. Pediatr Clin North Am 1996;43:933-947.

Steere AC: Lyme disease. N Engl J Med 2001;345:115-125.

Unkila-Kallio L, Kallio MJT, Eskola J, et al: Serum C-reactive protein, erythrocyte sedimentation rate, and white blood cell count in acute hematogenous osteomyelitis of children. Pediatrics 1994;93:59-62.

Dermatomyositis

Callen JP: Dermatomyositis. Lancet 2000;355:53-57.

Pachman LM: Juvenile dermatomyositis. Pathophysiology and disease expression. Pediatr Clin North Am 1995;42:1071-1098.

Rider LG, Miller FW: Classification and treatment of the juvenile idiopathic inflammatory myopathies. Rheum Dis Clin North Am 1997;23:619-655.

Other Causes of Arthritis

Arnold JMO, Teasell RW, MacLeod AP, et al: Increased venous alpha-adrenoceptor responsiveness in patients with reflux sympathetic dystrophy. Ann Intern Med 1993;118:619-621.

Bielory L, Gascon P, Lawley TJ, et al: Human serum sickness: A prospective analysis of 35 patients treated with equine anti-thymocyte globulin for bone marrow failure. Medicine 1988;67:40-57.

Calin A: Differentiating the seronegative spondyloarthropathies: How to characterize and manage Reiter's syndrome and reactive arthritis. J Musculoskel Med 1986;2:21-27.

Kunnamo I, Kallio P, Pelkonen, et al: Serum-sickness–like disease is a common cause of acute arthritis in children. Acta Paediatr Scand 1986; 75:964-969.

Larsson L-G, Baum J, Mudholkar GS, et al: Benefits and disadvantages of joint hypermobility among musicians. N Engl J Med 1993;329: 1079-1082.

Pinals RS: Polyarthritis and fever. N Engl J Med 1994;330:769-774.

Wilder RT, Berde CB, Wolohan M, et al: Reflex sympathetic dystrophy in children. J Bone Joint Surg Am 1992;74:910-919.

45 Gait Disturbances

George H. Thompson

Gait disturbances are common pediatric musculoskeletal complaints that produce significant concern in parents. Although most gait disturbances are benign and resolve with normal growth and development, others are pathologic in origin and necessitate treatment. It is important that the physician understands the various mechanisms and causes of gait disturbances (Table 45-1), their clinical features, appropriate diagnostic procedures, and treatment options.

GAIT CYCLE

The normal gait cycle is described by foot placement. The gait cycle begins with right heel strike, followed by left toe-off, left heel strike, and right toe-off, and ending with right heel strike. These five events describe one gait cycle and include two phases: stance and swing. The stance phase is the period of time during which one of the two feet is on the ground. The swing phase is the period during which a limb is being advanced forward without ground contact.

Measuring the duration of the gait cycle makes it possible to calculate the time required for each of the five phases. During normal gait, the duration of each phase is as follows: for weight acceptance, 11%; for single limb stance, 39%; for weight release, 11%; and for swing phase, 39%. Velocity, cadence, step length, stride length, and step width may be calculated from the timed and measured gait cycle.

DEVELOPMENT OF GAIT

Central nervous system maturation is necessary for the development of normal gait and accounts for the normal progression of developmental milestones. The normal milestones for locomotion include independent sitting at 6 months of age, crawling at about 9 months, walking without assistance at 12 to 15 months, and running at 18 months. A normal 1-year-old child has a wide-based stance and a rapid cadence with short steps; the elbows are flexed and reciprocal arm motion is not present. Foot strike occurs without an initial heel strike. A 2 year old child shows increased velocity, step length, and diminished cadence in comparison with a 1-year-old child. Most of the adult gait patterns are present in children by 3 years, with changes in velocity, stride, and cadence continuing to 7 years of age. The gait characteristics of a 7-year-old child are similar to those of the adult.

CLINICAL EVALUATION

The evaluation of a child with an abnormal gait begins with a carefully documented history and is followed by a thorough physical examination, with the physician paying special attention to clues identified by the history. Diagnostic studies, such as radiographs and laboratory tests, are ordered when appropriate.

HISTORY

The physician should inquire about the pregnancy and delivery, the age at which developmental milestones occurred, the presence of any systemic illnesses (chronicity, fever, weight loss, other organ system involvement, rash), and the family history for any congenital musculoskeletal abnormalities or syndromes. With regard to the gait disturbance, it is important to inquire when it was first observed, whether it is unilateral or bilateral, whether it is associated with any injuries or intercurrent systemic illness, and whether there has been a history of improvement or worsening with time.

PHYSICAL EXAMINATION

Many of the common gait disturbances can be diagnosed from the patient's clinical history. However, all children presenting with gait disturbance require careful evaluation of the musculoskeletal and neurologic systems.

General Musculoskeletal Examination

The musculoskeletal examination begins with the child ambulating in the examining room or adjacent hallway. The child must be adequately undressed and be observed from a distance while walking so that the trunk and lower extremities can be clearly visualized. The position of the thighs, knees, and lower legs, as well as the feet, should be observed during ambulation. Gait observation, plus the clinical history, allows diagnosis of most of the common gait disturbances such as torsional variations (in-toeing and out-toeing), toe-walking (equinus gait), and limping.

Limping is categorized as either painful (*antalgic*) or nonpainful (*Trendelenburg gait*), depending on the length of the stance phase. In an antalgic gait, the stance phase is shortened because the child decreases the time spent on the painful extremity. In a Trendelenburg gait, which is indicative of underlying proximal muscle weakness (muscular dystrophy) or hip instability (developmental hip dysplasia), the stance phase is the same for the involved and uninvolved sides, but the child leans over the involved side to shift the center of gravity over the involved extremity for balance. If the disorder is bilateral, it produces a waddling gait.

When the child is walking, the observer records the direction of the long axis of the foot with regard to the direction in which the child is walking. This defines the line of progression and is useful in the evaluation of in-toeing or out-toeing.

A careful musculoskeletal examination of both the upper and lower extremities is necessary. Although most of the findings in gait disturbances are confined to the lower extremities, it is important to assess the upper extremities and spine because they may be part of an underlying disease process. The range of motion of all joints should be assessed, and the joints should be palpated for evidence of tenderness, effusion, synovial thickening, and increased warmth. Joint range of motion may be limited by pain, effusions, or contractures.

Table 45-1. Mechanisms of Gait Disturbances
Mechanical
Trauma, fracture, sprain
Sports injury, overuse injury
Child abuse
Dysplastic lesions
Short leg
Osseous
Legg-Calvé-Perthes disease
Slipped capital femoral epiphysis
Osteomyelitis
Diskitis
Osteoid osteoma
Osgood-Schlatter disease
Articular
Developmental hip dysplasia
Septic arthritis
Toxic synovitis
Rheumatic disease (JRA, SLE)
Hemophilia-hemorrhage
Ankylosis of a joint
Neurologic
Guillain-Barré syndrome (other peripheral neuropathies)
Intoxication
Cerebellar ataxia
Brain tumor
Lesion occupying spinal cord space
Posterior spinal column disorders
Myopathy
Hemiplegia
Sympathetic reflex dystrophy
Cerebral palsy
Hematologic/Oncologic
Sickle cell pain crisis
Leukemia, lymphoma
Metastatic tumor
Primary bone tumor
Histiocytosis
Other
Soft tissue infection
Kawasaki disease
Conversion reaction
Gaucher disease
Phlebitis
Scurvy
Rickets
Peritonitis

Modified from Behrman R, Kliegman R (eds): Nelson Essentials of Pediatrics, 2nd ed. Philadelphia, WB Saunders, 1994, p 711.

JRA, juvenile rheumatoid arthritis; SLE, systemic lupus erythematosus.

Examination of the lower extremities should include measurement of lower extremity lengths and assessment of the hip, knee, ankle, and subtalar joints. The thighs, lower legs, and feet are inspected for evidence of asymmetry, soft tissue swelling, or injury. Palpation for areas of increased warmth or tenderness is performed. The shape of the foot is assessed for possible intrinsic deformity.

Lower Extremity Length Measurements

The most accurate clinical method of measuring lower extremity length is to have the child stand on a firm, level surface, with the examiner standing behind the child and placing index fingers over the lateral aspect of each of the child's iliac crests. The presence or absence of a pelvic obliquity can be observed. It is then possible to place blocks of various heights beneath the child's foot on the short side until the pelvis is level. The height of the block indicates the amount of lower extremity length discrepancy. Clinical measurements obtained by use of a tape measure can also be performed but are much less accurate. The most common method is performed by measuring from the anterior superior iliac spine to the distal aspect of the medial malleolus. These landmarks are sometimes difficult to palpate accurately, and there can be a considerable margin of error.

Joint Assessment

The range of motion of the hips, knees, ankles, and subtalar joints of both extremities must be assessed. Hip flexion is measured along with any flexion contractures. With the hip in extension, the degrees of abduction, adduction, internal rotation, and external rotation are measured, preferably with a goniometer, and recorded. Hip rotation is most accurately measured with the child in the prone position with the knees flexed. Knee flexion and extension, ankle dorsiflexion, and plantar flexion, as well as subtalar motion, must be assessed and recorded.

Spinal Evaluation

Spinal mobility should also be assessed because intraspinal abnormalities, such as diskitis and tumors, may initially be manifested as a gait disturbance. The child's ability to forward flex and to reverse lumbar lordosis is a sign of normal mobility (see Chapter 46). Areas of vertebral bone tenderness and muscle spasm are determined by direct palpation.

Neurologic Evaluation

Many gait disturbances have a neurologic cause or association. The neurologic examination should include muscle strength testing, sensory assessment (particularly the specific level of potential sensory deficits), deep tendon reflexes, and pathologic reflexes, such as the Babinski sign (up-going toes' extensor plantar response). Careful assessment of rectal tone and bladder distention may identify a spinal lesion.

RADIOGRAPHIC ASSESSMENT

The need for radiographic evaluation is based on the differential diagnosis. For many gait disturbances, radiographic assessment is not required. When necessary, plain radiographs of the lower extremities, pelvis, or spine are obtained first, followed by special diagnostic studies, such as scanograms for lower extremity length discrepancy, technetium bone scan for localization of occult lesions such as osteomyelitis, and computed tomography (CT) for assessment and localization of specific lesions. Magnetic resonance imaging (MRI) can be very helpful in the diagnosis of occult or soft tissue lesions (infection, tumor, metabolic disorder) and intraspinal pathologic processes.

LABORATORY TESTS

Tests such as complete blood cell count with differential; measurement of erythrocyte sedimentation rate; and C-reactive protein, rheumatoid factor, and antinuclear antibody determinations are indicated if an infectious, inflammatory, or immune disorder is suspected. Other tests may be indicated for the diagnosis of specific disorders. Electromyography, nerve conduction studies, muscle biopsies, and nerve biopsies are frequently necessary in the diagnosis of myopathic or neuropathic disorders (see Chapter 38). Determinations of creatine phosphokinase, aldolase, and aspartate transaminase levels are important in the evaluation of striated muscle function and should be ordered if an underlying myopathy or myositis is suspected.

GAIT DISTURBANCES

The three most common categories of gait disturbances of childhood are

- torsional variations (in-toeing and out-toeing)
- toe-walking (equinus gait)
- limping (antalgic and Trendelenburg gaits)

TORSIONAL VARIATIONS

Torsional variations—in-toeing and out-toeing of the lower extremities—are the most common gait disturbances that cause parents to seek advice from a physician. Most variations do not necessitate treatment because the disorder resolves with normal growth and development; however, they produce anxiety in parents, and the physician must have a clear understanding of the cause and natural history to appropriately reassure the family.

The common causes of in-toeing and out-toeing are listed in Table 45-2. The presence of in-toeing or out-toeing does not imply an abnormality of the foot; rather, it indicates only the direction in which the foot is pointing during ambulation. The causes of torsional variations can be located from proximal (hip) to distal (foot) in the involved extremity. Some causes, such as clubfeet, are obvious, whereas others are subtle.

NORMAL DEVELOPMENTAL ALIGNMENT

In utero position has important effects on the alignment of the lower extremities of infants. In the typical in utero position, the hips are flexed, abducted, and externally rotated; the knees are flexed; and the lower legs are internally rotated. The feet are in a supinated position against the posterolateral aspect of the opposite thigh. The musculoskeletal examination of an infant characteristically shows 20- to 30-degree hip flexion contractures, 50 to 60 degrees of abduction, 80 to 90 degrees of external rotation in extension, and minimal or no internal rotation. The knees have a 20- to 30-degree flexion contracture, and internal tibial torsion is present. These are normal findings. The increased external rotation of the hip is caused not by femoral retroversion but rather by a posterior hip capsule contracture, which begins to resolve at the time of independent ambulation.

The combination of external rotation at the hip and internal rotation of the lower leg produces a bowed appearance of the lower extremities in the weight-bearing position. This is not true bowing but rather a torsional combination. After ambulation, this physiologic bowing resolves over a 6- to 12-month period.

Physiologic genu valgum (knock-knees) is seen between 3 and 4 years of age. This is true genu valgum and not the result of torsional variations. This condition, too, resolves with growth, and normal adult knee alignment is obtained between 5 and 8 years of age. Assessment of the tibiofemoral angle (clinically and radiographically) in children between birth and 16 years of age reveals a mean varus alignment of 15 degrees in newborns. This decreases to approximately 10 degrees by 1 year of age. Neutral alignment occurs between 18 and 20 months of age. The maximum valgus of 12 degrees occurs by 3 to 4 years of age. The results are similar for boys and girls. By 7 years of age, the valgus alignment corrects to that of a normal adult (8 degrees in girls, 7 degrees in boys). Overall, 95% of cases of developmental physiologic genu varum and genu valgum resolve with growth. This is also true for children with more pronounced physiologic genu varus (16 to 35 degrees) or genu valgus (15 to 20 degrees), although in some children, the condition may not completely correct until adolescence.

TORSIONAL PROFILE

The torsional profile aids in the diagnosis and sequential follow-up of children with torsional variations (Fig. 45-1).

Foot Progression Angle

The foot progression angle represents the direction of the long axis of the foot with regard to the direction in which the child is walking (Fig. 45-2). Inward rotation is given a negative value and outward rotation a positive value. A normal foot progression angle in children and adolescence is 10 degrees (range, 3 to 20 degrees). The foot progression angle defines whether the gait is normal or if there is an in-toeing or out-toeing gait. The latter is considered abnormal when the foot progression angle exceeds 20 degrees. The recording of the angle allows a method for comparison during follow-up evaluations.

Hip Rotation

Hip rotation in extension is assessed with the child in the prone position and the knees together and flexed 90 degrees (Fig. 45-3). In this position, the hip is in neutral alignment. As the lower leg is rotated outwardly, internal rotation of the hip is produced, whereas inward rotation produces external rotation. The femoral neck normally makes a 135-degree angle with the femoral shaft. Typically, there is anterior angulation between the axis representing the femoral neck and the transcondylar axis of the distal femur. This angulation is known as *femoral anteversion*. Femoral anteversion decreases from approximately 40 degrees at birth to 15 degrees by maturity. A newborn hip typically externally rotates in extension to 80 to 90 degrees and has a limited internal rotation of 0 to 10 degrees. By 1 year of age, there is approximately 45 degrees of internal and external rotation. Hip rotation should be symmetrical. Asymmetrical rotation is

Table 45-2. Common Causes of In-Toeing and Out-Toeing	
In-Toeing	**Out-Toeing**
Medial (internal) femoral torsion	Lateral (external) femoral torsion
Medial (internal) tibial torsion	Lateral (external) tibial torsion
Metatarsus adductus	Calcaneovalgus feet
Talipes equinovarus (clubfoot)	Hypermobile pes planus

	Right	Left
Foot-progression angle (FPA)		
Hip rotation (extension)		
• Internal rotation		
• External rotation		
Thigh-foot angle (TFA)		
Foot shape		

Figure 45-1. Torsional profile for recording the measurements of the foot progression angle, hip rotation in extension, thigh-foot angle, and foot shape. This allows comparison between the right and left sides as well as with subsequent evaluations.

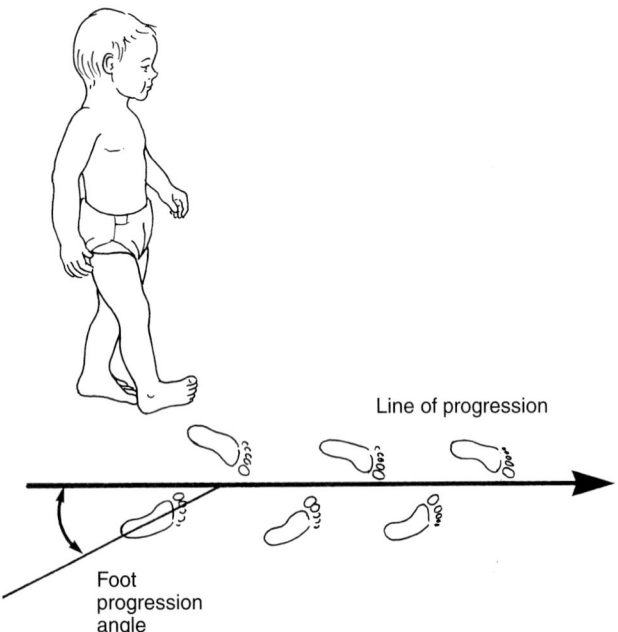

Figure 45-2. Foot progression angle. The long axis of the foot is compared with the direction in which the child is walking. If the foot points outward, the angle is positive. If the foot points inward, the angle is negative.

often indicative of a hip disorder and necessitates radiographs of the pelvis. The mean hip internal rotation in extension in older boys is 50 degrees (range, 25 to 65 degrees), and that in girls is 40 degrees (range, 15 to 60 degrees).

Thigh-Foot Angle

With the child in the prone position and the knees approximated and flexed 90 degrees, the long axis of the foot in the neutral or simulated weight-bearing position can be compared with the long axis of the thigh (Fig. 45-4). Inward rotation is given a negative value, whereas outward rotation is given a positive value. Inward rotation is indicative of internal tibial torsion, and outward rotation represents external tibial torsion. This angle must be accurately measured and recorded. The mean thigh-foot angle is 10 degrees (range, −5 to 30 degrees) from middle childhood through adult life. Infants have a mean thigh-foot angle of 5 degrees (range, −35 to 40 degrees) as a consequence of the normal in utero position.

Foot Shape

With the child again in the prone position, the shape of the foot is easily assessed (Fig. 45-5). This position is very helpful in the assessment of children with metatarsus adductus or a calcaneovalgus foot. The mobility of the ankle and subtalar joint can also be evaluated with the child in this position.

IN-TOED GAIT

Internal Femoral Torsion

Internal femoral torsion is the most common cause of in-toeing in children 2 years of age or older. It occurs more commonly in girls than boys (2:1). Most affected children have the common autosomal dominant condition generalized ligamentous laxity. Some authorities believe that femoral torsion is congenital, secondary to excessive or persistent infantile femoral anteversion, whereas others believe that it is acquired, secondary to abnormal sitting habits.

Clinical Examination. Clinical features of internal femoral torsion demonstrate that the entire lower extremity is inwardly rotated during gait. Characteristically, there is 80 to 90 degrees of internal rotation of the hip in the prone, extended position (Fig. 45-6). External rotation, as a consequence, is limited to 0 to 10 degrees. Features of generalized ligamentous laxity are present, including elbow, wrist, and finger hyperextension, thumb hyperabduction, knee hyperextension, and hypermobile pes planus. Involved children commonly sit in the "television" or "W"-style position. It is thought that this position allows the lower leg to act as a lever, thereby producing the torsional changes in the biologically plastic femora. This condition has also been called excessive or persistent femoral anteversion, implying an abnormality of the proximal femur. However, the torsion actually occurs throughout the femoral shaft and results in a change in the normal alignment between the hip and the knee.

Radiographic Evaluation. Radiographic evaluation of internal femoral torsion is not necessary. Results of anteroposterior radiography of the pelvis are normal, but there may be the appearance of a relatively vertical femoral neck angle, or coxa valga. However, if the radiograph is repeated with the hips in 15 degrees of abduction and 30 to 45 degrees internal rotation, the femoral neck angle is typically normal. CT or ultrasonography of the proximal and distal femur can be used to accurately measure the degree of torsion.

Treatment. The treatment of internal femoral torsion is predominantly by observation. Correction of abnormal sitting habits usually allows this variation to resolve with normal growth and development.

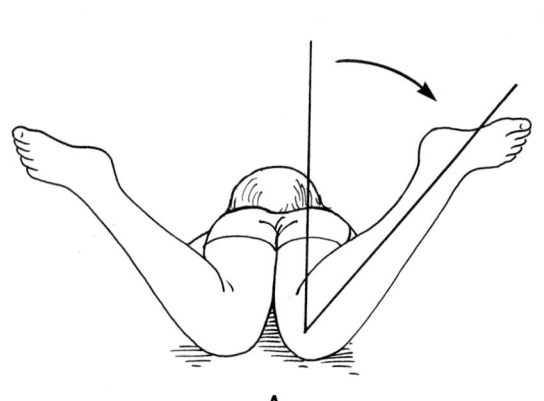

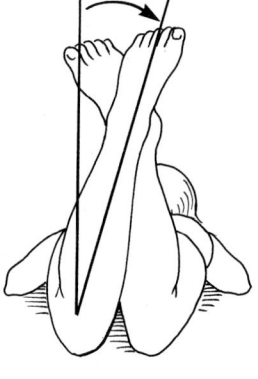

Figure 45-3. Hip rotation in extension. The child is in the prone position, with the knees flexed 90 degrees. The lower leg is vertically oriented. This is considered the neutral position. Outward rotation (A) of the leg produces internal hip rotation; inward rotation (B) produces external hip rotation.

A   B

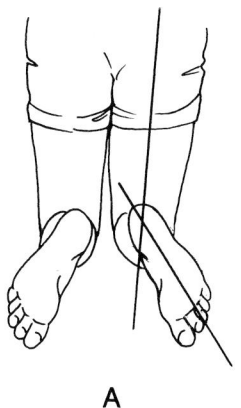
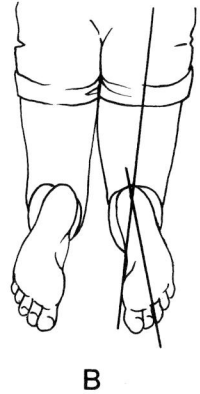
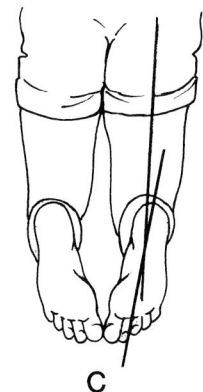

A **B** **C**

Figure 45-4. Thigh-foot angle. With the child in the prone position and the knees flexed and approximated, the long axis of the foot can be compared with the long axis of the thigh. The long axis of the foot bisects the heel and the third or middle toe. External tibial torsion (**A**) produces excessive outward rotation. Normal alignment (**B**) is characterized by slight external rotation. Internal tibial torsion produces inward rotation (**C**).

It takes 1 to 3 years for complete correction to occur, depending on the age of the child when the sitting habits are corrected. The correction of sitting habits can be very difficult in preschool-aged children, and improvement frequently does not occur until these children reach school age. The use of nighttime orthoses or daytime twister cables is of no value and may produce a compensatory external tibial torsion. The combination of internal femoral and compensatory external tibial torsion produces a genu valgum deformity. This can eventually result in patellofemoral malalignment, with patella subluxation or dislocation and pain.

Children 10 years of age or older may not have enough remaining musculoskeletal growth for spontaneous correction to occur. After these older children have been monitored up for 1 to 3 years without documentation of improvement or if there is significant cosmetic or functional disability, surgical intervention may be necessary. The procedures advocated include proximal femoral varus derotation osteotomy and simple derotation osteotomy of either the proximal or the distal femur. Sufficient derotation is performed to allow for equal internal and external hip rotation postoperatively.

It was once believed that internal femoral torsion was associated with bunions, back pain, degenerative osteoarthritis of the hip and knee, and decreased athletic ability. This is no longer accepted as true. The only significant long-term problem is abnormal gait and the potential for patellofemoral malalignment.

Internal Tibial Torsion

Internal tibial torsion is the most common cause of in-toeing in children younger than 2 years and is secondary to normal in utero positioning. This condition is commonly seen during the second year of life and may be associated with metatarsus adductus.

Clinical Examination. The degree of tibial torsion can be measured by the prone thigh-foot angle (torsional profile) (see Fig. 45-4). It can also be measured with the child supine and the knees flexed 90 degrees. The measurements should be recorded on each visit to the physician to document improvement.

Radiographic Evaluation. Radiographic assessment is of no value in the evaluation of internal tibial torsion. CT can be used to assess the degree of tibial torsion, but this is rarely necessary.

Treatment. Treatment of internal tibial torsion is predominantly conservative. This is a physiologic condition, and spontaneous

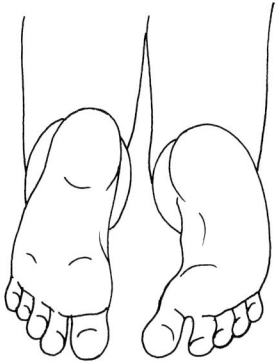

Figure 45-5. Foot shape. In the same position for measurement of the thigh-foot angle, the shape of the foot can also be evaluated. In this illustration, the left foot has normal alignment and the right foot demonstrates metatarsus adductus.

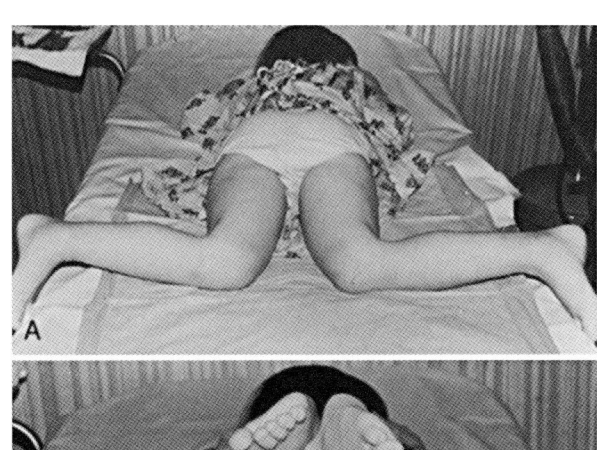
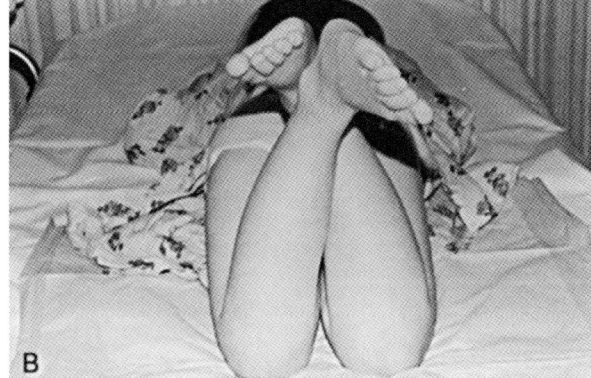

Figure 45-6. **A,** Clinical photograph of a 5-year-old girl demonstrating internal femoral torsion. She has approximately 80 degrees of internal rotation bilaterally. **B,** External rotation is limited to approximately 15 degrees, for a total arc of rotation of 90 to 95 degrees.

resolution with normal growth and development can be anticipated. Significant improvement usually does not occur until the child begins to pull up to standing and walk independently. Thereafter, it takes 6 to 12 months and occasionally longer for complete correction to occur. If there has been no documented improvement by 2 to 3 years of age, the use of a nighttime orthosis, such as a Denis Browne splint, may be considered. The effectiveness of night splints is controversial because of the lack of prospective studies on this issue. Persistent internal tibial torsion in an older child or adolescent is rare and may necessitate surgical derotation.

Metatarsus Adductus

Metatarsus adductus is a common problem of infants and young children. It occurs equally in boys and girls and is bilateral in approximately 50% of cases. Metatarsus adductus has hereditary tendencies and is more common in the firstborn than in later children, as a result of increased molding effect from the more rigid primigravida uterus and abdominal wall. Approximately 10% of children with metatarsus adductus have developmental dysplasia of the hip.

Clinical Examination. Clinically, the forefoot is adducted and occasionally supinated. The hindfoot and the midfoot are normal. The lateral border of the foot is convex, the base of the fifth metatarsal is prominent, and the medial border of the foot is concave. There is usually an increased interval between the first and second toes, with the great toe being held in an inwardly rotated or varus position. The ankle range of motion is normal. Forefoot mobility can vary from flexible to rigid. This parameter is assessed by stabilizing the hindfoot and midfoot in a neutral position and applying pressure over the first metatarsal head with the opposite hand. In the walking child with an uncorrected or partially corrected metatarsus adductus, there is an in-toed gait, abnormal shoe wear, and possible discomfort from shoe pressure.

Radiographic Evaluation. Radiographs of the foot are not necessary for routine metatarsus adductus because they do not demonstrate forefoot mobility. Anteroposterior and lateral weight-bearing radiographs demonstrate adduction of the metatarsals at the tarsometatarsal joint and an increased intermetatarsal angle between the first and second metatarsals. The midfoot and hindfoot are usually normal. Radiographs should be obtained if there are any suspected abnormalities of the midfoot or hindfoot.

Treatment. Treatment of metatarsus adductus is primarily conservative. The feet may be classified into three types of deformities, depending on forefoot flexibility:

Type I: The feet are flexible and can be placed into an overcorrected or abducted position. Voluntary correction can usually be elicited by stimulating the peroneal musculature by stroking the lateral border of the foot. These feet usually require no treatment.
Type II: These feet correct to the neutral position both passively and actively. The feet may benefit from a trial of modified shoes, such as straight or reversed last shoes. Commercially available orthoses may also be used. The shoes or orthoses are worn full time (22 hours per day) and the feet reevaluated at 4- to 6-week intervals. If the condition has improved, the treatment can be continued. If it has not improved, serial plaster long-leg or short-leg casts may be necessary.
Type III: These deformities are rigid and do not correct passively or actively. These feet are treated with serial plaster casts. The forefeet are manipulated before each cast application to stretch the medial soft tissue contractures. Short-leg walking casts are applied with the hindfoot held in the neutral position and the forefoot abducted. The casts are changed at 1- to 2-week intervals. Usually, complete correction can be obtained in 4 to 6 weeks,

depending on the age of the child and the severity of the deformity. The best results are obtained when the casting is initiated before 8 months of age. Once correction has been achieved, corrective shoes or orthoses may be used for an additional 2 to 3 months to maintain correction. A mild hallux varus may persist for several years after conservative treatment and may be of concern to the parents. This is commonly called the "searching toe" and eventually disappears with growth and development.

Significant metatarsus adductus persisting or manifesting after 4 years of age may necessitate surgical correction. Children 4 to 6 years of age with a fixed deformity undergo soft tissue releases. Serial casting is then carried out until forefoot correction has been obtained. This process usually requires 2 to 3 months. Children 6 years of age or older usually do not benefit from soft tissue releases alone and require metatarsal osteotomies to achieve satisfactory correction.

Talipes Equinovarus (Clubfoot)

A clubfoot represents a deformity not only of the foot but of the entire lower leg. Usually, a clubfoot is an obvious abnormality. It is classified into three groups:

1. The *congenital* clubfoot is usually an isolated abnormality.
2. The *teratologic* form is associated with a neuromuscular disorder, such as myelodysplasia (spina bifida), arthrogryposis multiplex congenita, or a syndrome complex.
3. *Positional* clubfoot is a normal foot that has been held in the deformed position in utero (as a result of oligohydramnios).

Congenital clubfoot, the most common type, is diagnosed and treated in infancy and usually does not produce a gait disturbance. Nevertheless, it is considered in the category of in-toeing because it can affect the alignment and function of the foot and lower leg in children. Persistent internal tibial torsion is common even after appropriate treatment. A mild (1.0- to 2.0-cm) lower extremity length inequality may be seen in adolescence, but this usually does not produce a limp or necessitate treatment. On occasion, residual muscle imbalance may cause the child to walk on the lateral border of the foot. This may produce discomfort and an antalgic gait. This problem is typically caused by a strong tibialis anterior muscle that is not opposed by its antagonists, the tibialis posterior and peroneus longus muscles. The problem can be corrected by centralizing the insertion of the tibialis anterior muscle to the mid-dorsum of the foot.

OUT-TOED GAIT

External Femoral Torsion

External femoral torsion, also known as *femoral retroversion,* is a very rare disorder unless it is associated with a slipped capital femoral epiphysis (SCFE).

Clinical Examination. Children with external femoral torsion demonstrate limitation of internal rotation and excessive external rotation when the hip is examined in the extended position. Typically, the hip externally rotates 70 to 90 degrees, whereas internal rotation is only 0 to 20 degrees. External femoral torsion is usually a bilateral disorder when it occurs idiopathically. If the deformity is unilateral, especially in an obese older child or a young adolescent, the presence of SCFE must be ruled out.

Radiographic Evaluation. Anteroposterior and Lauenstein (frog) lateral radiographs of the pelvis are necessary in any child or adolescent presenting with external femoral torsion, especially one who is obese, has nontraumatic anterior thigh or knee pain (referred pain), or has unilateral deformity. Approximately 20% of children with SCFE have simultaneous bilateral involvement. The typical changes of SCFE include widening of the physis and an abnormal relationship between the capital femoral epiphysis (CFE) and the femoral neck. The femoral head (CFE) appears to be slipped inferiorly and posteriorly, but, in actuality, the femoral neck is rotated anteriorly and superiorly.

Treatment. The treatment of idiopathic external femoral torsion is usually through observation. It is a very rare disorder that usually causes no significant functional impairment. If the femoral retroversion is caused by SCFE, the slip is treated surgically. The most common treatment today is in situ pinning with single or multiple cannulated screws.

On occasion, persistent femoral retroversion after SCFE can produce functional impairment, such as a severe out-toed gait and difficulty in approximating the knees in the sitting position. The latter can be very disabling to girls. Should this occur, a proximal femoral flexion, abduction, derotation osteotomy to restore the normal relationship between the femoral head and acetabulum and the distal femur is beneficial.

External Tibial Torsion

External tibial torsion is a relatively common disorder that is usually associated with a calcaneovalgus foot (Fig. 45-7). It is secondary to a normal variation of in utero positioning. In this condition, the plantar surface of the foot is against the wall of the uterus, forcing it into a hyperdorsiflexed, everted position. This results in the calcaneovalgus foot and, because of the externally rotated position, it also produces the external tibial torsion. When the alignment of the lower leg and the foot is combined with the normal increased external rotation of the hip in the newborn, it produces a very out-toed or externally rotated appearance of the lower extremity.

Clinical Examination. External tibial torsion is indicated by an abnormally positive thigh-foot angle (torsional profile) (see Fig. 45-4), typically 30 to 50 degrees.

Radiographic Evaluation. Radiographic assessment for external tibial torsion is not necessary.

Treatment. The treatment is observation. This condition follows the same clinical course as internal tibial torsion. Significant

improvement does not occur during the first year of life. With the onset of independent ambulation, spontaneous improvement begins to occur and is typically complete by 2 to 3 years of age.

Calcaneovalgus Foot

The calcaneovalgus foot is a relatively common finding in the newborn and is secondary to in utero positioning (see Fig. 45-7B). This condition is manifested by a hyperdorsiflexed foot with varying degrees of eversion and forefoot abduction. It is usually associated with external tibial torsion. These variations are typically unilateral but are occasionally bilateral.

Clinical Examination. The infant presents with an out-toed position of the involved extremity. The dorsum of the foot can easily be brought into contact with the anterior aspect of the lower leg, and the forefoot has an abducted appearance. The increased dorsiflexion should not be confused with the neonatal gestational age classification of Dubowitz. There is usually normal or almost normal ankle plantar flexion. External tibial torsion of 30 to 50 degrees is a common associated finding.

Three other conditions must be distinguished from a calcaneovalgus foot: (1) vertical talus, (2) posteromedial bow of the tibia, and (3) neuromuscular abnormalities, such as paralysis of the gastrocnemius muscle. The differentiation is usually made clinically with physical examination of the foot, lower leg, and neurologic systems and with appropriate radiographs.

Radiographic Evaluation. Simulated weight-bearing anteroposterior and lateral radiographs of the foot may be necessary to differentiate between the calcaneovalgus foot and a congenital vertical talus. In a calcaneovalgus foot, the radiographs either are normal or reveal an increase in hindfoot valgus. In the congenital vertical talus, the hindfoot is in equinus, whereas the midfoot and the forefoot are dorsally displaced, producing a rocker-bottom appearance. Anteroposterior and lateral radiographs of the tibia and fibula are necessary if there is bowing of the lower leg.

Treatment. In the typical calcaneovalgus foot, no treatment is necessary. The hyperdorsiflexion of the foot resolves during the first 3 to 6 months of life. On occasion, resistant feet may require passive stretching, taping, or casting into a plantar flexed position. Usually, by the time the child begins to pull to standing and walk independently, the calcaneovalgus condition has resolved. The external tibial torsion, however, persists and follows the same natural history as internal tibial torsion.

Hypermobile Pes Planus

Hypermobile, flexible, or pronated feet are flatfeet, a common cause of concern to parents. Children with this deformity are usually asymptomatic and have no limitation of activities. The family frequently thinks that the child is out-toeing because of the pronation of the midfoot and hindfoot, which may allow the forefoot to become abducted. Flexible flatfeet are also common in neonates and toddlers as a result of the associated laxity in the bone-ligament complexes of the feet and the abundant fat in the area of the medial longitudinal arch. The child usually demonstrates significant improvement by 6 years of age. In the older child, flexible flatfeet are usually secondary to generalized ligamentous laxity, an autosomal dominant condition. Most children and adolescents with flexible flatfeet or hypermobile pes planus are asymptomatic.

Clinical Examination. In the non–weight-bearing position in the older child with a flexible flatfoot, the normal medial longitudinal arch is visible, but in the weight-bearing position, the foot becomes

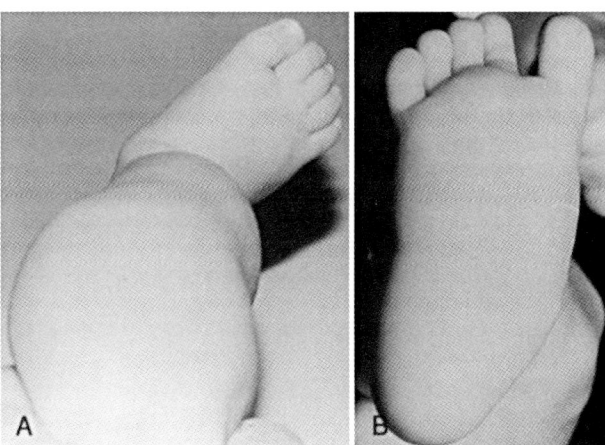

Figure 45-7. A, Clinical photograph of a 2-month-old girl demonstrating excessive external tibial torsion. This reverse or anterior thigh-foot angle shows approximately 50 degrees of external tibial torsion. B, A calcaneovalgus foot with forefoot abduction and increased hindfoot valgus in the same infant. There is also hyperdorsiflexibility of the foot in the ankle.

pronated with varying degrees of pes planus and hindfoot valgus. Instead of bearing weight over the lateral column of the foot, the weight is shifted medially, producing pronation. Subtalar motion is examined with the ankle in the neutral position and should be normal or slightly increased. Loss of subtalar motion may indicate a *rigid flatfoot*. Common causes of rigid flatfeet include tendo Achilles contracture, tarsal coalition, and neuromuscular disorders. Rigid flatfeet may also be a familial trait. Other joints, especially the elbows, hands, and knees, usually demonstrate generalized ligamentous laxity in patients with flexible flatfeet. Children with flexible flatfeet should be evaluated for external tibial torsion (torsional profile).

Radiographic Evaluation. Radiographs of asymptomatic flexible flatfeet are usually not indicated. Standing, anteroposterior, and lateral weight-bearing radiographs are obtained, if necessary. The most common indication is the presence of pain (Table 45-3). Anteroposterior radiographs reveal an increase in the talocalcaneal angle (>25 degrees) caused by the excessive hindfoot valgus. The lateral view shows distortion of the normal straight line relationship between the long axis of the talus and the first metatarsal and flattening of the normal medial longitudinal arch.

Treatment. Treatment of flexible flatfeet is conservative. Children with this problem do not predictably have symptoms related to their flatfeet; therefore, modified shoes and orthoses do not significantly alter the clinical or radiographic appearance of the feet. The diagnosis of flexible flatfeet is usually not possible until after 6 years of age. Treatment is indicated only for symptoms not attributable to other causes or to abnormal shoe wear. Feet that are symptomatic with vigorous physical activity usually respond readily to the use of commercially available medial longitudinal arch supports. Custom-made supports are usually more expensive and, in most cases, not more effective than commercially available supports. When the child has excessive heel valgus, pronation, or abnormal shoe wear that is unresponsive to a commercially or custom-made arch support, the use of a UCB (University of California, Berkeley) orthosis may be beneficial. This orthosis holds the hindfoot in the corrected position and restores the medial longitudinal arch. Surgery is rarely indicated. Lengthening of the calcaneus combined with medial cuneiform osteotomy can be effective.

EQUINUS GAIT (TOE-WALKING)

Toe-walking is probably the least common of the three categories of gait disturbances. Toe-walking can be a normal finding in children up to 3 years of age. Persistent toe-walking thereafter or acquired toe-walking at a later age is considered abnormal and necessitates careful evaluation. The differential diagnosis for persistent or acquired toe-walking includes

1. neuromuscular disorders, such as cerebral palsy, Duchenne muscular dystrophy, or spinal cord abnormality resulting from a tethered spinal cord or diastematomyelia
2. congenital tendo Achilles contracture (idiopathic toe-walking)
3. habitual toe-walking
4. lower extremity length discrepancy

The differentiation of toe-walking can usually be determined from the history and the physical examination. The examiner should establish the time at onset, the amount of time a child spends walking on his or her toes, whether it can be voluntarily corrected, and whether there has been improvement or worsening over time.

Neuromuscular Disorders

The neuromuscular disorder most likely to produce an equinus gait, either unilateral or bilateral, is cerebral palsy. The most common type of cerebral palsy is spastic diplegia, a disorder in which the lower extremities are more involved than the upper extremities. Prematurity is a common risk factor for spastic diplegia. It can be symmetrical or asymmetrical, with one side being slightly more involved than the other. Spastic diplegia tends to produce a bilateral equinus gait. Spastic hemiplegia, in which only one side is involved, is usually caused by birth trauma (asphyxia), perinatal stroke, or underlying congenital malformation and results in unilateral toe-walking.

Acquired or late-onset toe-walking is usually a result of a developing neuromuscular disorder, such as Duchenne muscular dystrophy. As muscle is replaced by fat and fibrous tissues, equinus and other contractures occur. There is usually a history of progressive clumsiness and frequent episodes of falling. The diagnosis of muscular dystrophy is usually made when the child is between 3 and 5 years of age. The diagnosis is confirmed by markedly elevated creatine phosphokinase levels and by muscle biopsy.

Table 45-3. **Differential Diagnosis of Foot Pain According to Age**

0-6 years	6-12 years	12-20 years
Poor-fitting shoes	Poor-fitting shoes	Poor-fitting shoes
Foreign body	Enthesopathy (JRA)	Stress fracture
Fracture	Foreign body	Puncture wound
Osteomyelitis*	Accessory navicular	Foreign body
Juvenile rheumatoid arthritis (JRA)	Pes cavus	Ingrown toenail
Leukemia	Tarsal coalition	Bunion
Drawing of blood	Hypermobile flatfoot	Metatarsalgia
Tumor†	Trauma (sprains)	Pes cavus
	Tumor†	Ganglion
	Osteomyelitis*	Plantar fasciitis
		Avascular necrosis of metatarsal (Freiberg infarction) or navicular bone (Köhler disease)
		Sever disease
		Achilles tendinitis
		Trauma (sprains)
		Plantar warts
		Tumor†

Modified from Behrman R, Kliegman R (eds): Nelson Essentials of Pediatrics, 2nd ed. Philadelphia, WB Saunders, 1994, p 726.

*Osteomyelitis may be hematogenous or secondary to a puncture wound.

†Soft tissue mass, osteoid osteoma, synovial sarcoma, lipoma, digital fibroma, hemangioma, subungual exostosis, Ewing sarcoma.

Clinical Examination. The examination of a child with toe-walking secondary to cerebral palsy reveals either a tendo Achilles contracture or a spastic equinus gait without contracture, as well as abnormal neurologic findings. These findings include increased muscle tone, spasticity, hyperactive deep tendon reflexes, and pathologic reflexes, such as a positive Babinski sign. Hamstring tightness, in addition to ankle equinus, may be a subtle sign of underlying mild cerebral palsy.

Children with Duchenne muscular dystrophy typically demonstrate pseudohypertrophy of the calves in addition to equinus contracture. They have proximal muscle weakness first, then generalized weakness, and perhaps (depending on the stage of progression) decreased or no upper extremity and knee-deep tendon reflexes. Ankle reflexes are usually preserved.

Radiographic Evaluation. Radiographic evaluation of a child with toe-walking is rarely necessary. CT or MRI of the brain and/or MRI of the spine is occasionally required during the evaluation of a possible neuromuscular disorder.

Other Testing. Dynamic electromyography and gait analysis studies can be helpful in distinguishing between toe-walking caused by mild cerebral palsy and that caused by a congenital tendo Achilles contracture. Serum muscle enzyme (creatine phosphokinase, aspartate transaminase, aldolase) levels and muscle biopsies are required for children with suspected Duchenne muscular dystrophy or other myopathies.

Treatment. The treatment of an equinus gait secondary to a neuromuscular disorder depends on an accurate diagnosis. The type of treatment depends on the severity of the involvement. In a spastic equinus gait without contracture, physical therapy and orthoses (daytime, nighttime, or both) may be beneficial. If a contracture has developed, serial casting may be performed in young children, whereas surgical lengthening of the tendo Achilles is usually necessary in older children.

Congenital Tendo Achilles Contracture (Idiopathic Toe-Walking)

Congenital tendo Achilles contracture or idiopathic toe-walking is a common cause of an equinus gait in young children, especially in bilateral cases. The foot cannot be dorsiflexed to the neutral or plantigrade position. The birth and developmental history and the neurologic findings are usually normal. However, mild developmental delays, especially in speech and in fine and gross motor skills, are seen in some children. A family history positive for tendo Achilles contracture, male predominance, and learning disabilities are common findings. Muscle biopsy samples have shown an increase in type I fibers, which suggests a neuropathic process.

Clinical Examination. Examination of the ankle shows a 10- to 15-degree fixed equinus contracture. The assessment of a tendo Achilles contracture should be performed with the hindfoot held in a slightly supinated position to bring the calcaneus beneath the talus. If this position is not used, dorsiflexion of the foot produces hindfoot valgus with the appearance of more dorsiflexion than is actually present. In congenital tendo Achilles contractures, no other musculoskeletal or neurologic abnormalities are present.

Radiographic Evaluation. Radiographs are not necessary unless an associated abnormality within the foot is thought to be present. Should this occur, anteroposterior and lateral weight-bearing radiographs of the foot should be obtained.

Treatment. The treatment of congenital tendo Achilles contracture consists of serial casting in young children. This method has a relatively high success rate, and the risk of recurrence after satisfactory correction is low. In older children or in younger children who have not responded to serial casting, surgical lengthening of the tendo Achilles is necessary. Postoperative orthoses are usually not required.

Habitual Toe-Walking

Habitual toe-walking occurs in a child who is walking on his or her toes voluntarily. Toe-walking occurs relatively commonly in young walkers. Their history and physical examination findings are entirely normal. This is a diagnosis of exclusion.

Clinical Examination. The findings in the examination of the child with habitual toe-walking are normal. The ankle has a full range of motion, and there is no evidence of an underlying neuromuscular disorder.

Radiographic Evaluation. Radiographic evaluation is not indicated.

Treatment. The treatment of habitual toe-walkers is observation. As the child becomes heavier and the central nervous system matures, the toe-walking should resolve. On occasion, an older child who has habitual toe-walking may benefit by a short course of short-leg walking casts. This may disrupt the toe-walking pattern and allow the child to develop a more normal gait. Habitual toe-walking is a very frustrating condition because no true abnormality is present, and the gait disturbance is voluntary. Fortunately, most habitual toe-walking ultimately resolves.

Lower Extremity Length Discrepancy

Lower extremity length discrepancy is a common cause for a unilateral equinus gait in older children and adolescents. Usually, mild discrepancies (1 to 2 cm) can be adequately compensated for during normal gait with minimal, if any, limping or toe-walking. Greater discrepancies may result in toe-walking. This is the child's preferred method of ambulation because the equinus equalizes leg lengths and prevents limping.

The differential diagnosis of a lower extremity length discrepancy is extensive (Table 45-4).

Clinical Examination. Examination of a child with a lower extremity length discrepancy shows shortness of the involved extremity; this can be measured by placing blocks of various heights beneath the foot until the pelvis is level. The range of motion of the joints, especially the hips, of the involved extremity must be assessed. The neurologic examination is also important. Children with subtle neurologic disorders, such as cerebral palsy, may also have a very mild lower extremity length discrepancy that contributes to an equinus gait.

Radiographic Evaluation. Children with a lower extremity length discrepancy require radiographic assessment. Lower extremity lengths can be measured radiographically by either an orthoroentgenogram or a scanogram. The orthoroentgenogram consists of overlapping exposures centered on the hips, knees, and ankles on a long cassette. The measurements of the lengths of the femur and tibia are made directly from the film. The advantage of this type of radiograph is that it shows associated angular deformities. A scanogram consists of three strip exposures of the hips, knees, and ankles on a standard-sized cassette with a radiographic ruler adjacent to the extremity. This is an accurate method of assessment, but it does not demonstrate angular deformities. CT techniques of

Table 45-4. Causes of Lower Extremity Length Discrepancy

Shortening	Lengthening
Congenital	**Congenital**
Hemiatrophy*	Hemihypertrophy*
Skeletal dysplasias	Local vascular malformation
Short femur	
Proximal focal femoral deficiency*	
Fibular, tibial hemimelia	
Developmental dysplasia of the hip*	
Tumor: Developmental	**Tumor: Developmental**
Neurofibromatosis	Neurofibromatosis
Multiple exostosis	Soft tissue hemangioma
Enchondromatosis (Ollier disease)	Arteriovenous malformation
Osteochondromatosis	Hemihypertrophy with Wilms tumor
Fibrous dysplasia (Albright syndrome)	Aneurysm
Punctate epiphyseal dysplasia	
Dysplasia epiphysealis hemimelia (Trevor disease)	
Radiation therapy before skeletal maturity (physeal arrest)*	
Resection of benign or malignant neoplasm	
Infection	**Infection: Inflammation**
Osteomyelitis*	Metaphyseal osteomyelitis
Septic arthritis	Rheumatoid arthritis
Tuberculosis	Hemarthrosis (hemophilia)
Trauma	**Trauma**
Physeal injury*	Metaphyseal, diaphyseal fracture
Failed joint replacement	Diaphyseal operations (bone grafts, osteotomy,
Atrophic nonunion	osteosynthesis, periosteal stripping)
Overlapping, malposition of fracture fragments*	
Burns	
Neuromuscular Disease	
Poliomyelitis	
Cerebral palsy*	
Myelomeningocele	
Peripheral neuropathy	
Focal cerebral lesions (hemiplegia)	
Other	
Legg-Calvé-Perthes disease*	
Slipped capital femoral epiphysis	

Adapted from Moseley C: Leg-length discrepancy. Pediatr Clin North Am 1986;33:1385; and Tachdjian M: Pediatric Orthopedics, 2nd ed. Philadelphia, WB Saunders, 1990.

Reprinted and modified from Behrman RE (ed): Nelson Textbook of Pediatrics, 14th ed. Philadelphia, WB Saunders, 1992, p 1702.

*Common.

measurement are the most accurate but not commonly used. Radiographs of the left hand and wrist for bone age are also obtained to assess when skeletal maturity will occur.

Treatment. The treatment of lower extremity length discrepancy depends on the function of the child and the magnitude of the discrepancy at skeletal maturity. Usually, discrepancies of 2 cm or less at maturity do not necessitate treatment. The normal mechanisms of gait allow compensation for these mild discrepancies without limping. Discrepancies between 2 and 5 cm are best managed by an appropriately timed epiphysiodesis (surgical closure of an epiphysis) of the distal femoral or proximal tibial epiphysis, or both, of the long extremity. Discrepancies greater than 5 cm may necessitate lengthening of the femur, tibia, or both, depending on the severity of the shortening and the location.

LIMPING

Limping, another common gait disturbance, is divided into antalgic or Trendelenburg gaits, depending on the presence or absence of pain and the duration of the stance phase between the normal and the abnormal sides. The differential diagnosis is extensive (Table 45-5). Most causes involve the lower extremity, but spinal disorders can also produce limping or difficulty walking, especially if there is spinal cord or peripheral nerve involvement. Painful (antalgic) gaits are predominantly caused by trauma, infection, neoplasia, and rheumatologic disorders. Trendelenburg gaits are generally caused by congenital, developmental, or neuromuscular disorders. Thus, antalgic gaits result from acute disorders, whereas Trendelenburg gaits usually result from chronic disorders. The type of gait, the presence or absence of systemic symptoms, and the anatomic location of the symptoms can usually be determined from the history and physical examination findings.

Table 45-5. Common Causes of Limping According to Age

Age	Antalgic (Painful)	Trendelenburg (Nonpainful)	Leg Length Discrepancy

Toddler (1-3 yr)	Infection
	  Septic arthritis
	    Hip
	    Knee
	  Osteomyelitis
	  Diskitis
	Occult trauma
	  Child abuse
	  Toddler's fracture
	Neoplasia
		Hip dislocation
		Neuromuscular disease
		  Cerebral palsy
			Negative

Child (4-10 yr)	Infection
	  Septic arthritis
	    Hip
	    Knee
	  Osteomyelitis
	  Diskitis
	Transient synovitis of the hip
	Legg-Calvé-Perthes disease
	Rheumatologic disorder
	  Juvenile rheumatoid arthritis
	Trauma
	Neoplasia (benign, malignant)
		Hip dislocation
		Neuromuscular disease
		  Cerebral palsy
			Positive

Adolescent (11+ yr)	Slipped capital femoral epiphysis Rheumatologic disorder Juvenile rheumatoid arthritis Trauma Neoplasia (benign, malignant)		Positive

Antalgic Gait

Congenital Origin

Tarsal Coalition. Tarsal coalition, also called *peroneal spastic flatfoot,* is a common foot disorder that is characterized by a painful, rigid valgus or pronation (flatfoot) deformity of the midfoot and hindfoot in association with peroneal muscle spasm but without true spasticity. This condition represents a congenital fusion or failure of segmentation between two or more tarsal bones. However, any condition that alters the normal motion of the subtalar joint may produce the clinical appearance of a tarsal coalition. Thus, congenital malformation, inflammatory disorders (e.g., juvenile rheumatoid arthritis), infection, neoplasms, and trauma involving the subtalar joint can manifest with pain, limping, or other symptoms similar to those of a tarsal coalition.

The most common coalitions occur between the calcaneus and navicular (calcaneonavicular) and the middle or medial facet between the talus and calcaneus (talocalcaneal). Coalitions can be fibrous, cartilaginous, or osseous. The incidence of tarsal coalition is approximately 1%, and it appears to be inherited as an autosomal dominant trait. Approximately 60% of calcaneonavicular and 50% of talocalcaneal coalitions are bilateral.

Clinical Examination. The onset of symptoms is insidious and usually occurs during late childhood or early adolescence. Although mild limitation of subtalar motion and a valgus or pronated hindfoot may have been present since early childhood, the onset of symptoms varies with the age at which the fibrous or cartilaginous coalition begins to ossify and further decrease motion. The talonavicular coalition ossifies between the ages of 3 and 5 years; the calcaneonavicular coalition, between 8 and 12 years; and the middle facet talocalcaneal coalition, between 12 and 16 years of age. The pain is typically felt laterally in the hindfoot and radiates proximally along the lateral malleolus and distal fibula into the peroneal muscle region. Symptoms are usually aggravated by sports or other vigorous activities and are relieved by rest. The foot is pronated in both the weight-bearing and the non–weight-bearing positions. Subtalar joint motion is diminished or absent, and attempts at motion produce pain.

Radiographic Evaluation. The diagnosis of tarsal coalition is made radiographically. The initial radiographs should include anteroposterior and lateral weight-bearing radiographs of the foot and an oblique radiograph. The latter is necessary in making the diagnosis of a calcaneonavicular coalition. Beaking of the anterior aspect of the talus in the lateral view suggests a talocalcaneal coalition. Axial views of the hindfoot can be useful in the diagnosis of a middle-facet talocalcaneal coalition. CT is the diagnostic procedure of choice for this coalition. CT should also be performed for all coalitions, because more than one coalition can occur.

Treatment. Treatment varies according to the type of coalition, the age of the patient, the extent of the coalition, and the presence or absence of degenerative osteoarthritis. Nonoperative treatment consists of cast immobilization, shoe inserts, or orthotics. Operative management usually involves excision of the coalition and interposition of muscle (calcaneonavicular), fat, or tendon (middle-facet talocalcaneal) to prevent re-formation of the coalition. Resections are effective in relieving pain, improving subtalar motion, and allowing resumption of normal activities. However, if significant degenerative osteoarthritis is present, a triple arthrodesis may be necessary. Only occasionally does nonoperative treatment yield complete relief of symptoms and restoration of normal function.

Developmental Origin

Legg-Calvé-Perthes Disease. Legg-Calvé-Perthes disease (LCPD) is idiopathic avascular necrosis (osteonecrosis) of the (CFE) and the associated complications in an immature, growing child. This disorder is caused by an interruption of the blood supply to the CFE. It occurs predominantly in boys (4:1 to 5:1) and is bilateral in approximately 20% of affected children. Children with LCPD have delayed skeletal or bone age, disproportionate growth, and mildly short stature. Secondary osteonecrosis is seen in patients with sickle cell anemia.

Clinical Examination. The clinical onset of LCPD typically occurs between 2 and 12 years of age, at a mean age of 7 years. Most children present with a limp and mild or intermittent pain in the anterior thigh or knee. This condition has been referred to as a "painless limp." Pertinent early physical findings include antalgic gait; muscle spasm with mild restriction of hip motion, especially abduction and internal rotation; proximal thigh atrophy; and mild short stature.

Radiographic Evaluation. The diagnosis is typically made from anteroposterior and Lauenstein (frog) lateral radiographs of the pelvis (Fig. 45-8). The radiographic characteristics can be divided into five distinct stages, depending on the interval from the onset of symptoms: (1) cessation of CFE growth, (2) subchondral fracture, (3) resorption or fragmentation, (4) reossification, and (5) healed, or

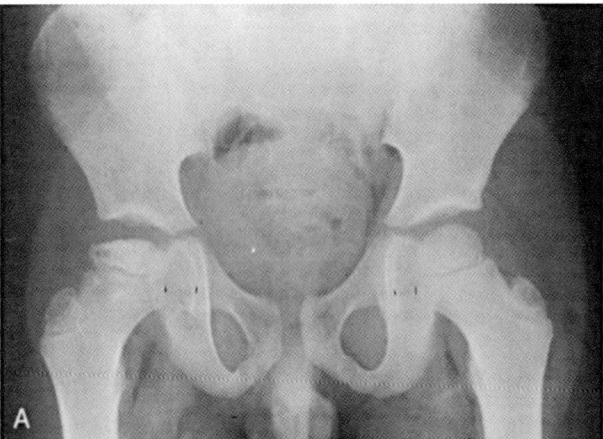

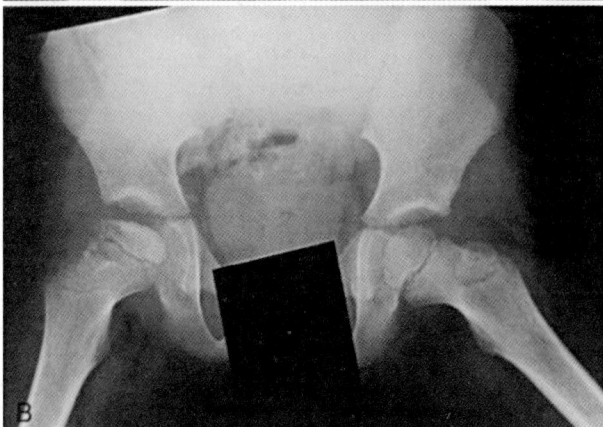

Figure 45-8. **A,** Anteroposterior radiograph of the pelvis demonstrating Legg-Calvé-Perthes disease (LCPD) of the right hip. The capital femoral epiphysis (CFE) is collapsing, and there is mild widening of the medial joint space. The left CFE is normal. **B,** Lauenstein (frog) lateral radiograph of the pelvis demonstrating limited hip abduction caused by LCPD.

residual. The symptoms are usually most pronounced during the phase of the subchondral fracture and fragmentation. A child with LCPD has a potential for collapse and extrusion of the femoral head, which results in a permanent deformity. If plain radiographs do not demonstrate LCPD in suspected cases, a bone scan or MRI is helpful.

Treatment. LCPD is a local, self-healing disorder. Prevention of femoral head deformity and secondary degenerative osteoarthritis in adulthood are the only indications for treatment. The four basic treatment goals are (1) elimination of hip irritability; (2) restoration and maintenance of a good range of hip motion; (3) prevention of CFE collapse, extrusion, or subluxation; and (4) attainment of a spherical femoral head at healing. Current treatment methods involve a concept of containment. The femoral head is contained within the acetabulum so that the latter acts as a mold for the reossifying CFE. This task may be accomplished by nonsurgical containment with abduction casts or orthosis or by surgical containment with proximal femoral varus osteotomy, pelvic osteotomy, or both. The long-term results favor operative containment, and satisfactory results occur in approximately 85% of cases.

Slipped Capital Femoral Epiphysis. SCFE is the most common adolescent hip disorder. It generally occurs in those who are obese and have delayed skeletal maturation and in those who are tall and thin and have had a recent growth spurt. It can also occur as a complication of an underlying endocrine disorder, such as hypothyroidism and pituitary disorders. When SCFE occurs before puberty, a hormonal abnormality or systemic disorder should be suspected. Studies of the histopathologic features of SCFE have indicated that mechanical factors are the ultimate cause of slippage. The initial abnormality is most likely secondary to endocrine changes during early adolescence. Obesity produces high shear forces across a weakened and obliquely oriented CFE, resulting in slippage.

Clinical Examination. The physical findings depend on the degree of slippage and the classification. The disorder is classified as either stable or unstable. In an unstable or acute SCFE, the CFE is separated from the femoral neck. This is extremely painful, and the adolescent is unable to stand or bear weight. In a stable or chronic SCFE, the most common type, the CFE and femoral neck are in continuity, and the slippage is occurring slowly by plastic deformation. The adolescent has an antalgic, out-toed gait. The hip range of motion demonstrates a lack of internal rotation and an increase in external rotation. Also, as the hip is flexed, it becomes progressively more externally rotated. Limitation of flexion and abduction in extension may also be present as a result of the deformity of the proximal femur.

Radiographic Evaluation. The diagnosis of SCFE is confirmed radiographically. Anteroposterior and Lauenstein (frog) lateral radiographs of the pelvis must be obtained (Fig. 45-9). Both hips should be visualized on each radiograph for simultaneous comparison. The earliest sign of SCFE is widening of the physeal plate without slippage. This is considered a *preslip condition*. If slippage occurs, the CFE remains in the acetabulum, whereas the femoral neck rotates anteriorly and superiorly, which results in varus and retroversion of the femoral head and neck. The severity of slippage can be classified by the degree of displacement of the CFE on the femoral neck.

Treatment. The goals of treatment are to prevent further slippage and minimize complications. These are achieved by performing an epiphysiodesis of the CFE. The technique selected depends on the classification and severity of slippage. The most common method is in situ internal fixation with a single or multiple cannulated screw.

Complications include chondrolysis and avascular necrosis of the CFE. These occur in approximately 5% of cases and can be another cause of limping.

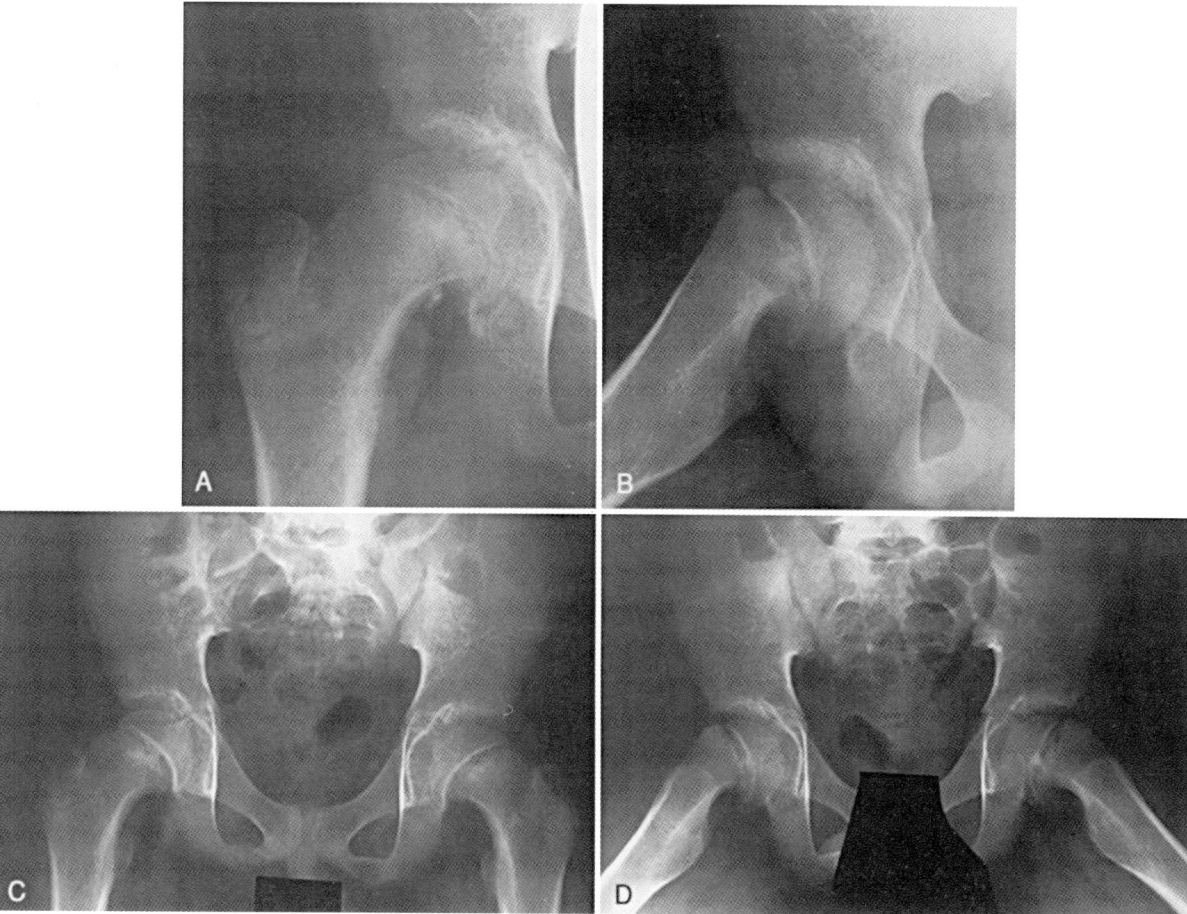

Figure 45-9. A, Anteroposterior radiograph of the right hip in a 13-year-old obese boy who had been limping and complaining of anterior thigh and knee pain for approximately 2 months. There is a mild stable or chronic slipped capital femoral epiphysis (SCFE). Klein's line, a line drawn along the superior aspect of the femoral neck, does not bisect the lateral portion of the CFE and thereby indicates slippage. Also, the physis is wide and irregular. B, Lauenstein (frog) lateral radiograph clearly demonstrates the slippage of the CFE with respect to the femoral neck. C, Anteroposterior radiograph of the pelvis demonstrates an asymptomatic mild stable or chronic left SCFE. It is always important to order radiographs of the pelvis rather than individual views of the right or left hip. D, Lauenstein (frog) lateral radiograph confirms bilateral SCFE.

Trauma

Sprains, Strains, and Contusions. *Sprains* are ligamentous injuries, whereas *strains* are muscle injuries. *Contusions* are the result of a direct injury and involve the skin and the subcutaneous tissues as well as underlying muscle.

Sprains are divided into three grades:

- grade I: mild with only slight stretching of the ligament
- grade II: a moderate injury with partial tearing of the ligament but normal stability
- grade III: a severe injury with ligamentous disruption and instability

Strains, sprains, and contusions of the lower extremities are among the most common injuries that produce limping. There is usually a history of trauma, and the location is readily apparent because of soft tissue swelling, ecchymoses, and pain. Most of these injuries occur during athletic activities, but they can also be the result of simple falls or other minor injuries.

Clinical Examination. In sprains, the physical examination typically reveals that the involved ligament is tender to direct palpation. There may be soft tissue swelling as well as ecchymoses. The range of motion of the involved joint is typically decreased because of pain. On occasion, a mild joint effusion or hemarthrosis may be present.

Strains involve the muscles, and there is usually tenderness to palpation, soft tissue swelling, and pain with joint motion as a result of stretching of the involved muscle. A palpable defect within the muscle is uncommon except in the most severe injuries. These injuries usually limit the excursion of the muscle and its associated joints.

Radiographic Evaluation. In children who sustain sprains, strains, or significant contusions, anteroposterior and lateral radiographs should be obtained. A word of caution regarding sprains is necessary. In children, ligaments are usually stronger than the adjacent physes. Therefore, a physeal injury may be present and may have the same clinical features as a sprain (Fig. 45-10). This is especially true with lateral ankle injuries. It is more likely that a Salter-Harris type 1 separation of the distal fibular epiphysis has occurred, rather than a true ligament injury. This condition should be suspected when there is more tenderness to palpation over the lateral malleolus than over the ligaments. If plain radiographs are normal, stress radiographs may be necessary to establish the diagnosis. This concept also applies to the knee.

Treatment. Treatment of sprains, strains, and contusions is usually symptomatic unless there is a grade III sprain or a physeal fracture. In the latter, cast immobilization is necessary.

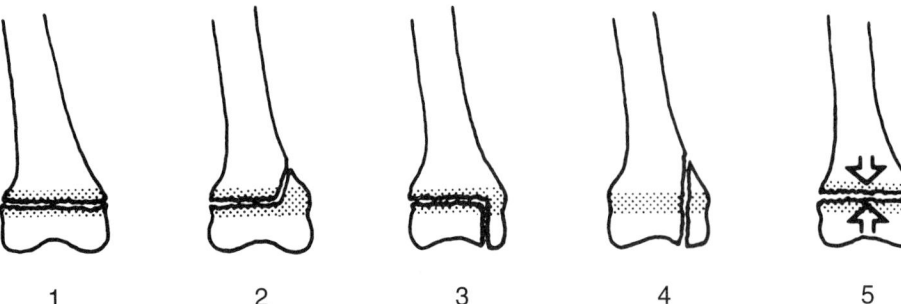

Figure 45-10. Salter-Harris classification of epiphyseal fractures. Types 1 and 2 are the most common. **1,** The epiphysis separates from the metaphysis. The germinal cells remain with the epiphysis, usually uninjured. Healing is rapid and growth is seldom arrested. **2,** Similar to type 1, except that a small piece of metaphysis breaks free to remain with the epiphysis. Healing is rapid and growth is usually normal. **3,** Separation passes a variable distance along the physis, then crosses the epiphysis. Accurate reduction of the intraarticular fracture is necessary to prevent later traumatic arthritis. Open reduction may be needed. Growth disturbances are not usually a problem. **4,** The fracture extends from the joint, across the physis, and into the metaphysis. This usually necessitates open reduction to prevent unilateral growth arrest and traumatic arthritis from malposition. **5,** This is a crushing injury that leads to death of the germinal cells of the physis and arrest of growth. This type is rare. (From Behrman RE [ed]: Nelson Textbook of Pediatrics, 14th ed. Philadelphia, WB Saunders, 1992, p 1722.)

Occult Fractures. Occult fractures of the tibia are a relatively common cause of limping or refusal to bear weight in very young children. They can also occur in the femur and fibula. These fractures can be the result of very innocuous trauma, such as tripping while walking, stepping on a toy, or falling from a height. Frequently, the injury may not have been observed, and the child cannot convey to the parents what happened. This can result in a very confusing appearance.

The most common occult fracture in early childhood is the "toddler's fracture" of the tibia. This is an oblique fracture of the distal third of the tibia without an associated fibula fracture. It most commonly occurs in children younger than 4 years of age. Occult tibia fractures can also occur in the metaphyseal regions, usually distally, but only rarely in the diaphysis. Diaphyseal fractures are more commonly the result of child abuse.

Clinical Examination. Physical findings in a child with an occult fracture can be very subtle. There is usually minimal, if any, soft tissue swelling. There is mild tenderness and perhaps increased warmth on palpation over the fracture. On occasion, the increased warmth may be indicative of osteomyelitis. Stress examination of the involved bone increases discomfort.

Radiographic Evaluation. Anteroposterior and lateral radiographs should be obtained (Fig. 45-11). The characteristic finding of a toddler's fracture is a faint oblique fracture line crossing the distal third of the tibia. On occasion, oblique radiographs may be helpful in revealing the fracture. Frequently, initial radiographs reveal no abnormality. If plain radiographs are normal, the child has no systemic symptoms, and an occult fracture of the tibia is suspected, simple immobilization in a long-leg cast is indicated. Another set of radiographs in 1 to 2 weeks usually reveals the fracture and evidence of healing. If, however, the child has systemic symptoms, such as low-grade fever, and if osteomyelitis is thought to be present, a bone scan should be obtained.

Treatment. An occult fracture, such as toddler's fracture, is treated with simple cast immobilization. The fractures typically heal satisfactorily within 2 to 4 weeks. A hip spica cast may be necessary for an occult fracture of the proximal femur.

Neoplasia

Neoplastic lesions of the musculoskeletal system in children are common. Fortunately, most are benign. Neoplastic lesions, benign or malignant, that involve bone, cartilage, or soft tissue of the spine, pelvis, and lower extremities can manifest as a mass, can cause pain, and can produce an antalgic gait. Leukemia or metastatic neuroblastoma of the bone marrow may produce deep bone pain and limp without objective findings on physical examination (no swelling or

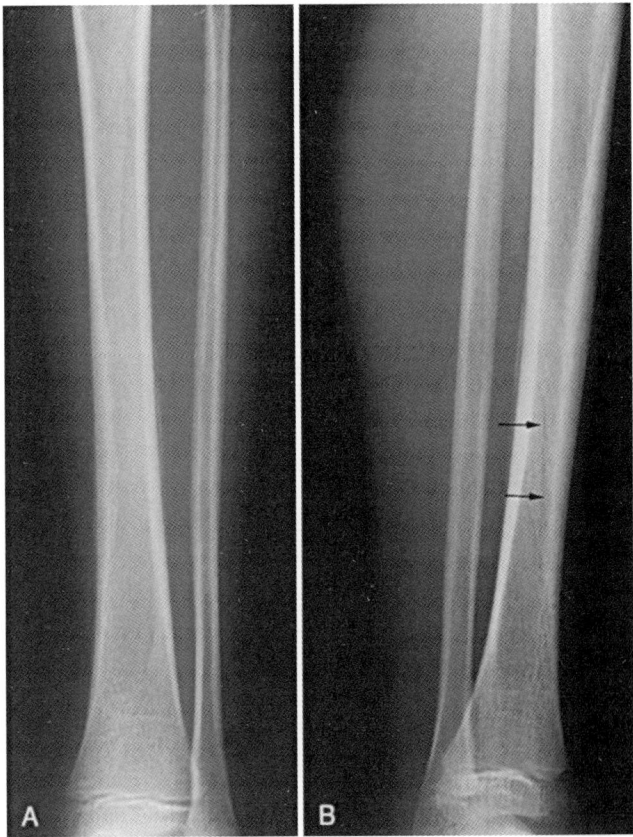

Figure 45-11. A, Anteroposterior radiograph of the lower leg of a 2-year-old girl who had been limping on the left lower leg for approximately 1 week. There was no observed trauma. No obvious abnormality is visible in this view. **B,** Lateral radiograph showing a faint oblique fracture line (*arrows*). This is characteristic of the "toddler's fracture." There is already early subperiosteal new bone or callus formation posteriorly.

tenderness). Night pain is a common characteristic of both benign and malignant primary or metastatic tumors. Osseous lesions can usually be diagnosed on plain radiographs, whereas for those of cartilage or soft tissue, MRI or other special imaging studies may be required for diagnosis.

Benign Neoplasms. The most common benign lesions that produce limping include a unicameral (simple) bone cyst and osteoid osteoma (Table 45-6). Other, less common benign lesions that can produce pain and limping include eosinophilic granuloma of bone, osteochondroma, and chondroblastoma. The latter lesion typically involves the epiphysis, especially of the proximal humerus.

In unicameral bone cysts, the symptoms are usually caused by a nondisplaced pathologic fracture. On occasion, a displaced fracture may occur. The most common location for a unicameral bone cyst is the proximal humerus, followed by the proximal femur. These can occur in any of the bones of the lower extremities, including the foot.

Osteoid osteomas have a highly vascularized nidus, which incites an intense, painful, inflammatory reaction. This results in sclerosis of the surrounding bone. The pain is typically worse at night and is characteristically relieved by aspirin.

Radiographic Evaluation. Most benign neoplasms are visible on anteroposterior and lateral radiographs of the symptomatic area. Characteristics of benign lesions include well-circumscribed lesions without periosteal new bone formation or soft tissue mass. If a lesion is suspected but not visible on plain radiographs, such as may occur in an osteoid osteoma, a technetium bone scan may be helpful. Further evaluation can be achieved with CT or MRI.

Treatment. The diagnosis and treatment of benign neoplasms are usually surgical. Biopsy is usually necessary to obtain a histologic diagnosis. Unicameral bone cysts can be managed by steroid injections or by curettage and bone grafting. With osteoid osteomas, resection is usually necessary to relieve symptoms. Other benign lesions are usually excised at the time of biopsy.

Malignant Neoplasms. Malignant lesions of the musculoskeletal system are relatively uncommon. Leukemia is the most common childhood malignancy and is frequently accompanied by musculoskeletal complaints, such as limping, fever, bone pain, pallor, bruising, and weight loss (Fig. 45-12). Common malignancies involving the musculoskeletal system include osteogenic sarcoma, Ewing sarcoma, and intraspinal tumors, such as astrocytomas (Table 45-7).

Table 45-6. Benign Bone Tumors and Cysts

Disease	Characteristics	Roentgenography	Treatment	Prognosis
Osteochondroma (osteocartilaginous exostosis)	Common; distal metaphysis of femur, proximal humerus, proximal tibia; painless, hard, nontender mass	Bony outgrowth, sessile or pedunculated	Excision, if symptomatic	Excellent; malignant transformation rare
Multiple hereditary exostoses	Osteochondroma of long bones; bone growth disturbances	Same as for osteochondroma	Same as for osteochondroma	Recurrences
Osteoid ostoma	Point tenderness; pain relieved by aspirin; femur and tibia; predominantly found in boys	Osteosclerosis surrounds small radiolucent nidus, 1 cm	Same as for osteochondroma	Excellent
Giant osteoid osteoma (osteoblastoma)	Same as for osteoid ostoma but more destructive	Osteolytic component; size greater than 1 cm	Same as for osteochondroma	Excellent
Enchondroma	Tubular bones of hands and feet; pathologic fractures, swollen bone; Ollier disease if multiple lesions are present	Radiolucent diaphyseal or metaphyseal lesion; may calcify	Excision or curettage	Excellent; malignant transformation rare
Nonossifying fibroma	Silent; rare pathologic fracture, onset in late childhood, adolescence	Incidental roentgenographic finding; thin sclerotic border, radiolucent lesion	None or curettage with fractures	Excellent; heals spontaneously
Eosinophilic granuloma	Onset at age 5-10 yr, skull, jaw, long bones; pathologic fracture; pain	Small, radiolucent without reactive bone; punched-out lytic lesion	Biopsy, excision rate; irradiation	Excellent; may heal spontaneously
Brodie abscess	Insidious local pain; limp; suspected as malignancy	Circumscribed metaphyseal osteomyelitis; lytic lesions with sclerotic rim	Biopsy; antibiotics	Excellent
Unicameral bone cyst (simple bone cyst)	Metaphysis of long bone (femur, humerus); pain, pathologic fracture	Cyst in medullary canal, expands cortex; fluid-filled unilocular or multilocular cavity	Currettage; steroid injection into lesion; bone graft	Excellent some heal spontaneously
Aneurysmal bone cyst	Same as for unicameral bone cyst; contains blood, fibrous tissue	Expands beyond metaphyseal cartilage	Curettage, bone graft	Excellent

From Thompson GH: Common orthopedic problems of children. In Behrman RE, Kliegman RM (eds): Nelson Essentials of Pediatrics, 2nd ed. Philadelphia, WB Saunders, 1994, p 744.

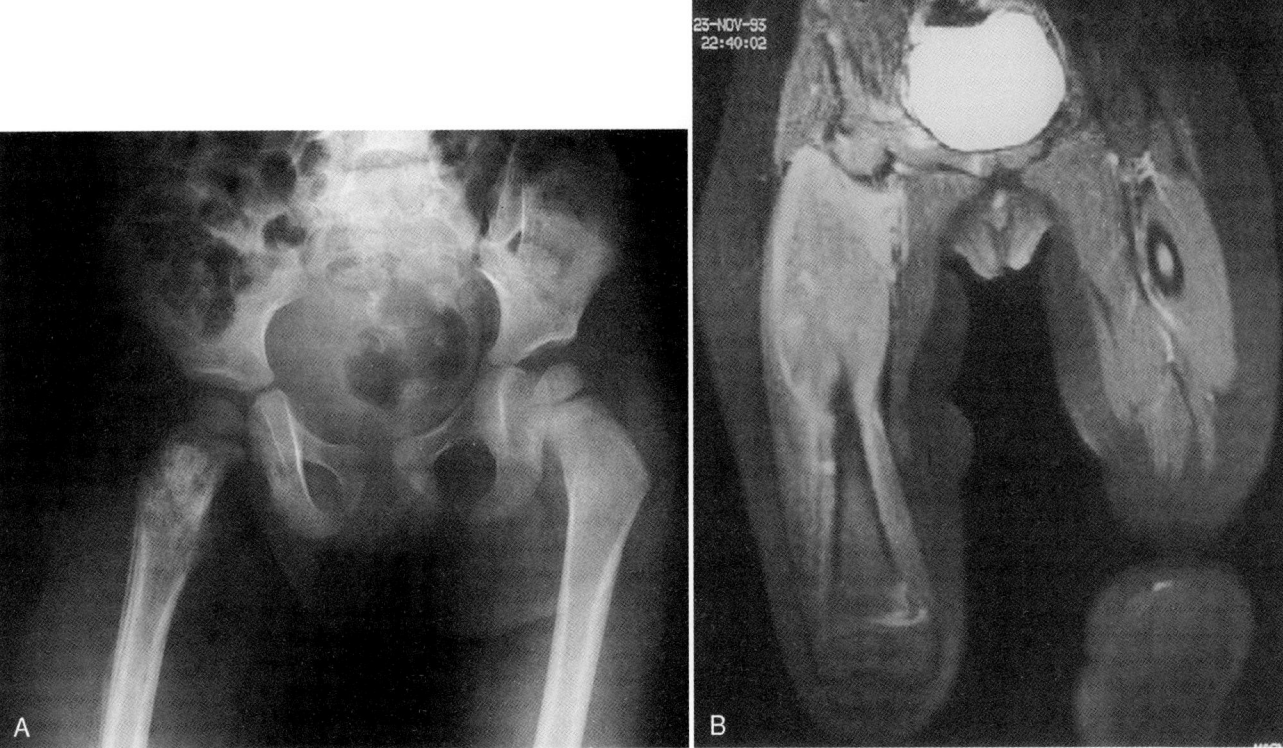

Figure 45-12. A, Anteroposterior pelvic radiograph of a 2-year-old girl who had been limping for 4 months. There is an extensive destructive lesion on the right proximal femur. B, A large soft tissue mass is demonstrated in MRI scan. The preoperative diagnosis was Ewing sarcoma, but at biopsy the diagnosis was acute lymphoblastic leukemia.

Intraspinal tumors tend to produce neurologic symptoms, such as muscle weakness, as the cause of limping. The other lesions may produce a mass, bone weakness, and possible pathologic fractures. Weight loss, fever, and pain are common associated complaints.

Clinical Evaluation. A careful musculoskeletal and neurologic examination is necessary for any child with a suspected neoplasm. In many cases, a mass, either in the involved bone or in adjacent soft tissues, may be palpable. These are typically tender and warm. These lesions are frequently adjacent to joints and may result in decreased range of motion. Neurologic evaluation may show evidence of muscle weakness or abnormal reflexes, suggestive of spinal cord or peripheral nerve involvement.

Radiographic Evaluation. Anteroposterior and lateral radiographs of the involved area usually reveal the presence of a neoplasm. Characteristics of a malignant osseous lesion include bone destruction, permeative or infiltrative appearance, periosteal new bone formation (Codman triangle), and an associated soft tissue mass (see Table 45-7). Radiographic abnormalities associated with acute leukemia include diffuse osteopenia, metaphyseal bands, periosteal new bone formation, geographic lytic lesions, sclerosis, and permeative distraction. Additional studies, such as a bone scan or MRI, may be helpful in localizing the lesion.

Treatment. Treatment of malignant lesions is complex. When they occur in the extremities, amputation or limb salvage procedures are usually performed. For intraspinal lesions, excision is required. On occasion, associated spinal fusions may be necessary to prevent

a postoperative spinal deformity. Chemotherapy and radiation are common adjunctive therapies.

Infection

Septic Arthritis/Osteomyelitis. Bone and joint infections are a common cause of limping in toddlers and children. When the infection is confined to the synovium of a joint, the condition is termed *septic arthritis.* If the primary focus of the infection is within bone, even if the joint is secondarily involved, the condition is termed *osteomyelitis.* Osteomyelitic processes can be acute, subacute, or chronic.

Acute osteomyelitis most commonly involves the femoral neck, the distal femoral metaphysis, and the proximal tibial metaphysis. Acute septic arthritis usually involves the hip, knee, or ankle. Children with these infections may be acutely ill.

Subacute osteomyelitis, which has a very distinct and different manifestation, occurs most commonly about the knee (Fig. 45-13). These children are usually afebrile and have night pain. Their hematologic studies yield normal findings. Radiographs show sclerotic metaphyseal lesions that occasionally cross the growth plate into the epiphysis. Culture specimens are positive only occasionally, and they invariably show *Staphylococcus aureus.* Sexually active adolescents may develop septic arthritis as a result of gonococcal infections.

Chronic osteomyelitis is exceedingly uncommon but is associated with open bone injuries after trauma (fractures, penetrating wounds).

Clinical Examination. Children with bone and joint infections may exhibit the clinical signs of bacteremia and infection, including elevations in temperature, white blood cell count, erythrocyte

Table 45-7. Comparison of Osteogenic and Ewing Sarcoma

	Osteogenic Sarcoma	Ewing Sarcoma
Age	Adolescence	Childhood and adolescence
Race	All races	White
Sex (M:F ratio)	1.5:1	1.5:1
Cell	Spindle cell, osteoid	Nonosseous, small round cell
Predisposition	Retinoblastoma	None
	Radiotherapy	
	Alkylating agents	
Site	Metaphysis, epiphysis; distal femur > proximal tibia > proximal humerus	Diaphysis, medullary cavity, cortical bone, soft tissue; femur > pelvis > tibia > humerus
Presentation	Local pain	Pain, fever, increased ESR, FUO, weight loss
Roentgenogram	Lytic, sclerotic	Mottled, lytic
	Sunburst pattern	Onion skin pattern
Differential diagnosis	Ewing sarcoma, osteomyelitis	Osteomyelitis, eosinophilic granuloma, lymphoma, neuroblastoma, rhabdomyocarcoma
Metastasis	Lung, bones	Lung, bones
	Skip lesions in the same bone	
Treatment	Surgery, chemotherapy	Surgery, radiotherapy
	Limb salvage if tumor is resectable and the patient is near adult height	Chemotherapy
Outcome	50%-60% survival	60% survival without metastasis; 5%-15% with metastasis, primary site dependent
Poor prognosis	Onset at age < 10 yr, large tumor size (>15 cm), symptoms < 2 months, metastasis	Pelvis, soft tissue tumor, increased LDH, metastasis, increased circulating PMNs, decreased circulating lymphocytes

Adapted from Behrman RE (ed): Nelson Textbook of Pediatrics, 14th ed. Philadelphia, WB Saunders, 1992, p 1312.

ESR, erythrocyte sedimentation rate; F, female; FUO, fever of unknown origin; LDH, lactate dehydrogenase; M, male; PMN, polymorphonuclear neutrophil.

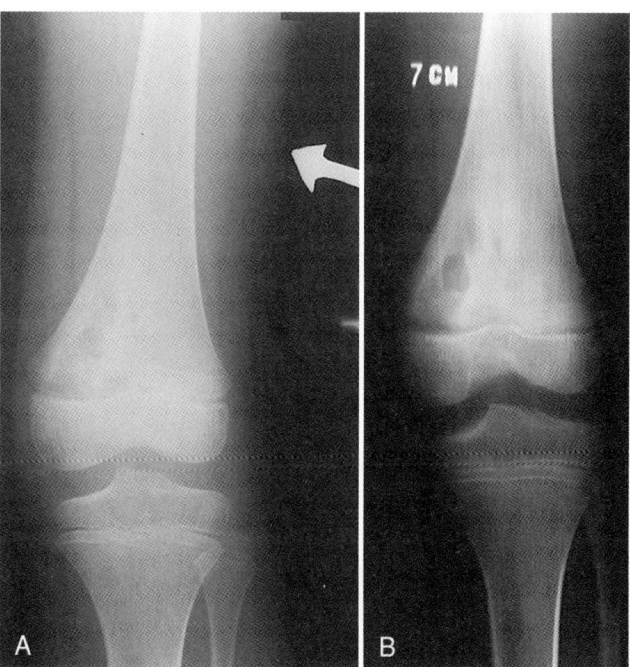

Figure 45-13. A, Anteroposterior radiograph of the distal femur in a 12-year-old girl with limping and nighttime knee pain for 6 months. There is a lucent lesion with surrounding sclerosis in the metaphysis. The lesion crosses the epiphysis; this is characteristic of a subacute osteomyelitis. B, Anteroposterior tomography clearly demonstrates the lucent nature of the lesion and its surrounding sclerosis.

sedimentation rate, and C-reactive protein level. Some infants present only with "pseudoparalysis." When the hip joint is involved, the child holds the hip in a position of flexion, abduction, and external rotation. This position unwinds the hip capsule and allows it to hold the greatest volume of intracapsular fluid. This initially decreases pressure, but as the pus continues to accumulate, even this position fails to relieve symptoms. A hip joint effusion is usually not palpable, but there may be overlying soft tissue swelling and tenderness.

Infections about peripheral joints, such as the knee, are more easily diagnosed. There is typically a joint effusion and perhaps soft tissue swelling, erythema, and increased warmth over the metaphysis if osteomyelitis is present. Osteomyelitis typically manifests with point tenderness over the involved site; with continued bone destruction and rupture of pus into the periosteum, tenderness becomes more diffuse. Infections can also occur about the ankle and foot. Infection of the foot is less common except as a sequela to puncture wounds through a tennis shoe, producing the classic *Pseudomonas aeruginosa* (or *S. aureus*) osteomyelitis-osteochondritis.

Radiographic Evaluation. Plain radiographs are not helpful in the early diagnosis (first 7 to 10 days) of osteomyelitis, inasmuch as they are usually normal, but must be obtained in the assessment of the child. After 10 to 14 days of active infection, bone destruction or periosteal bone elevation is seen. A bone scan or MRI can be very helpful in establishing an early diagnosis.

If a septic process about the hip is suspected, an ultrasound study may be beneficial in demonstrating an effusion. If this is present, arthrocentesis or hip aspiration is necessary. The synovial fluid analysis should include a cell count, measurement of protein and glucose levels, Gram stain, cultures, and sensitivity studies. Infections of peripheral joints, such as the knee, are more readily diagnosed by arthrocentesis.

If an osteomyelitis of a metaphyseal region is suspected, the subperiosteal space and bone may be directly aspirated with a large-bore needle. The material should be sampled for culture and sensitivity. If pus is not obtained, a bone scan or MRI can usually confirm infection.

Unfortunately, even in an acute infection, cultures from the joint or bone and blood are not always positive. *S. aureus* is the most common organism that produces osteomyelitis and the most common organism that produces septic arthritis in children 5 to 15 years of age. *Haemophilus influenzae* type b needs to be considered as a cause of septic arthritis in unimmunized children younger than 5 years. *Neisseria gonorrhoeae* infection is the most common cause of septic arthritis in sexually active adolescents. Neonatal osteoarticular infection is often caused by group B streptococcus or *S. aureus*, rarely by gram-negative organisms or *Candida* species. Patients with sickle cell anemia develop osteomyelitis as a result of *Salmonella* species or *S. aureus* infection and septic arthritis as a result of pneumococcal infection.

Treatment. Treatment of septic arthritis and osteomyelitis of the hip is always by surgical drainage (see Chapter 44) because the increased intracapsular pressure can tamponade the intracapsular vessels that supply the CFE, which results in avascular necrosis. Peripheral joints with septic arthritis, such as the knee and ankle, may be aspirated, treated with empirical antibiotics (nafcillin, methicillin, cefotaxime, ceftriaxone), and observed while the clinician is awaiting the results of cultures. The need for surgical drainage is based on the clinical response over a 24- to 48-hour period. If osteomyelitis is suspected but no pus is present within the metaphysis, this condition can also be treated empirically. When pus (abscess) is present, however, incision and drainage usually result in a more rapid resolution of infection and prevent secondary damage to the adjacent physeal plate.

Treatment of osteomyelitis takes 4 to 6 weeks; this may be accomplished by an initial regimen of intravenous antibiotics; once signs of improvement occur (decreased erythrocyte sedimentation rate, decreased leukocyte count, decreased pain, negative blood culture, and decreased fever, usually after 10 to 14 days), oral antibiotics may be substituted. The bacteria must be available for minimal inhibitory concentration (MIC) serum determination, the family should be highly compliant with the treatment regimen, and follow-up should be ensured.

Diskitis. See Chapter 46.

Rheumatologic Causes

Hip Monoarticular Synovitis. Transient monoarticular synovitis of the hip is the most common cause of limping in children. It can occur in all age groups, but the mean age at onset is 6 years; most patients are between 3 and 8 years of age. Hip monoarticular synovitis is characterized by acute onset of monoarthritic hip pain, an associated limp, and mild restriction of hip motion, especially abduction and internal rotation. The pain is felt in the groin, anterior thigh, or knee. Any child with nontraumatic anterior thigh or knee pain must be carefully evaluated for hip disease because these are the sites of referred pain. Septic arthritis and osteomyelitis must be excluded.

The cause of this disorder remains uncertain. Suspected causes include (1) active or recent systemic viral syndrome, (2) trauma, and (3) allergic hypersensitivity. Approximately 70% of affected children have had a nonspecific viral upper respiratory infection 7 to 14 days before the onset of symptoms.

Clinical Examination. The patient is usually ambulatory, and the hip is not held in the position of flexion, abduction, or external rotation unless a significant effusion has developed. The child walks with an antalgic (painful) gait on the involved side and is usually afebrile. Laboratory findings are usually within normal limits, but occasionally a minimal elevation of the white blood cell count or sedimentation rate may be seen.

Radiographic Evaluation. Anteroposterior and Lauenstein (frog) lateral radiographs of the pelvis are obtained to rule out the presence of other lesions. The radiographs in synovitis are normal. On occasion, ultrasonography of the hip may be useful in demonstrating a joint effusion. Bone scans may be necessary in difficult or unusual cases; in synovitis, these results are always normal.

Treatment. The treatment of monoarticular synovitis of the hip is symptomatic. Bed rest and avoidance of weight bearing until these symptoms resolve, followed by limited activities for 1 to 2 weeks thereafter, constitute the treatment of choice. The child's activities should be limited until the symptoms have completely resolved. A rapid return to normal activities may result in exacerbation.

When the diagnosis of monoarticular synovitis is in doubt, hip arthrocentesis may be necessary. The fluid that is aspirated shows a very low white blood cell count, and the cultures are negative.

Trendelenburg Gait

Developmental Origin

Developmental Dysplasia of the Hip. Developmental dysplasia of the hip is a very common disorder affecting infants (Fig. 45-14), but its presence after walking age is relatively uncommon. Unfortunately, no matter how careful the initial screening evaluation, a small number of children are seen each year with a late diagnosis of developmental dysplasia. When the problem occurs unilaterally, the child walks with a mild Trendelenburg gait or demonstrates toe-walking. With bilateral involvement, the child stands with an increased lumbar lordosis and has a waddling gait. There is functional impairment resulting from a lack of stability and associated muscle weakness, particularly in the hip abductors (gluteus medius).

Clinical Examination. The most common physical finding in the older child with a developmentally dislocated hip is limited hip abduction on the involved side. There may be a mild hip flexion contracture and apparent shortening of the extremity. The greater

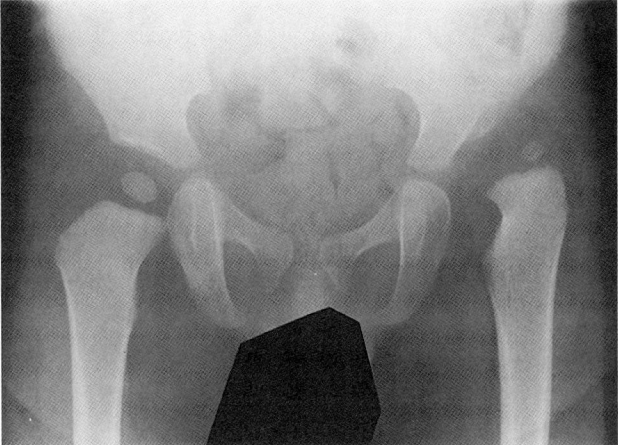

Figure 45-14. Anteroposterior radiograph of the pelvis of an 18-month-old girl demonstrating a developmental dislocation of the left hip. The acetabulum is severely dysplastic, and the femoral head is displaced laterally and superiorly. The Shenton line is markedly disrupted, and there is delayed ossification in the capital femoral epiphysis in comparison with the normal right hip.

trochanter lies above a line between the anterior-superior iliac spine and the ischial tuberosity (Nélaton line). In bilateral dislocations, the physical findings are more symmetrical but there is still limitation of hip abduction. Positive Trendelenburg signs are present on the involved side. The normal response to a Trendelenburg test occurs when the patient stands on the uninvolved leg and the abductor muscles are able to maintain balance by elevating the contralateral pelvis. A positive Trendelenburg sign, resulting from weakness, is demonstrated when the abductor muscles are unable to maintain pelvic balance and the patient compensates by leaning to the affected side.

Radiographic Evaluation. The diagnosis can be made from routine anteroposterior and Lauenstein (frog) lateral radiographs of the pelvis (see Fig. 45-14). Specialized studies, such as MRI and CT, are usually not necessary. Ultrasound study is not usually necessary in the older child because the CFE is ossified.

Treatment. Treatment of developmental dysplasia of the hip in the older child is usually surgical. The procedure consists of an open reduction of the hip with a pelvic osteotomy, femoral varus shortening and derotation osteotomy, or a combination of both. The procedure selected depends on the age of the child and the severity of the deformity of the acetabulum and proximal femur.

Lower Extremity Length Discrepancy. Lower extremity length discrepancy in older children and adolescents has been discussed earlier in this chapter.

Neuromuscular Origin

Cerebral Palsy. Children with a spastic hemiplegia or diplegia may have an associated painless limp caused by muscle spasticity and concomitant weakness of the antagonists. The history should focus on risk factors for cerebral palsy, prematurity, and other congenital anomalies external to the central nervous system, followed by a physical examination, with particular attention to the neurologic system. The neurologic examination reveals evidence of increased muscle tone, spasticity, hyperactive deep tendon reflexes, and pathologic reflexes, such as Babinski signs.

SUMMARY AND RED FLAGS

Conditions associated with limp must be divided into acute, painful lesions and chronic, painless lesions. Infection and trauma must be considered emergencies, as should conditions that are limb or articular threatening, such as septic arthritis and osteomyelitis of the hip, avascular necrosis, or SCFE. In addition, signs of spinal cord involvement (see Chapter 46) suggest acute processes that warrant immediate attention to prevent permanent paralysis.

Red flags include acute hip pain, fever with limp, neurologic manifestations (including bowel and bladder dysfunction), point tenderness, the presence of a mass, and signs of weight loss or hematologic abnormalities such as pallor or bruising.

REFERENCES

General

Sutherland DH, Olshen R, Cooper L, et al: The development of gait. J Bone Joint Surg Am 1980;62:336-353.

Rotational Abnormalities

Femoral/Tibial Torsion

Bruce RW Jr: Torsional and angular deformities. Pediatr Clin North Am 1996;43:867-881.

Dodgin DA, DeSwart RJ, Stefko RM, et al: Distal tibial/fibular derotation osteotomy for correction of tibial torsion: Review of technique and results in 63 cases. J Pediatr Orthop 1998;18:95-101.

Karol LA: Rotational deformities in the lower extremities. Curr Opin Pediatr 1997;9:77-80.

Ruwe PA, Gage JR, Ozonoff MB, et al: Clinical determination of femoral anteversion: A comparison of established techniques. J Bone Joint Surg Am 1992;74:820-830.

Strecker W, Keppler P, Gebhard F, et al: Length and torsion of the lower limbs. J Bone Joint Surg Br 1997;79:1019-1023.

Metatarsus Adductus

Asirvatham R, Stevens PM: Idiopathic forefoot-adduction deformity: Medial capsulotomy and abductor hallucis lengthening for resistant and severe deformities. J Pediatr Orthop 1997;17:496-500.

Bleck EE: Metatarsus adductus: Classification and relationship to outcomes of treatment. J Pediatr Orthop 1983;3:2-9.

Farsetti P, Weinstein SL, Ponseti IV: The long-term functional and radiographic outcomes of untreated and non-operatively treated metatarsus adductus. J Bone Joint Surg Am 1994;76:257-265.

Talipes Equinovarus (Clubfoot)

Alkjaer T, Pedersen EN, Simonsen EB: Evaluation of the walking pattern in clubfoot patients who received early intensive treatment. J Pediatr Orthop 2000;20:642-647.

Cuevas de Alba C, Guille JT, Bowen JR, et al: Computed tomography for femoral and tibial torsion in children with clubfoot. Clin Orthop 1998;353:203-209.

Ezra E, Hayek S, Gilai AN, et al: Tibialis anterior tendon transfer for residual dynamic supination deformity in treated clubfeet. J Pediatr Orthop B 2000;9:207-211.

Karol LA, Concha MC, Johnston CE: Gait analysis and muscle strength in children with surgically treated clubfeet. J Pediatr Orthop 1997;17:790-795.

Kuo KN, Hennigan SP, Hastings ME: Anterior tibial tendon transfer in residual dynamic clubfoot deformity. J Pediatr Orthop 2001;21:35-41.

Macnicol MF, Nadeem RD, Forness M: Functional results of surgical treatment in congenital talipes equinovarus (clubfoot): A comparison of outcome measurements. J Pediatr Orthop B 2000;9:285-292.

Roye BD, Vitale MG, Gelijins AC, et al: Patient-based outcomes after clubfoot surgery. J Pediatr Orthop 2001;21:42-49.

Calcaneovalgus Foot

Mosca, VS: Other conditions of the foot. In Morrissy RT, Weinstein SL (eds): Pediatric Orthopaedics, 5th ed. Philadelphia, Lippincott Williams & Wilkins, 2001, p 1178.

Hypermobile Pes Planus

Akrali O, Tiner M, Ozaksoy D: Effects of lower extremity rotation on prognosis of flexible flatfoot in children. Foot Ankle Int 2000;21:772-774.

Staheli LT, Chew DE, Corbet M: The longitudinal arch: A survey of 882 feet in normal children and adults. J Bone Joint Surg Am 1987;69:426-428.

Sullivan JA: Pediatric flatfoot: Evaluation and management. J Am Acad Orthop Surg 1999;7:44-53.

Wenger DR, Mauldin D, Speck G, et al: Corrective shoes and inserts as treatment for a flexible flatfoot in infants and children. J Bone Joint Surg Am 1989;71:800-810.

Equinus Gait (Toe-Walking)

Neuromuscular Disorders

Kelly IP, Jenkinson A, Stephens M, et al: The kinematic patterns of toe-walkers. J Pediatr Orthop 1997;17:478-480.

Rose J, Martin JG, Torburn L, et al: Electromyographic differentiation of diplegic cerebral palsy from idiopathic toe-walking: Involuntary coactivation of the quadriceps and gastrocnemius. J Pediatr Orthop 1999;19:677-682.

Congenital Tendo Achilles Contracture (Idiopathic Toe-Walking)

Eastwood DM, Dennett X, Shield LK, et al: Muscle abnormalities in idiopathic toe-walkers. J Pediatr Orthop B 1997;6:215-218.

Eastwood DM, Menelaus MB, Dickens DR, et al: Idiopathic toe-walking: Does treatment alter the natural history? J Pediatr Orthop B 2000; 9:47-49.

Sala DA, Shulman LH, Kennedy RF, et al: Idiopathic toe-walking: A review. Dev Med Child Neurol 1999;41:846-848.

Shulman LH, Sala DA, Chu ML, et al: Developmental implications of idiopathic toe-walking. J Pediatr 1997;130:541-546.

Stricker SJ, Angulo JC: Idiopathic toe-walking: A comparison of treatment methods. J Pediatr Orthop 1998;18:289-293.

Habitual Toe-Walking

Griffin PP, Wheelhouse WW, Shiavi R, et al: Habitual toe-walkers: A clinical and electromyographic gait analysis. J Bone Joint Surg Am 1977;59:97-101.

Lower Extremity Length Discrepancy

Dahl MT: Limb length discrepancy. Pediatr Clin North Am 1996;43:849-866.

Ballock RT, Wiesner GL, Myers MT, Thompson GH: Hemihypertrophy. Concepts and controversies. J Bone Joint Surg Am 1997;79:1731-1738.

Herzenberg JE, Paley D: Leg lengthening in children. Curr Opin Pediatr 1998;10:95-97.

Song KM, Halliday SE, Little DG: The effect of limb-length discrepancy on gait. J Bone Joint Surg Am 1997;79:1690-1698.

Stanitski DF: Limb-length inequality: Assessment and treatment options. J Am Acad Orthop Surg 1999;7:143-153.

Limping

General

Barkin RM, Barkin SZ, Barkin AZ: The limping child. J Emerg Med 2000; 18:331-339.

Connolly LP, Treves ST: Assessing the limping child with skeletal scintigraphy. J Nucl Med 1998;29:1056-1061.

Fischer SU, Beattie TF: The limping child: Epidemiology, assessment and outcome. J Bone Joint Surg Br 1999;81:1029-1034.

Lett AI, Skaggs DL: Evaluation of the acutely limping child. Am Fam Physician 2000;61:1011-1018.

Myers MT, Thompson GH: Imaging the child with a limp. Pediatr Clin North Am 1997;44:637-658.

Tarsal Coalition

Blakemore LC, Cooperman DR, Thompson GH: The rigid flatfoot: Tarsal coalitions. Foot Ankle Clin 1998;3:609-631.

Bohne WH: Tarsal coalition. Curr Opin Pediatr 2001;13:29-35.

Vincent KA: Tarsal coalition and painful flatfoot. J Am Acad Orthop Surg 1998;6:274-281.

Legg-Calvé-Perthes Disease

Guille JT, Lipton GE, Szoke G, et al: Legg-Calvé-Perthes disease in girls. A comparison of the results seen in boys. J Bone Joint Surg Am 1998;80:1256-1263.

Herring JA: The treatment of Legg-Calvé-Perthes disease. A critical review of the literature. J Bone Joint Surg Am 1994;76:448-458.

Herring JA, Neustadt JB, Williams JJ, et al: The lateral pillar classification of Legg-Calvé-Perthes disease. J Pediatr Orthop 1992;12:143-150.

Loder RT, Schwartz EM, Hensinger RN: Behavioral characteristics of children with Legg-Calvé-Perthes disease. J Pediatr Orthop 1993;13:598-601.

Martinez AG, Weinstein SL, Dietz FR: The weight-bearing abduction brace for the treatment of Legg-Perthes disease. J Bone Joint Surg Am 1992;74:12-21.

Meehan PL, Angel D, Nelson JM: The Scottish Rite abduction orthosis for the treatment of Legg-Perthes disease. J Bone Joint Surg Am 1992; 74:1-12.

Noonan KJ, Price CT, Kupiszewski SJ, et al: Results of femoral varus osteotomy in children older than nine years with Perthes' disease. J Pediatr Orthop 2001;21:198-204.

Salter RB, Thompson GH: Legg-Calvé-Perthes disease: The prognostic significance of the subchondral fracture and a two-group classification of the femoral head involvement. J Bone Joint Surg Am 1984;66:479-499.

Thompson GH, Price CT, Roy D, et al: Legg-Calvé-Perthes disease: Current concepts. Am Acad Orth Surg 2002;51:367-384.

Wall EJ: Legg-Calvé-Perthes disease. Curr Opin Pediatr 1999;11:76-79.

Weinstein SL: Natural history and treatment outcomes of childhood hip disorders. Clin Orthop 1997;344:222-242.

Slipped Capital Femoral Epiphysis

Carney BT, Weinstein SL, Noble J: Long-term follow-up of slipped capital femoral epiphysis. J Bone Joint Surg Am 1991;73:677-674.

Givon U, Bowen JR: Chronic slipped capital femoral epiphysis: Treatment by pinning in situ. J Pediatr Orthop B 1999;8:216-222.

Kennedy JG, Hresko MT, Kasser JR, et al: Osteonecrosis of the femoral head associated with slipped capital femoral epiphysis. J Pediatr Orthop 2001;21:189-193.

Loder RT, Richards BS, Shapiro PS, et al: Acute slipped capital femoral epiphysis: The importance of physeal stability. J Bone Joint Surg Am 1993;75:1134-1140.

Matava MJ, Patton CM, Luhmann S, et al: Knee pain as the initial symptom of slipped capital femoral epiphysis: An analysis of initial presentation and treatment. J Pediatr Orthop 1999;19:455-460.

Reynolds RA: Diagnosis and treatment of slipped capital femoral epiphysis. Curr Opin Pediatr 1999;11:80-83.

Weinstein SL: Natural history and treatment outcomes of childhood hip disorders. Clin Orthop 1997;344:222-242.

Wells D, King JD, Roe TF, et al: Review of slipped capital femoral epiphysis associated with endocrine disease. J Pediatr Orthop 1993;13:610-614.

Sprains/Strains

Saperstein AL, Nicholas SJ: Pediatric and adolescent sports medicine. Pediatr Clin North Am 1996;43:1013-1034.

Occult Fractures

Aronson J, Garvin K, Seibert J, et al: Efficiency of the bone scan for occult limping toddlers. J Pediatr Orthop 1992;12:38-44.

Mellick LB, Reesor K: Spiral tibial fractures of children: A commonly accidental spiral long bone fracture. Am J Emerg Med 1990;8: 234-237.

Tenenbien M, Reed MH, Black GB: The toddler's fracture revisited. Am J Emerg Med 1990;8:208-211.

Neoplasia

Copley L, Dormans JP: Benign pediatric bone tumors. Pediatr Clin North Am 1996;43:949-966.

Himelstein BP, Dormans JP: Malignant bone tumors of childhood. Pediatr Clin North Am 1996;43:967-984.

Tuten HR, Gabos PG, Keimar SJ, et al: The limping child: A manifestation of acute leukemia. J Pediatr Orthop 1998;18:625-629.

Septic Arthritis/Osteomyelitis

Blyth MJ, Kincaid R, Craigen MA, et al: The changing epidemiology of acute and subacute haematogenous osteomyelitis in children. J Bone Joint Surg Br 2001;83:99-102.

Kim HK, Alman B, Cole WB: A shortened course of parenteral antibiotic therapy in the management of acute septic arthritis of the hip. J Pediatr Orthop 2000;20:44-47.

Luhmann JD, Luhmann SJ: Etiology of septic arthritis in children: An update for the 1990's. Pediatr Emerg Care 1999;15:40-42.

Lyon RM, Evanich JD: Culture negative septic arthritis in children. J Pediatr Orthop 1999;19:655-659.

Newton PO, Ballock RT, Bradley JS: Oral antibiotics of bacterial arthritis. Pediatr Infect Dis J 1999;18:1102-1103.

Oudjhane K, Ozouz EM: Imaging of osteomyelitis in children. Radiol Clin North Am 2001;39:251-266.

Poyhia T, Azouz EM: MR imaging evaluation of subacute and chronic bone abscesses in children. Pediatr Radiol 2000;30:763-768.

Rasool MN: Primary subacute haematogenous osteomyelitis in children. J Bone Joint Surg Br 2001;83:93-98.

Sonnan GM, Henry NK: Pediatric bone and joint infections. Diagnosis and antimicrobial management. Pediatr Clin North Am 1996;43:933-947.

Waagner DC: Musculoskeletal infections in adolescents. Adolesc Med 2000;11:375-400.

Wall EJ: Childhood osteomyelitis and septic arthritis. Curr Opin Pediatr 1998;10:73-76.

Wang MN, Chen WM, Leck S, et al: Tuberculosis osteomyelitis in young children. J Pediatr Orthop 1999;19:151-155.

Hip Monoarticular Synovitis

Do TT: Transient synovitis as a cause of painful limps in children. Curr Opin Pediatr 2000;12:48-51.

Kocher MS, Zurakowski D, Kasser JR: Differentiating between septic arthritis and transient synovitis of the hip in children: An evidence-based clinical prediction algorithm. J Bone Joint Surg Am 1999;81:1662-1670.

Developmental Dysplasia of the Hip

DeKleuver M, Kooijman MA, Pavlov PW, et al: Triple osteotomy of the pelvis for acetabular dysplasia: Results at 8 to 15 years. J Bone Joint Surg Br 1997;79:225-229.

Kerry RM, Simonds GW: Long-term results of the late non-operative reduction of developmental dysplasia of the hip. J Bone Joint Surg Br 1998; 80:78-82.

Kim HT, Kim JI, Yoo CI: Diagnosing childhood acetabular dysplasia using the lateral margin of the sourcil. J Pediatr Orthop 2000;20:709-717.

Kim HT, Wenger DR: The morphology of residual acetabular deficiency in childhood hip dysplasia: Three-dimensional computed tomographic analysis. J Pediatr Orthop 1997;17:637-647.

Lin CJ, Romanus B, Sutherland DH, et al: Three-dimensional characteristic of cartilaginous and bony components of dysplastic hips in children: Three-dimensional computed tomography quantitative analysis. J Pediatr Orthop. 1997;17:152-157.

Olney B, Latz K, Asher M: Treatment of hip dysplasia in older children with a combined one-stage procedure. Clin Orthop 1998;347:215-223.

Vedantam R, Capelli AM, Schoenecker PL: Pemberton osteotomy for the treatment of developmental dysplasia of the hip in older children. J Pediatr Orthop 1998;18:254-258.

46 Back Pain in Children and Adolescents

John G. Thometz*

Persistent back pain in children necessitates a thorough evaluation to rule out disorders that can result in significant morbidity, such as infection or tumor. Back pain in younger children is unusual. The prevalence of complaints of low back pain increases with age, ranging from 1% at 7 years of age to about 20% by the teenage years. In adolescents, back pain is frequently mild and often resolves spontaneously. The complaints are often related to overactivity in sports, work, or a specific traumatic event. As noted in adults, back pain is not a disease but a symptom and is often associated in adolescents with headaches, emotional problems, daytime tiredness, and conduct disorders. Activity modification and rehabilitation or exercises for the spine are sufficient to prevent recurrent episodes of back pain. Severe or persistent back pain necessitates a thorough history, physical examination, and appropriate imaging studies to evaluate the child for potentially serious pathologic processes.

EVALUATION OF THE PEDIATRIC SPINE

Examination of the spine should be part of the routine physical examination in the healthy child and adolescent. Even in patients who present with back pain as a chief complaint, the most important diagnostic steps are a detailed history and a thorough and systematic examination (Table 46-1).

When findings on screening examinations are abnormal or when a patient presents with complaints of back pain, a more detailed examination is required. The spinal column, spinal cord, and spinal nerves are intimately related, and disorders affecting any one of these elements produce symptoms and signs in the others. Detailed examination of strength in the muscles of the spine and lower extremities (Fig. 46-1), sensation (Fig. 46-2), abdominal and lower extremity reflexes, anal sphincter tone, and perianal sensation should be performed when the primary examination suggests involvement of the neural structures that pass through the spinal column. Persistent or severe back pain is uncommon in young children and may be associated with serious underlying disease.

Interpretation of the results of patient evaluation requires an understanding of the normal sequence of growth and development of the spine, knowledge of normal spinal alignment, and an understanding of the age-related differential diagnosis of potential spinal disorders in children.

NORMAL GROWTH AND DEVELOPMENT OF THE SPINE

Formation of the vertebral column begins during the third week of gestation and is complete by the end of the first trimester. Further growth and primary ossification of the spinal column occurs during the second and third trimesters; however, the cartilaginous model of the spine is complete by week 12 of embryonic development.

Vertebral growth occurs in an orderly manner throughout childhood and adolescence. About 50% of vertebral column height is present by age 2 years. Acceleration of vertebral growth occurs during the adolescent growth spurt but contributes less to total height than does lower limb growth; the sitting heights of siblings in early and late adolescence are often remarkably similar. Spinal growth slows at menarche in girls and at the time of voice change in boys and is usually complete 2 to 3 years later. Developmental abnormalities of the column, such as idiopathic scoliosis, most commonly first appear just before the growth spurt. Alterations in spinal configuration caused by congenital deformities of vertebral segments change most rapidly during periods of rapid spinal growth: before age 2 years and at the time of the adolescent growth spurt.

There is a high association of genitourinary tract, cardiac, and neural abnormalities in patients with congenital abnormalities of the spine. Warning signs in patients with congenital spine deformities include leg-length inequality, foot-size asymmetry, high foot arches, hairy patches or hemangiomas or a mass over the spine, sacral dimpling, enuresis, toe walking, asymmetry or abnormality in the lower extremity deep tendon reflexes, and lower extremity weakness.

NORMAL SPINAL ALIGNMENT

The normal trunk is symmetric when viewed from the front or the back (Fig. 46-3). The shoulders and pelvis are parallel to each other and to the ground. The distance between the right and left elbows and the sides of the trunk is equal. When the trunk is viewed from the side, a series of curves is present (see Fig. 46-3). A convex anterior lordotic curve is present in the cervical region. The spine is concave anteriorly in a kyphotic pattern in the thoracic region. The normal lumbar spine is lordotic, and the sacrum and coccygeal regions are kyphotic. Normal adult sagittal alignment develops gradually; children younger than 10 years typically have less cervical lordosis and more lumbar lordosis than adults. Healthy children often are quite swaybacked. Injuries, infections, tumors, inflammation, and developmental abnormalities of the spine often produce alterations in these expected contours. Range of motion is demonstrated in Figure 46-4.

BACK PAIN OF BRIEF DURATION

Few children younger than 10 years sustain significant injuries of the spinal column or associated musculature in routine play and organized sports activities; extremity injuries are far more common. When the trunk is involved, contusions and abrasions are much more common than ligament sprains and muscle strains.

When a child presents with back pain of brief duration after a play or sports-related injury, a careful examination should be performed. If there are no other associated injuries and the screening examination shows no alterations in trunk configuration or lower extremity strength or sensation (see Figs. 46-1 and 46-2), no further workup is necessary. A brief period of rest for 1 to 2 days, followed by gradual

*This chapter is an updated and edited version of the chapter by Peter V. Scoles that appeared in the first edition.

Table 46-1. Guidelines for Primary Examination of the Back

History

Is there a history of back pain? If so, what is the
   Frequency?
   Duration?
   Relationship to activity?
   Antecedent trauma?
Is there associated pain in legs?
Is there incontinence or enuresis?
Is walking painful?
Have there been systemic signs of chronic illness?
Is there a family history of deformity?
Is there a family history of disk disease?

Physical Examination

General Appearance

Are the right and left sides of the trunk symmetric?
Are there hairy patches, nevi, sinuses, or dimpling over the
   midline of the spine?
Are the pelvis and shoulders level?
Is there normal kyphosis and lordosis?
On forward bending, is a rib hump present?

Motion

Can be patient easily bend forward and touch his or her toes?
Is normal hamstring flexibility present?

Lower Extremities

Are leg lengths equal?
Is strength normal in the major motor groups of the lower
   limbs?
Is sensation normal in the lower limbs?
Are reflexes normal at the knees and ankles?
Are pathologic reflexes present?

---

resumption of activities, is appropriate treatment. Routine radiographic evaluation is not necessary when the duration of symptoms is short and the physical examination findings are normal. Signs of systemic illness (fever, weight loss) or neurologic deficits warrant an immediate evaluation.

Acute back injuries occur more frequently in adolescence, as the size of participants and potential forces generated in recreational activities increase. If there are no other associated injuries and the screening examination findings are normal, no further radiologic workup is necessary. A period of rest followed by gradual resumption of activities is appropriate treatment. The importance of a comprehensive and balanced conditioning exercise program should be stressed to young athletes. Most sports-related injuries can be prevented by preparticipation conditioning, appropriate warm-up, careful supervision, and resting when fatigued.

Trauma sufficient to cause spine fractures may occur as a result of motor vehicle or bicycle accidents, falls, and diving and gymnastic injuries. The frequency and severity of spine trauma rises in later adolescence as exposure to potentially violent forces in sports and motor vehicles increases. In such cases, there is a clear relationship between the accident and the onset of symptoms. Injury to the spinal column should be suspected in all individuals whose level of consciousness is impaired after an accident, regardless of the presence or absence of symptoms.

Children with suspected acute spinal injury should be immobilized on backboards designed for children until definitive imaging studies can be performed and interpreted. Immobilization of the child's cervical spine on a solid backboard should be avoided. The child's occiput projects farther posteriorly than that of the adult, and flexion of the neck occurs if the child's neck is immobilized on a standard backboard. Spinal immobilization boards for children are readily available and have a cut-out section to accommodate the occiput. When such boards are not available, a blanket or firm mattress should be interposed between the trunk and the backboard to prevent neck flexion.

PERSISTENT BACK PAIN

Persistent or severe back pain is uncommon in young children but is more common in adolescents. The implications of severe or persistent back pain are more serious in younger patients than in adolescents. Persistent back pain in young children is not usually the result of congenital spinal deformity or developmental disorders of the spine. As a child enters and passes through the adolescent growth spurt, back pain may arise from a small number of congenital and developmental disorders of the spinal column. Degenerative

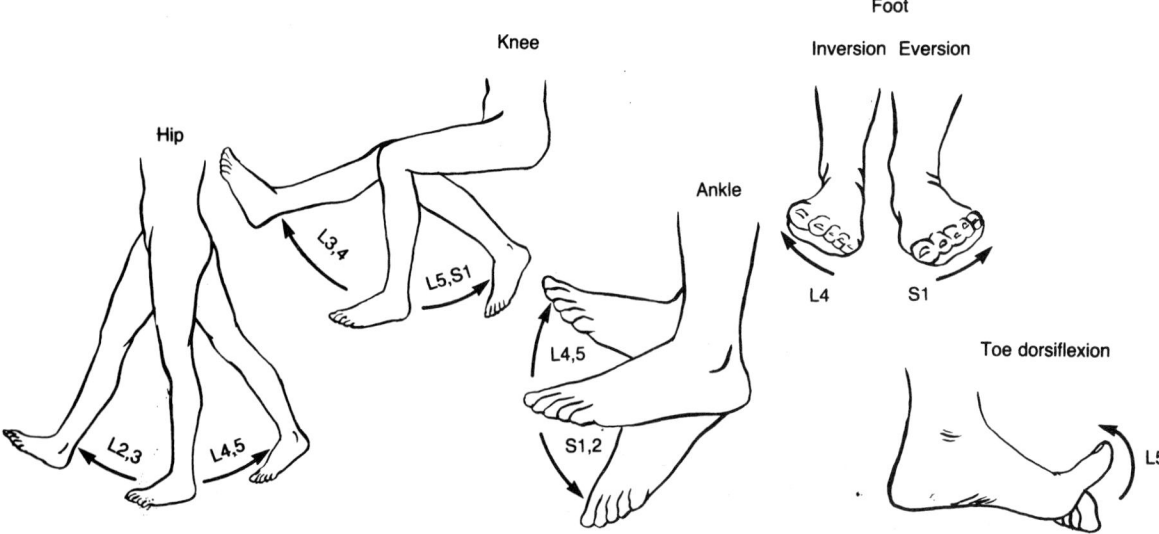

Figure 46-1. Motor control of the lower extremity. (From Reilly BM: Practical Strategies in Outpatient Medicine, 2nd ed. Philadelphia, WB Saunders, 1991, p 926.)

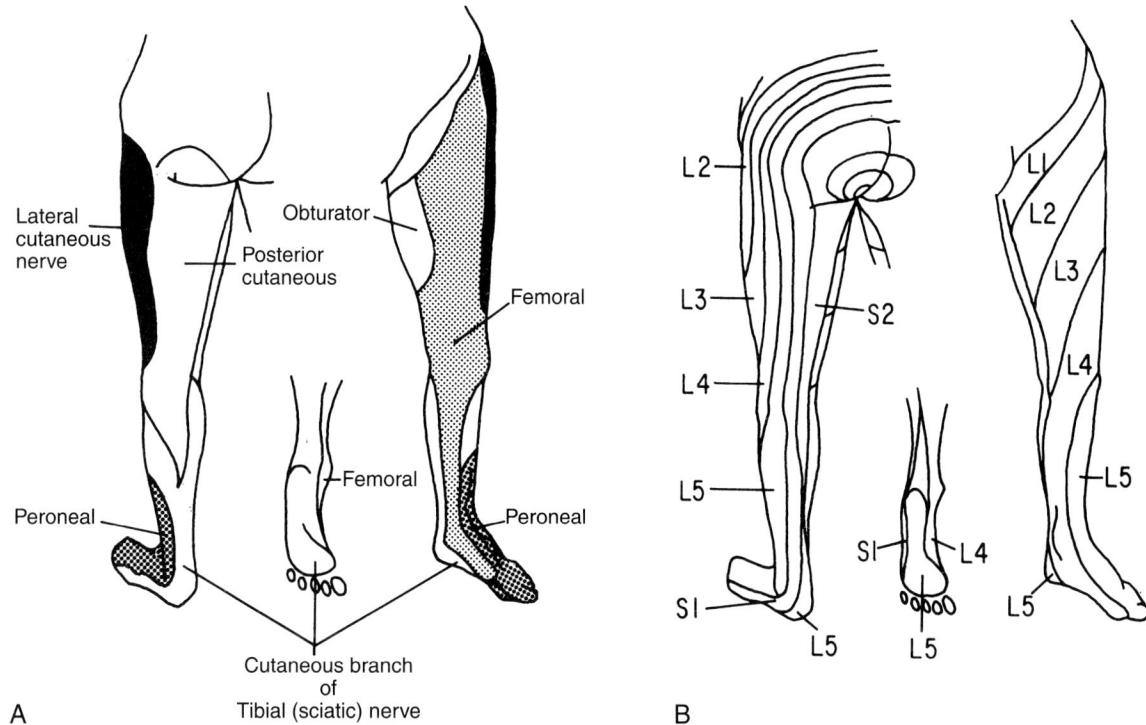

Figure 46-2. Sensory innervation of the lower extremity. **A,** Peripheral nerve innervation. **B,** Dermatomal (root) innervation. (From Reilly BM: *Practical Strategies in Outpatient Medicine,* 2nd ed. Philadelphia, WB Saunders, 1991, p 927.)

disorders of the spine such as intervertebral disk herniation are uncommon causes of back pain in childhood. In evaluating a patient, it is important to try to distinguish musculoskeletal-mechanical disorders from those with more generalized systemic signs or those suggestive of a neoplasia (Fig. 46-5).

The differential diagnosis of persistent back pain in children younger than 10 years includes intervertebral diskitis and vertebral body osteomyelitis, neoplasia of the vertebrae, primary neoplasia of the spinal cord, and metastatic neoplasia (Table 46-2). In older children and adolescents, congenital variations in the formation of the

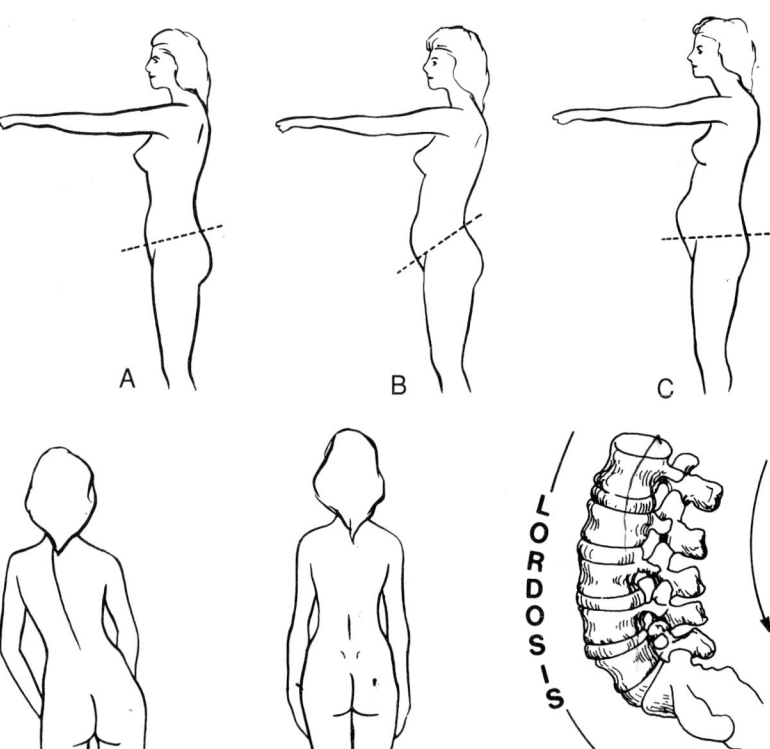

Figure 46-3. **A,** Normal posture with normal lumbar lordosis. **B,** Exaggerated lumbar lordosis caused by pelvic tilting. **C,** "Paunchy" posture. **D,** Spastic scoliosis caused by muscle spasm. **E,** Normal posture without scoliosis. **F,** The *normal orientation* of the lumbar spine is that of mild lordosis. Exaggerated lordosis may predispose the patient to mechanical back pain. (From Reilly BM: *Practical Strategies in Outpatient Medicine,* 2nd ed. Philadelphia, WB Saunders, 1991, p 908.)

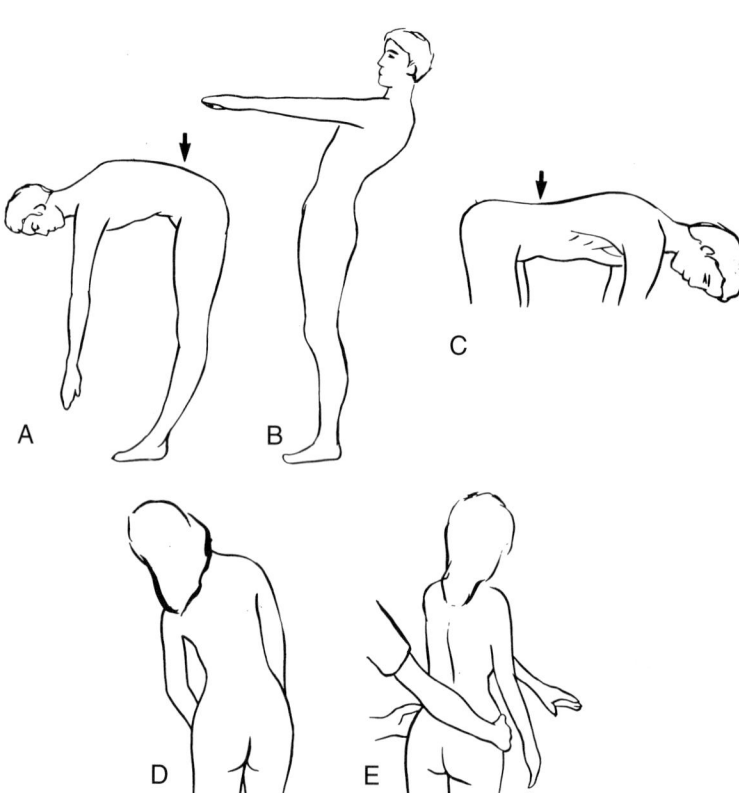

Figure 46-4. Back range of motion. **A,** Flexion. Note the normal reversal of lumbar lordosis during flexion *(arrow).* **B,** Extension. **C,** Persistent lordosis during back flexion as a result of muscle spasm *(arrow).* **D,** Lateral flexion. **E,** Lateral torsion (rotation). (From Reilly BM: Practical Strategies in Outpatient Medicine, 2nd ed. Philadelphia, WB Saunders, 1991, p 909.)

lower lumbar spine are sometimes responsible for chronic back pain (see Table 46-1). Developmental round back (kyphosis) is occasionally associated with midthoracic back pain in middle and late adolescence. Diskitis, skeletal neoplasia, and tumors of the spinal cord and nerves also occur in adolescence. In documenting the history, special attention must be given to the nature of the onset of symptoms, the presence of radiating pain in the legs, bowel and bladder function, associated abdominal pain, and the presence or absence of fever.

Although this issue is controversial, some authorities believe that school-aged children who carry an excessively heavy backpack are at risk for back pain and alterations of gait or posture. To alleviate this, it is recommended that the backpack be of appropriate size with wide padded straps and back padding. In addition, the weight limit of the pack should not exceed 10% to 15% of the child's body weight. The pack should be lifted with bending of the knees, and the straps should be adjusted so that the pack fits on the back and not below the waist.

SPECIFIC DIAGNOSIS

INTERVERTEBRAL DISKITIS

Intervertebral diskitis is the term applied to a number of processes that are characterized by back or leg pain and radiographically by narrowing of the intervertebral joint space between two adjacent vertebral segments (Figs. 46-6 and 46-7). Magnetic resonance imaging (MRI) studies suggest that diskitis may begin as a micro-abscess within the vertebral body adjacent to the vertebral endplate. The disk becomes infected from perforating vascular channels across the endplate. Vascular channels may also perforate the endplate on the opposite side of the disk, leading to involvement of the opposite vertebral body. In some patients, the symptoms resolve spontaneously without treatment. There is controversy as to whether antibiotic therapy is necessary in all patients with diskitis.

Most authorities believe that diskitis is a bacterial infection, usually caused by *Staphylococcus aureus.* Tuberculosis infection of the spine must also be considered in patients who have spent significant time outside the United States or in high-risk patients such as those who are immunocompromised. Surgical drainage, a critical component of effective treatment of other closed-space infections of the musculoskeletal system, is not usually required in most patients with intervertebral diskitis.

Clinical Findings

Three age-dependent patterns of presentation have been noted for intervertebral diskitis. Children younger than 3 years (the most common age) often present with irritability and refusal to walk or apparent dysfunction (limp, antalgic gait) of the lower extremities. Patients may have very tight hamstrings, loss of lumbar lordosis (the lumbar spine is the most common site), and refusal to allow passive motion of the lumbar spine. Patients between the ages of 3 and 8 years often have pain referred to the abdomen, particularly when the disk involves the lower thoracic spine. Adolescents with diskitis often have back pain; the discomfort often radiates into both legs. Additional features at all ages include low-grade fever; refusal to bear weight (sitting or standing); hyperlordosis; and, if intraspinal inflammation is present, decreased lower extremity muscle strength, decreased tone, and alterations of deep tendon reflexes. The erythrocyte sedimentation rate is usually elevated; the white blood cell count is usually normal but may be elevated in late cases. Early in the process, radiographs of the spine are often normal. Over a certain time, the disk space narrowing develops with subsequent erosion of the vertebral endplates (see Fig. 46-6). Traditionally, a bone scan has been recommended for assessment of diskitis. However, MRI is more sensitive than the bone scan. The MRI reveals the extent of the inflammatory process better and can delineate the degree of bone destruction (if any), the presence of abscess formation, or intraspinal inflammations (see Fig. 46-7).

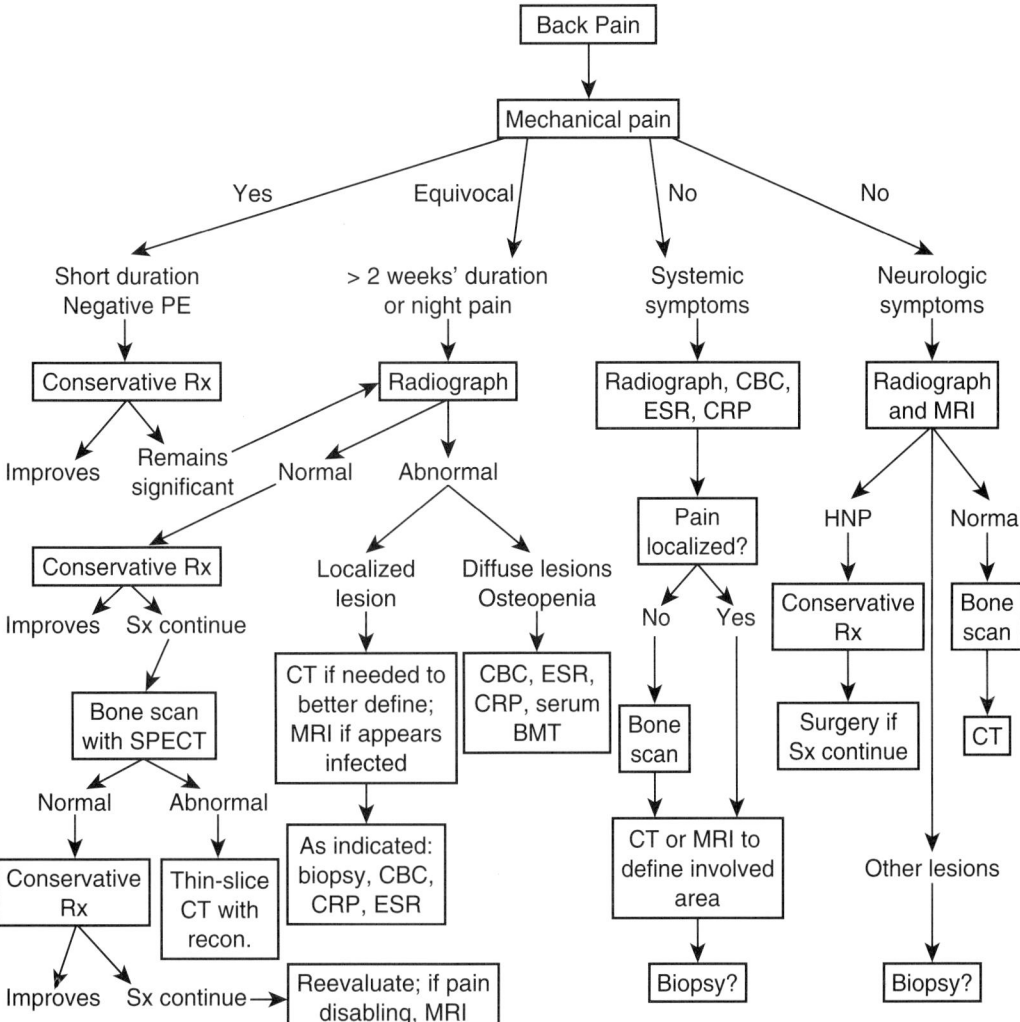

Figure 46-5. Approach to back pain in children. BMT, bone marrow testing; CBC, complete blood cell count; CRP, C-reactive protein; CT, computed tomography; ESR, erythrocyte sedimentation rate; HNP, herniated nucleus propulsus; MRI, magnetic resonance imaging; PE, physical examination results; recon., reconstruction; Rx, treatment; SPECT, single photon emission computed tomography; Sx, signs.

Treatment

The diagnosis of intervertebral diskitis should be suspected in young children with fever and unexplained back or leg pain and in previously healthy toddlers who become irritable and refuse to walk. Vertebral body osteomyelitis is a major consideration in the differential diagnosis and can usually be diagnosed with radiographs and MRI. After appropriate laboratory studies, including blood cultures, have been performed, treatment should be started. A bacterial cause is likely if fever, leukocytosis, and elevation of the sedimentation rate are present. Antibiotic therapy should be started in such cases, because *S. aureus* is the most commonly responsible organism. Knowing the antibacterial sensitivity patterns of community-acquired *S. aureus* helps the clinician choose the appropriate antibiotic (clindamycin, vancomycin, or methicillin). In immunocompromised hosts, broader spectrum antibiotic coverage is essential. If an organism is recovered, antibiotic coverage can be adjusted appropriately. Initial therapy should be intravenous; oral antibiotics can be considered as pain decreases and laboratory studies return to normal. A total of 4 to 6 weeks of therapy is recommended for patients with infectious intervertebral diskitis.

Immobilization of the spine is used for persistent symptoms. Patients without systemic signs of infection and in whom laboratory studies show no leukocytosis and only moderate elevation of the sedimentation rate are occasionally managed by antiinflammatory agents and rest.

Patients who remain ill or worsen after the initiation of rest and antibiotic treatment should undergo surgical biopsy and drainage. Biopsy should also be performed in patients in whom tuberculous intervertebral disk space infection is suspected (positive exposure history, positive purified protein derivative findings; see Chapter 2).

The evolution of radiographic findings lags behind clinical findings in intervertebral diskitis. Although patients with intervertebral diskitis may experience disk space narrowing and endplate erosion during the course of treatment, normal radiographs and bone scans at the time of initial evaluation do not preclude the diagnosis. Radiographic changes continue long after the inflammatory process has resolved. Progressive disk space narrowing, intervertebral disk space calcification, and spontaneous intervertebral arthrodesis are potential late findings.

Lack of focal increased isotope uptake on bone scans obtained 2 to 3 weeks after the onset of symptoms significantly lessens the likelihood of intervertebral diskitis. In such patients, careful study for other potential diagnoses is essential. Tumors of the spinal cord may manifest in a similar manner without causing the changes in

Table 46-2. **Differential Diagnosis of Back Pain**

Inflammatory Diseases

Diskitis*
Vertebral osteomyelitis (pyogenic, tuberculosis)
Spinal epidural abscess
Pyelonephritis*
Perinephric abscess
Pancreatitis
Paraspinal muscle abscess, myositis
Psoas abscess
Endocarditis
Pelvic osteomyelitis
Pelvic inflammatory disease

Rheumatologic Diseases

Pauciarticular juvenile rheumatoid arthritis*
Reactive arthritis
Ankylosing spondylitis
Psoriatic arthritis
Ulcerative colitis, Crohn disease
Fibrositis, fibromyalgia

Developmental Diseases

Spondylolysis (in adolescence)*
Spondylolisthesis (in adolescence)*
Scheuermann syndrome (in adolescence)*
Scoliosis
Spinal dysraphism

Mechanical Trauma and Abnormalities

Muscle strain/sprain*
Hip/pelvic anomalies
Herniated disk (rare)
Juvenile osteoporosis (rare)
Overuse syndromes (common with athletic training and in
  gymnasts and dancers)*
Vertebral stress fractures
Lumbosacral sprain*
Seat-belt injury
Trauma (direct injury; e.g., motor vehicle accident)*
Strain from heavy knapsacks

Neoplastic Diseases

Primary vertebral tumors (osteogenic sarcoma, Ewing
  sarcoma)
Metastatic tumor (neuroblastoma, rhabdomyosarcoma)
Primary spinal tumor (neuroblastoma, lipoma, cysts,
  astrocytoma, ependymoma)
Malignancy of bone marrow (ALL, lymphoma)
Benign tumors (eosinophilic granuloma, osteoid osteoma,
  osteoblastoma, bone cyst)

Other

Disk space calcification (idiopathic, ?S/P diskitis)
Conversion reaction
Sickle cell anemia*
Nephrolithiasis
Hemolysis (acute)
Hematocolpos
S/P lumbar puncture

Modified from Behrman R, Kliegman R (eds): Nelson Essentials of Pediatrics, 2nd ed.
Philadelphia, WB Saunders, 1994, p 711.

*Common.

ALL, acute lymphocytic leukemia; S/P, status post.

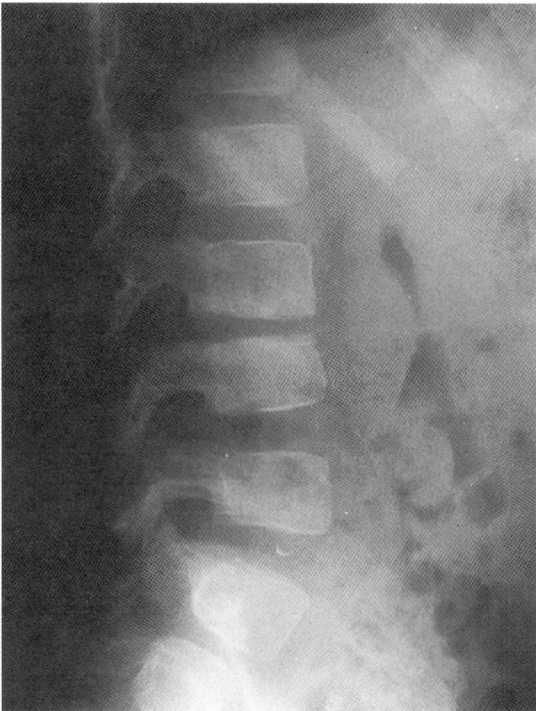

Figure 46-6. Intervertebral diskitis. There is loss of intervertebral disk space height between vertebral segments L3 and L4, with early endplate erosion on the anteroinferior surface of L3 and anterosuperior surface of L4.

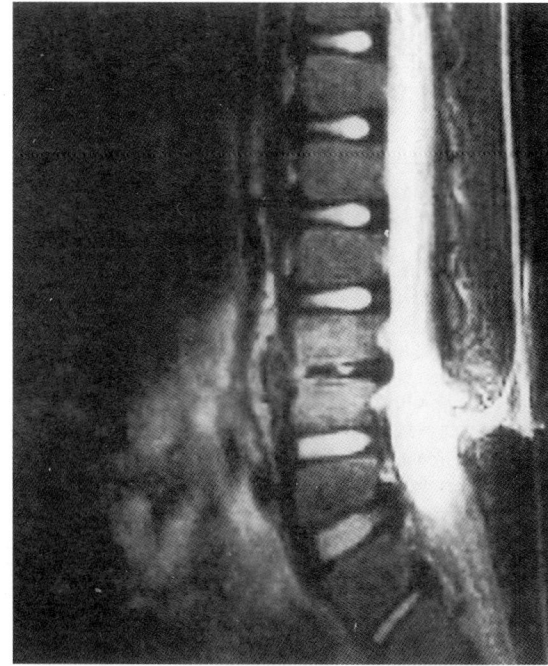

Figure 46-7. Intervertebral diskitis, magnetic resonance image. Note the increased marrow signal from the vertebral bodies adjacent to the narrowed L4 intervertebral disk. The normal bright signal is missing from the involved disk itself, and there is evidence of soft tissue abscess formation anterior to the involved disk space.

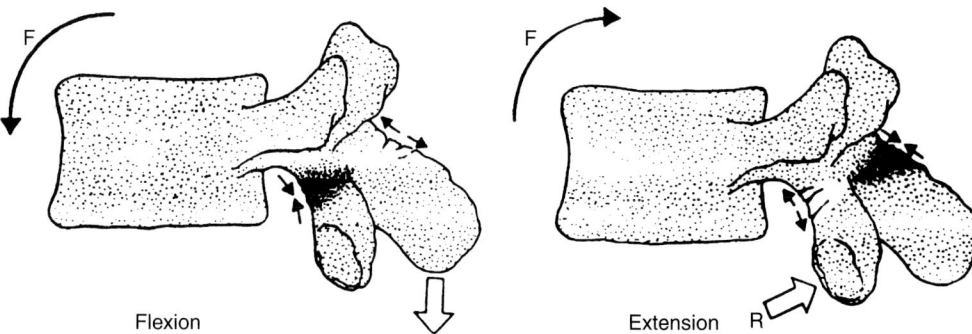

Figure 46-8. Stress leading to fracture of the pars interarticularis.

Flexion

Extension

the vertebral segments necessary to produce alterations on bone scanning. In such patients, MRI is invaluable.

SPONDYLOLYSIS AND SPONDYLOLISTHESIS

The most common abnormalities of the lower lumbar and lumbosacral spine—spina bifida occulta, at L5 or S1, and spondylolysis, usually at L5 to S1—are often noted as incidental radiologic findings in entirely asymptomatic individuals. A few individuals with spondylolysis (defect in the pars interarticularis without slippage) experience back pain and progressive slippage deformity, known as spondylolisthesis.

As a consequence of the normal lordotic tilt of the lumbar spine, shear forces are generated between the L5 and S1 vertebral segments. Forward displacement of L5 on S1 is normally prevented by the stable articulation of the superior facets of S1 and the inferior facets of L5. Defective formation of the posterior elements of the lumbosacral joint or defects in the bone connection between the body and the arch of the fifth lumbar vertebra render the anterior junction of L5 and S1 unstable and may lead to relative displacement.

Cause

Spondylolysis and spondylolisthesis in children and adolescents usually involve the fifth lumbar and first sacral units. Spondylolysis is not present at birth, but with growth and activity, it is seen by age 6 years in about 4% of children and 6% of adults. Spondylolysis appears to be less common in black persons and much more common in some North American Eskimo groups; the lowest incidence has been reported in black girls, and the highest in white boys. The male-to-female ratio is 2:1. The disorder appears to be multifactorial; both hereditary and mechanical factors have been implicated. Relatives of patients with spondylolysis are much more likely to be affected than are individuals in the general population, although the degree of slippage is not as well correlated.

Fatigue fracture of the posterior elements of L5 may be responsible for acutely painful spondylolysis in some preadolescent and adolescent athletes (Figs. 46-8 and 46-9). Activities that involve repeated trunk flexion and extension have been implicated; adolescent divers and gymnasts are reported to be susceptible to spondylolysis and spondylolisthesis. A high rate of spondylolysis has been reported in Scheuermann disease (thoracic kyphosis), which may be related to compensatory excessive lumbar lordosis. In addition, an increased incidence of spondylolisthesis has been noted among both patients with myelodysplasia and those with cerebral palsy.

Acute fracture-dislocation of vertebral units resulting from violent trauma in a strict sense is one form of spondylolisthesis, but because it differs so greatly from other types of spondylolisthesis in cause, presentation, and treatment, it is usually considered as a separate entity.

Presentation

Symptoms in patients with spondylolysis and spondylolisthesis are quite variable; many patients are asymptomatic. Some patients with minimal slips have extreme pain, while others with moderate to severe slips have little or no discomfort. Symptomatic patients complain of aching in the lumbar and lumbosacral regions. Buttock and posterior thigh pain may be present, but radicular symptoms of nerve root compression are usually absent unless the spondylolisthesis is severe. In severe cases, bowel and bladder dysfunction may also be present. Discomfort is usually increased by exercise and relieved by rest.

Signs vary with the severity of spondylolisthesis. Asymptomatic patients with slips of mild severity may have no outward manifestations of vertebral abnormality. Patients with moderate to severe slips usually have tenderness on palpation of the lumbar spine and increased lumbar lordosis. Spasm of the hamstring muscles may extend the sacral spine, causing the buttocks to seem flattened or heart-shaped in appearance. In severe slips, a step-off of L5 on S1 can be palpated. A flexible scoliotic deformity caused by paraspinal muscle spasm may be present.

Neurologic examination findings are usually normal in children with spondylolysis. Symptoms and signs of nerve root compression and mechanical instability are much more common in adult patients with progressive or severe untreated adolescent spondylolisthesis.

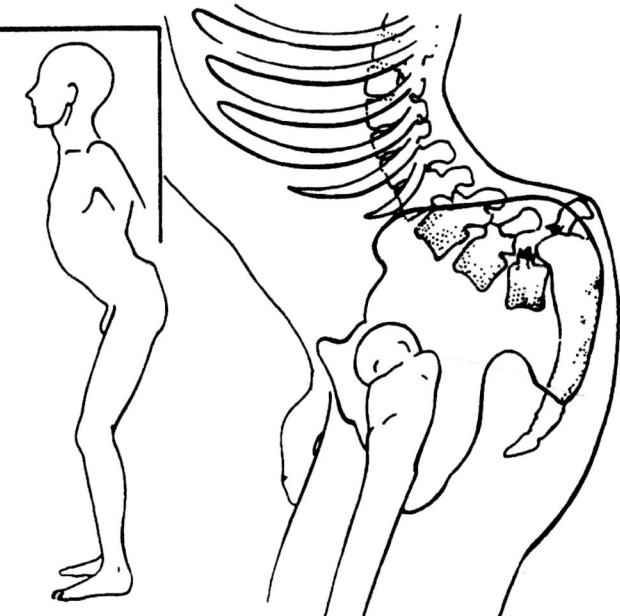

Figure 46-9. Clinical picture of severe spondylolisthesis.

Hamstring muscle spasm is a common finding in patients with symptomatic spondylolisthesis and at times may be the chief presenting problem. Affected patients are unable to flex far enough forward to touch their toes without bending their knees. When severe, hamstring spasm results in a loss of normal lumbar lordosis and produces a flattened appearance of the low back. Hamstring muscle spasm also interferes with gait; stride length is shortened, and patients run with a peculiar stiff-legged posture. The cause of hamstring spasm in spondylolisthesis is unclear; it does not appear to be caused by compression of spinal nerves, and it is rarely accompanied by other signs of nerve root compromise. Most authorities believe it is a result of abnormal strain on the hamstring muscles caused by mechanical instability of the lumbosacral junction.

Radiographic Assessment

If spondylolysis is suspected, radiographic assessment should consist of an anterior/posterior lateral right and left oblique views of the lumbar spine (Fig. 46-10). The oblique view of the lumbar spine illustrates the defect in the pars interarticularis. In cases of unilateral spondylolysis, there may be hypertrophy of the opposite pars or pedicle. A computed tomographic (CT) scan is helpful in determining the anatomy of the defect and can help assess the status of healing during treatment. CT scans also may identify sites of nerve root compression. The bone scan (single photon emission computed tomography scan) is sensitive in identifying the stress fracture before disruption is evident on radiographs. Immobilization at this point may heal the lesion. If the clinician suspects an associated herniated disk, MRI is indicated. The plain radiographs illustrate the degree of slippage. This must be documented to see whether progression is occurring over time. The most common classification system notes the position of the posterior border of the L5 vertebral body with regard to the S1 body. When the slip is less than 25% of the width of the first sacral body, the slip is considered mild. Slips exceeding 50% are considered severe. These cases are of concern in that the progression may proceed to the point at which L5 dislocates in front of the S1 vertebral body, which is called *spondyloptosis*.

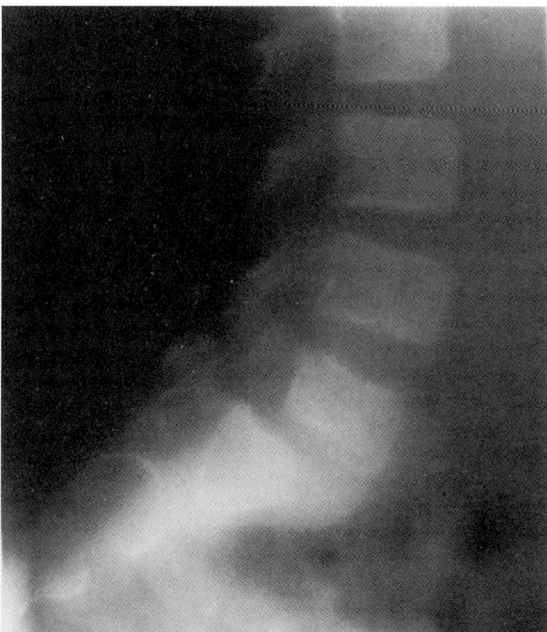

Figure 46-10. Spondylolisthesis. Slippage of L5 on the underlying body of S1 has occurred as a consequence of defective formation of the posterior elements of L5. In this case, slippage is moderate, measuring slightly more than 25% of the width of the S1 vertebral segment.

Treatment

In asymptomatic patients with a mild slip, no treatment is required; likelihood of progression is low. However, if significant progression occurs (even if a patient is asymptomatic), a posterolateral fusion is recommended. When a slip exceeds 50%, the likelihood of continued progression is high, and surgical stabilization should be performed. Both symptomatic and asymptomatic patients with this severe condition should undergo surgical stabilization.

Initial treatment of patients with symptomatic spondylolysis should be conservative. The examiner must also rule out other causes of back discomfort. Activity restriction with antiinflammatory medication is the initial treatment. When the pain is severe, a brace or corset is helpful. Then abdominal and paraspinal strengthening exercises are instituted to help relieve symptoms. Most patients with symptomatic spondylolysis or mild spondylolisthesis respond to conservative therapy and are able to return to sports. However, a small percentage of patients do not respond to conservative therapy; for these patients, surgical stabilization may be necessary. Patients with a severe slip who have a neurologic deficit that does not respond to conservative management also require surgical intervention. A fusion in situ (L5 to S1) is the most commonly performed surgical procedure for patients with a slip of less than 50%. Extension of the fusion to L4 is necessary to create a satisfactory fusion in patients with a more significant slip.

IDIOPATHIC KYPHOSIS

Abnormal increases in expected thoracic kyphosis in children and adolescents produce round back deformities (Fig. 46-11). These may be congenital, neuromuscular, or idiopathic in origin. Mild to moderate increases in kyphosis cause little deformity and few symptoms. Severe kyphosis is disfiguring, often causes back pain, and may lead to spinal cord compromise.

Round back posture is often encountered in otherwise healthy adolescents at school screening examinations. Affected patients are usually asymptomatic, although their parents often report poor posture. A history should be obtained and physical examination performed. Complaints of severe back pain or leg pain, enuresis, and findings of lower extremity weakness or increased reflex tone in patients with round back are ominous findings and warrant referral.

If accentuated kyphosis is present, radiographic follow-up is indicated. Two radiologic patterns are common. The majority of individuals, especially younger adolescents, have thoracic kyphotic curves of 20 to 45 degrees, with no underlying structural vertebral changes. Usually such curves correct easily on passive or active hyperextension. For such children, no treatment except for a thoracic hyperextension exercise program and periodic follow-up examination is necessary.

More severe kyphosis with accompanying structural changes in vertebral bodies at the apex of the deformity is present in a small subset of adolescents with kyphosis. Affected individuals often have kyphotic curves greater than 60 degrees and show little correction with hyperextension. Roentgenograms show vertebral wedging, endplate irregularity, and kyphosis (Fig. 46-12). *Scheuermann kyphosis* (an osteochondrosis) occurs in approximately 5% to 8% of the population, affecting boys 5 to 10 times more often than girls. The cause remains unclear but may be the result of disruption of growth of the anterior portion of the vertebral body and consequent wedging of multiple vertebral bodies. Back pain is usually mild; many affected patients have no pain at all. The deformity in most affected patients is minimal and only rarely is cosmetically unacceptable. Late neurologic complications are extremely rare.

Treatment depends on the degree of deformity and the age of the patient. Skeletally immature individuals with significant deformity

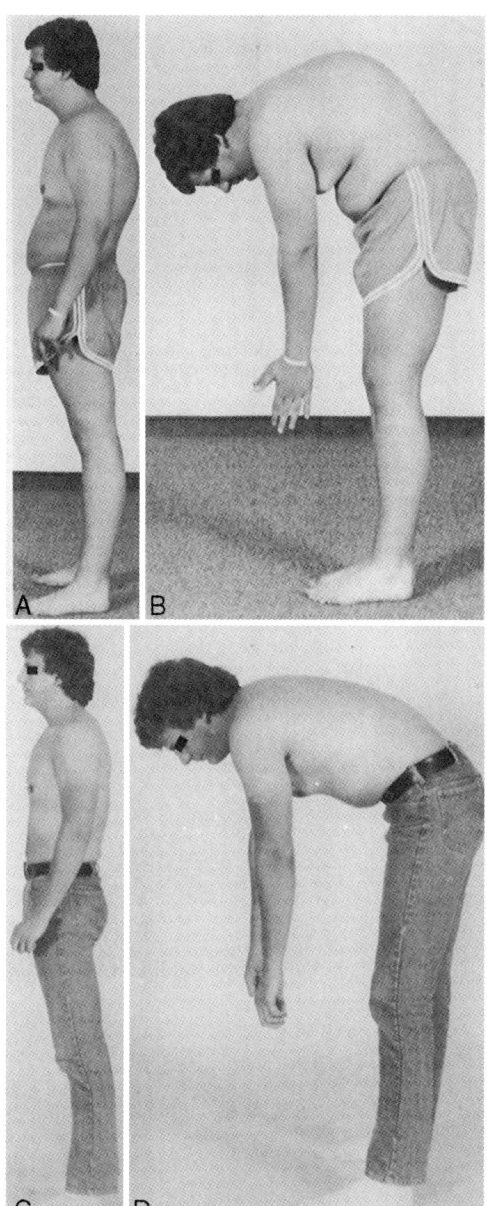

Figure 46-11. Preoperative (A and B) and postoperative (C and D) views of an adolescent boy with severe kyphosis secondary to Scheuermann disease. He required both anterior and posterior spinal fusion. He now has a markedly improved appearance and no further progression of the kyphosis. (From Renshaw TS: Pediatric Orthopedics. Philadelphia, WB Saunders, 1986, p 53.)

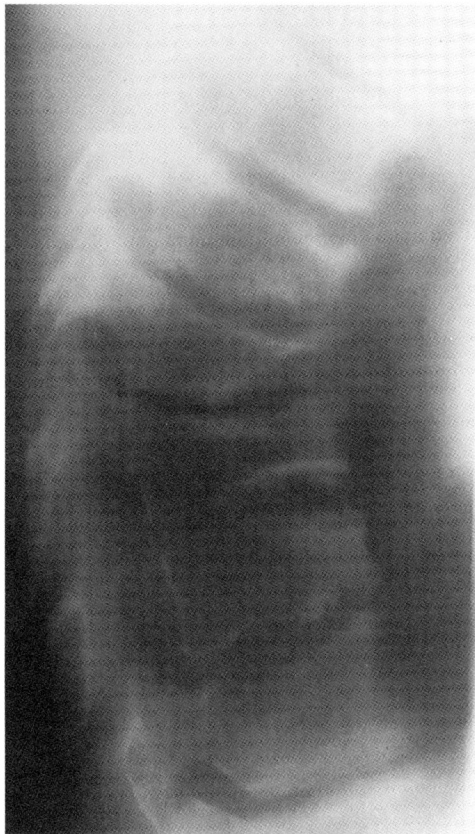

Figure 46-12. Scheuermann kyphosis. Lateral radiographs of the midthoracic spine in an asymptomatic 16-year-old boy with moderately severe kyphosis. There is severe wedging, loss of vertebral height, and endplate irregularity present on these films. His radiographic findings appear far worse than his symptoms and signs. If further collapse were to develop and the kyphosis became more severe, surgical intervention would be necessary.

may improve with a program of exercise and use of a Milwaukee or modified Boston brace. Bracing does not reverse a deformity, but it may prevent progression. Older patients with back pain usually respond to a back-strengthening exercise program. Patients with unacceptable deformity who are too old for brace treatment require surgical correction. Often this requires a combination of anterior release and posterior spinal instrumentation and fusion.

Congenital vertebral malformations that produce kyphotic deformities develop during the first trimester of gestation and, like other congenital abnormalities of the spine, are often associated with abnormalities of the genitourinary tract or the spinal cord. Kyphosis that results from congenital vertebral deformities is often obvious early in life and may be rapidly progressive (Fig. 46-13). The spinal

cord may become tented over the apex of the deformity, producing symptoms and signs of spasticity in the lower extremity and bladder. Progression of deformity is dangerous; congenital kyphosis is the spinal deformity most often associated with paraplegia. Patients should be promptly referred for orthopedic evaluation.

INTERVERTEBRAL DISK HERNIATION

Intervertebral disk rupture is much less common in children than in adults. Because most such patients are treated nonoperatively, the absolute incidence of the disorder is not known. In the United States, fewer than 1% of patients undergoing diskectomy are younger than 16 years. The frequency of symptomatic intervertebral disk herniation may be more common in Asian persons than in white persons, perhaps because of the smaller size of the spinal canal.

Some patients have a significant history of trauma. In other patients, congenital anomalies of the lumbar spine, such as transitional vertebra or spina bifida occulta, are noted. There may be a family history of low back pain or herniated disks. An autosomal dominant trait has been linked to the *COL 9A2* collagen IX gene.

The symptoms of a herniated lumbar disk in adolescents differ somewhat from those in adults; this may delay recognition. The initial complaint in adolescents is significant low back discomfort; it is only months later that the symptoms of leg discomfort become more noticeable or prominent. Pain typically is aggravated by activity and

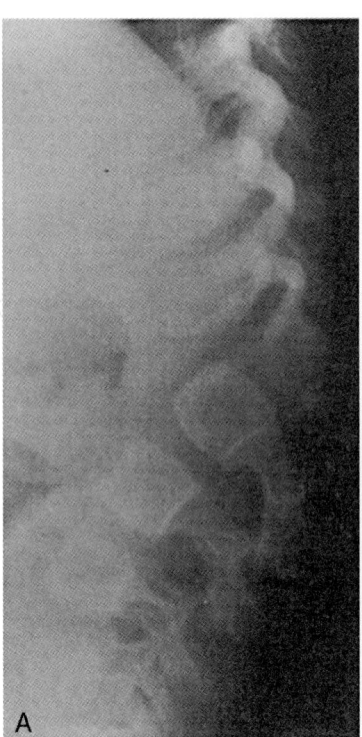
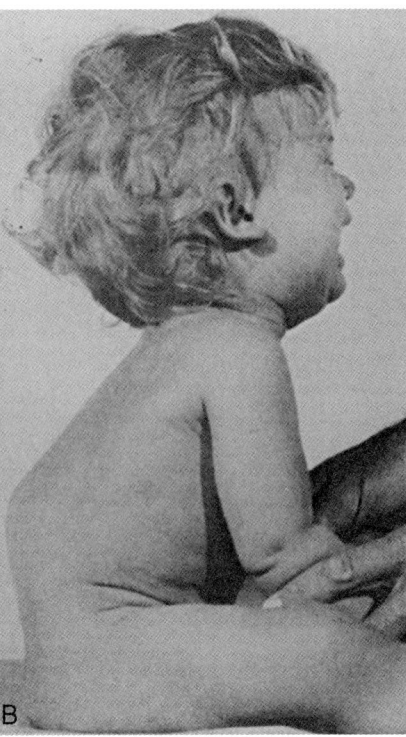

Figure 46-13. A, Congenital kyphosis secondary to failure of vertebral bodies to form at T12 and L1. **B,** The clinical appearance of the child. Thoracolumbar kyphosis is obvious. (From Renshaw TS: Pediatric Orthopedics. Philadelphia, WB Saunders, 1986, p 44.)

relieved with rest. Symptoms may be intermittent. The affected adolescent has poor back mobility, often with paravertebral muscle spasm. Lumbar lordosis may diminish, and there is a tendency to walk bent forward. Hamstring tightness with limited straight-leg raising is almost universal. Neurologic signs are less likely to be prominent in the adolescent with herniated disk than in the affected adult. Plain radiographs are needed as an initial study. These usually are normal other than for the loss of lumbar lordosis. The MRI is the procedure of choice for diagnosing a disk herniation. In rare cases, adolescents may develop a lesion that is a fracture of the posterior vertebral apophysis, which displaces posteriorly into the spinal canal and acts like a herniated disk. This is an avulsion fracture that is identified with either a CT scan or MRI. When a patient has severe symptoms, treatment should begin with bed rest, analgesics, and antiinflammatory agents. When the symptoms have begun to abate, physical therapy for lumbar and paraspinal strengthening is helpful. A lumbar corset may be helpful for patients who also have significant symptoms. Patients who present with progressive neurologic deficits require early surgical excision. Similarly, patients who fail to respond to a significant period of nonoperative management also require disk surgery.

The long-term results of a disk excision are good in 70% to 80% of the patients. Spinal fusion is not required unless the patient shows evidence of instability, which is quite rare.

SCOLIOSIS

Idiopathic scoliosis, a combination of lateral deviation and rotation of vertebral bodies, does not always produce back pain. When painful scoliosis is present, a careful search for the cause of the symptoms must be undertaken. Infection, tumor, a spinal cord syringomyelia or diastematomyelia (more common with left thoracic curves), and occult fractures may produce clinical findings that resemble idiopathic scoliosis but, in contrast to idiopathic scoliosis, cause significant chronic pain as well. Any patient with painful scoliosis should have a careful evaluation for other spinal anomalies causing the pain.

Etiology

Idiopathic scoliosis begins in the immature spine, although progression of preexisting curvatures may occur in adult life. The cause of idiopathic scoliosis remains unknown. Hormonal factors appear to play a role in curve progression, inasmuch as severe curves occur much more often in girls. Some studies have demonstrated abnormalities of proprioception and vibratory sensation in affected patients, which suggests that abnormalities of posterior column function may contribute to the development of curvature. Other investigators have implicated cerebellar or muscular (myopathy) dysfunction as a possible cause of spinal imbalance.

No clear genetic pattern has been established. Curves occur more frequently in individuals with affected first-degree relatives, but transmission is not mendelian. Although curvature is more likely to develop in the daughters of affected mothers than in other children, the magnitude of curvature in an affected individual is not related to the magnitude of curvature in relatives. It appears likely that a combination of genetic predisposition and other undefined factors is responsible for development and progression of idiopathic scoliosis.

Classification

Idiopathic curves are grouped into infantile (birth to 3 years), juvenile (4 to 10 years), and adolescent categories on the basis of age at onset of curvature. The infantile form differs enough from the other varieties to be considered a distinct entity. The distinction between juvenile and adolescent scoliosis is not as sharp.

Infantile Idiopathic Scoliosis

Infantile idiopathic scoliosis is rare in the United States, probably accounting for fewer than 1% of new cases of idiopathic scoliosis. It is more common in Europe. The majority of patients are boys, and most curves are convex toward the left rather than the right, as in the other varieties of idiopathic scoliosis. Some infants suspected of having idiopathic deformity actually have subtle congenital vertebral abnormalities. The diagnosis of idiopathic deformity is appropriate only when radiographic studies show no evidence of congenital vertebral anomalies (e.g., hemivertebra) and there are no signs of spinal dysraphism or of neuropathic or myopathic disorders.

Although many infantile curves resolve spontaneously, others progress relentlessly and are very difficult to treat effectively. Observation is appropriate until age 6 months in infants with idiopathic scoliosis, but prompt referral should be made if curves persist or increase during the period of observation.

Juvenile Idiopathic Scoliosis

Juvenile idiopathic scoliosis begins before the adolescent growth spurt. Some curves are probably undetected cases of infantile scoliosis. Others, particularly those that occur in older children, may be early manifestations of adolescent idiopathic scoliosis. Some curves remain small and, in fact, may resolve spontaneously. Others remain stable until the onset of the growth spurt and then progress unless treated. Still others progress steadily throughout childhood and adolescence. Some are associated with intraspinal anomalies (syrinx). There is no reliable method of predicting the behavior of juvenile curves at the time of diagnosis, but, in general, high-magnitude curves in young patients are more likely to increase with growth than are smaller curves in older children.

The majority of patients with juvenile curves greater than 30 degrees at the time of diagnosis require some form of active treatment. Treatment must begin at the time progression is first documented if severe deformity is to be prevented.

Adolescent Idiopathic Scoliosis

Most cases of idiopathic scoliosis in North America develop around the time of the adolescent growth spurt (Figs. 46-14 and 46-15). Often parents and children are unaware of the presence of curvature at outset. Nerve root impingement, intervertebral disk disease, and spinal cord compression are uncommon in young patients with idiopathic scoliosis. Large curves are more common in girls than in boys (7:1 ratio). Pain is so rare that children and adolescents with painful curves must be carefully studied in order to exclude neoplastic and inflammatory processes of the spinal column or neural canal. Idiopathic scoliosis is usually a painless disorder during childhood and adolescence. Severe structural curves may cause no pain until degenerative changes develop in adulthood.

School Screening Programs

School screening for spinal deformity is common in North America. Most programs concentrate on children in the late juvenile and early adolescent periods. The most common screening method employed is the forward-bend test, based anatomically on the vertebral rotation that accompanies lateral spinal deviation (see Fig. 46-14). Associated clinical findings include shoulder asymmetry, unequal distances between the medial borders of the elbows and the flanks, and apparent leg-length inequality or pelvic tilt. Breast asymmetry, caused by forward rotation of the chest wall on the side of the curve concavity and backward displacement of the chest wall on the convex side of the curve, is often present in affected girls.

The threshold for "identification" on screening examination is subjective, and it is not surprising that the incidence of spine asymmetry detected by school screening programs varies with the method of screening and the experience of the examiner. A range of 3% to 20% has been reported. Follow-up radiographic studies of children thought to have abnormal curvatures on school screening examinations indicate an incidence of scoliosis in screened children of less than 15% (range, 0.4% to 14%). The incidence of curves greater than 20 degrees at the time of primary screening is probably less than 0.5%. Simple devices such as the scoliometer determine spine

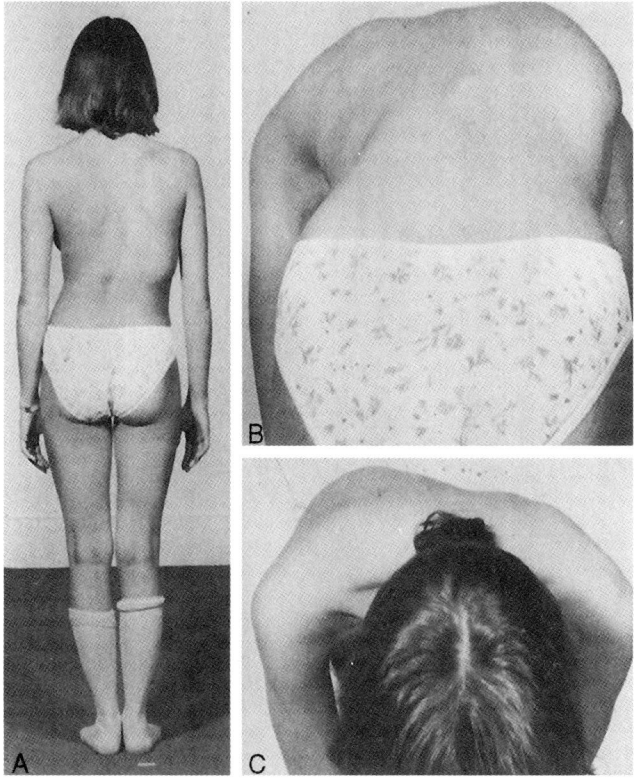

Figure 46-14. A, Adolescent idiopathic scoliosis, viewed from the back. Note the right-sided thoracic prominence. When the patient bends forward (B), the rib prominence is even more apparent. This is secondary to rotation of the ribs and spine. The rib prominence is also quite evident when viewed from the front (C). (From Renshaw TS: Pediatric Orthopedics. Philadelphia, WB Saunders, 1986, p 47.)

asymmetry by measuring the angle of trunk rotation at the apex of the rib hump. An angle of more than 7 degrees is an appropriate criterion for referral.

The first response to a positive school screening examination should be a repeated physical examination. If asymmetry is confirmed, a single standing posteroanterior spine film, including vertebral levels T1 to S1, should be obtained. Lateral films, bending films, and oblique views are not necessary. Referral is appropriate for skeletally immature children or adolescents with curves greater than 20 degrees.

Natural History

The natural history of curvature in patients with spine asymmetry is highly variable. Factors that appear to be associated with risk of progression include the magnitude of curvature at the time of detection, the chronologic and skeletal age of the patient, the pattern of curvature, and the menarcheal status. Immature patients with large-magnitude curves are far more likely to experience progression than are more mature patients with small curves. Progression of curves after skeletal growth is uncommon in idiopathic thoracic curves of less than 30 degrees at the end of growth but is likely to occur in patients with curves greater than 50 degrees at maturity.

Uncontrolled curve progression causes significant problems in adult life. Unacceptable deformity, back pain, chronic fatigue, and decreased work capacity are common. Premature degenerative arthritis and nerve root impingement caused by deformity and osteophytic spurring occur in patients with lumbar curves or double thoracic-lumbar curves. Asymptomatic decreased vital capacity is

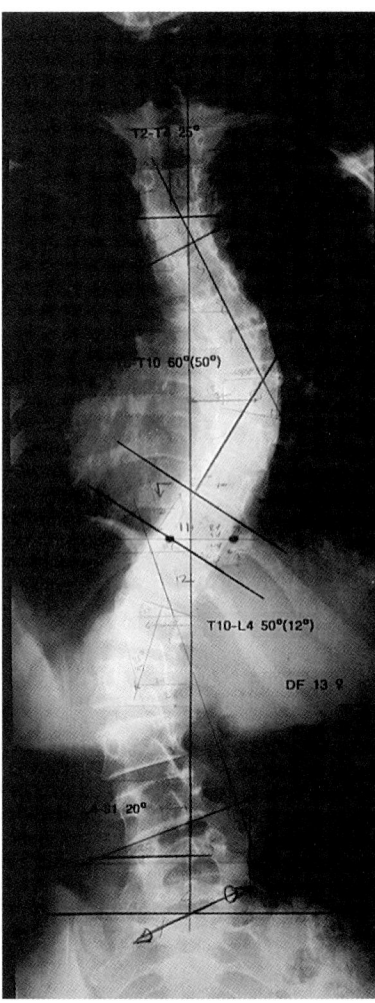

Figure 46-15. Adolescent idiopathic scoliosis. The patient, a 13-year-old girl, had a severe double-curve pattern with significant accompanying deformity but no pain. Surgical treatment was warranted to halt progression and restore spinal alignment.

common in patients with thoracic curves; symptomatic cardiopulmonary compromise (cor pulmonale) may develop in patients with curves greater than 80 degrees.

Treatment

The goals of treatment in idiopathic scoliosis are to bring a patient to skeletal maturity with a cosmetically acceptable, balanced, and stable curve that is unlikely to progress in adult life. Mature adolescents with curves less than 30 degrees need no treatment beyond initial evaluation. Further progression of curvature is unlikely to occur in these individuals. Patients with juvenile scoliosis and less mature adolescents with curves between 10 and 20 degrees should be monitored at 6-month intervals with single standing posteroanterior spine radiographs. If progression occurs, they should be referred for orthopedic care.

Active treatment is indicated for growing patients with curves greater than 30 degrees. Brace treatment remains the standard method of nonoperative treatment of idiopathic curvature. Surgical treatment is appropriate for patients with curves too severe for brace treatment. Documented progression in spite of nonoperative treatment is another indication for surgical intervention.

Improved instrumentation and internal fixation devices, intraoperative monitoring of spinal cord function, and autologous transfusion has improved the safety and efficacy of surgical correction. In most cases, patients can be out of bed within 3 to 4 days of surgery and are walking within 5 days of surgery. Return to school is usually possible within 3 weeks; most activities of normal life, including sports, can be resumed within 6 months. In many instances, no postoperative immobilization is required; in other cases, a removable lightweight plastic orthosis can be employed. Prolonged periods of immobilization in a plaster cast are uncommon.

TUMORS OF THE SPINAL COLUMN

Persistent back pain, muscle spasm, and abnormal trunk posture are ominous findings in children. Neoplastic disease must be considered in patients with no other obvious source of pain (see Table 46-2).

Primary Lesions of Bone

The most common primary bone tumors affecting the spinal column in children are osteoid osteoma (Fig. 46-16), osteoblastoma (Fig. 46-17), eosinophilic granuloma, and aneurysmal bone cysts (see Chapter 45). Although benign, these lesions may cause considerable back pain and local bone destruction. Osteogenic sarcoma, a malignant lesion of bone, occurs less commonly in the spine than in the long bones of children. Unexplained pain is the hallmark of spinal neoplasia and is usually the presenting complaint. At times, pain may be severe and unresponsive to nonnarcotic analgesics. In other instances, as in osteoid osteoma, the relief of symptoms that occurs with nonsteroidal antiinflammatory agents is so characteristic that it is considered a diagnostic finding. Paraspinal muscle spasm,

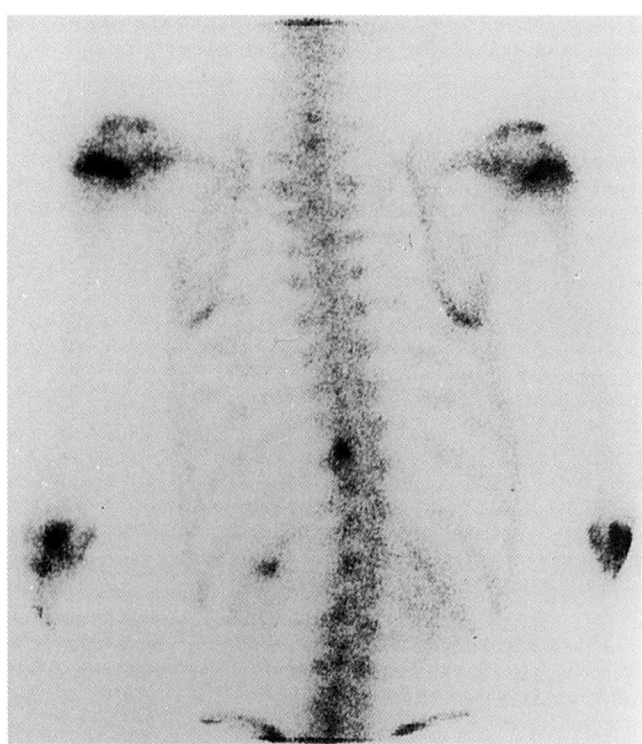

Figure 46-16. Osteoid osteoma of the spine. Technetium bone scanning shows increased uptake in the T10 vertebral body in a 15-year-old boy. Note the scoliosis that accompanies this painful lesion. The condition did not respond to antiinflammatory medications, and surgical excision was necessary.

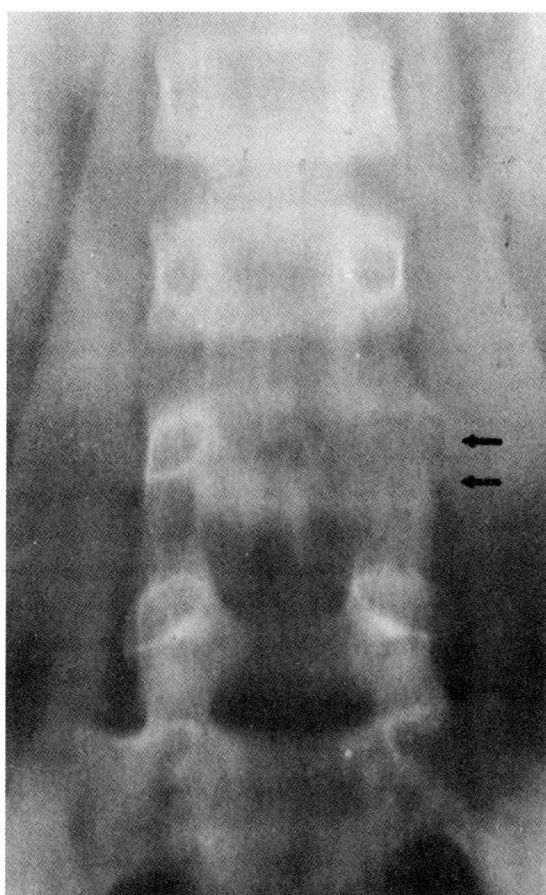

Figure 46-17. The patient presented with left-sided lumbar back pain. Note the destruction of the vertebral pedicle at L4 *(arrows)*. This proved to be an osteoblastoma. Children with back pain should be suspected of having a tumor of the spine or spinal cord until it is proven otherwise. (From Renshaw TS: Pediatric Orthopedics. Philadelphia, WB Saunders, 1986, p 57.)

tenderness in the soft tissues on the side of the spinal column, and alterations in spinal configuration are common. Scoliosis, loss of lumbar lordosis, or accentuations of thoracic kyphosis may be present.

Initial evaluation of patients with suspected spinal tumors should include standard anteroposterior and lateral radiographs of the spine (see Fig. 46-17). These may not show small lesions hidden in vertebral pedicles or posterior elements; other studies are often necessary. Technetium bone scanning is particularly useful (see Fig. 46-16). MRI and CT scans are usually necessary to localize lesions for surgical treatment. Prompt referral is essential when spinal neoplasia is suspected. The success of treatment depends in large part on early discovery and intervention.

Tumors of Neural Elements

Back pain, lower extremity weakness, and sphincter disturbances are common manifestations of neoplasms of the spinal cord. Although such lesions are rare, they must be suspected in children with unexplained back or leg pain, weakness, sensory or reflex abnormalities, bowel or bladder incontinence, or unexplained gait abnormalities. Neuroblastoma is the most common lesion, but sarcomas (including Ewing sarcoma, rhabdomyosarcoma, and hemangiosarcoma) and

astrocytomas or ependymomas also occur in the neural contents of the spinal canal.

In such patients, standard radiography often shows only loss of lordosis or scoliosis secondary to muscle spasm. MRI demonstrates the abnormality, but definitive diagnosis usually requires biopsy. The success of treatment is often related to promptness of diagnosis. Early referral of patients with unexplained back pain is essential for appropriate treatment.

Leukemia

Skeletal involvement is common in patients with leukemia; back pain or limb pain may be the presenting symptom in some children. Proliferation of abnormal hematopoietic tissue in the marrow of long bones or vertebral bodies causes pain and weakens their structure.

Clinical symptoms and signs in children with leukemic skeletal involvement may be confusing. Fever, localized pain and swelling, and elevations of the white blood cell count and erythrocyte sedimentation rate may be mistaken as signs of septic arthritis, osteomyelitis, or intervertebral disk space infection. The presence of abnormal white blood cells on the peripheral blood cell count or of thrombocytopenia increases the likelihood of bone marrow tumor rather than infection.

Osteopenia, periosteal elevation, and metaphyseal lucencies are common radiographic findings in leukemic involvement of long bones. These may be difficult to detect in patients with spinal involvement. Vertebral compression and wedging are sometimes present and may mimic acute fracture or, on occasion, osteomyelitis (Fig. 46-18). The absence of a history of trauma should alert the examiner to search for other causes of the radiographic abnormality. Preservation of intervertebral disk space height with collapse of adjacent vertebral segments is an indication that the vertebral bodies rather than the intervertebral disk are the sites of the abnormality. Technetium bone scanning is useful for detecting other areas of involvement, although it is not as reliable in leukemia as in other spinal lesions. MRI is useful for detecting areas of spinal involvement not visible on plain radiographs and for assessing the extent of intraspinal infiltrate or spinal cord compression present.

The diagnosis of leukemia can be established by bone marrow aspiration. Biopsy of involved vertebral segments is rarely necessary. Support of the spine in a custom-fabricated orthosis is useful for relieving pain and preventing further vertebral collapse during the initial phases of treatment. Prolonged brace treatment may be necessary to prevent vertebral compression fractures that may accompany the osteopenia resulting from steroid therapy. Surgical decompression and fusion may be required in rare cases of acute vertebral compression and spinal cord compromise.

SUMMARY AND RED FLAGS

Back pain in children may be referred pain from intraabdominal or retroperitoneal disease (see Table 46-2) or may represent direct involvement of the spinal cord, vertebral bodies, or paraspinal musculature. In most children with normal examination findings, back pain is benign, short-lived, and responsive to rest or nonsteroidal antiinflammatory agents.

Chronic persistent back pain, pain associated with lower extremity or bowel and bladder neurologic deficits, cutaneous lesions over the lumbar spine, systemic signs (as in inflammatory bowel disease, leukemia, osteomyelitis), acute pain, and tenderness with neurologic dysfunction after trauma are red flags. Signs of cord involvement are particularly ominous and are emergencies. Spinal cord involvement above T10 produces symmetric weakness, increased deep tendon reflexes, up-going toes, and an appropriate sensory loss; conus medullaris involvement (T10 to L2) produces symmetric weakness,

REFERENCES

Balagué F, Dudler J, Nordin M: Low-back pain in children. Lancet 2003;361:1403-1404.

Bell DF, Erlich MG, Zaleske DJ: Brace treatment for symptomatic spondylolisthesis. Clin Orthop 1988;236:192-198.

Brown R, Hussain M, McHugh K, et al: Discitis in young children. J Bone Joint Surg Br 2001;83:106-111.

Cassar-Pullicino VN, Eisenstein SM: Imaging in scoliosis: What, why and how? Clin Radiol 2002;57:543-562.

Conrad EU, Olszewki AD, Berger M, et al: Pediatric spinal cord tumors with spinal cord compromise. J Pediatr Orthop 1992;12:454-460.

Deyo RA, Weinstein JN: Low back pain. N Engl J Med 2001;344:363-370.

Edgar M: A new classification of adolescent idiopathic scoliosis. Lancet 2002;360:270-271.

Fernandez M, Carrol CL, Baker CJ: Discitis and vertebral osteomyelitis in children: An 18-year review. Pediatrics 2000;105:1299-1304.

Frennerd AK, Danielson BI, Nachemson AL: Natural history of symptomatic isthmic low-grade spondylolisthesis in children and adolescents: A seven year follow up study. J Pediatr Orthop 1991;11:209-213.

Hadley MN: Management of pediatric cervical spine and spinal cord injuries. Neurosurgery 2002;50:S85-S99.

Letts MH, Haasbeek J: Hematocolpos as a cause of back pain in premenarchal adolescents. J Pediatr Orthop 1990;10:731-732.

Lowe TG: Scheuermann disease. J Bone Joint Surg Am 1990;72:940-945.

Nussinovitch M, Sokolover N, Volovitz B, et al: Neurologic abnormalities in children presenting with diskitis. Arch Pediatr Adolesc Med 2002;156:1052-104.

Paassilta P, Lohinvia J, Goring HHH, et al: Identification of a novel common genetic risk factor for lumbar disk disease. JAMA 2001;285:1843-1849.

Pizzutillo PD, Hummer CD: Nonoperative treatment of painful adolescent spondylolysis or spondylolisthesis. J Pediatr Orthop 1989;9:538-540.

Prahinski JR, Polly DW Jr, McHale KA, et al: Occult intraspinal anomalies in congenital scoliosis. J Pediatr Orthop 2000;20:59-63.

Rogalsky RJ, Black GB, Reed MH: Orthopedic manifestations of leukemia in children. J Bone Joint Surg Am 1986;68:494-501.

Sachs B, Bradford D, Winter RB, et al: Scheuermann kyphosis. Follow-up of Milwaukee brace treatment. J Bone Joint Surg Am 1987;69:50-57.

Seitsalo SK, Osterman H, Hyvarinen K, et al: Progression of spondylolisthesis in children and adolescents. A long term followup of 272 patients. Spine 1991;16:417-421.

Sponseller PD: Sizing up scoliosis. JAMA 2003;289:608-609.

Watson KD, Papageorgiou AC, Jones GT, et al: Low back pain in schoolroom children: The role of mechanical and psychosocial factors. Arch Dis Child 2003;88:12-17.

Weinstein SL, Dolan LA, Spratt KF, et al: Health and function of patients with untreated idiopathic scoliosis. JAMA 2003;289:559-566.

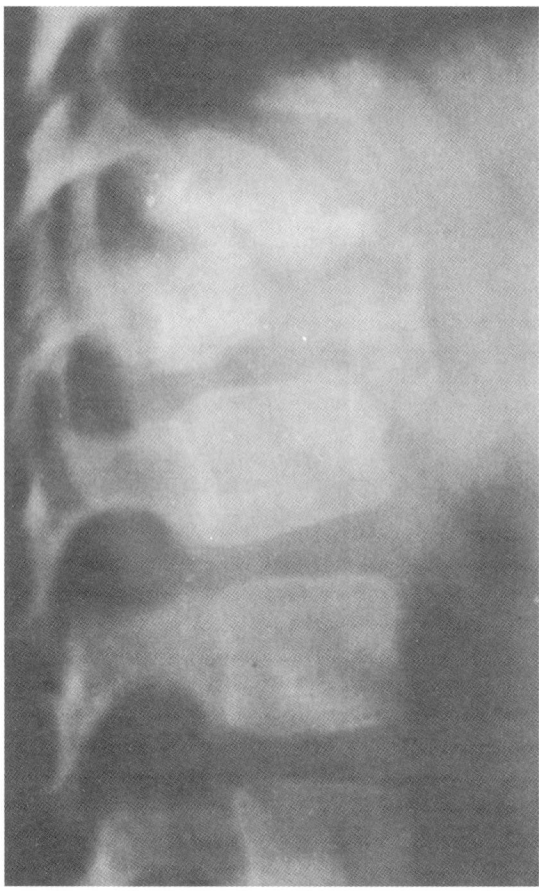

Figure 46-18. Osteomyelitis at T11 and T12. Note the destruction of the disk space and vertebral bodies with beginning of anterior ossification. In this patient, fusion occurred spontaneously, and the patient is now asymptomatic. (From Renshaw TS: Pediatric Orthopedics. Philadelphia, WB Saunders, 1986, p 59.)

increased knee and decreased ankle deep tendon reflexes, a saddle-type anesthesia, and up- or down-going toes on Babinski testing; and cauda equina involvement (below L2) produces asymmetric weakness, loss of deep tendon reflexes, and down-going toes. Such findings represent an acute emergency that warrants immediate imaging (MRI) and therapy, which may include high-dose corticosteroids, radiation therapy, or laminectomy to prevent permanent paralysis.

HEMATOLOGIC DISORDERS

47 Lymphadenopathy

John R. Schreiber   Brian W. Berman

Lymphadenopathy, defined as enlarged lymph nodal tissue measuring more than 1 cm in diameter, is common in children. Enlarged nodes are a feature of many illnesses because of the role of the nodes in filtering pathogens, the anatomy of the lymph node chains, and the cellular proliferation that occurs in nodal tissue after exposure to infectious agents or by infiltration with malignant cells. Most of the illnesses manifesting with enlarged lymph nodes represent common bacterial or viral infections that improve either spontaneously or after appropriate antimicrobial therapy. Some serious illnesses, particularly malignancy, can first manifest as lymphadenopathy. A thorough history, careful physical examination, and knowledge of the anatomy of tissues drained by lymph nodes, as well as of the type of adenopathy caused by various illnesses, often lead to the appropriate diagnosis without the need for complex diagnostic procedures.

MECHANISM OF LYMPHADENOPATHY

The lymphatic system consists of lymphatic vessels (afferent and efferent) that connect lymphatic tissues, including lymph nodes, to the peripheral circulation via postcapillary venules. The lymph nodes contain both B and T cells, which lie in a supportive framework within a connective tissue capsule (Fig. 47-1). The lymphatic fluid or "lymph"-containing antigens, bacteria, or other pathogens, as well as various lymphocytes and macrophages, enter through afferent lymphatic vessels; the cells within the node then interact with antigens. This interaction allows production of T cell and/or B cell humoral immune responses in the host's effort to clear the antigen or the pathogen. Efferent lymphatic vessels then carry lymph-containing antigen-sensitized lymphocytes from the nodes back to the peripheral circulation via the thoracic duct. Enlargement of the nodes can be caused by several factors. First, when nodes fulfill their normal function, hyperplasia occurs as a consequence of proliferation by nodal and newly arrived lymphoid cells. This proliferation is a response to antigenic stimulation. Such responses are particularly active in children, which explains the frequent observation of *lymphadenopathy* associated with some pediatric infections. Second, bacteria or their products that have traveled to the nodes may stimulate the arrival of inflammatory cells, such as neutrophils, and cause enlargement and symptoms of *lymphadenitis* (erythema and tenderness). Third, malignant cells either may arise in the node itself and proliferate, causing enlargement, or may arrive from distant cancerous sites and also infiltrate the nodal tissue. Finally, in rare genetic storage diseases, macrophages laden with abnormally metabolized lipids may lodge in lymph nodes, causing lymphadenopathy.

The regional areas drained by each lymph node group are also important in determining the cause of lymphadenopathy. The superficial cervical lymph nodes, for example, drain lymph from distinct areas of the head, neck, and throat (Fig. 47-2) and may enlarge if a local infection is present. These nodes, in turn, drain into the deep cervical nodes and eventually the thoracic duct. Because viral and bacterial pharyngitis and otitis media are common infections in children, the cervical and occipital areas, respectively, are some of the more common sites for lymphadenopathy in small children. In contrast, the inguinal nodes drain the areas surrounding and including the urethra, the vagina, and the penis and may be enlarged, particularly in adolescents with venereal diseases. The inguinal nodes also drain the distal extremities and may enlarge with soft tissue infections of the lower extremities.

HISTORY

The history is important in the evaluation of lymphadenopathy and often yields distinct clues to the appropriate diagnosis. First, the character and temporal course of the adenopathy are important. Rapid onset of unilateral lymphadenopathy in the groin after trauma to the lower extremity, for example, suggests infection originating in the traumatized extremity. In contrast, progressive enlargement of nodes noticed in several areas of the body that is accompanied by weight loss, fevers, night sweats, or other systemic illness is suggestive of diseases associated with involvement of multiple organ systems, such as lymphoma or tuberculosis. Second, the age of the child who has the enlarged lymph node or nodes is important in the consideration of the cause (Table 47-1).

Most neonates with adenopathy have been exposed to an infectious agent in utero (e.g., cytomegalovirus [CMV], syphilis, toxoplasmosis). In contrast, toddlers with adenopathy (depending on whether it is regional or diffuse) tend to have either focal infections that drain into the affected nodal chain (cervical chain lymphadenopathy with pharyngitis) (see Fig. 47-2) or a systemic viral infection that results in diffusely enlarged nodes. Similarly, malignancy manifested as adenopathy is rare in neonates but more common in toddlers and older children. The history should focus on presence of chronic illness, weight loss, systemic signs and symptoms, an immunodeficiency that would predispose to opportunistic infection, and the use of medications (procainamide, sulfasalazine, phenytoin, or tetracycline) that may be associated with lupus-like illnesses and adenopathy.

The family history may reveal the presence of infection, such as human immunodeficiency virus (HIV) or tuberculosis, in the parents or close relatives, or group A streptococcal infection or mononucleosis in a close contact. The family history should include place of birth, HIV risk (such as intravenous drug use), and travel history to determine whether the child is from or has been exposed to geographic areas with high rates of infections (e.g., tuberculosis in an incarcerated family member; travel to the Ohio River valley for histoplasmosis). Activities during travel are also important, such as the consumption of unprocessed cheeses or unpasteurized milk products, particularly from other countries that may contain pathogens, such as *Brucella* species or *Mycobacterium bovis.*

The social history may provide further clues. Is the child from a socioeconomic or immigrant ethnic group that has a more intense exposure to such infections as tuberculosis? Is there an adult in the household who is currently ill or taking medication? Is there an adult with a high risk of infection with tuberculosis (recent immigration from an endemic area, recent incarceration, known HIV infection,

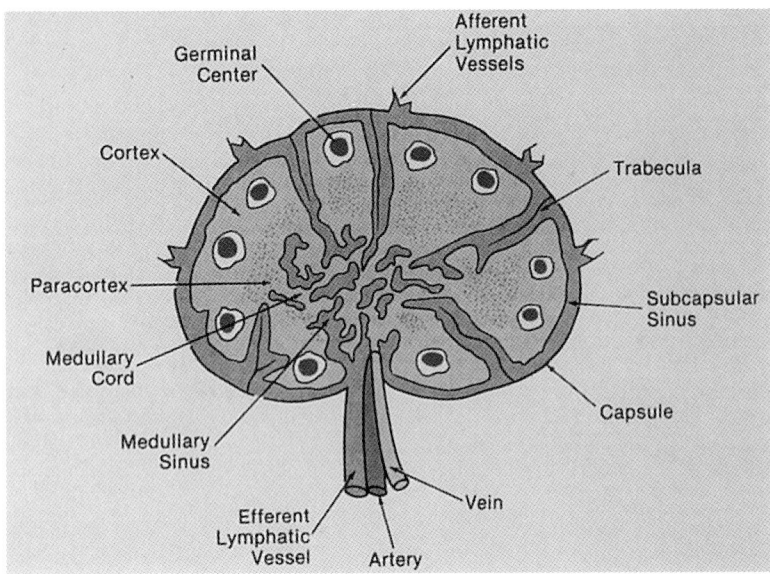

Figure 47-1. Diagrammatic representation of the structure of a lymph node. (From Faller DV: Diseases of the lymph nodes and spleen. In Wyngaarden JB, Smith LH, Bennett JC [eds]: Cecil Textbook of Medicine, 19th ed. Philadelphia, WB Saunders, 1992, p 979.)

homeless, intravenous drug use)? Does the family diet include raw meat that may predispose to acquisition of toxoplasmosis (a more common cause of toxoplasmosis than exposure to kitty litter in the United States)?

The presence of animals in the household or in households the child frequents may play a significant role in the lymphadenopathy. The presence of cats or, more often, kittens that scratch the child, for example, is often omitted from the parent's history of the patient unless such questions are specifically asked. Furthermore, some families may deny presence of household pets but forget to mention that the child plays with a neighbor's pet or with cats that are present in a barn or the neighborhood.

Adolescents should be questioned about sexual activity and other risk factors for HIV or other sexually transmitted diseases, such as

syphilis or lymphogranuloma venereum, a cause of diffuse or inguinal lymphadenopathy.

PHYSICAL EXAMINATION

Careful visual inspection yields an overall impression of size and distribution of significant lymphadenopathy as well as the presence of an associated infection. Overall physical appearance may indicate whether systemic signs, such as cachexia, are present. Palpation of the nodes, however, is necessary to appreciate the actual size and regions of lymphadenopathy. All areas in which lymphadenopathy is commonly present, including the cervical, auricular, axillary,

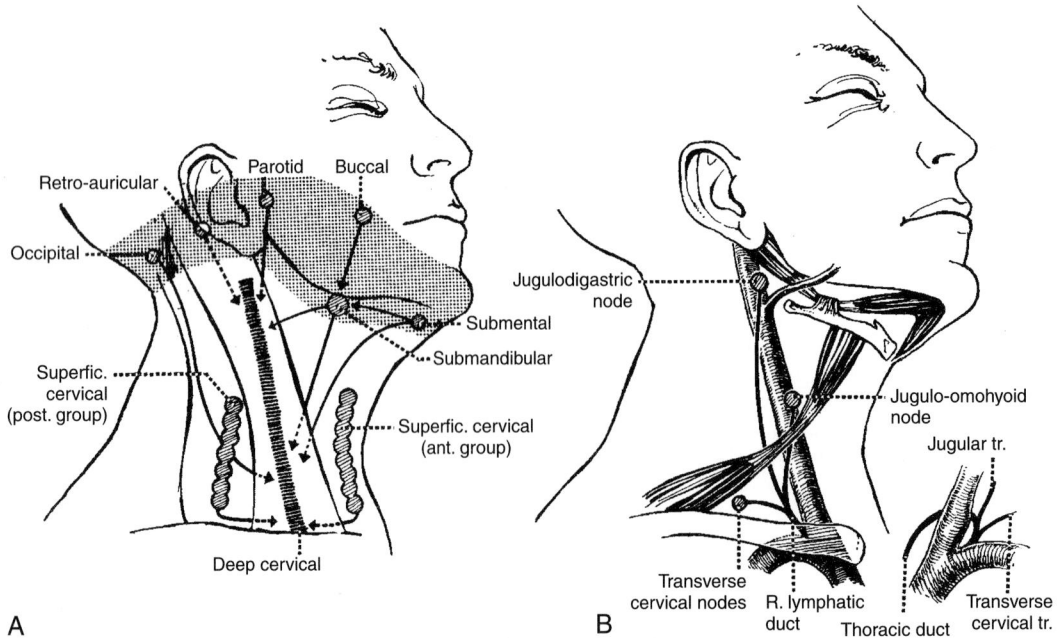

Figure 47-2. The superficial (**A**) and deep cervical (**B**) lymph nodes that drain the head and neck. ant., anterior; post., posterior; R., right; superfic., superficial; tr., tributary. (From O'Rahilly RO: Gardner-Gray-O'Rahilly Anatomy: A Regional Study of Human Structure, 5th ed. Philadelphia, WB Saunders, 1986, p 719.)

Table 47-1. Differential Diagnosis of Systemic Generalized Lymphadenopathy

Infant	Child	Adolescent
Common Causes		
Syphilis	Viral infection	Viral infection
Toxoplasmosis	EBV	EBV
CMV	CMV	CMV
HIV	HIV	HIV
	Toxoplasmosis	Toxoplasmosis
		Syphilis
Rare Causes		
Chagas disease (congenital)	Serum sickness	Serum sickness
Congenital leukemia	SLE, JRA	SLE, JRA
Congenital tuberculosis	Leukemia/lymphoma	Leukemia/lymphoma
Reticuloendotheliosis	Tuberculosis	Tuberculosis
Metabolic storage disease	Sarcoidosis	Sarcoidosis
Histiocytic disorders	Fungal infection	Fungal infection
	Plague	Plague
	Langerhans cell histiocytosis	Drug reaction (immune)
	Chronic granulomatous disease	
	Sinus histiocytosis	

CMV, cytomegalovirus; EBV, Epstein-Barr virus; HIV, human immunodeficiency virus; JRA, juvenile rheumatoid arthritis (as Still disease); SLE, systemic lupus erythematosus.

epitrochlear, inguinal, and supraclavicular areas, should be palpated because lymphadenopathy in certain regions is linked to systemic or local illness (Table 47-2).

Regional lymphadenopathy usually reflects pathologic processes within the lymphatic drainage distribution of that particular nodal chain. Enlarged cervical nodes commonly indicate the presence of infection in the oropharyngeal cavity. Similarly, posterior auricular nodes are seen with scalp infections and otitis media but are also common with rubella and some other viral illnesses such as parvovirus (fifth disease). The diagnosis of rubella or parvovirus infection is considered if there is a rash and fever in conjunction with posterior auricular nodes. The presence of supraclavicular nodes is usually pathologic and is a red flag for a serious illness such as malignancy. Supraclavicular nodes that are palpated on the right side often reflect a mediastinal tumor or invasive mediastinal infection, such as histoplasmosis. Supraclavicular nodes on the left side are often the result of metastatic spread of an abdominal tumor. The presence of either type of node mandates an urgent evaluation, including computed tomography (CT) or magnetic resonance imaging. Epitrochlear nodes, if unilateral, commonly indicate the hand or arm as a source of distal infection. Palpable bilateral epitrochlear lymph nodes usually reflect systemic illness, such as syphilis, sarcoidosis, or lymphoma. Inguinal node enlargement is common and is probably caused by the frequent occurrence of minor trauma and infections in a child's legs and feet. Significantly enlarged inguinal nodes, however, may be present with venereal diseases, such as syphilis, chlamydial urethritis, lymphogranuloma venereum, or with urinary tract infection, lymphoma, or abdominal tumors.

In addition to the location, the characteristic feel of the nodes often yields some clues as to the cause of the adenopathy:

- erythematous, tender, and warm: acute bacterial infection with suppurative adenitis
- tender, nonerythematous, and soft: viral infection or other systemic infection
- firm, hard, rubbery, and nontender: lymphoma or other infiltrating tumor
- hard, matted, immobile, and nontender: tumor, metastatic or local; fibrosis that follows acute infection

LABORATORY AND IMAGING EVALUATION

Many previously healthy children with acute lymphadenopathy require few, if any, laboratory or imaging studies. No laboratory testing may be required for well-appearing children whose acute, localized adenopathy can be attributed to an infection in the vicinity of the node. Patients with localized cutaneous bacterial infections causing adenopathy also may not need laboratory investigations before the initiation of antimicrobial therapy unless there is suspicion of bacteremia or invasive spread of the infection to underlying tissues.

Acute cervical adenopathy accompanying pharyngitis in children older than 18 months may necessitate a throat culture for group A streptococcus. The additional presence of hepatomegaly or splenomegaly should raise suspicion of Epstein-Barr viral (EBV) infections (mononucleosis). The clinician could obtain a complete blood cell count with white blood cell differential (to identify lymphocytosis and atypical lymphocytes) and EBV titers (or a monospot heterophile antibody test in children older than 10 years).

Supraclavicular adenopathy, acute cervical adenopathy accompanied by respiratory distress, or prolonged cervical adenopathy warrants anteroposterior and lateral radiographs of the neck and/or chest, a complete blood cell count with white blood cell differential, and placement of a purified protein derivative (PPD) tuberculosis skin test. CT with contrast is necessary in certain situations to fully delineate cervical adenopathy that is excessively large or that impinges on the airway, or to determine whether mediastinal adenopathy is present.

Children presenting with prolonged diffuse lymphadenopathy, hepatomegaly or splenomegaly, weight loss, night sweats, fevers, recurrent infections, or failure to thrive must be more thoroughly studied. Only after the complete blood cell count and differential and chest radiograph are analyzed should other diagnostic studies be considered. HIV, EBV, and CMV studies (culture, polymerase chain reaction, and serologic profiles) may be obtained for some children. Because the diagnoses of leukemia (through bone marrow aspiration, biopsy), lymphoma (through bone marrow aspiration, biopsy), systemic lupus erythematosus (through antinuclear antibody,

Table 47-2. Common Sites of Local Lymphadenopathy and Associated Diseases

Cervical

Oropharyngeal infection (viral or group A streptococcal, staphylococcal)
Scalp infection
Mycobacterial lymphadenitis (tuberculosis and nontuberculous mycobacteria)
Viral infection (EBV, CMV, HHV-6)
Cat-scratch disease
Kawasaki disease
Thyroid disease

Anterior Auricular

Conjuctivitis
Other eye infection
Oculoglandular tularemia

Posterior Auricular

Otitis media
Viral infection (especially rubella, parvovirus)

Supraclavicular

Malignancy or infection in the mediastinum (right)
Metastatic malignancy from abdomen (left)
Lymphoma
Tuberculosis

Epitrochlear

Hand infection, arm infection*
Lymphoma[†]
Sarcoid
Syphilis

Inguinal

Urinary tract infection
Venereal disease (especially syphilis or lymphogranuloma venereum)
Lower extremity suppurative infection
Plague

Hilar (Not Palpable, Found on Chest Radiograph or CT)

Tuberculosis[†]
Histoplasmosis[†]
Blastomycosis[†]
Coccidioidomycosis[†]
Leukemia/lymphoma[†]
Hodgkin disease[†]
Metastatic malignancy*
Sarcoidosis[†]

Axillary

Cat-scratch disease
Arm infection
Malignancy of chest wall
Leukemia/lymphoma
Brucellosis

*Unilateral.
[†]Bilateral.

CMV, cytomegalovirus; CT, computed tomography; EBV, Epstein-Barr virus; HHV-6, human herpesvirus 6.

double-stranded DNA antibodies), and cat-scratch disease (through biopsy and/or *Bartonella* serologic profile) require more invasive and expensive tests, the physician should first consider all aspects of the history and physical examination before ordering laboratory studies.

DIFFERENTIAL DIAGNOSIS

INFECTIONS OF THE OROPHARYNX

Pharyngeal infection is the most common cause of local lymphadenopathy in children (see Chapter 1). Many of these pharyngeal infections are associated with cervical lymphadenopathy; are viral in origin; and include adenovirus, parainfluenza, influenza, rhinovirus, and enterovirus as possible causes. EBV and CMV also commonly cause exudative pharyngitis and cervical lymphadenopathy. The chief complaint usually includes pain with swallowing (particularly pain with swallowing of acidic juices) and with talking, as well as tender, enlarged lymph nodes in the neck. Systemic manifestations, such as fever, muscle aches, and rhinorrhea, also may be present. An examination of the throat usually reveals a symmetric erythematous posterior pharynx with enlarged tonsils, often with exudates. Exudates can be seen with both viral and bacterial causes of pharyngitis and adenopathy, and thus do not reliably enable the examiner to discriminate between the two causes.

Herpes stomatitis (mucocutaneous involvement) or pharyngitis (oropharyngeal vesicles) is associated with bilaterally enlarged, tender, nonerythematous cervical nodes. Bacterial infection of the pharynx is also commonly associated with enlarged, tender cervical lymph nodes. Group A β-hemolytic streptococcus is the most common pathogen to cause such infections and is difficult to differentiate clinically from viral causes of pharyngitis and lymphadenopathy; thus, throat culture or rapid antigen detection is necessary. An associated sandpapery rash or beefy-red tonsils with palatal petechiae are not usually seen with viral pathogens and should make the examiner consider group A streptococci and toxin-mediated scarlet fever as a likely cause. Other bacteria also can cause pharyngitis and cervical adenopathy, including non–group A streptococci, as well as anaerobic organisms, such as *Fusobacterium* species. Anaerobic organisms can lead to painful oral gingivitis or stomatitis and pharyngitis (Vincent angina) that may progress to peritonsillar abscess. Asymmetry in the tonsils and the pharyngeal tissue surrounding the tonsils and uvula deviation away from the abscess may be seen with peritonsillar abscesses, along with unilateral tender, enlarged cervical lymph nodes. Another important syndrome that may occur after acute bacterial pharyngitis may manifest with high fever, and unilateral lateral neck swelling that may be confused with adenopathy. Such a constellation of findings, called *Lemierre syndrome,* is associated with septic thrombosis of the internal jugular vein, usually caused by invasion of the blood stream by *Fusobacterium* organisms, and should lead to prompt hospitalization, blood cultures, treatment with intravenous antibiotics, and imaging of the internal jugular vein via Doppler flow ultrasonography or CT with contrast enhancement.

Acute cervical lymphadenopathy or lymphadenitis (inflammation of the cervical lymph nodes with tender enlargement) is most likely to occur with group A streptococcal infection. *Staphylococcus aureus* infection and infection with oral bacteria, including non–group A streptococci and anaerobes such as *Fusobacterium* species, may also occur, presumably with the pharynx as the portal of entry. Other common sites for acute lymphadenitis are the submandibular nodes. Usually, these nodes quickly diminish in size after institution of antibiotics with appropriate coverage for these pathogens (e.g., amoxicillin/clavulanic acid, ampicillin/sulbactam, clindamycin).

Suppuration of the nodes with drainage is less common than adenitis and generally rules out viral infection as the primary cause. Acute suppurative cervical adenitis can be seen in infections of the face and scalp and is usually caused by group A streptococcal or *S. aureus* infection. Management of suppuration includes incision and drainage or, less often, excision of the suppurative node; Gram stain; bacterial, fungal, and mycobacterial cultures of the drainage; and institution of appropriate antimicrobial therapy (Fig. 47-3). Total

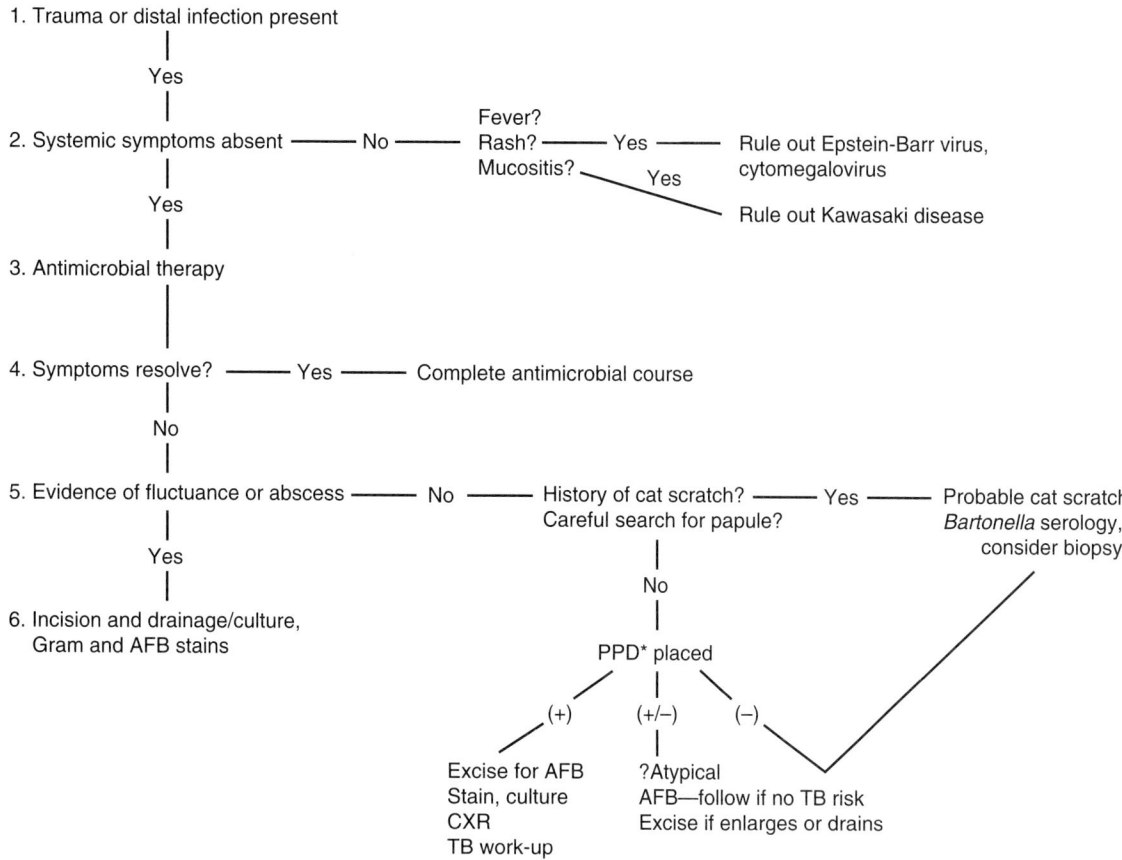

1. Trauma or distal infection present
   |
   Yes
   |
2. Systemic symptoms absent ——— No ——— Fever?
                                        Rash? ——— Yes ——— Rule out Epstein-Barr virus,
                                        Mucositis?   Yes   cytomegalovirus
   |
   Yes   Rule out Kawasaki disease
   |
3. Antimicrobial therapy
   |
4. Symptoms resolve? ——— Yes ——— Complete antimicrobial course
   |
   No
   |
5. Evidence of fluctuance or abscess ——— No ——— History of cat scratch? ——— Yes ——— Probable cat scratch
                                                 Careful search for papule?   *Bartonella* serology,
   | consider biopsy
   Yes   No
   | |
6. Incision and drainage/culture,   PPD* placed
   Gram and AFB stains |
                                          (+)   (+/−)   (−)
                                           | |
                                     Excise for AFB ?Atypical
                                     Stain, culture AFB—follow if no TB risk
                                     CXR   Excise if enlarges or drains
                                     TB work-up

* 5 mm induration if high risk or obvious close contact; 10 mm induration if younger than 4 years or chronic illness;
15 mm induration or more if 4 years or older without any risk factor.

Figure 47-3. Paradigm for the management of typical acute regional lymphadenopathy (e.g., cervical, axillary, inguinal) in children. AFB, acid-fast bacillus: tuberculosis (TB); CXR, chest radiograph; PPD, purified protein derivative.

excision should be performed if atypical mycobacterial infection is suspected, because draining fistulas may form if a needle biopsy or partial resection is performed. Fine-needle aspiration may reduce the risk of sinus formation.

INFECTIONS OF THE EXTREMITIES

Bacterial infections of the skin and soft tissues (erysipelas, abscess, cellulitis, fasciitis) of the extremities are common causes of localized lymphadenopathy and adenitis. These infections, primarily caused by group A β-hemolytic streptococci or *S. aureus,* may drain into and inflame single or multiple regional lymph nodes. Any laceration or insect bite that becomes superinfected may yield adenopathy "upstream" from the infected site. On occasion, penetrating injuries to the feet that occur in wet areas or through damp shoes may yield infections with other bacteria, such as *Pseudomonas aeruginosa.* These penetrating infections usually manifest with cellulitis or osteomyelitis; lymphadenopathy is noted during the physical examination. The most common sites of infection include the foot or leg, leading to unilateral inguinal lymphadenitis, and the hand or arm, causing axillary lymphadenitis or, less commonly, unilateral inflammation of the epitrochlear nodes.

EPSTEIN-BARR VIRUS INFECTION

Infection with EBV is a common cause of both regional and diffuse lymphadenopathy. This virus classically causes a "mononucleosis"

syndrome in adolescents (Fig. 47-4), consisting of acute pharyngitis that may have a prolonged course, with tender, firm cervical adenopathy (but sometimes with generalized adenopathy); malaise; fever; weight loss; and anorexia. Approximately 10% of patients become jaundiced; more than 80% have mild hepatitis that is clinically silent but can be documented with liver enzyme studies. Splenomegaly is present in more than 50% of patients and, in rare cases, progresses to splenic rupture. A small number of patients also have parapharyngeal lymphoid hyperplasia, which causes difficulty swallowing or breathing and can produce significant problems, leading to dehydration or airway obstruction. Small children with EBV infection often present with atypical symptoms or may be completely asymptomatic. Nonspecific rash (often after ampicillin or allopurinol therapy), fever, and mild cervical adenopathy may be the major symptoms on presentation, or the child may be significantly ill with high fever and pharyngitis. Young children with acute EBV infection are more likely to have hepatosplenomegaly, rash, and eyelid edema than are young adults.

The diagnosis of EBV infection in older children focuses on the characteristic clinical syndrome and a relative lymphocytosis seen in the differential white blood cell count (40% to 50%), which shows a substantial percentage of atypical lymphocytes (10% to 20%). Heterophile immunoglobulin M (IgM) antibodies, which are non–EBV directed and agglutinate sheep and horse red blood cells, are found in more than 80% of young adults with EBV and are at maximal titer 3 to 4 weeks after infection. Heterophile antibodies are rarely found in young children (younger than 5 years) with EBV

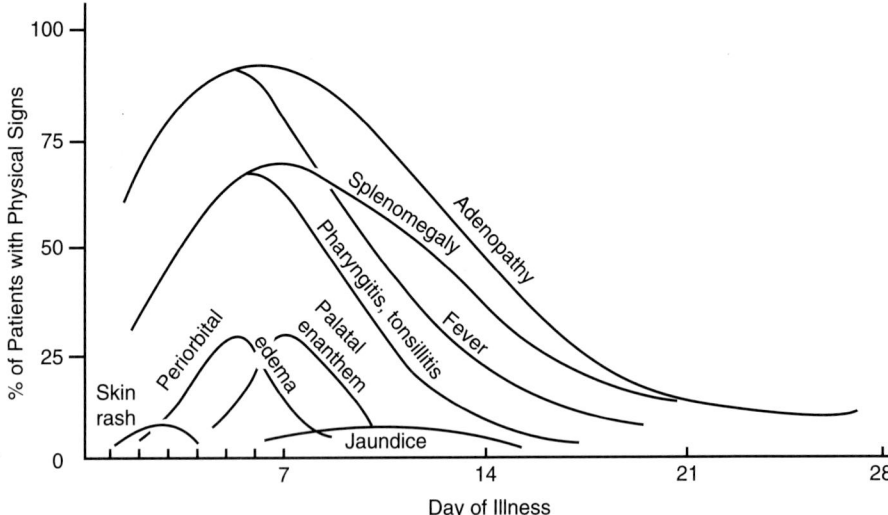

Figure 47-4. The clinical course of acute Epstein-Barr mononucleosis. Adenopathy occurs early in the infection and can persist for weeks. (Modified from Rapp CE, Hewston JF: Infectious mononucleosis and the Epstein-Barr virus. Am J Dis Child 1978;132:78.)

infections. In young children, antibody titers directed to specific EBV antigens are necessary to confirm the diagnosis (Fig. 47-5). IgM antibodies against viral capsid antigen (VCA) followed by immunoglobulin G (IgG) directed to VCA and early antigens (EAs) are the most common antibody profile. Antibodies to nuclear antigens develop weeks later and, if present with EA IgG, are indicative of infection in the recent past. Approximately 20% of children present after the VCA IgM has already declined. In these children, VCA and EA IgG are present.

Because group A streptococcal infection can present in a manner similar to, or be present simultaneously with, EBV infection, and because other viruses can initially cause pharyngitis and tender, enlarged cervical lymph nodes, differentiating these various causes of pharyngitis and lymphadenopathy is important. Acute streptococcal pharyngitis improves after institution of penicillin therapy; EBV infections do not, and they also have a more prolonged clinical course. In addition, severe malaise and splenomegaly do not occur with most bacterial or viral causes of pharyngitis and cervical lymphadenopathy. These findings prompt the clinician to consider EBV infection. Similarly, most viral causes of cervical adenopathy and pharyngitis (except CMV) are not associated with the brisk atypical lymphocytosis commonly seen with EBV infections, and they are not usually associated with abnormal liver function results.

CYTOMEGALOVIRUS INFECTION

CMV infection in children can be associated with a mononucleosis-like syndrome and lymphadenopathy. CMV mononucleosis is associated with fever and malaise similar to that seen in EBV; in contrast to EBV, however, CMV mononucleosis does not usually cause severe, exudative tonsillopharyngitis or the production of heterophil-specific or EBV-specific antibodies. CMV mononucleosis can be associated with an atypical lymphocytosis and diffuse lymphadenopathy in the normal host. Although CMV culture (especially from the urine) is frequently positive in children with CMV infection, many children, especially those in day care, are silently infected and excrete CMV in absence of clinical signs and symptoms. Therefore, CMV culture is less useful in the toddler age group. Women who are pregnant when they have primary CMV infections (often through sexual contact) are at risk of delivering a child with congenital CMV infection through transplacental infection or through contact with infected cervical secretions at the time of delivery. Infants with congenital CMV may have many complications and clinical findings, but lymphadenopathy is not a common finding. Identifying CMV in the urine of the neonate in the first week of life confirms congenital infection.

The diagnosis in older children is usually made serologically, in tests measuring both IgM and IgG antibodies directed to CMV or by obtaining a throat or blood specimen for culture (leukocyte) that is positive for CMV.

HUMAN HERPESVIRUS 6 INFECTION

Infection with the human herpesvirus 6 (HHV-6), in addition to causing roseola, has been associated with a mononucleosis-like syndrome with diffuse or cervical adenopathy in individuals who are seronegative for EBV and CMV. Human herpesvirus 7 may produce a similar clinical pattern as that seen in HHV-6. Elevated or rising titers of antibodies to HHV-6 have been found in patients with documented acute EBV and CMV infections. It is unclear whether these seroconversions represent false-positive results caused by antigens cross-reactive among EBV, CMV, and HHV-6 or whether the HHV-6 rising antibody titers may represent a reactivation of old HHV-6 disease.

CAT-SCRATCH DISEASE

Cat-scratch disease is caused by a small gram-negative bacillus, *Bartonella henselae* (formerly *Rochalimaea henselae*). *B. henselae* also causes bacillary angiomatosis in patients with HIV infection. Cat-scratch disease occurs several days after exposure to a scratch or, less commonly, a bite of a cat or kitten (more than 90% of patients with clinical cat-scratch disease report contact with cats). A papule at the site of the trauma usually develops, followed in 7 to 14 days by regional lymphadenopathy. Most patients with cat-scratch disease have a single enlarged, often tender lymph node. Axillary nodes are the most likely to be enlarged, probably because the upper extremities are the part of the body most likely to be scratched or bitten. The next most common sites are the neck and jaw, followed by the inguinal region. Although single nodes are most commonly affected, regional adenopathy may also occur. Generalized lymphadenopathy is extremely rare in the normal host.

Approximately half the patients have low-grade fever and malaise; a small number have high fevers (>39.5° C) and more severe systemic symptoms. In most patients, the swollen, inflamed nodes regress spontaneously within several weeks; approximately 10% progress to have purulent fluid drainage that is culture-negative by standard techniques. Uncommon complications include encephalopathy that resolves spontaneously; erythema nodosum; oculoglandular syndrome of Parinaud, in which the cat-scratch disease organism is inoculated into the eye and causes conjunctivitis and preauricular

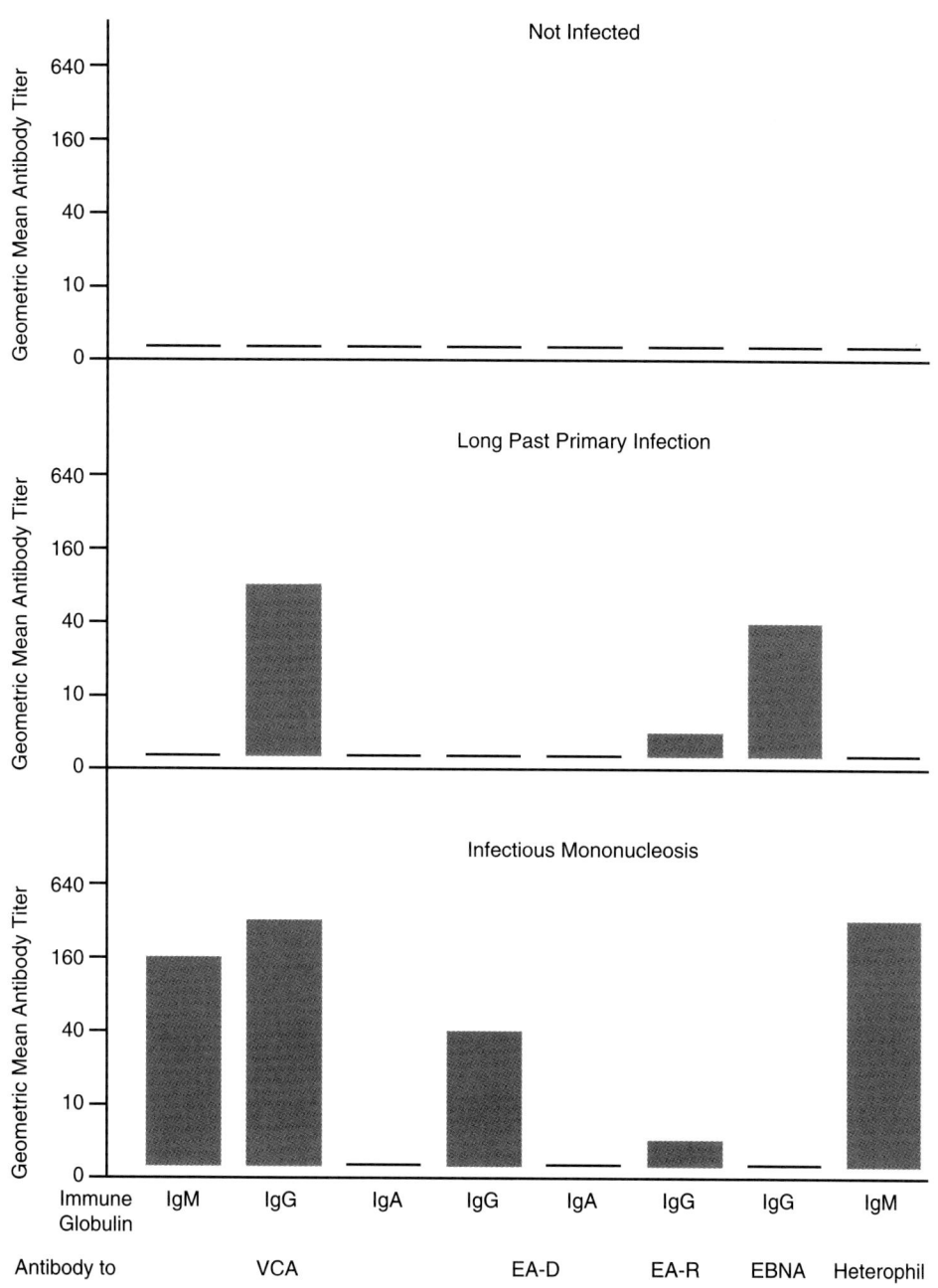

Figure 47-5. Serologic patterns in individuals not infected with Epstein-Barr virus (EBV) (*top*), infected with EBV in the past (*middle*), and acutely infected with EBV (*bottom*). EA, early antigen; EBNA, Epstein-Barr nuclear antigen; IgA, IgG, and IgM, immunoglobulins A, G, and M; VCA, viral capsid antigen. (From Henle W, Henle G: Serodiagnosis of infectious mononucleosis. Resid Staff Physician 1981;27:37.)

adenopathy; thrombocytopenia; hepatitis or splenitis with granulomas; transverse myelitis; and, in rare cases, osteolytic bone lesions.

The diagnosis is based on the history of contact with kittens or cats and the classic clinical manifestation, including a careful search for an entrance site papule. The "gold standard" for diagnosis is the pathologic sample of tissue from the involved node, which shows granulomas, central necrosis, and organisms seen on Warthin-Starry silver stain. The decision to perform a biopsy is usually reached when there is no clear history of a cat's scratch or when the presentation is atypical and cannot be differentiated from other, more serious illness, such as mycobacterial adenitis. Serologic tests for *Bartonella* species have good sensitivity and specificity and have proved useful in confirming the diagnosis of cat-scratch disease in children with appropriate history of exposure to cats and regional adenopathy.

The treatment of cat-scratch disease has not been adequately studied. Various antibiotics have been used in an uncontrolled manner. There are anecdotal reports of clinical improvement after administration of several antibiotics, including rifampin, gentamicin, ciprofloxacin, and trimethoprim-sulfamethoxazole. One prospective, randomized study of a small number of patients showed clinical benefit from azithromycin. Because cat-scratch disease is a self-limited illness in most children, most clinicians do not routinely use antimicrobial therapy.

CHRONIC GRANULOMATOUS DISEASE

Chronic granulomatous disease (see Chapter 51) comprises a group of rare inherited disorders of neutrophil function, characterized by recurrent pyogenic infections, which are often accompanied by lymphadenopathy and/or abscess formation. Most cases are inherited in an X-linked manner; 30% are autosomal recessive. Chronic granulomatous disease should be considered in a young child (often a boy) who presents with recurrent fever and infection, pneumonia, adenopathy, and abdominal pain. Family history often reveals another relative with the disease or recalls a death from an infection in a young child.

The diagnosis is made by neutrophil nitroblue tetrazolium testing or by chemiluminescent studies, which demonstrate the defective neutrophil oxidation. Common pathogens contain catalase and include *S. aureus* and *Aspergillus* species.

HUMAN IMMUNODEFICIENCY VIRUS

HIV infection may manifest with diffuse lymphadenopathy. Many HIV-infected children also have failure to thrive, poor weight gain, and evidence of other infections (oral thrush or opportunistic pneumonias such as that caused by *Pneumocystis carinii*). HIV-infected children are also more likely than normal hosts to have other infectious causes of lymphadenopathy, such as tuberculosis, or noninfectious causes, such as lymphoma. It is important to obtain a history of HIV risk factors. Regional lymphadenopathy is not a common manifestation of HIV infections unless the adenitis represents another bacterial or mycobacterial infection.

MYCOBACTERIAL INFECTIONS

Tubercular cervical adenitis is not common in the United States. In the past, it was often associated with ingestion of raw, contaminated milk and infection with *M. bovis*. Regional or diffuse lymphadenopathy caused by infection with *Mycobacterium tuberculosis* is also unusual in developed countries; however, it is increasing in frequency in children in the United States as a result of an increase in the number of adults actively infected. This increase is attributable to several issues, including immigration from endemic areas, reduction in tuberculosis control programs, the likelihood of HIV-infected individuals to have a high mycobacterial burden, noncompliance by infected individuals with multidrug treatment regimens, and drug resistance by the organism. Most adenitis caused by mycobacteria in the United States is caused by atypical strains that are not serious pathogens in the normal host.

Several historical and clinical criteria can be used to differentiate tuberculous adenitis from atypical mycobacterial infections. Most children with tuberculosis have a history of exposure to an adult with active tuberculosis. Infection with atypical mycobacteria is more common in the southern parts of the United States. Children with tuberculous adenitis may have hilar lymphadenopathy because the lungs are usually the source of primary infection. Evidence of extralymphatic disease also is common in children with tuberculosis; such disease includes pneumonia, pleural effusions, bone marrow suppression, liver function abnormalities, and miliary disease. Disseminated tuberculosis may manifest with diffuse lymphadenopathy, and it should be sought if pulmonary infiltrates and systemic symptoms are present. Such extralymphatic disease and diffuse lymphadenopathy are rare in normal children with adenitis caused by atypical mycobacteria but may occur in HIV-infected children infected with atypical mycobacteria.

The most common mycobacterial infection in children in the United States is infection of the lymph nodes with the atypical mycobacteria, primarily in the *Mycobacterium avium-intracellulare* complex as well as *Mycobacterium kansasii*, *Mycobacterium scrofulaceum*, and *Mycobacterium marinum*. The lymph nodes involved are unilateral and cervical in most infections, presumably because the organism enters via the oropharynx. Most frequently, a previously healthy child presents with unilateral lymphadenitis or adenopathy in the cervical, submandibular, or submaxillary region. Although fever may be present, other significant systemic symptoms are usually not present. In a small number of patients, the affected node spontaneously ruptures and drains before the visit to the physician. The drainage is not usually grossly purulent and may be a clue that atypical mycobacteria are the cause of the infected node.

The "gold standard" for diagnosis of lymphadenitis caused by atypical mycobacteria is acid-fast staining and culture of the excised node. Incision and drainage or needle aspiration of these nodes may lead to chronically draining sinus tracts, which may leave scars; thus, this method is contraindicated. Fine-needle aspiration may be beneficial. The usual clinical scenario involves a young, preschool-aged child with an enlarged cervical node that responds poorly to antibiotics. The child has no history of a cat's scratch and is otherwise clinically well. A tuberculin skin test (which should be placed in children with lymphadenopathy) (see Fig. 47-3) often yields 5 to 9 mm of induration because atypical mycobacteria have antigens cross-reactive to those of tuberculosis. This amount of induration is considered indeterminate for tuberculosis in low-risk patients and suggests that the adenopathy is caused by an atypical mycobacterium. Skin tests with antigens from the various atypical mycobacteria are very sensitive and specific for infection; however, these antigens are not consistently available. In rare cases, infection with atypical mycobacteria yields skin test results in the positive range of more than 15-mm induration, which mandates a more extensive workup that focuses on the possibility that the adenitis is caused by *M. tuberculosis* infection. Gradual resolution of lymphadenitis sometimes occurs in children with atypical mycobacterial infections. Excisional biopsy is not necessary if the diagnosis is made presumptively from skin test results of less than 10 mm of induration, if other infections are ruled out, if resolution occurs, and if the child is at low risk for infection with *M. tuberculosis* (see Chapter 2). If the node does not improve, continues to enlarge, or spontaneously drains, excision is recommended and is usually curative. Fine-needle aspiration (for culture and acid-fast staining) may also be used if the node is in an area where excision is impractical.

Chemotherapy with antitubercular drugs for atypical mycobacterial adenitis is controversial for several reasons. First, most of the atypical mycobacteria tend to be resistant to the usual antitubercular drugs, and multiple, potentially toxic regimens are required. Second, because this is a self-limited infection that sometimes resolves or can be cured with excision, long courses of chemotherapy seem unwarranted. Finally, although there have been no controlled trials, use of antitubercular therapy seems to have limited efficacy in comparison with excision. Antitubercular therapy should not be initiated without adequate cultures.

TOXOPLASMOSIS

Toxoplasma gondii is a protozoan organism that is a parasite of cats. Many other animals, including humans, can be incidentally and chronically infected hosts in which the parasite cannot complete its life cycle. Human acquisition of toxoplasmosis in childhood can result from contact with cat feces or soil that contains oocysts, which infect the child when they are ingested. Alternatively, the ingestion of raw or undercooked meat, particularly lamb and pork that contain tissue cysts, may lead to infection. Adults in the United States are more likely to be infected from ingestion of raw meat than from contact with oocysts in cat feces and soil. Finally, infection can be transmitted to the fetus, especially when a pregnant woman is acutely infected with toxoplasmosis. Although many of the fetal infections are asymptomatic, transplacental infection with toxoplasmosis can result in severe neurologic damage, chorioretinitis, aseptic meningitis, and significant systemic illness manifesting with the classic triad of hepatosplenomegaly, intracranial calcifications, and hydrocephalus. Although lymphadenopathy can occur in the newborn with congenital toxoplasmosis, it is a more common symptom of acute toxoplasmosis in older children and young adults.

The most common symptoms in children who acquire toxoplasmosis are lymphadenopathy, fever, malaise, myalgia, and pharyngitis. The nodes most commonly affected include anterior and posterior cervical and axillary, which may be tender; involvement is usually bilateral. The lymph node enlargement seen in toxoplasmosis is caused by reticular hyperplasia and inflammation. Most laboratory results are normal, but the white blood cell count may show an absolute lymphocytosis with atypical lymphocytes, which can cause confusion with EBV or CMV mononucleosis.

The diagnosis is made primarily with serologic studies. If tissue is available after biopsy, actual parasite forms can sometimes be demonstrated. Various diagnostic techniques can be used on the patient's serum, including indirect immunofluorescence, complement fixation, and enzyme-linked immunosorbent assay. A fourfold rise in IgG titer or the presence of IgM antibodies is diagnostic. In neonatal infections, tests measuring IgM have become more sensitive and specific. Antigen tests and cultures that grow the parasite are also available, but primarily on an investigational level.

Effective therapy consists of sulfonamides combined with pyrimethamine. Early treatment is especially important in the infant with congenital infection because treatment may improve neurologic outcome. Pregnant women newly infected with toxoplasmosis can be treated with spiramycin, which concentrates in the placenta and interrupts transplacental infection of the fetus; sulfonamides and pyrimethamine also eradicate the parasite from the fetus. These therapies significantly improve the previously poor outcome of the congenitally infected infant.

Treatment of older children with acute toxoplasmosis is more controversial. Many investigators do not treat immunologically normal individuals unless symptoms are persistent and severe. In contrast, individuals with T cell deficiencies, such as those with HIV infection, can develop severe disseminated toxoplasmosis, involving the central nervous system and retina. In these patients, prolonged therapy is mandatory.

SYPHILIS

Syphilis, caused by the spirochete *Treponema pallidum,* is common in the United States (see Chapter 29). Numerous factors caused a resurgent epidemic of syphilis in the 1980s and 1990s, including difficulty in eradicating the organism in patients with HIV, prostitution to obtain crack cocaine in the inner cities, and lack of attention to prenatal screening and syphilis control programs. Syphilis remains primarily a sexually transmitted disease. Pregnant women with syphilis who are untreated readily transmit the disease to the fetus, causing congenital syphilis. Congenital syphilis leads to significant sequelae.

The natural course of syphilis in adults includes three major clinical manifestations:

- *primary syphilis,* in which the individual develops a painless chancre at the site of inoculation
- *secondary syphilis,* in which the organism hematogenously disseminates to many organs
- *tertiary syphilis,* in which gummatous lesions develop in end organs, such as the brain, heart, and bones

Lymphadenopathy can be seen as one of the manifestations of syphilis in several situations. In primary syphilis, in which the inoculation site is usually the genital area, regional lymphadenopathy with painless, firm nodes occurs at the time that a chancre is observed. Thus, inguinal adenopathy in an adolescent who is sexually active mandates further examination and workup for sexually transmitted diseases such as syphilis. In secondary syphilis, the organism has disseminated, causing multiple organs to be involved with the infection. The classic manifestations are protean and usually include nonvesicular rashes. Lymphadenopathy, regional or generalized, is common and often includes epitrochlear nodes (a hint that syphilis may be the diagnosis if no other explanation is found on the examination of the extremity). Systemic symptoms may be present with fever, malaise, anorexia, and weight loss. Syphilis therefore should be at the top of the differential diagnosis in sexually active adolescents with rash and lymphadenopathy. Infants with congenital syphilis may also have generalized lymphadenopathy, although this finding is less common than other systemic symptoms, such as hepatosplenomegaly, snuffles, and periosteal reactive disease.

The diagnosis has been complicated by the inability to grow the organism in vitro. Darkfield examination of tissue from chancres or mucous lesions shows numerous spirochetes, but darkfield methods are often unavailable to routine laboratories. Serologic study continues to be the primary mode of diagnosis. Nontreponemal serologic studies rely on the production by the infected host of antibodies to nonspecific lipoidal host tissue antigens that arise as a result of infection with the spirochete. These tests include the Venereal Disease Research Laboratory (VDRL) test, the serologic test for syphilis, and the rapid plasma reagin (RPR) test. Levels of these antibodies decline after adequate treatment and are extremely useful in confirming eradication of the infection. False-positive reactions can occur, particularly in individuals with connective tissue disorders or mononucleosis. In contrast, the fluorescent treponemal antibody absorption test (FTA-ABS) measures antibodies directed specifically to *T. pallidum* and can be used as a confirmatory test in individuals with positive results on screening tests. These antibodies also usually remain present for the life of the infected individual, even if the patient receives adequate therapy. Thus, in contrast to the VDRL test, the FTA-ABS has little use in monitoring the efficacy of treatment.

The mainstay of treatment for syphilis remains penicillin, although doxycycline or tetracycline may be used in nonpregnant, HIV-negative adults with proven penicillin allergy. In all other situations, desensitization of penicillin-allergic individuals is suggested by the Centers for Disease Control and Prevention. Neonates may require relatively long courses of intravenous penicillin because of the difficulties in ruling out and treating presumed neurosyphilis. Infants should be treated for congenital syphilis if physical examination findings, laboratory findings, or radiographic data suggest disease; if the cerebrospinal fluid VDRL test result is reactive; if the VDRL titer is four or more times higher than the mother's titer; or if the mother had syphilis without documentation of appropriate treatment and declining VDRL titers. Treatment should also be considered if follow-up of the infant is likely to be inadequate or if an adequate workup is not possible. Aqueous crystalline penicillin intravenously for 10 days is the treatment of choice. However, if the cerebrospinal fluid test result is negative, some authorities recommend intramuscular procaine penicillin for 10 days instead or one dose of intramuscular benzathine penicillin with follow-up if risk factors are low but the diagnosis cannot be excluded.

Persons with HIV infection also require prolonged high-dose penicillin therapy because syphilis appears to be particularly difficult to eradicate in immunodeficient individuals.

ACUTE LEUKEMIA, LYMPHOMA, AND OTHER MALIGNANCIES

Lymphadenopathy is frequently among the presenting findings in patients with leukemia or lymphoma. Enlarged lymph nodes may be noted in an isolated, regional, or generalized distribution with or without systemic symptoms, such as fever, malaise, night sweats, weight loss, and anorexia. Malignant nodes are usually firm, rubbery, and nontender and may be matted. Unlike many of the acute lymphadenopathies caused by infectious agents, most lymph nodes that are malignant gradually increase in size over time. Approximately 50% of children with acute lymphoblastic leukemia have adenopathy at the time of diagnosis. Nodal disease may be either localized (often cervical) or generalized and is frequently accompanied by other signs and symptoms, including fevers, malaise, weight loss, pallor, bone pain, petechiae and bruising, splenomegaly, or hepatomegaly. The complete blood count usually demonstrates anemia, thrombocytopenia, leukocytosis or leukopenia, circulating blasts, or some combination thereof. Some patients, however, may have initial normal peripheral blood laboratory results. Acute myelogenous leukemia is less common in children but may manifest in a similar manner. Bone marrow biopsy and aspiration must be performed, and the findings are diagnostic.

Hodgkin disease often manifests with painless cervical or supraclavicular lymphadenopathy in older school-aged children and adolescents. Nodes are firmer than those seen in patients whose nodes are enlarged in reaction to infections. In a small number of children with Hodgkin disease, the size of the nodes may wax and wane for several months before a definitive diagnosis is made. Supraclavicular nodes usually indicate intrathoracic disease, which is present in 60% to 70% of patients at the time of diagnosis. Axillary or inguinal nodes may also be the sites of presenting lymphadenopathy. Approximately 30% of patients with Hodgkin disease have systemic symptoms at presentation, including fatigue, weight loss, fevers, night sweats, and poor appetite. Some patients with Hodgkin disease also have unusual symptoms, such as pruritus, hemolytic anemia, and chest pain after alcohol ingestion. Such systemic symptoms with lymphadenopathy are red flags for immediate workup for malignancy. Diagnosis is confirmed by biopsy of involved nodes and/or bone marrow aspiration if the tumor has spread to the bone marrow.

Non-Hodgkin lymphoma is a relatively common childhood malignancy and often manifests with mediastinal or pleural disease. Adenopathy in the supraclavicular, cervical, or axillary regions is usually present and may occur in the absence of chest involvement. Systemic symptoms are variable at the time of diagnosis. Lymph nodes, as with other malignancies, tend to be firm and rubbery. Their size may increase relatively rapidly over several weeks. Because lymphoblastic lymphoma may represent a variant of acute lymphoblastic leukemia, the signs and symptoms of leukemia and lymphoma may merge. Non-Hodgkin lymphoma of B cell origin (Burkitt and non-Burkitt lymphoma) in children in the United States usually originates in an intraabdominal site, and regional adenopathy, if present, is then in the inguinal or iliac regions. The African variety of Burkitt lymphoma often manifests as an expanding jaw mass.

Disseminated *neuroblastoma* may manifest as diffuse adenopathy in younger children. Such children often have primary adrenal or paraspinal masses with bone metastasis and have nonspecific systemic symptoms, abdominal mass, bone pain, and sometimes symptoms of spinal cord compression. *Other tumors,* such as rhabdomyosarcoma and thyroid cancer, manifest in rare cases with lymphadenopathy caused by local or disseminated metastasis.

SINUS HISTIOCYTOSIS

Sinus histiocytosis is a rare disorder characterized by massive lymphadenopathy in the cervical region; it is associated with fever, elevated sedimentation rate, leukocytosis, and polyclonal hypergammaglobulinemia. The symptoms tend to resolve spontaneously after several months, and the condition is probably caused by an immunoregulatory disorder. Diagnosis is made from biopsy of the involved nodes and pathologic examination.

MANAGEMENT STRATEGIES

REGIONAL LYMPHADENOPATHY

The typical child with acute regional lymphadenopathy (see Fig. 47-3) presents with enlarged nodes, commonly in the cervical region. A thorough history and careful physical examination should reveal whether nodes are definitively involved (in comparison with the parotid gland); whether infection is present at other sites, such as the pharynx; whether other causes (e.g., cat's scratch) exist for the adenopathy; and whether the nodes have the characteristics of malignancy. In many cases, no other abnormalities are found on examination, and systemic signs are minimal. Laboratory tests should include a complete blood cell count and differential as well as measurement of the erythrocyte sedimentation rate and the C-reactive protein. In the child with fever and a tender cervical lymph node, oral antibiotics (with activity against mouth flora, streptococci, and staphylococci) should be started; if the lymphadenopathy persists or worsens, intravenous antibiotics are indicated. A PPD test should be undertaken, and if the results are negative and symptoms resolve, it is reasonable to complete the antimicrobial course orally.

In contrast, if the lymphadenopathy continues or becomes frank lymphadenitis with erythema and tenderness despite antimicrobial therapy, further workup is indicated. Imaging the involved area is helpful but not always necessary. Although ultrasonography can reveal enlarged nodes or a fluid-filled abscess or cyst, CT with contrast enhancement of the area is the best method for defining the extent of inflamed nodes and whether an abscess is present. If an abscess is found, incision and drainage, followed by appropriate bacterial and mycobacterial cultures and stains, are appropriate. If atypical mycobacteria are suspected on the basis of a borderline positive PPD result or clinical presentation, excisional biopsy is preferred because incision and drainage often leads to draining sinus tracts that are difficult to heal. Enlarged nodes that do not recede in several weeks with appropriate antimicrobial therapy and without explanation (such as acute EBV infection) also should raise the suspicion of malignancy.

GENERALIZED LYMPHADENOPATHY

In the child with generalized lymphadenopathy, the cause may be infectious, immunologic, or malignant. Infectious causes, such as HIV, EBV, toxoplasmosis, secondary syphilis, and CMV infections, can generally be determined quickly through serologic testing. Noninfectious causes, such as systemic lupus erythematosus and serum sickness, can also generally be excluded by serologic studies and/or a careful history. If the generalized lymphadenopathy cannot be attributed to an infectious or other cause, and especially if there are systemic symptoms, malignancy should be considered. In addition, enlarging nodes that do not recede in several weeks, despite a diagnosis of a "viral" infection, should also raise concern for possible malignancy. An abnormal complete blood cell count demonstrating a depressed white blood cell, red blood cell, or platelet count or a chest radiograph or CT study demonstrating mediastinal adenopathy or pleural disease is highly suggestive of malignancy. Because serious disseminated infections, such as tuberculosis and histoplasmosis, can manifest in a similar manner, fine-needle aspiration or biopsy of an involved node or bone marrow aspiration is crucial. Excision of a node is preferred in some cases in order to obtain adequate tissue for pathologic study, stains, or cultures.

SUMMARY AND RED FLAGS

Lymphadenopathy is one of the most common manifestations of childhood diseases. Most often, localized adenopathy is associated with a bacterial infection in the vicinity of the node or with a viral pharyngitis. Even generalized adenopathy does not usually indicate a serious underlying disease. Adenopathy usually resolves either spontaneously or after appropriate antibiotic therapy. When adenopathy is accompanied by weight loss, recurrent fevers, night sweats, or other systemic signs or symptoms, a more serious cause must be vigorously sought. The presence of supraclavicular nodes is usually pathologic and is a red flag for serious illness. Obviously, adenopathy associated with hepatomegaly, splenomegaly, or an abdominal mass must be quickly investigated. Furthermore, if the adenopathy does not diminish or resolve after antibiotic therapy or after 3 weeks, a more thorough evaluation is necessary. In children with known immunodeficiencies, the cause of the adenopathy may be far more serious. These children are more prone to infections, and malignancies occur at a higher frequency in these children than in the general population.

REFERENCES

General References

Grossman M, Shiramizu B: Evaluation of lymphadenopathy in children. Curr Opin Pediatr 1994;6:68.

Kelly CS, Kelly RE Jr: Lymphadenopathy in children. Pediatr Clin North Am 1998;45:875.

Cervical Adenopathy

Alvarez A, Schreiber J: Lemierre's syndrome in adolescent children—Anerobic sepsis with internal jugular vein thrombophlebitis following pharyngitis. Pediatrics 1995;96:354.

Barton LL, Feigin RD: Childhood cervical lymphadenitis: A reappraisal. J Pediatr 1974;84:846.

Brook I: Aerobic and anaerobic bacteriology of cervical adenitis in children. Clin Pediatr 1980;19:693.

Peters TR, Edwards KM: Cervical lymphadenopathy and adenitis. Pediatr Rev 2000;21:399.

Epstein-Barr Viral Infections

Case Records of the Massachusetts General Hospital: Case 24-1994. N Engl J Med 1994;330:1739.

Cohen JI: Epstein-Barr virus infection. N Engl J Med 2000;343:481.

Rapp CE, Heweston JF: Infectious mononucleosis and the Epstein-Barr virus. Am J Dis Child 1978;132:78.

Sumaya CV, Ench Y: Epstein-Barr virus infectious mononucleosis in children: I. Clinical and general laboratory findings. Pediatrics 1985; 75:1003.

Cat-Scratch Disease

Bass JW, Freitas BC, Freitas AD, et al: Prospective randomized double blind placebo-controlled evaluation of azithromycin for treatment of cat-scratch diseases. Pediatr Infect Dis J 1998;17:447.

Bass JW, Vincent JM, Person DA: The expanding spectrum of *Bartonella* infections: II. Cat scratch disease. Pediatr Infect Dis J 1997;16:163.

Carithers HA: Cat-scratch diseases: An overview based on a study of 1,200 patients. Am J Dis Child 1985;139:1124.

Schutze GE: Diagnosis and treatment of *Bartonella henselae* infections. Pediatr Infect Dis J 2000;19:1185.

Human Immunodeficiency Virus

Baroni CD, Uccini S: The lymphadenopathy of HIV infection. Am J Clin Pathol 1993;99:397.

Mycobacterial Infections

Huebner RE, Schein MF, Cauthen GM, et al: Usefulness of skin testing with mycobacterial antigens in children with cervical adenopathy. Pediatr Infect Dis J 1992;11:450.

Wolinsky E: Mycobacterial lymphadenitis in children: A prospective study of 105 nontuberculous cases with long term follow-up. Clin Infect Dis 1995; 20:954.

Toxoplasmosis

Frenkel JK: Toxoplasmosis. Pediatr Clin North Am 1985;32:917.

Montoya JG, Remington JS: Studies on the serodiagnosis of toxoplasmic lymphadenitis. Clin Infect Dis 1995;20:781.

Sexually Transmitted Diseases

1998 Guidelines for treatment of sexually transmitted diseases. Centers for Disease Control and Prevention. MMWR Morb Mortal Wkly Rep 1998;47(RR-1):1.

Leukemia and Lymphoma

Shad A, Magrath I: Non-Hodgkin's lymphoma. Pediatr Clin North Am 1997;44:863.

Sinus Histiocytosis

Stones DK, Havenga C: Sinus histiocytosis with massive lymphadenopathy. Arch Dis Child 1992;67:521.

48 Pallor and Anemia

Brian W. Berman

Pallor, a perceptible reduction in the usual color and tone of the skin and/or mucosa, may result from alterations of cutaneous blood flow, anemia, or unknown mechanisms. Under normal circumstances, the pink appearance of the lips, mucosa, and, in white or Asian persons, skin is influenced by the nature and character of these tissues, the adequacy of vascular perfusion, and the concentration of hemoglobin. Pallor is a highly nonspecific finding that may be a manifestation of a wide diversity of diseases, or it may be normal for a given individual. Parental perception of pallor frequently generates considerable anxiety. Although pallor is most often intuitively associated with anemia by families as well as by physicians, an open-minded, broad diagnostic perspective is appropriate (Table 48-1).

Anemia is the condition in which hemoglobin concentration (or hematocrit) is more than two standard deviations below the mean. Anemia is clinically relevant only when the low hemoglobin concentration results in a decreased oxygen-carrying capacity in the blood. By definition, 2.5% of the general population have a hemoglobin or a hematocrit level below the defined limits of normal. This fact must be kept in mind in the evaluation of children with mild anemia for which no explanation can be identified. Hemoglobin concentration varies considerably with age and sex (Table 48-2). Newborns have relatively high levels of circulating hemoglobin, which is an intrauterine adaptation to a relatively hypoxic environment. During the first 2 months of life, hemoglobin production markedly diminishes as a physiologic nadir is reached. The mean hemoglobin level rises gradually during childhood for both boys and girls until puberty, when boys achieve a level approximately 20% higher than that of girls. The average hemoglobin level in black children is slightly lower (0.5 g/dL) than those in white or Asian children. It is appropriate to consider the hemoglobin concentration of a given patient in the context of age and sex.

Anemia occurs as the result of one (or a combination) of three pathophysiologic mechanisms:

- acute blood loss
- impaired production of erythrocytes
- increased destruction of red blood cells (RBCs), known as *hemolysis*

Under normal circumstances, the body's RBC mass is maintained at a level appropriate to support tissue oxygen needs through the oxygen-sensing regulatory stimulus of the hormone erythropoietin. Produced in the kidney, erythropoietin acts to stimulate the production of mature RBCs within the bone marrow. Over a 3- to 5-day period, RBC precursors mature into reticulocytes, which are released into the peripheral blood. In 24 to 48 hours, reticulocytes become mature RBCs, which then circulate in the peripheral blood for approximately 120 days. Senescent RBCs are removed from the circulation by reticuloendothelial cells within the spleen, liver, and bone marrow. A metabolic by-product of hemoglobin catabolism is bilirubin (see Chapter 20).

HISTORY

The child with pallor is not necessarily anemic. An assessment of sun exposure and familial patterns of complexion is crucial because many patients are, by nature, intrinsically pale. A careful evaluation of the medical history is fundamental in the assessment of the pale patient (Table 48-3). In addition, the examiner must determine the duration of the anemia, its association with other symptoms, and history of any chronic illness (weight loss, fever, malaise).

Table 48-1. Causes of Pallor in Children, Based on Etiologic Mechanism

   I. **Anemia**

  II. **Decreased Tendency of the Skin to Pigment**
    A. Physiologic (fair-skinned individuals)
    B. Limited sun exposure

 III. **Alteration of the Consistency of the Subcutaneous Tissue**
    A. Edematous states
        Increased intravascular hydrostatic pressure (e.g., congestive heart failure)
        Decreased intravascular oncotic pressure (hypoproteinemia)
        Increased vascular permeability (e.g., vasculitis)
    B. Hypothyroidism

  IV. **Decreased Perfusion of the Cutaneous/Mucosal Vasculature**
    A. Hypotension
        Cardiogenic shock (pump failure or rhythm disturbance)
        Hypovolemia (blood loss, dehydration)
        Anaphylaxis
        Sepsis
        Acute adrenal insufficiency
        Vasovagal syncope
    B. Vasoconstriction
        Increased sympathetic activity (hypoglycemia, pheochromocytoma)
        Neurologic complications (head trauma, seizures, migraine)

   V. **Chronic Medical Conditions**
    A. Malignant disease
    B. Atopy
    C. Chronic inflammatory disease
        Juvenile rheumatoid arthritis
        Inflammatory bowel disease
    D. Cardiopulmonary disease (including cystic fibrosis)
    E. Diabetes mellitus
    F. Congenital and acquired immunodeficiencies

From Reece RM: Manual of Emergency Pediatrics, 4th ed. Philadelphia, WB Saunders, 1992.

Table 48-2. Values (Normal Mean and Lower Limits of Normal) for Hemoglobin, Hematocrit, and MCV Determination

Age (yr)	Hemoglobin (g/dL)		Hematocrit (%)		MCV (fL)	
	Mean	*Lower Limit*	*Mean*	*Lower Limit*	*Mean*	*Lower Limit*
0.5-1.9	12.5	11.0	37	33	77	70
2-4	12.5	11.0	38	34	79	73
5-7	13.0	11.5	39	35	81	75
8-11	13.5	12.0	40	36	83	76
12-14						
Female	13.5	12.0	41	36	85	78
Male	14.0	12.5	43	37	84	77
15-17						
Female	14.0	12.0	41	36	87	79
Male	15.0	13.0	46	38	86	78
18-49						
Female	14.0	12.0	42	37	90	80
Male	16.0	14.0	47	40	90	80

From Nathan DC, Oski F: Hematology of Infancy and Childhood, 4th ed. Philadelphia; WB Saunders, 1993.

MCV, mean corpuscular volume.

Table 48-3. Historical Clues in Evaluation of Anemia

Variable	Comments
Age	Iron deficiency rare in the absence of blood loss before 6 mo in term or before doubling birth weight in preterm infants
	Neonatal anemia with reticulocytosis suggests hemolysis or blood loss; with reticulocytopenia, it suggests bone marrow failure
	Sickle cell anemia and β-thalassemia appear as fetal hemoglobin disappears (4-8 mo of age)
Family history and genetic considerations	X-linked: G6PD deficiency
	Autosomal dominant: spherocytosis
	Autosomal recessive: sickle cell, Fanconi anemia
	Family member with early age of cholecystectomy (bilirubin stones) or splenectomy; hemolysis
	Ethnicity (thalassemia with Mediterranean origin), (G6PD deficiency in blacks, Greeks, and Sephardic Jews)
	Race (β-thalassemia in whites; α-thalassemia in blacks and Asians; SC and SS in blacks)
Nutrition	Cow's milk diet and iron deficiency
	Strict vegetarian and vitamin B_{12} deficiency
	Goat's milk and folate deficiency
	Pica, plumbism, and iron deficiency
	Cholestasis, malabsorption, and vitamin E
Drugs	G6PD-susceptible agents
	Immune-mediated hemolysis (e.g., penicillin)
	Bone marrow suppression
	Phenytoin-increasing folate requirements
Diarrhea	Malabsorption of vitamins B_{12} and E and iron
	Inflammatory bowel disease and anemia of chronic disease or blood loss
	Milk protein allergy–induced blood loss
	Intestinal resection and vitamin B_{12} deficiency
Infection	*Giardia* and iron malabsorption
	Intestinal bacterial overgrowth (blind loop) and vitamin B_{12} deficiency
	Fish tapeworm and vitamin B_{12} deficiency
	Epstein-Barr virus, cytomegalovirus, and bone marrow suppression
	Mycoplasma and hemolysis
	Parvovirus and bone marrow suppression
	Chronic infection
	Endocarditis
	Malaria and hemolysis
	Hepatitis and aplastic anemia

Adapted from Scott JP: Hematology. In Behrman RE, Kliegman RM (eds): Nelson Essentials of Pediatrics, 2nd ed. Philadelphia, WB Saunders, 1994, p 519.

G6PD, glucose-6-phosphate dehydrogenase.

Dietary history is important as it relates to sources of iron. Infants, particularly those delivered prematurely and those consuming large amounts of cow's milk or formula without iron supplementation, are at risk for iron deficiency anemia, as are children and adolescents who consume little meat. Patients or breast-fed infants of mothers who follow a strict vegan diet may become deficient in vitamin B_{12}. A history of pica suggests possible lead toxicity, iron deficiency, or both.

A neonatal history of hyperbilirubinemia supports a possible diagnosis of congenital hemolytic anemia, such as hereditary spherocytosis, which is further supported by a family history of anemia, splenectomy, and/or cholecystectomy (resulting from gallstones caused by chronic hyperbilirubinemia).

Medication history is pertinent because certain drugs, including antimalarial agents and sulfonamide antibiotics, can induce oxidant-associated hemolysis in the patient deficient in glucose-6-phosphate dehydrogenase (G6PD), whereas other medications may cause immune hemolysis (penicillin) or decreased RBC production (chloramphenicol). Travel history may suggest exposure to infections, such as malaria.

PHYSICAL EXAMINATION

The general appearance of the child provides a clue as to the severity and chronicity of the problem. Severe anemia that develops slowly over weeks or months is often well tolerated. Vital signs (including orthostatic blood pressure), height, weight, and growth percentiles offer further insight into the severity of the problem. The findings of a thorough physical examination define the degree of pallor (conjunctiva, palms, skin), reveal the presence of underlying disease (all organ systems), and uncover signs of trauma. Isolated pallor in a well-appearing child who does not have evidence of systemic disease is usually much less ominous than that noted in a child with bruising, adenopathy, hepatosplenomegaly, or abdominal mass. Table 48-4 lists some clues that may assist in determining the underlying cause of the anemia.

Prominent cheekbones, dental malocclusion, and frontal bossing may occur in patients with chronic hemolytic anemias (sickle cell disease, thalassemia major) because of the expansion of bone marrow space. Tortuosity of conjunctival vessels occurs in the sickling syndromes. Splenomegaly is often present in children with congenital hemolytic anemia (see Chapter 19). Lymphadenopathy and hepatosplenomegaly may indicate the presence of infiltrative disease of the bone marrow and visceral organs, such as leukemia. Purpura in the anemic child is suggestive of associated thrombocytopenia, which may accompany aplastic anemia or leukemia.

Many congenital anomalies have been associated with hematologic syndromes. Patients with Fanconi anemia (constitutional aplastic anemia) are often short and hyperpigmented with hypoplastic "finger-like" thumbs, radial bone anomalies, and structural renal abnormalities. Patients with Diamond-Blackfan anemia (congenital hypoplastic anemia) are often short and have a "curious, intellectual" facial expression.

When pallor is related to chronic inflammation or infection or systemic disease, a diligent general physical examination may yield substantive information, such as hypertension and short stature in the child with chronic renal disease, joint inflammation in the child with rheumatologic disorders, digital clubbing in the child with advanced cyanotic cardiopulmonary diseases, and poor nutritional status in the child with inflammatory bowel disease.

Recent onset of pallor is suggestive of anemia. The child who has always appeared somewhat pale but has been otherwise well and is manifesting normal growth and development may merely be expressing an intrinsic constitutional characteristic. In such instances, the child and other family members often have light hair and skin complexion. An unremarkable general medical history and physical examination support a physiologic explanation for pallor.

Some children may appear pale as a result of limited sun exposure, as might occur during the winter in cooler climates.

Children with malignant disease or chronic illness (e.g., rheumatologic disorders, inflammatory bowel disease, chronic cardiopulmonary disorders, diabetes) may have a pale appearance that is unrelated or out of proportion to the degree of associated anemia. Atopic children often have distinctly pale mucosa as a result of local edema. Children with generalized edema caused by hypoproteinemia, congestive heart failure, or vasculitis often appear pale as a result of excess interstitial fluid within the mucosal or cutaneous tissues. Patients with hypothyroidism are pale because of myxedematous changes in the skin, subcutaneous tissue, and mucosa. The rare child with pheochromocytoma can appear pale on the basis of catecholamine-induced vasoconstriction.

LABORATORY EVALUATION

The initial laboratory test in a child with pallor should be a complete blood cell count (CBC) including a white blood cell (WBC) differential and platelet count. Anemia as a cause of pallor does not occur until the hemoglobin level falls below 8 to 9 g/dL. "False anemia" (resulting from laboratory error, sampling difficulty, or "statistical anemia") should be considered whenever a child is said to be anemic, particularly when laboratory findings do not seem consistent with clinical impressions. Capillary blood sampling can be associated with substantial error, depending on the difficulty in performing the procedure and the use of mechanical force necessary to promote blood flow. When laboratory or sampling errors are supected, it is always appropriate to obtain a repeated venipuncture sample. "Statistical anemia" relates to the fact that, by definition, 2.5% of the general population has hemoglobin levels below the lower limit of normal. This phenomenon should be considered when mild, unexplained normocytic anemia is identified in a healthy child.

Nearly all laboratories perform CBCs with the use of automated technology systems. Hemoglobin concentration (grams per deciliter), RBC count (cells per cubic millimeter), and mean corpuscular volume (MCV) (expressed in femtoliters [fL]) are directly measured. Hematocrit value, mean corpuscular hemoglobin, and mean corpuscular hemoglobin concentration are derived values and are less accurate. Other useful information reported includes RBC distribution width (RDW), WBC count (cells per cubic millimeter), and platelet count. Careful attention should be given to the hemoglobin value, the MCV, the RDW, the shape of the RBCs, and any abnormalities in the number of platelets or WBCs.

The reticulocyte count, reported as a percentage of total RBCs, is essential in categorizing anemia. An appropriately elevated reticulocyte count implies a response of the bone marrow to either hemolysis or acute or chronic blood loss. In cases of acute blood loss, the reticulocyte count is not elevated for 3 to 4 days. The reticulocyte count is therefore most helpful for cases in which the anemia has been present for more than a few days.

The MCV may provide very helpful information but must always be viewed in conjunction with a review of the peripheral blood smear, RDW, and reticulocyte count. A varied population of smaller and larger RBCs (e.g., reticulocytes) may yield a falsely normal MCV and be diagnostically misleading. *Microcytosis* may be associated with several commonly encountered anemias, including iron deficiency, thalassemia, lead toxicity, and anemia of chronic disease (Table 48-5). *Macrocytosis*, an unusual finding in children, is associated with vitamin B_{12} or folate deficiency, syndromes associated with elevated production of fetal-like RBCs (Fanconi anemia, Diamond-Blackfan anemia), and some cases of hypothyroidism (see Table 48-5). Normal standards for MCV are age related; a simple guideline is that the lower normal limit of MCV for children older than 6 months of age is 70 fL plus the patient's age in years until the adult standard of 80 to 100 fL is reached (see Table 48-2).

Table 48-4. **Physical Findings in the Evaluation of Anemia**

System	Observation	Significance
Skin	Hyperpigmentation	Fanconi anemia, dyskeratosis congenita
	Café-au-lait spots	Fanconi anemia
	Vitiligo	Vitamin B_{12} deficiency
	Partial oculocutaneous albinism	Chédiak-Higashi syndrome
	Jaundice	Hemolysis
	Petechiae, purpura	Bone marrow infiltration, autoimmune hemolysis with autoimmune thrombocytopenia, hemolytic uremic syndrome
	Erythematous rash	Parvovirus, Epstein-Barr virus
	Butterfly rash	SLE autoantibodies
Head	Frontal bossing	Thalassemia major, severe iron deficiency, chronic subdural hematoma
	Microcephaly	Fanconi anemia
Eyes	Microphthalmia	Fanconi anemia
	Retinopathy	Hemoglobin SS, SC disease
	Optic atrophy, blindness	Osteopetrosis
	Blocked lacrimal gland	Dyskeratosis congenita
	Kayser-Fleisher ring	Wilson disease
	Blue sclera	Iron deficiency
Ears	Deafness	Osteopetrosis
Mouth	Glossitis	B_{12} deficiency, iron deficiency
	Angular stomatitis	Iron deficiency
	Cleft lip	Diamond-Blackfan syndrome
	Pigmentation	Peutz-Jeghers syndrome (intestinal blood loss)
	Telangiectasia	Osler-Weber-Rendu syndrome (blood loss)
	Leukoplakia	Dyskeratosis congenita
Chest	Shield chest or widespread nipples	Diamond-Blackfan syndrome
	Murmur	Endocarditis: prosthetic valve hemolysis
Abdomen	Hepatomegaly	Hemolysis, infiltrative tumor, chronic disease, hemangioma, cholecystitis
	Splenomegaly	Hemolysis, sickle cell disease (early), thalassemia, malaria, lymphoma, Epstein-Barr virus, portal hypertension
	Nephromegaly	Fanconi anemia
	Absent kidney	Fanconi anemia
Extremities	Absent thumbs	Fanconi anemia
	Triphalangeal thumb	Diamond-Blackfan syndrome
	Spoon nails	Iron deficiency
	Beau line (nails)	Heavy metal intoxication, severe illness
	Mees line (nails)	Heavy metals, severe illness, sickle cell anemia
	Dystrophic nails	Dyskeratosis congenita
	Edema	Milk-induced protein-losing enteropathy with iron deficiency
Rectal	Hemorrhoids	Portal hypertension
	Heme-positive stool	Intestinal hemorrhage
Nerves	Irritable, apathy	Iron deficiency
	Peripheral neuropathy	Deficiency of vitamins B_1, B_{12}, and E, lead poisoning
	Dementia	Deficiency of vitamins B_{12} and E
	Ataxia, posterior column signs	Vitamin B_{12} and E deficiency
	Stroke	Sickle cell anemia, paroxysmal nocturnal hemoglobinuria

Adapted from Scott JP: Hematology. In Behrman RE, Kliegman RM (eds): Nelson Essentials of Pediatrics, 2nd ed. Philadelphia, WB Saunders, 1994, p 520.
SLE, systemic lupus erythematosus.

An individual with small RBCs may have a normal or near-normal hemoglobin level if the RBC count is increased, as occurs in patients with thalassemia minor, who often have RBC counts of more than 5×10^6. The mean corpuscular hemoglobin concentration reflects the concentration of hemoglobin per cell and would be expected to be low in patients with anemias in which RBCs are "underhemoglobinized," such as the hypochromic anemia of iron deficiency.

The RDW is derived from the histogram of RBC volumes. A normal RDW (11.5% to 14.5%) implies a uniform population of RBCs of similar size (in β-thalassemia trait, a uniform population of small cells exists; hence the MCV is low and the RDW is normal or minimally elevated). An elevated RDW is seen in iron deficiency (in which the population of small cells is variably sized; hence the MCV is low and the RDW is elevated) or some hemolytic anemias

(in which the RDW is elevated because of the presence of large reticulocytes) (Table 48-6).

Anemias are categorized on the basis of the adequacy of the reticulocyte response. The reticulocyte count, normally about 1% to 2%, is expressed as a percentage of the total number of RBCs; in some patients with moderate or severe anemia, the reticulocyte count may appear elevated, but in absolute terms, it may be insufficient. Therefore, the reticulocyte count must be corrected:

$$\text{corrected reticulocyte count} = \frac{\text{reticulocyte count} \times \text{hemoglobin}}{\text{(normal hemoglobin for age)}}$$

If the corrected reticulocyte count is greater than 2%, then the bone marrow is producing RBCs at an accelerated pace (Fig. 48-1).

Table 48-5. Causes of High or Low Mean Corpuscular Volume

Low mean corpuscular volume
Iron deficiency
Thalassemias
Lead toxicity
Anemia of chronic disease
Copper deficiency
Sideroblastic anemia
Hemoglobin E
High mean corpuscular volume
Normal newborn
Elevated reticulocyte count
Vitamin B_{12} or folate deficiency
Diamond-Blackfan anemia (congenital hypoplastic anemia)
Fanconi anemia
Aplastic anemia
Down syndrome
Hypothyroidism (occasionally)
Oroticaciduria
Lesch-Nyhan syndrome
Drugs (zidovudine, chemotherapy)
Chronic liver disease

Table 48-6. Red Blood Cell Distribution Width (RDW) in Common Anemias of Childhood

Anemia	MCV
Elevated RDW (Nonuniform Population of RBCs)	
Hemolytic anemia with elevated reticulocyte count	High
Iron deficiency anemia	Low
Anemias due to red blood cell fragmentation: DIC, HUS, TTP	Low
Megaloblastic anemias: vitamin B_{12} or folate deficiency	High
Normal RDW (Uniform Population of RBCs)	
Thalassemias	Low
Acute hemorrhage	Normal
Fanconi or aplastic anemia	High

DIC, disseminated intravascular coagulation; HUS, hemolytic uremic syndrome; MCV, mean corpuscular volume; RBC, red blood cell; TTP, thrombotic thrombocytopenic purpura.

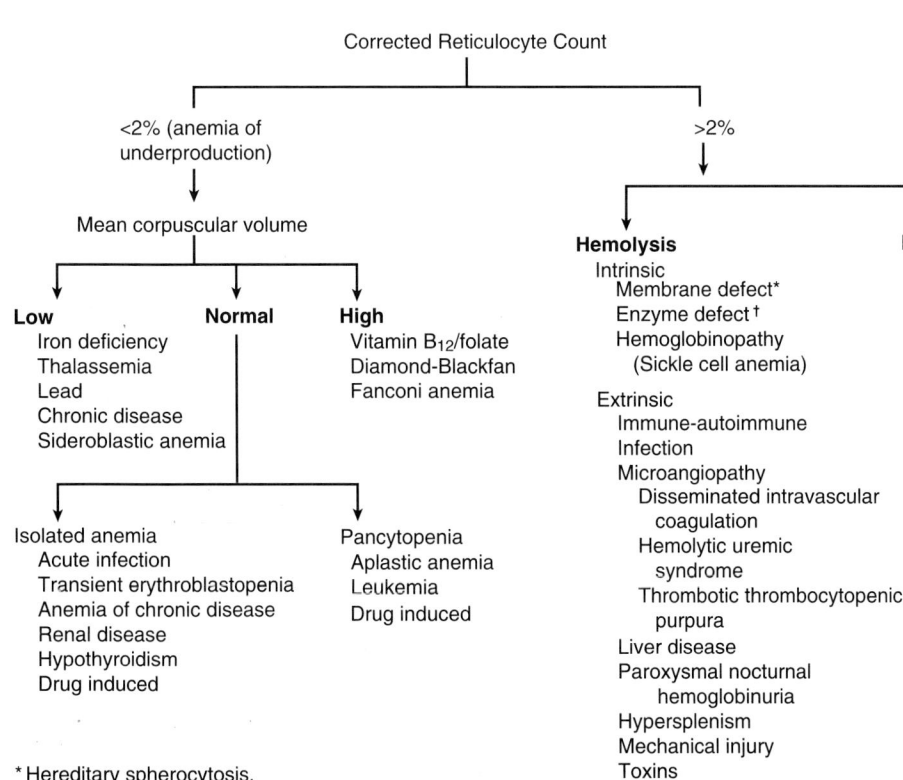

Figure 48-1. Diagnostic approach to anemia. *Hereditary spherocytosis, elliptocytosis, pyropoikilocytosis, stomatocytosis, or paroxysmal nocturnal hemoglobinuria. †Glucose-6-phosphate dehydrogenase, pyruvate kinase, or glucose phosphate isomerase deficiencies.

The WBC count, differential, and platelet count may provide extremely pertinent information. The presence of immature leukocytes on a smear, which may be associated with either a high or a low WBC count, is suggestive of leukemia. Leukopenia and thrombocytopenia occurring in a patient with anemia of underproduction are suggestive of aplastic anemia or infiltrative bone marrow disease, such as leukemia or neuroblastoma metastasis to the marrow.

Thrombocytosis may be present in patients with iron deficiency, blood loss, inflammatory disease, infection, malignancy, or asplenia.

The serum indirect bilirubin, lactate dehydrogenase, and urinary urobilinogen levels are elevated in patients with increased rates of RBC destruction. An elevated serum direct bilirubin level is seen only if hepatobiliary complications supervene (biliary tract stones, hepatitis). A low serum iron level, elevated total iron-binding capacity, and a low percentage of iron saturation (% saturation = serum iron/total iron binding capacity × 100) and/or decreased serum ferritin level are helpful in establishing a diagnosis of iron deficiency. Hemoglobin electrophoresis is necessary to define abnormal hemoglobins, such as sickle hemoglobin or hemoglobin C. Assessment of RBC enzyme levels (e.g., G6PD) may be necessary when infection- or medication-related hemolytic anemia is suspected in a male of Mediterranean or African descent. True macrocytic anemia may necessitate assessment of serum vitamin B_{12} and folate levels. Bone marrow aspirate and biopsy are appropriate whenever leukemia or aplastic anemia is seriously suspected.

If autoimmune hemolytic anemia is suspected because anemia, jaundice, reticulocytosis (may be absent if antibody reacts with reticulocytes), splenomegaly (not universally), and microspherocytes are noted, a direct Coombs test should be performed to detect the presence of an autoantibody on the RBC surface.

Abnormalities of RBC structure may be readily apparent on inspection of the peripheral blood smear and provide helpful diagnostic hints (Table 48-7, Fig. 48-2).

From a practical clinical perspective, it is best to consider the differential diagnosis of pallor in the context of the acuteness and severity of the clinical findings (Fig. 48-3). The well-appearing child may need only a CBC, which might provide reassurance to the parents. The pale child who appears mildly or moderately ill requires a laboratory evaluation for anemia as well as studies to detect any suspected underlying disease. The pale child who appears seriously ill requires urgent evaluation and appropriate therapeutic intervention. The only obligatory laboratory study is a CBC, with other laboratory assessments dictated on the basis of the suspected diagnosis (blood glucose, electrolyte, blood urea nitrogen [BUN], and creatinine measurements and blood culture). If hemorrhage or severe anemia is suspected, a type and cross-match must be sent to the blood bank; two large intravenous lines must be secured; and frequent serial evaluations of hemoglobin, blood pressure, pulse, perfusion, and end-organ function (central nervous system for mental status, renal function for urine output) must be assessed.

DIFFERENTIAL DIAGNOSIS OF ANEMIA

The classification of anemia is presented in Figure 48-1 and Figure 48-4.

Anemia Caused by Acute Blood Loss

Significant loss of blood on an acute or subacute basis leads to anemia. A period of about 24 hours may be required for full intravascular

---

Table 48-7. Peripheral Blood Morphologic Findings in Various Anemias

Microcytes	**Basophil Stippling**
Iron deficiency	Thalassemia
Thalassemias	Lead intoxication
Lead toxicity	
Anemia of chronic disease	**Red Blood Cell Fragments, Helmet Cells, Burr Cells**
	Disseminated intravascular coagulation
Macrocytes	Hemolytic-uremic syndrome
Newborns	Thrombotic thrombocytopenic purpura
Vitamin B_{12} or folate deficiency	Kasabach-Merritt syndrome
Diamond-Blackfan anemia	Waring blender syndrome
Fanconi aplastic anemia	Uremia
Liver disease	
Down syndrome	**Hypersegmented Neutrophils**
Hypothyroidism	Vitamin B_{12} or folate deficiency
Spherocytes	**Blasts**
Hereditary spherocytosis	Leukemia (All or AML)
Immune hemolytic anemia	Severe infection (rarely)
Sickled Cells	**Leukopenia/Thrombocytopenia**
Sickle cell anemias (SS disease, SC disease, S–β-thalassemia)	Aplastic or Fanconi anemia
	Leukemia
Elliptocytes	
Hereditary elliptocytosis	
Target Cells	
Hemoglobinopathies (especially hemoglobin C and thalassemia)	
Liver disease	

ALL, acute lymphocytic leukemia; AML, acute myeloid leukemia.

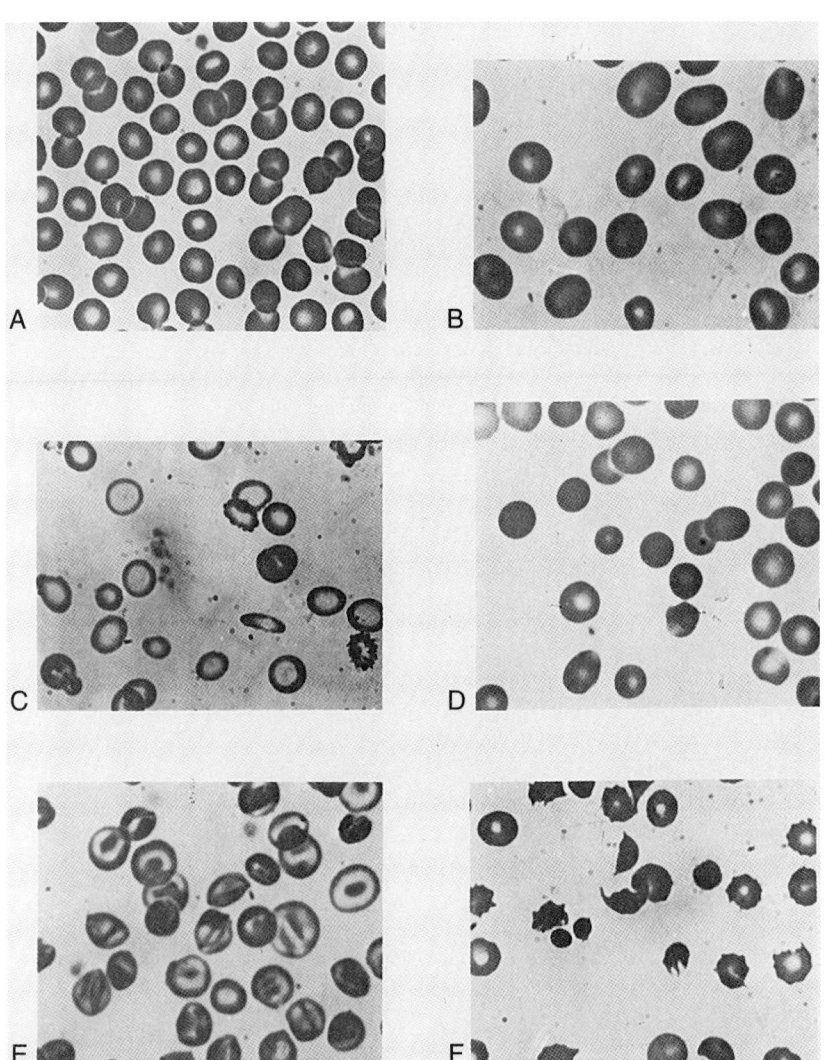

Figure 48-2. Morphologic abnormalities of the red blood cell. **A,** Normal. **B,** Macrocytes (folic acid deficiency). **C,** Hypochromic microcytes (iron deficiency). **D,** Spherocytes (hereditary spherocytosis). **E,** Target cells (hemoglobin CC disease). **F,** Schistocytes (hemolytic-uremic syndrome). (From Behrman RE, Kliegman RM [eds]: Nelson Essentials of Pediatrics, 2nd ed. Philadelphia, WB Saunders, 1994, p 521.)

equilibration after acute blood loss; the fall in hemoglobin level occurs gradually. In patients with severe acute blood loss, the primary concern is *intravascular volume,* which cannot be assessed by hemoglobin level. In this situation, the patient's condition is best assessed by measurement of blood pressure, heart rate, adequacy of peripheral perfusion (capillary refill time), and mental status. In most instances, an obvious history of blood loss is apparent (epistaxis, hematemesis, trauma), but severe occult blood loss may also occur. Large amounts of blood may accumulate in the gastrointestinal tract before the development of hematemesis, hematochezia, or melena. Intraabdominal bleeding may occur after trauma or may result from an ulcer (see Chapters 14 and 17) and may be associated with progressive anemia in the absence of an obvious source of blood loss. The clinical history coupled with the physical examination (including rectal examination) and tests for occult blood in the stool generally define the source of blood loss.

In anemia associated with blood loss, the RBC size and structure are normal, and after a period of 3 to 5 days, the reticulocyte count increases appropriately. If hemorrhage has ceased, the hemoglobin level may be expected to gradually rise unless supervening factors, such as iron deficiency, exist.

Severe hemorrhage associated with intravascular volume depletion warrants immediate intervention; RBC transfusions are necessary until hemorrhage has ceased. Less severe hemorrhage may not be associated with intravascular volume depletion and may merely manifest with moderate to severe anemia. Transfusions are necessary when the oxygen-carrying capacity of the blood is diminished to the point of impending tissue hypoxia; the need for transfusion therapy is based on clinical parameters, including the presence of fatigue, lightheadedness, tachycardia, dyspnea, and heart failure. If hemorrhage has ceased, if intravascular volume is replete, and if the patient is not manifesting signs of cardiorespiratory compromise, transfusion therapy can often be avoided. In such instances, it is appropriate to supply therapeutic doses of iron to ensure adequacy of the reticulocyte response (see Table 48-10).

Anemia Caused by Underproduction

Anemia caused by underproduction (see Figs. 48-1 and 48-4) is characterized by a suboptimal bone marrow response (a corrected reticulocyte count of <2%). The clinical context may be predictive of anemia of underproduction, as in the patient with chronic renal disease, chronic inflammatory or infectious disease, or hypothyroidism. Anemia of underproduction is evaluated on the basis of RBC size: microcytic, normocytic, or macrocytic.

Microcytic Anemias

Hemoglobin, the chief intracellular component of the RBC, is composed of heme (iron and protoporphyrin IX) and globin chains (α and β). Any factor that diminishes the availability or utilization of

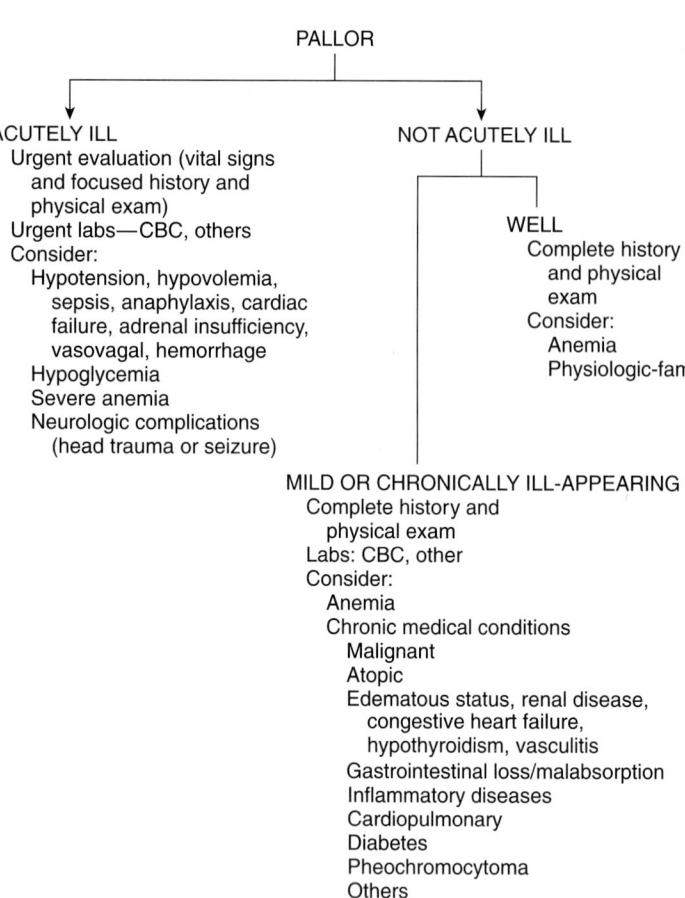

PALLOR

ACUTELY ILL
   Urgent evaluation (vital signs
      and focused history and
      physical exam)
   Urgent labs—CBC, others
   Consider:
      Hypotension, hypovolemia,
         sepsis, anaphylaxis, cardiac
         failure, adrenal insufficiency,
         vasovagal, hemorrhage
      Hypoglycemia
      Severe anemia
      Neurologic complications
         (head trauma or seizure)

NOT ACUTELY ILL

WELL
   Complete history
      and physical
      exam
   Consider:
      Anemia
      Physiologic-familial

MILD OR CHRONICALLY ILL-APPEARING
   Complete history and
      physical exam
   Labs: CBC, other
   Consider:
      Anemia
      Chronic medical conditions
         Malignant
         Atopic
         Edematous status, renal disease,
            congestive heart failure,
            hypothyroidism, vasculitis
         Gastrointestinal loss/malabsorption
         Inflammatory diseases
         Cardiopulmonary
         Diabetes
         Pheochromocytoma
         Others

Figure 48-3. Approach to the pale child. CBC, complete blood cell count.

any of these components results in microcytic anemia. The automated MCV represents the mean RBC volume and does not address variations in cell size. The RDW, however, does describe the variation in cell size and, if normal, defines a relatively uniform population of cells. Review of the peripheral blood smear also provides additional evidence regarding variability in cell size and shape. It is important to note that MCV is age related (see Table 48-2). When the diagnosis is not immediately apparent, it is helpful to carefully select from a variety of available laboratory studies (Table 48-8).

Iron Deficiency Anemia. Iron deficiency is the most common nutritional deficiency that causes anemia. Iron deficiency results when nutritional intake is insufficient to meet demands associated with growth and, in some instances, blood loss. Iron is a key component of the hemoglobin molecule; hence, its deficiency leads to anemia associated with underhemoglobinization (hypochromia) and small RBCs (microcytosis). At particular risk for the development of iron deficiency are infants, whose rapid growth and expanding blood volume impose considerable iron demands. Premature infants are at high risk because most in utero iron is transferred to the fetus during the last trimester of pregnancy and postnatal growth rate is rapid. Adolescent girls are at high risk because of menstrual blood loss and nutrition, which is often not optimal. When iron deficiency occurs outside of the setting of infancy or female adolescence, a pathologic source of blood loss must be strongly considered (especially occult gastrointestinal bleeding).

Nutritional sources of iron include iron-fortified infant formula (12 mg/L), iron-fortified infant cereal, breast milk (because of its high bioavailability), beef, fish, and fowl. Ascorbic acid (vitamin C) enhances the absorption of iron contained in vegetable products. The American Academy of Pediatrics recommends iron-fortified infant formula or breast milk until the age of 1 year and the introduction of foods rich in iron after 6 months of age. Low-iron formulas are not recommended. Cow's milk is a very poor source of nutritional iron, and, when ingested in large quantities by young infants, it is often a cause of occult gastrointestinal blood loss. Infants should receive no cow's milk until after 1 year of age and then not more than 24 ounces per day. Iron supplementation is necessary for preterm infants, most adolescent females, and pregnant women. Iron deficiency must be viewed as a systemic deficiency disorder, only one manifestation of which is anemia (Table 48-9).

Iron deficiency is usually detected by routine hemoglobin screening performed in children between 9 and 18 months of age and adolescent females who have been menstruating for more than 2 years. Screening for iron deficiency anemia is complicated by the fact that infants who currently have or recently had a viral illness often have mild transient anemia. The occurrence of mild anemia is two to three times higher in children who have experienced an infectious illness (including routine childhood illnesses) than in children who have been well in the preceding month.

Fewer than 2% of well-nourished 1-year-olds are anemic; hence, routine screening for iron deficiency can be reserved for a high-risk population, including preterm infants, infants fed cow's milk or nonfortified formula before the age of 1 year, older children who consume more than 24 ounces of cow's milk per day, menstruating adolescent girls, and all children of lower socioeconomic status.

Symptomatic iron deficiency is infrequent, but when it occurs, it is generally noted in infants who consume large amounts of cow's milk and have intestinal blood loss as a result of asymptomatic milk protein–induced enterocolitis. Such children may have pallor, irritability, fatigue, glossitis, blue sclera, and, in extreme cases, signs and symptoms of high-output cardiac failure (dyspnea, diaphoresis, pallor, tachycardia, gallop rhythm, and hepatomegaly). Blood loss may be intermittent; a negative stool test for blood does not rule out the diagnosis.

I. Acute blood loss with hemodilution

II. Anemia of RBC underproduction (i.e., inadequate reticulocyte count)
  A. Microcytic
    1. Iron deficiency
    2. Lead intoxication
    3. Thalassemia syndromes
    4. Anemia of chronic diseases
  B. Normocytic

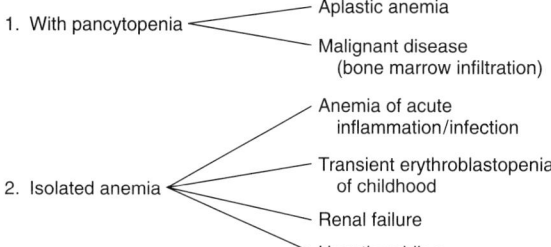

  C. Macrocytic

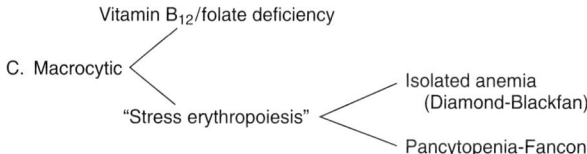

III. Anemia due to increased destruction = hemolysis (i.e., adequate reticulocyte count)
  A. Intrinsic RBC defect
    1. Hemoglobinopathies (sickle cell anemia, unstable hemoglobins)
    2. Membrane defects (hereditary spherocytosis, elliptocytosis)
    3. Enzymopathies (G6PD, pyruvate kinase deficiency)
  B. Extrinsic defects
    1. Immune hemolysis
    2. Infection (bacterial, viral, other)
    3. Microangiopathy (disseminated intravascular coagulation, hemolytic uremic syndrome, thrombotic thrombocytopenia purpura)
    4. Liver disease
    5. Paroxysmal nocturnal hemoglobinuria
    6. Hypersplenism
    7. Mechanical injury (e.g., burns)
    8. Toxins
    9. Nutritional (vitamin E deficiency)
    10. Metabolic (galactosemia)
    11. Wilson disease

Figure 48-4. Differential diagnosis of anemia. G6PD, glucose-6-phosphate dehydrogenase; RBC, red blood cell.

Mild anemia in otherwise well infants between 6 and 24 months of age, particularly in association with ingestion of large amounts of cow's milk, is most likely caused by iron deficiency. This is also true when mild anemia is detected in the healthy, menstruating adolescent. Empirical iron therapy is often prescribed in such circumstances (Table 48-10). If the hemoglobin level has normalized after 1 month of therapy, a presumptive diagnosis has been established, and the patient should receive an additional 2 to 3 months of *therapeutic* doses of iron to replete stores. An appropriate response to iron therapy is the diagnostic "gold standard."

Laboratory confirmatory studies are necessary when iron deficiency anemia is suspected in patients who are not at high risk for nutritional deficiency or in those in whom anemia is moderately severe. A serum ferritin level of less than 12 ng/dL or an iron saturation of less than 10% provides confirmation of the diagnosis.

Intravenous iron therapy is rarely necessary, although it may be useful in certain situations (iron malabsorption in patients with inflammatory bowel disease; children receiving hemodialysis). The optimal approach to iron deficiency anemia in infants and children is prevention.

Table 48-8. Laboratory Findings in Microcytic Anemia

	FEP	Fe	TIBC	Pb	HbA₂	Ferritin
Iron deficiency	↑	↓	↑	nl	nl	↓
α-Thalassemia	nl	nl	nl	nl	nl	nl
β-Thalassemia	nl	nl	nl	nl	↑	nl
Lead poisoning	↑	nl	nl	↑	nl	nl
Anemia of chronic disease	↑	↓	↓	nl	nl	nl or ↑

Adapted from Reece RM: Manual of Emergency Pediatrics, 4th ed. Philadelphia, WB Saunders, 1992.

Fe, iron; FEP, free erythrocyte protoporphyrin; HbA₂, hemoglobin A₂; nl, normal; Pb, lead; TIBC, total iron-binding capacity.

Thalassemia Syndromes. The thalassemia syndromes represent a heterogeneous group of inherited disorders of decreased globin production that lead to microcytic anemia, which is often mistaken for iron deficiency. The child with microcytic anemia who has no evidence of iron deficiency or lead toxicity probably has thalassemia.

β-Thalassemia Minor (Trait). Two genes, one inherited from each parent, code for the production of the β globin chains of hemoglobin. When one gene is affected by the β-thalassemia mutation, a moderate diminution in the production of the β globin chain occurs, resulting in mild microcytic anemia of underproduction. β-Thalassemia occurs most commonly in individuals of Mediterranean and African descent. Patients with β-thalassemia trait are asymptomatic, and the diagnosis is frequently made when anemia and microcytosis are noted at the time of routine screening for iron deficiency or incidentally when a CBC is obtained for the assessment of acute or chronic symptoms. Typically, patients have mild anemia and a low MCV. For an equivalent degree of anemia, the MCV is substantially lower than that seen in iron deficiency.

This phenomenon is reflected in the Mentzer index, calculated by dividing the MCV by the RBC count (in millions). An index of less than 13 is suggestive of thalassemia, whereas an index of more than 13 is generally seen in iron deficiency anemia. An MCV within the range of normal virtually excludes a diagnosis of β-thalassemia. A normal or mildly elevated RDW is usually seen in thalassemia and reflects a relatively uniform population of microcytic RBCs (as opposed to iron deficiency, wherein the RDW is uniformly elevated, reflecting the variation in cell size).

The peripheral blood smear demonstrates microcytosis, hypochromia, and target cells. Occasional fragments may be seen. The significance of β-thalassemia relates to (1) its confusion with iron deficiency (hence, patients may be treated unnecessarily with repeated courses of iron and undergo repeated unnecessary blood studies) and (2) its genetic implications. A mating between two individuals with β-thalassemia trait carries a 25% risk per pregnancy

Table 48-9. Nonhematologic Consequences of Iron Deficiency

Impairment of cognitive development
Pica
Epithelial abnormalities (gastrointestinal mucosal lesion, glossitis; spoon-shaped nails)
Exercise intolerance
Behavioral manifestations
Abnormal immune response (?)
Growth retardation
Impaired collagen synthesis (blue sclera)

Table 48-10. Therapy for Iron Deficiency

Infants and Children

4-6 mg/kg of elemental iron/day, given in divided doses 2 or 3 times/day (mild nutritional anemia deficiency in infants may be treated with a single daily dose of 3 mg/kg before breakfast)

Alternate therapy: iron polysaccharide, 5 mg/kg in a single daily dose

Adolescents

3 mg/kg/day of elemental iron (maximum, 200 mg) given in divided doses 2 or 3 times/day

Alternate therapy: iron polysaccharide, 150 mg/day as single dose

Available Iron Preparations

Ferrous sulfate drops: 15 mg of elemental iron/0.6 mL
Ferrous sulfate elixir: 44 mg of elemental iron/5 mL
Ferrous sulfate tablets: 65 mg of elemental iron/tablet
Iron polysaccharide: 100 mg of elemental iron per 5 mL or 150-mg tablets

Duration of Prescription

Continue *therapeutic dose* of iron for 2-3 months after hemoglobin level has corrected (to replete stores), after which maintenance nutritional needs must be met

of offspring with homozygous β-thalassemia (thalassemia major), an extremely serious disorder. Families with a child with a diagnosis of β-thalassemia minor should be appropriately screened and counseled. For purposes of screening, a normal age-adjusted MCV essentially excludes a diagnosis of β-thalassemia.

Homozygous β-Thalassemia. Homozygous β-thalassemia, also known as β-thalassemia major or Cooley anemia, results from the inheritance of the β-thalassemia mutation from each parent. This results in a severe deficiency of production of β globin chains. Excess α globin chains precipitate within developing erythroid elements in the marrow and lead to brisk intramarrow destruction of developing erythroid elements (ineffective erythropoiesis). As a result, patients with homozygous β-thalassemia present during infancy (6 to 12 months of age) with severe anemia and an inadequate reticulocyte count. The child with β-thalassemia major typically presents with fatigue, irritability, pallor, jaundice, and marked hepatosplenomegaly (caused by extramedullary hematopoiesis). Frontal bossing and prominent cheek bones (maxillary hyperplasia) may be noted and result from expansion of the marrow space in an attempt to compensate for severe anemia. Most patients are of Mediterranean (Italian or Greek) descent.

Laboratory findings include severe anemia and a decreased age-adjusted MCV. The peripheral blood smear is markedly abnormal, demonstrating severely underhemoglobinized RBCs, target cells, and wide variability in cell shape and size. Long-term transfusion therapy sufficient to suppress ineffective erythropoiesis (maintaining hemoglobin level higher than 10 g/dL) may be associated with relatively normal growth, development, and functional capabilities. Long-term deferoxamine iron chelation to prevent iron overload allows for prolonged survival and avoidance of transfusional hemosiderosis (hepatic, endocrine, and cardiac dysfunction), but it is a cumbersome treatment program that is associated with a substantial degree of poor compliance. Bone marrow transplantation, although associated with an approximate 10% risk of mortality, is curative and a potential treatment option for younger patients who have a human leukocyte antigen–identical, nonthalassemic sibling.

α-Thalassemia Syndromes. Four genes code for the α globin chains' hemoglobin: two on each chromosome 16. Progressive deletions of one, two, three, or four of these genes account for the variable laboratory and clinical findings associated with the α-thalassemia syndromes. Decreased α globin chain production leads to an excess of β globin chains, which tend to precipitate within developing RBCs in the bone marrow, leading to destruction. Mature RBCs are mildly hypochromic and microcytic and may appear to be targeted.

Deletion of one gene occurs in about 30% of African Americans, as well as in some individuals of Asian descent. This is known as the "silent carrier" state because it is not associated with anemia or microcytosis.

Deletion of two genes represents α-thalassemia minor. Such patients manifest mild anemia and microcytosis, with MCVs generally in the mildly decreased range (less microcytosis than is generally seen in β-thalassemia trait).

A three-gene deletion leads to hemoglobin H disease, which is associated with moderate hemolytic anemia, microcytosis, reticulocytosis, and splenomegaly.

A four-gene deletion represents hemoglobin Bart disease, in which the fetus is unable to produce any α chains; hence, nearly all in utero hemoglobin in such fetuses is Bart type (composed of four γ chains). Hemoglobin Bart has an extremely high oxygen affinity and leads to severe tissue hypoxemia and resultant fetal hydrops and death. On occasion, babies with hemoglobin Bart disease have been saved by extraordinary measures (intrauterine transfusion and early delivery), but they are then committed to lifelong transfusion support.

Hemoglobin H disease and hemoglobin Bart disease occur almost exclusively in individuals of Asian descent. This is because Asians and Africans have different chromosomal arrangements of the abnormal genes. When α-thalassemia minor (two-gene deletion) occurs in the Asian population, deletions may be *cis* (both genes deleted from the same chromosome) or *trans* (each chromosome missing one gene). In individuals of African descent, α-thalassemia minor (two-gene deletion) occurs only on the basis of a *trans* distribution; hence, a mating between two individuals with the African variety of α-thalassemia trait produces offspring with only two α genes deleted (α-thalassemia minor). A mating between two individuals of Asian descent who have α-thalassemia minor may produce an offspring with all four genes deleted (hemoglobin Bart disease). The implication of a diagnosis of α-thalassemia trait in individuals of African descent relates only to its confusion with iron deficiency. There are no serious genetic implications. Asians must be appropriately guided regarding the potential for transmission of serious hematologic disease if a mating between two individuals with α-thalassemia occurs.

Lead Poisoning. The occurrence of elevated serum and total body burdens of lead is a major public health problem, particularly in infants and young children from lower socioeconomic families living in old housing with lead-based paint. Elevated lead levels may decrease erythropoiesis because lead inhibits several enzymes along the path of protoporphyrin synthesis. Lead may also produce hemolysis.

Anemia is usually seen in association with lead levels of 60 to 70 µg/dL or higher. Anemia is mild, variably microcytic, and associated with prominent basophilic stippling of RBCs. Coexistent iron deficiency is common because both conditions are more prevalent in lower socioeconomic populations, and iron deficiency promotes increased lead absorption. The presence of mild microcytic anemia in children with mild to moderate lead burdens is usually due to concomitant iron deficiency. Lead chelation therapy is appropriate when lead levels are higher than 40 to 45 µg/dL. Additional features of marked lead toxicity include intestinal colic, lead lines in long bone radiographs, behavioral changes, renal tubular defects, and lead encephalopathy associated with increased intracranial pressures.

Anemia of Chronic Disease. In a wide variety of chronic inflammatory or infectious disorders, mild to moderate anemia may be present. The MCV is usually normal to mildly decreased. Chronic inflammation or infection impairs the transfer of iron from reticuloendothelial cells within the marrow to developing erythroid elements, which results in some degree of iron-deficient erythropoiesis, even though marrow stores of iron are quite adequate. Often the history and physical examination findings point to chronic illness, but occasional patients have no obvious manifestations of systemic disease. The presence of unexplained mild microcytic anemia should alert the clinician to the possibility of occult systemic disease. An elevated erythrocyte sedimentation rate is usually noted in patients with chronic inflammatory or infectious states. Anemia of chronic disease is characterized by no specific abnormalities on peripheral smear other than mild hypochromia and microcytosis. Serum ferritin level is often elevated as a result of the inflammatory state and is thus a poor reflection of iron status. Serum iron level and total iron-binding capacity are generally decreased, but the percentage of iron saturation is often within the low to normal range.

Rare Causes of Microcytic Anemia. *Sideroblastic anemias* are a group of very rare congenital (often X-linked) inherited diseases associated with impairment of protoporphyrin synthesis and variable microcytic anemia. The bone marrow examination demonstrates evidence of developing erythroid cells with excess iron deposited in mitochondria, which tend to form a circular appearance around the nucleus; hence the term *ringed sideroblast.*

Copper deficiency is another rare cause of microcytic anemia. Associated features include neutropenia and scurvy-like bone changes (periosteal elevation). Only under unusual circumstances, when prominent microcytic anemia is otherwise unexplained, should these rare disorders be considered.

Normocytic Anemia of Underproduction

When normocytic anemia of underproduction is identified in a patient, the key issue is whether anemia is occurring in isolation or is associated with other cytopenias (Fig. 48-5, Table 48-11; see Fig. 48-4). Normocytic anemia with an inadequate reticulocyte response and pancytopenia raises the possibility of serious primary or secondary bone marrow disease (see Table 48-11). The history and physical examination findings are often predictive of the presence of thrombocytopenia (easy bruising, petechiae, ecchymosis). Adenopathy and hepatosplenomegaly are suggestive of bone marrow infiltration caused by malignancy.

Acquired aplastic anemia is a rare disorder of childhood characterized by pancytopenia (neutropenia, anemia, thrombocytopenia) and a markedly hypoplastic bone marrow. Clinical manifestations may include pallor, fatigue, purpura, bleeding (cutaneous petechiae and ecchymosis, epistaxis, gingival oozing), and/or recurrent infection. The physical examination may reveal purpura and pale mucosa and skin. Adenopathy and hepatosplenomegaly are *not* features of this condition. The cause is often obscure but may be related to prior infection (hepatitis, Epstein-Barr virus), toxin exposure (benzene, other volatile compounds), or medications (chloramphenicol, anticonvulsants). Postinfectious, drug-related, or idiopathic acquired aplastic anemia is most likely mediated by immunologic mechanisms. The peripheral blood smear demonstrates normal-appearing RBCs, an absence of polychromasia, and few leukocytes and platelets. A bone marrow biopsy demonstrates hypoplasia involving all cell lines. Severe acquired aplastic anemia is most appropriately treated by bone marrow transplantation when a human leukocyte antigen–matched sibling marrow donor is available. Unrelated matched donors offer another possibility for bone marrow transplantation. If marrow transplantation is not feasible, immunosuppressive therapy, including antilymphocyte globulin, corticosteroids, and cyclosporine, has been used with variable success. Aplastic anemia should always be considered when anemia occurs in association with thrombocytopenia and leukopenia in the absence of adenopathy and hepatosplenomegaly.

Disorders associated with bone marrow infiltration, including *leukemia* and *metastatic malignancy,* often manifest with normocytic anemia of underproduction, thrombocytopenia, and either leukopenia or leukocytosis. Teardrop erythrocytes may be present in the peripheral smear. On occasion, the MCV is elevated. Many children with leukemia come to medical attention because of pallor, fatigue, and purpura. Limping and skeletal pain are also common with childhood leukemia. The physical examination often discloses pallor, purpura, adenopathy, and hepatosplenomegaly. Peripheral blood smear may show leukemic blasts. Bone marrow examination findings are diagnostic. Of childhood leukemia cases, 80% are lymphocytic (acute lymphocytic leukemia), and the remainder are myeloid. Modern chemotherapeutic treatment regimens have dramatically improved the long-term survival rates, so that more than two thirds of cases of acute lymphocytic leukemia are curable. Among some children with particularly favorable prognostic features, cure rates exceed 85%. Acute myeloid leukemia is a greater therapeutic challenge. Bone marrow transplantation, when available as an option, leads to a cure in about 65% of youngsters who have achieved a first remission. When transplantation is not an option, chemotherapy is curative in less than 50% of children.

When normocytic anemia of underproduction is isolated (unassociated with pancytopenia), several diagnostic entities must be considered. Mild anemia commonly accompanies *acute infections* (and inflammatory illness). Children are often incidentally found to be anemic several days to a few weeks after having childhood infectious illnesses, including viral upper respiratory tract infections, gastroenteritis, or undifferentiated febrile illnesses. Mild anemia has also been shown to occur 10 to 14 days after measles vaccination. Anemia reflects impaired erythrocyte production as a result of the bone marrow–suppressive and mild hemolytic effect of mediators of the immune/inflammatory response (including interleukins, interferons, tumor necrosis factor). Cessation of RBC production leads to a fall in hemoglobin concentration of about 1 g/dL per week. Mild anemia discovered during or shortly after acute illness does not necessitate an extensive evaluation; rather, a follow-up hemoglobin determination should be obtained several weeks later. Persistent anemia necessitates further evaluation.

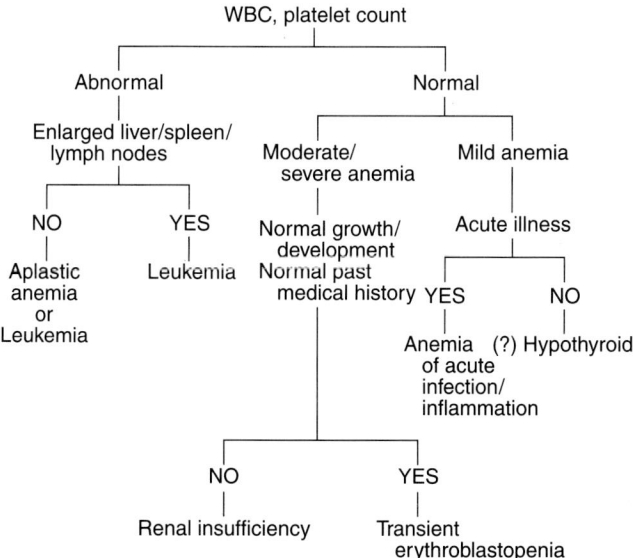

Figure 48-5. Diagnostic scheme of normochromocytic anemia of underproduction. WBC, white blood cell.

Table 48-11. **Differentiation of Red Blood Cell Aplasias and Aplastic Anemias**

Disorder	Age at Onset	Characteristics	Treatment
Congenital			
Diamond-Blackfan syndrome (congenital hypoplastic anemia)	Newborn–1 mo; 90% <1 yr age	Pure red cell aplasia, autosomal recessive, autosomal dominant or sporadic, elevated fetal hemoglobin, fetal i antigen present, macrocytic; some have thrombosis, short stature, webbed neck, cleft lip, triphalangeal thumb; late-onset leukemia	Prednisone, transfusion
Acquired			
Transient erythroblastopenia	6 mo–5 yr; 85% >1 yr age	Pure red blood cell defect; no anomalies, fetal hemoglobin, or i antigen; spontaneous recovery, normal MCV	Transfusion for symptomatic anemia
Idiopathic aplastic anemia (S/P hepatitis, drugs, unknown)	All ages	All cell lines involved; chloramphenicol, phenylbutazone, radiation	Bone marrow transplantation, antithymocyte globulin, cyclosporine, androgens
Familial			
Fanconi syndrome	Before 10 yr; mean, 8 yr	All cell lines; microcephaly, absent thumbs, café-au-lait spots, cutaneous hyperpigmentation, short stature; chromosomal breaks; high MCV and hemoglobin F; horseshoe or absent kidney; leukemic transformation; autosomal recessive trait	Androgens, corticosteroids, bone marrow transplantation
Paroxysmal nocturnal hemoglobinuria	After 5 yr	Initial hemolysis followed by aplastic anemia; increased complement-mediated hemolysis; thrombosis; iron deficiency	Iron, bone marrow transplantation, androgens, steroids
Dyskeratosis congenita	Mean for skin, 10 yr; mean for anemia, 17 yr	Pancytopenia; hyperpigmentation, dystrophic nails, leukoplakia; X-linked recessive; lacrimal duct stenosis; high MCV and fetal hemoglobin	Androgens, splenectomy, bone marrow transplantation
Familial hemophagocytic lymphohistiocytosis	Before 2 yr	Pancytopenia; fever, hepatosplenomegaly, hypertriglyceridemia, CSF pleocytosis	Transfusion (often lethal) VP-16, bone marrow transplantation
Infectious			
Parvovirus	Any age	Any chronic hemolytic anemia, typically sickle cell; new-onset reticulocytopenia	Transfusion
Epstein-Barr virus (EBV)	Any age; usually <5 yr	X-linked immunodeficiency syndrome, pancytopenia	Transfusion, bone marrow transplantation
Virus-associated hemophagocytic syndrome (CMV, HHV-6, EBV)	Any age	Pancytopenia; hemophagocytosis present in marrow	Transfusion, antiviral therapy, intravenous immunoglobulin

Adapted from Scott JP: Hematology. In Behrman RE, Kliegman RM (eds): Nelson Essentials of Pediatrics, 2nd ed. Philadelphia, WB Saunders, 1994, p 525.

CMV, cytomegalovirus; CSF, cerebrospinal fluid; HHV-6, human herpesvirus-6; MCV, mean corpuscular volume; S/P, status post; VP-16, etoposide.

Transient erythroblastopenia of childhood represents a temporary arrest of erythropoiesis, occurring predominantly in infants and toddlers, that is likely due to IgG antibodies that cross-react with early erythroid precursor cells. Patients present with pallor and fatigue, which occur gradually over several weeks to months. Because of the very gradual fall in hemoglobin level, most affected children are remarkably well compensated. Physical examination usually shows only marked pallor and mild tachycardia. Adenopathy and hepatosplenomegaly are *not* present. Congestive heart failure occurs only if anemia is very severe. The CBC demonstrates a normocytic anemia and profound reticulocytopenia. The WBC and platelet counts are normal in most patients; however, 25% of patients have mild neutropenia at the time of presentation. The peripheral blood smear is unremarkable. Recovery is spontaneous. Blood transfusion is indicated only for patients with severe, symptomatic anemia. Transient erythroblastopenia of childhood may be difficult to differentiate from congenital hypoplastic anemia (Diamond-Blackfan anemia), particularly in children younger than 1 year (see Table 48-11). In the latter condition, which represents a constitutional RBC aplasia syndrome, MCV and fetal hemoglobin levels are usually elevated for the patient's age.

The patient with previously undiagnosed chronic hemolytic anemia (sickle cell anemia, hereditary spherocytosis) may present with normocytic anemia and severe reticulocytopenia if *transient RBC hypoplasia* occurs on the basis of viral infection (most commonly with parvovirus B19). Because of a shortened RBC life span in patients with chronic hemolysis, a transient arrest of RBC production can cause severe anemia that evolves over several days.

Patients may have a history of neonatal jaundice and/or intermittent icterus, and they often have splenomegaly and an abnormal peripheral smear related to the underlying hemolytic disease.

Isolated anemia of underproduction occurs in children with *chronic renal disease* as a result of a deficiency of erythropoietin. Clinical and laboratory findings often suggest a diagnosis of renal insufficiency (poor growth, hypertension, edema, abnormal urinalysis, and elevated serum urea nitrogen and creatinine levels). The anemia of chronic renal disease can be successfully treated by recombinant human erythropoietin.

Macrocytic Anemia (see Figs. 48-1 and 48-4)

Congenital hypoplastic anemia (Diamond-Blackfan anemia) is a constitutional pure RBC aplasia syndrome that manifests during the first year of life with severe anemia and reticulocytopenia (see Table 48-11). The remainder of the CBC is otherwise unremarkable. Because synthesis of RBCs containing adult hemoglobin is markedly impaired, RBCs generally manifest fetal characteristics, including elevated MCV, increased levels of fetal hemoglobin, and the "i" surface antigen. Bone marrow aspirate demonstrates pure RBC aplasia. Two thirds of patients with congenital hypoplastic anemia initially respond to corticosteroid treatment; the remaining patients require long-term transfusion therapy. In patients who initially respond to steroid therapy, the anemia may become refractory over time. Bone marrow transplantation has been curative in selected steroid-resistant patients.

Fanconi anemia usually manifests with macrocytic anemia of underproduction and pancytopenia. It is a constitutional disorder frequently, but not invariably, associated with physical stigmata (see Table 48-11). Most patients do not present with overt hematologic manifestations until 4 or 5 years of age. Thumb and radial anomalies should alert the clinician to possible Fanconi anemia, even in the absence of cytopenias. RBCs tend to have fetal characteristics, including increased MCV and elevated fetal hemoglobin level. Patients usually respond initially to androgen therapy; however, mortality rates are high as a result of evolving resistance to treatment over time as well as a predisposition to myeloid leukemia and other malignancies. Bone marrow transplantation can be curative. Fanconi anemia is among the chromosomal breakage disorders wherein DNA is unusually fragile and susceptible to injury. The diagnostic laboratory abnormality is an increased chromosomal breakage when cells are cultured in the presence of a clastogenic agent, such as diepoxybutane.

Megaloblastic anemia (large RBCs with variable abnormalities of WBCs and platelets) caused by vitamin B$_{12}$ deficiency or folate deficiency is rare in children. In severe instances, pancytopenia may occur. In addition to large, ovoid RBCs, hypersegmented neutrophils (more than five lobes per cell) are often seen on the peripheral smear (Fig. 48-6). Platelets may be large. It is appropriate to suspect vitamin B$_{12}$ deficiency or folate deficiency in patients with otherwise unexplained macrocytic anemia. Documenting the presence of vitamin B$_{12}$ deficiency or folate deficiency requires an exhaustive etiologic search, including assessment of nutrition and gastrointestinal absorption. Nutritional vitamin B$_{12}$ deficiency may occur in breastfeeding infants of mothers on strict vegetarian diets that exclude milk and egg products.

Congenital pernicious anemia is a rare syndrome associated with vitamin B$_{12}$ malabsorption that is caused by gastric intrinsic factor deficiency. Children who have had resection of the terminal ileum, the site of absorption of vitamin B$_{12}$, may develop megaloblastic anemia. Vitamin B$_{12}$ malabsorption may occur with inflammatory disease involving the terminal ileum, such as Crohn disease or ulcerative colitis or in children who have had resection of the terminal ileum during infancy.

Unlike body stores of vitamin B$_{12}$, which may provide several years' reserve, folate stores are limited to several weeks' supply. Folate is ubiquitous in food sources; hence, nutritional deficiency is unusual.

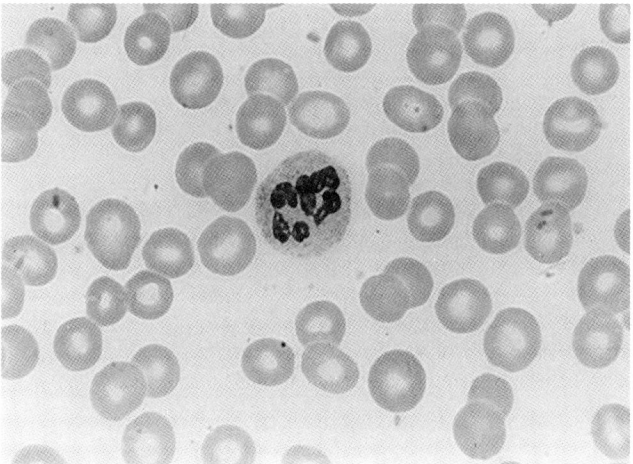

Figure 48-6. Hypersegmented polymorphonuclear leukocyte as seen in vitamin B$_{12}$ deficiency or folate deficiency.

Infants fed unsupplemented goat's milk may develop profound folate deficiency. Malabsorption of folate can occur in children who have limited small bowel absorptive capacity as a result of surgical resection or inflammatory disease. Patients with *chronic hemolytic anemia* (sickle cell disease) have an increased need for folate; they occasionally manifest folate deficiency if they are receiving no supplementation and endure a period of poor nutrition of several weeks' duration.

Anemia Caused by Increased Red Blood Cell Destruction. The *hemolytic disorders* (see Figs. 48-1 and 48-4) are characterized by shortened RBC survival and compensatory reticulocytosis. Usually, RBCs survive approximately 120 days in the circulation. New RBCs are manufactured at a rate equivalent to the destruction of senescent RBCs, so that under normal circumstances an appropriate hemoglobin level is maintained. Various factors, some intrinsic to the RBC, others extrinsic, can lead to accelerated RBC destruction. Several clinical and laboratory hallmarks are associated with hemolysis (Table 48-12). It is imperative that a technically adequate peripheral blood smear be examined whenever hemolysis is suspected. Although normal RBC structure does not exclude a diagnosis of hemolytic anemia, most hemolytic diseases are associated with

---

Table 48-12. Clinical and Laboratory Features Suggestive of Hemolytic Anemia

Pallor
Icterus
Splenomegaly
Gallstones
History of neonatal icterus
Positive family history of anemia, splenectomy, cholecystectomy
↑ Reticulocyte count
↑ RDW (due to ↑ reticulocyte count)
Abnormal RBC morphology
↑ Indirect bilirubin (normal direct bilirubin)
↓ Serum haptoglobin level
↑ Urinary urobilinogen level
Hemoglobinuria (+ dipstick test result for blood; no RBCs in urine)
↑ LDH level

LDH, lactate dehydrogenase; RBC, red blood cell; RDW, red blood cell distribution width.

Table 48-13. Hemolytic Anemia: Diagnostic Clues Based on Red Blood Cell Structure

Sickle cells: sickle cell disease
Target cells: hemoglobinopathies (HbC, HbS, thalassemia), liver disease
Schistocytes/burr cells/helmet cells/RBC fragments: microangiopathic hemolytic anemia—DIC, HUS, TTP
Spherocytes: hereditary spherocytosis, autoimmune hemolytic anemia
Cigar-shaped cells: hereditary elliptocytosis
"Bite" cells: G6PD deficiency
Poikilocytosis, microcytosis, fragmented erythrocytes, elliptocytes: hereditary pyropoikilocytosis

DIC, disseminated intravascular coagulation; G6PD, glucose-6-phosphate dehydrogenase; Hb, hemoglobin; HUS, hemolytic-uremic syndrome; RBC, red blood cell; TTP, thrombotic thrombocytopenic purpura.

morphologic abnormalities (Table 48-13). Depending on the cause of the hemolysis, RBCs may be removed from the circulation by reticuloendothelial cells (extravascular hemolysis) or may lyse within the circulation (intravascular hemolysis). In the latter circumstance, hemoglobin is released into the plasma and bound by the serum protein haptoglobin. In states of brisk intravascular hemolysis, haptoglobin may be depleted, and free hemoglobin may be filtered by the kidney and appear in the urine. Under such circumstances, the urine appears pink. A urinary dipstick test result is positive for blood, but the microscopic examination of the urinary sediment does not demonstrate intact RBCs.

Hemolysis Caused by Red Blood Cell Defects.
Disturbances of any of the three key components of the RBC—the membrane, enzymes, and hemoglobin—may lead to ongoing or intermittent hemolysis.

Hereditary Spherocytosis. The prototypic intrinsic membrane defect is *hereditary spherocytosis,* which is an inherited disorder (autosomal dominant or, in rare cases, recessive) occurring with a frequency of approximately 1 per 5000 live births. It is seen most typically in individuals of Northern European descent but may be identified in any population. The basic defect is an abnormality of a membrane protein (spectrin, protein 3, or ankyrin) that allows the RBC membrane to lose its redundancy and the usual biconcave disk shape, which results in a small, dense cell of spheroid configuration (see Fig. 48-2D). Hemolysis occurs because the spheroid RBCs are far less distensible and are unable to successfully traverse the microcirculation of the spleen. Characteristic clinical findings include anemia, reticulocytosis, and the presence of abundant microspherocytes on peripheral smear. Associated nonspecific findings of chronic hemolysis are often present, including pallor, icterus, and splenomegaly. The family history is often positive for anemia, splenectomy, or cholecystectomy.

Newborns with hereditary spherocytosis frequently develop jaundice within the first 24 hours after birth, often necessitating phototherapy and, occasionally, exchange transfusion. Diagnosis may be confirmed by an osmotic fragility test, which reflects the limited capacity of the RBC to expand when incubated in a hypotonic solution. The clinic spectrum of disease is broad. Some patients have mild, well-compensated hemolysis, and their condition is detected during their adult years after a diagnosis in one of their children. Other patients may have brisk hemolysis during infancy, necessitating intermittent transfusion support. Most patients have a disease course characterized by mild to moderate anemia, reticulocytosis, and splenomegaly. Patients are susceptible to exacerbations of anemia as a result of virus-induced hyperhemolysis or transient RBC hypoplasia. Parvovirus B19 may cause superimposed transient RBC hypoplasia of about 1 week's duration, resulting in moderate to severe anemia.

Splenectomy is performed in patients with moderate or severe disease. In patients who do not undergo splenectomy, gallstones nearly always develop as a result of chronic overproduction of bilirubin. When splenectomy is to be performed, it should be deferred until the patient is 5 to 7 years of age, except under extraordinary circumstances. The risk of potentially fatal postsplenectomy infection is markedly decreased if splenectomy is performed after the early years of life. Before splenectomy is performed, it is critical that all patients be immunized with the pneumococcal, *Haemophilus influenzae* b, and meningococcal vaccines. Preventive penicillin or amoxicillin therapy (250 mg twice daily) is recommended in all patients who have undergone splenectomy. Although controversial, antibiotic prophylaxis continued indefinitely is recommended by many authorities. Others recommend prophylaxis for 5 years and keeping antibiotics at home to be used for acute febrile illness while under medical supervision. After splenectomy, children who develop high fever should be evaluated for the possibility of bacteremia (usually caused by *Streptococcus pneumoniae,* less often by *H. influenzae,* meningococci, staphylococci, or gram-negative bacteria). Appropriate cultures and liberal use of empirical parenteral antibiotic therapy are indicated because a high fatality rate is associated with untreated bacteremia in splenectomized patients.

Hereditary Elliptocytosis. Hereditary elliptocytosis represents a heterogeneous group of inherited disorders characterized by variable chronic hemolysis and abundant elliptical RBCs on peripheral smear. The clinical and laboratory findings are similar to those seen in hereditary spherocytosis. Splenectomy is appropriate in patients with moderate to severe hemolytic disease.

Hereditary Pyropoikilocytosis. Hereditary pyropoikilocytosis is an autosomal recessive membrane disorder that manifests in the newborn period and is characterized by marked jaundice and anemia, reticulocytosis, and striking aberrations of RBC structure (see Table 48-13). Hemolysis lessens with advancing age.

Glucose-6-Phosphate Dehydrogenase Deficiency. The most common RBC enzyme defect is G6PD deficiency. An X-linked disorder, G6PD deficiency occurs most commonly in individuals of African and Mediterranean descent and should always be considered in the differential diagnosis of acute hemolytic anemia in boys. Deficiency of G6PD activity renders hemoglobin susceptible to oxidant insult, which leads to precipitation of hemoglobin, membrane damage, and, ultimately, RBC destruction. Oxidant injury may occur because of intercurrent infection or ingestion of various substances, including medications, toxins, and foods (Table 48-14).

The African variety of G6PD mutant, G6PD A, is not associated with chronic hemolysis but usually manifests as mild, acute hemolytic anemia related to specific precipitating factors. Rarely is hemolysis sufficiently severe to warrant transfusion therapy. Patients are often incidentally found to be anemic with evidence of an appropriate reticulocyte response. A peripheral blood smear may demonstrate "bite" cells as portions of the RBC (precipitates of hemoglobin) are removed by reticuloendothelial cells (Fig. 48-7). G6PD enzyme assay is necessary for the establishment of a diagnosis, but the test must be performed on a sample that has been depleted of reticulocytes because newly released RBCs have large amounts of G6PD. The Mediterranean variety of G6PD deficiency tends to be more severe and may be associated with chronic hemolysis, as well as with superimposed acute events caused by infection or medication, leading to symptomatic anemia and the occasional need for transfusion therapy.

Pyruvate Kinase Deficiency. Pyruvate kinase deficiency is an uncommon autosomal recessive disorder characterized by chronic hemolytic anemia. Patients may have anemia, reticulocytosis,

Table 48-14. Factors Known to Promote Hemolysis in Patients with G6PD Deficiency

Viral or bacterial infection
Fava beans
Vitamin C (large doses)
Mothballs (naphthalene)
Benzene and other volatiles
Medications
    Sulfonamides*
    Antimalarial drugs†
    Nitrofurantoin
    Nalidixic acid
    Chloramphenicol
    Vitamin K analogues
    Methylene blue
    High-dose aspirin
    Stibophen
    Niridazole
    Probenecid
    Dimercaprol (BAL)
    Toluidine blue
    Phenylhydrazine

*Sulfanilamide, sulfapyridine, sulfadimidine, sulfacetamide, sulfafurazole, salicylazo-sulfapyridine (Azulfidine), dapsone, sulfoxone, septrin.

†Primaquine, pamaquine, chloroquine (use with caution).

G6PD, glucose-6-phosphate dehydrogenase.

variable splenomegaly, and a peripheral blood smear that may demonstrate spiculated RBCs. Specific enzyme assay can be performed by specialized laboratories. Moderate or severe hemolytic disease often improves after splenectomy. Some patients require intermittent transfusion support. Iron overload out of proportion to transfusion needs can result from intestinal iron hyperabsorption (stimulated by brisk erythroid bone marrow activity).

Hemoglobinopathies. Hemoglobinopathies usually occur as a result of a single amino acid substitution in the globin chain. Hemoglobinopathies are among the most common causes of chronic hemolytic disease. Sickle cell syndromes are the most frequently encountered disorders of hemoglobin.

Sickle Hemoglobinopathy Syndromes

The sickle hemoglobinopathy syndromes are a group of genetically determined disorders encountered most frequently in individuals of Central African descent and should be considered in the differential diagnosis of anemia in any African-American child. These disorders occur less frequently in individuals of Mediterranean or Arabic background.

Sickle cell anemia (SS disease) is an autosomal recessive disorder characterized by a single amino acid substitution of the β globin chain (valine for glutamic acid in the number 6 position). Sickle hemoglobin has a tendency to form insoluble fibers within the RBC on deoxygenation, which may ultimately lead to the formation of the characteristic crescent-shaped sickled erythrocyte (Fig. 48-8). Sickle hemoglobin may occur in the doubly heterozygous state in patients with hemoglobin C or β-thalassemia and give rise to a disorder generally less severe than SS disease. Approximately 1 per 400 African Americans has sickle cell disease.

Sickle cell trait (the heterozygous state) occurs in about 8% of African Americans and is rarely associated with clinical disease except under states of unusually severe arterial hypoxemia. Spontaneous hematuria may occasionally occur in sickle trait as a result of the induction of sickling in the extremely hypertonic environment of the renal medulla. Patients with sickle cell trait are distinctly *not* anemic and have a *normal* peripheral blood smear.

The diagnosis of sickle cell anemia is usually straightforward. Children are variably anemic with reticulocytosis. The peripheral blood smear demonstrates characteristic sickled erythrocytes (see Fig. 48-8). The hemoglobin solubility test (sickle preparation, Sickledex) result is positive in patients older than 6 months of age

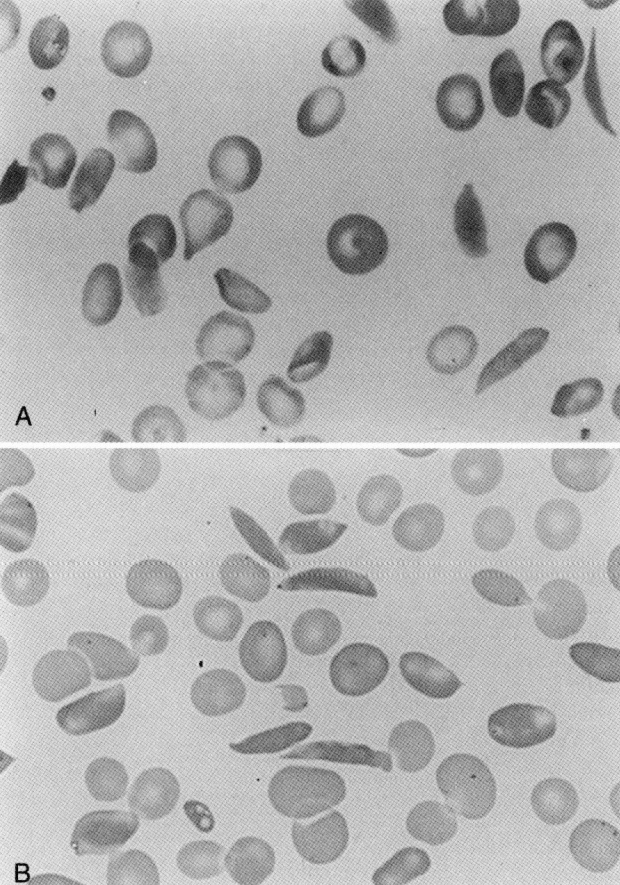

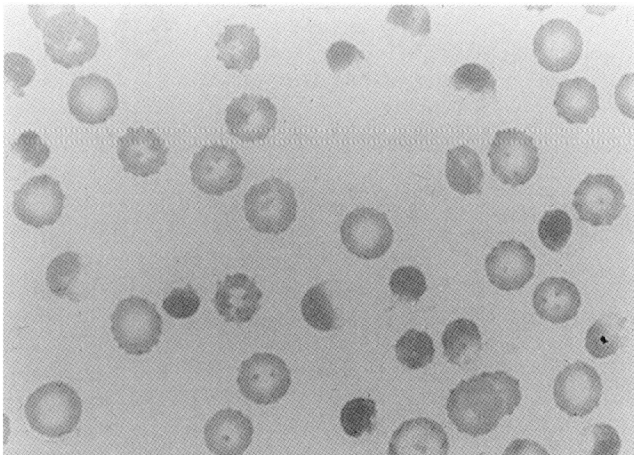

Figure 48-7. "Bite" cells and burr cells as seen in G6PD deficiency hemolysis.

Figure 48-8. Sickle cell anemia. A and B, Sickled erythrocytes and target cells.

Table 48-15. Hemoglobin Electrophoresis Diagnosis of Sickle Hemoglobinopathy

Disease	Hemoglobin Type
Normal	A
SS disease	S (*no* hemoglobin A)
S trait	A + S (about equal proportions)
SC disease	S + C (about equal proportions)
S–β-thalassemia	S > A (S predominant hemoglobin)

with sickle cell trait *and* disease. The definitive diagnosis must be established by hemoglobin electrophoresis (Table 48-15). Diagnosis in newborns is routinely and accurately performed in most locations within the United States as a component of state-mandated neonatal screening programs.

The clinical manifestations of sickle hemoglobinopathy include (1) chronic hemolytic anemia, (2) vasoocclusion resulting in ischemic injury to tissue, and (3) susceptibility to infection (Table 48-16). Infants younger than 4 to 6 months usually show no clinical manifestations, because of naturally high levels of fetal hemoglobin. By 1 to 2 years of age, most affected patients have had a specific sickling-related manifestation.

Patients may appear variably pale and icteric, depending on the degree of hemolysis. Enlargement of the spleen is routinely seen between 6 and 36 months of age in patients with SS disease and may persist into adolescence in some patients with milder variants (SC disease, S-thalassemia). Autoinfarction from microvascular occlusion ultimately leads to fibrosis of splenic tissue by age 3 to 4 years in most patients with homozygous SS disease. Maxillary hyperplasia and dental malocclusion occur commonly as a result of compensatory bone marrow expansion. Gallstones occur regularly and may lead to symptoms of cholelithiasis, acute cholecystitis, biliary tract obstruction, and/or pancreatitis. Many patients have delayed growth and pubertal development but ultimately achieve normal adult height. Exacerbation of anemia can occur as a result of infection-induced hyperhemolysis (in which case the patient may present with *increasing* jaundice, tachycardia, progressive anemia) or transient virus-induced bone marrow suppression (manifesting as progressive pallor, fatigue, tachycardia, and *decreased* jaundice). Hyperhemolytic episodes may also occur in male patients with concomitant G6PD deficiency. RBC transfusions are necessary when progressive anemia is accompanied by significant clinical symptoms.

The "painful crisis" is the most classic vasoocclusive manifestation of the sickle hemoglobinopathy syndromes. Pain most often affects the extremities, axial skeleton, or abdomen. The hand-foot syndrome (dactylitis) is characterized by pain, swelling, and erythema involving the metacarpal and metatarsal bones in infants and young children. Painful events are highly variable with regard to frequency and severity. Most events are unprecipitated; others may be related to infection, cold exposure, exercise, or trauma. Infarction of cortical bone may lead to localized extremity swelling, which may be difficult to differentiate from osteomyelitis. Abdominal pain may be confused with other intraabdominal processes, including appendicitis, cholecystitis, and perforated viscus. Sickle-associated abdominal pain (which may produce a rigid abdomen) often occurs in the context of skeletal pain, and bowel sounds are usually preserved, which helps differentiate the pain from that caused by an acute surgical complication. Chest pain may accompany pneumonia, pulmonary infarction, or fat embolus from infarcted bone marrow. Parenteral analgesic therapy is required when pain is severe (Table 48-17). Patients receiving parenteral narcotic therapy require careful monitoring of level

Table 48-16. Clinical Manifestations of Sickle Cell Anemia*

Manifestation	Comments
Anemia	Chronic: onset, 3-4 mo of age; folate therapy may be required for chronic hemolysis; hematocrit usually 18%-26%
Aplastic crisis	Parvovirus infection, reticulocytopenia; acute and reversible
Sequestration crisis	Massive splenomegaly, shock; treat with transfusion
Hemolytic crisis	May be associated with G6PD deficiency
Dactylitis	Hand-foot swelling in early infancy
Painful crisis	Microvascular painful vasoocclusive infarctions of muscle, bone, bone marrow, lung, intestines
Cerebral vascular accidents	Large- and small-vessel sickling and thrombosis (stroke); necessitates chronic transfusion
Acute chest syndrome	Infection, infarction, hypoventilation, bone marrow emboli, severe hypoxemia, infiltrate, dyspnea, rales
Chronic lung disease	Pulmonary fibrosis, restrictive lung disease, cor pulmonale
Priapism	Causes eventual impotence; treat with transfusion, oxygen, or corpora cavernosa to spongiosa shunt, local injection of α-adrenergic agents
Ocular	Retinopathy
Gallbladder disease	Bilirubin stones; cholecystitis
Renal	Hematuria, papillary necrosis, renal-concentrating deficit; nephropathy
Cardiomyopathy	Heart failure (fibrosis)
Leg ulceration	Seen in older patients
Infections	Functional asplenia, defects in properdin system; pneumococcal bacteremia, meningitis, and arthritis; deafness from meningitis in 35%; *Haemophilus influenzae* sepsis, *Salmonella,* and *Staphylococcus aureus* osteomyelitis; severe *Mycoplasma* pneumonia; *Escherichia coli* urinary tract infection; transfusion-acquired (HIV; hepatitis A, B, C, D, and E; EBV; CMV)
Growth failure, delayed puberty	May respond to nutritional supplements
Psychological problems	Narcotic addiction, dependence unusual; chronic illness

Adapted from Scott JP: Hematology. In Behrman RE, Kliegman RM (eds): Nelson Essentials of Pediatrics, 2nd ed. Philadelphia, WB Saunders, 1994, p 530.

*Clinical manifestations with sickle cell trait are unusual but include renal papillary necrosis (hematuria), sudden death on exertion, intraocular hyphema extension, and sickling in unpressurized airplanes.

CMV, cytomegalovirus; EBV, Epstein-Barr virus; G6PD, glucose-6-phosphate dehydrogenase; HIV, human immunodeficiency virus.

Table 48-17. Treatment of Severe Vasoocclusive Painful Crisis in Sickle Cell Anemia
Correct Dehydration
Maintenance rate plus correction for abnormal fluid losses and fever
5% dextrose in water plus ½ normal saline solution
No potassium chloride unless serum K⁺ < 3.5 mEq/L
Analgesics
Narcotics
Meperidine, 0.75-1.0 mg/kg IV, or morphine sulfate, 0.1-0.15 mg/kg IV, every 2 hr (*not* PRN)
plus
Nonsteroidal antiinflammatory agents
Ibuprofen or naproxyn sodium PO
or
Ketorolac 1.0 mg/kg (max, 60 mg) IV × 1 then 0.5 mg/kg/dose (max, 30 mg) IV q6h (*not* PRN)
Monitor
CNS: level of alertness
Respiratory status (respiratory rate and effort, pulse oximetry)
Vital signs (pulse, BP, temperature)
Incentive Spirometry to Prevent Acute Chest Syndrome

BP, blood pressure; CNS, central nervous system; IV, intravenously; PO, orally; PRN, as necessary.

of consciousness, respiratory status, and vital signs because narcotics may induce excessive sedation and/or decreased ventilatory effort, thus contributing to the development of the acute chest syndrome.

Acute Chest Syndrome

This syndrome represents an acute febrile pulmonary illness with new radiographic infiltrates with or without pleural effusions. Signs of respiratory distress may appear rapidly (within 2 to 6 hours) and include increased respiratory rate and effort, flaring, and grunting in association with progressive hypoxemia. It is unclear in most cases whether the primary event represents pneumonia, intrapulmonary vasoocclusive sickling, hypoventilation induced by narcotic analgesia or pain (splinting), or fat embolus, but local and systemic hypoxemia may promote further sickling with rapid expansion of infiltrates. The acute chest syndrome represents a major cause of mortality in children and adolescents and requires aggressive supportive respiratory care, broad-spectrum antibiotic (cefotaxime with vancomycin if resistant pneumococci are common in the patient's community, plus erythromycin) coverage, and, if symptoms are progressive, transfusion (simple or partial exchange) therapy. Many patients also respond to β-agonist aerosols (albuterol) and parenteral steroids, in part because asthma may be a common precipitant of acute chest syndrome. The incidence of acute chest syndrome may be reduced in patients with a vasoocclusive crisis by incentive spirometry to prevent atelectasis.

Acute Splenic Sequestration

This disorder results from vascular occlusion of splenic sinusoids, leading to the trapping of blood within the substance of the spleen. Rapid enlargement of the spleen and progressive anemia occur. Patients may present with severe hypovolemic shock. Infants and young children are susceptible to this potentially lethal complication before autoinfarction of the spleen occurs. Transfusion therapy is necessary for moderate to severe events.

Stroke

Stroke occurs in approximately 10% to 15% of patients with sickle hemoglobinopathy and may manifest with focal seizures, hemiparesis, gait disturbances, aphasia, or alterations in consciousness. Most strokes occur as a result of large cerebral vessel occlusion involving the carotid vessels. Subarachnoid and intracerebral hemorrhage occasionally occur in affected children. Patients with stroke require urgent evaluation, exchange transfusion and supportive therapy, and chronic transfusion to prevent recurrence. All children with sickle cell disease who have a seizure or focal neurologic symptoms or signs must be evaluated for possible stroke. Magnetic resonance imaging coupled with magnetic resonance angiography allows for rapid noninvasive assessment of brain and large cerebral vessel disease. An additional 10% to 20% of children have "silent" brain infarctions, presumably due to microvascular occlusion. Cognitive deficits are common in these children.

Priapism

Priapism, a persistent, painful penile erection caused by venous occlusion, occurs in teenagers and young adults and may lead to long-term impotence. In addition to analgesic and fluid therapy, local injection of α-adrenergic agents within 4 hours of presentation often leads to detumescence. Persistent priaprism may require exchange transfusion.

Infection

Infection is the leading cause of death in young children with sickle cell disease. Dysfunction of the spleen, beginning at about 4 to 6 months of age, renders patients susceptible to overwhelming infection (sepsis, meningitis) caused by encapsulated organisms, particularly *S. pneumoniae* and, less commonly, *H. influenzae* type b. Children older than 5 years of age are at less risk of infection, but when infection does occur, gram-negative organisms account for about half of all episodes. *Escherichia coli* urinary tract infections and *Salmonella* infections (bacteremia, gastroenteritis, osteomyelitis) are also observed in children with sickle cell disease. Osteomyelitis may also occur as a result of *Staphylococcus aureus* infection and should be suspected in the patient who presents with focal skeletal pain and fever.

Preventive penicillin (or amoxicillin) therapy (in patients younger than 3 years, 125 mg twice daily; in those older than 3 years, 250 mg twice daily) beginning at 3 months of age has dramatically decreased the incidence of serious infection and mortality. All patients with sickle cell disease who present with fever of higher than 101° to 102° F should be considered bacteremic until proven otherwise, even if they do not appear ill. Untreated bacteremia may rapidly lead to septic shock and death. Broad-spectrum antibiotic therapy (cefotaxime, ceftriaxone; vancomycin if penicillin-resistant pneumococci are suspected) to eradicate susceptible organisms should be promptly instituted pending culture results.

Prognosis and Treatment

The course of sickle hemoglobinopathy is quite variable; a small percentage of patients account for a disproportionately large number of complications. Mortality during the first decade of life has dramatically declined as a result of comprehensive approaches to care, which include neonatal diagnosis, extensive family education, preventive antibiotic therapy, and access to medical care providers who are knowledgeable in the treatment of this disorder. Newer treatment modalities are being investigated, including bone marrow transplantation, which is curative but carries a risk of morbidity and mortality. Daily oral hydroxyurea therapy, which increases fetal hemoglobin levels and alters red cell–endothelium interactions, leads to a reduction in vasoocclusive complications. Hydroxyurea should be considered in moderate to severely afflicted patients. The outlook for patients with sickle hemoglobinopathy has improved markedly since

1980. Among children for whom the condition is diagnosed in the neonatal period and comprehensive care is provided, the 10-year survival rate is higher than 98%. The doubly heterozygous states for sickle and hemoglobin C (SC) disease and sickle (S) disease with β-thalassemia represent sickling syndromes of a generally lesser degree of severity than SS disease. Severe complications do, however, occur in patients with SC disease and S–β-thalassemia (including sepsis and acute chest syndrome); hence, comprehensive care and aggressive therapy for complications are justified.

Hemoglobin E

Hemoglobin E is seen with considerable frequency among individuals of Asian descent. Hemoglobin E trait is characterized by mild anemia and mild microcytosis. There are no significant clinical implications. The diagnosis is confirmed by hemoglobin electrophoresis. When hemoglobin E occurs in the double heterozygous state with β-thalassemia, patients often have a moderately severe thalassemic syndrome; hence, genetic counseling is advisable.

Acquired Autoimmune Hemolytic Anemia. This condition is diagnosed infrequently in children and adolescents and may occur as a transient, postviral process or in conjunction with underlying immunologic dysfunction (immunodeficiency, human immunodeficiency virus [HIV] infection, lymphoid malignancy). Patients may present with pallor and, if hemolysis is brisk, with fatigue, tachycardia, and icterus. Splenomegaly is variably present. The degree of anemia is highly variable, and the reticulocyte count is elevated in most patients; however, a minority of patients present with a low reticulocyte count, because of immune destruction of reticulocytes. The peripheral smear demonstrates microspherocytes; results of the direct Coombs test are positive. Patients with autoimmune hemolytic anemia should be studied for evidence of immunologic dysfunction, infection, and malignancy (immunoglobulin levels, T and B lymphocyte counts, HIV and Epstein-Barr virus studies, chest radiography). The characteristics of the antibody types are noted in Table 48-18. Warm antibodies (usually IgG) may be idiopathic or associated with lymphoma, HIV or Epstein-Barr virus infections, rheumatologic disorders, or, most likely, a nonspecific infectious phenomenon. Cold antibodies (usually IgM) may also be seen in response to viral infections, to *Mycoplasma pneumoniae* and syphilis infections, or to autoimmune disorders. Aggressive therapy is appropriate because life-threatening hemolysis is known to occur. If no underlying disease is uncovered, corticosteroids (prednisone, 2 mg/kg/day in divided doses) should be administered, and the patient should be observed closely. Intravenous immunoglobulin (1 to 2 g/kg) and high-dose steroids (methylprednisolone, 30 mg/kg intravenously to a

1-g maximum dose) should be considered in severe cases. Recombinant antibodies directed to B lymphocytes have been effective in refractory cases. Transfusion therapy is used only if absolutely necessary, because cross-matching of blood may be difficult.

ANEMIA IN THE NEONATE

It is appropriate to view neonatal anemia in the context of three possible pathophysiologic pathways (Table 48-19): (1) acute blood loss, (2) anemia of underproduction, and (3) anemia associated with increased destruction. Familial genetic disorders may manifest in the neonatal period or any time during infancy (Table 48-20).

The full-term infant has a normal hemoglobin value (hemoglobin, 15 to 21 g/dL; hematocrit, 45% to 65%) that is substantially higher than that in older infants and young children. This finding represents a functional adaptation to the relatively hypoxic in utero environment. The reticulocyte count is elevated to about 7% to 8% during the first 3 days of life, after which there is an abrupt cessation of erythropoiesis until 2 months of age, when a physiologic hemoglobin nadir of about 9.5 to 10 g/dL is reached. This physiologic anemia of infancy is exaggerated in preterm infants, whose hemoglobin levels may fall to approximately 7 g/dL at about 1 to 1.5 months of age. This fall in hemoglobin value represents a physiologic response to the oxygen-rich extrauterine environment.

NEONATAL ANEMIA CAUSED BY BLOOD LOSS

Anemia caused by blood loss is often obvious. It occurs in placenta previa, abruptio placentae, or large cephalohematoma. Other instances of hemorrhage may be occult and include intracranial and intrahepatic hematomas. Internal hemorrhage is much more likely to occur in difficult, traumatic deliveries. Twin-twin transfusion may occur, leading to anemia in one infant and polycythemia in the other. Fetal-maternal hemorrhage, although common, is sufficiently severe to cause anemia in only a small percentage of neonates. The Kleihauer-Betke test may detect the presence of fetal RBCs in the maternal circulation but may yield false-negative results, particularly in mothers with type O blood who have antibodies against infant A, B, or AB blood cells. Fetal-maternal hemorrhage must always be suspected when otherwise unexplained anemia occurs in a newborn.

The time course and extent of blood loss determine the clinical presentation. If blood loss has been mild or chronic, infants may appear normal or may be somewhat pale and tachycardic. In the event of severe acute blood loss, the newborn may present with signs

Table 48-18. Characteristics of Antibodies in Immune Hemolytic Anemia

	Warm-Antibody Disease	Cold Agglutinin Disease	Paroxysmal Cold Hemoglobinuria	Drug-Related Immune, Type I	Drug-Related Immune, Type II
Antibody isotype	IgG (rarely IgA)	IgM	IgG	IgG	IgM, IgG
Optimum temperature of reaction	37° C	0° C	0° C	37° C	37° C
Direct Coombs test	IgG ± C3	C3 only	C3 only	IgG only	C3 only
Agglutination in saline	None (rarely +)	++++	+	0 to +	0 to ++ (with drug)
Lysis by complement in vitro	Rare	Poor	Well	None	Sometimes well
Clinical severity	Mild to very severe	Mild to moderate	Moderate to severe	Mild to moderate	Mild to severe
Response to prednisone	Often	None	Often	If needed	Not needed
Response to splenectomy	Often	Rare	None	Not needed	Not needed

From Disorders of red cells. In Andreoli TE, Carpenter CJ, Bennett JC, Plum F (eds): Cecil Essentials of Medicine (4th ed). Philadelphia, WB Saunders, 1997, p 389.

IgA, IgG, and IgM, immunoglobulins A, G, and M.

Table 48-19. Anemia in the Neonate
Blood Loss (common)
Placenta previa
Abruptio placentae
Twin-twin transfusion
Fetal-maternal hemorrhage (acute versus chronic)
Neonatal hemorrhage
Decreased RBC Production (unusual)
Diamond-Blackfan anemia
Congenital leukemia
Transient myeloproliferative syndrome in Down syndrome
Osteopetrosis
Hemolysis
Intrinsic RBC defect (uncommon)
Membrane (hereditary spherocytosis or elliptocytosis)
Enzyme (G6PD, PK)
Hemoglobin (α or γ chain abnormality)
Extrinsic RBC defect
Immune (ABO, Rh, minor group incompatibilities) (common)
Infection (intrauterine infection, bacterial, viral, protozoal)
DIC
Kasabach-Merritt syndrome
Galactosemia

DIC, disseminated intravascular coagulation; G6PD, glucose-6-phosphate dehydrogenase; PK, pyruvate kinase; RBC, red blood cell.

of acute illness, including lethargy, tachycardia, hypotension, and respiratory distress. The hemoglobin value is a poor index of the severity of acute blood loss because equilibration of fluid compartments may take 24 to 36 hours. Blood loss as a cause of anemia should always be suspected in cases of obstetric complications, multiple births, or difficult and traumatic delivery. In cases of severe blood loss, emergency transfusion therapy is appropriate. In the neonate who is hemodynamically stable but has experienced significant blood loss, a more conservative approach is recommended.

NEONATAL ANEMIA CAUSED BY DECREASED RED BLOOD CELL PRODUCTION

Anemia caused by decreased RBC production in the newborn is unusual. Infants with congenital hypoplastic anemia (Diamond-Blackfan anemia) are, at worst, mildly anemic during the newborn period. Congenital leukemia is a rare disorder characterized by infiltration of the bone marrow, leading to anemia, thrombocytopenia, and leukocytosis in association with hepatosplenomegaly and, occasionally, cutaneous leukemic infiltrates manifesting as blue papular lesions ("blueberry muffin" spots). Infants with Down syndrome may present with a clinical and hematologic picture identical to that of congenital leukemia, which is a transient myeloproliferative process that spontaneously remits over several months. Infantile osteopetrosis (marble bone disease), a disorder characterized by a limited ability to degrade bone, usually does not cause pancytopenia until a few months after birth.

NEONATAL ANEMIA CAUSED BY INCREASED RED BLOOD CELL DESTRUCTION

Anemia caused by increased RBC destruction (hemolytic anemia) places the neonate at risk for indirect hyperbilirubinemia as a result of the limited hepatic bilirubin-conjugating ability during the first weeks of life. Even relatively small increases in the rate of RBC

destruction can lead to marked increases in serum bilirubin level (see Chapter 20). All infants who have elevations of indirect bilirubin levels above the normal range during the first 3 days of life should be evaluated for possible hemolysis, with a hemoglobin level, reticulocyte count, peripheral blood smear, maternal and infant blood type assessments, and direct Coombs test.

Intrinsic disorders of the erythrocyte may manifest in the neonate. Infants with *hereditary spherocytosis* or *elliptocytosis* may develop anemia and extreme hyperbilirubinemia that necessitates phototherapy and, in some cases, exchange transfusion. A peripheral blood smear and the family history may be helpful in identifying an intrinsic RBC membrane defect.

G6PD deficiency can occur in newborn boys (rarely girls) of African or Mediterranean descent. Because of the increased susceptibility of neonatal RBCs to oxidant injury, anemia, reticulocytosis, and hyperbilirubinemia may occur without an obvious precipitating oxidant insult. *Hemoglobinopathies* rarely manifest during the neonatal period. β Globin chain defects, such as sickle cell syndromes and thalassemia, are not clinically apparent until about 4 months of age, because of the predominance of fetal hemoglobin in the perinatal period.

Severe α-thalassemia (hemoglobin Bart disease) can affect the fetus. Such infants develop severe in utero anemia, with resultant hydrops, because of the limited ability of hemoglobin Bart to release oxygen to tissues.

Isoimmune hemolytic anemia is the most common cause of anemia in the newborn. It is caused by incompatibility between maternal and fetal blood groups, including Rh, ABO, or minor blood group antigens. In Rh incompatibility, the mother is Rh negative and the infant is Rh positive (inherited from the father). If the mother has been exposed to Rh-positive blood cells through prior pregnancy, miscarriage, therapeutic abortion, or mismatched blood transfusion, immunoglobulin G antibodies may develop, which traverse the placenta and cause immune destruction of fetal Rh-positive cells. In such instances, hemolysis occurs in utero and in the neonatal period. In severe circumstances, the fetus may be extremely anemic, which results in heart failure, hydrops fetalis, and death. In less serious instances, infants may be born quite anemic and develop brisk hyperbilirubinemia, which can lead to *kernicterus* (bilirubin encephalopathy). The severity of Rh immune hemolytic disease increases with successive pregnancies. This disorder is uncommon, because of the routine practice of administering Rh immune globulin to Rh-negative mothers who are 28 to 30 weeks' pregnant and within 72 hours of delivery (and after spontaneous or therapeutic abortion). Prenatal management of the affected fetus may include spectrophotometric assessment of amniotic fluid as an assessment of fetal bilirubin level, and, in high-risk situations, serial fetal hemoglobin levels obtained by ultrasonographically guided aspiration of umbilical cord blood (cordocentesis). When the fetus demonstrates progressive in utero severe anemia, intrauterine intravascular blood transfusion therapy has been shown to decrease the risk of fetal demise. Management of the neonate relates largely to the severity of the hemolysis. Hyperbilirubinemia must be treated aggressively with phototherapy and, if severe, exchange transfusion. RBC transfusions are appropriate for symptomatic anemia.

On occasion, anemia is detected several weeks after Rh hemolysis and may be associated with a profoundly depressed reticulocyte count. This late anemia is of uncertain origin, but inappropriately low erythropoietin levels have been noted. Symptomatic infants may require transfusion therapy. Affected infants have been successfully treated with human recombinant erythropoietin.

Immune incompatibility in the ABO system is common and usually occurs when mothers whose blood type is O have newborns whose blood type is A or B. The degree of hemolysis is usually much less severe than in Rh disease. Fetal hydrops is extremely rare. Most babies with ABO incompatibility manifest jaundice (indirect hyperbilirubinemia) during the first 1 to 2 days after birth. Hemoglobin levels are often within the normal to mildly anemic

Table 48-20. Genetic Disorders Associated with Anemia

Syndrome	Genetic Characteristics	Hematologic Phenotype
Diamond-Blackfan syndrome	Autosomal recessive (AR); sporadic mutations and autosomal dominant (AD) inheritance have been described	Steroid-responsive hypoplastic anemia after 5 months of age
Fanconi pancytopenia	AR, probably abnormalities in multiple genes (at least five genetic subtypes have been identified)	Steroid-responsive hypoplastic anemia, some macrocytic red blood cells, shortened
		Cells are hypersensitive to DNA
Aase syndrome	AR, possible AD	Steroid-responsive hypoplastic anemia that macrocytic improves with age
Pearson syndrome	Mitochondrial DNA abnormalities, X-linked or AR	Hypoplastic sideroblastic anemia unresponsive to pyridoxine
Lethal osteopetrosis	AR, caused by defective resorption of immature bone	Hypoplastic anemia due to marrow encroachment
Congenital dyserythropoietic anemias (CDA)	AR	Type I: megaloblastoid erythroid and nuclear chromatin bridges between cells Type II: hereditary erythroblastic multinuclearity and positive acidified serum test results (HEMPAS) Type III: erythroblastic multinuclearity and macrocytosis
Peutz-Jeghers syndrome	AD	Iron deficiency anemia from chronic blood loss
Dyskeratosis congenita	X-linked recessive, locus on Xq28, some cases with AD inheritance	Hypoplastic anemia usually present between 5 and 15 years of age
X-linked α-thalassemia/mental retardation (ATR-X and ATR-16) syndromes	ATR-X: X-linked recessive, mapped to Xq13.3; ATR-16: mapped to 16p13.3, deletions of α globin locus	ATR-X: hypochromic, microcytic anemia, mild form of hemoglobin H disease ATR-16: more significant hemoglobin, H disease and anemia are present
Thrombocytopenia with absent radii (TAR) syndrome	AR	Hemorrhagic anemia, possibly hypoplastic anemia as well
Osler hemorrhagic telangiectasia syndrome	AD, mapped to 9q33-34	Hemorrhagic anemia

From Ohls RK: Evaluation and treatment of anemia in the neonate. In Christensen RD (ed): Hematologic Problems of the Neonate. Philadelphia, WB Saunders, 2000, p 153.

range, but moderate anemia occasionally occurs. The reticulocyte count is usually mildly elevated, and the peripheral blood smear may show microspherocytes. The blood types of mother and infant are different (type O mother with type A or B infant). Results of the Coombs test are usually weakly or moderately positive, but false-negative results do occur.

Treatment is generally directed toward hyperbilirubinemia and may require phototherapy. Intravenous immunoglobulin therapy has been helpful in some selected patients. Exchange transfusion is rarely necessary. Anemia occasionally necessitates blood transfusion.

Immune incompatibility may also occur on the basis of minor blood groups, such as the Duffy or Kell antigen systems. Clinical and laboratory findings are similar to those in ABO hemolytic disease, except that the direct Coombs test result is usually strongly positive.

Other causes of hemolytic anemia in the newborn include bacterial sepsis, and, less often, intrauterine infection (cytomegalovirus, toxoplasmosis, herpes, rubella, and syphilis). Intrauterine infectious syndromes can cause mild to moderate hemolytic anemia of several months' duration. Such infants may demonstrate physical stigmata, including small size for gestational age, microcephaly, chorioretinitis, hepatosplenomegaly, intracranial calcifications, and "celery stalking" of the long bones on radiographic study.

Microangiopathic hemolytic anemia can occur in the newborn as a result of *disseminated intravascular coagulation* (DIC). In the neonate, DIC is usually caused by serious infection, hypoxemia resulting from respiratory distress syndrome in the preterm infant, or ischemic tissue injury related to birth asphyxia. Newborns with

hemolysis resulting from infection or DIC are often extremely ill and require RBC transfusion support.

Microangiopathic hemolytic anemia and consumptive thrombocytopenia can occur in the *Kasabach-Merritt syndrome,* which is associated with *cavernous hemangiomas* and localized intravascular coagulation. Some infants have obvious expansive cutaneous and subcutaneous lesions, but occult visceral hemangiomas, particularly in the liver, can occur. The peripheral blood smear demonstrates evidence of RBC fragments and burr cells. Kasabach-Merritt syndrome may necessitate treatment with plasma and platelet transfusions (if consumptive coagulopathy is severe). Corticosteroids and interferon therapy have been helpful in some affected infants.

The diagnostic approach to anemia in the neonate requires a careful assessment of maternal, prenatal, and perinatal history, as well as the clinical status of the neonate (Fig. 48-9). CBC, reticulocyte count, peripheral blood smear, maternal and infant blood types, and direct Coombs tests are virtually always necessary laboratory studies. Other studies must be dictated by the clinical and initial laboratory findings.

SUMMARY AND RED FLAGS

Anemia is a common finding in children. A complete and thorough evaluation of clinical findings (history and physical examination) is the most important element in the establishment of a diagnosis and in defining appropriate therapy.

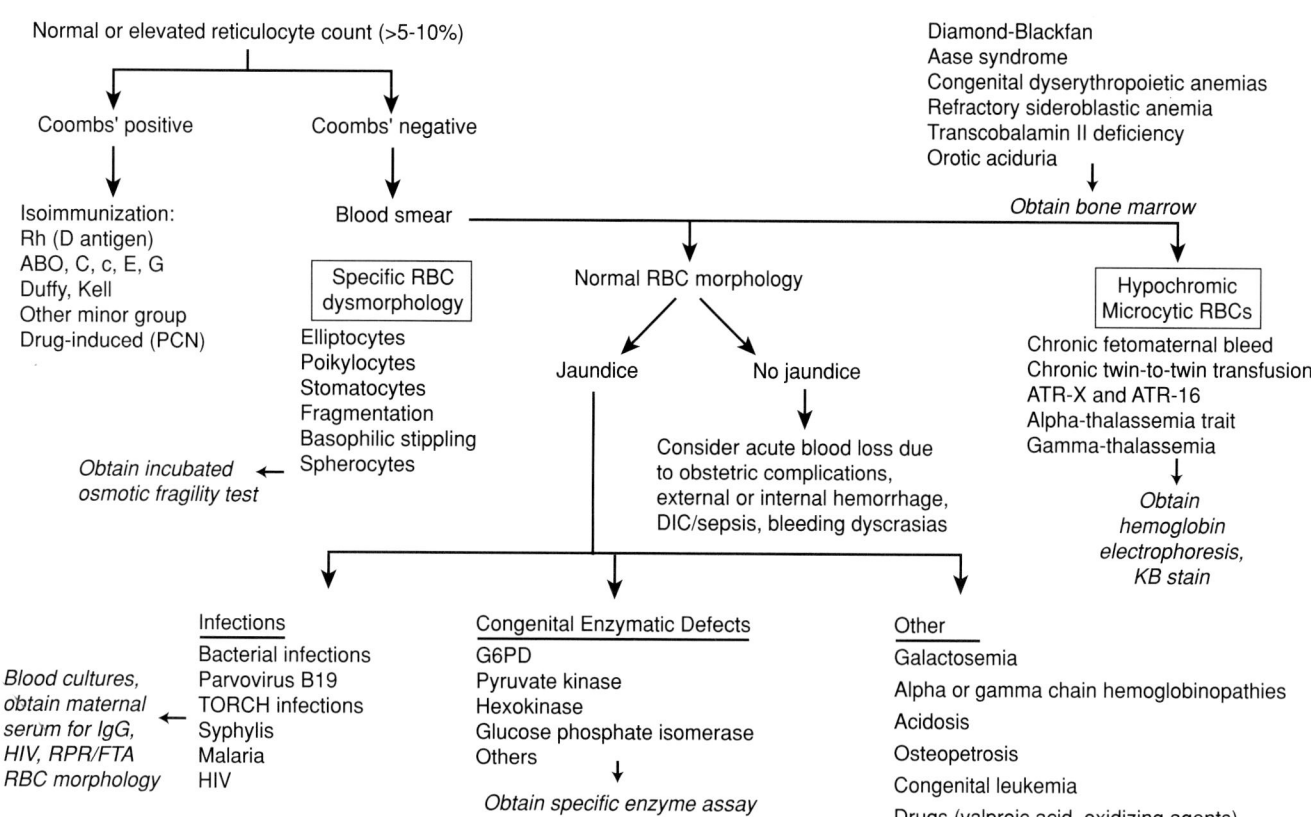

Figure 48-9. Differential diagnosis of neonatal anemia. The physician first seeks information from the family, maternal, and labor and delivery histories and then obtains initial laboratory tests: hemoglobin, reticulocyte count, blood type, direct Coombs' test, peripheral smear, red blood cell (RBC) indices, and bilirubin concentration. Results are used to navigate the diagnostic flow chart. ATR-16, α-thalassemia retardation syndrome, chromosome 16–linked; ATR-X, α-thalassemia retardation syndrome, X-linked; DIC, disseminated intravascular coagulation; FTA, fluorescent treponemal antibody test; G6PD, glocose-6-phosphate dehydrogenase; HIV, human immunodeficiency virus; KB, Kleihauer-Betke; PCN, penicillin; RPR, rapid plasma reagin test; TORCH, toxoplasmosis, other infections, rubella, cytomegalovirus, and herpes simplex. (From Ohls RK: Evaluation and treatment of anemia in the neonate. In Christensen RD [ed]: Hematologic Problems of the Neonate. Philadelphia, WB Saunders, 2000, p 162.)

Table 48-21. Red Flags
Anemia Accompanied By
Abnormal vital signs (tachycardia, hypotension, hypertension)
Neutropenia and/or thrombocytopenia
High MCV with normal RDW
Blasts on the peripheral smear
Firm adenopathy
Bruising or bleeding
Weight loss, failure to thrive
Shortness of breath, fatigue
Fever
Hypoxia
Organomegaly
Edema
Oliguria-anuria
Bloody diarrhea
Red urine (hemoglobinuria)
Family history of anemia

MCV, mean corpuscular volume; RDW, red blood cell distribution width.

Anemia may be a primary event reflecting intrinsic hematologic disease, or it may be a manifestation of a wide variety of disorders involving virtually any organ system. Anemia must always be fully evaluated, in view of the potential diagnostic and therapeutic implications. Patients who appear acutely ill should have a more thorough and prompt evaluation because acute blood loss must be treated quickly. If acute blood loss is not suspected, acute hemolysis or splenic sequestration of RBCs must be considered.

Anemia is often a sign of underlying acute or chronic disease. In such cases, anemia is not usually an isolated finding. Therefore, symptoms such as shortness of breath, extreme pallor, weight loss, fevers, lethargy, and fatigue should prompt a thorough evaluation of the patient.

On physical examination, the findings of abnormal vital signs, failure to thrive, bleeding or bruising, adenopathy, or organomegaly should lead the examiner to suspect that a potentially serious underlying disorder is present (Table 48-21).

When a CBC is obtained, a low hemoglobin value accompanied by any abnormality of MCV, WBC, or platelet count should be taken seriously and should be more thoroughly investigated.

REFERENCES

Workup of Anemia

Bessman JD, Jilmer PR, Gardner FH: Classification of red cell disorders by MCV and RDW. Am J Clin Pathol 1983;80:322.

Hermiston ML, Mentzer WC: A practical appproach to the evalution of the anemic child. Pediatr Clin North Am 2002;49:877.

Hoffman R, Benz EJ, Shattil SJ, et al: Hematology: Basic Principles and Practice, 3rd ed. New York, Churchill Livingstone, 2000.

Kline NE: A practical approach to the child with anemia. J Pediatr Health Care 1996;10:99.

Kohli-Kumar M: Screening for anemia in children: AAP recommendations—a critique. Pediatrics 2001;108:E56.

Nathan DG, Orkin SH, Ginsburg D, Look AT: Nathan and Oski's Hematology of Infancy and Childhood, 6th ed. Philadelphia, Saunders, 2003.

Novak RW: Red blood cell distribution within pediatric microcytic anemias. Pediatrics 1987;80:251.

Segel GB, Hirsh MG, Feig SA: Managing anemia in a pediatric office practice: Part 1. Pediatr Rev 2002;23:75.

Segel GB, Hirsh MG, Feig SA: Managing anemia in a pediatric office practice: Part 2. Pediatr Rev 2002;2:111.

Walters MC, Abelson HT: Interpretation of the complete blood count. Pediatr Clin North Am 1996;43:599.

Anemia with Acute and Chronic Disease

Abshire TC: The anemia of inflammation. A common cause of childhood anemia. Pediatr Clin North Am 1996;43:623.

Cowin HL, Krantz SB: Anemia of the critically ill: "Acute" anemia of chronic disease. Crit Care Med 2000;28:3098.

Fitzsimons EJ, Brock JH: The anaemia of chronic disease. BMJ 2001;322:811.

Means RT Jr: Advances in the anemia of chronic disease. Int J Hematol 1999;70:7.

Hemolytic Anemia

Beutler E: Glucose-6-phosphate dehydrogenase deficiency. N Engl J Med 1991;324:169.

Davidson RN, Wall RA: Prevention and management of infections in patients without a spleen. Clin Microbiol Infect 2001;7:657.

Lynch AM, Kapila R: Overwhelming postsplenectomy infection. Infect Dis Clin North Am 1996;10:693.

Sackey K: Hemolytic anemia: Part 1. Pediatr Rev 1999;20:152.

Sackey K: Hemolytic anemia: Part 2. Pediatr Rev 1999;20:204.

Trivedi DH, Bussel JB: Immunohematologic disorders. J Allergy Clin Immunol 2003:S669.

Hypoplastic Anemia

Cherrick I, Karayalcin G, Lanzkowsky P: Transient erythroblastopenia of childhood. Prospective study of fifty patients. Am J Pediatr Hematol Oncol 1994;16:320.

DaCosta L, Thiebant-Noel W, Fixler J, et al: Diamond-Blackfan anemia. Curr Opin Pediatr 2001;13:10.

Farhi DC, Luebbers EL, Rosenthal NS: Bone marrow biopsy findings in childhood anemia: Prevalence of transient erythroblastopenia of childhood. Arch Pathol Lab Med 1998;122:638.

Krijanovski OI, Sieff CA: Diamond-Blackfan anemia. Hematol Oncol Clin North Am 1997;11:1061.

Iron Deficiency

Abelson HT: Complexities in recognizing and treating iron deficiency anemia. Arch Pediatr Adolesc Med 2001;155:332.

Alter BP: Bone marrow failure syndromes in children. Pediatr Clin North Am 2002;49:973.

American Academy of Pediatrics Committee on Nutrition: Iron fortification of infant formulas. Pediatrics 1999;104:119.

Bogen DL, Duggan AK, Dover GJ, et al: Screening for iron deficiency anemia by dietary history in a high-risk population. Pediatrics 2000;105:1254.

Cheng TL: Iron deficiency anemia. Pediatr Rev 1998;19:321.

Kwiatkowski JL, West TB, Heidary N, et al: Severe iron deficiency anemia in young children. J Pediatr 1999;135:514.

Lozoff B, Wolf AW, Jimenez E: Iron-deficiency anemia and infant development: Effects of extended oral iron therapy. J Pediatr 1996;129:382.

Walters T, Pino P, Pizarro F, Lozoff B: Prevention of iron deficiency anemia: Comparison of high and low iron formulas in healthy infants after six months of life. J Pediatr 1998;132:635.

Wharton BA: Iron deficiency in children: Detection and prevention. Br J Haematol 1999;106:270.

Sickle Cell Disease

Fixler J, Styles L: Sickle cell disease. Pediatr Clin North Am 2002;49:1193.

Kinney TR, Sleeper LA, Wang WC, et al: Silent cerebral infarcts in sickle cell anemia: A risk factor analysis. The Cooperative Study of Sickle Cell Disease. Pediatrics 1999;103:640.

Quinn CT, Buchanan GR: The acute chest syndrome of sickle cell disease. J Pediatr 1999;135:416.

Rucknagel DL: Progress and prospects for the acute chest syndrome of sickle cell anemia. J Pediatr 2001;138:160.

Schatz J, Brown RT, Pascual JM, et al: Poor school and cognitive functioning with silent cerebral infarcts and sickle cell disease. Neurology 2001;56:1109.

Section on Hematology/Oncology Committee on Genetics, American Academy of Pediatrics: Health supervision for children with sickle cell disease. Pediatrics 2002;109:526.

Vichinsky EP, Neumayr LD, Earles AN, et al: Causes and outcomes of the acute chest syndrome in sickle cell disease. National Acute Chest Syndrome Study Group. New Engl J Med 2000;342:1855.

Walters MC, Storb R, Patience M, et al: Impact of bone marrow transplantation for symptomatic sickle cell disease: An interim report. Multicenter investigation of bone marrow transplantation for sickle cell disease. Blood 2000;95:1998.

Wang W, Enos L, Gallagher D, et al: Neuropsychologic performance in school-aged children with sickle cell disease: A report from the Cooperative Study of Sickle Cell Disease. J Pediatr 2001;139:391.

Wethers DL: Sickle cell disease in childhood: Part II. Diagnosis and treatment of major complications and recent advances in treatment. Am Fam Physician 2000;62:1309.

Woodard P, Lubin B, Walters CM: New approaches to hematopoietic cell transplantation for hematological diseases in children. Pediatr Clin North Am 2002;4:989.

Yaster M, Kost-Byerly S, Maxwell LG: The management of pain in sickle cell disease. Pediatr Clin North Am 2000;47:699.

49 Neck Masses in Childhood

David J. Beste*

There are various paradigms for diagnosing neck masses. The dichotomous approaches are acquired versus congenital, inflammatory versus noninflammatory, and neoplastic versus nonneoplastic. Multifactorial approaches are based on anatomy, age at presentation, and historical and physical characteristics of the mass. Systemic features (fever, weight loss), airway compromise, recognizable clinical patterns of symptoms and signs, and the nature of progression of the mass also help determine a diagnosis.

The presence of a new neck mass in a child is stressful for the parents, for a child old enough to understand the implications, and for the physician. After noting a cervical mass, parents worry about the possibilities of serious infection, surgery, or a diagnosis of cancer. The physician who understands and acknowledges these concerns can better care for the emotional needs of the family while evaluating and treating the child.

Diagnosis of neck masses relies on pattern recognition. Important factors in pattern recognition of neck masses are (1) anatomic position (Table 49-1, Fig. 49-1), (2) presence of signs of inflammation, (3) associated symptoms (fever, night sweats, weight loss, upper airway symptoms), and (4) temporal development of the mass and symptoms.

HISTORY

Most often, a child presenting with an inflammatory mass has an obvious explanation. If a cervical mass is inadvertently found on physical examination, a redirected history (such as a prior or current sore throat) is necessary to elicit the cause.

The child's age provides some evidence for origin of the cervical mass. The presence of a mass in the neonatal period is most likely of congenital origin. Fibromatosis colli, branchial cleft or pouch anomalies (especially if a sinus tract is present), vascular and lymphatic malformations, or dermoids may manifest early. In infants and toddlers, the most common masses are cellulitic or abscessed lymph nodes. Hemangiomas enter their rapid growth phase, and some branchial cleft anomalies, pilomatrixoma, and lymphatic and vascular malformations become evident in toddlers. The incidence of malignant neuroblastoma peaks among children younger than 1 year of age. Children have a high incidence of lymphadenitis, but a rare chronic lymphadenitis may be a childhood lymphoma, whose incidence peaks among children younger than 14 years. Branchial cleft anomalies and thyroglossal duct cysts occur throughout childhood. The incidences of some rare malignancies, such as salivary tumors, peak during adolescence. Localized lymphadenitis is rare in adolescents, but mononucleosis is common and may be accompanied by generalized lymphadenitis and systemic features (see Chapter 47).

Table 49-1. Childhood Neck Masses Associated with Cervical Regions*

Submental
Lymphadenitis
  Viral
  Bacterial
Thyroglossal duct cyst

Submandibular
Lymphadenopathy
  Viral
  Bacterial
    Atypical mycobacterial
Lymphatic malformation
Submandibular gland sialadenitis
Kimura disease

Jugulodigastric
Lymphadenopathy, superficial cellulitis
  Viral
  Bacterial
    Abscess
Lymphadenitis, deep cellulitis
  Viral
  Bacterial
    Abscess
Hemangioma
Cat-scratch disease (superficial or deep)
First branchial anomaly
Kimura disease
Langerhans histiocytosis

Preauricular
Lymphadenopathy
  Atypical mycobacterial
Hemangioma
First branchial cleft anomaly
Parotid sialadenitis
Parotid neoplasm

Postauricular
Dermoid
Langerhans histiocytosis

Hyoid
Thyroglossal duct cyst
Dermoid
Lymphadenitis
  Viral
  Bacterial

Continued

---

*This chapter is an updated and edited version of the chapter by Robin E. Miller and Michael L. Nieder that appeared in the first edition.

Table 49-1. Childhood Neck Masses Associated with Cervical Regions*—cont'd

Suprasternal

Lymphatic malformation
Thyroid goiter
Thyroid nodule
  Cystic
  Solid
    Papillary carcinoma
    Medullary carcinoma
Hemangioma
Neurofibromatosis

Supraclavicular

Lymphatic malformation
Neuroblastoma
Vascular malformation

Posterior Cervical Triangle

Lymphadenitis
  Viral
  Bacterial
    Abscess
Lymphatic malformation
Cat-scratch disease
Neurofibromatosis

Midsternocleidomastoid

Second branchial cleft anomaly
Fibromatosis colli
Fourth branchial cleft anomaly

*In decreasing frequency (see Fig. 49-1 for location of each region).

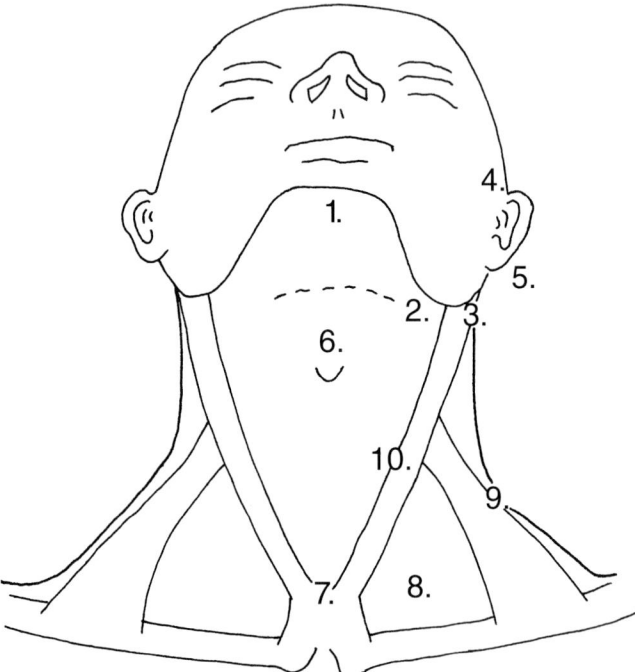

Figure 49-1. Regions of the head and neck. 1, submental; 2, submandibular; 3, jugulodigastric; 4, preauricular; 5, postauricular; 6, hyoid; 7, suprasternal; 8, supraclavicular; 9, posterior cervical triangle; 10, midsternocleidomastoid. (See Table 49-1 for neck masses associated with each region.)

The character and duration of any prodromal illness is important because most childhood neck masses are usually inflammatory from local head and neck lesions, or they may be part of a more generalized illness. A history of localized pain, dysphagia, or swelling in the head and neck region and systemic manifestations of fever, cough, rash, or gastrointestinal symptoms need to be evaluated. Viral and bacterial upper aerodigestive diseases are a common source of cervical lymphadenopathy and lymphadenitis. Lymph node enlargement is the appropriate response to these infections, but a change in the size or character of the nodes, musculoskeletal symptoms, or new aerodigestive symptoms may signal a secondary complication involving the cervical nodes.

The rapid onset of an inflammatory mass in an otherwise previously healthy child may result from the secondary infection of a preexisting congenital lesion. Sometimes there is a history of a fullness, dimple, or small mass; these signs may be subtle or nonexistent. Congenital lesions such as hemangioma, lymphatic and vascular malformations, and branchial cleft anomalies may not become evident until infected. The rapid progression is surprising and draws immediate attention to the area.

A history of exposure to animals provides important information regarding tularemia, cat-scratch disease and some mycobacterial diseases. A history of travel to a developing nation may be suggestive of tuberculous cervical lymphadenitis. Ethnic heritage is important in the diagnosis of Kimura disease, and a family history of similar neck masses is invaluable for diagnosis of some syndromes.

A history of high fever suggests an inflammatory (autoimmune, reactive lymphadenopathy) or infectious origin. Malignancy or a granulomatous process should be considered when fever is accompanied by constitutional symptoms such as night sweats and weight loss. In general, slowly enlarging lesions are more likely to be benign.

Masses that are painless and that enlarge very rapidly are suggestive of malignancy, whereas masses associated with infections are sometimes quite painful. Presence of the mass since birth, a prior lesion in a similar position, or a finding of chronic drainage from the region is indicative of congenital cysts or clefts.

Recent upper respiratory illnesses (otitis, tonsillitis, pharyngitis) should be noted, as should any recent trauma or other infection in the head and neck region. A dental history can be particularly revealing because toothaches, bleeding gums, prior dental problems, and mouth trauma, with resultant odontogenic abscesses, are often associated with cervical lymphadenopathy. Information regarding all relevant exposures to illness, including tuberculosis contacts and travel history, must be sought. The patient and family should be queried about pertinent risk factors for human immunodeficiency virus such as intravenous drug abuse, high-risk sexual activity, and previous transfusions. Contact with cats, which serve as vectors for both cat-scratch disease and toxoplasmosis, should be identified. A history of pica could also be linked with toxoplasmosis.

A detailed review of systems can be extremely helpful. Symptoms such as palpitations, heat intolerance, or weight loss should be noted, because hyperthyroidism can result not only in midline goiter but also in lymphadenopathy (Table 49-2). Similarly, manifestations of hypothyroidism should be noted (Table 49-3). The age-related causes of hypothyroidism are noted in Table 49-4.

Symptoms associated with connective tissue disease (rashes, joint pain, and stiffness) are important to consider. Symptoms indicating extrinsic compression of the trachea, esophagus, or recurrent laryngeal nerve (vocal cord paralysis) must be identified, because progression of the mass could result in life-threatening airway compromise. In addition to pain, such symptoms might include dyspnea, orthopnea, dysphagia, or stridor.

Other serious conditions associated with neck masses include the various types of immunodeficiency syndromes. It is important

Table 49-2. Clinical Manifestations of Hyperthyroidism

Increased catecholamine effects	Nervousness
	Palpitations
	Tachycardia
	Atrial arrhythmias
	Systolic hypertension (wide pulse pressure)
	Tremor
	Brisk reflexes
	Hyperdynamic precordium
Hypermetabolism	Increased sweating
	Shiny, warm, smooth skin
	Heat intolerance
	Fatigue
	Weight loss with increased appetite
	Increased bowel movement (hyperdefecation)
Myopathy	Weakness
	Periodic paralysis
	Cardiac failure, dyspnea
Miscellaneous	Proptosis, stare, exophthalmos, lid lag
	Hair loss
	Inability to concentrate
	Personality change (emotional lability)
	Goiter
	Thyroid bruit
	Onycholysis
	Acute thyroid storm (hyperpyrexia, tachycardia, coma, high-output heart failure, shock)

From Styne DM, Sperling MA, Chernausek SP: Endocrine disorders. In Behrman RE, Kliegman RM (eds): Nelson Essentials of Pediatrics, 2nd ed. Philadelphia, WB Saunders, 1994, p 632.

Table 49-3. Symptoms and Signs of Hypothyroidism*

Ectodermal	Poor growth
	Dull facies: thick pale lips, large tongue, depressed nasal bridge, periorbital edema
	Dry, scaly skin
	Sparse, brittle hair
	Diminished sweating
	Carotenemia
	Vitiligo
Circulatory	Sinus bradycardia/heart block
	Cold extremities
	Cold intolerance
	Pallor
	ECG changes: low-voltage QRS complex
Neuromuscular	Muscle weakness
	Hypotonia with constipation, potbelly
	Myxedema coma (CO_2 narcosis, hypothermia)
	Pseudohypertrophy of muscles
	Myalgia
	Physical and mental lethargy
	Delayed relaxation of reflexes
	Paresthesia (nerve entrapment: carpal tunnel syndrome)
	Umbilical hernia
	Hearing loss
	Cerebellar ataxia
Metabolic	Myxedema (tongue, face, extremities)
	Serous effusions (pleural, pericardial, ascites)
	Hoarse voice (cry)
	Weight gain (in adolescent)
	Menstrual irregularity
	Arthralgia
	Elevated CPK
	Macrocytosis (anemia)

From Styne DM, Sperling MA, Chernausek SP: Endocrine disorders. In Behrman RE, Kliegman RM (eds): Nelson Essentials of Pediatrics, 2nd ed. Philadelphia, WB Saunders, 1994, p 631.

*Other features in infants and children: delayed bone maturation; long bone growth delay and epiphyseal dysgenesis; delayed dentition; elevated cholesterol; elevated prolactin; and, occasionally, "precocious puberty."

CPK, creatine phosphokinase; ECG, electrocardiogram.

to obtain a history of recurrent infections (thrush, sinopulmonary infections, cellulitis, recurrent cutaneous abscesses). A mass that becomes more painful with eating (and with associated dry mouth [xerostomia]), although found not only in patients with immunodeficiencies or autoimmune disorders, could represent infection of a salivary gland.

PHYSICAL EXAMINATION

The majority of pediatric cervical adenopathies can be examined adequately by examination and palpation during the standard examination. If the physical examination is limited, full palpation and inspection may not be possible without sedation or a general anesthesia. Persistence or returning at another time can be successful with some uncooperative children. When a child is cooperative, there are two intraoral techniques that are useful for an improved delineation of cervical masses: inspection (and palpation) of Waldeyer's ring and the bimanual palpation of the floor of the mouth.

Anatomic location gives a great deal of useful information about the causes of masses (see Table 49-1 and Fig. 49-1). As a rule, masses arise from tissue that is native to their location. Rests of ectopic tissue or metastases are rare. Moreover, a mass firmly fixed to an organ or structure is most likely to result from a neoplasm or

infection of that tissue. In children, extension of a mass to adjacent structures occurs infrequently.

DIAGNOSTIC TESTING

For any unusual case, discussion with the radiologist before diagnostic imaging provides better information to answer the clinician's questions. The radiologist can offer the best imaging modality for the patient's clinical situation, as well as focus the imaging technique to the likely pathologic process and reduce the procedure's duration. Computed tomographic (CT) scans are generally faster and thus less likely to require sedation for the child. CT scans are generally better in assessing bone involvement. Magnetic resonance imaging (MRI) is particularly good at assessing soft tissue involvement. However, MRI is more difficult because of the longer scanning duration, the physical constraints of the magnet, and the noise, all of which increase the apprehension of children. Experienced pediatric radiology and anesthesia staff can routinely overcome the obstacles associated with MRI.

Table 49-4. Causes of Hypothyroidism in Infancy and Childhood

Age	Manifestation	Cause
Newborn	No goiter	Thyroid gland dysgenesis,* panhypopituitarism, TSH deficiency, TSH unresponsiveness
	Goiter	Inborn defect in hormone synthesis (iodine trapping defect, iodine organification defect [peroxidase deficiency: Pendred syndrome], iodotyrosine deiodination defect, thyroglobulin synthesis defect)
		Maternal goitrogens, including propylthiouracil, methimazole, iodides, amiodarone, radioiodine
		Severe iodide deficiency (endemic)
1-10 yr	No goiter	Thyroid gland dysgenesis, TSH deficiency, TSH unresponsiveness
		Cystinosis
		Hypothalamic-pituitary insufficiency
	Goiter	Inborn defect in hormone synthesis or effect
		Hashimoto thyroiditis: chronic lymphocytic thyroiditis*
		Goitrogenic drugs
		Endemic cretinism (iodine deficiency)
10-18 yr	No goiter	Hypothalamic-pituitary disorders (neoplasms, eosinophilic granuloma, other granulomatous processes, therapeutic CNS irradiation, idiopathic)
	Goiter	Hashimoto thyroiditis*
		Inborn defect in hormone synthesis or effect
		Goitrogenic drugs (lithium, amiodarone, foods)
		Surgical after thyrotoxicosis or thyroglossal duct cysts

*Most common for age group indicated.

CNS, central nervous system; TSH, thyroid-stimulating hormone.

BENIGN NECK MASSES

ACUTE INFLAMMATORY/ INFECTIOUS CERVICAL MASSES

The most common benign neck mass is lymphadenopathy associated with a viral upper respiratory tract infection (see Chapter 47). Secondary bacterial lymphadenitis also commonly occurs after a viral infection. The area of primary infection determines which nodes are involved. The posterior cervical nodes are the primary nodes for the nose and nasopharynx. The oropharynx drains to the jugulodigastric nodes, medial and anterior to the superior sternocleidomastoid muscle. The posterior nasopharynx and oropharynx also drain to the retropharyngeal and parapharyngeal spaces. The anterior medial perioral area drains to the submental nodes, and the lateral perioral and intraoral areas drain to the submandibular spaces (see Table 49-1 and Fig. 49-1).

The parapharyngeal space, the deep cervical fascial space, is the least understood site of cervical lymphadenopathy. Deeply situated in the neck, it is not easily examined by visual inspection or palpation. It contains multiple lymph nodes, important vascular structures (the internal carotid artery and internal jugular vein), and important nervous structures (vagus, glossopharyngeal and hypoglossal nerves, sympathetic chain). The parapharyngeal space drains lymph from the lateral skull base, from as far laterally as the external auditory canal and as far medially as the nasopharynx. Its medial wall drains from the adenoids superiorly to the tonsils inferiorly. Inflammatory or neoplastic processes may cause lymphadenopathy in this space. The tonsil on the affected side can be deviated medially by the mass effect in a parapharyngeal space. Manifesting with jugulodigastric nodes, fullness, or a mass in the region of the parotid tail, parapharyngeal space infections are usually rather extensive before they are identified.

The retropharyngeal space is a potential outpouching of the parapharyngeal space, which may cause the posterior pharyngeal wall to bulge on the affected side. A swelling or an abscess in the retropharyngeal space cannot extend beyond the midline because of the median raphe. Moreover, the retropharyngeal space extends inferiorly to the mediastinum; therefore, infection in this space can progress to mediastinitis.

Viral and Bacterial Lymphadenitis

In viral lymphadenitis, a concurrent upper respiratory illness is usually present. The nodes reliably enlarge in the jugulodigastric and posterior cervical locations. The lymphadenitis usually produces only mild local inflammatory signs and is treated with symptomatic support, observation, and parental reassurance.

Bacterial lymphadenitis commonly occurs after a viral upper respiratory infection or a bacterial infection of the primary drainage site of these nodes. Bacterial lymphadenitis is recognized by the pronounced inflammation that it produces. Tenderness to palpation and severe overlying cellulitis are its hallmarks. The nodes are commonly in the superficial cervical fascial spaces. Early treatment with oral antibiotics during the cellulitic stage of lymphadenitis may prevent progression to severe cellulitis or abscess. Progressive local inflammation may signal abscess formation. Pointing—local skin erythema with fullness and subsequent necrosis with underlying softening and fluctuance—is a sign for incision and drainage of the involved nodes. Isolated superficial node abscess may still be treated on an outpatient basis after incision and drainage.

An infection with multiple nodal sites involved, severe systemic signs of infection, or deep cervical involvement warrants hospitalization and treatment with intravenous antibiotics. The presence of severe systemic signs or generalized cervical inflammation calls for early imaging. If the child has respiratory distress, tracheal deviation, or submandibular fullness with tongue elevation, emergency airway management may be necessary. If severe symptoms are not present, a 24-hour trial of intravenous antibiotic is appropriate. If fever or systemic or local inflammatory signs do not respond within 24 hours, CT imaging with contrast material is useful for evaluating the extent of involvement and establishing the presence of abscesses. Early consultation with the pediatric head and neck surgeon is essential.

Deep cervical infections and parapharyngeal space infections are relatively frequent but are not as easily identified on examination. Fullness and inflammation in the retromandibular area in association with jugulodigastric nodes and fullness of the affected tonsil without inflammation are signs of a parapharyngeal space infection. Torticollis or avoidance of neck rotation may be suggestive of isolated or combined retropharyngeal space involvement. CT imaging is not sensitive enough to distinguish between nodes with small abscesses and nodes with cellulitis or necrosis. A pediatric head and neck surgeon may help prevent fruitless surgery in this instance.

Mycobacterial Lymphadenitis

The most common mycobacterial cervical lymphadenitis is the atypical tuberculosis, resulting from either *Mycobacterium avium* or *Mycobacterium intracellulare* infection. Atypical mycobacterial disease usually manifests as an asymptomatic unilateral mass located anywhere from the preauricular area extending through the tail of the parotid to the submaxillary space. This area overlies the facial nerve trunk and its branches. These nodes are usually painless, nontender, and without warmth. Systemic signs of inflammation are usually absent. The infection begins with an increase in the size of the superficial nodes, followed by pointing until they adhere to the overlying skin. The skin becomes erythematous, and painless necrosis results in a draining fistula. The fistula itself may drain for many months before the infection burns out. On occasion, several nodes may enlarge, sometimes in different nodal areas. Individual nodes may progress through the stages of inflammation, necrosis, and fistula at varying rates. Evaluation by imaging techniques is not generally useful, because the nodes are usually superficial and readily palpable. Imaging should be used if the masses do not follow the typical natural history or if other symptoms develop.

Tuberculin skin testing is positive about 50% of the time. The diagnosis is usually made by biopsy, because cultures do not reliably demonstrate the organisms. Secondary infection by opportunist bacterial organisms may obfuscate the primary infectious cause. A mycobacterial RNA reverse transcriptase in situ polymerase chain reaction test to detect mycobacterial RNA in excised tissue may improve diagnosis when commercially available.

Cervical tuberculous lymphadenitis is rare in the United States but is still seen in developing countries. Any bilateral chronic lymphadenitis should be evaluated for cervical tuberculous lymphadenitis with tuberculin skin testing and a chest radiograph.

Cat-Scratch Disease

The usual manifestation of cat-scratch disease is a nontender papule that occurs 3 to 10 days after inoculation of the pathogen. There may be a history of scratches by or exposure to flea-infested kittens, which are the major reservoir of *Bartonella henselae*. Two weeks later, the papule develops, and regional lymph nodes become enlarged.

Available diagnostic testing includes indirect fluorescent antibody assay and enzyme immunoassay. Nodal aspiration specimens can be sent for polymerase chain reaction for *B. henselae* bacilli. Diagnostic imaging by CT scan or MRI may be useful for determining the extent of lymphadenopathy. Biopsies should be sent for Warthin-Starry staining. Although antibiotic treatment with macrolides is effective in immunocompromised patients, treatment is not thought to shorten the clinical course in immunocompetent children. However, surgical curettage of the necrotizing granulomas seems to shorten the duration of individual draining fistulas without the risks of extensive dissection in an inflamed neck.

NECK MASSES IN PATIENTS UNDERGOING BONE MARROW TRANSPLANTATION OR CHEMOTHERAPY

A new neck mass in a child undergoing chemotherapy or bone marrow transplantation is a major concern. Extension or recurrence of the primary malignancy, presence of an infection, or development of a lymphoproliferative disorder may alter the patient's prognosis and therapy; early diagnosis is essential. Early imaging evaluation by CT scan or MRI is useful for determining the extent of the mass and/or the nodal involvement. In immunocompromised patients, infections may manifest without the usual inflammatory signs and symptoms.

Bone marrow, lung, and visceral transplant recipients are at risk for Epstein-Barr virus infection, which causes post-transplantation lymphoproliferative disorder. This disorder has a high mortality rate, approaching 30% in some series. Cervical lymphadenopathy may be the presenting symptom, but tonsillar, adenoidal, and pharyngeal symptoms (i.e., sore throat, exudative tonsillitis, and airway obstruction) are uniformly present. Diagnosis is made by cervical node biopsy or tonsillectomy, with or without adenoidectomy. Adenotonsillectomy to relieve airway symptoms and discomfort can also provide a histologic diagnosis. Prompt recognition may enhance treatment with a combination of immunosuppression reduction, antiviral therapy, and, in resistant cases, chemotherapy.

KIMURA DISEASE

Asymptomatic, unilateral chronic cervical lymphadenopathy in Asian boys is suspect for Kimura disease. This benign condition is characterized by peripheral eosinophilia and elevated immunoglobulin E levels. Biopsies should be performed to rule out malignancy. Histologic specimens show a massive eosinophilic infiltration of the nodal architecture. This benign condition necessitates no therapy unless the adenopathy creates functional disability.

CONGENITAL MASSES

THYROGLOSSAL DUCT CYSTS

A midline neck mass between the submental area and the cricoid is suspect for a thyroglossal duct (TGD) cyst (Figs. 49-2 and 49-3). The incidence of TGD cysts is highest during the second decade of life, but they may appear from infancy to adulthood. These masses usually have a gradual onset with slow growth and rarely regress or resolve spontaneously. TGD cysts may also manifest with acute onset of infection or abscess. In these cases, drainage and culture for aerobic, anaerobic, and mycobacterial organisms are suggested. Empirical treatment for gram-positive skin pathogens is suggested until the culture results are available. A draining sinus often results from an infected TGD cyst.

The differential diagnosis for midline neck masses includes anterior hyoid lymph nodes and dermoid cysts. Anterior hyoid lymph nodes frequently have a source of the inflammation that drains to those nodes (acne of the anterior chin). These lymph nodes resolve after the inciting infection or inflammatory process resolves. Dermoid cysts are uncommon and do not vary in size. Often the exact nature of the lesion is not known until the time of surgical excision.

Diagnostic imaging is controversial. Thyroid scan or ultrasonography to document the existence of normal thyroid tissue is advocated by some authorities. Very rare instances of surgical excision of a TGD cyst have resulted in permanent hypothyroidism.

Surgical excision is the treatment of choice. Excision of the TGD cyst prevents the risk of infection and eliminates the rare occurrence of thyroid malignancy with the cyst. Infected TGD cysts should be treated with appropriate antibiotics before excision. Preoperative infections are highly likely to recur, resulting in further scarring and making resection more difficult and extensive. Infrequent recurrences may complicate an appropriately performed excision. Repeated wide local resection is then advocated in this situation.

BRANCHIAL CLEFT ANOMALIES

Branchial cleft anomalies may appear at any age from the neonatal period to adulthood. These masses are usually in the area anterior and medial to the sternocleidomastoid muscles. Although these

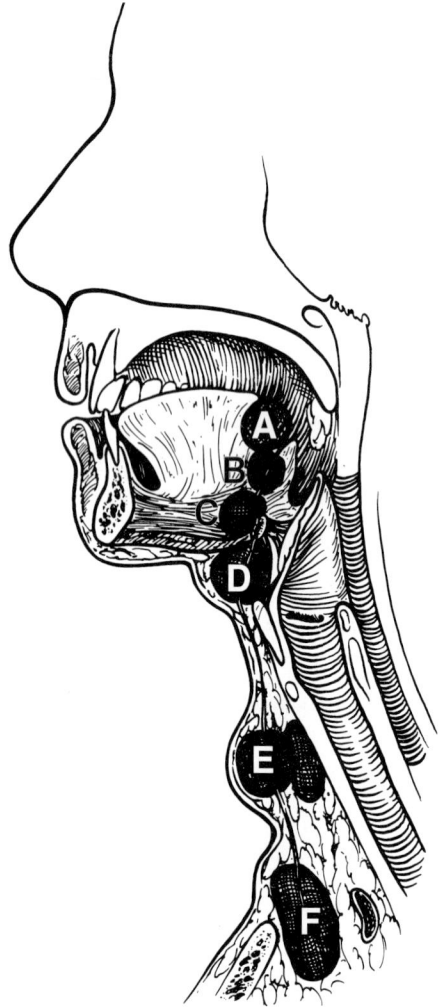

Figure 49-2. Thyroglossal duct cysts. These cysts can be located anywhere from the base of the tongue to behind the sternum. **A** and **B**, lingual (rare); **C** and **D**, adjacent to hyoid bone (common); **E** and **F**, suprasternal fossa (rare). (From Welch K, Randolph JG, Ravitch MM, et al: Pediatric Surgery. Chicago, Year Book Medical Publishers, 1986, p 549.)

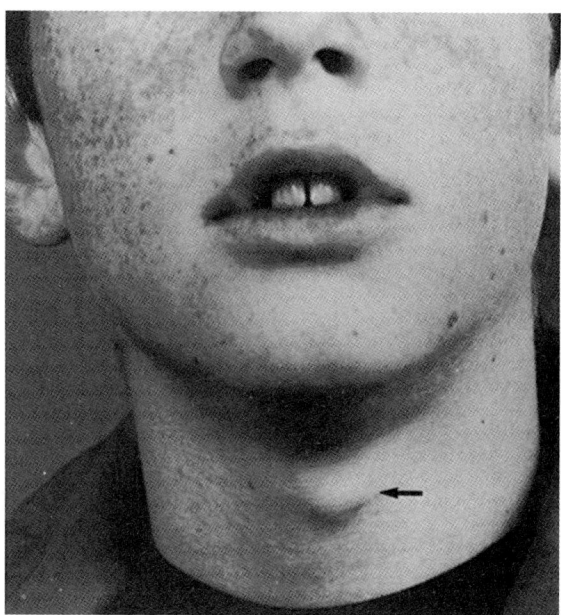

Figure 49-3. Thyroglossal duct cyst (*arrow*) located in the midline of the neck. (From Lusk RP: Neck masses. In Bluestone CD, Stool SE [eds]: Pediatric Otolaryngology, 2nd ed, vol 2. Philadelphia, WB Saunders, 1990, p 1298.)

anomalies are usually unilateral, second branchial cleft sinus or cysts are occasionally bilateral (Fig. 49-4).

First branchial cleft anomalies manifest with a sinus tract anterior or inferior to the lobule of the ear. Sometimes this tract extends as far anteriorly as the midportion of the mandible. These tracts usually end near the external auditory canal; they are thought to represent a duplication of the external auditory canal. They may have a fistulous opening in the cartilaginous canal or end blindly on the bony canal. A radiographic sinogram is not recommended as a routine evaluation because of the increased infection risk. Any sinus tract infection has the potential for facial nerve damage or paresis because the sinus tract is intimately intertwined with the facial nerve. Surgery is the treatment of choice.

Second branchial cleft anomalies may manifest as asymptomatic pits, soft cysts, inflamed masses, or draining sinuses. Sinuses may drain small amounts of mucous with upper respiratory infections or may drain regularly. Once infected, recurrent infections of the mass or sinus are the rule, because sterilization of this space is unlikely to occur.

When second branchial cleft anomalies are associated with familial hearing loss, preauricular pits, and ocular findings, a diagnosis of *branchial-oto-renal syndrome* is probable. This autosomal dominant disorder has variable penetrance; therefore, not all the syndrome components may be present in each family member. Genetic testing is available.

Second branchial cleft anomalies are uniformly located at the anterior border of the middle third of the sternocleidomastoid muscle (Fig. 49-5). The diagnosis is usually made on clinical grounds. The use of imaging modalities is rarely beneficial. Imaging can be very helpful when the anomaly is infected or is in an unusual anatomic location (Fig. 49-6). Sinograms are rarely beneficial and are invasive, and sedation or general anesthesia may be needed to obtain them. There is a risk of causing a new infection of the sinus tract, and dye may not reliably delineate the full extent of any tract.

The natural history of these lesions is to remain or grow until they are surgically excised. Unless a lesion is symptomatic, surgical excision is best deferred until an infant is at least 6 months of age. Delaying treatment of asymptomatic stable branchial cleft anomalies is reasonable, but intermittent examinations are prudent. A child with a minimally draining sinus may defer treatment until 5 years of age. However, growing cystic lesions and previously infected lesions are best expeditiously excised. The occurrence of squamous cell carcinoma in branchial cleft anomalies is very controversial and is not thought to be grounds for immediate excision. Recurrence rates of second branchial cleft anomalies are very low when the anomalies are completely excised. In all cases, the cyst should be excised with the entire tract to reduce the risk of recurrence.

Fourth branchial cleft anomalies are much less common. Manifesting occasionally as a lower cervical sinus, more often as a mass or cyst, and frequently as an acutely inflamed mass over the lateral thyroid, these lesions are more of a diagnostic challenge. Fourth branchial cleft anomalies have a high predilection for being left-sided. They may be confused with thyroid masses, lymphatic malformations, or second branchial cleft anomalies or confused with abscessed cervical nodes when infected. Involvement of the thyroid with abscess formation is very common and almost diagnostic.

The natural history of these lesions is to persist; a draining sinus or recurrent inflammatory masses often develop until surgical excision is completed. Diagnostic imaging by ultrasonography, CT scan with contrast material, or MRI imaging can be very informative. A discussion with the radiologist before ordering imaging can provide the most efficient use of these procedures, but multiple imaging

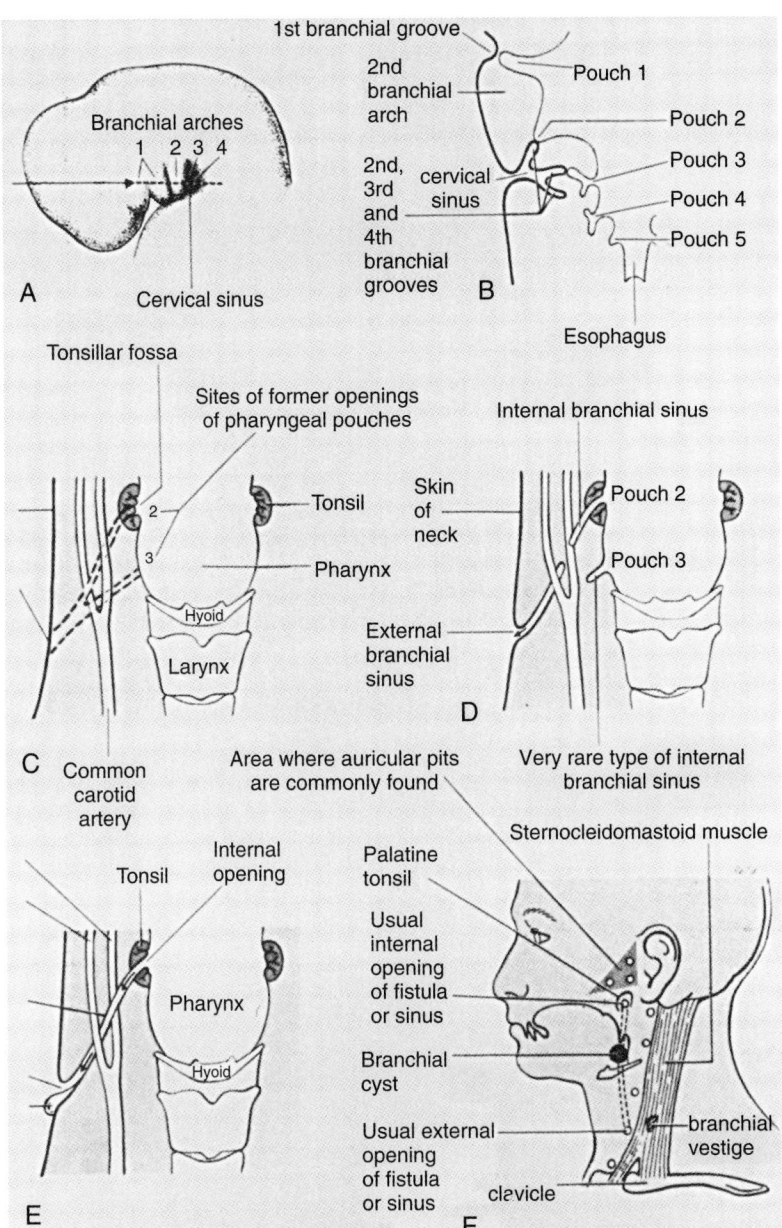

Figure 49-4. A, The head and neck region of a 5-week embryo. B, Horizontal section through the embryo illustrating the relationship of the cervical sinus to the branchial arches and pharyngeal pouches. C, The adult neck region, indicating the former sites of openings of the cervical sinus and the pharyngeal pouches. The broken lines indicate possible courses of branchial fistulas. D, The embryologic basis of various types of branchial sinuses. E, A branchial fistula resulting from persistence of parts of the second branchial cleft and the second pharyngeal pouch. F, Possible sites of branchial cysts and openings of branchial sinuses and fistulas. A branchial vestige is also illustrated. (From Moore KL: The Developing Human: Clinically Oriented Embryology. Philadelphia, WB Saunders, 1977.)

techniques may be necessary. Direct laryngoscopy often reveals a sinus originating in the pyriform sinus and is diagnostic.

VASCULAR LESIONS

Vascular lesions are a common cause of pediatric head and neck masses. They manifest as soft to firm, nontender masses that may be present at birth or may evolve gradually. Expansion to adjacent sites or multiple sites is common; lesions may involve not just the deep cervical organs but also the head or thorax. Airway symptoms or dysphagia necessitates evaluation for extension to the oropharynx, hypopharynx, and larynx or for secondary lesions in those areas.

Vascular lesions have been classified as vascular tumors (including hemangiomas) and vascular malformations such as capillary malformations, arterial and venous malformations, and lymphatic malformations. Vascular tumors are not present at birth but grow rapidly, whereas vascular malformations are present at birth and grow gradually at the same rate as the affected patient. Suspected vascular lesions can be evaluated with ultrasonography, which can distinguish vascular tumors from vascular malformations and lymphatic malformations. Although ultrasonography is useful for determining the character of the lesions, CT scan is useful for determining the extent of the lesions before treatment. MRI and magnetic resonance angiography are additionally useful for determining extent of the lesion.

Hemangioma

Hemangiomas manifest as firm, doughy masses, most frequently in the parotid area. They are compressible, but slow, constant pressure may be necessary to compress them. Hemangiomas occur three times more frequently in girls than in boys and grow rapidly over the first several months of life. A quiescent period follows, sometimes for years, and then involution usually begins. About 30% of hemangiomas involute by 3 years of age; 50% by 5 years; and 80% to 90% by 10 years. Some residual evidence of the lesion, such as thinning of the skin or subcutaneous fat, hypopigmentation, or scarring, usually remains.

Severe or "malignant" hemangiomas, which threaten life or organ function, rarely occur as isolated cervical masses but appear more

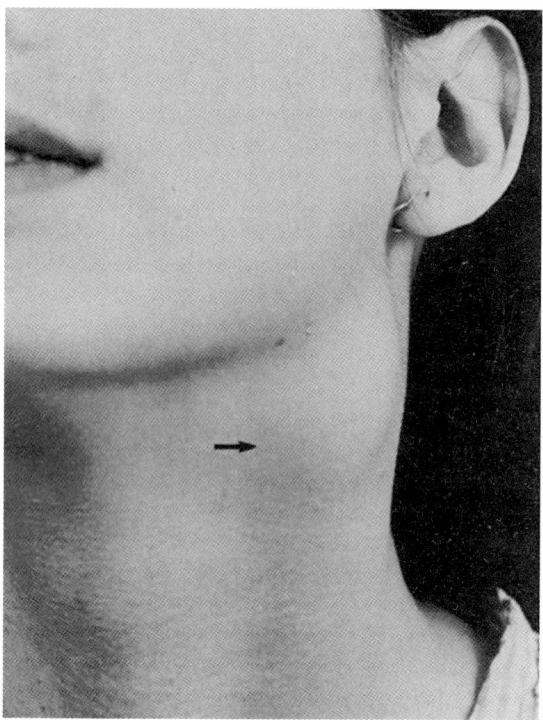

Figure 49-5. Branchial cleft cyst (*arrow*) along the anterior border of the sternocleidomastoid muscle. (From Lusk RP: Neck masses. In Bluestone CD, Stool SE [eds]: Pediatric Otolaryngology, 2nd ed, vol 2. Philadelphia, WB Saunders, 1990, p 1298.)

commonly in the face. Recurrent bleeding may occur with ulceration of a superficial cervical hemangioma. Corticosteroid therapy (prednisone) in the dose range of 2 to 3 mg/kg/day may be remedial for these lesions. Symptomatic cervical hemangiomas that fail to involute may be surgically excised, sometimes preceded by embolization. Additional therapies such as recombinant interferons alfa-2a and alfa-2b and interstitial neodymium:yttrium-aluminum-garnet photocoagulation are in the early stages of investigation. Flashlamp-pulsed dye lasers are effective for superficial cutaneous vascular lesions.

Stridor may signal another site of hemangioma, particularly of the subglottis. Evaluation by lateral soft tissue radiograph or by laryngoscopy is diagnostic.

Vascular Malformations

Vascular malformations may be categorized as low-flow lesions, such as venous and capillary lesions, and high-flow lesions, such as arteriovenous and arterial malformation. Treatment for high-flow lesions is usually embolization and excision. Low-flow malformations may be sclerosed, and subsequent excision may be necessary. Superficial cutaneous lesions and capillary malformations such as port wine stains respond well to flashlamp-pulsed dye laser therapy.

Lymphatic Malformations

Lymphatic malformations manifest as soft masses anywhere in the neck but most frequently in the submandibular triangle. These lesions are not usually tender but can be very painful when inflamed. The extent of cervical involvement varies greatly. Transillumination of the mass, although not diagnostic, sometimes provides differentiation

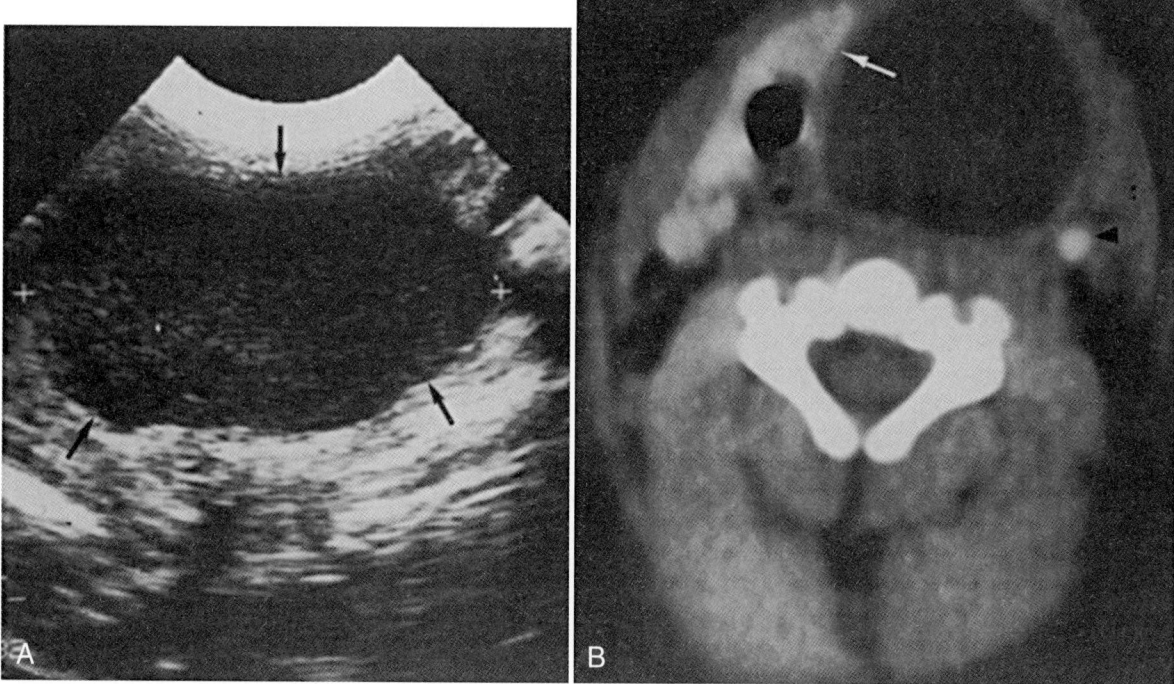

Figure 49-6. **A,** The longitudinal coronal sonogram of a 2-week-old boy with a nontender left-sided neck mass (*arrows*) that is uniformly hypoechoic with good through transmission. **B,** The computed tomographic scan reveals low attenuation of the mass anteromedial to the carotid (*arrowhead*) sheath. The trachea and the esophagus are displaced to the right. The epicenter of this branchial cleft cyst is inferior to the left lobe of the thyroid gland (*arrow*), which is elevated and displaced to the right. (From Lima JA, Graviss ER: Methods of examination. In Bluestone CD, Stool SE [eds]: Pediatric Otolaryngology, 2nd ed, vol 2. Philadelphia, WB Saunders, 1990, p 1290.)

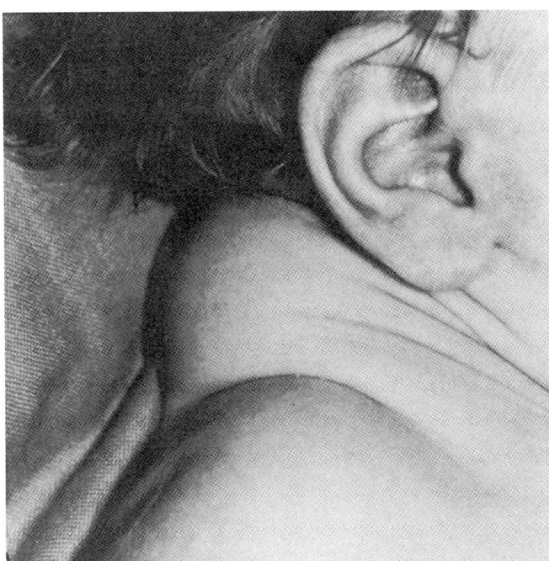

Figure 49-7. Lymphangioma of neck in a 2-week-old patient. (From Clary RA, Lusk RP: Neck masses. In Bluestone CD, Stool SE [eds]: Pediatric Otolaryngology, 3rd ed, vol 2. Philadelphia, WB Saunders, 1996, p 1494.)

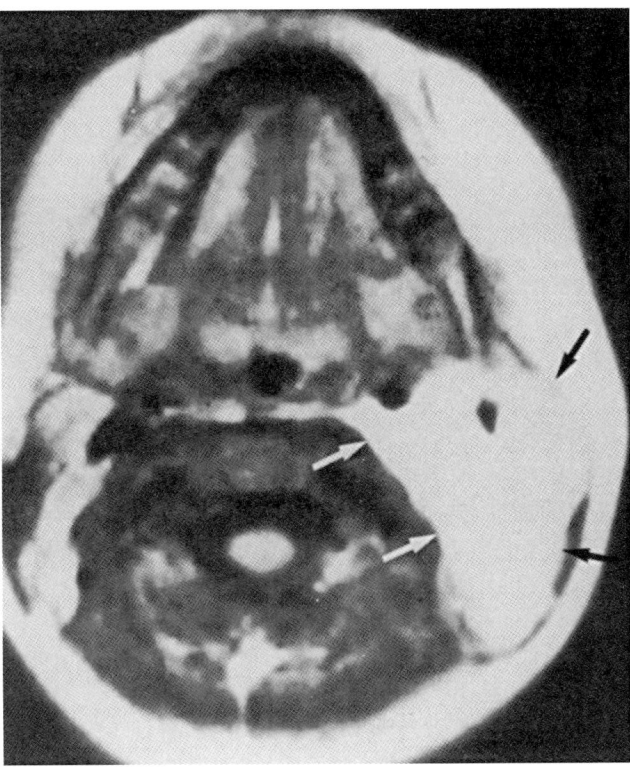

Figure 49-8. Magnetic resonance imaging clearly delineates the extent of the lymphangioma of the patient in Figure 49-7. *Arrows* mark the borders of the lymphangioma. (From Clary RA, Lusk RP: Neck masses. In Bluestone CD, Stool SE [eds]: Pediatric Otolaryngology, 3rd ed, vol 2. Philadelphia, WB Saunders, 1996, p 1494.)

from other vascular masses. Transillumination involves placing a light source on the mass in a darkened room; when positive, the entire mass seems to glow.

Lymphatic malformations do not have readily discernible margins because they are extensions of the normal lymphatic vessel anatomy (Fig. 49-7). The lymph vessels extend from muscles, organs, and nerves that form the lymphatic mass. Currently, these lymphatic malformations are described as macrocystic if individual cystic spaces are larger than 1 cm in diameter or as microcystic if the spaces are smaller than 1 cm. Cervical lymphatic malformations with very large cystic spaces are sometimes called *cystic hygromas.* MRI is the best imaging method for determining the type and extent of malformations (Fig. 49-8).

The natural history of lymphatic malformations is to grow slowly at the same rate as the surrounding tissues. Spontaneous regression is very rare. Infections may cause a previously asymptomatic cervical malformation to rapidly increase in size, causing severe airway compromise or dysphagia. Antibiotic coverage for the infection, corticosteroids, and careful observation in a critical care unit may be necessary, especially for neonates.

Benefits of surgical excision or sclerosis must be weighed against the risks of injury to the surrounding tissues. The resulting functional deficit may outweigh the benefits of surgical excision. Even after a successful surgical excision, surrounding smaller but abnormal and unrecognized lymphatic vessels can expand because of rerouting in the lymphatic flow. Within hours after near complete excision, the malformation can permanently or temporarily blossom to presurgical magnitude.

A staging system by de Serres and colleagues based on anatomic infrahyoid or suprahyoid disease was found to correlate with efficacy of excision and complications. Rates of complications, including cranial nerve injury, wound infection, seroma formation, malocclusion, speech delay, cosmetic deformity, and persistent disease, ranged from 17% in stage I disease to 100% in stage V disease.

OK432, a lyophilized low-virulence Su strain of group A *Streptococcus,* offers an improvement in sclerosis therapy with little damage to surrounding tissues. It is less effective with microcystic lesions, with lesions with massive craniofacial involvement, and in cases with previous surgery. Therapeutic trials are currently under way and seem promising.

SALIVARY MASSES

Inflammatory

Acute sialadenitis is rarely seen today because of mumps vaccination. When it is seen, it usually manifests with severe pain and inflammation of the parotid or submandibular glands. Acute bacterial sialadenitis (acute suppurative parotitis) is usually a complication of dehydration caused by another illness. Clinical diagnosis can be made from the localized inflammation, but bacterial culture from the affected salivary duct is confirmatory. Milking the tender affected gland can express purulent drainage for intraoral collection. *Staphylococcus aureus* is the most common pathogen. Treatment involves hydration, antibiotics, and sialagogues to increase salivary flow.

Chronic and recurrent sialadenitis in children is now more common than acute sialadenitis. The parotid gland is the most common site, and the disorder manifests with minimal inflammation and diffuse or localized parotid gland enlargement. Imaging by sialography is not necessary for diagnosis and increases the risk of an acute infection. Culture-directed intravenous antibiotic therapy has been effective against both chronic and recurrent parotitis. If the condition is chronically symptomatic with acute exacerbations, a superficial parotidectomy may be necessary.

Noninflammatory

Ranulas are mucoceles of the sublingual salivary gland. Appearing in the anterior submandibular space, the mass has ill-defined edges and is best evaluated by intraoral inspection and bimanual palpation. The clinician does this with one hand palpating the floor of the patient's mouth while simultaneously the other hand palpates the patient's submandibular space. Imaging with CT scan or MRI can be helpful, but differentiating a ranula from macrocystic lymphatic malformations can still be difficult.

Bilateral submandibular gland enlargement may result from cystic fibrosis or Sjögren's syndrome. Unilateral enlargement always raises the possibility of a neoplasm.

A salivary mass is more likely to be a carcinoma in a child than in an adult. Fifty-nine percent of salivary masses are hemangiomas, 28% are lymphangioma, and 13% are salivary neoplasms. The incidence of salivary neoplasm is increased by childhood radiation treatment for adenotonsillar hypertrophy.

If the presence of hemangioma or lymphatic malformation is unclear, ultrasonography is the most efficient method of differentiating these lesions. Other imaging modalities can be useful if delineation of the lesion's magnitude is of concern. If a malignancy is suspected, fine-needle aspiration may be performed during a CT scan. A questionable or negative result of fine-needle aspiration does not preclude surgical biopsy.

The presence of an asymptomatic solid solitary mass in any of the major or minor salivary glands is very suspect for malignancy. Most of these malignancies occur in later childhood or adolescence, and the parotid gland is the most common site. The most common manifestation of a salivary neoplasm is a rapidly growing mass in the preauricular or infra-auricular area. If a parotid salivary neoplasm is suspected, the biopsy of choice is a superficial parotidectomy with facial nerve dissection. This provides an appropriate excisional specimen with margins that carries less risk for facial nerve paralysis.

MYOFIBROMATOSIS

Fibromatosis colli is common in neonates. Manifesting as smooth, oval, and nontender masses, they involve the middle third of the sternocleidomastoid muscle. The fibrosis can shorten the sternocleidomastoid muscle and cause torticollis. In rare cases, fibromatosis colli is associated with plagiocephaly or craniofacial anomalies. Therapy consists of passive range-of-motion exercises stretching the sternocleidomastoid muscle. Parents can often perform the therapy; a physical therapist may be necessary in severe cases. Imaging with ultrasonography or with CT scan may be diagnostic but is rarely necessary. Consultation with a surgeon is warranted if the mass is not limited to the sternocleidomastoid muscle, is enlarging, or is inflamed.

PILOMATRIXOMA

Pilomatrixoma, formerly called *calcifying epithelium of Malherbe,* occurs most commonly in the head and neck of children younger than 2 years. It is a benign growth of the hair cortex cells or the hair follicle of the sebaceous glands, and it manifests as a hard mass attached to the skin, the bulk of the mass being subcutaneous. Usually it is a solitary lesion, but there may be other noncontiguous or secondary lesions. The subcutaneous portion of the mass is mobile and is blue or blue-black mixed with white areas. The mass is frequently misidentified as a hemangioma because of its blue color. It grows slowly until excised. If infected, it drains, and recurrent infections commonly develop until it is excised. Surgical excision with conservation of the surrounding tissue is the treatment of choice, and recurrences are infrequent.

THYROID MASSES

For a patient with a thyroid mass, the clinician must ask questions regarding symptoms of hypothyroidism or hyperthyroidism (see Tables 49-2 and 49-3). If there is a history of radiotherapy to the neck or a family history of endocrine tumors, a solitary mass is highly suspect for carcinoma. Multiple endocrine neoplasia type 2 is an autosomal dominant or, in rare cases, a sporadic disease in which patients develop medullary carcinoma of the thyroid. A careful

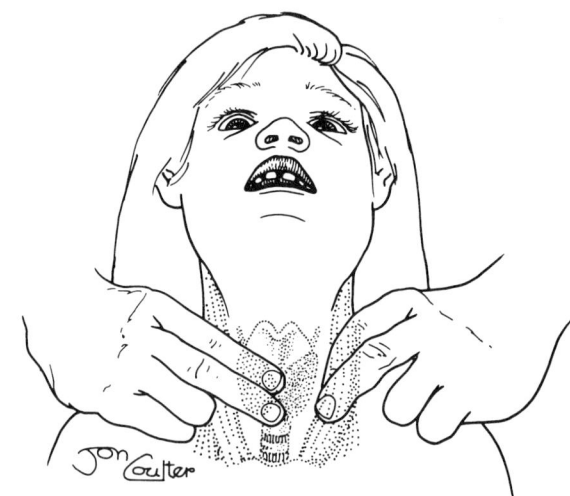

Figure 49-9. Palpation of the thyroid gland. The examiner stands behind the patient. A slight retraction of the sternocleidomastoid muscle away from the midline with one of the examiner's hands permits the examiner's other hand to outline the surface of the lobe. (From Lima JA, Graviss ER: Methods of examination. In Bluestone CD, Stool SE [eds]: Pediatric Otolaryngology, 2nd ed, vol 2. Philadelphia, WB Saunders, 1990, p 1284.)

family history of primary hyperparathyroidism can delineate the autosomal dominant or recessive types and is important for determining prognosis.

In a careful physical examination, the clinician attempts to differentiate diffuse goiter from solitary or multiple nodules (Fig. 49-9). Thyroxine (T_4), triiodothyronine (T_3), and thyroid-stimulating hormone are tested to evaluate thyroid function in patients with diffuse goiters (Table 49-5). Results of these tests are routinely normal in thyroid malignancies.

If a solitary mass is present, then ultrasound evaluation determines whether the lesion is cystic or solid. Cystic masses can be aspirated during the ultrasound study and sent for cytologic evaluation. Radionucleotide scanning determines the presence of hyperfunctioning ("hot") nodules or hypofunctioning ("cold") nodules. Cold nodules are very suspect for malignancy. The prevalence of carcinoma in solitary thyroid nodules is 15% to 40%; therefore, biopsy must be definitive. The use of surgical biopsy, by hemithyroidectomy, is generally recommended over fine-needle aspiration biopsy.

MALIGNANT NECK MASSES

Approximately 25% of pediatric malignancies involve the head and neck. However, unlike adult cervical malignancies, the majority of these do not originate in the head or neck. Mesenchymal derivatives make up 90% of pediatric cervical malignancies.

LYMPHOMA

Lymphomas are the third most common pediatric malignancy, constituting 12% of new pediatric tumors annually. The manifestation is typically that of a chronic lymphadenopathy with minimal local symptoms.

Hodgkin lymphomas in children most typically manifest as asymptomatic masses involving the cervical or supraclavicular nodes. Less frequently, axillary or inguinal nodes are the presenting symptom; subdiaphragmatic disease is rare. Biopsy of the mass is suggested. Staging is also modified by the presence of preoperative fevers, night sweats, and weight loss. The presence of these symptoms significantly worsens the prognosis.

Table 49-5. Laboratory Test Results in Various Types of Thyroid Function Abnormalities in Children

	Serum Total T$_4$	Free T$_4$	Serum TSH	Serum T$_3$ Resin Uptake	Serum TBG
Primary hypothyroidism	↓	↓	↑	↓	N
Hypothalamic (TRH) hypothyroidism	↓	↓	N	↓	N
Pituitary (TSH) hypothyroidism	↓	↓	N	↓	N
TBG deficiency	↓	N	N	↑	↓
TBG excess	↑	N	N	↓	↑

From Endocrine disorders. In Behrman RE, Kliegman RM (eds): Nelson Essentials of Pediatrics, 2nd ed. Philadelphia, WB Saunders. 1994, p 629.

T$_3$, triiodothyronine; T$_4$, thyroxine; TBG, thyroxine-binding globulin; TRH, thyrotropin-releasing hormone; TSH, thyroid-stimulating hormone.

↓, decreased; ↑, increased; N = normal.

Pediatric non-Hodgkin lymphomas are diffuse, aggressive, and frequently widespread at initial diagnosis. Non-Hodgkin lymphomas make up 60% of pediatric lymphomas and generally occur as abdominal or thoracic masses. In Africa and the Middle East, Burkitt lymphomas are most frequent and seem to have a different natural history than in the United States and Europe. Endemic lymphomas frequently occur in the mandibular or oropharyngeal lymph nodes.

Staging of the lymphomas requires open biopsy of the affected nodes. Molecular studies, immunophenotypic cell markers, and karyotypic cell markers can then be identified.

RHABDOMYOSARCOMA

Rhabdomyosarcoma is the most common soft tissue sarcoma of childhood. Within the head and neck, this lesion originates in the nasopharynx (chronic sinusitis, nasal discharge), ear, or orbit (proptosis) and may manifest with serosanguineous drainage from the nose or ear that is refractory to medical therapy. Typically, it is accompanied by painless enlargement of cervical nodes. Therefore, a thorough examination of the nasopharynx is warranted in patients with cervical adenopathy. The median age at diagnosis is approximately 6 years.

Rhabdomyosarcoma is a very aggressive tumor, and treatment involves a combination of modalities, including surgery, chemotherapy, and radiation. Because total excision is an extremely important factor in determining prognosis, early diagnosis is very important.

NEUROBLASTOMA

Neuroblastomas arise from postganglionic sympathetic cells. In the neck, the cervical sympathetic chain is the site of origin. These tumors manifest as firm masses in the lower neck lateral to the trachea in infants younger than 1 year. Horner syndrome (unilateral ptosis, miosis, and ipsilateral facial anhydrosis) may develop as a result of cervical or thoracic sympathetic chain neuroblastoma. In 35% of affected children, regional metastasis is detected at presentation. As expected, children with isolated distant nodal involvement have a better prognosis than do those with disseminated metastatic involvement. Treatment is multimodal; surgery is usually required in all patients. Subsequent radiotherapy or chemotherapy is based on clinical and biologic features.

DIAGNOSTIC APPROACH

The clinician should first try to establish the most likely broad diagnostic category by history and physical examination. Only when a diagnosis is suspected should the clinician attempt to narrow the differential by using the appropriate diagnostic testing. It is particularly important to decide which patients can be observed or managed medically by the primary care physician and which should be referred to a hematologist/oncologist, otolaryngologist, or pediatric surgeon. The physical examination is often the most valuable diagnostic tool.

A general approach to the patient with a neck mass is presented in Figure 49-10. First, the clinician must decide whether the history and physical findings are suggestive of a congenital lesion. If they are, then after initiating treatment of any associated infection, the patient should be referred to a surgical specialist immediately. If the lesion is not congenital, the next step should be to determine whether the lesion appears inflamed or infected. If it is inflamed or infected, associated systemic infections (upper respiratory) or local infections (dental abscess, scalp lesion) should be sought. If pharyngitis is present, a throat culture should be considered to rule out group A streptococcal infection. If the culture result is negative and symptoms persist, the physician should consider a viral infection with Epstein-Barr virus or cytomegalovirus (CMV), and appropriate serologic testing may be done. Toxoplasmosis or cat-scratch disease can be contemplated as well. A complete blood cell count with differential may be helpful at this point, because Epstein-Barr virus is often associated with an atypical lymphocytosis. If the inflamed lesion becomes fluctuant, referral should be made for incision and drainage.

The diagnosis of Kawasaki disease should be considered in any patient with an inflammatory node that does not suppurate and for which there is not an immediate explanation (see Chapter 55). For patients whose signs and symptoms do not fit these criteria, other systemic disorders should be considered. The patient and family should be questioned for human immunodeficiency virus risk factors and tested if appropriate. Signs and symptoms of connective tissue disease should be sought and a chest radiograph obtained. If the patient is found to have a history remarkable for recurrent infections, further workup for immunodeficiencies should be considered (see Chapter 51). If after all of these steps are taken the diagnosis remains unknown, the lesion may be monitored expectantly for 2 to 3 weeks. If regression of the mass has not occurred by the time of follow-up, further evaluation should be pursued.

If on examination the mass does not appear to be inflammatory, and if it is located in the supraclavicular or posterior cervical region, a complete blood cell count should be performed and a chest radiograph obtained. Because of the high incidence of malignancy associated with these findings, an immediate referral should be made for incisional biopsy. If the lesion is overlying the thyroid, and if the manifestation is not consistent with thyroglossal duct cyst, thyroid function tests and a thyroid scan should be performed, and referral for fine-needle aspiration or excisional biopsy should be made.

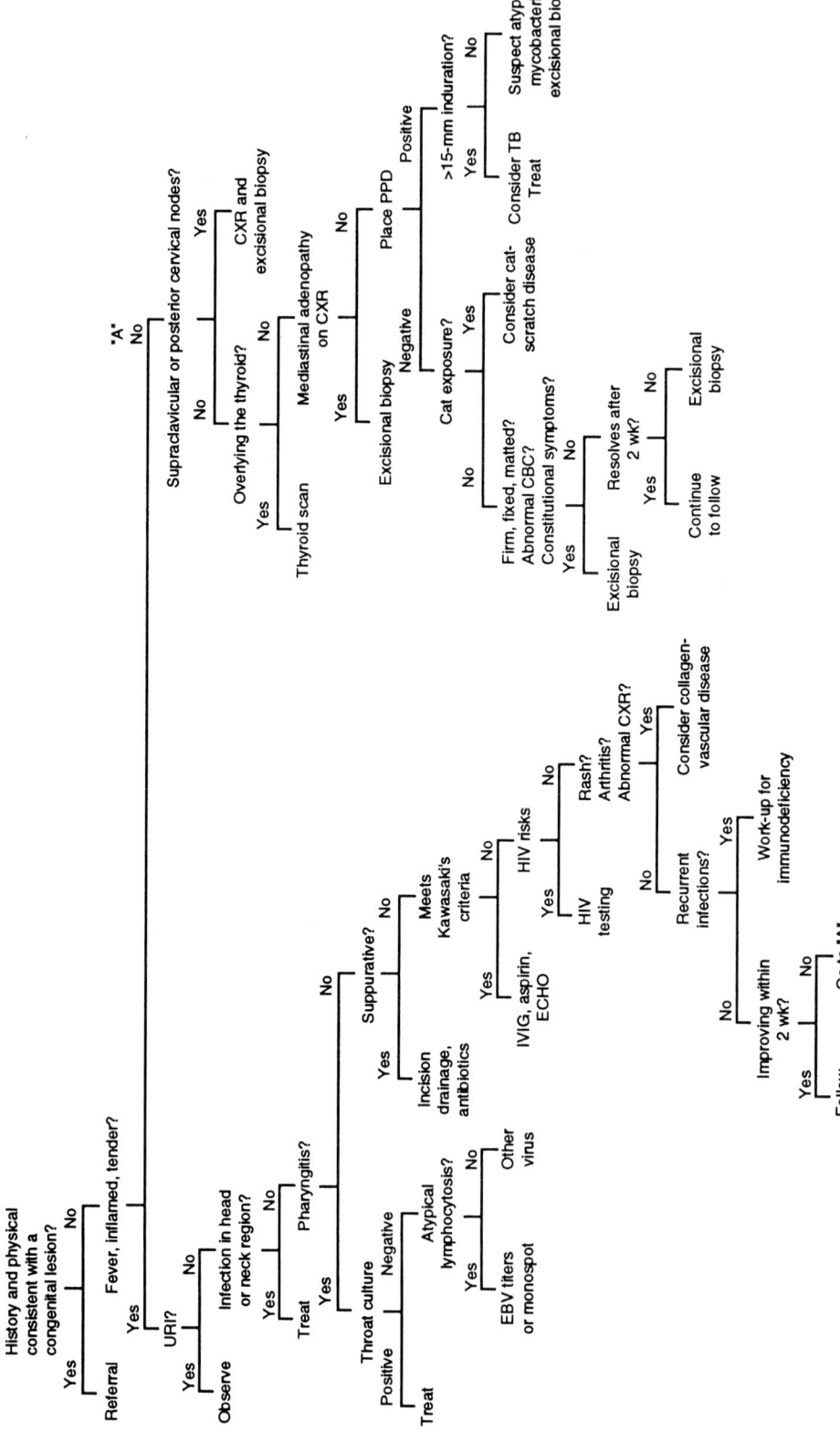

Figure 49-10. Diagnostic decision tree for childhood neck masses. CBC, complete blood count; CXR, chest radiograph; EBV, Epstein-Barr virus; ECHO, echocardiogram; HIV, human immunodeficiency virus; IVIG, intravenous immune globin; PPD, purified protein derivative; TB, tuberculosis; URI, upper respiratory infection.

For lesions lying outside of these regions, a purified protein derivative test should be part of the initial workup. In patients whose skin tests yield positive results, with more than 5 to 15 mm of induration (depending on risk group), tuberculosis is the most likely diagnosis (see Chapter 2). If the patient is at low risk for tuberculosis and the skin test yields a "positive" reaction with less than 15 mm of induration, infection with atypical mycobacteria should be suspected. These cases should be referred for excisional biopsy or curettage, and the material should be obtained for culture of acid-fast bacteria. If the patient is found to be anergic, immunodeficiencies and malignancies should be suspected.

If the purified protein derivative test does not yield a reaction, the diagnosis of cat-scratch disease may be entertained. Patients with a history of cat exposure and physical findings consistent with this diagnosis may be observed for a period of 2 to 3 weeks. If the nodes continue to enlarge, excisional biopsy with Warthin-Starry staining of the biopsy specimen is appropriate. In patients with noninflammatory nodes, especially with a history of cat exposure, toxoplasmosis should also be considered, and titers may be obtained.

In the patient whose clinical picture is not consistent with cat-scratch disease and whose diagnosis has not been established during the evaluation just described, the possibility of malignancy must be strongly considered. The clinician should consider several questions that indicate red flags:

- Are the nodes firm, matted, or fixed to underlying tissue?
- Are there associated constitutional symptoms?
- Are there abnormalities on the complete blood count that would suggest malignancy or on the chest radiograph that would suggest mediastinal adenopathy or mass?

If the answer to any of these questions is yes, immediate referral should be made for excisional biopsy. If none of the answers is yes, the mass may again be monitored with serial measurements for 2 to 3 more weeks. Masses that continue to increase in size and those that do not regress over the next several weeks should be examined through biopsy.

SUMMARY AND RED FLAGS

Diagnosis of childhood cervical masses is challenging and satisfying. The basic clinical history and physical examination skills are reliably successful in this area. The differential diagnosis can be limited on the basis of anatomic, inflammatory, and historical information. The likelihood of successful treatment is high in children.

Red flags include signs of airway compromise; dysphagia; supraclavicular adenopathy; a solid, solitary mass in a salivary gland; a cold thyroid nodule; matted or fixed nodes; and fever, night sweats, or weight loss associated with a neck mass (Table 49-6).

Table 49-6. "Red Flags": Signs and Symptoms Suspect for Malignancy or Decompensation

Supraclavicular adenopathy
Adenopathy in posterior triangle without evidence of scalp inflammation
Nodes fixed to underlying tissue
Size > 3 cm
Matting of nodes into single indistinct mass
Slow, steadily progressive painless enlargement
Signs of airway obstruction
Constitutional symptoms in association with above:
    Fever
    Weight loss
    Night sweats

REFERENCES

Bacterial Lymphadenitis

Sichel JY, Gomori JM, Saah D, Elidan J: Parapharyngeal abscess in children: The role of CT for diagnosis and treatment. Int J Pediatr Otorhinolaryngol 1996;35:213-222.

Mycobacterium Lymphadenitis

April MM, Garelick JM, Nuovo GJ: Reverse transcriptase in situ polymerase chain reaction in atypical mycobacterial adenitis. Arch Otolaryngol Head Neck Surg 1996;122:1214-1218.

Cat-Scratch Disease

Kacker A, Kuhel WI, Hoda RS: Quiz Case 2: Cat-scratch disease. Arch Otolaryngol Head Neck Surg 2000;126:677-682.

Neck Masses in Patients Undergoing Bone Marrow Transplantation or Chemotherapy

Posey LA, Kerschner JE, Conley SF: Posttransplantation lymphoproliferative disease in children: Otolaryngologic manifestations and management. South Med J 1999;92:1079-1082.

Kimura Disease

Chusid MJ, Rock AL, Sty JR, et al: Kimura's disease: An unusual cause of cervical tumor. Arch Dis Child 1997;77:153-154.

Thyroglossal Duct Cysts

Buchino JJ, Fallat ME, Montgomery VL: Pathological case of the month. Papillary carcinoma of the thyroid in a thyroglossal duct remnant. Arch Pediatr Adolesc Med 1999;153:999-1000.
Sullivan DP, Liberatroe LA, April MM, et al: Epidermal inclusion cyst versus thyroglossal duct: Sistrunk or not? Ann Otol Rhinol Laryngol 2001;110:340-344.

Branchial Cleft Cyst, Sinus, Vestige

Milbrath MM, Beste DJ, Sty JR: Comparative imaging: Thyroid abscess. Clin Nucl Med 1990;15:197.

Vascular Lesions

Clymer MA, Fortune D, Reinisch L, et al: Interstitial Nd: YAG photocoagulation for vascular malformations and hemangiomas in childhood. Arch Otolaryngol Head Neck Surg 1998;124:431-436.
Fishman SJ. Mulliken JB: Vascular anomalies. A primer for pediatricians. Pediatr Clin North Am 1998;45:1455-1477.
Jackson IT, Careno R, Potparic Z, Hussain K: Hemangiomas, vascular malformations and lymphovenous malformations: Classification and methods of treatment. Plast Reconstr Surg 1993;91:1216-1230.
Mulliken JB, Glowacki J: Hemangiomas and vascular malformations in children: A classification based on endothelial characteristics. Plast Reconstr Surg 1982;69:412-422.

Lymphatic Malformations

de Serres LM, Sie KC, Richardson MA: Lymphatic malformations of the head and neck. A proposal for staging. Arch Otolaryngol Head Neck Surg 1995;121:577-582.

Salivary Masses

Bentz BG, Hughes CA, Ludemann JP, et al: Masses of the salivary gland region in children. Arch Otolaryngol Head Neck Surg 2000;126:1435-1439.
Pershall KE, Koopmann CF Jr, Coulthard SW: Sialadenitis in children. Int J Pediatr Otorhinolaryngol 1986;11:199-203.

Myofibromatosis

Jaber M, Goldsmith AJ: Sternocleidomastoid tumor of infancy: Two cases of an interesting entity. Int J Pediatr Otorhinolaryngol 1999;47:269-274.

Pilomatrixoma

Duflo S, Nicollas R, Roman S, et al: Pilomatrixoma of the head and neck in children: A study of 38 cases and a review of the literature. Arch Otolaryngol Head Neck Surg 1998;124:1239-1242.

Thyroid Masses

Alter CA. Moshang T Jr: Diagnostic dilemma. The goiter. Pediatr Clin North Am 1991;38;567-578.

Lymphoma

Hudson MM, Donaldson SS: Hodgkin's disease. Pediatr Clin North Am 1997;44:891-906.
Shad A, Magrath I: Non-Hodgkin's lymphoma. Pediatr Clin North Am 1997;44:863-890.

Rhabdomyosarcoma

Blatt J, Snyderman C, Wollman MR, et al: Delayed resection in the management of non-orbital rhabdomyosarcoma of the head and neck in childhood. Med Pediatr Oncol 1997;28:294-298.
Coene IJ, Schouwenburg PF, Voute PA, et al: Rhabdomyosarcoma of the head and neck in children. Clin Otolaryngol Allied Sci 1992;17:291-296.
Raney RB, Asmar L, Vassilopoulou-Sellin R, et al: Late complications of therapy in 213 children with localized, nonorbital soft-tissue sarcoma of the head and neck: A descriptive report from the Intergroup Rhabdomyosarcoma Studies (IRS)–II and –III. IRS Group of the Children's Cancer Group and the Pediatric Oncology Group. Med Pediatr Oncol 1999;33:362-371.

Neuroblastoma

Castleberry RP: Biology and treatment of neuroblastoma. Pediatr Clin North Am 997;44:919-935.

50 Bleeding and Thrombosis

J. Paul Scott

Hemostasis is a process that maintains normal blood flow through healthy vessels but, when a vessel is damaged, rapidly generates a clot at the site of vascular injury. In addition to flow, the major components of the hemostatic mechanism are the platelets, the anticoagulant proteins, the procoagulant proteins, and various components of the vascular wall. Normal hemostasis is an interactive process in which each element cooperates closely to generate a rapid, cohesive, focused reaction. An abnormality of one element destabilizes the system, but significant clinical symptoms often manifest only when two components are affected. Typical examples include the patient with hemophilia who bleeds after sustaining trauma and the antithrombin III-deficient woman in whom thrombosis develops during pregnancy. The astute clinician is aware of situations that may exacerbate preexisting conditions. Pretreatment of known predisposing conditions can prevent complications, as exemplified by infusion of factor VIII concentrate before and after surgery to a patient with hemophilia A to prevent excessive bleeding.

Table 50-1 shows common bleeding symptoms and the most common disorders that trigger these symptoms.

THE COAGULATION CASCADE

Two opposing systems generate local clots but limit the clot to the area of vascular damage. Figure 50-1 shows the sequence of activation of coagulation. The cascade is capable of rapid response because generation of a small number of activated factors at the "top" of the cascade leads to thousands of molecules of thrombin. Deficiencies of proteins at or below factors XI or VII in the coagulation cascade sequence result in clinical bleeding symptoms, whereas deficiencies of factor XII, prekallikrein, and high-molecular-weight kininogen do not. The coagulation mechanism is continuously generating a small amount of thrombin, probably through autocatalysis of factor VII to factor VIIa. If there is trauma, tissue factor and factor VII combine to activate factor X to factor Xa both directly and indirectly via factor IX. Factor Xa then forms a complex on a membrane surface (provided by the activated platelet) with factor V and calcium, which results in more thrombin generation. Platelets stick to areas of vessel injury, thus restricting thrombin generation and clot formation to the area of damage.

Thrombin exerts positive feedback on the system by acting on factor XI to trigger the intrinsic system, cleaving factors V and VIII to activate them, further accelerating thrombin generation, aggregating platelets, and activating factor XIII. In this model, coagulation is always "turned on" and, therefore, reacts faster than if it were static and suddenly had to initiate a series of reactions to trigger clot formation. This dynamic concept underscores the impact of deficiencies in anticoagulant proteins, inasmuch as the system is continuously generating thrombin. A deficiency of an inhibitory enzyme or a cofactor removes part of the "brakes" on the system and causes increased thrombin generation.

COAGULATION INHIBITORS

Four key systems interact to inhibit the coagulation mechanism:

- antithrombin (AT)
- protein C/S system
- fibrinolytic system
- tissue factor pathway inhibitor (TFPI)

ANTITHROMBIN

AT is a member of the serine protease inhibitor family (serpins) that inhibits thrombin, factor Xa, and, less efficiently, factors IXa and XIa. When AT is bound to heparin, this reaction is accelerated 1000-fold. AT is the active anticoagulant operative during heparin therapy; if AT is deficient, heparin therapy may fail. Heparin-like molecules are synthesized by endothelial cells and interact with AT on the vessel wall to inhibit coagulation. Both congenital and acquired AT deficiencies are associated with a predisposition toward thrombosis. AT is consumed during clotting.

Table 50-1. Common Causes of Clinical Bleeding Symptoms

Mucocutaneous Bleeding

Acute
  Immune thrombocytopenic purpura
  Child abuse
  Trauma
  Poisoning with anticoagulants (rat poison)
Chronic/insidious
  von Willebrand disease
  Platelet function defect
  Marrow infiltration/aplasia

Deep/Surgical Bleeding

Hemophilia
Vitamin K deficiency
von Willebrand disease

Generalized Bleeding

Disseminated intravascular coagulation
Vitamin K deficiency
Liver disease
Uremia

Procoagulants

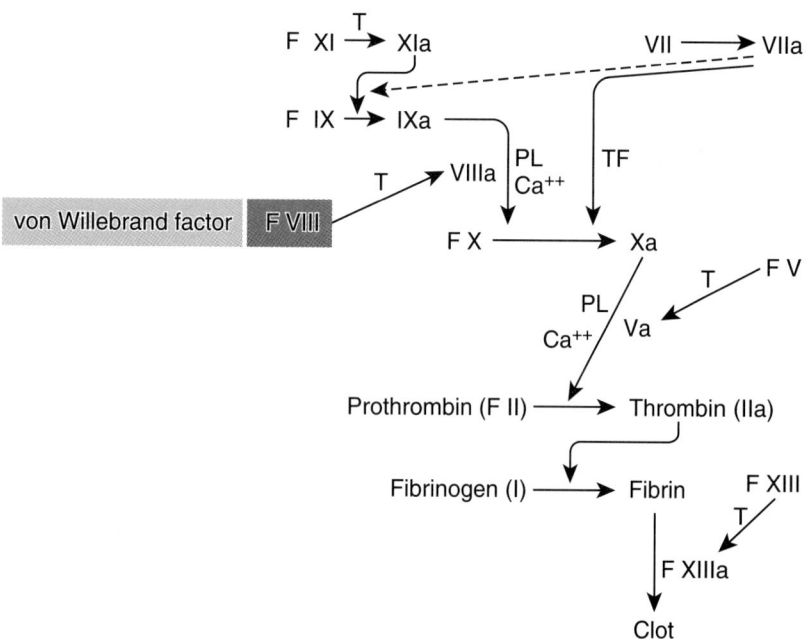

Figure 50-1. The coagulation cascade and the critical positive feedback role of factor IIa (thrombin) (T) on multiple aspects of the coagulation cascade. In addition, thrombin aggregates platelets and thereby contributes to platelet plug formation. The *dotted line* connecting factor VIIa with factor IX depicts the physiologic pathway of factor IX activation in vivo. Factor VIII circulates bound to von Willebrand factor. After activation by thrombin, factor VIIIa can participate with factor IXa in the activation of factor X. Factor XIIIa cross-links fibrin and stabilizes the fibrin clot. Ca^{2+}, calcium; PL, platelet phospholipid surface; TF, tissue factor. (Modified from Montgomery RR, Scott JP: Hemorrhage and thrombotic diseases. In Behrman RE, Kliegman RM, Jenson HB [eds]: Nelson Textbook of Pediatrics, 16th ed. Orlando, Fla, WB Saunders, 1999, p 1505.)

PROTEIN C/PROTEIN S SYSTEM

The protein C/protein S system is complex and limits clot extension by inactivating the rate-limiting coenzymes of the coagulation cascade, factors VIII and V. To prevent extension of the clot, the anticoagulant mechanism must limit thrombin formation to areas of vascular damage. The protein C/protein S system accomplishes this goal.

As a first step, thrombin binds to the protein thrombomodulin on intact endothelial cells. Thrombomodulin-bound thrombin then converts protein C into its activated form, activated protein C (APC). APC then combines with protein S to inactivate factors VIII and V.

In addition, APC may also promote fibrinolysis. In such a manner, thrombin itself is inactivated when bound to thrombomodulin and simultaneously augments the anticoagulant response by generating APC. APC limits the amount of thrombin that can be generated subsequently.

ATIII, protein C, and protein S are important inhibitors of clotting because deficiencies of each of these proteins, either inherited or acquired, are associated with an increased risk of thrombosis. A mutation in factor V (factor V Leiden) that makes it less susceptible to proteolysis by APC (resistance to APC) is the most common hereditary predisposition to thrombosis.

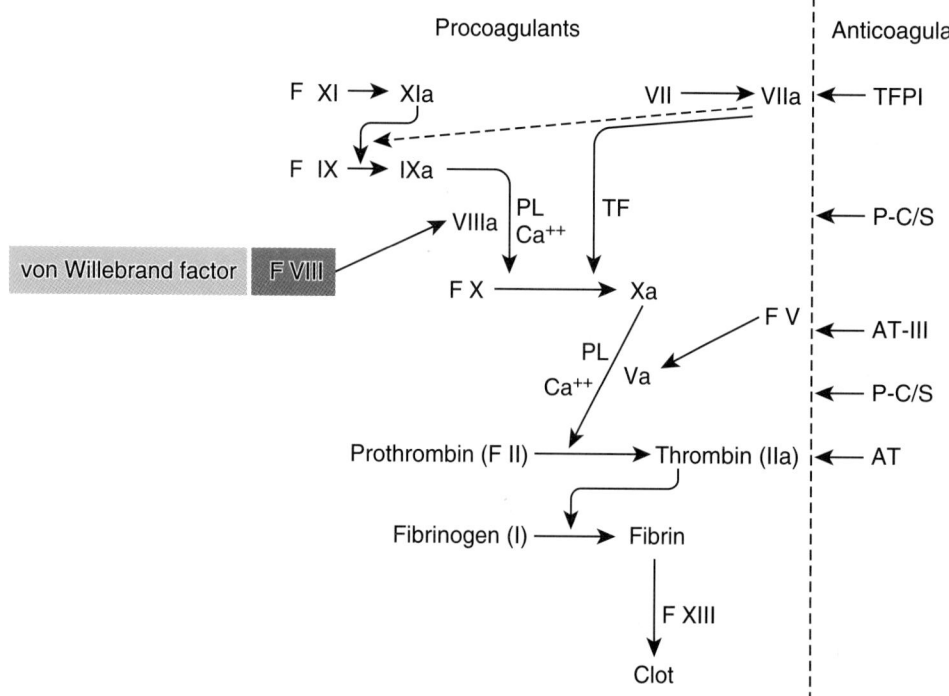

Figure 50-2. The major sites of action of the physiologic anticoagulants. Antithrombin (AT) irreversibly binds and inactivates factor Xa and thrombin. Thrombin binds to endothelial thrombomodulin and activates protein C. The activated protein C/protein S complex (P-C/S) proteolyses and inactivates factors Va and VIIIa. The tissue factor pathway inhibitor (TFPI) binds to the complexes of factor VIIa–tissue factor–factor Xa and inactivates factor VIIa. Ca^{2+}, calcium; PL, platelet phospholipid surface; TF, tissue factor. (Modified from Montgomery RR, Scott JP: Hemorrhage and thrombotic diseases. In Behrman RE, Kliegman RM, Jenson HB [eds]: Nelson Textbook of Pediatrics, 16th ed. Orlando, Fla, WB Saunders, 1999, p 1505.)

TFPI is an inhibitor of factor VIIa. Because a pathologic deficiency state of TFPI has not been discovered, the role of TFPI as a physiologic inhibitor of coagulation is unclear at present (Fig. 50-2).

FIBRINOLYTIC SYSTEM

The fibrinolytic system dissolves and removes clots from the vascular system so that normal flow through vessels can be restored. Endothelial cells synthesize two activators of plasminogen: tissue-type plasminogen activator (TPA) and urokinase, both of which convert plasminogen to plasmin, the enzyme that degrades fibrin.

Normally, plasminogen activator and its inhibitor, plasminogen activator inhibitor, are synthesized in equimolar amounts and are released from endothelial cells in parallel, leading to minimal amounts of active fibrinolysis. Increased activation or damage to the vascular system can alter this balance and result in increased TPA release, thus generating plasmin and lysing local clots.

When fibrin is degraded by plasmin, fibrin degradation products (FDPs) are formed. These can be measured in the clinical laboratory by immunologic assays that detect the presence of proteolysed fibrin(ogen) (FDPs) or that measure the breakdown products of plasmin action on cross-linked fibrin (D-dimer). Plasminogen activator has been synthesized in a recombinant form (rTPA) and is an effective pharmacologic fibrinolytic agent in vivo.

THE PLATELET-ENDOTHELIAL CELLS AXIS

Clotting is initiated when platelets adhere to damaged endothelium (Fig. 50-3). In areas of vascular damage, the adhesive protein, von Willebrand factor (vWF), binds to the exposed subendothelial collagen matrix and undergoes a conformational change. vWF then binds to its platelet receptor, glycoprotein Ib, and activates platelets. Activated platelets secrete adenosine diphosphate (ADP), which induces nearby circulating platelets to aggregate. Platelet-to-platelet cohesion is mediated by the binding of fibrinogen to its platelet receptor, glycoprotein IIb/IIIa. Therefore, both vWF and fibrinogen play essential roles in normal platelet function in vivo. Simultaneously with the platelet adhesion-aggregation response, coagulation is being activated. The platelet membrane brings the reactants of the cascade into close proximity, promoting rapid, effective factor catalysis and accelerating the reactions 1000-fold faster than would occur in the absence of the appropriate surface.

Normally, endothelial cells provide an antithrombotic surface through which blood flows without interruption. Nevertheless, the endothelial cell is capable of a rapid change in function and character so that it can augment coagulation after stimulation with a variety of modulating agents, including lymphokines and cytokines, as well as noxious agents such as endotoxin and infectious viruses (Fig. 50-4). Widespread alteration of endothelial cell function can shift and dysregulate the hemostatic response and promote activation of clotting. This is probably the mechanism by which sepsis induces the clinical syndrome of disseminated intravascular coagulation (DIC).

DEVELOPMENTAL HEMOSTASIS

Hemostatic disorders in newborns are common, more so than at any other pediatric age. The neonate is relatively deficient in most procoagulant and anticoagulant proteins. Platelet function may also be impaired. Blood flow characteristics in the newborn are unique because of the high hematocrit, small-caliber vessels, low blood pressure, and special areas of vascular fragility. Table 50-2 presents the normal values for coagulation screening tests and procoagulant proteins in preterm and full-term infants, as well as in older children. Table 50-3 presents age-specific values for the anticoagulant and fibrinolytic proteins.

Levels of factors V and VIII, fibrinogen, vWF, and platelets become normal by 28 weeks of gestation. Protein S levels are also

Blood Vessel

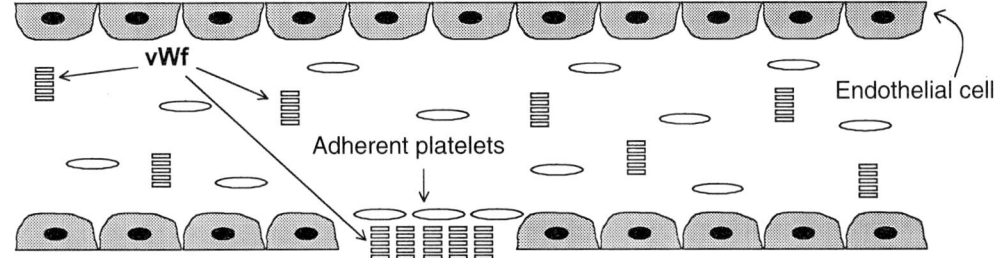

Adherence of platelets to damaged endothelium is vWf-dependent

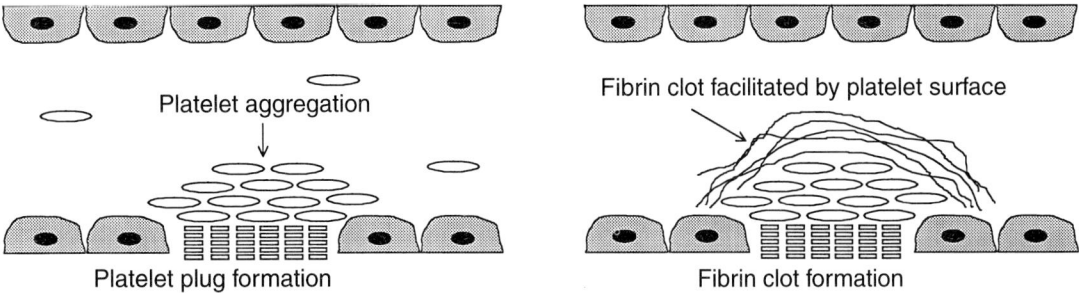

Figure 50-3. The endothelial cell–platelet–von Willebrand factor (vWF) interaction that results in initiation of the normal platelet plug by the adhesion of platelets to damaged endothelium, mediated by vWF with subsequent formation of the platelet plug and fibrin clot. (Courtesy of R. R. Montgomery.)

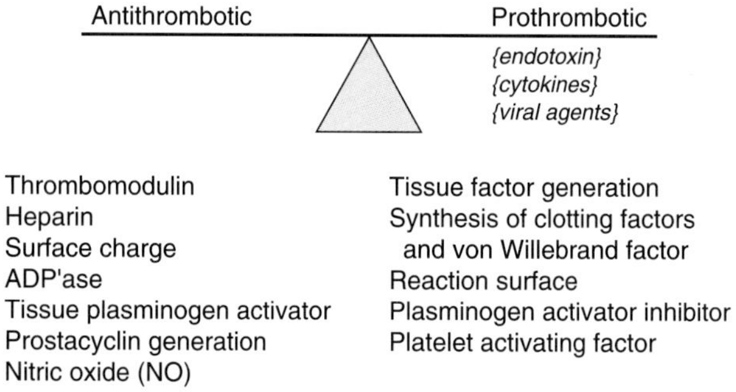

Antithrombotic	Prothrombotic
	{endotoxin}
	{cytokines}
	{viral agents}
Thrombomodulin	Tissue factor generation
Heparin	Synthesis of clotting factors
Surface charge	and von Willebrand factor
ADP'ase	Reaction surface
Tissue plasminogen activator	Plasminogen activator inhibitor
Prostacyclin generation	Platelet activating factor
Nitric oxide (NO)	

Figure 50-4. Endothelial balance. The pivotal role of the endothelium in maintaining a balance between antithrombotic and prothrombotic activities, as influenced by endotoxins, viruses, and immunomodulatory cytokines. ADPase, adenosine diphosphatase; NO, nitric oxide.

normal at birth, but levels of other anticoagulant proteins, especially protein C, ATIII, and plasminogen, are low in full-term infants and are even lower in premature neonates. The levels of most procoagulant and anticoagulant proteins increase throughout gestation; therefore, the most immature infant has the lowest levels of these proteins and is at the highest risk of either bleeding or thrombotic complications. The hemostatic balance of neonates, especially premature neonates, is precarious and easily shifted toward bleeding, thrombosis, or both.

Vitamin K deficiency is a particular problem of the newborn. Vitamin K is a fat-soluble vitamin that induces the post-translational γ-carboxylation of the vitamin K–dependent substances (factors II, VII, IX, and X; protein C; and protein S). This carboxylation step occurs after the protein is synthesized in the liver and must occur for the vitamin K–dependent coagulation factor to bind calcium, the bridge to the membrane surface on which these proteins form complexes with other members of the clotting cascade and catalyze subsequent reactions. Vitamin K deficiency effectively renders these proteins unable to bind to a surface. Most of the vitamin K in adults originates from the diet and from bacterial production in the intestine. The breast-fed neonate is at high risk for vitamin K deficiency because human milk is relatively deficient in vitamin K, the neonatal liver itself is immature, and the newborn's gut requires several days to develop normal bacterial flora.

Severe vitamin K deficiency in neonates, *hemorrhagic disease of the newborn* (HDN), occurs in breast-fed infants who have not received intramuscular vitamin K prophylaxis. Such infants may experience diffuse bleeding and even central nervous system hemorrhage at 3 to 5 days of life. HDN is an extraordinarily rare event in the United States because of nearly universal neonatal administration of vitamin K. In the evaluation of bleeding in a newborn, the clinician should confirm that vitamin K has been administered. Patients with disorders of the gastrointestinal tract, those taking broad-spectrum antibiotics, those born of mothers who received phenobarbital or phenytoin during pregnancy (very-early-onset HDN), and those with cholestasis and malabsorption (late-onset HDN) are at higher risk for vitamin K deficiency.

CLUES FROM THE HISTORY AND PHYSICAL EXAMINATION

HISTORY

Table 50-4 is an outline of historical questions that are important for the diagnosis of bleeding disorders. To obtain a meaningful history, it is critical to obtain quantifiable, precise information: a documented need for postsurgery transfusion because of excessive bleeding, nosebleeds that necessitate cautery, and large (>2 inches in diameter) or raised bruises in areas not usually associated with trauma. Although easy bruising and nosebleeds are common in children, the presence of large bruises at multiple sites, prolonged nosebleeds, and hematoma formation are rare in otherwise well children, but are seen in 20% to 38.5% of children with a bleeding disorder. Evaluation of children with an isolated history of easy bruising in a commonly traumatized area yields few findings of disease, whereas there is a much higher likelihood of pathologic processes with a history of large bruises at multiple sites. Epistaxis that is *prolonged* (>15 to 30 minutes), especially without trauma or a history of allergy or infection, that requires cautery or packing, or that results in iron deficiency is more likely to be caused by a hemostatic deficiency or an anatomic problem. Some helpful questions include "What was the biggest bruise you ever had, and what caused it?"; "Which finger do you pick your nose with?"; and "Have you ever noted little red dots [petechiae] on your skin?"

A personal or family history of gynecologic bleeding is often valuable. Menorrhagia causing iron deficiency anemia, bleeding after childbirth, or need for transfusion or early hysterectomy because of bleeding is often inappropriately assumed to have anatomic causes ("dysfunctional uterine bleeding"). The clinician must ascertain the number of pads used per day, in addition to the length and the frequency of each menstrual cycle (see Chapter 30). If the majority of women in a family have an underlying bleeding disorder, then that family's "normal menstrual periods" may be quite abnormal. Many adolescent girls with menorrhagia caused by an underlying bleeding disorder respond to oral contraceptive agents; therefore, improvement in bleeding symptoms after starting oral contraceptive agents does not rule out a bleeding disorder.

Historical information is equally important in deciding who requires evaluation for a predisposition to thrombosis. Virtually all pediatric patients in whom a blood clot develops in the absence of major vascular instrumentation need careful laboratory screening for a prothrombotic state (a hereditary or acquired disorder that predisposes to clotting). The only patients for whom there is insufficient evidence to judge whether studies need to be performed are neonates with catheters in place in whom venous or arterial thrombi develop in association with the catheter. Even in these situations, a detailed family history should be documented for early-onset stroke; early myocardial infarction; and blood clots in the veins, arteries, or lungs.

PHYSICAL EXAMINATION

The most important determination is whether the patient appears acutely or chronically ill, including vital signs and growth parameters. The nose should be examined for ulcers or anatomic bleeding sites, and the heart should be examined for the presence of murmurs (as occur in anemia and endocarditis). Joints should be examined for chronic arthropathy (as occurs in hemophilia) or joint laxity (as occurs in Ehlers-Danlos syndrome), and the extremities are examined for thumb or radial anomalies (thrombocytopenia–absent radius syndrome, which occurs in Fanconi anemia). The abdomen and lymph nodes should be examined for the presence of hepatosplenomegaly and adenopathy.

The examination of the skin should include a search for pallor, hematomas, petechiae, ecchymoses, telangiectasias, poor wound healing (large or abnormal scars), lax (loose) skin, and varicose veins (possible deep venous thrombosis). *Petechiae* are pinpoint, flat, dark red lesions caused by capillary bleeding into the skin. *Ecchymoses* are larger lesions (bruises) that are flat and usually not palpable. *Hematomas* are accumulations of blood in the skin or deeper tissues; in the skin, hematomas are raised and palpable. Bruises should be described in detail, including whether hematomas are associated with bruises and whether petechiae are present. Petechiae and ecchymoses are usually painless.

Purpura refers to any group of disorders characterized by the presence of dark-red, purplish, or brown lesions of the skin and mucous membranes. The discoloration is caused by the leakage of red blood

Table 50-2. Reference Values for Coagulation Tests in Healthy Children*

Test	19-27 Weeks' Gestation[†]	28-31 Weeks' Gestation[†]	30-36 Weeks' Gestation	Full Term	1-5 Years	6-10 Years	11-18 Years	Adult
PT (sec)	—	15.4 (14.6-16.9)	13.0 (10.6-16.2)	13.0 (10.1-15.9)	11 (10.6-11.4)	11.1 (10.1-12.0)	11.2 (10.2-12.0)	12 (11.0-14.0)
INR	—	—	1.0 (0.61-1.7)	1.00 (0.53-1.62)[‡]	1.0 (0.96-1.04)	1.01 (0.91-1.11)	1.02 (0.93-1.10)	1.10 (1.0-1.3)
APTT (sec)	—	108 (80-168)	53.6 (27.5-79.4)[‡§]	42.9 (31.3-54.3)[‡]	30 (24-36)	31 (26-36)	32 (26-37)	33 (27-40)
Fibrinogen	1.00 (±0.43)	2.56 (1.60-5.50)	2.43 (1.50-3.73)[†§]	2.83 (1.67-3.99)	2.76 (1.70-4.05)	2.79 (1.57-4.0)	3.0 (1.54-4.48)	2.78 (1.56-4.0)
Bleeding time (min)	—	—	—	—	6 (2.5-10)[‡]	7 (2.5-13)[‡]	5 (3.8)[‡]	4 (1-7)
Factor II	0.12 (±0.02)	0.31 (0.19-0.54)	0.45 (0.20-0.77)[‡]	0.48 (0.26-0.70)[‡]	0.94 (0.71-1.16)[‡]	0.88 (0.67-1.07)[‡]	0.83 (0.61-1.04)[‡]	1.08 (0.70-1.46)
Factor V	0.41 (±0.10)	0.65 (0.43-0.80)	0.88 (0.41-1.44)[§]	0.72 (0.34-1.08)[‡]	1.03 (0.79-1.27)	0.90 (0.63-1.16)[‡]	0.77 (0.55-0.99)[‡]	1.06 (0.62-1.50)
Factor VII	0.28 (±0.04)	0.37 (0.24-0.76)	0.67 (0.21-1.13)[‡]	0.66 (0.28-1.04)[‡]	0.82 (0.55-1.16)[‡]	0.86 (0.52-1.20)[‡]	0.83 (0.58-1.15)[‡]	1.05 (0.67-1.43)
Factor VIII procoagulant	0.39 (±0.14)	0.79 (0.37-1.26)	1.11 (0.5-2.13)	1.00 (0.50-1.78)	0.90 (0.59-1.42)	0.95 (0.58-1.32)	0.92 (0.53-1.31)	0.99 (0.50-1.49)
vWf	0.64 (±0.13)	1.41 (0.83-2.23)	1.36 (0.78-2.10)	1.53 (0.50-2.87)	0.82 (0.60-1.20)	0.95 (0.44-1.44)	1.00 (0.46-1.53)	0.92 (0.50-1.58)
Factor IX	0.10 (±0.01)	0.18 (0.17-0.20)	0.35 (0.19-0.65)[‡§]	0.53 (0.15-0.91)[‡§]	0.73 (0.47-1.04)[‡]	0.75 (0.63-0.89)[‡]	0.82 (0.59-1.22)[‡]	1.09 (0.55-1.63)
Factor X	0.21 (±0.03)	0.36 (0.25-0.64)	0.41 (0.11-0.71)[‡]	0.40 (0.12-0.68)[‡]	0.88 (0.58-1.16)[‡]	0.75 (0.55-1.01)[‡]	0.79 (0.50-1.17)	1.06 (0.70-1.52)
Factor XI	—	0.23 (0.11-0.33)	0.30 (0.08-5.2)[‡§]	0.38 (0.40-0.66)[‡]	0.30 (0.08-0.52)[‡§]	0.38 (1.10-0.66)	0.74 (0.50-0.97)[‡]	0.97 (0.56-1.50)
Factor XII	0.22 (±0.03)	0.25 (0.05-0.35)	0.38 (0.10-0.66)[‡§]	0.53 (0.13-0.93)[‡]	0.93 (0.64-1.29)	0.92 (0.60-1.40)	0.81 (0.34-1.37)[‡]	1.08 (0.52-1.64)
PK	—	0.26 (0.15-0.32)	0.33 (0.09-0.89)[‡]	0.37 (0.18-0.69)[‡]	0.95 (0.65-1.30)	0.99 (0.66-1.31)	0.99 (0.53-1.45)	1.12 (0.62-1.62)
HMWK	—	0.32 (0.19-0.52)	0.49 (0.09-0.89)[‡]	0.54 (0.06-1.02)[‡]	0.98 (0.64-1.32)	0.93 (0.60-1.30)	0.91 (0.63-1.19)	0.92 (0.50-1.36)
Factor XIIIa	—	—	0.70 (0.32-1.08)[‡]	0.79 (0.27-1.31)[‡]	1.08 (0.72-1.43)	1.09 (0.65-1.51)	0.99 (0.57-1.40)	1.05 (0.55-1.55)
Factor XIIIb	—	—	0.81 (0.35-1.27)[‡]	0.76 (0.30-1.22)[‡]	1.13 (0.69-1.56)[‡]	1.16 (0.77-1.54)[‡]	1.02 (0.60-1.43)	0.98 (0.57-1.37)

Data from Andrew M, Paes B, Johnston M: Development of the hemostatic system in the neonate and young infant. Am J Pediatr Hematol Oncol 1990;12:95–104; and Andrew M, Vegh P, Johnston M, et al: Maturation of the hemostatic system during childhood. Blood 1992;80:1998–2005.

*All factors except fibrinogen are presented as units/mL (fibrinogen in mg/mL), where pooled normal plasma contains 1 unit/mL. All data are expressed as the mean followed by the upper and lower boundaries encompassing 95% of the normal population.

[†]Levels for 19-27 weeks and 28-31 weeks are from those of adults.

[‡]Values are significantly different from those of adults.

[§]Values are significantly different from those of full-term infants.

APTT, activated partial thromboplastin time; HMWK, high-molecular-weight kininogen; INR, international normalized ratio; PK, prekallikrein; PT, prothrombin time; vWf, von Willebrand factor.

Table 50-3. Reference Values for the Inhibitors of Coagulation in Healthy Children in Comparison with Adults*

Inhibitor	19-27 Weeks' Gestation[†]	28-31 Weeks' Gestation[†]	30-36 Weeks' Gestation	Full Term	1-5 Years	6-10 Years	11-18 Years	Adult
ATII	0.24 (±0.03)[‡]	0.28 (0.20-0.38)[‡]	0.38 (0.14-0.62)[‡§]	0.63 (0.39-0.87)[‡]	1.11 (0.82-1.39)	1.11 (0.90-1.31)	1.06 (0.77-1.32)	1.0 (0.74-1.26)
Protein C	0.11 (±0.03)[‡]	—	0.28 (0.12-0.44)[‡§]	0.35 (0.17-0.53)[‡]	0.66 (0.40-0.92)[‡]	0.69 (0.45-0.93)[‡]	0.83 (0.55-1.11)[‡]	0.96 (0.64-1.28)
Protein S								—
Total (U/mL)	—	—	0.26 (0.14-0.38)[‡§]	0.36 (0.12-0.60)[‡]	0.86 (0.54-1.18)	0.78 (0.41-1.14)	0.72 (0.52-0.92)	0.81 (0.61-1.13)
Free (U/mL)	—	—	—	—	0.45 (0.21-0.69)	0.42 (0.22-0.62)	0.38 (0.26-0.55)	0.45 (0.27-0.61)
Plasminogen (U/mL)	—	—	1.70 (1.12-2.48)[‡]	1.95 (1.25-2.65)[‡]	0.98 (0.78-1.18)	0.92 (0.75-1.08)	0.86 (0.68-1.03)	0.99 (0.77-1.22)
TPA (ng/mL)	—	—	8.48 (3.00-16.70)	9.6 (5.0-18.9)	2.15 (1.0-4.5)[‡]	2.42 (1.0-5.0)[‡]	2.16 (1.0-4.0)[‡]	1.02 (0.68-1.36)
α_2AP (U/mL)	—	—	0.78 (0.40-1.16)	0.85 (0.55-1.15)	1.05 (0.93-1.17)	0.99 (0.89-1.10)	0.98 (0.78-1.18)	1.02 (0.68-1.36)
PAI-1	—	—	5.4 (0.0-12.2)[‡]	6.4 (2.0-15.1)	5.42 (1.0-10.0)	6.79 (2.0-12.0)[‡]	6.07 (2.0-10.0)[‡]	3.60 (0-11.0)

Data from Andrew M, Paes B, Johnston M: Development of the hemostatic system in the neonate and young infant. Am J Pediatr Hematol Oncol 1990;12:95-104; and Andrew M, Vegh P, Johnston M, et al: Maturation of the hemostatic system during childhood. Blood 1992;80:1998-2005.

*All values are expressed in units/mL, where pooled plasma contains 1 unit/mL, with the exception of free protein S, which contains a mean of 0.4 unit/mL. All values presented as the mean by the upper and lower boundaries encompassing 95% of the population.

[†]Levels for 19-27 weeks and 28-31 weeks are from multiple sources and cannot be analyzed statistically.

[‡]Values are significantly different from those of adults.

[§]Values are significantly different from those of full-term infants.

α_2AP, α_2-antiplasmin; ATIII, antithrombin-III; PAI-1, plasminogen activator inhibitor type 1; TPA, tissue plasminogen activator.

| **Table 50-4.** History of a Bleeding Disorder |

I. **History of Disorder**
  A. *Onset* of symptoms
    1. Age
    2. Acute versus lifelong
    3. Triggering event
    4. Timing of bleeding after injury: immediate versus delayed
  B. *Sites* of bleeding
    1. **Mucocutaneous***
      a. Epistaxis
        (1) Duration, frequency, seasonal tendency
        (2) Associated trauma (nose picking, allergy, infection)
        (3) **Resultant anemia, emergency department evaluation, cautery**
      b. Oral (gingiva, frenulum, tongue lacerations, bleeding after tooth brushing, after dental extractions requiring sutures/packing)
      c. Bruising (number, sites, size, **raised** [other than extremities], spontaneous versus trauma, knots within center, skin scarring)
      d. Gastrointestinal bleeding
    2. **Deep**
      a. Musculoskeletal
        (1) Hemarthroses, unexplained arthropathy
        (2) Intramuscular hematomas
      b. Central nervous system hemorrhage
      c. Genitourinary tract
    3. **Surgical**
      a. Minor (sutures, lacerations, poor or delayed wound healing)
      b. Major
        (1) Tonsillectomy and adenoidectomy
        (2) Abdominal surgery

  C. **Perinatal history**
      a. Superficial (bruising, petechiae)
      b. Deep
        (1) Circumcision
        (2) Central nervous system bleeding
        (3) Gastrointestinal bleeding
        (4) Cephalohematoma
        (5) Unexplained anemia or hyperbilirubinemia
        (6) Delayed cord separation, bleeding after cord separation
      c. Vitamin K administration
      d. Maternal drugs
  D. **Obstetric/gynecologic bleeding**
    1. Menorrhagia
      (1) Onset, duration, amount (number of pads), frequency, persistence after childbirth
      (2) **Resultant anemia, iron deficiency**
    2. Bleeding at childbirth (onset, duration, **transfusion requirement,** history of traumatic delivery, recurrences with subsequent pregnancies, spontaneous abortions)
  E. **Medications**
      a. Aspirin and nonsteroidal antiinflammatory drugs
      b. Anticoagulants
      c. Antibiotics
      d. Anticonvulsants
  F. **Diet**
      a. Vitamin K
      b. Vitamin C

II. **Family History**
  Draw family tree. The items just listed should be applied to immediate family members, especially a history of easy bruising, epistaxis, excessive bleeding after surgery, menorrhagia, excessive bleeding after childbirth, or a family history of others with diagnosed or suspect bleeding disorders. Attempt to deduce inheritance pattern.

*Significant historical information is presented in boldface type.

cells from affected vessels. Purpuric lesions can be caused by abnormalities of the platelets, of coagulation proteins, or of vessel walls.

COAGULATION SCREENING TESTS

After obtaining a history and performing a physical examination, the clinician must determine the need for a hemostatic evaluation. The presence of significant symptoms should warrant such an evaluation. The history is likely to be the most sensitive screening tool for a significant bleeding disorder, although the history is often nonspecific. Its use in a very young child, especially before toddler age, is limited, and attention must shift to the perinatal history and the family history.

For patients who are to be evaluated for a bleeding disorder because of clinical clues or planned surgery, the initial screening studies should assess the clotting factors and platelet and vessel wall interaction, including vWF function. No set of screening tests is complete and capable of detecting the panorama of hemorrhagic disorders, but the screen should include

- prothrombin time (PT)
- partial thromboplastin time (PTT)
- functional fibrinogen level or thrombin time
- platelet count

- bleeding time
- vWF function (ristocetin cofactor activity)

There are no satisfactory tests to *screen* for a thrombotic tendency.

PROTHROMBIN TIME AND PARTIAL THROMBOPLASTIN TIME

The PT and PTT (Fig. 50-5) are measures of all the coagulation factors except factor XIII. Fibrinogen function should be measured as fibrinogen activity or thrombin time. The bleeding time provides an indirect measure of platelet number, platelet function, and the platelet–vessel wall interaction. The PTT is the screening test that checks for deficiency of all clotting factors except factors VII and XIII. The PTT can be prolonged either by a deficiency of a clotting factor or by the presence of an agent in the plasma that delays the clotting time (an inhibitor). The PT is especially sensitive to deficiencies of factor VII.

To test for an inhibitor, one part of the patient's plasma is mixed with one part of pooled normal plasma obtained from 20 to 50 healthy adults. Pooled normal plasma provides a 100% level of each clotting factor. If mixed 1:1 with plasma that is deficient in one or several factors, the mixture should possess at least a 50% level of each factor and the PTT should correct to the normal range. If an inhibitor is present, the PTT usually does not correct to normal. The

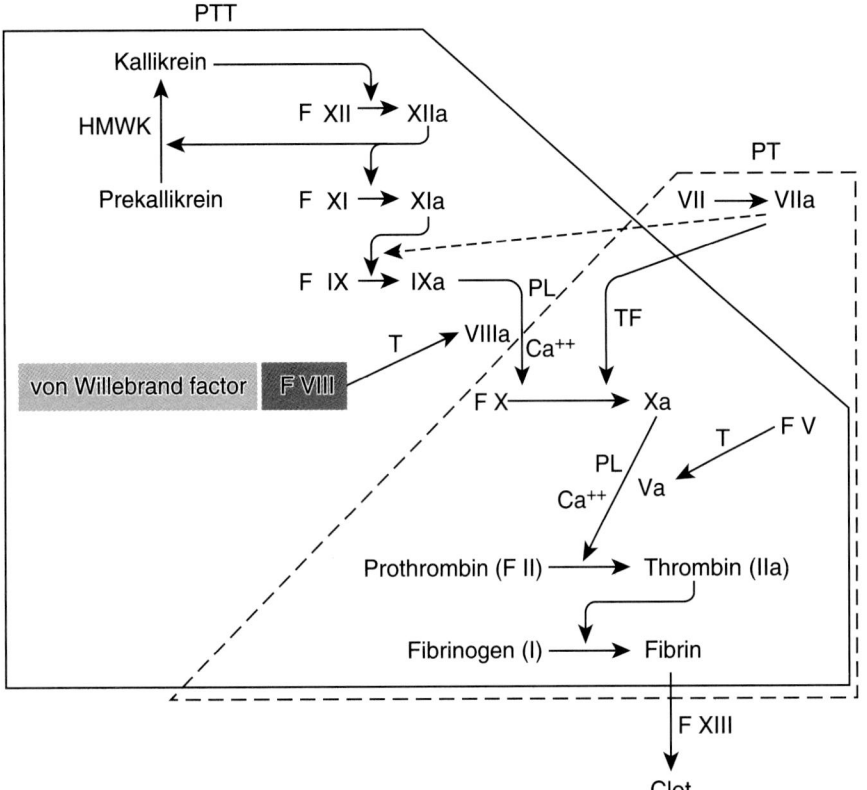

Figure 50-5. Elements of the coagulation cascade measured by the prothrombin time (PT) and the partial thromboplastin time (PTT). Note that prekallikrein (PK), high-molecular-weight kininogen (HMWK), and factor XII are shown in this figure and not in the depiction of the coagulation cascade in Figure 50-1, because a deficiency of PK, HMWK, or factor XII can cause a prolongation of the PTT. However, a deficiency of any of these proteins alone is not associated with a clinical bleeding disorder. Ca^{2+}, calcium; PL, platelet phospholipid surface; TF, tissue factor. (Modified from Montgomery RR, Scott JP: Hemorrhage and thrombotic diseases. In Behrman RE, Kliegman RM, Jenson HB (eds): Nelson Textbook of Pediatrics, 16th ed. Orlando, Fla, WB Saunders, 1999, p 1505.)

most common types of inhibitors include anticoagulants, such as heparin, and autoantibodies directed against either specific clotting factors (factor VIII inhibitors) or the phospholipid substances used in the PTT (lupus-type anticoagulants).

The PTT is especially sensitive to deficiencies of factors VIII, IX, and XI (hemophilia A, B, and C, respectively). A prolonged PTT in an asymptomatic child is most commonly caused by factor XII deficiency or by a lupus-type anticoagulant. The PTT can yield a false result

1. when poor venipuncture technique, by adding tissue factor to the blood, activates clotting and artifactually shortens the PTT
2. when insensitive laboratory reagents fail to detect clinically significant deficiencies (commonly in factor IX)
3. when the citrate concentration is not corrected for blood with a high hematocrit (in neonates and in patients with cyanotic congenital heart disease), leading to a prolonged PTT

BLEEDING TIME

The bleeding time is measured by placing a blood pressure cuff on the patient's arm and inflating it to 40 mm Hg; lower pressures have been used for infants. An incision of predetermined length and depth is made on the volar surface of the arm below the antecubital fossa using a standardized automated device. The wound is blotted with filter paper, and the time until the blood stops oozing is measured with a stopwatch.

The bleeding time is an indirect measure of platelet number and a more direct measure of platelet function, vascular integrity, and platelet interaction with the vascular subendothelium. As such, the bleeding time should be abnormal in patients with thrombocytopenia, platelet function abnormalities, abnormal collagen (Ehlers-Danlos syndrome), and von Willebrand disease. Unfortunately, because of its insensitivity and high level of variability, the bleeding time is a relatively poor tool for detecting the milder forms of these hemostatic disorders and cannot be used to rule out von Willebrand disease

and mild or moderate platelet function deficits. Figures 50-6 to 50-8 provide an approach to evaluate the patient with an isolated prolongation of the PT, PTT, or bleeding time, respectively.

THROMBIN TIME AND REPTILASE TIME

The thrombin time and reptilase time are tests that measure the conversion of fibrinogen to fibrin. The thrombin time is sensitive to heparin effect, whereas the snake venom reptilase time remains normal in the presence of heparin. Both the thrombin time and the reptilase time are prolonged by uremia, by dysfibrinogenemia, by

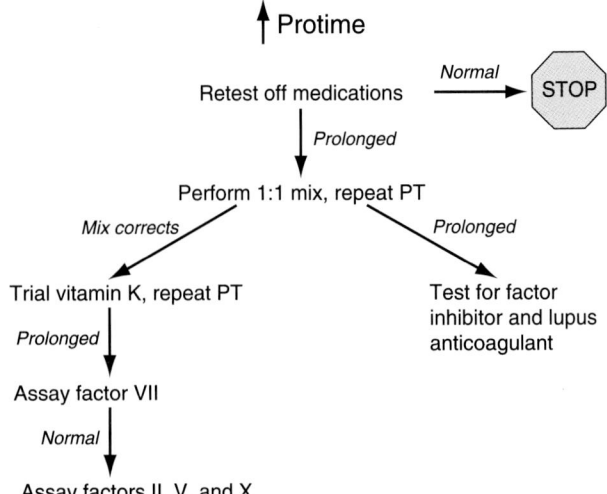

Figure 50-6. Flow diagram for the evaluation of an isolated prolongation of the prothrombin time (PT).

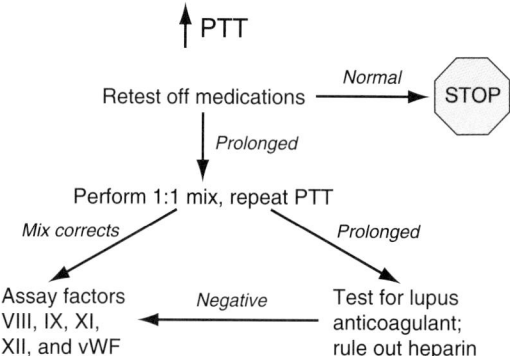

Figure 50-7. Flow diagram for the evaluation of a patient with a prolonged partial thromboplastin time (PTT). To rule out heparin effect, the thrombin time is compared with the reptilase time. If the thrombin time is significantly longer than the reptilase time, heparin is present in the sample. vWF, von Willebrand factor.

low fibrinogen levels (<75 mg/dL), and by FDPs formed by the action of plasmin on fibrin(ogen).

Both FDPs and D-dimer represent products formed when the fibrinolytic enzyme plasmin degrades fibrin. FDPs are a measure of plasmin action on fibrin and fibrinogen and should be less specific than the D-dimer assay, which measures the proteolytic breakdown products of cross-linked fibrin.

MUCOCUTANEOUS BLEEDING

Mucocutaneous bleeding occurs within the skin or mucous membranes. Common complaints include prolonged, frequent nosebleeds; gum bleeding; prolonged bleeding after tooth extraction; menorrhagia; and easy bruising with or without petechiae formation. Mucocutaneous bleeding is usually associated with abnormalities of platelet number or function, of platelet cofactors, or of the vessel wall.

The well-appearing child who presents with the *acute onset* of petechiae and purpura, often in association with nosebleeds or bleeding gums, and otherwise normal examination findings typically has *acute immune thrombocytopenic purpura* (ITP). The majority of affected children have an antecedent viral illness. After exposure to the viral infection, an antibody that binds to the platelet membrane develops, leading to the premature destruction of the antibody-coated platelets in the spleen.

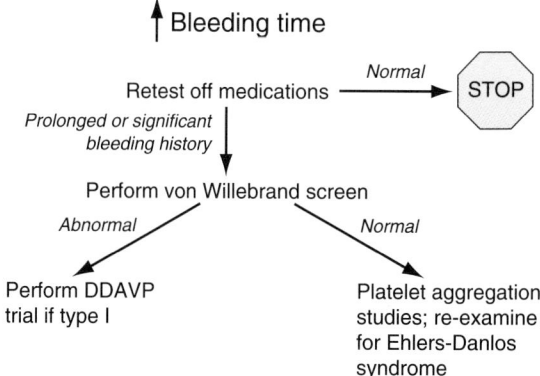

Figure 50-8. Evaluation for an isolated prolongation of bleeding time. DDAVP, desmopressin.

The peak ages for the presentation of ITP are 1 to 4 years of age and adolescence, but ITP occurs throughout childhood and adolescence. Girls are more commonly affected in adolescence but not in childhood. The workup of a child with thrombocytopenia should include a careful history aimed at detecting symptoms (weight loss, fever, bone pain, anorexia) of other preexisting illnesses (leukemia, systemic lupus erythematosus [SLE], endocarditis, human immunodeficiency virus [HIV]), exposures to drugs or toxins, and a personal or family history of thrombocytopenia. The physical examination must be detailed and include a search for signs of malignancy (lymphadenopathy, hepatosplenomegaly), chronic illness, and congenital malformations. When evaluating the complete blood cell count (CBC), the clinician should ensure that the hemoglobin, white blood cell count, differential, indices, and smear are normal, which would make the diagnosis of a hematologic malignancy or other marrow failure syndrome unlikely. The presence of large platelets on the smear or measured as a high mean platelet volume suggests accelerated thrombopoiesis and increased platelet destruction. The differential diagnosis of thrombocytopenia is noted in Table 50-5.

After the presumptive diagnosis of ITP, requisite laboratory studies other than the CBC, smear, and platelet count can be debated. Some authorities would obtain a Coombs test to rule out a simultaneous autoimmune hemolytic anemia, but the significance of this finding in a patient with normal hemoglobin is undefined. The role of studies for platelet antibodies is unclear; there are no data indicating that these studies are either diagnostic or prognostic in children. If the child is male, is young, and has a history of eczema or recurrent infection, immunoglobulin levels to rule out Wiskott-Aldrich syndrome are indicated (see Chapter 51). Similarly, in older children, especially girls as they approach adolescence, an antinuclear antibody test to rule out SLE manifesting as thrombocytopenia is warranted. Some clinicians would perform an antinuclear antibody test on all patients with new diagnoses, whereas others would defer the study, because fewer than 2% of affected adults and children are found to have SLE after presenting with acute ITP. In contrast, a much higher percentage of individuals with SLE have thrombocytopenia at some time during their illness (see Chapter 44). An antinuclear antibody test is more likely to yield positive results in children with chronic ITP. HIV infection occasionally manifests as ITP.

In the past, a bone marrow aspiration would be performed before any treatment for ITP. However, the diagnostic yield of bone marrow examination in a child with normal findings on a careful physical examination (no lymphadenopathy or hepatosplenomegaly) and a completely normal CBC, other than isolated thrombocytopenia, is negligible.

Once a diagnosis of ITP is made, several therapeutic options are available, including simple observation and education. The family should be advised that the child must avoid activities that increase the risk of head injury. Treatment should be reserved for children at high risk for clinical bleeding (platelet count < 10,000/mm³ to 20,000/mm³ and children with petechiae and mucosal hemorrhages). Some authorities argue that patients with mucous membrane purpura are at higher risk and definitely require treatment. The major cause of mortality in ITP is related to intracranial hemorrhage, which has been observed in fewer than 0.5% to 1% of patients. Table 50-6 provides a perspective on treatment alternatives for ITP. Treatment of acute ITP remains controversial. Whom to treat, when to treat, and what agent to use remain open questions. Options for initial therapy for patients in need of treatment include intravenous immune globulin (IVIG), prednisone, and intravenous anti-D antibody. IVIG may induce a faster rise in platelet count and may produce a higher response rate than intravenous anti-D antibody. Intravenous anti-D antibody is less expensive than IVIG and appears to have fewer side effects than prednisone. Intravenous anti-D antibody often causes hemolysis and a reduction in the hematocrit. Transfusion of platelets should be reserved for life-threatening bleeding, because transfused platelets are rapidly destroyed.

Table 50-5. **Differential Diagnosis of Thrombocytopenia in Children**

I. Destructive Thrombocytopenias
Primary Platelet Consumption Syndromes

Immunologic
> Idiopathic thrombocytopenia purpura
> Drug-induced thrombocytopenia
> Infection-induced thrombocytopenia (human immunodeficiency virus)
> Post-transfusion purpura
> Autoimmune or lymphoproliferative disorders
> Neonatal immune thrombocytopenias
> Allergy and anaphylaxis
> Post-transplantation thrombocytopenia

Nonimmunologic
> Chronic microangiopathic hemolytic anemia and thrombocytopenia
> Hemolytic-uremic syndrome
> Thrombotic thrombocytopenic purpura
> Catheters, prostheses, or cardiopulmonary bypass
> Congenital or acquired heart disease

Combined Platelet and Fibrinogen
  Consumption Syndromes
Disseminated intravascular coagulation
Kasabach-Merritt syndrome
Other causes of local consumption coagulopathy

Miscellaneous Causes

Specific to the neonate
> Phototherapy
> Perinatal aspiration syndromes
> Persistent pulmonary hypertension
> Rhesus alloimmunization
> Status post exchange transfusion
> Polycythemia
> Metabolic inborn errors of metabolism
> Maternal HELLP syndrome

Glomerular disease
Preeclampsia
Fatty acid–induced thrombocytopenia

II. Impaired or Ineffective Production
Congenital and Hereditary Disorders

Primary hematologic processes
> TAR syndrome
> Other congenital thrombocytopenias with megakaryocytic hypoplasia
> Fanconi aplastic anemia
> Bernard-Soulier syndrome*
> May-Hegglin anomaly*
> Wiskott-Aldrich syndrome*
> Miscellaneous hereditary thrombocytopenias (X-linked or autosomal)*
> Mediterranean thrombocytopenia

Associated with trisomy 13 or 18

Metabolic inborn errors
> Methylmalonic acidemia
> Ketotic glycinemia
> Holocarboxylase synthetase deficiency
> Isovaleric acidemia
> Some mitochondrial disorders

Acquired Disorders
Aplastic anemia
  Marrow infiltrative processes
  Drug- or radiation-induced
  Nutritional deficiency states (iron, folate, or
    vitamin B_{12})

III. Sequestration
  Hypersplenism
  Hypothermia

Modified from Schultz Beardsley D: Platelet abnormalities in infancy and childhood. In Nathan DG, Oski FA (eds): Hematology of Infancy and Childhood, 4th ed. vol 2. Philadelphia, WB Saunders, 1993, p 1566.

*These hereditary thrombocytopenias can be associated with normal or increased bone marrow megakaryocytes.

HELLP, hypertension, elevated liver enzymes, low platelets; TAR, thrombocytopenia–absent radius.

Table 50-6. Common Treatment Alternatives for Childhood Acute Immune Thrombocytopenic Purpura (ITP)

	Pro	Con	Cost Analysis for 15-kg 3-Year-Old
IVIG	Intravenous	Expensive	Author's hospital: 1 g/kg initial dose, 4-hr infusion as outpatient: $2350
Prednisone	Rapid onset of action Bone marrow not required Noninfectious High frequency of response	Frequently needs multiple doses Does not alter long-term outcome IV line in place for several hours	
	Inexpensive Oral Effective in 75%-80% of patients	Corticosteroid side effects May need multiple courses No effect on long-term outcome	2-week course of 2 mg/kg: $7.00
	Relatively rapid onset action	? Requires bone marrow aspiration	Procedure and histologic examination: $800-$1000
IV Anti-D Antibodies	Less expensive Relatively rapid onset of action Highly effective before splenectomy	IV administration Mild fall in hemoglobin; in rare cases, severe intravascular hemolysis Ineffective after splenectomy	1 dose, 50 µg/kg: $1070
Splenectomy	Curative in 80% of patients	Expensive, invasive Impairs host defense against encapsulated organisms Reserved for chronic, severe ITP Spontaneous remissions of ITP may occur late	$10,000-$20,000

IV, intravenous; IVIG, intravenous immune globulin.

Ten percent to 20% of children with ITP have persistence of thrombocytopenia for more than 6 months (chronic ITP). These patients are more likely to be older (adolescent) girls or to have had an insidious onset of symptoms. The clinician must look carefully for predisposing causes, including SLE, HIV infection, or medications. The treatment of chronic ITP is evolving and includes repeated doses of IVIG or intravenous anti-D antibody. Because of improved medical therapy, splenectomy is limited to patients with severe, refractory chronic ITP.

NEONATAL THROMBOCYTOPENIA

Thrombocytopenia is common, especially in sick newborns. The differential diagnosis of neonatal thrombocytopenia includes most of the causes seen in older children, in addition to those peculiar to the newborn (Fig. 50-9, in the shaded areas; see also Table 50-5). When evaluating the thrombocytopenic newborn, the physician must know the perinatal history. The physician should ask about the mother's health during this and previous pregnancies, including any history of current or previous low platelets or of children dying of hemorrhage. A maternal history of fever, viral infection (cytomegalovirus, rubella), sexually transmitted diseases (syphilis, HIV), medications, toxemia, or collagen-vascular disease (SLE) is informative. The family history should be evaluated for bleeding disorders, recurrent infections, or malignancies, especially in children.

During examination of the newborn, the most important element to determine is the child's general well-being. The examiner should look especially for signs of systemic illness, as well as lymphadenopathy, hepatosplenomegaly, mass lesions, hemangiomas, bruits, and congenital anomalies, especially of the radial bones.

The examiner should carefully evaluate the hemoglobin, the white blood cell count, and the differential for the presence of abnormal cells (blasts). Red blood cell structure should be examined for signs of microangiopathy. Small platelets (low mean platelet volume) suggest abnormal thrombopoiesis, whereas large platelets are found with accelerated platelet destruction. Mechanistically, thrombocytopenia can be caused by synthetic failure, sequestration, or destructive processes. The destructive processes are most common and are either immune or nonimmune in origin. Nonimmune causes of platelet consumption—for example, DIC, sepsis, congenital infections, or thrombotic events—are usually associated with obvious clinical findings. When evaluating the ill-appearing child or neonate for thrombocytopenia, the examiner should perform coagulation studies to detect fibrinogen consumption (fibrinogen level, D-dimer, FDPs). Neonates with immune-mediated platelet destruction usually appear healthy.

After the clinician obtains a thorough history, performs a careful physical examination, and evaluates the CBC, the initial step in management of the child with thrombocytopenia depends on the cause and severity of the thrombocytopenia. In the neonate with severe thrombocytopenia (platelet count $< 30,000/mm^3$ to $40,000/mm^3$) delivered vaginally, an ultrasound study of the head should be done to rule out intracranial bleeding. Platelet transfusion for thrombocytopenia can serve both as a therapeutic tool for stopping the bleeding and as a diagnostic maneuver. In patients with decreased platelet synthesis, survival of transfused platelets should be normal, whereas in thrombocytopenic states caused by platelet destruction, transfused platelets should be cleared rapidly. For this reason, platelet transfusions are usually contraindicated in thrombocytopenic states caused by accelerated platelet destruction, as in ITP and hemolytic-uremic syndrome. The yield and survival of the transfused platelets should be monitored with serial platelet counts after transfusion.

Antibody-mediated thrombocytopenia in the neonate is caused by transfer of maternal immunoglobulin G antibodies that react with the neonate's platelets. A mother with active ITP or a history of previous ITP is at risk for delivering a thrombocytopenic baby. There is no definitive, noninvasive method to determine the newborn's risk of thrombocytopenia, although the actual risk of severe bleeding during delivery appears low. In contrast, children born to mothers who are

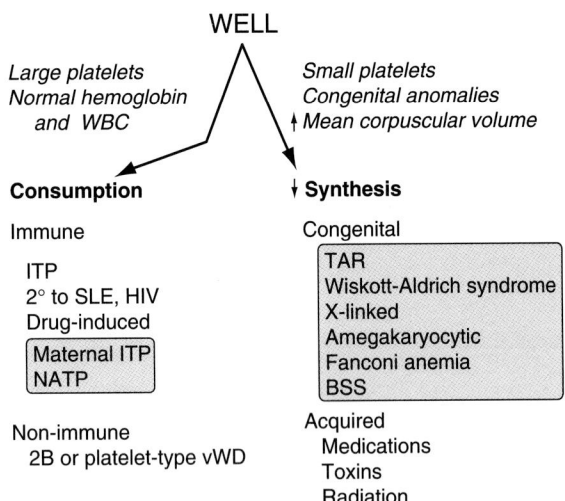

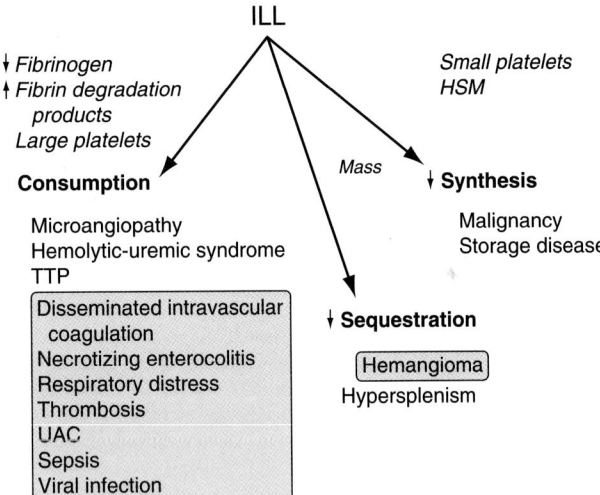

Figure 50-9. Differential diagnosis of childhood thrombocytopenic syndromes. The syndromes are initially separated by their clinical appearance. Clues leading to the diagnosis are presented in *italics*. The mechanisms and common disorders leading to these findings are shown in the lower part of the figure. Disorders that commonly affect neonates are listed in the *shaded boxes*. BSS, Bernard-Soulier syndrome; HIV, human immunodeficiency virus; HSM, hepatosplenomegaly; ITP, idiopathic immune thrombocytopenic purpura; NATP, neonatal alloimmune thrombocytopenic purpura; SLE, systemic lupus erythematosus; TAR, thrombocytopenia–absent radius (syndrome); TTP, thrombotic thrombocytopenic purpura; UAC, umbilical artery catheter; vWD, von Willebrand disease; WBC, white blood cell; 2°, secondary.

sensitized to paternal alloantigens present on the fetal platelets have a higher risk of perinatal hemorrhage and symptomatic thrombocytopenia. *Neonatal alloimmune thrombocytopenic purpura* (NATP), the platelet equivalent of maternal Rh isoimmunization, differs from Rh disease in that firstborn children are commonly affected. The importance of this diagnosis is that it is commonly associated with prenatal intracranial hemorrhage with a resultant high rate of morbidity and mortality (15%). Therefore, recognition of the diagnosis in the first pregnancy can have a major impact on the management of subsequent pregnancies. Transfusion of washed maternal platelets that lack the paternal alloantigen toward which the maternal antibody is directed will correct the platelet count and prevent further bleeding. Random donor platelets are rapidly destroyed. Newborns with NATP

can be easily differentiated from thrombocytopenic newborns of mothers with ITP on the basis of the mother's platelet count. Mothers with ITP are thrombocytopenic unless they have had a splenectomy. Mothers of infants with NATP have normal platelet counts.

Although the initial diagnosis of NATP is usually made by studying the reaction of maternal sera against paternal platelets, prenatal diagnosis is performed with molecular biologic techniques to detect the allelic differences between the mother and the fetus by analysis of various fetal DNA sources. After prenatal diagnosis, treatment of the mother with IVIG has been shown to raise the fetal platelet count and prevent fetal bleeding. In addition, postnatal treatment of the neonate with IVIG and corticosteroids may be helpful after restoration of a normal platelet count by transfusion of washed maternal platelets. All blood products administered to the neonate with thrombocytopenia should be radiated to prevent graft-versus-host disease, because some patients may have a congenital immunodeficiency syndrome manifested by thrombocytopenia.

CHILD ABUSE

The most common cause of remarkable bruising and bleeding with normal hemostatic screening studies is child abuse (see Chapter 36).

CHRONIC/INSIDIOUS ONSET OF MUCOCUTANEOUS BLEEDING

When symptoms of skin and mucous membrane bleeding are lifelong, the most common cause is *von Willebrand disease*. Congenital platelet function defects, congenital thrombocytopenic syndromes, and abnormalities of the vessel wall are less common. Von Willebrand disease, the deficiency of vWF, is the most common hereditary bleeding disorder, with a prevalence of approximately 1% of all children.

The inheritance of von Willebrand disease is usually autosomal dominant. vWF is a large multimeric protein that functions as the bridge between platelets and damaged vessel walls; therefore, deficient or dysfunctional vWF causes delayed formation of the platelet plug (see Fig. 50-3). In addition, vWF serves as a carrier protein for factor VIII. A profound deficiency of vWF is associated with low levels of factor VIII, so that the patient with severe von Willebrand disease has the clinical manifestations of both von Willebrand disease and hemophilia.

The presentation of von Willebrand disease is highly variable. Mucocutaneous bleeding or no symptoms are the most common findings. Because neonatal vWF levels are often elevated after vaginal delivery, the onset of clinical symptoms for mild and moderate von Willebrand disease is usually during the toddler stage or later. The only presenting complaint may be abnormal preoperative coagulation studies. The laboratory diagnosis of the disease is particularly challenging because there is no single test that optimally measures vWF function.

The PTT and bleeding time were thought to be adequate screening tests to detect von Willebrand disease. The disease can be detected in 92% of affected individuals with a battery that includes the PTT, bleeding time, and vWF activity, but in only 58% of such patients is either the PTT or the bleeding time abnormal. Physician judgment is critical, and the need for additional workup is defined by the clinical clues, including the patient's personal history of bleeding, the family history, and the potential for surgery.

The diagnosis of von Willebrand disease is further complicated by the observation that vWF is a labile protein and levels can be increased by stress, medication, trauma, pregnancy, and difficult venipuncture. In addition, vWF levels are blood type–dependent, and thus levels must be interpreted on the basis of the patient's blood type. It remains unclear whether there is a physiologically different hemostatic level of vWF for different blood groups. Age has been shown to influence vWF levels in adults, but this has not been adequately investigated in children. Furthermore, there are multiple variants of von Willebrand disease. As a result, the clinician should perform repeated studies if there is a high index of suspicion or abnormal positive screening tests, or both.

Von Willebrand disease can be classified as type 1 (classic disease with mild or moderate deficiency), type 2 (a dysproteinemia), or type 3 (severe disease: virtual absence of vWF and low levels of factor VIII). The treatment of the disease is dependent on the type and the response to 1-deamino(8-D-arginine) vasopressin (DDAVP). DDAVP is a synthetic vasopressin analog that induces the release of vWF and factor VIII. Levels of these factors rise threefold to fourfold after a dose of 0.3 µg/kg. For most cases of von Willebrand disease, DDAVP is the treatment of choice. A therapeutic trial with measurements of vWF before and both 1 hour and 4 hours after DDAVP administration should be performed to document the efficacy of DDAVP before surgery. Patients with rare variant forms of von Willebrand disease (type 2A, type 2B, and platelet type) may have no response or an adverse response to DDAVP; therefore, full studies to identify the subtype are needed before a trial of DDAVP. These studies correlate functional levels of vWF with the amount of protein measured antigenically (the vWF antigen), the multimeric size of the protein (vWF multimers), and the aggregation response of the patient's platelet-rich plasma to high and low concentrations of ristocetin.

Most patients with mild and moderate type 1 von Willebrand disease have a satisfactory response to DDAVP; hemostasis for most surgical procedures can be provided with daily doses of DDAVP on consecutive days. For severely affected patients or those with variant forms of the disease noted previously (type 2A, type 2B, platelet type), treatment should be individualized. Some patients with type 2A respond to DDAVP. Severely affected patients with von Willebrand disease and those with the 2B variant should receive a clotting factor concentrate containing a full complement of normal vWF multimers (Humate-P) in doses similar to those outlined for factor VIII in Table 50-7.

PLATELET FUNCTION DEFECTS

For patients with mucocutaneous bleeding but a normal platelet count and normal vWF studies, platelet aggregation studies should be performed to evaluate for a primary or secondary platelet function defect. A large number of medications alter platelet function and may induce an acquired abnormality of platelet function. A careful history to elicit exposure to medications and to determine whether clinical symptoms correlate with exposure to specific drugs is critical. Common medications that alter platelet functions are aspirin, nonsteroidal antiinflammatory drugs, alcohol, penicillin in high doses, and valproic acid.

Most primary platelet function defects cause relatively mild mucocutaneous bleeding symptoms. In these disorders, there is most commonly an abnormality of the storage granules or release mechanism within the platelet, causing delayed or diminished response to agonists that induce platelet aggregation, such as collagen. Platelet function defects, like most other hemostatic defects, are accentuated by medications that impair platelet function. In rare instances, a patient demonstrates impressive petechiae and hematomas at birth because of an absence of one of the essential platelet membrane receptors for the adhesive proteins vWF or fibrinogen. These disorders, *Glanzmann thrombasthenia* (deficiency of glycoprotein IIb/IIIa, the fibrinogen receptor) and *Bernard-Soulier syndrome* (deficiency of glycoprotein Ib, the von Willebrand receptor), represent the most severe types of platelet function defects. The platelet count is normal in Glanzmann thrombocytopenia, but patients with Bernard-Soulier syndrome usually have thrombocytopenia with remarkably large platelets. Patients with mild or moderate platelet function defects often respond to DDAVP, but more severe bleeding may necessitate platelet transfusions.

CHRONIC THROMBOCYTOPENIC SYNDROMES

Patients with long-standing thrombocytopenia usually present with mucocutaneous bleeding. Mechanisms of the thrombocytopenia include impaired marrow synthesis, sequestration, and increased destruction (see Fig. 50-9). These can be acquired or congenital.

In general, the congenital thrombocytopenic syndromes usually manifest at the time of birth or early in infancy. These syndromes may be associated with congenital anomalies (thrombocytopenia–absent radius syndrome and Fanconi anemia) or as part of a complex hereditary syndrome (Wiskott-Aldrich syndrome with small platelets, eczema, and immunodeficiency) in addition to thrombocytopenia. Small platelets are a frequent finding in many of the syndromes associated with decreased platelet production. During the physical examination of patients with suspected congenital thrombocytopenia, the clinician must search not only for the signs of bleeding but also for subtle congenital anomalies, including abnormal growth parameters; the presence of skin lesions; and anomalies of the limbs, axial skeleton, and urinary tract.

The acquired causes of thrombocytopenia resulting from decreased production usually have an insidious onset of symptoms and are often associated with other abnormalities in the blood count. The *aplastic syndromes* (congenital aplastic anemia and acquired aplastic anemia) are associated with the gradual onset of thrombocytopenia, usually in association with a falling granulocyte count and anemia (see Chapter 48). Platelets are small, and the mean corpuscular volume is usually elevated.

Table 50-7. Characteristics of Factors VIII and IX and Respective Modes of Treatment for Bleeding Episodes Caused by Hemophilia A or B

	Factor VIII	Factor IX
Yield	1.5%-2%/U/kg infused	0.7%-1.0%/U/kg infused
Half-life	8-12 hr	18-24 hr
Therapeutic level		
Life and limb threatening	80%-100%	80%-100%
Routine: hemarthrosis	40%	30%
Dose computation	Level desired × weight (kg) × 0.5	Level desired × weight (kg) × 1.3
Therapeutic alternatives	DDAVP*	Recombinant factor IX concentrate
	Recombinant factor VIII concentrate	Monoclonal factor IX concentrate
	Monoclonal factor VIII concentrate	Prothrombin complex concentrate (PCC)†

*After adequate levels have been demonstrated.

†Repeated doses are associated with thromboembolic risk.

DDAVP, 1-deamino(8-D-arginine) vasopressin.

Infiltration of the marrow by malignant cells or storage cells interferes with normal thrombopoiesis and commonly results in thrombocytopenia. Common malignancies associated with thrombocytopenia include acute lymphoblastic leukemia, lymphomas, histiocytosis X, and metastatic solid tumors (neuroblastoma). Abnormalities of other blood elements, as well as findings of adenopathy, hepatosplenomegaly, or masses, are clues to the presence of an infiltrative disorder.

Disorders of the vessel walls may present either acutely or chronically. *Vasculitic disorders* often manifest with lesions of the skin and mucous membranes that appear hemorrhagic and are associated with clinical symptoms related to involvement of other organ systems (gastrointestinal, renal, central nervous system). Paradoxically, patients with these disorders usually have normal coagulation studies and normal platelet counts. Henoch-Schönlein purpura is an example; it manifests with a purpuric rash, including both petechiae and larger palpable purpuric lesions of the lower extremities and buttocks, often found in association with arthritis, cramping abdominal pain, and focal glomerulonephritis (see Chapters 55 and 56).

Petechiae and ecchymoses are also common symptoms of disorders of the collagen matrix. Patients with Ehlers-Danlos syndrome have lax joints, hyperelastic skin, and abnormal wound healing. These patients frequently present with ecchymoses and rarely with petechiae. Hemostatic studies are often nondiagnostic, other than that the bleeding time is usually prolonged. The diagnosis is made on the basis of clinical findings, although platelet aggregation studies may be mildly abnormal.

DEEP BLEEDING

Bleeding into the tissues of the muscles or joints is characteristic of hemophilia. The presentation of the patient with hemophilia varies with severity, age, and exposure to trauma. Surprisingly, only one third of boys with hemophilia bleed excessively at circumcision, and neonatal intracranial bleeding is rare despite the trauma of a vaginal delivery. After the neonatal period, children with hemophilia usually present as toddlers with either intramuscular hematomas or hemarthroses. In the toddler stage, the most commonly affected joints are the ankles and elbows; the knees, hips, and shoulders are affected later. The affected children, who are usually boys, usually bruise easily, and hematomas frequently develop over areas of common trauma (the forehead, arms, and legs, especially over the pretibial area). Other common bleeding sites include the frenulum and sites of venipuncture. Sites of life-threatening bleeding include the central nervous system (the most common cause of death from hemorrhage); the mouth and throat, resulting in airway obstruction; and the retroperitoneal area or gastrointestinal tract, leading to exsanguination.

Red flags for the diagnosis of hemophilia are

- persistent bleeding after circumcision
- hemarthrosis/intramuscular hematoma
- bleeding frenulum

The deficiency of factor VIII (hemophilia A) or factor IX (hemophilia B) causes bleeding because delayed thrombin formation results in a large, friable clot. Often there is an initial hemostatic plug that breaks down hours after the injury (secondary bleeding). Because factors VIII and IX are necessary for normal wound healing, patients with inadequate replacement or untreated hemophilia frequently have poorly healed wounds.

Hemophilia A occurs in 1 per 10,000 live births and hemophilia B in about 1 per 40,000. The PTT is prolonged and should correct on 1:1 mix with normal plasma. Specific assays for factors VIII and IX should be performed to identify the deficient factor. Severity is determined by the level of the deficient clotting factor. Severe hemophilia is defined as less than 1% factor activity, moderate as 1% to 5% activity, and mild as greater than 5% activity. These factor levels correlate approximately with clinical symptoms: Patients with severe deficiency bleed spontaneously; patients with moderate deficiency bleed with minor trauma; and patients with mild deficiency bleed only after significant trauma, and their condition may go undiagnosed for many years.

Because hemophilia A and hemophilia B are transmitted as X-linked traits, the family history may be informative if there is a history of male maternal relatives with a bleeding disorder. Approximately 33% of affected patients have new mutations and therefore have a negative family history. In rare cases, bleeding complications have occurred in female carriers, especially at surgery; thus, all carriers should have factor levels measured. According to the *Lyons hypothesis* (random inactivation of the X chromosome), some carriers should be symptomatic because they represent the lower end of the predicted bell-shaped distribution of factor levels for female carriers.

Treatment of hemophilia requires prompt replacement or correction of the deficient factor with the safest available material. Table 50-7 provides dosing information and therapeutic alternatives for factors VIII and IX deficiency. Treatment of bleeding episodes should be continued until the wound has healed. Recombinant factor VIII or IX concentrate appears to be the current optimal treatment product, with monoclonally purified factor as a second choice. For patients with mild hemophilia A who respond to DDAVP with adequate levels, DDAVP is the treatment of choice. Even when recombinant material is available, all children with bleeding disorders should receive hepatitis B vaccine. Prophylaxis with factor concentrates has revolutionized the care of children with hemophilia by preventing chronic arthropathy and muscular atrophy. Patients with hemophilia should be monitored at comprehensive treatment centers that are experienced in the medical, social, physical, and financial impact of hemophilia care.

The common complications of hemophilia treatment can be divided into those of immunologic origin and those caused by infectious organisms. In 15% to 25% of patients with hemophilia A and a smaller percentage of patients with hemophilia B, inhibitors to clotting factor replacement material develop. These inhibitors, usually immunoglobulin G antibodies, lead to rapid inactivation and clearance of infused replacement material. The presence of an inhibitor should be suspected and tested for in any patient with hemophilia who does not respond appropriately to factor replacement. The treatment of patients with inhibitors is problematic and should be relegated to experts in hemophilia care. The management of acute bleeding episodes may require administration of an activated clotting factor concentrate to "bypass" the inhibitor.

Infectious complications of hemophilia therapy were once exceedingly common but, fortunately, have been curtailed by donor screening, sophisticated viral inactivation processes, and chemical purification techniques used in the preparation of plasma-derived replacement material. Recombinant factor concentrates represent the culmination of these efforts. Older patients treated before 1983 with concentrates were exposed to HIV, hepatitis C, and sometimes to hepatitis B and the δ agent. Most patients exposed to HIV became infected and manifested the spectrum of signs and symptoms of HIV infection. Viral inactivation techniques in conjunction with intense donor screening for hepatitis C antibody has greatly decreased the risk of hepatitis C exposure. Nevertheless, chronic non-A, non-B hepatitis is a common finding in older patients with hemophilia who were treated with concentrates.

SURGICAL BLEEDING

Aside from technical causes, most surgical bleeding results from a failure to recognize a preexisting coagulopathy. Von Willebrand disease and primary or secondary platelet dysfunction are the most common causes of bleeding after ear, nose, and throat surgery. Significant hemorrhaging after general surgery is often a manifestation of previously undiagnosed mild or moderate hemophilia or vitamin K deficiency.

When elective surgery is planned, the decision to perform preoperative hemostatic screening is influenced by the patient's age (and therefore previous exposure to trauma), personal and family histories of bleeding, and type of surgery. Certain surgical procedures (tonsillectomy, scoliosis repair, central nervous system surgery) provide major challenges to hemostasis, having a high frequency of bleeding complications. In contrast, most general surgical procedures (e.g., hernia repair) rarely involve clinical bleeding. The diagnostic yield of preoperative studies before tonsillectomy and adenoidectomy remains controversial. In studies, the frequency of detecting significant hemostatic abnormalities in children with no prior diagnosis of a hemostatic disorder before tonsillectomy has varied from 0.5% to 11.5%.

GENERALIZED BLEEDING

Generalized bleeding is a manifestation of a major disorder of hemostasis, usually caused by a deficiency of multiple factors in association with deficient or dysfunctional platelets. Generalized bleeding occurs most commonly in the context of DIC in seriously ill patients. In rare cases, rat poison (warfarin) intoxication produces such bleeding.

DISSEMINATED INTRAVASCULAR COAGULATION

DIC is a generalized consumption of clotting factors, anticoagulant proteins, and platelets triggered by a life-threatening illness and usually accompanied by ischemia, hypoxia, and shock (Table 50-8). DIC may be either a hemorrhagic or a thrombotic disorder, or both, inasmuch as the clinical manifestations of this generalized coagulopathy are highly variable. Laboratory studies usually demonstrate a prolonged PT, decreased fibrinogen level, and decreased platelet level (these are the most reliable indicators of DIC), in addition to increased FDP (and elevated D-dimer) levels and a prolonged PTT.

Several mechanisms can trigger acute DIC, including widespread endothelial damage induced directly or indirectly by infectious organisms and release of procoagulant material after trauma. Virtually any life-threatening illness can trigger DIC. In acute DIC, activation of the clotting mechanism leads to consumption of clotting factors (I, II, V, VIII), anticoagulant proteins (C, S, antithrombin, plasminogen), and platelets. In the syndrome known as *purpura fulminans,* microvascular thromboses develop in the skin, causing painful purpuric lesions that progress to localized necrotic lesions. Table 50-9 presents laboratory findings in DIC in comparison with those in other acquired coagulopathies that potentially could be confused with DIC. Because DIC is virtually always seen in a child with a life-threatening illness, the clinical diagnosis is usually made on the basis of the child's clinical appearance in association with laboratory abnormalities. Clotting factor and anticoagulant protein levels are confirmatory but seldom necessary to reach a diagnosis of DIC. The only diagnosis difficult to differentiate from DIC in the laboratory is that of severe hepatic disease with impending liver failure. Nevertheless, the patient with severe liver disease is markedly jaundiced; thrombocytopenia is relatively mild.

The treatment of DIC focuses on the cause of the DIC, on the altered homeostasis that sustains the coagulopathy, and on the bleeding or thrombotic complications that ensue. Shock itself plays a critical role in DIC because shock reduces the reticuloendothelial clearance of activated clotting factors and complexes. Reduced hepatic blood flow causes decreased synthesis of depleted clotting and anticoagulant proteins.

To summarize the treatment of DIC:

1. Treat the initiating and propagating events.
2. Optimize cardiorespiratory status by improving perfusion and correcting acidosis.
3. Replace deficient platelets, clotting factors, and anticoagulant proteins (Table 50-10). Specific indications for replacement are

Table 50-8. Causes of Disseminated Intravascular Coagulation

Infection
Meningococcemia (purpura fulminans)
Other gram-negative bacteria (*Haemophilus* species, *Salmonella* species, *Escherichia coli*)
Gram-positive bacteria (group B streptococci, staphylococci)
Rickettsiae (Rocky Mountain spotted fever)
Virus (cytomegalovirus, herpes, hemorrhagic fevers)
Malaria
Fungus

Tissue Injury
Central nervous system trauma (massive head injury)
Multiple fractures with fat emboli
Crush injury
Profound shock or asphyxia
Hypothermia or hyperthermia
Massive burns

Malignancy
Acute promyelocytic leukemia
Acute monoblastic or myelocytic leukemia
Widespread malignancies (neuroblastoma)

Venom or Toxin
Snake bites
Insect bites

Microangiopathic Disorders
"Severe" thrombotic thrombocytopenic purpura or hemolytic-uremic syndrome
Giant hemangioma (Kasabach-Merrit syndrome)

Gastrointestinal Disorders
Fulminant hepatitis
Severe inflammatory bowel disease
Reye syndrome

Hereditary Thrombotic Disorders
Antithrombin deficiency
Homozygous protein C deficiency

Neonatal Disorders
Maternal toxemia
Group B streptococcal infections
Abruptio placentae
Severe respiratory distress syndrome
Necrotizing enterocolitis
Congenital viral disease (cytomegalovirus, herpes)
Erythroblastosis fetalis

Miscellaneous Disorders
Severe acute graft rejection
Acute hemolytic transfusion reaction
Severe collagen-vascular disease
Kawasaki disease
Heparin-induced thrombosis
Infusion of "activated" prothrombin complex concentrates
Hyperpyrexia/encephalopathy, hemorrhagic shock syndrome

Modified from Montgomery RR, Scott JP: Hemostasis: Disease of the fluid phase. In Nathan DG, Oski FA (eds): Hematology of Infancy and Childhood, 4th ed. vol 2. Philadelphia, WB Saunders, 1993, p 1639.

Table 50-9. Differential Diagnosis of Coagulopathies that Can Be Confused with Disseminated Intravascular Coagulation (DIC)

	Prothrombin Time	Partial Thromboplastin Time	Fibrinogen	Platelets	Fibrinogen Degradation Products	Clinical Keys
DIC	↑	↑	↓	↓	↑	Shock (see Table 50-8)
Liver failure	↑	↑	↓	Normal or ↓	↑	Jaundice
Vitamin K deficiency	↑	↑	Normal	Normal	Normal	Malabsorption, liver disease
Sepsis without shock	↑	↑	Normal	Normal	↑ or normal	Fever

variable and depend on the patient's clinical condition and severity of bleeding.

The following are rough guidelines for treatment:

- fresh-frozen plasma, 10 to 15 mL/kg every 6 to 12 hours, to provide clotting factors
- platelets, one bag/5 kg for platelet count less than 50,000/mm^3
- cryoprecipitate, one bag/5 kg for fibrinogen level less than 100 mg/dL
- anticoagulant therapy for major vessel thrombosis

The efficacy of anticoagulant therapy in DIC has not been proved in controlled prospective studies. Heparin has been used for the treatment of purpura fulminans, acute promyelocytic leukemia, and thromboses that develop in conjunction with DIC. Most patients with DIC have a coagulopathy that consumes procoagulant proteins and causes clinical oozing or bleeding; in a small percentage of patients, however, thrombosis develops. In these patients, anticoagulant therapy may decrease morbidity and should be administered in a manner similar to that for those patients who have major vascular thrombosis (Table 50-11). Deficient clotting factors and platelets should be transfused to prevent further development of thrombosis or bleeding during anticoagulation. In rare cases of partially compensated DIC, heparin therapy has been used to slow the coagulopathy, but no studies have documented the benefits of heparin in such circumstances. Finally, in some patients with DIC and poor peripheral perfusion, particularly those in whom the extremities are cool and cyanotic, low-dose heparin (5 to 10 units/kg/hour) has been tried to prevent small- and large-vessel thromboses. In DIC associated with severe sepsis, coagulation and the inflammatory response are activated. The protein C/S system interacts with both of these. Activated protein C has anti-inflammatory and antithrombotic properties. Drotrecogin alfa (recombinant activated protein C) reduces mortality and leads to a more rapid recovery of cardiorespiratory function in severe sepsis with organ dysfunction in adults. Clinical trials in children with DIC and sepsis are ongoing.

NEONATAL PURPURA FULMINANS

The neonate who presents with multiple purpuric lesions over the buttocks, trunk, extremities, and face (nose, ears) that change from dark red to purple and black over a few minutes in association with abnormal neurologic findings or an abdominal mass presents a special case.

Although the differential diagnosis of these findings should include both sepsis with DIC and a generalized viral infection, the key finding in such a child is the presence of painful petechiae and purpura (purpura fulminans). The most likely diagnosis with this presentation is homozygous protein C deficiency. After viral and bacterial cultures, diagnostic studies should include CBC, platelet count, and coagulation screening for DIC, as well as measurements of protein C, protein S, ATIII, and plasminogen.

To confirm this diagnosis, the clinician must differentiate DIC from congenital protein C deficiency. DIC is characterized by the consumption of clotting factors, anticoagulant proteins, and platelets. Although protein C levels fall in DIC, patients with congenital protein C deficiency have strikingly low levels of protein C.

Table 50-10. Commonly Used Hemostatic Agents*

Component	Contents	Usual Dose	Comments/Disadvantages
FFP (unit)	1 U/mL of each clotting factor	10-15 mL/kg	Large volume
Cryoprecipitate (bag)	100 units factor VIII/bag 150 mg fibrinogen/bag Factor XIII, fibronectin	0.2 bag/kg	Infectious risk
Platelets (unit)	5.0-7.0 × 10^{10} platelets in 30-60 mL of plasma	0.2 U/kg	Infectious risk
Factor concentrates (units)	Units as labeled	Factor VIII, 20-50 μ/kg*	Recombinant
		Factor IX, 30-130 μ/kg*	
DDAVP	4 μg/mL	0.3 μg/kg/dose	Increases factor VIII and vWf threefold to fourfold; Useful for platelet function defects, uremia, liver disease Rare hyponatremia
AT concentrate	Units as labeled	$\dfrac{\text{Desired-baseline AT} \times \text{wt}}{1.4}$	Plasma-derived, virus inactivated

*Key points to transfusion: (1) Determine deficiency state. (2) Use appropriate dose and material. (3) Measure response 1-2 hours and 24 hours after transfusion.

AT, antithrombin; FFP, fresh-frozen plasma; DDAVP, 1-deamino(8-D-arginine) desmopressin; vWF, von Willebrand factor.

Table 50-11. Comparison of Antithrombotic Agents

	Fibrinolytic Therapy	Standard Heparin*	Warfarin
Indication	Recent onset of life- or limb-threatening thrombus	Thrombus of indeterminate age	Long-term oral anticoagulation
Dose	rTPA, 0.1-0.2 mg/kg/hr IV	50 U/kg/bolus, 20-25 U/kg/hr by continuous infusion	0.1-0.2 mg/kg/day PO
Adjustment	Increase dose for lack of clinical effect	↑ dose by 5%-10% q6h until adequate level or PTT achieved	Daily until stable INR achieved
Course	1-72 hr	5-14 days	Weeks to months
Monitors	"Lytic state" ↑ FDP or D-dimer (rTPA) ↑ thrombin time (UK)	PTT, 2-2½ × control value Thrombin time infinity Heparin level, 0.3-0.7 IU/mL	INR, 2.0-3.0
Mechanism	Activation of plasminogen to plasmin	Accelerates AT-dependent inactivation of factors IIa (thrombin) and Xa	Impairs vitamin K–dependent carboxylation of factors II, VII, IX, X
Risk of bleeding	Medium/high	Low	Low

*For low-molecular-weight (LMW) heparin, the dose is 1.0 mg/kg q12h (1.6 mg/kg for neonates and infants) subcutaneously. Check LMW heparin level 3 hours after the fourth dose with the goal of achieving a LMW heparin level of 0.5-1.0 IU/mL. LMW heparin may be used for long-term outpatient anticoagulation. Aspirin is the only commonly used antiplatelet agent, and the usual dose is 80 mg/day (one baby aspirin daily). There is no need to monitor aspirin therapy.

AT, antithrombin; FDP, fibrin degradation product; INR, international normalized ratio; IV, intravenously; PO, per os (orally); PTT, partial thromboplastin time; rTPA, recombinant tissue-type plasminogen activator; UK, urokinase.

Anticoagulant proteins are routinely consumed in situations of widespread activation of the clotting mechanism. Therefore, mildly depressed levels of protein S, ATIII, and plasminogen would be expected when there is generalized intravascular coagulation. In congenital protein C deficiency, the protein C level is strikingly lower than that of the other anticoagulant proteins, which increases the likelihood that the deficiency of protein C represents the primary cause of the coagulopathy. To determine whether the deficiency is hereditary, the next step is to obtain blood samples from the parents to measure levels of the deficient protein or proteins. In homozygous deficiencies, the levels of both parents should be reduced. Deficiency of protein C, protein S, or AT usually manifests as venous thromboembolic disease in adulthood and is inherited as a codominant trait. Congenital severe, symptomatic protein C deficiency is usually inherited in an autosomal recessive manner from asymptomatic parents.

Therapy must be instituted promptly to replace the deficient anticoagulant protein with fresh-frozen plasma. Fresh-frozen plasma contains all of the clotting factors in an unconcentrated form. Protein C has a short half-life and may need to be infused every 6 to 12 hours to maintain measurable levels. This, unfortunately, leads to problems with fluid and protein overload if repeated doses of plasma are necessary. Protein C concentrate is undergoing clinical trials, and when it is available, the patient should be treated with protein C concentrate to correct the deficiency. The patient should also undergo anticoagulation with heparin to limit further thromboses. A striking improvement after administration of protein C, either as plasma or as concentrate, is strong evidence of the diagnosis. Warfarin therapy has been effective in managing such patients on a chronic basis.

OTHER CAUSES OF GENERALIZED BLEEDING

A coagulopathy is a common complication of severe *liver disease,* resulting from deficient production of multiple clotting factors and anticoagulant proteins in association with increased FDPs formed as a result of hyperfibrinolysis. FDPs inhibit platelet function.

Uremia results in a diffuse bleeding diathesis, with mucosal bleeding (epistaxis, gastrointestinal bleeding) as a major manifestation. The major underlying mechanism in uremic bleeding appears to be increased nitric oxide generation, leading to abnormal platelet function. Many patients with bleeding caused by uremia or liver disease respond to DDAVP.

Vitamin K deficiency manifests as generalized bleeding into the skin, gastrointestinal tract, and central nervous system. Children at highest risk are breast-fed neonates, malnourished individuals, those receiving broad-spectrum antibiotics, those with cholestatic liver disease and subsequent vitamin K malabsorption, and those who have ingested rat poison/warfarin. The treatment of patients with vitamin K deficiency is parenteral vitamin K. The response is usually rapid, but in emergency situations, transfusion of fresh-frozen plasma corrects the coagulopathy faster. Differentiation of some of these syndromes from DIC is presented in Table 50-9.

THROMBOSIS

Thromboembolic disease in pediatrics has a bimodal age distribution. Venous and arterial thrombi are common in newborns, especially in premature neonates, because of the combination of low levels of anticoagulant proteins, decreased blood flow, elevated blood viscosity because of high hematocrit, and, in particular, because of the placement of intravascular catheters for monitoring and nutrition. The second peak of thromboembolic disease, usually venous in character, is in adolescence, when patients with primary deficiencies of anticoagulant proteins typically present and when secondary disorders (e.g., vasculitis, pregnancy, malignancy, surgery, major trauma, inflammatory bowel disease, and infection) induce a higher frequency of venous thrombosis.

Abnormalities of protein C or protein S may be identified in 25% of the children with deep venous thrombosis. Furthermore, in 40% to 60% of patients with familial or recurrent thrombotic disease, factor V Leiden is the cause of the prothrombotic condition. This structural abnormality of factor V renders it resistant to proteolysis by APC. The prothrombin G20210A mutation is a mutation in the 3′ untranslated end of the prothrombin mRNA that results in higher circulating levels of prothrombin. In young adults with thromboses, the most common hereditary abnormalities are (in order) factor V Leiden, the prothrombin 20210 mutation, and deficiencies of protein C, protein S and antithrombin. There are significant racial differences in the frequency distribution of these mutations. Because factor V Leiden and prothrombin 20210 mutations are common, combined defects are not unusual.

VENOUS THROMBOEMBOLIC DISEASE

Diagnostic Approach

Venous thromboembolic disease classically manifests with a warm, swollen, tender extremity or affected organ. The differential diagnosis in such cases includes trauma, infection, stasis without thrombosis, lymphedema, and neoplasm. In children and adolescents, thrombi may develop within major internal organs with distinctive clinical manifestations, including sagittal sinus thrombosis with resultant increased intracranial pressure; hepatic vein thrombosis with the Budd-Chiari syndrome; portal vein thrombosis associated with splenomegaly and varices; and renal vein thrombosis with a resultant abdominal mass, hematuria, and proteinuria. Long-term central venous access is associated with a significant risk of asymptomatic venous thrombosis. Pulmonary emboli may manifest as "atypical" pneumonia that results in shortness of breath and hypoxemia in the absence of fever. The hypoxemia may occur in the presence of minimal findings on routine chest radiographs.

The clinician should obtain a careful history for antecedent trauma, infection, or other predisposing causes of thromboembolic disease (Table 50-12). The abdomen and extremities should be carefully examined for mass lesions leading to venous stasis. The presence of a bruit or hemihypertrophy of the affected limb is a clue to an arteriovenous malformation. In addition, masses within the bone, abdominal tumors, and lymphatic obstruction should be considered. Initial laboratory studies should include a CBC, platelet count, and evaluation for DIC, as well as cultures of the blood if the patient is febrile. During the process of a localized thrombosis, there may be consumption of clotting factors, but rarely is the consumption significant enough in older children and adults to induce abnormal results on routine coagulation screening tests (platelets, PT, PTT, fibrinogen). Tests for fibrin breakdown (FDPs, D-dimer) may be positive. Unfortunately, these tests are nonspecific and not necessarily diagnostic of vascular thrombosis. Studies in adults have indicated that a negative assay for D-dimer has a strong negative predictive value for pulmonary embolus, especially when combined with an algorithm for risk assignment. The diagnostic approach to a patient with suspected venous thrombosis is presented in Figure 50-10.

Specific Diagnostic Studies

Venography remains the "gold standard" for the diagnosis of venous thromboembolic disease. Doppler flow studies, various forms of plethysmography, and compression ultrasonography have been used with variable results.

Doppler studies detect the flow of red blood cells through the artery or vein being examined. Plethysmography measures the change in blood volume within the extremity that occurs with respiration. If there is obstruction to flow, the normal physiologic variation is diminished.

Compression ultrasonography simply assesses the ability of the ultrasound probe to fully compress (completely lose the image of the lumen) when pressure is applied to the probe overlying the vessel in question. Fluid-filled vessels are readily compressible, whereas those in which a clot is present in the lumen are not. When these

---

Table 50-12. Hypercoagulable States
Primary Disorders (Congenital)
Factor V Leiden (activated protein C resistance)
Prothrombin 20210 mutation
Protein C deficiency
Protein S deficiency
Antithrombin deficiency
Plasminogen deficiencies
Homocystinuria
Dysfibrinogenemia
Secondary Disorders (Acquired)
Coagulopathies
Lupus anticoagulant (antiphospholipid syndrome)
Nephrotic syndrome
Oral contraceptives
Malignancy
Therapy with activated prothrombin complex concentrates
Pregnancy
Autoimmune disorders
Platelet Disorders
Diabetes mellitus
Myeloproliferative disorders
Thrombocythemia
Paroxysmal nocturnal hemoglobinuria
Flow and Vessel Disorders
Polycythemia-hyperviscosity
Marfan syndrome
Vasculitis
Vessel grafts
Vascular stasis
Trauma
Indwelling catheters
Surgery
Immobilization

Adapted from Schafer A: The hypercoagulable states. Ann Intern Med 1985;102:814; and from Behrman RE, Kliegman RM (eds): Nelson Essentials of Pediatrics, 2nd ed. Philadelphia, WB Saunders, 1994, p 56.

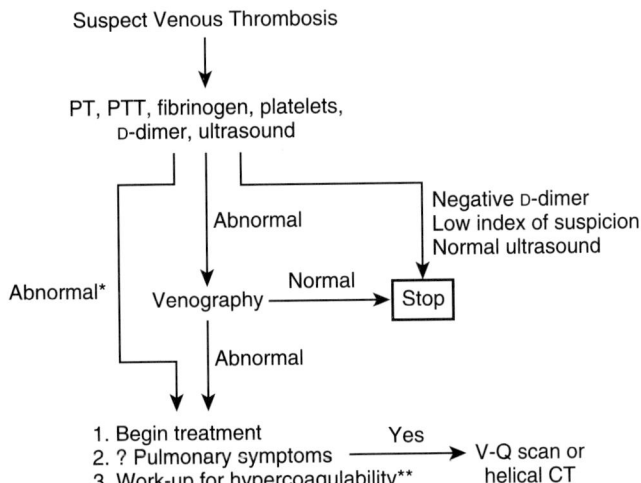

Figure 50-10. Flow diagram for the approach to a patient with venous thromboembolic disease. For patients with clinical findings indicative of thrombosis, positive D-dimer assay and positive compression or Doppler ultrasound study for deep vein thrombosis, some authors would treat without confirming the diagnosis by venography. **See Table 50-12. CT, computed tomography; PT, prothrombin time; PTT, partial thromboplastin time; V-Q, ventilation-perfusion.

findings have been compared with venography, variable results have been obtained, which is suggestive of significant differences in the techniques employed. Although repetitive Doppler studies and plethysmography appear to be relatively sensitive and specific, their sensitivity and specificity in children have not been documented. Before committing a child to long-term anticoagulant therapy, it may be best to document the presence of thrombosis by the most accurate tool currently available, contrast venography.

After a diagnosis of deep vein thrombosis has been made, the clinician must assess the risk of propagation and embolization of the thrombus. Calf vein thrombi rarely embolize and therefore are usually treated symptomatically. More proximal thrombi have a much higher likelihood of propagation and embolization and thus mandate systemic anticoagulation. If the patient has respiratory symptoms of any sort, a ventilation-perfusion scan to evaluate for pulmonary emboli is warranted. Although ventilation-perfusion scanning for pulmonary emboli has been the standard for many years, helical computed tomographic scanning may be equally useful with the added benefit of providing anatomic detail to the analysis. Patients with symptoms indicative of pulmonary emboli require closer monitoring and more vigorous therapy (see Chapter 3). If pulmonary embolus is strongly suspected, anticoagulation with heparin should be started before the diagnostic evaluation is completed.

Once a diagnosis of thrombosis has been made, the clinician should

- measure levels of anticoagulant proteins: protein C, protein S, antithrombin, plasminogen
- perform molecular analysis for factor V Leiden and prothrombin 20210 mutations
- measure plasma homocysteine
- perform anticardiolipin antibody and lupus anticoagulant assays to evaluate for the antiphospholipid syndrome

Levels of protein C, AT, and plasminogen may be depleted after development of deep vein thrombosis, pulmonary emboli, or both. As such, low levels do not necessarily imply a congenital deficiency. If low levels are found, studies should be performed on the parents to establish the inheritance of the deficiency, because all these are inherited as autosomal codominant traits. The patient's levels should be reevaluated several months after the acute event; the clinician should remember that warfarin reduces functional levels of all the vitamin K–dependent proteins, including proteins C and S.

The lupus anticoagulant causes a prolonged PTT that fails to correct on mixing with normal plasma because of the presence of an antibody that reacts with the phospholipid reagent in the PTT. The lupus anticoagulant does not bind in vivo to the platelet membrane; thus, the whole blood clotting time is normal. Paradoxically, the lupus anticoagulant is associated with venous and arterial thromboembolic disease and spontaneous abortions but is usually not a cause of clinical bleeding.

If these study findings are negative, the thrombin time should be measured or a comparison of functional and antigenic levels of fibrinogen should be done to detect a *dysfibrinogenemia.*

ARTERIAL THROMBOSIS

Arterial thrombi are rare in older children and adolescents and are frequently a manifestation of a systemic disorder resulting in vascular damage or embolic disease (sickle cell anemia, Kawasaki disease, bacterial endocarditis, periarteritis nodosa, cocaine ingestion). Homocystinuria can manifest with arterial thromboses. The presence of an intraarterial catheter is an obvious nidus for thrombosis.

Neck trauma that is often mild can cause carotid or vertebral artery dissection or aneurysms. These dissections or aneurysms can result in emboli to the brain. A history of neck trauma (which may be minor) should be sought in older children who present with arterial stroke.

ANTICOAGULANT THERAPY

Heparin

Heparin is the most commonly used agent for the initial treatment of venous or arterial thrombosis. Heparin functions as an anticoagulant by binding to ATIII and accelerating the ATIII-dependent inactivation of thrombin and factor Xa, as well as of factors IXa and XIa. Although most studies of heparin pharmacokinetics have been performed in adults, there are important differences in the pharmacologic features of heparin in children and especially neonates. Thirty-nine percent of children achieve a prolongation of the PTT within the target range after a bolus dose of 50 U/kg. Children younger than 1 year required an average of 28 U/kg/hour to maintain a therapeutic level of the PTT. In contrast, most children older than 1 year are satisfactorily maintained on 20 U/kg/hour of heparin. One protocol recommends an initial bolus of 50 U/kg of heparin, with 20 to 25 U/kg/hour for a minimum of 5 days to maintain a PTT of approximately 2 to 2½ times the control value. The heparin dose should be adjusted every 4 to 6 hours until a satisfactory level is attained. Reports in adults suggest that the heparin level is superior for monitoring heparin therapy. Studies have documented an increased risk of recurrent thrombi in patients who failed to achieve adequate anticoagulant levels promptly. Heparin levels are especially useful in premature and full-term newborns who may have a "normal" prolonged PTT. A therapeutic range of 0.3 to 0.6 U/dL appears to be effective.

Low-molecular-weight (LMW) heparin provides an alternative to standard heparin therapy. Pediatric experience with LMW heparin given subcutaneously is similar to that in adults. LMW heparin given to infants and children with thromboses appears to be as effective as standard heparin, with a similar or reduced risk of bleeding. LMW heparin requires much less laboratory monitoring. The therapeutic dose of the LMW heparin enoxaparin in pediatrics is 1.6 mg/kg for neonates and 1.0 mg/kg every 12 hours for older children.

For long-term anticoagulant therapy, warfarin can be started soon after the institution of heparin therapy; 5 days of heparin therapy is as good as longer courses of treatment for routine venous thrombotic disease.

Fibrinolytic Therapy

Fibrinolytic therapy is indicated for serious and potentially life-threatening thrombosis. Fibrinolytic therapy provides for more rapid lysis of clots than does standard anticoagulant treatment with heparin, and it is clinically effective in both arterial and venous clots. Because bleeding complications are many times higher than those with heparin in older individuals, the clinical severity of the clot must justify the use of lytic therapy. For smaller thrombi or those in nonvital locations, heparin is safe and effective. Lytic therapy is best used early in the evolution of the thrombus. If the clot has been long-standing, it is unlikely that fibrinolytic therapy will be efficacious.

The presence of any intracranial process, recent major surgery, or recent significant bleeding is an absolute contraindication to fibrinolytic therapy and a relative contraindication to heparin treatment. In patients with a normal cranial sonogram (or computed tomography) and complete occlusion of the aorta or evidence of compromise of major organ function, fibrinolytic therapy has been safely and successfully administered with very careful monitoring. Table 50-11 outlines dose and monitoring studies for two commonly used fibrinolytic agents: recombinant TPA and urokinase. Fibrinolytic therapy appears to result in a more rapid return of pulmonary artery flow after pulmonary emboli and may decrease the likelihood of postphlebitic syndrome after deep vein thrombosis.

Warfarin

Warfarin (Coumadin) is the anticoagulant of choice for long-term oral therapy. Warfarin acts by blocking the vitamin K–dependent post-translational modification of factors II, VII, IX, and X and of protein C and protein S. The usual dose is 0.05 to 0.2 mg/kg/day. Younger children appear to require higher doses to achieve a therapeutic level of the international normalized ratio (INR).* If warfarin therapy is started early in the course of heparin therapy for thrombotic disease, effective oral anticoagulant effect is often achieved by day 5, at which time levels of all the vitamin K–dependent factors should be depressed by warfarin.

Early in the course of treatment with warfarin, the PT is affected first because factor VII has the shortest half-life of the vitamin K–dependent procoagulants and factor VII levels fall briskly after warfarin treatment. The aim of warfarin therapy for venous thromboembolic disease is to achieve a stable INR of 2.0 to 3.0.

For prevention of embolization from prosthetic valves, an INR of 3.0 to 4.0 is preferable. Patients with protein C or protein S deficiency are at risk for warfarin-induced skin necrosis when warfarin therapy is initiated, particularly if high doses are used. These individuals should be given heparin before warfarin is started, and they should not receive a loading (high) dose of warfarin.

SUMMARY AND RED FLAGS

Bleeding and thrombotic problems are often familial but may be acquired. A family history and personal history that quantitate bleeding episodes are of utmost help in planning an evaluation. Red flags include anemia; signs of end-organ bleeding or vascular occlusion, particularly the central nervous system; signs of a systemic disorder (pancytopenia, hypotension, rash, weight loss, chronic fever, liver-renal-pulmonary system involvement); and signs of hemorrhagic shock.

REFERENCES

General

Andrew M: The relevance of developmental hemostasis to hemorrhagic disorders of newborns. Semin Perinatol 1997;21:70-85.

Burk CD, Miller L, Handler SD, et al: Preoperative history and coagulation screening in children undergoing tonsillectomy. Pediatrics 1992;89:691-695.

Esmon CT: Blood coagulation. In Nathan DG, Orkin SH (eds): Nathan and Oski's Hematology of Infancy and Childhood, 6th ed. Philadelphia, Saunders, 2003.

Montgomery RR, Scott JP: Hemorrhage and thrombotic diseases. In Behrman RE, Kliegman RM, Jenson HB (eds): Nelson Textbook of Pediatrics, 17th ed. Philadelphia, Saunders, 2004.

Nosek-Cenkowska B, Cheang MS, Pizzi NJ, et al: Bleeding and bruising symptomatology in children with and without bleeding disorders. Thromb Haemost 1991;65:237-241.

Coagulopathy

Levi M, Ten Cate H: Disseminated intravascular coagulation. N Engl J Med 1999;341:586-592.

Lusher JM: Inhibitor antibodies to factor VIII and factor IX: Management. Semin Thromb Hemost 2000;26:179-188.

Manco-Johnson MJ: Antiphospholipid antibodies in children. Semin Thromb Hemost 1998;24:591-598.

Mannucci PM, Tuddenham EG: The hemophilias—From royal genes to gene therapy. N Engl J Med. 2001;344:1773-1779.

Monagle R, Andrew ME: Acquired disorders of hemostasis. In Nathan DG, Orkin SH (eds): Nathan and Oski's Hematology of Infancy and Childhood, 6th ed. Philadelphia, Saunders, 2003.

Montgomery RR, Gill JC, Scott JP: Hemophilia and von Willebrand disease. In Nathan DG, Orkin SH (eds). Nathan and Oski's Hematology of Infancy and Childhood, 6th ed. Philadelphia, Saunders, 2003.

Werner EJ, Abshire TC, Giroux DS, et al: Relative value of diagnostic studies for von Willebrand disease. J Pediatr 1992;121;34-38.

Yeowell HN, Pinnell SR: The Ehlers-Danlos syndromes. Semin Dermatol 1993;12:229-240.

Platelets

Beardsley DS, Nathan DG: Platelet abnormalities in infancy and childhood. In Nathan DG, Orkin SH (eds). Nathan and Oski's Hematology of Infancy and Childhood, 5th ed. Philadelphia, WB Saunders, 1998.

Bolton-Maggs PH: Idiopathic thrombocytopenic purpura. Arch Dis Child 2000;83:220-222.

George JN, Woolf SH, Raskob GE, et al: Idiopathic thrombocytopenic purpura: A practice guideline developed by explicit methods for the American Society of Hematology. Blood 1996;88:3-40.

Halperin D, Doyle JJ: Is bone marrow examination justified in idiopathic thrombocytopenic purpura? Am J Dis Child 1988;142:508-512.

Kuhne T, Imbach P: Chronic immune thrombocytopenic purpura in childhood. Semin Thromb Hemost 1998;24:549-553.

Udom-Rice I, Bussel JB: Fetal and neonatal thrombocytopenia. Blood Rev 1995;9:57-64.

Thrombosis

David M, Andrew M: Venous thromboembolic complications in children. J Pediatr 1993;123:337-346.

Leys D, Lucas C, Gobert M, et al: Cervical artery dissections. Eur Neurol 1997;37:3-12.

Manco-Johnson MJ: Disorders of hemostasis in childhood: Risk factors for venous thromboembolism. Thromb Haemost 1997;78:710-714.

Seligsohn U, Lubetsky A: Genetic susceptibility to venous thrombosis. N Engl J Med 2001;344:1222-1231.

Weinmann E, Salzman E: Deep-vein thrombosis. N Engl J Med 1994;331:1630.

Wells PS, Anderson DR, Rodger M, et al: Excluding pulmonary embolism at the bedside without diagnostic imaging: Management of patients with suspected pulmonary embolism presenting to the emergency department by using a simple clinical model and D-dimer. Ann Intern Med 2001;135:98-107.

Therapy

Andrew M, Michelson AD, Bovill E, et al: Guidelines for antithrombotic therapy in pediatric patients. J Pediatr 1998;132:575-588.

Bernard GR, Vincent JL, Laterre PF, et al: Efficacy and safety of recombinant human activated protein C for severe sepsis. N Engl J Med 2001;344:699-709.

Dix D, Andrew M, Marzinotto V, et al: The use of low molecular weight heparin in pediatric patients: A prospective cohort study. J Pediatr 2000;136:439-445.

Mannucci PM: Desmopressin (DDAVP) in the treatment of bleeding disorders: The first 20 years. Blood 1997;90:2515-2521.

Merli G, Spiro TE, Olsson CG, et al: Subcutaneous enoxaparin once or twice daily compared with intravenous unfractionated heparin for treatment of venous thromboembolic disease. Ann Intern Med 2001;134:191-202.

Nowak-Gottl U, Auberger K, Halimeh S, et al: Thrombolysis in newborns and infants. Thromb Haemost 1999;82(Suppl 1):112-116.

---

*The INR corrects the PT for institutional differences in reagents and instruments. When a patient is taking a stable warfarin dosage, the INR is calculated by a ratio of the patient's PT to the control PT raised to a correction factor (the International Sensitivity Index) that allows for comparison of different PT reagents and machines in different laboratories. For all patients receiving chronic warfarin therapy, their anticoagulant therapy should be measured as the INR. The INR level should be maintained between 2.0 and 3.0 for effective, safe anticoagulant therapy. An INR exceeding 3.0 has been associated with increased risk of bleeding without improved therapeutic effects for patients with venous thromboembolic disease.

INFECTIOUS DISORDERS

51 Recurrent Infection

Laurence A. Boxer   R. Alexander Blackwood

The immune system's function is to prevent and retard the local establishment or systemic dissemination of bacteria, viruses, fungi, and protozoa. The immune system has four primary components:

1. *Antibody-mediated immunity* (B cell immunity) is mediated by bone marrow–derived lymphocytes (B cells) and plasma cells (further differentiated B cells), which release antibodies (immunoglobulins) into secretions, plasma, and interstitial spaces after activation.
2. *Cell-mediated immunity* (T cell immunity) is mediated by thymus-derived lymphocytes (T cells) in the blood and peripheral lymphoid tissue. Although T cells do not produce immunoglobulin, they are necessary for B cell function. T cells in conjunction with antigen-presenting cells such as macrophages regulate the selective activation of specific clones of B cells and the production of antigen-specific antibodies.
3. The *phagocytic system* consists of tissue macrophages, as well as bloodborne monocytes and neutrophils. In response to specific signals, phagocytes ingest and kill invading microorganisms. Tissue macrophages also serve as antigen-presenting cells for T cell–B cell subsets.
4. The *complement system* acts synergistically with the remainder of the immune system to amplify resistance to microbial infection both directly (complement-mediated cytolysis) and indirectly (recruitment of phagocytic cells).

Defects of these systems produce definable immunodeficiency states and produce characteristic infections (Table 51-1).

The differential diagnosis for patients with recurrent infections is formidable, in view of the complexity of the immune system (Table 51-2). Similarities may exist in the manifestations of neutrophil, immunoglobulin, and complement disorders. Children with "frequent infections" must be carefully evaluated. Often these patients ultimately have no identifiable underlying immunologic defect. They frequently have respiratory allergy or other risks for recurrent infections (Table 51-3). Most patients with recurrent infections do not have an underlying identifiable immunodeficiency. Because of the low probability of identifying a discrete immune defect, the primary physician faces the difficult decision about the extent of the evaluation and which patients merit a complete evaluation.

Immunologic evaluation should be initiated for at least one of the following: (1) more than two systemic bacterial infections (sepsis, meningitis, osteomyelitis); (2) three serious respiratory infections (pneumonia, sinusitis) or bacterial infections (cellulitis, draining otitis media, lymphadenitis) per year; (3) the presence of an infection at an unusual site (hepatic or brain abscess); (4) infections with unusual pathogens (*Aspergillus* pneumonia, disseminated candidiasis, or infection with *Serratia marcescens*, *Nocardia* species, *Burkholderia cepacia*); (5) infections of unusual severity; and (6) dissemination of recurrent mycobacterial infections.

The clinician should remember that (1) respiratory allergy, such as asthma or allergic rhinitis, can mimic respiratory infections, and (2) a single chronic infection may wax and wane with intermittent, inadequate treatment and may manifest as a series of infections. Nevertheless, many nonimmune disorders are characterized by an increased susceptibility to infection; these must also be considered (see Table 51-3).

HISTORY AND PHYSICAL EXAMINATION

HISTORY

The clinician must determine (1) the frequency, location, severity, and complications of the infections; (2) the accuracy of how infections were documented; (3) the presence or absence of a symptom-free interval; (4) the microbiologic features of any isolate; and (5) the response to antibiotic therapy.

Perinatal History. Exposure to a maternal viral infection (human immunodeficiency virus [HIV], cytomegalovirus, herpes simplex virus, rubella) during gestation or a history of prematurity, blood transfusions, respiratory distress syndrome (with bronchopulmonary dysplasia), or other neonatal illnesses may be discovered. Infants previously placed on respirators may develop chronic obstructive lung disease (bronchopulmonary dysplasia), predisposing them to recurrent pulmonary infections; blood transfusions predispose to HIV or other bloodborne pathogens (see Table 51-3). Although screening of blood for HIV antibody has reduced the number of infections with HIV, other opportunistic infections may be acquired after infusion of blood or blood products. Most perinatal HIV infections are seen in children whose mother or mother's partner has engaged in high-risk behavior (i.e., multiple sex partners or use of cocaine or intravenous drugs). Symptomatic perinatal cytomegalovirus infection is associated with low birth weight. It is also seen in babies born to cytomegalovirus-seronegative mothers who have been hospitalized for more than 4 weeks or who have received multiple blood transfusions or a single transfusion with a total volume exceeding 50 mL; in neonates who received blood from a seropositive donor; and in infants in day care centers. Attention should be paid to the time of umbilical cord separation. Infants with a history of delayed umbilical cord separation and recurrent episodes of sepsis or pneumonia should be evaluated for the leukocyte adhesion deficiency. Additional clues to the diagnosis are noted in Table 51-4.

Recurrent Infections or Signs of Immunologic Disorders in Other Family Members. Specific patterns of inheritance have been determined for a variety of immunologic defects. In addition, common patterns of exposure may become evident; a history of blood transfusion or a lifestyle that suggests promiscuity, bisexuality, or illicit drug use predisposes to exposure to acquired immunodeficiency syndrome. A family history of unexplained infant deaths may be attributable to inherited disorders of immunity. Additional clues are noted in Table 51-4.

Table 51-1. Risk Factors and Related Pathogens Affecting Immunocompromised Patients

I. Humoral Defects

A. *Antibody Deficiency (B Cell Defects)*

1. Bacteria
Staphylococcus aureus (sepsis, sinopulmonary infection)
Haemophilus influenzae (sepsis, meningitis, arthritis, sinopulmonary infection)
Streptococcus pneumoniae (sepsis, meningitis, arthritis)
Pseudomonas aeruginosa (sepsis, pneumonia)
Mycoplasma species (arthritis, pneumonia)
Salmonella species (enteritis)
Campylobacter species (enteritis)
2. Viruses
Enterovirus, including polio vaccine (encephalitis, paralysis, myositis, arthritis)
Rotavirus (enteritis)
3. Protozoa
Giardia lamblia (enteritis)

B. *Complement Deficiencies*

1. C1, C2, C3, C4, factor B
Streptococcus pyogenes
S. pneumoniae, S. aureus, H. influenzae, Neisseria meningitidis, Klebsiella species (sepsis, meningitis, arthritis)
2. C5-8, properdin deficiency
N. meningitidis, N. gonorrhoeae (meningitis, sepsis, arthritis)

II. Combined B and T Cell Defects (Congenital, Acquired Immunodeficiency Syndrome, Immunosuppression, Malignancies)

A. *Bacteria*

Listeria monocytogenes (sepsis, meningitis)
Salmonella (sepsis)
Mycobacterium tuberculosis (pneumonia, disseminated disease)
Atypical mycobacteria (*Mycobacterium avium, Mycobacterium intracellulare*) (sepsis, pneumonia, disseminated disease)
Nocardia species (pneumonia, CNS infection)
Legionella species (pneumonia)

B. *Fungi*

Cryptococcus neoformans (sepsis, meningitis)
Histoplasma capsulatum (pneumonia, disseminated disease)
Coccidioides immitis (pneumonia, meningitis)

C. *Viruses*

Varicella-zoster (cutaneous and CNS infection, pneumonia, hepatitis)
Cytomegalovirus (bone marrow infection, pneumonia, retinitis, esophagitis, colitis, CNS infection)
Herpes simplex (CNS infection, pneumonia, esophagitis, hepatitis, disseminated disease)
Epstein-Barr virus (lymphoma)
Measles (pneumonia, encephalitis)
Polyomavirus BK (hemorrhagic cystitis, ureteric stenosis, renal insufficiency)
Polyomavirus JC (progressive multifocal leukoencephalopathy)

D. *Protozoa*

Pneumocystis carinii (pneumonia, rare extrapulmonary spread)
Toxoplasma gondii (CNS infection, myocarditis)
Cryptosporidium species (enteritis)

E. *Helminth*

S. stercoralis (enteritis, pneumonia, sepsis, meningitis)

III. Neutropenia (Severe Chronic Neutropenia, Aplastic Anemia, Myelosuppression, Myelophthisis, Myelosuppressive Agents, Bone Marrow Transplantation)

A. *Bacteria*

Escherichia coli (sepsis, pneumonia, pyelonephritis)
Klebsiella pneumoniae (sepsis, pneumonia)
P. aeruginosa (sepsis, pneumonia, cutaneous lesions)
Mixed anaerobic and aerobic enteric bacteria (typhlitis, perianal abscess)
S. aureus (sepsis, cellulitis, soft tissue infection)
Staphylococcus epidermidis (line infection)
Corynebacterium JK strain (sepsis)
α-Hemolytic streptococci (sepsis)

B. *Fungi*

Candida species (sepsis, pneumonia, ophthalmitis, liver and spleen abscesses)
Aspergillus species (sepsis, pneumonia, sinusitis, CNS infection, cutaneous lesions)
Mucor (pneumonia, sinusitis, CNS infection)
Fusarium species (sepsis, cutaneous lesions, pneumonia)
Alternaria species (sepsis, cutaneous lesions)

IV. Phagocytic Dysfunction

A. *Chronic Granulomatous Disease*

1. Bacteria (soft tissue, lymphadenitis, pneumonia, osteomyelitis)
Catalase positive organisms, e.g., *S. aureus, Serratia marcescens, Burkholderia cepacia, Nocardia* species
2. Fungi (pneumonia, liver infection, soft tissue), *Candida* species, *Aspergillus* species

B. *Other Phagocyte Defects (Leukocyte Adhesion Deficiency, Hyperimmunoglobulin E, Chédiak-Higashi Syndrome, Specific Granule Deficiency, Rac-2 Deficiency)*

1. Bacteria (soft tissue, pneumonia, lymphadenitis)
Pseudomonas species, *S. aureus, E. coli, Klebsiella, Enterobacteria* species
2. Fungus (pneumonia)
Candida infection if diabetic

V. Splenic Dysfunction (e.g., Asplenia, Sickle Cell Anemia)

A. *Bacteria*

S. pneumoniae (sepsis, meningitis)
H. influenzae type b (sepsis, meningitis)
N. meningitidis (sepsis, meningitis)
Capnocytophaga canimorsus

B. *Protozoa*

Babesiosis
Malaria

CNS, central nervous system.

Table 51-2. Cause and Mechanism of Recurrent Infection in Immunodeficiency States

Disorder	Pathogen	Deficiency
Primary Immunodeficiencies		
Humoral immunodeficiency syndromes (predominantly B cell defects)	Bacterial pathogens, enteroviruses	Reduced phagocytic efficiency, failure of lysis and agglutination of bacteria, inadequate neutralization of bacterial toxins
Cellular immunodeficiency syndromes (predominantly T cell defects)	CMV, VZV, *Strongyloides stercoralis; Mycobacterium, Listeria, Nocardia, Cryptococcus,* and *Candida* species; *Pneumocystis carinii*	Absence of or impaired delayed hypersensitivity response; absence of T cell cooperation for B cell synthesis of antibodies to T cell–specific antigens
Severe combined immunodeficiency syndrome	Many bacteria, fungi, and viruses	Absence of T cell and B cell responses
Wiskott-Aldrich syndrome	Gram-negative enteric organisms, CMV, HSV, staphylococci; *Streptococcus pneumoniae, Haemophilus influenzae, P. carinii*	Decreased antibody production to carbohydrate antigens
Ataxia-telangiectasia	Sinopulmonary infections with saprophytes	T helper cell deficiency, immunoglobulin deficiency
Splenic insufficiency or absence	*Salmonella* species, *S. pneumoniae,* gram-negative organisms	Defective opsonization, defective clearing of organisms
Neutropenia (ANC <500/mm^3)	Pyogenic bacteria or fungi, *Pseudomonas* species, *Staphylococcus aureus*	Decreased neutrophil numbers
Chédiak-Higashi syndrome	*S. aureus, Candida albicans,* gram-negative organisms	Defective neutrophil bactericidal activity secondary to impaired chemotaxis and degranulation
Specific granule deficiency	*S. aureus,* gram-negative organisms	Defective neutrophil bactericidal activity
Leukocyte adhesion deficiency	Gram-negative organisms, *Pseudomonas aeruginosa, S. aureus*	Impaired neutrophil bactericidal activity secondary to impaired chemotaxis, and adhesion to endothelium and phagocytosis of C3bi-coated microorganisms from lack of CD11/CD18 complex on neutrophils
Hyperimmunoglobulin E syndrome	*S. aureus*	Defective neutrophil chemotaxis; impaired opsonization of *S. aureus*
Chronic granulomatous disease	Catalase-positive organisms, e.g., *S. aureus, Serratia* species, *Burkholderia cepacia, Nocardia* species, *Candida* species, *Aspergillus* species	Impaired neutrophil bactericidal activity secondary to impaired production of hydrogen peroxide
Myeloperoxidase deficiency	*Candida* species in diabetic patients	Failure to kill *Candida* organisms efficiently by neutrophils
Complement deficiencies (C1, C2, C3, C4, and factor B)	*Streptococcus pyogenes, S. pneumoniae, S. aureus, H. influenzae, Klebsiella* species	Defective chemotaxis and opsonization of microbes
C5-C8 and properdin deficiencies	*Neisseria meningitidis, Neisseria gonorrhoeae*	Defective membrane attack mechanism
Secondary Immunodeficiencies		
AIDS	CMV, VZV, adenovirus, HBV, *Giardia lamblia, Entamoeba histolytica, Mycobacterium avium–intracellulare, Toxoplasma gondii, Mycobacterium tuberculosis, Cryptococcus neoformans, P. carinii; Campylobacter, Candida, Isospora, Aspergillus, Nocardia, Strongyloides,* and *Cryptosporidium* species	Retrovirus infections transmitted by bodily fluid impair T cell response, reduced T helper cell numbers
Cancer	VZV, HSV, *Escherichia coli; Pseudomonas, Klebsiella, Listeria, Cryptococcus, Pneumocystis,* and *Mycobacterium* species	Neutropenia, lymphopenia, impaired cellular immunity
Immunosuppression	HSV, VZV, CMV, EBV, hepatitis virus, *Pseudomonas* species, *E. coli; Klebsiella, Acinetobacter, Serratia, Candida, Aspergillus, Mucor,* and *Cryptococcus* species	Dependent on agent used, leads often to impaired cellular immunity and neutropenia
Transplantation	CMV, HSV, VZV, hepatitis virus, *S. aureus; Pseudomonas, Klebsiella, Candida, Aspergillus, Nocardia,* and *Pneumocystis* species; EBV	Probably related to use of immunosuppressive agents
Malnutrition	Measles, HSV, VZV, *Mycobacterium* species	Impaired T cell function, reduction in complement activity

Modified from Feigin RD, Innis JW: Opportunistic infections in the compromised host. In Oski FA, DeAngelis CD, Feigin RD, Warshaw JB (eds): Principles and Practice of Pediatrics. Philadelphia, JB Lippincott, 1990, p 1039.

AIDS, acquired immunodeficiency syndrome; ANC, absolute neutrophil count; CMV, cytomegalovirus; EBV, Epstein-Barr virus; HBV, hepatitis B virus; HSV, herpes simplex virus; VZV, varicella-zoster virus.

Table 51-3. Infections in Patients without Primary Immunodeficiency Syndromes

Predisposing Causes	Organism and Type of Infection
Alteration of Mucocutaneous Barriers	
Indwelling Catheter	
Central venous catheter (Broviac, Hickman)	*Staphylococcus aureus; Staphylococcus epidermidis;* and *Bacteroides, Candida, Pseudomonas* species: bacteremia, fungemia
Urinary catheter	*Escherichia coli, Enterococcus* species, *Staphylococcus saprophyticus:* pyelonephritis
Tenckhoff catheter (continuous ambulatory peritoneal dialysis)	*S. epidermidis, S. aureus, E. coli, Pseudomonas aeruginosa, Candida* species: peritonitis
Cerebrospinal fluid shunts	*S. epidermidis, S. aureus,* diphtheroid, *Bacillus* species: meningitis
Aspirated pulmonary foreign body	*S. aureus,* anaerobes: pneumonia, pulmonary abscess, empyema
Burns	*P. aeruginosa, S. epidermidis, Candida* species: cutaneous lesions, sepsis
Inhalation Therapy: Contaminated Solutions	*P. aeruginosa, Serratia marcescens, Legionella* species: pneumonia
Surgical Wounds	
Abdominal	Gram-negative bacteria, *S. aureus, S. epidermidis, Candida* species: peritonitis
Nongastrointestinal	*S. aureus, S. epidermidis,* streptococci, gram-negative bacteria: wound abscess, sepsis
Fistula-Sinus Communications	
Neurocutaneous fistula	*S. aureus, S. epidermidis, E. coli:* meningitis
Neuroenteric fistula	Gram-negative bacteria: meningitis
Otic, facial sinus-meningeal sinus tract	*Pneumococcus:* meningitis
Facial sinus fracture (CSF rhinorrhea)	*Pneumococcus:* meningitis
Intravenous Drug Abuse	*S. aureus, P. aeruginosa,* streptococci: endocarditis, osteomyelitis Hepatitis B, C, D viruses: AIDS
Prosthetic Devices	
Cardiac valves	*S. epidermidis,* streptococci, *S. aureus,* diphtheroid, *Candida* species: endocarditis
Pacemaker	*S. epidermidis, S. aureus, Candida* species: subcutaneous pocket or endocardial infection
Chronic Disease	
Malnutrition	Measles; tuberculosis; herpes simplex virus; bacterial, parasitic, and viral diarrhea, gram-negative bacteria: sepsis, pneumonia
Cystic fibrosis	*S. aureus, Haemophilus influenzae,* mucoid *P. aeruginosa, Burkholderia cepacia:* pneumonia
Diabetes mellitus	Urinary tract infections, *Mucor,* and other fungi: sinus-orbital infection
Nephrotic syndrome	*Pneumococcus, E. coli:* peritonitis
Uremia	*S. aureus,* gram-negative bacteria, fungi: sepsis, soft tissue infection
Cirrhosis, ascites	*Pneumococcus, E. coli:* peritonitis
Prolonged broad-spectrum antibiotic therapy	*Candida* species, *Enterococcus* species, multidrug-resistant gram-negative or gram-positive bacteria: sepsis
Spinal cord injury	Gram-negative or gram-positive bacteria: pneumonia, pyelonephritis, pressure sores, abscesses, osteomyelitis
Sickle cell anemia	*Pneumococcus:* sepsis, meningitis, osteoarticular infection *Salmonella* species, *S. aureus:* osteomyelitis
Congenital heart disease	*S. aureus,* streptococcus viridans group: endocarditis
Urinary tract anomaly	*E. coli, S. saprophyticus, Enterococcus* species: pyelonephritis
Kartagener syndrome (dysmotile cilia)	*H. influenzae, Moraxella catarrhalis, Pneumococcus:* pneumonia, sinusitis
Eczema	*S. aureus, Streptococcus* species, varicella, herpes simplex, molluscum: cutaneous infection, cellulitis
Protein-losing enteropathy (lymphangiectasia)	*Pneumococcus:* sepsis, peritonitis *Giardia* species: diarrhea
Periodontitis	*Fusobacterium* species: cellulitis, facial space infection
Chronic blood product transfusion	CMV; EBV; parvovirus; HHV-6; hepatitis A (rare), B, C, D virus; West Nile virus: syphilis, bacteremia (*P. aeruginosa*) HIV, parvovirus: Chagas disease, malaria; direct inoculation →primary disease

Modified from Behrman RE (ed): Nelson Textbook of Pediatrics, 16th ed. Philadelphia, WB Saunders, 2000, p 788.

AIDS, acquired immunodeficiency syndrome; CMV, cytomegalovirus; CSF, cerebrospinal fluid; EBV, Epstein-Barr virus; HIV, human immunodeficiency virus; HHV-6, human herpesvirus–6.

Table 51-4. Clinical Aids to the Diagnosis of Immunodeficiency

Suggestive of B Cell Defect

Recurrent bacterial infections of the upper and lower respiratory tracts

Recurrent skin infections, meningitis, osteomyelitis secondary to encapsulated bacteria (*Streptococcus pneumoniae, Haemophilus influenzae, Staphylococcus aureus, Neisseria meningitidis*)

Paralysis after vaccination with live attenuated poliovirus

Reduced levels of immunoglobulins

Suggestive of T Cell Defect

Systemic illness after vaccination with any live virus or BCG

Unusual life-threatening complication after infection with benign viruses (giant cell pneumonia with measles; varicella pneumonia)

Chronic oral candidiasis after 6 months of age

Chronic mucocutaneous candidiasis

Graft-versus-host disease after blood transfusion

Reduced lymphocyte counts for age

Suggestive of Combined Immunodeficiency Disease

Marked lymphopenia for age

Low level of immunoglobulins

Absence of lymph nodes and tonsils

Small thymus

Chronic diarrhea

Failure to thrive

Recurrent infections with opportunistic organisms

Congenital Syndromes with Immunodeficiency of T and B Cells

Acrodermatitis enteropathica: dermatitis, alopecia, diarrhea

Ataxia-telangiectasia: ataxia, telangiectasia

Autoimmune polyglandular syndrome: hypofunction of one or more endocrine organs, chronic mucocutaneous candidiasis

Cartilage hair hypoplasia: short-limbed dwarfism, sparse hair, neutropenia

Centromeric instability syndrome: dysmorphic facies, ataxia, and developmental delay

Wiskott-Aldrich syndrome: thrombocytopenia, male gender, eczema

Congenital Syndromes with Phagocyte Disorders

Chédiak-Higashi syndrome: oculocutaneous albinism, nystagmus, recurrent bacterial infections, peripheral neuropathies

Chronic granulomatous disease: recurrent infection with catalase-positive organisms including *Burkholderia cepacia, S. aureus*

Leukocyte adhesion deficiency: recurrent bacterial infections, gingivitis, delayed separation of the umbilical cord, neutrophilia

Rac-2 deficiency: recurrent life-threatening bacterial infections, neutrophilia, normal expression of leukocyte integrins and/or L-selectin

Suggestive of Macrophage Dysfunction

Disseminated atypical mycobacterial infection, recurrent *Salmonella* infection

Fatal infection after BCG vaccination

Suggestive of Asplenia

Ivemark syndrome: bilateral right-sidedness sequence, bilateral three-lobed lungs, bilateral morphologic right atria, complex congenital heart disease, Howell-Jolly bodies on blood smear

BCG, bacille Calmette-Guérin.

Exposure to Tobacco or Marijuana. The incidence of respiratory disease is increased in children exposed to cigarette smoke or other noxious fumes (wood-burning stove) in the home.

Exposure to Animals; Chemicals; Farms; or Plants at Home, School, or Day Care. Often, respiratory and dermatologic findings are seen as a result of exposure to environmental allergens and toxins. Specific bacteriologic and parasitic exposures are associated with certain pets (*Salmonella* organisms and iguanas or turtles; psittacosis and birds; *Bartonella* organisms and cats).

Family History of Allergic Diseases. A child who has one allergic parent or two allergic parents is predisposed to allergic reactions by 25% and 50%, respectively.

Travel to Foreign Countries, Camp, or Rural Areas. A travel history may suggest exposure to unusual organisms that are regionally endemic, such as certain parasites and specific insect or animal bites, or to contaminated water.

Changes in the Daily Routine or Sleeping Arrangements. A move to a new house or to a new nursery school or exposure to a new babysitter, pet, or housekeeper may suggest possible allergic and infectious risks.

Recurrent Episodes of High Fever with Purulent Secretions. The presence of fever and purulent secretions is suggestive of bacterial infection, which could be caused by broad categories of immunodeficiencies (see Table 51-1). The presence of serious bacterial infections without phagocyte recruitment (pus formation) is suggestive of an inability of neutrophils to migrate to sites of infection (chemotactic disorders).

Health of the Patient between Infections. If the patient is generally healthy between infections, demonstrating adequate appetite, growth, and development, the patient is unlikely to have an underlying serious systemic illness.

Location and Severity. If the episodes are similar in location and severity, the patient may have an allergy or local mechanical problems, such as an anatomic obstruction or foreign bodies.

History of Skull Fracture, Dermal Sinus Tracts, or Dermoids or Insertion of a Central Nervous System Shunt (see Table 51-3). Any direct communication to the cerebrospinal fluid that bypasses the blood-brain barrier predisposes patients to central nervous system infection. Basilar skull fractures and dermal sinus tracks or fistulae may communicate with the subarachnoid space or neural tissue. Other conditions predisposing patients to opportunistic infection of the central nervous system include penetrating foreign body, cerebrospinal fluid shunts, myelomeningocele, and encephalocele. Local infections (treated or untreated) of the sinuses or of the middle ear may spread to contiguous structures to form cerebral abscesses or subdural-epidural empyema. Intravenous drug abuse, bacterial endocarditis, heart disease with right-to-left shunt, lymphoma, leukemia, immunosuppression, acquired immunodeficiency syndrome, and organ transplantation are associated with an increased risk of central nervous system infections.

Recurrent Pulmonary Infections. Independent of any other underlying conditions, endotracheal intubation predisposes the patient to recurrent pulmonary infections with nosocomial organisms. Additional risks for recurrent pneumonitis are noted in Table 51-5.

Table 51-5. Differential Diagnosis of Recurrent Pneumonitis

Hereditary Disorders

Cystic fibrosis
Sickle cell disease
α_1-Antitrypsin deficiency
Familial Mediterranean fever

Disorders of Immunity

Collagen disease (SLE, JRA)
Acquired immunodeficiency syndrome
Selective IgG class deficiencies
Common variable immunodeficiency syndrome
Severe combined immunodeficiency syndrome
Allergic alveolitis (dusts [farmer's lung], molds [allergic aspergillosis], excreta [pigeon breeder's lung])
Complement deficiencies
Chronic asthma

Disorders of Leukocytes

Hyperimmunoglobulin E syndrome
Chédiak-Higashi syndrome
Leukocyte adhesion deficiency
Chronic granulomatous disease

Disorders of Cilia

Immotile cilia syndrome
Kartagener syndrome

Damage by Physical Agents

Lipoid pneumonia
Kerosene pneumonia
Smoke inhalation

Iatrogenic Pulmonary Damage

Drugs (bleomycin, nitrofurantoin)
Radiation pneumonitis
Graft-versus-host disease

Recurrent Aspiration

Gastroesophageal reflux
Tracheoesophageal fistula
Cleft palate
Neuromuscular disorders
Familial dysautonomia

Neoplasm

Primary
Metastatic
Histiocytosis X

Anatomic Disorders

Sequestration
Bronchopulmonary dysplasia
Lobar emphysema
Bronchiectasis
Pulmonary lymphangiectasis
Pulmonary hemosiderosis
Vascular ring
Atelectasis (mucus plug, foreign body)

Others

Sarcoidosis
Desquamative interstitial pneumonitis
Sickle cell acute chest syndrome

IgG, immunoglobulin G; JRA, juvenile rheumatoid arthritis; SLE, systemic lupus erythematosus.

PHYSICAL EXAMINATION

The physical examination may provide important clues (see Table 51-4). Height and weight measurements identify failure to thrive or recent weight loss. Chronic respiratory infections are suggested by scarred tympanic membranes, postnasal drip, and cervical adenopathy. Transverse nasal creases, circles under the eyes, and posterior pharyngeal "cobblestoning" suggest respiratory allergy. Recurrent cough, wheezing, digital clubbing, and chest deformity are suggestive of pulmonary disease. Auscultation of the apex of the heart in the right side of the thorax (dextrocardia) may be accompanied by ciliary motility abnormalities or asplenia. Lymphadenopathy, hepatosplenomegaly, pallor, wasting, and recent weight loss are suggestive of systemic disease. Absence of lymph tissue (tonsils, lymph nodes, or thymus on chest radiograph) is suggestive of T cell, B cell, or combined cellular immunity deficiency states. Parotid enlargement with lymphadenopathy and hepatosplenomegaly is suggestive of HIV infection.

When a discrepancy exists between the severity of an illness as reported by the parent and the child's physical appearance, it is often prudent to delay a detailed evaluation until more objective evidence of recurrent fevers, severe respiratory disease, or unusual skin manifestations are documented by repeat examinations during acute episodes.

DIAGNOSTIC CATEGORIES

The information obtained from the history and physical examination is usually sufficient to make a tentative classification:

1. The patient who is probably healthy.
2. The atopic or allergic patient.
3. The patient with a nonimmunologic defect in host defense (see Table 51-3).
4. The patient with hereditary fevers.
5. The immunodeficient patient (see Tables 51-1 and 51-2).

THE PATIENT WHO IS PROBABLY HEALTHY

Many children have repeated minor infections. Although nearly all patients with well-characterized phagocytic or immune abnormalities have recurrent respiratory infections, the converse is seldom true. At least 50% of children with a complaint of recurrent infections are probably healthy and have a relatively brief history of repeated infections or a single prolonged illness from which recovery has been delayed. Most upper respiratory tract infections last less than 7 days; duration of longer than 14 days is unusual. Most children younger than 1 year who have a large family or who attend day care develop respiratory or gastrointestinal infections about six times during the first year of life.

The healthy child has normal growth and development before the illness and usually a normal physical examination finding. The onset of the recurrent infection may coincide with entry into day care, preschool, or kindergarten. Such children usually have appropriate-sized tonsils and lymph nodes. Minimal laboratory tests that might include a complete blood cell count and erythrocyte sedimentation rate measurement are used to exclude rheumatic disorders; culture and radiographs of the affected area may provide additional data. With reassurance of the parents, these children recover spontaneously. Simple measures, rather than a complex set of laboratory studies, are often the only treatment required.

THE ALLERGIC PATIENT

Approximately 30% of children with recurrent respiratory sinopulmonary symptoms can be categorized as atopic (allergic on a hereditary basis) children and have normal growth and development. Episodes of recurrent illness are nonfebrile, with poor response to antibiotics and accompanied by upper respiratory symptoms, such as coughing, sneezing, or wheezing. The family history includes atopy; the patient's history includes food intolerance, colic, blotchy skin, or infantile eczema. The physical examination of allergic school-aged children may reveal the typical characteristics of pallor; dark circles under the eyes; open mouth with dry lips; coated tongue; evidence of nasal obstruction; transverse nasal crease; boggy, pale nasal mucosa; mucus in the pharynx; posterior pharyngeal "cobblestoning"; and postnasal drip. Other features may include cervical lymphadenopathy and an increase in the chest anteroposterior diameter, pectoral hypertrophy, chest asymmetry, chronic sinusitis, chronic respiratory obstruction, dry skin, eczema, and dermatographism.

The laboratory evaluation of the allergic child should include a complete blood cell count, erythrocyte sedimentation rate measurement, nasal smear for eosinophils, spirometry before and after bronchodilator use, sinus radiographs or computed tomography, with or without a chest radiograph, and quantitation of immunoglobulins, including a measurement of immunoglobulin E (IgE) level. An IgE level exceeding 50 IU/mL in an infant younger than 1 year or an IgE level exceeding 100 IU/mL in a child older than 1 year is suggestive of an allergic disorder.

THE PATIENT WITH AN ANATOMIC ABNORMALITY OR CHRONIC ILLNESS: NONIMMUNOLOGIC DEFECT IN HOST DEFENSE

Approximately 10% of children with recurrent infections have an underlying chronic disease or a structural defect that predisposes them to recurrent infections (see Table 51-3). Many chronic illnesses may directly or indirectly alter immune function, resulting in recurrent infections. Malnutrition and specific vitamin deficiencies may alter immune cell function. Protein-losing enteropathies may lead to hypocomplementemia and hypogammaglobulinemia. Structural or anatomic defects often result in recurrent infections that are generally localized to the affected organ system. Eustachian tube abnormalities (as in cleft palate) result in recurrent or chronic otitis media; congenital heart disease results in an increased risk of endocarditis; and posterior urethral valves, vesicoureteral reflux, or ureteral pelvic junction obstruction results in recurrent urinary tract infections. Pneumonitis may result from congenital malformations (tracheo-esophageal fistulas or sequestration), from aspiration of a foreign body (peanut, small toys) or chronic aspiration (gastroesophageal reflux), and from bronchopulmonary dysplasia (see Table 51-5). Chronic illnesses that result in recurrent pulmonary infections of nonimmunologic origin include cystic fibrosis, immotile cilia syndrome, or α_1-antitrypsin deficiency.

Children with anatomic abnormalities appear ill, with poor growth; they may initially appear normal. Patients with recurrent pneumonia usually have chronic cough with rales and digital clubbing; others may have failure to thrive, chronic diarrhea, abdominal distention, hepatosplenomegaly, muscle wasting, and pallor. Most children with a possible nonimmunologic cause for recurrent infection should undergo laboratory tests such as a complete blood cell count, chest radiograph or computed tomography, sweat chloride test, and cultures of involved sites. Tests for quantitative immunoglobulin should also be performed to rule out an antibody deficiency. Possible nonimmunologic diagnoses for recurrent infections are listed in Tables 51-3 and 51-5.

THE PATIENT WITH HEREDITARY FEVERS

Hereditary fevers are a heterogeneous group of rare inflammatory disorders that manifest with recurrent fevers and organ-localizing inflammation and symptoms. *Familial Mediterranean fever,* an autosomal recessive disorder, manifests with recurrent fevers,

serositis (peritoneum, pleura), and joint involvement, and occurs predominantly in individuals of Sephardic Jewish, Arabic, Armenian, and Turkish descent. Episodes last 12 to 72 hours. The responsible gene is localized to chromosome 16p13.3 and encodes for marenostrin/pyrin, a protein predominantly expressed in myeloid cells. A dramatic response to colchicine is observed. TNF-receptor–associated periodic syndrome (*Hibernian fever*), an autosomal dominant disorder, manifests with similar clinical features. The major differences include autosomal dominance, slightly older age at onset, non-Mediterranean descent, longer duration of fever, and preponderance of abdominal symptoms. TNF-receptor–associated syndrome is caused by a mutation in the gene encoding tumor necrosis factor receptor type 1, located at chromosome 12p13. *Hyperimmunoglobulinemia D* (hyper-IgD) *and periodic fever syndrome* is an autosomal recessive disorder characterized by recurrent episodes of fever with lymphadenopathy, abdominal pain, hepatomegaly, splenomegaly, and joint and skin involvement in association with elevated IgD levels (>141 mg/L). In addition, elevated serum immunoglobulin A (IgA) has been found in 82% of individuals with hyper-IgD and periodic fever syndrome. The gene for hyper-IgD and periodic fever syndrome is on chromosome 12q24. A syndrome of *periodic fever associated with aphthous stomatitis, pharyngitis, and cervical adenitis* manifests in children younger than 5 years. Spontaneous remission occurs in these patients with increased age; exacerbations usually respond to prednisone (1 to 2 mg/kg/day).

THE IMMUNODEFICIENT PATIENT

Approximately 10% of children with recurrent infection have an immunodeficiency. Frequently, the onset of infections occurs between the ages of 6 and 12 months. The infections often vary in type, location, and severity, although pneumonias predominate (see Table 51-1). Unusual organisms and unexpected complications are often present. Such children may respond to antibiotics but become ill when the medications are discontinued. Failure to thrive is often noted (see Chapter 13).

DIAGNOSTIC APPROACH TO THE PATIENT WITH RECURRENT INFECTIONS

Patients with pyogenic infections involving multiple sites or organ systems should be investigated for an immunodeficiency. Children with two or more severe infections by 9 months of age and older children with frequent infections and growth failure should also be evaluated. Recurrent pulmonary infection, hepatic abscesses, and perirectal abscesses alert the clinician to consider possible neutrophil dysfunction and opsonic defects involving antibody or complement production.

A number of physical findings may be present in the child with immunodeficiency. Skin abnormalities include alopecia, eczema, pyoderma, and telangiectasia. Evidence of hematologic disease, such as pallor, petechiae, jaundice, and mouth ulceration, is associated with immunodeficiencies. Absent or diminished tonsils or lymph nodes are indicative of cellular immunodeficiency. Generalized lymphadenopathy and splenomegaly may be suggestive of HIV disease, a phagocyte disorder, or a possible associated hematologic disorder (Tables 51-6 and 51-7; see Table 51-4).

The initial and advanced laboratory evaluations for a suspected immunodeficiency are outlined in Figure 51-1. Because 80% of patients with primary immunodeficiency have an antibody deficiency, tests for antibody function and immunoglobulin levels are appropriate. Patients with a convincing history of recurrent infections should undergo other tests for immunodeficiency, even if the initial screening test results are normal. Subsequent testing must be individualized, based on the results of the investigations for each

Table 51-6. Clinical Patterns in Some Primary Immunodeficiencies

Features	Diagnosis
Newborns and Infants: Aged ≤6 Months	
Hypocalcemia, heart disease, unusual facies, small jaw	DiGeorge syndrome
Cyanosis, heart disease, midline liver	Congenital asplenia
Delayed umbilical cord separation, leukocytosis, recurrent infections	Leukocyte adhesion deficiency syndrome
Diarrhea, pneumonia, thrush, failure to thrive	Severe combined immunodeficiency
Maculopapular rash, alopecia, lymphadenopathy, hepatosplenomegaly	Severe combined immunodeficiency with graft-versus-host disease
Melena, draining ears, eczema	Wiskott-Aldrich syndrome
Oculocutaneous albinism, recurrent infections, neutropenia	Chédiak-Higashi syndrome
Recurrent pyogenic skin infections, pneumonia	Rac-2 deficiency
Recurrent pyogenic infections, sepsis	C3 deficiency
Chronic gingivitis, recurrent aphthous ulcers and skin infections, severe neutropenia	Severe congenital neutropenia
Mouth ulcers, neutropenia, autoimmune hemolytic anemia, recurrent infections	Immunodeficiency with hyper-IgM syndrome
Infants and Children: Aged 6 Months–5 Years	
Severe progressive infectious mononucleosis	X-linked lymphoproliferative syndrome (Duncan disease)
Paralytic disease after oral polio immunization	X-linked agammaglobulinemia
Recurrent cutaneous and systemic staphylococcal infections, coarse facial features	Hyperimmunoglobulin E syndrome
Persistent thrush, nail dystrophy, endocrinopathies	Chronic mucocutaneous candidiasis
Recurrent deep-seated skin abscesses	Specific granule deficiency
Lymphadenopathy, dermatitis, pyloric-antral obstruction, pneumonias, small bone osteomyelitis	Chronic granulomatous disease
Short stature, fine hair, severe varicella infection	Cartilage hair hypoplasia with short-limbed dwarfism
Children > Age 5 Years and Adults	
Progressive dermatomyositis with chronic ECHO virus encephalitis	X-linked agammaglobulinemia
Sinopulmonary infections, neurologic deterioration, telangiectasis	Ataxia-telangiectasia
Recurrent *Neisseria* meningitis	C5, C6, C7, and C8 deficiency
Sinopulmonary infections, malabsorption, splenomegaly, autoimmunity	Common variable immunodeficiency

Modified from Conley ME, Stiehm ER: Immunodeficiency disorders: General consideration. In Stiehm ER (ed): Immunologic Disorders in Infants and Children, 4th ed. Philadelphia, WB Saunders, 1996, p 212.

ECHO, enteric cytopathogenic human orphan virus; IgM, immunoglobulin M.

patient. A neutrophil count below 500/mm^3 might indicate severe congenital neutropenia, cyclic neutropenia, idiopathic neutropenia, marrow failure, or replacement of marrow by leukemia or a tumor if other hematopoietic cell lines are affected. Once initial immunoglobulin level screening is completed, other tests may include specific antibody responses to vaccines (tetanus, rubella, pneumococcal); immunoglobulin G (IgG) subclass levels for IgG1, IgG2, IgG3, and IgG4; and delayed hypersensitivity skin tests. Table 51-6 presents the characteristic clinical features of some of the primary immunodeficiencies.

LYMPHOCYTE DISORDERS

Lymphocyte disorders are a heterogeneous group of primary disorders involving both cell-mediated and humoral immunity. Disorders affecting T cell function (cell-mediated immunity) tend to be more severe than primary B cell disorders; combined deficits carry the poorest prognosis.

Children with altered T lymphocyte function have recurrent infections (see Tables 51-1 and 51-7) or unusual responses to usually benign infectious agents, or they develop infections with unusual organisms. *Pneumocystis carinii,* cytomegalovirus, measles, and varicella often cause fatal pneumonitis in these patients. Pneumonitis occurring with any of these agents should alert the clinician to a potential immunodeficiency. Affected children also have a higher incidence of malignancy and autoimmune disorders. A partial list of primary disorders of lymphocyte function is shown in Table 51-7; their evaluation is described in Figure 51-1.

DISORDERS OF ANTIBODY PRODUCTION

X-LINKED AGAMMAGLOBULINEMIA

Bruton agammaglobulinemia, an X-linked recessive disorder characterized by an arrest in B cell differentiation, leaves affected children severely deficient in serum immunoglobulins and at serious risk for recurrent life-threatening infections. The affected gene product encoded at chromosome Xq22 is a cytoplasmic protein tyrosine kinase (Bruton tyrosine kinase [BTK]), which is essential for pre–B cell growth into mature B cells; its mutation accounts for the absence

Table 51-7. Disorders of Lymphocyte Function

Disorder	Genetics	Onset	Manifestations	Pathogenesis	Associated Features
Bruton agammaglobulinemia	X-linked (Xq21.3-q22)	Infancy (6-9 months)	Recurrent high-grade infections, sinusitis, pneumonia, meningitis	Arrest in B cell differentiation (pre-B–B level; initiation of BTK)	Lymphoid hypoplasia
Common variable immunodeficiency	Not known	Second to third decade	Sinusitis, bronchitis, pneumonia, chronic diarrhea	Arrest in B cell to plasma cell differentiation	Autoimmune disease, RA, SLE, Graves disease, ITP, malignancy
Transient hypogamma-globulinemia of infancy	Not known	Infancy (4-9 months)	Recurrent viral and pyogenic infections	Delayed development of plasma cell maturation	Frequent in families with immunodeficiencies
IgA deficiency	Not known	Variable	Sinopulmonary infections; Gastrointestinal infections; may be unaffected	Failure of IgA expressing B cell differentiation	IgG subclass deficiency, common variable immunodeficiency, autoimmune diseases
IgG subclass deficiency	AR (14q32.3)	Variable	Variable (unaffected to recurrent sinopulmonary infections and gastrointestinal infections)	Defect in isotype IgG production secondary to mutation of genes encoding the μ chain on 14q32.3	IgA deficiency
Immunodeficiency with increased IgM	X-linked (Xq26.3-q27.1)	2-3 years	Recurrent pyogenic infections (otitis media, sinusitis, tonsillitis, pneumonia)	Defect in IgG and IgA synthesis secondary to abnormal gene encoding CD40 ligand on T cells	Hematologic autoimmune disease
Immunodeficiency with increased IgM	AR (12p13)	2-3 years	Recurrent pyogenic infections (otitis media, sinusitis, tonsillitis, pneumonia)	Mutation of activation-induced cytidine deaminase gene that controls signaling in B cells	Hematologic autoimmune disease
DiGeorge anomaly	Not hereditary microdeletion (22 q11.2)	Early infancy	Variable	Hypoplasia of third and fourth pharyngeal pouch	Hypoparathyroidism, micrognathia, hypertelorism, congenital heart disease
Wiskott-Aldrich syndrome	X-linked (Xp11.22)	Early infancy	Recurrent otitis media, pneumonia, meningitis with encapsulated organisms	Control of assembly of actin filaments	Recurrent infections, atopic dermatitis, platelet dysfunction, thrombocytopenia
Ataxia-telangiectasia	AR (11q22.3)	2-5 years	Sinopulmonary infections	Defect in DNA repair and control of cell cycle	Neurologic and endocrine dysfunction, malignancy, telangiectasias
Cartilage-hair hypoplasia (short-limbed dwarf)	AR (9p13)	Birth	Variable infections	Mutation in the RMRP gene disrupting RNAse MRP RNA affecting multiple organs	Metaphyseal dysplasia, short extremities, neutropenia
Severe combined immunodeficiency (SCID)	X-linked (Xq13.1-q21.1)	1-3 months	Candidiasis, all types of infections (bacterial, viral, fungal, protozoal)	IL-2Rγ depletion (severe T cell depletion), T cell negative, B cell positive, natural killer cell negative	Severe graft-versus-host disease from maternal fetal transfusions
	AR (5p13)	1-3 months	Same as previous entry	T cell-negative, B cell-positive, natural killer cell-positive, SCID secondary to IL-7 receptor α-chain mutation on 5p13	Graft-versus-host disease from blood transfusions
	AR (1q31-q32)	1-3 months	Same as previous entry	T cell-negative, B cell-positive, natural killer cell-positive, SCID secondary to mutant CD45 phosphatase (which encodes for tyrosine kinase signaling protein, known as CD45 deficiency	Same as previous entry
	AR (11q23)	1-3 months	Same as previous entry	T cell-negative, B cell-positive, natural killer cell-positive, SCID secondary to mutations in CD 3 genes	Same as previous entry

Continued

Table 51-7. Disorders of Lymphocyte Function—cont'd

Disorder	Genetics	Onset	Manifestations	Pathogenesis	Associated Features
	AR	1-3 months	Same as previous entry	T cell–negative, B cell–positive, natural killer cell–negative, SCID secondary to mutant Janus-associated kinase 3 gene on 19p13.1	Same as previous entry
	AR (Omenn syndrome)	1-3 months	Same as previous entry	T cell–negative, B cell–negative, natural killer cell–positive, SCID associated with deficiencies of recombinase-activating gene proteins secondary to RAG1 or RAG2 gene on 6q21.3	Same as previous entry
	AR (20q13.2-q13.11) (ADA deficiency)	1-3 months	Same as previous entry	Enzyme deficiency results in dATP-induced T cell toxicity	Multiple skeletal abnormalities, chondroosseous dysplasia
	AR (PNP deficiency) (14q13.1)	1-3 months	Same as previous entry	Enzyme deficiency results in dGTP-induced T cell toxicity	Neurologic disorders, severe graft-versus-host disease from blood transfusions
	AR (reticular dysgenesis)	1-3 months	Same as previous entry	Defective maturation of common stem cell affecting myeloid and lymphoid cells	Agammaglobulinemia, alymphocytosis, agranulocytosis
Class II MHC deficiency	AR (16p13)	Early infancy	Persistent diarrhea secondary to cryptosporidiosis, bacterial pneumonia, *P. carinii* pneumonia, septicemia, viral and candida infections; patients are not at risk for graft-versus-host disease	Three mutations affect subunits of RFX, a multiprotein transcription factor complex that binds the X-box motif of the MHC class II promoter, which controls expression of MHC class II molecules; a fourth mutation involves MHC class II transactivator (CIITA), which is a molecule that controls the inducibility of expression of class II MHC genes	Few CD4+ T cells normal or CD8+ T cells elevated MHC class II antigens are lacking on B cells and monocytes Immune responses are impaired
Class I MHC deficiency	AR (6q21.3)	1-3 months	Similar to MHC class II deficiency	Mutations affecting either TAP1 or TAP2 genes within MHC locus on chromosome 6 that encodes the peptide-transporter proteins called transporters associated with antigen processing (TAPs); TAPs transport peptide antigens from the cytoplasm to join the α chain of MHC class I molecules and β₂ microglobulin; if the complex cannot be completed because of a lack of peptide antigens, MHC class I complex is destroyed in the cytoplasm	Deficiency of CD8+ T cells, normal number of CD4+ cells
CD8 lymphopenia	AR (2q12)	Early infancy	Infections similar to those in SCID	Mutations in gene encoding ζ-associated protein 70 (ZAP-70), a tyrosine kinase important in T cell signaling	Normal or elevated CD4+ T cells, no CD8+ T cells, normal natural killer cells, normal B cells, normal immunoglobulin levels

ADA, adenosine deaminase; AR, autosomal recessive; BTK, Bruton tyrosine kinase; dATP, deoxyadenosine triphosphate; dGTP, deoxyguanosine triphosphate; IgA, IgG, and IgM, immunoglobulins A, G, and M; IL-2Rγ, interleukin-2 receptor γ chain; IL-7, interleukin-7; ITP, idiopathic thrombocytopenic purpura; MHC, major histocompatibility complex; PNP, purine nucleoside phosphorylase; RA, rheumatoid arthritis; RAG1 and RAG2, recombinase-activating genes 1 and 2; SLE, systemic lupus erythematosus.

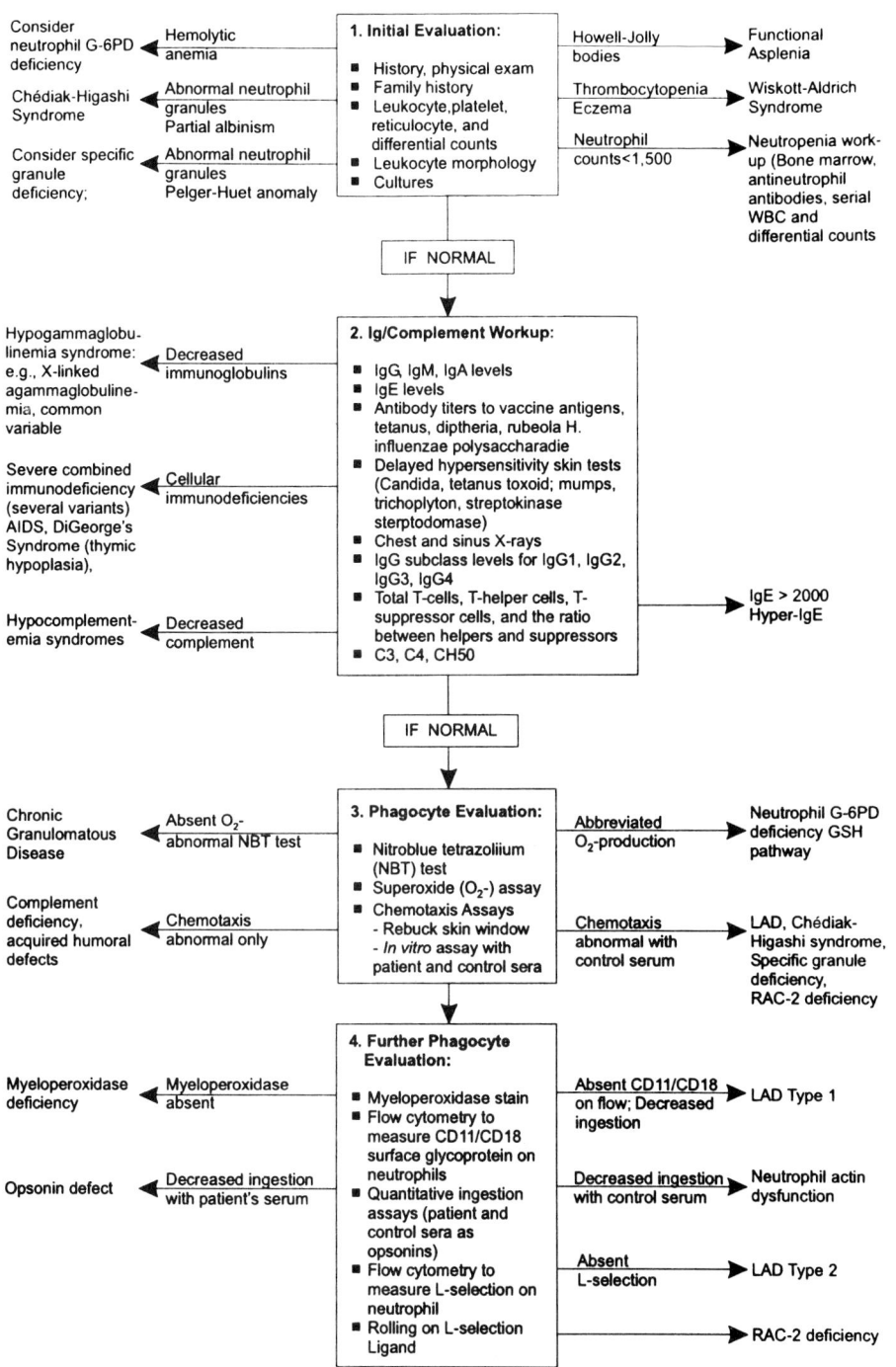

Figure 51-1. Algorithm for the work-up of a patient with infections. AIDS, acquired immunodeficiency syndrome; G6PD, glucose-6-phosphate dehydrogenase; GSH, reduced glutathione; IgA, IgE, IgG, and IgM, immunoglobulins A, E, G, and M; LAD, leukocyte adhesion deficiency syndrome; NBT, nitroblue tetrazolium; WBC, white blood cell. (Modified from Boxer LA: Quantitative abnormalities of granulocytes. In Beutler E, Lichtman MA, Coller BS, et al [eds]: Williams Hematology, 6th ed. New York, McGraw-Hill, 2001, p 847.)

of circulating B cells in these patients. The mutant BTK gene has been found in myeloid cells, which may account for the intermittent neutropenia associated with this condition. More than 400 different mutations in the BTK gene have been identified.

Although some affected children are asymptomatic until the age of 2 years, most show symptoms in infancy between 6 and 9 months of age, when transplacentally derived maternal antibodies disappear. They develop repeated infections (recurrent otitis media, sinusitis, pneumonia, meningitis) with highly pathogenic bacteria, such as pneumococci, staphylococci, streptococci, and *Haemophilus* species. They handle most simple viral infections well; immunizations do not cause problems except for live polio vaccine, which has

resulted in paralysis. Exposure to other enteroviruses has led to chronic diarrhea, hepatitis, pneumonitis, and persistent meningoencephalitis.

Affected patients have marked hypoplasia of lymphoid tissue (adenoids, tonsils, lymph nodes) with absence of germinal centers and rare plasma cells. The diagnosis can be suspected if serum IgG, immunoglobulin M (IgM), and IgA levels are less than 5% of age-adjusted control values in a patient with normal T cell function. On occasion, children with X-linked agammaglobulinemia present with an elevated IgA or IgG level but do not respond to immunizations with specific antibody production. Treatment includes aggressive antibiotic management of infections and replacement of immunoglobulin, although chronic pulmonary and gastrointestinal diseases may occur (Table 51-8).

COMMON VARIABLE IMMUNODEFICIENCY

Common variable immunodeficiency (CVID) is a heterogeneous group of disorders characterized by the development of severe hypogammaglobulinemia, which results in chronic respiratory infections (sinusitis, bronchitis, pneumonia) and severe gastrointestinal disease. CVID is associated with a celiac disease–like syndrome, which occurs in up to 60% of patients. These patients experience heavy bacterial overgrowth of the small bowel, jejunal villous atrophy, and intestinal nodular lymphoid hyperplasia. The bacteria overgrowth in the gut often leads to diarrhea, steatorrhea, malabsorption, and protein-losing enteropathy. Patients can also develop noncaseating granulomas of the liver, spleen, lungs, and skin. *Giardia lamblia* infection is common in these patients and may play a role in the gastrointestinal problems because many such patients experience improvement with metronidazole. As in X-linked agammaglobulinemia, the most common manifestations of CVID are chronic infections of the upper and lower respiratory tracts. Hematologic abnormalities include immune-mediated thrombocytopenia, anemia, leukopenia, and systemic lupus erythematosus. There appears to be an increased susceptibility to lymphoreticular malignancies and carcinoma of the stomach in affected adults.

Patients with CVID have low circulating levels of IgG, IgM, and IgA but normal to increased numbers of circulating B cells with greatly reduced numbers of plasma cells in the intestinal lamina propria. B cells fail to respond to normal maturational signals.

TRANSIENT HYPOGAMMAGLOBULINEMIA OF INFANCY

The fetus is capable of producing IgM or IgG by the 20th week of gestation when adequately stimulated; under normal conditions, however, neonatal levels of IgG are a reflection of prior maternal immunity via transplacental passage of maternal IgG. Significant antibody production does not normally begin until the second or third month of life. Because maternal antibodies have a half-life of approximately 30 days, the infant may develop a variable physiologic hypogammaglobulinemia between the ages of 4 and 9 months. If profound in extent or duration, this transient hypoglobulinemia may lead to recurrent viral and pyogenic infections. Infants with such infections are capable of making specific antibodies (tetanus, diphtheria toxoids), they respond to immunizations, and they have normal numbers of circulating B and T cells. Lymph nodes are small, and germinal centers are reduced in size and number. The abnormality may be caused by decreased maturation of B cells to antibody-producing plasma cells. Most patients do not require gamma globulin therapy and achieve normal immunoglobulin levels between 12 and 36 months of age.

IMMUNOGLOBULIN A DEFICIENCY

IgA deficiency is the most common primary immunodeficiency. The mode of transmission appears to be variable: either autosomal recessive or autosomal dominant with variable penetrance. The defect causes an arrest in B cell maturation. Patients with IgA deficiency may be asymptomatic or may present with recurrent sinopulmonary and gastrointestinal infections. IgA deficiency is also often associated with IgG2 or IgG4 subclass deficiency, which worsens the prognosis. There is also a high incidence of autoimmune disorders and an association with CVID.

Most patients with IgA deficiency do not require treatment other than antibiotic management of their infections. Blood products that include immunoglobulins are often contraindicated because patients may develop antibodies against IgA, possibly precipitating anaphylactic reactions.

IMMUNOGLOBULIN G SUBCLASS DEFICIENCY

Four different subclasses of IgG (IgG1 [65% of total IgG], IgG2 [25%], IgG3 [5% to 10%], and IgG4 [5%]) have been identified. Different types of antigens elicit a particular subclass of IgG

Table 51-8. Management of Infections in the Host Compromised by B and T Lymphocyte Defects

Immunodeficiency Syndrome	Management	Prevention of Infection
Humoral defects (predominant B cell deficiency)	Intravenous immunoglobulin, 0.4 g/kg Bacterial and viral culture Incision and drainage of abscess Bactericidal antibiotics based on culture and sensitivity of microorganism Intraventricular immunoglobulin for echovirus, encephalitis, pleconaril, antiviral therapy	Maintenance intravenous immunoglobulin, 0.3-0.5 g/kg q3-4wk Avoid live virus vaccines in patient and relatives Respiratory care, postural drainage, monitor for cor pulmonale Chronic antibiotic prophylaxis is controversial
Cellular defects (predominant T cell deficiency)	Bacterial, viral, fungal, protozoal culture, microscopy, and stains Incision and drainage of abscess Biopsy, bronchoalveolar lavage if indicated Antibacterial, antiviral, antifungal, antiprotozoal therapy as appropriate for culture, sensitivity, stains, and symptoms Intravenous immunoglobulin if helper T lymphocyte–associated antibody deficiency or SCID is present	Prophylactic trimethoprim-sulfamethoxazole for *Pneumocystis carinii* No live virus vaccines or BCG Careful screening for tuberculosis Irradiated blood products decrease risk of GVH CMV-negative blood products Varicella-zoster immune globulin used for those with varicella exposure Immunologic reconstitution Bone marrow transplantation Fetal thymus transplantation for DiGeorge symptoms Polyethylene glycol ADA enzyme infusion ADA genetic reconstitution

ADA, Adenosine deaminase enzyme; BCG, bacille Calmette-Guérin; CMV, cytomegalovirus; GVH, graft-versus-host disease, which increases risk of infection; SCID, severe combined immunodeficiency.

response (e.g., protein antigens tend to elicit an IgG1 response, whereas carbohydrates elicit an IgG2 response). In children younger than 2 years, it is difficult to elicit an antibody response to carbohydrate antigens (reflected by the necessity of protein conjugation for pneumococcal and *Haemophilus influenzae* vaccine).

The spectrum of IgG subclass deficiency is variable. Some patients do well, whereas others have recurrent upper and lower respiratory infections, otitis media, sinusitis, and gastroenteritis, with both bacteria and viruses. In some children, immune function improves with age, often reaching normal levels by the age of 7 or 8 years. Total IgG level is usually normal, and only on examination of IgG subclasses can the defect be detected. Determination of antibody titers to polysaccharide antigens (*Streptococcus pneumoniae, Neisseria meningitidis*) aids in the assessment of immunologic function and the specific need for medical intervention. Many children with subclass deficiency do well with no treatment; others respond to prophylactic antibiotics; and still others require intravenous immune globulin replacement.

IMMUNODEFICIENCY WITH INCREASED IMMUNOGLOBULIN M LEVEL

Immunodeficiency with increased IgM level is a heterogeneous group of disorders characterized by normal or increased concentrations of IgM and IgD but decreased levels or absence of IgG, IgA, and IgE (see Table 51-7). The most common form of these disorders is X-linked hyper-IgM syndrome. Patients with these disorders are more susceptible to *P. carinii* pneumonia and to recurrent pyogenic infections. This is because of deficiency of the T cell surface molecule, CD154 (or CD40 ligand). This membrane glycoprotein is essential for T cell initiation of B cell isotype switching and CD80 and CD86 upregulation. Failure to upregulate B cell activity results in diminished B cell–derived costimulatory molecules, defective purging of autoreactive thymocytes, increased incidence of autoimmune disease, defective recognition of tumor cells, and increased incidence of cancer. An autosomal recessive form of this disorder may be caused by an intrinsic B cell defect in CD40-mediated signaling.

X-LINKED LYMPHOPROLIFERATIVE DISEASE (DUNCAN SYNDROME)

X-linked lymphoproliferative disease is a rare genetic disorder characterized by immunodysregulation in response to Epstein-Barr virus (EBV). The usual manifestation is a fulminant, often fatal infection with EBV. Survivors of primary EBV infection often develop acquired hypogammaglobulinemia, B cell lymphoma, aplastic anemia, vasculitis, and lymphomatoid granulomatosis. The gene responsible for X-linked lymphoproliferative disease has been localized to chromosome Xq25. It encodes for a ligand-receptor pair on B and T cell that results in their coregulation. Mutations are thought to result in the uncontrolled proliferation of B cells after EBV infection.

COMBINED DISORDERS OF T AND B CELLS

T lymphocytes are the effectors for cell-mediated immunity. T lymphocytes differentiate in the thymus and serve as regulators of the humoral and the cell-mediated immune system; they modulate the activities of nonlymphocytic cells, such as monocytes. Patients with combined defects in T and B cell function have infections or other problems that are more severe than those in patients with only antibody deficiency.

DiGEORGE SYNDROME

DiGeorge syndrome is characterized by a constellation of clinical features that include dysmorphic facies, hypoparathyroidism, congenital heart defects, and deficiency in cell-mediated immunity (see Table 51-7). The clinical anomalies are caused by the maldevelopment of structures that are derived from the first through the sixth branchial pouches during embryogenesis, resulting in variable hypoplasia of the thymus, parathyroid glands, face, ears, aortic arch, and heart. Congenital heart defects include truncus arteriosus, ventricular septal defect, interrupted aortic arch, and tetralogy of Fallot. Hypocalcemia with tetany is often the initial problem in the first and second month after birth. Facial abnormalities include microstomia, hypertelorism, and low-set ears. A majority of the cases of DiGeorge syndrome are associated with a microdeletion at chromosome 22q11.2, although a deletion at a second loci at chromosome 10p13 results in a similar clinical picture. Both chromosomal anomalies can be diagnosed with fluorescent in situ hybridization.

The degree of immunodeficiency is highly variable and related to the extent of residual thymic function. Some patients have infections with opportunistic organisms (*P. carinii*, viruses, and fungi), whereas others exhibit normal immune function. Serum immunoglobulin levels are appropriate, but antibody response to specific antigenic challenges varies. Intradermal delayed hypersensitivity may be absent, decreased, or normal, whereas lymph node paracortical areas and thymus-dependent regions of the spleen show variable degrees of cell depletion, depending on the degree of thymic deficiency. The total lymphocyte count may vary from severely depressed to normal, but T cell levels are usually depressed. No correlation has been shown between severity of congenital defects and the severity of immunodeficiency, although immune function often improves with age. The management of DiGeorge syndrome is described in Table 51-8.

WISKOTT-ALDRICH SYNDROME

Wiskott-Aldrich syndrome, an X-linked recessive disorder mapped to chromosome Xp11.22, is characterized by abnormalities in lymphocyte, platelet, and phagocyte function (see Table 51-7). The gene product encodes for a protein that controls the assembly of actin filaments and intracellular vesicle transport in lymphocytes and megakaryocytes. Wiskott-Aldrich syndrome is characterized by this triad: (1) recurrent infections involving encapsulated bacteria and opportunistic pathogens, (2) hemorrhage secondary to thrombocytopenia and platelet dysfunction, and (3) atopic dermatitis. Presenting in early infancy with pneumonia, otitis media, and meningitis, patients are susceptible to infection with encapsulated organisms. Later, they develop fungal and *P. carinii* infections but are also at risk for disseminated herpes simplex and cytomegalovirus infections. Patients have selective defects in multiple areas of their immune system. Initial serum IgG levels are typically normal, with elevated IgA and IgE and decreased IgM levels. Patients initially respond normally to protein antigens, such as tetanus, but serum antibody levels diminish over time. Their antibody response to polysaccharide antigens is extremely poor, and blood-group isohemagglutinins are absent. The serum half-life of immunoglobulin also appears to be decreased. There are abnormalities in cellular immunity manifested by anergy and diminished response to mitogen stimulation. They may exhibit moderately reduced numbers of CD3+, CD4+, and CD8+ T cells.

Thrombocytopenia characterized by small platelets is a unique feature. Prolonged bleeding at circumcision or profuse bloody diarrhea is observed. Many children with this disorder succumb to bleeding disorders or infection; 12% die of secondary lymphomas. Bone marrow or cord blood transplantation from a human leukocyte antigen–identical sibling or a human leukocyte antigen–matched unrelated donor has corrected the immunologic and platelet abnormalities in patients with Wiskott-Aldrich syndrome.

ATAXIA-TELANGIECTASIA

Ataxia-telangiectasia is an autosomal recessive disorder characterized by neurologic dysfunction, endocrine abnormalities, oculocutaneous telangiectasia, immunodeficiency, and a high rate of malignancy (see Table 51-7). The defective gene, located on chromosome 11q22.3, encodes for a phosphatidylinositol 3-kinase involved in intracellular signal transduction and DNA repair. Cerebellar ataxia is usually the first presenting sign, occurring when the child begins to walk. The patient's neurologic status often worsens, and choreoathetosis, involuntary myoclonic jerks, and oculomotor abnormalities develop. Telangiectasias first appear in the bulbar conjunctivae between 2 and 5 years of age and later spread to areas of trauma. Endocrine abnormalities, such as insulin-resistant diabetes mellitus, and hypogonadism are common. There is a 15% risk of malignancy; non-Hodgkin lymphoma is the most common.

Patients with ataxia-telangiectasia are extremely sensitive to ionizing radiation, as a result of alteration in DNA repair. This accounts for the high incidence of chromosomal translocations involving chromosomes 7 and 14 at the site of T cell receptor genes and immunoglobulin heavy-chain genes. The degree of immunodeficiency is quite variable; both B cell and T cell abnormalities occur. The most common B cell abnormalities include IgA deficiency (75% of patients), IgE deficiency (85%), and monomeric IgM (80%). IgG subclass deficiency occurs in about 50%; IgG2 and IgG4 deficiencies are the most common. T cells show abnormal, delayed-type hypersensitivity reaction, proliferative response to mitogens, and allograft rejection. The thymus is abnormally small, and although circulating T lymphocyte numbers appear to be normal, peripheral lymphoid tissue reveals depletion in resident T cells. Patients with ataxia-telangiectasia have sinopulmonary infections. Administration of blood products that include immunoglobulins can lead to anaphylactic reactions because IgA-deficient patients often produce autoantibodies to IgA.

CARTILAGE-HAIR HYPOPLASIA (SHORT-LIMBED DWARFISM)

Cartilage-hair hypoplasia is an autosomal recessive disease characterized by metaphyseal dysostosis; sparse, thin hair; and variable immunodeficiency (see Table 51-7). Lymphocyte numbers may be normal or dramatically depressed. Proliferative responses to mitogens are generally depressed; immune function may deteriorate with time. The immunodeficiency can range from mild to severe; in most affected patients, it is relatively mild, and patients benefit most from replacement immunoglobulin. Patients may have moderate to severe neutropenia, making them susceptible to both viral and bacterial infections.

SEVERE COMBINED IMMUNODEFICIENCY SYNDROMES

Severe combined immunodeficiency (SCID) is a heterogeneous group of disorders characterized by profound abnormalities in B cell and T cell function. In the first few months after birth, patients present with recurrent pneumonia, failure to thrive, and chronic diarrhea. They often have candidiasis of the mouth, esophagus, face, and diaper area, in addition to other infections (bacterial, viral, fungal, protozoal). Adenovirus and cytomegalovirus frequently progress into chronic pneumonitis; disseminated, life-threatening varicella and measles infections occur; and live-virus vaccines can result in a fatal infection such as disseminated mycobacterial infection with bacille Calmette-Guérin. Severe graft-versus-host disease frequently develops after blood transfusions that contain live donor lymphocytes.

Most patients exhibit severe deficits in immunoglobulin synthesis that range from agammaglobulinemia to isolated subclass deficiencies; responses to specific antigens are usually impaired. B cells may be absent or increased, but T cell abnormalities are always present. T cell numbers are generally fewer than 10% of normal in more than 80% of patients. Patients are anergic, and T cells show decreased proliferative responses to mitogens, decreased cytotoxicity, and decreased immunoregulatory activity. Residual host natural killer cell activity may account for graft failure in patients with SCID who are treated with haploidentical bone marrow transplantation.

X-LINKED RECESSIVE SEVERE COMBINED IMMUNODEFICIENCY

X-linked recessive SCID is the most common form of SCID (approximately 46% of the cases) and is characterized by T cell and natural killer cell depletion in the presence of normal numbers of B cells (see Table 51-7). The abnormal gene has been mapped to the Xq13 region encoding for the γ chain that is common to five interleukin molecules (interleukins-2, -4, -7, -9, and -15). The interleukin-2 receptor is necessary for thymic maturation of T cells; its deficiency explains T cell depletion. T cell depletion in conjunction with diminished levels of several cytokine receptors arising from a single mutated gene further explains how T cells, B cells, and natural killer cells can all be affected. Female carriers can be identified because lymphocytes and natural killer cells exhibit nonrandom inactivation of the X chromosome. The management of X-linked recessive SCID is noted in Table 51-8. Isolated deficiencies in the α subunits of the interleukin-2 and interleukin-7 (5p13) receptor that clinically manifest with SCID have also been identified.

DEFICIENCY OF JANUS-ASSOCIATED KINASE-3

Janus-associated kinase 3 (Jak 3) is the only signaling molecule known to associate with the γ chain of interleukin receptors (see Table 51-7). This disorder resembles X-linked recessive SCID with regard to susceptibility to infections and transfusion-related graft-versus-host disease. Affected patients also have low levels of T cells and natural killer cells but elevated levels of B cells. Natural killer cell numbers remain low even after successful bone marrow transplantation.

DEFICIENCY OF CD45

CD45 is a transmembrane tyrosine phosphatase, found exclusively on hematopoietic cells, which regulates *src* tyrosine kinases (required for signal transduction of T and B cell receptors). Deficiency of CD45 manifests clinically as SCID with low numbers of T cells but normal B cells (see Table 51-7). Although serum immunoglobulin levels may be normal initially, they decrease with time, and there is a diminished response to specific antigen challenge.

CD8 LYMPHOPENIA

ζ-Associated protein 70 (ZAP-70) is a tyrosine kinase that plays an essential role in the positive and negative selection of maturing T cells (see Table 51-7). The gene encoding ZAP-70 is located at chromosome 2q12; its deficiency results in CD8 lymphopenia. The severity of the immunodeficiency is variable; however, affected patients generally have normal or elevated CD4$^+$ T cells and essentially no CD8$^+$ T cells.

OMENN SYNDROME

This form of SCID is characterized by the absence of functional T cells and B cells (see Table 51-7). The circulating lymphocytes are predominantly natural killer cells. Mutation in recombinase-activating gene 1 or 2 (RAG1 and RAG2) leads to impaired rearrangement of B cell receptor and T cell receptor genes. Affected patients develop a generalized erythroderma and desquamation, diarrhea, hepatosplenomegaly, hypereosinophilia, and hyper-IgE. Omenn syndrome is fatal unless corrected by bone marrow transplantation.

RETICULAR DYSGENESIS

Reticular dysgenesis is the most severe form of SCID. It is characterized by agammaglobulinemia, lymphopenia, and neutropenia; erythroid and platelet precursor numbers are normal. Affected patients die shortly after birth of overwhelming infection unless they are treated successfully with bone marrow transplantation (see Table 51-8).

DEFICIENCY OF MAJOR HISTOCOMPATIBILITY COMPLEX MOLECULES (BARE LYMPHOCYTE SYNDROME)

The expression of cell surface major histocompatibility complex (MHC) molecules is important for cell-cell recognition; the failure to express these molecules is associated with SCID. Deficiencies have been described in the expression of both class I and class II MHC molecules (see Table 51-7). Deficiency in class II MHC molecules is more common, accounting for 5% of cases of SCID. It is also more severe because class II molecules are required for the positive selection of T helper cells in the thymus, for T cell recognition of antigen-presenting cells, and for T helper cell interactions with B cells. Deficiency in class I MHC molecules results in decreased numbers of CD8+ T cells but normal numbers of CD4+ T cells, whereas deficiency in class II MHC molecules results in low numbers of CD8+ T cells and normal or elevated numbers of CD8+ T cells. The defect is not in the class II MHC gene itself but in genes regulating the transcription of class II MHC genes. A similar defect exists for class I MHC gene expression. Patients with these forms of SCID have altered T helper/suppressor interaction, as well as altered antigen presentation.

ADENOSINE DEAMINASE DEFICIENCY

Adenosine deaminase deficiency, an autosomal recessive trait, results in an inability to catalyze the conversion of adenosine and deoxyadenosine to inosine and deoxyinosine, respectively. The gene is located on chromosome 20q13.2-q13.11, and its deficiency results in the accumulation of deoxyadenosine, which is phosphorylated to deoxy–adenosine triphosphate (deoxy-ATP) (see Table 51-7). Deoxy-ATP is toxic to lymphocytes, leading to their demise and to subsequent SCID. Patients with this enzyme deficiency have different degrees of agammaglobulinemia and lymphopenia. In addition, they often have associated chondroosseous dysplasia with multiple skeletal abnormalities. Treatment is described in Table 51-8.

PURINE NUCLEOSIDE PHOSPHORYLASE DEFICIENCY

Purine nucleoside phosphorylase (PNP) is the enzyme (chromosome 14q11) that follows adenosine deaminase in the purine salvage pathway and catalyzes the conversion of inosine and guanosine to hypoxanthine and guanine, respectively (see Table 51-7). PNP deficiency leads to the intracellular buildup of deoxy-guanosine triphosphate (deoxy-GTP). Like deoxy-ATP, deoxy-GTP is toxic to T cells, resulting in T cell lymphopenia, whereas the number of B cells remains normal. Serum immunoglobulin and isohemagglutinin levels are normal. Specific antibody production is impaired because T helper function is abnormal. In patients with SCID, a low serum uric acid level is suggestive of PNP deficiency.

COMPLEMENT SYSTEM DEFICIENCIES

The complement system has an integral role in the regulation of the immune system and its response to infectious agents. As the complement cascade is activated and progresses, all areas of the immune system are affected: C4a and C2a regulate vascular permeability, C3b and C3bi regulate phagocytosis, C5a mediates the release of cytokines from monocytes and is chemotactic for neutrophils, and C9 complex formation mediates cell lysis.

Activation of the *classic pathway* begins with fixation of C1, by way of Clq to the crystallized fragment receptor of an antigen-antibody complex. A conformational shift results in the activation of C1s, which activates C4 and then C2. The C142 complex acts as a C3 convertase, which activates C3 from C3b, whereas in the *alternative pathway,* BbC3b activates C3. C3bi, an important opsonin, is formed by cleavage of C3b by C3b inactivator. C3b formation results in the sequential activation of C5 through C9. C9 activation results in the formation of the *membrane attack complex,* consisting of 12 to 18 C9 molecules that form a transmembrane channel, resulting in cell lysis. Teichoic acid from bacterial cell wall, endotoxic lipopolysaccharides, and aggregates of immunoglobulin, especially IgA, are potent activators of the alternative pathway. Although protein deficiencies or abnormalities have been identified for all 11 components in the classical complement pathway, the severity and the type of infection varies because of the considerable overlap between the two pathways (Table 51-9).

In addition, C1 inhibitor deficiency is an autosomal dominant disorder that results in dysregulation of the classic complement pathway. Activation of the classic pathway results in angioneurotic edema secondary to the uncontrolled formation of C4a and C2a, two vasoactive proteins. After minor trauma, affected patients develop swelling and edema without urticaria, pain, or erythema. The swelling usually lasts 24 to 48 hours before subsiding spontaneously. Angioedema involving the larynx or upper airways can be life-threatening, and involvement of the bowel leads to abdominal pain, vomiting, and diarrhea. Affected children often do not come to medical attention until after puberty; androgens such as danazol or stanozolol are effective at preventing attacks.

SECONDARY COMPLEMENT DEFICIENCIES

IgG binds to C1q, protecting it from rapid catabolism; therefore, children with hypogammaglobulinemia develop partial C1q deficiency. Patients with chronic membranoproliferative glomerulonephritis and partial lipodystrophy may develop nephritic factor, an antibody that protects the C3bBb complex from inactivation, resulting in the consumption of C3 and a relative C3-deficient state. These patients are at risk for developing pyogenic infections, including meningitis, if their serum C3 levels fall below 10% of normal levels. Patients with acute postinfectious glomerulonephritis and systemic lupus erythematosus may develop an antibody similar to nephritic factor, which protects the C3 convertase of the classic pathway.

Most newborns are relatively deficient in all components of the classic pathway, as well as in factor B and properdin in the alternative pathway; their ability to generate serum-derived chemotactic factors and opsonization is markedly diminished. Complement activity is even lower in premature infants. Malnutrition and anorexia nervosa may lead to decreased levels of all components of complement, whereas cirrhosis of the liver is associated with decreased synthesis of C3.

Immune complex disease (systemic lupus erythematosus, postinfectious nephritis) can result in increased complement consumption and relative deficiency. Increased complement consumption has also been demonstrated in lepromatous leprosy, bacterial endocarditis, malaria, dengue fever, acute hepatitis B, and infectious mononucleosis. Burn injuries can induce massive activation of complement, which accounts at least partially for the increased risk of infection in burned patients. In patients with erythropoietic protoporphyria or porphyria cutanea tarda, hypocomplementemia develops because certain wavelengths of light activate complement, which results in abnormal consumption.

DIAGNOSIS AND MANAGEMENT

The most useful screening test is the total hemolytic complement activity (CH_{50}). The CH_{50} measures the ability of all 11 components

Table 51-9. Genetic Deficiencies of Complement Components

Component	Genetics	Associated Clinical Findings	
		Associated Diseases	*Recurrent Infections*
C1q	Autosomal recessive	SLE, MPGN, vasculitis	Septicemia, meningitis, pyoderma, dermatitis
C1s	Autosomal recessive	SLE	Recurrent pneumonia, meningitis
C1r	Autosomal recessive	SLE, CGN, vasculitis	Recurrent pneumonia, meningitis
C1 inhibitor	Autosomal dominant	Hereditary angioedema, SLE	
C4	Autosomal recessive	SLE, HSP, Sjögren syndrome	Recurrent pneumonia, meningitis
C2	Autosomal recessive	SLE, HSP, ITP, CGN, dermatomyositis, vasculitis, MPGN	Recurrent septicemia, especially pneumococcal; meningitis; pneumonia
C3	Autosomal recessive	SLE, MPGN, vasculitis	Severe pyogenic infection caused by meningococci and pneumococci
C5	Autosomal recessive	SLE	Disseminated gonococcal and meningococcal disease, pyoderma, meningitis
C6	Autosomal recessive	SLE, MPGN, Sjögren syndrome, Raynaud phenomenon	Disseminated gonococcal and meningococcal disease
C7	Autosomal recessive	SLE, scleroderma, ankylosing spondylitis, rheumatoid arthritis, Raynaud phenomenon	Disseminated gonococcal and meningococcal disease
C8	Autosomal recessive	SLE	Disseminated gonococcal and meningococcal disease
C9	Autosomal recessive		Meningococcal meningitis, extragenital gonococcal infections
Factor D	X-linked/autosomal recessive		Recurrent sinusitis, bronchitis, DGI
Factor I	Autosomal recessive		Pyogenic infections, septicemia
Factor H	Autosomal recessive	Hemolytic-uremic syndrome	Pyogenic infections, septicemia
Properdin	X-linked		Septicemia
Factor B	Autosomal recessive		Meningococcal meningitis

CGN, chronic glomerulonephritis; DGI, disseminated gonococcal infection; HSP, Henoch-Schönlein purpura; ITP, idiopathic thrombocytopenia purpura; MPGN, membranoproliferative glomerulonephritis; SLE, systemic lupus erythematosus.

of the classic pathway to lyse antibody-coated red blood cells. This assay does not identify abnormalities in the alternative pathway, but with factor H and I deficiency, increased consumption of C3 is identified by a decrease in CH_{50}. The alternative pathway can be screened by use of a hemolytic assay in which rabbit erythrocytes serve as both the activating surface and the target. Measurements of C3 and C4 can help distinguish complement deficiencies. Although deficiency in several of the complement components results in an increased susceptibility to meningococcal disease, the routine screening of infected patients has a low yield. However, the incidence of complement deficiency in individuals with meningococcal disease caused by uncommon serogroups is significantly higher, warranting an evaluation of the complement cascade (terminal complement and properdin deficiency being most common). In hereditary angioneurotic edema, C4 levels are generally low, but C3 levels are normal. Low C3 and C4 levels are seen when the classic pathway is activated, whereas activation of the alternative pathway characteristically results in low C3 levels and normal C4 levels.

No specific therapy exists for any of the genetic disorders of complement. Replacement factors are not available. Some patients with angioedema respond to androgen therapy, especially in short-term use. For patients at increased risk for infection as a result of other deficiencies in the complement system, appropriate immunizations and aggressive management of infections are the bulwark of therapy.

PHAGOCYTE DISORDERS

Neutrophils are important in protecting the skin, mucous membrane, and the lining of the respiratory and gastrointestinal tracts. They form the first line of defense against microbial invasion. During the critical first 2 to 4 hours after tissue invasion by pathogenic organisms, the arrival of phagocytic cells at the site of infection is crucial for the containment of the infection, limiting the size of the local lesion, and preventing dissemination.

To arrive at the site of inflammation and be effective, phagocytic cells must attach (adhere) to the vascular endothelium near the site of invasion or inflammation. Once attached to the endothelium, they pass through the vessel wall (diapedesis), move in a unidirectional manner toward the site of inflammation (chemotaxis), adhere to and ingest the offending organisms (phagocytosis), and activate biochemical pathways important in intracellular microbial killing (degranulation and oxidative metabolism). Microbial killing is accomplished by two mechanisms: (1) respiratory burst and (2) degranulation. The respiratory burst consists of the de novo synthesis of highly toxic and often unstable derivatives of molecular oxygen (respiratory burst oxidase). Degranulation is the process by which lysosomal granules, containing preformed polypeptide antibiotics and proteases, fuse with the phagocytic vacuoles containing the ingested microbes.

Patients whose neutrophils have defects in adhesion or cell motility generally have cutaneous abscesses with common pathogens such as *Staphylococcus aureus* or have mucous membrane lesions caused by agents such as *Candida albicans* or oral anaerobic bacterial flora. Individuals with defects in the interferon γ–interleukin-12 axis are more susceptible to infections with atypical mycobacteria. If the defect in adhesion and chemotaxis is profound, lesions may contain few, if any, neutrophils. Disorders of phagocyte microbicidal activity (chronic granulomatous disease) are associated with cutaneous abscesses, lymphadenitis, pulmonary infections, and gastrointestinal problems, such as antral obstruction. Affected patients tend to have more deep-seated and chronic infections involving the liver and lung (Table 51-10).

DISORDERS OF MACROPHAGE FUNCTION

DEFECTS IN THE INTERFERON γ–INTERLEUKIN-12 AXIS

The interferon γ–interleukin-12 axis is crucial to host defense against intracellular pathogens, including *Mycobacteria, Listeria,* and *Salmonella* organisms. Dendritic cells and macrophages produce interleukin-12 in response to bacterial pathogens (see Table 51-10). Various defects with this axis have been described with both autosomal dominant and recessive inheritance patterns. Interleukin-12, in turn, stimulates the secretion of interferon γ by T cells and natural killer cells. Interferon α release binds to macrophage stimulating the production of tumor necrosis factor α and augmenting the respiratory burst that promotes bacterial killing.

The classic members of this group of disorders involve mutations in the interferon γ receptor, the signaling chain of the interferon γ receptor, the interleukin-12 receptor, or interleukin-12 itself. The interferon-γ receptor contains two chains (ligand-binding and signaling). Complete absence of either chain causes the most severe disease, manifesting early in infancy, often with disseminated atypical mycobacterial infection, recurrent *Salmonella* infection, or fatal infection after bacille Calmette-Guérin vaccination. Partial receptor chain loss causes milder disease, often in early childhood, but nonetheless with increased susceptibility to nontuberculous mycobacterial disease. Deficiencies in the production of interferon γ have been described, as have defects in interleukin-12 production and in the interleukin-12 receptor expression. Many affected patients have increased susceptibility to nontuberculous mycobacteria but show some response to treatment with interferon γ.

DISORDERS OF NEUTROPHIL NUMBERS

CYCLIC NEUTROPENIA

Cyclic neutropenia is an autosomal dominant disorder characterized by periodic episodes of profound neutropenia (absolute neutrophil counts <200 cells/cm^3), generally lasting 3 to 6 days and occurring in 21-day cycles (see Table 51-10). During the episodes of neutropenia, individuals develop aphthous ulcers, gingivitis, stomatitis, and cellulitis. Death from overwhelming infection with *Clostridium perfringens* occurs in about 10% of patients. During periods of neutropenia, the bone marrow demonstrates arrest in granulocyte maturation at the myelocyte stage. Mutations in the neutrophil elastase 2 (hydrolytic enzyme involved in bacterial killing) gene (ELA2) have been identified.

SEVERE CONGENITAL NEUTROPENIA

Severe congenital neutropenia is an autosomal recessive disorder characterized by severe persistent neutropenia (absolute neutrophil count <500 cells/cm^3) and recurrent bacterial infections (see Table 51-10). Affected patients often have increased plasma concentrations of granulocyte colony–stimulating factor (G-CSF) as well as circulating eosinophils and monocytes. Their bone marrow demonstrates failure of myeloid cell maturation from promyelocytes to myelocytes. Approximately 90% of these patients have mutations in the neutrophil elastase gene (see previous section on cyclic neutropenia). Three-dimensional molecular modeling suggests that most, if not all, of the mutations associated with cyclic neutropenia occur near the active site of the elastase gene and binding pocket for the enzyme's natural inhibitors. In contrast, the mutations responsible for severe congenital neutropenia would be predicted to alter molecular folding. These abnormalities potentially affect the storage of neutrophil elastase in primary granules of the neutrophil and may contribute to accelerated apoptosis of myeloid precursors found in the bone marrow of both groups of patients.

SHWACHMAN-DIAMOND SYNDROME

Shwachman-Diamond syndrome is a rare autosomal recessive disorder characterized by exocrine pancreatic insufficiency, skeletal abnormalities, bone marrow dysfunction, and recurrent infections (see Table 51-10). Neutropenia develops in all affected patients (cyclic or recurrent); pancytopenia develops in 10% to 25%.

GLYCOGEN STORAGE DISEASE TYPE 1B

Hypoglycemia, hepatosplenomegaly, and failure to thrive in infants characterize this autosomal recessive disorder (see Table 51-10). Neutropenia is a hallmark of this disorder. The marrow appears normal despite a severe reduction of blood neutrophils. The genetic defect maps to chromosome 11q23 and is attributed to an intracellular transport protein defect for glucose-6-phosphatase translocase, which shuttles glucose-6-phosphate from the cytoplasm to the endoplasmic reticulum.

DYSKERATOSIS CONGENITA

This disorder may be inherited both in an X-linked manner and in an autosomal dominant and recessive manner (see Table 51-10). It is associated with epiphora, learning disorders, pulmonary disease, hyperhidrosis, dental caries, short stature, and the development of pancytopenia. The gene for the X-linked form is located at q28 and encodes for dyskerin, a multifunctional protein possibly involved in ribosomal RNA biosynthesis, ribosomal subunit assembly, and the telomerase complex. The disorder arises from defective telomerase maintenance.

CHRONIC IDIOPATHIC NEUTROPENIA

Several disorders, some congenital, others acquired, cause selective neutropenia in both children and adults (see Table 51-10). Patients with chronic idiopathic neutropenia have normal and near normal erythrocyte, reticulocyte, lymphocyte, and platelet counts and normal or increased blood monocyte counts and immunoglobulin levels. Marrow examinations show a spectrum of abnormalities, from normal cellularity to selective hypoplasia of the neutrophilic series. The clinical course of the individual patient often correlates with the extent of neutropenia. In general, patients with the lowest levels of blood neutrophils and the fewest neutrophil precursors in the bone marrow have the most frequent problems.

TREATMENT OF CONGENITAL NEUTROPENIAS

The mainstay of treatment of all congenital neutropenias is recombinant human granulocyte colony–stimulating factor (rhG-CSF). Approximately 10% of patients with the diagnosis of severe congenital neutropenia and Shwachman-Diamond syndrome develop myelodysplasia/acute myelogenous leukemia. These two disorders constitute a preleukemia syndrome; malignant transformation was seen before the availability of rhG-CSF. It may be that the use of rhG-CSF permits patients to live longer and thereby facilitates the risk for malignant transformation. No cases of malignant transformations have been observed in patients with either cyclic or idiopathic neutropenia.

DISORDERS OF NEUTROPHIL ADHESION

CONGENITAL LEUKOCYTE ADHESION DEFICIENCY

Leukocyte adhesion deficiency is a group of disorders of leukocyte function that is characterized by recurrent soft tissue infections, delayed wound healing, and severely impaired pus formation. Leukocyte adhesion deficiency type 1 is a rare autosomal recessive

Table 51-10. Phagocyte Dysfunction

Disorder	Cause	Impaired Function	Clinical Consequence
Severe Neutropenia Disorders			
Cyclic neutropenia	Mutations in ELA2, encoding neutrophil elastase on chromosome 19p13.3	21-Day oscillations in neutrophil and monocyte counts	Recurrent pyogenic infections during neutropenia intervals; recurrent fevers; chronic gingivitis
Severe congenital neutropenia	Mutation in ELA2 encoding neutrophil elastase on chromosome 19p13.3	Developmental arrest of bone marrow myeloid cells at the promyelocyte stage	Recurrent pyogenic infection; chronic gingivitis; risk for developing MDS/AML
Shwachman-Diamond syndrome	Mutation at 7q11. Protein function unknown	Bone marrow stem cell defect associated with impaired neutrophil production	Intermittent neutropenia that may progress to aplastic anemia or MDS/AML
		Associated with pancreatic exocrine insufficiency and skeletal abnormalities	
Glycogen storage disease type 1B	Autosomal recessive; gene maps to 11q23, leading to intracellular transport protein defect for glucose	Impaired production of neutrophils as well as chemotactic defect; hypoglycemia	Recurrent pyogenic infection; gingivitis
Dyskeratosis congenita	Inherited either as X-linked (common) or as autosomal dominant or recessive Defect for X-linked inheritance maps to Xq28	Impaired neutrophil production associated with epiphora, pulmonary infections, hyperhidrosis, dental caries, and short stature	Recurrent pyogenic infections; may progress to pancytopenia
Cartilage-hair hypoplasia (short-limbed dwarfism)	Autosomal recessive	Impaired production of neutrophils; depressed cellular immunity associated with short limbs, thin hair	Recurrent pyogenic and viral infections
Chronic idiopathic neutropenia	Variable causes	Impaired production of neutrophils	Gingivitis, recurrent pyogenic infections
Degranulation Abnormalities			
Chédiak-Higashi syndrome	Autosomal recessive; disordered coalescence of lysosomal granules Gene found at 1q42-45; the encoded protein has structural features homologous to those of a vesicular sorting protein	Decreased neutrophil chemotaxis, degranulation and bactericidal activity; platelet storage pool defect; impaired NK function, failure to disperse melanosomes	Neutropenia; recurrent pyogenic infections, propensity to develop marked hepatosplenomegaly in the accelerated phase; pigment dilution in skin and fundus
Specific granule deficiency	Autosomal recessive; abnormal regulation of various myeloid granule genes by a mutation in transacting factor, CCAAP/enhances binding protein epsilon	Impaired chemotaxis and bactericidal activity; bilobed nuclei in neutrophils; reduced content of neutrophil defensins, gelatinase, collagenase, vitamin B$_{12}$-binding protein, lactoferrin	Recurrent deep-seated abscesses
Adhesion Abnormalities			
Leukocyte adhesion deficiency	Autosomal recessive; absence of CD11/CD18 surface adhesive glycoprotein (β$_2$ integrins) on leukocyte membranes most commonly arising from failure to express CD18 messenger RNA	Decreased binding of C3bi to neutrophils and impaired adhesion to ICAM1 and ICAM2	Neutrophilia; recurrent bacterial infection associated with absence of pus formation
Leukocyte adhesion deficiency type 2	Autosomal recessive; absence of neutrophil sialyl-Lewis X	Decreased adhesion to activated endothelium expressing ELAM	Neutrophilia; recurrent bacterial infections without pus
Neutrophil actin dysfunction	Altered polymerization of neutrophil cytoplasmic actin; perhaps arising from the presence of an inhibitor to F-actin formation	Impaired neutrophil adhesion, chemotaxis, and bacterial killing	Neutrophilia; recurrent bacterial infections without pus
Disorders of Cell Motility			
Enhanced Motile Responses			
Familial Mediterranean fever	Autosomal recessive gene on chromosome 16 that encodes for a protein called *pyrin*; pyrin may modify neutrophil activation	Excessive accumulation of neutrophils at inflamed sites that may be the result of the neutrophil response to chemokines generated by dysregulated monocytes	Recurrent fever, peritonitis, pleuritis, arthritis, and amyloidosis

Condition	Mechanism	Cellular defect	Infections
Depressed Motile Responses			
Defects in the generation of chemotactic signals	IgG deficiencies; C3 and properdin deficiency can arise from genetic or acquired abnormalities; mannose binding protein deficiency predominantly in neonates	Deficiency of serum chemotaxis and opsonic activities	Recurrent pyogenic infections
Intrinsic defects of the neutrophil (e.g., leukocyte adhesion deficiency, Chédiak-Higashi syndrome, specific granule deficiency, neutrophil actin dysfunction, neonatal neutrophils)	In the neonatal neutrophil, there is diminished ability to express β_2-integrins and there is a qualitative impairment in β_2-integrin function	Diminished chemotaxis	Propensity to develop pyogenic infections
Direct inhibition of neutrophil mobility (e.g., drugs)	Ethanol, glucocorticoids, cyclic AMP	Impaired locomotion and ingestion; Impaired adherence	Possible cause of frequent infections; neutrophilia seen with epinephrine is the result of cyclic AMP release from endothelium
Immune complexes	Bind to crystallized fragment receptors on neutrophils in patients with rheumatoid arthritis, systemic lupus erythematosus, other inflammatory states	Impaired chemotaxis	Recurrent pyogenic infections
Hyperimmunoglobulin E syndrome	Autosomal dominant; variable expression of a soluble inhibitor from mononuclear cells affecting neutrophil chemotaxis; high levels of antistaphylococcal IgE	Impaired chemotaxis at times; impaired IgG opsonization of *Staphylococcus aureus*	Recurrent skin and sinopulmonary infections
Defects of Microbicidal Activity			
Chronic granulomatous disease (CGD)	X-linked and autosomal recessive; failure to express functional gp91phox in the phagocyte membrane in p22phox (autosomal recessive) Other autosomal recessive forms of CGD arise from failure to express protein p47phox or p67phox	Failure to activate neutrophil respiratory burst; failure to failure to kill catalase-positive microbes	Recurrent pyogenic infections with catalase-positive microorganisms
G6PD deficiency	Less than 5% of normal activity of G6PD	Failure to activate NADPH-dependent oxidase	Infections with catalase positive microorganisms
Myeloperoxidase deficiency	Autosomal recessive; failure to process modified precursor protein arising from missense mutation	H_2O_2-dependent antimicrobial activity not potentiated by myeloperoxidase	None
Rac-2 deficiency	Autosomal dominant; dominant negative inhibitor by mutant protein of Rac-2–mediated functions	Absent receptor mediated O_2 generation and chemotaxis; Impaired neutrophil rolling on endothelium	Neutrophilia; recurrent bacterial infections
Deficiencies of glutathione reductase and glutathione synthetase	Failure to detoxify H_2O_2	Excessive formation of H_2O_2	Minimal problems with recurrent pyogenic infections
Impaired Macrophage Function			
Defects in the interferon γ–interleukin-12 axis	Interferon γ receptor ligand–binding chain, interferon γ receptor–signaling chain, interleukin-12 receptor β_1 chain, interleukin-12p40 deficiency The interferon γ receptor abnormalities may be inherited in an autosomal dominant or recessive manner.	Impaired killing of microorganisms; fatal BCG infection secondary to inability to either produce interleukin-12 by dendritic cells and macrophages, which is necessary to induce secretion of interferon γ by T cells and NK cells or secondary to depressed bactericidal activity of macrophages lacking normal function of interferon γ receptor	Infection with atypical mycobacteria, *Salmonella* organisms, and *Listeria* organisms
Impaired Spleen Function			
Splenic absence or dysfunction	Congenital absence of spleen, removal of spleen, vascular occlusion of spleen	Removal or impaired function of splenic macrophages	Propensity for infection with encapsulated bacteria

Modified from Boxer LA: Quantitative abnormalities of granulocytes. In Beutler E, Lichtman MA, Coller, BS, et al (eds): Williams Hematology, 6th ed. New York, McGraw-Hill, 2001, p 836.

AML, acute myelogenous leukemia; AMP, adenosine monophosphate; BCG, bacille Calmette-Guérin; ELA2, neutrophil elastase 2 gene; ELAM, expression of leukocyte adhesion molecule 1; G6PD, glucose-6-phosphate dehydrogenase; H_2O_2, hydrogen peroxide; IgE and IgG, immunoglobulins E and G; MDS, myelodysplasia; NADPH, nicotinamide adenine dinucleotide phosphate; NK, natural killer.

disorder characterized by marked neutrophilia even in the absence of a specific infection (ranging from 15 to 60×10^9 cells/L). Patients have a decreased or no expression of a family of leukocyte surface glycoproteins, designated CD11/CD18 complex (also referred to as the β_2 integrin family of leukocyte adhesive proteins) (see Table 51-10). These proteins include LFA-1 (CD11a/CD18), Mac-1 (CD11b/CD18), and P150,95 (CD11c/CD18), expressed on lymphocytes, monocytes/macrophages, and neutrophils, respectively. Diminished or absent surface expression of these proteins accounts for a profound impairment of neutrophil and monocyte adhesion-dependent functions in vitro, including cell migration and complement-mediated phagocytosis. Activated neutrophils of patients with the most severe clinical form of leukocyte adhesion deficiency express fewer than 0.3% of the normal amount of the β_2 integrins, whereas those of the patients with the moderate phenotype may express 2% to 7% of normal numbers of β_2 integrin molecules.

Leukocyte adhesion deficiency type 2 manifests with growth retardation, dysmorphic features, and neurologic deficits in association with an increased susceptibility to infection, because the neutrophils are unable to emigrate into tissues. Affected patients have an apparent defect in the generation of transport in guanosine diphosphate L-fructose, resulting in defective fucosylation of L-selectin and neutrophils, which leads to impaired neutrophil rolling on endothelial cells.

Rac-2 is the predominant GTPase in human neutrophils, and it is integral to the function of the actin cytoskeleton. Deficiency in Rac-2 is associated with decreased neutrophil chemotaxis, superoxide generation, and decreased degranulation in response to formyl peptides.

DISORDERS OF NEUTROPHIL MOTILITY

Depressed neutrophil chemotaxis has been observed in a wide variety of clinical conditions (see Table 51-10). Patients with chemotactic disorders may be infected by various microorganisms, including fungi as well as gram-positive or gram-negative bacteria. *S. aureus* is the most common pathogen. The skin, gingival mucosa, and regional lymph nodes are typically involved. Respiratory tract infections are common; sepsis is rare. Delayed or inappropriate signs and symptoms of inflammation are common. With mild chemotactic disorders, the cells can be demonstrated to move slowly in chemotactic assays; they accumulate in sufficient numbers to produce pus. Patients with neutrophils that have profound defects in chemotaxis are usually identified through other phagocytic assays, such as monitoring of adhesion and phagocytosis.

HYPERIMMUNOGLOBULIN E SYNDROME

The hyperimmunoglobulin E (Job) syndrome is characterized by markedly elevated levels of serum IgE, chronic dermatitis, and serious recurrent bacterial infections (see Table 51-10). The skin infections are remarkable for their absence of surrounding erythema, leading to the formation of "cold abscesses." Neutrophils and monocytes from patients with this syndrome exhibit a variable but at times profound chemotactic defect that appears extrinsic to the neutrophil. Clinical manifestations of hyperimmunoglobulin E begin as early as 1 to 8 weeks of age. Hyperimmunoglobulin E syndrome is characterized by a chronic eczematoid rash. The rash is typically papular and pruritic, involving the face and extensor surfaces of arms and legs. Skin lesions frequently are sharply demarcated and usually lack surrounding erythema. By 5 years of age, all patients have had a history of recurrent skin abscesses and recurrent pneumonias with pneumatoceles, along with chronic otitis media and sinusitis. Patients may also develop septic arthritis, cellulitis, or osteomyelitis. The major pathogen is *S. aureus.* Other associated features include coarse facial features, manifested by a broad nasal bridge, prominent

nose, dental abnormalities, and irregular proportional cheeks and jaw. Growth retardation is found in a small number of affected patients and appears to be related to the presence of chronic illness.

Serum IgE levels exceed 2500 IU/mL. Unlike atopic patients, who rarely have similar elevated IgE levels, patients with hyperimmunoglobulin E syndrome have immediate-type hypersensitivity to *S. aureus* and *C. albicans,* depressed antibody response to diphtheria and tetanus vaccine, and decreased lymphocyte proliferative response to *C. albicans.* Usually, patients with hyperimmunoglobulin E syndrome have normal concentrations of IgG, IgA, and IgM but elevated blood and sputum eosinophil counts. They also exhibit increased osteoclastic activity by monocytes, which results in osteoporosis and an increased incidence of fractures. The molecular basis is unknown. There is growing evidence that a defective interferon γ–interleukin 12 pathway leads to the preferential activation of T helper 2 cells and increased IgE synthesis. In addition, a predisposition to bacterial infections may arise from production of a chemotactic inhibitor, released by mononuclear cells, that inhibits normal neutrophil and monocyte chemotaxis. Treatment is supportive.

DISORDERS OF DEGRANULATION

CHÉDIAK-HIGASHI SYNDROME

Chédiak-Higashi syndrome is a rare autosomal recessive disorder that is characterized by partial ocular cutaneous albinism, neutropenia, and morphologic disorder in which all leukocytes contain giant cytoplasmic granules (see Table 51-10). Chédiak-Higashi syndrome affects all granule-bearing cells. Giant azurophil and specific granules are found in circulating neutrophils. Many of the abnormal myeloid precursors die in the marrow, which results in a moderate neutropenia with white cell counts of about 2.5×10^9 cells/L. Despite normal ingestion of particles and active oxygen metabolism, these neutrophils kill microorganisms slowly. This delay reflects a slow but inconsistent delivery of dilute amounts of hydrolytic enzymes from the giant granules into the phagosomes. Monocytes from patients with Chédiak-Higashi syndrome have the same functional derangements. Recurrent infections affect the skin, respiratory tract, and mucous membranes and are caused by both gram-positive and gram-negative bacteria as well as by fungi; *S. aureus* is the most common organism. Natural killer function also is impaired. Despite normal platelet counts, patients with Chédiak-Higashi syndrome have prolonged bleeding times, which is related to a platelet storage pool abnormality. Neuropathy, which can be sensory or motor, may be present; ataxia may be a prominent feature.

A propensity for lymphohistiocytic proliferation, known as the *accelerated phase,* occurs in the reticuloendothelial systems of patients with Chédiak-Higashi syndrome, which intensifies the already existing neutropenia and leads to pancytopenia. This proliferation is associated with recurrent bacterial and viral infections and fever and usually results in death. The onset of the accelerated phase may be related to the inability to contain and control the EBV infection and leads to features that simulate viral-mediated hemophagocytic syndrome. Treatment of the accelerated phase requires bone marrow transplantation.

SPECIFIC GRANULE DEFICIENCY

Specific granule deficiency is a rare disorder that affects both sexes and is probably inherited as an autosomal recessive disease (see Table 51-10). Clinically, patients with this disorder have recurrent infections involving the skin and lungs. *S. aureus* is the most common pathogen, although *C. albicans* and a variety of gram-negative bacteria have also been isolated. Specific granule–deficient neutrophils lack proteolytic activity in the tertiary granules, vitamin B_{12}–binding protein, lactoferrin, and collagenase in the specific granules and lack the bactericidal proteins known as defensins in the primary granules. Neutrophils from affected patients have abnormal chemotaxis and a mild defect in bactericidal activity.

The diagnosis of specific granule deficiency is suggested by the presence of neutrophils that are devoid of specific granules but contain azurophilic granules on the blood smear. The diagnosis can be confirmed by demonstration of a severe deficiency in either lactoferrin or vitamin B_{12}–binding proteins by immunoperoxidase staining or by quantitation of the proteins. The nuclei of the neutrophils are also bilobed. An acquired form of specific granule deficiency can be observed in burned patients or in individuals with myelodysplasia. Treatment is supportive.

DISORDERS OF NEUTROPHIL OXIDATIVE METABOLISM

CHRONIC GRANULOMATOUS DISEASE

Chronic granulomatous disease (CGD) is a rare disease with an incidence of approximately 4 per 1 million. In CGD, phagocytosis by neutrophils and monocytes is normal; however, their ability to kill catalase-positive microorganisms is severely depressed or absent because of a defect in the generation of antimicrobial oxygen metabolites (see Table 51-10). CGD is caused by mutations involving one of several genes that encode a component of nicotinamide adenine dinucleotide phosphate (NADPH) oxidase.

Several laboratory tests are used to classify the forms of CGD. The initial diagnosis is usually made through the nitroblue tetrazolium dye test, in which the yellow water-soluble tetrazolium dye is not reduced to a blue and soluble formazan pigment because of the failure of the CGD neutrophil to generate superoxide anion.

The inability of phagocytes to generate superoxide anion is caused by the absence of one of the components of the NADPH oxidase system. Approximately 65% of affected children lack the membrane-bound component of the oxidase cytochrome b_{558}. The gene for this protein is located on the X chromosome. Not surprisingly, the family histories of children with the X-linked variety of CGD often include male maternal relatives who died of infections at a young age. Virtually all other patients with CGD lack one of the two identified cytosolic factors, either a 47-kD protein or a 67-kD protein. These deficiencies are inherited in an autosomal recessive manner.

Although the clinical manifestation is variable, several clinical features suggest the diagnosis of CGD (Tables 51-11 and 51-12). Any patient with recurrent lymphadenitis should be considered to have CGD. Patients with bacterial hepatic abscesses, osteomyelitis at multiple sites or in the small bones of the hands and feet, a family history of recurrent infections, or unusual catalase-positive microbial infections require evaluation. The onset of clinical signs and symptoms may occur from early infancy to young adulthood, and the attack rate and severity of infections are variable. The most common pathogen is *S. aureus*. Infection with *S. marcescens, B. cepacia, Aspergillus* species, *C. albicans,* or *Salmonella* species occurs frequently. Pneumonia, lymphadenitis, and skin infections are the most common infections encountered. Infections are characterized by microabscesses and granuloma formation. Patients may develop the sequelae of chronic infection, including anemia of chronic disease, lymphadenopathy, hepatosplenomegaly, hypergammaglobulinemia, chronic purulent dermatitis, restrictive lung disease, gingivitis, hydronephrosis, and gastrointestinal narrowing (see Table 51-12).

Treatment includes bactericidal antibiotics and drainage for infections or abscesses, prophylactic trimethoprim-sulfamethoxazole, and long-term continuous interferon γ therapy. Steroids and antibiotics are used to treat granulomatous obstructing lesions of the gastrointestinal or urinary tract.

Table 51-11. Clinical Sites of Infection in Chronic Granulomatous Disease*

Disorder	Percentage of Affected Patients with Disorder
Pneumonia	77%
Dermatitis	68%
Lymphadenitis	60%
Hepatic abscess	39%
Osteomyelitis	32%
Persistent diarrhea	18%
Septicemia	17%
Perirectal abscess	14%
Urinary tract infection	~10%
Gastric antrum narrowing	Rare
Pericarditis	Rare
Meningitis	Rare

Based on data from Forrest CB, Forehand JR, Axtell RA, et al: Clinical features and current management of chronic granulomatous disease. Hematol Oncol Clin North Am 1988;2:2.

*The incidence of this disease is 4:1,000,000.

Glucose-6-phosphate dehydrogenase (G6PD) deficiency can accentuate the clinical spectrum in CGD. Leukocytes from patients with CGD have normal G6PD activity. However, a few individuals with apparent CGD whose neutrophils demonstrate markedly diminished (<5%) or no G6PD activity have been described. These patients also have the hemolytic anemia classically associated with G6PD deficiency. Neutrophils in severe G6PD deficiency progressively develop an attenuated respiratory burst as a result of the depletion of intracellular NADPH, the primary substrate for the respiratory burst to oxidase.

Table 51-12. Chronic Conditions Associated with Chronic Granulomatous Disease In Order of Frequency

Lymphadenopathy
Hepatomegaly
Splenomegaly
Hypergammaglobulinemia
Anemia of chronic disease
Underweight
Chronic diarrhea
Short Stature
Gingivitis
Dermatitis
Pulmonary fibrosis
Ulcerative stomatitis
Gastric antral narrowing
Granulomatosis ileocolitis
Chorioretinitis
Urinary outlet obstruction
Lupus syndromes
Idiopathic thrombocytopenia purpura
Behçet syndrome
Glomerulonephritis

From Boxer LA: Management: White cell disorders. In Furie B, Atkins MB, Mayer RJ, Cassileth PA (eds): Clinical Practice of Hematology and Oncology: Presentation, Diagnosis, and Treatment. Philadelphia, Elsevier, 2003.

MYELOPEROXIDASE DEFICIENCY

Myeloperoxidase deficiency is the most common hereditary disorder of neutrophil function; its incidence is 1 per 2000. Myeloperoxidase is an enzyme that catalyses the production of intraphagosomal hypochlorous acid; myeloperoxidase deficiency causes a diminished rate of microbial killing in neutrophils after ingestion (see Table 51-10). Although killing of the bacteria is slower than normal, eventually effective killing of bacteria occurs. Most patients with this genetic disorder are not at increased risk of developing pyogenic infections and require no therapy. However, a few patients with concurrent diabetes mellitus and myeloperoxidase deficiency have developed severe infection with *C. albicans.*

ASPLENIA

The spleen plays a particularly important role in attenuating infection, especially during the first year of life before specific immunity to certain bacteria has developed. The spleen exclusively filters unopsonized bacteria, such as pneumococci and *H. influenzae.* Bacterial clearance is rapidly followed by the development of some humoral immunity, which may be detectable within days after exposure. In addition to its function of removing microbes, the spleen also produces antibodies. Individuals without spleens (anatomic or functional) are subject to a severe form of sepsis that is rapid in onset and can lead to sudden death if it is not recognized and treated promptly (see Tables 51-1 and 51-10). Pneumococci are responsible for more than 50% of such infections; *H. influenzae, S. aureus,* group A streptococci, gram-negative enteric bacilli, and meningococci have also been identified (see Table 51-1).

The diagnosis of anatomic or functional asplenia is suggested by the presence of red blood cell inclusions, particularly Howell-Jolly bodies on peripheral blood smear. The diagnosis is confirmed when no spleen is noted on ultrasonography of the abdomen or by the failure of uptake of technetium 99–sulfur colloid, which is normally taken up by the entire reticuloendothelial system. Pitted or pocked erythrocytes are also noted in asplenic patients.

Functional asplenia occurs in children with sickle cell disease, initially as a result of vascular occlusion by the sickle cells in the splenic circulation. Congenital absence of the spleen may occur alone or as part of an *asplenia syndrome* with congenital heart disease (see Chapters 10 and 11). The usual presentation in the asplenia syndrome is that of a cyanotic newborn, often with respiratory distress and a midline liver. Clues to the presence of the asplenia syndrome are often found on the chest radiograph. This condition should be considered when the cardiac position is distorted with that of the stomach and liver, especially if pulmonary vascular markings are very diminished as a result of pulmonary atresia or if pulmonary edema secondary to obstructive pulmonary veins is present.

The risk of fulminant infection in patients who have undergone splenectomy (from surgery or trauma) or in those with functional asplenia or congenital asplenia is highest in the first few years. The risk is lower in older children and in adults, probably because they have developed opsonizing antibodies through previous exposure. The management of functional or anatomic asplenia lies mainly in prevention. When splenectomy becomes necessary, partial protection against life-threatening infections can be obtained by immunizing patients with conjugated and polyvalent pneumococcal, *H. influenzae* type b, and meningococcal vaccines. Booster immunization may be needed because of waning immunity with time. Prophylactic antibiotics may be given continuously in a single daily dose for 1 to 3 years or up to the age of 16 years (some authorities suggest longer periods or even for life) after splenectomy in children who are not old enough to complain of mild symptoms. Parents of older asplenic children are advised to have their children seen by a physician or to administer the antibiotics at the first sign of a febrile respiratory illness.

SUMMARY AND RED FLAGS

Recurrent benign infections are common, especially in large families or in day care settings, in which children may manifest 6 to 10 upper respiratory tract infections or gastroenteritis episodes a year. These infections usually last less than 1 week. The child continues to grow and develop normally, and his or her activities are not restricted.

Red flags include absent lymphoid tissue, failure to thrive, digital clubbing, chronic diarrhea, prolonged infections, infections with unusual organisms, repeated serious infections, eczematous dermatitis, a family history of early childhood deaths (presumably from infection), and other diseases associated with increased risks for infection (sickle cell anemia, malignancy, asplenia).

REFERENCES

Family History and Physical Examination

Stiehm ER: They're back: Recurrent infections in pediatric practice. Contemp Pediatr 1990;7:20.

Diagnostic Approach

Buckley RH: Primary immunodeficiency diseases due to defects in lymphocytes. N Engl J Med 2000;343:1313.
Conley ME, Stiehm ER: Immunodeficiency disorders: General consideration. In Stiehm ER (ed): Immunologic Disorders in Infants and Children, 4th ed. Philadelphia, WB Saunders, 1996, p 212.
Ochs HD, Smith CIE, Puck JM: Primary Immunodeficiency Diseases: A Molecular and Genetic Approach. New York, Oxford University Press, 1999.
Strober W, Eisenstein E, Jaffe JS, et al: Immunologic and genetic studies in common variable immunodeficiency. Ann Intern Med 1993;118:720.
Wengler GS, Allen RC, Parolini O, et al: Nonrandom X chromosome inactivation in natural killer cells from obligate carriers of X-linked severe combined immunodeficiency. J Immunol 1993;150:700.

Complement System Deficiency

Colten HR, Rosen FS: Complement deficiencies. Annu Rev Immunol 1992;10:809.
Frank MM: Complement deficiencies. Pediatr Clin North Am 2000;47:1339.
Puck JM: Primary immunodeficiency diseases. JAMA 1997;278:1835.
Ratnoff WD: Inherited deficiencies of complement in rheumatic diseases. Rheum Dis Clin North Am 1996;22:75.
Walport MJ: Inherited complement deficiency: Clues to the physiological activity of complement in vivo. Q J Med 1993;86:355.
Whaley K, Schwaeble W: Complement and complement deficiencies. Semin Liver Dis 1997;17:297.

Phagocyte Disorders

Boxer LA: Qualitative abnormalities of granulocytes. In Beutler E, Lichtman MA, Coller BS, et al (eds): Williams Hematology, 6th ed. New York, McGraw-Hill, 2001, p 835.
Lekstrom-Himes JA, Gallin JI: Immunodeficiency diseases caused by defects in phagocytes. N Engl J Med 2000;343:1703.

Neutropenia

Dale DC, Bonilla MA, Davis MW, et al: A randomized controlled phase III trial of recombinant human G-CSF for treatment of severe chronic neutropenia. Blood 1993;81:2496.
Dale DC, Person RE, Bolyard AA, et al: Mutations in the gene encoding neutrophil elastase in congenital and cyclic neutropenia. Blood 2000; 96:2317.

Chronic Granulomatous Disease

Forrest CB, Forehand JR, Axtell RA: Clinical features and current management of chronic granulomatous disease. Hematol Oncol Clin North Am 1998;2:253.
Johnston RB Jr: Clinical aspects of chronic granulomatous disease. Curr Opin Hematol 2001;8:17.

Winkelstein JA, Marino MP, Johnston RB Jr, et al: Chronic granulomatous disease. Report on a national registry of 368 patients. Medicine 2000;79:155.

Macrophage Dysfunction

Gately MK, Renzetti LM, Magram J, et al: The interleukin-12/interleukin-12-receptor system: Role in normal and pathologic immune responses. Annu Rev Immunol 1998;16:495.

Waghorn DJ: Overwhelming infection in asplenic patients: Current best practice preventive measures are not being followed. J Clin Pathol 2001; 54: 2214.

Leukocyte Adhesion Deficiency

Arnaout MA: Dynamics and regulation of leukocyte–endothelial cell interactions. Curr Opin Hematol 1993;1:113.

Fischer A, Lisowska-Grospierre B, Anderson DC, Springer TA: Leukocyte adhesion deficiency: Molecular basis and functional consequences. Immunodefic Rev 1988;1:39.

Chédiak-Higashi Syndrome

Boxer LA, Smolen JE: Neutrophil granule constituents and their release in health and disease. Hematol Oncol Clin North Am 1988;2:101.

Ganz T, Metcalf JA, Gallin JI, et al: Microbicidal/cytotoxic proteins of neutrophils are deficient in two disorders: Chédiak-Higashi syndrome and "specific" granule deficiency. J Clin Invest 1988;82:552.

Specific Granule Deficiency

Boxer LA, Coates TD, Haak RA, et al: Lactoferrin deficiency associated with altered granulocyte function. N Engl J Med 1982;307:404.

Johnston JJ, Boxer LA, Berliner N: Correlation of mRNA levels with protein defects in specific granule deficiency. Blood 1992;80:2088.

Disorders of Neutrophil Motility

Boxer LA, Allen JM, Baehner RL: Diminished polymorphonuclear leukocyte adherence: Function dependent on release of cyclic AMP by endothelial cells after stimulation of β-receptors by epinephrine. J Clin Invest 1980;66:268.

Weston BW, Axtell RA, Todd RF III, et al: Clinical and biologic effects of granulocyte-colony stimulating factor in the treatment of myelokathexis. J Pediatr 1991;188:229.

Hyperimmunoglobulin E Syndrome

Jeppson JD, Jaffe HS, Hill HR: Use of recombinant human interferon gamma to enhance neutrophil chemotactic responses in Job syndrome of hyperimmunoglobulin E and recurrent infections. J Pediatr 1991;3:383.

Leung DYM, Geha RS: Clinical and immunologic aspects of the hyperimmunoglobulin E syndrome. Hematol Oncol Clin North Am 1988;2:81.

Myeloperoxidase Deficiency

Nauseef WM: Myeloperoxidase deficiency. Hematol Pathol 1990;4:165.

Asplenia

Briden ML, Patullo AL: Prevention and management of overwhelming postsplenectomy infection—An update. Crit Care Med 1999;27:836.

Cesko I, Hajdu J, Toth T, et al: Ivemark syndrome with asplenia in siblings. J Pediatr 1997;130:822.

Gikonyo DK, Tandon R, Lucas RF Jr, et al: Scimitar syndrome in neonates: Report of four cases and review of the literature. Pediatr Cardiol 1986;6:193.

Reid M: Splenectomy, sepsis, immunisation and guidelines. Lancet 1994;344:970.

Rose V, Izukawa T, Moes CAF: Syndromes of asplenia and polysplenia: A review of cardiac and noncardiac malformation in 60 cases with special reference to diagnosis and prognosis. Br Heart J 1975;37:840.

Spelman D: Prevention of overwhelming sepsis in asplenic patients: Could do better. Lancet 2001;357:2002.

52 Meningismus and Meningitis

Peter L. Havens*

A stiff neck (nuchal rigidity) may have many causes (Table 52-1), but *meningitis* must always be considered. *Meningismus,* also called *meningism,* is not the same as stiff neck; it also includes other signs of meningeal irritation (headache, Kernig and Brudzinski signs) (Fig. 52-1). Patients with meningitis usually do not complain solely of a stiff neck; most have fever, alterations of consciousness, or seizures. Alternatively, most patients who have only a stiff neck do not have meningitis. In meningitis, the stiffness is caused by inflammation of the cervical dura and reflex spasm of the extensor muscles of the neck. Consequently, there is pain and limitation of motion on *flexion* of the neck. Lateral movement of the neck may be normal and pain-free. Meningeal irritation may also be found in other conditions (tumor, subarachnoid hemorrhage); however, when it is found, especially in the presence of fever, meningitis must be confirmed or excluded.

The child with a stiff neck may have torticollis, with the head drawn to one side and rotated and the chin pointing to the contralateral side. Spasm of the strap muscles of the neck may be found. Usually the neck can be flexed, but rotation or lateral movement is limited and causes pain. Torticollis is rarely a manifestation of meningitis (Table 52-2).

A child may present with a painful neck that is not stiff. In this instance, the neck can be moved, albeit with pain, in all directions. This finding is seen in children with a variety of disorders, including lymphadenitis, cervical spine injuries, and acute strains of the neck musculature.

The disease process causing a stiff neck may originate in any of the structures of the neck: cervical dura, muscles, ligaments, bones, fascia, lymph nodes, glands, or viscera. With this knowledge, a complete history can be documented, a physical examination and laboratory investigation performed, and an appropriate differential diagnosis formulated.

BACTERIAL MENINGITIS

CLINICAL PRESENTATION

Bacterial meningitis is usually a disease of infants and young children. The attack rate is highest between the ages of 3 and 8 months; 66% of cases occur in children younger than 5 years of age. Bacterial meningitis is seen during all seasons; however, there may be a seasonal correlation between the presence of preceding respiratory pathogens (viral, mycoplasmal) in the upper respiratory tract and the subsequent development of bacterial meningitis. Bacterial meningitis usually occurs sporadically. Clusters of cases have been noted in day care centers and other closed communities. Bacterial meningitis occurs more frequently in children with traumatic fractures of the cribriform plate or paranasal sinuses (pneumococci); in children who have undergone neurosurgical procedures (*Staphylococcus aureus, Staphylococcus epidermidis, Corynebacterium* species); in children

with congenital or acquired immunodeficiencies (pneumococci, *Listeria monocytogenes,* meningococci); in children with anatomic or functional asplenia (pneumococci, meningococci); and in children with sickle hemoglobinopathies (pneumococci). There may be a genetic predisposition in some groups to the development of meningitis, inasmuch as there is an increased incidence of *Haemophilus influenzae* type b meningitis in Navajo Indians and Eskimos.

Bacterial meningitis manifests in two patterns. In the first, the symptoms develop slowly over several days, the initial symptoms being those of gastroenteritis or an upper respiratory infection. The signs and symptoms of meningitis develop subsequently. In the second pattern, the disease develops suddenly and quickly, the first indications of illness being the signs and symptoms of sepsis syndrome and meningitis.

The manifestations of meningitis depend on the child's age. In infants, the findings are usually nonspecific and may be subtle; they include vomiting, diarrhea, irritability, lethargy, poor appetite, respiratory distress, seizures, hypothermia, and jaundice. Only 50% of affected infants have fever; some present only with fever. It is uncommon for affected young infants to have a stiff neck; only 30% have a bulging fontanelle.

Older children present with more specific meningeal signs. They complain of a headache that is described as being severe, generalized, deep-seated, and constant. They also complain of nausea, vomiting, anorexia, and photophobia. On examination, they demonstrate irritability, mental confusion or altered consciousness, nuchal rigidity, and, occasionally, hyperesthesia and ataxia.

The clinician demonstrates *nuchal rigidity* by feeling resistance and observing a painful response while flexing the patient's neck. The stiffness may not be recognized until the end of flexion. The neck usually can be rotated without symptoms. In the child who is crying and tensing the muscles, nuchal rigidity may be demonstrated if the examiner places one hand under the occiput of the supine patient and lifts the child. If the neck does not flex, it is stiff. Alternatively, a sitting child may be observed following an object as it falls to the floor. The child who flexes the neck to look at the object does not have nuchal rigidity. In the presence of meningitis, flexion of the neck causes spontaneous flexion of the legs at the hips and knees, the *Brudzinski sign* (see Fig. 52-1). The *Kernig sign* is elicited

Table 52-1. Differential Diagnosis of a Stiff Neck
Meningitis: bacterial, aseptic
Upper lobe pneumonia
Torticollis
Neck trauma (accidental, intentional, overuse)
Inflammatory: cervical spinal cord myelitis, atlantoaxial subluxation, demyelinating encephalomyelitis
Neck inflammation (lymphadenopathy, lymphadenitis, thyroiditis, deep neck cellulitis, jugular thrombophlebitis)
Retropharyngeal abscess, epiglottitis

*This chapter is an updated and edited version of the chapter by Jay H. Mayefsky that appeared in the first edition.

955

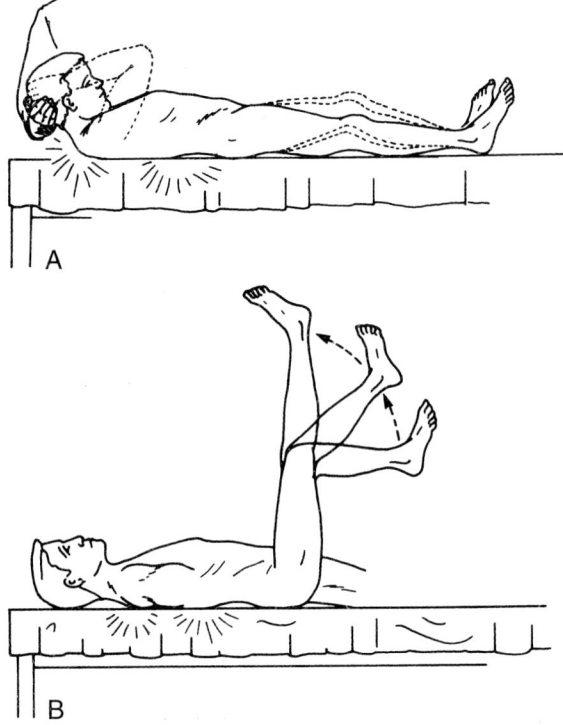

Figure 52-1. *A,* Brudzinski sign. The patient lies supine, and the head is passively elevated from the table by the examiner. The patient complains of neck and low back discomfort and attempts to relieve the meningeal irritation by involuntary flexion of the knees and hips. *B,* Kernig sign. The patient lies supine, with the hips and knees flexed. The knees are then gradually extended. Complaints of pain in the lower back, neck, and/or head are suggestive of meningeal irritation. (From Reilly BM: Practical Strategies in Outpatient Medicine, 2nd ed. Philadelphia, WB Saunders, 1991, p 95.)

Table 52-2. Differential Diagnosis of Torticollis
Congenital
Muscular torticollis
Positional deformation
Hemivertebra (cervicosuperior dorsal spine)
Unilateral atlantooccipital fusion
Klippel-Feil syndrome
Unilateral absence of sternocleidomastoid muscle
Pterygium colli
Trauma
Muscular injury (cervical muscles)
Atlantooccipital subluxation
Atlantoaxial subluxation
C2-C3 subluxation
Rotary subluxation
Fractures
Inflammation
Cervical lymphadenitis
Retropharyngeal abscess
Cervical vertebral osteomyelitis
Rheumatoid arthritis
Spontaneous (hyperemia, edema) subluxation with adjacent head and neck infection (rotary subluxation syndrome)
Upper lobe pneumonia
Neurologic
Visual disturbances (nystagmus, superior oblique paresis)
Dystonic drug reactions (phenothiazines, haloperidol, metoclopramide)
Cervical cord tumor
Posterior fossa brain tumor
Syringomyelia
Wilson disease
Dystonia musculorum deformans
Spasmus nutans
Other
Acute cervical disk calcification
Sandifer syndrome (gastroesophageal reflux, hiatal hernia)
Benign paroxysmal torticollis
Bone tumors (eosinophilic granuloma)
Soft-tissue tumor
Hysteria

From Behrman RE (ed): Nelson Textbook of Pediatrics, 16th ed. Philadelphia, WB Saunders, 2000, p 2090.

when the patient lies supine and, with the knee flexed, the leg is flexed at the hip. The knee is then extended. A positive sign is present if this movement is limited by contraction of the hamstrings and causes pain. Absence of nuchal rigidity is found in 1.5% of older children with meningitis; it may be absent in children who have overwhelming infections (meningococcemia), are deeply comatose, or who have focal or global neurologic impairment.

As many as 15% of children with bacterial meningitis initially present in a comatose or semicomatose state (see Chapter 40). Focal neurologic signs are found in 15% of children at some point during their illness. These signs include hemiparesis, quadriparesis, cranial nerve palsies, endophthalmitis, visual field defects, cortical blindness, ataxia, deafness, and vestibular nerve dysfunction. Because of the short duration and inconsistent development of increased intracranial pressure, papilledema is usually not seen at presentation. When it is present, venous sinus thrombosis, subdural effusion, or an intracranial abscess must be considered. Seizures occur before hospital admission in up to 20% of affected patients.

Children with meningitis may also present with cutaneous findings. Although commonly associated with meningococcal disease, purpura, petechiae, or a diffuse nonspecific maculopapular rash may be present in meningitis caused by any of the common bacterial pathogens. Meningitis has also been reported in 8% of toddlers with coincident buccal (facial) cellulitis and in 1% of children with periorbital cellulitis (10% if there is bacteremia). This creates a problem for the practitioner, who must decide whether to perform a lumbar puncture on a child with facial cellulitis. When the child is younger than 2 to 3 years of age, has meningeal signs, or appears severely ill or if *H. influenzae* type b infection is suspected, the child should be evaluated for meningitis.

Bacterial meningitis has been reported in children with septic arthritis. This has been assumed to be caused by simultaneous infection after a bacteremia. Reactive arthritis caused by immune complex deposition is also seen with bacterial meningitis. This arthritis affects one large joint and appears 5 to 7 days after treatment for meningitis has started. In general, arthritis occurring acutely with meningitis should be assumed to be infectious (see Chapter 44).

Various eye disorders have also been described with acute bacterial meningitis, including transient cataracts, paralysis of the extraocular muscles, pupillary dysfunction, dendritic ulcers, endophthalmitis, and conjunctivitis.

DIAGNOSTIC STUDIES

Lumbar Puncture and Cerebrospinal Fluid Analysis

The definitive diagnosis of meningitis is based on examination of the cerebrospinal fluid (CSF). The CSF is usually obtained via a lumbar puncture (spinal tap). The lumbar puncture is performed by introducing a small-bore, short-beveled, spinal needle with a stylet into

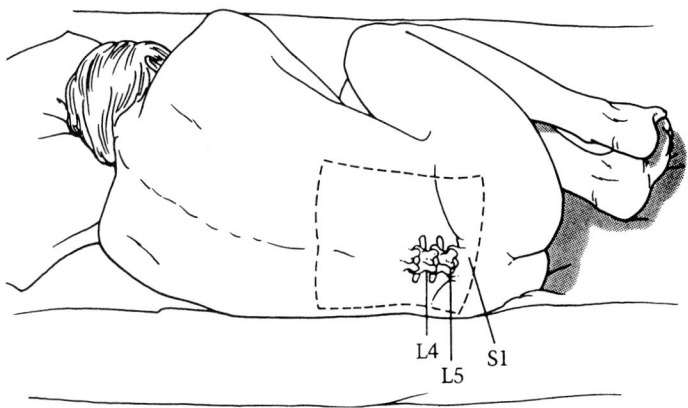

Figure 52-2. Lateral decubitus position for a lumbar puncture. L4-L5 position is determined by a vertical line drawn between the superior iliac crests. (From Davidson RI: Lumbar puncture. In Vander Salm TJ, Cutler BS, Wheeler HB [eds]: Atlas of Bedside Procedures, 2nd ed. Boston, Little, Brown, 1992, p 443.)

the subarachnoid space at the L3-L4 or L4-L5 level (Figs. 52-2 to 52-4). A needle with a stylet is used to minimize the risk of introducing a nest of epidermal cells into the subarachnoid space that may later grow into a cord-compressing epidermoid tumor. Approximately 3 mL of fluid is removed for analysis.

There are a few contraindications for the performance of a lumbar puncture. The first is cardiorespiratory compromise. Performance of the lumbar puncture requires that the child be held in flexion to open the intervertebral spaces. In seriously ill children or children with significant underlying cardiac or pulmonary disease, this positioning may be enough to cause respiratory compromise. The lumbar puncture may need to be postponed, be performed cautiously with continuous oxygen saturation monitoring, or performed with the patient in the sitting position.

Second, children with increased intracranial pressure from a focal central nervous system (CNS) lesion, such as brain abscess or tumor, or from illnesses associated with cerebral edema, such as Reye syndrome or severe herpes encephalitis, have a high risk of cerebral herniation after a lumbar puncture. Therefore, if signs or symptoms of increased intracranial pressure are present, the lumbar puncture should be postponed until the increased pressure is lowered with appropriate treatment (hyperventilation, mannitol). If a lumbar puncture is delayed, appropriate antibiotic therapy should be initiated without further delay. Signs of increased intracranial pressure include ptosis, anisocoria, sixth cranial nerve palsy, Cushing triad (hypertension, bradycardia, irregularities of respiration), and papilledema.

Third, a lumbar puncture should not be done if the spinal needle must pass through an area of infection on its way to the subarachnoid space. To do so might introduce pathogens into the CNS that could cause meningitis.

Epidural hematomas causing lower limb paralysis may be a complication of lumbar punctures in children with bleeding disorders. Therefore, in children with hemophilia, disseminated intravascular coagulopathy, or thrombocytopenia, lumbar puncture should be postponed until the bleeding disorder is corrected, and extra care should be taken to avoid a traumatic lumbar puncture. Such children should be monitored after the procedure for the development of neurologic deficits. Empirical therapy may be started while the coagulopathy is corrected.

Other, more rare complications of lumbar puncture include cortical blindness from compression of the posterior cerebral artery against the tentorium cerebelli, causing ischemic infarction of the occipital lobes. Cervical spinal cord infarction, with respiratory arrest and flaccid tetraplegia, may occur if intracranial hypertension causes herniation of the cerebellar tonsils through the foramen magnum with resulting compression of the anterior spinal artery or its penetrating branches. Post–lumbar puncture headache may occur in up to 10% of older children and adults; it is presumably caused by persistent CSF leakage at the lumbar puncture site.

The CSF is examined for red blood cells (RBCs), white blood cells (WBCs) and differential, glucose, protein, and the presence (by culture, by Gram stain or other stain, or by antigen or DNA testing for specific agents) of pathogenic organisms. Opening pressure measurements are obtained with the head of the bed flat and with the child relaxed and in the lateral decubitus position with the back no longer tightly flexed. Normal values in children and adults are less than 150 mm H_2O; values of 150 to 200 mm H_2O are questionably elevated; and an opening pressure higher than 200 mm H_2O is definitely abnormal. Opening pressure is less than 50 mm H_2O in premature infants and less than 100 mm H_2O in normal newborns. Opening pressure measurements are elevated if the lumbar puncture is performed with the patient in the sitting position and if the patient is combative or performing the Valsalva maneuver. Obstructive hydrocephalus, hyperventilation, or removal of fluid can all lead to lowering of the measurement. Children with bacterial meningitis usually have a mean opening pressure of 180 ± 70 mm H_2O.

Normal CSF is clear and colorless (Table 52-3). Blood in the CSF indicates a traumatic lumbar puncture or a CNS hemorrhage. Differentiation between the two can be achieved by centrifugation of the CSF sample. When blood has been present in the CSF for several hours, the CSF is xanthochromic after centrifugation. However, if the blood was recently mixed with CSF, as in the case of a traumatic tap, the supernatant is clear. Xanthochromic CSF can also be caused by icterus or an elevated CSF protein concentration. Obtaining a RBC count on tubes 1 and 3 may also differentiate the two conditions, because the count is unchanged in CNS hemorrhage but may decline in traumatic taps.

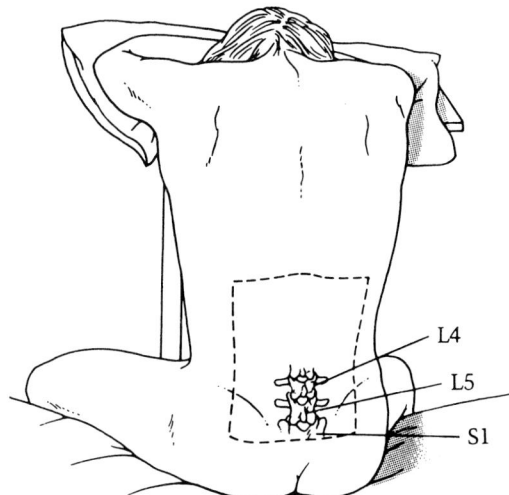

Figure 52-3. Sitting position for a lumbar puncture. (From Davidson RI: Lumbar puncture. In Vander Salm TJ, Cutler BS, Wheeler HB [eds]: Atlas of Bedside Procedures, 2nd ed. Boston, Little, Brown, 1992, p 443.)

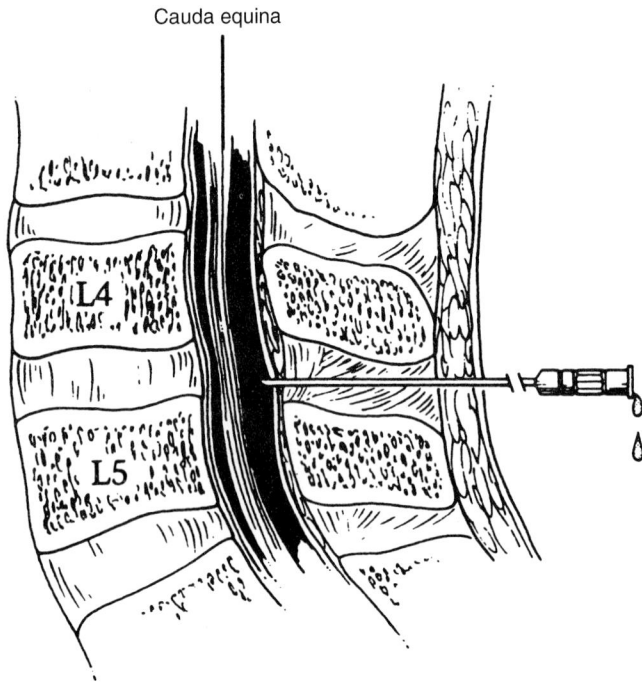

Cauda equina

Figure 52-4. The needle and stylet are advanced into the subarachnoid space. On penetration into the space, the examiner often feels a give or pop after moving through the dura. After the needle enters into the subarachnoid space, the clinician removes the stylet and collects the cerebrospinal fluid. (From Davidson RI: Lumbar puncture. In Vander Salm TJ, Cutler BS, Wheeler HB [eds]: Atlas of Bedside Procedures, 2nd ed. Boston, Little, Brown, 1992, p 447.)

The normal values for WBCs in the CSF are shown in Table 52-3. Most children with bacterial meningitis have a WBC count of at least 1000/mm³ in their CSF, but, in general, more than 6/mm³ in children after the neonatal period is considered abnormal. An absolute neutrophil count exceeding 3/mm³ (neutrophils may be as high as 35%) is also considered abnormal and evidence of a bacterial infection. Although there are case reports of children with proven (usually rapidly fulminant meningococcal) bacterial meningitis who do not have CSF pleocytosis, the CSF of 98% of children with meningitis has pleocytosis and more than 50% neutrophils. It takes at least 400 WBCs/mm³ to turn CSF turbid. Therefore, even though the CSF obtained may be clear to the naked eye, the sample must be examined under the microscope. Neonates may have 0 to 30 (mean, 9) WBCs in the CSF, with up to 60% polymorphonuclear neutrophils.

On occasion, the spinal needle is advanced too far and passes through the subarachnoid space and penetrates the richly vascularized ventral epidural space. Blood is thereby introduced into the subarachnoid space, and the CSF appears bloody. This occurrence is often called a *traumatic tap*. It is then difficult to know whether the WBCs seen on examination of the CSF are caused by CSF

Table 52-3. Cerebrospinal Fluid Findings in Central Nervous System Disorders

Condition	Pressure (mm H₂O)	Leukocytes (mm³)	Protein (mg/dL)	Glucose (mg/dL)	Comments
Normal	50-80	<5, ≥75% lymphocytes	20-45	>50 (or 75% serum glucose)	—
Common Forms of Meningitis					
Acute bacterial meningitis	Usually elevated (100-300)	100-10,000 or more; usually >1000; PMNs predominate	Usually 100-500	Decreased usually <40 (or <66% serum glucose)	Organisms usually seen on Gram stain and recovered by culture; latex agglutination of CSF usually positive
Partially treated bacterial meningitis	Normal or elevated	5-10,000; PMNs usual, but mononuclear cells may predominate if pretreated for extended period of time	Usually 100-500	Normal or decreased	Organisms may be seen on Gram stain; latex agglutination of CSF may be positive; pretreatment may render CSF sterile
Viral meningitis or meningoencephalitis	Normal or slightly elevated (80-150)	Rarely >1000 cells; Eastern equine encephalitis and lymphocytic choriomeningitis (LCM) may have cell counts of several thousand; PMNs early, but mononuclear cells predominate through most of the course	Usually 50-200	Generally normal; may be decreased to <40 in some viral diseases, particularly mumps (15%-20% of cases)	HSV encephalitis is suggested by focal seizures or by focal findings on CT or MRI scans or EEG; enteroviruses and HSV infrequently recovered from CSF; HSV and enteroviruses may be detected by PCR of CSF

Table 52-3. Cerebrospinal Fluid Findings in Central Nervous System Disorders—cont'd

Condition	Pressure (mm H₂O)	Leukocytes (mm³)	Protein (mg/dL)	Glucose (mg/dL)	Comments
Uncommon Forms of Meningitis					
Tuberculous meningitis	Usually elevated	10-500; PMNs early, but lymphocytes predominate through most of the course	100-3000 may be higher in presence of spinal block	<50 in most cases; decreases with time if treatment is not provided	Acid-fast organisms almost never seen on smear; organisms may be recovered in culture of large volumes of CSF; *Mycobacterium tuberculosis* may be detected by PCR of CSF
Fungal meningitis	Usually elevated	5-500; PMNs early, but mononuclear cells predominate through most of the course; cryptococcal meningitis may have no cellular inflammatory response	25-500	<50; decreases with time if treatment is not provided	Budding yeast may be seen; organisms may be recovered in culture; cryptococcal antigen (CSF and serum) may be positive in cryptococcal infection
Syphilis (acute) and leptospirosis	Usually elevated	50-500; lymphocytes predominate	50-200	Usually normal	Positive CSF serologic findings; spirochetes not demonstrable by usual techniques of smear or culture; darkfield examination may be positive
Amebic (*Naegleria*) meningoencephalitis	Elevated	1,000-10,000 or more; PMNs predominate	50-500	Normal or slightly decreased	Mobile amebae may be seen by hanging-drop examination of CSF at room temperature
Brain and Parameningeal Abscesses					
Brain abscess	Usually elevated (100-300)	5-200; CSF rarely acellular; lymphocytes predominate; if abscess ruptures into ventricle, PMNs predominate and cell count may reach >100,000	75-500	Normal unless abscess ruptures into ventricular system	No organisms on smear or culture unless abscess ruptures into ventricular system
Subdural empyema	Usually elevated (100-300)	100-5000; PMNs predominate	100-500	Normal	No organisms on smear or culture of CSF unless meningitis also present; organisms found on tap of subdural fluid
Cerebral epidural abscess	Normal to slightly elevated	10-500; lymphocytes predominate	50-200	Normal	No organisms on smear or culture of CSF
Spinal epidural abscess	Usually low, with spinal block	10-100; lymphocytes predominate	50-400	Normal	No organisms on smear or culture of CSF
Chemical (drugs, dermoid cysts, myelography dye)	Usually elevated	100-1000 or more; PMNs predominate	50-100	Normal or slightly decreased	Epithelial cells may be seen within CSF by use of polarized light in some children with dermoids
Noninfectious Causes					
Sarcoidosis	Normal or slightly elevated	0-100; mononuclear	40-100	Normal	No specific findings
Systemic lupus erythematosus with CNS involvement	Slightly elevated	0-500; PMNs usually predominate; lymphocytes may be present	100	Normal or slightly decreased	No organisms on smear or culture; LE preparation may be positive; positive neuronal and ribosomal P protein antibodies in CSF
Tumor, leukemia	Slightly elevated to very high	0-100 or more; mononuclear or blast cells	50-1,000	Normal to decreased (20-40)	Cytologic findings may be positive

Adapted from Behrman RE (ed): Nelson Textbook of Pediatrics, 16th ed. Philadelphia: WB Saunders, 2000, p 759.

CSF, cerebrospinal fluid; CT, computed tomography; EEG, electroencephalogram; HSV, herpes simplex virus; LE, lupus erythematosus cell; MRI, magnetic resonance imaging; PCR, polymerase chain reaction; PMN, polymorphonuclear neutrophil.

pleocytosis or are peripheral blood WBCs contaminating the CSF. To aid in this determination, the ratio of WBCs to RBCs in the CSF is compared with the ratio of WBCs to RBCs in the patient's peripheral blood. A higher ratio in the CSF indicates the presence of CSF pleocytosis. When the CSF ratio is at least 10 times higher than the blood ratio, bacterial meningitis is indicated, with a sensitivity of 88% and a specificity of 90%. Conversely, the negative predictive value for the presence of bacterial meningitis of a less than 10-fold difference between the ratios is 99%. Traumatic taps usually do not alter the CSF glucose, Gram stain, or culture findings, which are often abnormal with bacterial meningitis. When there is doubt about the validity of the cell count after a bloody tap, the lumbar puncture should be repeated after several hours by introducing the spinal needle one intervertebral space above the original tap site.

In normal CSF, the glucose concentration is two-thirds that of serum glucose concentration. The CSF glucose concentration is low in most infected infants and younger children and in 45% of school-aged children with bacterial meningitis. In children older than 2 months of age, a CSF/serum glucose ratio of less than 0.4 is 80% sensitive and 98% specific for the presence of bacterial meningitis. The presence of RBCs in a CSF sample that is promptly analyzed does not affect the glucose concentration.

The normal CSF protein concentration is less than 45 mg/dL in children older than 2 months. The mean CSF protein concentration is 90 (range, 20 to 170) in full-term infants and 115 (range, 65 to 150) in preterm infants.

The CSF protein concentration is elevated in more than 90% of younger children with bacterial meningitis but in only 60% of infected school-aged children. Every 1000 RBCs in the CSF (from a traumatic tap) increases the protein concentration by 1 mg/dL.

The presence of bacterial pathogens in the CSF should be investigated. Microscopic examination of a Gram-stained sample of the fluid is performed first. The sensitivity of this test is directly related to the number of organisms in the CSF and is inversely related to the age of the patient. The Gram stain identification of certain organisms, such as *H. influenzae,* may be problematic. A decision whether to treat a child for bacterial meningitis should not be based on the Gram stain alone; the definitive diagnosis is based on the CSF culture. Rapid diagnostic tests for bacterial antigens in CSF, including countercurrent immunoelectrophoresis and latex particle agglutination, suffer from variations in sensitivity and specificity that limit their value in clinical practice.

Some patients will have been treated with antibiotics before the lumbar puncture is performed. When the CSF from such a child is examined, organisms may not be seen on Gram stain or recovered on culture. However, abnormalities of CSF cell count, protein concentration, and glucose concentration usually continue to suggest the diagnosis of bacterial meningitis. In this setting, presumptive treatment for bacterial meningitis is initiated. If an organism is identified by culture or antigen detection, definitive antibiotic treatment is administered. If no organism is identified, the decision to continue treatment depends on the clinical suspicion of bacterial meningitis and the exclusion of other causes of aseptic meningitis (Tables 52-4 and 52-5).

Computed Tomography

Routine computed tomography (CT) of the head is not indicated in children with suspected meningitis. Even though most children with bacterial meningitis have increased intracranial pressure, most CT scans are normal. In addition, most lumbar punctures do not result in cerebral herniation in patients with meningitis. CT should be reserved for children who show *clinical signs* of herniation or cerebral edema and for those who may have an intracranial mass causing signs and symptoms similar to meningitis. In these children, a blood specimen should be obtained for culture, broad-spectrum parenteral antibiotics started, CT performed when the patient is stable, and a lumbar puncture performed subsequently when appropriate. Even in the management of the child with proven meningitis, CT is not routinely indicated because it seldom provides information that leads to a specific intervention and adds little to the prediction of long-term outcome. CT aids in the evaluation of focal neurologic signs, in children in whom a brain abscess or subdural empyema is suspected, and in patients in whom cerebral edema is suspected.

Other Laboratory Tests

Usually, the peripheral blood WBC and platelet counts are elevated with bacterial meningitis. A low WBC count and thrombocytopenia may also be seen; these are associated with overwhelming infection and a poor outcome. The sensitivity (70%), specificity (54%), and negative predictive value (81%) of the differential WBC count are too low to render the differential WBC examination useful in making the diagnosis of bacterial meningitis.

Blood cultures may be useful in identifying the bacterial pathogen of meningitis. However, a negative blood culture may be found in up to 33% of children with meningococcal meningitis, 20% of children with pneumococcal cases, and 10% of patients with *H. influenzae* type b meningitis. These numbers increase with prior antibiotic therapy. In addition, there is a negative correlation between the length of illness before diagnosis and the rate of positive blood cultures.

TREATMENT

The mainstay of treatment for bacterial meningitis is antibiotic therapy. Antibiotics should be started as soon as possible after the lumbar puncture is performed and samples are obtained for culture. In most instances, antibiotic therapy is initiated before the etiologic agent is definitively identified. Empirical therapy should be directed toward all the common pathogens for the age of the patient. Later, when the bacterium is identified and antibiotic sensitivities are determined, the most appropriate drug or combination of drugs should be used (Table 52-6).

In newborns, bacterial meningitis is most frequently caused by group B streptococci, *Escherichia coli* and other gram-negative organisms (*Klebsiella, Enterobacter, Salmonella*), and *L. monocytogenes.* In older infants and children, the usual pathogens are *Streptococcus pneumoniae, Neisseria meningitidis,* and in the unvaccinated child, *H. influenzae* type b.

Either penicillin G (450,000 U/kg/day) plus gentamicin or ampicillin (300 to 400 mg/kg/day) plus gentamicin is used in combination for treatment of meningitis caused by group B streptococci or *L. monocytogenes.* Cefotaxime or ceftriaxone, plus an aminoglycoside or ampicillin, is used for treatment of meningitis caused by gram-negative enteric organisms. Ampicillin is used for treatment of β-lactamase–negative *H. influenzae,* but ceftriaxone or cefotaxime is more often used if organisms are β-lactamase producers. Penicillin or ampicillin is used for meningitis caused by susceptible *N. meningitidis,* and cefotaxime or ceftriaxone is used for penicillin-resistant meningococcal meningitis. Ceftriaxone is not used in children younger than 1 month because of its long half-life. Use of aminoglycosides requires monitoring plasma concentrations to ensure therapeutic benefit and avoid ototoxicity and nephrotoxicity.

Penicillin or ampicillin is used for treatment of meningitis caused by penicillin-susceptible *S. pneumoniae,* but treatment of penicillin-resistant pneumococcus requires cefotaxime or ceftriaxone. Vancomycin is used for treatment of meningitis caused by pneumococcus that is resistant to both penicillin and cefotaxime or in patients with severe β-lactam hypersensitivity. Vancomycin is not recommended as monotherapy for patients with pneumococcal meningitis; rifampin is added for treatment of penicillin- and cefotaxime-resistant organisms. Meropenem may be used in treatment of pneumococcal meningitis in select instances in children older than 3 months, when other therapies cannot be used because of drug resistance in the organism or patient hypersensitivity to other therapies.

Empirical treatment of the patient with bacterial meningitis is chosen on the basis of the organisms most likely to be causing the infection and the likelihood that those organisms are antibiotic

Table 52-4. Clinical Conditions and Infectious Agents Associated with Aseptic Meningitis

Viruses

Enteroviruses (coxsackievirus, echovirus, poliovirus, enterovirus)
Arboviruses: Eastern equine, Western equine, Venezuelan equine, St. Louis encephalitis, Powassan and California encephalitis, West Nile virus, Colorado tick fever
Herpes simplex (types 1, 2)
Human herpesvirus type 6
Varicella-zoster virus
Epstein-Barr virus
Parvovirus B19
Cytomegalovirus
Adenovirus
Variola (smallpox)
Measles
Mumps
Rubella
Influenza A and B
Parainfluenza
Rhinovirus
Rabies
Lymphocytic choriomeningitis
Rotaviruses
Coronaviruses
Human immunodeficiency virus type 1

Bacteria

Mycobacterium tuberculosis
Leptospira species (leptospirosis)
Treponema pallidum (syphilis)
Borrelia species (relapsing fever)
Borrelia burgdorferi (Lyme disease)
Nocardia species (nocardiosis)
Brucella species
Bartonella species (cat-scratch disease)
Rickettsia rickettsiae (Rocky Mountain spotted fever)
Rickettsia prowazekii (typhus)
Ehrlichia canis
Coxiella burnetii
Mycoplasma pneumoniae
Mycoplasma hominis
Chlamydia trachomatis
Chlamydia psittaci
Chlamydia pneumoniae
Partially treated bacterial meningitis

Bacterial Parameningeal Focus

Sinusitis
Mastoiditis
Brain abscess
Subdural-epidural empyema
Cranial osteomyelitis

Fungi

Coccidioides immitis (coccidioidomycosis)
Blastomyces dermatitidis (blastomycosis)
Cryptococcus neoformans (cryptococcosis)
Histoplasma capsulatum (histoplasmosis)
Candida species
Other fungi (*Alternaria, Aspergillus, Cephalosporium, Cladosporium, Dreschlera hawaiiensis, Paracoccidioides brasiliensis, Petriellidium boydii, Sporotrichum schenckii, Ustilago* species, *Zygomycetes*)

Parasites (Eosinophilic)

Angiostrongylus cantonensis

Gnathostoma spinigerum
Baylisascaris procyonis
Strongyloides stercoralis
Trichinella spiralis
Toxocara canis
Taenia solium (cysticercosis)
Paragonimus westermani
Schistosoma species
Fasciola species

Parasites (Noneosinophilic)

Toxoplasma gondii (toxoplasmosis)
Acanthamoeba species
Naegleria fowleri
Malaria

Postinfectious

Vaccines: rabies, influenza, measles, poliovirus
Demyelinating or allergic encephalitis

Systemic or Immunologically Mediated

Bacterial endocarditis
Kawasaki disease
Systemic lupus erythematosus
Vasculitis, including polyarteritis nodosa
Sjögren syndrome
Mixed connective tissue disease
Rheumatoid arthritis
Behçet syndrome
Wegener granulomatosis
Lymphomatoid granulomatosis
Granulomatous arteritis
Sarcoidosis
Familial Mediterranean fever
Vogt-Koyanagi-Harada syndrome

Malignancy

Leukemia
Lymphoma
Metastatic carcinoma
Central nervous system tumor (e.g., craniopharyngioma, glioma, ependymoma, astrocytoma, medulloblastoma, teratoma)

Drugs

Intrathecal injections (contrast media, serum, antibiotics, antineoplastic agents)
Nonsteroidal antiinflammatory agents
OKT3 monoclonal antibodies
Carbamazepine
Azathioprine
Intravenous immune globulins
Antibiotics (trimethoprim-sulfamethoxazole, sulfasalazine, ciprofloxacin, isoniazid)

Miscellaneous

Heavy metal poisoning (lead, arsenic)
Foreign bodies (shunt, reservoir)
Subarachnoid hemorrhage
Postictal state
Postmigraine state
Mollaret syndrome (recurrent)
Intraventricular hemorrhage (neonate)
Familial hemophagocytic syndrome
Post neurosurgery
Dermoid-epidermoid cyst

Compiled from Cherry JD: Aseptic meningitis and viral meningitis. In Feigin RD, Cherry JD (eds): Textbook of Pediatric Infectious Diseases, 4th ed. Philadelphia, WB Saunders, 1998, p 450; and from Davis LE: Aseptic and viral meningitis. In Long SS, Pickering LK, Prober CG (eds): Principles and Practice of Pediatric Infectious Disease. New York, Churchill Livingstone, 1997, p 329.

Table 52-5. Characteristics of the Most Common Causes of the Aseptic Meningitis Syndrome

Organism	Age Group	Season	Prodrome	Clinical Characteristics	Epidemiologic Characteristics	Agent Diagnosis	Serology
Common							
Enteroviruses	Infants, young children	Summer, fall	None, or mild GI or pharyngitis syndrome for 1-3 days	Exanthem, myopericarditis, conjunctivitis, pleurodynia, hand-foot-mouth disease, herpangina, myositis, hepatitis	Epidemic	Culture or PCR of CSF, blood, throat, stool	Enterovirus serologic study
Arboviruses	Children, elderly	Summer, early fall	Fever, rash, malaise for 1-5 days	Encephalitis or aseptic meningitis	Geographic area, contact with insect vector, encephalitis in community or animals	PCR of CSF	IgM, paired IgG
Herpes simplex type 2	Young adults	Year round	Genital vesicles for 1-7 days	Associated primary herpes lesions	Sexual exposure	Culture of genital lesions; PCR of CSF	IgM, paired IgG
Borrelia burgdorferi	Children, adults	Spring to late fall	Erythema migrans; secondary symptoms weeks to months later	Facial palsy or other cranial nerve palsy; radiculitis; heart block	Endemic area, deer tick exposure (often unrecognized)	PCR of CSF	IgG, IgM: EIA with Western blot confirmation
Less Common							
Mumps	5- to 9-year-olds	Late winter–spring	Parotitis, orchitis: 2-10 days	Parotitis, orchitis, oophoritis, pancreatitis	Exposure to mumps or vaccination	Culture of CSF, throat	IgM, paired IgG
HIV	Young adults	Year round	Fever, arthralgias, maculopapular rash, pharyngitis, adenopathy	Same as prodrome; meningitis may occur 1-5 days into the illness	2-6 weeks after sexual or blood exposure	Blood PCR for HIV, RNA, or DNA	IgG (EIA) negative at this stage
Lymphocytic choriomeningitis virus	Older children, young adults	Fall, early winter	Fever and flulike syndrome, 5-21 days	Orchitis, alopecia	Exposure to mice, hamsters	Culture of CSF, blood	IgG
Mycobacterium tuberculosis	Infants (primary infection), young adults (reactivation)	Year round	Fever	Pneumonia, basilar inflammation with cranial nerve palsy and intracranial hypertension	History of tuberculosis or exposure, HIV risk factors	Culture CSF for mycobacteria	None
Leptospira	Young adults	Late summer, early fall	Hepatitis and hematuria, 1-7 days	Conjunctivitis, splenomegaly, jaundice, nephritis, rash	Exposure to animals, water contaminated with animal urine	Culture of blood, CSF, urine	Paired IgG
Fungal	Premature infant, young adult	Year round	Fever	Basilar inflammation on CT or MRI, cranial nerve findings	Endemic area (blastomycosis, histoplasmosis) Immunodeficiency (cryptococcosis) Prematurity (candidal disease)	Culture of CSF for fungus, meningeal biopsy	Specific IgG
Mycoplasma organisms	Children, young adults	Fall, winter	Fever, malaise, sore throat, cough	Cough, rash, hemolytic anemia	Family or community epidemic	PCR of CSF, nasopharyngeal secretions	IgM

Modified from Connolly KJ, Hammer SM: The acute aseptic meningitis syndrome. Infect Dis Clin North Am 1990;4:599-622; and from Davis LE: Aseptic and viral meningitis. In Long SS, Pickering LK, Prober CG (eds): Principles and Practice of Pediatric Infectious Disease. New York, Churchill Livingstone, 1997, p 331.

CSF, cerebral spinal fluid; CT, computed tomography; EIA, enzyme immunoassay; GI, gastrointestinal; HIV, human immunodeficiency virus; IgG and IgM, immunoglobulins G and M; MRI, magnetic resonance imaging; PCR, polymerase chain reaction.

Table 52-6. Antibiotics Used for the Treatment of Bacterial Meningitis*

Drug	Neonates		Infants and Children
	0-7 Days	*8-28 Days*	
Amikacin[†‡]	15-20 divided q12h	20-30 divided q8h	20-30 divided q8h
Ampicillin	200-300 divided q8h	300 divided q4h or q6h	300 divided q4-6h
Cefotaxime	100 divided q12h	150-200 divided q8h or q6h	200-300 divided q8h or q6h
Ceftriaxone[§]	—	—	100 divided q12h or q24h
Ceftazidime	150 divided q12h	150 divided q8h	150 divided q8h
Gentamicin[†‡]	5 divided q12h	7.5 divided q8h	7.5 divided q8h
Meropenem	—	—	120 divided q8h
Nafcillin	100-150 divided q8h or q12h	150-200 divided q8h or q6h	150-200 divided q4h or q6h
Penicillin G	250,000-450,000 divided q8h	450,000 divided q6h	450,000 divided q4h or q6h
Rifampin	—	—	20 divided q12h
Tobramycin[†‡]	5 divided q12h	7.5 divided q8h	7.5 divided q8h
Vancomycin[†‡]	30 divided q12h	30-45 divided q8h	60 divided q6h

Modified from Klein JO: Antimicrobial treatment and prevention of meningitis. Pediatr Ann 1994;23:76.

*Dosages in mg/kg (U/kg for penicillin G) per day.

[†]Smaller doses and longer dosing intervals, especially for aminoglycosides and vancomycin for very-low-birth-weight neonates, may be advisable.

[‡]Monitoring of serum levels is recommended to ensure safe and therapeutic values.

[§]Use in neonates is not recommended because of inadequate experience in neonatal meningitis.

resistant. The age of the patient, vaccination history (conjugate *H. influenzae* type b vaccine and conjugate *S. pneumoniae* vaccine), prior antibiotic use (which may select for penicillin-resistant pneumococci), and prevalence of antibiotic resistance in the patient's community are considered. In children from birth to 4 weeks of age, ampicillin (or penicillin) and cefotaxime or, less often, ampicillin (or penicillin) and an aminoglycoside are used. After 4 weeks of age, *L. monocytogenes* is uncommon as a cause of bacterial meningitis, and empirical treatment with cefotaxime or ceftriaxone plus vancomycin is appropriate. When organism identification and antibiotic susceptibility are known, antibiotic therapy is changed accordingly.

The duration of antibiotic treatment for bacterial meningitis has not been studied thoroughly. The commonly accepted length of treatment for *H. influenzae* and pneumococcal meningitis is 7 to 10 days, but longer therapy may be appropriate for some patients with a complicated course. A 5- to 7-day regimen is adequate for most children with meningococcal meningitis. Gram-negative enteric meningitis is treated for 3 weeks after the spinal fluid is sterile. In the newborn, group B streptococcal and *Listeria* meningitis are treated for 14 to 21 days.

Control of spread of the organisms causing bacterial meningitis is important. If ampicillin was used for therapy, the child with *H. influenzae* type b meningitis receives oral rifampin in a dosage of 20 mg/kg/day in one dose for 4 days (maximum dose, 600 mg/day) to eradicate nasopharyngeal carriage of the organism. Rifampin is administered before the child is discharged from the hospital. In addition, if there are any household members younger than 48 months who are not fully immunized against *H. influenzae* or are immunosuppressed, or if there is a child younger than 12 months even if the primary vaccine series has been given, all members of the household should receive rifampin prophylaxis. If the child is in attendance more than 25 hours a week in a day care center where all children are younger than 2 years of age and two cases of invasive *H. influenzae* type b disease have occurred within 60 days, all attendees and personnel should receive rifampin. If there are incompletely vaccinated children younger than 2 years in the day care center, they too should receive rifampin, even when only one case of invasive *H. influenzae* disease has occurred. In addition, they must receive any missing doses of the vaccine. Pregnant women are not treated with rifampin.

To prevent spread of meningococcal meningitis, prophylaxis to eradicate nasopharyngeal carriage should be given to the patient; all household, day care, and nursery contacts; and persons who have contact with the patient's oral or nasopharyngeal secretions and medical personnel who have had intimate contact with the patient's nasopharyngeal secretions within 7 days before antibiotic therapy. Prophylaxis is with oral rifampin (10 mg/kg [maximum dose, 600 mg] every 12 hours for four doses); intramuscular ceftriaxone (125 mg in children younger than 12 years and 250 mg in older children and adults); or oral ciprofloxacin (500 mg as a single oral dose to nonpregnant persons older than 18 years). Meningococcal vaccine may be considered for contacts in special circumstances but only when the infection is caused by a vaccine serotype.

The morbidity associated with bacterial meningitis is from neuronal damage caused both by the invasiveness of the infecting organism and by the host inflammatory response. When β-lactam antibiotics are given to control organism invasiveness, release of toxins from dying bacteria actually may increase the host inflammatory response and resultant tissue damage. In vitro and animal studies show that dexamethasone inhibits production of tumor necrosis factor α and interleukin-1 when given before exposure to bacterial endotoxin. In view of these beneficial cellular effects, dexamethasone use might be expected to uniformly improve the clinical outcome in pediatric patients with bacterial meningitis. Perhaps because the effectiveness of dexamethasone is greatest when given before endotoxin exposure, these potential benefits have not been uniformly identified in children. However, there is adequate data from randomized controlled trials to support the use of dexamethasone in children with meningitis caused by *H. influenzae* and to consider its use in patients with meningitis caused by *S. pneumoniae*.

For patients with *H. influenzae* meningitis, dexamethasone administration reduces the rate of moderate or more severe bilateral hearing loss; dexamethasone on a schedule of 0.15 mg/kg/dose intravenously every 6 hours for 4 days is recommended. A regimen of 0.4 mg/kg/dose given every 12 hours in four doses (2 days) may be equally effective. Dexamethasone is most effective at reducing hearing loss if the first dose is given before administration of antibiotics. Antibiotic therapy should not be delayed for this purpose. Dexamethasone is associated with mild gastrointestinal bleeding; some practitioners recommend concurrent use of medications to decrease gastric acid production for the duration of therapy.

For patients with *S. pneumoniae* meningitis, adjunctive therapy with dexamethasone has not been shown in randomized controlled trials to be of benefit in preventing neurologic complications (including hearing loss). However, metaanalysis of multiple trials supports its use, and the American Academy of Pediatrics recommends that its use be "considered" in this setting. The dose is the same as used in *H. influenzae* meningitis. Because dexamethasone use is associated with rapid decrease in fever and meningeal inflammation, it may lead to an impression of clinical improvement in the absence of CSF sterilization. Consideration should be given to repeating a lumbar puncture after 24 hours of therapy to document sterilization of the CSF. Dexamethasone decreases meningeal inflammation and may therefore limit penetration of antibiotics into CSF; however, when cefotaxime, ceftriaxone, vancomycin, or rifampin is used in the high doses recommended for treatment of bacterial meningitis, their CSF concentrations remain adequate for treatment of most cases of meningitis caused by penicillin-resistant *S. pneumoniae*.

There are no data to suggest that patients with meningitis caused by *N. meningitidis* will benefit from treatment with corticosteroids.

Dexamethasone use has not been studied for patients with meningitis younger than 2 months of age or for patients with meningitis caused by group B streptococcus or gram-negative enteric organisms. Dexamethasone does not have a proven benefit if given more than 1 hour after administration of the first dose of antibiotics.

CLINICAL COURSE

The child with bacterial meningitis must be observed very carefully during the first few days of the illness, when life-threatening complications may occur. The complications may result from septicemia, such as septic shock or disseminated intravascular coagulation, or from meningitis itself. The most serious complication is cerebral edema leading to increased intracranial pressure and herniation (see Chapter 40). Consequently, vital signs and the child's mental status must be monitored frequently, and the child should be transferred to an intensive care unit should these problems arise.

Fever normally persists for 3 to 5 days and for as long as 9 days in 13% of children. Dexamethasone therapy usually suppresses fever, which may recur after this steroid is discontinued. Prolonged or recurrent fever is often associated with a subdural effusion, infections at other sites such as joints or the lungs, thrombophlebitis secondary to intravenous lines, abscess formation from intramuscular injections, or drug-related fever. A secondary rise in fever is usually caused by a nosocomial viral infection or a subdural effusion. If no source for an abnormally prolonged or secondary fever is found, a repeat lumbar puncture to assess the response to antibiotics should be considered. This is especially relevant if there is suspicion of antimicrobial resistance.

Occipital-frontal circumference is measured at baseline and daily, to identify progressive intracranial hypertension or subdural effusion in infants. Baseline and serial neurologic evaluations are performed, because alterations of mental status, seizures, and focal neurologic deficits may be found during the course of the illness. These result from direct neuronal damage by inflammatory mediators and from disruption of normal cerebral blood flow by cerebral edema, vasculitis, thrombosis, and loss of cerebral autoregulation. The presence of focal neurologic abnormalities on admission can be associated with long-term neurologic deficits.

Twenty percent to 30% of affected children may have seizures during the first few days of the illness. These seizures should be treated with benzodiazepines, fosphenytoin, or phenobarbital because of the risk of cerebral injury from prolonged seizures. When these seizures are generalized and easily controlled, they are not associated with permanent neurologic deficits or subsequent seizures. Anticonvulsant medication may be discontinued at the time of discharge in uncomplicated cases. Seizures that are difficult to control or that persist or develop after the first few days of hospitalization, as well as focal seizures, are more often associated with later neurologic sequelae. The presence of seizures should prompt investigation for possible causes such as hyponatremia, hypocalcemia, or venous sinus thrombosis.

Secondary subdural effusions are found in approximately 30% of children with bacterial meningitis. Such effusions may be detected by ultrasonography; CT or magnetic resonance imaging (MRI) is more commonly used. These effusions are most often asymptomatic, do not contain live organisms, and alone do not indicate a poor prognosis. Subdural effusions are caused by intense meningeal inflammation. Such inflammation can be associated with arteritis and venulitis, which is further associated with focal neurologic deficits and seizures. However, the subdural effusion itself is not directly responsible for these complications and is just a sign of the intensity of the inflammation present. Drainage of a subdural effusion in a patient with bacterial meningitis is warranted only when there is evidence that the effusion is causing intracranial hypertension or focal brain compression.

Meticulous attention is paid to fluid management in children with bacterial meningitis. Because of potential changes in mental status and the possibility of vomiting and aspiration in patients with intracranial hypertension and depressed sensorium, patients are not usually fed by mouth early in the hospitalization.

Historically, patients with bacterial meningitis were treated with a fluid restriction of two thirds of their calculated maintenance, to prevent the development of the syndrome of inappropriate secretion of antidiuretic hormone (SIADH), complications of which include free water retention and hyponatremia, which can lead to seizures and worsening cerebral edema. SIADH is defined by the presence of increased total body water and hyponatremia with corresponding serum and extracellular fluid hypoosmolality. SIADH is accompanied by high urine sodium concentrations, inappropriate elevation of urine osmolality, and normally functioning kidneys and adrenal glands, and volume depletion is absent. SIADH probably occurs in fewer than 10% of patients with meningitis.

At the time of hospital admission, most children with meningitis have intravascular volume depletion and compensatory, appropriately elevated antidiuretic hormone. The hypovolemia is caused by increased fluid losses from vomiting and fever, sepsis-induced capillary leakage, and decreased oral intake. Restriction of fluid intake results in perpetuation of hypovolemia and possible reduction of cerebral perfusion.

The initial evaluation of a child with meningitis includes a clinical assessment of intravascular volume and the following laboratory tests: serum electrolytes, urine electrolytes, and urine specific gravity. Children in shock require vigorous fluid resuscitation with isotonic solutions. Such children must be monitored carefully. In addition, the use of intravenous colloid and vasopressors (dopamine, epinephrine) may decrease fluid requirements while maintaining systemic and cerebral perfusion.

If an affected child shows signs of intravascular volume depletion, he or she should receive deficit fluid replacement with isotonic crystalloid and full maintenance fluids calculated to restore euvolemia over 24 hours. Some practitioners use half normal saline, lactated Ringer solution, or normal saline for the maintenance fluids, in hopes of preventing further hyponatremia, cerebral edema, and worsening intracranial hypertension.

Fluid management is tailored to each patient. Electrolytes must be monitored frequently, and volume status must be reevaluated with accurate monitoring of intake and output and serial measurements of body weight. Careful monitoring allows identification of the unusual occurrence of SIADH, diabetes insipidus, or cerebral salt wasting. In the unusual child with increased total body water and serum sodium concentration less than 135 mEq/L, with high urine sodium concentration and high urine osmolality, SIADH may be suspected, and fluids should be restricted to two-thirds maintenance level. The child should be observed closely, and as the sodium normalizes, the fluids may be liberalized. If hyponatremic seizures occur, hypertonic saline (3% NaCl) should be administered.

OUTCOME

The case fatality rate for children with bacterial meningitis is generally less than 5% to 10%. Neurologic abnormalities may be present in up to 50% of children at the time of hospital discharge, but many

Table 52-7. Sequelae of Bacterial Meningitis

Death
Cranial nerve dysfunction (usually transient)
Hemiparesis
Quadriparesis
Spinal cord infarction
Brain infarction
Hypertonia
Hypotonia
Ataxia (cerebellar or vestibular)
Permanent seizure disorder
Sensorineural hearing loss
Cortical blindness
Obstructive hydrocephalus
Diabetes insipidus
Transient cataracts
Transverse myelitis
Pericardial effusion (immune complex or septic)
Joint effusion (immune complex or septic)
Polyarteritis
Behavioral problems
Language delay
Mental retardation

findings resolve over the ensuing 1 to 2 years, and long-lasting sequelae are less common (Table 52-7). Death and neurologic sequelae are more common in neonates, young infants, and children with meningitis caused by *S. pneumoniae* or *E. coli*. Sensorineural hearing loss, from bacterial infection and damage to the cochlea, is the most common readily identifiable neurologic sequela, occurring in up to 30% of children after meningitis with *S. pneumoniae* and in 5% to 10% of children with meningitis caused by *H. influenzae* or *Neisseria meningitides*. Hearing loss is more likely to occur in children with initial CSF glucose concentration less than 20 mg/dL. Vestibular damage with balance disturbance may be found as well. All children with bacterial meningitis should undergo hearing testing before hospital discharge.

BACTERIAL MENINGITIS IN CHILDREN WITH INTRAVENTRICULAR SHUNTS

Between 20% and 30% of individuals with ventriculoperitoneal shunts experience a shunt infection at some time during their lives. The majority (70%) of these infections occur within 2 months of the initial surgery; 80% occur within 6 months.

Children with shunt infections differ from other children with bacterial meningitis. The most common pathogens in children with shunts are *S. epidermidis* (coagulase-negative staphylococci) and, less often, *S. aureus* (coagulase-positive staphylococci). Only 30% have meningeal signs. The others may instead present with erythema along the subcutaneous tract of the shunt, fever, nausea, vomiting, malaise, headache, abdominal pain (from infected CSF irritating the peritoneum), and signs of increased intracranial pressure (especially papilledema). Diagnosis is best made by percutaneous needle aspiration of the shunt, not by lumbar puncture. The degree of CSF pleocytosis is usually much less than in children without shunts. The number of WBCs in the CSF of patients with shunt infections may average less than 100. The CSF glucose concentration is only mildly depressed, and the protein concentration is often normal.

The usual treatment for a shunt infection includes appropriate systemic antibiotics, supportive care, removal of the infected shunt, external ventricular drainage, and in some cases, intraventricular antibiotics.

RECURRENT BACTERIAL MENINGITIS

Recrudescence is the reappearance of bacterial meningitis during the therapy of the initial episode. Poor penetration of antibiotics to the site of infection or antibiotic resistance (acquired, selected) should be suspected. *Relapse* occurs between 3 days and 3 weeks after successful therapy and usually represents persistent infection in sequestered sites (subdural empyema, ventriculitis, cerebral abscess, mastoiditis, cranial osteomyelitis, orbital infection). Relapse may be secondary to inadequate choice, duration, or dosage of antibiotics.

Recurrent bacterial meningitis is defined as reappearance of bacterial meningitis after convalescence. It is most commonly associated with developmental anatomic abnormalities, but it can also be secondary to traumatic or surgical CSF fistula, congenital or acquired immunodeficiency, or unrecognized parameningeal focus of infection (Table 52-8).

In patients with CSF fistula and recurrent bacterial meningitis, *S. pneumoniae*, α-hemolytic streptococci, and *H. influenzae* type b are most commonly associated with cranial defects such as skull fracture, cribriform plate defect, middle or inner ear dysplasia, or encephalocele. The most commonly recognized site of fistula is the middle ear, with a defect in the stapes footplate. Many patients with congenital fistulous communication between the CNS and the middle ear are deaf, and they may have Mondini dysplasia of the semicircular canals and cochlea visible on CT scan.

E. coli, *S. aureus*, *Enterococcus* organisms, and *Bacteroides fragilis* are most commonly associated with lumbosacral defects such as dermoid cyst, midline dermal sinus tract, or myelomeningocele.

In patients with immunodeficiency, pneumococcal infections are associated with hypogammaglobulinemia or the absence of

Table 52-8. Conditions Associated with Recurrent Bacterial Meningitis

Congenital Cerebrospinal Fluid (CSF) Fistula
Stapes footplate fistula
Oval window fistula
Cochlear aqueduct defect
Giant apical air cell syndrome
Basiethmoidal or cribriform plate defect
Cranial or spinal dermal sinus
Meningocele
Encephalocele
Neurenteric cyst
Klippel-Feil syndrome

Traumatic or Surgical CSF Fistula
Skull fracture involving paranasal sinuses, cribriform plate, petrous bone
Postoperative (particularly after nasal surgery)

Immunodeficiency
Immunoglobulin deficiency
Complement component deficiency
Hemoglobinopathy
Congenital or acquired asplenia
Leukemia
Lymphoma

Parameningeal Infection
Mastoiditis
Sinusitis
Skull bone osteomyelitis

Idiopathic

Adapted from Kline MW: Review of recurrent bacterial meningitis. Pediatr Infect Dis J 1989;8:630.

complement components C2, C3, and C3b inhibitor. Repeated meningococcal infections are more probably associated with deficiencies in the terminal complement components C5, C6, C7, C8, and C9 (see Chapter 51).

Evaluation of the patient with recurrent bacterial meningitis includes a thorough family history for recurrent infections, examination of midline structures from anus to epiglottis, evaluation of hearing, and fine-cut cranial CT or MRI to evaluate middle and inner ear anatomy or lumbosacral anatomy as guided by the history and examination.

Definitive treatment involves antibiotic therapy for the acute infection, followed by surgical repair of the fistula or treatment for the immunodeficiency.

ASEPTIC MENINGITIS, ENCEPHALITIS, AND MENINGOENCEPHALITIS

Aseptic meningitis is an inflammatory process of the meninges, most often characterized by acute signs and symptoms of meningeal irritation; CSF pleocytosis, usually with a predominance of mononuclear cells; a normal or, less frequently, elevated CSF protein concentration; normal or, less often, low CSF glucose concentration; and no organisms demonstrable by Gram stain or bacterial cultures. There are many causes of aseptic meningitis (see Table 52-4). The most common cause is viral infection; up to 90% of cases are caused by enteroviruses and arbovirus. The definitive diagnosis is made by identifying the organism in the CSF. However, this is not always possible, and other causes must be excluded by history, presence or absence of associated symptoms, and appropriate laboratory tests (see Table 52-5).

VIRAL MENINGITIS

Enteroviral meningitis occurs most often during the summer and early fall months. Transmission is via the fecal-oral route, and young children exhibit increased transmission of the viruses and more severe disease in comparison with other age groups. Initially, patients may have a respiratory tract infection, a nonspecific febrile illness or vomiting and diarrhea. Viral infection of the meninges occurs 7 to 10 days after initial exposure. The clinical course may be biphasic. Virus from the oropharynx can be cultured only during the first 5 to 7 days of the illness but may be excreted in stool for 6 to 8 weeks.

Children with viral meningitis present with fever, nuchal rigidity, irritability, headache, and vomiting. Less common symptoms are anorexia, drowsiness, photophobia, myalgia, and malaise. As in bacterial meningitis, affected young infants often lack meningeal signs. In addition, children may have an altered sensorium, but focal neurologic signs are rare. Seizures are more common in infants.

The number of WBCs in the CSF varies from zero to several thousand (see Table 52-3). Up to 75% of initial (early in the illness) CSF specimens contain a predominance of polymorphonuclear cells. Mononuclear cells predominate by 2 days after the onset of symptoms. Of children with enteroviral meningitis, 18% may have decreased CSF glucose concentrations, whereas 12% may have elevated CSF protein. When the clinician is in doubt as to whether a patient has viral or bacterial meningitis and the patient does not appear ill, it may be worthwhile to withhold antibiotics and repeat the lumbar puncture after several hours.

Treatment of viral meningitis is supportive. Admission to the hospital may be required while bacterial meningitis is being ruled out and for intravenous hydration. Analgesics and antipyretics may also be indicated. The lumbar puncture performed to diagnose viral meningitis is often helpful in ameliorating the acute symptoms. The mechanism for this is not clear.

The outcome is quite good for patients in whom common viral pathogens cause aseptic meningitis. Sequelae in older children are rare. Adverse outcomes are more common (but unusual) in children who have viral meningitis during the first year of life. Speech and language development may be affected. Treatment and outcome for the other types of aseptic meningitis depend on the underlying cause (see Table 52-5).

TUBERCULOUS MENINGITIS

Tuberculous meningitis is an important treatable cause of aseptic meningitis. During the primary pulmonary tuberculous infection and subsequent lymphohematogenous spread to extrapulmonary sites, tubercle bacilli produce local microscopic granulomas in the CNS and meninges. If this primary CNS infection is not contained by host defense mechanisms (T lymphocytes, monocytes), or if host defense mechanisms fail at a later period, tuberculous meningitis may result. Meningitis occurs weeks to months after the primary pulmonary process.

The symptoms of tuberculous meningitis are insidious and subacute (weeks to months). Stage 1 is a prodrome with nonspecific manifestations (apathy, poor school function, irritability, weight loss, fever, night sweats, nausea); stage 2 is heralded by the onset of neurologic signs (headache, cranial neuropathy, nuchal rigidity, signs of increased intracranial pressure); and stage 3 manifests with altered levels of consciousness (lethargy, stupor, coma). Meningismus is not present in all patients.

The diagnosis is supported by a history of contacts with adults with known active tuberculosis, a chronic cough, or human immunodeficiency virus (HIV) disease or by a history of immigration, poverty, or homelessness. In addition, the patient's chest radiograph is consistent with active or, more often, quiescent tuberculosis (parenchymal-hilar node calcifications, infiltrates, hilar adenopathy, and, in rare cases, endobronchial or cavitary lesions), and the patient's tuberculin skin test yields a positive result (see Chapter 2). Cranial CT or MRI may show the most intense meningeal inflammation around the base of the brain or inflammatory mass lesions (tuberculomas). The CSF results (see Table 52-3) include profound hypoglycorrhachia, a high CSF protein, lymphocyte- or monocyte-predominant cells (usually 500 cells/mm^3), increased opening pressure, and, on occasion, tubercle organisms on acid-fast staining. Polymerase chain reaction (PCR) amplification of *Mycobacterium tuberculosis* DNA aids in making a more rapid diagnosis than does culture of CSF, sputum, or gastric aspirates, which traditionally requires 2 to 6 weeks. The differential diagnosis depends on the stage of the illness (Table 52-9).

Treatment includes supportive care for coma and increased intracranial pressure, including the use of intravenous corticosteroids. Antituberculous therapy includes the use of isoniazid (10 to 20 mg/kg/day), rifampin (10 to 20 mg/kg/day), pyrazinamide (20 to

---

Table 52-9. Differential Diagnosis of Tuberculous Meningitis

Fungal meningitis (cryptococcosis, histoplasmosis, blastomycosis, coccidioidomycosis)
Neurobrucellosis
Neurosyphilis
Neuroborreliosis
Focal parameningeal infection (sphenoid sinusitis, endocarditis)
Pyogenic brain abscess
Central nervous system (CNS) toxoplasmosis
Partially treated bacterial meningitis
Neoplastic meningitis (lymphoma, carcinoma)
Cerebrovascular accident
CNS sarcoidosis

Modified from Leonard JM, Des Prez RM: Tuberculous meningitis. Infect Dis Clin North Am 1990;4:769-787.

Table 52-10. Classification of Encephalitis by Cause and Source

I. **Infections: Viral**
  A. Spread: person to person only
    1. Mumps: frequent in an unimmunized population; often mild
    2. Measles: may have serious sequelae
    3. Enteroviruses: frequent at all ages; more serious in newborns
    4. Rubella: uncommon; sequelae rare except in congenital rubella
    5. Herpesvirus group
      a. Herpes simplex (types 1 and 2, possibly 6): relatively common; sequelae frequent; devastating in newborns
      b. Varicella-zoster virus: uncommon; serious sequelae not rare
      c. Cytomegalovirus, congenital or acquired: may have delayed sequelae in congenital type
      d. Epstein-Barr virus (infectious mononucleosis): not common
    6. Pox group
      a. Vaccinia and variola: uncommon, but serious CNS damage occurs
    7. Parvovirus (erythema infectiosum): not common
    8. Influenza A and B
    9. Adenovirus
    10. Other: reoviruses, respiratory syncytial, parainfluenza, hepatitis B
  B. Arthropod-borne agents
    Arboviruses: spread to humans by mosquitoes or ticks; seasonal epidemics depend on ecology of the insect vector; the following occur in the United States:

Eastern equine	California
Western equine	Powassan
Venezuelan equine	Dengue
St. Louis	Colorado tick fever
West Nile	

  C. Spread by warm-blooded mammals
    1. Rabies: saliva of many domestic and wild mammalian species
    2. Herpesvirus simiae ("B" virus): monkeys' saliva
    3. Lymphocytic choriomeningitis: rodents' excreta

II. **Infections: Nonviral**
  A. Rickettsial: in Rocky Mountain spotted fever and typhus; encephalitic component from cerebral vasculitis
  B. *Mycoplasma pneumoniae:* interval of some days between respiratory and CNS symptoms
  C. Bacterial: tuberculous and other bacterial meningitis; often has encephalitic component
  D. Spirochetal: syphilis, congenital or acquired; leptospirosis; Lyme disease
  E. Cat-scratch disease
  F. Fungal: immunologically compromised patients at special risk: cryptococcosis; histoplasmosis; aspergillosis; mucormycosis; candidosis; coccidioidomycosis
  G. Protozoal: *Plasmodium, Trypanosoma, Naegleria,* and *Acanthamoeba* species; *Toxoplasma gondii*
  H. Metazoal: trichinosis; echinococcosis; cysticercosis; schistosomiasis

III. **Parainfectious: Postinfectious, Allergic**
  Patients in whom an infectious agent or one of its components plays a contributory role in etiology, but the intact infectious agent is not isolated in vitro from the nervous system; it is postulated that in this group, the influence of cell-mediated antigen-antibody complexes plus complement is especially important in producing the observed tissue damage
  A. Associated with specific diseases (these agents may also cause direct CNS damage; see I and II

Measles	Rickettsial infections
Rubella	Influenza A and B
Mumps	Varicella-zoster
Mycoplasma pneumoniae	

  B. Associated with vaccines

Rabies	Measles
Vaccinia	Yellow fever

IV. **Human Slow-Virus Diseases**
  Accumulating evidence that viruses frequently acquired earlier in life, not necessarily with detectable acute illness, participate in later chronic neurologic disease (similar events also known to occur in animals)
  A. Subacute sclerosing panencephalitis; measles; rubella?
  B. Creutzfeldt-Jakob disease (spongiform encephalopathy)
  C. Progressive multifocal leukoencephalopathy
  D. Kuru (Fore tribe in New Guinea only)
  E. Human immunodeficiency virus

V. **Unknown: Complex Group**
  This group constitutes more than two thirds of the cases of encephalitis reported to the Centers for Disease Control and Prevention, Atlanta, Georgia; the yearly epidemic curve of these undiagnosed cases suggests that the majority are probably caused by enteroviruses and/or arboviruses

  There is also a miscellaneous group that is based on clinical criteria: Reye syndrome is one current example; others include the extinct von Economo encephalitis (epidemic during 1918-1928); myoclonic encephalopathy of infancy; retinomeningoencephalitis with papilledema and retinal hemorrhage; recurrent encephalomyelitis (? allergic or autoimmune); pseudotumor cerebri; and epidemic neuromyasthenia (Iceland disease)

  An encephalitic clinical pattern may follow ingestion or absorption of a number of known and unknown toxic substances; these include ingestion of lead and mercury and percutaneous absorption of hexachlorophene as a skin disinfectant and gamma benzene hexachloride as a scabicide

Modified from Behrman RE (ed): Nelson Textbook of Pediatrics, 14th ed. Philadelphia, WB Saunders, 1992, p 667.
CNS, central nervous system.

40 mg/kg/day), and streptomycin (20 to 40 mg/kg/day) for 2 months on a daily basis, followed by 10 months of daily isoniazid and rifampin. Other therapy may be needed for resistant organisms.

ENCEPHALITIS

Encephalitis is inflammation of the brain parenchyma, whereas meningoencephalitis is inflammation of the brain accompanied by inflammation of the meninges. Manifestations of encephalitis may result primarily from direct invasion by the causative organism (primary encephalitis) or may be caused predominantly by the inflammatory response to the agent (postinfectious or parainfectious). Encephalopathy is used to describe CNS illness unaccompanied by inflammation (for example, lead poisoning or pseudotumor cerebri). Meningoencephalitis is distinguished from aseptic meningitis by evidence of brain parenchymal involvement, including behavior or personality changes; altered level of consciousness (including agitation or coma); generalized seizures; focal neurologic signs, including focal seizures and focal motor defects (hemiparesis or ataxia); or movement disorders (Table 52-10).

Enteroviruses and arboviruses cause most cases of encephalitis in children. Enterovirus encephalitis, uncommon without meningeal involvement, is suggested by epidemic occurrence and presence of typical prodrome or associated findings (see Table 52-5); prompt diagnosis is by PCR for enterovirus in CSF, blood, throat, or stool specimens. A CSF or blood specimen is preferred, because PCR may identify enterovirus in throat and especially stool for weeks after the primary infection has resolved. Arbovirus encephalitis is suggested by mosquito or tick exposure and epidemic occurrence and is diagnosed by findings of arbovirus immunoglobulin M in CSF or blood or by paired serologic findings for immunoglobulin G.

Infections with *herpes simplex virus* (HSV) *type 1,* the most common cause of endemic encephalitis, occur throughout the year. In neonates, HSV encephalitis usually occurs between 7 and 21 days of age; may produce focal or generalized CNS disease; and may occur with or without conjunctivitis, oral mucosal involvement, vesicles on skin, or disseminated disease (hepatitis, pneumonia, septic appearance). After the neonatal period, HSV encephalitis is usually isolated to the CNS and classically produces necrotizing encephalitis with a focus in the temporal lobe. Symptoms in persons with HSV encephalitis range broadly: from those suggesting mild aseptic meningitis to presence of status epilepticus and coma and then death. In addition to neutrophils and monocytes, CSF examination may show increased numbers of erythrocytes and elevated protein. CT, MRI, and an electrencephalogram may suggest a temporal lobe focus. Specific diagnosis is by PCR of CSF for herpes simplex DNA. CSF culture is usually negative. In the appropriate clinical setting, presumptive therapy with intravenous acyclovir, 60 mg/kg/day given every 8 hours, is indicated while the results of PCR of CSF for HSV are awaited. Adequate hydration to avoid acyclovir-induced renal failure and close monitoring of absolute neutrophil count is crucial. A 3-week regimen of high-dose intravenous acyclovir is recommended for proven cases of HSV encephalitis.

POSTINFECTIOUS ENCEPHALITIS

Postinfectious encephalitis, also called *acute disseminated encephalomyelitis* (ADEM), is an immune-mediated inflammation of the CNS most commonly found in children older than 2 years. CNS illness begins 4 to 21 days after viral or bacterial infections, vaccination, or drug or plasma administration. Symptoms include fever, headache, neck stiffness, anorexia, vomiting, and mental status changes (psychosis, coma, seizures), and there are focal neurologic signs. CSF may be normal or may show elevated pressure, lymphocytic pleocytosis, and mildly elevated protein concentration. MRI shows discrete areas of increased signal on T2-weighted images, particularly at the gray-white junction. The biphasic clinical course and

typical MRI appearance allows distinction from acute encephalitis. ADEM is distinguished from the first episode of multiple sclerosis by the occurrence of ADEM in younger children, the lack of recurrence on follow-up, and results of appropriate CSF studies. Most patients recover full function. Corticosteroid therapy may lead to more rapid clinical improvement. Intravenous immune globulin and plasmapheresis have been used in severe cases.

ADEM in children younger than 2 years with severe, generalized CNS illness is sometimes referred to as *acute toxic encephalopathy* and is associated with increased risk of residual neurologic deficits. When ADEM is accompanied by RBCs in the CSF (usually 10 to 500 RBCs/mm^3), it is sometimes called *acute hemorrhagic leukoencephalopathy.*

CHRONIC OR RECURRENT ASEPTIC MENINGITIS

Recurrent aseptic meningitis may represent *Mollaret meningitis,* probably caused by HSV, which can be diagnosed by identifying HSV DNA in CSF by PCR. In Mollaret syndrome, brief episodes of meningitis alternate with asymptomatic periods. Headache, nuchal rigidity, fever, nausea, and vomiting are presenting symptoms. CSF examination reveals pleocytosis that initially is predominantly polynuclear but switches to mononuclear after the first day. The protein concentration is elevated, and the glucose concentration is depressed. The CSF returns to normal in a few days. After several years, the illness may suddenly disappear.

Children with hypogammaglobulinemia, or after bone marrow transplantation, may develop chronic or recurrent meningitis with enteroviruses, which can be diagnosed by specific PCR on CSF. Pleconaril, an antiviral agent, is useful for treatment of these patients.

Chronic meningitis is defined by 4 weeks of headache of subacute onset, fever, and stiff neck, often associated with signs of encephalitis such as confusion, disorientation, or lethargy. CSF may show pleocytosis, elevated protein concentration, and low glucose concentration (Table 52-11). Evaluation includes a thorough history and physical examination, CT or MRI of the head and spine, and other tests as indicated.

CLINICAL CLUES TO OTHER CAUSES OF NUCHAL RIGIDITY

The other conditions that manifest with neck stiffness are listed in Table 52-12. They may be differentiated from meningitis by the presence of specific neurologic signs or symptoms; the presence of signs and symptoms characteristic of another disease; the absence of signs and symptoms other than a stiff and painful neck; a history of predisposing factors; and findings of a thorough head and neck examination.

STIFF NECK ASSOCIATED WITH NEUROLOGIC SIGNS AND SYMPTOMS

When a child presents with a stiff neck and a neurologic deficit, the nature of the deficit directs the proper evaluation. For example, in a child who presents with altered sensorium, encephalitis or a CNS hemorrhage is considered. Cranial nerve involvement suggests basilar meningitis or intracranial hypertension, including intracranial masses. Weakness or pain in the upper extremities may be caused by pressure on the cervical nerve roots and may occur with an abscess, tumor, or trauma to the cervical spine. Ascending paralysis associated with a stiff neck is characteristic of Guillain-Barré syndrome. Muscular rigidity and dystonic movements are present in dystonia musculorum deformans, spasmodic torticollis, and Huntington chorea.

Table 52-11. Cerebrospinal Fluid Formula in Chronic Meningitis and Related Syndromes*

Lymphocytic, low glucose	
<50-100 WBCs[†]	Carcinoma
	Sarcoidosis
	Subarachnoid hemorrhage
50-500 WBCs	Tuberculosis
	Fungal
	Syphilis
	Parasitic (toxoplasmosis, cysticercosis)
	Viral (lymphocytic choriomeningitis, mumps meningoencephalitis)
Lymphocytic, normal glucose	
<50-100 WBCs[†]	Sarcoidosis
	Chronic benign lymphocytic meningitis
	Vasculitis
	Intracranial mass lesions
	Multiple sclerosis
50-500 WBCs	Most fungal, viral, and parasitic infections
	Chemical meningitis
Pleocytosis with neutrophilic predominance	Bacteria (*Nocardia, Actinomyces, Brucella* species)
	Fungi (*Blastomyces, Coccidioides, Aspergillus, Zygomycetes, Cladosporium, Pseudoallescheria* species)
	Systemic lupus erythematosus
	Chemical meningitis
	Discharge from epidermoid tumors or craniopharyngioma
	Intrathecal drugs, contrast agents
Pleocytosis with eosinophilic predominance	Hodgkin disease
	Parasites (*Angiostrongylus cantonensis, Cysticercus* species, *Gnathostoma spinigerum*)
	Tuberculosis
	Coccidioides
	Chemical meningitis (e.g., ibuprofen, foreign bodies)

From Tucker T, Ellner JJ: Chronic meningitis. In Scheld WM, Whitley RJ, Durack DT (eds): Infections of the Central Nervous System. New York, Raven Press, 1991, p 704.

*Note that categorization is based on the typical cerebrospinal fluid findings. Exceptions may occur.

[†]Usually <50; occasionally 50-100.

WBCs, white blood cells.

Ocular torticollis is caused by either superior oblique muscle weakness or congenital nystagmus. Torticollis and neck stiffness develop in the infant to compensate for abnormal eye movement. A good eye examination helps to make this diagnosis.

STIFF NECK ASSOCIATED WITH OTHER DISEASES

Neck stiffness is common in generalized viral and bacterial illnesses, such as influenza A or staphylococcal toxic shock syndrome. Neck stiffness may be caused by spread of inflammation to the soft tissues of the neck, as in pharyngitis; deep neck infections; or upper lobe pneumonia. Spasm of the neck muscles caused by tetanus or reflux esophagitis may occur. In juvenile rheumatoid arthritis, neck stiffness may result from cervical spine involvement.

NECK PAIN

A child's unwillingness to move the neck because of pain may be confused with nuchal rigidity. An examination of the neck for muscle spasm and muscle or bone tenderness; a history of trauma, unusual positioning of the neck, or exposure to a draft; radiation of pain to shoulder and arm muscles; and the ability of the examiner to flex and rotate the child's neck, plus the absence of other signs and symptoms, help to make the diagnosis. If a cervical subluxation, fracture, or dislocation is suspected, the neck should be immobilized and appropriate radiographs obtained.

Treatment is directed to the underlying cause. For the most common causes (minor trauma and myositis), analgesic and antiinflammatory medication, along with local heat and a soft cervical collar, constitutes the appropriate treatment.

HISTORY OF PRIOR INFECTION

Acute disseminated encephalomyelitis may occur a few days to weeks after a nonspecific infection, vaccine, or other exposure.

Atlantoaxial subluxation occurring 1 week to 1 month after an upper respiratory tract infection or upper neck inflammatory process is called *Grisel syndrome*. The cause may be softening and stretching, or distention, of spinal ligaments secondary to inflammation. It is most common in children between the ages of 6 and 12 years. Patients present with reduced range of motion in the neck and tenderness over the upper third of the cervical spine in the absence of cervical myalgia. The subluxation can be seen on radiographs of the cervical spine. Treatment includes reducing the subluxation and neck immobilization (cervical collar or traction) for variable periods of time.

CONGENITAL CAUSES

There are several congenital causes of nuchal rigidity. They are caused by inborn errors of metabolism resulting in muscle stiffness or neurologic disorders, congenital anomalies of bone, perinatal problems, and primary neurologic disorders. They are diagnosed from age at onset and associated signs and symptoms.

One common cause is *congenital torticollis* (see Table 52-2). The infant presents in the weeks after birth with limited range of motion in the neck and a fibrous mass in the body of one sternocleidomastoid muscle. The head is tilted toward the affected side, and the chin is rotated to the opposite side. The mass initially increases in size and then resolves in 2 to 6 months, leaving a fibrotic and shortened sternocleidomastoid muscle. Treatment includes massage and stretching

Table 52-12. **Causes of Nuchal Rigidity Other than Meningitis Categorized by Presentation**

Neurologic Signs and Symptoms	Signs and Symptoms of a Specific Disease	Neck Pain	History of Prior Infection	Other
Encephalitis	Upper lobe pneumonia	Cervical spine or rib	Acute disseminated	*Congenital*
Guillain-Barré syndrome	Epiglottitis	osteomyelitis	encephalomyelitis	Ligamentous laxity of
Acute cerebellar ataxia	Pharyngitis-tonsillitis	Diskitis	Atlantoaxial	transverse ligament
Brain abscess	Otitis media-mastoiditis	Osteoid osteoma	dislocation	Hemivertebrae
Epidural abscess	Tuberculosis	Eosinophilic		Klippel-Feil syndrome
Dystonia musculorum	Cat-scratch disease	granuloma		Sprengel deformity
deformans	Herpes zoster	Intraspinal tumor		Arnold-Chiari
Spasmodic torticollis	Tetanus	Osseous tumor of		malformation
Paroxysmal torticollis	Trichinosis	cervical spine		Basilar impression
Huntington chorea	Chagas disease	Rhabdomyosarcoma		Congenital torticollis
Cervical cord	Diphtheria	Lymphoma		Congenital absence of
syringomyelia	Rabies	Facet syndrome		transverse ligament
Chiari crisis: brainstem	Wilson disease	Disk syndrome		Congenital absence or
herniation	Fibrodysplasia ossificans	Acute cervical myalgia		hypertrophy of
Multiple sclerosis	progessiva	Myositis (due to		cervical muscles
Poliomyelitis	Spasmus nutans	draft or positioning)		Intrauterine constraint
Tic and Tourette syndrome	Benign paroxysmal	Fibromyalgia		Hereditary stiff baby
Vestibular dysfunction	vertigo	Tension headache		syndrome
	Reflux esophagitis	Functional torticollis		Infantile Gaucher
Vascular Abnormalities	(Sandifer syndrome)	Calcification of disks		disease
Subarachnoid hemorrhage	Black widow spider bite	Neuritis of spinal		Maple syrup urine
Cerebral aneurysms	Scorpion sting	accessory nerve		disease
Venous and venous sinus	Kawasaki syndrome	Esophageal foreign		Glutaricaciduria
thrombosis	Systemic lupus	body		Cerebral palsy
	erythematosus	Clavicular fracture		Kernicterus
Neoplasms	Sarcoidosis	Cervical spine trauma		
Posterior fossa tumors	Vogt-Koyanagi-			*Intoxications*
Brainstem tumors	Harada syndrome			Phenothiazines
Tumors of 3rd ventricle	Juvenile rheumatoid			Strychnine
Intraspinal tumor	arthritis			Lead
Leaking				Methanol
craniopharyngioma	*Deep Neck Infections*			Vitamin A
Superior oblique muscle	Lateral pharyngeal space			
weakness	Retropharyngeal space			
Congenital nystagmus	Masticator space			
	Visceral space			
Cervical Spine Trauma	Ludwig angina			
Subluxation	Dental infection			
Dislocation	Carotid sheath and			
Fractures	jugular vein thrombosis			
Sprain	Sialoadenitis			
Disc injury	Parotitis			
	Bezold abscess			
	(mastoiditis)			
	Congenital cysts and			
	fistulas			
	Primary deep cervical			
	adenitis			

of the affected muscle and results in resolution of the disorder in 70% of cases.

RED FLAGS

Stiff neck is not synonymous with meningismus, but in a patient with a stiff neck, meningitis must be considered. Patients with meningitis usually have additional symptoms and red flags (fever, headache, irritability, altered mental status). Petechiae and purpura should suggest overwhelming meningococcal or other cause of bacterial meningitis. Affected infants with meningitis are more likely than other patients to have subtle and nonspecific symptoms. Clinical clues to

other causes of stiff neck are listed in Table 52-12. If a cervical spine injury is suspected, the neck should be immobilized until appropriate radiographs are obtained.

REFERENCES

Bacterial Meningitis

Ahmed A: A critical evaluation of vancomycin for treatment of bacterial meningitis. Pediatr Infect Dis J 1997;16:895.
American Academy of Pediatrics Committee on Infectious Diseases: Treatment of bacterial meningitis. Pediatrics 1988;81:904.
Arditi M, Mason EO Jr, Bradley JS, et al: Three-year multicenter surveillance of pneumococcal meningitis in children: Clinical characteristics, and

outcome related to penicillin susceptibility and dexamethasone use. Pediatrics 1998;102:1087.

Baraff LJ, Lee SI, Schriger DL: Outcomes of bacterial meningitis in children: A meta-analysis. Pediatr Infect Dis J 1993;2:389.

Bonadio WA: The cerebrospinal fluid: Physiologic aspects and alterations associated with bacterial meningitis. Pediatr Infect Dis J 1992;11:423.

Bonsu B, Harper MB: Fever interval before diagnosis, prior antibiotic treatment, and clinical outcome for young children with bacterial meningitis. Clin Infect Dis 2001;32:566.

Brown LW, Feigin RD: Bacterial meningitis: Fluid balance and therapy. Pediatr Ann 1994;23:93.

Carraccio CL, Lomonico MP, Fisher MC: Limp as a presenting sign of meningitis. Pediatr Infect Dis J 1990;9:673.

de Gans J, Van de Beek D: Dexamethasone in adults with bacterial meningitis. N Engl J Med 2002;347:1549.

Dodge PR:. Neurological sequelae of acute bacterial meningitis. Pediatr Ann 1994;23:101.

Feigin RD, McCracken GH, Klein JO: Diagnosis and management of meningitis. Pediatr Infect Dis J 1992;11:785.

Freedman SB, Marrocco A, Pirie J, et al: Predictors of bacterial meningitis in the era after *Haemophilus influenzae.* Arch Pediatr Adolesc Med 2001;155:1301.

Friedland IR, Paris MM, Rinderknecht S, et al: Cranial computed tomographic scans have little impact on management of bacterial meningitis. Am J Dis Child 1992;146:1484.

Friedland IR, Shelton S, Paris M, et al: Dilemmas in diagnosis and management of cephalosporin-resistant *Streptococcus pneumoniae* meningitis. Pediatr Infect Dis J 1993;12:196.

Funderburk JG, Steele RW: A child with recurrent meningitis. Clin Pediatr 1998;37:259.

Geiseler PJ, Nelson KE: Bacterial meningitis without clinical signs of meningeal irritation. South Med J 1982;75:448.

Givner LB, Kaplan SL: Meningitis due to *Staphylococcus aureus* in children. Clin Infect Dis 1993;16:766.

Gumerlock MK, Spollen LE, Nelson MJ: Cervical neurenteric fistula causing recurrent meningitis in Klippel-Feil sequence: Case report and literature review. Pediatr Infect Dis J 1991;10:532.

Kanegaye JT, Soliemanzadeh P, Bradley JS: Lumbar puncture in pediatric bacterial meningitis: Defining the time interval for recovery of cerebrospinal fluid pathogens after parenteral antibiotic pretreatment. Pediatrics 2001;108:1169.

Kaplan SL, Catlin FI, Weaver T, et al: Onset of hearing loss in children with bacterial meningitis. Pediatrics 1984;73:575.

Kessler SL, Dajani AS: *Listeria* meningitis in infants and children. Pediatr Infect Dis J 1990;9:61.

Klein JO: Antimicrobial treatment and prevention of meningitis. Pediatr Ann 1994;23:76.

Law DA, Aronoff SC: Anaerobic meningitis in children: Case report and review of the literature. Pediatr Infect Dis J 1992;11:968.

Lieb G, Krauss J, Collmann H, et al: Recurrent bacterial meningitis. Eur J Pediatr 1996;155:26.

Madagame ET, Havens PL, Bresnahan JM, et al: Survival and functional outcome of children requiring mechanical ventilation during therapy for acute bacterial meningitis. Crit Care Med 1995;23:1279.

McIntyre PB, Berkey CS, King SM, et al: Dexamethasone as adjunctive therapy in bacterial meningitis: A meta-analysis of clinical trials since 1988. JAMA 1997;278:925.

Meirovitch J, Kitai-Cohen Y, Keren G, et al: Cerebrospinal fluid shunt infections in children. Pediatr Infect Dis J 1987;6:921.

Nagata M, Hara T, Aoki T, et al: Inherited deficiency of ninth component of complement: An increased risk of meningococcal meningitis. J Pediatr 1989;114:260.

Pomeroy SL, Holmes SJ, Dodge PR, et al: Seizures and other neurologic sequelae of bacterial meningitis in children. N Engl J Med 1990;323:1651.

Radetsky M: Duration of treatment in bacterial meningitis: A historical inquiry. Pediatr Infect Dis J 1990;9:2.

Radetsky M: Duration of symptoms and outcome in bacterial meningitis: An analysis of causation and the implications of a delay in diagnosis. Pediatr Infect Dis J 1992;11:694.

Saez-Llorens X, McCracken GH: Antimicrobial and anti-inflammatory treatment of bacterial meningitis. Infect Dis Clin North Am 1999;13:619.

Schuchat A, Robinson K, Wenger JD, et al: Bacterial meningitis in the United States in 1995. N Engl J Med 1997;337:970.

Snedeker JD, Kaplan SL, Dodge PR, et al: Subdural effusion and its relationship with neurologic sequelae of bacterial meningitis in infancy: A prospective study. Pediatrics 1990;86:163.

Tesoro LJ, Selbst SM: Factors affecting outcome in meningococcal infections. Am J Dis Child 1991;145:218.

Unhanand M, Mustafa MM, McCracken GH, et al: Gram-negative enteric bacillary meningitis: A twenty-one-year experience. J Pediatr 1993; 122:15.

Ward E, Gushurst CA: Uses and technique of pediatric lumbar puncture. Am J Dis Child 1992;146:1160.

Wong M, Schlaggar BL, Buller RS, et al: Cerebrospinal fluid protein concentration in pediatric patients. Arch Pediatr Adolesc Med 2000;154:827.

Aseptic Meningitis and Encephalitis

Achard JM, Lallement PY, Veyssier P: Recurrent aseptic meningitis secondary to intracranial epidermoid cyst and Mollaret's meningitis: Two distinct entities or a single disease? A case report and nosologic discussion. Am J Med 1990;89:807.

Ahmed A, Brito F, Goto C, et al: Clinical utility of the polymerase chain reaction for diagnosis of enteroviral meningitis in infancy. J Pediatr 1997;131:393.

Aufricht C, Tenner W, Stanek G: Aseptic meningitis in the decennium of *Borrelia burgdorferi* infection (Lyme disease). Pediatrics 1991;87:268.

Auxier GG: Aseptic meningitis associated with administration of trimethoprim and sulfamethoxazole. Am J Dis Child 1990;144:144.

Baker RC, Lenane AM: The predictive value of cerebrospinal fluid differential cytology in meningitis. Pediatr Infect Dis J 1989;8:329.

Bia FJ, Barry M: Parasitic infections of the central nervous system. Neurol Clin 1986;4:171.

Dagan R, Jenista JA, Menegus MA: Association of clinical presentation, laboratory findings, and virus serotypes with the presence of meningitis in hospitalized infants with enterovirus infection. J Pediatr 1988;113:975.

Dorfman DH, Glaser JH: Congenital syphilis presenting in infants after the newborn period. N Engl J Med 1990;323:1299.

Golden SE: Aseptic meningitis associated with *Ehrlichia canis* infection. Pediatr Infect Dis J 1989;8:335.

Gutierrez K, Abzug MJ: Vaccine-associated poliovirus meningitis in children with ventriculoperitoneal shunts. J Pediatr 1990;117:424.

Harrison SA, Risser WL: Repeat lumbar puncture in the differential diagnosis of meningitis. Pediatr Infect Dis J 1988;7:143.

Ito Y, Ando Y, Kimura H, et al: Polymerase chain reaction–proved herpes simplex encephalitis in children. Pediatr Infect Dis J 1998;17:29.

Kimberlin DW, Lin CY, Jacobs RF, et al: Natural history of neonatal herpes simplex virus infections in the acyclovir era. Pediatrics 2001;108:223.

Kimberlin DW, Lin CY, Jacobs RF, et al: Safety and efficacy of high-dose intravenous acyclovir in the management of neonatal herpes simplex virus infections. Pediatrics 2001;108:230.

Kitai I, Navas L, Rohlicek C, et al: Recurrent aseptic meningitis secondary to an intracranial cyst: A case report and review of clinical features and imaging modalities. Pediatr Infect Dis J 1992;11:671.

Negrini B, Kelleher KJ, Wald ER: Cerebrospinal fluid findings in aseptic versus bacterial meningitis. Pediatrics 2000;105:316.

Newton RW: Tuberculous meningitis. Arch Dis Child 1994;70:364.

Rao SP, Teitlebaum J, Miller ST: Intravenous immune globulin and aseptic meningitis. Am J Dis Child 1992;146:539.

Rust RS: Multiple sclerosis, acute disseminated encephalomyelitis, and related conditions. Semin Pediatr Neurol 2000;7:66.

Sabetta JR, Andriole VT: Cryptococcal infection of the central nervous system. Med Clin North Am 1985;69:33.

Sugiura A, Yamada A: Aseptic meningitis as a complication of mumps vaccination. Pediatr Infect Dis J 1991;10:209.

Waecker NJ, Connor JD: Central nervous system tuberculosis in children: A review of 30 cases. Pediatr Infect Dis J 1990;9:539.

Whitley RJ, Cobbs CG, Alford CA, et al: Diseases that mimic herpes simplex encephalitis. Diagnosis, presentation, and outcome. JAMA 1989; 262:234.

Wilhelm C, Ellner JJ: Chronic meningitis. Neurol Clin 1986;4:115.

Other Causes of Nuchal Rigidity

Abbassioun K: Fever, meningeal reaction and increased intracranial pressure. Clin Pediatr 1971;10:332.

Beniz J, Forster DJ, Lean JS, et al: Variations in clinical features of the Vogt-Koyanagi-Harada syndrome. Retina 1991;11:275.

Bredenkamp JK, Maceri DR: Inflammatory torticollis in children. Arch Otolaryngol Head Neck Surg 1990;116:310.

Kiwak KJ: Establishing an etiology for torticollis. Postgrad Med 1984;75:126.

Krueger DW, Larson EB: Recurrent fever of unknown origin, coma, and meningismus due to a leaking craniopharyngioma. Am J Med 1988;84:543.

Lund L, Nielsen D, Andersen ES: Meningismus as main symptom in toxic shock syndrome. Acta Obstet Gynecol Scand 1988;67:395.

Reik L: Disorders that mimic CNS infections. Neurol Clin 1986;4:223.

Rizzo JD, Rowe SA: Meningism in a ten-month-old infant during OKT3 therapy. J Heart Transplant 1990;9:727.

Stein MT, Trauner D: The child with a stiff neck. Clin Pediatr 1982;21:559.

Welinder NR, Hoffmann P, Hakansson S: Pathogenesis of non-traumatic atlanto-axial subluxation (Grisel's syndrome). Eur Arch Otorhinolaryngol 1997;254:251.

53 Bites

Martha S. Wright

Bites and stings by animals and insects are common causes of human injury. The spectrum of diseases after these injuries is broad; the recognizable clinical syndromes result from direct trauma, effects of toxins, immune phenomena, and transmitted infections.

MAMMALIAN BITES

Approximately 4.5 million mammalian bites occur each year in the United States and account for 2% of all emergency department visits. Children are at particular risk for significant injury; 70% of dog bite-related fatalities occur in victims younger than 10 years. Between 1% and 15% of all children are injured by animal bites each year.

TYPES OF BITES

Dog. Dog bites account for 80% to 90% of animal bite wounds. Demographic studies reveal that German shepherds, pit bulls, rottweilers, huskies, and mixed breeds are implicated in a disproportionate number of attacks and that the typical pediatric victim is a boy between 5 and 9 years old who provoked a family or neighborhood dog. In young children, 60% to 80% of bites involve the head and neck; in older children and adults, the extremities are most commonly injured.

The animal's large teeth and strong jaw muscles are responsible for the observed patterns of injuries. Dogs tear and crush tissue, producing lacerations, abrasions, and avulsions. Wound infection occurs in 3% to 18% of bites, and other complications such as sepsis, septic arthritis, meningitis, osteomyelitis, tenosynovitis, endophthalmitis, rabies, and tetanus have been reported. In children, scarring and disfigurement may result because of the predilection for bites to the face.

Cat. Cats are responsible for about 10% of reported animal bites annually. Victims of cat bite are more frequently female and are older than dog bite victims (mean age, 19.5 years). In more than 50% of cases, an unknown or stray animal bites a child. The cat's sharp teeth and claws and relatively weak jaw forces predispose the victim to scratches and puncture wounds that may penetrate bone. In adults, more than 80% of cat bites are inflicted on the upper extremities and hands; in children, a third of bites occur on the face and neck. Complications are similar to those seen after dog bites, although wound infections are more common and occur in 29% to 50% of cat bites. In addition, cats are the leading domestic carrier of rabies. Furthermore, cat bites and scratches may lead to cat-scratch disease (see Chapter 47).

Human. Human bites are much less common than dog and cat bites but can be associated with significant complications. More than 50% of human bites occur during fights in children older than 10 years of age. Other causes of "tooth-skin" contact include sports events, play activities, and child abuse. In contrast to injury patterns seen in adults, in whom deep hand lacerations and avulsions predominate, the types of injuries noted in children are usually abrasions involving the hands (knuckles), face, and neck. Wound infection, tenosynovitis, osteomyelitis, amputation, and transmission of various infectious pathogens, including hepatitis B and syphilis, are known complications of human bites.

Rodent. Rat bites are a problem primarily among laboratory workers and children living in poverty. Children younger than 10 years are at greatest risk and account for up to 70% of rat bites. The characteristic rat bite is a puncture wound on the finger or hand that occurs during sleep or during attempts to handle the animal. Rat bites may result in wound infection in fewer than 10% of cases and in transmission of a variety of diseases, including plague (bubonic, pneumonic, septicemic, and meningeal), rat-bite fever, leptospirosis, melioidosis, and tetanus. Rabies transmission by rodents has not been reported in the United States.

DIAGNOSTIC STRATEGIES

Patient care is focused according to the type and immunization status of the animal responsible for the bite, report of unusual behavior in the animal, the time and circumstances of the injury, the immunization status of the victim, and any other victim characteristics that would predispose to infection (splenectomy, immunosuppression).

The physical examination should include careful inspection and exploration of the bite wound, with special attention to altered neurovascular function and joint capsule integrity. Laboratory tests are rarely indicated in the initial evaluation of the acute noninfected wound. Pretreatment cultures in this setting have a low predictive value for causative organisms in wounds that subsequently become infected. Wounds with evidence of infection, however, should be cultured both aerobically and anaerobically. Radiologic studies may be indicated if concern exists for fracture or the presence of a foreign body (e.g., a tooth).

TREATMENT STRATEGIES

The differential diagnosis of a mammalian bite wound is rarely in question. Instead, the dilemma is how to proceed with treatment. Current literature lacks large prospective studies to support many of the recommendations made for wound preparation, laceration repair, and use of prophylactic antibiotics. The aims of management include prevention of infection, maintenance and restoration of function of the injured area, and promotion of wound healing. These goals are effectively accomplished by meticulous wound care combining copious irrigation and débridement of devitalized tissue. Tetanus immunization status should be updated according to standard guidelines. With the exception of bites to the hand and cat bites, surgical closure can be accomplished safely without apparent increase in infection risk. Delayed primary closure is recommended for hand bites.

Epidemiologic studies have identified several types of bites that appear to carry higher than average risk for infection. These include

Table 53-1. Risk Factors for Bite Wound Infections
Hand/foot wounds
Genital area bites
Penetration of bone, joint, tendon sheath structure
Puncture wounds
Crush injuries
Delay in treatment > 24 hours
Cat bites
Immunosuppression (including asplenia)
Presence of foreign material

Table 53-2. Microorganisms Associated with Mammalian Bite Wound Infections

Common	Uncommon
Dogs	
Mixed infection	*Acinetobacter* species
Pasteurella multocida	*Aeromonas hydrophila*
Staphylococcus aureus	α, β, γ Streptococci
Staphylococcus epidermidis	*Bacteroides* species
	Brucella canis
	Capnocytophaga canimorsus (formerly DF-2)
	Enterobacter cloacae
	Enterococcus species
	Escherichia coli
	Klebsiella species
	Moraxella species
	Peptococcus species
	Peptostreptococcus species
	Pseudomonas species
Cats	
P. multocida	*Acinetobacter* species
S. aureus	*Bacteroides* species
	Corynebacterium species
	Enterobacter cloacae
	Fusobacterium species
	Streptococcus species
	S. epidermidis
Humans	
α, β, γ Streptococci	*Enterococcus* species
Bacteroides species	*Eubacterium* species
Corynebacterium species	*Klebsiella pneumoniae*
Eikenella corrodens	*Neisseria* species
Fusobacterium species	*Peptococcus* species
Mixed infection	*Pseudomonas* species
Peptostreptococcus species	*Veillonella* species
S. aureus	

cat puncture wounds; closed-fist and other hand injuries from humans, dogs, or cats; and all bites in immunocompromised patients (Table 53-1). Rodent bites, most minor dog bites, and abrasions or minor lacerations caused by any species in an immunocompetent victim are at no higher risk for infection than other nonbite wounds.

The use of prophylactic antibiotics in both high-risk and low-risk bite wounds has been studied, but consensus regarding efficacy is lacking because of study limitations. These studies suggest that prophylactic antibiotics in uninfected, low-risk, carefully prepared wounds do not decrease the likelihood of infection. Most experts recommend the use of prophylactic antibiotics for high-risk wounds and facial bites, although the evidence on which these recommendations are based is limited by studies with small sample sizes and inconsistent findings.

All infected wounds necessitate antibiotic therapy. Recommended antibiotics include those whose spectrum can address the expected organisms (Table 53-2). Penicillin is active against *Streptococcus* species, the gram-negative anaerobic rod *Eikenella corrodens,* and *Pasteurella multocida,* the infecting agent in 50% to 80% of cat bites and in 15% to 36% of dog bites. Semisynthetic penicillins and first- and second-generation cephalosporins are used to treat *Staphylococcus* species. Dicloxacillin in combination with penicillin; amoxicillin/clavulanate; and, in the penicillin-allergic patient, erythromycin are effective. Amoxicillin/clavulanate has the disadvantage of associated gastrointestinal side effects but eliminates the need for two drugs and is palatable in suspension. The broad-spectrum intravenous agents cefotaxime, ceftriaxone, imipenem/cilastin, and ticarcillin/clavulanate are currently recommended for severe wound infections or septic complications (Table 53-3).

Concern for rabies infection causes many people to seek medical attention after an animal bite. Risk for rabies is greatest after exposure to wild animals, particularly raccoons, skunks, and bats. Most postexposure rabies prophylaxis given in the United States follows dog and cat bites. Treatment guidelines are outlined in Tables 53-4 and 53-5.

RED FLAGS

Dog bite wounds to the head and face in young children have been associated with brain injury and meningitis. Compressive forces of 400 pounds per square inch generated by a dog's jaws can easily fracture an infant's skull. A computed tomographic scan of the head is useful in the assessment of the integrity of the skull and facial bones.

P. multocida typically produces a rapidly progressive, painful cellulitis that develops within 24 hours of the bite. Infections that develop after 24 hours are more frequently caused by *Staphylococcus* or *Streptococcus* species.

Closed-fist injuries contaminated with human oral flora can result in severe, disabling soft tissue infection and osteomyelitis. These wounds necessitate scrupulous wound care, and patients may benefit from evaluation by a hand surgeon.

SNAKEBITE

Of the 45,000 snakebites reported each year in the United States, approximately 8000 are caused by venomous snakes, and a disproportionate number are seen in 5- to 19-year-old male patients. Only 10 to 15 deaths are recorded yearly, but no data are available on morbidity or resulting disability. Most of these attacks occur in the

Table 53-3. Antibiotic Regimens for Bite Wound Therapy

Oral Regimens	Parenteral Regimens
Amoxicillin/clavulanate	Ampicillin/sulbactam
Ciprofloxacin and clindamycin	Ciprofloxacin and clindamycin
Azithromycin	Azithromycin
Penicillin and dicloxacillin	Penicillin and nafcillin
TMP/SMX and clindamycin	TMP/SMX and clindamycin
Cefuroxime	Cefuroxime
Doxycycline and dicloxacillin	Ceftriaxone
	Doxycycline and nafcillin

Adapted from Smith PF, Meadowcroft AM, May DB: Treating mammalian bite wounds. J Clin Pharm Ther 2000;25:85.

TMP/SMX, trimethoprim/sulfamethoxazole.

Table 53-4. Rabies Postexposure Prophylaxis Guide: United States, 1999

Animal Type	Evaluation and Disposition of Animal	Postexposure Prophylaxis Recommendations
Dogs, cats, and ferrets	Healthy and available for 10 days' observation	Persons should not begin prophylaxis unless animal develops clinical signs of rabies*
	Rabid or suspected rabid	Immediately vaccinate
	Unknown (e.g., escaped)	Consult public health officials
Skunks, raccoons, foxes, and most other carnivores; bats	Regarded as rabid unless animal proven negative by laboratory tests[†]	Consider immediate vaccination
Livestock, small rodents, lagomorphs (rabbits and hares), large rodents (woodchucks and beavers), and other mammals	Consider individually	Consult public health officials. Bites of squirrels, hamsters, guinea pigs, gerbils, chipmunks, rats, mice, other small rodents, rabbits, and hares almost never require antirabies postexposure prophylaxis

From the Centers for Disease Control and Prevention: Human rabies prevention: United States 1999. MMWR Morb Mortal Wkly Rep 1999;48(RR-1):1.

*During the 10-day observation period, begin postexposure prophylaxis at the first sign of rabies in a dog, cat, or ferret that has bitten someone. If the animal exhibits clinical signs of rabies, it should be euthanized immediately and tested.

[†]The animal should be euthanized and tested as soon as possible. Holding for observation is not recommended. Discontinue vaccine if immunofluorescence test results of the animal are negative.

southeastern and southwestern United States between April and September, although the two families of indigenous poisonous snakes, Crotalidae (pit vipers) and Elapidae, are distributed throughout the continental United States (Table 53-6).

DIAGNOSTIC STRATEGIES

The first diagnostic challenge is to ascertain whether a poisonous snake inflicted the bite and then to determine whether envenomation occurred. Poisonous snakes can be differentiated from nonpoisonous snakes by directly inspecting the (preferably dead) snake or by a witness's description. Nonpoisonous snakes have round pupils, small teeth instead of fangs, a rounded snout, and no rattle on the tail (Fig. 53-1). Other information that influences the patient's management includes time elapsed since the bite, therapy rendered in the field, development of symptoms, and victim characteristics such as tetanus immunization status.

Inspection of the bite site usually confirms envenomation. Twenty percent of pit viper bites are "dry" and necessitate nothing

Table 53-5. Rabies Postexposure Prophylaxis Schedule: United States, 1999

Vaccination Status	Treatment	Regimen*
Not previously vaccinated	Wound cleansing	All postexposure treatment should begin with immediate thorough cleansing of all wounds with soap and water. If available, a virucidal agent such as a povidone-iodine solution should be used to irrigate the wounds
	RIG	Administer 20 IU/kg body weight. If anatomically feasible, *the full dose should be infiltrated around the wound(s)* and any remaining volume should be administered IM at an anatomic site distant from vaccine administration. Also, RIG should not be administered in the same syringe as vaccine. Because RIG might partially suppress active production of antibody, no more than the recommended dose should be given
	Vaccine	HDCV, RVA, or PCEC, 1.0 mL IM (deltoid area[†]), one each on days 0[‡], 3, 7, 14, and 28
Previously vaccinated[§]	Wound cleansing	All postexposure treatment should begin with immediate thorough cleansing of all wounds with soap and water. If available, a virucidal agent such as a povidone-iodine solution should be used to irrigate the wounds
	RIG	RIG should *not* be administered
	Vaccine	HDCV, RVA, or PCEC, 1.0 mL IM (deltoid area[†]), one each on days 0[‡] and 3

From the Centers for Disease Control and Prevention: Human rabies prevention: United States 1999. MMWR Morb Mortal Wkly Rep 1999;48(RR-1):1.

*These regimens are applicable for all age groups, including children.

[†]The deltoid area is the only acceptable site of vaccination for adults and older children. For younger children, the outer aspect of the thigh may be used. Vaccine should never be administered in the gluteal area.

[‡]Day 0 is the day the first dose of vaccine is administered.

[§]Any person with a history of preexposure vaccination with HDCV, RVA or PCEC; prior postexposure prophylaxis with HDCV, RVA, or PCEC; or previous vaccination with any other type of rabies vaccine and a documented history of antibody response to the prior vaccination.

HDCV, human diploid cell vaccine; IM, intramuscularly; PCEC, purified chick embryo cell vaccine; RIG, rabies immune globulin; RVA, rabies vaccine adsorbed.

Table 53-6. Characteristics of Snakes Indigenous to the United States

	Crotalidae	Elapidae

Representative species	Rattlesnakes (*Crotalus, Sistrurus* species)
	Copperhead (*Agkistrodon contortrix*)
	Water moccasin (*Agkistrodon piscivorus*)
		Coral snakes
		  Eastern: *Micrurus fulvius*
		  Arizona: *Micruroides euryxanthus*

Geographic location	Rattlesnakes: throughout United States Copperhead: Southeast, northeast, west to Texas Water moccasin: Southeast to southern Illinois	Eastern coral snake: Midatlantic and southeastern states east of Mississippi Arizona coral snake: Arizona and New Mexico

Physical characteristics	Triangular-shaped head
	Elliptical pupils
	Two curved maxillary fangs
	Pits located on side of head between eye and
	  nostril
	Some species with "rattles"
		Round head
		2-ft length
		Typical color pattern: black snout with alternating
		  red and black bands; bands bordered by narrow
		  yellow rings
		Two maxillary fangs

Percentage of all snakebites in United States	99%	1%
Clinical characteristics of envenomation		
Local	Intense pain Fang marks (1-2 cm apart) Erythema Swelling Hemorrhagic vesicles Cutaneous necrosis	Minimal pain and swelling Small puncture marks (7-8 mm apart)
Systemic	Coagulopathy, hemolytic anemia Seizures, coma Weakness, paralysis Shock, hypotension Respiratory failure, pulmonary edema Oliguria, hematuria, hemoglobinuria	Malaise Bulbar palsies Generalized weakness Paralysis Respiratory failure
Antivenin	Antivenin (Crotalidae) polyvalent (Wyeth) Fab AV (CroFab) (Savage Laboratories)	Antivenin for *M. fulvius*

more than wound care. An envenomated pit viper wound, however, is immediately painful, with erythema and swelling developing at the site in minutes (Fig. 53-2). Over the next several hours, vesicles and hemorrhagic bullae develop as the swelling increases, in some cases involving the entire limb and ipsilateral trunk. In addition to wound inspection, a complete physical assessment of the patient is necessary. Crotalidae venoms are snake-specific combinations of hemotoxic, neurotoxic, nephrotoxic, and cardiotoxic peptides and necrotizing proteinases that can cause multiple organ system dysfunction. Severity may be judged by the features in Table 53-7. Coral snake venom contains a potent neurotoxin that causes the gradual onset of weakness and flaccid paralysis. These symptoms occur in the absence of local tissue destruction or pain at the bite site.

Laboratory evaluation of the patient with an envenomated snakebite should include complete blood cell count, coagulation studies, type and crossmatch, serum electrolyte measurements, blood urea nitrogen/creatinine measurement, and urinalysis.

DIFFERENTIAL DIAGNOSIS

The symptoms exhibited after a snakebite may overlap those of other clinical entities and cause considerable confusion in the absence of history of snakebite. Pit viper envenomation can mimic septic shock, severe hemolytic anemia, hemolytic-uremic syndrome, and necrotic arachnidism. The weakness and flaccid paralysis of coral snake envenomation are similar to the neurologic manifestations seen in botulism, polio, Guillain-Barré syndrome, transverse myelitis, and spinal cord compression syndromes.

TREATMENT STRATEGIES

The goals of therapy are treatment of systemic and local venom effects, venom inactivation, and prevention of long-term disability. An approach combining supportive care, conscientious wound management, and the appropriate use of antivenin (Fig. 53-3) is the most successful. Very little information on methods of treatment exist, and many of the current recommendations are based on anecdotal reports.

After snakebite, the patient should be transported rapidly to a medical facility. Validated first aid measures, such as splinting and elevation of the injured extremity, continuous suction over the wound with appropriate equipment (The Extractor pump, Sawyer Products, Safety Harbor, Fla.), and application of constriction bands (2- to 4-cm bands placed loosely above the bite to restrict lymphatic flow while allowing arterial and venous blood flow), should be instituted. Suction, if begun within 5 to 10 minutes of a bite, removes 30% to 50% of radiolabeled venom in animal models. There remains some controversy related to the use of constricting bands and suction. Fang mark incisions are no longer advocated, as these do not hasten venom removal and can cause additional tissue and tendon damage if improperly performed. Tourniquets are contraindicated.

In a medical facility, assessments of the wound and major organ function are the first priorities. Treatment of cardiovascular and respiratory dysfunction must be performed urgently. After stabilization, wound care should proceed with irrigation, loose dressing, splinting for comfort, and tetanus immunization. Prophylactic use of broad-spectrum antibiotics is not routinely recommended. Fasciotomies are rarely necessary despite the impressive nature of the swelling, and their use should be based on an objective direct measure of elevated compartment pressure. Previously recommended therapies, including

Venomous Snakes   **Nonvenomous Snakes**

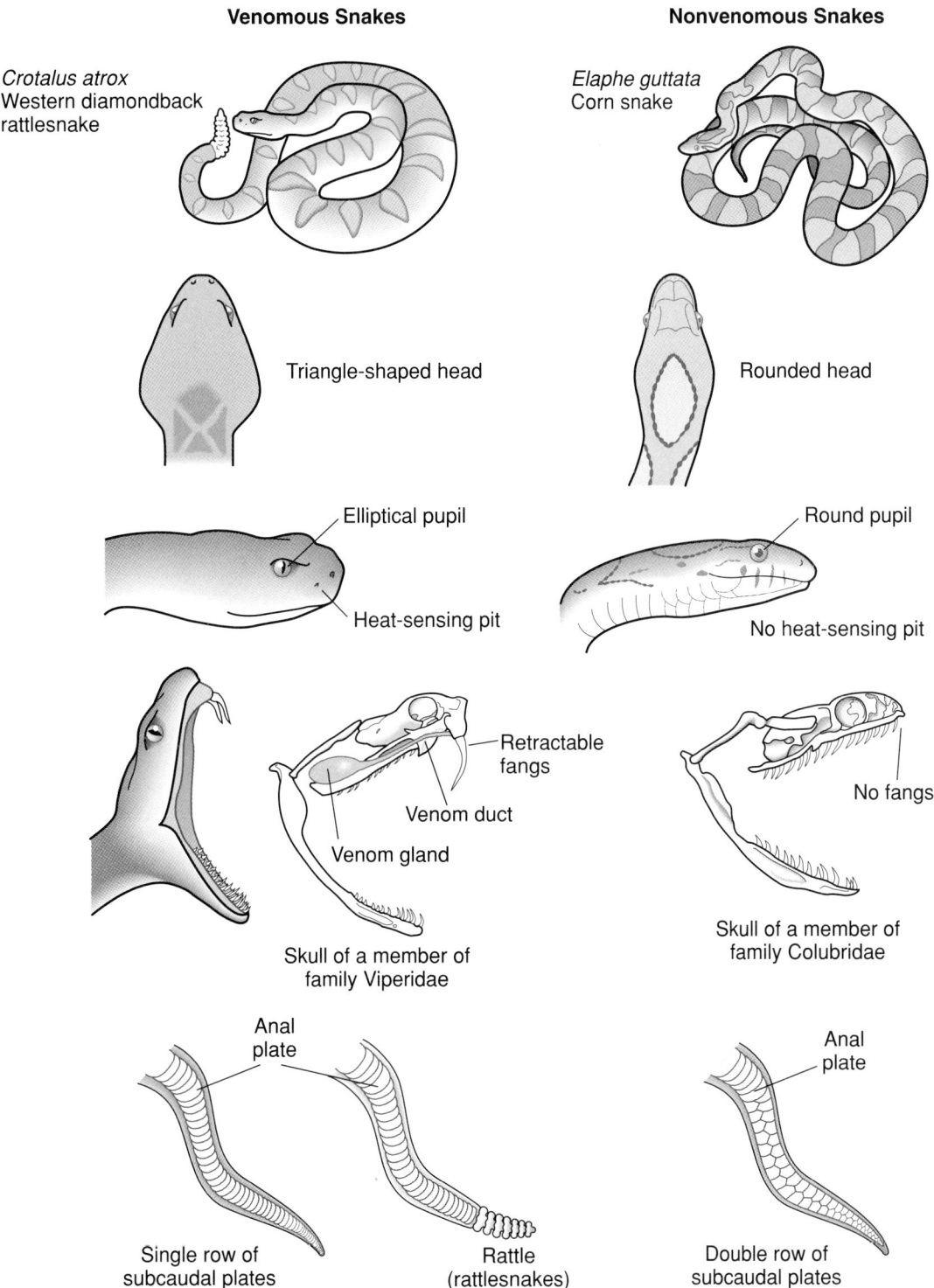

Figure 53-1. Comparison of venomous snakes (pit vipers) and nonvenomous snakes in the United States. (Redrawn from Gold BS, Dart RC, Barish RA: Bites of venomous snakes. N Engl J Med 2002;347:347.)

early wide excision of the wound and use of steroids, do not improve outcome, and cryotherapy and electroshock therapy have proved harmful.

Treatment with antivenin depends on the type of snakebite and the clinical manifestations (see Fig. 53-3). Options include a single polyvalent horse-serum–based antivenin that is effective against all indigenous crotaline species (Antivenin [Crotalidae] polyvalent,

Wyeth-Ayerst, Philadelphia, PA) and sheep serum–derived (ovine) polyclonal, polyvalent antibody fragment (Fab) affinity-purified antivenom (FabAV [CroFab], Savage Laboratories, Melville, NY). Dosage of the horse-serum–based product is based on wound appearance, presence of systemic symptoms, and laboratory test abnormalities (see Table 53-7 and Fig. 53-3). The sheep-serum–derived product is delivered at a standard initial dose of

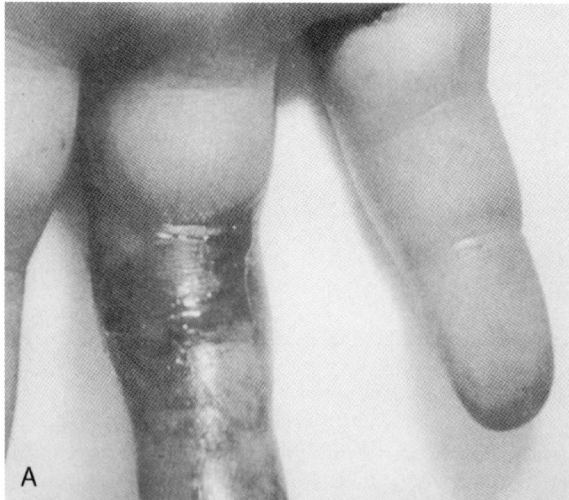
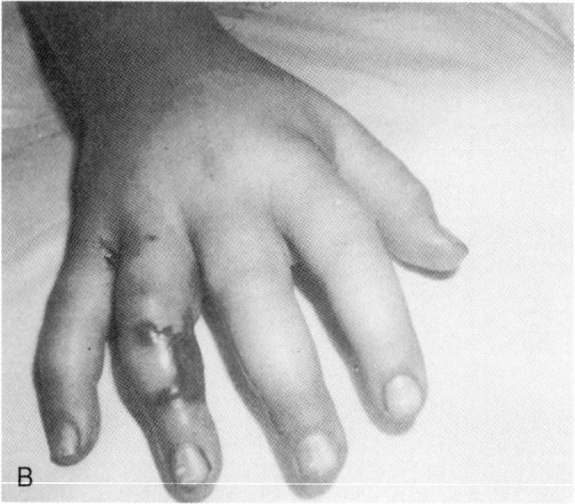

Figure 53-2. A, Crotalid envenomation; photograph taken 60 minutes after bite. Marked swelling and ecchymosis are apparent. Fang marks are barely visible. B, In the same patient, the back of the hand shows extensive swelling. (From Wolf MD: Envenomation. In Holbrook PR [ed]: Textbook of Pediatric Critical Care. Philadelphia, WB Saunders, 1993, p 1028.)

4 to 6 vials and then re-dosed hourly until the envenomation symptoms have stopped progressing. The primary risk associated with the use of antivenin is acute hypersensitivity reaction, including anaphylaxis; serum sickness may occur after treatment. The incidence of these reactions appears to be significantly lower with the sheep-serum–derived product.

Antivenin treatment after known or suspected Eastern coral snakebite is advocated, regardless of the wound characteristics. Administration of three to five vials of *Micrurus fulvius* antivenin given intravenously after skin testing neutralizes the maximum amount of venom injected by this snake and should be given before the progression of neurologic signs. There is no antivenin available for the treatment of Arizona coral snake bites. Questions about therapy should be addressed to a poison control center at 800-222-1222.

RED FLAGS

Coral snakes and some pit vipers, such as the Mojave rattler, can cause unimpressive cutaneous reactions but life-threatening systemic effects. Snakebites in children are generally more severe than in adults because children receive a larger dose of venom per body weight. These patients should be monitored closely in intensive care

settings. Knowledge of locally indigenous snakes is helpful for making decisions to use antivenin after pit viper bites.

MARINE ANIMAL BITES

The exact incidence of injuries to children from marine animals is not known, but geographic proximity to the marine environment and family leisure activities along the coasts increase the chance of exposure to and injury by these creatures.

TYPES OF BITES

Stingray. A deep puncture wound of the lower extremity in a person wading in a warm tidal pool is the typical injury. The aptly named stingray is responsible for more human stings than any other marine vertebrate, accounting for as many as 2000 injuries per year. When disturbed in its location on the sandy bottoms of secluded bays and lagoons, the stingray reflexively whips its tail upward, jabbing a serrated, retropointed spine into the victim (Fig. 53-4). A heat-labile venom containing serotonin, phosphodiesterase, and 5'-nucleotidase is injected into the wound.

The spine creates a lacerated puncture wound on the lower extremity that is contaminated by debris, slime, and spinous fragments. Abdominal and chest wounds can occur and are associated with major organ damage. Pain at the site is intense, worsening over 30 to 90 minutes and lasting as long as 2 days. Systemic signs and symptoms such as nausea, seizures, hypotension, and muscle cramps frequently develop, whereas arrhythmias, paralysis, and death, although reported, are rare.

Jellyfish. Of the 100 species of coelenterates that are hazardous to humans, the majority are located in the Indo-Pacific oceans. In the United States, significant injuries are seen after contact with the Atlantic (*Physalia physalis*) and the Pacific (*Physalia utriculus*) Portuguese man-of-war and the lion's mane (*Cyanea capillata*). Found in the warm coastal waters during the summer months, these large jellyfish inject venom into the victim from nematocysts that line their 75-foot-long tentacles.

The components of the venom are species-specific and affect the cardiovascular, autonomic, and central nervous systems by destabilizing cell membranes and altering calcium channel function. Tentacles and nematocysts leave evidence of a jellyfish attack on the skin in a characteristic "whip mark" pattern associated with urticaria, erythema, and vesiculation. Children are more likely to experience systemic effects, such as fever, chills, muscle spasms, hypotension, paralysis, and centrally mediated respiratory failure, because of the injection of a larger dose of venom in relation to body weight.

Anemones, Corals. Hard and soft corals and anemones found along the United States coasts present minimal risk of serious envenomation to snorkelers and swimmers. Although these animals possess nematocysts that sting, the venom is rarely responsible for more than a burning sensation and a pruritic wheal at the site of injury. The greater risk for morbidity arises from abrasions and lacerations caused by contact with the rough exoskeletons of hard corals that become infected with organisms from the marine or cutaneous environment.

Echinoderms. Sea urchins and starfish species indigenous to United States coastal waters are not dangerously venomous like their tropical relatives, but they do present a risk for puncture wounds to the curious child who unwittingly steps on or handles these animals. Puncture wounds from the spines are intensely painful, erythematous, and edematous. Wound tattooing from the purple or black spines may

Table 53-7. Guidelines for Assessing the Severity of North American Pit Viper Envenomations*

Type of Signs or Symptoms	Severity of Envenomation		
	Minimal	*Moderate*	*Severe*
Local	Swelling, erythema, or ecchymosis confined to the site of the bite	Progression of swelling, erythema, or ecchymosis beyond the site of the bite	Rapid swelling, erythema, or ecchymosis involving the entire body part
Systemic	No systemic signs or symptoms	Non–life-threatening signs and symptoms (nausea, vomiting, perioral paresthesias, myokymia, and mild hypotension	Markedly severe signs and symptoms (hypotension [systolic blood pressure <80 mm Hg], altered sensorium, tachycardia, tachypnea, and respiratory distress
Coagulation	No coagulation abnormalities or other important laboratory abnormalities	Mildly abnormal coagulation profile without clinically significant bleeding; mild abnormalities on other laboratory tests	Markedly abnormal coagulation profile with evidence of bleeding or threat of spontaneous hemorrhage (unmeasurable INR, APTT, and fibrinogen; severe thrombocytopenia with platelet count <20,000/mm^3); results of other laboratory tests may be severely abnormal

From Gold BS, Dart RC, Barish RA: Bites of venomous snakes. N Engl J Med 2002;347:347-356.

*The ultimate grade of severity of any envenomation is determined on the basis of the most severe sign, symptom, or laboratory abnormality (e.g., systolic blood pressure of <70 mm Hg in the absence of local swelling should be graded as a severe envenomation).

APTT, activated partial thromboplastin; INR, international normalized ratio.

result. Systemic effects are exceedingly rare and are similar to those seen after jellyfish envenomation. Late complications include granuloma formation, delayed inflammatory reactions, and infection.

DIAGNOSTIC STRATEGIES

Information regarding the circumstances of the injury may help identify the offending animal. The victim's tetanus status and immunocompetence should be ascertained. Inspection of the wound for the characteristics previously described guides therapy. Attention to cardiovascular and neurologic parameters is important because systemic effects of venoms typically affect these organ systems.

DIFFERENTIAL DIAGNOSIS

The differential diagnosis of these injuries is frequently complicated by the victim's inability to identify the animal. However, the type of wound produced, the location of the wound, and the systemic symptoms after the bite or sting may narrow the diagnostic focus. Painful puncture wounds and lacerations are produced by stingrays, echinoderms, and a variety of poisonous fish, including scorpionfish and stonefish. Cutaneous urticaria and vesicle formation, especially in a linear pattern, are usually the result of contact with jellyfish, anemones, or soft coral.

TREATMENT STRATEGIES

Treatment is directed at maintaining cardiovascular and neurologic stability, pain control, and venom inactivation. Specific interventions may be based on wound characteristics if the offending organism cannot be conclusively identified (Fig. 53-5). Wound care should be performed to prevent secondary infection, and tetanus immunization should be given if necessary. The efficacy of prophylactic antibiotics in otherwise healthy patients is unproven. Antibiotics are indicated, however, for infected wounds and wounds in immunocompromised patients who are at high risk for overwhelming infection with *Vibrio* species. Broad-spectrum agents should cover the expected organisms

(Table 53-8). Trimethoprim-sulfamethoxazole is a reasonable choice for children, and tetracycline or ciprofloxacin is used in older patients.

ARTHROPOD BITES

Of the one million species in the insect kingdom, the order Hymenoptera and the class Arachnida contain the few members that pose the greatest medical threat to humans.

HYMENOPTERA

Honeybees, wasps, yellow jackets, and fire ants are found throughout the United States and are responsible for the largest number of insect bites brought to medical attention. These insects envenomate their victim with immunoreactive substances that cause annoying local reactions and can trigger synthesis of immunoglobulin E (IgE) antibodies that can mediate systemic anaphylaxis on subsequent reexposure. Non-IgE immune-mediated reactions may also follow exposure to Hymenoptera venom and include a serum sickness–like syndrome, Guillain-Barré syndrome, acute glomerulonephritis, thrombocytopenic purpura, and transverse myelitis.

Bees. Bees attack their victims with barbed stingers that remain in the wounds and must be removed carefully to prevent further envenomation. A bee sting causes immediate pain and gradual development of local swelling, erythema, and pruritus. Systemic reactions, including nausea, vomiting, diarrhea, and fever, have been noted in adults after attacks by swarms.

Wasps, Hornets, Yellow Jackets. These insects have smooth stingers that can be used repeatedly to inject venom. Local and systemic reactions are similar to those seen after bee stings.

Fire Ants. Fire ants are found throughout the southern United States. These insects swarm from their hill when disturbed and

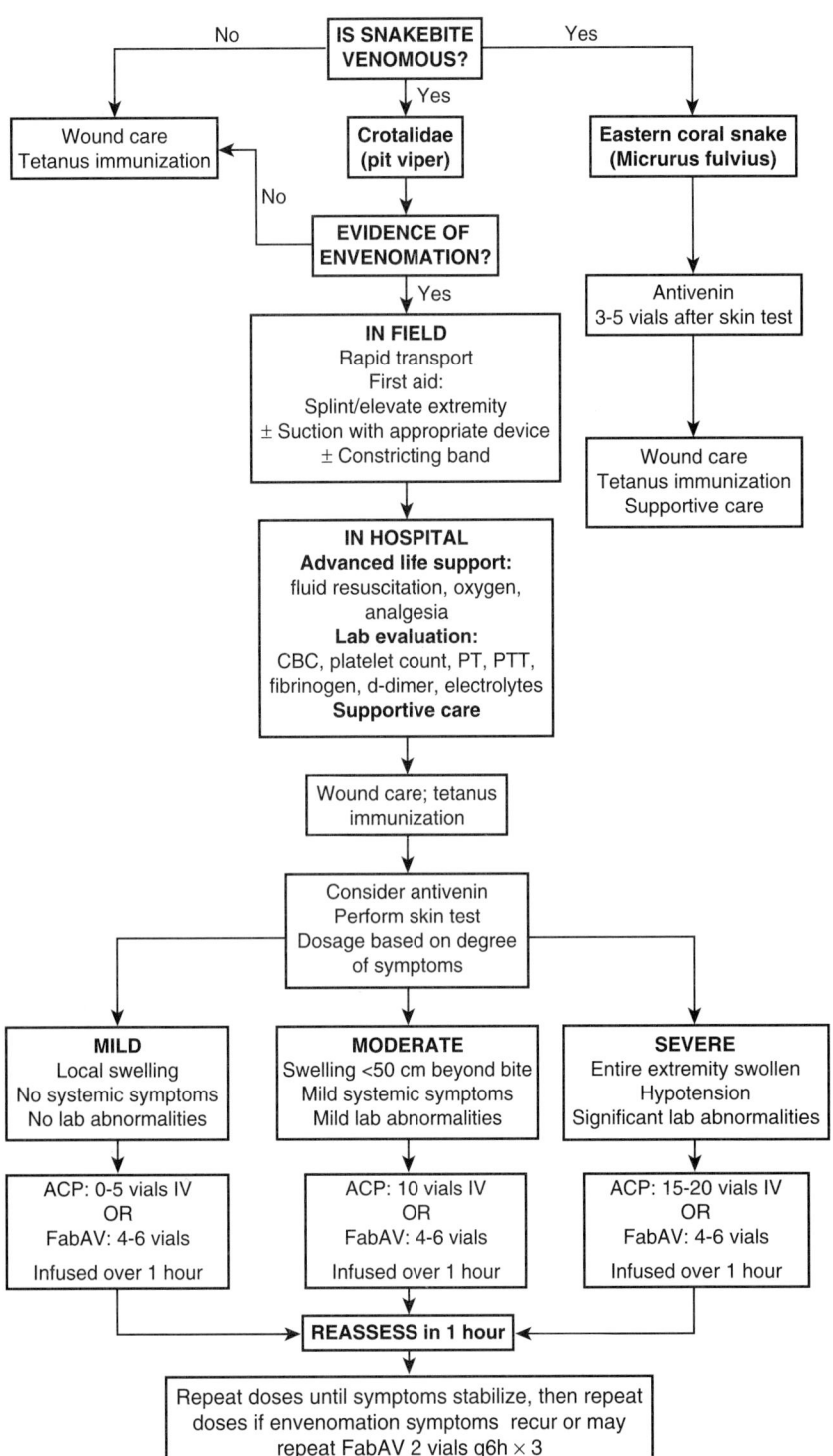

Figure 53-3. Treatment of snakebite. Symptoms of moderate envenomation include weakness, paresthesias, tachycardia and hypotension; laboratory findings include hemoconcentration, low fibrinogen level and thrombocytopenia. Symptoms of severe envenomation include hypotension, shock, hemorrhage and respiratory distress; laboratory findings include anemia, acidosis and coagulopathy. ACP, Antivenin (Crotalidae) polyvalent, Wyeth-Ayerst, Philadelphia, PA; CBC, complete blood cell count; FabAV, Polyvalent, ovine-derived, polyclonal antibody fragment antivenin (CroFab), Savage Laboratories, Melville, NY; PT, prothrombin time; PTT, partial thromboplastin time.

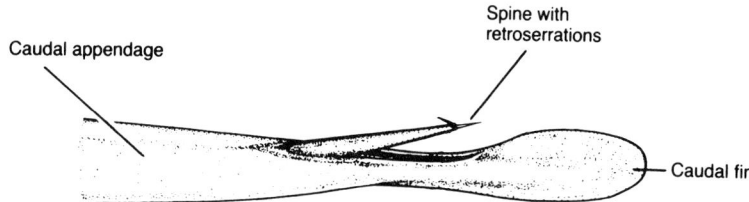

Figure 53-4. Venomous apparatus of the stingray. Venom is stored in acini below the skin of the caudal appendage and is released after puncture by the spine. (Adapted from Kreuzinger R: In Halstead BW [ed]: Poisonous and Venomous Marine Animals of the World. Princeton, NJ, Darwin Press, 1978. Reprinted from Wolf MD: Envenomation. In Holbrook PR [ed]: Textbook of Pediatric Critical Care. Philadelphia, WB Saunders, 1993, p 1037.)

attack the victim en masse, injecting venom that causes severe pain and burning. Each ant sting produces a small erythematous wheal surrounding a sterile pustule.

Diagnostic Strategies

Knowledge of previous allergic reactions, insect type, time and circumstances of the sting, and development of symptoms guides patient treatment. After Hymenoptera stings, patients should be assessed for cardiovascular and respiratory dysfunction and other signs of anaphylaxis.

Differential Diagnosis

Anaphylaxis is the syndrome resulting from antigen-triggered, IgE-mediated release of histamine and other vasoactive substances from mast cells. Sixty to 80 deaths from insect sting–induced anaphylaxis occur yearly, mostly in adults. Between 0.5% and 5% of the United States population has had a significant allergic reaction to bee stings, but up to 80% of all deaths from such stings are reported in persons with no history of hypersensitivity.

The clinical syndrome of anaphylaxis develops within 30 minutes of a sting and is characterized by symptoms in two or more organ systems (Table 53-9). Death results either from hypoxemia secondary to airway obstruction or from cardiac failure secondary to shock. The differential diagnosis of anaphylaxis includes asthma, hereditary angioneurotic edema, vasovagal syncope, other types of distributive shock, upper airway infections, sepsis, and scombroid fish poisoning.

Treatment Strategies

Anaphylaxis therapy is directed at relieving airway edema (epinephrine, intubation) or bronchospasm (epinephrine, β-agonist aerosols [albuterol]) and at improving perfusion (intravenous fluids, epinephrine). This is followed by relieving the other systemic effects of histamine (antihistamines H₁ and H₂ blockers) and other mediators (corticosteroids), suppressing further histamine release and mediator synthesis, and blocking histamine tissue receptors (H₁ and H₂ receptor antagonists) (Fig. 53-6). In mild cases, patient comfort and relief from pruritus are achieved with antihistamines. In severe cases, however, cardiovascular and respiratory support may be required. Patients experiencing bee sting anaphylaxis should be skin tested and offered desensitization therapy. Progressive desensitization is highly effective at preventing future anaphylactic reactions.

Red Flags

Anaphylaxis can have a biphasic course in which the patient's initial histamine-related symptoms resolve but return several hours later. These late symptoms are caused by synthesized mediators, such as prostaglandins, leukotrienes, and kinins. When the clinician is planning the disposition (hospitalization or home care) for a patient after an acute anaphylactic reaction, the potential for symptom recurrence should be considered.

ARACHNIDA

Spiders. In the United States, only two spiders have been responsible for fatal outcomes: the black widow (*Latrodectus mactans*) and the brown recluse (*Loxosceles reclusa*). All spiders are venomous, but only the black widow and a handful of others, of which the brown recluse is the best known, are capable of causing serious symptoms.

Black Widow. The black widow spider is a nonaggressive insect that lives under rocks and in woodpiles throughout the continental United States. Only the female black widow spider, which injects a potent neurotoxin at the time of the bite, is poisonous to humans. This spider measures 15 to 18 mm, has a shiny black body, and has the characteristic red hourglass-shaped marking on her abdomen (Fig. 53-7).

Although the bite itself is usually painless, patients may describe a vague burning sensation at the site. Within an hour after envenomation, severe muscle spasms of the abdomen, back, and chest; hypertension; and descending paresthesia, especially in the soles of the feet, develop. Cholinergic symptoms may be present and include diaphoresis, increased salivation, lacrimation, vomiting, and diarrhea. These symptoms, caused by venom-mediated synaptic acetylcholine and norepinephrine release, generally resolve in 24 to 48 hours, although malaise and dysphoria may persist for 2 to 4 weeks.

Because the spider is rarely recovered and the bite may be undetected, the diagnosis is usually based on clinical features. The observed symptom complex must be differentiated from appendicitis, peritonitis, electrolyte disturbances, and cholinergic crisis from organophosphate poisoning or other toxins.

Treatment is directed at circulatory support, analgesia, and muscle spasm relief. Benzodiazepines and opioid analgesics appear to be most effective in managing the pain. Calcium gluconate has been recommended in a number of anecdotal reports for pain relief; however, the effect is transient and inconsistent, and there is little experience with pediatric envenomation. Antivenin is available (Merck, Sharpe, and Dohme) for patients with life-threatening hypertension or pain that is unrelieved by narcotics. A single dose of one vial is recommended after skin testing for patients younger than 12 years and older than 65 years, because persons in these age groups tend to be the most severely affected.

Brown Recluse. The brown recluse spider is the most familiar representative of a group of spiders responsible for the syndrome known as "necrotic arachnidism." These spiders inject enzyme-rich venom that causes extensive local skin necrosis and a variety of systemic symptoms.

The brown recluse spider is found in the southeastern and midwestern United States, especially Missouri, Arkansas, Oklahoma, and Kansas, where it can be found in dark areas under rocks and in woodpiles. It is not aggressive, but it bites defensively when disturbed. This brown spider displays a characteristic violin-shaped marking on its dorsal cephalothorax (Fig. 53-8).

The bite of a necrotizing spider frequently goes unnoticed by the victim for several hours, after which local itching, redness, and pain

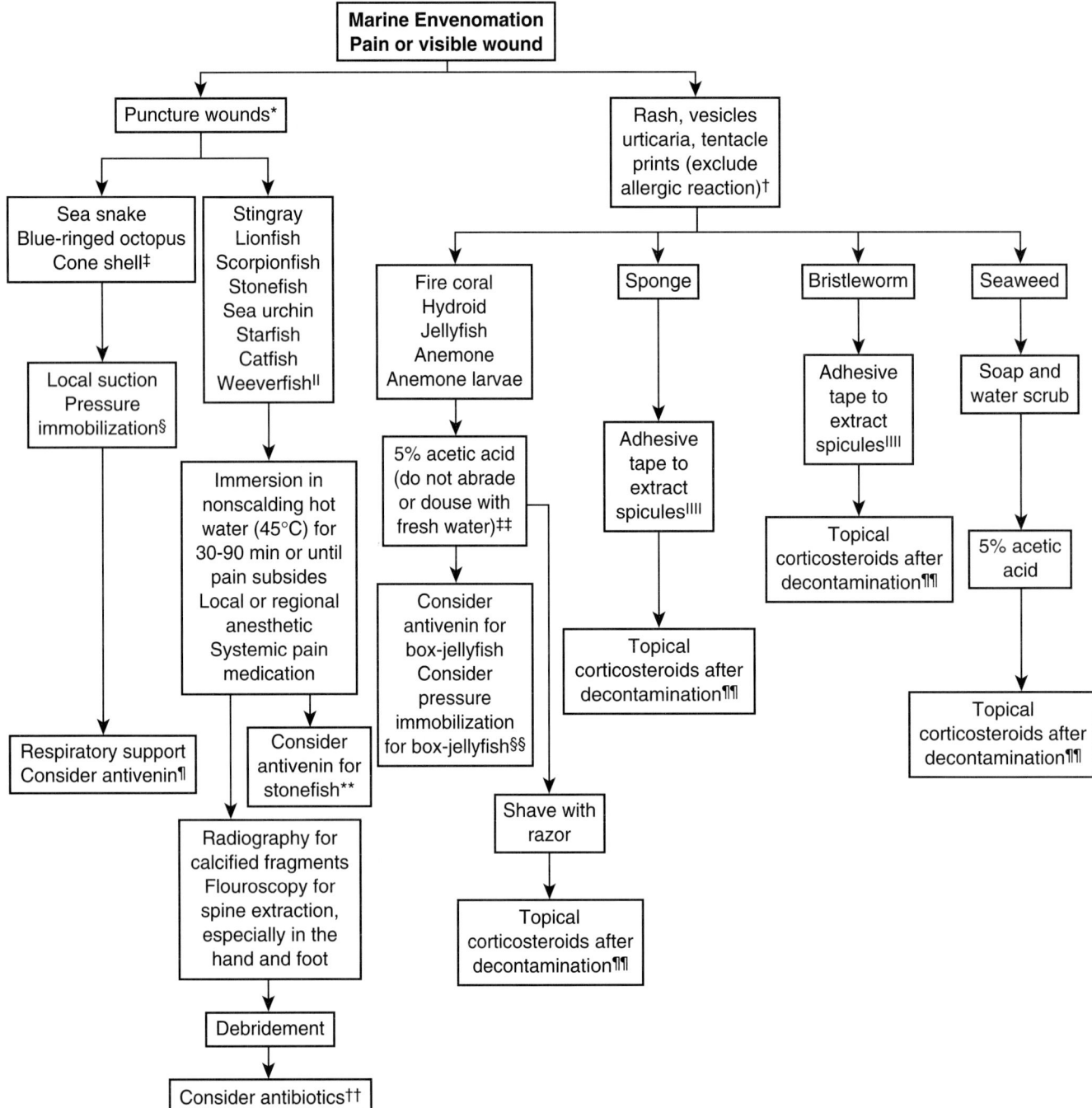

Figure 53-5. An algorithmic approach to marine envenomations. *A gaping laceration, particularly of the lower extremity, with cyanotic edges suggests a stingray wound. Multiple punctures in an erratic pattern with or without purple discoloration or retained fragments are typical of a sea urchin sting. One to eight (usually two) fang marks are usually present after a sea snake bite. A single ischemic puncture wound with an erythematous halo and rapid swelling suggests scorpionfish envenomation. Blisters often accompany a lionfish sting. Painless punctures with paralysis suggest the bite of a blue-ringed octopus; the site of a cone shell sting is punctate, painful, and ischemic in appearance. †Wheal and flare reactions are nonspecific. Rapid (within 24 hours) onset of skin necrosis suggests an anemone sting. "Tentacle prints" with cross-hatching or a frosted appearance are pathognomonic for box-jellyfish (*Chironex fleckeri*) envenomation. Ocular or intraocular lesions may be caused by fragmented hydroids or coelenterate tentacles. An allergic reaction must be treated promptly. ‡Sea snake venom causes weakness, respiratory paralysis, myoglobinuria, myalgias, blurred vision, vomiting, and dysphagia. The blue-ringed octopus injects tetrodotoxin, which causes rapid neuromuscular paralysis. §If *immediately* available (which is rarely the case), local suction can be applied, without incision, by means of a plunger device, such as the Extractor (Sawyer Products, Safety Harbor, Fla.). As soon as possible, venom should be sequestered locally with a proximal venous-lymphatic occlusive band of constriction or (preferably) the pressure immobilization technique, in which a cloth pad is compressed directly over the wound by an elastic wrap that should encompass the entire extremity at a pressure of 9.33 kPa (70 mm Hg) or less. Incision and suction are not recommended. ¶Early ventilatory support has the greatest influence on outcome. The minimal initial dose of sea snake antivenin is one to three vials; up to 10 vials may be required.

Continued

Figure 53-5, cont'd. ‖‖The wounds range from large lacerations (stingrays) to minute punctures (stonefish). Persistent pain after immersion in hot water suggests a stonefish sting or a retained fragment of spine. The puncture site can be identified by forcefully injecting 1% to 2% lidocaine or another local anesthetic agent without epinephrine near the wound and observing the egress of fluid. The clinician should not attempt to crush the spines of sea urchins if they are present in the wound. Spine dye from already-extracted sea urchin spines will disappear (be absorbed) in 24 to 36 hours. **The initial dose of stonefish antivenin is one vial per two puncture wounds. ††The antibiotics chosen should cover *Staphylococcus, Streptococcus,* and microbes of marine origin, such as *Vibrio.* ‡‡Five percent acetic acid (vinegar) is a good all-purpose decontaminant and is mandated for the sting from a box-jellyfish. Alternatives, depending on the geographic region and indigenous jellyfish species, include isopropyl alcohol, bicarbonate (baking soda), ammonia, and preparations containing these agents. §§The initial dose of box-jellyfish antivenin is one ampule intravenously or three ampules intramuscularly. ¶¶If inflammation is severe, steroids should be given systemically (beginning with at least 2 mg/kg/day [maximum, 100 mg] of prednisone or its equivalent) and the dosage tapered over a period of 10 to 14 days. ‖‖‖An alternative is to apply and remove commercial facial peel materials, followed by topical soaks of 30 mL of 5% acetic acid (vinegar) diluted in 1 L of water for 15 to 30 minutes several times a day until the lesions begin to resolve. Surface desquamation should be anticipated in 3 to 6 weeks. (Reprinted with permission from Auerbach PS: Marine envenomations. In Auerbach PS [ed]: Wilderness Medicine: Management of Wilderness and Environmental Emergencies, 3rd ed. St. Louis: Mosby-Yearbook, 1995, p 1327.)

develop. Over the next several days, the center of the lesion turns black, and a slowly healing ulcer remains after the eschar sloughs. Nausea, vomiting, fever, headache, arthralgias, and myalgias are common features. Severe hemolytic anemia, seizures, renal failure, and shock are rarely reported. Children are bitten more frequently than adults and are more likely to have severe manifestations, especially hemolytic anemia. Diagnosis may be aided by an enzyme-linked immunosorbent assay for *Loxosceles* toxin.

Treatment requires conscientious wound care with skin grafting as necessary, tetanus prophylaxis, and management of systemic symptoms. Specific modalities, such as local steroid injection, systemic corticosteroids, early wide excision of the lesion, local infiltration with phentolamine, and use of oral dapsone, which decreases the local infiltration of neutrophils into the envenomated area, have been advocated, but none have proven beneficial in affecting the outcome. Systemic steroids may be useful in the management of hemolytic anemia.

Scorpions. Of the 650 species of scorpions in the world, only one species dangerous to humans is found in the United States. The bark scorpion, or *Centruroides exilicauda,* makes its home in Arizona, Texas, southern California, and northern Mexico and is responsible for the majority of deaths reported from scorpion envenomation. The scorpion contains a potent neurotoxin in specialized glands at the base of its tail. Humans are stung when they disturb the scorpions in their hiding places under rocks and logs or in clothing and shoes. Children weighing less than 45 kg are especially vulnerable to the effects of the venom.

Scorpion venom causes acetylcholine and catecholamine release and calcium channel dysfunction. After a sting, there is vague discomfort, tingling, and hyperesthesia at the site. Within 60 minutes, hyperactivity, restlessness, roving eye movements, tachycardia, and hypertension as well as cholinergic symptoms of salivation, lacrimation, vomiting, bronchorrhea, and wheezing develop and persist for as long as 36 hours (Table 53-10).

Table 53-8. Microorganisms Associated with Infection in Marine-Acquired Wounds

Aeromonas hydrophila
Bacteroides fragilis
Chromobacterium violaceum
Clostridium perfringens
Erysipelothrix rhusiopathiae
Escherichia coli
Mycobacterium marinum
Pseudomonas aeruginosa
Salmonella enteritidis
Staphylococcus aureus
Streptococcus species
Vibrio parahaemolyticus
Vibrio vulnificus

Adapted from Auerbach PS: Marine envenomations. N Engl J Med 1991;325:486.

Table 53-9. Clinical Manifestations of Anaphylaxis

Skin	**Gastrointestinal**
Urticaria	Nausea
Flushing	Vomiting
Angioedema	Diarrhea
Pruritus	
Pulmonary	**Neurologic**
Bronchospasm	Disorientation
Upper airway obstruction	Feeling of impending doom
Cardiovascular	
Hypotension	
Dysrhythmias	
Shock	

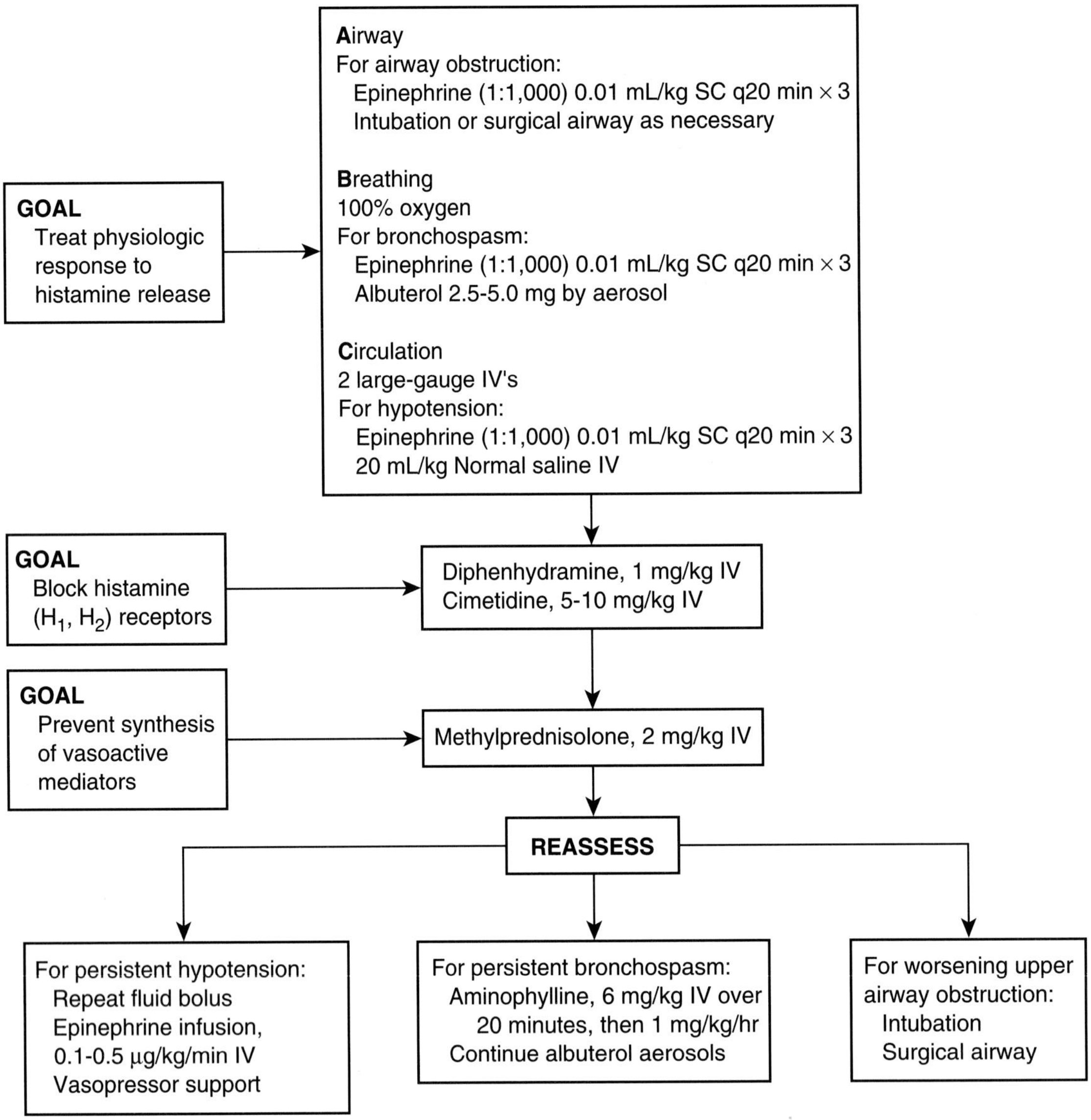

Airway
For airway obstruction:
  Epinephrine (1:1,000) 0.01 mL/kg SC q20 min × 3
  Intubation or surgical airway as necessary

Breathing
100% oxygen
For bronchospasm:
  Epinephrine (1:1,000) 0.01 mL/kg SC q20 min × 3
  Albuterol 2.5-5.0 mg by aerosol

Circulation
2 large-gauge IV's
For hypotension:
  Epinephrine (1:1,000) 0.01 mL/kg SC q20 min × 3
  20 mL/kg Normal saline IV

GOAL
Treat physiologic response to histamine release

GOAL
Block histamine (H_1, H_2) receptors

Diphenhydramine, 1 mg/kg IV
Cimetidine, 5-10 mg/kg IV

GOAL
Prevent synthesis of vasoactive mediators

Methylprednisolone, 2 mg/kg IV

REASSESS

For persistent hypotension:
  Repeat fluid bolus
  Epinephrine infusion, 0.1-0.5 µg/kg/min IV
  Vasopressor support

For persistent bronchospasm:
  Aminophylline, 6 mg/kg IV over 20 minutes, then 1 mg/kg/hr
  Continue albuterol aerosols

For worsening upper airway obstruction:
  Intubation
  Surgical airway

Figure 53-6. Treatment of anaphylaxis. IV, intravenously; SC, subcutaneously.

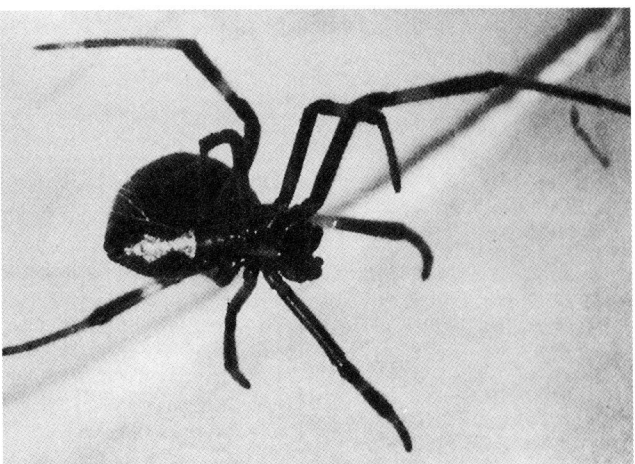

Figure 53-7. The female black widow spider has a shiny, black, globular body with a red hourglass-shaped mark on the abdomen. (From Paton BC: Bites—Human, dog, spider and snake. Surg Clin North Am 1963;43:537.)

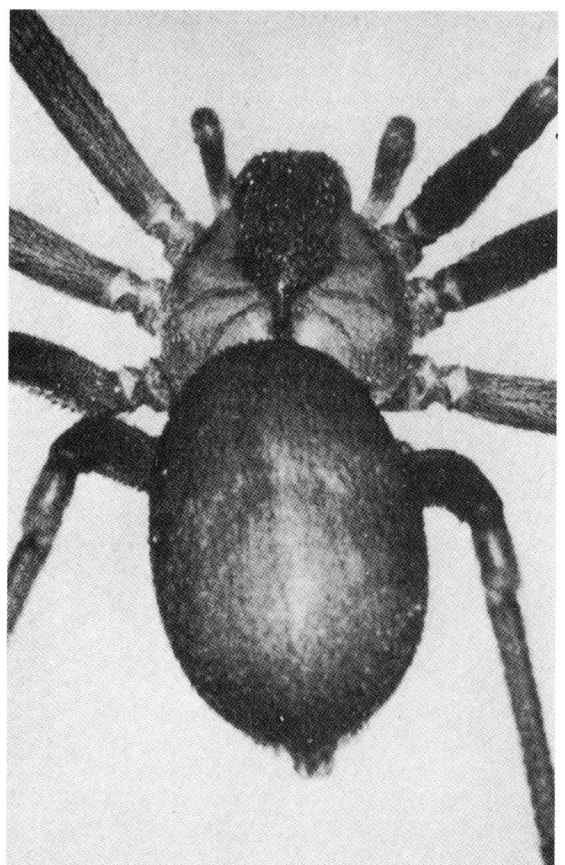

Figure 53-8. The brown recluse spider is 10 to 15 mm long, is light tan to dark brown in color, and has a species-specific dorsal, dark, violin-shaped band. (From Dillaha CJ, Jansen GT, Honeycutt WM, Hayden CR: North American loxoscelism. Necrotic bite of the brown recluse spider. JAMA 1964;188:33.)

Table 53-11. Tickborne Diseases in the United States

Disease	Agent	Region
Lyme disease	*Borrelia burgdorferi*	Northeast, Wisconsin, Minnesota, California
Relapsing fever	*Borrelia* species	West
Tularemia	*Francisella tularensis*	Arkansas, Missouri, Oklahoma
Rocky Mountain spotted fever	*Rickettsia rickettsii*	Southeast, West, south central United States
Q fever	*Rickettsia burnetii*	Southwest, West
Ehrlichiosis	*Ehrlichia chaffeensis*	South central, South, Atlantic, upper midwest
Colorado tick fever	*Coltivirus* species	West
Babesiosis	*Babesia* species	Northeast

Adapted from Spach DH, Liles WC, Campbell GL, et al: Tickborne diseases in the United States. N Engl J Med 1993;329:936.

Table 53-10. Scorpion Envenomation

Grade 1:	Local discomfort and paresthesia
Grade 2:	Pain and paresthesia extend up the extremity
Grade 3:	Motor hyperkinesis
	Cranial nerve dysfunction
	Dysphagia
	Roving eyes
	Facial paresthesia
	Restlessness
Grade 4:	Cranial nerve dysfunction
	Drooling, uncontrollable eye movements
	Fasciculations, facial and distal muscles
	Neuromuscular hyperactivity
	Opisthotonos
	Convulsions
	Wheezing
	Hyperthermia
	Cyanosis

From Wolf MD: Envenomation. In Holbrook PR (ed): Textbook of Pediatric Critical Care. Philadelphia, WB Saunders, 1993, p 1024.

Marked agitation and restlessness are the most prominent clinical features but may suggest other causes, such as encephalitis, phenothiazine toxicity, movement disorders, or seizures.

Treatment is directed at supporting cardiorespiratory function and pain control. Young children frequently require hospitalization, monitoring, and sedation. Goat serum antivenin is available in Arizona but has not been approved by the Food and Drug Administration.

Ticks. Ticks threaten human health in their role as vectors for a variety of rickettsial, bacterial, and spirochetal diseases (Table 53-11) and through the toxin-mediated syndrome of tick paralysis. These arthropods inhabit grassy fields and woodlands throughout the United States. The bite itself is rarely cause for alarm although granuloma formation is known to occur at the site and certain spirochetal diseases may produce characteristic lesions (erythema migrans in Lyme disease; see Chapter 44). In general, tick bites go unnoticed, and only about 50% of patients with proven tickborne diseases relate a tick bite history.

Tick paralysis is characterized by motor weakness or acute ataxia that progresses into an ascending flaccid paralysis. As the result of a neurotoxin elaborated at the bite site that blocks acetylcholine release at the neuromuscular junction, clinical symptoms disappear when the tick is removed. These neurologic symptoms must be distinguished from those of Guillain-Barré syndrome, poliomyelitis, spinal cord compression syndromes, and botulism (see Chapter 38).

REFERENCES

Mammalian Bites

Abrahamian FM: Dog bites: Bacteriology, management and prevention. Curr Infect Dis Rep 2000;2:446.

American Academy of Pediatrics: Bite wounds. In Pickering LK (ed): 2003 Red Book Report of the Committee on Infectious Diseases, 26th ed. Elk Grove Village, Ill, American Academy of Pediatrics, 2003, p 182.

Brogan TV, Bratton SL, Dowd MD, Hegenbarth MA: Severe dog bites in children. Pediatrics 1995;96:947.

Centers for Disease Control and Prevention: Human rabies prevention: United States, 1999: Recommendations of the Advisory Committee on Immunization Practices. MMWR Morb Mortal Wkly Rep 1999; 48(RR-1):1.

Cummings P: Antibiotics to prevent infection in patients with dog bite wounds: A meta-analysis of randomized trials. Ann Emerg Med 1994;23:535.

Fleisher GR: The management of bite wounds. N Engl J Med 1999;340:138.

Glaser C, Lewis P, Wong S: Pet-, animal- and vector-borne infections. Pediatr Rev 2000;21:219.

Goldstein EJC: Current concepts on animal bites: Bacteriology and therapy. Curr Clin Trop Infect Dis 1992;19:99.

Jones N, Khoosal M: Infected dog and cat bites. N Engl J Med 1999;340:1841.

Ordog GJ, Balasubramanium S, Wasserman J: Rat bites: 50 cases. Ann Emerg Med 1985;14:126.

Sacks JJ, Kresnow M, Houston B: Dog bites: How big a problem? Inj Prev 1996;2:52.

Sacks JJ, Sinclair L, Gilchrist J, et al: Breeds of dogs involved in fatal human attacks in the United States between 1979 and 1998. J Am Vet Med Assoc 2000;217:836.

Smith PF, Meadowcroft AM, May DB: Treating mammalian bite wounds. J Clin Pharm Ther 2000;25:85.

Talan DA, Citron DM, Abrahamian FM, et al: Bacteriologic analysis of infected dog and cat bites. N Engl J Med 1999;340:85.

Weiss HB, Friedman DI, Coben JH: Incidence of dog bite injuries treated in emergency departments. JAMA 1998;279:51.

Snake Bites

Bond GR: Snake, spider and scorpion envenomation in North America. Pediatr Rev 1999;20:147.

Dart RC, Siefert SA, Carroll L, et al: Affinity-purified, mixed monospecific crotalid antivenom ovine Fab for the treatment of crotalid venom poisoning. Ann Emerg Med 1997;30:33.

Gold BS, Dart RC, Barish RA: Bites of venomous snakes. N Engl J Med 2002;347:347.

Kunkel DB, Curry SC, Vance MV, et al: Reptile envenomations. J Toxicol Clin Toxicol 1984;21:503.

Offerman SR, Bush SP, Moynihan JA, et al: Crotaline Fab antivenom for treatment of children with rattlesnake bites. Pediatrics 2002;110:968.

Tanzen DA, Ruha AM, Graeme KA, et al: Epidemiology and hospital course of rattlesnake envenomations cared for at a tertiary referral center in central Arizona. Acad Emerg Med 2001;8:177.

Wagner CW, Golladay ES: Crotalid envenomation in children: Selective conservative management. J Pediatr Surg 1989;24:128.

Walter FG, Bilden EF, Gibly RL: Envenomations. Crit Care Clin 1999; 15:353.

Marine Animal Bites

Auerbach PS: Marine envenomations. In Auerbach PS (ed): Wilderness Medicine: Management of Wilderness and Environmental Emergencies, 3rd ed. St. Louis, Mosby-Yearbook, 1995, pp 1327.

Brown CK, Shepherd SM: Marine trauma, envenomations, intoxications. Emerg Med Clin North Am 1992;10:385.

Isbister GK: Venomous fish stings in tropical northern Australia. Am J Emerg Med 2001;19:561.

Arthropod Bites

Bond GR: Antivenin administration in *Centruroides* scorpion stings: Risks and benefits. Ann Emerg Med 1992;21:788.

Eitzen EM, Seward PN: Arthropod envenomations in children. Pediatr Emerg Care 1988;4:266.

Gomez HF, Krywko DM, Stoecker WV: A new assay for the detection of *Loxosceles* species (brown recluse) spider venom. Ann Emerg Med 2002;39:469.

Isbister GK, Gray MR: A prospective study of 750 definite spider bites, with expert spider identification. QJM 2002;95:723.

Lee JM, Greenes DS: Biphasic anaphylaxis reactions in pediatrics. Pediatrics 2000;106:762.

Likes K, Banner W, Chavez M: *Centruroides exilicauda* envenomation in Arizona. West J Med 1987;141:634.

Rauber A: Black widow spider bites. J Toxicol Clin Toxicol 1983;21:473.

Spach DH, Liles WC, Campbell GL, et al: Tick-borne disease in the United States. N Engl J Med 1993;329:936.

Valentine MD, Lichtenstein LM: Anaphylaxis and stinging insect hypersensitivity. JAMA 1987;258:2882.

Wright SW, Wrenn KD, Murray L, et al: Clinical presentation and outcome of brown recluse spider bites. Ann Emerg Med 1997;30:28.

54 Fever of Unknown Origin

Andrea C. S. McCoy   Stephen C. Aronoff

Fever in the pediatric population is usually grouped into four categories:

- fever in the neonate
- fever with localizing signs
- fever without localizing signs
- fever of unknown origin (FUO)

Subcategories of FUO include classic FUO, nosocomial FUO, neutropenic FUO, FUO with human immunodeficiency virus (HIV) infection, and periodic (episodic) fevers.

DEFINITIONS

The core temperature is a balance between the heat generated from the body's metabolic processes and the heat-dissipating mechanisms. Heat is generated by inefficient cellular metabolism. The body is cooled by a combination of heat loss by radiation, conduction, evaporation, and convection. Cooling takes place mainly by radiation and evaporation from the skin. The lungs also contribute to cooling but to a lesser degree.

An elevation in temperature is a result of fever or hyperthermia. *Fever* is the physiologic adjustment of the normal regulating mechanism in the hypothalamic set point, resulting in an elevated body temperature. *Hyperthermia* is failure of the body's cooling mechanisms to dissipate excessive heat production (malignant hyperthermia, heat stress, heat stroke). Fever often results from the direct action of systemically produced cytokines (interleukin-β, tumor necrosis factor α) on the hypothalamus. These proteins are synthesized as the response to inflammation, infection, or malignancy, and they elevate the hypothalamic set point.

In adults, FUO is defined as an illness lasting more than 3 weeks, a fever higher than 38.3° C (101° F) on several occasions, and uncertainty of diagnosis after a 1-week study in the hospital. In pediatrics, the definition is variable, because the duration of elevated temperature ranges from 8 days to 3 weeks (average, 2 weeks). This may be dependent on the age of the patient, with shorter periods of fever in young infants and more traditional adult standards in adolescent patients. For this discussion, FUO is defined as an oral or rectal temperature higher than 38° C (100.4° F) at least twice a week for more than 3 weeks, a noncontributory history and physical examination, a normal chest roentgenogram, and normal findings on urinalysis in an immunologically normal host. In accordance with this definition, the differential diagnosis for FUO in children is large (Table 54-1).

Four pediatric case series are summarized in Table 54-2. An infectious origin accounted for 33% to 52% of cases; the others resulted from autoimmune diseases (6% to 20%), neoplasias (2% to 13%), and miscellaneous or undiagnosed causes (11% to 67%). In adults, infections account for about 25%; malignancy (hematologic and solid), for 15%; inflammatory conditions, for 24%; and miscellaneous conditions, for 7%. Thirty percent resolve without a diagnosis.

Infection is the most common cause of FUO in children of all ages, and respiratory infections account for 50% of these infections. Often these illnesses represent atypical manifestations of common childhood bacterial or viral diseases rather than unusual or uncommon disorders (see Table 54-1). Infections occur twice as often in children younger than 6 years, whereas connective tissue disease occurs more often in children older than 6 years of age. The mortality rate in adult studies is higher than that in pediatric series (32% versus 9%), largely because of untreatable primary diseases (cancer) rather than undiagnosed lethal diseases.

EVALUATION

The evaluation of a child with FUO centers on a detailed history and physical examination. The history documentation should be repeated, because parents often remember important details after the initial interview. The physical examination findings may also change during the course of the investigation, revealing important clues (Fig. 54-1).

HISTORY

The history should include the time of day of the fever, who measured the temperature, and the instrument that was used to measure the temperature. Unlike rectal measurements, axillary temperatures and aural or forehead measurements with liquid crystal thermometers do not always match core temperature. Increased temperatures after exercise and in the afternoon often represent normal variations. The appearance of the child while febrile is also important. Increased temperature without sweating might be seen in a child with ectodermal dysplasia or factitious temperature.

The pattern of fever should be noted. Sustained fever, intermittent fever, and relapsing fever have been associated with different disease states.

Sustained or *remittent fever* remains elevated with little variation during the day and has been associated with typhoid fever, tularemia, malarial infections, and rickettsial diseases such as typhus and Rocky Mountain spotted fever.

Intermittent fever normalizes at least once a day and is associated with tuberculosis, abscesses, lymphomas, juvenile rheumatoid arthritis (JRA), and some forms of malaria.

Children with *relapsing fever* have afebrile days between febrile episodes. Relapsing fever has been associated with rat-bite fever, *Borrelia* species infection, malaria, brucellosis, subacute bacterial endocarditis, African trypanosomiasis, lymphomas, and Lyme disease.

Saddle-back or *double-hump fever* lasts a few days, is followed by an afebrile day or two, and then returns. It has been associated with some viruses and dengue fever.

Double quotidian fever (two fever spikes each day) occurs in kala-azar, malaria, and gonococcal endocarditis.

Periodic fevers occur as acute febrile episodes separated by prolonged afebrile, healthy periods. Diseases to consider include cyclic neutropenia, familial Mediterranean fever, hyperimmunoglobulin D syndrome, Muckle-Wells syndrome, tumor necrosis factor receptor superfamily IA–associated periodic fever syndrome (TRAPS), and the syndrome of periodic fever, aphthous stomatitis, pharyngitis, and

Table 54-1. Causes of Fever of Unknown Origin in Children

Infections

Bacterial Diseases

Specific organism causing systemic disease
   Bartonellosis
   Brucellosis
   Campylobacter species infection
   Cat-scratch disease
   Gonococcemia (chronic)
   Meningococcemia (chronic)
   Salmonellosis
   Streptobacillus moniliformis infection
   Tuberculosis
   Tularemia
Localized infections
   Abscesses: abdominal, dental, hepatic, pelvic, perinephric, rectal, subphrenic, splenic, periappendiceal
   Cholangitis
   Endocarditis
   Mastoiditis
   Osteomyelitis
   Pneumonia
   Pyelonephritis
   Sinusitis
   Thrombophlebitis
   Urinary tract infection

Spirochete

Borrelia (borreliosis: *Borrelia recurrentis, Borrelia burgdoferi*)
Leptospirosis
Lyme disease
Spirillium minor infection
Syphilis

Viral Diseases

Cytomegalovirus
Hepatitis
Human immunodeficiency virus (and its opportunistic-associated infections)
Infectious mononucleosis (Epstein-Barr virus)
Unidentified presumed virus

Chlamydial Diseases

Lymphogranuloma venereum
Psittacosis

Rickettsial Diseases

Ehrlichiosis
Q fever
Rocky Mountain spotted fever

Fungal Diseases

Blastomycosis (nonpulmonary)
Coccidioidomycosis (disseminated)
Histoplasmosis (disseminated)

Parasitic Diseases

Extraintestinal amebiasis
Babesiosis
Giardiasis
Malaria
Toxoplasmosis
Trypanosomiasis
Visceral larva migrans

Autoimmune Hypersensitivity Diseases

Drug fever

Hypersensitivity pneumonitis
Juvenile rheumatoid arthritis (systemic onset, Still disease)
Polyarteritis nodosa
Rheumatic fever
Serum sickness
Systemic lupus erythematosus
Undefined vasculitis

Neoplasms

Atrial myxoma
Ewing sarcoma
Hepatoma
Hodgkin disease
Leukemia
Lymphoma
Neuroblastoma

Granulomatous Diseases

Granulomatous hepatitis
Sarcoidosis
Crohn disease

Familial-Hereditary Diseases

Anhidrotic ectodermal dysplasia
Cyclic neutropenia
Deafness, urticaria, amyloidosis syndrome
Fabry disease
Familial dysautonomia
Familial Hibernian fever
Familial Mediterranean fever
Hyperimmunoglobulin D syndrome
Hypertriglyceridemia
Ichthyosis
Muckle-Wells syndrome
Tumor necrosis factor receptor superfamily IA–associated periodic fever syndrome (TRAPS)

Miscellaneous

Behçet syndrome
Central fever
Chronic active hepatitis
Diabetes insipidus (central and nephrogenic)
Factitious fever
Habitual fever
Hemophagocytic syndromes
Histiocytosis syndromes
Hypothalamic-central fever
Immunodeficiency disorders
Infantile cortical hyperostosis
Inflammatory bowel disease
Kawasaki disease
Neurenteric cyst
Pancreatitis
Postoperative (pericardiotomy, craniectomy) status
Pulmonary embolism
Recurrent (periodic) fever, aphthous stomatitis, pharyngitis, adenitis (PFAPA)
Spinal cord injury crisis
Thyrotoxicosis

Undiagnosed Fever

Persistent
Recurrent
Resolved

Modified from Behrman RE (ed): Nelson Textbook of Pediatrics, 14th ed. Philadelphia, WB Saunders, 1992, p 653.

Table 54-2. **Comparison of Four Pediatric Fever of Unknown Origin Studies**

	McClung	Pizzo et al	Lohr and Hendley	Steele
Year reported	1972	1975	1977	1991
Definition of fever	>38.9° C	>38.5° C	>38.3° C	≥38° C
Duration of fever on multiple occasions	3-wk outpatient or 1-wk inpatient	>2 wk	3-wk outpatient or 1-wk inpatient	3 wk
No. of patients	99	100	54	109
Diagnosis (%)				
Infection	47 (47)	52 (52)	18 (33)	24 (22)
Autoimmune disease	11 (11)	20 (20)	8 (15)	7 (6)
Inflammatory bowel disease	3 (3)		3 (6)	1 (1)
Neoplasm	8 (8)	6 (6)	7 (13)	2 (2)
Miscellaneous	19 (19)	10 (10)	8 (15)	2 (2)
No diagnosis made	11 (11)	12 (12)	10 (19)	73 (67)

adenitis (PFAPA). Many periodic fever syndromes are inherited as autosomal dominant disorders (familial Mediterranean fever, hyperimmunoglobulin D syndrome, TRAPS, Muckle-Wells syndrome).

Unfortunately, neither the fever pattern nor the duration is specific for a particular cause. Fevers lasting for more than 1 year are not usually infectious; factitious fever, collagen-vascular or granulomatous disorders, familial diseases, or malignancies need to be considered in these patients.

A history of rash is important for diagnosing Lyme disease, JRA, and acute rheumatic fever (see Chapter 55). A history of pica is associated with visceral larva migrans and toxoplasmosis. Exposure to domestic and wild animals should be identified to exclude zoonoses (see Chapters 53 and 55). The food history should be detailed and should include water sources, use of game meats, cooking practices, and consumption of unpasteurized, raw milk.

Domestic or foreign travel is critically important in the establishment of a differential diagnosis. Areas visited, accommodations, activities, prophylactic treatments, animal and insect exposures, and water and food sources should be reviewed. Coccidioidomycosis, histoplasmosis, malaria, Lyme disease, and Rocky Mountain spotted fever have regional distributions. Emigrant children are at increased risk for endemic diseases and *Mycobacterium tuberculosis*.

Previous medical records should be reviewed. Weight loss is important for diagnosing many chronic diseases such as lymphoma, tuberculosis, and inflammatory bowel disease. Poor weight gain and growth, with or without gastrointestinal symptoms, may be the only historical clue to inflammatory bowel disease (see Chapter 15). HIV risk factors in the parents and child should be reviewed. Past and current medications should also be reviewed. Family history may give clues to familial Mediterranean fever and other familial disorders (see Table 54-1). The review of systems may reveal heat intolerance, palpitations, tremors, and declining quality of schoolwork in a child with hyperthyroidism. A history of severe head trauma may be associated with hypothalamic dysfunction and central fevers.

PHYSICAL EXAMINATION

Whenever possible, the patient should be examined during a febrile episode. A high fever in the absence of an increased pulse may be present in a patient with factitious fever. To verify this diagnosis, the temperature of immediate voided urine may be recorded. Tremor, high heart rate, palpitations, exophthalmos, lid lag, eyelid retraction, and smooth, flushed skin with diaphoresis are suggestive of hyperthyroidism.

Eyes

The ophthalmologic examination should include assessment of acuity, extraocular motion, visual field integrity, and gaze, as well as

inspection of external structures and funduscopic examination (see Chapter 43). Conjunctivitis, iritis-uveitis-scleritis, or both may be seen in a variety of infectious conditions, including Epstein-Barr virus (EBV) infection, leptospirosis, rickettsial infection, and cat-scratch disease. Conjunctivitis, uveitis, or both occur with Kawasaki disease, systemic lupus erythematosus (SLE), polyarteritis nodosa, and rheumatoid arthritis. Sarcoidosis may be associated with conjunctival and uveal tract nodules. A thorough funduscopic evaluation (and, if needed, slit-lamp examination) should be performed. Sarcoidosis may be accompanied by vascular occlusions, hemorrhages, vascular sheathing, and preretinal inflammatory exudates. Cytomegalovirus (CMV) produces chorioretinitis associated with white infiltrates near vessels and confluent depigmented areas. Histoplasmosis causes small atrophic spots and, in rare cases, focal granulomas of the retina and choroid. *Toxoplasma gondii* is a common cause of recurrent retinochoroiditis. Retinal changes also occur with bacterial endocarditis. Tuberculosis can cause formation of choroidal tubercles and also ulcerative palpebral conjunctival lesions. Slit-lamp examination may also reveal iridocyclitis in JRA, Behçet syndrome, and inflammatory bowel disease.

Ears, Nose, and Throat

The frontal and maxillary sinuses should be transilluminated and palpated for tenderness. The nares should be inspected for inflamed mucosa and purulent discharge. Tympanic membranes should be viewed and insufflated (see Chapter 4). The mouth should be checked for lesions, inflammation, and tooth tenderness. Behçet syndrome is rare in children; it may manifest with oral aphthous lesions. Inspection of teeth and gums may reveal a dental abscess. Exudative and nonexudative pharyngitis is associated with EBV infection, tularemia, leptospirosis, and CMV. PFAPA syndrome is characterized by periodic fever, aphthous stomatitis, pharyngitis, and cervical adenopathy. *Candida* infection in the mouths of children older than 2 years may result from immunodeficiency such as HIV or from the use of inhaled steroids.

Neck

The neck should be examined for adenopathy or thyroid enlargement (see Chapter 49). The rest of the lymphatic system should be carefully examined. A single tender node may be seen with cat-scratch disease. Generalized adenopathy can be seen in CMV infection, EBV infection, and systemic JRA (see Chapter 47).

Heart, Lungs, and Abdomen

Careful auscultation of the heart and lungs is essential. A mitral or aortic regurgitant murmur may be the initial finding of endocarditis

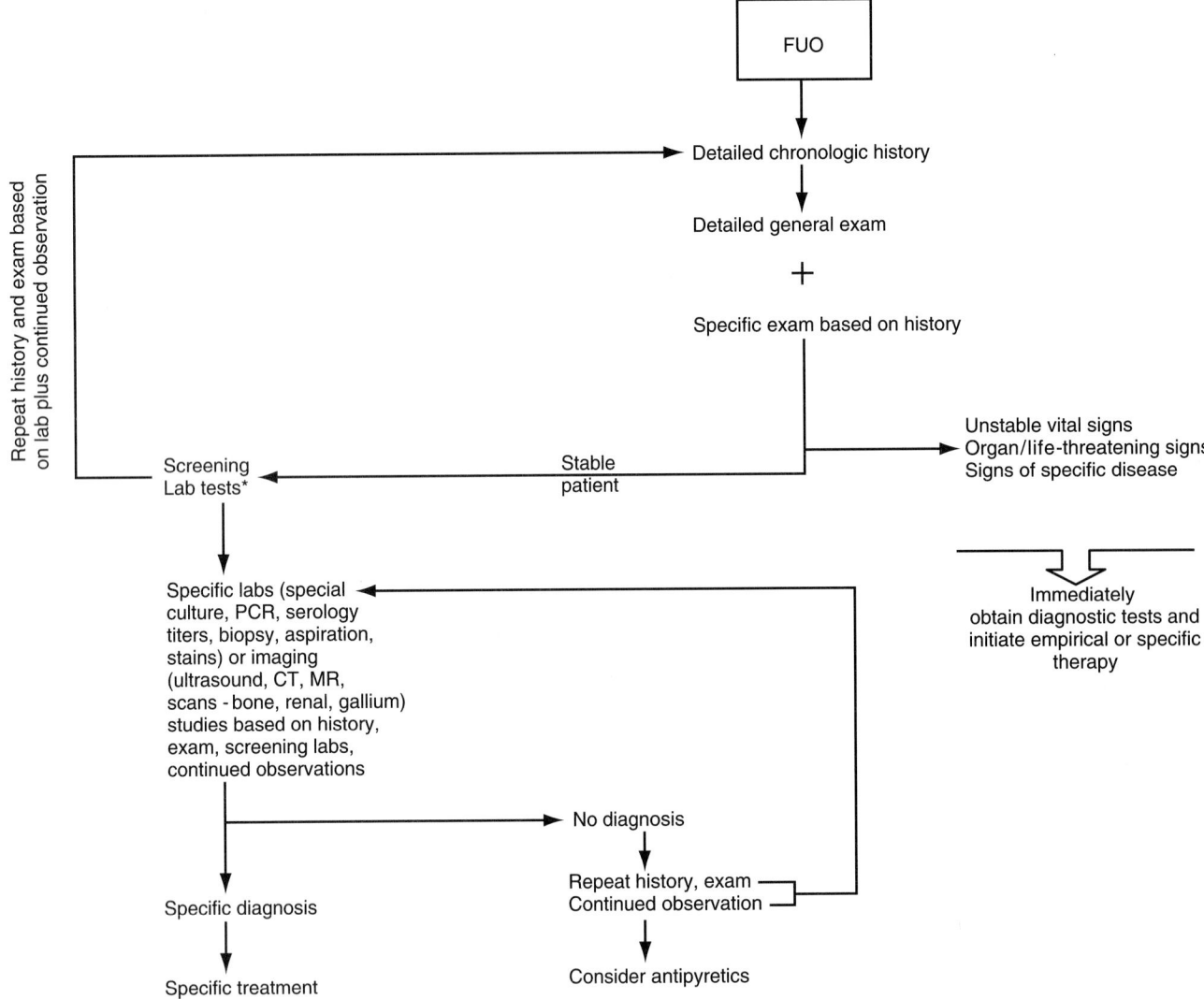

Figure 54-1. Approach to the evaluation of fever of unknown origin (FUO) in children. *Screening laboratory tests (labs) include a complete blood cell count, measurement of erythrocyte sedimentation rate, urinalysis, blood and urine cultures, and a chest radiograph. CT, computed tomography; MR, magnetic resonance; PCR, polymerase chain reaction.

or of carditis in children with acute rheumatic fever. A pericardial friction rub may also suggest JRA, SLE, rheumatic fever, malignancy, or viral pericarditis. The abdomen must be carefully palpated for evidence of masses (see Chapter 22) or hepatosplenomegaly (see Chapters 18 and 19). Abdominal tenderness may be present with abdominal abscesses, hepatosplenomegaly, and inflammatory bowel disease. A rectal examination should be performed, and stool should be tested for occult blood. Sexually active girls should have a pelvic examination. Pain on movement of the uterus during the pelvic examination may indicate pelvic inflammatory disease.

Musculoskeletal Evaluation

The musculoskeletal examination should include assessments of strength and of active and passive range of motion and evaluation for warmth, tenderness, or swelling of joints. Irritability and pain on palpation over a bone or disuse pseudoparalysis may be the first clue to osteomyelitis. Bone pain may also result from neoplastic infiltration of the bone marrow or sickle cell anemia. Unexplained fever, arthralgias, and arthritis may be present with acute rheumatic fever, Lyme disease, Kawasaki disease, SLE, periarteritis nodosa, and Behçet

syndrome (see Chapter 44). Myalgias may be present with rickettsial diseases, periarteritis nodosa, Takayasu arteritis, and dermatomyositis, and they occur quite commonly with viral diseases such as influenza.

Skin

The skin must be inspected for evidence of rashes, lesions, and petechiae (see Chapter 55). JRA may manifest with an evanescent, salmon-colored macular rash over the trunk and joints that may appear and disappear rapidly and be evident only during febrile periods. Dermatomyositis is characterized by a heliotropic rash of the upper eyelids and an erythematous eruption (vasculitis) over the extensor surfaces (Gottron sign). SLE may manifest with a butterfly rash over the nose and malar regions, signs of photosensitivity in sun-exposed areas, or vasculitis. The rash of Kawasaki disease is erythematous and may manifest in many forms. In Rocky Mountain spotted fever, there are macular erythematous spots on the palms and soles that develop into petechiae on wrists and ankles. Endocarditis may be associated with splinter hemorrhages or Janeway lesions (painless, small, erythematous or hemorrhagic lesions on the palms and soles).

Lyme disease usually manifests with erythema migrans. This rash begins at the site of the tick bite and is erythematous with a pale center. The rash radiates out from the bite in a circular manner and persists for weeks; satellite secondary lesions may also appear.

Tularemia, salmonellosis, listeriosis, and EBV infections may feature generalized maculopapular rashes.

LABORATORY AND SPECIAL STUDIES

Laboratory evaluation should proceed in a stepwise, focused manner with emphasis on identifying serious illnesses with defined interventions (see Fig. 54-1). Initial studies should include a complete blood cell count with differential, erythrocyte sedimentation rate (ESR) measurement, blood cultures, urinalysis, urine culture, tuberculin skin tests with controls (anergy panel), and chest radiograph. Because EBV infection is common in childhood, viral-specific antibody titers may also be obtained at the initial evaluation (see Chapter 47). Further studies should be directed by information obtained from detailed histories and physical examinations. Specific serologic studies aid in the diagnosis of CMV; toxoplasmosis; brucellosis; tularemia; hepatitis A, B, and C; and leptospirosis. Biopsies of lymph nodes, the skin, the liver, or bone marrow may be indicated. Radiologic studies that may be of benefit if directed by the history, physical examination findings, and initial laboratory study results include sinus films or computed tomography (CT), abdominal ultrasonography, abdominal (contrast) CT or magnetic resonance imaging (MRI), gallium or indium scans, upper gastrointestinal series with small bowel follow-through, and technetium bone scanning. Aspiration of presumed abscess material or fluid collections (pleural, ascitic) is best performed under CT or ultrasound guidance.

The complete blood cell count with differential is neither specific nor diagnostic. There may be a predominance of neutrophils on the smears of patients with collagen-vascular disease or bacterial infections and in some viral infections. Approximately 30% of patients have abnormal white blood cell counts; 46% may have a "left shift," lymphocytosis, atypical lymphocytes, or blasts. Except for leukemic blasts, abnormalities are not specific for disease categories.

An elevated ESR indicates inflammation. The ESR is usually (70% to 90% of the time) high in children with FUO caused by infectious pathogens, malignancies, and collagen-vascular diseases. Of patients with an ESR less than 10 mm/hour, 90% have a self-limited or viral disease.

Urinalysis and urine culture identify occult infections, particularly in young girls. The urinalysis may also be abnormal in patients with endocarditis and collagen-vascular and other inflammatory disorders.

Unexpected consolidations, calcifications, interstitial changes, perihilar adenopathy, or cardiomegaly (heart failure, pericarditis) may be found on chest radiographs. Chest films are abnormal in 10% to 15% of patients with FUO.

Specialized radiologic studies performed without specific diagnostic clues from the history, physical examination findings, or initial laboratory evaluation results have a surprisingly low yield. In one report, abnormal findings were discovered in 8 of 43 abdominal ultrasonograms, 3 of 14 abdominal CT scans, 5 of 11 indium scans, 1 of 4 gallium scans, and 2 of 15 technetium bone scans. Positron-emission tomography is another potential technique for investigating FUO.

CAUSE

INFECTION

Infections identified in large series of children with FUO include subacute bacterial endocarditis, urinary tract infections, sinusitis, abscesses, osteomyelitis, and rheumatic fever (postinfectious process) (see Table 54-2).

Subacute Bacterial Endocarditis

Subacute bacterial endocarditis is rare in children, but its incidence increases with advancing age and history of preexisting heart disease (see Chapter 11). Murmurs or a change in the characteristic of the prior murmur may not be initially evident. Vegetations also may not be visible initially by transthoracic echocardiography; a transesophageal approach is much more sensitive. Serial blood cultures with anaerobic and aerobic media are necessary for definitive diagnosis.

Urinary Tract Infection

Both upper and lower urinary tract infections may be asymptomatic, and leukocytes may not always be present in urine (see Chapter 23). Sterile pyuria may be present with tuberculosis, Kawasaki disease, reactive arthritis, interstitial nephritis, nongonococcal urethritis, viral cystitis, and collagen-vascular syndromes. Renal ultrasonography may show areas of decreased echogenicity, enlarged echogenic kidneys, and renal or perinephric abscesses. Kidneys may be enlarged with acute pyelonephritis. With an enhanced CT scan, infected parenchyma may show nonenhancing lucency. Nuclear medicine renal scans also identify active areas of infection and old scars.

Sinusitis

Factors that decrease the size and patency of the ostium or impair the mucociliary transport system predispose a child to sinusitis. Ethmoid and maxillary sinuses are present at birth. The frontal sinuses usually appear near 5 or 6 years of age but may be asymmetric or absent. Sphenoid sinuses may be seen radiographically by 9 years of age (see Chapter 32). Prolonged nasal congestion, headache, purulent nasal discharge, sore throat, daytime cough, tender teeth, and halitosis may be present in children with sinusitis. Radiographic sinus series or CT studies may be helpful. Rhinoscopy may show purulent material at the ostium of an infected sinus. Infectious complications of sinusitis include dural space empyema or brain abscesses.

Abscesses

Hepatic, renal, perinephric, pelvic, and subphrenic abscesses may be present with FUO. Internal jugular thrombophlebitis may manifest with prolonged fever and severe neck pain. Liver abscess may manifest with right upper quadrant tenderness and hepatomegaly. Blood cultures and liver function study results are often normal. The diagnosis may be made with MRI, CT, ultrasonography, or an indium-labeled white blood cell scan. Perinephric abscesses may yield normal intravenous pyelograms, whereas CT or ultrasonography is diagnostic. CT or ultrasound guidance may be used to direct percutaneous drainage of most abscesses. Pelvic abscesses should be suspected in children with FUO who have abdominal, rectal, or pelvic tenderness.

Osteomyelitis

Osteomyelitis usually follows bacteremia, but it sometimes follows penetrating injury. Tenderness to palpation over the infected site is common. Technetium scans show early changes (1 week), whereas abnormalities in plain films appear later (2 weeks). MRI is another valuable imaging modality. The blood or bone culture is often positive, and the ESR is often elevated.

Rheumatic Fever

Acute rheumatic fever may cause FUO; the diagnosis is made by fulfillment of the modified Jones criteria (see Chapter 11). Initially, a child may present with polyarthralgia and an increased ESR. Elbows, wrists, knees, and ankles are frequently involved. The later migratory nature of the true arthritis differentiates rheumatic fever from JRA.

Bacterial Syndromes

Bacterial syndromes that cause FUO in children include agents of

- Lyme disease
- cat-scratch disease
- rat-bite fever
- tularemia
- brucellosis
- leptospirosis
- chronic bacteremias (meningococcus, gonococcus)

Lyme Disease

Lyme disease is caused by the spirochete *Borrelia burgdorferi* and is transmitted by the *Ixodes dammini* and *Ixodes pacificus* ticks. The usual manifestation is with erythema migrans, an erythematous, annular, expanding rash with central clearing. The rash resolves 1 to 30 days (usually 2 weeks) after exposure. Patients may exhibit fever, chills, fatigue, headaches, malaise, myalgias, arthralgias, and lymphadenopathy. Two to 8 weeks after exposure, facial nerve palsy, peripheral neuropathy, cardiac conduction defects, myocarditis, and aseptic meningitis may occur. Months to years after exposure, arthritis and chronic neurologic symptoms can be seen (see Chapter 44). Diagnosis is usually made clinically and verified with antibody titers and Western blot. Polymerase chain reaction has limited availability.

Cat-Scratch Disease

Cat-scratch disease is a febrile illness associated with cats (usually kittens) and, more rarely, dogs. *Bartonella henselae,* which may be transmitted by the cat flea and by cat saliva, is the etiologic agent. After a scratch or bite, a papule forms and may persist from days to months. Regional lymphadenopathy with one or more nodes occurs proximal to the skin site 1 to 9 weeks after inoculation. The node or nodes become enlarged and tender and may have overlying erythema. The lymphadenopathy usually resolves after 2 months but may last up to 3 years. Affected children may have adenopathy with fever, headache, malaise, anorexia, sore throat, and conjunctivitis (see Chapter 47).

Rat-Bite Fever

Rat-bite fever is a relapsing fever caused by *Streptobacillus moniliformis* or *Spirillum minus*. *S. moniliformis* is a pleomorphic gram-negative bacillus transmitted by rat bite or by contaminated food or water. In 1 to 10 days after exposure, patients may exhibit fever, chills, malaise, and muscle aches. A rash may form on the extremities; arthralgias and arthritis may occur. Endocarditis is a late manifestation. Diagnosis is made by blood culture. A fourfold increase in antibody titers may also be seen. Treatment is with penicillin.

Tularemia

Francisella tularensis is the causative agent of tularemia. The disease is spread by contact with wild animals, such as rabbits and squirrels, and by insects that bite these animals, such as mosquitoes, ticks, and deer flies, as well as by contaminated water. A maculopapular nodule forms at the portal of entry and later becomes ulcerated. The child may present with fever, chills, and headache. Lymphadenopathy, pharyngitis, conjunctivitis, hepatosplenomegaly, and pneumonia may also occur. Diagnosis is made by serologic study. Treatment is with streptomycin or gentamicin.

Brucellosis

Brucellosis is caused by gram-negative coccobacilli: *Brucella abortus, Brucella melitensis, Brucella suis,* or *Brucella canis.* The microorganisms are found in sheep, goats, cattle, swine, and dogs. Infection may occur by airborne spread or by ingestion of meat or milk. The child may present with fever, chills, malaise, arthralgias, or myalgias. Pneumonia, cardiac involvement, and central nervous system (CNS) involvement occur in rare cases. Diagnosis is made by special culture techniques and serologic study.

Leptospirosis

Leptospirosis is caused by members of the spirochete genus *Leptospira.* Infection is spread by contact with the urine of wild or domestic animals. In 1 to 2 weeks after exposure, patients experience the abrupt onset of fever, chills, malaise, myalgias, and headache. Conjunctival suffusion and rash are common findings. Liver, renal, and CNS involvement may also occur. Diagnosis is made by special culture techniques and microscopic agglutination.

Fungal Infections

Fungal causes of FUO include

- Blastomycosis
- Histoplasmosis
- Coccidioidomycosis
- Cryptococcoses

Blastomyces dermatitidis is a saprophytic fungus with both yeast and mycelial forms found in the soil in North America. Infections with this fungus may be disseminated or pulmonary. The diagnosis is made by visualization of single-budding yeast in clinical material, culture on Sabouraud agar, or serologic tests. Amphotericin B is used for treatment of severe, life-threatening disease; oral imidazole therapy has been employed for milder infections.

Histoplasma capsulatum is a yeast found in soil in the Ohio River valley that causes pulmonary and disseminated disease. Diagnosis is made by the demonstration of the microorganism in biopsy specimens or by complement-fixing antibody. Treatment is with amphotericin B or itraconazole.

Coccidioides immitis is found in soil in the southwestern United States. Infections in humans are associated with a febrile pulmonary disease characterized by cough, rash, and chest pain. Diagnosis is usually made serologically. Disseminated infections are treated with amphotericin B or fluconazole.

Cryptococcus neoformans is often found in pigeon droppings and can cause a variety of diseases. The diagnosis is made by culture or by identification of encapsulated yeast in collected specimens. Treatment is with amphotericin B in combination with flucytosine.

Chlamydial Infection

Psittacosis and lymphogranuloma venereum are chlamydial causes of FUO. *Chlamydia psittaci* may be transmitted by infected birds and produces respiratory illness with fever. Cardiac, liver, CNS, and thyroid involvement are rare. Diagnosis is made serologically. *Chlamydia trachomatis* is a sexually transmitted organism that causes urogenital infections, perihepatitis, invasive lymphadenopathy (lymphogranuloma venereum), neonatal conjunctivitis, and neonatal pneumonia. Diagnosis is by cell culture and rapid antigen tests. Treatment is with erythromycin, azithromycin, or doxycycline.

Q Fever

Q fever is caused by *Coxiella burnetii* and manifests with headache, fever, chills, malaise, and, on occasion, respiratory symptoms.

Hepatic, cardiac, and CNS involvement may occur. Rash is usually not seen. Domestic farm animals, cats, rodents, and marsupials may be infected. Pasteurization destroys the organism in milk. Treatment is with doxycycline, fluroquinolones, or chloramphenicol.

Rocky Mountain Spotted Fever

Rocky Mountain spotted fever manifests with fever, headache, intense myalgias, and abdominal symptoms. A characteristic rash is usually present by the sixth day of illness. The rash covers the palms, wrists, soles, and ankles and progresses from macular to petechial. The disease can last up to 3 weeks. Many end organs, including the heart, kidneys, and CNS, can be involved. Transmission of the causative agent, *Rickettsia rickettsii,* occurs by tick bite. Diagnosis is made by serologic study. Treatment is with doxycycline.

Ehrlichiosis

Human ehrlichioses are caused by *Ehrlichia chaffeensis, Anaplasma phagocytophilia,* and *Ehrlichia ewingii* and are transmitted by the Lone Star tick or the black legged deer tick. The illness is usually seen in the southeastern and upper midwestern United States and has a manifestation similar to that of Rocky Mountain spotted fever. The patient presents with headache, myalgias, fever, chills, nausea, vomiting, weight loss, thrombocytopenia, and leukopenia. Rash is inconsistent but may be seen after 1 week. Pulmonary and renal complications can occur. Mental status changes are less frequent. Doxycycline is used for treatment. Diagnosis is confirmed by isolation of the organism, serologic study, and polymerase chain reaction.

Cytomegalovirus Infection

CMV may cause a mononucleosis-like syndrome in children. Generalized or cervical adenopathy may be seen along with fatigue, malaise, fever, hepatosplenomegaly, and abdominal pain (see Chapter 47). A morbilliform rash may also be present. Retinitis, hepatitis, colitis, and pneumonia may occur in children with impaired immune systems. The virus is transmitted by contact with secretions. Infection is diagnosed by culture (nasopharyngeal, blood, urine) or by the detection of specific immunoglobulin G and immunoglobulin M antibodies.

Infectious Mononucleosis

Infectious mononucleosis is typically caused by EBV and may manifest with fever, exudative pharyngitis, malaise, and fatigue (see Chapter 47). The appearance of rash is usually preceded by ampicillin therapy. Tender lymphadenopathy and hepatosplenomegaly may occur. The diagnosis may be made by nonspecific tests (heterophile antibody or Monospot) in older patients, but these studies are unreliable for young children. Specific antibody tests against viral capsid antigen, early antigen, and nuclear antigen are recommended in younger children. Treatment is supportive.

Human Immunodeficiency Virus Infection

Infection with HIV or associated opportunistic infections or associated malignancies is another cause of FUO in children.

Parasites

FUO in children may be caused by parasitic infections, including (1) babesiosis, (2) toxoplasmosis, and (3) toxocariasis.

Babesiosis is caused by *Babesia microtia* and is a parasite of rodents transmitted to humans by tick bite. Infection may result in fever, chills, nausea, vomiting, night sweats, myalgias, and arthralgias. Identification of the organism in a thick smear of red blood cells is diagnostic.

T. gondii is a protozoan parasite. Children become infected from eating contaminated, undercooked meat or from exposure to the feces of domestic cats. If acquired in adulthood, the disease is usually asymptomatic and self-limited. Toxoplasmosis is a mononucleosis-like illness (see Chapter 47).

Toxocariasis (visceral larva migrans) results from ingestion of larvae of *Toxocara canis* or from *T. cati* shed in dog and cat feces, respectively. Infection results in fever, intense eosinophilia, hepatomegaly, and hypergammaglobulinemia. Lung, heart, and CNS involvement is rare. The eye may become infected. Diagnosis is presumed with increased eosinophils and hypergammaglobulinemia. Elevated titers of antibodies to A and B blood groups are often seen. Treatment is largely supportive.

In a child who has traveled outside the United States, consideration must be given to the areas traveled, water sources, and activities. Some causes of FUO after travel to a foreign country include malaria, hepatitis, typhoid fever, tuberculosis, amebic liver abscess, and filariasis.

Malaria

Malaria is transmitted by the bite of an infected mosquito carrying *Plasmodium falciparum, Plasmodium vivax, Plasmodium ovale,* or *Plasmodium malariae.* The patient experiences chills, rigors, fever, diaphoresis, and headaches. The incubation period varies among species, from 1 week to several months. Demonstration of the parasite on thick peripheral blood smear is diagnostic. Treatment is given according to the species involved and the area where the patient was exposed.

Hepatitis

Hepatitis A may be contracted by ingestion of contaminated food or water. Hepatitis B and C viruses are transmitted through blood products or sexual contact. Diagnosis is by serologic testing. Symptoms can include fever, malaise, jaundice, hepatomegaly, nausea, and anorexia. Hepatitis B and C can become chronic (see Chapter 20).

Typhoid Fever

Typhoid fever is caused by infection with *Salmonella typhi.* After ingestion of contaminated water or food, incubation lasts from 1 to 6 weeks. Persistent fever, rose spots, and glomerulonephritis are clinical hallmarks of typhoid fever. Diagnosis is by blood or, in rare cases, bone marrow culture. Treatment is with ceftriaxone or cefotaxime.

Tuberculosis

Tuberculosis may manifest as FUO in children (see Chapters 2 and 47). Affected children may have pulmonary or extrapulmonary disease. The signs and symptoms of pulmonary disease may vary greatly: from weight loss, skin test conversion, and low-grade fever to mass effect from mediastinal lymphadenopathy and fulminant disseminated pulmonary involvement with miliary infiltrates or, in rare cases, cavitation. Nonpulmonary tuberculosis more commonly manifests as FUO, in as much as positive chest radiograph findings and pulmonary signs may initiate an early workup for tuberculosis. Hematogenous spread may cause liver, heart, or renal involvement. Ingested bacilli may result in gastrointestinal tuberculosis. The diagnosis requires demonstration of acid-fast bacilli from sputum, gastric aspirate, or the affected organ. Skin testing may yield negative results even with positive controls.

Amebic Infection

Intestinal infection with *Entamoeba histolytica* may produce invasion of the mucosal lining and spread to other organs such as the liver. Amebic liver abscess may manifest with fever, weight loss, right upper quadrant pain, and anorexia. The patient may have painful hepatomegaly without splenomegaly. The abscess may be localized with abdominal ultrasonography. Diagnosis is by serologic study. Treatment is with metronidazole.

Filariasis

Filariasis may result from the bite of a mosquito infected with *Wuchereria bancrofti, Brugia malayi,* or *Brugia timori.* Disease results from inflammation and obstruction of lymph channels by the developing nematode. Patients may present with fever, myalgias, lymphadenitis, and lymphangitis. Diagnosis is made by observing microfilariae in blood or adult worms in tissue biopsy material.

RHEUMATOLOGIC CAUSES OF FEVER OF UNKNOWN ORIGIN

Collagen-vascular diseases as a cause of FUO are more common in children older than 6 years. Establishing the diagnosis is often difficult and may take months. JRA, polyarteritis, SLE, and Behçet syndrome may all manifest as FUO (see Chapter 44).

Juvenile Rheumatoid Arthritis

JRA is a diagnosis that requires time to identify all of its manifestations and to exclude other entities. JRA is defined by arthritis (swelling or both pain and limitation of motion) of unknown origin that begins in a child younger than 16 years and persists for a minimum of 6 weeks. JRA is divided into three subtypes: systemic, polyarticular, and pauciarticular. The systemic form (Still disease) often manifests with prolonged high fever. Affected children often have a daily fever and may have a fine macular rash, arthralgias, arthritis, hepatosplenomegaly, or pericardial involvement. Polyarticular JRA may manifest with arthritis, low-grade fever, morning stiffness, anorexia, and weight loss.

Polyarteritis

Polyarteritis is a necrotizing vasculitis that may manifest with myalgia, arthralgia, fever, vasculitic skin lesions, and abdominal pain. Cardiac, CNS, and renal involvement may also occur. The ESR usually is markedly elevated. Biopsy and the presence of antibodies to proteinase 3 and myeloperoxidase (antineutrophil cytoplasmic antibodies) are helpful. Treatment is with prednisone or cyclophosphamide.

Systemic Lupus Erythematosus

SLE may manifest with fever, photosensitivity, mouth sores, weight loss, rash, myalgias, malaise, and hepatosplenomegaly. Patients may also have serositis and renal involvement. Laboratory tests that are helpful include lupus erythematosus cell preparation and those for antinuclear antibody, anti-Smith antibody, anti–ribonuclear protein antibody, anti-Ro (Sjögren syndrome type A) antibody, and anti-La (Sjögren syndrome type B) antibody.

Behçet Disease

Behçet disease is very rare in children but may manifest with FUO. Patients may have aphthous stomatitis, arthritis, genital ulcers, uveitis, and erythema nodosum.

Neoplasms

Hodgkin disease, lymphoma, neuroblastoma, and leukemia may all manifest as FUO. In young children, leukemia, neuroblastoma, and lymphoma should be suspected, whereas in adolescents, Hodgkin disease and Ewing sarcoma are more common as causes of FUO.

Hodgkin Disease

Hodgkin disease may manifest with firm, nontender adenopathy, fever, night sweats, and weight loss. Diagnosis is made through biopsy. Treatment is with radiation and chemotherapy.

Lymphoma

Non-Hodgkin lymphoma may manifest as painless adenopathy, cough or dyspnea from a mediastinal mass, abdominal mass, nerve compression, bone pain, fever, and weight loss. Diagnosis is by biopsy. Treatment depends on site and extent of tumor. Surgery, radiation, and chemotherapy may be used.

Neuroblastoma

Neuroblastoma may manifest as abdominal, thoracic, or pelvic masses; spinal cord compression; bone pain; hypertension; hepatomegaly; diarrhea; and fever (see Chapter 22). Diagnosis is aided by radiologic studies and urinary catecholamine measurements and is confirmed by biopsy. Surgery, radiation, and chemotherapy are used for treatment.

Leukemia

Both acute lymphocytic leukemia and acute nonlymphocytic leukemia may manifest with lethargy, pallor, bleeding, fever, bone pain, lymphadenopathy, and arthralgias. Diagnosis is made by blood smear and bone marrow aspirate with biopsy. Treatment is with chemotherapy.

MISCELLANEOUS CAUSES OF FEVER OF UNKNOWN ORIGIN

Familial Mediterranean Fever

Familial Mediterranean fever is an autosomal recessive trait seen in Sephardic Jews and people of Middle Eastern descent. The fever may be accompanied by joint, abdominal, and chest pain. Mutations in the gene encoding pyrin have been identified. Prophylactic treatment is with colchicine.

Anhidrotic Ectodermal Dysplasia

Anhidrotic ectodermal dysplasia is an X-linked recessive disorder associated with decreased ability to sweat, dental abnormalities, and sparse hair. Eyebrows and eyelashes may be absent. Fever may result from inability of the body to cool itself. Diagnosis is made by skin biopsy that shows absence of eccrine glands.

Drug Fever

Drug fever is a diagnosis of exclusion. Some drugs are more likely than others to cause drug fever (α-methyldopa, quinidine, penicillins). There is no characteristic fever pattern. There is a highly variable lag time between the initiation of the drug and the onset of fever, and there is an infrequent association with rash or eosinophilia. Some drugs may cause fever by virtue of physiologic side effects. Anticholinergic drugs may decrease sweating and diminish the body's ability to cool itself. Chronic salicylate intoxication can cause increased heat production by uncoupling oxidative phosphorylation.

Kawasaki Disease

Kawasaki disease may manifest with a variety of signs, including rash; lymphadenopathy; conjunctival hyperemia; strawberry tongue; erythematous lips; swelling of hands and feet; arthralgia; arthritis; myocarditis; late desquamation of hands, feet, and perineal area; and sterile pyuria (see Chapter 55). Fever may be high and spiking. Diagnosis is by fulfillment of clinical criteria. The ESR may be greatly elevated. White blood cells may be increased in number with left shift; platelets are also elevated in number. Treatment is with intravenous gamma globulin and aspirin.

Inflammatory Bowel Disease

Inflammatory bowel disease (ulcerative colitis, Crohn disease) may manifest with FUO. Ulcerative colitis may manifest with bloody diarrhea, fever, fecal urgency, and straining (see Chapter 15). Pyoderma gangrenosum, arthritis, and erythema nodosum can also be seen. Diagnosis is made by radiographic studies and colonoscopy. Treatment is supportive and includes topical or systemic steroids or enteric antiinflammatory agents. Crohn disease (regional enteritis) may manifest with abdominal pain, fever, anorexia, and growth failure. Diarrhea may develop later. Arthritis, erythema nodosum, and finger clubbing may also occur. Diagnosis is by radiographic studies. The ESR is usually elevated. Treatment is with prednisone, immunosuppressive drugs and cytotoxic drugs.

Pheochromocytoma

Pheochromocytomas are rare catecholamine-secreting tumors; 10% occur in children. These tumors manifest with paroxysmal or sustained hypertension, headache, excessive sweating, fever, hyperglycemia, and palpitations. The tumors are usually in the adrenal medulla, but 35% of those occurring in children are multiple or extraadrenal. Diagnosis is made with 24-hour urinary metanephrine collection. Localization of tumor is by CT, MRI, or iodine 131–metaiodobenzylguanidine scanning. Treatment consists of surgical removal.

Thyrotoxicosis

Hyperthyroid states may manifest with FUO. Children usually have multiple symptoms, such as irritability, tremor, eyelid lag, and exophthalmos. Diagnosis is made from thyroid function studies.

Factitious Fever

Factitious fever may be a form of Munchausen syndrome or Munchausen syndrome by proxy (see Chapter 36). A variety of techniques have been used to falsely elevate a recorded temperature. A mercury thermometer may be rubbed between hands or placed near a light bulb. Hot liquids may be placed in the mouth before an oral temperature is taken. Hot rectal douches have also been reported to raise a rectally taken temperature. Even with pathologic fevers, there is some circadian rhythm to the temperature curve; with factitious fever there is no rhythm. In addition, there is usually no vasoconstriction, sweating, tachypnea, or tachycardia. If factitious fever is suspected, the temperature should be obtained while the patient is observed. The temperature of freshly voided urine can also be recorded.

Other patients may produce actual diseases that cause true fevers, such as by injecting infected pyogenic material subcutaneously or intravenously or by taking toxic levels of thyroid hormone. Once the diagnosis is documented, psychiatric care is indicated.

Patients in Whom No Diagnosis Is Made

If no diagnosis is made, most patients are clinically well and asymptomatic on follow-up. Some may be determined to be healthy from the start; most are in good health at follow-up, whereas few have symptoms at the end of evaluation. Some may have relapses of fever for a few months. JRA, inflammatory bowel disease, and PFAPA syndrome may not be immediately diagnosed but usually manifest typical symptoms and signs within 2 years of the onset of the FUO.

SUMMARY AND RED FLAGS

Workup of patients with FUO should proceed in a stepwise manner. It should be kept in mind that many patients with FUO have unusual, atypical, or complicated manifestations of common childhood illness, mainly infectious. Initial evaluation should include blood and urine cultures, chest radiograph, complete blood cell count with differential, ESR measurement, purified protein derivative testing with controls, and EBV titers (see Fig. 54-1). Further testing should be done only if directed by findings from the history and physical examinations. The outcome of undiagnosed patients appears to be favorable in general.

Red flags include weight loss, night sweats, focal findings on examination, signs of organ system (bone marrow, liver, kidney) dysfunction or failure, and unstable vital signs suggestive of sepsis. Only in this last category should a rapid diagnostic approach be performed and empirical antibiotic therapy initiated. In most situations, immediate or empirical antimicrobial therapy is not indicated. However, once the diagnosis of FUO is suspected and the fever pattern documented, the febrile response may be attenuated with antipyretic agents.

REFERENCES

Brusch JL, Weinstein L: Fever of unknown origin. Med Clin North Am 1988;72:1247-1261.

Feder HM Jr: Periodic fever, aphthous stomatitis, pharyngitis, adenitis: A clinical review of a new syndrome. Curr Opin Pediatr 2000;12:253-256.

Gartner JC Jr: Fever of unknown origin. Adv Pediatr Infect Dis 1992;7:1-24.

Lohr JA, Hendley JO: Prolonged fever of unknown origin. Clin Pediatr 1977;16:768-773.

Mackowiak PA, LeMaistre CF: Drug fever: A critical appraisal of conventional concepts. Ann Intern Med 1987;106:728-733.

Majeed HA: Differential diagnosis of fever of unknown origin in children. Curr Opin Rheumatol 2000;12:439-444.

McAllister WH, Kushner DC, Babcock DS, et al: Fever without source. American College of Radiology Appropriateness Criteria. Radiology 2000;215(Suppl):829-832.

McCarthy PL: Fever without apparent source on clinical examination. Curr Opin Pediatr 2003;15:112-120.

McClung MC: Prolonged fever of unknown origin in children. Am J Dis Child 1972;124:544-550.

Miller ML, Szer I, Yogev R, et al: Fever of unknown origin. Pediatr Clin North Am 1995;42:999-1115.

Mourad O, Palda V, Detsky AS: A comprehensive evidence-based approach to fever of unknown origin. Arch Intern Med 2003;163:545-551.

Petersdorf RG, Beeson PB: Fever of unexplained origin: Report on 100 cases. Medicine 1961;40:1-30.

Pizzo PA, Lovejoy FH, Smith DH: Prolonged fever in children: Review of 100 cases. Pediatrics 1975;55:468-473.

Provencher DE, Cahill RA, Good RA, et al: Fever of unknown origin and neutropenia in a young boy. Ann Allergy Asthma Immunol 2002;89:448-451.

Rakover Y, Adar H, Tal I, et al: Behçet disease: Long-term follow-up of three children and review of the literature. Pediatrics 1989;83:986-992.

Saxe SE, Gardner P: The returning traveler with fever. Infect Dis Clin North Am 1992;6:427-439.

Steele RW, Jones SM, Lowe BA, et al: Usefulness of scanning procedures for diagnosis of fever of unknown origin in children. J Pediatr 1991;119:526-530.

Talano JAM, Katz BZ: Long-term follow-up of children with fever of unknown origin. Clin Pediatr 2000;39:715-717.

Thomas KT, Feder HM, Lawton AR, et al: Periodic fever syndrome in children. J Pediatr 1999;135:15-21.

Vanderschueren S, Knockaert D, Adriaenssens T, et al: From prolonged febrile illness to fever of unknown origin. Arch Intern Med 2003;163:1033-1041.

55 Fever and Rash

Robert M. Lembo

Fever and rash are each protean manifestations of disease. Their coexistence suggests a relatively narrow spectrum of pathologic entities for diagnostic consideration. This spectrum includes local or disseminated infection with a wide range of microbial pathogens; toxin-mediated disorders, including those associated with bacterial superantigen production; and the vasculitides, including hypersensitivity disorders (see Chapter 56). The essential elements for accurate diagnosis include a detailed history, a careful systematic observation of the patient for evidence of toxicity, and a thorough physical examination. Because this approach lacks perfect sensitivity, the laboratory may play an important role in the diagnostic process.

ASSESSMENT

HISTORY

Key elements are summarized in Table 55-1. Information about the features of the rash includes when it occurred in relation to the fever, its evolution or progression, and its anatomic distribution. Essential information from the epidemiologic and social history should include exposure to known ill contacts; recent travel or exposure to individuals from different geographic areas; exposure to pets, wildlife, or insects; recent immunizations; a detailed list of medications; blood transfusion; and, for the adolescent patient, intravenous drug use and sexual activity.

The medical and family history should be used to assess the overall health of the patient over time, as well as that of family members, to determine the possibility of underlying primary or acquired immunodeficiency or diseases associated with autoimmunity or chronic inflammation. A history of increased susceptibility to infection, as manifested by chronic or recurrent infectious illnesses after infancy, such as pneumonia, sinusitis, bronchitis, otitis media, diarrhea, and bacteremia, is an important indicator of underlying immunodeficiency disease (see Chapter 51). In addition, the occurrence of an unusually severe infection or an infection with a pathogen of low virulence (e.g., *Pneumocystis carinii*) should raise suspicion of an immunodeficiency state. A history of hemolytic anemia, leukopenia, thrombocytopenia, or arthritis suggests an autoimmune disorder or malignancy, which may also be associated with impairment in immune function (see Chapter 44).

In a thorough systems review, the clinician should assess the probability of a subacute or chronic underlying infectious, inflammatory, or malignant disease by inquiring about anorexia, nausea, vomiting, weight loss, night sweats, fatigue, cough, and exercise intolerance. The clinician should seek symptoms suggesting multisystem disease, such as myalgias, arthralgia, headache, precordial pain or pain with inspiration, abdominal pain, jaundice, skin photosensitivity, peripheral edema, alopecia, Raynaud phenomenon, and hematuria. In patients with symptoms that indicate the presence of multisystem disease, a thorough survey of the functional status of the central, peripheral, and autonomic nervous systems is clinically relevant. Specific inquiries into visual disturbances, photophobia, disordered mentation, neck stiffness, paraesthesia, weakness, or seizure activity are essential and may reveal potentially life-threatening infection within the central nervous system or a systemic vasculitis involving the nervous system, such as systemic lupus erythematosus (SLE) or polyarteritis nodosa.

EXAMINATION

Key elements of the physical examination are summarized in Table 55-2 (see also Chapters 56 and 57). The physical examination is used to refine the probability of underlying serious illness, as estimated by the history and the Acute Illness Observation Score, an observation scale containing six items (quality of cry, reaction to parent, state variation, color, hydration, and response to social overtures). The score is especially useful in evaluating infants younger than 24 months.

A critical first step is an assessment of the patient's vital signs. The highest point of the fever is an important indicator of underlying serious illness. Approximately 7% of children younger than

---

Table 55-1. Essential Elements of the History in the Clinical Assessment of Fever and Rash

Demographic Data
Age
Gender
Ethnicity
Season
Geographic area

Exposures
Ill contacts (home, day care, school, workplace)
Sexual contacts
Travel
Pets, wildlife, insects (especially ticks)
Medications and drugs
Transfusions
Immunizations

Features of Rash
Temporal associations (onset relative to fever)
Progression and evolution
Location and distribution
Pain or pruritus

Associated Symptoms
Focal (suggesting organ-specific illness)
Systemic (suggesting generalized or multisystem illness)

Prior Health Status
Medical and surgical history
Growth and development
Recurrent infectious illnesses

Family History

syndrome, dengue hemorrhagic shock syndrome, hemorrhagic fever with renal syndrome caused by *Hantavirus,* and the hemorrhagic shock–encephalopathy syndrome must also be considered in this context. Hypertension may be noted in association with vasculitic disorders involving small to medium-sized arteries, such as polyarteritis and SLE.

The clinical characteristics of the rash are helpful in establishing an etiologic diagnosis. A morphologic nomenclature of cutaneous manifestations helps the clinician with differential diagnosis, documentation, and communication (Figs. 55-1 to 55-8; see Chapter 56). An *exanthem* is defined as a skin eruption occurring as a sign of a generalized disease. An *enanthem* is an eruption on the mucous membranes that occurs in the context of generalized disease. Exanthems and enanthems may be macular, maculopapular, vesicular, urticarial, petechial, or diffusely erythematous. Because a wide variety of infectious agents, including viruses, bacteria, and the rickettsiae, can cause exanthems and enanthems, very few of these eruptions are pathognomonic (Table 55-3). Tables 55-4 and 55-5 summarize the clinical features of several common bacterial and viral exanthems.

Certain skin lesions may be clues to potentially life-threatening infections. The presence of fever and a petechial rash, especially in a child younger than 24 months, is of particular concern. Between 2% and 20% of affected patients have an underlying bacterial infection and, depending on the clinical setting, 0.5% to 10% have sepsis caused by *Neisseria meningitidis.* Other affected patients may have infection with enteroviruses, particularly enteric cytopathogenic human orphan (ECHO) virus 9, *Streptococcus pneumoniae, Haemophilus influenzae* type b, *Rickettsia rickettsii,* and, occasionally in the western United States, *Yersinia pestis;* bacterial endocarditis; or a noninfectious vasculitis. Although patients with concurrent cough or emesis and petechiae confined to areas above the nipple line may be at lesser risk for bacteremia or invasive infectious disorders, this manifestation does not preclude life-threatening illness.

Purpura

Larger areas of bleeding into the skin produce purpura. Diffuse purpuric lesions may be noted in a wide variety of disorders. These include infectious diseases associated with organisms with a predilection for vascular endothelium, such as *N. meningitidis* and *R. rickettsii;* virus-associated diseases, such as dengue hemorrhagic fever and the hemorrhagic fever with renal syndrome caused by the *Hantavirus;* uncommon bacterial diseases, such as Brazilian purpuric fever caused by *Haemophilus aegyptius;* and the hemorrhagic shock–encephalopathy syndrome. Purpura are also associated with disseminated intravascular coagulation (DIC) and profound thrombocytopenia, such as in idiopathic thrombocytopenic

24 months with a fever of 40° C (104° F) or greater (with or without a rash) at the time of initial presentation are bacteremic. The sensitivity and specificity of this finding for bacteremia in this age group are approximately 57% and 75%, respectively. Therefore, for purposes of clinical decision making, all children with hyperpyrexia should be considered to be at high risk for bacteremia or other serious bacterial infections.

The presence of tachycardia and tachypnea with a stable blood pressure in any patient with fever and rash suggests the presence of sepsis. Evidence of alteration in mental status suggests either the sepsis syndrome associated with major alterations in organ system perfusion or primary meningoencephalitis. The presence of hypotension usually indicates septic shock, which may lead to multiorgan dysfunction syndrome. Other disorders such as toxic shock

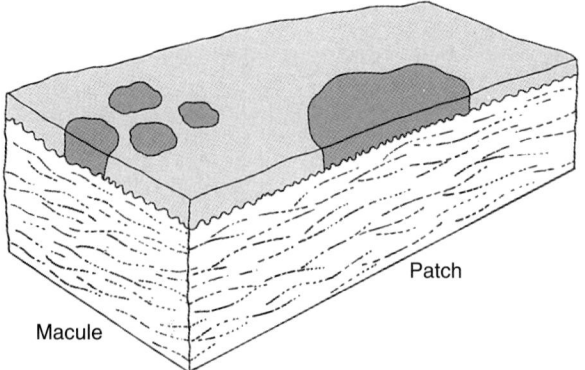

Figure 55-1. Primary lesions: flat, nonpalpable. (From Swartz MH: *Textbook of Physical Diagnosis: History and Examination.* Philadelphia, WB Saunders, 1989, p 92.)

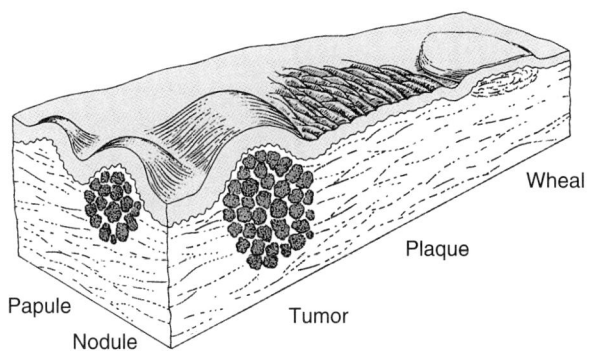

Figure 55-2. Primary lesions: palpable, elevated, solid masses. (From Swartz MH: Textbook of Physical Diagnosis: History and Examination. Philadelphia, WB Saunders, 1989, p 92.)

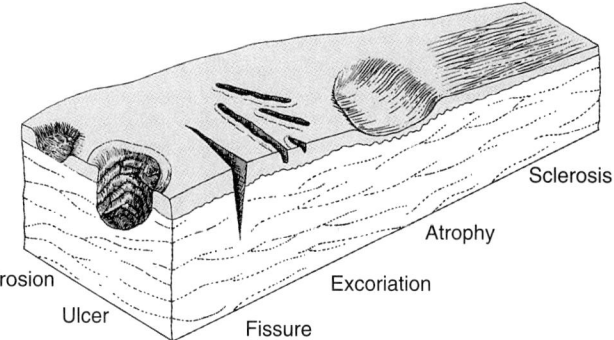

Figure 55-5. Secondary lesions below the skin plane. (From Swartz MH: Textbook of Physical Diagnosis: History and Examination. Philadelphia, WB Saunders, 1989, p 82.)

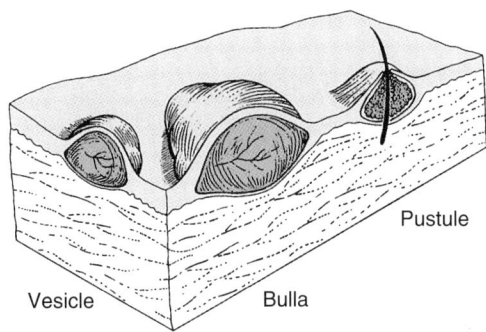

Figure 55-3. Primary lesions: palpable, elevated, fluid-filled masses. (From Swartz MH: Textbook of Physical Diagnosis: History and Examination. Philadelphia, WB Saunders, 1989, p 93.)

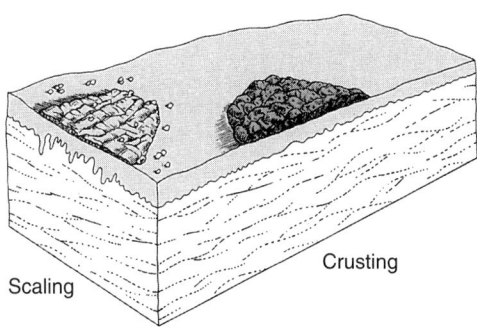

Figure 55-6. Secondary lesions above the skin plane. (From Swartz MH: Textbook of Physical Diagnosis: History and Examination. Philadelphia, WB Saunders, 1989, p 82.)

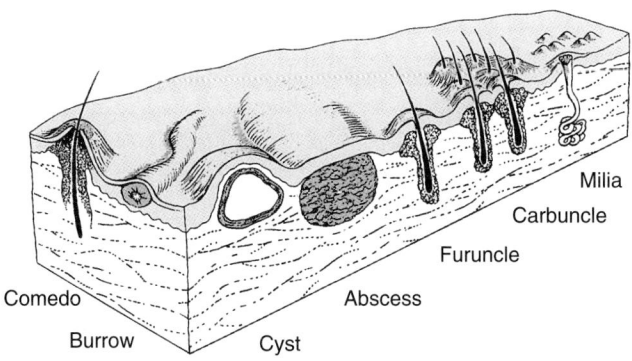

Figure 55-4. Special primary lesions. (From Swartz MH: Textbook of Physical Diagnosis: History and Examination. Philadelphia, WB Saunders, 1989, p 81.)

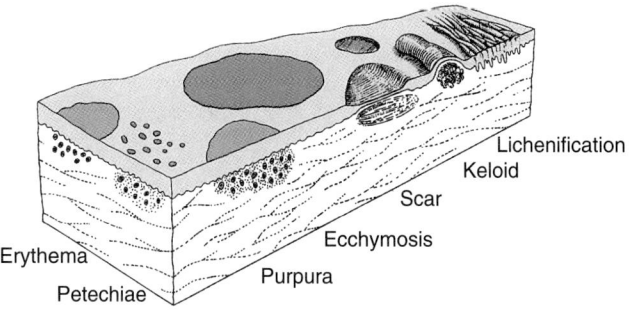

Figure 55-7. Other important dermatologic terms. (From Swartz MH: Textbook of Physical Diagnosis: History and Examination. Philadelphia, WB Saunders, 1989, p 95.)

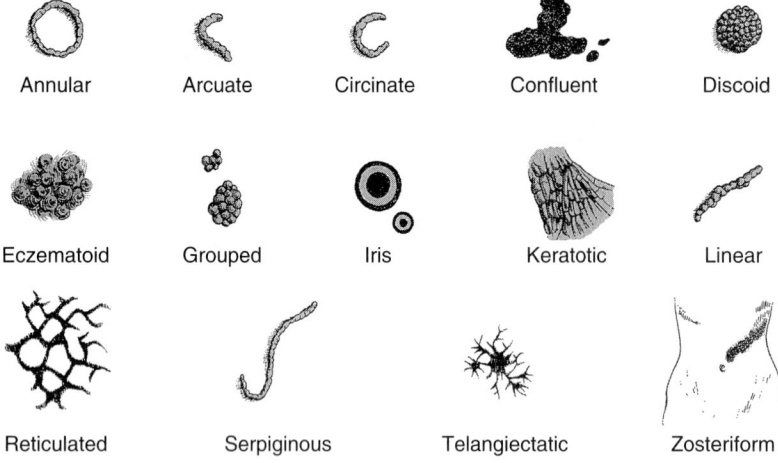

Figure 55-8. Descriptive dermatologic terms. (From Swartz MH: Textbook of Physical Diagnosis: History and Examination. Philadelphia, WB Saunders, 1989, p 96.)

Lesion	Description	Example
Annular	Ring shaped	Ringworm
Arcuate	Partial rings	Syphilis
Bizarre	Irregular or geographic pattern not related to any underlying anatomic structure	Factitial dermatitis
Circinate	Circular	
Confluent	Lesions run together	Childhood exanthems
Discoid	Disc shaped without central clearing	Lupus erythematosus
Discrete	Lesions remain separate	
Eczematoid	An inflammation with a tendency to vesiculate and crust	Eczema
Generalized	Widespread	
Grouped	Lesions clustered together	Herpes simplex
Iris	Circle within a circle; a bull's-eye lesion	Erythema multiforme (iris)
Keratotic	Horny thickening	Psoriasis
Linear	In lines	Poison ivy dermatitis
Multiform	More than one type of shape or lesion	Erythema multiforme
Papulosquamous	Papules or plaques associated with scaling	Psoriasis
Reticulated	Lace-like network	Oral lichen planus
Serpiginous	Snake-like, creeping	Cutaneous larva migrans
Telangiectatic	Relatively permanent dilatation of the superficial blood vessels	Osler-Weber Rendu disease
Universal	Entire body involved	Alopecia universalis
Zosteriform*	Linear arrangement along a nerve distribution	Herpes zoster

*Also known as dermatomal.

purpura (see Chapter 50). Purpura can occur in the noninfectious vasculitides, such as Henoch-Schönlein purpura (see Chapter 56). Discrete, raised purpuric lesions (palpable purpura) distributed predominantly over the buttocks and lower extremities are typical for this disorder. All febrile patients presenting with diffuse or discrete purpuric lesions must be considered to be at risk for bacteremia (Fig. 55-9).

Purpura followed by subsequent necrosis of skin is referred to as *purpura fulminans,* which has been reported after relatively benign infections such as varicella or with more serious disorders (meningococcemia).

Urticarial Rashes

See Chapter 56.

Vesicular Rashes

Vesicular rashes (sharply demarcated, raised lesions containing clear fluid), bullae (vesicles exceeding 1 cm in diameter), or pustules (raised lesions containing cloudy fluid composed of serum and inflammatory cells) may be suggestive of focal or disseminated infection with various pathogens (see Fig. 55-3). Localized vesicles may signify infection with herpes simplex virus type 1 or 2 (especially if the vesicles are grouped on an erythematous base) or varicella-zoster virus (especially if grouped vesicles are distributed in a dermatomal pattern) (Fig. 55-10) or infection with nonviral pathogens, such as *Rickettsia akari* (the cause of rickettsialpox) and *Rickettsia tsutsugamushi* (the cause of scrub typhus). Localized pustules and bullae are usually suggestive of pyodermas caused by *Staphylococcus aureus,* but pustular lesions distributed on the palms

Text continued on page 1006

Table 55-3. Differential Diagnosis of Fever and Rash

Lesion	Pathogen or Associated Factor
Maculopapular or Macular Rash	*Viruses*
	Measles (confluent), rubella (discrete), roseola (human herpesvirus-6),* fifth disease (parvovirus),* Epstein-Barr virus,* enteroviruses,* hepatitis B virus (papular acrodermatitis or Gianotti-Crosti syndrome), human immunodeficiency virus, dengue virus, adenovirus
	Bacteria
	Rheumatic fever (group A streptococcus), scarlet fever, erysipelas, *Arcanobacterium haemolyticus*, secondary syphilis, leptospirosis, *Pseudomonas*, meningococcal infection (early), *Salmonella*, Lyme disease, *Mycoplasma pneumoniae*,* *Listeria monocytogenes*, *Brucella melitensis*
	Rickettsia
	Early Rocky Mountain spotted fever, typhus (scrub, endemic), ehrlichiosis (monocytic)
	Other
	Kawasaki disease,* *Coccidioides immitis*
Diffuse Erythroderma	*Bacteria*
	Scarlet fever (group A streptococcus),* other streptococci, toxic shock syndrome (*Staphylococcus aureus*),* staphylococcal scarlet fever, Ehrlichiosis (*Ehrlichia chaffeensis*)
	Fungi
	Candida albicans
Urticarial Rash	*Viruses*
	Epstein-Barr virus, hepatitis B, human immunodeficiency virus, enteroviruses
	Bacteria
	Mycoplasma pneumoniae, group A streptococci, *Shigella*, meningococcus, *Yersinia*
	Other
	Various parasites, insect bites, food-drug allergens (usually afebrile)
Vesicular, Bullous, Pustular	*Viruses*
	Herpes simplex,* varicella-zoster,* coxsackieviruses A and B,* ECHO virus, parvovirus B19
	Bacteria
	Staphylococcal scalded skin syndrome, staphylococcal bullous impetigo, group A streptococcal crusted impetigo, gonococcemia*
	Other
	Toxic epidermal necrolysis, erythema multiforme (Stevens-Johnson syndrome),* rickettsialpox
Petechial-Purpuric	*Viruses*
	Atypical measles, congenital rubella, cytomegalovirus, enterovirus, human immunodeficiency virus, hemorrhagic fever viruses, hemorrhagic varicella, EBV, hepatitis B
	Bacteria
	Sepsis (meningococcal,* gonococcal, pneumococcal,* *Haemophilus influenzae**), endocarditis, rat-bite fever (*Spirillum minus* or *Streptobacillus moniliformis*), *Pseudomonas aeruginosa*
	Rickettsiae
	Rocky Mountain spotted fever,* epidemic typhus, ehrlichiosis
	Other
	Vasculitis, thrombocytopenia, Henoch-Schönlein purpura,* malaria
Erythema Nodosum	*Viruses*
	EBV, hepatitis B
	Bacteria
	Group A streptococcus, tuberculosis, *Yersinia*, cat-scratch disease
	Fungi
	Coccidioidomycosis, histoplasmosis
	Other
	Sarcoidosis, inflammatory bowel disease, estrogen-containing oral contraceptives, systemic lupus erythematosus, Behçet disease
Distinctive Rashes	
Ecthyma gangrenosum	*Pseudomonas aeruginosa*
Erythema chronicum migrans	Lyme disease
Necrotic eschar	Aspergillosis, mucormycosis
Erysipelas	Group A streptococcus
Koplik spots	Measles

Modified from Prince A: Infectious diseases. In Behrman RE, Kliegman RM (eds): Nelson Essentials of Pediatrics, 2nd ed. Philadelphia, WB Saunders, 1994, p 299.
*Common.

EBV, Epstein-Barr virus; ECHO, enteric cytopathogenic human orphan.

Table 55-4. Common Bacterial Exanthems

Disease	Cause	Age	Season	Transmission	Incubation (Days)	Prodrome
Scarlet fever	Group A streptococcus	School age	Fall, winter, spring	Direct contact, droplets	1-4	Sore throat, headache, abdominal pain, cervical lympha- denopathy, fever, 0-2 days, acute onset
Scalded skin syndrome (see Fig. 55-11)	*S. aureus* producing exfoliative toxin	Neonates and infants	Any	Colonization, contact	Unknown	None
Toxic shock syndrome	*S. aureus* producing toxic shock syndrome toxins	Usually adolescent girls if menstrual; others variable	Any	Colonization, contact	Variable, often 1-5	Myalgias, or preceding viral croup or pneumonia if biphasic May be secondary to wound infection
Meningococcemia (see Fig. 55-9)	*Neisseria meningitidis*	Any (<5 yr)	Winter/spring, follows influenza epidemics	Close, prolonged contact	5-15	Fever, malaise, myalgia, 1-10 days
Rocky Mountain spotted fever	*Rickettsia rickettsii*	Any (>5 yr) Male > female	Summer	Carrier ticks	3-12	Fever, myalgia, headache, malaise, ill appearance, 2-4 days
Rickettsialpox	*Rickettsia akari*	Any	Any	Blood-sucking mite	7-14	Fever, chills, headache, malaise, 4-7 days

DIC, disseminated intravascular coagulation; IVIG, intravenous immune globulin.

Features and Rash Structure	Enanthem	Complications	Prevention	Comments
Diffuse erythema with "sandpaper" feel and "goose flesh" appearance; accentuation of erythema in flexural creases (Pastia lines); circumoral pallor, lasts 2-7 days; may exfoliate	Palatal petechiae, strawberry tongue	Peritonsillar abscess, rheumatic fever, glomerulo-nephritis	Prevent rheumatic fever with penicillin within 10 days of onset of pharyngitis; treat with penicillin	Similar rash may be noted with *Arcanobacterium haemolyticum* in adolescents; group A streptococci may also produce toxic shock or true bacteremic shock syndromes in addition to cellulitis, lymphangitis, and erysipelas; *Staphylococcus aureus* may produce a scarlatiniform rash
Sudden onset, tender erythroderma progressing to diffuse flaccid bullae; significant perioral, perinasal peeling; eventual diffuse exfoliation (positive Nikolsky sign), possibly fever, conjunctivitis, rhinorrhea	Unusual	Shock	Treat with intravenous nafcillin, or vancomycin if methicillin-resistant *S. aureus*	—
Diffuse sunburn-like erythroderma; hypotension (may be orthostatic), diarrhea, emesis, mental confusion; late desquamation	Conjunctivitis	Shock, multisystem organ dysfunction Systemic inflammatory response syndrome	Treat with intravenous nafcillin (vancomycin if resistant), clindamycin plus intravenous fluids, plus dopamine, possible IVIG or steroids; prevent by frequent changes of tampon	—
Erythematous, nonconfluent, discrete papules (early); petechiae, purpura, ecchymosis present on trunk, extremities, palms, soles	Petechiae	Shock, meningitis, pericarditis, arthritis, endophthalmitis, gangrene, DIC	Contacts: rifampin; general: vaccine; treat with ceftriaxone, cefotaxime, penicillin (if sensitive)	*Neisseria gonorrhoeae*, pneumococcus, *Haemophilus influenzae* type b, group A streptococci may produce similar clinical manifestations
Early maculopapular, then petechial or, rarely, purpuric; present on extremities, palms and soles, trunk	Petechiae variable	Shock, myocarditis, encephalitis, pneumonia	Remove ticks as soon as possible; use tick repellants; treat with doxycycline	*Ehrlichia chaffeensis* and other rickettsiae may produce similar illnesses with or without a rash
At primary bite site, eschar; secondary papulovesicles in same stage throughout illness; fewer vesicles than in chickenpox (5-30); present on trunk and proximal extremities	Unknown	Usually none	Treat with doxycycline	Often confused with chickenpox; may be more common than expected, especially in crowded urban settings with poor housing

Table 55-5. Common Viral Exanthems

Disease	Cause	Age	Season	Transmission	Incubation (Days)	Prodrome
Measles (rubeola)	Measles virus	Infants, adolescents	Winter/spring	Respiratory droplet	10-12	High fever, cough, coryza, conjunctivitis, 2-4 days
Rubella (German measles) (minor measles) (see Fig. 55-13)	Rubella virus	Infants, young adults	Winter/spring	Respiratory droplet	14-21	Malaise, low-grade fever (<101° F), posterior auricular, cervical, occipital adenopathy, 0-4 days
Roseola (exanthem subitum)	Human herpesvirus type 6 or herpesvirus type 7	Infants (6 mo-2 yr)	Any	Unknown; saliva of asymptomatic carrier?	5-15 (?)	Irritability, high fever 3-4 days, cervical, occipital adenopathy
Fifth disease (erythema infectiosum) (see Fig. 55-12)	Parvovirus B19	Prepubertal children, schoolteachers	Winter/spring	Respiratory droplets; blood transfusion, placenta	5-15	Headache, malaise, myalgia; often afebrile
Chickenpox (varicella) (see Fig. 55-10)	Varicella-zoster virus	1-14 yr	Late fall, winter, early spring	Respiratory droplet	12-21	Fever
Enteroviruses	Coxsackievirus, ECHO virus, and others	Infants, young children	Summer/fall	Fecal-oral	4-6	Variable: irritable, fever, sore throat, myalgias, headache
Mononucleosis	Epstein-Barr virus	Children, adolescents	Any	Close contact, saliva, blood transfusion	28-49	Fever, adenopathy, eyelid edema, sore throat, hepatosplenomegaly, malaise; lymphocytosis
Gianotti-Crosti syndrome (papular acrodermatitis of childhood)	Hepatitis B virus, Epstein-Barr virus, other	1-6 yr	Any	Variable; fecal, sexual, blood products for hepatitis B	Unknown; 50-180 days for hepatitis B	Usually none except for specific viral disease; arthritis-arthralgia for hepatitis B

CNS, central nervous system; ECHO, enteric cytopathogenic human orphan; HBIG, hepatitis B virus immune globulin; HIV, human immunodeficiency virus; VZIG, varicella-zoster immune globulin.

Features and Rash Structure	Enanthem	Complications	Prevention	Comments
Maculopapular (confluent), begins on face, spreads to trunk; lasts 3-6 days Brown color develops; fine desquamation; toxic, uncomfortable appearance, photophobia; rash may be absent in HIV infection	Koplik spots on buccal mucosa before rash	Febrile seizures, otitis, pneumonia, encephalitis, laryngotracheitis, thrombocytopenia; delayed subacute sclerosing panencephalitis	General: measles vaccine at 12-15 months, and again by 12 yr Exposure: measles vaccine if within 72 hr; immune serum globulin if within 6 days (must then wait 5-6 mo to vaccinate)	Reportable to public health department; epidemics reported, contagious 3 days before symptoms and to 4 days after rash
Discrete, nonconfluent, rose-colored macules and papules, begins on face and spreads downward; lasts 1-3 days	Variable erythematous macules on soft palate	Arthritis, thrombocytopenia, encephalopathy; fetal embryopathy	General: rubella vaccine at 12-15 months and again by 12 yr; exposure: possibly immune serum globulin	Reportable to public health department; epidemics reported, contagious 2 days before symptoms and 5-7 days after rash
Discrete macules on trunk, neck; sudden-onset rash with defervescence; lasts 0.5-2 days; some patients have no rash	Variable erythematous macules on soft palate	Single or recurrent febrile seizures; hemophagocytic syndrome; encephalopathy; dissemination (e.g., liver, CNS, lung) in immunosuppressed patients	None	No epidemics
Local erythema of cheeks (slapped-cheek appearance); lacy pink red erythema of trunk and extremities, ±pruritus; rash may lag prodrome by 3-7 days; lasts 2-4 days, may recur 2-3 wk later	None	Arthritis, aplastic crisis in patients with chronic hemolytic anemia (e.g., sickle cell), fetal anemic hydrops, vasculitis, Wegener granulomatosis	Isolation of patients with aplastic crisis but not normal host with fifth disease	Epidemics reported; once rash is present, the normal host is not contagious; patients with aplastic crisis often have no rash
Pruritic papules, vesicles in various stages; 2-4 crops and then crusts; distributed on trunk and then face, extremities; lasts 7-10 days; recurs years later in dermatomal distribution (zoster, shingles)	Oral mucosa, tongue	Staphylococcal or streptococcal skin infection, arthritis, cerebellar ataxia, encephalitis, thrombocytopenia, Reye syndrome (with aspirin), myocarditis, nephritis, hepatitis, pneumonia; dissemination in immunocompromised patients; fetal embryopathy	VZIG for exposed immunosuppressed patients, susceptible pregnant women, preterm neonates, and infants at birth whose mother developed varicella 5 days before and 2 days after birth; active immunization possible with live attenuated vaccine	Acyclovir therapy for immunosuppressed and possibly normal patients (controversial); contagious 1-2 days before rash and 5 days after rash (usually no longer contagious when all lesions are crusted and no new lesions appear)
Hand-foot-mouth: vesicles in those locations; others: nonspecific, usually fine, nonconfluent, macular or maculopapular rash, rarely petechial, urticarial, or vesicular; lasts 3-7 days	Yes	Aseptic meningitis, hepatitis, myocarditis, pleurodynia, paralysis: usually in younger patients	None	Rash may appear with fever or after defervescence; rash may be present in <50% of enteroviral illnesses; epidemics possible, contagious up to 2 wk
Maculopapular, or morbilliform on trunk, extremities; may be confluent; often elicited by simultaneous administration of ampicillin or allopurinol; rash in 15% and in 50% with drug-induced form; lasts 2-7 days	Variable	Anemia, thrombocytopenia, aplastic anemia, hepatitis; rarely, hemophagocytic syndrome, lymphoproliferative syndrome	None	Cytomegalovirus and toxoplasmosis also produce mononucleosis-like illnesses; monospot or heterophile test results negative
Papules, papulovesicles, discrete or confluent; face, arms, extremities, often spares trunk; lasts 4-10 days	Variable	As per specific disease	Hepatitis B: HBIG plus vaccine	—

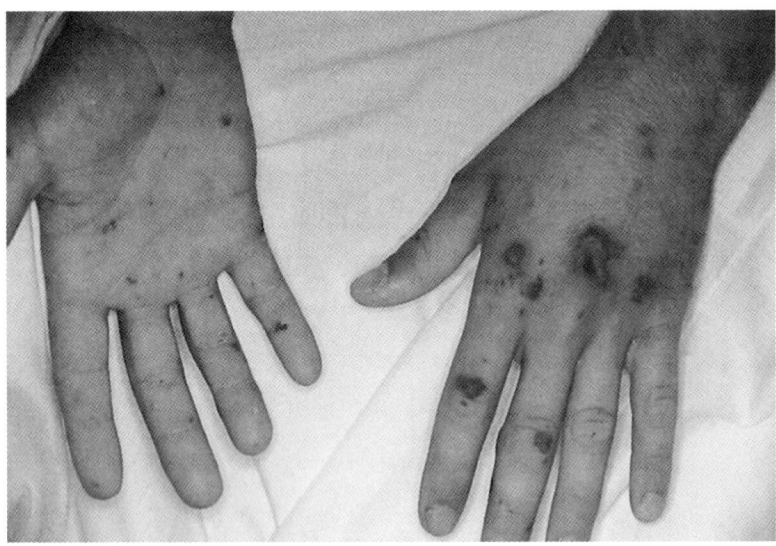

Figure 55-9. Purpuric lesions with sharply marginated borders on the hands of a patient with meningococcemia. (Courtesy of Department of Dermatology, Yale University School of Medicine.)

and soles in the context of fever may represent infective emboli with microabscess formation (Janeway lesions), which are often caused by *S. aureus* bacteremia.

Vesicles distributed in a more generalized pattern, especially with a concentration of lesions over the head and trunk, are suggestive of primary varicella-zoster virus infection (chickenpox), whereas a more generalized pattern with a concentration over the extremities is suggestive of enteroviral infection, especially with coxsackievirus A16 (hand-foot-mouth disease). The clinician evaluating the sexually active patient, especially a menstruating girl, presenting with asymmetric generalized pustules or vesicopustular lesions should also consider disseminated infection with *Neisseria gonorrhoeae.* Diffuse vesiculobullae may be noted in Stevens-Johnson syndrome, a hypersensitivity syndrome with significant constitutional symptoms.

Nodules

Nodules (discrete, raised, firm, well-demarcated lesions without fixation to the overlying skin) (see Fig. 55-2) may be associated with a number of underlying infectious or inflammatory disorders, such as polyarteritis and, rarely in children, Sweet syndrome (febrile neutrophilic dermatosis). Red, pink, or plum-colored nodules distributed in a seemingly random manner over the skin surface may represent leukemic infiltrates.

Erythema nodosum (erythematous and painful nodules usually distributed over the extremities) may be associated with bacterial infectious agents, such as group A β-hemolytic streptococcus; *S. pneumoniae; Yersinia* species; mycobacterial infections; fungal

infections with *Candida* species, *Histoplasma capsulatum, Cryptococcus neoformans,* or *Coccidioides immitis;* or drug reactions, especially in response to sulfonamides. Nonerythematous and nontender subcutaneous nodules may also be noted in patients with acute rheumatic fever, polyarticular juvenile rheumatoid arthritis (JRA), and dermatomyositis.

Ulcers

Ulcers are depressed lesions in which the epidermis and some or all of the dermis has been destroyed (see Fig. 55-5). In immunocompromised hosts, infection with herpes simplex virus may manifest with shallow erosive or ulcerative lesions. In immunocompetent hosts, cutaneous ulcerations may be noted in noninfectious disorders associated with vasculitis, such as SLE, polyarteritis nodosa, and Henoch-Schönlein purpura.

Pyoderma gangrenosum and *ecthyma gangrenosum* are painful cutaneous ulcerative lesions with an erythematous, raised edge. The lesion usually begins as a papule and breaks down rapidly with central necrosis. It may be seen in immunocompromised patients with systemic infections with bacterial pathogens, such as *Pseudomonas aeruginosa* and *Stenotrophomonas maltophila* (ecthyma). In immunocompetent patients, the lesion may manifest in the context of inflammatory bowel disease (pyoderma gangrenosum) or rheumatoid arthritis. Digital ulcerations may be noted in patients with small-vessel vasculitis, such as SLE. Oral ulcerations may be noted in those with herpes simplex or coxsackievirus (hand-foot-mouth disease) or as a manifestation of Behçet disease or inflammatory bowel disease.

Erythema

Diffuse erythema is probably associated with toxin-mediated disorders characterized by superantigen production (see Tables 55-3 and 55-4). Nonspecific T cell stimulation caused by superantigen production results in several acute rash-fever disorders, such as the staphylococcal scalded skin syndrome (Fig. 55-11), streptococcal scarlet fever, staphylococcal or streptococcal toxic shock syndrome, and, possibly, Kawasaki disease.

Localized erythema in the context of acute fever is strongly suggestive of cellulitis or abscess. The presence of warmth, tenderness, and associated lymphangitis is highly indicative. Organisms causing cellulitis or abscess formation are usually inoculated directly into the skin as a result of trauma. However, bacteremic localization is well

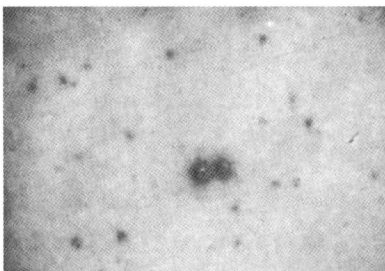

Figure 55-10. Skin lesions of chickenpox. Note the varying stages of development (macules, papules, and vesicles) present at the same time. (Courtesy of P. F. Lucchesi, M.D.)

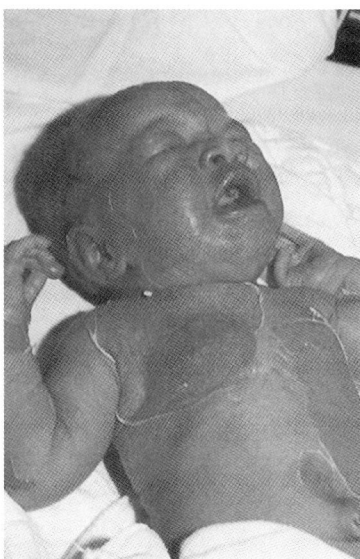

Figure 55-11. Infant with staphylococcal scalded skin syndrome. (From Behrman RE [ed]: Nelson Textbook of Pediatrics, 16th ed. Philadelphia, WB Saunders, 2000.)

described among young children with preseptal or facial cellulitis associated with *H. influenzae* type b or *S. pneumoniae*.

Patients with SLE may present with an isolated erythematous malar rash (butterfly rash), which is exacerbated by exposure to sunlight. The acute onset of intense "slapped-cheek" erythema of the face suggests erythema infectiosum, a recognizable exanthem caused by parvovirus B19, and should be differentiated easily from the malar rash of SLE, which usually manifests other characteristics, such as hyperkeratosis and follicular plugging. In addition, patients with erythema infectiosum tend to have a maculopapular lacelike rash over the arms, which may spread to the buttocks and thighs (Fig. 55-12; see Table 55-5).

Patients with dermatomyositis may have localized lilac-colored lesions over the eyelids (heliotrope rash), which may be associated with periorbital edema. Such patients characteristically, but not invariably, have an erythematous, scaly eruption on the face, neck, knees, elbows, and phalanges. When the rash is localized over the knuckles, it resembles dripped wax and has been referred to as *Gottron papules*.

Toxic Epidermal Necrolysis

Toxic epidermal necrolysis, an exfoliative dermatosis characterized by diffuse cutaneous erythema and full-thickness necrosis of the epidermis resembling a scald injury, may be an extremely severe form of erythema multiforme major. It is usually associated with exposure to drugs and differs histopathologically from staphylococcal scalded skin syndrome, which also manifests clinically with diffuse erythema and blistering, in its cleavage plane (see Table 55-4). In scalded skin syndrome, blistering is produced more superficially by disruption of the epidermal granular cell layer in response to one of two staphylococcal epidermolytic toxins (ET-A or ET-B). This results in easy disruption of skin with firm rubbing (Nikolsky sign).

Nonspecific Maculopapular Eruptions

Most fever-rash syndromes are characterized by nonspecific maculopapular eruptions that rarely assist the clinician in decision making. Although some experienced clinicians believe that characterizing the maculopapular eruption as *rubelliform* (generalized discrete maculopapular rash) or *morbilliform* (generalized confluent maculopapular rash) is of help diagnostically, prospective evaluation of this classification scheme indicates that the clinical features of the rash at presentation are unhelpful in defining the causative agent.

Star Complex

A valuable cluster of associated findings is the complex of sore throat (pharyngitis), elevated temperature, moderate to severe arthritis, and rash (STAR complex), which may be pruritic or urticarial, in the absence of signs of carditis, serositis, meningitis, adenopathy, or reticuloendothelial hyperplasia on physical examination. Short-duration (<3 weeks) STAR complex is associated usually with an infection caused by known viral agents, such as rubella (Fig. 55-13), parvovirus B19, hepatitis B virus, adenovirus, Epstein-Barr virus, and the enteroviruses; Lyme disease; or serum sickness associated with exposure to cefaclor, penicillin, or the combination of trimethoprim and sulfamethoxazole. STAR complex of intermediate duration (3 to 6 weeks) is suggestive of acute rheumatic fever, and that of long duration (>6 weeks) is suggestive of systemic JRA.

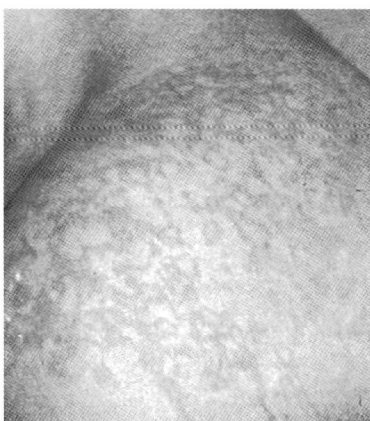

Figure 55-12. Erythema infectiosum. (From Korting GW: Hautkrankheiten bei Kindern und Jugendlichen, 3rd ed. Stuttgart, Germany, FK Schattauer Verlag, 1982.)

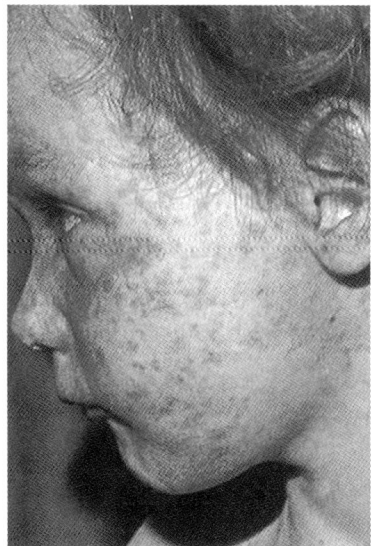

Figure 55-13. Rash of rubella (German measles). (From Korting GW: Hautkrankheiten bei Kindern und Jugendlichen, 3rd ed. Stuttgart, Germany, FK Schattauer Verlag, 1982.)

Other Clusters of Findings

Clusters of findings on examination that are of diagnostic importance include the following:

1. the *mucocutaneous-lymph node cluster* (bilateral conjunctival injection, palmar-plantar erythema/indurative edema of the hands and feet, erythema of the oropharyngeal mucosa/"strawberry" tongue, cervical lymphadenopathy), which is suggestive of Kawasaki disease, toxic shock syndrome, Stevens-Johnson syndrome, streptococcal scarlet fever, Rocky Mountain spotted fever, dengue, and leptospirosis
2. the *reticuloendothelial cell hyperplasia cluster* (hepatosplenomegaly with or without generalized adenopathy), which is suggestive of (1) disseminated infectious disease caused by bacteria (*Salmonella typhi* or other enteric fever pathogens), virus (cytomegalovirus, human immunodeficiency virus–1 [HIV-1], Epstein-Barr virus), rickettsia (*R. tsutsugamushi* in "scrub typhus"), protozoa (malaria), or fungus (*H. capsulatum, C. immitis*); (2) disseminated malignancy; (3) sarcoidosis; (4) histiocytic syndromes; or (5) collagen-vascular disease
3. the *mononucleosis-like syndrome cluster* (exudative pharyngitis and regional adenopathy with or without splenomegaly), which is suggestive of (1) infection with group A streptococcus, *Francisella tularensis,* Epstein-Barr virus, toxoplasmosis, cytomegalovirus, or coxsackievirus or (2) hypersensitivity reactions caused by drugs such as phenytoin.

The presence of isolated lower respiratory tract findings (decreased breath sounds, rales, expiratory wheezing) indicate underlying pulmonary infection with an organism such as measles, respiratory syncytial virus, adenovirus, *Mycobacterium pneumoniae,* or *Legionella pneumophila.* Although sarcoidosis, collagen-vascular disease, and systemic vasculitis (Wegener granulomatosis, Henoch-Schönlein purpura) may involve the lower respiratory tract, isolated pulmonary findings are infrequently indicative of these disorders.

Joint Manifestations

Pain, swelling, tenderness, and limited range of motion involving one joint or multiple joints, or that migrate from joint to joint, or discrete pain at the insertion of tendons, ligaments, or fascia (enthesopathy) indicates a primary infectious illness, a "reactive" (immunologically mediated) disorder, or a systemic inflammatory condition (see Chapter 44). Primary infectious illnesses associated with this finding include *N. gonorrhoeae, Borrelia burgdorferi,* parvovirus, and rubella, including vaccine-associated strains. Reactive disorders, such as reactive arthritis (arthritis/enthesitis, conjunctivitis, urethritis), may be associated with infection caused by enteric pathogens, such as *Salmonella* and *Shigella* organisms, or genital pathogens, such as *N. gonorrhoeae* or *Chlamydia* species, but may also include diseases of unknown origin, such as inflammatory bowel disease, in which the rash is usually erythema nodosum. Systemic inflammatory conditions include Kawasaki syndrome, polyarteritis, SLE, systemic-onset JRA, acute rheumatic fever, and familial Mediterranean fever.

Cardiac Manifestations

Isolated cardiac manifestations may accompany acute rheumatic fever, bacterial endocarditis, or systemic-onset JRA (see Chapter 11). The presence of tachycardia out of proportion to the severity of the fever may be indicative of the carditis accompanying acute rheumatic fever, although this is not an invariable finding. A precordial friction rub is suggestive of pericarditis, which is noted frequently in patients with JRA. The presence of a new murmur or a changing murmur on auscultation is suggestive of bacterial endocarditis, whereas the detection of the apical systolic murmur of mitral regurgitation or the diastolic murmur of aortic insufficiency is suggestive

of acute rheumatic fever. A gallop rhythm on auscultation indicates underlying myocarditis, which may accompany coxsackievirus infection, rheumatic disease, or Kawasaki disease.

Ocular Manifestations

Isolated ocular manifestations, such as conjunctival injection and frank conjunctivitis, may be suggestive of infection with measles or adenovirus, leptospirosis, Kawasaki disease, erythema multiforme, or reactive arthritis. Anterior uveitis (redness with accompanying photophobia or pain or change in vision) may indicate Kawasaki disease, systemic JRA, sarcoidosis, ulcerative colitis or, uncommonly, an infection such as leptospirosis (see Chapter 44). Retinal hemorrhages seen on funduscopy may indicate bacterial endocarditis.

Neurologic Manifestations

Neurologic findings accompanying fever and rash may be indicative of specific infectious or immunologically mediated disorders. Mental status findings suggestive of recent-onset psychosis may indicate cerebritis, which can accompany SLE. Significant alteration in mental status accompanied by seizure or focal motor impairment or cerebellar dysfunction may be suggestive of primary infectious encephalitis associated with arbovirus, herpes simplex, measles, varicella-zoster virus, rickettsia, or *M. pneumoniae* infection. Nuchal rigidity, the Kernig sign, or the Brudzinski sign indicates meningeal irritation, which may accompany infection caused by the enteroviruses; bacteria such as *S. pneumoniae, N. meningitidis,* or *H. influenzae* type b; fungi such as *H. capsulatum* and spirochetes such as *B. burgdorferi;* or inflammation caused by underlying SLE, sarcoidosis, or Kawasaki disease (see Chapter 52). Cranial nerve palsies, ataxia, or peripheral neuropathy may accompany infection with *B. burgdorferi* early in the course of Lyme disease (especially Bell palsy), or it may indicate an underlying vasculitis, such as SLE. Movement abnormalities, particularly chorea, may be suggestive of either SLE or acute rheumatic fever.

LABORATORY TESTS

The history and physical examination together determine the prior probability of a specific disease. In the context of a very high or very low prior probability of a specific disease, laboratory testing adds very little useful information. Thus, laboratory testing is most useful when the prior probability of disease is equivocal.

The clinician should perform a Gram stain of any ulcerative, pustular, petechial, or purpuric lesion. The identification of bacteria suggests pyogenic infection, which may be localized or disseminated. The presence of only polymorphonuclear white blood cells in fluid of pustular lesions does not exclude bacterial infection from consideration, especially disseminated infection with *N. gonorrhoeae.* Specimens of these lesions or any fluid from a pustule should also be obtained for bacterial culture.

Vesicular and bullous lesions in a febrile child with an uncertain diagnosis should be unroofed, scraped at the base, and submitted for microscopic examination after Tzanck preparation (see Chapter 56). The presence of multinucleated giant cells or eosinophilic intranuclear inclusions indicates infection with herpesvirus or varicella-zoster virus. The sensitivity of the Tzanck preparation for cutaneous herpes simplex infection is 64%, and the specificity is 86%. Because the sensitivity of the procedure is low, a negative result does not exclude the diagnosis of herpes simplex infection. Thus, to isolate the virus, a specimen of the lesion should also be obtained for culture or polymerase chain reaction (PCR). The diagnostic yields of both the viral culture and the Tzanck preparation are also a function of the type of lesion sampled. The rates of viral recovery from culture and positive microscopy are highest when vesicular lesions are sampled (100% and 67%, respectively) and lowest when crusted ulcers are sampled (33% and 17%, respectively). More reliable rapid diagnostic techniques are available, including PCR or direct fluorescent antibody staining of vesicle scrapings and enzyme immunoassay for detection of herpes simplex virus antigens.

Punch biopsy for light and electron microscopy and immunohistologic studies should be considered for diagnostic purposes for patients presenting with fever and bullous lesions that are clearly not typical pyodermas; fever and nodular lesions; or lesions suggestive of vasculitis (palpable purpura, livedo reticularis). A punch biopsy with indirect immunofluorescent antibody staining may also be useful for patients with petechial lesions, especially in an acral distribution, for the early diagnosis (at days 4 to 8 of illness) of infection with *R. rickettsii*. This procedure has a sensitivity of 53% and a specificity of 100%. The low sensitivity of the test may be related to the rickettsiostatic effect of antimicrobial treatment before presentation, but it indicates clearly that decision making in the acute care setting is limited by the high rate of false-negative classifications expected with this procedure.

Diagnosing a systemic infectious illness may necessitate the use of specific bacterial, viral, or fungal culture techniques; paired acute- and convalescent-phase serologic study; antigen detection systems; or molecular techniques such as PCR. Culture techniques are most specific when normally sterile tissue or body fluids are sampled and inoculated directly into liquid or solid media. Interpretation of bacterial cultures obtained from nonsterile sites, such as the tonsils and nasopharynx, are subject to increased rates of false-positive results because of recovery of organisms that colonize these areas.

Serologic techniques are potentially useful in establishing a diagnosis of a specific infection by demonstrating a fourfold rise in titer between samples obtained during the acute and convalescent phases of illness. Detection of a recent infection with group A streptococci may be accomplished by demonstrating a fourfold rise in antibodies to streptolysin-O (ASO titer) or by demonstrating the presence of other extracellular antigens produced by the streptococci (deoxyribonuclease B, hyaluronidase, streptokinase, nicotinamide adenine dinucleotidase) with the Streptozyme agglutination test. On occasion, during the acute phase of illness, a single titer that exceeds a certain threshold value (ASO titer > 1:333 or complement fixation titer > 1:256 for *M. pneumoniae*) may strongly suggest a specific diagnosis at presentation.

Antigen detection systems are useful for rapid diagnosis. A solid phase detection system, such as enzyme-linked immunosorbent assay (ELISA), has the advantage of being independent of the need for intact cellular material but is affected by antigen or antibody cross-reactivity in the sample (which limits specificity) and by poor antigen-antibody affinity (which limits sensitivity). Nonetheless, ELISA is the preferred technique for the serologic diagnosis of a wide spectrum of infectious agents, including *B. burgdorferi* (the causative agent of Lyme disease) and hepatitis B virus.

Latex particle agglutination is an alternative solid phase antigen detection system that does not require intact cellular material and whose advantages include rapidity of use and ease of interpretation. Latex particle agglutination is used for the rapid identification of patients with group A streptococcal pharyngitis or with invasive disease caused by encapsulated bacteria, such as *S. pneumoniae*, *H. influenzae* type b, *N. meningitidis*, group B streptococci, and *Escherichia coli* BK1. Latex particle agglutination is limited by factors similar to those affecting ELISA. Latex agglutination tests for group A streptococci have specificities of more than 90%, which facilitates their use for clinical confirmation of infection, but their sensitivities are only 60% to 90%, which limits their use in excluding infection.

Confirmation of infection with the rickettsiae is probably best accomplished through serologic techniques demonstrating a fourfold increase in titer, because culture systems are not widely available. Alternatively, culture, immunoblot, or PCR techniques rather than serologic tests best confirm many specific viral pathogens.

The identification of patients with noninfectious systemic illness caused by underlying collagen-vascular disease, immune complex disease, or vasculitis is best accomplished through serologic techniques combined with other indirect laboratory evidence of active inflammation or tissue injury (see Chapter 44).

DIAGNOSIS AND DECISION MAKING

Accurate diagnosis depends on careful synthesis of selected data obtained from the clinical assessment. Because most children with acute episodes of fever and rash have a common, self-limited infectious disease, a specific diagnosis can often be established simply by pattern recognition alone (e.g., visual recognition of the common exanthema of childhood or the specific lesion of erythema chronicum migrans) or with minimal use of adjunctive testing (a rash consistent with scarlet fever accompanied by a positive latex agglutination test for group A streptococcal antigen). Because the spectrum of infectious pathogens is broad, however, presenting complaints or features of the rash may be atypical and, on occasion, the diagnosis may not yield easily to simple pattern recognition. In these situations, empirical use of the laboratory may prove useful to the clinician.

In series of febrile children presenting for evaluation of generalized erythematous rashes of various patterns that were not indicative of a specific disorder by history or examination, an infectious cause could be established in 65% after a limited set of laboratory tests. The tests consisted of a throat culture for streptococci (including non–group A streptococci) and serologic studies to detect rubella, measles, hepatitis A and B virus, Epstein-Barr virus, parvovirus B19, and *M. pneumoniae*. This strategy was based on physician knowledge of the age-specific and/or seasonal incidence of infectious pathogens in the population studied. It may be preferable to "watchful waiting" and serial clinical follow-up when the patient is judged to be at risk for a treatable illness associated with significant subsequent morbidity (e.g., streptococcal infection leading to acute rheumatic fever) or when specific information is necessary to advise parents of the risk of contagion to other children, to immunocompromised contacts, or to pregnant women.

The subset of patients with fever and rash who appear toxic, have unstable vital signs or altered mental status, or manifest a petechial or purpuric component to their rash must have a comprehensive evaluation and a diagnosis confirmed as quickly as possible to detect potentially life-threatening underlying infection. The diagnostic approach to the child with fever and a petechial or purpuric rash includes a complete blood cell count with a differential white blood cell count, a coagulation profile, and cultures of throat, blood, and cerebrospinal fluid (CSF). If the patient has normal mental status, no nuchal rigidity, and no toxicity, a lumbar puncture may not be needed. Patients older than 36 months with primary complaints of sore throat and fever and clinical evidence of pharyngitis may be evaluated more conservatively, with a complete blood cell count and differential and a throat swab for rapid streptococcal antigen detection and culture.

Patients with a normal platelet count and coagulation profile but with a total peripheral white cell count exceeding 15,000/mm³ or less than 5000/mm³, an absolute band count exceeding 500 cells/mm³, or a CSF examination demonstrating more than 7 cells/mm³ in the context of fever and petechiae or purpura have up to a 48% likelihood of invasive bacterial or rickettsial infection and thus should be admitted to a hospital for appropriate antimicrobial therapy. Patients with thrombocytopenia and an abnormal coagulation profile should be admitted for further evaluation and treatment of DIC, which may have an underlying infectious or inflammatory cause. Patients with thrombocytopenia and a normal coagulation profile may have infection with tickborne rickettsial pathogens, *Ehrlichia chaffeensis*, Epstein-Barr virus, an autoimmune disease such as SLE, or a primary hematologic-oncologic disorder, such as idiopathic thrombocytopenic purpura or leukemia associated with an intercurrent infection; such patients should be evaluated for these disorders. However, irrespective of the suspected underlying cause, all such patients with platelet counts less than 50,000/mm³ should be admitted to the hospital for observation and consultation with a hematologist. Furthermore, many authorities recommend treating all patients with parenteral antibiotics if they manifest fever without a focus and petechiae that cannot be explained by significant and repeated coughing or emesis.

In certain instances, the diagnostic approach to disorders manifesting with fever and rash is wholly dependent on an aggregation of nonspecific signs, symptoms, and laboratory results. These disorders either have many underlying causes manifesting with overlapping features or have unknown causes for which no confirmatory tests have yet been devised. Diagnosis by formalized aggregation, termed *syndromic diagnosis,* must be considered an essential part of the comprehensive approach to the patient with fever and rash. Although syndromic diagnosis is based on explicit clinical criteria, some of the clusters of signs, symptoms, and laboratory findings were established originally for epidemiologic purposes (case definition) to facilitate exploration of an underlying cause. As such, although they are usually quite specific, these criteria may be less sensitive when they are applied in the acute care setting for the purposes of clinical diagnosis.

Syndromic diagnosis is applicable to the following disorders: toxic shock syndrome, acute rheumatic fever (see Chapter 11), SLE (see Chapter 44), Kawasaki disease, erythema multiforme, hypersensitivity reactions (serum sickness), and dermatomyositis (see Chapter 44).

TOXIC SHOCK SYNDROME

The diagnosis of toxic shock syndrome is confirmed from criteria established by the Centers for Disease Control and Prevention. The criteria include

1. temperature higher than 39.2° C
2. diffuse macular erythroderma
3. desquamation localized predominantly on palms and soles during convalescence
4. hypotension, defined as systolic blood pressure less than the fifth percentile for age among children or adolescents, or orthostatic hypotension
5. evidence of multisystem involvement as manifested by dysfunction in more than three organ systems (gastrointestinal: diarrhea, vomiting; musculoskeletal: myalgia, elevated creatine phosphokinase; hyperemic: vagina, pharynx, conjunctiva; renal: sterile pyuria, blood urea nitrogen or creatinine levels > twice normal; liver: bilirubin or aspartate or alanine aminotransferase level > twice normal; hematologic: thrombocytopenia; CNS: altered mental status).
6. negative evidence of underlying bacterial infection, as indicated by sterile cultures of blood, urine, and cerebrospinal fluid, and a throat culture negative for significant growth of group A streptococci
7. negative diagnostic studies for measles virus, the rickettsiae, and the leptospirae

Because toxic shock syndrome is probably the result of superantigen production by either staphylococci or streptococci, both menstrual and nonmenstrual cases have been described, and a history of tampon use is of limited assistance to the pediatric clinician. Affected younger children present with symptoms of acute-onset hyperpyrexia and complaints of myalgia, headache or dizziness, sore throat, or gastrointestinal upset manifested by vomiting, abdominal pain, or diarrhea. A cofocus of infection (tracheitis, pneumonia, wound, nasal packing) may be identified on examination, which may be the only clue that the patient has nonmenstrual toxic shock syndrome.

KAWASAKI DISEASE

Kawasaki disease, also known as the *mucocutaneous lymph node syndrome,* is an acute, febrile illness of unknown origin that has a worldwide distribution and tends to affect young children (predominantly

younger than 5 years), irrespective of race. Ninety percent of affected patients are younger than 8 years at diagnosis. The recurrence rate is 4%. The major morbid sequelae are aneurysms of the coronary arteries, noted in up to 25% of untreated patients.

Six criteria have been established for the diagnosis of Kawasaki disease:

1. fever of more than 38° C persisting for more than 5 days
2. bilateral, bulbar, nonexudative conjunctival injection
3. polymorphous rash, which may be accentuated in the perineal or perianal region
4. changes in the extremities, including indurative edema of the hands or feet and palmar or plantar erythema or desquamation, especially in the periungual region
5. changes in the oral mucosa, including cracking or fissuring of the lips, strawberry tongue, and diffuse oropharyngeal erythema
6. enlargement of a single or of multiple cervical lymph nodes to more than 1.5 cm in diameter (Figs. 55-14 to 55-19)

The presence of fever and at least four of the remaining five criteria is sufficient for clinical confirmation in a patient who has no clinical or laboratory evidence of another disease, such as a common infectious exanthema, Epstein-Barr virus infection, scarlet fever, toxic shock syndrome, leptospirosis, rickettsiosis, JRA, measles, drug reaction, polyarteritis, or the Stevens-Johnson syndrome.

Older children may have presenting features such as vomiting, diarrhea, arthralgias, arthritis, headache, and sore throat that may initially obscure the diagnosis. Associated findings in Kawasaki disease include aseptic meningitis, urethritis, jaundice, hepatitis, and hydrops of the gallbladder. Supportive but nondiagnostic laboratory data include peripheral blood leukocytosis, mild nonhemolytic anemia, thrombocytosis (platelet count > 650,000/mm³ in the second or

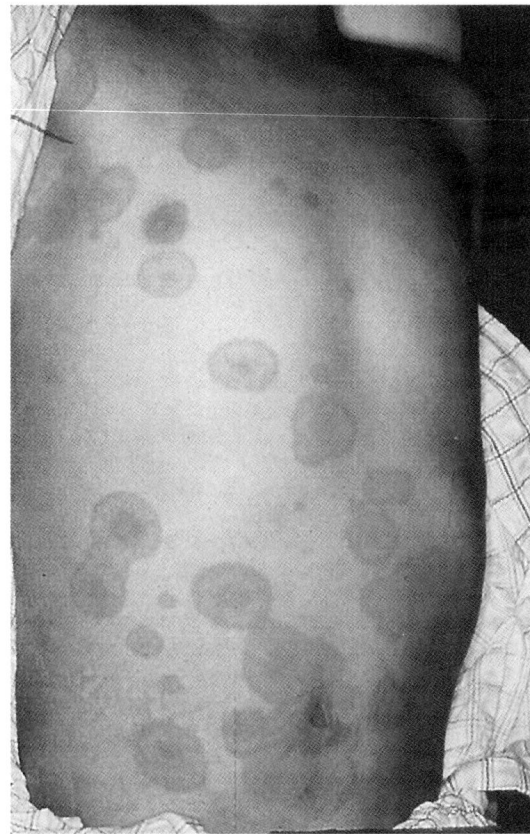

Figure 55-14. Erythema multiforme in a child with Kawasaki disease (mucocutaneous lymph node syndrome). (Courtesy of Tomisaku Kawasaki, M.D.)

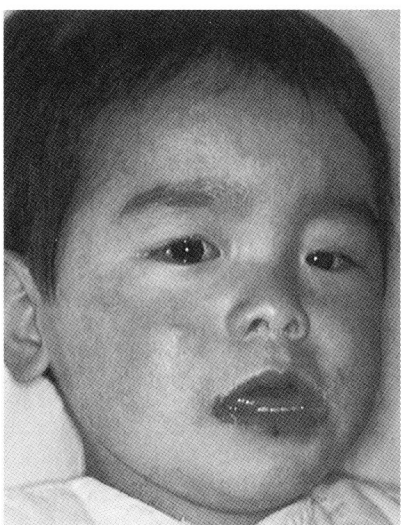

Figure 55-15. Kawasaki disease. Note characteristic facies with congestion of the bulbar conjunctivae and hemorrhagic crusts and erosions of the lips. (Courtesy of Tomisaku Kawasaki, M.D.)

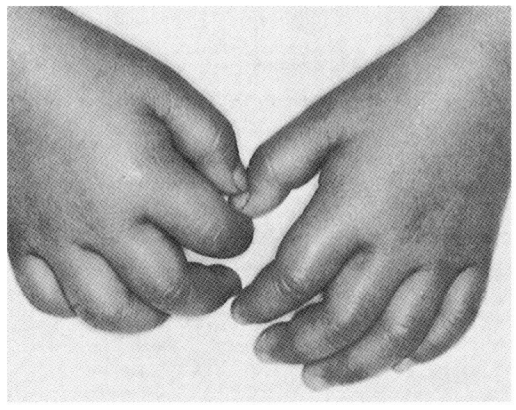

Figure 55-16. Indurative edema of the hands in Kawasaki disease. (Courtesy of Tomisaku Kawasaki, M.D.)

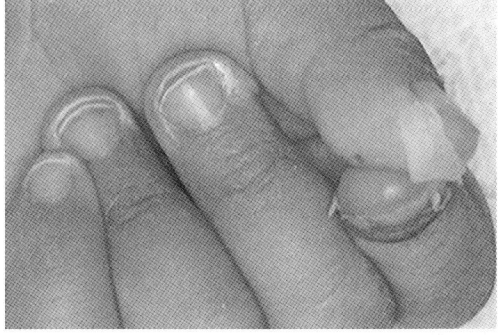

Figure 55-17. Desquamation of the fingers in a patient with Kawasaki disease, convalescent stage. (Courtesy of Tomisaku Kawasaki, M.D.)

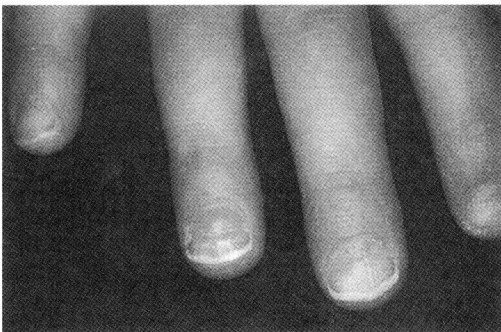

Figure 55-18. Beau lines, a horizontal groove on the nails of a patient with Kawasaki disease, convalescent stage. (From Hurwitz S: Clinical Pediatric Dermatology: A Textbook of Skin Disorders of Childhood and Adolescence, 2nd ed. Philadelphia, WB Saunders, 1993, p 549.)

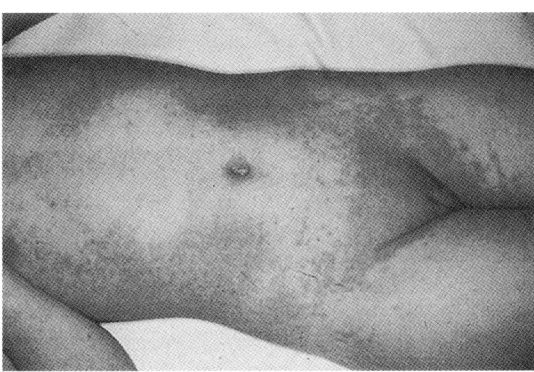

Figure 55-19. A scarlet fever–like rash in a child with Kawasaki disease. (Courtesy of Tomisaku Kawasaki, M.D.)

third week of disease), elevated sedimentation rate (ESR) or C-reactive protein level, elevated bilirubin or hepatic transaminase levels, hypoalbuminemia, hyponatremia, and sterile pyuria. Electrocardiography may demonstrate prolonged PR or QT intervals or nonspecific changes in the ST-T waves, whereas echocardiography may reveal pericardial effusion, decreased myocardial contractility, or valvar insufficiency early and coronary artery ectasia or aneurysms later in the course of illness. The disease phases, complications, and pathologic correlates are summarized in Table 55-6.

Because cardiovascular sequelae similar to those in classic Kawasaki disease have been found in young patients (especially those younger than 6 months) who present with incomplete or atypical features of this disorder, patients with prolonged febrile illnesses (>5 days) should be considered at high risk. They should be monitored by serial clinical examination, electrocardiography, and echocardiography for any evidence of cardiovascular dysfunction or early coronary artery abnormalities.

ERYTHEMA MULTIFORME

Erythema multiforme is a hypersensitivity syndrome that manifests skin lesions, with or without mucosal involvement (see Chapter 56). The lesions are erythematous and demonstrate polymorphous characteristics. The basic lesions are macular, urticarial, and vesiculobullous and are symmetrically distributed, especially over the palms, soles, and extensor surfaces of the extremities. The primary lesion is an erythematous macule or urticarial lesion in which a central papule, vesicle, or fine petechiae develop. Subsequently, the central portion clears, and a target ("iris") lesion, with concentric rings of

Table 55-6. Kawasaki Disease: Disease Phases, Complications, and Degree of Arteritis in Untreated Patients

	Acute	Subacute	Convalescent	Chronic
Clinical findings	Duration (1-11 days) Fever, conjunctivitis, oral changes, extremity changes, irritability, rash, cervical lymphadenopathy, high ESR	Duration (11-21 days) Irritability persists Prolongation of fever may occur Normalization of most clinical findings Palpable aneurysms may develop	Duration (21-60 days) Most clinical findings resolve Aneurysmal dilatation of peripheral vessels may persist Conjunctivitis may persist	Duration (? yr)
Complications	Early arthritis Myocarditis Pericarditis Mitral insufficiency Congestive heart failure Iridocyclitis Meningitis Sterile pyuria	Cononary aneurysms Late-onset arthritis Mitral insufficiency Gallbladder hydrops Fingertip and toe desquamation Thrombocytosis Coronary thrombosis with infarction	Arthritis may persist Coronary and peripheral aneurysms may persist Acute-phase reactant normalization	Angina pectoris, coronary stenosis, or myocardial insufficiency may develop
Arterial correlates	Perivasculitis, vasculitis of capillaries, arterioles, venules Inflammation of intima of medium and large arteries	Aneurysms, thrombi, stenosis of medium-sized arteries, panvasculitis, edema of vessel wall Myocarditis less prominent	Vascular inflammation decreases	Scar formation Intimal thickening
Cause of death	Myocarditis	Myocardial infarction Rupture of aneurysm Myocarditis	Myocardial infarction Ischemic heart disease	Myocardial infarction

Modified from Hicks RV, Melish ME: Kawasaki syndrome. Pediatr Clin North Am 1986;33:1151. Reprinted from Behrman RE (ed): Nelson Textbook of Pediatrics, 14th ed. Philadelphia, WB Saunders, 1992, p 630.

ESR, erythrocyte sedimentation rate.

alternating erythema and cyanosis, is apparent (see Fig. 55-14). The presence of these characteristic lesions on the skin and, at most, one mucosal surface (usually the oral mucosa) in an acutely febrile child is characteristic of erythema multiforme minor. Recurrent erythema multiforme minor has been associated with herpes simplex virus infection.

The presence of these characteristic skin lesions and involvement of two or more mucosal surfaces is characteristic of erythema multiforme major, a more severe form of this hypersensitivity syndrome (Stevens-Johnson syndrome). The key feature that distinguishes this syndrome is the presence of blistering lesions, which may involve the lips, eyes, nasal mucosa, genitalia, or rectum (Figs. 55-20 and 55-21). Extensive ocular involvement, including corneal ulceration, uveitis, and panophthalmitis, may develop. Pulmonary and renal involvement has also been reported. Erythema multiforme major has been associated with *M. pneumoniae* infection and exposure to drugs, including penicillins, sulfonamides, and anticonvulsants.

SERUM SICKNESS

Serum sickness is a systemic hypersensitivity reaction resulting from immune complex deposition in or around blood vessels that causes tissue damage through complement activation and may follow the administration of foreign proteins or drugs. Because other disorders, such as SLE, are characterized by immune complex–type hypersensitivity, serum sickness manifests clinical features that are nonspecific and include complaints of abdominal pain, nausea, vomiting, malaise and arthralgia, polyarticular arthritis and tender lymphadenopathy associated with fever, and an urticarial or erythematous palmar or plantar serpiginous rash. Uncommon findings include

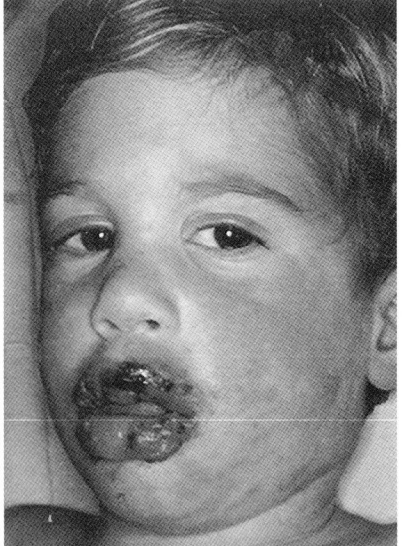

Figure 55-20. Stevens-Johnson syndrome (bullous erythema multiforme). Mucous membrane involvement with severe swelling and hemorrhagic crusting of the lips. (From Hurwitz S: Clinical Pediatric Dermatology: A Textbook of Skin Disorders of Childhood and Adolescence, 2nd ed. Philadelphia, WB Saunders, 1993, p 527.)

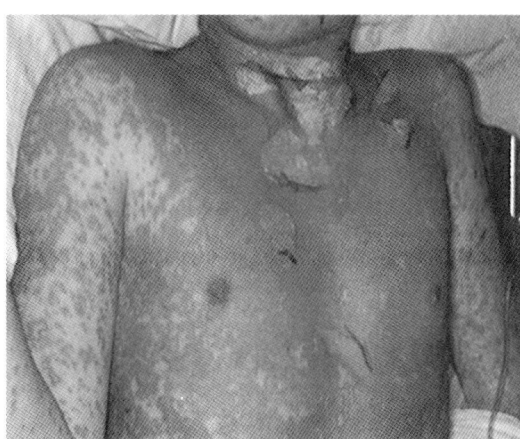

Figure 55-21. Stevens-Johnson syndrome. Confluent erythema, target lesions, blisters, and exfoliation of the epidermis are present. (From Hurwitz S: Clinical Pediatric Dermatology: A Textbook of Skin Disorders of Childhood and Adolescence, 2nd ed. Philadelphia, WB Saunders, 1993, p 528.)

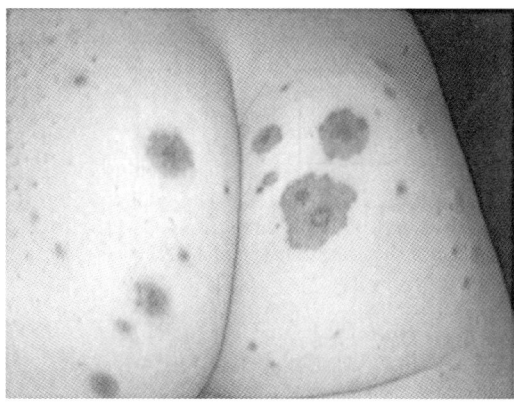

Figure 55-22. Henoch-Schönlein purpura (anaphylactoid purpura). Hemorrhagic macules, papules, and urticarial lesions appear in a symmetric distribution over the buttocks of a young child. (From Hurwitz S: Clinical Pediatric Dermatology: A Textbook of Skin Disorders of Childhood and Adolescence, 2nd ed. Philadelphia, WB Saunders, 1993, p 540.)

peripheral neuropathy, angioedema, and clinical evidence of myoperi-carditis. Critical to the diagnosis of serum sickness is a history of exposure to drugs or heterologous protein antitoxins given from 1 day to 2 weeks before the onset of illness; antibiotics such as the peni-cillins, sulfonamides, and cephalosporins; anticonvulsants such as phenytoin; antihypertensives such as hydralazine and propranolol; and antivenins. Characteristically, illness associated with a primary exposure evolves less rapidly than illness associated with a second-ary exposure; this reflects the time required for immune complexes generated in response to the exposure to reach a critical level for clinical manifestations to develop.

Laboratory testing plays a minor direct role in the diagnosis of serum sickness. Eosinophilia is helpful when noted on the peripheral blood smear or when the level of total hemolytic complement in serum is found to be depressed. Although glomerulonephritis may occur, it is usually clinically silent or mild, and urinalysis demon-strates cylindruria or minimal, but not heavy, proteinuria. This latter finding, if present on urinalysis, should suggest an alternative diag-nosis. Serologic laboratory testing may be of assistance in excluding other, more specific disorders that mimic serum sickness, such as SLE, rubella, hepatitis B, and Epstein-Barr virus. A watchful waiting approach may support the diagnosis, inasmuch as the syndrome should resolve within approximately 4 weeks if exposure to the pur-ported offending agent has been curtailed. Persistence of findings beyond this period indicate another disorder associated with immune complex–mediated vasculitis (see Chapters 44 and 56).

OTHER DISORDERS

Certain disorders manifesting with fever and rash can be approached as diagnoses of exclusion or as diagnoses necessitating tissue confir-mation. These disorders are generally encountered with low fre-quency in pediatric practice, but all are well described and have associated morbidities, and thus accurate and timely diagnosis is imperative. Diagnoses of exclusion include systemic-onset (chronic) JRA (see Chapter 44), and Henoch-Schönlein purpura. Representa-tive diagnoses usually necessitating tissue confirmation are sarcoido-sis and other vasculitides, such as polyarteritis nodosa or Wegener granulomatosis.

Henoch-Schönlein purpura is a vasculitic syndrome of unknown origin that affects vessels in the skin, joints, gastrointestinal tract, and kidneys. The clinical manifestations include a rash, which initially is urticarial and then frequently evolves into a maculopapu-lar eruption; after this eruption, petechiae and then purpuric plaques

distributed predominantly on the buttocks and over the lower extremities develop (Fig. 55-22). These plaques usually are raised from the skin surface, which gives the rash its characteristic feature of "palpable purpura." Associated findings that are variably present include arthralgias and arthritis; edema of the feet, hands, face, scro-tum, and scalp; melena, which may accompany intussusception; and an abnormal urinalysis that demonstrates hematuria and proteinuria.

Laboratory testing is of use to the clinician in excluding the infec-tious or hematologic causes of purpura. Specifically, the results of both the platelet count and the coagulation profile are normal, and blood cultures are sterile. A Gram stain of the lesion is not usually needed, but the results are negative, and skin biopsy demonstrates the characteristic leukocytoclastic vasculitis involving the vessels in the dermis. This finding is not specific for Henoch-Schönlein pur-pura, nor is it required for clinical confirmation.

MANAGEMENT

Treatment of patients with fever and rash includes both anticipatory guidance and specific interventions. Anticipatory guidance alone usually suffices for patients who have a clearly identifiable, acute, self-limited, and noninvasive infectious disorder. Parents should be informed of the probable duration of illness, the expected evolution of clinical manifestations, potential complications and how to recog-nize them, and when to recontact the physician (passive surveillance) (see Tables 55-4 and 55-5). Active surveillance by the physician to detect complications through follow-up telephone contact or a return visit may be appropriate when there is concern that the caretakers may not be reliable observers or when the patient manifests a higher level of clinical toxicity than anticipated. Among patients in whom the diagnosis is nonspecific, the strategy of active surveillance is clinically prudent.

Therapeutic interventions may be supportive, empirical, or defin-itive. *Supportive interventions* are appropriate for all patients but especially for those with recognizable derangements in physiologic homeostasis at presentation. These interventions are aimed at preventing or replacing fluid losses; maintaining adequate systemic oxygenation, ventilation, and perfusion; and supporting metabolism through maintenance of adequate levels of blood glucose. For most patients, fluid maintenance or replacement may be achieved via the enteral route, but for patients with altered mental status or car-diovascular instability, the parenteral approach is more appropriate.

The use of antipyretics as supportive therapy for patients with fever remains controversial. Arguments in favor of such therapy include decreasing symptomatic discomfort associated with the febrile state and reducing the undesirable metabolic and cardiopulmonary effects. A concern exists, however, regarding the choice of antipyretic agents for treating fever and rash. Reye syndrome has been reported in association with aspirin consumption among patients with varicella or other viral illnesses. In view of the high likelihood that patients with an acute fever-rash illness have an underlying viral illness, aspirin should be avoided for antipyresis; acetaminophen should be used instead. In patients with fever and rash caused by systemic inflammatory disorders (JRA, SLE), aspirin or, more often, other nonsteroidal antiinflammatory agents (ibuprofen, naproxen, tolmetin) play an important role in both control of fever and modulation of disease activity.

Empirical therapy is employed when the diagnosis of a treatable disorder associated with unacceptable rates of morbidity or mortality is suspected but when confirmation is lacking, either because more specific test results are pending at the time of presentation or no specific tests exist to guide management further. Empirical therapy with antibiotics is an appropriate strategy for patients with focal cutaneous infection, such as cellulitis and erythema chronicum migrans, for patients with petechial or purpuric rash who are thought to have invasive infectious disorders, or for patients who appear toxic or manifest signs of cardiovascular instability.

Cellulitis is associated with a broad spectrum of bacterial organisms in immunocompetent hosts. The most common organisms directly inoculated after local trauma (even microscopic, less obvious trauma) are coagulase-positive *S. aureus* and group A streptococci. The most common organisms acquired through bacteremic localization unassociated with trauma in children younger than 4 years of age (preseptal or buccal cellulitis) are *S. pneumoniae* and, less commonly, *H. influenzae* type b. In immunocompromised hosts, *P. aeruginosa* and the gram-negative enteric rods are also frequently recovered. Empirical treatment of the immunocompetent host with cellulitis should include either an antistaphylococcal penicillin or a first-generation cephalosporin. A third-generation cephalosporin, such as ceftriaxone or cefotaxime, should be given for secondary cellulitis believed to be related to a primary bacteremia. The immunocompromised host should be treated empirically with a combination of an aminoglycoside and a third-generation cephalosporin with activity against *P. aeruginosa,* such as ceftazidime. Bacteremic patients may require a complete 7- to 10-day course of parenteral therapy.

Empirical treatment of the patient with fever and petechiae or purpura should be directed at correcting underlying DIC (see Chapter 50), if present, and at providing broad-spectrum antimicrobial therapy against both gram-positive and gram-negative bacteria. If epidemiologic evidence or clinical features are suggestive of infection with a *Rickettsia* species, the antimicrobial regimen should include doxycycline in a dosage of 4 mg/kg/day, not to exceed 100 mg/day for children younger than 9 years of age. Doxycycline at this dosage is preferred over chloramphenicol for treatment of Rocky Mountain spotted fever and ehrlichiosis, even for children younger than 8 years, and minimizes the risk of staining dentition. Ongoing monitoring of coagulation status, platelet counts, and renal function is essential.

The empirical choice of antimicrobial agents is guided by the age of the patient and the presence of any underlying focus of infection, such as meningitis. Young infants (younger than 2 months) are frequently infected by group B streptococcus, gram-negative enteric rods, and, to a lesser extent, *Listeria monocytogenes* or the encapsulated pathogens, such as *S. pneumoniae, H. influenzae* type b, *N. meningitidis,* and *N. gonorrhoeae.* Disseminated herpes simplex infection or herpes meningoencephalitis should be considered in the neonate (younger than 1 month) presenting with a vesicular rash and laboratory evidence of DIC, or with a sterile CSF pleocytosis. Older infants, children, and adolescents are frequently infected by the encapsulated pathogens and by *Salmonella* species.

For very young infants (<30 days), the combination of intravenous ampicillin and an aminoglycoside or, more often, a third-generation cephalosporin, such as cefotaxime, constitutes appropriate empirical therapy (see Chapters 52 and 57). Parenteral administration of acyclovir should be considered if herpes simplex is a possibility. For older patients, parenteral monotherapy with a third-generation cephalosporin, such as ceftriaxone or cefotaxime, usually suffices. However, because of the increasing frequency of infection with penicillin-resistant *S. pneumoniae,* vancomycin should be added to the regimen if pneumococcal meningitis is suspected (see Chapters 52 and 57).

Patients for whom a diagnosis is established by pattern recognition, case finding, syndromic aggregation, biopsy, or exclusion may receive *definitive interventions,* as available, if the treatment benefits outweigh the risks. Because definitive interventions may not always be curative, they include prescription of antimicrobial agents, antiinflammatory drugs, or immunosuppressants.

Toxic shock syndrome should be treated intravenously with a β-lactamase–resistant penicillin at the maximal dosage appropriate for the patient's age. Toxin and cytokine production should be curtailed with a bacterial protein synthesis inhibitor such as clindamycin.

Intravenous immunoglobulin reduces T cell production of interleukin-6 and tumor necrosis factor α and may be used as adjunctive therapy for streptococcal toxic shock syndrome to neutralize bacterial exotoxins.

Group A streptococcal infections or associated disorders, such as acute rheumatic fever, should be treated with penicillin. Standard therapy for pharyngitis associated with scarlet fever or acute rheumatic fever is penicillin given orally or as an intramuscular injection of benzathine penicillin (see Chapters 1 and 11).

Infections with herpes simplex virus or varicella-zoster virus may be treated with oral or intravenous acyclovir. Intravenous therapy is particularly appropriate for immunocompromised or immunosuppressed patients (see Chapter 29). The benefits of acyclovir therapy for herpes simplex virus or varicella-zoster virus in immunocompetent hosts are less clear.

Pharmacologic interventions in the systemic inflammatory disorders of unknown origin include antiinflammatory agents, such as the nonsteroidal agents and corticosteroids. Antiinflammatory therapy with prednisone has been reported to be beneficial in reducing mortality rates among patients with acute rheumatic fever who manifest severe carditis (congestive heart failure), systemic-onset JRA, SLE, dermatomyositis, and the vasculitides. Patients with acute rheumatic fever who do not have carditis, Henoch-Schönlein purpura, Stevens-Johnson syndrome, or serum sickness may also benefit symptomatically from antiinflammatory therapy, but the efficacy of such therapy in the reduction or prevention of morbidity remains controversial. Steroids may increase the risk of infection.

Immunosuppressant or modulating agents include intravenous immune globulin (IVIG), cyclosporine, azathioprine, and cyclophosphamide. Although the latter drugs may be used adjunctively with corticosteroids as interventions for SLE or the necrotizing vasculitides, IVIG administration is considered a definitive intervention in all patients with Kawasaki disease to reduce coronary aneurysm formation. The most effective treatment regimen for patients with Kawasaki disease of less than 10 days' duration is one dose of IVIG (2 g/kg) given over 12 hours and adjunctive aspirin therapy (80 to 100 mg/kg/day) to control inflammation until the patient is afebrile, followed by a reduction in daily aspirin dosage to 3 to 5 mg/kg for a total of 6 to 8 weeks to prevent thrombotic complications. Because 10% of patients may have persistent fever (>48 hours) or recrudescence of fever after the one-dose IVIG regimen, repeated treatment with IVIG is recommended. Alternatively, high-dose intravenous corticosteroid therapy (methylprednisolone, 30 mg/kg/day) for 1 to 3 days may be employed to control systemic inflammation. Patients requiring repeated treatment tend to have greater initial cardiac involvement, including pericardial effusion, ventricular dysfunction, and coronary artery ectasia, but have outcomes similar to those of patients not requiring repeat treatment.

SUMMARY AND RED FLAGS

Most childhood episodes of fever and rash represent benign, self-limited viral illnesses with little or no sequelae. *Red flags* include toxic appearance; unstable vital signs or meningismus; fever without a focus in children older than 2 years in association with petechiae or purpura; manifestations of treatable diseases with significant sequelae (rheumatic fever, Kawasaki disease, Rocky Mountain spotted fever, Stevens-Johnson syndrome, SLE, JRA); and contagious illnesses, which are of concern for either immunocompetent or immunosuppressed patients.

REFERENCES

American Academy of Pediatrics: Lyme disease. In Report of the Committee on Infectious Diseases, 25th ed. Elk Grove Village, Ill, American Academy of Pediatrics, 2000, pp 374-379.

American Heart Association Committee on Rheumatic Fever, Endocarditis, and Kawasaki Disease: Guidelines for long-term management of patients with Kawasaki disease. Circulation 1994;89:916-922.

Baker RC, Sequin JH, Leslie N, et al: Fever and petechiae in children. Pediatrics 1989;84:1051-1055.

Balfour HH, Rotbart HA, Feldman S, et al: Acyclovir treatment of varicella in otherwise healthy adolescents. J Pediatr 1992;120:627-633.

Baraff LJ, Bass JW, Fleisher GR, et al: Practice guidelines for the management of infants and children 0 to 36 months of age with fever without source. Pediatrics 1993;92:1-12.

Bialecki C, Feder HM, Grant-Kels JM: The six classic childhood exanthems: A review and update. J Am Acad Dermatol 1989;21:891-903.

Boh DD, Millikan LE: Vesiculobullous diseases with prominent immunologic features. JAMA 1992;268:2893-2898.

Burns J, Wiggins J, Toews W, et al: Clinical spectrum of Kawasaki disease in infants younger than 6 months of age. J Pediatr 1986;109:759-763.

Eichenfield LF, Honig PJ: Blistering disorders in childhood. Pediatr Clin North Am 1991;38:959-976.

Font J, Cervera R, Espinosa G, et al: Systemic lupus erythematosus in childhood. Ann Rheum Dis 1998;57:456-459.

Frieden IJ, Resnick SD: Childhood exanthems: Old and new. Pediatr Clin North Am 1991;38:859-887.

Goodyear HM, Laidler PW, Price EH, et al: Acute infectious erythemas in children: A clinico-microbiological study. Br J Dermatol 1991;124:433-438.

Han RK, Silverman ED, Newman A, McCrindle BW: Management and outcome of persistent or recurrent fever after initial intravenous gamma globulin therapy in acute Kawasaki disease. Arch Pediatr Adolesc Med 2000;154:694-699.

Han RK, Sinclair B, Newman A, et al: Recognition and management of Kawasaki disease. Can Med Assoc J 2000;162:807-812.

Hurwitz S: Erythema multiforme: A review of its characteristics, diagnostic criteria, and management. Pediatr Rev 1990;11:217-222.

Jacobs RF, Schutze GE: Ehrlichosis in children. J Pediatr 1997;131:184-192.

Jones EM, Callen JP: Collagen vascular disease of childhood. Pediatr Clin North Am 1991;38:1019-1039.

Jundt JW, Creager AH: STAR complexes: Febrile illnesses associated with sore throat, arthritis, and rash. South Med J 1993;86:521-528.

Kingston ME, Mackey D: Skin clues in the diagnosis of life-threatening infections. Rev Infect Dis 1986;8:1-11.

Levy M, Koren G: Atypical Kawasaki disease: Analysis of clinical presentation and diagnostic clues. Pediatr Infect Dis J 1990;9:122-126.

Malane MS, Grant-Kels JM, Feder HM, et al: Diagnosis of Lyme disease based on dermatologic manifestations. Ann Intern Med 1991;114:490-498.

Manders SM: Toxin-mediated streptococcal and staphylococcal disease. J Am Acad Dermatol 1998;39:383-398.

Mandl KD, Stack AM, Fleisher GR: Incidence of bacteremia in infants and children with fever and petechiae. J Pediatr 1997;131:398-404.

McCarthy PL, Sharpe MR, Spiesel SZ, et al: Observation scales to identify serious illness in febrile children. Pediatrics 1982;70:802-809.

Newburger JW, Takahashi M, Beiser AS, et al: A single intravenous infusion of gamma globulin as compared with four infusions in the treatment of acute Kawasaki syndrome. N Engl J Med 1991;324:1633-1639.

Schlossberg D: Fever and rash. Infect Dis Clin North Am 1996;10:101-110.

Solomon AR, Rasmussen JE, Varani J: The Tzanck smear in the diagnosis of cutaneous herpes simplex. JAMA 1984;251:633-635.

Stockheim JA, Innocentini N, Shulman ST: Kawasaki disease in older children and adolescents. J Pediatr 2000;137:250-252.

Walker DH, Cain BB, Olmstead PM: Laboratory diagnosis of Rocky Mountain spotted fever by immunofluorescent demonstration of *Rickettsia rickettsii* in cutaneous lesions. Am J Clin Pathol 1978;69:619-623.

Weiner LB: Management of young children with fever and rash. Pediatr Infect Dis J 1991;10:416-417.

56 Rashes and Skin Lesions

Amy Jo Nopper   Manju E. George*

Approximately 20% to 30% of pediatric office visits involve a primary or secondary dermatologic complaint. In addition to the myriad of primary skin disorders, other disorders of the skin are frequently markers of underlying systemic disease, including many hereditary disorders.

HISTORY, PHYSICAL EXAMINATION, AND DIAGNOSTIC PROCEDURES

HISTORY

Obtaining a careful and focused history is necessary to establish diagnoses of pediatric skin disorders. It may be helpful to examine the patient first and then proceed with a relevant line of questioning. Important questions to ask include the following:

1. When did the eruption begin?
2. How did the eruption evolve (distribution, spread, change in structure of individual lesions)?
3. Are the lesions pruritic or painful?
4. Have there been previous similar episodes?
5. Are there associated systemic symptoms?
6. Are there exacerbating or alleviating factors?
7. Has treatment been rendered? If so, what effect has it had?
8. Are there affected family members or close contacts?
9. Is there a family history of skin disease?

PHYSICAL EXAMINATION

It is necessary to identify the primary skin lesion, secondary skin lesions or changes, size, color, distribution, and configuration of the lesions. Several specific signs are pathognomonic for certain diseases. Examination of the hair, nails, and mucosal surfaces should be included. Palpation of cutaneous lesions provides additional information, such as firmness, tenderness, mobility, temperature, and ability to blanch with pressure. Precise morphologic descriptions are critical for establishing a differential diagnosis (see also Chapter 55).

Primary Lesions

Macules and Patches. Macules are flat, circumscribed lesions that are detected because of a change in color. Pink or red macules may be caused by inflammation or vasodilatation. Brown, black, or white lesions may be caused by alterations in melanin synthesis. Purple hues may represent extravasation of blood into the skin. Macules greater than 1 cm in diameter are usually described as patches.

Papules, Nodules, Plaques, and Tumors. *Papules* are circumscribed, palpable, elevated solid lesions. Typically less than 0.5 to 1 cm in diameter, these lesions may be epidermal or dermal in origin and may be flat-topped or dome-shaped. Papules that are 0.5 to 2 cm in diameter are described as nodules. *Nodules* are epidermal, dermal, or subcutaneous lesions that may, in some cases, evolve from preexisting papules. *Plaques* are elevated flat-topped lesions, larger than 1 cm in diameter, and often formed by coalescence of papules. *Tumors* are larger nodules greater than 2 cm in diameter that are usually solid and well circumscribed.

Vesicles and Bullae. Vesicles are elevated fluid-filled lesions. Bullae are large vesicles, usually greater than 1 cm in diameter. The tenseness or flaccidity of the blister indicates whether the level of separation is intraepidermal or subepidermal (Fig. 56-1 and Table 56-1).

Pustules. Pustules are white or yellow well-circumscribed lesions that contain purulent material. Pustules do not always signify an infectious cause.

Wheals. Wheals are edematous, elevated lesions that are transient in nature and variable in shape and size. They may be white or erythematous and often have central pallor.

Telangiectases. These are ectatic, dilated superficial blood vessels of the skin that typically blanch when pressure is applied.

Secondary Lesions

Secondary lesions may represent the natural evolution of primary lesions or changes that result from external manipulation, such as scratching.

Crusts. Crusts represent serum, pus, blood, or exudate that has dried on the skin surface.

Scales. Scales appear as yellow, white, or brownish flakes on the skin surface that represent desquamation of stratum corneum.

Erosions. Erosions are moist, erythematous, circumscribed lesions that result from partial or complete loss of the epidermis. They often result from rupture of a blister. Erosions do not involve the dermis or subcutaneous tissue; therefore, they heal without scarring.

Ulcers. Ulcers are deeper than erosions and penetrate the dermis or fat and usually heal with scarring.

Lichenification. Lichenification, or thickening of the skin, usually results from chronic scratching or rubbing. Accentuation of skin markings or hyperpigmentation is observed.

Fissures. A fissure is a linear crack in the epidermis extending to the dermis.

*This chapter is an updated and edited version of the chapter by Linda G. Rabinowitz that appeared in the first edition.

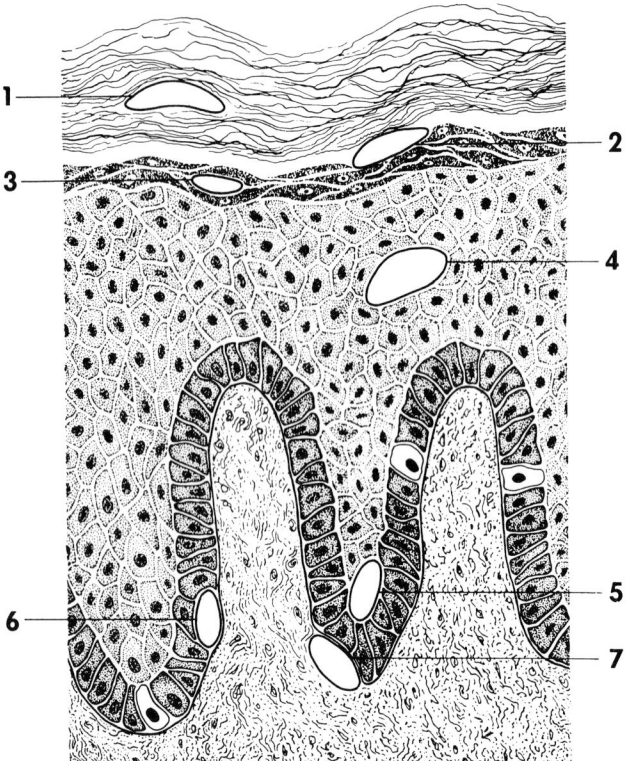

Figure 56-1. Blister cleavage sites in the skin. *1,* Intracorneal. *2,* Subcorneal. *3,* Granular layer. *4,* Intraepidermal. *5,* Suprabasal. *6,* Junctional (between the basal cell membrane and basement membrane). *7,* Subepidermal. (From Esterly NB: The skin. In Behrman RE [ed]: Nelson Textbook of Pediatrics, 14th ed. Philadelphia, WB Saunders, 1992, p 1640.)

Table 56-1. Sites of Blister Formation of Selected Vesiculobullous Diseases

Site of Cleavage	Clinical Example
Intracorneal	Miliaria crystallina
Granular layer	Bullous impetigo
	Staphylococcal scalded skin syndrome
	Pemphigus foliaceus
Intraepidermal	Dermatophytosis
	Insect bites
	Incontinentia pigmenti
	Scabies
	Viral blisters
Suprabasal	Pemphigus vulgaris
Basal cell layer	Epidermolysis simplex
Junctional	Junctional epidermolysis bullosa
Subepidermal	Toxic epidermal necrolysis
	Dermatitis herpetiformis
	Recessive dystrophic epidermolysis bullosa
	Dominant dystrophic epidermolysis bullosa
	Linear IgA disease of childhood

IgA, immunoglobulin A.

Atrophy. Atrophy represents loss of substance of the skin. Epidermal atrophy is characterized by loss of skin markings, increased wrinkling, and transparency with visibility of underlying vasculature. Dermal or subcutaneous atrophy results in depression of the skin with minimal, if any, epidermal changes.

Excoriations. Excoriations are linear erosions on the skin caused by scratching.

DIAGNOSTIC TECHNIQUES

Potassium Hydroxide Test

A common diagnostic procedure is the potassium hydroxide (KOH) preparation. This simple and rapid test can confirm the diagnosis of dermatophyte or candidal infections. Scale is scraped with a curved blade onto a microscope slide. Hair or nail fragments can also be examined. A glass coverslip is then placed on the slide after 1 to 2 drops of 10% to 20% KOH are added. The slide is heated gently but not boiled, which can result in KOH crystallization and subsequent difficulty in interpretation. Dermatophyte infections are confirmed by identifying fungal hyphae, which appear as long, branching septate filaments. Pseudohyphae or budding spores are characteristic of candidiasis. Short, broad hyphae and clusters of budding cells, resembling "spaghetti and meatballs," are diagnostic of tinea versicolor.

Tzanck Smear

A Tzanck smear is useful for diagnosis of varicella-zoster virus and herpes simplex virus (HSV) infections. The smear is prepared by unroofing a blister with a curved blade and gently scraping the blister base and underside of the roof. The material is spread in a thin layer onto a glass slide. The slide is air-dried and stained with Giemsa or Wright stain. Identification of multinucleated giant cells, a syncytium of epidermal cells with multiple overlapping nuclei, establishes the diagnosis. These cells may have 2 to 15 nuclei and are much larger than other inflammatory cells. Although a positive result of Tzanck preparation is confirmatory, a negative test result does not rule out herpes viral infection. Viral specimens should be obtained for culture to differentiate HSV from varicella-zoster virus infections.

Scabies Test

A scabies preparation exhibiting the mite, egg, or feces (scybala) confirms the diagnosis of scabies infestation. The mite is most often found within burrows (serpiginous or elongated papules), which may have a vesicle or pustule at one end. A drop of mineral oil should be applied to the lesion so that the scraped material adheres to the blade. The site is then scraped firmly with a curved blade, which occasionally induces minimal bleeding. The material is applied to a microscope slide, another drop of mineral oil is added, and a glass coverslip is placed. Mites are eight-legged arachnids that are easily identified under low magnification. Eggs are frequently observed as smooth ovals approximately half the size of the mite. Feces are smaller than ova and appear as red-brown pellets, often in clusters.

Gram Stain

A Gram stain can be useful in the diagnosis and treatment of suspected bacterial infections. After the site is disinfected, the pustule or blister roof is carefully removed with a needle or straight blade. The contents of the pustule are removed in a sterile manner and spread thinly onto a glass slide. The specimen is air-dried or heat-fixed, stained, and examined microscopically. Results help determine which antibiotic, if any, is indicated. Bacterial cultures are typically obtained simultaneously.

Table 56-2. Wood Lamp Examination Findings

Fluorescence	Clinical Appearance	Organisms/Disease
Coral, red, pink	Brown or red thin plaques in groin, axillae, or toe webs	Erythrasma (*Corynebacterium minutissimum*)
Pale green	Hypopigmented or hyperpigmented macules and plaques on trunk	Tinea versicolor (*Pityrosporum orbiculare, Pityrosporum ovale, Malassezia furfur*)
Bright yellow-green	Infection of the toe web space; often in burn patients	*Pseudomonas aeruginosa*
Yellow-green	Scaling of scalp with patchy hair loss	Tinea capitis (*Microsporum canis, Microsporum audouinii*) Not *Trichophyton tonsurans*

Wood Lamp Examination

A Wood lamp emits low-intensity ultraviolet light at 365 nm and is useful for accentuating pigmentary alterations and detecting several fungal or bacterial infections. The examination is performed in a darkened room, and the lamp is held 4 to 6 inches from the patient's skin. Characteristic color changes are outlined in Table 56-2.

Skin Biopsy

A skin biopsy can be performed when a clinical diagnosis is unclear. Histologic evaluation of a small skin specimen may reveal changes in the epidermis, dermis, or subcutaneous tissue that confirm or rule out specific disorders. Direct immunofluorescence testing can be extremely helpful in the diagnosis of collagen-vascular and auto-immune bullous diseases (Table 56-3).

NEONATAL DERMATOLOGY

Many entities unique to newborns are caused by physiologic phenomena in response to the infant's transition to the new environment. Most such entities are benign and self-limited. There are also specific skin disorders that are seen primarily in this age group, including congenital infections that require prompt recognition and intervention.

Table 56-3. Immunofluorescent Findings in Immune-Mediated Cutaneous Diseases

Disease	Involved Skin	Uninvolved Skin	Direct IF	Indirect IF	Other Antibodies
Dermatitis herpetiformis	Negative	Positive	Granular IgA ± C in papillary dermis	None	IgA antiendomysial antibody and tissue transglutaminase antibody with celiac disease
Bullous pemphigoid	Positive	Positive	Linear IgG and C band in BMZ, occasionally IgM, IgA, IgE	IgG to BMZ in 70%	None
Pemphigus vulgaris	Positive	Positive	IgG in intercellular spaces of epidermis between keratinocytes	IgG to intercellular space, desmoglein 3	None
Pemphigus foliaceus	Positive	Positive	IgG to desmosomal glycoprotein, desmoglein 1	Same as direct IF	None
Herpes gestationis	Positive	Positive	C3 at BMZ, occasionally IgG	IgG anti-BMZ	None
Linear IgA bullous dermatosis (chronic bullous dermatosis of childhood)	Positive	Positive	Linear IgA at BMZ, occasionally C	Low titer, rare IgA, anti-BMZ	None
Discoid lupus erythematosus	Positive	Negative	Linear IgG, IgM, IgA, and C3 at BMZ (lupus band)	None	Antinuclear antibody (ANA) negative
Systemic lupus erythematosus	Positive	Variable: exposed to sun, 30%-50%; nonexposed, 10%-30%	Linear IgG, IgM, C3 at BMZ (lupus band)	None	ANA Anti-Ro (SSA) Anti-RNP Anti-DNA Anti-Sm
Henoch-Schönlein purpura	Positive	Negative	IgA around vessel walls	None	IgA rheumatoid factor, occasionally

From Esterly NB: The skin. In Behrman RE (ed): Nelson Textbook of Pediatrics, 14th ed. Philadelphia, WB Saunders, 1992, p 1623.

BMZ, basement membrane zone at the dermoepidermal junction; C, complement; IF, immunofluorescence; IgA, IgE, IgG, and M, immunoglobulins A, E, G, and M.

PHYSIOLOGIC CHANGES OF THE SKIN

Acrocyanosis

The normal newborn usually displays a bluish-purple discoloration of the hands, feet, and lips. Referred to as *acrocyanosis,* this typically occurs in association with crying or cold stress. It results from increased peripheral arteriolar tone, which leads to vasospasm and subsequent venous pooling. Acrocyanosis should be differentiated from central cyanosis, which is noted on mucosal surfaces (see Chapter 10). Physiologic acrocyanosis gradually resolves spontaneously during the neonatal period.

Cutis Marmorata

Cutis marmorata is also associated with neonatal cold stress. Characterized by symmetric reticulated cyanosis involving the trunk and extremities, this marbled appearance usually resolves upon rewarming of the infant. When this vascular pattern is seen in older infants or children, it may be associated with Down syndrome, Cornelia de Lange syndrome, or hypothyroidism.

Cutis marmorata should be differentiated from *cutis marmorata telangiectatica congenita* (CMTC), a condition also referred to as *congenital phlebectasia.* The persistent cutis marmorata of CMTC is characteristically asymmetric, often segmental, mottled or marble-like, and more localized than physiologic cutis marmorata. In addition, the reticulated mottling of CMTC is darker in color and does not resolve with rewarming. Although CMTC improves with age, the abnormal vascular pattern is more persistent than that seen in physiologic cutis marmorata. It may be an isolated entity or may have distinct associations, including atrophy of the affected extremity, ulcerations, or coexistent vascular malformations and tumors.

Harlequin Color Change

The harlequin color change is a distinctive condition observed in infants lying on their sides. It is characterized by marked erythema on the dependent side of the infant's body with simultaneous blanching of the nondependent side. This phenomenon occurs more often in premature infants but may be observed in full-term newborns. The change may be caused by autonomic immaturity, which results in altered peripheral vascular tone.

Although it typically occurs within the first 3 weeks of life, harlequin color change is most often noted at 2 to 5 days of age. The changes develop abruptly and usually resolve within 20 minutes.

COMMON NEONATAL DERMATOSES

Miliaria

Miliaria results from sweat retention and is exacerbated by heat and humidity. Affected newborns are frequently in incubators or receiving phototherapy. Keratinous plugging of the eccrine ducts and subsequent release of eccrine sweat into the surrounding skin produce two distinct clinical manifestations with different sites of eccrine duct obstruction. In *miliaria crystallina,* obstruction occurs just below the stratum corneum, resulting in superficial, noninflammatory 1- to 2-mm vesicles. In *miliaria rubra,* or "prickly heat," obstruction occurs in the mid-epidermis. This is associated with an inflammatory response exhibited by vesicles, papules, or papulovesicles surrounded by a rim of erythema. The lesions occur in clusters on the trunk, face, scalp, and intertriginous regions. Neither type of miliaria warrants therapy, but improvement occurs with cooling of the skin and avoidance of excessive warmth and moisture.

Milia

Milia are pinpoint white or yellow papules that are present in 40% to 50% of neonates. Located predominantly on the face, they may also be seen in the oral cavity, where they are referred to as *Epstein's pearls* (palate) or *Bohn's nodules* (gingiva). The lesions represent keratin-filled epidermal inclusion cysts, which usually resolve spontaneously during the first few weeks of life. Unusually widespread or persistent lesions may be associated with defects such as hereditary trichodysplasia, oral-facial-digital syndrome, or particular subtypes of epidermolysis bullosa.

Neonatal Acne

Neonatal acne (neonatal cephalic pustulosis) develops in approximately 20% of newborns. Typically, it is not present at birth but appears during the first month after birth. Characterized by papules, pustules, and closed or open comedones located on the face or trunk, this condition usually resolves within the first several months of life. Therapeutic intervention is rarely required. It is believed that both maternal and endogenous androgens play a role. It remains unclear whether these infants are at greater risk for severe adolescent acne.

Sebaceous Gland Hyperplasia

Sebaceous gland hyperplasia is characterized by the presence of multiple flesh- to yellow-colored tiny papules primarily on the nose and cheeks of full-term infants. The increased sebaceous cell size and number as well as sebaceous gland volume may result from maternal androgen stimulation. Spontaneous resolution occurs within the first 4 to 6 months of life.

Seborrheic Dermatitis

Seborrheic dermatitis, common during infancy, typically manifests within the first several weeks after birth. Characterized by erythema and a yellow, greasy scale, it usually resolves spontaneously within several months. The eruption occurs at sites where sebaceous glands are concentrated, such as the face, chest, and posterior auricular and intertriginous areas. "Cradle cap" is seborrhea that is confined to the scalp. Involvement of the diaper area is characterized by salmon-colored patches that arise in skin folds and spread to the genitalia, suprapubic area, and upper medial thighs. Unlike atopic dermatitis, this eruption is not very pruritic. Secondary candidal or bacterial infection is common.

The diagnosis is established clinically. The presence of greasy yellow scale and salmon-colored patches, involvement of the scalp and intertriginous areas, early onset, and lack of pruritus or atopic history help distinguish seborrheic from atopic dermatitis. However, some infants have an overlap of seborrheic dermatitis and atopic dermatitis. Seborrheic dermatitis should also be differentiated from psoriasis or Langerhans cell histiocytosis, in which the lesions, often in a seborrheic distribution, are typically purpuric, erosive, or crusted. Skin biopsy findings, as well as hepatosplenomegaly, purpura, lymphadenopathy, anemia, thrombocytopenia, external otitis, interstitial pneumonia, and osseous lesions, further distinguish histiocytosis from seborrheic dermatitis.

Treatment of the scalp consists of mild keratolytic shampoos, such as those containing ketoconazole, selenium sulfide, or zinc pyrithione. Mineral oil may be helpful in removing thick, adherent scale. The scalp and diaper dermatitis may be treated with low-potency topical corticosteroids and barrier ointments. Topical antifungal or antibacterial agents should be used for coexisting candidiasis or impetigo.

Diaper Dermatitis

Diaper dermatitis is one of the most common dermatologic disorders of infants and toddlers. A differential diagnosis, including characteristic clinical features, is seen in Table 56-4. It comprises a group of inflammatory conditions that involve the lower abdomen, genitalia,

Table 56-4. Diaper Dermatitis

Disease	Clinical Manifestation	Other Features	Treatment
Friction	Inner surface of thighs, genitalia, buttocks, abdomen Mild erythema with a shiny glazed surface, occasional papules	Course waxes and wanes, aggravated by talc	Responds well to frequent diaper changes, avoidance of diapers, simple drying measures
Irritant	Confined to convex surfaces of buttocks, perineal area, lower abdomen, proximal thighs Sparing of intertriginous creases	Exacerbated by excessive heat, moisture, sweat retention	Gentle cleansing Lubricants (petrolatum) Barrier pastes (zinc oxide) Low-potency corticosteroids
Allergic contact	Often confined to the convex surfaces in direct contact with the offending agent, with sparing of the intertriginous skin Mild cases: diffuse erythema, papules, vesicles, edema, scaling Severe cases: papules, vesicles, psoriasiform lesions, annular plaques, secondary erosions, ulcerations, infiltrated nodules	May complicate an irritant dermatitis or arise de novo Often attributable to topical antibiotics or to preservatives, plus emulsifiers in topical baby products	Removal of offending agent Judicious use of low-potency topical corticosteroids Barrier ointments
Seborrheic	Salmon-colored patches with greasy, yellow scale Involves intertriginous areas Fissures, maceration, weeping occasionally seen	May involve axillae, scalp "Cradle cap" Infants remain healthy and asymptomatic Significant hypopigmentation may be prominent in black infants	Low-potency topical corticosteroids Anticandidal agents for coexistent infection
Candidiasis	Typically involves skin creases Bright-red eruption, well demarcated; may have white scale at borders Characteristic satellite papules and pustules	Occasionally associated with oral thrush Occurs commonly after treatment with antibiotics	Aluminum acetate dressings Topical anticandidal medications, including nystatin and clotrimizole (Lotrimin)
Intertrigo	Well-demarcated areas of maceration and oozing Intergluteal region and fleshy folds of the thigh	Often associated with miliaria	Avoidance of excessive heat Cool clothing
Psoriasis	Bright red, scaly, well demarcated May persist for months or recur frequently Less responsive to topical therapy	Red scaly lesions may be present on trunk or extremities Nail changes	Low-potency topical corticosteroids Emollients
Staphylococcal infection	Characterized by many thin-walled pustules on erythematous bases that leave a collarette of scale after rupturing	—	Antistaphylococcal therapy
Acrodermatitis enteropathica	Early lesions are vesicular and pustular More often, well-demarcated, dry, scaly, crusty lesions in periorificial distribution are seen	Irritability or listlessness Failure to thrive, alopecia, diarrhea	Secondary to zinc deficiency Treat with zinc replacement
Langerhans cell histiocytosis	Often mimics candidiasis Persistent seborrhea-like eruption; clusters of infiltrated papules, which are often hemorrhagic or purpuric Ulceration may be seen	Involvement of axillae and retroauricular skin Reddish-yellow papules and patches on the head and neck Anemia, thrombocytopenia, hepatosplenomegaly, osseous lesions	Chemotherapy for systemic disease

upper thighs, and buttocks. Clinical manifestations include erythema, edema, erosions, vesicles, and pustules. Secondary changes of postinflammatory hyperpigmentation or hypopigmentation are common.

Irritants are common causes of diaper rash. Although urinary ammonia was thought to be the primary factor in the development of diaper dermatitis, feces now appear to play a more important role. Fecal ureases, by converting urea to ammonia, cause elevation of skin pH, which, in turn, increases fecal protease and lipase activity. These proteases and lipases cause disruption of the epidermal barrier. Skin wetness, friction, maceration, and contact with feces, urine, and microbes further compromise epidermal integrity. This results in increased permeability of the skin to irritants such as soaps, powders, and detergents. Diaper dermatitis may begin as early as 1 to 2 months of age but may become a chronic or recurrent problem in older infants as well.

OTHER NEONATAL DERMATOSES

Erythema Toxicum Neonatorum

Erythema toxicum neonatorum is a benign condition that occurs in 30% to 70% of white full-term infants. Erythema toxicum occurs less frequently in premature infants. The eruption is characterized by blotchy, erythematous macules or patches with central papules, pustules, or vesicles that give the infant a "flea-bitten" appearance (Fig. 56-2). The lesions develop most commonly between the second and fourth days after birth; however, they may appear during the first 2 to 3 weeks. They are self-limited and usually resolve within several days. Typical sites of involvement include the face, trunk, and proximal extremities. There may be very few to hundreds of lesions.

A Giemsa or Wright stain of the intralesional contents reveals sheets of eosinophils with a relative absence of neutrophils. Peripheral eosinophilia may be present in up to 20% of affected infants. Erythema toxicum is occasionally confused with transient neonatal pustular melanosis, congenital cutaneous candidiasis, impetigo neonatorum, milia, herpes simplex, or miliaria rubra (prickly heat).

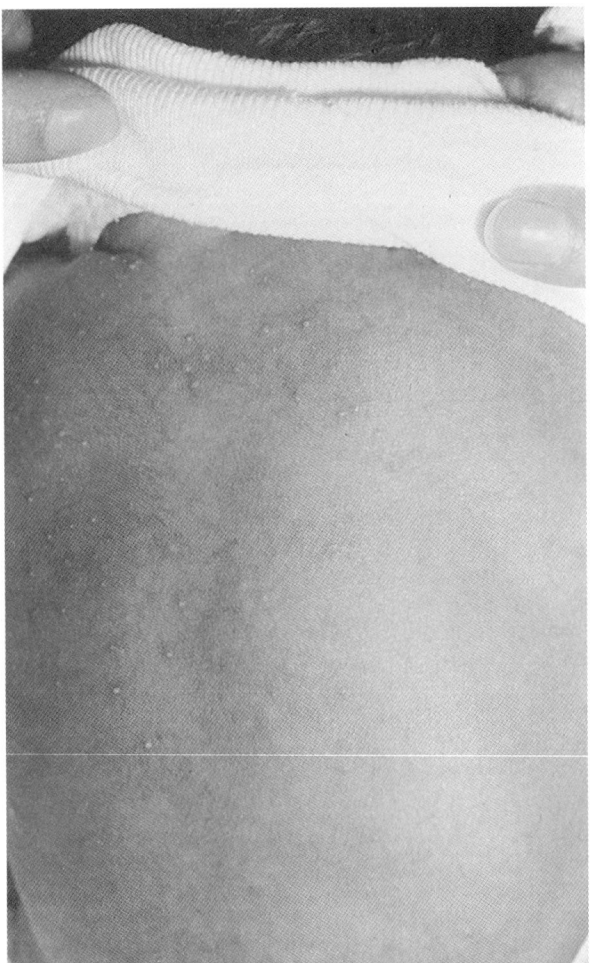

Figure 56-2. White papules surrounded by erythema are characteristic of erythema toxicum.

Transient Neonatal Pustular Melanosis

Transient neonatal pustular melanosis, seen in up to 4% of neonates, occurs more often in African American infants. Typically present at birth, the initial lesions are 2- to 5-mm pustules distributed over the face, neck, and upper chest and, less often, on the sacrum, trunk, thighs, palms, and soles. In contrast to the lesions of erythema toxicum, there is no erythema surrounding each pustule, and Wright stain of pustular contents reveals many neutrophils. In both disorders, the pustules are sterile and should be distinguished from those seen in potentially serious infections caused by HSV, *Staphylococcus aureus,* or candidal species.

The superficial pustules of transient neonatal pustular melanosis rupture spontaneously within the first few days after birth, leaving hyperpigmented macules that have collarettes of fine scale. It is common to see only hyperpigmented macules at birth. These brown spots slowly fade over several weeks to months.

Neonatal Lupus Erythematosus

Neonatal lupus erythematosus is a unique annular erythematous eruption of the neonatal period. Lesions of neonatal lupus are often scaly, annular plaques that usually occur in a photodistribution. Lesions characteristically involve the face and scalp and may affect the periorbital and malar areas, creating a "raccoon eyes" appearance. Other manifestations may include transient hypopigmentation with epidermal atrophy or telangiectasias. Cutaneous lesions may be present at birth but often appear within the first 2 to 3 months of life. The lesions are often exacerbated by sun exposure. The majority of skin findings are transient, lasting up to 6 to 9 months.

Cutaneous findings or congenital heart block are present individually in approximately 50% (each) of affected infants. An overlap of both is present in approximately 10% of affected infants. The major morbidity and mortality of neonatal lupus result from congenital heart block. The heart block is believed to be caused by fibrosis of the atrioventricular node from intrauterine inflammation caused by the transfer of anti-Ro and anti-La antibodies.

The diagnosis of neonatal lupus includes examination of anti-Ro, anti-La, and anti-U1RNP autoantibodies in both the infant and the mother. Studies have shown that mothers of approximately 95% of infants with neonatal lupus have anti-Ro antibodies. Skin biopsy is usually not necessary. Direct immunofluorescence yields positive findings of granular deposits of immunoglobulin G, C3, and immunoglobulin M at the dermoepidermal junction in approximately 50% of the cases. Workup should include platelet count and liver function tests, because approximately 5% to 10% of affected infants have liver disease or thrombocytopenia.

Mothers with high titers of anti-Ro antibodies or with systemic lupus erythematosus have a higher risk of delivering an infant with neonatal lupus and should be counseled appropriately. Despite high antibody titers, fewer than half of mothers of affected infants are symptomatic at the time of delivery. In most of these mothers, evidence of connective tissue disease, usually Sjögren's syndrome or subacute cutaneous lupus develops over time. These mothers should be monitored closely in subsequent pregnancies with fetal heart rate monitoring and echocardiograms. The risk of recurrence of congenital heart block in subsequent pregnancies may be as high as 15% to 25%.

Differential diagnosis should include annular erythema of infancy, tinea corporis, and cutis marmorata telangiectatica congenita (CMTC). Treatment consists of photoprotection and topical steroids. Most cutaneous changes resolve spontaneously by 6 to 9 months of age as a result of a gradual decrease in maternal antibodies.

Acropustulosis of Infancy

Acropustulosis of infancy is a condition that may present at birth or during the first few weeks or months afterward. The disorder is characterized by recurrent eruptions of pruritic pustules or vesicles involving the hands and feet. On occasion, involvement includes other sites such as the trunk or abdomen. The lesions frequently begin in crops, which typically last approximately 1 week, and resolve with desquamation, followed by postinflammatory hyperpigmentation.

Acropustulosis is often confused with infantile scabies; family history and examination of scrapings of the involved area may help differentiate between these two diagnoses. Scrapings of lesions in acropustulosis often demonstrate neutrophils. Bacterial infection should also be ruled out by wound cultures. Treatment is symptomatic and consists of control of pruritus with low- to mid-potency topical corticosteroids and antihistamines. Parents should be advised that lesions tend to occur episodically until approximately 2 to 3 years of age.

Eosinophilic Pustular Folliculitis

Eosinophilic pustular folliculitis is another disorder of infancy characterized by recurrent crops of vesicles and pustules. Lesions are often present on the forehead and scalp. The condition tends to occur in a cyclic pattern and is very pruritic. Scraped material from the pustules subjected to Wright stain demonstrates a large number of eosinophils but no evidence of infectious organisms. A complete blood cell count may show peripheral eosinophilia. In rare cases, skin biopsy may be necessary. Histopathologic study demonstrates a perifollicular and dermal infiltrate of eosinophils, as well as lymphocytes and histiocytes. Because the clinical condition is very similar to infantile acropustulosis, some authors contend that eosinophilic pustular folliculitis may be part of the same clinical spectrum. This condition is not associated with systemic disease, and treatment is symptomatic with topical corticosteroids and antihistamines. Eosinophilic pustular folliculitis usually resolves spontaneously by 2 to 3 years of age.

Subcutaneous Fat Necrosis

Subcutaneous fat necrosis is a condition of otherwise healthy infants that is sometimes associated with preceding trauma, cold injury, or hypoxia. This disorder occurs primarily in full-term and postmature infants. Single or multiple erythematous to violaceous, indurated, tender nodules or plaques arise on the buttocks, thighs, back, cheeks, and arms. In rare cases, lesions liquefy, ulcerate, and drain an oily substance. The diagnosis can be confirmed by the characteristic histopathologic findings of fat lobules containing pathognomonic needle-shaped clefts surrounded by a mixed inflammatory infiltrate of lymphocytes, histiocytes, and foreign body giant cells. Intact lesions heal spontaneously within several months, whereas ulcerated lesions may heal more slowly and result in scarring. All patients should be screened for potentially life-threatening hypercalcemia, which may accompany this disorder. Early in the course of this disorder, the serum calcium may be normal, but several weeks later it may rise.

DEVELOPMENTAL DEFECTS

Nevus Sebaceous

Nevus sebaceous (an epidermal nevus) of Jadassohn is an asymptomatic, well-circumscribed, hairless plaque of sebaceous gland derivation. Typically present at birth, these lesions are variable in size, usually solitary, and located on the scalp, face, and neck. During infancy, they are yellowish-orange smooth, velvety, or waxy plaques. These nevi tend to thicken and become verrucous during puberty.

Because up to 15% of these lesions develop secondary benign or malignant neoplasms during adolescence or adulthood, prophylactic surgical excision is recommended before puberty.

MARKERS OF CRANIAL AND SPINAL DYSRAPHISM

Dermoid Cysts

Dermoid cysts are nontender, noncompressible, firm, congenital subcutaneous nodules found along sites of closure of embryonic clefts. Dermoids are lined by stratified squamous epithelium that contains mature adnexal structures. Although these lesions are often noted in newborns, they may not be detected until later in infancy or in childhood after the lesion enlarges or becomes inflamed. Lesions are often described as rubbery and may be blue to skin-colored in appearance. A tuft of hair may be seen protruding from an orifice in the dermoid. Dermoid cysts are often found in the head and neck region, often the lateral portion of an eyebrow.

The most important concern with dermoid cysts is the potential for an intracranial connection. Up to 25% of midline or nasal dermoid cysts may have an intracranial connection; all midline head and spinal lesions should be imaged. If a connection is present, the patient is at risk for infection because the dermoid cyst and sinus can serve as a portal of entry for bacteria. These patients should be referred to neurosurgery for removal and repair. Dermoid cysts that are not midline, including those commonly seen at the lateral brow area, should also be excised because of the potential risk of infection. After surgical excision, lesions do not usually recur.

Aplasia Cutis Congenita

Aplasia cutis congenita is a heterogeneous group of disorders in which there is a congenital absence of skin (Fig. 56-3). This disorder may involve the epidermis, dermis, and subcutaneous tissues. The most common type of aplasia cutis is membranous aplasia cutis. These lesions are well-demarcated, small, oval, 1- to 5-cm defects on the vertex of the scalp. They are easily identified by their classic "punched-out" appearance and may have an atrophic surface with a glistening, membrane-like surface at birth. In older children, these lesions resemble scars. If the lesion is associated with a hair collar or midline in location, the clinician should evaluate for the potential of cranial dysraphism.

The defect is usually solitary; however, in a minority of patients, multiple sites may be affected. Aplasia cutis can also occur on the

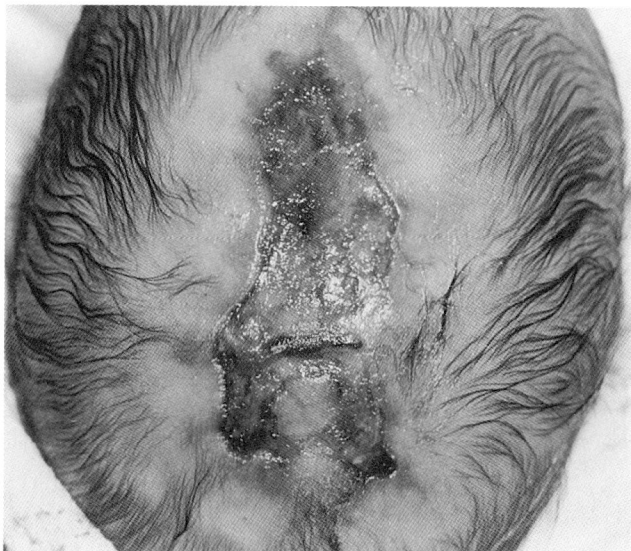

Figure 56-3. Congenital absence of skin (aplasia cutis congenita) on the scalp of a neonate.

trunk and limbs, where the defects are often bilateral and symmetric. Congenital absence of the skin of the lower extremities can be associated with certain types of epidermolysis bullosa. Aplasia cutis in the lumbosacral area is of particular importance because it may be associated with spinal dysraphism.

Lesions of membranous aplasia cutis usually necessitate no further investigation, and gradual epithelialization typically occurs spontaneously. However, large, deep, or widespread lesions with underlying bone defects may necessitate surgical intervention.

Hair Collar Sign

The term *hair collar sign* is a designation for hypertrichosis that usually either partly or completely encircles a congenital scalp lesion (Fig. 56-4). Usually the ring of hair is denser, darker, and coarser in texture than the normal scalp hair. A hair collar sign surrounding a congenital scalp nodule is a strong marker for cranial dysraphism, including encephaloceles and meningoceles. However, this sign is not entirely specific, inasmuch as it may be found encircling lesions of aplasia cutis. If a hair collar sign is seen in combination with a capillary malformation, the risk of cranial dysraphism is increased substantially. Therefore, all congenital midline scalp nodules, particularly those with a hair collar sign and underlying vascular stain, should be imaged to evaluate for an intracranial connection. A magnetic resonance imaging (MRI) scan is the "gold standard," but it occasionally misses a small intracranial connection.

Hypertrichosis of the Lumbar Area

Lumbosacral hypertrichosis may be a normal variant, especially in certain ethnic groups. However, hypertrichosis in this area in association with other stigmata indicative of a neurologic defect is highly suggestive of spinal dysraphism. The area may be poorly circumscribed, and the hair can be light or dark. The hypertrichosis is often present at birth. Complete neurologic examination should be performed. There are no defined parameters to determine further evaluation of isolated hypertrichosis. If a spinal defect is suspected, further evaluation by ultrasonography or MRI of the spine is necessary.

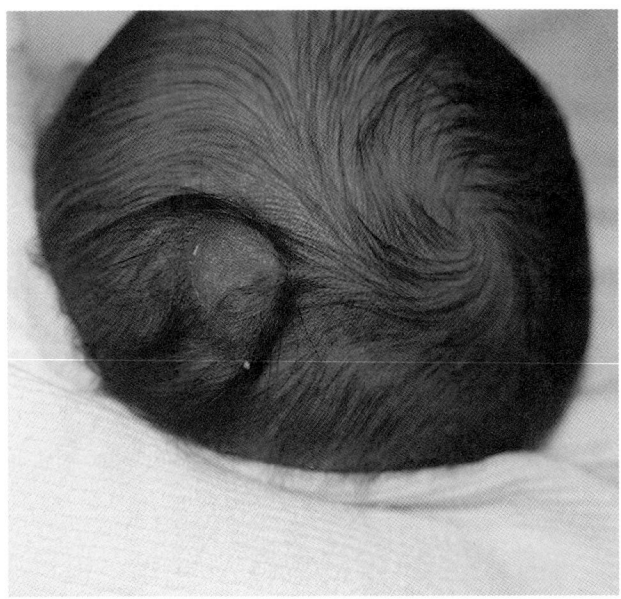

Figure 56-4. A classic hair-collar sign.

Sacral Dimples

Lumbosacral dimples are common findings in neonates. Large, deep dimples that are located in the superior portion of the gluteal crease should be radiologically imaged to rule out dermal sinuses communicating directly with the spinal canal. These dimples should not be probed because of the potential communication with the spinal canal. Sacral dimples seen in association with other cutaneous findings such as hypertrichosis, vascular birthmarks, a mass, or deviated gluteal cleft carry particularly high risk for spinal dysraphism. Imaging should be performed with ultrasonography of the lumbar spine in infants younger than 6 months and with MRI of the spine in infants older than 6 months of age.

Hemangiomas and Capillary Malformations of Lumbosacral Area

Hemangiomas that overlie the midline of the back are strong markers for spinal dysraphism, most often lipomyelomeningocele, intraspinal lipoma, or a tethered cord. Hemangiomas that are larger than 4 cm and overlap the midline appear to carry greater risk for spinal dysraphism. Ultrasonography or MRI should be performed. The risk of spinal dysraphism is increased when hemangioma is seen in association with other cutaneous findings such as sacral dimples, hypertrichosis or a deviated gluteal cleft.

Hemangiomas of the diaper area, lumbosacral spine, and skin creases may be problematic because they are prone to ulceration. Ulcerated lesions should be treated aggressively with topical barrier ointments and antibiotic ointment as indicated for any breakdown or erosions. For ulcerations that are deep or slow to heal, pulsed dye laser therapy may accelerate healing.

A solitary midline capillary malformation of the back without additional clinical findings may be a marker for spinal dysraphism, but this association is less clear. All affected infants should be evaluated for additional neurocutaneous stigmata. If a lumbosacral capillary malformation is detected with other cutaneous markers of spinal dysraphism, imaging is warranted.

DERMATOLOGIC DISORDERS IN OLDER INFANTS AND CHILDREN

SCALING DISORDERS

The term *papulosquamous* refers to conditions in which the primary lesions are papules or plaques associated with scale. These disorders are typically benign but can be chronic and therapeutically challenging.

Pityriasis Rosea

Pityriasis rosea is an acute, common, self-limited eruption that has no gender predilection. Although the precise cause is unknown, a viral origin is suspected because there have been reports of epidemics, clusters of cases among closely related individuals, and low recurrence rates. Furthermore, a prodrome of malaise, headache, and respiratory symptoms is occasionally observed.

The eruption usually begins with a solitary oval, pink scaly plaque, approximately 3 to 5 cm in diameter, that is typically located on the trunk or proximal extremities. Referred to as the *herald patch*, this finding is observed in 50% to 70% of cases. When the herald patch has an elevated red border and central clearing, it resembles tinea corporis. Performing a KOH preparation can differentiate these two conditions. Within 1 to 2 weeks after appearance of the herald patch, numerous small, pink scaly papules or plaques arise over the trunk and proximal extremities, sparing the face and distal extremities. The lesions classically have a fine cigarette paper–like peripheral collarette of scale. These oval 0.5- to 2-cm lesions have their long axis oriented along skin lines and, when present on the trunk, result in a "Christmas-tree" pattern. Young children, particularly African Americans, may have an "inverse" type of pityriasis rosea, with most lesions distributed on the distal extremities, face, neck, and intertriginous regions. Other variants seen in children demonstrate lesions that are papular, vesicular, pustular, purpuric, or lichenoid.

Pityriasis rosea is most severe during the first month and gradually abates over the ensuing 12 to 14 weeks. Some cases resolve within a few weeks. Therapy is unnecessary; however, topical corticosteroids or oral antihistamines help relieve pruritus. In addition, pityriasis rosea improves significantly with exposure to ultraviolet light. Postinflammatory hypopigmentation or hyperpigmentation may persist for several months, especially in dark-skinned patients. Other dermatoses that resemble pityriasis rosea include secondary syphilis, guttate psoriasis, drug eruptions, dermatophyte infections, seborrheic dermatitis, nummular eczema, Mucha-Habermann disease, and cutaneous T cell lymphoma. In sexually active adolescents, a rapid plasma reagin test should be obtained to rule out the possibility of secondary syphilis. Persistence of the eruption after 3 to 4 months necessitates a search for another diagnosis.

Psoriasis

Psoriasis is characterized by well-demarcated, erythematous scaly papules and plaques located most often on the scalp, elbows, knees, genitalia, and lumbosacral regions. The course is more chronic and unpredictable than that of pityriasis rosea. Psoriasis occurs in approximately 1% to 3% of the population and is estimated to manifest before the age of 20 years in about 25% of patients. It affects both sexes equally in adulthood, but childhood psoriasis is more prevalent in girls. It is uncommon in Native Americans and African Americans. The cause is multifactorial, but there is a genetic predisposition in many affected individuals. There is a family history of psoriasis in approximately 30% of cases.

Psoriasis encompasses a broad spectrum of clinical manifestations, ranging from mild, asymptomatic, virtually undetectable disease to extensive, chronic, debilitating disease. The course is usually marked by recurrent flares and remissions and is often exacerbated by stress, trauma, infection, climate, hormonal factors, and particular medications. The lesions are caused by a marked increase in epidermal cell proliferation and turnover; turnover is increased fourfold to sevenfold in comparison with normal skin.

Although morphologic variations exist, the classic lesions of psoriasis are well-demarcated erythematous papules or plaques with a silvery-white scale (Fig. 56-5). The lesions usually begin as small erythematous papules that gradually enlarge and coalesce to form plaques up to several centimeters in diameter. The micaceous (mica-like) scale of the psoriatic plaque is more adherent centrally than peripherally. Removal of this scale results in multiple small bleeding points. This is referred to as the *Auspitz sign* and is secondary to disruption of the dilated blood vessels that are located high in the papillary dermis. Although this finding is seen in psoriasis, it is not pathognomonic.

The *Koebner phenomenon,* another characteristic feature of psoriasis, is an isomorphic response (development of new or larger lesions) occurring at sites of injury or trauma such as scratching, sunburn, or surgery. The Koebner phenomenon is also observed in lichen planus, lichen nitidus, vitiligo, and verrucae. Psoriatic lesions tend to be distributed symmetrically. Although extensor surfaces are typically involved, a variant of psoriasis, known as *inverse psoriasis,* affects flexural surfaces, such as the axillae and groin.

Scalp lesions are present in most children with psoriasis. Diffuse, thick white scale may be accompanied by erythema. In contrast to seborrhea, psoriasis often extends beyond the hairline, affecting the forehead, ears, and neck. The lesions are variably pruritic and are generally not associated with hair loss. Scalp psoriasis tends to be more resistant to therapy than is seborrheic dermatitis.

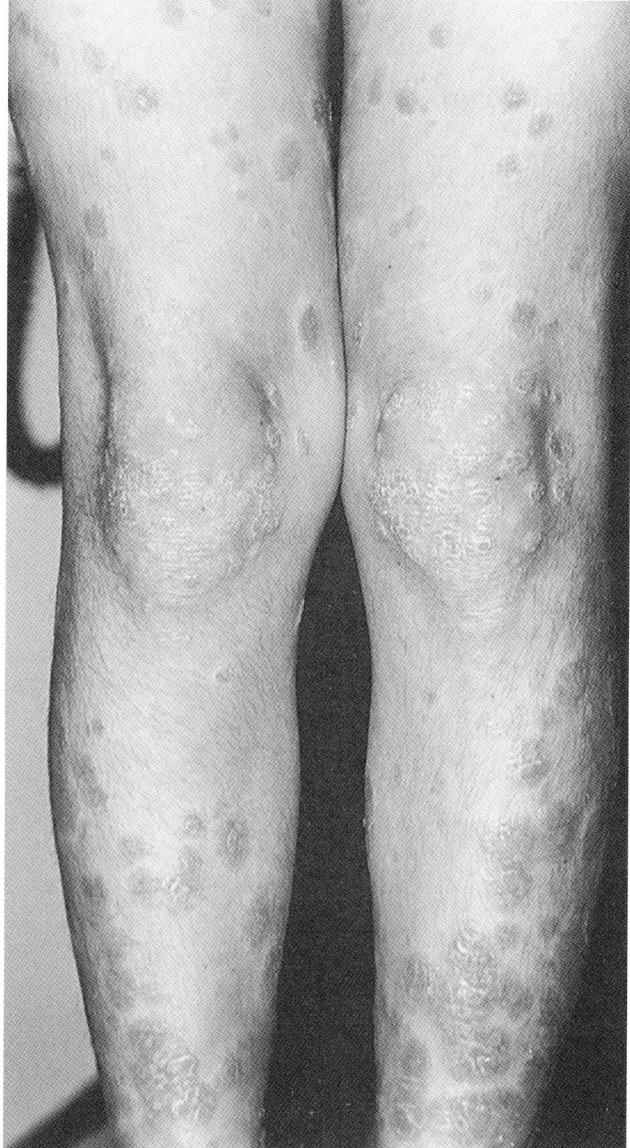

Figure 56-5. Well-demarcated erythematous, scaly plaques of psoriasis.

Nail abnormalities are seen in 25% to 50% of patients with psoriasis. Nail pits are the most common finding, identified by multiple pinpoint depressions that are irregularly distributed over the nail plate. Although nail pitting is characteristic of psoriasis, it is not a pathognomonic sign; it is also associated with atopic dermatitis, alopecia areata, and trauma. Other nail changes include separation of the nail plate from the nail bed (onycholysis), subungual hyperkeratosis, discoloration, crumbling, and "oil spots" on the nail plate. Yellowish-brown spots on the nail, thought to be caused by glycoprotein accumulation, characterize this latter finding, which is seen more often in older patients.

Guttate psoriasis, characterized by numerous droplike lesions, is a variant commonly seen in children and young adults. The round to oval, pinkish-red, somewhat scaly papules arise in crops and are widely distributed, particularly on the trunk. Two thirds of affected patients have a history of an upper respiratory tract infection, usually streptococcal in origin, that was present 1 to 3 weeks before the onset of lesions. Clinical improvement is seen after appropriate antibiotic therapy. Guttate psoriasis, in contrast to large-plaque psoriasis, is unlikely to become a chronic condition.

Psoriasis is usually diagnosed from the clinical appearance of skin lesions. However, when the diagnosis is unclear, a skin biopsy may be helpful. Differential diagnosis of psoriasis includes seborrheic dermatitis, dermatophytosis, pityriasis rosea, lichen planus, atopic dermatitis, and subacute cutaneous lupus erythematosus.

The course of psoriasis is marked by recurrent flares and remissions. Although it is unpredictable, there appears to be a subset of individuals whose disease gradually improves over time. Various therapeutic modalities are available and may range from simple topical regimens to aggressive systemic management.

For mild cases, topical corticosteroids, tar, anthralin, and emollients may be sufficient. Moderate- to high-potency topical corticosteroids are usually effective within 2 to 3 weeks of the beginning of therapy. However, remissions may be temporary because tachyphylaxis often develops. Care should be taken with the chronic, generalized application of topical corticosteroids in children, because systemic absorption may occur. Tar solutions and shampoos may be helpful for removal of scale from the scalp, especially when used in conjunction with topical corticosteroid preparations.

Other useful topical medications include salicylic acid, anthralin, tazarotene, and calcipotriene. Salicylic acid can be combined with topical corticosteroids, emollients, or oils to enhance scale removal. Anthralin is a tricyclic hydrocarbon that, when applied daily for 15 to 30 minutes and then washed away thoroughly, can be highly effective. A topical synthetic vitamin D_3 derivative, calcipotriene (Dovonex), is a promising therapeutic alternative. This agent must be used cautiously in smaller children because it may lead to decreased vitamin D levels.

Ultraviolet light therapy is generally effective. This can be in the form of natural sunlight or ultraviolet B (UVB) light therapy via a light box. Care must be taken, however, to avoid sunburn, which can result in exacerbation of the disease. For moderate to severe cases, daily use of crude coal tar in combination with UVB therapy, referred to as *Goeckerman therapy,* can result in complete clearing and long-term remissions after 2 to 4 weeks of treatment. Narrowband (311-nm) UVB therapy has been increasingly used and may be superior to conventional UVB therapy. In recalcitrant or severe debilitating psoriasis, photochemotherapy (psoralen plus ultraviolet A), oral retinoids, methotrexate, and cyclosporine can be used. Unfortunately, side effects limit their usefulness in children. The use of oral corticosteroids should be avoided, because withdrawal may result in severe erythroderma or flares of the disease.

Pityriasis Lichenoides

Pityriasis lichenoides can manifest in two forms: pityriasis lichenoides et varioliformis acuta (PLEVA) or pityriasis lichenoides chronica. These diseases most commonly affect children between ages 5 and 15. Both diseases are believed to be part of the same clinical spectrum. PLEVA is characterized by multiple, 2- to 4-mm, nonpruritic, variably scaly erythematous macules and papules that may progress to vesicular, necrotic, or crusted lesions. The lesions often involve the trunk but may spread to the extremities. One key feature is that lesions are usually present in different stages. The eruption typically occurs in crops, the condition may resolve spontaneously within several months, or recurrences and relapses may occur episodically for several years.

Pityriasis lichenoides chronica is characterized by pink to brown papules with central adherent scale, found primarily in the trunk and proximal extremities. The clinical course is variable, and the lesions may last from months to years. After the papule recedes, postinflammatory hypopigmentation or hyperpigmentation may occur. Sequelae are uncommon, and the lesions usually heal without a scar. Pityriasis lichenoides chronica may initially resemble pityriasis rosea. The most important differential diagnosis to consider in patients with pityriasis lichenoides chronica is cutaneous T cell lymphoma (mycosis fungoides). These conditions can have very similar clinical features, and the patient with a persistent eruption

should have a skin biopsy. Treatment with oral erythromycin for 4 to 6 weeks has shown benefit in some children.

Lichen Planus

Lichen planus occurs in patients of all ages but is less commonly seen in children than in adults. It is characterized by the "five Ps": *p*urple, *p*olygonal, *p*lanar, *p*ruritic *p*apules. The primary lesion is a shiny, violaceous, flat-topped papule, often with angulated borders, measuring from 2 mm to no more than 1 cm in diameter. The lesions are very pruritic and demonstrate the Koebner phenomenon, which results in development of new lesions (often in a linear configuration) at sites of scratching. Distribution may be localized or generalized, and lesions may number from few to numerous. Sites of predilection include the volar wrists, forearms, legs, genitalia, and mucous membranes. A reticulated pattern of delicate white lines or streaks (*Wickham striae*), seen on the buccal mucosa or skin, aids in confirming the diagnosis.

Nail changes are seen in approximately 10% of patients. These include longitudinal ridging, generalized nail destruction, red or brown discoloration, subungual hyperkeratosis, and thinning of the nail plate. Pterygium formation results from the overgrowth of fibrous tissue, which extends from the proximal nail fold to the tip of the nail, obliterating the nail plate. Medications that can produce a lichenoid eruption that is indistinguishable from lichen planus include β blockers, antituberculous agents, tetracycline, furosemide, dapsone, phenothiazines, and carbamazepine.

It is often possible for the experienced clinician to diagnose lichen planus strictly on clinical grounds. If necessary, a skin biopsy specimen can reveal specific findings. The clinical differential diagnosis includes psoriasis and drug eruptions. If oral lesions are present, the clinician must consider the possibility of aphthous stomatitis, erythema multiforme, herpes simplex, or leukoplakia.

Topical corticosteroids are the treatment of choice in most cases. Lichen planus usually resolves spontaneously over 1 to 2 years, but some cases may persist for many years. Generalized eruptions may respond to a short course of systemic corticosteroids. Oral antihistamines provide symptomatic relief.

Ichthyosis

The ichthyoses are a group of inherited disorders characterized by scaling of the skin. The term *ichthyosis* was initially chosen to describe the fish scale–like appearance of the skin. This reference is offensive to some patients; thus, the ichthyoses are also referred to as *disorders of cornification.* The pathogenesis of these conditions appears to be multifactorial.

The ichthyoses can be divided into four main subtypes based on mode of inheritance, clinical features, histologic findings, and biochemical markers (Table 56-5). The most common of these subtypes, *ichthyosis vulgaris,* has a prevalence of 1 in 300, is transmitted in an autosomal dominant manner, and is the mildest form of ichthyosis. The scaling of ichthyosis vulgaris usually appears after 3 months of age. Approximately 50% of affected patients have concomitant atopic dermatitis. The scales are fine and white and appear to be pasted on. Sites of involvement include the extensor surfaces of the limbs and the trunk, whereas flexural surfaces are characteristically spared. Ichthyosis vulgaris usually worsens during winter months but tends to improve with age.

Emollients and keratolytics are the mainstay of therapy. Ichthyosis vulgaris can usually be managed with lubricants such as petroleum jelly and α-hydroxy acids (lactic and glycolic acid) or urea-containing preparations that improve binding of water to the epidermis. In addition, salicylic acid is a useful keratolytic agent but may result in irritation or burning. Salicylism has been noted following systemic absorption. These side effects may also be noted with use of urea, lactic acid, and glycolic acid. Systemic retinoids are reserved for treatment of severe forms because of the potential for serious side effects.

Table 56-5. Ichthyoses

Subtype	Mode of Inheritance	Gene Defect	Clinical Features	Histologic Findings
Ichthyosis vulgaris	Autosomal dominant	Decreased filaggrin	Fine, whitish, adherent scales Increased involvement of extensor surfaces Face and diaper area usually spared	Absence of granular layer Small, poorly formed keratohyaline granules

X-linked ichthyosis	X-linked	Steroid sulfatase deficiency	Brown, large, adherent scales increased on extensor surfaces
			Relative sparing of flexures, palms, and soles
			Associated findings:
			  Comma-shaped corneal opacities
			  Cryptorchidism
				Increased or normal granular layer
				Hyperkeratosis with acanthosis

Lamellar ichthyosis	Autosomal recessive	Transglutaminase 1 gene mutations in many patients	Collodion baby at birth (translucent membrane encasing body) Generalized large, dark, platelike scales Fissuring between scales Ectropion, eclabium Mild erythroderma Scarring alopecia Nail dystrophy	Massive orthohyperkeratosis Mild/moderate acanthosis
Congenital ichthyosiform erythroderma	Autosomal recessive	Markedly accelerated epidermal turnover rate	Collodion baby at birth Generalized erythroderma with fine, white scale Corneal dystrophy, nail dystrophy, and sparse hair may be present	Nonspecific Mild thickening of stratum corneum Foci of parakeratosis

The presence of a collodion membrane at birth is sometimes seen in normal infants but may be the first sign of underlying ichthyosis, particularly *lamellar ichthyosis.* This type of ichthyosis is inherited in an autosomal recessive manner and is clinically manifested by large platelike scales and ectropion and eclabium (Fig. 56-6). *Congenital ichthyosiform erythroderma* is another type of ichthyosis that may manifest with a collodion membrane at birth. These infants often have underlying erythroderma with finer and lighter scales.

Seborrheic Dermatitis

Seborrheic dermatitis is characterized by an erythematous, scaly, symmetrical eruption that occurs most often in hair-bearing and intertriginous regions. Seborrhea of infancy is discussed in the section on neonatal dermatology. In adolescents, yellowish, greasy scale of the scalp, eyebrows, nasolabial folds, nasal bridge, posterior auricular regions, and midchest may be accompanied by mild erythema. Immunodeficiency disorders and neurologic dysfunction may be associated with severe, recalcitrant seborrheic dermatitis.

Therapy consists of low-potency topical corticosteroids. Antiseborrheic shampoos containing selenium sulfide, salicylic acid, zinc pyrithione, and tar are helpful for controlling scaling. Ketoconazole cream or shampoo (Nizoral) can be used in patients who are not responding to topical corticosteroid preparations. Although patients usually respond well to therapy, recurrences are common.

Atopic Dermatitis

Atopic dermatitis (eczema) is a chronic condition characterized by pruritus, a personal or family history of atopy, and an age-dependent distribution. It is common during infancy and childhood. Ninety percent to 95% of affected individuals have signs before the age of 5 years.

Typical lesions are red crusted or scaly plaques consisting of tiny vesicles or papules. Some individuals have follicular accentuation,

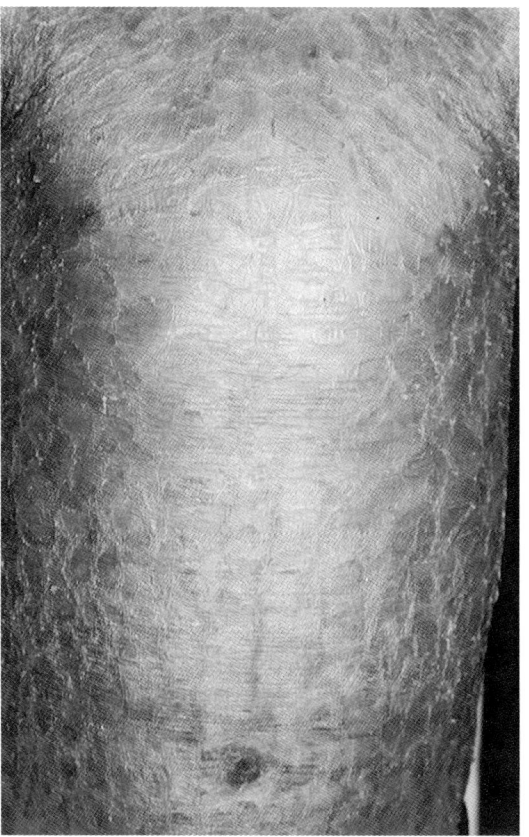

Figure 56-6. Large platelike scales seen in lamellar ichthyosis, an autosomal recessive disorder.

particularly on the trunk, manifested by a goosebump-like texture. Lichenification (thickened skin with exaggerated skin markings) is a feature of chronic atopic dermatitis and results from repeated rubbing and scratching. Excoriations are secondary lesions caused by scratching. Postinflammatory pigmentary changes are frequently noted, especially in dark-skinned individuals. Associated findings are noted in Table 56-6. The distribution of the lesions tends to be age dependent. The *infantile* form typically begins between 2 and 6 months of age. The cheeks, face, scalp, trunk, and extensor surfaces of the arms and legs are characteristically involved. The diaper region is usually spared because the skin is well hydrated from occlusive diapers. The differential diagnosis is noted in Table 56-7.

Childhood atopic dermatitis occurs between the ages of 2 and 10 years. The neck, wrists, ankles, and flexural surfaces of the extremities are predominant sites of involvement (Fig. 56-7). After puberty, atopic dermatitis has a predilection for the face, neck, hands, and feet. The clinical features of the skin lesions are not specific to this condition, inasmuch as other eczematous eruptions (contact dermatitis, seborrheic dermatitis) have a similar appearance. Laboratory tests are of limited value, and histologic findings reveal a nonspecific spongiotic dermatitis. The distribution of lesions, age at onset, and history are most important for establishing the diagnosis. Obtaining a complete personal and family history of atopic diatheses is necessary.

Secondary infections are the most common complication. Individuals with atopic dermatitis have increased colonization with *S. aureus.* Most affected children need occasional treatment with antibiotics to eradicate secondary infection. The presence of pustules, extensive excoriations, or weeping and crusted lesions suggests the need for antibiotic therapy. Topical therapy with mupirocin may be sufficient for limited areas; however, widespread involvement may necessitate the use of oral antimicrobial agents. The increase in methicillin-resistant *S. aureus* infections has limited therapeutic options in some patients. Secondary infection with HSV is referred to as *eczema herpeticum,* or *Kaposi varicelliform eruption* (Fig. 56-8). This occurs after inoculation of the eczematous skin with the HSV. Transmission may occur during routine child care from a caretaker with a herpetic fever blister. The hallmark of this condition is the rapid development of numerous umbilicated vesicles and pustules. Later in the course, multiple erosions are seen. The infection may be associated with fever and other constitutional symptoms, and expedient treatment with acyclovir is required. Hospitalization may be necessary in young infants or severely affected individuals. Recurrences of eczema herpeticum can be problematic.

Diagnosis

The differential diagnosis is presented in Table 56-7.

Treatment

Management of atopic dermatitis is noted in Table 56-8. Topical corticosteroids continue to be important in the management of atopic dermatitis because they have the advantage of decades of clinical use, in addition to a well-established side effect profile. Possible adverse effects from prolonged or high-potency topical corticosteroid use include cutaneous atrophy, telangiectases, propensity for easy bruising, development of contact dermatitis (rare, usually secondary to vehicle), and effects from systemic absorption (growth retardation, electrolyte abnormalities, hyperglycemia, hypertension, and increased susceptibility to infection).

To minimize the side effects of topical corticosteroid, the following instructions should be noted:

1. Avoid use of high-potency corticosteroids on the face, diaper area, and intertriginous skin. Lotrisone is a combination of clotrimazole and clobetasol dipropionate. Because clobetasol dipropionate is a class I ultrapotent topical corticosteroid, this agent should not be used in small infants or in the diaper or intertriginous areas.
2. Avoid extended use of high-potency preparations.
3. Avoid use of high-potency preparations with occlusion.
4. Avoid administration of large quantities of corticosteroids with unlimited refills (only a quantity sufficient to last between appointments should be prescribed).
5. Avoid indiscriminate use of topical corticosteroids on all cutaneous eruptions. They may exacerbate some conditions such as tinea corporis or acne.

Topical immunomodulators are an important therapeutic option in the treatment of atopic dermatitis. Topical tacrolimus (Protopic) is an immunosuppressive agent that has been approved for the treatment of moderate to severe atopic dermatitis in children older than 2 years. Tacrolimus is a macrolide calcineurin inhibitor with immunomodulatory effects. This agent should be reserved for children with moderate to severe atopic dermatitis because of the potential side effects, including the potential for secondary superinfection and systemic toxicity. Infectious events that may occur with increased frequency and severity include herpes simplex, molluscum contagiosum, and warts. Documented toxic effects in transplant recipients who used this agent orally include hypertension, hyperglycemia, neurotoxicity, and nephrotoxicity. Patients with extensive skin involvement, erythroderma, or widespread erosions are at particular risk for toxic levels of tacrolimus. Any child with severe atopic dermatitis on topical tacrolimus would probably benefit from a pediatric dermatologist's input.

Table 56-6. Atopic Dermatitis: Associated Findings	
Ichthyosis vulgaris	Affects 20% of patients with atopic dermatitis
	Primarily involves legs and trunk
Keratosis pilaris	Asymptomatic hyperkeratotic follicular papules found mainly on extensor surface of upper arms and anterior thighs, also facial in children
Pityriasis alba	Hypopigmented patches on the cheeks and occasionally upper body
Hyperlinear palms/ soles	Common physical finding in atopic individuals
Dennie-Morgan fold	A double line found under the lower eyelids
	Not pathognomonic
Lichen spinulosus	More commonly seen in darker skin
	Pruritic grouped hyperkeratotic follicular spires
Eye findings	Keratoconjunctivitis, cataracts, keratoconus (abnormally shaped cornea), retinal detachment (rare)
Dyshidrotic eczema	Firm vesicles found on the palms and soles, lateral aspects of digits
	Frequently associated with hyperhidrosis
Nummular eczema	Well-demarcated, scaly, coin-shaped lesions usually on the lower extremities
	Associated with xerosis
	Occasionally exudative lesions
Juvenile plantar dermatosis	Painful erythema, scaling, cracking, and fissuring of feet
	Often associated with hyperhidrosis
	Improvement after puberty

Table 56-7. Differential Diagnosis of Atopic Dermatitis

Condition	Similarities	Differences
Seborrheic dermatitis	Scaly plaques Erythroderma may be seen when severe	Earlier onset Pruritus minimal or absent Well-demarcated lesions Characteristic yellowish-salmon greasy lesions with intertriginous distribution
Contact dermatitis		
Primary irritant	Common in infants, young children May have similar distribution depending on the irritant (i.e., cheeks, chin, neck)	Usually less pruritic and less eczematoid Diaper area distribution uncommon in atopic dermatitis
Allergic	Pruritic Erythematous, papulovesicular eruption	Well circumscribed Uncommon in first few months of life Involutes spontaneously on removal of offending agent
Psoriasis	Scaly, red lesions	Deeper red-violaceous hue Thick micaceous scale Characteristic nail changes Sharply demarcated lesions Distinct distribution Pruritus may be less intense
Scabies	Frequent eczematous changes secondary to scratching, rubbing, or irritating therapy Can be very difficult to distinguish in infancy	Presence of hyperpigmented nodules Presence of burrows Isolation of mite from skin scrapings Acute onset Affected household members
Langerhans cell histiocytosis	Scaly, erythematous eruption Usually begins during first year of life	Primarily children <3 yr of age Presence of purpuric papules Associated hematologic abnormalities, hepatosplenomegaly
Acrodermatitis enteropathica	Vesiculobullous eczematoid lesions Onset during infancy	Acral, periorificial distribution Associated features: failure to thrive, diarrhea, alopecia, nail dystrophy Low serum zinc levels
Wiskott-Aldrich syndrome	Severe eczematous dermatitis	X-linked recessive disorder Associated features of thrombocytopenia, defects in cellular and humoral immunity, bloody diarrhea
Phenylketonuria	Eczematous eruption	Hereditary Mental retardation, seizures, diffuse hypopigmentation, blond hair, photosensitivity Elevated blood phenylalanine levels
Hyper-IgE syndrome	Symptoms begin in first 3 mo of life Eczematous dermatitis involving the face and extensor surfaces Personal or family history of atopy	Coarse facial features, irregularly proportioned jaw and cheeks, broad nasal bridge, prominent nose, severe oral mucositis Lifelong history of severe streptococcal or staphylococcal infections of the skin, limbs, joints Exceptionally high serum IgE levels Diminished neutrophil chemotaxis

IgE, Immunoglobulin E.

Pimecrolimus (Elidel) is another immunomodulatory agent that has also been approved for children older than 2 years with mild to moderate atopic dermatitis. Pimecrolimus is also a macrolide calcineurin inhibitor with a similar mechanism of action to tacrolimus. Pimecrolimus was specifically developed for the treatment of inflammatory skin diseases. However, as an immunomodulatory agent with a potential for side effects, it should be used with caution, especially in infants and preferably in coordination with recommendations of a pediatric dermatologist.

Systemic corticosteroids should not be used for routine management of atopic dermatitis. Atopic dermatitis is a chronic condition, and systemic corticosteroids provide a "quick fix" but only a short-term remedy. Short-term use of these agents often causes a significant rebound effect. Patients who receive systemic corticosteroids for other systemic diseases should be warned of this effect and the importance of topical corticosteroids and thick emollients as they are weaned off systemic steroids. The risks of systemic corticosteroids clearly outweigh the benefits, and these agents should be reserved only for severe cases in which aggressive topical therapy, including wet wraps, has failed.

LUMPS AND BUMPS

The presence of cutaneous or subcutaneous nodules and tumors can present a diagnostic challenge. They are also a source of great concern to parents, who fear the possibility of malignancy. Fortunately, most

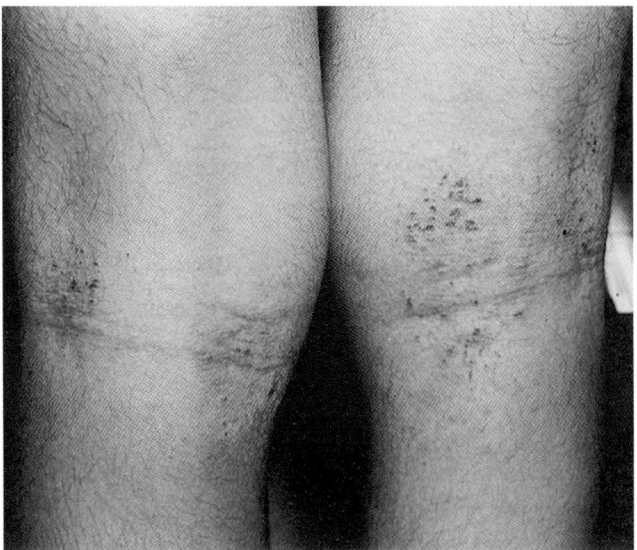

Figure 56-7. Excoriations in the popliteal fossae, a common site of involvement of childhood atopic dermatitis.

nodules and tumors in children are benign, and cutaneous malignancies are rare (Table 56-9).

GRANULOMA ANNULARE

Granuloma annulare is characterized by skin-colored to mildly erythematous dermal papules and nodules that may expand and coalesce into rings. These asymptomatic annular plaques measure 1 to 4 cm in diameter and appear most commonly on the dorsal hands and feet or extensor surfaces of the extremities (Fig. 56-9). The centers of these lesions usually appear normal but are occasionally hyperpigmented or violaceous in color. The overlying epidermis is unaffected. Multiple lesions are common, particularly in children. Granuloma annulare may be seen in all age groups, but at least 40% of cases occur before 15 years of age. The cause is unclear. Some cases have been associated with preceding trauma, such as insect bites.

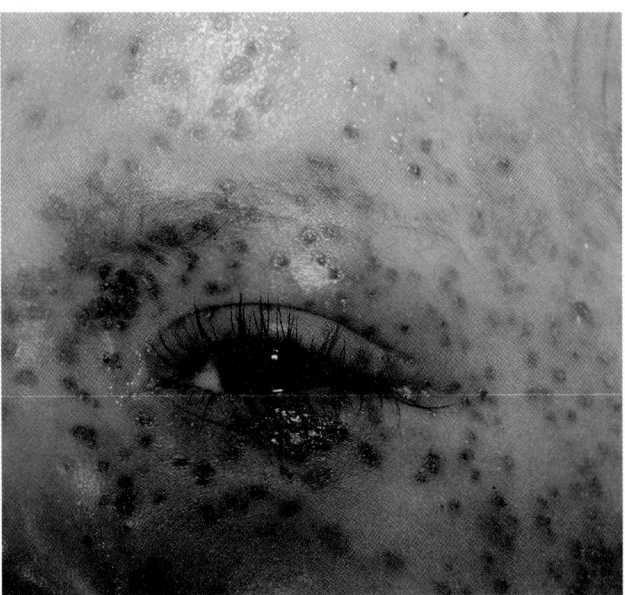

Figure 56-8. Eczema herpeticum infection in a patient with atopic dermatitis.

Histologically, there is dermal infiltration of lymphocytes and histiocytes surrounding degenerated collagen. Some authorities postulate that the condition may result from a cell-mediated immune response. In children, this condition is rarely associated with diabetes, as has been reported in adults.

The differential diagnosis of granuloma annulare includes tinea corporis, sarcoidosis, rheumatoid nodules, necrobiosis lipoidica diabeticorum, annular lichen planus, secondary syphilis, and leprosy. The eruption is most commonly confused with that of tinea corporis, but tinea has epidermal changes such as scaling, vesiculation, or pustules.

There are several variants of granuloma annulare. Generalized granuloma annulare is characterized by many asymptomatic papules symmetrically distributed. The ringlike lesions may coalesce into reticulated or circinate forms. The features of subcutaneous granuloma annulare are single or multiple deep nodules on the extremities, buttocks, and scalp. This entity is most frequently mistaken for rheumatoid nodules; however, the latter are usually larger and seen in the setting of rheumatoid arthritis.

Granuloma annulare resolves spontaneously over several months to years. Although more than 50% of cases clear within 2 years, recurrences are common. Treatment is generally unnecessary, but the use of topical or intralesional corticosteroids may hasten resolution.

SOLITARY MASTOCYTOMA

A mastocytoma is a solitary skin-colored to light red or tan papule or plaque that is often located on the trunk, extremities, or neck. Some lesions may have a yellow or pink hue. The lesion may appear at birth or within the first few months of life. Histopathologic study reveals the dermis densely infiltrated with mast cells. The characteristic finding on physical examination is that stroking the lesion causes histamine release that results in tense edema within the lesion and an erythematous flare, known as the Darier sign. A skin biopsy and special stains for mast cells may confirm the clinical diagnosis. Symptoms such as pruritus or flushing, when present, are usually mild. Treatment is not usually necessary unless the patient has symptoms of excessive histamine release. The condition is self-limited and resolves spontaneously over several years. The lesions do not need to be excised.

URTICARIA PIGMENTOSA

Urticaria pigmentosa is characterized by the development of multiple reddish-brown to tan macules or papules (mastocytomas), usually within the first 8 to 12 months of life (Fig. 56-10). The lesions may vary in size from a few millimeters to several centimeters. Some lesions may not become pigmented until the child is approximately 6 months of age. Therefore, early lesions of urticaria pigmentosa may resemble recurrent urticaria until pigmentation is noted. The Darier sign, or urtication of the lesions upon rubbing, is seen in urticaria pigmentosa. At times, these lesions may produce enough histamine release to cause flushing, diarrhea, vomiting, tachycardia, and hypotension.

Antihistamines should be used in any patient experiencing prominent histamine effects. Patients should be monitored closely for any symptoms that suggest systemic mastocytosis. In rare cases, other organs may be involved, including the intestines, bone, liver, spleen, and bone marrow. Intestinal involvement may be manifested by chronic diarrhea. The liver and spleen should be palpated for hepatosplenomegaly, and the patient should be monitored for any symptoms of bone involvement. Routine bone marrow and hematologic examinations are not required. Systemic manifestations are more common in adults; however, infants or children with significant systemic symptoms may require further evaluation. In most infants, the condition remits spontaneously by puberty. Children who present at an older age tend to have a more persistent condition that is less likely to remit spontaneously. Parents should be counseled about the avoidance of mast cell degranulating agents (Table 56-10).

Table 56-8. **Management of Atopic Dermatitis**

Therapeutic Modality	Indications and Recommendations
Bathing	Recommended daily for 10-15 min with warm, not hot, water. May use fragrance-free bath oils. Hydrates the skin.
Soaps	Mild, fragrance-free cleansers, such as Dove, Basis, Aveenobar, Olay, Cetaphil, or Aquanil, are essential
Emollients	Best applied immediately after bathing/showering. Should be used as often as possible. Petroleum jelly is ideal emollient: contains no water, additives, or preservatives and prevents evaporative water loss from skin. Thick creams such as Eucerin, Nivea, Aquaphor, Vanicream, and Cetaphil are some alternatives.
Compresses	Indicated for acute weeping lesions of atopic dermatitis. Helps cool and dry the skin, reduces inflammation. Use cool tap water or aluminum acetate solutions for 20 min, 2-4 times daily. Follow with topical corticosteroid application when appropriate.
Topical corticosteroids	Indicated to reduce pruritus and inflammation. Potency of topical corticosteroid determined by age of patient, site of involvement, severity of dermatitis, and duration of therapy. Facial and intertriginous skin should be treated with low-potency preparations. Apply before emollient. Use lowest potency that is effective. Monitor closely for potential side effects, such as striae and cushingoid features.
Topical immunomodulators	Tacrolimus and pimecrolimus very effective for moderate to severe disease.
Antihistamines	Controversial whether effective in this condition. If helpful, recommend oral, not topical, administration. May help some patients sleep. Hydroxyzine (2 mg/kg/day) often more effective than diphenhydramine (5 mg/kg/day). May induce drowsiness. Nonsedating antihistamines include cetivizine and fexotenadine.
Antibiotics	Patients have increased colonization with *Staphylococcus aureus*. Use if multiple excoriations, crusts, or pustules suggest secondary infection or if severe or resistant eczema is present. Treat with antistaphylococcal antibiotics. *Caution*: 1. Increased erythromycin and methicillin resistance in many regions of United States. 2. Do not use erythromycin with the nonsedating antihistamines: increased risk of cardiac arrhythmia.
Ultraviolet light	Useful for severe, uncontrollable atopic dermatitis. May administer ultraviolet B light (UVB), or ultraviolet A light in conjunction with oral 8-methoxypsoralen (PUVA).
Tars	Useful for chronic, dry, lichenified lesions, not for acute dermatitis.
Environmental conditions	Environmental factors may influence the severity of the dermatitis. Some helpful measures: Avoid fragrances in all topicals and laundry products. Avoid wool, feathers, dust exposure. Reduce house dust mites. Eliminate animal dander. Use plastic mattress covers. Reduce stress/anxiety. Increase environmental humidity to reduce skin evaporative losses. Avoid smoking.

JUVENILE XANTHOGRANULOMA

Juvenile xanthogranulomas (JXGs) are papules, nodules, or plaques within the skin that are solitary or multiple; well demarcated; rubbery to firm; and yellow, orange, or red. One of the most distinct clinical features of a JXG is its characteristic yellow color. On examination, overlying telangiectasias may be visualized. Lesions are of variable size, usually 1/2-2 cm, and are most commonly located on the head and neck region. The differential diagnosis should include Spitz nevus, solitary mastocytoma, and occasionally nevus sebaceous. Biopsy demonstrates the characteristic histopathologic features of lipid-laden histiocytes and Touton giant cells. Most JXGs are asymptomatic, but occasionally they cause pruritus or pain. The lesions may be present at birth or within the first years of life. JXGs are usually benign, and therapy is generally not required. After a brief period of growth, the lesion often stabilizes and involutes spontaneously in months to years.

Multiple lesions may prompt a search for the rare possibility of extracutaneous involvement. Lesions may be found in the iris, and a JXG is the most common cause of anterior chamber hemorrhage in children. The incidence of ocular disease in JXGs is approximately 0.3% to 0.4%. Ophthalmologic examination is recommended if a JXG is present near the eye or with multiple lesions. Involvement has also been described in the testes, lungs, liver, spleen, and heart. In a patient with multiple JXGs, the clinician should evaluate for

symptoms of organ involvement. JXGs are not related to diet, high lipid levels, or diabetes insipidus. Interestingly, JXGs appear to be seen in increased frequency in patients with neurofibromatosis type 1. An increased risk of juvenile chronic myelogenous leukemia has been reported in the setting of patients with both neurofibromatosis type 1 and JXGs.

DISORDERS OF PIGMENTATION

These conditions are often cosmetically disfiguring and persistent. They can be markers of serious systemic diseases. Pigmentary disorders may be localized or generalized; congenital or acquired; and transient, stable, or progressive (Tables 56-11 and 56-12).

CONGENITAL DISORDERS OF HYPOPIGMENTATION AND DEPIGMENTATION

Piebaldism

Piebaldism, or partial albinism, is characterized by circumscribed areas of depigmentation in the newborn. The leukoderma is usually located on the frontal scalp and is associated with a white forelock; however, the depigmented patches characteristically involve the trunk, upper arms, and legs. Hyperpigmented or normally pigmented

Table 56-9. Lumps and Bumps: Distinguishing Features

Diagnosed Lesion	Usual Onset	Color	Size	Site	Comments	Therapy
Epidermal cyst	Birth, childhood, adolescence	Skin-colored	1-3 cm	Face, scalp, neck, trunk	Potential for inflammation and infection	Elective excision vs observation
Dermoid cyst	Birth	Skin-colored	1-4 cm	Face, scalp, lateral eyebrow	When midline, may have sinus tract	Elective excision
Pilomatricoma	Any age, 50% before adolescence	Skin-colored Reddish-blue Bluish-gray	0.5-3 cm	Head, neck	Malignant transformation possible but rare	Elective excision vs observation
Dermatofibroma	Adulthood 20% before age 20 yr	Skin-colored Tan, brown, black	0.3-1 cm	Extremities	May follow trauma	Elective excision vs observation
Neurofibroma	Occasionally at birth Usually childhood or adolescence	Usually skin-colored Also pink, blue	2 mm to several centimeters	Any body site	May be associated with neurofibromatosis May see café au lait spots	Elective excision vs observation
Juvenile xanthogranuloma	Birth Childhood	Yellow to reddish-brown	0.5-4 cm	Head, neck, trunk, proximal extremities	Extracutaneous lesions involving eye	Ophthalmology consult; resolves spontaneously
Keloids	Peak between puberty and age 30	Pink to violaceous	Variable	Any site of injury Commonly earlobes after piercing	Often tender or pruritic Familial tendency	Difficult Intralesional steroids Excision
Granuloma annulare	Childhood Adolescence	Skin-colored to red	1-4 cm	Distal extremities	May be generalized in approximately 15% of cases	Observe, self limited Topical steroids if needed
Lipoma	Puberty Adulthood	Skin-colored	Variable May be >10 cm	Any, but usually neck, shoulders, back, abdomen	Malignant change very rare	Observe Excision
Solitary mastocytoma	Birth Early infancy	Skin-colored to light brown or tan Occasionally pink or yellowish hue	1-5 cm	Any site, but most often on arms, neck, trunk	Positive Darier sign, urticarii with stroking	Usually resolves spontaneously; antihistamines may be helpful
Erythema nodosum	Usually >10 yr of age Peak in third decade	Begin bright to deep red, then develop a brownish-red to violaceous bruise-like appearance	1-5 cm	Symmetric distribution over pretibial region, legs Occasionally arms	Tender Association with many infectious agents (group A streptococci, tuberculosis, mycoplasma), inflammatory diseases (sarcoidosis, inflammatory bowel disease), medications (birth control pills)	Thorough evaluation and treatment of underlying cause Antiinflammatory agents Bed rest/elevation of legs

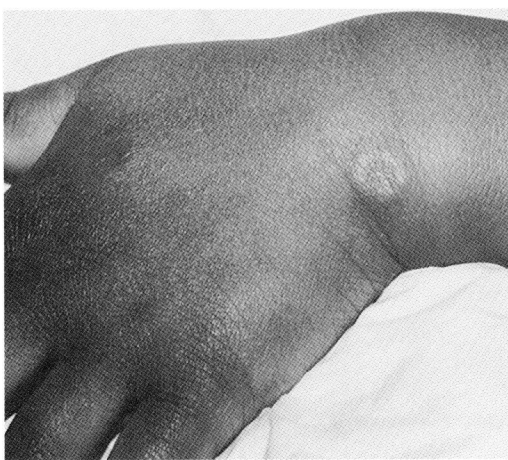

Figure 56-9. Ring of confluent dermal papules, typical of granuloma annulare.

Table 56-10. Mast Cell Degranulating Agents to Avoid in Urticaria Pigmentosa
Aspirin
Opiates: morphine, codeine
Alcohol
Polymyxin B (topical antibiotics)
Thiamine
Quinine
IV contrast dyes for radiology procedures
Certain anesthetic agents

IV, intravenous.

macules or patches may occur within the depigmented patches. This rare condition is transmitted in an autosomal dominant pattern. The disorder is usually present at birth but may not be recognized because of the light color of neonatal skin. A Wood lamp may enhance the contrast between depigmented and normal skin.

Piebaldism is a stable condition throughout life, and most affected individuals are otherwise normal. There are, however, several rare syndromes associated with partial albinism. Sun protection and cosmetic camouflage of the depigmented skin are the mainstays of therapy.

Waardenburg Syndrome

Waardenburg syndrome is a rare autosomal dominant disorder associated with piebaldism. It is characterized by a white forelock, areas of leukoderma, congenital sensorineural deafness, heterochromia of the irides, and lateral displacement of the medial canthi. Other features may include a flattened nasal bridge, confluent eyebrows, hypoplasia of the nasal alae, speech impairment that may or may not be related to presence of a cleft lip or palate, and various skeletal abnormalities.

Albinism

Albinism is manifested by diffuse congenital hypopigmentation or depigmentation of the skin, hair, and eyes. This heterogeneous group of disorders is composed of approximately 10 types of oculocutaneous albinism and five forms of ocular albinism. Most types of oculocutaneous albinism are inherited in an autosomal recessive pattern. The variants of ocular albinism are transmitted in an X-linked or autosomal recessive mode of inheritance.

The various forms of albinism can usually be diagnosed by findings on physical examination. These features include absent or reduced pigmentation of skin and hair and ophthalmologic findings such as foveal hypoplasia, nystagmus, photophobia, transillumination of the irides, fundal depigmentation, and decreased visual acuity. Patients should be monitored closely by ophthalmologists and evaluated for hearing loss. In white persons, the skin is usually milk white and the hair is white, blond, or light brown. The pupils are usually pink, and the irides are blue or gray. In African Americans, the skin may appear tan or white and is frequently freckled. The hair is usually blond or red, and the eyes are blue or hazel.

Treatment of albinism includes photoprotection and sun avoidance. Individuals are predisposed to severe actinic damage and should be monitored closely for the development of actinic keratoses, basal cell carcinomas, squamous cell carcinomas, and melanomas.

Tuberous Sclerosis

Ash leaf spots are hypopigmented macules, sometimes present at birth or within the first few months or years of life, that allow early identification of individuals with tuberous sclerosis. Although occasionally observed in normal infants, the characteristic lesions are present in up to 90% of patients with tuberous sclerosis. They are usually 2 to 3 cm in size and are located on the trunk and extremities. The macules may be lancet-shaped or may have a confetti-like or irregularly shaped appearance (Fig. 56-11). Wood lamp examination may facilitate identification. Although tuberous sclerosis is an autosomal dominant disorder, spontaneous mutations are responsible for up to 50% of new cases. Other cutaneous findings include facial angiofibromas (adenoma sebaceum), periungual or subungual fibromas, gingival fibromas, shagreen patches (connective tissue

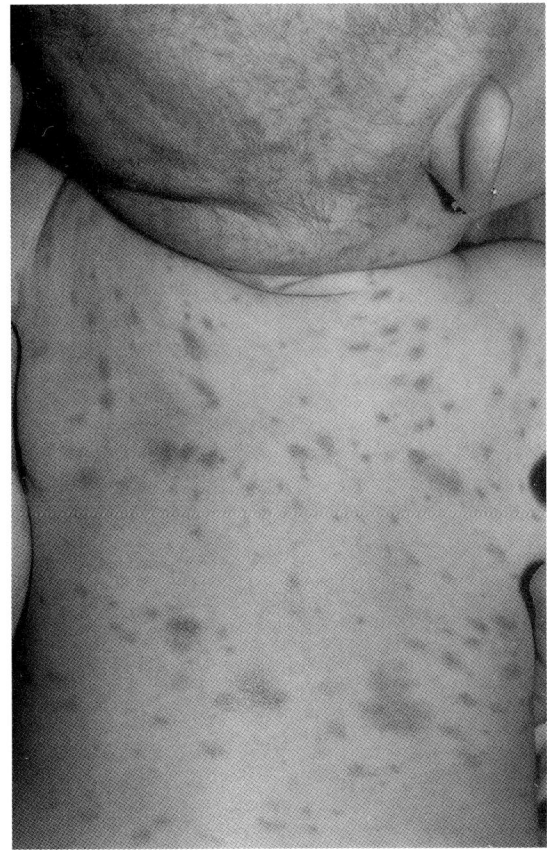

Figure 56-10. Urticaria pigmentosa.

Table 56-11. Congenital and Acquired Disorders of Hypopigmentation and Depigmentation

Disorder	Congenital versus Acquired	Hypopigmented or Depigmented	Clinical Features
Piebaldism (partial albinism)	Congenital	Depigmented	Autosomal dominant inheritance Leukoderma of frontal scalp White forelock Usually involves face, neck, ventral trunk and/or flank areas Within areas of depigmentation, may have areas of normal or hyperpigmentation Special variant includes Waardenburg syndrome, associated with sensorineural deafness
Nevus depigmentosus	Congenital	Hypopigmented	Well-circumscribed hypopigmented patch (not depigmented as name suggests) May be isolated or segmental in distribution Usually present at birth or early infancy Wood lamp examination may aid in diagnosis Often found on trunk/proximal extremities
Hypomelanosis of Ito	Congenital	Hypopigmented	Whorls and streaks of hypopigmentation that follow lines of Blaschko Usually present at birth or manifesting within first years of life Possible systemic associations, including central nervous system, eye, and musculoskeletal abnormalities
Nevus anemicus	Congenital	Hypopigmented	Rubbing or temperature change causes erythema of surrounding skin Often unilateral, often on trunk Not accentuated by Wood lamp examination Asymptomatic
Ash leaf spot	Congenital	Hypopigmented	Hypopigmented macules/patches often present at birth Wood lamp examination may aid in diagnosis Solitary lesion often not of clinical significance; at least 3 must be present to meet one criteria for tuberous sclerosis Full examination for other signs of tuberous sclerosis
Pityriasis alba	Acquired	Hypopigmented	Postinflammatory hypopigmentation Poorly demarcated, hypopigmented, slightly scaly patches often located on cheeks Repigmentation usually occurs
Vitiligo	Acquired	Depigmented	Complete loss of pigment in involved areas May be segmental in distribution, especially in children Hyperpigmentation may be present at borders of lesion: trichrome variant Infrequently associated with autoimmune disorders, including hypothyroidism

hamartomas), and fibrous plaques (typically on the forehead). Systemic manifestations include seizures, mental retardation, cardiac rhabdomyomas, renal angiomyolipomas and cysts, retinal nodular hamartomas, and pulmonary cysts. Imaging studies of the brain may demonstrate cortical tubers or subependymal nodules, which are pathognomonic for tuberous sclerosis.

ACQUIRED DISORDERS OF HYPOPIGMENTATION OR DEPIGMENTATION

Postinflammatory Hypopigmentation

Postinflammatory hypopigmentation is a common form of acquired hypopigmentation and may follow any inflammatory skin condition, including bullous disorders, infections, eczema, psoriasis, pityriasis rosea, secondary syphilis, insect bites, acne, pityriasis lichenoides chronica, and burns. More frequently detected in dark-skinned individuals, the clinical findings consist of irregularly shaped hypopigmented patches of variable size, often with a mottled appearance, located at sites of preceding inflammation. Postinflammatory

hypopigmentation usually resolves gradually over several months, and no treatment is necessary other than photoprotection.

Pityriasis Alba

Pityriasis alba may be postinflammatory hypopigmentation in atopic patients and is characterized by oval but poorly demarcated, slightly scaly, hypopigmented macules or patches located on the face, upper trunk, or extensor surfaces of the arms. The lesions generally vary from 0.5 to 2 cm in diameter, are often multiple, and are usually asymptomatic. Pityriasis alba may resemble tinea versicolor or tinea corporis but can be differentiated by its negative KOH results. The hypopigmentation typically persists for several months to years. Although no therapeutic intervention is required, the use of emollients and low-potency topical corticosteroids may be effective.

Vitiligo

Vitiligo is an acquired disorder characterized by complete loss of pigment of the involved skin. The condition often manifests during

Table 56-12. **Congential and Acquired Disorders of Hyperpigmentation**

Freckles (ephelides)	Acquired	Small, tan to brown, 1- to 5-mm macules
		Increase in number and pigmentation in summer and spring during exposure to sunlight
		Seen in fair-skinned individuals in sun-exposed areas
Lentigines	Acquired	Uniform, dark, brown/black 2- to 5-mm macules
		No seasonal variation or change with sun exposure
		Involve any part of the body, including mucous membranes
Café au lait spots	Congenital/ acquired	May be seen at birth or later in life
		Tan to brown discrete macules or patches; usually round or oval
		Six or more lesions larger than 5 mm in prepubertal persons and larger than 15 mm in postpubertal persons to meet criteria for neurofibromatosis
		Other stigmata of neurofibromatosis may appear only later in childhood
		Neurofibromatosis lesions: smooth, well-demarcated borders resembling "coast of California"
		McCune-Albright syndrome: larger lesions with more jagged, not as well-demarcated borders resembling "coast of Maine"
Dermal melanocytosis (Mongolian spot)	Congenital	Brown, blue-gray patches often seen in the lower trunk and lumbosacral area; may involve shoulders and extremities
		Seen usually in African Americans, Asians, Native Americans
		Usually fades later in life
		Benign with no known extracutaneous findings
Nevus of Ota	Congenital/ acquired	50% present at birth, 50% during second decade
		Unilateral blue-gray pigmentation in trigeminal nerve distribution
		Commonly involves ipsilateral sclera
		May increase in size and color with time
Nevus of Ito	Congenital/ acquired	Patchy blue-gray pigmentation of shoulder, supraclavicular area and deltoid areas
		May increase in size and color with time
Congenital melanocytic nevus	Congenital	Tan, brown/dark brown macules, patches, or plaques seen at birth or early infancy
		Variable color and texture
		Small (<2 cm), medium (2-20 cm), large (>20 cm)
		Large or multiple (>3) nevi carry risk of neurocutaneous melanosis or melanoma
Nevus spilus (speckled lentiginous nevus)	Congenital/ acquired	Well-demarcated, hyperpigmented patch with smaller, darker macules and papules within larger patch
		May look like a "chocolate chip cookie"
		May be extensive and segmental in distribution
		Small risk of malignant transformation; follow clinically
Acquired melanocytic nevi	Acquired	May start as hyperpigmented macules (junctional melanocytic nevi); over time, may become elevated papules (compound melanocytic nevi)
		Peaks in number during 2nd-3rd decade of life
		Abnormalities in color, borders, size, symmetry may suggest malignant transformation
Melanoma	Acquired	Variegation in color, texture or border of congenital and acquired melanocytic nevus
		Rare in childhood; risk correlated with family history and sun exposure in childhood

childhood and is believed to occur in genetically predisposed persons. Many authorities believe that vitiligo is an autoimmune process with circulating antibodies that destroy melanocytes. There is an increased incidence of autoimmune diseases in affected individuals and their families. The incidence of vitiligo in persons with diabetes mellitus is also higher than that of the general population. The onset of vitiligo may be precipitated by sunburn or other trauma.

Physical findings are usually sufficient for establishing the diagnosis. Well-demarcated depigmented macules and patches that are often bilateral and symmetric are distributed on the extremities, on the periorificial areas, and within skin folds. In some cases, depigmentation may have a segmental distribution. This variant is seen more commonly in children than in adults.

The clinical course is unpredictable. Spontaneous complete repigmentation is unusual; however, partial repigmentation may be seen during the summer months, especially within lesions of less than 2 years' duration. Repigmentation proceeds gradually and is more likely to occur in children than in adults. Treatment options include daily application of topical corticosteroids, which may be effective in patients with more limited disease. For more cosmetically disfiguring vitiligo in motivated, compliant patients, photochemotherapy may provide the best chance of repigmentation. Psoralen can be

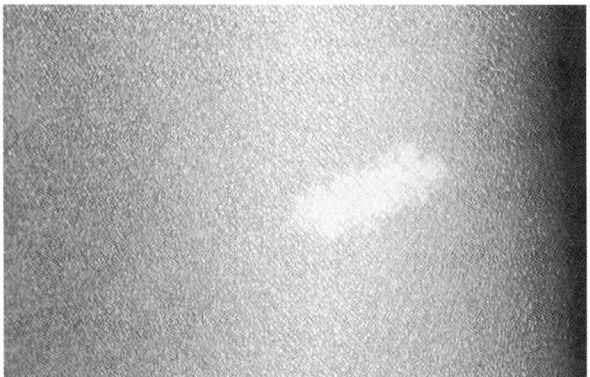

Figure 56-11. Ash leaf macule of tuberous sclerosis.

administered either topically or systemically, and ultraviolet A light can be provided by natural sunlight or via an ultraviolet light box. This form of therapy is often effective in children or young adults, especially for lesions of recent onset. Care must be taken to avoid burning, because this can further exacerbate disease activity. Narrow-band UVB therapy (311 nm) has also shown promise. Photochemotherapy usually requires several months until appreciable improvement is noted. Other interventions may consist of camouflage with cosmetics and careful photoprotection at sites of depigmentation in order to prevent development of cutaneous malignancy. Bleaching agents are another option in individuals with depigmentation of greater than 50% of their cutaneous surface.

DISORDERS OF HYPERPIGMENTATION
(see Table 56-12)

Epidermal Melanocytic Lesions

Lentigines

Lentigines are 1- to 5-mm macules that are darker than freckles and may occur on any cutaneous site, including the mucous membranes. Lentigines have no seasonal variance, and those that manifest during early childhood often disappear during adulthood. A lentigo may be clinically indistinguishable from a junctional nevus (mole); however, these lesions are histologically distinct.

Several syndromes are associated with multiple lentigines. *Lentiginosis profusa* is an entity characterized by multiple deeply pigmented macules that are usually present at birth or early infancy.

These individuals have no associated systemic or developmental abnormalities, unlike children with the *LEOPARD syndrome,* which also manifests during infancy. As the acronym suggests, these children may have multiple *l*entigines, *e*lectrocardiograph abnormalities, *o*cular hypertelorism, *p*ulmonic stenosis, *a*bnormal genitalia, growth *r*etardation, and neural *d*eafness. Multiple lentigines located on the mucous membranes, especially the vermilion border of the lips and buccal mucosa, should alert the clinician to the possibility of *Peutz-Jeghers syndrome,* which is characteristically associated with intestinal polyposis and subsequent risk of malignant transformation and intussusception. *Solar lentigines* occur in sun-exposed areas in older children.

Café au Lait Macules

Café au lait macules are well-circumscribed tan macules that usually measure less than 0.5 cm and may be as large as 15 to 20 cm in diameter. The lesions are found on any cutaneous site and may be present at birth or appear during early childhood. Although café au lait spots are seen in 10% to 20% of normal individuals, the presence of many macules should raise the clinical suspicion of neurofibromatosis (Table 56-13). The presence of six or more café au lait spots (>0.5 cm in prepubertal children; >1.5 cm in postpubertal children) fulfills one of the diagnostic criteria for neurofibromatosis type 1. Although the lesions are not pathognomonic, they are present in most patients with neurofibromatosis and tend to be larger and more numerous. Café au lait spots have also been associated with tuberous sclerosis, McCune-Albright syndrome, Turner syndrome, Bloom syndrome, ataxia-telangiectasia, Russell-Silver syndrome, Fanconi

Table 56-13. Neurocutaneous Syndromes

Syndrome	Mode of Inheritance	Cutaneous Findings	Systemic Findings
Tuberous sclerosis	Autosomal dominant	Ash leaf macules Angiofibromas (adenoma sebaceum) Shagreen patches Periungual/subungual fibromas Gingival fibromas	CNS involvement (seizures, mental retardation, cortical tubers) Cardiac rhabdomyomas Retinal gliomas Renal carcinoma or hamartoma Renal or pulmonary cysts Skeletal abnormalities
Neurofibromatosis (NF) (NF1 >85% cases)	Autosomal dominant	Café au lait macules (> 6 measuring ≥ 1.5 cm) in adults and > 0.5 cm in children Axillary, inguinal freckling (Crowe sign) Neurofibromas Blue-red macules and pseudoatrophic macules (involuted neurofibromas) Lisch nodules (melanocytic hamartomas of the iris)	Acoustic neuroma in NF2 Optic glioma may result in exophthalmos, decreased visual acuity Mental retardation (rarely) Seizure disorders (rarely) Tumors (astrocytomas) Hyperactivity, macrocephaly Learning disabilities, speech delay Osseous defects (up to 50%) Intestinal neurofibromas Endocrine disorders
Incontinentia pigmenti	X-linked dominant	Phase 1: inflammatory vesicles/bullae in crops over trunk and extremities, may persist weeks to months Phase 2: irregular linear verrucous lesions on ≥ 1 extremity, resolves spontaneously within several months Phase 3: brown to blue-gray hyperpigmentation, swirl-like formations on extremities and trunk; increases in intensity through second year of life, then remains stable for many years Phase 4: streaked hypopigmented lesions	Eosinophilia CNS involvement (seizures, spasticity, ↓ IQ) in 30% Spastic abnormality Ophthalmic changes (strabismus, cataracts, optic atrophy, retinal damage) Alopecia Skeletal abnormalities Dental abnormalities

CNS, central nervous system; IQ, intelligence quotient.

anemia, epidermal nevus syndrome, Gaucher disease, and Chédiak-Higashi syndrome.

Dermal Melanocytic Lesions

Dermal Melanocytosis (Mongolian Spots)

Dermal melanocytosis, also known as mongolian spots, are large, poorly demarcated, slate-gray to blue-black patches usually located over the buttocks or lumbosacral region of normal infants. The condition occurs in approximately 80% to 90% of black infants, 75% of Asian infants, and 10% of white neonates. Mongolian spots may be single or multiple and frequently measure up to 10 to 20 cm in diameter. This benign disorder is present at birth, usually fades during early childhood, and necessitates no therapeutic intervention. In rare cases, the lesions may persist into adulthood and may benefit from therapy with lasers that treat dermal pigmentation. These lesions should not be confused with bruising or child abuse.

The *nevus of Ota* and *nevus of Ito* are special variants of dermal melanocytosis seen most commonly in Asian and black individuals. In contrast to mongolian spots, these conditions tend to persist throughout adulthood. The nevus of Ota is a slate-gray to blue-black macular lesion located in the distribution of the trigeminal nerve. The condition is usually unilateral and involves the forehead, temple, periorbital region, nose, and cheek. Pigmentation of the sclera occurs in about 50% of affected individuals. The disorder may be cosmetically disfiguring, and laser treatment may be promising in some cases. The nevus of Ito is a similar process occurring in the distribution of the lateral supraclavicular and brachial nerves. The condition is usually unilateral and involves the shoulder, neck, upper arm, scapular, and/or deltoid regions. It may be seen alone or in conjunction with the nevus of Ota.

Postinflammatory Hyperpigmentation

Postinflammatory hyperpigmentation is the most common cause of acquired hyperpigmentation in children. This pigmentary alteration can follow any inflammatory insult and is seen commonly after insect bites, diaper dermatitis, acne, drug reactions, or other skin trauma. The clinical features are usually more striking in darkly pigmented individuals and often may be more pronounced than the original inflammatory lesions. The increased pigmentation usually resolves gradually over several months to years.

Melanocytic Nevi and Melanoma

Congenital Melanocytic Nevi

Congenital melanocytic nevi are pigmented macules, papules, patches or plaques that are present at birth or early infancy in approximately 1% of children. The lesions are often tan at birth and become darker and hairier during infancy and childhood (Fig. 56-12). Congenital nevi can be divided into small (<2 cm), medium (2 to 20 cm), and giant (>20 cm) lesions on the basis of their final adult size. In neonates and infants, lesions larger than 9 cm on the head and larger than 6 cm on the body constitute giant congenital melanocytic nevi. Most nevi are small to medium in size. The incidence of giant melanocytic nevi is approximately 1 in 20,000 live births.

The malignant potential of congenital nevi remains an area of great controversy. The risk of malignant transformation is significantly lower in affected black patients: Before 19 years of age, it is 1 in 10,000, and the maximum risk increases to 1 in 3700 between the ages of 15 and 35 years. The risk of malignant transformation in the general population for small and medium congenital nevi is unknown, and there are no universal guidelines for their management. Some experts advocate prophylactic excision of these lesions, whereas others advocate close observation of the nevi. Most dermatologists

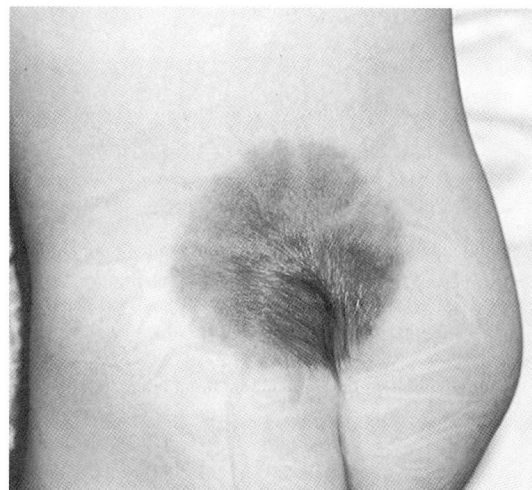

Figure 56-12. Hairy congenital melanocytic nevus. Magnetic resonance image of the lumbosacral spine was normal.

agree that removal of these nevi can wait until later childhood, when local anesthesia and outpatient surgery are feasible.

The risk of malignant transformation of giant congenital nevi is another controversial issue, and the lifetime risk is probably between 5% and 10%. These large lesions warrant close observation and serial photography. Careful annual or semiannual examinations with palpation of the nevi is essential, as melanoma can arise from deep portions of the nevi with little or no apparent surface alterations. Most authors suggest that giant congenital nevi be completely removed early in infancy or childhood because the risk of malignant transformation appears to be substantial in the first decade of life. Removal may require extensive grafting as well as soft tissue expansion procedures.

Neurocutaneous Melanosis

Neurocutaneous melanosis is defined as the presence of giant (>20 cm) and/or multiple (more than three) congenital melanocytic nevi, not necessarily giant, in association with benign or malignant melanocytic infiltration of the leptomeninges. Clinically symptomatic neurocutaneous melanosis substantially worsens the prognosis of large or giant congenital melanocytic nevi, and most affected patients die within 3 years of the onset of initial neurologic symptoms. The most frequent clinical manifestations include hydrocephalus, seizures, papilledema, headaches, increase in head circumference, paresis, and mental retardation.

MRI (contrast) of the head and spine is suggested in newborns with giant congenital melanocytic nevi, particularly in the posterior axial distribution and especially if satellite nevi are present. MRI abnormalities of the brain have been identified in asymptomatic patients with giant or multiple congenital melanocytic nevi. The most common imaging abnormalities in asymptomatic patients seen were T1 shortening in the cerebellum, temporal lobes, pons, and medulla. Radiologic findings can be very subtle and may be missed by radiologists unfamiliar with this entity. Controversy exists with regard to the need for baseline and follow-up imaging in asymptomatic patients, inasmuch as the implications of these studies are unclear.

Acquired Melanocytic Nevi

Acquired melanocytic nevi arise during early childhood as 1- to 2-mm hyperpigmented macules occurring most often on sun-exposed skin.

These flat moles usually represent junctional nevi, in which nests of nevus cells are located along the dermoepidermal junction. Over time, some nevus cells may spread into the dermis, forming compound melanocytic nevi, which clinically appear somewhat larger and more papular than junctional nevi. In some nevi, the nevus cells may become restricted to the dermis. These intradermal nevi are usually fleshy or even pedunculated in appearance. Located usually on the head, neck, or upper trunk, these nevi may clinically resemble skin tags.

There is a gradual increase in the number of nevi during childhood and adolescence. The average individual acquires approximately 20 to 40 melanocytic nevi. This number peaks at 25 years of age. In general, fair-skinned persons have a greater number of nevi than do darkly pigmented persons.

Melanoma

Although melanomas are very rare in childhood, their incidence in adults is increasing. The overall lifetime risk of melanoma in white persons in the United States is currently approximately 1 in 75 individuals. Melanoma can arise de novo or from preexisting congenital or acquired melanocytic nevi. It appears that congenital nevi possess a greater risk of malignant transformation. Nevi should therefore be observed for specific changes that may be indicative of malignancy. These alterations include

1. rapid growth of the nevi
2. changes in texture, including nodularity, crusting, ulceration, bleeding, or loss of normal skin lines
3. changes in pigmentation, especially the development of red, white, or blue hues
4. border irregularity, especially notched or scalloped edges
5. symptoms of itching, tenderness, or pain

In general, melanomas occur more frequently in light-pigmented individuals and in those with a family history of melanoma. Melanomas usually appear as darkly pigmented nodular masses larger than 6 mm in diameter. They are often asymmetric and tend to have irregular borders and surface characteristics. Melanomas must be differentiated from other benign pigmented lesions, including congenital and acquired melanocytic nevi, blue nevi, Spitz nevi, vascular lesions such as hemangiomas and pyogenic granulomas, and pigmented lesions caused by trauma. Suspect lesions should be referred to a dermatologist.

The mortality rate of melanoma is estimated to be between 10% and 20%. The prognosis depends on the thickness of the lesion. For lesions less than 0.75 mm in depth, the prognosis is excellent. Surgical excision is the treatment of choice. Patients should be educated on the importance of photoprotection with broad-spectrum (ultraviolet A and B) sunscreens. Sunscreen ingredients that offer this protection include titanium dioxide and zinc oxide.

REACTIVE ERYTHEMAS

MORBILLIFORM DRUG ERUPTION

Morbilliform (measles-like) eruptions are the most common cutaneous manifestations of drug-induced eruptions in children. In this eruption, fine erythematous macules and papules are distributed over the trunk. The rash often spreads centripetally from the trunk to the extremities. Lesions may coalesce into large plaques and are usually pruritic. Morbilliform drug eruptions are often difficult to differentiate from viral exanthems. It is believed that concomitant viral infections may predispose susceptible individuals to develop an allergic morbilliform drug eruption.

Although this eruption is usually self-limited, it may be an early manifestation of a more severe reaction such as Stevens-Johnson syndrome (SJS), toxic epidermolysis necrosis, or anticonvulsant hypersensitivity syndrome. Worrisome signs and symptoms of these entities may include high fever, mucous membrane involvement, lymphadenopathy and other systemic involvement. Signs of visceral involvement may include elevated hepatic transaminases, hematologic changes, or renal manifestations. Many agents, including common antibiotics, can trigger a morbilliform drug eruption. These drugs include penicillins, sulfonamides, thiazides, sulfonylureas, nonsteroidal antiinflammatory drugs (NSAIDs), aromatic anticonvulsants, and gold. Treatment includes prompt diagnosis with discontinuation of the offending drug and symptomatic care with antihistamines and emollients. The rash may last an average of 1 to 2 weeks and sometimes progresses despite discontinuation of the offending medication.

FIXED DRUG ERUPTION

A fixed drug eruption is characterized by the sudden development of solitary or multiple, well-demarcated, annular, erythematous, or hyperpigmented plaques. One of the distinguishing features is persistent postinflammatory hyperpigmentation, which may last weeks to months after the eruption subsides. The size of the lesion may vary, and the sites of predilection include the lips, trunk, legs, arms, and genitals. In some cases, the lesion may have a central bulla. When numerous blisters occur, the condition may resemble erythema multiforme. In this case, skin biopsy may prove helpful, although it may still be difficult to differentiate the two disorders histologically.

Systemic symptoms are rare, although the patient may complain of local pruritus or a burning sensation. Discontinuation of the offending drug causes a decrease in intensity of the erythema and edema; repeated challenge with the same agent causes a reappearance of the lesion in the same location as previously and may produce new lesions. Future outbreaks may be progressively more severe. The most common agents inducing fixed drug eruption include barbiturates, sulfonamides, phenolphthalein, tetracyclines, paracetamol, salicylates, NSAIDs, and even certain foods that contain yellow dye No. 5. Treatment is aimed at discontinuation and avoidance of the offending agent.

HYPERSENSITIVITY REACTIONS

URTICARIA

Urticaria is a common eruption in childhood. This condition is characterized by transient, edematous, erythematous, often annular plaques (Fig. 56-13). Central clearing may be seen but is not always present.

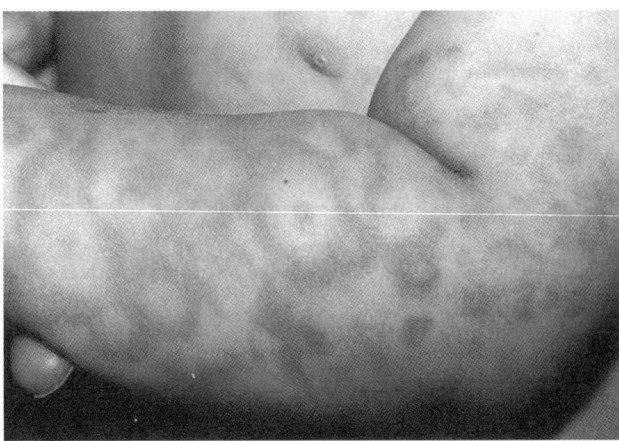

Figure 56-13. Giant annular urticaria with large, bizarre shapes.

The eruption is often sudden and pruritic, and each lesion rarely lasts longer than a few hours. Although the lesions are transient, they may continue to appear in new locations, and the entire urticarial episode may last hours to years.

Giant annular urticarial lesions are usually large, up to 20 to 30 cm, and polycyclic. A centrally bruised appearance is common within these lesions. Lesions may be of different sizes with bizarre shapes and patterns. Affected patients are often irritable and may have edema of the hands, eyelids, or feet. *Angioedema* is a form of urticaria that manifests with marked edema affecting deeper tissue planes and frequently involves the lips, dorsum of the hand or feet, scalp, scrotum, or periorbital tissue.

Giant annular lesions are often confused with the target lesions of erythema multiforme. However, there are key features by which to differentiate the two disorders. Urticarial lesions, by definition, are transient and last less than 24 hours, whereas lesions in erythema multiforme are fixed and usually last 1 to 2 weeks in the same anatomic location. Outlining the lesions with a marker may help determine whether the lesions are fixed or transient. Another differentiating feature is that the lesions in erythema multiforme usually have a dusky, necrotic center or blister. Skin biopsy may also aid in differentiating between the two disorders (Table 56-14).

Urticaria may be defined as either acute or chronic. *Acute* urticaria lasts less than 6 weeks. When hives continue to develop for more than 6 weeks, urticaria is considered to be chronic. Acute urticaria is often caused by drugs (particularly antibiotics), foods (milk, nuts, eggs, fish), infections (including group A streptococci, *Mycoplasma* organisms, Epstein-Barr virus, and many other pathogens), or physical stimuli (cold, exercise, vibration) (Table 56-15).

The cause of *chronic* urticaria is typically difficult to determine. A thorough history and a careful physical examination are the most helpful tools for determining the cause. Causes include infections (chronic otitis media, sinusitis, dental infections, urinary tract infections, hepatitis), thyroid disease, and medications. There is no routine battery of laboratory tests that should be obtained for the evaluation of urticaria. However, evaluation for chronic infection and other causes as suggested by the history and physical examination findings should be pursued. Serial history documentation and physical examinations should be performed.

Urticaria is usually self-limited. Treatment of pruritus consists of elimination of identifiable causes and administration of antihistamines. Hydroxyzine and diphenhydramine are often used but produce drowsiness. Nonsedating antihistamines are popular, but prescribers must be aware of potential interactions with concurrent medications. H_1 and H_2 blockers may be combined as needed. Systemic steroids are usually not indicated, unless there is airway involvement or anaphylaxis.

Table 56-15. Types of Urticaria

Due to ingestants (IgE mechanism in some cases)
  Foods, particularly fish, shellfish, nuts, eggs, and peanuts; food additives (tartrazine, azo dyes, benzoates)
  Drugs (penicillin, aspirin, sulfonamides, codeine)
Due to contactants (IgE mechanism in some cases)
  Plant substances (e.g., stinging nettle)
  Animal: insect (tarantula hairs, Portuguese man-of-war, cat scratch, moth scales)
  Drugs applied to the skin
  Animal saliva
Due to injectants (IgE mechanism in some cases)
  Drugs (particularly penicillin), transfused blood, therapeutic antisera, insect stings and bites (papular urticaria), allergenic extracts
Due to inhalants (IgE mechanism)
  Pollens, danders, and ? molds
Due to infectious agents (mechanism unknown)
  Parasites
  Viruses (e.g., hepatitis, infectious mononucleosis)
  Bacteria (streptococcus, mycoplasma)
  ? Fungi
Due to physical factors (mechanism mostly unknown)
  Cold urticaria
  Pressure urticaria
  Solar urticaria
  Aquagenic urticaria
  Local heat urticaria
  Dermographism
  Exercise-induced
  Vibratory angioedema
Episodic angioedema with eosinophilia (? a distinct entity)
Cholinergic urticaria (a distinct entity)
Associated with systemic diseases (mechanism mostly unknown)
  Collagen-vascular (systemic lupus erythematosus, cryoglobulinuria, Sjögren syndrome)
    Cutaneous vasculitis
    Serum sickness–like disease
  Malignancy (leukemia-lymphoma)
  Hyperthyroidism, hypothyroidism
  Urticaria pigmentosa (systemic mastocytosis)
Associated with genetic disorders (various mechanisms)
  Familial cold urticaria
  Hereditary angioedema
  Amyloidosis with deafness and urticaria
  C3b inactivator deficiency
Chronic urticaria and angioedema (mechanism unknown)
Psychogenic urticaria (existence as an entity uncertain)

Adapted from Behrman RE (ed): Nelson Textbook of Pediatrics, 14th ed. Philadelphia, WB Saunders, 1992, p 600.

IgE, immunoglobulin E.

Table 56-14. Urticaria versus Erythema Multiforme

Urticaria	Erythema Multiforme
Transient lesions: usually hours	Fixed lesions: lasting several days in same location
Asymmetric, variable, and bizarre shapes	Usually round or oval
No epidermal change: may have central clearing	Epidermal change: usually central necrosis, duskiness, blistering or crusting
Continued appearance of new lesions	All lesions present within first few days
Associated edema of hands/feet, eyelids	No edema
Generalized	Acral distribution

ERYTHEMA MULTIFORME MINOR

Erythema multiforme minor is a distinct hypersensitivity eruption that is often triggered by HSV infection (Table 56-16). This self-limited condition lacks internal organ involvement and has minimal complications. In this entity, usually zero to one mucous membrane is involved; the one most commonly involved is the orolabial mucosa. Discrete oral lesions may be present, and large bullous lesions are occasionally seen on the lips. Typically, lesions appear 1 to 3 weeks after a herpetic infection. Erythema multiforme minor may not be

Table 56-16. Potential Causes of Erythema Multiforme-like Reactions

Infectious Agents	Antibiotics
Herpes simplex 1, 2*	Penicillin
Mycoplasma pneumoniae†	Sulfonamides†
Tuberculosis	Isoniazid
Group A streptococcus	Tetracyclines
Hepatitis B vaccine	**Anticonvulsants**
BCG vaccine	Phenytoin†
Yersinia species	Phenobarbital†
Enteroviruses	Carbamazepine†
Histoplasmosis	
Coccidioidomycosis	**Other Drugs**
Chemicals	Phenylbutazone
	Captopril
Terpenes	Etoposide
Perfumes	Aspirin
Nitrobenzene	**Other**
Specific Diseases	Radiation therapy
Leukemia	
Lymphoma	

Modified from Esterly NB: The skin. In Behrman RE (ed): Nelson Textbook of Pediatrics, 14h ed. Philadelphia, WB Saunders, 1992, p 1641.

*Recurrent erythema multiforme.

†Erythema multiforme major (Stevens-Johnson syndrome: toxic epidermal necrolysis).

BCG, bacille Calmette-Guérin.

preceded by a clinically recognizable herpetic lesion, but polymerase chain reaction and in situ hybridization techniques have demonstrated HSV DNA and antigens in the lesions of erythema multiforme minor.

The clinical picture in erythema multiforme minor may be variable. The typical lesion in erythema multiforme minor is an erythematous papule with a dusky, purpuric, or necrotic center. The lesions are described as targetoid with concentric zones of color change: a dusky center or blister, a peripheral ring of pale edema, and an erythematous halo. Some lesions may not demonstrate the characteristic concentric changes, and the appearance of the lesions may be variable, depending on the stage at which the lesion is visualized. The Koebner phenomenon may be seen with lesions occurring in areas of injury. In erythema multiforme minor, the lesions are acrally distributed and may appear on the dorsa of the hands, feet, palms, and soles. Lesions tend to be grouped, particularly around the elbows and knees (see Table 56-14).

The disease is usually self-limited and necessitates supportive treatment with analgesics, topical steroids, and antihistamines. Systemic steroids are not indicated. Lesions often heal within 1 to 3 weeks and may leave residual hyperpigmentation. In children with recurrent HSV-associated erythema multiforme minor, acyclovir may prove helpful.

ERYTHEMA MULTIFORME MAJOR

For many years, the terms *erythema multiforme major* and *Stevens-Johnson syndrome* (SJS) have been used synonymously. However, there is controversy as to whether they are the same entity. Erythema multiforme major appears to be an infection-triggered hypersensitivity reaction. Many agents are reported to be associated with erythema multiforme major, but *Mycoplasma pneumoniae* has been reproducibly associated with this entity.

The cutaneous lesions of erythema multiforme major tend to be similar to those of erythema multiforme minor. Lesions are often targetoid and bullous and may demonstrate concentric color changes, indistinguishable from the lesions of erythema multiforme minor. However, patients with erythema multiforme major have

involvement of at least two mucous membranes. The mucous membranes most commonly involved are the conjunctiva and oral mucosa. Patients with erythema multiforme major associated with mycoplasmal infection usually have lesions in a predominantly acral distribution, and the eruption tends not to be as generalized as in SJS.

Histopathologic study of the lesions usually demonstrates a perivascular lymphocytic infiltrate with individual keratinocyte necrosis. There may be vacuolar degeneration of the basal layer, spongiosis, papillary dermal edema, and junctional or subepidermal cleft formation. In general, patients with erythema multiforme major tend to have increased inflammation and decreased epidermal necrosis in comparison with patients with SJS.

Treatment of erythema multiforme major is symptomatic and aimed at alleviating painful mucosal erosions. Liquid antacids or topical glucocorticoid or anesthetic preparations may be used. Systemic corticosteroids are usually not justified and may be associated with a more frequent and longer course of disease. Most children suffer an uncomplicated course with minimal complications.

STEVENS-JOHNSON SYNDROME/TOXIC EPIDERMAL NECROLYSIS COMPLEX

Most authorities consider SJS and toxic epidermal necrolysis (TEN) to be part of a continuum of disease. In general, they are severe reactions most often elicited by drugs with frequent internal organ involvement and an increased incidence of complications and sequelae. However, SJS and TEN differ in the severity of body surface involvement. In SJS, there is less than 10% body surface involvement; with 10% to 30% body surface involvement, the condition is labeled *SJS/TEN overlap;* and TEN refers to cases with more than 30% body surface involvement.

SJS is a unique hypersensitivity reaction. Although many factors have been implicated in the origin of SJS/TEN, medications are the most common causes in children. In particular, sulfonamides, aromatic anticonvulsants (phenytoin, carbamazepine, lamotrigine phenobarbital), and NSAIDs are cited as the some of the most common triggers. The nature of the reaction is not clearly understood, but it is believed to be a cytotoxic immune reaction aimed at the destruction of keratinocytes expressing drug-related antigens.

SJS usually begins with a nonspecific prodrome followed by generalized blisters, erosions, erythema, and hemorrhagic crusting of mucous membranes of the mouth, nose, eyes, and/or genitalia (Fig. 56-14). At least two mucous membranes must be involved to establish this diagnosis. Lesions are usually roundish, irregularly shaped, and less targetoid with numerous erythematous to violaceous macules and papules with dusky centers. The macules may then quickly progress to bullae with skin necrosis. Involvement usually

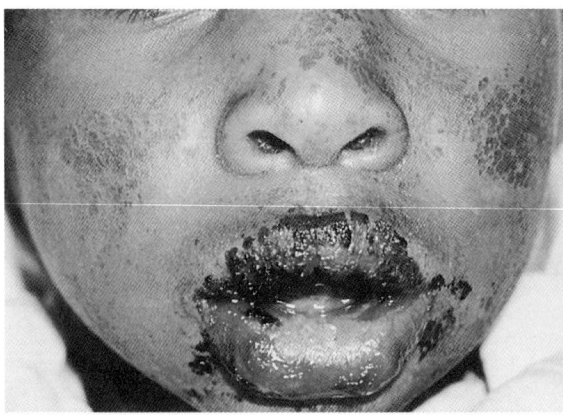

Figure 56-14. Erosions and crusting of the lips in Stevens-Johnson syndrome.

begins more proximally, with a predilection for the face, chest, and neck. The distal extremities are often spared. There is a striking tendency for coalescence, reminiscent of a diffuse erythema. The eruption in SJS is more generalized and tends to be more truncally distributed than that of erythema multiforme major.

Histopathologic findings in SJS are characterized by prominent epidermal necrosis with minimal inflammation. Epidermal injury and subepidermal separation may be observed. Spongiosis and dermal edema are usually absent.

TEN is the most severe hypersensitivity reaction, with an estimated mortality rate of 5% to 20%. Clinically, patients experience tender erythema of the skin that progresses rapidly to blistering and subsequent denudation. Malaise and prolonged fever often accompany these skin changes. Sheets of necrotic epidermis may slough off and leave denuded patches in areas of pressure, such as the back and shoulders. Mucous membranes are typically involved, and lesions are similar to those seen in SJS with flaccid, hemorrhagic blisters. In severe cases of TEN, sheets of necrotic epidermis may include skin appendages such as fingernails and toenails.

Extracutaneous involvement often includes fever, weakness, and arthralgia. SJS/TEN may be complicated by dehydration, electrolyte imbalance, and bacterial infection. TEN is often accompanied by a systemic toxic state with increased morbidity and mortality. Generalized lymphadenopathy and hepatosplenomegaly may be present. Internal organ involvement, manifesting as tracheal and bronchial symptoms, dehydration, shock, myocarditis, confusion, and coma, can be prominent in TEN. Late complications often include postinflammatory hypopigmentation or hyperpigmentation and, in more extensive cases, scarring.

Supportive therapy is the mainstay of treatment; few physicians believe that systemic corticosteroids are helpful in SJS/TEN, although this remains a topic of controversy. Removal of the triggering factor is of utmost importance. Careful ophthalmologic monitoring is necessary, because corneal scarring may lead to blindness. Maintenance of hydration and prevention of secondary bacterial infection are goals of treatment. Affected patients are cared for as if they sustained a severe burn; fluid and electrolyte balance, temperature control, protein loss, and prevention of infection are serious concerns. Affected children usually require initial management in a pediatric intensive care unit or burn center.

Although there are no case-control studies to date, intravenous immune globulin (IVIG) may prove helpful in the treatment of patients with TEN. The mechanism of action of IVIG is believed to be a blockade of Fas-mediated keratinocyte death.

With meticulous supportive care, most children survive; however, there is a high mortality rate. Poor prognostic factors include advanced age (elderly patients), neutropenia, impaired renal function, and extensive skin lesions. Recovery is slow; skin lesions require several weeks to heal, depending on extent of involvement. Scarring and stricture formation may occur at mucosal sites.

ALLERGIC CONTACT DERMATITIS

Allergic contact dermatitis is an example of a type IV delayed hypersensitivity reaction. This T cell–mediated immune response occurs after contact of the responsible antigen with the skin. The reaction becomes apparent 7 to 14 days after the first antigenic exposure. Future contact with the same antigen provokes an inflammatory response within hours to 1 to 3 days.

Acute contact dermatitis is usually characterized by the sudden onset of erythema, vesiculation, edema, and intense pruritus. Chronic contact dermatitis results in the development of lichenification, scaling, and hyperpigmentation and possible bacterial infection. *Poison ivy* is the most common cause of allergic contact dermatitis (*Rhus* dermatitis) in the United States. Direct contact of the skin with the sap of poison ivy, oak, or sumac may result in dermatitis. Contact with clothing or pets that have been exposed to the plant resin or smoke from the fire of such plants being burned are other forms of exposure. The eruption is usually seen as linear vesicles and papules or plaques. The spread to body sites is caused by exposure to the plant resin, not by the blister fluid. Therefore, scratching affected skin or contact with affected individuals should not result in spreading of the eruption. Other common forms of allergic contact dermatitis result from exposure to cosmetics, fragrances, hair dyes, and nickel.

Nickel dermatitis often results from prolonged contact with the nickel in jewelry or belt buckles. The eczematous changes are usually localized to the sites of contact, including the earlobes, neckline, wrists, and waistline. One case series observed that most children with allergic contact dermatitis in response to nickel presented with a generalized lichenoid papular id reaction, in addition to erythematous subumbilical and periumbilical papules and plaques at the site of nickel exposure. This case series demonstrated a high percentage of children presenting with a lichenoid eruption of the elbows and knees, at sites distant to nickel exposure, which resembled an id reaction.

The diagnosis of contact dermatitis can usually be determined from history and clinical examination findings. The distribution of linear or well-demarcated areas may be helpful in confirming the diagnosis. When allergic contact dermatitis is suspected but the responsible agent is unclear, patch testing with a selected group of antigens may provide useful information. Prevention of future exposure to inciting antigens is necessary.

Usually, treatment with topical corticosteroids, emollients, and antihistamines is sufficient to control the eruption. However, widespread dermatitis or severe involvement of the face may necessitate administration of systemic corticosteroids. A 2- to 3-week course of prednisone, with a taper to prevent rebound reactions, usually results in complete resolution. Wet compresses with aluminum acetate aid in the drying of weeping, vesicular lesions and provide symptomatic relief.

BULLOUS LESIONS

STAPHYLOCOCCAL SCALDED SKIN SYNDROME

Staphylococcal scalded skin syndrome (SSSS) (Table 56-17) is an exfoliative dermatitis produced by staphylococcal epidermolytic toxins. The condition is most common in children younger than 5 years but is also seen in adults. The condition may be localized or generalized, and approximately 80% to 85% of childhood SSSS is secondary to infection with *S. aureus* group II, usually phage type 71. Most cases have been associated with exfoliative toxin A; a minority of SSSS cases are secondary to exfoliative toxin B. *Bullous impetigo* is considered a localized form of SSSS. On the other end of the spectrum, SSSS can be a generalized, rapidly progressive disorder.

The diagnosis of SSSS should be considered in children with generalized tender erythema. A positive *Nikolsky sign,* the ability to laterally spread a blister or slough the skin with the application of light tangential pressure, is seen in most cases. The initial sites of involvement are usually the face, neck, groin, and axillae. It is common for the disease process to start periorificially. Flaccid bullae, sheets of desquamating skin, or moist red erosions that heal within several days may be present. Healing, without residual scarring, occurs within 1 to 2 weeks, as the level of cleavage is beneath the stratum corneum within the granular layer. In contrast to SJS or TEN, the mucosal surfaces are usually unaffected. The diagnosis is usually established from the clinical presentation. *S. aureus* may be isolated from a minority of blood cultures. The organism is more likely to be isolated from distant sites, such as the nares, throat, and conjunctivae, than from the bullae themselves. In some children, the toxin may be produced by an underlying infection, such as pneumonia, osteomyelitis, or septic arthritis.

Oral antibiotics may be indicated in localized SSSS. Children with widespread involvement usually require hospitalization, treatment

Table 56-17. **Vesiculobullous Eruptions**

Entity	Clinical Clues
I. Hereditary	
A. Epidermolysis bullosa (AR, AD)	Bullae at birth in more severe forms Localized or widespread Dystrophic nails in some forms Bullae induced by trauma, friction; may occur spontaneously Mucosal involvement in severe forms
B. Incontinentia pigmenti (X-linked recessive)	Crops of blisters at birth or early infancy Often linear May have coexistent streaky hyperpigmentation Eosinophilia Associated CNS, dental, ocular, cardiac, skeletal abnormalities Girls affected; boys may have Klinefelter syndrome
C. Porphyria cutanea tarda (AD or acquired)	On dorsal hands, other sun-exposed skin Heal with milia formation Increased fragility of skin Hypertrichosis
D. Epidermolytic hyperkeratosis (bullous congenital ichthyosiform erythroderma) (AD)	Verruciform scales in flexural surfaces Bullae within first week after birth Hyperkeratosis after third month Collodion membrane at birth in some cases
II. Autoimmune	
A. Linear IgA disease (chronic bullous disease of childhood)	Onset usually before age 6 yr Sites of predilection: perioral, periocular, lower abdomen, buttocks, anogenital region Annular or rosette configuration of tense blisters: "cluster of jewels" Mucous membranes commonly involved Spontaneous remission DIF shows linear deposits of IgA at DEJ
B. Bullous pemphigoid	Large, tense subepidermal bullae Lower abdomen, thighs, face, flexural areas Oral lesions common; rare in children DIF shows linear deposits of C3 and IgG at DEJ
C. Pemphigus vulgaris	Flaccid bullae, persistent erosions Seborrheic distribution Mucosal involvement very common, usually the initial manifestation Positive Nikolsky sign DIF with intercellular (desmosomal) deposits of IgG, C3
D. Pemphigus foliaceus	Small flaccid bullae or shallow erosions with scaling, crusting Back, scalp, face, upper chest, abdomen; photodistribution Oral lesions uncommon May resemble a generalized exfoliative dermatitis DIF shows intercellular deposition of IgG, C3 in superficial epidermis
E. Dermatitis herpetiformis	Intensely pruritic Associated with gluten-sensitive enteropathy Extensor surfaces of elbows, knees, buttocks, shoulders, neck Hemorrhagic lesions on palms and soles DIF shows granular deposition of IgA in dermal papillae
III. Infectious	
A. Bacterial	
1. Staphylococcal scalded skin syndrome (SSSS)	Generalized, tender erythema Positive Nikolsky sign Occasionally associated with underlying infection such as osteomyelitis, septic arthritis, pneumonia Desquamation, moist erosions observed More common in children <5 yr of age
2. Bullous impetigo	Localized SSSS
B. Viral	
1. Herpes simplex virus	Grouped vesicles on erythematous base May be recurrent in same site: lips, eyes, cheeks, hands Reactivated by fever, sunlight, trauma, stress Positive Tzanck smear, herpes culture

Table 56-17. **Vesiculobullous Eruptions—cont'd**

Entity	Clinical Clues
2. Varicella	Crops of vesicles on erythematous base: "dewdrops on rose petal" Highly contagious Multiple stages of lesions may be present simultaneously Associated with fever Positive Tzanck smear, varicella-zoster culture
3. Herpes zoster	Grouped vesicles on erythematous base, limited to one or several adjacent dermatomes Usually unilateral Burning, pruritus Positive Tzanck smear, varicella-zoster culture Thoracic dermatomes most commonly involved in children
4. Hand-foot-mouth syndrome (coxsackievirus)	Prodrome of fever, anorexia, sore throat Oval blisters in acral distribution, usually few in number Shallow oval oral lesions on erythematous base Highly infectious Peak incidence: late summer, fall
C. Fungal	
1. Tinea corporis	Annular scaly plaques, usually with central clearing Pustule formation common Positive KOH, fungal culture
2. Tinea pedis	Vesicles and erosions on instep Interdigital fissuring Positive KOH, fungal culture
D. Scabies	Burrow formation Interdigital web spaces, genitalia, ankles, lower abdomen, wrist Intensely pruritic; vesicles on palms and soles Very contagious Positive scabies preparation
IV. Hypersensitivity	
A. Erythema multiforme major (Stevens-Johnson syndrome)	Prodrome of fever, headache, malaise, sore throat, cough, vomiting, diarrhea Involvement of two mucosal surfaces; hemorrhagic crusts on lips usually present Target lesions progress from central vesiculation to extensive epidermal necrosis; sheets of denuded skin may be present Associated with infection, drugs
B. Toxic epidermal necrolysis	Possible extension of Stevens-Johnson syndrome involving >30% of body surface Severe exfoliative dermatitis Affects older children, adults Frequently related to drugs (e.g., sulfonamides, anticonvulsants) Positive Nikolsky sign
V. Extrinsic	
A. Contact dermatitis	Irritant or allergic Distribution dependent on the irritant/allergen Distribution helpful in establishing diagnosis
B. Insect bites	Occur occasionally after flea or mosquito bites May be hemorrhagic bullae Often in linear or irregular clusters Very pruritic
C. Burns	Irregular shapes and configurations May be suggestive of abuse Vary from first to third degree; bullae with second and third degree
D. Friction	Usually on acral surfaces May be related to footwear Often activity related
VI. Miscellaneous	
A. Urticaria pigmentosa	Positive Darier sign Coexistent pigmented lesions Usually manifests during infancy Dermatographism commonly seen
B. Miliaria crystallina	Clear, 1 to 2-mm superficial vesicles occurring in crops, rupturing spontaneously Intertriginous areas, especially neck and axillae

AD, autosomal dominant; AR, autosomal recessive; CNS, central nervous system; DEJ, dermoepidermal junction; DIF, direct immunofluorescence; IgA and IgG, immunoglobulins A and G; KOH, potassium hydroxide.

with intravenous antibiotics, and supportive management. The skin should be handled very carefully, and adhesive bandages should be avoided. Pain control is frequently necessary. Underlying infection should be suspected and investigated on an individual basis. The prognosis is good in immunocompetent children.

EPIDERMOLYSIS BULLOSA

Epidermolysis bullosa is a heterogeneous group of inherited blistering disorders characterized by spontaneous and post-traumatic bulla formation. It is estimated to occur in approximately 1 in 50,000 births; the severe variants are seen less frequently. There are several distinct variants that are distinguished by the inheritance pattern, cutaneous manifestations, histologic findings, and ultrastructural abnormalities.

In *epidermolysis bullosa simplex,* the level of blister cleavage is intraepidermal. This form results from a defect in the basal cell keratins 5 and 14, which have been localized to chromosomes 12 and 17, respectively, and are necessary for epidermal integrity. Most of the simplex forms are relatively mild and are autosomal dominant conditions. Bullae formation may be localized or generalized, but it is usually worst in areas of frequent trauma, such as the hands, feet, and joints.

In the localized *Weber-Cockayne variant,* blisters are usually confined to the hands and feet and develop after significant friction or trauma. This form may not become apparent until adolescence or adulthood and may manifest after strenuous activities such as hiking, military training, or golf. There are also generalized forms of epidermolysis bullosa simplex in which the bullae are much more extensive and usually apparent at birth and during early infancy. In general, the various subtypes are characterized by bullae that heal without scarring, mild or no nail changes, and minimal mucosal involvement. There are usually no associated extracutaneous manifestations.

In *junctional epidermolysis bullosa,* the cleavage plane occurs at the level of the lamina lucida of the dermoepidermal junction. This variant results from defects in the protein laminin 5, which is localized to the anchoring filaments, which are fibrillar structures within the lamina lucida. The junctional form is transmitted in an autosomal recessive mode of inheritance. There is a wide spectrum of subtypes, including Herlitz and non-Herlitz types, ranging from moderate involvement to a more severe, potentially fatal variant. There is a specific subset of junctional epidermolysis bullosa associated with pyloric atresia resulting from altered expression of $\alpha_6\beta_4$ integrin. Ureterovesical obstruction may produce recurrent UTIs. Most forms are clinically apparent at birth.

In general, there are widespread bullae that heal with atrophy, not scarring. Dysplastic nails, severe oral lesions, and enamel dysplasia are usually seen. The most severe variant has been referred to as *epidermolysis bullosa letalis of Herlitz.* Often fatal by 2 years of age, this variant is characterized by exuberant granulation tissue on the face and around the mouth. Extracutaneous manifestations include pyloric atresia, chronic anemia, and laryngeal involvement that often necessitates tracheostomy.

In *dystrophic epidermolysis bullosa,* tissue separation occurs below the dermoepidermal junction at the level of the lamina densa. The lamina densa is made up of anchoring fibrils composed of type VII collagen. Individuals with the dystrophic form have qualitative or quantitative abnormalities caused by mutations in the gene for type VII collagen. Dystrophic epidermolysis bullosa is further separated into variants that may be inherited in either an autosomal dominant or recessive pattern. They are usually apparent at birth; there is a wide array of clinical manifestations, but the condition is generally characterized by nail dystrophy and generalized blisters that heal with scarring and milia formation. In the more severe recessive dystrophic form, affected individuals usually have severe interdigital scarring, which results in syndactyly between fingers and eventual encasement of fingers and thumbs known as the *mitten deformity.* Severe mucosal involvement is a constant feature of recessive

dystrophic epidermolysis bullosa, and esophageal stenosis and obstruction are significant causes of morbidity and mortality. Chronic malnutrition, growth failure, and increased susceptibility to infection may lead to sepsis and death in this epidermolysis bullosa subset. Affected patients have multiple extracutaneous manifestations, as well as a very high frequency of aggressive and recurrent squamous cell carcinomas. The dominant dystrophic forms are usually more localized and have a better prognosis than does recessive dystrophic epidermolysis bullosa.

It is usually impossible to distinguish the variants of epidermolysis bullosa on the basis of clinical manifestations alone; skin biopsies are generally necessary. Transmission electron microscopy remains the gold standard for diagnosis. Immunofluorescent antigenic mapping is helpful in determining the precise level of blister formation; epidermolysis bullosa–specific monoclonal antibodies may provide further data.

Treatment modalities are dependent on the severity of the particular variant. In general, the emphasis is on wound care, prevention of infection, and prevention of mechanical factors likely to induce blister formation. Topical antibiotics and nonadhesive semipermeable dressings may be necessary for recalcitrant wounds. All adhesives should be avoided. In patients with the severe variants of epidermolysis bullosa, a multidisciplinary approach is imperative and should focus on preventive care. All affected patients should undergo genetic counseling.

PURPURA AND PETECHIAE

Purpura results from leakage of blood from vessels into the skin or mucous membranes (Table 56-18) (see Chapter 50). Purpuric lesions do not blanch when pressure is applied. Small lesions that are

---

Table 56-18. Causes of Purpura

Infections	Drugs
Rocky Mountain spotted fever	Aspirin
Sepsis	Corticosteroids
Subacute bacterial endo-	Penicillins
carditis	Sulfonamides
Streptococcal infection	Thiazides
Gonococcemia	**Other**
Meningococcemia	Scurvy
Hepatitis	Trauma
Echovirus 9	Cryoglobulinemia
Atypical measles	Henoch-Schönlein purpura
Collagen-Vascular Diseases*	PLEVA
Lupus erythematosus	Polyarteritis nodosa
Dermatomyositis	Malignancy
Rheumatoid arthritis	
Hematologic Disorders	
Idiopathic thrombocytopenic purpura	
Acute lymphocytic leukemia	
Aplastic anemia	
DIC	
Clotting factor deficiencies	
Warfarin or heparin use	

*Usually livedo pattern.

DIC, disseminated intravascular coagulation; PLEVA, pityriasis lichenoides et varioliformis acuta.

pinpoint-sized or a few millimeters in diameter are called *petechiae*. Large lesions may be referred to as *ecchymoses*. Raised or palpable purpura is diagnostic of vasculitis and can be seen in conditions such as Henoch-Schönlein purpura, lupus erythematosus, and Rocky Mountain spotted fever. Inflammation and destruction of blood vessel walls are responsible for the raised quality of these lesions. Nonpalpable purpura can be seen with platelet abnormalities, leukemia and other thrombocytopenic conditions (see Chapter 50), capillaritis (pigmented purpuras), scurvy, viral exanthems, and physical exertion. Petechiae on the upper body (above the nipple line) can result from crying, vomiting, or coughing. Careful clinical examination is important for detecting these lesions and establishing a proper diagnosis.

HENOCH-SCHÖNLEIN PURPURA

Henoch-Schönlein (anaphylactoid) purpura is a small-vessel vasculitis that usually occurs in children and young adults (Table 56-19). The skin, joints, kidneys, and gastrointestinal tract can be involved. It is an immune complex B–mediated disorder that typically demonstrates perivascular immunoglobulin A deposition in affected tissues. The antigens responsible for this hypersensitivity reaction may be bacteria or viruses, but drugs and foods have been implicated as well. Streptococcal infections frequently precede the onset of Henoch-Schönlein purpura, although the precise nature of the immunologic reaction is unclear.

The dermatologic features include purpuric macules, papules, or urticarial lesions that have a predilection for the buttocks and extensor aspects of the extremities. Hemorrhagic bullae and ulcerations can also be present. In affected infants, edema of the hands, feet, genitalia, and face may be seen. Systemic involvement is present in approximately two thirds of affected patients. Gastrointestinal features include vomiting, colicky abdominal pain, nausea, diarrhea, bleeding, and, in rare cases, intussusception (see Chapter 14). Arthritis or arthralgias are most often noted in the elbows and knees. There may be purpura overlying the affected joints. Joint effusions are rare. Renal involvement is the most serious complication and can be manifested by hematuria and/or hypertension (see Chapter 25).

The clinical course is characterized by acute onset of cutaneous lesions, often associated with fever and malaise. Attacks usually last for several weeks. Recurrences are common, but spontaneous resolution almost always occurs.

The diagnosis of Henoch-Schönlein purpura is usually made on clinical grounds, but a skin biopsy confirms the presence of leukocytoclastic vasculitis. Direct immunofluorescence staining of the skin biopsy specimen reveals immunoglobulin A and C3 deposition around the blood vessels in the superficial dermis.

Treatment includes supportive care and analgesics for joint pains. Systemic corticosteroids may be indicated when there is significant gastrointestinal pain or renal involvement, but this treatment remains controversial.

Systemic corticosteroids are generally not indicated for skin involvement alone. The prognosis is excellent in the pediatric population. Mortality is rare and is usually caused by severe renal involvement.

VASCULAR BIRTHMARKS

Vascular birthmarks can be classified into two groups: hemangiomas and vascular malformations (Fig. 56-15). Hemangiomas are the most common of the vascular tumors, and their behavior is characterized by a growth phase (endothelial proliferation), followed by a plateau or stabilization phase and then an involutional phase. Vascular malformations are usually apparent at birth and tend to be stable developmental abnormalities of any combination of vessels, including capillaries, veins, arteries, and lymphatic vessels. Differentiating features of hemangiomas and vascular malformations are listed in Table 56-20.

HEMANGIOMAS

Hemangiomas are the most common benign tumors occurring in children. These lesions develop in 10% to 12% of white infants by 1 year of age. Girls are affected apprsoximately three times as often as boys. The incidence is higher in premature infants. The natural

Table 56-19. Types of Vasculitis and Associated Skin Lesions

Type of Vasculitis	Blood Vessels Involved	Type of Skin Lesion
Leukocytoclastic or hypersensitivity angiitis: Henoch-Schönlein purpura, cryoglobulinemia, hypocomplementemic vasculitis	Dermal capillaries, venules, and occasional small muscular arteries in internal organs	Purpuric papules, hemorrhagic bullae, cutaneous infarctions
Rheumatic vasculitis: systemic lupus erythematosus, rheumatoid vasculitis	Dermal capillaries, venules, and small muscular arteries in internal organs	Purpuric papules: ulcerative nodules; splinter hemorrhages; periungual telangiectasia and infarctions
Granulomatous vasculitis		
Churg-Strauss allergic granulomatous angiitis	Dermal small and larger muscular arteries and medium muscular arteries in subcutaneous tissue and other organs	Erythematous, purpuric, and ulcerated nodules, plaques, and purpura
Wegener granulomatosis	Small venules, arterioles of dermis, and small muscular arteries	Ulcerative nodules, peripheral gangrene
Periarteritis: classic type limited to skin and muscle	Small and medium muscular arteries in deep dermis, subcutaneous tissue, and muscle	Deep subcutaneous nodules with ulceration; livedo reticularis; ecchymoses
Giant cell arteritis: temporal arteritis, polymyalgia rheumatica, Takayasu disease	Medium muscular arteries and larger arteries	Skin necrosis over scalp

From Wyngaarden JB, Smith LH (eds): Cecil Textbook of Medicine, 18th ed. Philadelphia, WB Saunders, 1988.

Vascular Birthmarks

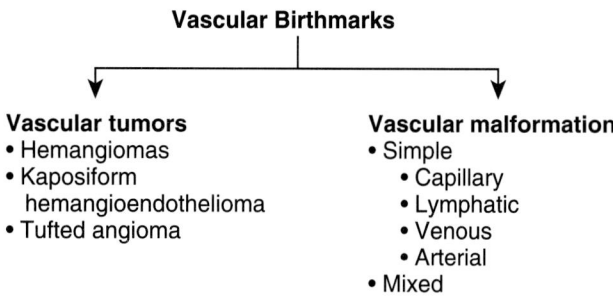

Vascular tumors
- Hemangiomas
- Kaposiform
  hemangioendothelioma
- Tufted angioma

Vascular malformations
- Simple
  - Capillary
  - Lymphatic
  - Venous
  - Arterial
- Mixed

Figure 56-15. Classification of vascular birthmarks (based on 1996 classification at International Society for Study of Vascular Anomalies— Vascular Tumors).

course of hemangiomas includes proliferative and involutional phases that end in complete, spontaneous regression in most cases.

Classification

There are three types of hemangiomas:

- *Superficial* hemangiomas, once referred to as *strawberry marks,* are the most common type (~50% to 60%); they are bright red with well-demarcated borders (Fig. 56-16).
- *Deep* hemangiomas, called *cavernous* in the past, are the least common of the three types (~10% to 15%); they are violaceous to skin-colored. These lesions involve the deep reticular dermis and subcutaneous tissue.
- *Mixed* hemangiomas (~30%) possess both superficial and deep components (Fig. 56-17).

Most hemangiomas occur on the head and neck, but any area of the body may be involved. Hemangiomas may be indistinguishable from port-wine stains in the early weeks of life. Lesions must be followed closely during the first few weeks after birth to determine whether a proliferative phase is present. Although the cause of hemangiomas is not clear, their natural course has been well documented. Hemangiomas may be present at birth but typically appear by 3 to 4 weeks of life. The initial lesion may be a white macule with central threadlike telangiectases or a red macule resembling a port-wine stain. A peripheral zone of pallor representing vasoconstriction may be noted at this stage. Within the first few months of life, the macule becomes raised and enlarges. During the first 6 months of life, hemangiomas proliferate at a rapid rate. After 6 months, the lesions grow at a slower rate. Involution may begin as early as the first year of life and is heralded by a color change from bright cherry red to dull red-violet. Deep hemangiomas start to lose their blue-violet hue. In time, the central portion of the superficial hemangioma

Table 56-20. Differentiation of Hemangiomas versus Vascular Malformations

Hemangiomas	Vascular Malformations
40% recognized at birth	90% recognized at birth
Vascular tumors with rapid postnatal growth and slow involution	Static malformation of dysplastic vessels that grows proportionally with child
Rapid endothelial cell turnover and proliferation	Normal endothelial cell turnover
Increased incidence in girls (approximately 3:1–5:1)	Girl-to-boy ratio of 1:1

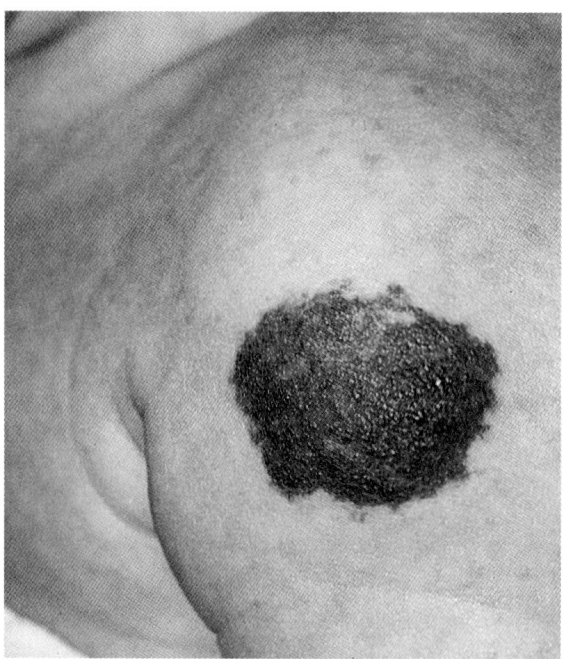

Figure 56-16. A superficial hemangioma early in its proliferative phase.

develops a grayish-white color that eventually extends to the periphery of the lesion. Lesions on the lips and nose and deep hemangiomas usually involute more slowly. It is not possible to predict precisely how long a hemangioma will take to involute. Statistically, 50% of lesions are gone by 5 years of age, 70% by 7 years, and more than 90% by 9 years. By 10 to 12 years of age, 95% to 97% of hemangiomas have disappeared. Once resolved, residual skin changes such as hypopigmentation, atrophy, and telangiectasias may be present in up to 10% to 20% of affected patients.

Hemangiomas have many potential complications and associations (Table 56-21). For most hemangiomas, no treatment is needed. Management of hemangiomas is based on a variety of factors. These include the size of the lesion, location of the lesion, age of the patient, rate of growth/involution at the time of presentation, and risk

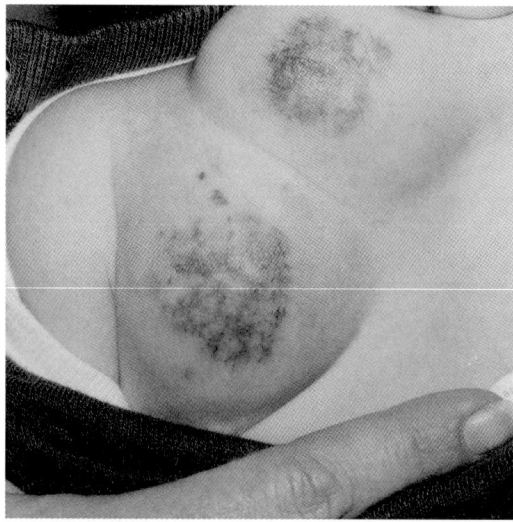

Figure 56-17. A mixed hemangioma with prominent deep component.

Table 56-21. Complications and Syndromes of Hemangiomas

Location	Complication
Lips/perineal/lumbosacral area	Ulceration
	Seen in rapidly growing lesions, especially of oral mucosa and genital area
	Risk of infection, scarring, hemorrhage; can be very painful
	Treatment consists of topical/oral antibiotics, barrier ointments, occlusive dressings; pulsed dye laser often beneficial
High output, extensive lesions	Congestive heart failure; hypothyroidism
	Extensive lesions with a large vascular supply may compromise cardiac function
"Beard" distribution	Respiratory/airway compromise
	Monitor for stridor
	Symptomatic subglottic hemangiomas may occur in 50%-60% of patients with extensive "beard" involvement
	Often manifests within first 2-3 months of life
Periorbital distribution	Associated ocular complications in up to 80% of patients
	Screening by ophthalmologist to rule out astigmatism or amblyopia
Ear lesions	Location can cause obstruction of auditory canal or decreased auditory conduction
	Monitor for otitis media or speech delay
Lumbosacral hemangiomas	High risk of spinal dysraphism; imaging of all midline lumbosacral hemangiomas should be considered
	Increased risk with other lumbosacral abnormalities (e.g., hypertrichosis, dimple, tags)
	Associated urogenital/anogenital anomalies may be present
Large, extensive cervicofacial hemangiomas	PHACES syndrome
	P: Posterior fossa malformations
	H: Hemangiomas of cervicofacial region
	A: Arterial anomalies (especially intracranial)
	C: Cardiac anomalies/coarctation of aorta
	E: Eye anomalies
	S: Sternal anomalies/abdominal clefting, ectopia cordis
Benign neonatal hemangiomatosis	Multiple cutaneous hemangiomas *without* evidence of visceral involvement
	History taking/physical examination should be performed thoroughly to rule out systemic involvement; further studies dependent on clinical presentation
	Benign clinical course with involution of hemangiomas within first year
Disseminated neonatal hemangiomatosis	Multiple cutaneous hemangiomas *with* evidence of visceral involvement
	Liver most commonly affected; also can affect lungs, gastrointestinal tract, eyes, mouth, and tongue
	Workup necessary to determine extent of systemic involvement; aggressive treatment usually needed

or presence of complications. Systemic corticosteroids can be used in a dosage of 2 to 3 mg/kg/day for extensive, disfiguring lesions or for lesions that compromise function of vital organs. Steroids are continued for several months and are gradually tapered. Examples of such lesions include midface or periorbital lesions, which may cause airway or vision compromise. These lesions warrant close clinical observation during the rapid growth phase of early infancy. Additional therapeutic modalities include intralesional steroids, pulsed dye laser therapy, surgery, embolization, and sclerosing agents. Interferon-alfa has also been used for treatment of serious and life-threatening hemangiomas, but there have been concerns arising from reports of spastic diplegia.

Kasabach-Merritt Phenomenon

Kasabach-Merritt phenomenon is defined as a rapidly growing vascular tumor in association with thrombocytopenia, hemolytic anemia, and consumptive coagulopathy. In the past, this association was thought to occur with infantile hemangiomas. Studies show that Kasabach-Merritt phenomenon is associated with distinct vascular lesions: namely, kaposiform hemangioendothelioma or tufted angioma. Clinical examination findings, lesion histologic findings, and the behavior of associated vascular tumors differ from those of conventional infantile hemangiomas. These lesions are often firm and

violaceous with a shiny texture and may proliferate for several years. This condition can be life-threatening and may warrant aggressive multimodal therapeutic modalities, including high-dose systemic corticosteroids, compression therapy, embolization, irradiation, interferon-alfa, chemotherapy (namely, vincristine), and surgical excision.

VASCULAR MALFORMATIONS

Salmon Patches (Nevus Simplex)

Salmon patches are the most common vascular lesions in infancy. These lesions consist of ectatic capillaries and are present at birth in about 40% of infants. These pink to red macules can be located on the nape of the neck, glabella, forehead, upper eyelids, and nasolabial regions.

No treatment is necessary, because most of these fade by 1 to 2 years of age. Persistent lesions can be treated successfully with the pulsed dye laser if cosmetically disturbing.

Port-Wine Stains

Port-wine stains (also known as capillary malformations or *nevus flammeus*) occur in 0.3% of all newborns. They are present at birth and represent progressive ectasia of the superficial vascular plexus.

These lesions do not undergo spontaneous resolution. They are usually unilateral and segmental but can be bilateral. The face and neck are the most commonly affected sites. Port-wine stains are typically pink to red during infancy and darken to reddish-purple hues with advancing age. Affected adults frequently have thickened, nodular port-wine stains that may be associated with soft tissue hypertrophy. Port-wine stains occur as isolated cutaneous lesions or in conjunction with other abnormalities.

Sturge-Weber syndrome includes ipsilateral association of a facial port-wine stain always involving the V1 distribution of the trigeminal nerve, eye abnormalities (primarily glaucoma), and vascular malformations of the ipsilateral leptomeninges and brain (Fig. 56-18). The incidence of Sturge-Weber syndrome is approximately 5% to 10% in infants with a port-wine stain of the V1 distribution of the trigeminal nerve. Consequences of Sturge-Weber syndrome may include seizures, developmental delay, hemiplegia, and glaucoma. Neuroimaging may be helpful in demonstrating the characteristic calcifications of the leptomeninges and the abnormal cerebral cortex, although these changes may be quite subtle with early studies. Newborns at risk for Sturge-Weber syndrome should have careful clinical follow-up.

Other syndromes associated with port-wine stains include Klippel-Trenaunay syndrome and Parkes-Weber syndrome. Klippel-Trenaunay syndrome is characterized by a capillary malformation (or mixed capillary/venous/lymphatic malformation), varicose veins, and soft tissue and/or bone overgrowth of the affected limb. Parkes-Weber syndrome is the association of arteriovenous malformations, limb overgrowth, and the variable presence of lymphedema and multiple arteriovenous shunts. Klippel-Trenaunay syndrome is a slow-flow capillary-venous malformation, whereas Parkes-Weber syndrome is a fast-flow arterial-venous malformation. Both entities can result in overgrowth and hypertrophy of the affected limb; however, Parkes-Weber syndrome usually results in increased morbidity and clinical consequences.

Treatment of a port-wine stain is best accomplished with the pulsed dye laser. Several treatments are generally required over months to years to achieve desired fading. Many experts believe that early initiation of pulsed dye laser therapy results in superior cosmetic results.

Venous and Lymphatic Malformations

Venous and lymphatic malformations are slow-flow vascular malformations that are often present at birth. Venous malformations are bluish, poorly demarcated, compressible masses. The characteristic bluish hue is caused by the presence of ectatic venous channels in the dermis. Often there may be associated swelling with changes in position or activity. Venous malformations can be segmental or more generalized, and radiologic imaging may assist in determining the extent of the lesion. Evaluation for central nervous system abnormalities with cranial imaging is recommended for patients with venous malformations of the face, to rule out developmental intracranial venous abnormalities that usually are asymptomatic. Many lesions manifest with pain caused by muscle involvement or with episodes of thrombosis or hematoma. Other associated risks include bone abnormalities (thinning, demineralization, or hypoplasia) and chronic localized intravascular coagulation. Treatment is aimed at correcting disfigurement or functional impairments. Therapy can include sclerotherapy, deep laser surgery, compression, and surgical excision. In many cases, it may be best to not intervene and to treat symptomatically.

Lymphatic malformations, previously referred to as lymphangiomas, are usually skin-colored masses that may have superficial clear or hemorrhagic vesicles that occasionally leak lymphatic fluid. These lesions can be classified as macrocystic, microcystic, or mixed. Macrocystic malformations often occur on the head and neck and are frequently diagnosed by prenatal ultrasonography. When such a large lymphatic malformation occurs on the head and neck region, it is often referred to as *cystic hygroma.* Microcystic malformations are usually more superficial lesions with a "fish egg" appearance (hemorrhagic and clear vesicles) that intermittently leak lymphatic fluid. This characteristic lesion was previously referred to as *lymphangioma circumscriptum.* These lesions usually become more evident in childhood rather than infancy. Large lymphatic malformations may impinge on vital structures and cause severe compromise in the neonatal period. Cellulitis is a potential complication of lymphatic malformations and may require prophylactic antibiotics if recurrent. Surgical therapy of these lesions is often difficult and may result in recurrences and complications. Treatment includes sclerotherapy and surgery in select lesions.

Cutis Marmorata Telangiectatica Congenita

CMTC manifests as an erythematous to dark, bluish-purple, reticulated vascular birthmark that does not resolve with physiologic warming. This disorder is characteristically more segmental and asymmetric than is physiologic cutis marmorata. The clinical findings are most often noted within the first few days of life. Associated features may include cutaneous atrophy and ulcerations. CMTC has also been reported to be associated with additional abnormalities, including body asymmetry, other vascular malformations, psychomotor or mental retardation, and glaucoma (with lesions in the V1/V2 trigeminal nerve distribution). Findings similar to CMTC have also been observed in infants with neonatal lupus, and this diagnosis should be considered. The clinical course of CMTC is characterized by gradual fading within the first 1 to 2 years of life, and treatment is generally not required.

Pyogenic Granuloma

Pyogenic granulomas are acquired vascular lesions that arise from the connective tissue of the skin or mucous membranes. These vascular nodules may be associated with antecedent trauma and represent a reactive, proliferative process. They are usually solitary, but multiple lesions occur in rare cases. Arising as small red papules, pyogenic granulomas grow rapidly and can ulcerate, leading to profuse bleeding. Histologically, these lesions resemble hemangiomas of infancy. In contrast to hemangiomas, however, they rarely regress spontaneously and may recur. Treatment involves destruction by pulsed dye laser therapy, electrodesiccation, surgical removal, or cryotherapy.

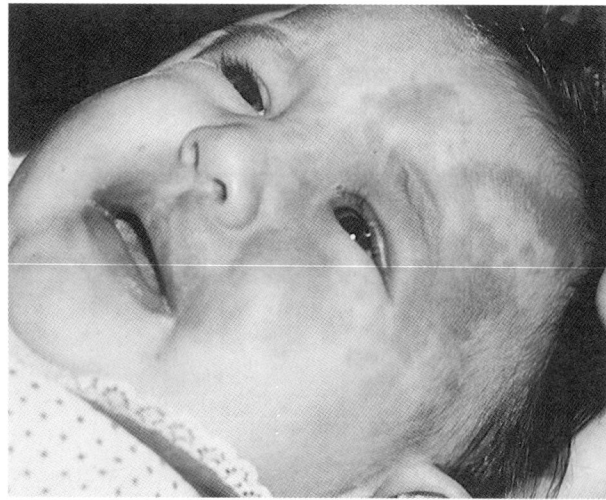

Figure 56-18. Port-wine stain of the face.

Spider Angioma (Nevus Araneus)

Telangiectases are dilated capillaries that appear as red linear stellate or punctate lesions. There are many causes of primary telangiectasias (spider angiomas, Osler-Weber-Rendu syndrome, CMTC) and secondary telangiectasias, such as collagen-vascular diseases. Spider angiomas are the most common of the telangiectasias. In the pediatric age group, these lesions are typically not associated with systemic disease.

Spider angiomas are seen most often on the face, trunk, and upper extremities. They are acquired lesions that usually develop after 2 years of age. Small vessels radiate from a central punctum (arteriole), giving the appearance of a "spider." When pressure is applied to the central punctum, the lesion blanches. Treatment, if desired, consists of gentle electrodesiccation or pulsed dye laser therapy. In some cases, spider angiomas clear without treatment.

ALOPECIA

Alopecia (hair loss) is the most common hair abnormality seen in children.

HISTORY AND PHYSICAL EXAMINATION

An accurate history alone can often lead to a presumptive diagnosis. Information regarding duration of loss, rate of shedding, drug intake, trauma, family history of hair disorders, symptoms such as pruritus or burning, breakage, and hair care is particularly important. The scalp should be examined for the pattern and distribution of hair loss, erythema, scaling, scarring, pustules, and crusts. Abnormal or broken hairs, as well as texture, length, and color, should be noted. Associated abnormalities of the teeth, nails, and sweat glands may occur. Hair pulls (gentle pulling on small tufts of hair) and microscopic examination of removed hairs should be performed. Appropriate tests (KOH, fungal culture, scalp biopsy) may be necessary to confirm the clinical suspicions.

CLASSIFICATION

Classification of alopecia is somewhat arbitrary, but it is helpful to determine whether hair loss is acquired or congenital and localized or diffuse. Congenital alopecia usually results from aplasia cutis, intrauterine injury, or nevus sebaceous. Five common disorders responsible for most cases of childhood hair loss are (1) alopecia areata, (2) tinea capitis, (3) traction alopecia, (4) trichotillomania, and (5) telogen effluvium.

Alopecia Areata

Alopecia areata is a common disorder that affects all ages, particularly children. Although the exact pathogenesis is unclear, it is generally thought to be an autoimmune condition associated with lymphocytic inflammation around hair follicles. There is a family history of alopecia areata for approximately 20% of affected individuals. Clinically, there is acute onset of hair loss that is occasionally preceded by burning or itching of the scalp. Well-demarcated, localized areas of alopecia result, and the scalp is usually normal without epidermal changes. The exclamation point hairs are pathognomonic and are caused by breakage of abnormally growing hairs. Exclamation point hairs, when pulled out, appear as a tapered or attenuated bulb secondary to atrophy of that portion. When the disease is active, dystrophic anagen hairs can be easily pulled from the periphery of lesions. Nail pitting, often seen in rows, is seen in some cases.

Although the course is unpredictable, about half of affected patients have a recurrence. Factors that portend a poor prognosis for regrowth include extensive loss, early onset, nail involvement, atopic background, and an ophiasis pattern (involvement of the temporal and occipital hairline). Treatment consists of topical, intralesional corticosteroids; topical minoxidil; anthralin; sensitization to contact allergens; and psoralen plus ultraviolet A light. Other helpful measures include camouflage, hairpieces, and support groups. In some cases, hair regrows without medical intervention.

Tinea Capitis

Tinea capitis (ringworm) is another common cause of alopecia in children, although it may not always be associated with hair loss or breakage. The "seborrheic" type of tinea capitis is manifested by diffuse scaling without scalp inflammation. Alopecia is often not noted, but broken hairs are occasionally present. This type of alopecia is frequently misdiagnosed as dandruff. Tinea capitis can also manifest as localized scaly patches, kerions, and "black-dot" patches. This latter type features hairs that have broken at the surface of the scalp, resulting in a black-dot appearance. *Kerions* are boggy, inflammatory plaques on the scalp that are caused by hypersensitivity to the offending dermatophyte (Fig. 56-19). Pustules and drainage are common, but the purulent material is often sterile. Cervical lymphadenopathy, fever, and elevated white blood cell counts may accompany kerions. The differential diagnosis of tinea capitis should include psoriasis, alopecia areata, trichotillomania, folliculitis, and seborrheic dermatitis.

The most common etiologic agent of tinea capitis is *Trichophyton tonsurans,* a dermatophyte that produces endothrix infections. Because spores are not present on the surface of the hair shafts, Wood lamp examination is not useful. If, however, the infection is caused by *Microsporum canis* or another dermatophyte that produces an ectothrix infection, Wood lamp examination results in positive fluorescence. Fungal cultures should be performed in all suspected cases of tinea capitis. Fungal culture can be performed with standard toothbrush and Petri dish. KOH preparations can be useful if positive, but false-negative results are possible. Some children may be asymptomatic carriers.

Traditional therapy consists of oral griseofulvin for 6 to 8 weeks. The standard dose is 15 to 20 mg/kg/day of microsized preparations, and this can be given in single or divided doses. Griseofulvin should be administered with fat-containing foods, because fat is required for optimal absorption. Selenium sulfide 2.5% shampoo or 2% ketoconazole shampoo should be used to decrease surface spores and reduce spread to other individuals. On occasion, there is a secondary bacterial infection that necessitates antibiotic therapy. Kerions respond to griseofulvin; in severe cases, systemic corticosteroids may be added to decrease inflammation and reduce the risk of scarring. Antifungal agents that may be useful include fluconazole,

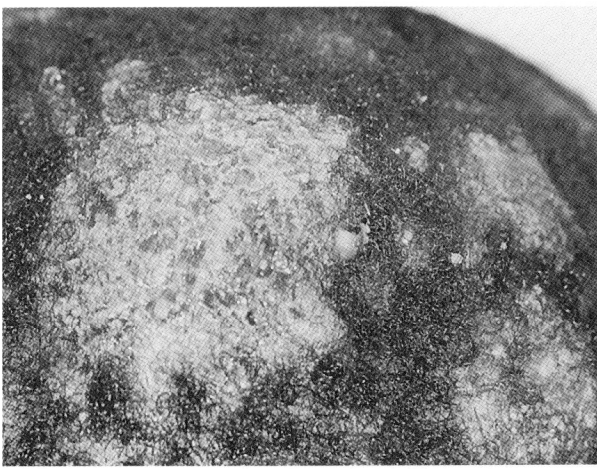

Figure 56-19. Boggy, purulent, crusted plaques typical of kerions.

itraconazole, and terbinafine. Incision and drainage are not indicated. A follow-up fungal culture may be obtained to confirm adequacy of treatment.

Traction Alopecia

Traction alopecia is seen in individuals whose hair is tightly braided or pulled into ponytails for long periods of time. Chronic tension on the hair shafts leads to breakage and gradual hair loss. Damaging hairstyle procedures such as straightening and waving may also result in hair breakage if performed improperly. On clinical examination, the clinician sees linear areas of hair loss at the part line or throughout the scalp. The alopecia is reversible in most cases. However, if the traction is maintained for years, the alopecia may become permanent secondary to scarring. Treatment is aimed at avoiding all tension-producing trauma. The patient should be advised to stop all hair chemical procedures, wear loose styles with no braids, avoid wearing heavy objects in the hair and ponytails, and handle hair as naturally and gently as possible.

Trichotillomania

In trichotillomania, individuals pull, break, or twist hair from the scalp, eyebrows, eyelashes, and/or pubic hair. In younger children, this form of hair pulling is usually a harmless habit that is outgrown. Trichotillomania in older children and adolescents may represent a more serious psychological problem with a less favorable prognosis. Psychiatric assistance may be required, and the disorder may be refractory to treatment. On physical examination, there are hairs of varying length in bizarre, often geometric, patterns. The occiput is often spared. Hairs have blunt tips because of mechanical breakage. Scalp biopsy may be necessary if the diagnosis is unclear. Treatment is aimed at identifying underlying psychological stressors. Supportive therapy and psychological and/or psychiatric evaluation is usually needed.

Telogen Effluvium

Telogen effluvium is characterized by excessive shedding of telogen (resting) hairs. This may result from medications, febrile illness, crash diets, parturition, surgical procedures or anesthesia, endocrine disorders, or severe emotional stress. A large number of growing hairs enter the resting phase, resulting in a threefold to fivefold increase in the number of resting hairs. Gradually, these numerous telogen hairs are shed over 6 to 24 weeks. Affected individuals notice sparser scalp hair 2 to 4 months after they have been exposed to the inciting factor. The prognosis for this type of diffuse alopecia is excellent. Patient education is important, as is reassurance that regrowth can be expected within approximately 6 months. Women who have telogen effluvium after parturition may experience partial regrowth of hair. No treatment is indicated.

INFECTIONS AND INFESTATIONS

IMPETIGO

Impetigo is the most frequently diagnosed bacterial skin infection. It is a contagious superficial skin infection, occurring most often in infancy and early childhood. The two major pathogens, *S. aureus* and group A β-hemolytic streptococcus (*Streptococcus pyogenes*), can cause lesions at any body site.

Classification

Nonbullous Impetigo

Nonbullous impetigo accounts for the majority of cases and is secondary to infection with either of the aforementioned pathogens.

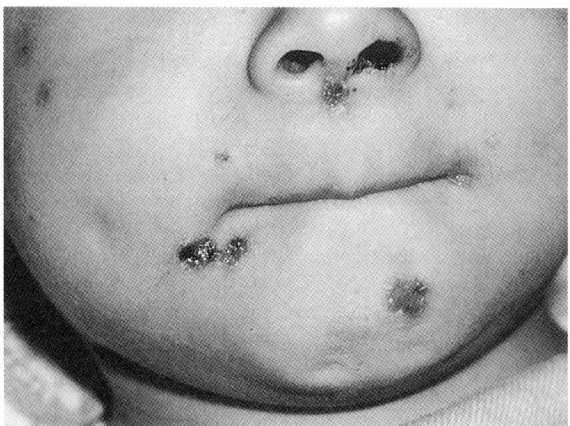

Figure 56-20. Multiple honey-colored crusted lesions of impetigo.

Clinically, the lesions of nonbullous impetigo caused by either organism are indistinguishable. The lesions typically arise on the face or extremities, after trauma such as insect bites, cuts, and abrasions or after varicella infection. The primary lesion is usually a vesicle or a pustule that develops secondary changes of honey-colored crusting, the clinical hallmark of this condition. In general, the lesions are smaller than 2 cm and may be single or multiple (Fig. 56-20). Surrounding erythema is often absent. Although patients are generally asymptomatic, regional lymphadenopathy is sometimes present.

The differential diagnosis includes HSV infections, nummular eczema, varicella, kerions, and scabies. Nonbullous impetigo usually resolves spontaneously within 2 weeks. It is highly contagious, however, and should therefore be treated with appropriate antimicrobial agents to decrease outbreaks.

Bullous Impetigo

Bullous impetigo is always caused by *S. aureus,* usually phage type 71 coagulase-positive organisms or a related group 2 phage type. It develops on intact skin and is a localized form of SSSS. The initially transparent flaccid bullae are more likely to occur on covered body sites such as the trunk and perineum than are the lesions of nonbullous impetigo. They do, however, occur on the face and extremities as well. Intact vesicles or bullae may be observed, or moist, erythematous shallow erosions may be the sole clinical finding after disruption of the bullae. Bullous impetigo should be differentiated from allergic contact dermatitis, burns, erythema multiforme, and inflammatory bullous diseases.

Treatment

Impetigo may be treated with topical or oral antibiotics. Topical antibiotics are inferior to oral agents in the treatment of cutaneous infections, with the exception of mupirocin (Bactroban). Mupirocin is bactericidal at concentrations that result from topical administration and has been found to be comparable or even superior to oral erythromycin in several studies. Furthermore, this topical antibiotic has fewer side effects than oral erythromycin. The major adverse effect is an allergic contact sensitivity to the propylene glycol in its vehicle. Treatment guidelines recommend application two times daily for 7 to 10 days.

There are many oral antibiotics with good antistreptococcal and antistaphylococcal activity. Some of the more cost-effective choices include cephalexin and dicloxacillin. The incidence of erythromycin-resistant strains of *S. aureus* has increased dramatically in many regions of North America, and this agent should be reserved for regions in which resistance is not yet a problem. Oral antibiotics should be used when there is widespread involvement or evidence of soft tissue involvement. A 7-day course is usually satisfactory. Recurrent impetigo is often secondary to carriage of *S. aureus*. Although intranasal carriage is common, colonization can also involve the axillae and perineum. Intranasal application of mupirocin daily for 5 days may eradicate the organism; however, recolonization occurs over time.

Complications

Potential but rare complications of impetigo include pneumonia, cellulitis, osteomyelitis, septic arthritis, and septicemia. More specifically, streptococcal infections can result in scarlet fever, guttate psoriasis, lymphadenitis, and lymphangitis. Furthermore, nephritogenic strains can result in post-streptococcal glomerulonephritis (see Chapter 25). The latency period after impetigo is approximately 3 weeks. Treatment does not prevent post-streptococcal glomerulonephritis but does prevent the spread of the organism to other people.

MOLLUSCUM CONTAGIOSUM

Molluscum contagiosum, caused by a large DNA poxvirus, is most often seen in children and adolescents. The characteristic well-circumscribed, skin-colored to pearly papules usually arise in crops on the face, trunk, and extremities but have a predilection for the axillary, antecubital, and crural regions (Fig. 56-21). Generally ranging in size from 1 to 5 mm, these asymptomatic papules have a central umbilication, often with a central core. In some individuals, eczematous changes develop at sites of the molluscum lesions, probably representative of a delayed hypersensitivity response. This so-called "molluscum dermatitis" may be localized or more extensive, is not an uncommon finding, and, in fact, may be more prominent on examination than the molluscum papules, which are occasionally missed. The associated eczematous dermatitis may resemble nummular eczema or tinea corporis. Molluscum lesions often become inflamed or appear infected shortly before spontaneous involution. The diagnosis is made by the clinical appearance of the lesions. However, skin biopsies or microscopic examination of the core of the lesions can confirm the diagnosis by revealing molluscum bodies, which are masses of virus-infected epidermal cells. The condition should be differentiated from warts, closed comedones, and milia.

Molluscum contagiosum is both contagious and autoinoculable. The incubation period ranges from 2 weeks to 6 months, and multiple family members are often affected. Immunosuppressed persons are at risk for more aggressive disease, especially patients infected with human immunodeficiency virus infection. Patients with pre-existing atopic dermatitis are also at greater risk for widespread molluscum lesions because of altered cutaneous T cell immunity.

Treatment options include curettage, liquid nitrogen, topical retinoids, and imiquimod cream. Topical cantharidin is effective and relatively painless, and it is thus a good choice for treating children. It is applied to individual lesions and washed off when blistering occurs, usually within 4 hours. Most pediatric dermatologists avoid application of cantharidin to facial or genital lesions because of concerns of a possible aberrant reaction. As with other poxvirus infections, these lesions occasionally result in scarring or pits as the lesions resolve.

WARTS

Warts are intraepidermal tumors caused by human papillomavirus, a small DNA virus. They may be present in up to 10% of the general population. There are more than 80 types of human papillomavirus. The virus produces four major types of warts: common, flat, plantar, and genital (condyloma acuminatum). The incubation period generally varies from 1 to 6 months, depending on the size of the inoculum, the site of infection, and the host's immune status. The duration of the wart is variable as well; approximately 65% of the lesions resolve spontaneously within 2 years. Warts can be spread between persons and between body sites by direct or indirect contact. Most warts are located on the fingers, hands, and elbows because trauma to these sites promotes inoculation of the virus.

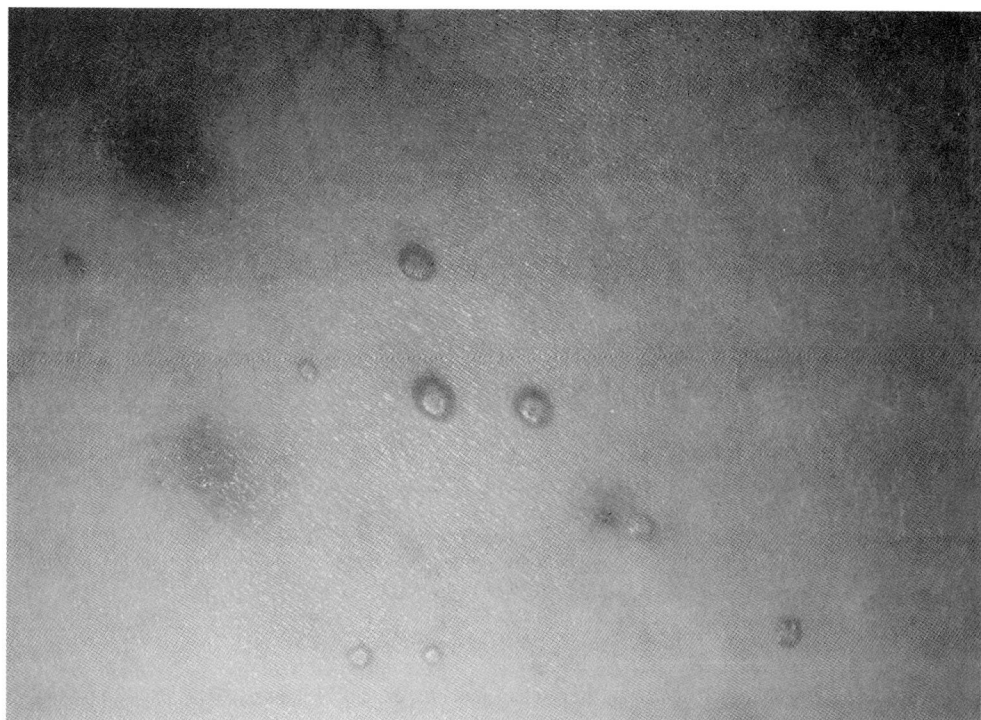

Figure 56-21. The characteristic umbilicated lesions of molluscum contagiosum.

Warts also display the Koebner phenomenon, which results in linear configurations of lesions at sites of shaving or scratching.

Classification

Common Warts

Verruca vulgaris, or the common wart, is found most commonly on the dorsal surface of the hands or fingers, although it may be located at any body site. The lesions may be solitary or multiple and measure from several millimeters to more than 1 cm. Varying in color from yellowish tan to grayish black, the common wart has a distinct rough, papillated surface (Fig. 56-22). Punctate thrombosed capillaries, clinically manifested by black dots, may be seen on the surface.

Flat Warts

Verrucae plana, or flat warts, are 2- to 5-mm flat-topped papules that are typically skin-colored, tan, or brown. They are distributed on the face, neck, and extremities. They often appear grouped, especially when the Koebner phenomenon has occurred secondary to shaving or other trauma. These lesions are most often confused with lichen planus or lichen nitidus, because these disorders also feature flat-topped papules.

Plantar Warts

Verrucae plantaris, or plantar warts, develop on the weight-bearing areas of the toes, heels, and midmetatarsal region. The lesions are pushed into the skin in such a manner that the verrucous surface is even with the surrounding skin. These warts are often very tender and may produce significant discomfort with ambulation. Plantar warts may be difficult to distinguish from corns and calluses.

Genital Warts

Condylomata acuminata, or genital warts, are fleshy papillomatous growths found on the genitalia. Their growth can be exuberant in some patients, resulting in cauliflower-like masses. In early or mild cases, the only physical finding may be subtle skin-colored, flat-topped papules. These genital warts should be differentiated from moist papular or nodular lesions of secondary syphilis (condylomata lata). Although nonvenereal transmission may occur, the presence of genital warts in young children is usually associated with sexual abuse (see Chapter 29).

Treatment

Treatment is designed to be cytodestructive and varies, depending on type of wart, site of the lesion, age and immune status of the patient,

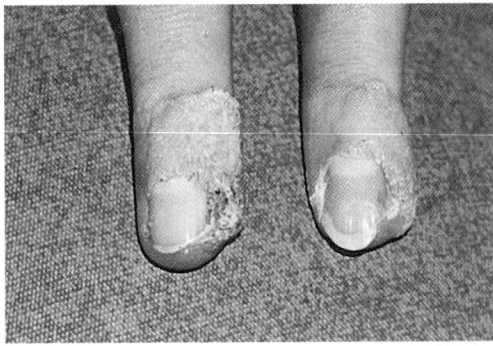

Figure 56-22. Periungual warts are common in children and are often difficult to treat.

and extent of involvement. Topical treatment includes keratolytic preparations, such as salicylic and lactic acid. Salicylic acid is available in a variety of paints and plasters that can be applied daily for several weeks and leads to maceration of the infected skin, which can then be easily removed. Cantharidin can be applied in the office setting and washed off several hours later, after blisters have formed; it is not for facial or genital warts. It results in effective and relatively painless eradication of the wart virus. Liquid nitrogen, or cryotherapy, is another effective modality, but its burning sensation may limit its usefulness in small children. However, pretreatment with eutectic mixture of topical anesthetics may be helpful. Podophyllin is reserved for the treatment of genital warts because it is most effective on mucosal surfaces. Cimetidine has been reported to lead to resolution of common warts; however, these studies remain controversial. Imiquimod (Aldara) has been approved for the treatment of genital warts, although it is not approved by the U.S. Food and Drug Administration for use in children. Extremely recalcitrant warts may necessitate surgical or laser (pulsed dye or carbon dioxide) treatment. Multiple or serial treatments may be necessary, and recurrences are common. A conservative approach is often best for this self-limited infection, because the treatment may be worse than the condition. Prolonged periods of applying duct tape to the wart (plantar, finger) has also resulted in resolution.

HERPES SIMPLEX VIRUS

HSV is a large DNA virus that is divided into two major antigenic subtypes. Type 1 (HSV-1) has been traditionally associated with oral and nongenital herpes infections; type 2 (HSV-2) is generally responsible for genital infection. The clinical lesions are indistinguishable but can be differentiated by serologic tests. HSV infections are categorized as either primary or recurrent. Primary manifestations usually follow an incubation period of approximately 1 week. They range from subclinical infections to localized or generalized vesicular eruptions to life-threatening systemic infections. Primary herpetic infections can involve any cutaneous or mucosal surface.

The classic clinical manifestation consists of grouped umbilicated vesicles on an erythematous base. The lesions usually begin as papules, which evolve into vesicles or, sometimes, pustules within approximately 48 hours. The vesicles rupture and form a crust over the next 5 to 7 days and generally heal within 2 weeks. The cutaneous eruption is often accompanied by fever, regional lymphadenopathy, or flulike symptoms (see Table 56-17).

After the primary infection, the virus remains dormant until reactivated. Recurrent infections are characterized by localized vesicular eruptions and symptoms such as itching or burning at the same site. Recurrent HSV infections are usually less severe than primary herpes. Reactivation of the virus may be triggered by sunburn, cutaneous trauma, febrile illnesses, menstruation, or emotional stress. Oral acyclovir, if administered during the prodromal period before the onset of lesions, may abort or shorten recurrent episodes.

Herpetic gingivostomatitis is typically seen in infants and toddlers. Multiple vesicles and subsequent erosions develop on the lips, gingivae, anterior portion of the tongue, or hard palate. The condition is very painful and is often accompanied by inability to eat and drink. Fever, irritability, and cervical lymphadenopathy are frequently observed. The fever typically resolves within 3 to 5 days, whereas the oral lesions may persist for up to 2 weeks. The eruption may resemble aphthous ulcers, which are usually more localized and are not accompanied by systemic symptoms. Enteroviruses may produce similar oral manifestations; however, they tend to spare the gingivae and often affect the posterior pharynx.

The diagnosis of HSV infection can be established by a positive Tzanck smear, a viral culture, or immunofluorescent staining. Treatment is supportive, with an emphasis on pain control and fluid replacement. Oral acyclovir may hasten resolution of the lesions and shorten the course of the illness.

Neonatal herpes is a potentially fatal infection, often with severe central nervous system involvement. Intravenous acyclovir and vigilant supportive care are required. Immunocompromised children who develop a herpetic infection should receive intravenous acyclovir and be monitored carefully for evidence of pulmonary, hepatic, and central nervous system involvement.

Another high-risk group consists of children with underlying atopic dermatitis who, if exposed to HSV, are susceptible to rapid spread of herpetic blisters. This condition, referred to as *eczema herpeticum* or *Kaposi varicelliform eruption,* may be accompanied by fever and malaise. Oral or intravenous acyclovir and supportive care are indicated.

VARICELLA

Varicella (*chickenpox*) is a common, very contagious, but usually self-limited infection caused by the varicella-zoster virus. Since the introduction of the varicella vaccine, mild and atypical variants of this disease have been common.

Incubation

Transmitted by close contact and respiratory droplets, varicella has an incubation period of 10 to 21 days. The cutaneous manifestation in healthy children is characterized by crops of lesions (usually two or three crops of 50 to 100 lesions each) that initially appear as 2- to 3-mm red macules and then evolve through papular, vesicular, and finally pustular stages within approximately 24 hours. The vesicular stage has traditionally been described as resembling "dewdrops on a rose petal." It is common to see lesions in various stages at the same anatomic site. All vesicles become crusted and resolve over several days. Chickenpox usually heals without scarring, except for lesions that have been excoriated or secondarily infected. The eruption is usually accompanied by fever, intense pruritus, and malaise (see Table 56-17).

When the diagnosis is unclear, confirmatory tests include immunofluorescent staining and viral culture. A positive Tzanck smear supports the diagnosis but is not specific for varicella. Symptomatic treatment consists of oral antihistamines, aluminum acetate soaks (Domeboro), oatmeal baths, calamine lotion, and cool compresses. Lesions should be observed for signs of secondary bacterial infection. Immunocompromised individuals or those receiving systemic corticosteroids usually require intravenous acyclovir. Some pediatricians advocate the use of oral acyclovir for healthy children in whom varicella develops or who have sibling contacts. Oral acyclovir, if given, should be administered within 24 hours of onset of the eruption.

High-risk individuals (immunosuppressed, immunocompromised, those with malignancies) who have been exposed to varicella should receive gamma globulin prophylaxis as soon as possible. If varicella develops in a pregnant woman within 5 days before delivery or in a mother 48 hours after delivery, the infant should also be treated with gamma globulin prophylaxis.

HERPES ZOSTER

Similar to HSV, the varicella-zoster virus remains dormant in the dorsal root ganglia after initial infection. Reactivation of the virus results in the clinical manifestations of herpes zoster, or shingles. The infection usually manifests as a linear or bandlike papulovesicular eruption affecting one or several dermatomes (Fig. 56-23; see Table 56-17). Commonly, there is a prodrome of burning, pruritus, or pain of the affected skin that may last several days before the appearance of cutaneous lesions. Vesicles become crusted, and all lesions resolve within a few weeks. The most common dermatomes involved are within the thoracic regions. Up to 10 satellite lesions may be encountered outside the primary dermatomes in uncomplicated zoster. An increased number of satellite lesions is observed in generalized zoster, which carries a greater risk of systemic involvement. Widespread vesicles should raise the suspicion of an underlying immunodeficiency disorder.

Immunocompromised patients, especially children with lymphoreticular malignancies, are at increased risk for zoster and should be treated with either oral or intravenous acyclovir. As in HSV infections, lesions of the nasal tip are suggestive of ocular involvement. Ocular complications occur in approximately 50% of the patients with ophthalmic zoster. The potential for deep keratitis, uveitis, secondary glaucoma, and loss of vision warrants prompt ophthalmologic evaluation. Patients with zoster should avoid contact with high-risk individuals who are susceptible to development of varicella.

SCABIES

Scabies is an extremely common eruption. It occurs in persons of all ages and results from infestation of the superficial layers of skin by the human mite *Sarcoptes scabiei.* The infestation is highly contagious and is therefore seen frequently among individuals living in crowded conditions. Humans are the only source of the mite,

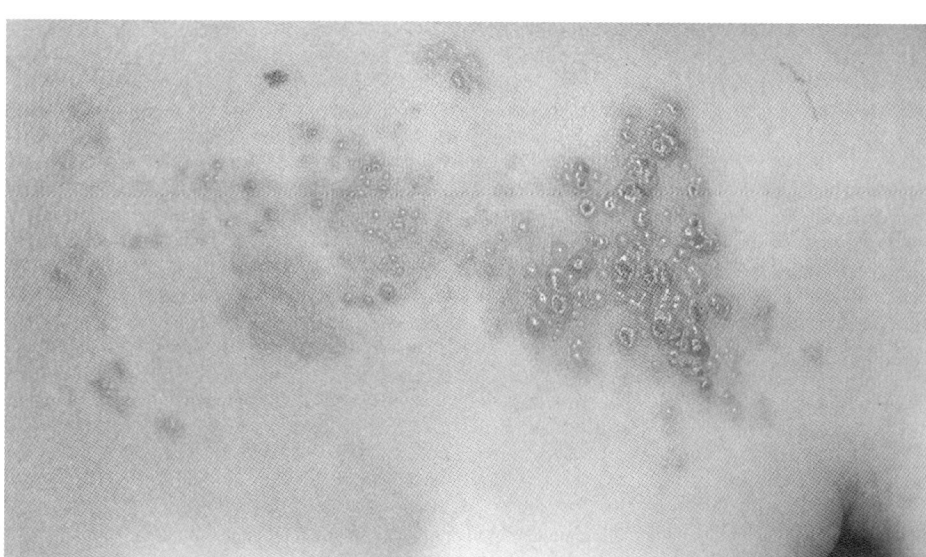

Figure 56-23. A dermatomal distribution of umbilicated vesicles is characteristic of herpes zoster.

which can be passed from one person to another. Fomites can also play an important role in transmission. In previously unexposed individuals, the incubation period varies from 2 to 6 weeks. The incubation period is significantly shortened in individuals who have been previously exposed to the mite.

Although the morphologic appearance of scabies can vary dramatically, the hallmark lesion is the burrow. A burrow is a serpiginous or linear papule caused by movement of the mite through the epidermis. Although considered to be characteristic of scabies, the burrow is apparent in only a minority of patients. Other typical lesions include papules, vesicles, and pustules, the distribution of which is age dependent. Nodules may appear during active infection and may persist for several weeks to months after treatment. These persistent nodules are referred to as post-scabitic nodules and may be a manifestation of an ongoing hypersensitivity response. In infants, the distribution is generalized and involves the scalp, face, neck, axillae, palms, and soles (Fig. 56-24). Because the eruption is extremely pruritic, secondary infection and eczematization are common, leading to misdiagnoses of impetigo and atopic dermatitis. In affected older children, adolescents, and adults, the lesions characteristically involve the volar aspects of the wrists, ankles, interdigital web spaces, buttocks, genitalia, groin, abdomen, and axillae. Unlike infantile scabies, the lesions always spare the head.

The diagnosis can be confirmed by scraping the newer lesions, ideally a burrow, with a blade after the application of mineral oil. The scraping may be viewed microscopically, and the presence of mites, ova, or feces is considered diagnostic. Although the yield may be low, particularly in children, suspect lesions should be scraped and an attempt to identify the mite should be made. In prolonged cases of scabies, which have been appropriately treated, the diagnosis of acropustulosis of infancy needs to be considered.

Topical 5% permethrin cream (Elimite) is the treatment of choice. It has been highly effective in eradicating the mite and is safer than topical lindane (Kwell). Permethrin cream is applied to the body and thoroughly washed off after 8 to 12 hours. This treatment may be repeated 1 to 2 weeks later. Lindane is not recommended as first-line treatment for scabies because of its potential for neurotoxicity. Six percent sulfur should be used in infants younger than 4 to 6 weeks and in pregnant women.

It is critical that all household members as well as close contacts be treated simultaneously to prevent reinfestation. All linens and clothes should be washed and dried in an electric dryer, because heat kills the mite. Bulkier linens, such as bedspreads, and stuffed toys can be placed in plastic bags for several days. Mites do not survive without a human host for more than 2 to 3 days. The topical antiscabietic agents can cause an irritant dermatitis that may last for several weeks and may improve with emollients and judicious use of topical corticosteroids.

PEDICULOSIS

Lice are ectoparasitic insects. *Pediculus humanus capitis,* the head louse, causes the most common form of louse infestation. This occurs more often in white persons; girls are more susceptible than boys. Because the head louse can survive for more than 2 days off the host's scalp, the condition can be transmitted via shared hats, combs, brushes, and even clothing or bedding. On physical examination, the nits (ova) can be found close to the scalp on the proximal hair shafts. They appear as small, oval, whitish bodies approximately 0.5 mm in length. They adhere tightly to the hair shaft and are not easily removed. The nits can be more readily identified by their fluorescence under a Wood lamp. Microscopic examination of the proximal hair shaft may further aid in recognition of the nits. The infestation is characterized by intense pruritus, especially at night.

Treatment of pediculosis capitis consists of topical application of 1% permethrin (Nix) shampoo applied to the scalp for 5 to 10 minutes, rinsed, and repeated 1 week later. Permethrin (5%) is used for recalcitrant cases. A recent study demonstrated that Ovide lotion (0.5% malathion) was a fast-killing and particularly effective ovicide. It is extremely important to wash and dry (on a hot cycle) all exposed bedding and clothing. All combs and brushes should be soaked with the pediculicide for 15 minutes, and all items that cannot be machine washed with hot water or dry-cleaned should be placed in plastic bags for 2 weeks. Family members and other close contacts should be examined and subsequently treated if there is any evidence of pediculosis.

CANDIDIASIS

Candidal species, particularly *Candida albicans,* may be considered part of the normal cutaneous flora in most individuals. However, predisposing factors such as endocrinologic disorders, genetic disorders, immunosuppressive conditions, and the administration of systemic corticosteroids or antibiotics may allow for overgrowth of this organism and subsequent infection. *Candidiasis* refers to an acute or chronic infection of the skin, mucous membranes, or internal organs caused by this pathogenic yeast. Other conditions, such as warmth, moisture, and disruption of the epidermal barrier, further promote invasion and overgrowth. Cutaneous candidiasis can have a variety of clinical manifestations, depending on the site of infection. Some of the most common manifestations include (1) oral candidiasis (thrush), (2) candidal diaper dermatitis, (3) vulvovaginitis, and (4) paronychia.

Oral candidiasis is a common condition of infancy and in immunosuppressed individuals. It is characterized by painful inflammation of the oral cavity with multiple, often confluent, white plaques on an intensely erythematous base. The condition is often acquired during vaginal delivery and passage through an infected vaginal canal; however, it is often not apparent until the second week after birth. The disorder usually responds to treatment with oral nystatin suspension, which is applied to the oral mucosa four times daily until 2 days after the lesions have completely resolved. Oral fluconazole (Diflucan) is another therapeutic option for more extensive or resistant cases. Extensive involvement or failure to respond to treatment may suggest an underlying immunodeficiency disease. Cutaneous lesions in the intertriginous and diaper areas are frequently coexistent with thrush.

Candidal paronychia manifests with erythema and edema of the proximal and lateral nail folds, which is usually not associated with tenderness, in contrast to acute bacterial paronychia. The nail is often dystrophic, crumbly, and thick. The condition is seen commonly in thumb suckers. Treatment with topical antifungal creams with yeast coverage, applied nightly under occlusion for several weeks, usually results in clinical resolution.

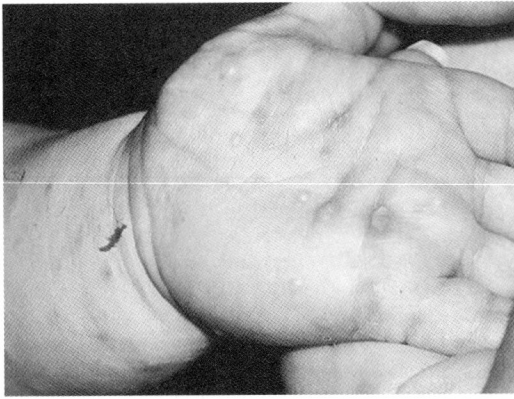

Figure 56-24. Lesions of the palms and soles are typical of scabies in infants.

DERMATOPHYTOSES

Classification

The dermatophytes are a group of fungi that infect the hair, skin, and nails and result in a collection of clinical syndromes referred to as *dermatophytoses*. The clinical conditions are referred to as *tinea* (or ringworm), and the affected body site determines the name of the entity. This group of infections is caused by species of *Trichophyton, Microsporum,* and *Epidermophyton.* Dermatophyte infections are usually confined to the epidermis.

Tinea Capitis

Tinea capitis is discussed in the section on alopecia.

Tinea Corporis

Tinea corporis is characterized by one or multiple annular erythematous patches that can occur anywhere on the body (Fig. 56-25). The lesions typically have a papular scaly border and demonstrate central clearing. Vesiculation and pustulation, especially peripherally, are commonly observed. The borders are usually sharply demarcated. Identification of fungal hyphae by KOH examination of scrapings of the lesion's scaly border confirms the diagnosis. Psoriasis, nummular eczema, secondary syphilis, the herald patch of pityriasis rosea, and the annular plaques of granuloma annulare may resemble tinea corporis (Fig. 56-26).

Tinea Pedis

Tinea pedis is diagnosed most often in postpubertal adolescents. The clinical manifestation is variable, but multiple vesicles or erosions on the insteps are characteristic. Other findings include fissures and

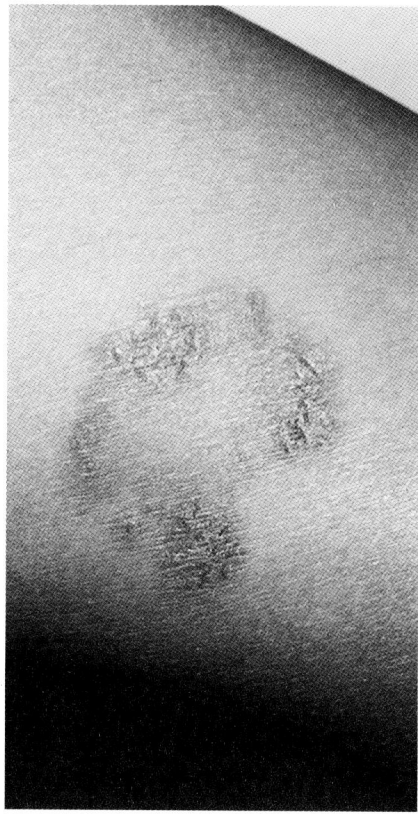

Figure 56-26. Nummular eczema, also seen as scaly, red, annular patches or plaques, can mimic tinea corporis.

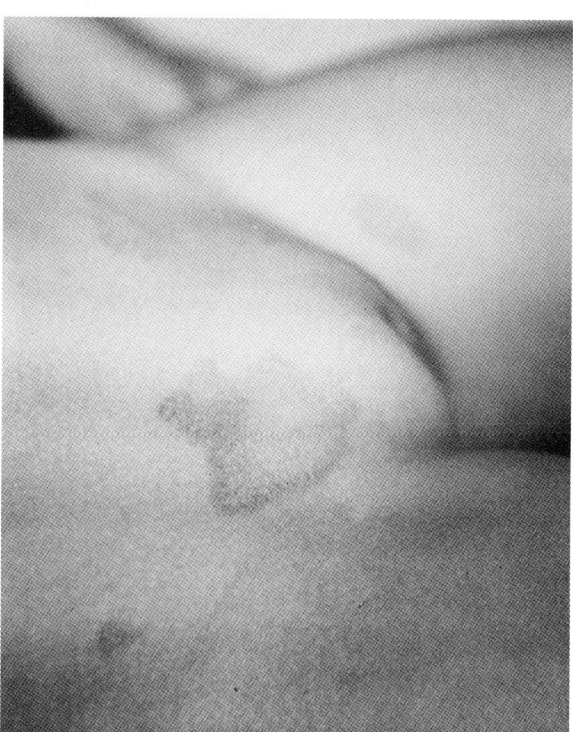

Figure 56-25. Annular erythematous, scaly plaques with central clearing are seen in tinea corporis.

maceration of the web spaces and "moccasin foot" tinea pedis, in which there is generalized scaling of one or both soles with extension onto the lateral aspect of the foot. The differential diagnosis includes atopic or contact dermatitis, juvenile plantar dermatosis, psoriasis, and scabies. The clinician should have increased suspicion for tinea pedis if unilateral involvement is present. A positive KOH scraping or fungal culture rules out these other entities.

Tinea Faciei

Tinea faciei, a dermatophyte infection of the face, is commonly seen in children. Erythematous, scaly, and often in a malar distribution, the condition may resemble lupus erythematosus but is less symmetrical. Atopic, contact, and seborrheic dermatitis may have similar cutaneous manifestations. Again, the diagnosis can be confirmed by a positive KOH scraping or fungal culture.

Tinea Cruris

Tinea cruris, uncommon before adolescence, is an erythematous, scaly eruption involving the inguinal creases and medial thighs. The eruption is usually symmetric, and sometimes the margins are papular. This infection may resemble candidiasis, in which there is also scrotal erythema. *Erythrasma,* an uncommon superficial bacterial infection caused by *Corynebacterium minutissimum,* may also mimic tinea cruris. The coral red fluorescence seen on Wood lamp examination is diagnostic of erythrasma, which can be further differentiated from tinea cruris by a negative KOH preparation and fungal culture.

Treatment

Tinea infections of the skin can usually be successfully managed with topical antifungal agents such as clotrimazole, econazole, ciclopirox, tolnaftate, or terbinafine creams or lotions. These medications are applied twice daily for approximately 2 to 4 weeks. They should be continued for several days after clinical resolution is apparent. Widespread eruptions or treatment failures may necessitate systemic antifungal therapy, such as griseofulvin, fluconazole, itraconazole, or terbinafine.

Tinea Versicolor

Occurring more frequently in adolescents and adults, tinea versicolor is a superficial fungal infection characterized by multiple, slightly scaly macules and patches located on the upper trunk, neck, proximal extremities, and, on occasion, the face. The macular lesions vary in hue (pink, tan, brown, white), hence the name "versicolor." In darkly pigmented or tanned individuals, the macules appear hypopigmented; in fair-skinned persons or during winter months, the lesions usually appear tan-brown. Tinea versicolor is caused by *Pityrosporum orbiculare*, also called *Malassezia furfur*, a dimorphic fungus that is a skin saprophyte. It is generally present in its yeast form, which does not produce a rash. When proliferation of the filamentous form occurs, the organism produces the characteristic lesions of tinea versicolor. Usually asymptomatic or only slightly pruritic, tinea versicolor is primarily a cosmetic disturbance that occurs most commonly in warm and humid environments.

Although the diagnosis is established by the distinctive clinical presentation, a KOH scraping of the fine scale reveals multiple round spores and short, curved hyphae, giving the characteristic "spaghetti and meatballs" appearance typical of this disorder. Wood lamp examination may demonstrate yellow, orange, or blue-white fluorescence, further supporting the diagnosis. The organism is lipophilic and requires olive oil overlay on routine fungal media to grow in culture. The differential diagnosis includes postinflammatory pigment alteration, pityriasis alba, vitiligo, contact dermatitis, seborrheic dermatitis, and pityriasis rosea. Tinea versicolor is a chronic condition. Although usually responsive to therapy, recurrences are common. Application of 2.5% selenium sulfide shampoo to the affected skin 15 to 20 minutes daily for 1 to 2 weeks, or overnight application on a weekly basis for 1 to 2 months, can be very effective. Other topical treatments include broad-spectrum antifungal creams or lotions; however, the expense of widespread application may be prohibitive.

In extremely widespread or recalcitrant cases, or in immunosuppressed individuals, treatment with fluconazole, itraconazole, or terbinafine may be indicated. After successful treatment, the lesions remain temporarily hypopigmented or hyperpigmented.

ACNE VULGARIS

Acne is a very common condition in adolescents, but all age groups can be affected. Open and closed comedones, inflammatory papules, pustules, and nodules are characteristic primary lesions (Fig. 56-27). Scarring and sinus tracts are present in moderate to severe forms. Androgens stimulate the sebaceous follicles, leading to hyperkeratosis of the follicular epithelium. The microscopically plugged follicle is clinically apparent as a comedo. Sebaceous gland contents (sebum) accumulate, and if the follicle walls rupture, releasing sebaceous material into the surrounding dermis, inflammatory papules and pustules result. *Propionibacterium acnes*, an anaerobic follicular diphtheroid, contributes to the inflammatory process.

DIAGNOSIS

The diagnosis of acne is a clinical one; skin biopsies and other diagnostic studies are not necessary. In some cases, endocrinologic evaluation may be needed to further elucidate the hormonal factors contributing to formation of acne lesions. Drug-induced acne can be seen in all age groups; the offending drugs include glucocorticoids, androgens, hydantoin, and isoniazid.

TREATMENT

Treatment of acne varies, depending on the types of lesions present and individual tolerance to acne medication. Patients should be instructed to use mild cleansers and oil-free, noncomedogenic moisturizers, sunscreen, and makeup. Antibacterial soaps and cleansers may help reduce surface bacteria. Topical medications include benzoyl peroxide, retinoids, antibiotics and combination products. Benzoyl peroxide has antibacterial and mild comedolytic effects. Tretinoin acts specifically on comedones, causing decreased new comedo formation and fragmentation and expulsion of existing comedones. Benzoyl peroxide products can be used as an adjunct to tretinoin therapy, but tretinoin is more effective in reducing and preventing abnormal keratinization of the follicular canal.

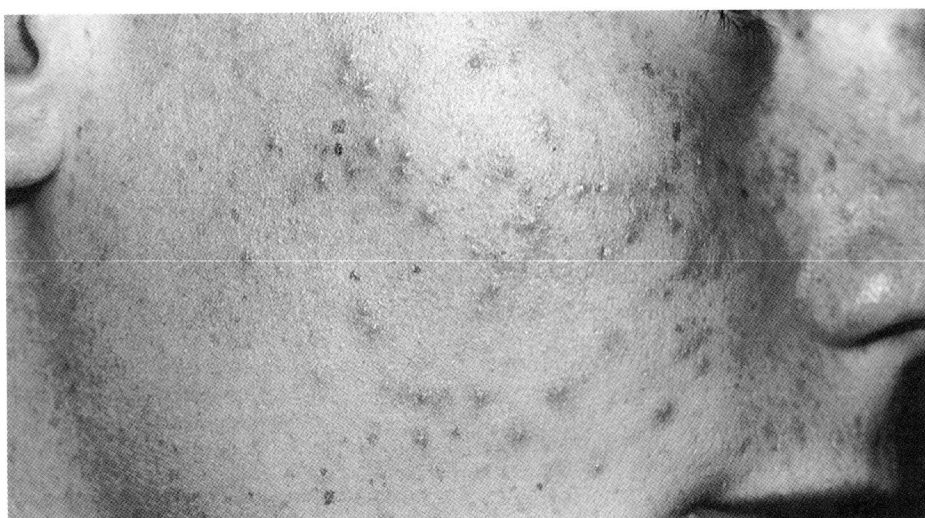

Figure 56-27. Inflammatory papules and pustules of acne vulgaris.

Products such as adapalene (Differin) have proved to be less irritating than tretinoin. Tazarotene is a strong topical retinoid that can be used for patients with extensive comedones in acne that is unresponsive to tretinoin.

Inflammatory acne requires use of antibiotics, either topically or systemically. Doxycycline, minocycline, tetracycline, and erythromycin are some of the more frequently used oral antibiotics. More recently, azithromycin has been used as well, especially in those patients in whom photosensitivity is a problem. Numerous topical antibiotic preparations are available; most contain either erythromycin or clindamycin. Benzoyl peroxide and erythromycin (Benzamycin) and benzoyl peroxide and clindamycin (Benzaclin) are combination topical preparations.

Nodular acne or recalcitrant severe inflammatory acne is best treated with isotretinoin, a synthetic vitamin A derivative. Any patient needing oral isotretinoin or other retinoid therapy should be referred to a dermatologist because of the potential side effects. Side effects such as cheilitis, dry skin and mucous membranes, vertebral hyperostoses, reversible alopecia, and elevated triglyceride levels may be seen. Depression is a controversial side effect but nonetheless should be monitored for during monthly visits. Visual complaints and headaches may also occur. Teratogenicity has been well documented; there is a 25-fold increased risk of fetal malformations from isotretinoin. Pregnancy testing is mandatory for all women of childbearing potential, and two forms of contraception must be used by all sexually active patients taking this drug. Patients must sign a consent form reviewing all these side effects and concerns before initiating therapy. The risks, benefits, and possible side effects must be discussed with each patient (and parent), and treatment must be individualized. Monthly visits and monthly laboratory evaluation should be performed.

REFERENCES

General Overview

Dohil MA, Baugh WP, Eichenfield LF: Vascular and pigmented birthmarks. Pediatr Clin North Am 2000;47:783-812.

Drolet BA: Cutaneous signs of neural tube dysraphism. Pediatr Clin North Am 2000;47:813-824.

Eichenfield LF, Frieden IJ, Esterly NB: Textbook of Neonatal Dermatology. Philadelphia, WB Saunders, 2001, pp 117-136, 137-178, 324-353, 353-369, 370-394.

Harper J, Oranje A, Prose N: Textbook of Pediatric Dermatology. London, Blackwell Sciences, 2000, pp 629-636, 1743-1752.

Hurwitz S: Clinical Pediatric Dermatology. Philadelphia, WB Saunders, 1993.

Schachner LA, Hansen RC: Pediatric Dermatology. New York, Churchill Livingstone, 1995, pp 915-949.

Neonatal

Albright A, Gartner J, Weiner E: Lumbar cutaneous hemangiomas as indicators of tethered spinal cords. Pediatrics 1989;83:977-980.

Buyon JP: Neonatal lupus. Curr Opin Rheumatol 1996;8:485-490.

Carrascosa JM, Riberia M, Bielsa I, et al: Cutis marmorata telangiectatica congenita or neonatal lupus? Pediatr Dermatol 1996;13:230-232.

Drolet BA, Clowry L, McTigue K, Esterly NB: The hair collar sign: Marker for cranial dysraphism. Pediatrics 1995;96:309-313.

Drolet BA, Prendiville J, Golden J, et al: Membranous aplasia cutis with hair collars. Arch Dermatol 1995;131:1427-1431.

Enjolras O, Boukobza M, Jdid R: Cervical occult spinal dysraphism: MRI findings and the value of a vascular birthmark. Pediatr Dermatol 1995;12:256-259.

Garcia-Patos V, Pujol RM, de Moragas JM: Infantile eosinophilic folliculitis. Dermatology 1994;1989:133-138.

Hebert AA, Esterly NB: Bacterial and candidal cutaneous infections in the neonate. Dermatol Clin 1986;4:3-20.

Humeau S, Bureau B, Litoux P, et al: Infantile acropustulosis in six immigrant children. Pediatr Dermatol 1995;12:211-214.

Krafchik BR: Neonatal lupus erythematosus. Adv Exp Med Biol 1999;455:23-26.

Kriss VM, Desal NS: Occult spinal dysraphism in neonates: Assessment of high-risk cutaneous stigmata on sonography. AJR Am J Roentgenol 1998;171:1687-1692.

Lee LA, Frank MB, McCubbin VR, Reichlin M: Autoantibodies of neonatal lupus erythematosus. J Invest Dermatol 1994;102:963-966.

Thorton CM, Eichenfield LF, Shinall EA: Cutaneous telangiectasias in neonatal lupus erythematosus. J Am Acad Dermatol 1995;33:19-25.

Vicente J, Espana A, Idoate M, et al: Are eosinophilic pustular folliculitis of infancy and infantile acropustulosis the same entity? Br J Dermatol 1996;135:807-809.

Weston WL, Morelli JG, Lee LA: The clinical spectrum of anti-Ro positive cutaneous neonatal lupus erythematosus. J Am Acad Dermatol 1999;41:675-681.

Atopic Dermatitis and Other Scaling Disorders

Eichenfield LF, Lucky AW, Boguniewicz M, et al: Safety and efficacy of pimecrolimus cream (ASM 981) 1% in the treatment of mild to moderate atopic dermatitis in children and adolescents. J Am Acad Dermatol 2002;46:495-504.

Paller A, Eichenfield LF, Leung DYM, et al: A 12-week study of tacrolimus ointment for the treatment of atopic dermatitis in pediatric patients. J Am Acad Dermatol 2001;44:S47-S57.

Rabinowitz LG, Esterly NB: Atopic dermatitis and ichthyosis vulgaris. Pediatr Rev 1994;15:220-226.

Nodules and Tumors

Chang MW, Frieden IJ, Good W: The risk of intraocular juvenile xanthogranuloma: Survey of current practices and assessment of risk. J Am Acad Dermatol 1996;34:445-449.

Zvulunov A, Barak Y, Metzker A: Juvenile xanthogranuloma, neurofibromatosis, and juvenile chronic myelogenous leukemia. Arch Dermatol 1995;131:904-908.

Disorders of Pigmentation

DeDavid M, Orlow SJ, Porvost N, et al: Neurocutaneous melanosis: Clinical features of large congenital melanocytic nevi in patients with manifest central nervous system melanosis. J Am Acad Dermatol 1996;35:529-538.

Kadonaga JN, Frieden IJ: Neurocutaneous melanosis: Definition and review of the literature. J Am Acad Dermatol 1991;24:747-755.

Pinto FJ, Bolognia JL: Disorders of hypopigmentation in children. Pediatr Clin North Am 1991;38:991-1017.

Ruiz-Maldonado R, del Rosario Barona-Mazuera M, Hidalgo-Galvan LR, et al: Giant congenital melanocytic nevi, neurocutaneous melanosis and neurological alterations. Dermatology 1997;195:125-128.

Shpall S, Frieden I, Chesney M, Newman T: Risk of malignant transformation of congenital melanocytic nevi in blacks. Pediatr Dermatol 1994;11:204-208.

Steiner J, Adamsbaum C, Desguerres I, et al: Hypomelanosis of Ito and brain abnormalities: MRI findings and literature review. Pediatr Radiol 1996;26:763-768.

Hypersensitivity Reactions

Bruce F: Could it be a drug eruption? Aust Fam Physician 1997;26:689-695.

Gianetti A, Malmusi M, Girolomoni G: Vesiculobullous drug eruptions in children. Clin Dermatol 1993;11:551-555.

Manders SM: Serious and life-threatening drug eruptions. Am Fam Physician 1995;51:865-871.

Schopf E, Stuhmer A, Rzany B, et al: Toxic epidermal necrolysis and Stevens-Johnson syndrome. An epidemiological study from West Germany. Arch Dermatol 1991;127:839.

Sharma V, Beyer D, Paruthi S, Nopper AJ: Prominent pruritic periumbilical papules: Allergic contact dermatitis to nickel. Pediatr Dermatol 2002;9:106-109.

Sharma VK, Dhar S: Clinical pattern of cutaneous drug eruptions among children and adolescents in North India. Pediatr Dermatol 1995;12:178-183.

Straussberg R, Harel L, Ben-Amitai D, et al: Carbamazepine-induced Stevens-Johnson syndrome treated with IV steroids and IVIG. Pediatr Neurol 2000;22:231-233.

Viard I, Wehrli P, Bullani R, et al: Inhibition of toxic epidermal necrolysis by blockade of CD95 with human intravenous immunoglobulin. Science 1998;282:490-493.

Vesiculobullous Lesions

Feldman SR: Bullous dermatoses associated with systemic disease. Dermatol Clin 1993;11:597-608.

Fine JD, Bauer EA, Briggaman RA, et al: Revised clinical and laboratory criteria for subtypes of inherited epidermolysis bullosa. J Am Acad Dermatol 1991;24:119-135.

Rabinowitz LG, Esterly NB: Inflammatory bullous diseases in children. Dermatol Clin 1993;11:565-581.

Vascular Birthmarks

Burrows PE, Laor T, Paltiel H, Robertson RL: Diagnostic imaging in the evaluation of vascular birthmarks. Dermatol Clin 1998;16:455-488.

Drolet BA, Esterly NB, Frieden IJ: Hemangiomas in children. N Engl J Med 1999;341:173-181.

Enjolras O, Mulliken JB: Vascular tumors and vascular malformations (new issues). Adv Dermatol 1997;13:375-423.

Enjolras O, Wassef M, Mazoyer E, et al: Infants with Kasabach-Merritt syndrome do not have "true" hemangiomas. J Pediatr 1997;30:631-640.

Frieden IJ, Reese V, Cohen D: PHACE syndrome: The association of posterior fossa malformations, hemangiomas, arterial anomalies, coarctation of the aorta and cardiac defects, and eye abnormalities. Arch Dermatol 1996;132:307-311.

Sahn EE: Vesiculopustular diseases of neonates and infants. Curr Opin Pediatr 1994;6:442-446.

Uitto J, Christiano AM: Inherited epidermolysis bullosa. Dermatol Clin 1993; 11:549-563.

Wagner A: Distinguishing vesicular and pustular disorders in the neonate. Curr Opin Pediatr 1997;9:396-405.

Alopecia

Atton A, Tunnessen W: Alopecia in children: The most common causes. Pediatr Rev 1990;12:25-30.

Muller SA: Trichotillomania. Dermatol Clin 1987;5:595-601.

Stroud JD: Hair loss in children. Symposium on Pediatric Dermatology. Pediatr Clin North Am 1983;30:641-657.

Infections and Infestations

Darmstadt GL, Lane AT: Impetigo: An overview. Pediatr Dermatol 1994;11:293-303.

Kahn RM, Goldstein EJ: Common bacterial skin infections. Postgrad Med 1993;93:175-182.

Meinking TL, Entzel P, Villar ME, et al: Comparative efficacy of treatments of pediculosis capitis infestations: Update 2001. Arch Dermatol 2001;137:287-292.

57 Fever without Focus

Kristine G. Williams   David M. Jaffe

Fever is one of the most common reasons for a child to visit a physician. Two thirds of all children visit a physician for fever before they reach the age of 2 years. In 20% of febrile children, history and physical examination do not reveal an apparent source of infection.

Fever is part of an integrated, nonspecific response of the body to various disease states such as infection, neoplasm, immune-mediated conditions, and inflammatory disorders. A child with fever of recent onset with no adequate historical or physical explanation for the fever is said to have *fever without focus* (FWF) or *fever without localizing signs*. Bacterial pathogens account for 3% to 5% of these cases. The remaining patients have a self-limited viral illness. The challenge is to identify which children have fever caused by bacterial pathogens, in order to avoid the morbidity and mortality associated with delayed treatment or lack of treatment.

Distinct but related disease processes are *occult bacteremia, serious bacterial illness* (SBI), and *fever of unknown origin* (FUO) (see Chapter 54). Occult bacteremia is the presence of pathogenic bacteria in the blood of a child who does not appear ill and has no clear focus of infection. With the exception of otitis media, the child with occult bacteremia does not have a focal bacterial infection. SBI consists of the sequelae of occult bacteremia: meningitis, sepsis, bone and joint infections, urinary tract infections (UTIs), pneumonia, and enteritis. A child with fever for at least 8 days and no apparent focus of infection after initial evaluation has FUO (see Chapter 54).

The distinction between FWF and FUO is important for several reasons. First, the differential diagnoses are different. Second, the child with FWF is generally in need of a more urgent evaluation. Third, unlike those with FUO, some patients with FWF may be best managed with expectant antibiotic treatment. Finally, most patients with FWF who do not appear ill can be managed as outpatients while many children with FUO require inpatient evaluation.

PATHOPHYSIOLOGY OF FEVER

Temperature is controlled by the thermoregulatory center, located in the preoptic area of the anterior hypothalamus. The thermoregulatory center receives input from peripheral receptors and the temperature of the blood bathing the hypothalamus and acts on autonomic, endocrine, and behavioral mechanisms to maintain the body temperature at a particular set point. Fever results when the hypothalamic set point is elevated above the normal range. The hypothalamic set point normally maintains body temperature around 37° C, but there can be significant variation among individuals. Normal temperatures range from 36° C to 37.8° C, depending on the time of day, with the peak in the afternoon (5 PM to 7 PM) and the trough in the early morning (2 AM to 6 AM). Although the circadian rhythm is not well established in infancy, it becomes more reliable by the second year of life.

The febrile response not only produces an elevation in body temperature but also causes physiologic changes that enhance the individual's ability to eliminate infection. Production of acute-phase reactants and alterations in metabolism and endocrine function are examples of these changes. Acute-phase reactants—proteins that are produced in response to infection or injury—include ceruloplasmin, C-reactive protein, haptoglobin, amyloid A, complement, and fibrinogen. Hormones and cytokines, some of which are endogenous pyrogens, regulate production of acute-phase proteins.

Exogenous pyrogens, such as bacteria or endotoxins, generate the production of endogenous pyrogens, which play a vital role in prostaglandin-related set point elevation and regulation of acute-phase responses (Fig. 57-1).

Fever results when the thermoregulatory set point is elevated above the normal set point. To reconcile the new set point and the current body temperature, the hypothalamus generates physiologic changes involving endocrine, metabolic, autonomic, and behavioral processes. These physiologic alterations produce physical changes or behaviors that are indicative of a febrile response. Diversion of blood from peripheral vessels to central vessels causes coolness of the extremities but helps increase core temperature. Shivering increases metabolic activity and heat production. The affected patient may feel cold and seek a warmer environment or add clothing to feel warmer and prevent heat loss. Once these processes have resulted in increasing the core temperature to match the elevated set point, the thermoregulatory center works to maintain the temperature as it does during normothermia. The thermoregulatory point is reset once the infection is resolved. The hypothalamus then produces physiologic changes to *decrease* the core temperature; these include sweating, dilation of cutaneous blood vessels, and the sensation of feeling hot, which may lead to behaviors such as removing clothing or seeking a cooler environment.

Fever has both positive and negative effects. High body temperatures may impair the reproduction and survival of some invading microorganisms by decreasing required nutrients, such as free iron, or by increasing immunologic responses such as phagocytosis. However, at extremely high temperatures, immunologic responses may be impaired. Fever increases the basal metabolic rate by 10% to 12% for each degree Celsius elevation of temperature. This increases oxygen consumption, carbon dioxide production, and fluid and caloric needs. Fluid requirements increase 100 mL/m^2/day for each 1° C rise in temperature above 37.8° C.

Heat illness must be distinguished from fever as a cause for elevated body temperature. In heat illness, there is an unregulated rise in body temperature, despite the fact that the hypothalamic set point is normal. It can result from excessive heat production or inadequate heat dissipation. Temperatures may reach extreme heights and can result in multiorgan dysfunction and death. Restoration of normal body temperature in heat illness is mandatory. Administration of drugs such as ibuprofen and acetaminophen, which restore the hypothalamic set point to normal, is useless. The most effective therapy for heat illness is external cooling (Table 57-1).

Other causes of high body temperature are noted in Table 57-2.

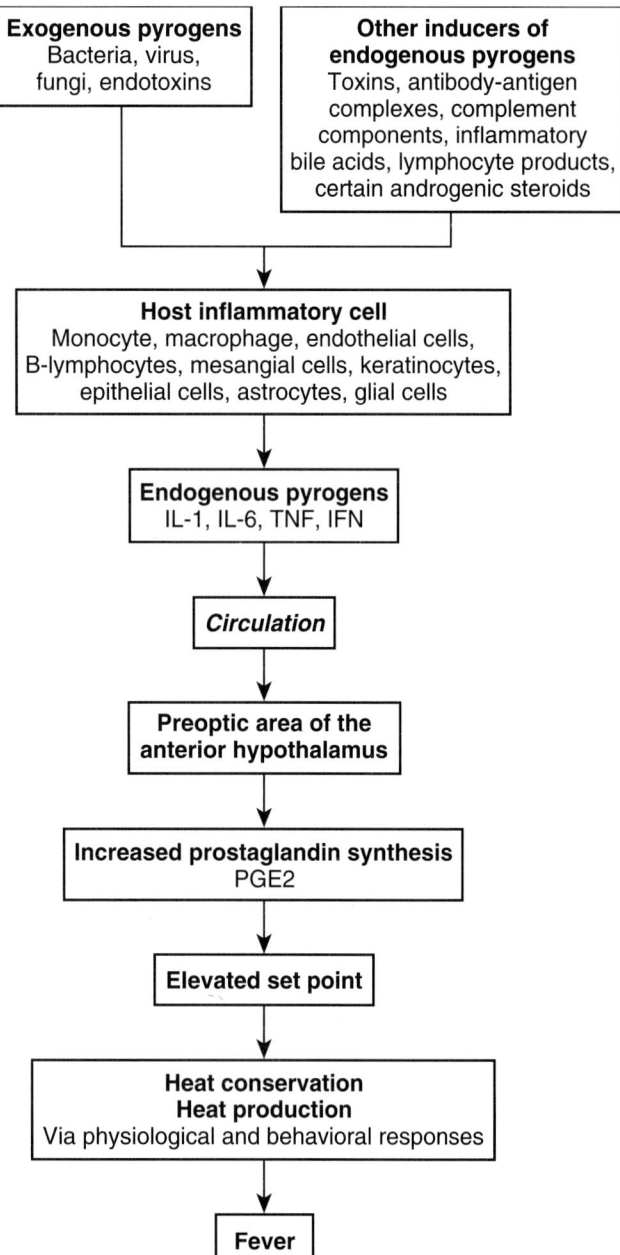

Figure 57-1. Proposed pathways by which exogenous pyrogens produce fever. IFN, interferon; IL-1 and IL-6, interleukin-1 and interleukin-6; PGE₂, prostaglandin E₂; TNF, tumor necrosis factor. (Data from Cimpello LB, Goldman DL, Khine H: Fever pathophysiology. Clin Pediatr Emerg Med 2000;1:84-93.)

DATA COLLECTION

HISTORY

When a child has FWF, the caregiver usually reports the presence of fever with no associated signs or symptoms, except perhaps mild, nonpurulent rhinorrhea. A detailed history may reveal a potential source for infection. A complete history addresses several important issues: (1) onset and duration of fever; (2) degree of temperature; (3) by what method and in which anatomic site the temperature was taken; (4) medications given, including antipyretics and home remedies; (5) environmental exposures; (6) associated symptoms;

(7) ill contacts; and (8) recent immunizations. Inquiry into the child's medical history may reveal important information such as recurrent febrile illnesses, primary or acquired immunodeficiency, or medications, such as chemotherapy, that alter host defenses.

FEVER: TEMPERATURE MEASUREMENT

Measuring temperature accurately is essential for the appropriate management of febrile children. Accurate temperature measurement must take into account both reliability and validity of the measurement tool. There are many sources of error in the clinical setting that may influence reliability. Individual patient characteristics that may affect reliability include normal temperature variation, exertion, ingestion of hot or cool liquids, and bundling of infants. Environmental issues such as poor instrument calibration or ambient temperature can affect temperature measurement. Measurement variation, including probe placement and length of time for equilibration, also threaten reliability.

Glass thermometers are the standard tools for temperature measurement. The thermometer should be inserted to a depth of 2 to 3 cm into the rectum in a supine or prone restrained infant. Three minutes is considered adequate time for equilibration of a rectal measurement. The most widely accepted definition of fever is rectal temperature of 38° C (100.4° F) or higher. It is important to consider that infants, especially those younger than 2 months of age, may have a blunted febrile response to infection. Hence, lack of fever should not be used as a criterion for ruling out infection in infants. Although rectal temperature measurement is the "gold standard," it should be avoided in neutropenic, immunocompromised patients, in whom rectal manipulation may seed the blood with bacteria.

There is a certain amount of ambiguity about the effect of bundling on infant temperatures. One small study based in a hospital nursery found that healthy newborns 1 to 3 days old who were bundled in 5 blankets and placed in a 26.6° C room had a mean increase in rectal temperature of 0.56° C over 2½ hours. Rectal temperatures of 2 of the 12 bundled infants reached 38° C. In a larger study of healthy infants between 11 and 95 days of age, skin and rectal temperatures were compared in control (diaper and terry coverall) and bundled infants in open cribs where room temperature was 72° to 75° F. In bundled infants, in comparison with control infants, there was a significant rise in skin temperature but not in rectal temperature. In the evaluation of newborns with elevated body temperatures, physicians should consider bundling and environmental conditions. However, a rectal temperature above 38° C is unlikely to result exclusively from bundling, especially in infants beyond the first few days after birth.

Oral thermometry can be considered for cooperative patients, and axillary temperatures, although considered imprecise and inaccurate, are convenient. Studies have found correlation between axillary and rectal temperature measurements in neonates, but the temperatures are not interchangeable. In older infants and children, the sensitivity for fever detection in the axilla is below 50%. Thus, when detection of fever is critical for diagnosis and management, axillary temperatures should not be used.

The tympanic membrane thermometer contains a probe that gathers infrared energy emitted through the tympanic membrane and converts the amount of emitted energy to a temperature. It can be used in an oral- or rectal-equivalent mode that involves a preset internal calibration. Tympanic temperatures are thought to reflect the temperature of blood flowing toward the hypothalamus because of the proximity of the tympanic membrane to the internal carotid artery. Issues such as speed, comfort, and infection control have contributed to increased use. The majority of studies find tympanic membrane thermometers to be inaccurate in children; a few support their use. Although ambient temperature has been shown to influence readings, the presence of otitis media or cerumen does not. In young infants in whom rectal temperature has been used as the "gold standard," investigators have found significant differences

Table 57-1. Characteristics of Fever in Comparison with Heat illness

	Examples	Mechanism of Temperature Elevation	Need to Reduce Body Temperature to Normal	Treatment
Fever	Infection, malignancy, trauma	Centrally thermoregulated in response to elevation of setpoint in PAOH	Optional	Acetaminophen or ibuprofen
Heat illness	Hyperthyroidism, atropine poisoning, heat stroke, malignant hyperthermia	Increased heat production or decreased heat loss	Mandatory	External cooling

From Lorin M: Fever: Pathogenesis and treatment. In Feigin RD, Cherry JD (eds): Textbook of Pediatric Infectious Diseases. Philadelphia, WB Saunders, 1998, p 91.

PAOH, preoptic region of the anterior hypothalamus.

between tympanic and rectal temperatures, even when used with the calibration mode. This may result from difficulty inserting the ear-piece fully into the ear canal of small patients. It is probably wise not to rely on tympanic temperature measurement in neonates, young infants, and other patients in whom small differences in temperatures would be important in terms of evaluation and treatment.

A common problem is how to manage the child whose caregiver states that the child had a tactile "fever" at home. In a retrospective study of infants younger than 2 months hospitalized for possible sepsis, 224 of 244 infants (92%) with reported fever per rectum by thermometer had fever on presentation or during the subsequent 48 hours of hospitalization. Only 22 of 48 (46%) infants with reported tactile fever had fever on presentation or during the subsequent 48 hours of hospitalization. Other studies have shown subjective fever assessment to have sensitivity between 73% and 81% and specificity between 76% and 86%. Thus, although caregivers are not perfect at detecting fevers, a history of subjective fever should not be ignored. Infants with a history of tactile fever who are afebrile on presentation and who have a normal clinical examination may not require further evaluation.

PHYSICAL EXAMINATION

Because by definition FWF is nonfocal, the clinician must rely on history and observation to gain a sense of the seriousness of illness. The child with fever appears either extremely ill or not ill. Extremely ill–appearing children are typically lethargic or irritable. They may show signs of shock, including weak peripheral pulses, tachycardia, poor perfusion, respiratory distress, mottling, cyanosis, or decreased mental status (Table 57-3). After thorough clinical and laboratory evaluation, such children should be admitted to the hospital for expectant antibiotic treatment.

Infants and children with FWF who do not appear extremely ill create the most confusion in terms of evaluation and management.

Temperature

Clinicians often use the height of the temperature as a marker of degree of illness. In fact, the risk of occult bacteremia is low in children with temperatures less than 39° C and increases as the temperature exceeds 39° C. Although the best predictors of occult bacteremia are the child's clinical appearance and complete blood cell count results, the clinician may use the temperature as an independent indicator of risk of bacteremia.

Some investigators have shown a correlation between the height of a fever and the probability of a serious bacterial infection. Others have found that children with hyperpyrexia are subject to more diagnostic procedures, but that they do not have a higher frequency of SBI or occult bacteremia. Although most studies of hyperpyrexia do not have large sample sizes, temperature exceeding 41.1° C may be associated with a greater occurrence of meningitis, bacteremia, and pneumonia.

Observational Scales

The physician's ability to make a hypothesis about the child's degree of illness, on the basis of observation, is critical in the evaluation of febrile children. An objective scoring measure may be used in an effort to assess serious illness in young febrile children. The Acute Illness Observation Scale (AIOS) (Table 57-4), also known as the Yale Observation Score, is a six-item predictive model graded on a

Table 57-2. Causes of Hyperthermia

Excessive Heat Production

Exertion
Heat stroke (exertion)
Malignant hyperthermia (anesthesia induced)
Neuroleptic malignant syndrome
Catatonia
Tetanus
Status epilepticus
Delirium
Endocrine disorders (hyperthyroidism, pheochromocytoma)
Drugs (cocaine, amphetamines, ephedrine, phencyclidine, tricyclic antidepressants, LSD, lithium, thyroid hormone, salicylates)

Diminished Heat Dissipation

Heat stroke
Occlusive dressings
Dehydration
Extensive burns (including severe sunburn)
Anhidrotic ectodermal dysplasias
Anticholinergic-like drugs (atropine, antihistamines, phenothiazines, tricyclic antidepressants)
Autonomic neuropathy
Spinal cord level paralysis (spinal crisis)
Possible overbundling (especially in a warm environment)
Therapeutic hyperthermia

Hypothalamic Dysfunction*

Stroke
Encephalitis
Granulomatous processes (sarcoid, tuberculosis, eosinophilic)
Trauma
Central: idiopathic
Phenothiazines
Hemorrhage

*Usually associated with hypothermia.
LSD, lysergic acid diethylamide.

Table 57-3. Definitions of Related Infectious and Shock States

Infection: Microbial phenomenon characterized by an inflammatory response to the presence of microorganisms or the invasion of normally sterile host tissue by those organisms

Bacteremia: The presence of viable bacteria in the blood

Systemic Inflammatory Response Syndrome: The systemic inflammatory response to a variety of severe clinical insults; the response is manifested by two or more of the following conditions:
 Temperature >38° C or <36° C
 Heart rate >90 beats/min*
 Respiratory rate >20 breaths/min* or PaCO$_2$ <32 mm Hg
 WBCs >12,000 cells/min3, <4000 cells/mm^3, or >10% immature (band) forms

Sepsis: The systemic response to infection; this systemic response is manifested by two or more of the following conditions as a result of infection:
 Temperature >38° C or <36° C
 Heart rate >90 beats/min*
 Respiratory rate >20 breaths/min* or PaCO$_2$ <32 mm Hg
 WBCs >12,000 cells/mm^3, <4000 cells/mm^3, or >10% immature (band) forms

Severe Sepsis: Sepsis associated with organ dysfunction, hypoperfusion, or hypotension; hypoperfusion and perfusion abnormalities may include, but are not limited to, lactic acidosis, oliguria, or an acute alteration in mental status

Septic Shock: Sepsis with hypotension, despite adequate fluid resuscitation, along with the presence of perfusion abnormalities that may include, but are not limited to, lactic acidosis, oliguria, or an acute alteration in mental status; patients who are on inotropic or vasopressor agents may not be hypotensive at the time that perfusion abnormalities are measured

Hypotension: A systolic blood pressure of <90 mm Hg* or a reduction of >40 mm Hg from baseline in the absence of other causes for hypotension

Multiple Organ Dysfunction Syndrome: Presence of altered organ function in an acutely ill patient such that homeostasis cannot be maintained without intervention

From American College of Chest Physicians/Society of Critical Care Medicine Consensus Conference: Definitions for sepsis and organ failure and guidelines for the use of innovative therapies in sepsis. Crit Care Med 1992:20:864.

*Adult standards for vital signs; adjust accordingly for children norms.

PaCO$_2$, arterial partial pressure of carbon dioxide; WBC, white blood cell.

scale of 1 to 5. Use of the AIOS in conjunction with the history and physical examination has a higher sensitivity for identifying serious illness than history and physical examination alone. However, the AIOS has not been shown to provide sufficient data to identify serious illness in 4- to 8-week-old infants. The inadequacy of the AIOS in detecting serious illness in this age group may be related to the fact that very young infants have not yet developed many of the social gestures used in this scale.

LABORATORY DATA

When there is no focus of infection, clinical appearance alone may not adequately distinguish the child with occult bacterial illness from one with a self-limited viral infection. Laboratory tests are used to substantiate clinical suspicion and to help identify children at high risk for serious illness.

COMPLETE BLOOD CELL COUNT

There is a direct relationship between the white blood cell (WBC) count and the prevalence of bacteremia in febrile children. In one study of children aged 3 to 36 months who had a temperature exceeding 39.5° C, the prevalence of bacteremia varied by WBC count: 42.9% for a WBC count exceeding 30,000/mm^3, 16.6% for a WBC count of 15,000/mm^3 to 30,000/mm^3, and 2.8% for a WBC count of 10,000/mm^3 to 15,000/mm^3. No patients with a WBC count less than 10,000/mm^3 had bacteremia.

Despite its direct relationship with bacteremia, using a WBC count to identify children with bacteremia has limitations. A WBC count less than 15,000/mm^3 and even leukopenia may be found in children with *Neisseria meningitidis* bacteremia. A minority of children with occult nontyphoidal *Salmonella* bacteremia have been found to have a WBC count exceeding 15,000/mm^3. A WBC count exceeding 15,000/mm^3 and an absolute band count exceeding 500/mm^3 are not predictive of bacteremia in infants younger than 8 weeks.

The receiver operating characteristic curve is a graphic representation of the trade-off between sensitivity and specificity of a given test. One large, prospective trial employed the receiver operating characteristic curve to quantify accuracy of the height of temperature and WBC count as a predictor of bacteremia in children 3 to 36 months of age with FWF. Investigators found that a WBC count of 10,000/mm^3 has a sensitivity of 92% and a specificity of 43%, whereas a WBC count of 20,000/mm^3 has a sensitivity of 38% and a specificity of 92%. As the WBC count increases, the risk of not identifying patients who have bacteremia increases, but the risk of misidentifying patients without bacteremia decreases.

Band counts have not been found to be predictive of occult bacteremia, because they may be elevated in patients with viral illnesses. Receiver operating characteristic curves for WBC, absolute neutrophil (ANC), and absolute band counts show that ANC is the most predictive of occult bacteremia, followed by WBC count. The risk of occult pneumococcal bacteremia (OPB) for patients with ANCs exceeding 10,000 cells/mm^3 is 7.8%. For patients with ANCs less than 10,000 cells/mm^3, the risk of OPB is only 0.8%. ANC retains its predictive power even after adjusting for confounding variables such as age, temperature, WBC count, and absolute band count (Fig. 57-2).

ANTIGEN TESTING

Latex agglutination and enzyme immunoassay antigen testing are rapid and exist for many of the organisms causing SBI in children, including *Streptococcus pneumoniae* and *Haemophilus influenzae* type b. Although they are sensitive for determining *H. influenzae* type b bacteremia, these tests do not have sufficient sensitivity for routine clinical practice for detection of OPB. In addition, there is a substantial false-positive rate for latex agglutination testing of urine for *N. meningitidis*. The overall utility of latex agglutination tests for detection of pneumococcal or meningococcal bacteremia is low, and these tests do not add substantially to more routine laboratory testing, such as the complete blood cell count and blood culture.

POLYMERASE CHAIN REACTION

Studies have focused on polymerase chain reaction (PCR) methods as a means of detecting *H. influenzae, N. meningitidis,* and *S. pneumoniae* bacteremia, as well as common viruses. Most of these studies show that PCR has a relatively high sensitivity in comparison to blood culture for *S. pneumoniae* bacteremia. However, PCR results

Table 57-4. Acute Illness Observation Scale

Observation Item	1 Normal	3 Moderate Impairment	5 Severe Impairment
Quality of cry	Strong with normal tone *or* Content and not crying	Whimpering *or* Sobbing	Weak *or* Moaning *or* High-pitched
Reaction to parent stimulation	Cries briefly, then stops *or* Content and not crying	Cries off and on	Continual cry *or* Hardly responds

State variation	If awake → stays awake
	
	or
	If asleep and
	  stimulated →wakes
	  up quickly
		Eyes close
		  briefly → awakens
		or
		Awakes with prolonged
		  stimulation
			Falls a sleep
			
			or
			Will not rouse

Color	Pink	Pale extremities *or* Acrocyanosis	Pale *or* Cyanotic *or* Mottled *or* Ashen
Hydration	Skin normal, eyes normal *and* Mucous membranes moist	Skin, eyes normal *and* Mouth slightly dry	Skin doughy *or* Skin tented *and* Dry mucous membranes *and/or* Sunken eyes
Response (talk, smile) to social overtures	Smiles *or* Alert (≤2 mo)	Brief smile *or* Alert briefly (≤2 mo)	No smile; face anxious, dull, expressionless *or* No alertness (≤2 mo)

From McCarthy PL, Sharpe MR, Spiesel SZ, et al: Observation scales to identify serious illness in febrile children. Pediatrics 1982;70:802.

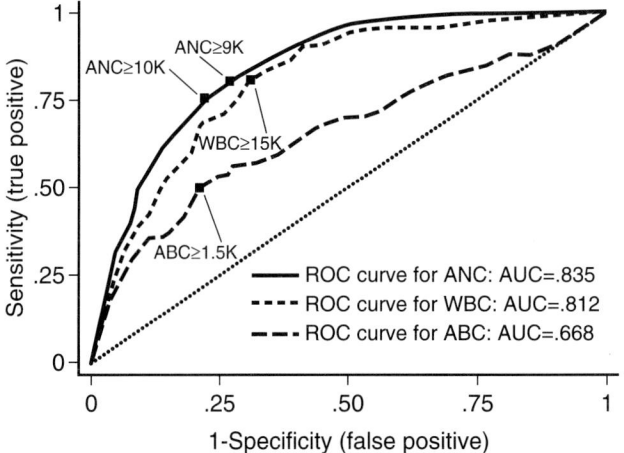

Figure 57-2. Receiver operating curve (ROC) comparing WBC count, ANC, and ABC. ABC, absolute band count; ANC, absolute neutrophil count; AUC, area under the curve; WBC, white blood cell. (Data from Kupperman N, Fleisher GR, Jaffe DM: Predictors of occult pneumococcal bacteremia in young febrile children. Ann Emerg Med 1998; 31:679-687.)

are also positive in a relatively large percentage of patients with negative blood culture results. PCR has been found to have a high degree of sensitivity and specificity in patients with known *N. meningitidis,* but it has not been studied for unknown or unsuspected cases. PCR may be useful in identifying the cause of fever as a common respiratory virus such as respiratory syncytial virus, influenza viruses, parainfluenza viruses, enteroviruses, or herpes simplex virus.

BLOOD CULTURES

Blood cultures are the "gold standard" for determination of bacteremia. Although blood cultures do not provide immediate results, current methods allow for continuous monitoring of bacterial growth. Blood cultures are easy to perform and provide essential information in the course of patient follow-up because they identify patients with bacteremia who are at risk for SBI. Preliminary blood culture results are typically available within 24 hours, with positive identification of organisms within 48 hours.

False-negative blood culture results may be due to prior treatment with antibiotics, missing an episode of bacteremia if it is intermittent, and inoculation of too little blood into the culture media. Alternatively, too much blood inoculated into the blood culture bottle may yield a false-negative result because of ongoing killing of bacteria by neutrophils. Three to 5 mL of blood should be added to each blood culture bottle. False-positive results may be due to inadequate skin preparation, leading to contamination with skin flora.

LUMBAR PUNCTURE

Lumbar puncture is indicated if the patient is younger than 28 days or if diagnosis of sepsis or meningitis is considered, regardless of the child's age. Normal cerebrospinal fluid (CSF) findings, including chemistry, cell count with differential, Gram stain, and culture, help exclude the diagnosis of meningitis. Fewer than 1% of children with normal preliminary CSF results have a positive culture; in most of these, the pathogen is *N. meningitidis.* Thus, even in the presence of normal preliminary CSF results, close follow-up is essential (see Chapter 52).

URINALYSIS AND URINE CULTURE

Although urine culture is the "gold standard" for the diagnosis of a UTI, urinalysis helps identify children with occult UTI. Studies have compared enhanced urinalysis (uncentrifuged urine for cell count and Gram stain) and dipstick with the urine culture. Enhanced urinalysis findings of pyuria (>10 WBCs/mm³) *and* bacteriuria (bacteria on any 10 oil immersion fields) supports presumptive treatment, whereas the finding of bacteriuria *or* pyuria supports presumptive treatment if the clinician has a high suspicion for UTI. Enhanced urinalysis may be difficult and time consuming to perform. In contrast, urine dipstick is a quick and simple test. Findings of moderate leukocyte esterase or positive nitrite support presumptive treatment pending the culture results (see Chapter 23). Children should have a catheterized urine specimen obtained, unless they are toilet-trained and can supply a clean voided specimen. Suprapubic aspiration is acceptable but requires technical expertise, and parents often perceive it as unsuitably invasive. However, it may be the only alternative for boys with severe phimosis. The use of plastic receptacles attached to the perineum should be discouraged, because contamination from skin and fecal flora commonly occurs.

CHEST RADIOGRAPHS

Chest radiographs are most often normal in children who have FWF. Respiratory signs or symptoms, such as tachypnea, retractions, rales, wheezing, rhonchi, nasal flaring, grunting, cough, or hypoxia, may predict chest radiograph findings consistent with pneumonia. In practice, pneumonia can often be diagnosed solely on the basis of the clinical findings of fever, tachypnea, and rales; chest radiographs are not always necessary. However, chest radiographs may be useful in evaluating for the presence of pleural effusion or other complications of pneumonia. Chest radiographs should be considered for infants younger than 2 months because such patients may have infiltrates consistent with bacterial pneumonia despite negative physical examination findings. A chest radiograph should also be considered for infants and children with temperature exceeding 39° C, a WBC count exceeding 20,000 cells/mm³, and no source found on physical examination.

STOOL ANALYSIS AND CULTURE

Analysis and culture of stool are important if diarrhea is present. Bacterial enteritis is indicated by the presence of blood, mucus, or more than 5 WBCs/high-power field (hpf). If these screening tests are positive, a stool culture should be obtained. Because some institutions do not routinely perform stool analyses, a stool culture should be considered for a child with a history of diarrhea associated with fever, blood, or mucus.

DIFFERENTIAL DIAGNOSIS

In 20% of children with a fever, history and physical examination reveal no apparent source. Most of the children who present with FWF are subsequently determined to have a self-limited viral infection (Table 57-5). These children may be in the prodromal phase of a variety of viral infections such as enterovirus, influenza, or roseola. However, 2% to 5% may have occult bacteremia, and 5% to 7% may have bacterial infection of the urinary tract or other site.

Table 57-5. Differential Diagnosis of Fever without Focus

	Example	3 to 36 Months	0 to 3 Months
Common			
Viral infections	Viremia, exanthem	Enterovirus, parainfluenza adenovirus, RSV, CMV, roseola, fifth disease, influenza, other viruses	Same as in 3-36 months plus HSV
Bacterial infections	Occult bacteremia	*Streptococcus pneumoniae, Haemophilus influenzae, Neisseria meningitidis, Salmonella* species	Same as in 3-36 months plus group B streptococci, gram-negative organisms, *Listeria monocytogenes*
	Urinary tract infection	*Escherichia coli, Klebsiella* species, other gram-negative organisms	Same as in 3-36 months
	Other site	Unlikely without signs	Meningitis (same as above bacterial organisms), salmonellosis
Rarer			
Connective tissue diseases		Rheumatic fever, SLE, sarcoidosis, JRA	
Malignancies		Leukemia, lymphoma, neuroblastoma, Ewing sarcoma	
Poisoning		Atropine, salicylates, cocaine, anticholinergics	

CMV, cytomegalovirus; HSV, herpes simplex virus; JRA, juvenile rheumatoid arthritis; RSV, respiratory syncytial virus; SLE, systemic lupus erythematosus.

Noninfectious conditions manifesting with FWF are extremely rare. Historical clues (recurrences, chronicity) or systemic signs usually indicate malignancy and connective tissue disorders. If the history and physical examination are not suggestive, these diagnoses need not be pursued. Heat-related illness or drug ingestion may be considered if supported by the history. Fever caused by immunization may not be accompanied by other signs or symptoms, but the history should suggest immunization as the cause. More specifically, fever from diphtheria-pertussis-tetanus vaccine usually has an onset within 12 to 24 hours and may last up to 48 hours. Measles-mumps-rubella vaccine may cause fever 7 to 10 days after injection and may be associated with a faint rash. The pneumococcal vaccine may cause fevers during the first 72 hours after the primary series.

In one prospective analysis to identify pathogens causing FWF in children younger than 3 months, a cause was determined in 50% of patients through the use of multiple cultures and antibody titers for bacteria and viruses. Viral agents were identified in 40% of patients and represented 73% of identifiable pathogens. The majority of the viruses were nonpolio enteroviruses; the rest were parainfluenza, respiratory syncytial virus, adenovirus, and cytomegalovirus. A detailed investigation to identify a viral pathogen is not necessary unless FWF evolves into FUO or fever with end-organ involvement, as in hepatitis or meningitis.

URINARY TRACT INFECTIONS

UTIs are almost always occult in children younger than 2 years because the symptoms, except for fever, are nonspecific or nonexistent. UTI occurs in 2% of febrile children younger than 5 years. The prevalence is higher in white patients, especially white infant girls with FWF, who have up to a 30% risk of UTI. This racial difference is possibly caused by differences in blood group antigens on the surface of uroepithelial cells that may affect the ability of *Escherichia coli* to adhere. The prevalence of UTI in girls younger than 12 months is 6.5% and in boys the same age is 3.3%. Girls aged 1 to 2 years have a prevalence of 8.1%, in comparison with 1.9% in boys of the same age. In uncircumcised boys, the rate of UTI is 5 to 20 times that of UTI in circumcised boys. Urine specimens should be obtained from the following children with FWF: those with a history of UTI, those with a history of urinary tract anomalies or vesicoureteral reflux, all infants younger than 2 months, boys younger than 1 year (especially if uncircumcised), and girls younger than 2 years.

There is an age-associated risk of bacteremia, particularly in infants. The incidence of bacteremia in patients younger than 1 month is 21%. In infants aged 1 to 2 months, 2 to 3 months, and 3 to 6 months, the incidence is 13%, 4%, and 8%, respectively. There may be a referral bias of sicker patients accounting for this prevalence, but the possibility of bacteremia is large enough to recommend obtaining a blood culture in children younger than 6 months with suspected UTI.

OCCULT BACTEREMIA

Occult bacteremia is defined by the presence of a positive blood culture for pathogenic bacteria in a febrile patient who does not appear extremely ill and who has no focus for infection, excluding otitis media. About 90% of bacteremia is caused by *S. pneumoniae. N. meningitidis*, nontyphoidal *Salmonella,* and other bacteria such as *Staphylococcus aureus* and group A streptococci account for the remainder of cases. The incidence of *H. influenzae* type b bacteremia has decreased dramatically because of childhood immunization.

Natural History

Most untreated *S. pneumoniae* bacteremia resolves spontaneously; approximately 25% of patients have continued fever with persistent bacteremia or other complications. The estimated risk of meningitis in patients with occult pneumococcal bacteremia is 3% to 6%. Other serious, uncommon complications include cellulitis, osteomyelitis, and pneumonia.

N. meningitidis bacteremia is frequently associated with serious sequelae. Children with *N. meningitidis* bacteremia are much more likely to progress to meningitis than are those with *S. pneumoniae* bacteremia. In a 10-year retrospective review of unsuspected meningococcemia, 12 of the 25 cases of meningococcemia occurred in children who appeared well enough at initial presentation not to raise concern for serious, invasive disease. Of these 12 patients, 4 of whom were initially untreated and 8 of whom were treated with oral antimicrobial agents, 3 (25%) developed meningitis and 2 died (17%).

Nontyphoidal *Salmonella* bacteremia is often accompanied or preceded by enteritis. In some instances, particularly in young infants, the diarrhea is mild or even absent. The prevalence of *Salmonella* bacteremia among patients with *Salmonella* enteritis has been reported to be between 2% and 45%; fever is not always present. *Salmonella* infection seldom causes serious complications in patients with normal host defenses and resolves spontaneously. Infants younger than 3 months and immunocompromised individuals are exceptions. They should be treated with antibiotics because nontyphoidal *Salmonella* bacteremia may cause meningitis, sepsis, and death in these groups. In children older than 3 months who are otherwise healthy, serious sequelae are much less common. The most common complication of nontyphoidal Salmonella bacteremia is persistent bacteremia. Empirical parenteral antibiotic therapy may lower this risk (Table 57-6).

OCCULT PNEUMOCOCCAL BACTEREMIA

Ten percent to 25% of children with OPB who are not treated with antibiotics at the time of initial evaluation develop serious bacterial infections, including cellulitis, pneumonia, osteomyelitis, and sepsis. Meningitis may develop in 3% to 6% of these children. In a large retrospective study of 382 children with OPB not treated with antibiotics, 17% of 48 patients not receiving empiric antibiotics had persistent bacteremia at follow-up and 10% (of 48) developed focal complications, including 1 case of meningitis. Studies have shown that early diagnosis and treatment with antibiotics may decrease the risk of many complications, possibly even meningitis.

Studies have attempted to stratify patients according to risk of OPB so that practitioners might have a guide for anticipatory use of laboratory studies and antibiotics. Independent predictors of OPB in children aged 3 to 36 months with fever of 39° C or higher who were treated as outpatients include ANC, temperature, and age younger than 2 years. Children between 2 and 3 years of age with temperature less than 39.5° C have a 1.1% risk of OPB. The ANC becomes important in determining the risk of OPB in children aged 2 to 3 years with temperature exceeding 39.5° C and in those aged 3 to 24 months with temperature exceeding 39° C. The risk of OPB in these patients is 0.8% if ANC is less than 10,000/mm^3 and 8.3% if the ANC exceeds 10,000/mm^3 (Table 57-7).

If the clinician does not have access to the ANC, using the complete blood cell count alone is an alternative method of stratification. In the same study sample, patients with WBC counts exceeding 15,000 cells/mm^3 had a 6% risk of pneumococcal bacteremia, in comparison with 0.7% for those with WBC counts less than 15,000 cells/mm^3.

PNEUMOCOCCAL VACCINE

A 7-valent protein-polysaccharide pneumococcal conjugate vaccine is licensed for use in the United States and is recommended for routine use in all infants and children younger than 2 years of age, with doses given at 2, 4, and 6 months of age and a booster at 12 to 15 months. The four-dose regimen is highly efficacious against invasive disease and somewhat efficacious against otitis media and

Table 57-6. Antibiotic Therapy for Diseases Commonly Associated with Fever without Focus

Disease	Antibiotic	Dosage	Duration
Suspected Bacteremia			
Age: <1 week (hospitalized)	Ampicillin + cefotaxime	Ampicillin: 75-150 mg/kg/day IV in divided doses q8h Cefotaxime: 100 mg/kg/day IV in divided doses q12h	Until cultures negative
Age: 1-4 weeks (hospitalized)	Ampicillin + cefotaxime (or ceftriaxone)	Ampicillin: 100-200 mg/kg/day in divided doses q6h Cefotaxime: 150 mg/kg/day in divided doses q8h (Ceftriaxone: 75 mg/kg/day in divided doses q12-q24h)	Until cultures negative
Age: >4 weeks	Ceftriaxone	50-100 mg/kg IM/IV q12-q24h	See Figures 57-3 and 57-4
OPB	Amoxicillin	25-50 mg/kg/day PO in divided doses t.i.d.	10 days
Penicillin-Resistant OPB	Amoxicillin	80-90 mg/kg/day PO in divided doses b.i.d.	10 days
Salmonella **Bacteremia**			
Age: <3 months	Cefotaxime	100-200 mg/kg/day IV/IM in divided doses q8h	7-10 days
Age: >3 months	Amoxicillin	50 mg/kg/day PO in divided doses t.i.d.	5-7 days
Pneumonia	Amoxicillin*	25-50 mg/kg/day PO in divided doses t.i.d. (use high dose if penicillin resistance suspected)	10 days
	or Erythromycin	40 mg/kg/day PO in divided doses q.i.d.	10 days
Urinary Tract Infection	TMP/SMX	8-10 mg/kg/day of TMP component PO in divided doses b.i.d.	7-14 days
	or Amoxicillin	25-50 mg/kg/day PO in divided doses t.i.d.	7-14 days

*Some recommend cefotaxime for all salmonella bacteremias; sensitivities must be tested for each episode of bacteremia.

b.i.d., twice a day; IM, intramuscularly; IV, intravenously; OPB, occult pneumococcal bacteremia; PO, per os (orally); q.i.d., four times a day; SMX, sulfamethoxazole; t.i.d., three times a day; TMP, trimethoprim.

pneumonia. It is unknown how effective the vaccine is for children who have been given fewer than four doses or for older children.

In this era of reduced pneumococcal and *H. influenza* one must reevaluate the strategies for the management of febrile 3- to 36-month-old children. If the rate of bacteremia is 1.5%, one reasonable diagnostic strategy is to send a blood culture and empirically treat with antibiotics those children with a white blood cell count of 15×10^9 or greater. If widespread use of vaccines reduces the overall rate of occult bacteremia to 0.5%, clinical judgment may be an appropriate, cost-effective strategy for fully vaccinated children.

Table 57-7. Risk of Occult Pneumococcal Bacteremia by Age, Temperature, and ANC

Age	Temperature	ANC (cells/mm³)	Risk of Bacteremia
2-3 years	<39.5° C	—	1.1%
3-24 months *or* 2-3 years	≥39° C ≥39.5° C	<10,000	0.8%
3-24 months *or* 2-3 years	≥39° C ≥39.5° C	≥10,000	8.3%

ANC, absolute neutrophil count.

EVALUATION AND MANAGEMENT

CHILDREN YOUNGER THAN 3 MONTHS

Febrile infants younger than 12 weeks who appear extremely ill have an incidence of SBI of 17.3%, including 10.7% for bacteremia and 3.9% for meningitis. The probability of SBI in febrile infants younger than 12 weeks who do not appear extremely ill is 8.6%. The rate of *bacteremia* in all febrile infants younger than 2 months of age is between 2% and 3%. The relatively high incidence of bacterial disease probably results from a combination of factors unique to this age group: decreased opsonin activity; decreased macrophage function; decreased neutrophil function; poor immunoglobulin G antibody response to encapsulated bacteria; and susceptibility to bacterial pathogens such as group B streptococci, gram-negative enteric organisms, and *Listeria monocytogenes*.

In young infants, clinical evaluation alone is inadequate for excluding serious bacterial infections. Management of febrile infants younger than 28 days includes a sepsis evaluation and hospitalization for parenteral antimicrobial therapy pending culture results. The reasoning for this conservative approach lies in the difficulty in evaluating the behavioral state of neonates, the rapid evolution of bacterial infections, the immature neonatal immune system, and the possibility of life-threatening viral meningoencephalitis caused by herpes simplex viruses and enteroviruses. Sepsis evaluation should include culture of the CSF, blood, and urine; a complete blood cell count with differential; examination of the CSF for cells, protein, and glucose; and urinalysis. A chest radiograph also should be considered.

A combination of clinical evaluation and laboratory studies can be used to define a specific population of infants aged 29 to 60 days who do not appear extremely ill and are at low risk for SBI. Infants at low risk for SBI are those who are previously healthy with no focus of bacterial infection on physical examination and who have negative laboratory screening results. A number of prospective studies have contributed to the development of specific low-risk screening criteria. The age groups included vary by study, ranging from 0 to 90 days to 29 to 56 days. Because there are differences in study criteria used to define infants at low risk for SBI, the most conservative values have been used in the guidelines presented in this chapter. In general, negative laboratory screening results consist of a WBC count of 5,000 to 15,000/mm³; fewer than 1500 bands/mm³ or a band-to-neutrophil ratio of less than 0.2; fewer than 10 WBCs/hpf and no organisms on urinalysis; and fewer than 8 WBCs/hpf and no organisms on CSF examination. Some experts also include a negative chest radiograph and, when diarrhea is present, a stool examination with fewer than 5 WBCs/hpf (Fig. 57-3). The mean probability of serious bacterial infection in infants younger than 90 days who fulfill the low-risk criteria is 1.4%.

Most experts suggest that febrile infants 28 to 60 days old who meet the low-risk criteria and have access to close follow-up can be managed as outpatients after they receive ceftriaxone. Blood, urine, and CSF cultures should be obtained before empirical antibiotic treatment so that viral and bacterial causes may be distinguished. An alternative strategy is to manage such infants as outpatients, without empirical antibiotic therapy, after blood, CSF, and urine cultures are obtained. Although most of the original studies on outpatient management of febrile infants included infants aged 2 to 3 months, many experts now agree that infants aged 2 to 3 months can be managed safely according to the guidelines for infants and children aged 3 to 36 months (Fig. 57-4).

Regardless of whether the clinician chooses to treat the patient with empirical antibiotics, all "low-risk" infants should be reevaluated within 24 hours. Those who appear ill or who have positive culture results should be admitted for parenteral antibiotics. If a child appears well and all culture results are negative, close follow-up should be continued and a return visit made in 24 hours. Infants with occult bacteremia caused by penicillin-sensitive *S. pneumoniae* who are afebrile and appear well can be managed as outpatients with oral amoxicillin and careful follow-up. Infants with a UTI should be hospitalized. Once culture and sensitivity results of urine and blood cultures are known, an infant who is afebrile, does not appear extremely ill, and is not bacteremic may be treated with oral antibiotics and close follow-up.

CHILDREN AGED 3 TO 36 MONTHS

The risk of bacteremia for children in this age group with FWF and temperature exceeding 39° C is about 3%. The organisms most commonly associated with bacteremia are *S. pneumoniae* and *N. meningitidis.* If the temperature is less than 39° C, the risk of bacteremia is less than 1%. Well-appearing children with no focus of infection and a rectal temperature less than 39° C do not need screening studies.

Blood cultures are important in the management of children with FWF, because those with occult bacteremia can be identified. When blood cultures are drawn, it is important to establish a communication system between the laboratory and the physician and between the physician and the family, in the event that the cultures are positive.

The following strategy is suggested to clarify the approach to a child between the ages of 3 and 36 months with FWF who does not appear ill (see Fig. 57-4).

According to the study upon which these recommendations are based, use of this strategy would result in administration of antibiotics to 24% of children 3 to 36 months with temperatures exceeding 39° C. Approximately 76% of cases of OPB would be correctly identified. If all patients are reevaluated regardless of whether they received expectant antibiotic therapy, the risk of serious sequelae should decrease in the approximately 24% of patients in whom OPB is missed on initial screening.

Examination and culture of the CSF are the only tests to exclude the diagnosis of meningitis. They should be considered in any child

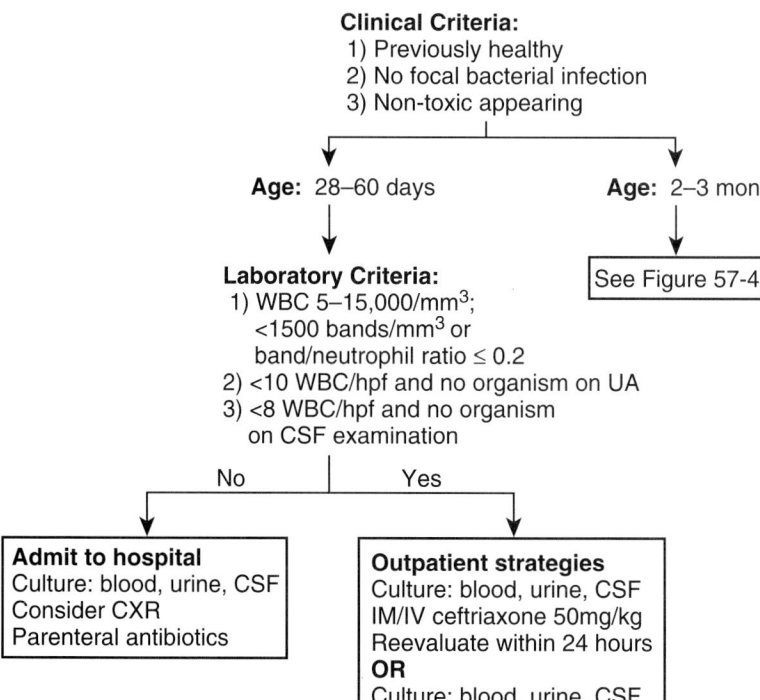

Figure 57-3. *Algorithm for management of infants aged 28 to 90 days with fever without focus who do not appear extremely ill. CSF, cerebrospinal fluid; CXR, chest radiograph; hpf, high-power field; IM, intramuscular; IV, intravenous; UA, urinalysis; WBC, white blood cell.*

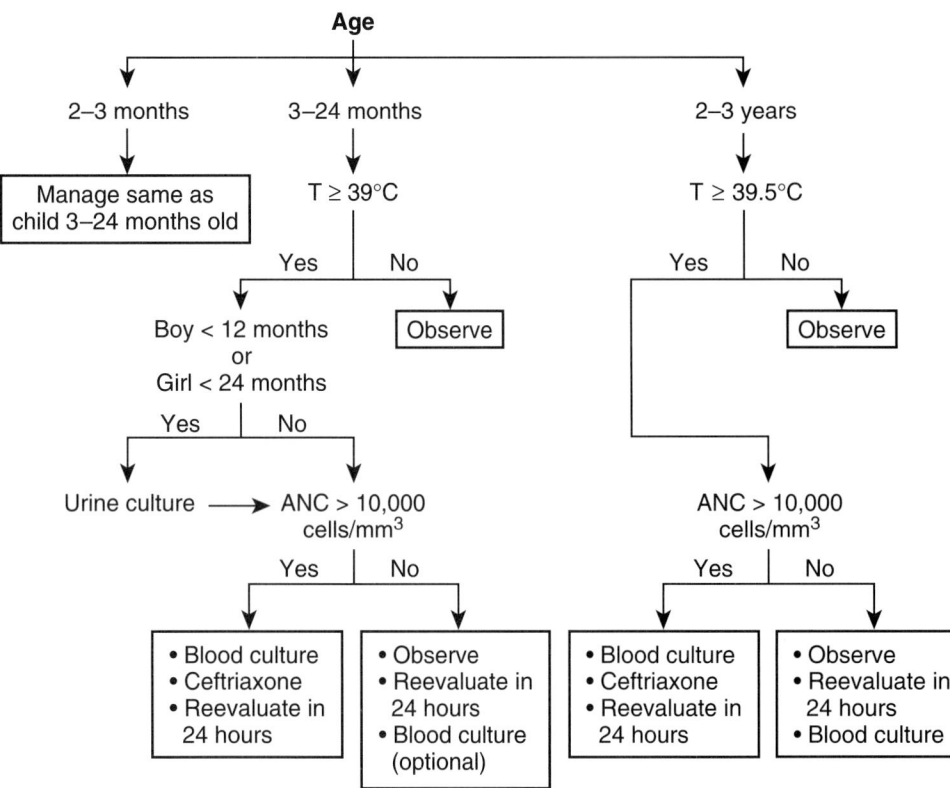

Figure 57-4. Algorithm for management of children aged 3 to 36 months with fever without focus who do not appear extremely ill. ANC, absolute neutrophil count; T, temperature.

in whom the diagnosis of sepsis or meningitis is suspected on the basis of the history, observation, and physical examination findings. Approximately 1% of children with normal initial CSF findings have a positive CSF culture, usually resulting from *N. meningitidis.* Outpatient management is acceptable for those with a low probability of meningitis, good follow-up, and reliable caregivers. Blood cultures should be obtained for all children in whom sepsis or meningitis is suspected. Expectant treatment with ceftriaxone should be considered.

A febrile child with moderate leukocyte esterase or positive nitrite findings on urine dipstick testing of an appropriately collected specimen should be treated presumptively for a UTI. Urine cultures should be obtained for any patient with a suspected UTI. The choice of antibiotics should be guided by knowledge of the common pathogens that cause UTIs and by patterns of antibiotic sensitivity in the community. For outpatient treatment, trimethoprim-sulfamethoxazole, or amoxicillin may be used (see Table 57-6). Hospitalization should be considered for the child who is vomiting, is dehydrated, or appears ill; for those in whom compliance is likely to be poor; and for any patient with underlying renal or urologic anomalies.

The mean probability of an infiltrate on chest radiograph is 3.3% in children with FWF. Most children with infiltrate on chest radiograph who do not appear ill are presumed to have viral pneumonia. Children with higher fevers, leukocytosis, or low pulse oximetry readings may be at increased risk of bacterial pneumonia, and a chest radiograph should be considered. In fact, in one prospective cohort study of children younger than 5 years with temperature exceeding 39° C and WBC count exceeding 20,000/mm³, pneumonia was found on chest radiographs of 26% of those without clinical evidence of pneumonia. In this same sample, radiographic evidence of pneumonia was found in 40% of patients with clinical findings suggestive of pneumonia. A chest radiograph should be considered at follow-up for ill-appearing children with a positive blood culture, no focus of infection, and persistent fever.

In summary, management of children aged 3 to 36 months with fever is based on experience and numerous study results:

- *Child who appears extremely ill on initial evaluation or on follow-up:* Admit to the hospital for parenteral antibiotics after appropriate laboratory evaluation.
- *Well-appearing child aged 3 to 24 months with temperature less than 39° C or aged 2 to 3 years with temperature less than 39.5° C:* No diagnostic tests need to be initiated. The caregiver should be instructed to take the child back to the physician if the fever persists for more than 48 hours or if the child's condition deteriorates.
- *Child aged 3 to 24 months with temperature exceeding 39° C or aged 2 to 3 years with temperature exceeding 39.5° C:* Urine culture is suggested for boys younger than 12 months and for girls younger than 2 years. A complete blood cell count and blood culture should be obtained. Ceftriaxone should be given if the ANC exceeds 10,000 cells/mm³ or if the WBC count exceeds 15,000 cells/mm³. Children should be reevaluated in 24 hours. If the child is afebrile and well on follow-up and the cultures show no growth, no further therapy is necessary.
- *Child with positive blood culture:* Reevaluation should occur in any child whose blood culture is presumptively positive. If the blood is found to contain *N. meningitidis* or *H. influenzae* (which has been rare since the advent of *H. influenzae* b immunization), a CSF sample and a repeat blood culture should be obtained, and the child should be admitted to the hospital for parenteral antibiotics, pending the results of the cultures. The child with OPB who appears well and is afebrile can be managed as an outpatient with parenteral ceftriaxone followed by oral antibiotics according to the sensitivity of the organism. Because of the concern of pneumococcal resistance to penicillin, a second dose of intramuscular ceftriaxone may be given until penicillin sensitivity is documented. If the culture is positive for nontyphoidal *Salmonella* organisms and the child is younger than 3 months, full sepsis evaluation and intravenous antibiotics are recommended.

Oral antibiotics and close follow-up is recommended for older children.

- *Child with positive urine culture:* If the child is afebrile and appears well, treatment with oral antibiotics is recommended, according to the sensitivity of the organism (see Table 57-6).

CHILDREN OLDER THAN 36 MONTHS

Evaluation and management of ill-appearing children older than 36 months with FWF are similar to those of younger children. An important exception is that blood cultures are not routinely ordered to screen for occult bacteremia. The clinician can observe and reevaluate a well-appearing older child with temperature exceeding 39° C without first obtaining blood cultures. Close attention should be paid to environmental exposures and ill contacts, because of the high likelihood of increased contacts in this school-aged cohort.

PHARMACOLOGIC THERAPY

ANTIPYRETIC THERAPY

When fever is caused by an alteration in the hypothalamic set point, as in infection, therapy to inhibit prostaglandin production and reset the thermostat may be appropriate, particularly because children experience symptomatic improvement with fever reduction. Acetaminophen is the standard agent used in this setting. The dosage is 10 to 15 mg/kg per dose given every 4 hours, with a maximum single dose of 650 mg. Aspirin is not recommended, because of its association with Reye syndrome. Ibuprofen is a nonsteroidal antiinflammatory agent that is effective in reducing fever. The dosage is 5 to 10 mg/kg every 6 to 8 hours. It is safe for most patients, except for those with renal disease or severe dehydration. Gastrointestinal upset is reported in 10% to 15% of patients.

External cooling is another method of controlling fevers. In febrile patients, external cooling may be of limited effectiveness because it causes cutaneous vasoconstriction and shivering, both of which contribute to maintaining or raising the core temperature. Studies have shown that the combination of sponging and administration of antipyretic drugs lowers temperature slightly more rapidly during the first 30 minutes but that overall there is no difference in the final temperature reduction. In addition, febrile children have been found to have significantly more discomfort when external cooling is added to antipyretic therapy.

CEFTRIAXONE

Ceftriaxone is useful for outpatient therapy because adequate tissue levels are achieved for 24 hours with a single intramuscular dose and because it is active against the typical pathogens causing SBI. The usual dose is 50 to 75 mg/kg/day when given intramuscularly. It is estimated that the risk of anaphylaxis is 10% to 15% in patients with penicillin allergy.

Cases of cephalosporin treatment failure in penicillin-resistant and cephalosporin-resistant *S. pneumoniae* meningitis have been reported. The efficacy of ceftriaxone therapy for outpatient management of occult bacteremia may change if the prevalence of these resistant strains increases.

Antibiotic therapy should be adjusted according to in vitro susceptibility and patient response to treatment. Penicillin-resistant *S. pneumoniae* may be a concern for patients who have recently been treated with antibiotics, attend day care, or live in communities with high rates of penicillin resistance. High-dose oral amoxicillin (80 to 90 mg/kg/day) is recommended for patients with nonmeningeal infections presumed to be caused by resistant pneumococcal bacteria.

SUMMARY AND RED FLAGS

Because of its vague nature, the subject of FWF is confusing and the literature is often conflicting. Because of the high volume of febrile infants and children who present to physician's offices and emergency departments, it is important to have a reliable system for individual patient evaluation and management. Although the majority of patients with FWF have a self-limited viral illness, 3% to 5% have an invasive (bacteremic or nonbacteremic) bacterial infection. Because of the potential for morbidity and mortality from the organisms that cause invasive disease, identification of patients at high risk is essential. Although there is no single, rapid test that correctly categorizes all patients, the combination of careful clinical evaluation and appropriate laboratory screening criteria can help identify a level of risk in children of different ages. The reduction of bacteremias due to *H. influenzae* and vaccine serotype pneumococcus requires a careful reevaluation of our approach to management of the febrile child.

Red flags include a history of immunodeficiency or other chronic medical illness, toxic appearance, signs of shock (see Table 57-3), petechiae or purpura (see Chapter 55), poor responsiveness and other signs of altered mental status, and neutropenia (see Chapter 58).

REFERENCES

General

Cheng TL, Partridge JC: Effect of bundling and high environmental temperature on neonatal body temperature. Pediatrics 1993;92:238-240.

Cimpello LB, Goldman DL, Khine H: Fever pathophysiology. Clin Pediatr Emerg Med 2000;1:84-93.

Corneli HM: Beyond the fear of fever. Clin Pediatr Emerg Med 2000;1:94-101.

Grover F, Berkowitz CD, Lewis RJ, et al: The effects of bundling on infant temperature. Pediatrics 1994;94:669-673.

Mackowiak PA, Wasserman SS, Levine MM: A critical appraisal of 98.6° F, the upper limit of the normal body temperature, and other legacies of Carl Reinhold August Wunderlich. JAMA 1992;268:1578-1580.

McCarthy PL, Dolan TF Jr: Hyperpyrexia in children. Am J Dis Child 1976;130:849-851.

Schmitt BD: Fever phobia. Am J Dis Child 1980;134:176-181.

Wittler R, Cain K, Bass J: A survey about management of febrile children without source by primary care physicians. Pediatr Infect Dis J 1998;17:271-277.

Laboratory

Bachur R, Perry H, Harper M: Occult pneumonias: Empiric chest radiographs in febrile children with leukocytosis. Ann Emerg Med 1999;33:166-173.

Jaffe D, Fleisher G: Temperature and total white blood cell count as indicators of bacteremia. Pediatrics 1991;87:670-674.

Procop G, Hartman J, Sedor F: Laboratory tests in evaluation of acute febrile illness in pediatric emergency room patients. Am J Clin Pathol 1997;107:114-121.

Measurement

Baker MD, Avner JR, Bell LM: Failure of infant observation scales in detecting serious illness in febrile 4- to 8-week-old infants. Pediatrics 1990;85:1040-1043.

Bonadio WA, Hegenbarth M, Zachariason M: Correlating reported fever in young infants with subsequent temperature patterns and rate of serious bacterial infections. Pediatr Infect Dis J 1990;9:158-160.

Bonadio WA, Hennes H, Smith D, et al: Reliability of observation variables in distinguishing infectious outcome of febrile young infants. Pediatr Infect Dis J 1993;12:111-114.

Brennan DF, Falk JL, Rothrock SG, et al: Reliability of infrared tympanic thermometry in the detection of rectal fever in children. Ann Emerg Med 1995;25:21-30.

Childs C, Harrison R, Hodkinson C: Tympanic membrane temperature as a measure of core temperature. Arch Dis Child 1999;80:262-266.

Craig J, Lancaster G, Williamson P, et al: Temperature measured at the axilla compared with the rectum in children and young people: Systematic review. BMJ 2000;320:1174-1178.

Doezema D, Lunt M, Tandberg D: Cerumen occlusion lowers infrared tympanic membrane temperature measurement. Acad Emerg Med 1995;2:17-19.

Hooker EA, Smith SW, Miles T, et al: Subjective assessment of fever by parents: Comparison with measurement by non-contact tympanic thermometer and calibrated rectal glass mercury thermometer. Ann Emerg Med 1996;28:313-317.

Johnson KJ, Bhatia P, Bell EF: Infrared thermometry of newborn infants. Pediatrics 1991;87:34-38.

McCarthy PL, Lembo RM, Fink HD, et al: Observation, history, and physical examination in diagnosis of serious illnesses in febrile children less than or equal to 24 months. J Pediatr 1987;110:26-30.

McCarthy PL, Sznajderman SD, Lustman-Finding K, et al: Mothers' clinical judgment: A randomized trial of the Acute Illness Observation Scales. J Pediatr 1990;116:200-206.

Petersen-Smith A, Barber N, Coody DK, et al: Comparison of aural infrared with traditional rectal temperatures in children from birth to age three years. J Pediatr 1994;125:83-85.

Stewart JV, Webster D: Re-evaluation of the tympanic thermometer in the emergency department. Ann Emerg Med 1992;21:158-161.

Yetman RJ, Coody DK, West MS, et al: Comparison of temperature measurements by an aural infrared thermometer with measurements by traditional rectal and axillary techniques. J Pediatr 1993;122:769-773.

Evaluation and Management

Baker M: Evaluation and management of infants with fever. Pediatr Clin North Am 1999;46:1061-1072.

Baker M, Avner J: Management of fever in young infants. Clin Pediatr Emerg Med 2000;1:102-108.

Baraff L: Management of fever without source in infants and children. Ann Emerg Med 2000;36:602-614.

Baraff LJ, Bass JW, Fleisher GR, et al: Practice guideline for the management of infants and children 0 to 36 months of age with fever without a source. Pediatrics 1993;92:1-12.

Occult Bacteremia

Alpern ER, Alessandrini EA, Bell LM, et al: Occult bacteremia from a pediatric emergency department: Current prevalence, time to detection, and outcome. Pediatrics 2000;106:505-510.

Bandyopadhyay S, Bergholte J, Clackwell CD, et al: Risk of serious bacterial infection in children with fever without a source in the post–*Haemophilus influenzae* era when antibiotics are reserved for culture-proven bacteremia. Arch Pediatr Adolesc Med 2002;156:512-517.

Dashefsky B, Teele DW, Klein JO: Unsuspected meningococcemia. J Pediatr 1983;102:69-72.

Edwards K, Griffin M: Great expectations for a new vaccine. N Engl J Med 2003;349:1312-1314.

Isaacman D: The occult bacteremia controversy. Clin Pediatr Emerg Med 2000;1:109-116.

Isaacman D, Shults J, Gross T, et al: Predictors of bacteremia in febrile children 3 to 36 months of age. Pediatrics 2000;106:977-982.

Klein J: Management of the febrile child without a focus of infection in the era of universal pneumococcal immunization. Pediatr Infect Dis J 2002;21:584-588.

Kupperman N: Occult bacteremia in young febrile children. Pediatr Clin North Am 1999;46:1073-1109.

Kupperman N, Fleisher G, Jaffe D: Predictors of occult pneumococcal bacteremia in young febrile children. Ann Emerg Med 1998;31:679-687.

Lee GM, Fleisher GR, Harper MB: Management of febrile children in the age of the conjugate pneumococcal vaccine: A cost-effectiveness analysis. Pediatrics 2001;108:835-844.

Whitney C, Farley M, Hadler J, et al: Decline in invasive pneumococcal disease after the introduction of protein-polysaccharide conjugate vaccine. N Engl J Med 2003;348:1737-1746.

Urinary Tract Infection

American Academy of Pediatrics: Practice parameter: The diagnosis, treatment, and evaluation of the initial urinary tract infection in febrile infants and young children. Pediatrics 1999;103:843-852.

Bachur R, Harper MB: Reliability of the urinalysis for predicting urinary tract infections in young febrile children. Arch Pediatr Adolesc Med 2001;155:60-65.

Goldsmith B, Campos J: Comparison of urine dipstick, microscopy, and culture for the detection of bacteriuria in children. Clin Pediatr 1990;29:214-218.

Hoberman A, Wald E, Reynolds E, et al: Is urine culture necessary to rule out urinary tract infection in young febrile children? Pediatr Infect Dis J 1996;15:304-309.

Hoberman A, Wald E, Reynolds E, et al: Pyuria and bacteriuria in urine specimens obtained by catheter from young children with fever. J Pediatr 1994;124:513-519.

Nelson D, Gurr M, Schunk J: Management of children with urinary tract infections. Am J Emerg Med 1998;16:643-647.

Shaw K, McGowan K, Gorelick M, et al: Screening for urinary tract infection in infants in the emergency department: Which test is best? Pediatrics 1996;101:E1. (Available at Hyperlink http://www.pediatrics.org/cgi/content/full/101/6/e1; accessed October 29, 2003)

Antipyretic Therapy

Axelrod P: External cooling in the management of fever. Clin Infect Dis 2000;31:S224-S229.

Bonadio W, Bellomo T, Brady W, et al: Correlating changes in body temperature with infectious outcome in febrile children who receive acetaminophen. Clin Pediatr 1993;32:343-346.

Friedman A, Barton L: Efficacy of sponging vs acetaminophen for reduction of fever. Sponging Study Group. Pediatr Emerg Care 1990;6:6-7.

Mackowiak P: Diagnostic implications and clinical consequences of antipyretic therapy. Clin Infect Dis 2000;31:S230-S233.

Mackowiak P: Physiologic rationale for suppression of fever. Clin Infect Dis 2000;31:S185-S189.

Torrey S, Henretig F, Fleisher G, et al: Temperature response to antipyretic therapy in children: Relationship to occult bacteremia. Am J Emerg Med 1985;3:190-192.

Yamamoto L, Wigder H, Fligner D, et al: Relationship of bacteremia to antipyretic therapy in febrile children. Pediatr Emerg Care 1987;3:223-227.

Antibiotic Therapy

Gilbert DN, Moellering RC, Sande MA: The Sanford Guide to Antimicrobial Therapy 2001. Hyde Park, Vt, Antimicrobial Therapy, 2001.

Nelson JD, Bradley JS: Nelson's Pocket Book of Pediatric Antimicrobial Therapy. Philadelphia, Lippincott Williams & Wilkins, 2000.

Siberry GK, Iannone R: Formulary: The Harriet Lane Handbook. St. Louis, Mosby, 2000.

58 Fever and Neutropenia

Philip A. Pizzo

Neutropenia is the condition of a decreased number of circulating neutrophils. The absolute neutrophil count (ANC) is calculated by multiplying the white blood cell count by the percentage of polymorphonuclear leukocytes and band forms. An ANC of less than 1000 cells/mm^3 in white infants between the ages of 2 weeks and 1 year and an ANC of less than 1500 cells/mm^3 in older children is considered to represent neutropenia. African-American children tend to normally have ANCs that are 200 to 600 cells/mm^3 lower than those of white children.

An ANC less than 500 cells/mm^3 is associated with an increased risk for infection; this risk is highest with profound neutropenia (ANC < 100 cells/mm^3) or prolonged neutropenia (>1 week).

The risk for infection is particularly heightened when there are additional problems with the host defense matrix, such as altered physical defense barriers (e.g., oral or gastrointestinal mucositis, central venous catheters). Patients who present with an ANC between 500 and 1000 cells/mm^3 but whose ANC is expected to fall below 500 cells/mm^3 within the following 24 to 48 hours are also at risk for an infection and should be promptly evaluated and treated. *Fever* is usually defined as a single oral temperature of at least 38.5° C or three successive readings of at least 38° C in a 24-hour period.

This chapter concentrates on patients who have repeated or prolonged episodes of neutropenia that are most often caused by cancer therapy–induced myelosuppression. Numerous congenital and other acquired disorders cause neutropenic states (Table 58-1, Fig. 58-1). Patients with these disorders often have recurrent mucocutaneous infections with *Staphylococcus aureus* or group A streptococci; those with severe and prolonged neutropenia tend to develop bacterial sepsis (see Chapter 51). Patients with chemotherapy-induced neutropenia have other disorders of host defense, such as mucosal breakdown from mucositis, monocytopenia, lymphopenia, and qualitative B and T lymphocyte defects. Much of the current understanding and approach to neutropenia with fever in children has been developed in patients with malignancies and chemotherapy-induced neutropenia.

DIAGNOSIS

Patient history, physical examination, and laboratory investigations are the mainstays of the diagnosis and monitoring of chemotherapy-induced neutropenia in patients with fever. These assessments should be performed at least once daily during the period of fever and neutropenia (Table 58-2). In addition to the degree and duration of neutropenia, other aspects of the patient's cellular and humoral immune defense, as well as the reason for the neutropenia (iatrogenic versus congenital versus infectious), also greatly influence the risk for infection. The onset of fever in a neutropenic patient should be considered an emergency. Rapid therapy is mandatory to prevent the development of or to treat high-grade bacteremia caused by an invasive organism that may quickly produce sepsis, shock, and death. Antibiotic treatment may initially be empirical and then modified by findings obtained through repeated assessments. Negative laboratory or radiographic findings do not exclude an infectious focus for the fever, because the diminished inflammatory response resulting from the neutropenia may alter the classic signs and symptoms of infection. Pain, tenderness, and induration may nevertheless be present in soft tissue infections. When such symptoms are present in profoundly neutropenic patients who are afebrile, it is equally important to evaluate and treat such patients as if they were infected. Certain organisms, such as *Clostridium septicum,* can result in life-threatening infections in neutropenic patients in the absence of fever.

HISTORY

The history follows traditional guidelines (Table 58-3). For accurate detection of fever, oral temperatures should be checked at least three times daily. Patients at risk for neutropenia should understand the importance of fever and should be seen by a physician within 2 hours of its onset. More than a third of affected patients may present with other infectious or noninfectious conditions (e.g., dehydration, systemic hypotension, inadequate pain control, bleeding), which complicate the presentation.

The *duration of neutropenia* is crucial in the evaluation. It is also important to note whether this is the first occurrence of fever during the current episode of neutropenia or whether the patient has a recurrent or persistent fever (described later). Determining the nature and timing of the antecedent chemotherapy is important. Certain cytotoxic agents are only mildly myelosuppressive, and recovery from neutropenia is relatively rapid. Other drug combinations (or even use of fewer myelosuppressive agents in patients who have received high-dose chemotherapy) cause a profound and prolonged dose-dependent neutropenia. Furthermore, particular infectious syndromes can be associated with certain chemotherapeutic agents. Cytosine arabinoside typically causes oral mucositis, which is associated with an increased frequency of *Streptococcus mitis* infections. It is also important to recognize that the concurrent use of other medications can be a cofactor in the development of neutropenia (e.g., the use of antibiotics such as trimethoprim-sulfamethoxazole or the use of therapeutic antiviral agents for treatment of human immunodeficiency virus [HIV] infection). The use of a bone marrow–stimulating cytokine, such as granulocyte-macrophage colony–stimulating factor or granulocyte colony–stimulating factor, can reduce the expected duration and depth of neutropenia. Chronic steroid therapy not only increases the risk for infection but also may blunt the ability of the patient to develop a fever in response to an infection.

Questions regarding the patient's medical history should include information about previous episodes of fever and neutropenia; their course, duration, and complications; and whether a specific organism was isolated. The underlying illness also influences the choice and dosage of empirical antibiotic therapy (e.g., imipenem-cilastatin should be avoided by a patient with a brain tumor because of the risk of seizures).

Patients with HIV disease are often severely immunocompromised in addition to being neutropenic. They appear to be at a higher risk for certain opportunistic infections. They may suffer chronic or

Table 58-1. Etiologic Factors in Neutropenia

Congenital Neutropenias

Kostmann syndrome (severe congenital autosomal recessive neutropenia)

Chronic benign (idiopathic) neutropenia (occasionally familial and autosomal dominant)

Fanconi anemia

Schwachman syndrome (chronic moderate neutropenia, pancreatic insufficiency)

Cartilage-hair hypoplasia (moderate neutropenia, short-limb dwarfism, abnormal cellular immunity, fine hair)

Dyskeratosis congenita (neutropenia in 1/3 of patients, nail dystrophy, leukoplakia, skin hyperpigmentation)

Neutropenia associated with metabolic disturbances (organic acidemias)

Reticular dysgenesis

Cyclic neutropenia

Neutropenia with agammaglobulinemia and dysgammaglobulinemia

Acquired Neutropenias

Aplastic anemia

Reticuloendothelial sequestration (hypersplenism)

Infections (sepsis, HIV infection, tuberculosis, acute viral or rickettsial infections)

Autoimmune or neonatal isoimmune neutropenia, systemic lupus erythematosus

Bone marrow infiltration and replacement with malignant cells (leukemia, neuroblastoma)

Drug induced (chemotherapy for cancer treatment, immunosuppression for other diseases, antibiotics, [especially sulfa drugs], anticonvulsants, antipsychotics, antithyroid agents, cardiovascular agents, antihistamines, NSAID, AZT, antivirals)

Radiation therapy

Osteopetrosis

AZT, zidovudine; HIV, human immunodeficiency virus; NSAID, nonsteroidal antiinflammatory drug.

recurrent bacterial or viral infections, even after an adequate course of antibiotic therapy has been completed. Patients with cancer or aplastic anemia are at much higher risk for developing invasive fungal infections with *Aspergillus* species or *Candida* species, especially when the duration of neutropenia is protracted (e.g., >14 days).

An exposure history is important in determining the pathogens most likely to be involved. A hospitalized patient usually becomes colonized with multidrug-resistant organisms common to that environment. The balance of the patient's own endogenous flora is often shifted toward more resistant and virulent bacteria. Infections with gram-positive bacteria, especially with coagulase-negative staphylococci resistant to β-lactam antibiotics, are common. The number of infections with *Pseudomonas aeruginosa* has decreased. If a fever occurs while the patient is an outpatient, it is important to know whether other close contacts have been sick. However, most infections in the immunocompromised host arise from the patient's endogenous flora and cannot be avoided.

An in-depth review of systems can reveal minor complaints that may help determine the cause of the fever. Information about perianal tenderness or pain associated with defecation is not usually volunteered by patients but can be indicative of perianal cellulitis or abscess. The presence of any foreign bodies (e.g., central venous catheters, intraventricular reservoirs or shunts, prosthetic devices,

patches after cardiac surgery) must be noted and considered when antimicrobial therapy is chosen.

PHYSICAL EXAMINATION

A meticulous physical examination must be repeated daily as long as the patient is febrile and neutropenic. Particular attention must be directed to common but often occult sites of infection, such as the oral cavity, the periungual area, and the perianal area. Examination of the perirectal area should usually be limited to careful inspection and external palpation. A careful rectal examination should be performed only when symptoms strongly suggest a localized infection (e.g., tenderness or fluctuance). The area around the exit site of a central venous catheter should be inspected and palpated daily; attention must be given to skin lesions and tenderness around the fingernails and toenails.

LABORATORY EVALUATION

Cultures of blood, urine, and any site of presumed infection are essential. Despite cultures, the cause of the fever may not be identified initially in nearly 70% of patients.

Therapy in chemotherapy-induced neutropenia with fever must never be delayed because of the lack of a proven infectious organism. Therapy is initiated empirically in such cases. Some centers recommend routine surveillance cultures in patients with prolonged neutropenia, with the rationale that most organisms causing infections in the immunocompromised host arise from the endogenous flora or are acquired in the hospital. The predictive yield of these cultures is low, and they are rarely justified. Possible exceptions include cultures from the anterior nares to diagnose colonization with methicillin-resistant *S. aureus* or *Aspergillus* species in centers where outbreaks or a high prevalence of those infections have been observed.

At least two sets of blood specimens should be obtained for culture from all patients. If a central venous catheter is present, a culture from each lumen is warranted. Although anaerobic bacteria cause only about 5% of documented bacteremic episodes, aerobic and anaerobic cultures are important. Cultures for bacteria and fungi and a specimen with Gram stain should be obtained from any infectious site, including the exit site of a central venous catheter. If a lesion is chronically infected, special stains and cultures for *Mycobacterium* organisms should be performed as well. Diarrheal stool should be assessed for *Clostridium difficile* toxin, bacteria, viruses, and parasites. Urine culture and analysis are part of the routine evaluation. Pyuria may be absent in the neutropenic patient with a urinary tract infection.

The value of viral cultures or polymerase chain reaction in the initial evaluation of the febrile neutropenic patient is less defined. For patients with respiratory symptoms, specimens should be obtained to look for respiratory viruses, and for patients with mucositis, even if they are presumed to have chemotherapy-induced stomatitis, specimens should be obtained to look for herpes simplex virus infection. Specimens of vesicular skin lesions should be obtained to detect herpes viruses, and a DFA (direct fluorescent antibody) should be performed. The initiation of empirical antibacterial therapy should not, however, be postponed because of the possibility of a viral cause.

Deep-seated tissue infections can be diagnostically and therapeutically challenging. Infections of the liver and spleen (e.g., hepatosplenic candidiasis) are sometimes difficult to visualize with radiographic methods when a patient is neutropenic. When such infections are highly suspected, a computed tomography (CT)–directed, open, or laparoscopic biopsy can be considered. Pulmonary lesions can have an infectious (bacterial or fungal) origin or an embolic origin, or they can represent a complication of the underlying disease (metastases). Unfortunately, endoscopy can be

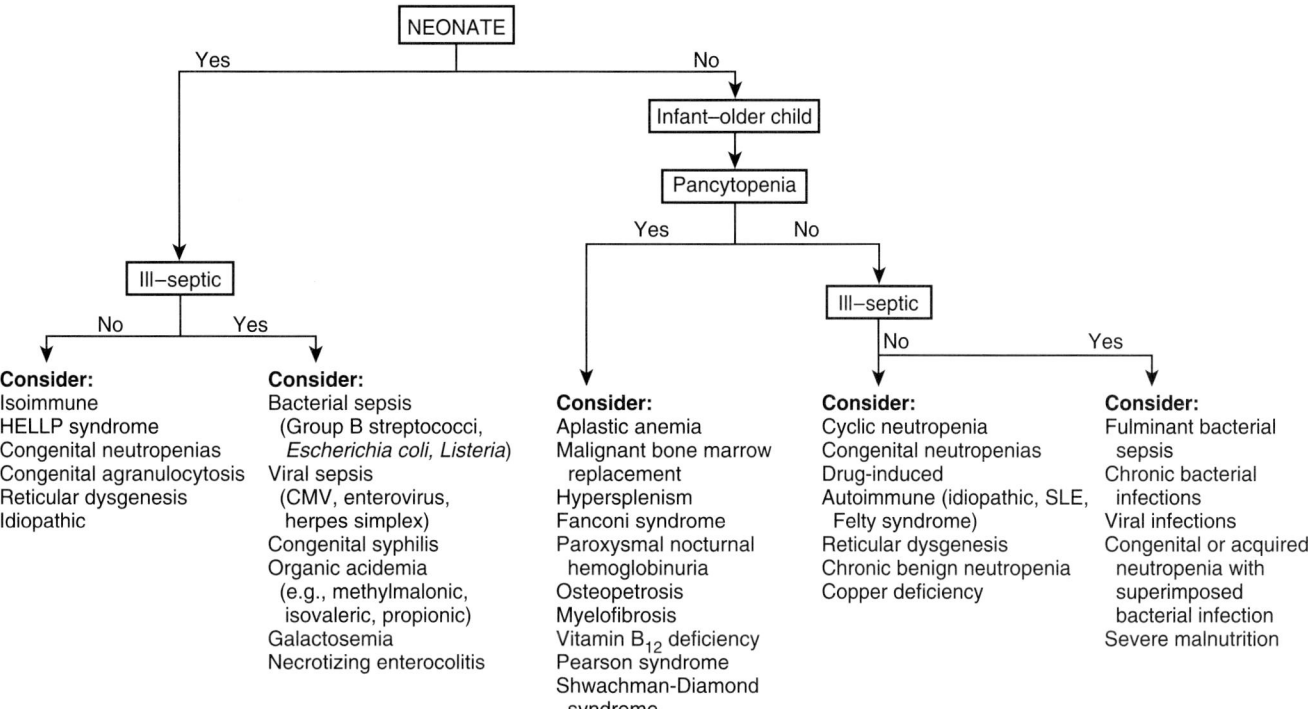

Figure 58-1. Diagnostic approach to neutropenia. CMV, cytomegalovirus; HELLP, preeclampsia-induced neutropenia with hemolysis, elevated liver enzymes, and low platelets; SLE, systemic lupus erythematosus.

associated with a high risk of bacteremia in the neutropenic patient who may also have friable mucosa. The presence of mucositis and thrombocytopenia often makes surgical interventions and biopsies less feasible. A definitive diagnosis of deep tissue infections may need to be postponed until the neutropenia has resolved.

IMAGING

A radiograph is usually obtained at presentation (especially in patients with pulmonary symptoms or those anticipated to have protracted neutropenia [i.e., >10 to 14 days]) and thereafter as clinically indicated or at least weekly in the patient with persistent neutropenia. Radiologic findings may be subtle but become more prominent once the neutrophil count recovers. This phenomenon occurs even when the patient is clinically improving. Chest radiographs are usually normal in patients without respiratory symptoms but can be useful in the diagnosis of pulmonary aspergillosis. Chest CT can be helpful in patients with normal chest radiographs, especially in the setting of prolonged fever. Ultrasonography, CT, and magnetic resonance imaging are used to identify the presence of hepatosplenic candidiasis, but the results can remain inconclusive until the granulocyte count recovers.

Bone scans with technetium 99m may be helpful in a symptomatic patient, but their interpretation can be difficult in patients with bone metastases. Because of the diminished inflammatory response, a gallium scan is usually not helpful.

DIFFERENTIAL DIAGNOSIS

Two important factors must be considered in the differential diagnosis of fever and neutropenia: age and underlying immune status of the patient (Table 58-4; see Fig. 58-1 and Table 58-1).

NEUTROPENIA IN THE CHILD WITHOUT IMMUNODEFICIENCY

Neonates

Neonatal neutropenia occurs most frequently during the first week of life; 43% of such episodes are reported on the day of birth. Fewer than 40% of these neonates have an identifiable infectious cause (see Table 58-4). An elevated temperature is not always present in the infected neonate; indeed, septic neonates often demonstrate hypothermia. Empirical antibiotic therapy is often initiated for 2 to 3 days and stopped if cultures remain negative. If the neutropenia is prolonged, there is an increased risk of infections with nosocomial, endogenous, or fungal organisms, as seen in children with neonatal isoimmune neutropenia. This form of neutropenia results from the presence of maternal immunoglobulin G antineutrophil antibodies after the mother becomes sensitized to the paternal antigens on the fetal neutrophil. This condition is analogous to hemolytic disease of the newborn. The organisms recovered in neonates vary according to several factors: onset of fever and neutropenia (first day after birth versus later), degree of general supportive care necessary (regular well-baby nursery versus intensive care unit), and duration of neutropenia.

Primary acquired autoimmune neutropenia in infancy is associated with a higher incidence of infections, particularly otitis media, upper respiratory tract infections, and benign skin infections; routine antibiotic therapy is usually sufficient.

Older Children

The risk for infectious complications in well-appearing children with transient neutropenia and without an underlying immune defect is low but increases with the duration of neutropenia. In a study of 119 otherwise immunocompetent patients with a median duration of neutropenia of 13 days (range, 1 to 491 days), only four patients

Table 58-2. Evaluation of the Febrile Neutropenic Patient with Chemotherapy-Induced Neutropenia

	Time of Evaluation	Comment
History and physical examination	Daily	See Table 58-3 for history
Laboratory studies		
Complete blood cell count with differential	At pretreatment evaluation and then daily	Less frequently in patients with known protracted neutropenia (after bone marrow transplantation, aplastic anemia)
Chemistry profile, electrolyte levels	At pretreatment evaluation and then at least weekly	To monitor kidney and liver function
Drug levels	Within 36 hours of initiation of certain antibiotics	In patients receiving aminoglycosides, vancomycin, or flucytosine
Blood cultures	Daily until negative Daily until patient is afebrile Daily if there is a new fever	Blood cultures should be drawn from each port if a multilumen central venous line is used Peripheral cultures at least initially and once daily if there is a new fever
Urine culture	At pretreatment evaluation With any urinary tract symptoms	—
Throat culture	At pretreatment evaluation	—
Cultures of sites of infection	At pretreatment evaluation	Exit site of central venous catheters, skin lesions, drainage fluid
Radiographic Studies		
Chest radiograph	At pretreatment evaluation Weekly with persistent fever With new fevers or symptoms	At initial evaluation in all patients, regardless of symptoms (complaints can be minimal)
Only in Selected Patients		
Lumbar puncture	Not routinely necessary except in special patient populations	Indicated in febrile (neutropenic) newborns and infants Indicated in patients with intraventricular foreign bodies (shunt, reservoir) if no evidence of increased intracranial pressure present In symptomatic patients (headache, meningismus)
Virus cultures/PCR	At pretreatment evaluation in symptomatic patients In patients with protracted fever of unknown origin	URI symptoms: respiratory viruses Prolonged fever: cytomegalovirus, herpes simplex, HHV-6 Skin lesions: herpes simplex, varicella-zoster Hematuria: adenovirus
Sputum examination	Daily in intubated patients Limited yield in most nonintubated patients	Induced sputum or bronchoalveolar lavage may be helpful in patient with chronic lung infections or HIV infection and respiratory symptoms
Endoscopy	Avoid if possible during neutropenia	Empirical treatment often preferable
Other radiographic evaluations (MRI, CT, ultrasonography)	Indicated in selected patients or clinical settings	CT of lung is more sensitive than plain chest films to detect fungal lesions CT or MRI of liver and/or spleen helpful in diagnosing hepatosplenic candidiasis (see Chapter 19) Sinus films or CT in patients with symptoms or fever for >7 days Esophagogram in patients with symptoms (mucositis, odynophagia, retrosternal pain)

Nuclear medicine evaluations:
  Indium white blood cell scan
  Gallium scan
		Only with specific localizing symptoms
		Often unreliable because of the lack of an inflammatory response

Bone scan		—

CT, computed tomography; HHV-6, human herpes virus 6; HIV, human immunodeficiency virus; MRI, magnetic resonance imaging; PCR, polymerase chain reaction; URI, upper respiratory infection.

(whose neutropenia lasted more than 30 days) developed an infectious complication (stomatitis in two, cellulitis in one, pneumonia in one). In another study, of 68 immunocompetent children with transient neutropenia, 5 of the 17 children who appeared ill at presentation had a serious bacterial infection (bacteremia or meningitis), but none of the 51 well-appearing children had an infectious focus.

NEUTROPENIA IN THE CHILD WITH AN IMMUNODEFICIENCY

Fever in the immunocompromised neutropenic patient is often of undetermined origin; evaluation and therapy must follow an empirical approach. The spectrum of likely infections varies according to the underlying disease, especially in the patient with prolonged

Table 58-3. Important Aspects of the History in the Febrile Neutropenic Patient

Chief complaint	Complaints are often minimal and frequently focused on the rapid onset of general malaise
History of current illness	Duration of fever, duration of neutropenia
	Current drugs (especially prophylactic antibiotics and cytokines)
	Date and type of last chemotherapy
Medical history	Previous episodes of fever and neutropenia (were any complications defined?)
	Underlying illness: its duration, stage, and treatment
Family history	Exposure history (other members of family sick?)
Review of systems	Headaches? Sinus pain? Earache? Rhinorrhea?
	Sore throat? Mouth ulcers? Pain with swallowing?
	Cough? Chest pain?
	Abdominal pain (constant, colicky, localized)?
	Tenderness in perirectal area?
	Diarrhea (mucoid, bloody, watery?)
	Dysuria? Frequency? Vaginal discharge?
	Tenderness around exit site of central venous catheter?
	Other skin lesions? Joint pain? Fingernail-toenail pain?
	Foreign bodies present?

Table 58-4. Fever and Neutropenia in the Child without Underlying Immunodeficiency

Neonate

Infectious Cause (40%)

Bacterial infections, onset of neutropenia on first day after birth, duration 2-4 days (35%)

Symptoms: sepsis, shock, respiratory distress, meningitis

Organisms: group B streptococci, *Escherichia coli, Klebsiella* species, *Listeria monocytogenes,* enterococci, *Haemophilus influenzae, Streptococcus pneumoniae*

Postnatal viral infections, onset of neutropenia on day 3 after birth, prolonged duration; more common in neonates who have undergone multiple transfusions (20%)

Symptoms: hepatitis, thrombocytopenia, respiratory distress

Organisms: most commonly cytomegalovirus, HSV

Associated with necrotizing enterocolitis in premature neonates, onset of neutropenia on day 20 after birth, duration 1-2 weeks (35%)

Organisms: often none recovered; possible association with *Clostridium perfringens, E. coli, Staphylococcus epidermidis,* rotavirus

Idiopathic (40%)

Isoimmune Cause (Neutrophil Count Normalized by 7 Weeks of Age)

Symptoms: mostly cutaneous infections

Organisms: *Staphylococcus aureus, E. coli,* α-hemolytic streptococci

Other Causes:

Maternal preeclampsia, postoperatively, post–exchange transfusion

Infant and Child

Transient Neutropenia, Autoimmune Neutropenia

Symptoms: severe infectious complications are rare; otitis media, skin infections, upper respiratory tract infections are most common

Organisms: *H. influenzae, S. pneumoniae, S. aureus,* group A streptococci

HSV, herpes simplex virus.

neutropenia. In the patient with an unknown source of fever (Table 58-5), diagnostic studies may be quite helpful.

S. aureus and coagulase-negative staphylococci are the most commonly recovered isolates (Table 58-6). The most common gram-negative organisms in neutropenic cancer patients are *Escherichia coli* and *Klebsiella pneumoniae;* the incidence of infections caused by *Enterobacter* species, however, appears to be rising. This is particularly worrisome because these organisms can induce bacterial β-lactamase production and rapidly develop resistance to cephalosporins and penicillins. It is unclear why the frequency of infections with *P. aeruginosa* has decreased in cancer patients since 1990. Children with HIV infection, especially if they have an indwelling central venous catheter, have a relatively high incidence of infections with this organism. Anaerobes are usually found only in patients with polymicrobial infections, especially if extensive mucosal damage (necrotizing gingivitis, perianal cellulitis) is present.

Patients with cancer and prolonged neutropenia and especially children with aplastic anemia are at risk for fungal infections (see Table 58-6). An aggressive search for possible foci should be initiated in the patient with prolonged (>5 to 7 days) neutropenia and persistent or recurrent fevers. The patient is also at risk for fungal infections if prolonged and repeated periods of neutropenia occurred in the past.

Candida species can cause a local infection (thrush, esophagitis), fungemia, or deep tissue infection (hepatosplenic candidiasis). Risk factors for the development of candidemia are previous bacteremia, prolonged neutropenia, fever, and administration of antimicrobial agents. *Candida* species recovered from blood should never be considered a contaminant, because it can be the only manifestation of an invasive infection. Hepatosplenic candidiasis can be very difficult to document until the neutrophil count recovers. This infection should be suspected in the patient with low-grade, recurrent fevers and a rise in serum alkaline phosphatase levels. Infection with *Aspergillus* species is a major concern in patients with aplastic anemia, relapsed leukemia, or with bone marrow transplants before engraftment. Invasive pulmonary aspergillosis is associated with a mortality rate as high as 95%. A common extrapulmonary site of aspergillosis or mucormycosis is the paranasal sinuses; an infection at this site can progress to the central nervous system and be fatal.

SPECIFIC SYMPTOMS

Subtle complaints or seemingly trivial findings on physical examination may indicate the presence of an infectious focus. Important findings not to be missed and red flags are listed in Table 58-7.

Table 58-5. Fever of Unknown Origin in the Immunocompromised Neutropenic Patient

	Organism	Evaluation
Cancer or Aplastic Anemia		
Early during neutropenia	Bacteria	Cultures, CXR
Prolonged neutropenia (≥7 days)	Bacteria, fungi (*Candida, Aspergillus*); less commonly viruses and/or parasites	Cultures; CXR; sinus films; CT of chest; CT, MRI, or ultrasound study of abdomen
Bone Marrow Transplantation	Bacteria (gram-positive and gram-negative) during the period of neutropenia *Streptococcus pneumoniae* infection in the chronic period (>100 days after allogeneic transplant) Herpes simplex early after transplantation; CMV approximately 50 days after transplantation; and varicella-zoster virus approximately 100 days after transplantation Fungi (*Candida, Aspergillus*) during the immediate posttransplantation period	Cultures (including surveillance cultures); CXR; sinus films; CT of chest; CT, MRI, or ultrasound study of abdomen
HIV Infection	Bacterial (gram-positive, gram-negative) Viral (CMV, HIV) Mycobacterial, including *Mycobacterium avium–intracellulare* and *Mycobacterium tuberculosis* Fungal (*Cryptococcus, Candida, Aspergillus*)	Cultures of blood and bone marrow, CXR, sinus films, CT of chest and abdomen

CMV, cytomegalovirus; CT, computed tomography; CXR, chest x-ray; HIV, human immunodeficiency virus; MRI, magnetic resonance imaging.

Headaches

Infections of the central nervous system are relatively uncommon in children with cancer, and a routine lumbar puncture in patients with fever and neutropenia is therefore not warranted except in affected young infants. However, if symptoms are suggestive of a central nervous system process, evaluation of the cerebrospinal fluid should include a Gram stain, routine bacterial and fungal cultures, and cryptococcal antigen determination, in addition to cell count with cytologic study and measurement of protein and glucose levels. Patients with intraventricular devices are at an increased risk for infections with bacteria that commonly colonize the skin (coagulase-positive and coagulase-negative staphylococci, *Corynebacterium* species, and enterococci). In one study, *Propionibacterium acnes* was the most common pathogen, sometimes producing no clinical symptoms. *Listeria monocytogenes* can cause meningitis in patients with impaired T lymphocyte function; patients often present with low-grade fevers and personality changes. In the severely immunosuppressed patient, regardless of neutrophil count, the presence of infections with fungal (*Cryptococcus* species), viral (herpes simplex virus, varicella-zoster virus, cytomegalovirus, Epstein-Barr virus), or parasitic (*Toxoplasma gondii*) pathogens should be considered. A brain abscess can occur rarely in such patients.

Ears and Nose

The most likely pathogens to cause ear infections in children with fever and neutropenia are the same as in the immunocompetent host (*Streptococcus pneumoniae*, nontypeable *Haemophilus influenzae*, *Moraxella* species). In addition, the gram-positive and gram-negative organisms that colonize the oropharynx and nasopharynx must be considered.

Sinusitis is often accompanied by only mild localized tenderness or minimal (often nonpurulent) nasal discharge. Bacterial infections are usually caused by the same organisms as in the immunocompetent host. Fungal infections are an additional concern in the patient with prolonged neutropenia (*Aspergillus* species, *Mucor* species, *Fusarium* species). In addition to the radiologic studies (sinus plain

films, CT, and/or magnetic resonance imaging), the diagnosis must often be established through a sinus aspirate or biopsy. Because such infections may extend intracranially, an aggressive diagnostic approach is mandatory. Surgical débridement and early institution of antifungal therapy are essential for patient survival.

Mouth or Throat Pain, Pain with Swallowing

Although mucositis can be caused by chemotherapy, it is necessary to exclude herpes simplex virus and *Candida albicans* infections. Gingivitis or periodontitis is usually caused by a mixed infection with aerobic and anaerobic pathogens. Esophagitis (cytomegalovirus, herpes simplex virus, *Candida* species) can manifest as retrosternal pain, dysphagia, odynophagia, emesis, or refusal to eat and drink.

Cough, Chest Pain, Abnormal Chest Radiograph

Infections of the respiratory tract are common in the immunocompromised patient. Symptoms and findings on physical examination can be minimal. Symptoms often worsen transiently, even with appropriate antibiotic treatment, when the neutrophil count is recovering. Although bacterial and viral infections are the most common pathogens, fungal organisms or parasites are occasionally recovered. Most symptoms can be caused by any of these microorganisms, but some should prompt immediate attention:

1. *Chest pain:* Although a noninfectious process (pulmonary embolus) can be responsible, an infection with *Aspergillus* species should be suspected.
2. *Nonproductive cough, chest pain, or effusion on chest radiograph:* These symptoms may be caused by infection with *Legionella* or *Mycoplasma* species (direct fluorescent antibody test or culture on special media is necessary for the diagnosis). In addition, infection with *S. pneumoniae* or gram-negative bacteria (e.g., *P. aeruginosa*) must also be considered.
3. *Hypoxemia and diffuse interstitial infiltrate on chest radiograph:* *Pneumocystis carinii* should be seriously considered in the hypoxic patient with minimal or diffuse findings on chest

Table 58-6. Predominant Organisms in the Cancer Patient with Fever and Neutropenia

Organism	Comment
Gram-Positive Bacteria	
Staphylococcus aureus	Methicillin-resistant organisms have emerged
Coagulase-negative staphylococci	Predominant pathogen in many centers, often associated with an infected intravascular catheter
α-Hemolytic streptococci	Oral mucositis; bacteremia can be associated with adult respiratory distress syndrome
Enterococci	Increased incidence, perhaps from the use of third-generation cephalosporins, which do not cover enterococci
	Vancomycin-resistant enterococci have emerged
Corynebacterium group JK	Arises often from cutaneous defects (intravascular catheter, cellulitis)
	More common after prolonged neutropenia and hospitalization
Clostridium difficile	Common infection after antibiotic therapy, may be nosocomial
Gram-Negative Bacteria	
Enterobacteriaceae (*Escherichia coli, Klebsiella pneumoniae*)	Predominant gram-negative organisms
Pseudomonas aeruginosa	Decreased incidence in cancer patients, but possibly increasing in HIV-infected patients
Enterobacter species, *Citrobacter, Serratia* species	Less common but potentially serious because of the risk of developing resistance to β-lactam antibiotics
Anaerobes	Often as part of polymicrobial infection, especially in the oral cavity, gastrointestinal tract, and perianal area
Fungi	
Candida species	Most common; thrush, esophagitis, candidemia, hepatosplenic candidiasis, endophthalmitis
Aspergillus species	Incidence varies with center; sinusitis and pulmonary infections in patients with prolonged profound neutropenia
Cryptococcus species	Solitary pulmonary lesions can be misdiagnosed as metastasis; patients with prolonged immunosuppression (HIV infection, aplastic anemia) are at risk for meningitis
Mucor species	Can cause invasive, necrotic sinusitis; orbital infections; erosive palate lesions; with central nervous system involvement in the patient with prolonged neutropenia (aplastic anemia)
Histoplasma capsulatum, Blastomyces dermatidis, Coccidioides immitis	Pulmonary or disseminated disease in immunocompromised hosts (in endemic areas)
Trichosporon beigelii, Fusarium species	Less common; can cause disseminated disease
Viruses	
Herpes simplex virus	Oral gingivostomatitis, esophagitis
Varicella-zoster virus	Not specifically associated with neutropenia; rather, associated with underlying immune status
Cytomegalovirus	In bone marrow transplant recipients and patients with aplastic anemia; can be associated with serious infection (especially pneumonitis, hepatitis, colitis)
Parasites	
Pneumocystis carinii, Strongyloides stercoralis, Cryptosporidium species	Not specifically associated with neutropenia; rather, associated with underlying immune status

HIV, human immunodeficiency virus.

radiographs. However, the patient with HIV infection rarely presents with the "typical" radiographic picture.

Bacterial pathogens predominate in patients with pneumonia whose neutropenia lasts less than 14 days, whereas fungal and other opportunistic infections are more commonly seen with prolonged neutropenia and lymphopenia. A chest radiograph may not initially show an infiltrate, even if the patient has clinical evidence of pneumonia. However, if an infiltrate is present, the distinction between patchy or diffuse infiltrates may help guide the differential diagnosis (Table 58-8, Fig. 58-2). Bronchoalveolar lavage or even an open-lung biopsy should be considered if the patient fails to respond to empirical antimicrobial therapy.

Abdominal Pain, Diarrhea, Perirectal Tenderness

Acute or subacute right lower quadrant pain and fever (especially in patients with acute leukemia) may indicate the presence of *typhlitis,*

a necrotizing cellulitis involving the cecum. The etiologic organisms include anaerobes and gram-negative bacilli, most notably clostridia and *P. aeruginosa.* These organisms may also cause pneumatosis intestinalis, noted on abdominal radiographs as cystic, gas-filled submucosal or subserosal bleblike lesions. In patients whose symptoms are progressing despite optimal antibiotic therapy, surgical intervention may be necessary.

Diarrhea with or without colicky abdominal pain is often caused by infection with *C. difficile,* a pathogen that produces toxins in association with prior or concurrent antibiotic therapy. *C. difficile* can be diagnosed with culture and toxin assay.

Mild abdominal pain, persistent low-grade fever, and a rising alkaline phosphatase level in a patient with prolonged periods of neutropenia (>7 days) may indicate hepatosplenic candidiasis. Radiographic studies may be unrevealing while the patient remains neutropenic, but CT, magnetic resonance imaging, or ultrasonography may help establish the diagnosis with neutrophil recovery, especially in patients who still remain febrile.

Table 58-7. Symptoms Not to Be Missed and Red Flags

Symptom	Consider
With Short Duration Neutropenia (<7 Days)	
Sinus tenderness	Bacterial sinusitis
Oral and esophageal mucositis	Infection with herpes simplex virus or *Candida* species
Pulmonary infiltrate	Bacteria or viral pneumonia
Abdominal pain	Typhlitis
Tenderness around exit site of catheter	Exit site or tunnel infection
Crepitus	Gas gangrene
Diarrhea	*Clostridium difficile* colitis
Perirectal tenderness	Anaerobic mixed cellulitis
With Prolonged Duration Neutropenia (>10 Days)	
Sinus tenderness, stuffy nose	Fungal sinusitis
Oral and esophageal mucositis	Infection with herpes simplex virus or *Candida* species
Chest pain with patchy infiltrate	Pulmonary aspergillosis
Abdominal pain with rising alkaline phosphatase level and leukocytosis at time of neutrophil recovery	Hepatosplenic candidiasis
Small, erythematous skin lesions	Disseminated candidiasis
Crepitus	Gas gangrene
Diarrhea	*C. difficile* colitis
Perirectal tenderness	Mixed cellulitis

Minor fissures, erosions, or ulcerations in the perianal area can result in a cellulitis, most commonly with gram-negative organisms, *S. aureus,* and anaerobes. During episodes of neutropenia, symptoms and findings may be minimal (tenderness, mild erythema, and, in rare cases, fluctuance). These symptoms can become more prominent when the neutrophil count rises. The progression of the symptoms and signs does not necessarily indicate that the current treatment is inadequate. In addition to receiving systemic antibiotics, the patient should be treated with sitz baths and stool softeners, and close attention should be paid to personal hygiene.

Urinary Tract Complaints

Urinary tract infections are relatively uncommon in children with fever and neutropenia, although the risk is increased in children with an obstructive urologic process, a neurogenic bladder dysfunction, or an indwelling bladder catheter. The diagnosis is complicated by the fact that neutropenic patients do not usually have pyuria, even in the presence of an active infection. In addition to bacterial infections, the urinary tract can also become infected with *C. albicans,* either as a superficial mucositis in the bladder or as part of a disseminated infection. The presence of pseudohyphae in the urine is not diagnostic of invasive disease.

Miscellaneous Symptoms and Complaints

Musculoskeletal infections are unusual in patients with cancer and can be difficult to diagnose because of the lack of an inflammatory response and the possibility of a complication associated with the underlying disease. Pain from leukemic infiltrates or metastases

Table 58-8. Common Pathogens Causing Pulmonary Infiltrates in the Febrile Neutropenic Patient*

Localized Infiltrate	Diffuse Infiltrate
Bacteria	**Bacteria**
Common: *Streptococcus pneumoniae, Haemophilus influenzae*	Common: *S. pneumoniae, H. influenzae*
Rare: *Klebsiella* species, *Pseudomonas* species, *Staphylococcus aureus, Mycobacterium* species, *Nocardia* species	Rare: *Legionella, Chlamydia, Nocardia, Mycobacterium* species
	Mycoplasma
Fungi	**Fungi**
Common: *Aspergillus, Cryptococcus, Histoplasma* species	Common: *Aspergillus* species, *Pneumocystis carinii, Cryptococcus* species, *Histoplasma* species
Rare: Zygomycetes, *Candida* species	Rare: Zygomycetes, *Candida* species
	Parasites
	Toxoplasma gondii, Strongyloides species
Viruses	**Viruses**
Herpes simplex virus, varicella-zoster virus	Herpes simplex virus, varicella-zoster virus, cytomegalovirus, measles virus, influenza virus, parainfluenza virus, respiratory syncytial virus, adenovirus

*Pathogens listed in order of frequency.

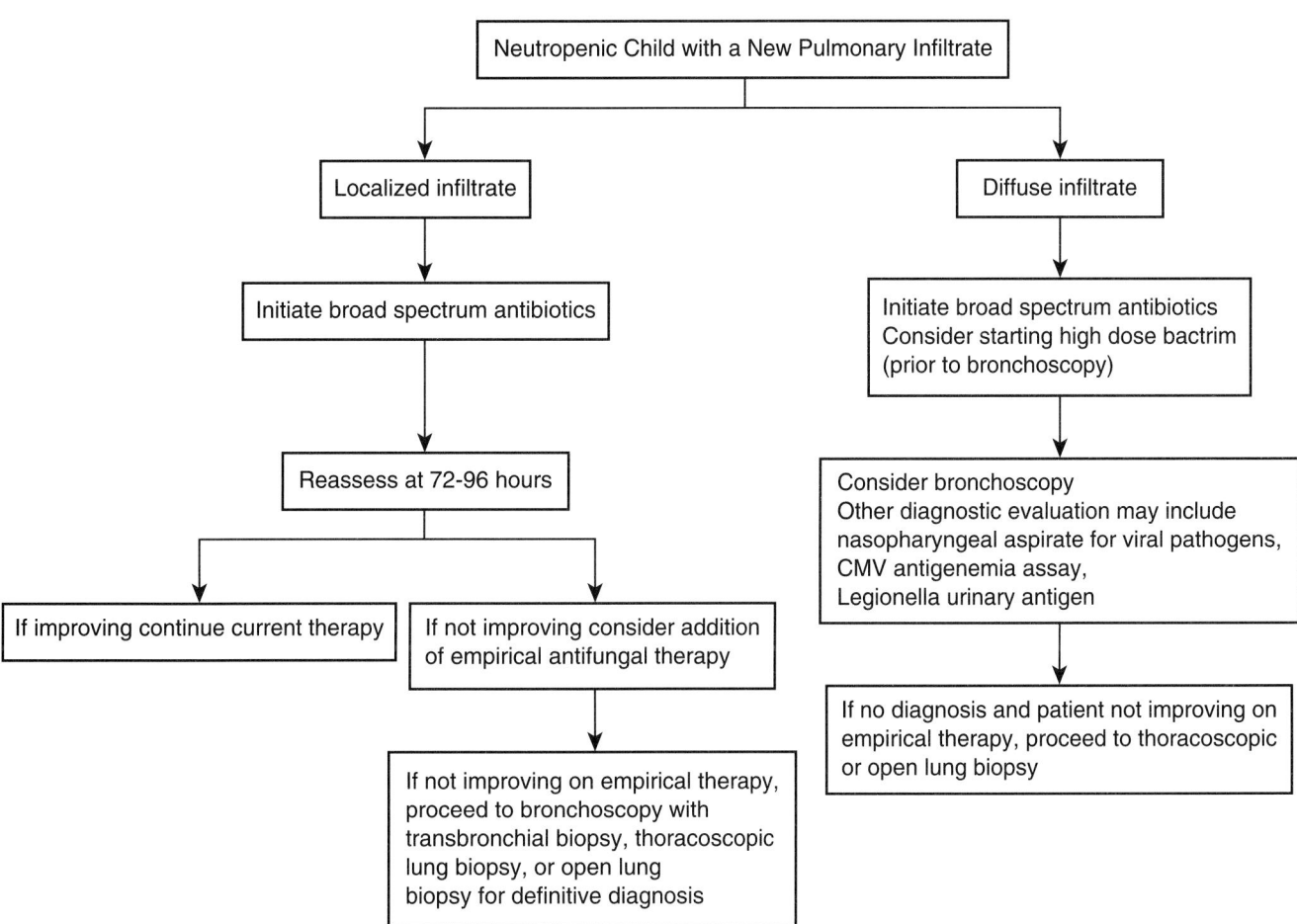

Figure 58-2. Algorithm for the management of the child with neutropenia and a pulmonary infiltrate. CMV, cytomegalovirus. (From Pizzo PA, Poplack DG [eds]: Principles and Practice of Pediatric Oncology, 4th ed. Philadelphia, Lippincott Williams & Wilkins, 2002, p 1244.)

must be distinguished from signs of infection. Immediate surgical intervention and antibiotic therapy are necessary if crepitus and soft tissue tenderness are present, because these symptoms suggest an infection with *Clostridium* organisms or toxin-producing *Bacillus cereus.*

Localized cutaneous infections can occur, primarily because the integrity of the epidermis is often iatrogenically disrupted by needle punctures, surgery, and radiation. Although uncommon, tropical myositis has been observed in immunocompromised children with cancer or HIV infection. Special attention should be paid to the exit site of central venous catheters because even extensive central catheter tunnel infections sometimes manifest with only minimal erythema and swelling. Such infections are usually characterized by tenderness along the subcutaneous tract of the catheter. Pathogens most commonly isolated include staphylococci, streptococci, and *Candida* species. In addition, the skin can become infected as part of a systemic infection with bacteria (*P. aeruginosa*), fungi (*Candida* species), or viruses (herpes simplex virus, varicella-zoster virus).

TREATMENT STRATEGIES

An important aspect of the treatment of the febrile neutropenic immunosuppressed patient is prompt initiation of empirical broad-spectrum antibiotics immediately after a careful evaluation.

Decisions about which antibiotics to use initially or to add to the regimen depend on the duration of the neutropenia and the patient's clinical and laboratory manifestations (Fig. 58-3, Table 58-9). An empirical regimen should include coverage for both gram-positive and gram-negative bacteria, including *P. aeruginosa*. The specific regimen used depends on the dominant isolates and the sensitivity pattern at the patient's treatment center. Common regimens include the use of either a third-generation cephalosporin (ceftazidime or cefepime) or a carbapenem (imipenem-cilastin or meropenem) alone or in combination with an aminoglycoside or another β-lactam antibiotic (Table 58-10). Whether vancomycin should be added to the initial empirical therapy or reserved until a specific isolate has been debated. In a randomized study of 550 episodes of fever and neutropenia, no treatment failures were observed when vancomycin was added only after a gram-positive infection had been documented. In centers where there is a high frequency of methicillin-resistant *S. aureus,* enterococci, or severe viridans streptococci (e.g., *S. mitis*), it is appropriate to include vancomycin in the initial antibiotic regimen.

Modifications to the initial empirical treatment are often required for patients with continued fever and neutropenia (see Table 58-9). Reasons to modify the initial regimen include the lack of a clinical response (e.g., persistent or new fever after a week of empirical therapy or evidence that the patient's condition is deteriorating); the isolation of a pathogen that is not optimally covered by the current regimen; the development of specific findings on physical examination;

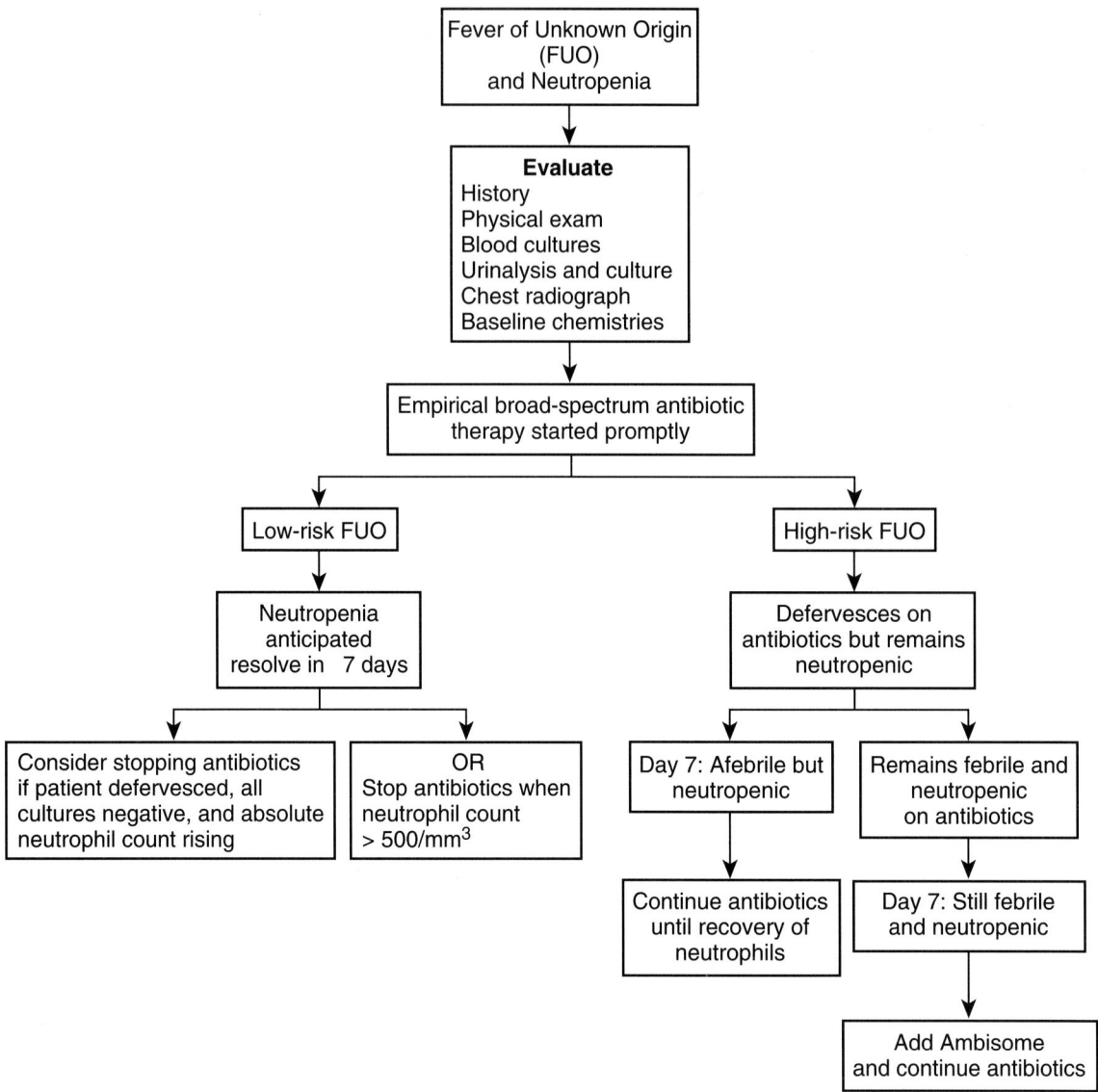

Figure 58-3. Algorithm for the initial management of the child who has unexplained fever and neutropenia. (From Pizzo PA, Poplack DG [eds]: Principles and Practice of Pediatric Oncology, 4th ed. Philadelphia, Lippincott Williams & Wilkins, 2002, p 1255.)

or the emergence of a fungal, viral, or parasitic infection. The antimicrobial drugs most often added include

- vancomycin for *Staphylococcus epidermidis,* methicillin-resistant *S. aureus, Corynebacterium* species, or α-hemolytic streptococci
- aminoglycosides for *P. aeruginosa, Enterobacter* species, *Serratia* species, or *Citrobacter* species because these organisms are more likely to break through single-agent coverage as a result of inducible β-lactamases or mutations
- clindamycin or metronidazole, when the initial regimen does not have adequate antianaerobic coverage and a site of presumably mixed infection is defined (e.g., necrotizing gingivitis, perianal abscess)
- amphotericin B or a liposomal formulation (e.g., AmBisome) for suspected or proven fungal infection in patients who remain febrile and neutropenic for 7 or more days
- acyclovir for suspected or proven herpesvirus infection
- ganciclovir for cytomegalovirus infection

Indwelling central venous catheters can be associated with local infections (exit site infection, tunnel infection), bacteremia, or fungemia. The incidence of infectious complications appears to be similar in patients with externalized catheters (Hickman, Broviac) or subcutaneously implanted devices (port-A-Cath, MediPort), and such infections can occur regardless of whether the patient is neutropenic. An exit site infection can usually be managed without removal of the catheter, except for infections with *Mycobacterium* or *Aspergillus* species. However, tunnel infections usually persist unless the catheter is removed. Most bacteremias can be treated without removal of the catheter, if three important caveats are considered:

1. The catheter has to be removed if *Candida* species or *Bacillus* species is isolated, if there is evidence of a tunnel infection, or if cultures remain persistently positive, despite adequate therapy.
2. Antibiotics must be given through *all* lumens of the catheter in a rotating manner, and specimens should be drawn for culture from all lumens as well.
3. If the placement of a new catheter is necessary, this should be performed only after at least 24 to 48 hours of antibiotic therapy have been completed and preferably when the patient is no longer neutropenic.

Table 58-9. Modifications of Initial Antimicrobial Regimen for Febrile Neutropenic Cancer Patients

Status or Symptom	Modifications of Primary Regimen
Fever	
Persistent for >5 days	Add empirical antifungal therapy
Recurrence after ≥5 days in patient with persistent neutropenia	Add empirical antifungal therapy
Persistent or recurrent fever at time of recovery from neutropenia	Evaluate liver and spleen with computed tomography, ultrasonography, or magnetic resonance imaging for hepatosplenic candidiasis, and evaluate need for antifungal therapy
Blood Stream	
Cultures before antibiotic therapy	—
Gram-positive organism	Add vancomycin pending further identification
Gram-negative organism	Maintain regimen if patient is stable and isolate is susceptible
	If *Pseudomonas aeruginosa, Enterobacter, Serratia,* or *Citrobacter* organism is isolated, add an aminoglycoside or, if resistant to cephalosporin, add a carbapenem
Organism isolated during antibiotic therapy	
Gram-positive organism	Add vancomycin
Gram-negative organism	Change to new combination regimen (e.g., meropenem plus gentamicin or vancomycin, or gentamicin plus piperacillin)
Head, Eyes, Ears, Nose, Throat	
Necrotizing or marginal gingivitis	Add specific antianaerobic agent (clindamycin or metronidazole) to empirical therapy
Vesicular or ulcerative lesions	Suspect herpes simplex infection; culture and begin acyclovir therapy
Sinus tenderness or nasal ulcerative lesions	Suspect fungal infection with *Aspergillus* or *Mucor* species
Gastrointestinal Tract	
Retrosternal burning pain	Suspect infection with *Candida* species, herpes simplex virus, or both; add antifungal therapy and, if no response, acyclovir; bacterial esophagitis is also a possibility; for patients who do not respond within 48 hr, endoscopy should be considered
Acute abdominal pain	Suspect typhlitis, as well as appendicitis, if pain in right lower quadrant; add specific antianaerobic coverage to empirical regimen and monitor closely for need for surgical intervention
Perianal tenderness	Add specific antianaerobic drug to empirical regimen and monitor need for surgical intervention, especially when patient is recovering from neutropenia
Respiratory Tract	
New focal lesion in patient recovering from neutropenia	Observe carefully, because this may be a consequence of inflammatory response in concert with neutrophil recovery
New focal lesion in patient with continuing neutropenia	*Aspergillus* species is the chief concern; perform appropriate cultures and consider biopsy; if patient is not a candidate for procedure, administer high-dose amphotericin B (1.5 mg/kg/day) or liposomal formulation
New interstitial pneumonitis	Attempt diagnosis by examination of induced sputum or bronchoalveolar lavage; if not feasible, begin empirical treatment with trimethoprim-sulfamethoxazole or pentamidine; consider noninfectious causes and the need for open-lung biopsy if condition has not improved after 4 days of therapy

From Pizzo PA, Poplack DG (eds): Principles and Practice of Pediatric Oncology, 4th ed. Philadelphia, Lippincott Williams & Wilkins, 2002, p 1260.

The duration of empirical therapy without positive cultures or without findings on physical examination depends on the recovery of the neutrophil count (see Fig. 58-3). For most proven infections, an adequate duration of treatment is a total of 10 to 14 days after the first negative culture. Therapy should be monitored with blood levels when indicated (vancomycin, aminoglycosides); kidney and liver function should be evaluated regularly so that antibiotic dosages can be adjusted.

PREVENTIVE STRATEGIES

Three approaches have been explored to prevent infections in neutropenic patients.

Preventing Exogenous Infections. The most important preventive strategy remains careful hand washing by all caregivers. Various isolation methods have been studied, but the results are controversial. The use of high-efficiency particulate air-filtered or laminar air-flow rooms is expensive, and their use is probably limited to patients who are anticipated to have a very prolonged neutropenia (e.g., a patient who has undergone bone marrow transplantation or other profound immunosuppression).

Preventing Endogenous Infections. Most infections are derived from endogenous flora. Several studies have evaluated regimens attempting "gut decontamination" with oral nonabsorbable antibiotics; most have failed to demonstrate a clear benefit. However, specific indications for prophylaxis exist, including the use of

Table 58-10. Commonly Used Antimicrobial Agents for Pediatric Cancer Patients

Class	Agent	Spectrum	Daily Dose (Maximum)	Comments
Antibiotics				
Third-generation cephalosporin	Ceftazidime	Enteric bacteria, some gram-positive aerobes; no anaerobic coverage	100 mg/kg divided q8h (6 g/day)	Only ceftazidime covers *Pseudomonas aeruginosa*
Fourth-generation cephalosporin	Cefepime	Enteric bacteria, gram-positive aerobes	150 mg/kg divided q8h (4 g/day)	Active against some *P. aeruginosa, Enterobacter, Serratia* species resistant to ceftazidime; broader gram-positive spectrum
Carbapenems	Imipenem	Most gram-negative and gram-positive aerobes, including *P. aeruginosa,* enterococci; excellent anaerobic coverage	60-100 mg/kg divided q6h (4 g/day)	*Stenotrophomonas maltophilia* and *Burkholderia cepacia* not covered; add aminoglycoside for *P. aeruginosa*
	Meropenem	Similar to imipenem	60-120 mg/kg divided q8h (3 g/day)	Less likely than imipenem to cause seizures
Extended-spectrum penicillins	Piperacillin, azlocillin, mezlocillin	Enteric aerobes, including *P. aeruginosa, Enterobacter, Serratia;* anaerobes	300 mg/kg divided q4h (21 g/d)	Must be paired with an aminoglycoside for coverage of *P. aeruginosa*
	Piperacillin/ tazobactam	Similar to piperacillin; increased activity versus some gram-negative and anaerobes	300 mg/kg divided q6h (18 g/day)	Not adequate as monotherapy; for *P. aeruginosa,* aminoglycoside should be added
Monobactam	Aztreonam	Exclusively gram-negative aerobes, including *P. aeruginosa*	100-150 mg/kg divided q6h (8 g/day)	Limited spectrum requires pairing with gram-positive agent; not cross-reactive with β-lactams so can be used by penicillin- or cephalosporin-allergic patients
Glycopeptide	Vancomycin	Exclusive gram-positive	25-40 mg/kg divided q6-12h (4 g/day)	No need to add vancomycin routinely for empirical coverage for fever and neutropenia
	Linezolid	Exclusively gram-positive, including vancomycin-resistant enterococci, methicillin-resistant *Staphylococcus aureus,* and penicillin- and cephalosporin-resistant pneumococci	10 mg/kg q12h	Excellent oral bioavailability
	Quinupristin/ dalfopristin	Exclusively gram-positive, similar to linezolid	7.5 mg/kg q8h	Venous irritation; should be given via central venous catheter
Antifungals				
Amphotericin	Amphotericin B	Very broad antifungal activity including *Candida, Aspergillus, Zygomycetes, Cryptococcus Histoplasma* species	0.5 mg/kg/day for empirical therapy; higher doses (1.0-1.5 mg/kg) are necessary for aspergillosis	Significant nephrotoxicity may be reduced by saline hydration before daily infusion
	Lipid formulations (liposomal amphotericin B, amphotericin B lipid complex, amphotericin B colloidal dispersion)	Same spectrum as nonlipid formulation	3 mg/kg for empirical therapy, ≥5 mg/kg for aspergillosis	Significantly less nephrotoxicity with equal efficacy
Azoles	Ketoconazole	*Candida albicans, Cryptococcus* species, *Histoplasma* species	5-10 mg/kg/day orally	Gastric acidity required for absorption
	Fluconazole	*C. albicans,* but not *Candida krusei* and some *Candida glabrata; Cryptococcus* species	6-12 mg/kg/day	Gastric acidity required for absorption

Table 58-10. Commonly Used Antimicrobial Agents for Pediatric Cancer Patients—cont'd

Class	Agent	Spectrum	Daily Dose (Maximum)	Comments
	Itraconazole	*Aspergillus, Histoplasma, Blastomyces* species	6-8 mg/kg/day	Absorption erratic but increased by taking drug with meals
	Voriconazole	*Aspergillus, Candida* but not *Zygomycetes*	4-8 mg/kg b.i.d.	Some consider this treatment of choice for initial empirical therapy
Antiviral				
Antiherpetics	Acyclovir	HSV, VZV	HSV: 750 mg/m^2 divided q8h; VZV: 1,500 mg/m^2 divided q8h	Intravenous dose VZV is twice that for HSV; hydration should be ensured when high doses are given
	Ganciclovir	CMV, HSV, VZV	CMV: 5 mg/kg q12h for 14 days then 5 mg/kg/day for maintenance	Granulocytopenia is the major dose-limiting toxicity; not routinely used for HSV and VZV, but dose used for CMV should be effective for the other herpesviruses
	Foscarnet	HSV, VZV, CMV (including most acyclovir- and ganciclovir-resistant strains)	CMV: 60 mg/kg/day q8h for 14 days, then 90-120 mg/kg/day for maintenance;VZV, HSV:40 mg/kg q8h	Nephrotoxicity is dose-limiting effect; renal function and electrolytes require close monitoring
Anti-PCP agents	Trimethoprim-sulfame-thoxazole	*Pneumocystis carinii, Entamoeba histolytica;* also covers routine gram-positive and gram-negative bacteria, plus *S. maltophilia, B. cepacia*	20 mg/kg/day for PCP treatment	May cause bone marrow suppression in high doses
	Pentamidine	*P. carinii*	4 mg/kg/day for treatment	Adverse effects include pancreatitis, hypoglycemia, hypocalcemia, infusional hypotension
	Dapsone	*P. carinii*	2 mg/kg/day (for prophylaxis)	High incidence of hemolytic reactions, can also cause methemoglobinemia
	Atovaquone	*P. carinii*	30 mg/kg/day (1500 mg/day)	Suspension formulation has better bioavailability

From Pizzo PA, Poplack DG (eds): Principles and Practice of Pediatric Oncology, 4th ed. Philadelphia, Lippincott Williams & Wilkins, 2002, p 1246.

CMV, cytomegalovirus; HSV, herpes simplex virus; PCP, *Pneumocystis carinii* pneumonia, VZV, varicella-zoster virus.

trimethoprim-sulfamethoxazole for the prevention of *P. carinii* pneumonia in patients with leukemia or acquired immunodeficiency syndrome and the use of acyclovir and ganciclovir for the prevention of herpes simplex virus and cytomegalovirus infections, respectively, in the patient undergoing bone marrow transplantation. Fluoroquinolone prophylaxis is not recommended because of the emergence of resistant organisms.

Improving the Host Defense. Immunizations play an important role in the prevention of infections in the immunocompetent host, but active immunization is usually unsuccessful or unreliable in the immunocompromised patient. Passive immunization with intravenous immunoglobulins has no proven benefit in preventing infection in patients with neutropenia, but it may be of benefit in children with HIV infection. Hematopoietic growth factors (cytokines) shorten the duration of neutropenia. In addition, cytokines and certain cytotoxic agents (cyclophosphamide) are currently being investigated for their ability to increase the number of circulating progenitor cells that can be harvested and infused during times of neutropenia.

SUMMARY AND RED FLAGS

The early initiation of empirical broad-spectrum antibiotic therapy, combined with the careful monitoring of physical findings and an aggressive diagnostic approach, has significantly decreased the rates of morbidity and mortality from fever and neutropenia. Modifications of the current approach may be necessary as the spectrum of pathogens changes or as strategies that improve host defense mechanisms become more effective. Nonetheless, simple measures, such as hand washing and educating the patient and caregivers about contacting the physician in the event of fever continue to be some of the most important interventions.

All episodes of fever and neutropenia are medical emergencies and necessitate immediate evaluation, treatment, and hospitalization of the patient. Red flags include hypotension, poor capillary perfusion, reduced level of consciousness, and petechiae, which suggest fulminant bacterial infection and the items noted in Table 58-7.

REFERENCES

Neonatal Neutropenia

Aprikyan AA, Liles WC, Park JR, et al: Myelokathexis, a congenital disorder of severe neutropenia characterized by accelerated apoptosis and defective expression of *bcl-x* in neutrophil precursors. Blood 2000;95:320-327.

Baley ME, Stork EK, Warketin PI, et al: Neonatal neutropenia: Clinical manifestations, cause, and outcome. Am J Dis Child 1988;142:1161.

Funke A, Berner R, Traichel B, et al: Frequency, natural course, and outcome of neonatal neutropenia. Pediatrics 2000;106:45-51.

Neutropenia in Older Children

Alter BP: Aplastic anemia, pediatric aspects. Oncologist 1996;1:361-366.

Bruin MC, von dem Borne AE, Tamminga RY, et al: Neutrophil antibody specificity in different types of childhood autoimmune neutropenia. Blood 1999;94:1792-1802.

Feder HM Jr: Periodic fever, aphthous stomatitis, pharyngitis, adenitis: A clinical review of a new syndrome. Curr Opin Pediatr 2000;12:253-256.

Haddy TB, Rana SR, Castro O: Benign ethnic neutropenia: What is a normal absolute neutrophil count? J Lab Clin Med 1999;133:15-22.

Jonsson OG, Buchanan GR: Chronic neutropenia during childhood: A 13-year experience in a single institution. Am J Dis Child 1991;145:232-235.

Logue GL, Shastri KA, Laughlin M, et al: Idiopathic neutropenia: Antineutrophil antibodies and clinical correlations. Am J Med 1991;90:211-216.

Roilides E, Marshall D, Venzon D, et al: Bacterial infections in human immunodeficiency virus type 1–infected children: The impact of central venous catheters and antiretroviral agents. Pediatr Infect Dis J 1991;10:813.

Shastri KA, Logue GL: Autoimmune neutropenia. Blood 1993;81:1984-1995.

Visser G, Rake JP, Fernandes J, et al: Neutropenia, neutrophil dysfunction, and inflammatory bowel disease in glycogen storage disease type Ib: Results of the European Study on Glycogen Storage Disease Type I. J Pediatr 2000;137:187-191.

Young NS: Agranulocytosis. JAMA 1994;271:935-938.

Fever and Neutropenia in Cancer Patients

Dichter JR, Levine SJ, Shelhamer JH: Approach to the immunocompromised host with pulmonary symptoms. Hematol Oncol Clin North Am 1993;4:887.

Fergie JE, Patrick CC, Lott L: *Pseudomonas aeruginosa* cellulitis and ecthyma gangrenosum in immunocompromised children. Pediatr Infect Dis J 1991;10:496-500.

Gorelick MH, Owen WC, Seibel NL, et al: Lack of association between neutropenia and the incidence of bacteremia associated with indwelling central venous catheters in febrile pediatric cancer patients. Pediatr Infect Dis J 1991;10:506-510.

Pizzo PA: Fever in immunocompromised patients. N Engl J Med 1999;341:893-900.

Pizzo PA: The compromised host. In Goldman L, Bennett JC (eds): Cecil Textbook of Medicine, 21st ed. Philadelphia, WB Saunders, 2000, pp 1569-1580.

Shelhamer JH, Toews GB, Masur H, et al: Respiratory disease in the immunosuppressed patient. Ann Intern Med 1992;117:415-431.

Treatment of Fever and Neutropenia in Cancer Patients

Bow EJ, Ronald AR: Antibacterial chemoprophylaxis in neutropenic patients: Where do we go from here? Clin Infect Dis 1993;17:333-337.

Buchanan GR: Approach to the treatment of the febrile cancer patient with low-risk neutropenia. Hematol Oncol Clin North Am 1993;5:919.

Dale DC, Liles WC: Return of granulocyte transfusions. Curr Opin Pediatr 2000;12:18-22.

Freifeld AG: The antimicrobial armamentarium. Hematol Oncol Clin North Am 1993;4:813.

Freifeld A, Marchigiani D, Walsh T, et al: A double-blind comparison of empirical oral and intravenous antibiotic therapy for low-risk febrile patients with neutropenia during cancer chemotherapy. N Engl J Med 1999;29:305-311.

Freifeld AG, Walsh T, Marshall D, et al: Monotherapy for fever and neutropenia in cancer patients: A randomized comparison of ceftazidime versus imipenem. J Clin Oncol 1995;13:165-176.

Hughes WT, Armstrong D, Bodey GP, et al: Guidelines for the use of antimicrobial agents in neutropenic patients with unexplained fever. Clin Infect Dis 2002;34:730-751.

Jain Y, Arya LS, Kataria R: Neutropenic enterocolitis in children with acute lymphoblastic leukemia. Pediatr Hematol Oncol 2000;17:99-103.

Katz JA, Mustafa MM: Management of fever in granulocytopenic children with cancer. Pediatr Infect Dis J 1993;12:330-339.

Mueller BU, Pizzo PA: Cytokines and biological response modifiers in the treatment of infection. Cancer Treat Res 1998;96:201-222.

Mullen CA, Petropoulos D, Roberts WM, et al: Outpatient treatment of fever and neutropenia for low risk pediatric cancer patients. Cancer 1999;86:126-134.

Ozer H, Armitage JO, Bennett CL, et al: 2000 Update of recommendations for the use of hematopoietic colony-stimulating factors: Evidence-based, clinical practice guidelines. American Society of Clinical Oncology Growth Factors Expert Panel. J Clin Oncol 2000;18:3558-3585.

Riikonen P, Saarinen UM, Makipernaa A, et al: Recombinant human granulocyte-macrophage colony–stimulating factor in the treatment of febrile neutropenia: A double blind placebo-controlled study in children. Pediatr Infect Dis J 1994;13:197-202.

Rubin M, Hathorn JW, Marshall D, et al: Gram-positive infections and the use of vancomycin in 550 episodes of fever and neutropenia. Ann Intern Med 1988;108:30.

Viscoli C, Moroni C, Boni L, et al: Ceftazidime plus amikacin versus ceftazidime plus vancomycin as empiric therapy in febrile neutropenic children with cancer. Rev Infect Dis 1991;13:397-404.

Walsh TJ, Lee J, Lecciones J, et al: Empiric therapy with amphotericin B in febrile granulocytopenic patients. Rev Infect Dis 1991;13:496-503.

Winston DJ, Ho WG, Bruckner DA, et al: Beta-lactam antibiotic therapy in febrile granulocytopenic patients. Ann Intern Med 1991;115:849-859.

ENDOCRINE/METABOLIC DISORDERS

59 Disorders of Puberty

Mitchell E. Geffner*

Puberty is defined by both biologic and social standards. Puberty is the time when there is an increase in sex steroid production, resulting in physical changes such as breast development in girls and testicular enlargement in boys, as well as maturation of processes required for future fertility. Puberty, also known as adolescence, is the time when children make the transition to adult patterns of behavior, which involve maturity, responsibility, and sexuality.

NORMAL PUBERTAL DEVELOPMENT

TERMINOLOGY

Various terms are used to discuss puberty (Table 59-1). *Bone age* refers to the degree of epiphyseal calcification, width, and proximity to adjacent metaphyses and is a marker of physical maturity that normally corresponds to chronologic age. *Dental age* generally correlates with bone age. Bone age is usually determined from a radiograph of the left hand and wrist, with comparison to gender appropriate standards in Greulich and Pyle's bone age atlas. In infants and toddlers, a more accurate assessment of bone age can be determined from a radiograph of the hemiskeleton, with primary attention to epiphyses of the long bones. Delayed or advanced bone age occurs in many conditions; bone age is strongly influenced by sex steroid production. The timing of the onset of puberty is usually more closely linked to the bone age than to the chronologic age when the two are significantly discordant. Regardless of chronologic age, linear growth ceases when the bone age reaches 15 years in girls and 18 years in boys.

ANATOMY

Puberty is controlled by the production of gonadotropin-releasing hormone (GnRH) in the anterior hypothalamus. GnRH-containing cell bodies project axons to the median eminence, where they terminate on the hypothalamic portal vessels. This system is referred to as the GnRH pulse generator. After GnRH reaches the anterior pituitary gland via the portal vasculature, it stimulates the production of both follicle-stimulating hormone (FSH) and luteinizing hormone (LH) by the gonadotroph cells. In girls, both FSH and LH are required for estrogen production by ovarian granulosa cells. The regulated secretion of FSH and LH is also required for follicle growth, ovulation, and maintenance of the corpus luteum. In boys, FSH regulates spermatogenesis by Sertoli cells within the seminiferous tubules, and LH activates Leydig cells to produce testosterone. Androgens cause development of male internal and external reproductive organs and secondary sexual characteristics in both sexes by binding to receptor proteins in the cells of target tissues. Sex steroids also exert a negative feedback effect on the pituitary gland and hypothalamus.

PHYSIOLOGY

Perinatal Period and Infancy

Maternal estrogens stimulate breast development in both male and female fetuses. Maternal estrogens also stimulate uterine developmental and endometrial growth; at birth, withdrawal of the high levels of maternal estrogen and placental progesterone causes the infant endometrium to regress or even slough and manifests as vaginal bleeding (see Chapter 30).

At birth, levels of LH and FSH in both sexes rise markedly and remain elevated for several months. In the girl, FSH stimulates ovarian granulosa cells to produce 17β-estradiol sufficient to maintain prenatal breast development for up to 8 months of life. Estrogen-induced vaginal cornification is generally evident as abundant vaginal discharge at birth and is maintained as long as estrogens are produced. Ovarian size from birth to 3 months ranges from 0.7 to 3.6 cm³, decreasing to 2.7 cm³ by 12 months and to 1.7 cm³ by 24 months; this size persists until the onset of puberty. Ultrasound studies of the ovaries in normal infants show many microcysts.

Male breast development regresses rather quickly after birth. Elevated LH levels after birth stimulate Leydig cell production of testosterone for 6 to 12 months, leading to further genital development. Penis length increases from 3 to 5 cm in the full-term newborn to 4.5 to 6 cm by 2 to 3 years.

Childhood

By 2 years of age, serum gonadotropin levels decrease, and thus serum sex steroid levels also decrease, frequently to levels undetectable by conventional assays.

Beginning approximately at ages 6 to 7 years in girls and 7 to 8 years in boys, adrenal androgen production begins to increase and can be detected by the presence of increasing concentrations of the weak adrenal androgen dehydroepiandrosterone (DHEA) and its sulfated derivative, DHEA sulfate (DHEAS). Despite these serum levels, there is initially no secondary sexual (pubic or axillary) hair development.

Adolescence

Beginning on average at about 10.5 years in girls and 11.5 years in boys, there is the return of activity of the hypothalamic GnRH pulse generator, leading to increased serum levels of FSH and LH. The trigger mechanism for this resurgence is unknown, but it may be linked to attainment of a critical body mass or fat mass. Leptin, a hormone produced by fat cells, may be the connection between weight (fat mass) and pubertal events. In early puberty, the activity of the hypothalamic GnRH pulse generator is mostly evident overnight (sleep-entrained), with pulses increasing in number and amplitude and eventually occurring every 60 to 90 minutes. Over time, this process begins to occur during the daytime; there is always greater gonadotropin secretion at night. Because of the longer half-life of sex steroids, serum levels of estradiol and testosterone

*This chapter is an updated and edited version of the chapter by Ruth P. Owens that appeared in the first edition.

Table 59-1. Puberty Terminology	
Gonadarche:	Maturation of the gonads under the control of the hypothalamus and pituitary gland
Thelarche:	Presence of breast development in girls
Gynecomastia:	Presence of breast development in boys
Adrenarche or pubarche:	Development of male hormone–regulated secondary sexual characteristics, including pubic hair, axillary hair, apocrine (underarm) odor, and acne, in both sexes
Menarche:	Time of the first menstrual period
Spermarche:	Time when a boy is first able to produce sperm

Table 59-3. Androgen Effects
Psychological changes
Skin and hair oils, sweat odors
Areolar growth and pigment
Sexual skin pigment and folding
Phallic growth
Voice change
Sexual hair growth
Hairline recession
Statural growth
Muscle mass/strength

show little, if any, diurnal variation. Testosterone levels may be slightly higher in the morning with advancing puberty. There is central sensitivity to the negative feedback effects of sex steroids, leading to significant elevations of gonadotropins when sex steroid production is impaired. The function of the hypothalamic GnRH pulse generator can be accelerated in the setting of obesity, and LH and FSH secretion can revert to the prepubertal pattern in the setting of significant weight loss, as occurs in girls with anorexia nervosa.

Usually within 6 months of the onset of this heightened GnRH pulse generator activity in girls, there is also increasing production of androgens by the adrenal glands, the major source of male hormones in girls. In boys, the testes are the main source of androgens, although male adrenarche also begins about 6 months after gonadarche.

SEX STEROID EFFECTS

In response to FSH, both testes and ovaries enlarge, starting gonadarche. Ovarian granulosa cells produce 17β-estradiol, which causes estrogen effects that generally occur in a fixed order (Table 59-2). Growth increase is one of the early effects of estrogen. Growth is stimulated by estrogen-stimulated increased production of growth hormone and insulin-like growth factor 1. Estrogen along with growth hormone and thyroid hormones increases bone mineralization and growth.

In response to LH, testicular Leydig cells produce testosterone, which is converted to dihydrotestosterone, leading to androgen effects that generally occur in the same order (Table 59-3).

Note that growth is not stimulated early by rising testosterone; in fact, during the phase when testosterone levels are beginning to rise, growth is usually slowed perceptibly from a prepubertal height velocity of perhaps 5 cm/year to a velocity as slow as 4 cm/year for 12 to 18 months. As levels of testosterone increase closer to 400 ng/dL and testis volume increases to between 10 and 12 cm^3, boys make the transition to rapid growth. Rapid growth for boys thus occurs for about 2 years in middle puberty, and slower growth continues for 2 to 3 more years.

Table 59-2. Estrogen Effects
Vaginal and urethral cornification
Breast development, often asymmetric
Growth
Fat development
Uterine development
Menarche: 2 to 2½ years after breast buds

Benign adolescent gynecomastia occurs in as many as 40% to 60% of normal boys; enough estrogen relative to the amount of testosterone is produced so that breast development occurs. This usually starts in early to middle puberty (peak age, 13 years), before adult male concentrations of testosterone are achieved. It typically starts on one side and resolves within 2 years. Gynecomastia is more common in obese boys, although true breast tissue in this setting is often difficult to distinguish from fat tissue.

CHRONOLOGY OF PUBERTY

Girls

Girls begin puberty at an average age of 10.5 years (range, 8 to 13 years; mean ±2.5 standard deviations). There are data suggesting that female puberty begins at an earlier age and that African American girls begin puberty about 1 year earlier than white girls, but this is not universally accepted. In 85% of girls, the first clinically detectable sign of puberty is breast development, although ovarian enlargement, which is not clinically detectable in a strict sense, occurs first. Breast buds appear as small nodules either directly underneath the nipples or slightly off center, causing the areolae and nipples to be pushed out and sometimes cause minor, transient discomfort as the skin around the nipple is stretched. Breast development may be unilateral and asymmetric in its earliest stages. Pubic hair usually begins to develop within the next 6 months; in approximately 15% of girls, pubic hair precedes breast development. Such discordance has no clinical significance. The female adolescent growth spurt commences near the onset of thelarche, generally spanning a 2-year period between the ages of 11 and 13 years. Axillary hair generally begins, on average, between 12 and 13 years. Menarche, a rather late event in female puberty, occurs, on average, between 12.2 and 12.8 years. It is often preceded by a whitish, non–foul-smelling vaginal discharge (physiologic leukorrhea) for up to 6 months. At the time of menarche, an adolescent girl has reached 96.5% of her adult height potential. However, this may not be true in clinical situations in which menarche occurs at a younger bone age than is typical for the average adolescent girl. Menstrual cycles for the first 2 years after menarche are often anovulatory and irregular.

Boys

Boys begin puberty at an average age of 11.5 years (range, 9 to 14 years; mean ±2.5 standard deviations). The first clinically detectable sign of puberty is testicular enlargement, a fact generally unknown to patients and their parents. From birth to the start of puberty, male testicular volumes range between 1 and 2 mL as determined by the use of an orchidometer (a series of ellipsoid models of varying volumes). Stretched penile length (measured with a rigid tape measure on the dorsum of the penis from the pubic symphysis to the tip of the nonerect penis without considering any foreskin tissue) averages about 3.5 cm (range, 2.8 to 4.2 cm) at birth and grows by an average of 2.5 cm until the start of puberty. The onset of male puberty is considered to have begun when at least one of the two testicles reaches 3 mL in volume. It takes approximately 5 to 6 years for the testicles to reach the average adult volume of 20 mL. Approximately 75% to 80% of the adult testicle consists of seminiferous tubules; Leydig cells make up the remainder.

Within 6 months after the start of testicular enlargement, pubic hair can be found; pubic hair precedes testicular enlargement in approximately 15%. The presence of pubic hair is incorrectly considered the first evidence of puberty in boys by both patients and parents. This is followed by the development of axillary hair at approximately 14 years of age. During this period, penile enlargement also occurs, reaching a mean adult length of 12.4 ±1.6 cm at 20 years of age. The male adolescent growth spurt typically occurs between the ages of 13 and 15 years, commencing when the testicular volumes reach 12 mL. By age 15 years, a boy has attained 98% of his final adult height. The ability of adolescent boys to produce sperm, as evidenced by detection of spermatozoa in urine samples, begins between 13.5 and 15 years.

CLINICAL STAGING OF PUBERTY

Standardized staging of pubertal development in both sexes allows for comparison between children, as well as longitudinal monitoring of individual children.

Breast development in girls, genitalia in boys, and pubic hair in both sexes are scored according to five-stage systems originally devised by James M. Tanner and referred to as Tanner stages 1 to 5. Axillary hair in both sexes is rated by a three-stage system referred to as stages 1 to 3. Puberty itself is not staged, because different components of puberty may occur at different stages.

Girls

For breast development, Tanner stage 1 refers to no breast development; Tanner stage 2, to the presence of just breast buds (one or two); Tanner stage 3, to the beginning of formation of the peripheral mound with elevation of the breast; Tanner stage 4, to a further increase in breast size, with the formation of the so-called "double contour," in which the areola and papilla are both raised off the surface of the whole breast; and Tanner stage 5, to adult size, with a return to the single contour in which the surface of the areola is again flush with that of the breast. It may be difficult to differentiate between Tanner stages 3 and 5 without personally observing the patient traverse through Tanner stage 4, because the only difference between these two stages is breast size (determined mostly by fat content). Thus, small breasts, especially in an older adolescent girl, should not necessarily be construed as Tanner stage 3, especially if she has already menstruated, which typically occurs when the breasts have reached Tanner stage 4 and/or if women in the family typically have small breasts.

Boys

For external genitalia, Tanner stage 1 refers to the prepubertal state (testes ≤ 2 mL in volume); Tanner stage 2, to slight enlargement of the testes and scrotum; Tanner stage 3, to lengthening of the penis and further enlargement of the testes and scrotum; Tanner stage 4, to continued penile growth in both length and width with development of the glans; and Tanner stage 5, to adult appearance. An alternative, simplified, and equally accurate approach involves only sizing of the testicles, whereby 3 mL represents the start of puberty, 12 mL correlates with the start of the growth spurt, and 20 mL is the average adult size. In some cases, the appearance of pubic hair does not occur until the testicular volumes reach 12 to 15 mL. Testicular volumes may differ at all stages between sides but not usually by more than

one size on a standard orchidometer. It is important not to confuse a hydrocele with an enlarged testis.

Girls and Boys

Tanner staging of pubic hair is similar in both sexes. Tanner stage 1 is defined by having no pubic hair. Tanner stage 2 is characterized by the presence of a few, countable strands of curly, coarse, pigmented hair either in the mons area or perilabially in girls or at the base of the penis and/or on the scrotum in boys. Lighter, peach fuzz–like hair in the pubic region is not pubic hair. On occasion, especially in individuals from ethnic populations from Mediterranean countries or Northern India, there may be an extension of coarse body hair (hypertrichosis) to the pubic region that is very difficult to discern from pubic hair. Tanner stage 3 refers to the presence of coarser, darker, and curlier hairs, the number of which is no longer countable, which have spread more laterally. Tanner stage 4 refers to a thick, fully triangular pattern of hair growth, without spread to the thighs. Finally, Tanner stage 5 refers to the adult pattern in which there is spread of hair to the medial thighs. The designation Tanner stage 6 is used to describe hair growing up the linea alba, referring to the so-called male escutcheon.

Axillary hair is the simplest component of puberty to quantify. Stage 1 refers to absence of any hair. Stage 2 refers to a countable number of curly, coarse, pigmented strands in at least one armpit. Stage 3 refers to the adult complement, which is merely more hair than is present in stage 2. For the individual with shaved axillae, it is safe to assume either stage 2 or stage 3 hair is present.

FAMILY PATTERNS

The timing of puberty is affected by familial patterns; both parents' history is important in assessing the child with early or late puberty. The following information is useful for establishing the parental effect:

- year of mother's menses
- year father began shaving on a daily basis
- age when parents stopped growing

PRECOCIOUS PUBERTY

DEFINITION

The onset of puberty, at least in girls, may be occurring earlier than in the past; therefore, the definition of precocious puberty has been modified to refer to the appearance of any feature of puberty before 7 years of age in African American girls (and perhaps even before 6 years), before 8 years of age in white girls (and perhaps even before 7 years), and before 9 years of age in boys (regardless of race). If this conservative definition is applied, it remains important to consider pathologic causes in children who present with signs of puberty in the age range between the new and former definitions. The family pattern must also be considered; early onset of puberty is frequently familial.

NORMAL VARIANTS

Idiopathic Isolated Premature Thelarche

This common condition is the development of breast tissue in girls before 8 years of age in white children and 7 years of age in African American children, with no other manifestations of puberty (Fig. 59-1). Elevated serum estrogen levels for age have been difficult to demonstrate, although higher levels than in age-matched normal girls have been measured by an ultrasensitive estradiol assay. Development of

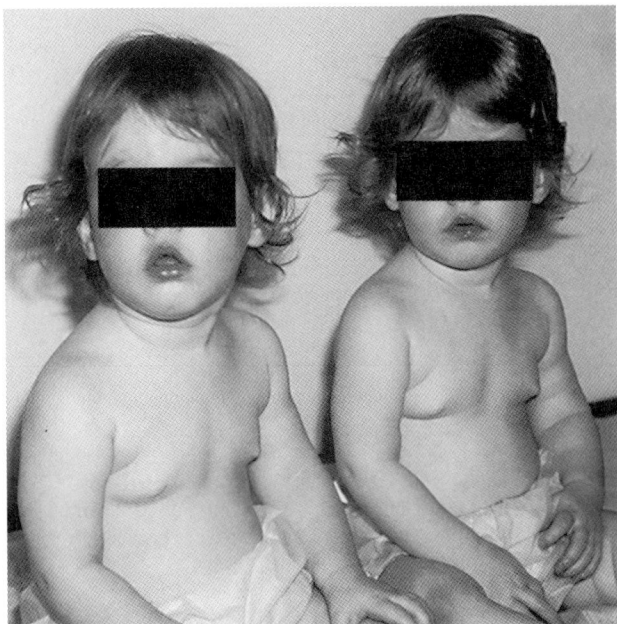

Figure 59-1. Two-year-old twin sisters with idiopathic isolated premature thelarche manifested by isolated breast development to Tanner stage 3.

breast tissue commonly begins between 2 and 3 years of age; it may be present from birth. The observed tissue may be asymmetric, unilateral, or bilateral. When asymmetric or unilateral, parents are typically concerned about the possibility of malignancy, an extremely rare occurrence in childhood. The early breast tissue frequently regresses without intervention, but it may persist. If it persists, the degree of development does not usually exceed Tanner stage 3. The bone age, if determined, is not advanced, and there is no associated growth spurt. If these simple clinical criteria are met, no hormonal studies or additional radiologic procedures are necessary.

Physiologic breast enlargement occurs in neonates from placental transfer of estrogens. Most marked in the first weeks of life, it usually regresses by 1 to 2 months.

Idiopathic Isolated Precocious Adrenarche

This common normal variant is characterized by the development of pubic hair, axillary hair and odor, and/or a small amount of acne in white girls before the age of 8 years, in African American girls before the age of 7 years, and in boys before the age of 9 years. It appears to result from early production of adrenal androgens. Precocious adrenarche occurs much more commonly in girls than in boys and develops most often in obese and/or African American girls and in brain-injured children. There is no associated evidence of virilization (no growth spurt, no significant advancement of bone age, no increase in muscle bulk, no voice deepening, and no temporal hair recession). In girls, there is no associated clitoromegaly and no evidence of estrogen-mediated components of puberty; in boys, there is no testicular enlargement. If a child presents at a very young age, it is generally presumed that an organic cause will be found. However, in infant boys with isolated scrotal hair, typically no cause is found, and the hair subsequently falls out. In most cases of idiopathic precocious adrenarche, serum levels of DHEA and/or DHEAS are in the pubertal ranges. If these criteria are met, no additional laboratory studies are indicated. This pubertal variant was considered benign and self-limited, but data suggest that, at least in girls with associated low birth weight, it may be an early manifestation of polycystic ovary disease.

ISOSEXUAL CENTRAL PRECOCIOUS PUBERTY

Central sexual precocity results from activation of the hypothalamic-pituitary-gonadal axis at an earlier-than-normal age (Fig. 59-2). Isosexual development refers to pubertal changes appropriate for the sex of the child, such as breast budding in girls and testicular enlargement in boys. This is to be distinguished from contrasexual development, in which the pubertal features in girls are mediated by male hormones (clitoromegaly) and those in boys are mediated by female hormones (breast development).

Causes of isosexual precocious puberty are listed in Table 59-4. The majority of cases in girls, who are at least 10-fold more likely to be affected than boys, are idiopathic, whereas only a small percentage of affected boys have no definable cause. Ovarian size, as seen on a sonogram, is generally a reflection of ovarian estrogen production. In true central puberty, pituitary gonadotropins cause both ovaries to increase in size.

In true male central puberty, testes enlarge and androgen production increases. The size of testes enlargement sufficient to determine puberty is debatable. In general, prepubertal testes are less than 2 cm³ in volume and 2 cm in length. A testis 3 cm³ in volume and 2.5 cm in length is enlarging. If on examination *both* testes are enlarged and androgen signs are present, testosterone levels are increasing. If pituitary gonadotropins are increasing or if LH levels increase markedly after GnRH stimulation, the diagnosis is central precocious puberty.

Hypothalamic hamartomas, which may be associated with ectopic secretion of GnRH or transforming growth factor α, are common causes of precocious puberty. Approximately 3% of children with

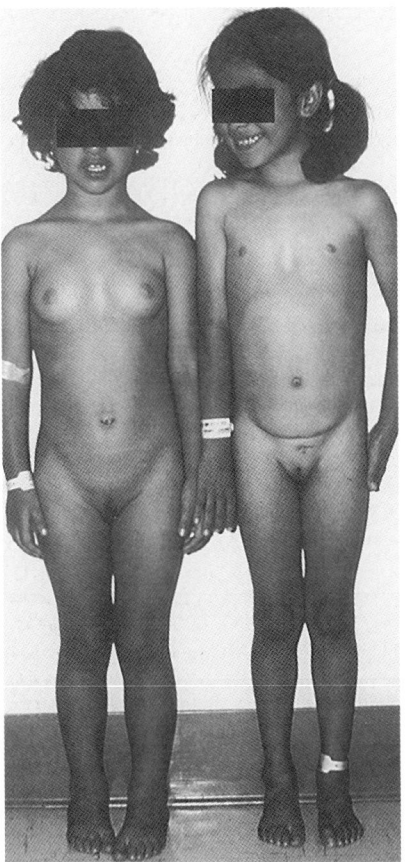

Figure 59-2. Three-year-old girl (left) with isosexual central precocious puberty characterized by both breast and pubic hair development, and tall stature, contrasted to a normal 5-year-old prepubertal girl (right).

Table 59-4. Causes of Isosexual Central Precocious Puberty

Idiopathic
Hypothalamic hamartomas
Other brain tumors (astrocytomas, ependymomas, gliomas, pinealomas)
Congenital defects (hydrocephalus, cysts, septooptic dysplasia)
Previous infection of the central nervous system (meningoencephalitis)
Major head trauma
Neurodevelopmental disability
Neurofibromatosis (with or without a hypothalamic optic glioma)
Untreated or undertreated peripheral causes of puberty (congenital virilizing adrenal hyperplasia)
Hypothyroidism (prolonged and untreated or undertreated)

Table 59-5. Causes of Precocious Pseudopuberty

Androgen Overproduction: Girls

Ovarian arrhenoblastomas
Gonadoblastomas
Ovarian hyperthecosis
Ovarian granulosa cell tumors

Androgen Overproduction: Boys

Leydig cell tumors
Human chorionic gonadotropin–secreting tumors (hepatoblastomas and germ cell tumors)
McCune-Albright syndrome
Familial testotoxicosis

Androgen Exposure or Overproduction: Girls and Boys

Nonclassical (late-onset) adrenal hyperplasia
Androgen-secreting adrenal tumors
Generalized glucocorticoid resistance
Some cases of Cushing syndrome
Teratoma
Exogenous anabolic steroid abuse

Estrogen Overproduction: Girls

Ovarian cysts
Ovarian granulosa cell tumors (isolated or as part of Peutz-Jeghers syndrome)
McCune-Albright syndrome
Exogenous sources
Aromatase excess

Estrogen Overproduction: Boys

Certain adrenal tumors
Sertoli cell tumors (usually in the setting of Peutz-Jeghers syndrome)
Exogenous sources
Aromatase excess

neurofibromatosis type I develop central precocity, usually caused by a hypothalamic optic glioma.

Central precocious puberty in the setting of untreated or undertreated peripheral causes of puberty, such as congenital virilizing adrenal hyperplasia, is caused by premature activation of the GnRH pulse generator, presumably as a result of continuous central nervous system exposure to high levels of androgens (or androgens aromatized to estrogens). Precocious puberty is common in the setting of long-standing untreated primary hypothyroidism, although the mechanism is not clear. It is clinically distinguished by the usual manifestations of hypothyroidism, including delayed growth and bone age.

PRECOCIOUS PSEUDOPUBERTY

Precocious pseudopuberty refers to gonadal or adrenal sex-steroid secretion not resulting from activation of the hypothalamic-pituitary-gonadal axis (pituitary-independent). It is caused by excessive production of or exposure to either androgens or estrogens (Table 59-5).

Androgen Exposure or Overproduction

Anabolic steroids have been taken by boys and girls to improve muscle development and athletic performance. In boys, if anabolic steroids are taken at the age of puberty, secondary sexual development will progress, but the testes will remain small. In girls, anabolic steroids can produce clitoral enlargement (particularly in diameter), complexion problems, and hirsutism, as well as emotional upsets.

Girls

Ovarian tumors producing androgens (*thecoma*) and sometimes also estrogen may be palpable on physical examination and are usually easily seen on a pelvic sonogram. *Arrhenoblastoma,* a virilizing ovarian tumor, is rare in children. *Gonadoblastomas,* which are not always virilizing, typically occur in phenotypic girls who have a Y chromosome (see Chapter 31). *Granulosa cell tumors* usually cause estrogen overproduction but occasionally cause virilization.

Adrenal tumors can be detected with ultrasonography or computed tomography. Androgens produced by adrenal tumors are not suppressed by dexamethasone. Excessive adrenal androgens may be produced as a result of late-onset or nonclassical adrenal hyperplasia and can be suppressed by dexamethasone (see Chapter 31). Such an enzymatic deficiency is mild, inasmuch as it does not cause ambiguity of genitalia; however, it is associated with an increasing growth rate and advanced bone age and may begin any time after birth.

Boys

If *both testes are slightly increased* in volume and testosterone levels are increased but LH and FSH levels are low, there are two possibilities: Either the testes are being stimulated by human chorionic gonadotropin (hCG), which acts like LH and does not increase volume, as with FSH, or the testes are functioning autonomously. β-hCG levels must be determined, and if they are increased, tumors producing hCG must be found and removed; such tumors may include hepatoma, hepatoblastoma, teratoma, and chorioepithelioma.

If *both testes are producing testosterone autonomously without gonadotropin stimulus,* the condition of *testotoxicosis* is probable. Children with this autosomal-dominant disorder have signs of puberty by 4 years of age (Fig. 59-3). Testosterone production and Leydig cell hyperplasia occur in the setting of prepubertal serum LH levels, because of gain-of-function mutation in the gene for the LH receptor, resulting in its constitutive activation. Affected boys and men are fertile. Girls who carry this mutation do not develop precocious puberty.

If *one testis* is *enlarged,* a Leydig cell adenoma in that testicle is probably producing excess testosterone; the tumor must be removed. The high levels of testosterone have suppressed LH and FSH, and the other testicle remains small. Depending on age, a testicular prosthesis may be inserted to replace the removed testicle.

If androgen signs are developing steadily but *neither testis has enlarged,* the androgen is presumed to be either from the adrenal glands or from an exogenous source. An adrenal source is either a

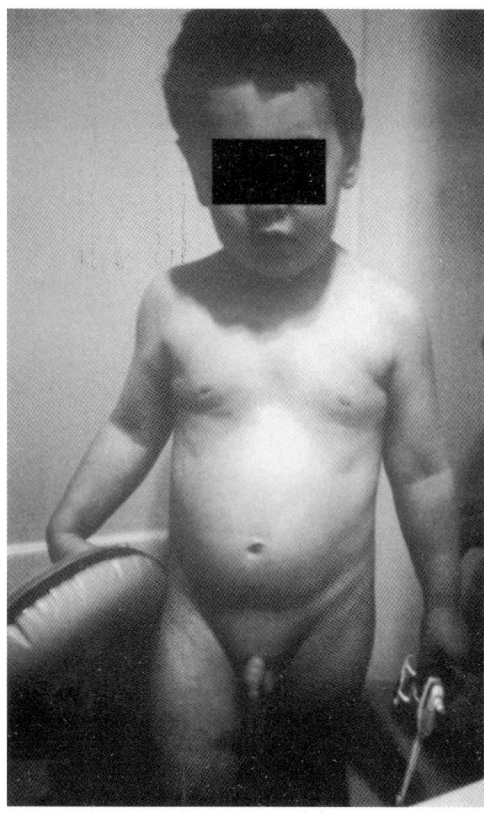
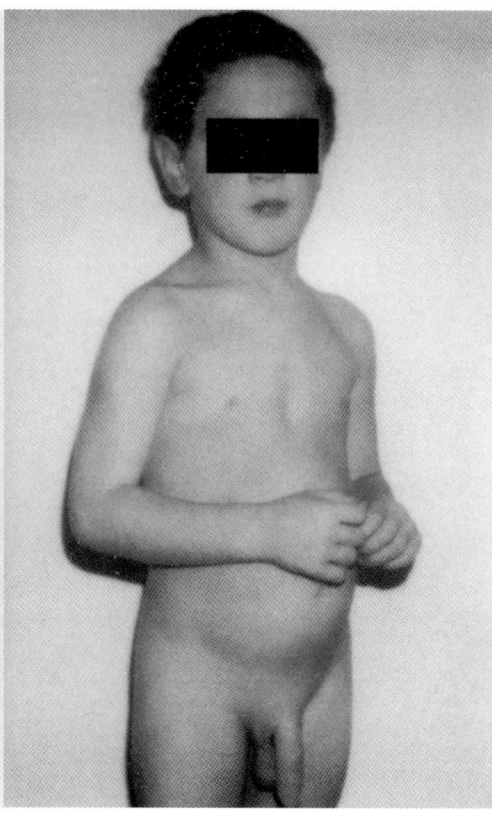

Figure 59-3. Boy with familial testotoxicosis associated with significant penile enlargement, moderate pubic hair growth, and mild-moderate testicular enlargement over a 1.75-year period. **Left,** At 2 years of age. **Right,** At 3.75 years of age.

tumor or a steroid synthesis enzymatic deficiency that leads to excessive adrenal androgen production. An adrenal tumor would have affected growth whenever the gland started to function, but not necessarily beginning at birth. A defect in steroid synthesis caused by an enzymatic deficiency (usually 21-hydroxylase) may be congenital, as in congenital adrenal hyperplasia (see Chapter 31), and the excess androgen production resulting from the enzymatic deficiency would have been produced from the time of birth, leading to increased growth velocity from early life. Children with congenital adrenal hyperplasia may have severe adrenal crises during an illness or surgery. A late-onset or nonclassical form of adrenal hyperplasia may also occur. A tumor can be identified by computed tomography or ultrasonography and must be removed.

Estrogen Overproduction

The most common cause of premature progressive breast development is *simple premature thelarche*. In this case, a pelvic ultrasound study may show prepubertal ovaries varying from 1 to 3 cm³ in volume with many small follicular cysts. Some cysts may be larger (persistent follicular cysts). Estradiol is produced by the granulosa cells lining the follicles and causes vaginal discharge and breast development. Estradiol may cause uterine development as well but generally does *not* cause increased growth velocity. LH and FSH levels are low. The follicular cysts regress spontaneously (90% of the time) within a few weeks to months, and the vaginal cornification is lost within 1 week of cyst regression. The breast tissue then softens but can remain for months. Thus, this premature thelarche of persistent follicular cysts is usually benign and self-limited; 10% of the cysts may persist and enlarge. Some follicular cysts may become large enough to threaten ovarian torsion and to necessitate surgical treatment (see Chapter 22).

Granulosa cell tumors are usually isolated occurrences but may occur as part of Peutz-Jeghers syndrome (oral melanosis and intestinal polyps). Aromatase is the enzyme that is responsible for conversion of androgen to estrogen; aromatase excess is an autosomal dominant disorder.

McCune-Albright Syndrome

This disorder (Fig. 59-4) consists of the clinical triad of polyostotic fibrous dysplasia, hyperpigmented macules (café au lait spots) with irregular borders ("coast of Maine"), and multiple autonomous endocrinopathies (most commonly gonadotropin-independent precocious puberty, but also hyperthyroidism, acromegaly, and hypercortisolemia). Precocious puberty occurs much more commonly in girls than in boys. Patients have a mutation in their $G_s a$ gene that occurs early in embryogenesis and results in constitutive activation of adenylyl cyclase only in affected tissues. This activation leads to the autonomous function of involved tissues, resulting, in the case of affected endocrine glands, in unregulated production of hormone. Precocity in girls, often heralded by menstrual bleeding, frequently occurs before 2 years of age. The ovaries are enlarged and have many follicular cysts; the patient has elevated levels of estradiol. Later, when the GnRH pulse generator is activated, the patient may transition from gonadotropin-independent to central precocious puberty.

Vaginal Bleeding

The usual progression of puberty in girls dictates that breast and uterine development begin about 2 years before the menses. When the rate of pubertal progression is accelerated, menses may start as early as 1 to 1½ years after thelarche; if the rate is slow, menses may start perhaps 3 to 4 years after thelarche. In any case, vaginal bleeding is always a much later sign than breast development, and whenever vaginal bleeding occurs too early—especially if it ever occurs before breast development starts—it must be investigated thoroughly (see Chapter 30).

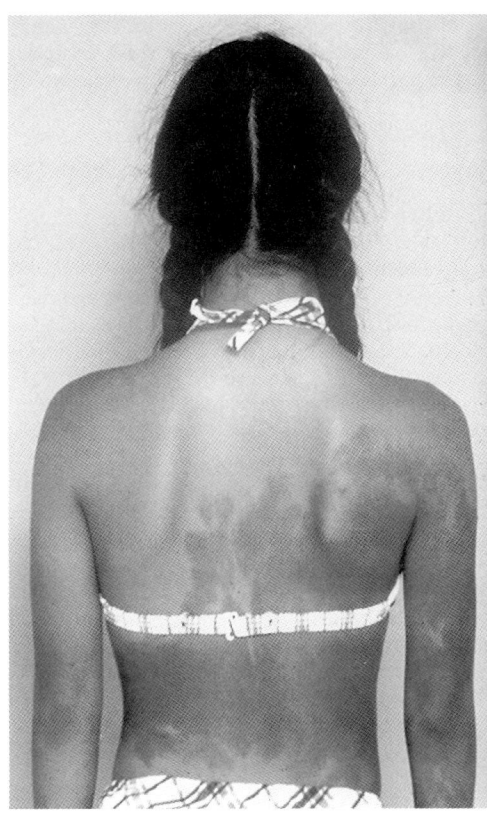 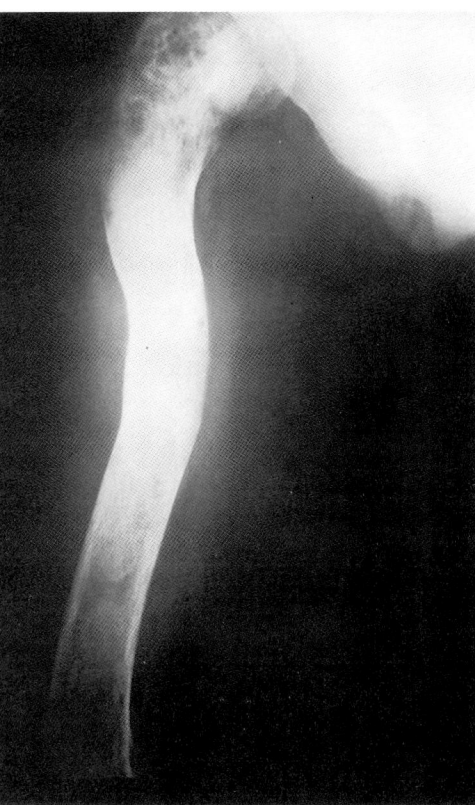

Figure 59-4. Twelve-year-old girl with McCune-Albright syndrome with café au lait spot with irregular border ("coast of Maine") on the back (**left**) and representative lesion of fibrous dysplasia involving the left humerus (**right**).

Gynecomastia

Breast tissue frequently develops in boys during midpuberty, when the production of estrogen from testosterone in the testes temporarily overbalances the testosterone effects. Only rarely does breast tissue develop in younger boys, inasmuch as young boys do not respond to transient gonadotropin stimulation with estrogen production. Differential diagnosis includes estrogen-producing tumors (gonadal or adrenal), exogenous estrogen, hCG-producing tumors, aromatase excess, certain types of male pseudohermaphroditism, and Klinefelter syndrome. Certain medications and illicit drugs are associated with gynecomastia. A prolactinoma should be considered, especially in the setting of galactorrhea.

Evaluation of gynecomastia in prepubertal boys may include karyotyping and measurement of gonadotropins, estradiol, testosterone, hCG, and prolactin level. Imaging is dictated by the results.

DIAGNOSTIC APPROACH TO PRECOCIOUS PUBERTY

In the initial evaluation of the child with precocious puberty, the clinician attempts to determine

- whether the process is a normal variant or pathologic
- the rate of progression of the pubertal changes
- whether the process originates centrally or peripherally

Initial evaluation should include

- medical history: growth patterns; excessive responses to illness (adrenal crisis); exposure to exogenous sex steroids; history of hydrocephalus, meningitis, or encephalitis
- review of symptoms: growth records, head size since birth, vision problems, headache, age at onset of androgen signs (behavior changes, need for increased hair washing because of oiliness, need for deodorant), age at onset of estrogen signs (vaginal discharge, breast budding, underpants size), café au lait spots ("Coast of Maine" in McCune-Albright syndrome or "Coast of California" in neurofibromatosis)
- family history: timing of maternal and paternal growth and pubertal development; siblings and cousins with early development; neurofibromatosis
- physical examination: vital signs, height, weight, head circumference, tooth age, café au lait spots, neurofibromata, pubic and axillary hair, body odor, skin and hair oils, visual fields, optic disks, breast development, vaginal cornification/discharge, penis/clitoris size, scrotal/labial development, testicular volume, pubic hair stages, facial asymmetry or bone abnormalities (McCune-Albright syndrome), neurologic status, affect or mood, intellectual ability

The first test is usually a determination of bone age; if the bone age is not significantly advanced (within 20% of the chronologic age in months) and not associated with an increase in height velocity, the results suggest a normal variant, a slowly progressive process, or a process of relatively short duration. If the bone age is significantly advanced, a workup is mandatory (Table 59-6). Clinical and laboratory findings in sexual precocity are listed in Table 59-7.

For girls with breast development, pelvic ultrasonography and determination of central precocity are the initial diagnostic tests. Because of the pulsatile secretion of serum gonadotropins, random measurements of LH and FSH even by ultrasensitive immunochemiluminescent assay (ICMA) are occasionally low even in the setting of central activation. If this occurs and there is clinical suspicion nonetheless of maturation of the GnRH pulse generator, a GnRH stimulation test should be performed. With central precocity, as with normal puberty, endogenous GnRH that "primes" the gonadotrophs is being produced, so that after administration of a single pharmacologic dose of GnRH, there is copious release of LH. If, on the other hand, the precocity has a peripheral basis, the high levels of circulating estradiol, through central negative feedback, prevent the gonadotrophs from releasing LH in response to the exogenous GnRH bolus.

Table 59-6. Diagnostic Approach to Precocious Puberty

Girls with Breast Development, with or without Androgen Effects

Random serum FSH and LH measurement by ICMA; estradiol measurement

GnRH stimulation test (if random FSH and LH levels uninformative)

Pelvic ultrasonography

   Prepubertal ovaries: ultrasonography (or other radiologic imaging) to image adrenal glands and question about exogenous sources

   One enlarged ovary: either functioning ovarian cyst or solid granulosa-cell tumor

   Bilaterally enlarged ovaries for age: GnRH test to distinguish between central precocity (usual) or McCune-Albright syndrome (rare)

Head MRI with contrast medium (if central precocity is confirmed biochemically and is progressive)

Girls with Contrasexual Androgen Effects (Virilization)

Serum total testosterone (provides an index of the severity of the process)

17-Hydroxyprogesterone (for CAH)

ACTH stimulation test (for CAH) (optional)

24-hour urine free cortisol and creatinine (for Cushing syndrome)

Abdominal/pelvic MRI (if testing suggests either adrenal or ovarian tumor)

Boys with Isosexual Precocity

Prepubertal testes: ultrasonography (or other radiologic imaging) of adrenal glands; question about exogenous sources

One enlarged testis: ultrasonography (or other radiologic imaging) of this testis for androgen-producing tumor

Bilaterally enlarged testes for age: GnRH test to distinguish between central precocity and other causes (familial testotoxicosis, hCG-producing tumor, CAH with adrenal rests, or hypothyroidism)

If central precocity is confirmed biochemically, head MRI with contrast

Tests to Consider, in Either Sex, Depending on Clinical Presentation'

Serum hCG

Prolactin

T₄ and TSH

ACTH, adrenocorticotropic hormone; CAH, congenital adrenal hyperplasia; FSH, follicle-stimulating hormone; GnRH, gonadotropin-releasing hormone; hCG, human chorionic gonadotropin; ICMA, immunochemiluminescent assay; LH, luteinizing hormone; MRI, magnetic resonance imaging.

If a girl with advanced bone age presents only with contrasexual androgenic effects (specifically, evidence of virilization), measurement of gonadotropins and estradiol is not indicated. Measurement of serum 17-hydroxyprogesterone is the diagnostic test for 21-hydroxylase deficiency, the most common enzyme abnormality associated with nonclassical or late-onset adrenal hyperplasia (see Chapter 31). On occasion, an adrenocorticotropic hormone (ACTH) stimulation test may need to be performed to determine the specific enzymatic deficiency. Screening for Cushing syndrome with a 24-hour urine collection with measurement of free cortisol (and creatinine to document completeness of collection) may also be indicated if the appropriate "Cushingoid" body habitus is present. Magnetic resonance imaging of the head is not usually indicated in the evaluation of virilization in girls.

For boys, the testicular examination guides the evaluation. Testotoxicosis and hCG-producing tumors cause some testicular enlargement but less than expected for the degree of virilization.

TREATMENT OF PRECOCIOUS PUBERTY

General Issues

Not all cases of precocious puberty necessitate treatment. Cases of idiopathic precocious thelarche and adrenarche should be monitored, because their manifestations are not typically progressive and there is no significant early onset of the other components of puberty or short stature. In addition, not all children with central precocious puberty require treatment, inasmuch as a significant number of cases are either slowly progressive and/or transient. Unless there is rapid progression and/or significant psychosocial difficulties, most children with central precocity should be observed for a 3- to 6-month period before pubertal reversal therapy is initiated. The reasons that favor treatment include preservation of acceptable final height, prevention of psychological trauma (menstruation at an early age), reversal of mature physical appearance to decrease the risk of pregnancy in girls (because other people assume that affected children are older than they appear), and reduction of aggressiveness and preoccupation with sexuality. Serious psychological effects of early puberty are not usually encountered. If a decision is made to reverse puberty, the goal of therapy is to inhibit secretion and/or effects of estrogens in girls and androgens in boys.

Central Precocious Puberty

The goal of therapy is to inhibit secretion of gonadotropins and reduce production of sex steroids, by the administration of GnRH analogs with a prolonged duration of action (Table 59-8). This causes downregulation of pituitary GnRH receptors, preventing the response to endogenous GnRH and thus decreasing LH and FSH secretion. Several doses of GnRH are necessary to produce the antagonistic response, because the treatment initially stimulates the axis and only later results in downregulation. Accurate verification of adequate suppression of the axis typically requires repeat GnRH testing, although random LH-ICMA levels may be sufficient.

Therapy is stopped at about 11 years in girls and 12 years in boys so that puberty can resume. Successful GnRH agonist treatment is associated with a stabilization of androgen effects in boys and estrogen effects in girls; there is no effect on androgen-mediated events in girls. Complete reversal of physical changes to the prepubertal state is unusual. Height velocity and the rate of bone age maturation should slow; on some occasions, height velocity actually becomes subnormal. This is not necessarily problematic as long as bone age maturation slows commensurately. Final height is optimized with earlier initiation of therapy. Once GnRH analog therapy is discontinued, reactivation of the hypothalamic-pituitary-gonadal axis occurs within 12 months. Long-term fertility data in individuals treated with GnRH analogs as children are limited, but there are reports of successful childbearing in this population.

Large tumors in the hypothalamic-pituitary region are surgically removed. Hypothalamic hamartomas are benign and tend to grow very slowly; therefore, surgery is usually not recommended.

Precocious Pseudopuberty

Treatment is directed at the underlying cause (Table 59-9). The precocious puberty of McCune-Albright syndrome is treated with inhibitors (testolactone or anastrozole) of aromatase, the enzyme that converts androgen to estrogen. The results of this approach are variable, and sometimes a GnRH agonist must be added if central puberty is also present. Ketoconazole is an effective therapy for familial testotoxicosis because it has the desirable and reversible side

Table 59-7. Clinical and Laboratory Findings in Sexual Precocity

	Serum Gonadotropin Concentration	LH Response to GnRH	Serum Sex Steroid Concentrations	Gonadal Size	Miscellaneous
True Precocious Puberty (Premature Reactivation of Hypothalamic GnRH pulse Generator	Prominent LH pulses, initialy during sleep	Pubertal	Pubertal values of testosterone or estradiol	Normal pubertal testicular enlargement or ovarian and uterine enlargement (by sonography)	MRI scan of brain to rule out CNS tumor or other abnormality
McCune-Albright syndrome	Prepubertal	Prepubertal	Pubertal	Enlarged	Skeletal survey
Incomplete Sexual Precocity (Pituitary Gonadotropin Independent)					
Boys					
Chorionic gonadotropin–secreting tumor	High hCG	Prepubertal	Pubertal values of testosterone	Slight to moderate uniform enlargement of testes	Hepatomegaly suggests hepatoblastoma; CT scan of brain if chorionic gonadotropin–secreting CNS tumor suspected
Leydig cell tumor	Prepubertal	Prepubertal	Very high testosterone	Irregular asymmetric enlargement of testes	
Familial testotoxicosis	Prepubertal	Prepubertal	Pubertal values of testosterone	Testes symmetric and larger than 2.5 cm but smaller than expected for pubertal development; spermatogenesis occurs	Familial; probably sex-limited, autosomal dominant trait
Premature adrenarche	Prepubertal	Prepubertal	Prepubertal testosterone; DHEAS or urinary 17-ketosteroid values appropriate for pubic hair stage 2	Testes prepubertal	Onset usually after 6 yr of age; more frequent in brain-injured children
Girls					
Granulosa cell tumor (follicular cysts may present similarly)	Low	Prepubertal	Very high estradiol	Ovarian enlargement on physical examination, MRI, CT, or sonography	Tumor often palpable on abdominal examination
Follicular cyst	Low	Prepubertal	Prepubertal to very high estradiol values	Ovarian enlargement on physical examination, MRI, CT, or sonography	Single or repetitive episodes; exclude McCune-Albright syndrome (skeletal survey)
Feminizing adrenal tumor	Low	Prepubertal	High estradiol and DHEAS values	Ovaries prepubertal	Unilateral adrenal mass
Premature thelarche*	Prepubertal	Prepubertal	Prepubertal or early pubertal estradiol	Ovaries prepubertal	Onset usually before 3 yr of age
Premature adrenarche	Prepubertal	Prepubertal	Prepubertal estradiol; DHEAS or urinary 17-ketosteroid values appropriate for pubic hair stage 2	Ovaries prepubertal	Onset usually after 6 yr of age: more frequent in brain-injured children

Modified from Yen SSC, Jaffe RB (eds): Reproductive Endocrinology, 3rd ed. Philadelphia, WB Saunders, 1991, p 543.

*Same pattern evident with exogenous estrogen administration.

CNS, central nervous system; CT, computed tomography; DHEAS, dehydroepiandrosterone; LH, luteinzing hormone; GnRH, gonadotropin-releasing factor; hCG, human chorionic gonadotropin; MRI, magnetic resonance imaging.

Table 59-8. GnRH Analogs Used to Treat
Precocious Puberty

Leuprolide acetate (Lupron Depot) given as an intramuscular
   injection every 3-4 wk*
Leuprolide acetate (Lupron) given as a daily subcutaneous
   injection
Nafarelin acetate (Synarel) given b.i.d. by intranasal route

*Preferred because of infrequent dosing.
b.i.d., twice a day.

effect of interfering with sex steroid synthesis; spironolactone is an
androgen receptor blocker.

DELAYED OR ABSENT PUBERTY

Delayed puberty is the failure of development of any pubertal feature
by 13 years of age in girls or by 14 years of age in boys. A lower
cutoff may be appropriate in a child with a strong familial pattern of
early puberty.

DIFFERENTIAL DIAGNOSIS

Delay or absence of puberty is caused by

- constitutional delay: a variant of normal
- hypogonadotropic hypogonadism: low gonadotropin levels as
  a result of a defect of the hypothalamus and/or pituitary gland
  (Table 59-10)
- hypergonadotropic hypogonadism: high gonadotropin levels as a
  result of a lack of negative feedback because of a gonadal problem
  (Table 59-11)

   Girls may have isolated absence of adrenarche with normal breast
development (see later discussion).

Constitutional Delay of Growth and Puberty

This is the most common cause of delayed puberty and is thought to
be a normal variant. It is usually diagnosed in boys, probably as a
result of ascertainment bias of referral patterns. The exact cause is
unknown, but approximately 50% of affected patients have a
first-degree relative with delayed puberty and/or late growth. This
tendency can occur in a child of the same gender as the affected

Table 59-9. Treatment of Precocious Pseudopuberty

Tumors
   Surgical removal
   Chemotherapy and/or radiation as indicated
Illicit or unintentional administration of exogenous estrogens
   or androgens should be uncovered and eliminated
Familial testotoxicosis: ketoconazole or spironolactone and
   testolactone
Adrenal hyperplasia: exogenous glucocorticoid
Hypothyroidism: levothyroxine
McCune-Albright syndrome: testolactone or anastrozole
GnRH agonist therapy may need to be added to any of above
   medical therapies if central puberty becomes superimposed
   at an early age

GnRH, gonadotropin-releasing hormone.

Table 59-10. Causes of Delayed Puberty:
Hypogonadotropic Hypogonadism

**Hypothalamic Pulse Generator and/or Pituitary
Disorders**
Tumors
Trauma (accidental or surgical)
Congenital malformations
Radiation
Infection (meningoencephalitis)
Increased intraventricular pressure (hydrocephalus)
Chronic disease
Malnutrition (anorexia nervosa)
Hypothyroidism
Hyperprolactinemia
Excessive exercise (girls)
Kallmann syndrome
Isolated gonadotropin deficiency

Pituitary Disorders
Mutation of GnRH receptor gene
Mutations of genes encoding pituitary transcription
   factors (*Prop-1*)
X-linked congenital adrenal hypoplasia (*DAX-1* gene
   mutation)
LH-β subunit mutation
FSH-β subunit mutation

Gonadotropin Deficiency Associated with Obesity
Prader-Willi syndrome (see Chapters 38 and 60)
Bardet-Biedel syndrome
Mutations of either the leptin or the leptin receptor gene
Mutation of the prohormone convertase (*PC1*) gene

FSH, follicle-stimulating hormone; GnRH, gonadotropin-releasing hormone;
LH, luteinizing hormone.

parent or in a child of the opposite gender. An affected child typically
presents in early adolescence, when peers are beginning to develop
and having growth spurts but the patient is not. The patient's height
is usually at or below the third percentile (see Chapter 60). In the
classical case, the affected child had a normal length at birth, a

Table 59-11. Delayed Pubertal Development Resulting
from Primary Gonadal Defects

Congenital Primary Gonadal Failure
Turner syndrome
Congenital anorchia
Klinefelter syndrome
Gonadal dysgenesis (XX, XY, and others)
Syndromes associated with genital ambiguity
Testicular regression
Lipoid adrenal hypoplasia (StAR gene defect)
P450c17 or 17α-OHase deficiency
Mutations of the LH receptor
Mutations of the FSH receptor

Acquired Causes of Gonadal Failure
Autoimmunity
Galactosemia
Chemotherapeutic agents (cyclophosphamide)
Radiation therapy to the pelvis
Trauma to the testes

FSH, follicle-stimulating hormone; LH, luteinizing hormone; StAR, steroidogenic acute
regulatory protein.

slowdown in height velocity between 6 months and 2 years of age that resulted in short stature, and a normal or near-normal height velocity thereafter along the child's current height percentile. The physical examination findings are unremarkable and, depending on the age, the child may have delayed puberty. The cardinal diagnostic result is a bone age that is moderately delayed in comparison with chronologic age. There may also be a history of delayed dentition. Without intervention, final adult height usually reaches or approximates the target height range. However, children with constitutional delay may have a blunted pubertal growth spurt in relation to their peers and, therefore, may not reach their genetic target height range.

Hypogonadotropic Hypogonadism

A variety of central nervous system insults may disrupt production of gonadotropins. The GnRH pulse generator may be disrupted by an interfering substance, such as excess prolactin (with or without hypothyroidism), or by stress, chronic illness, malnutrition, or excessive physical activity. The hypothalamic arcuate nucleus may be damaged by trauma, radiation, infection, infiltration, increased intracranial pressure, or surgery. The most common mass lesions are craniopharyngiomas, gliomas, and cysts. Congenital conditions or malformations may have allowed enough GnRH for infantile development but not enough for pubertal needs.

Kallmann Syndrome

This is the combination of impaired or absence of sense of smell and gonadotropin deficiency. Other features include color blindness, atrial septal defects, and renal structural anomalies (unilateral renal agenesis). The X-linked form is caused by a mutation of the *KAL* gene; there are autosomal recessive and autosomal dominant forms.

LH and FSH deficiencies may also be isolated or caused by multiple pituitary hormone deficiencies. The latter condition may be a result of pituitary damage from trauma, radiation, infection, sickle cell disease, compression by infiltrate or tumor, or autoimmune processes. In differentiating primary pituitary deficiency from that secondary to hypothalamic deficiency, the clinician should remember that all pituitary hormones *except* prolactin are stimulated by hypothalamic-releasing hormones; prolactin is inhibited by hypothalamic prolactin inhibitory factor. Therefore, if all pituitary hormones, *including* prolactin, are deficient, the problem is in the pituitary gland. If prolactin levels are present or even elevated but the other pituitary hormones are deficient, the problem is above the pituitary gland, in the stalk or hypothalamus.

Hypergonadotropic Hypogonadism: Boys

If the testes are small, they may have been damaged by torsion, sickle cell disease, infection, autoimmune disease, chemotherapy, or radiation and may not be able to respond to LH and FSH stimulation. If the bone age is greater than 10 years and the hypothalamus has probably matured, the serum LH and FSH may then be high.

When the testis size is prepubertal and LH is present but testosterone is not increasing, there may be a problem with the LH receptor.

Klinefelter Syndrome

This occurs in 1:500 boys and is often associated with a 47,XXY karyotype; common features include reduced intelligence, adolescent gynecomastia (often pronounced), and small, firm testes. The testes rarely exceed 5 mL in volume (approximately 25% of the average adult volume). Patients, often tall and thin, may have delayed puberty. Virilization may be incomplete, the phallus is often smaller than average, and infertility near 100%.

Hypergonadotropic Hypogonadism: Girls

In this condition, the ovary may be unable to synthesize estrogen (an inherited metabolic defect, possibly associated with excess adrenal mineralocorticoid and hypertension), the ovary may not be formed well (dysgenesis), or the ovary may have been damaged by any of the factors listed for testicular damage and by galactosemia.

The ovary may be intact but may not be stimulated by gonadotropins. Gonadotropins are present but not effective if there is an FSH receptor problem.

Turner Syndrome

The two most common features of Turner syndrome (see Chapter 60) are short stature (involving the limbs to a greater degree than the trunk) and ovarian failure (Fig. 59-5). Diagnosis in the neonatal period is possible because of the presence of lymphedema and a webbed neck. Additional features include shield chest, increased carrying angle (cubitus valgus), short fourth metacarpal, hypoplastic nails, renal anomalies, and coarctation of the aorta. Approximately 50% of affected girls have no stigmata except short stature and, thus, are typically identified later. About 20% may have spontaneous puberty with functioning ovaries for at least a short period of time, but the infertility rate is greater than 99%.

Girl with Delayed or Absent Adrenarche

If a girl has advanced breast development but no androgen signs, she may have a deficiency of androgen receptors, as occurs in androgen insensitivity syndrome (*testicular feminization*) (see Chapter 31). In girls, the androgens come predominantly from the adrenal glands (adrenarche). If the bone age has not passed 8 years, when DHEAS

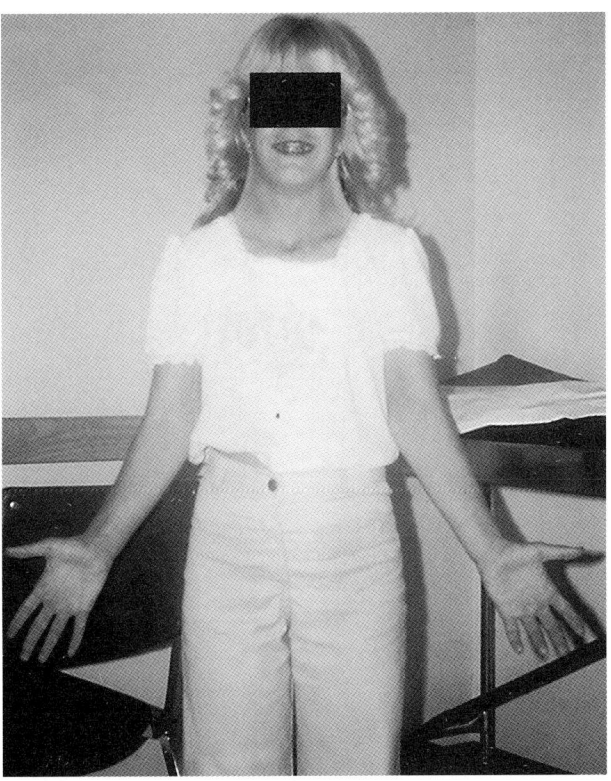

Figure 59-5. Sixteen-year-old girl with Turner syndrome (45,XO), characterized by short stature, absence of thelarche, webbed neck, and increased carrying angles.

generally increases, adrenarche may simply be delayed (*delayed adrenarche*). If bone age is advanced, however, there is a deficiency in androgen production. There may be an inherited problem in androgen synthesis from an enzyme deficiency, or the adrenal may be damaged secondary to autoimmune, infectious, or hypoxic injury. In these latter conditions, other signs of adrenal insufficiency would be evident (see Chapter 31).

DIAGNOSTIC APPROACH TO DELAYED PUBERTY

A normal growth rate with delayed, but not absent puberty, and a family history of "late blooming" suggests the diagnosis of constitutional delay of growth and puberty, which is the most commonly encountered cause (Table 59-12). A bone age that correlates with the patient's pubertal status confirms the clinical impression; no other testing is necessary.

Initial evaluation should include

- medical history: trauma, illness, medications, radiation, infection, malnutrition, autoimmune problems, sickle status, stresses, growth records, galactosemia
- review of symptoms: vision problems, headache, vomiting, ability to detect odors, age at onset of androgen signs, age at onset of estrogen signs, small genitalia at birth, signs of adrenal insufficiency

such as hyperpigmentation, need for deodorant, need to wash hair more frequently
- family history: timing of maternal and paternal growth and pubertal development; siblings and cousins with delayed development
- physical examination: signs of chronic disease, temperature, blood pressure, height, weight, head circumference, dental age, tanning (hyperpigmentation), pubic and axillary hair, body odor, skin and hair oils, visual fields, optic disks, ability to detect odors, breast development, vaginal cornification/discharge, penis size, scrotal development, testicular volume, pubic hair stages, neurologic status, affect or mood, intellectual ability, dysmorphic features

Initial laboratory evaluation screens for chronic disease (complete blood cell count, chemistry profile, sedimentation rate), hypothyroidism (free thyroxine and thyroid-stimulating hormone), and hyperprolactinemia (prolactin level). If growth is slow, the clinician should measure insulin-like growth factor 1 levels and consider growth hormone testing. The clinician should measure testosterone levels in boys and estradiol levels in girls.

Measurements of random FSH and LH and results of a GnRH stimulation test differentiate between hypogonadotropic hypogonadism and primary gonadal failure (Figs. 59-6 and 59-7). Elevated gonadotropin levels support a diagnosis of primary gonadal failure. Chromosomal karyotyping is then performed.

Table 59-12. Differential Diagnostic Features of Delayed Puberty

	Stature	Serum Gonadotropins	GnRH Test: LH Response	Serum Gonadal Steroids	Serum DHEAS	Karyotype	Olfactions
Constitutional Delay in Growth and Puberty	Short for chronologic age, usually appropriate for bone age	Prepubertal, later pubertal	Prepubertal, later pubertal	Low, later normal	Low for chronologic age, appropriate for bone age	Normal	Normal
Hypogonadotropic Hypogonadism							
Isolated gonadotropin deficiency	Normal; absent pubertal growth spurt	Low	Prepubertal or no response	Low	Appropriate for chronologic age	Normal	Normal
Kallmann syndrome	Normal; absent pubertal growth spurt	Low	Prepubertal or no response	Low	Appropriate for chronologic age	Normal	Anosmia or hyposmia
Idiopathic multiple pituitary harmone deficiencies	Short stature and poor growth since early childhood	Low	Prepubertal or no response	Low	Usually low	Normal	Normal
Hypothalamo-pituitary tumors	Decrease in growth velocity of late onset	Low	Prepubertal or no response	Low	Normal or low for chronologic age	Normal	Normal
Primary Gonadal Failure							
Turner syndrome (gonadal dysgenesis) and variants	Short stature since early childhood	High	Hyper-response for age	Low	Normal for chronologic age	45,X or variant	Normal
Klinefelter syndrome and variants	Normal to tall	High	Hyper-response at puberty	Low or normal	Normal for chronologic age	47,XXY or variant	Normal
Familial XX or XY gonadal dysgenesis	Normal	High	Hyper-response for age	Low	Normal for chronologic age	XX or XY	Normal

From Styne DM, Grumbach MM: Disorders of puberty in the male and female. In Yen SSC, Jaffe RB (eds): Reproductive Endocrinology, 3rd ed. Philadelphia, WB Saunders, 1991, p 513.
DHEAS, dehydroepiandrosterone sulfate; GnRH, gonadotropin-releasing hormone; LH, luteinizing hormone.

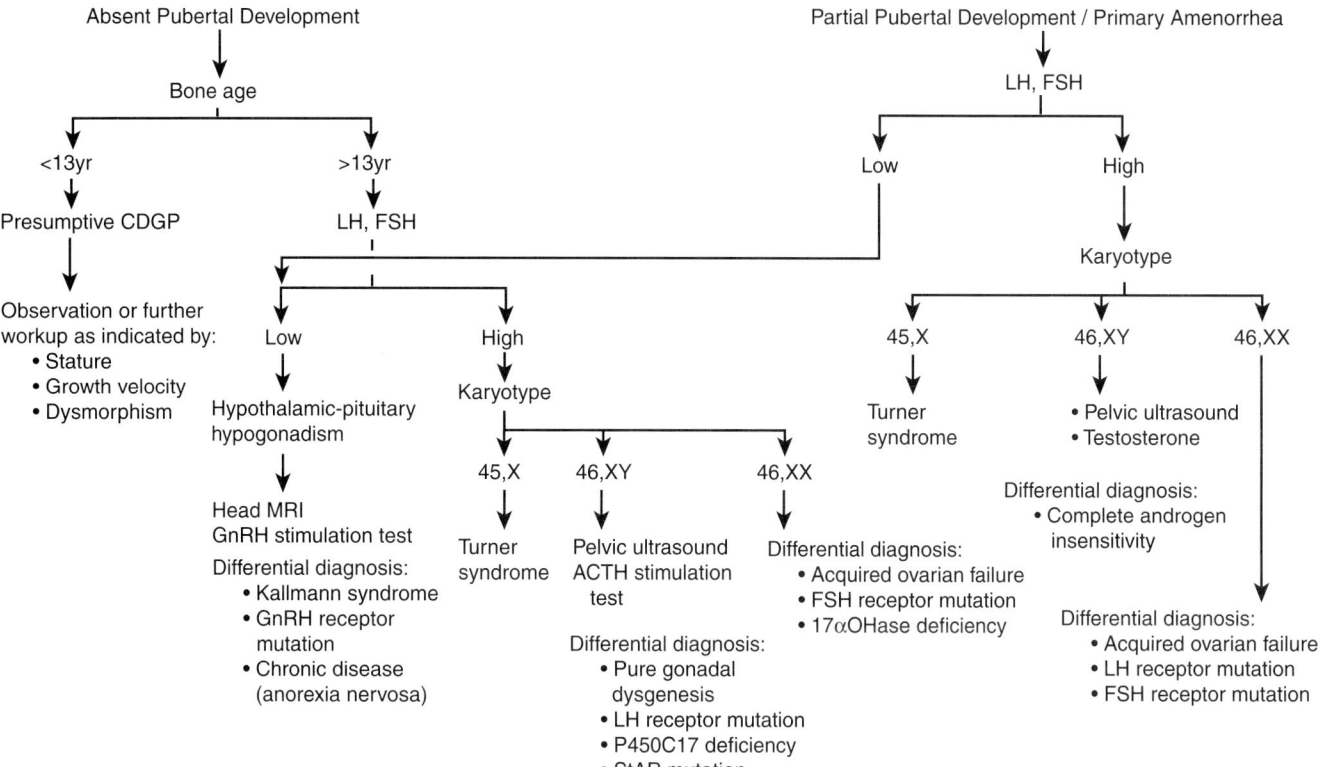

Figure 59-6. Diagnostic approach to delayed puberty in girls. ACTH, adrenocorticotropic hormone; CDGP, constitutional delay of growth; FSH, follicle-stimulating hormone; GnRH, gonadotropin-releasing hormone; LH, luteinizing hormone; MRI, magnetic resonance imaging; StAR, steroidogenic acute regulatory protein; US, ultrasonography. (From DeGroot L J, Jameson J L [eds]: Endocrinology, 4th ed. Philadelphia, WB Saunders, 2001, p 2023.)

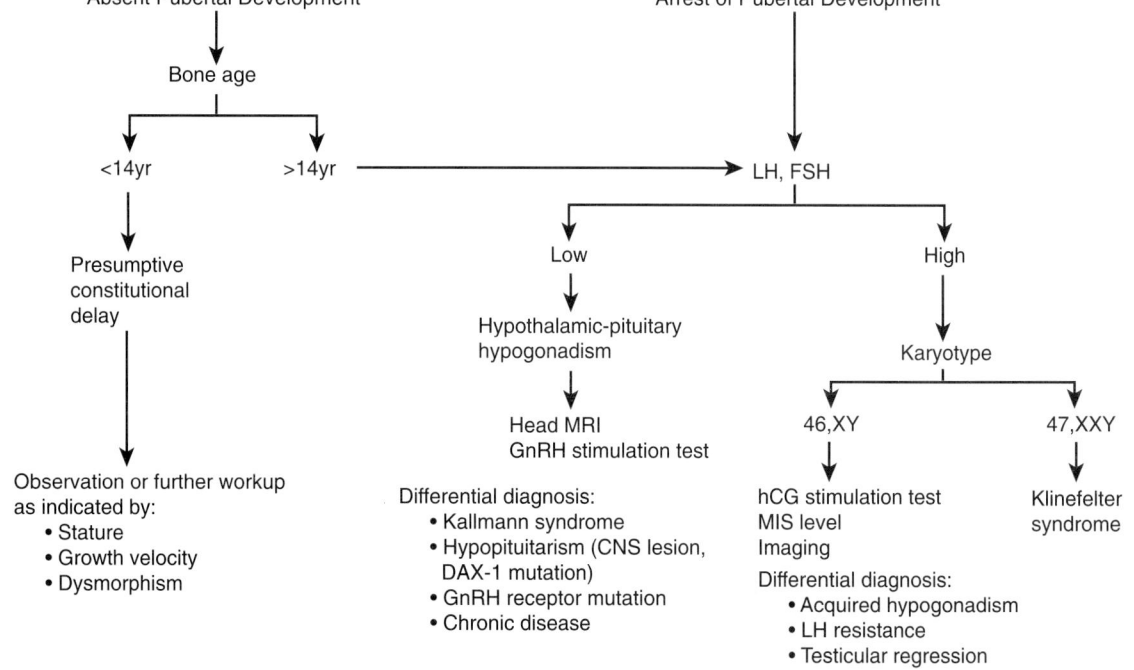

Figure 59-7. Diagnostic approach to evaluation of delayed puberty in boys. CNS, central nervous system; FSH, follicle-stimulating hormone; GnRH, gonadotropin-releasing hormone; hCG, human chorionic gonadotropin; LH, luteinizing hormone; MIS, müllerian-inhibiting substance; MRI, magnetic resonance imaging. (From DeGroot L J, Jameson J L [eds]: Endocrinology, 4th ed. Philadelphia, WB Saunders, 2001, p 2023.)

GnRH stimulation testing, with measurement of serum LH levels over 1 to 2 hours, is often employed. Its rationale is based on the fact that a child in puberty has a significant rise in serum LH over baseline. Unfortunately, the GnRH test is not helpful in distinguishing between constitutional delay and hypogonadotropic hypogonadism because, in both cases, the LH response is blunted secondary to lack of endogenous GnRH priming of the gonadotrophs. However, the child with constitutional delay eventually develops an appropriate pubertal response to GnRH stimulation testing.

If Kallmann syndrome is being considered, a magnetic resonance imaging scan may show abnormalities in the olfactory region. If a 46,XX girl has unexplained ovarian failure, antiovarian antibodies are obtained. An hCG stimulation test and a serum level of mullerian-inhibiting substance (secreted by Sertoli cells) are useful for determining whether functional testicular tissue is present.

TREATMENT OF DELAYED PUBERTY

If delayed puberty is merely physiologic, there is no medical necessity for initiating sex steroid replacement. "Watchful waiting" is usually the appropriate course of action. However, adolescent boys with constitutional delay of growth and puberty who are short, underdeveloped, and psychologically compromised frequently benefit from a short course of testosterone therapy. This is usually given as long-acting intramuscular testosterone, at a dosage of 50 to 100 mg every 3 to 4 weeks for a course ranging between 3 and 12 months. Treatment is generally begun at about 13 years of age and, if possible, when the testes are about 6 to 8 mL in volume. These doses stimulate height and weight gain, allow adequate virilization (increased pubic and axillary hair growth and penile enlargement), and do not typically suppress pituitary FSH and LH secretion, thereby allowing simultaneous endogenous pubertal progression (testicular enlargement). This narrows the physical gap between the patient and peers, without causing undue advancement of bone age. Acne is the principal side effect, and the adult height is not altered. It is the hope that at the conclusion of treatment, the boy will continue to grow and develop rapidly with the testosterone treatment perceived as a "jump starter" of spontaneous puberty. A short course of low-dose anabolic steroids, such as oxandrolone or fluoxymesterone, has also been employed in prepubertal and pubertal boys, and low-dose estradiol has been used in prepubertal and pubertal girls with constitutional delay.

Treatment of hypogonadism is aimed at mimicking normal physiology with stepwise replacement of testosterone in boys and estrogen and progesterone in girls. For boys with hypogonadism,

low-dose parenteral testosterone is initiated at 50 mg every 3 to 4 weeks, with increases in 50-mg increments made over a 2 to 3-year period. Most adult men receive 200 mg every 3 to 4 weeks, which is based on the daily adult male testosterone production rate of 6 mg. Some adult men are treated with 300 mg every 2 weeks. Adult men can use testosterone by patch, which is often associated with local irritation, or by gel.

For girls, daily estrogen therapy is given for 1 year. This can be either in the form of conjugated estrogens (Premarin) at 0.3 mg daily for the first 6 months and 0.625 mg daily for the second 6 months, or with an analogous schedule of ethinyl estradiol replacement. This duration does not place the uterus at undue risk for hyperplasia and malignancy, but at the end of 1 year, progesterone must be added. One commonly used regimen is a shift of the conjugated estrogen dose to days 1 to 23 of the calendar month with addition of medroxyprogesterone acetate (Provera) on days 10 to 23. With this approach, withdrawal bleeding generally occurs between day 23 and the end of the month, although there can be some variability in the timing between patients. Alternatively, at the 1-year point, the conjugated estrogens can be abandoned in favor of a more conventional oral contraceptive or substituted with a weekly estrogen patch used in conjunction with oral medroxyprogesterone acetate. If a girl prefers not to menstruate, the full benefits of hormone replacement can be achieved with continuous conjugated estrogen and medroxyprogesterone acetate therapy, as is present in Prempro.

Patients of either sex with hypogonadotropic hypogonadism are potentially fertile, but sex-steroid therapy alone is ordinarily not sufficient to initiate gametogenesis, although there are rare cases in boys in which testosterone replacement alone has stimulated spermatogenesis. The general approach to fertility induction in either sex involves addition of either cyclical gonadotropin therapy or pump-driven GnRH therapy at the age of desired conception. Finally, if hypogonadotropic hypogonadism is present as one component of hypopituitarism, it is critical to adequately replace all deficient hormones. In contrast, patients with primary hypogonadism have intrinsic gonadal damage and are normally infertile.

SUMMARY AND RED FLAGS

Early, late, or asynchronous puberty can indicate underlying pathology. Red flags related to puberty are listed in Table 59-13. Important findings not to miss are listed in Table 59-14.

Table 59-14. Things Not to Miss with Regard to Puberty

Dysmorphic features
Unusual thinness or obesity
Cutaneous findings
Penis or clitoris diameter and length
Size of testes in patients with gynecomastia
Other endocrine deficiencies or excesses

Table 59-13. Red Flags Related to Puberty

Pubertal changes in African American girls beginning before age 6 years (excluding isolated thelarche from birth to 2 years of age)
Pubertal changes in white girls beginning before age 7 years (excluding isolated thelarche from birth to 2 years of age)
Pubertal changes in all boys beginning before 9 years of age
Absence of pubertal changes in girls by 13 years of age
Absence of pubertal changes in boys by 14 years of age
Neurologic signs and symptoms (headaches, visual disturbances)
Vaginal bleeding before breast development
Significantly asymmetric gonadal size in either sex (boys, by clinical examination; girls, by pelvic ultrasonography)
Testicular underdevelopment
Girls with advancing breast development but no androgen signs
Galactorrhea
Pelvic mass

REFERENCES

Normal Pubertal Development

Bourguignon J-P: The neuroendocrinology of puberty. Growth Gen Hormones 1995;11:1.
Caprio M, Fabbrini E, Isidori AM, et al: Leptin in reproduction. Trends Endocrinol Metab 2001;12:65.
Conte FA, Grumbach MM, Kaplan SL: A diphasic pattern of gonadotropin secretion in patients with the syndrome of gonadal dysgenesis. J Clin Endocrinol Metab 1975;40:670.

Herman-Giddens ME, Slora EJ, Wasserman RC, et al: Secondary sexual characteristics and menses in young girls seen in office practice: A study from the Pediatric Research Office Settings network. Pediatrics 1997;99:505.

Kaiserman KB, Nakamoto JM, Geffner ME, McCabe ERB: Minipuberty of infancy and adolescent pubertal function in adrenal hypoplasia congenita. J Pediatr 1998;133:300.

Kaplowitz PB, Oberfield SE: Reexamination of the age limit for defining when puberty is precocious in girls in the United States: Implications for evaluation and treatment. Drug and Therapeutics and Executive Committees of the Lawson Wilkins Pediatric Endocrine Society. Pediatrics 1999;104:936.

Nakamoto JM: Myths and variations in normal pubertal development. West J Med 2000;172:182.

Pyle SI, Waterhouse, AM, Greulich WW: A Radiographic Standard of Reference for the Growing Hand and Wrist. Prepared for the United States National Health Examinaton Survey. Cleveland Press of Case Western Reserve University, Year Book Medical Publishers, Chicago, 1971.

Rosenfield RL, Bachrach LK, Chernausek SD, et al: Current age of onset of puberty. Pediatrics 2000;106:622.

Precocious Puberty

Blanco-Garcia M, Evain-Brion D, Roger M, Job JC: Isolated menses in prepubertal girls. Pediatrics 1985;76:43.

Clemons RD, Kappy MS, Stuart TE, et al: Long-term effectiveness of depot gonadotropin-releasing hormone analogue in the treatment of children with central precocious puberty. Am J Dis Child 1993;147:653.

Diamond FB, Shulman DI, Root AW: Scrotal hair in infancy. J Pediatr 1989;114:999.

Eckert KL, Wilson DM, Bachrach LK, et al: A single-sample, subcutaneous gonadotropin-releasing hormone test for central precocious puberty. Pediatrics 1996;97:517.

Fenton C, Tang M, Poth M: Review of precocious puberty part I: Gonadotropin-dependent precocious puberty. Endocrinologist 2000; 10:107.

Feuillan PP, Jones JV, Barnes K, et al: Reproductive axis after discontinuation of gonadotropin-releasing hormone analog treatment of girls with precocious puberty: Long term follow-up comparing girls with hypothalamic hamartoma to those with idiopathic precocious puberty. J Clin Endocrinol Metab 1999;84:44.

Ibáñez L, Dimartino-Nardi J, Potau N, Saenger P: Premature adrenarche—Normal variant or forerunner of adult disease? Endocr Rev 2000; 21:671.

Kosugi S, Van Dop C, Geffner ME, et al: Characterization of heterogeneous mutations causing constitutive activation of the luteinizing hormone receptor in familial male precocious puberty. Hum Mol Genet 1995;4:183.

Léger J, Reynaud R, Czernichow P: Do all girls with apparent idiopathic precocious puberty require gonadotropin-releasing hormone agonist treatment? J Pediatr 2000;137:819.

Jung H, Carmel P, Schwartz MS, et al: Some hypothalamic hamartomas contain transforming growth factor alpha, a puberty-inducing growth factor, but not luteinizing hormone-releasing hormone neurons. J Clin Endocrinol Metab 1999;84:4695.

Merke DP, Cutler GB Jr: Evaluation and management of precocious puberty. Arch Dis Child 1996;75:269.

Schwindinger WF, Levine MA: McCune-Albright syndrome. Trends Endocrinol Metab 1993;4:238.

Tang M, Fenton C, Poth M: Review of precocious puberty part II: gonadotropin-independent precocious puberty. Endocrinologist 2000; 10:397.

Delayed or Absent Pubertal Development

Achermann JC. Jameson JL: Advances in the molecular genetics of hypogonadotropic hypogonadism. J Pediatr Endocrinol Metab 2001;14:3.

Argente J: Diagnosis of late puberty. Horm Res 1999;51(Suppl 3):95.

Brook CGD: Treatment of late puberty. Horm Res 1999;51(Suppl 3):101.

Katzman DK, Golden NH, Neumark-Sztainer D, et al: From prevention to prognosis: Clinical research update on adolescent eating disorders. Pediatr Res 2000;47:709.

Kulin H: Delayed puberty. J Clin Endocrinol Metab 2000;81:3460.

Seminara SB, Oliveira LMB, Beranova M, et al: Genetics of hypogonadotropic hypogonadism. J Endocrinol Invest 2000;23:560.

60 Short Stature

Leona Cuttler

Short stature is a symptom, not a disease. It may represent a normal variant or may be a signal of serious physical or emotional illness. Because linear growth is a crucial component of childhood, growth is in many ways an index of childhood well-being. Illnesses, even those not involving aberrations of growth-regulating hormones, often interfere with growth. Therefore, the measurement and charting of heights sequentially on standardized growth charts constitute a central part of a child's medical evaluation.

DEFINITION OF SHORT STATURE

The definition of short stature depends on both statistical and cultural variables. Heights below the first, third, or fifth percentile for age and sex are often used to distinguish short children from others. Similarly, the child who is more than 2 or 2.5 standard deviations below the mean for age may be considered to have short stature. Implicit in all such definitions is the understanding that height is a normally distributed characteristic; therefore, a proportion of normal individuals have heights below each of these arbitrary cutoff points. The greater the deviation from the mean, the more likely the short stature reflects an underlying pathologic process. In addition to actual height, poor linear growth can also be defined as a subnormal rate of growth or as stature that is inappropriately low for the child's genetic endowment (Figs. 60-1 and 60-2).

Whichever definition is utilized in the evaluation of short stature, the physician's diagnostic task is generally to distinguish normal children with short stature from those who have short stature as a result of an underlying medical condition; the more the child's height or growth rate deviates from age-related norms and family growth patterns, the greater is the likelihood of an underlying medical condition (Table 60-1).

Cultural variables may also influence the degree to which a height is perceived as a medical problem. For example, historically, boys at the third or fifth percentile have been more likely to be evaluated for short stature than have girls of equivalent height in relation to peers.

Short stature should be distinguished from "failure to thrive." The latter term refers primarily to poor *weight* gain in infants and young children (although linear growth may be secondarily affected), whereas short stature refers primarily to subnormal linear growth throughout childhood and adolescence (see Chapter 13).

NORMAL PATTERNS OF GROWTH

FETAL GROWTH AND BIRTH SIZE

Fetal growth and birth size normally reflect mainly maternal factors, including maternal or uterine size, parity and multiparity, nutrition, and uteroplacental blood flow. Many congenital disorders that markedly stunt postnatal growth (gonadal dysgenesis, congenital growth hormone [GH] deficiency) have a small effect on prenatal growth and birth size. Heredity, which plays a major role in postnatal growth, generally does not influence birth size. Birth size usually does not predict the eventual growth pattern in most children. An exception is the baby who is small for gestational age (as a result of intrauterine growth retardation). Disorders causing smallness for gestational age may affect fetal cell number by reduced innate growth (chromosomal disorders [trisomies D and E] or syndromes [Russell-Silver]), infection (congenital rubella, cytomegalovirus), or toxins (alcohol) (Table 60-2). Some infants with intrauterine growth retardation (caused by nutritional problems or poor placental function) may show catch-up growth (a period of rapid growth that occurs spontaneously after relief from a condition that had suppressed the rate of growth), although 10% to 20% remain shorter than expected beyond infancy and early childhood.

POSTNATAL GROWTH PATTERNS

The rate of linear growth is greatest in infancy (see Fig. 60-2). During infancy, genetic or familial influences begin to exert a profound effect on height. These influences cause approximately 66% of normal infants to shift linear growth percentiles during the period from birth to 18 to 24 months. By 24 months, these shifts are complete and most children have entered a specific "growth channel" or linear growth percentile in relation to peers. After infancy, there is a strong tendency for normal children to maintain their growth channel; significant deviation from this channel is often an indication of illness.

Linear growth rate slows somewhat in childhood, between infancy and adolescence. The average rate of growth is approximately 6 cm (2.4 inches) per year during middle childhood; sustained rates below 4.5 to 5 cm (1.8 to 2 inches) per year are considered abnormal. Figure 60-2 illustrates norms for growth velocity at each age. Just before puberty, growth rates tend to slow to a nadir. In children with average tempo of puberty, the nadir may reach as low as 3.8 cm (1.5 inches) per year in boys and 4.2 cm (1.7 inches) per year in girls (third percentile).

Growth accelerates again at puberty. The timing of the pubertal growth spurt differs between girls and boys. Girls generally begin pubertal development at 10 to 11 years of age (e.g., in the study by Tanner and colleagues, mean = 10.8 years, SD = 1 year); breast enlargement is generally the first sign of puberty. Cross-sectional data suggest the possibility of earlier onset of puberty (as well as racial differentials) (see Chapter 59). In girls, the pubertal growth spurt starts coincidentally with breast development and peaks before menarche. For girls with an average tempo of puberty, mean peak growth velocity (8 to 9 cm [3.1 to 3.5 inches] per year) is reached at 11 to 12 years of age. After menarche, the growth rate declines. In boys, testicular enlargement is generally the first sign of puberty and occurs at approximately 11.5 years on average (range, 9 to 14.3 years). In boys with an average tempo of pubertal development, peak growth velocity occurs at approximately 13 to 14 years, with an average rate of 10.3 cm (4 inches) per year. The ultimate taller stature of boys relative to girls results, in part, from the longer period of prepubertal growth and from the higher peak growth velocity during puberty.

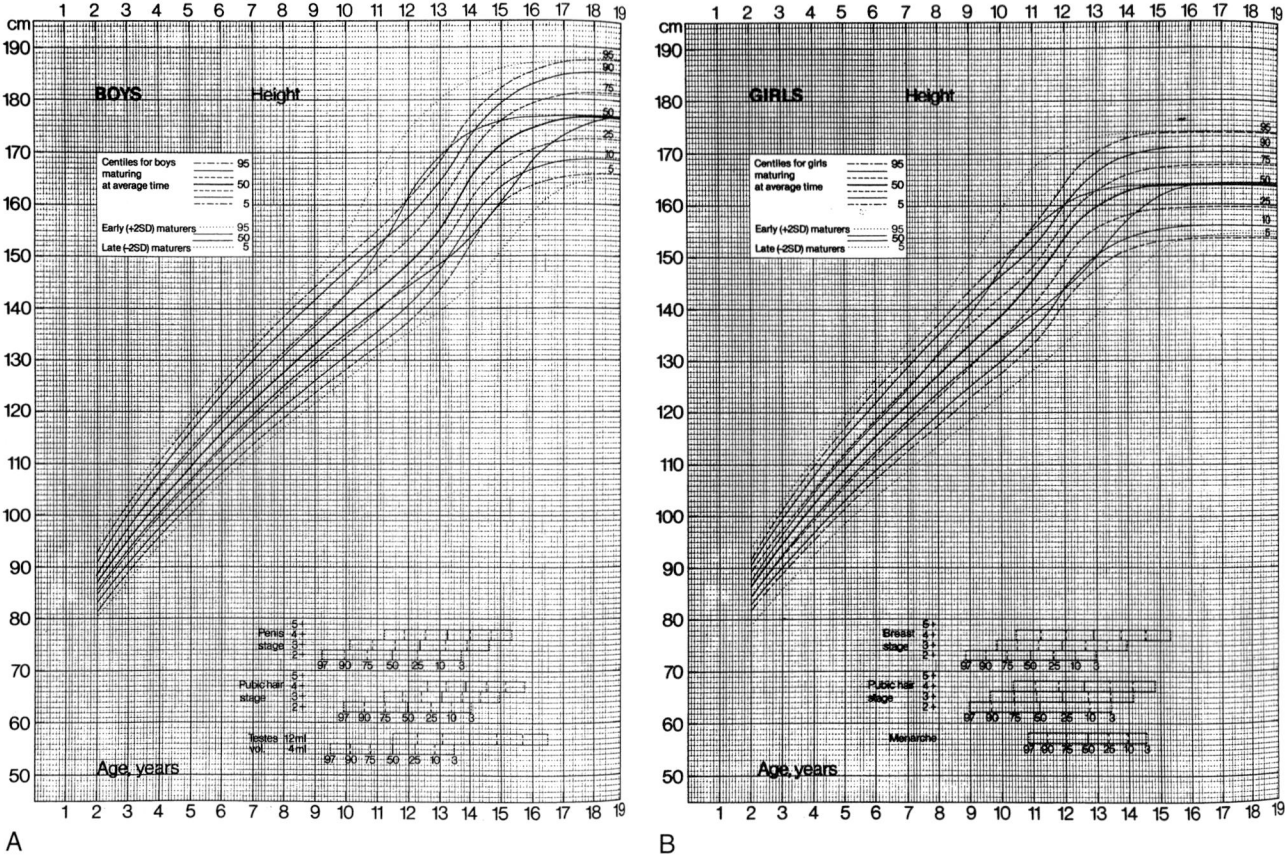

Figure 60-1. **A,** Height attained for American boys. Lines with early growth increment refer to the 50th centile (*solid*) and 95th centile (*dashed*) for boys 2 standard deviations (SD) early in growth tempo; lines with gradual and delayed increment refer to the 50th centile (*solid*) and 5th centile (*dashed*) for boys 2 SD late in growth tempo. **B,** Height attained for American girls. Lines with early growth increment refer to the 50th centile (*solid*) and 95th centile (*dashed*) for girls 2 SD early in growth tempo; lines with gradual and delayed increment refer to the 50th centile (*solid)* and 5th centile (*dashed*) for girls 2 SD late in growth tempo. (Redrawn from Tanner J, Davies P: Clinical longitudinal standards for height and height velocity in North American children. J Pediatr 1985;107:317-329.)

There are large variations in the timing of puberty—and therefore in growth rates—among individuals of the same age. Therefore, growth rates during adolescence should be assessed with longitudinally derived norms rather than with cross-sectional data (see Fig. 60-2). In late puberty, growth decelerates and eventually ceases when the epiphyses have fused. After menarche, girls generally grow approximately 7 cm (2.8 inches) before reaching adult height. On average, growth is nearly complete by age 15 and 16 years in girls and boys, respectively, but there are significant individual variations.

Because of these characteristic patterns of growth during childhood and adolescence, the rate of growth (centimeters per year or inches per year) is a key variable in evaluating a short child. Growth rates may vary somewhat with season and can be affected by transient illness, but a child should maintain a relatively set growth channel on the linear growth percentile charts after 2 to 3 years of age. A child whose rate of growth is consistently at the third percentile cannot sustain a height parallel to the normal curve (i.e., falls below the previous growth channel). A persistently slow rate of growth in relation to age-appropriate norms is alarming and is likely to reflect an underlying medical disorder.

MEASURING A CHILD

Stature is evaluated as supine length until 2 years of age and as standing height thereafter (Fig. 60-3). For measurement of supine length, an infant lies on an inflexible ruled horizontal surface, at one end of which one person holds the infant's head in contact with a fixed board; a second person extends the infant's leg as much as possible and brings a movable plate in contact with the infant's heels. Recumbent measurements average 1 cm (0.4 inch) more than standing height. After 2 years of age, children are measured standing and barefoot with a device such as a Harpenden stadiometer; a vertical metal bar is affixed to an upright board or wall, and height is measured at the top of the head by a sliding perpendicular plate or block. In contrast to these techniques, measurements of length using pen marks at the head and foot of infants are often grossly inaccurate, as are height measurements using a flexible metal rod atop a standard weight scale.

With the use of optimal techniques, the variation in measurement among observers is less than 0.3 cm (0.1 inch). It is then possible to determine changes in height over 3- to 4-month intervals to estimate the annualized growth rate. However, because of normal seasonal variations in growth rates, a longer interval between measurements (6 to 12 months) is more reliable.

Measurements are interpreted in terms of age-related norms for North American children. Heights (or, for infants, length) are plotted on standard growth charts for North American children (see Fig. 60-1). Calculated growth rates (centimeters per year or inches per year) should be evaluated in relation to age-related norms with growth velocity charts for North American children (see Fig. 60-2). These respective measurements enable assessment of the child's height in relation to age-specific norms and the child's growth rate in relation to age-matched peers. In addition, height may be plotted on charts

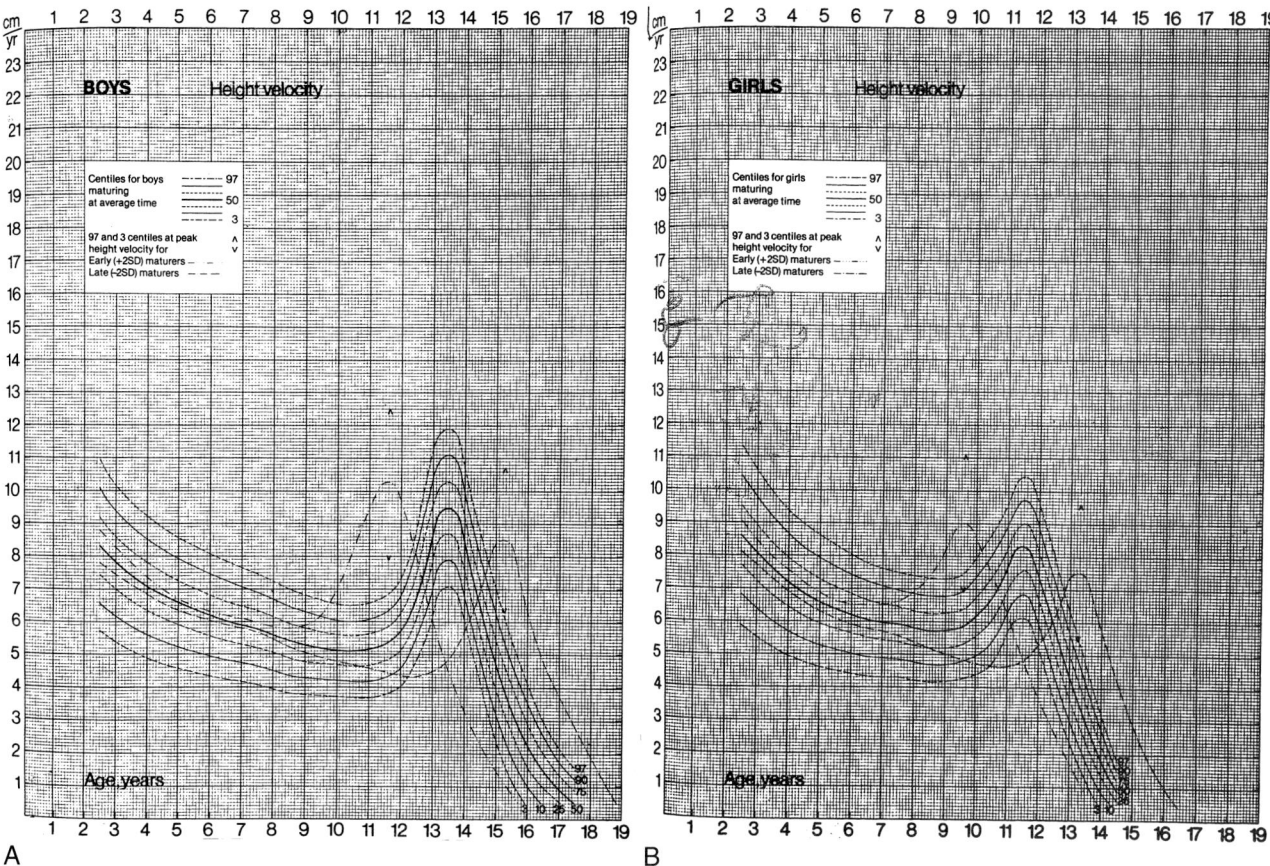

Figure 60-2. A, Height velocity for American boys. Lines with early velocity refer to the 50th centile for boys 2 standard deviations (SD) early in growth tempo; lines with late or gradual velocity refer to the 50th centile for boys 2 SD late in growth tempo. ^ and v, 97th and 3rd centiles for peak velocities of early and late maturers, respectively. B, Height velocity for American girls. Lines with early velocity refer to the 50th centile for girls 2 SD early in growth tempo; lines with late or gradual velocity refer to the 50th centile for girls 2 SD late in growth tempo. ^ and v = 97th and 3rd centiles for peak velocities of early and late maturers, respectively. (Redrawn from Tanner J, Davies P: Clinical longitudinal standards for height and height velocity in North American children. J Pediatr 1985;107:317-329.)

relating the child's stature to midparental height in order to assess the child's height in relation to his or her genetic potential.

Other useful measurements in the assessment of the child's growth include the upper-to-lower segment ratio (U/L) (Fig. 60-4), the arm span, and the head circumference. The U/L is determined by measuring the lower segment (vertical distance between the symphysis pubis and the floor, with the child standing) and the upper segment (difference between the lower segment and height). The normal U/L is age-dependent (see Fig. 60-4) and differs among races. Disorders associated with short stature and abnormal body proportions include hypothyroidism (high U/L), certain skeletal dysplasias (high U/L), and radiation-induced spinal damage (low U/L). *Arm span* is the distance between the outstretched middle fingertips with the child standing against a flat board or wall; disorders associated with short stature and abnormal arm span include certain skeletal dysplasias.

Weight should be considered in relation to a child's stature. Undernutrition is generally caused by nonendocrine factors; less commonly, it is caused by endocrinopathies such as poorly controlled diabetes mellitus or hyperthyroidism. Obesity in childhood is usually exogenous, reflecting in part overeating and sedentary habits rather than endocrine disturbances. Exogenous obesity is generally associated with an accelerated growth rate. In contrast, endocrine disorders that do cause obesity (Cushing syndrome, hypothyroidism, and, in some instances, GH deficiency) as well as certain syndromes associated with obesity (Prader-Willi and Laurence-Moon-Biedl syndromes) are usually associated with slow growth. Therefore, the obese child who has a slow growth velocity is likely to have a serious underlying condition.

FACTORS THAT INFLUENCE LINEAR GROWTH IN CHILDHOOD

FAMILIAL AND GENETIC FACTORS

Both parental height and parental pattern of growth are key influences on a child's growth pattern. This strong familial influence on height is not detectable at birth but is manifested by 2 to 3 years of age. The correlation between child height and midparental height is 0.5 by 2 years of age. This trend becomes more pronounced with age; the correlation coefficient of adult height with midparental height is 0.7.

In addition to the influence of actual height, parents' patterns of growth are often repeated in their children. In particular, many men who were "late bloomers" with delayed onset of puberty and delayed but normal growth spurts have sons with a similar growth pattern. In addition to these normal familial or genetic influences on growth, other genetic disorders may interfere with growth (see Table 60-1).

Table 60-1. Causes of Short Stature

Variations of Normal	**Syndromes of Short Stature**
Constitutional	Turner Syndrome (gonadal dysgenesis)
Familial short stature	Noonan syndrome (pseudo–Turner syndrome)
Endocrine Disorders	Autosomal trisomy 13, 18, 21
GH deficiency	Prader-Willi syndrome
Congenital	Laurence-Moon-Biedl syndrome
Isolated GH deficiency or panhypopituitarism	Autosomal abnormalities
With midline defects	Dysmorphic syndromes (Russell-Silver, de Lange)
Pituitary agenesis	Pseudohypoparathyroidism
Genetic defects for GH, transcription factors (Pit-1), or	**Chronic Disease**
GHRH receptor	Cardiac disorders
Acquired	Left-to-right shunt
Hypothalamic/pituitary tumors	Congestive heart failure
Histiocytosis X	Pulmonary disorders
CNS infections and granulomas	Cystic fibrosis
Head and trauma (birth and later)	Gastrointestinal disorders
Hypothalamic/pituitary radiation	Malabsorption (e.g., celiac disease)
CNS vascular accidents	Disorders of swallowing
Hydrocephalus	Inflammatory bowel disease
Autoimmune	Hepatic disorders
Psychosocial dwarfism: emotional deprivation	Hematologic disorders
(functional GH deficiency)	Sickle cell anemia
Amphetamine treatment for hyperactivity (?)	Thalassemia
Laron dwarfism (GH insensitivity)	Renal disorders
Hypothyroidism	Renal tubular acidosis
Glucocorticoid excess	Chronic uremia
Endogenous	Immunologic disorders
Exogenous	Chronic infection
Diabetes mellitus under poor control	AIDS
Diabetes insipidus (untreated)	**Malnutrition**
Hypophosphatemic vitamin D–resistant rickets	Kwashiorkor, marasmus
Bone Dysplasias	Iron deficiency
Osteochondrodystrophies	Zinc deficiency
	Anorexia caused by chemotherapy of neoplasms

Modified from DM: Growth disorder. In Fitzgerald PA (ed): Handbook of Clinical Endocrinology. Norwalk, Conn: Appleton & Lange, 1992, p 73-99.

AIDS, acquired immunodeficiency syndrome; CNS, central nervous system; GH, growth hormone; GHRH, growth hormone–releasing hormone.

BIRTH SIZE

See earlier section on fetal growth and birth size.

NUTRITION

Adequate intake and metabolic utilization of nutrients are essential for normal growth. Poor nutritional intake or utilization first affects weight, and only when severe and prolonged does it affect height.

GENERAL WELL-BEING

Because growth is a barometer of a child's health, general well-being and freedom from serious illness are necessary for a child to achieve his or her genetic growth potential. Chronic illnesses that are not primarily problems of stature often interfere with growth secondarily, and short stature may be the presenting feature of such conditions as inflammatory bowel disease, celiac disease, and renal disease.

PSYCHOLOGICAL FACTORS

Under normal circumstances, emotional and psychological factors do not have a great effect on growth. However, emotional distress under certain circumstances can interfere with growth (e.g., deprivation dwarfism).

ENDOCRINE INFLUENCES

GH is essential for normal growth in childhood and adolescence. Its secretion from the pituitary gland is determined by a finely balanced interplay of stimulatory and inhibitory influences. The hypothalamic peptides GH-releasing factor and somatostatin (somatotropin release inhibiting factor) stimulate and inhibit GH secretion, respectively. GH is secreted episodically; peak secretion occurs during sleep. It exerts its growth-promoting effect through stimulating the production of insulin-like growth factor I (IGF-I) as well as through a direct effect on bone. IGF-I, in turn, has a negative feedback effect to dampen pituitary GH release. Other factors (including transcription factors such as Pit-1 and Prop-1) and hormones (including ghrelin and thyroid hormone) also influence the production and secretion of GH. Deficiency of GH in a child markedly impairs height and growth rate.

Thyroid hormone is also essential for normal postnatal linear growth. *Glucocorticoids,* in excess, stunt growth. Deficiency of glucocorticoids generally does not adversely affect growth if the child is otherwise healthy. *Sex steroids* (estradiol in girls and testosterone

Table 60-2. Potential Causes of Intrauterine Growth Retardation (IUGR)

Nutrition (in Mothers)

Adolescents, especially those who are not married
Women with low prepregnancy weights
Women with inadequate weight gain during pregnancy
Women who have low income or problems purchasing food
Women with a history of frequent conceptions
Women with a history of having infants of low birth weight
Women with diseases that influence nutritional status:
    diabetes, tuberculosis, anemia, drug addiction, alcoholism,
    or mental depression
Women known to be dietary faddists or with frank pica
Low maternal weight at mother's birth

Chronic Disease

Chronic maternal hypertension
Nephritis
Essential hypertension
Pregnancy-induced hypertension
Advanced maternal diabetes mellitus
Lupus anticoagulant
Severe cyanotic congenital heart disease
Eisenmenger complex
Sickle cell anemia
Diminished environmental oxygen saturations at high altitudes

Drugs

Amphetamines
Antimetabolites (e.g., aminopterin, busulfan, methotrexate)
Bromides
Cigarettes (carbon monoxide, thiocyanate, nicotine)
Cocaine
Ethanol (acetaldehyde)
Heroin
Hydantoin
Isotretinoin
Methadone
Methylmercury
Phencyclidine
Polychlorinated biphenyls (PCBs)
Propranolol
Steroids (prednisone)
Toluene
Trimethadione (Tridione)
Warfarin

Placental Disorders

Twins (implantation site)
Twins (vascular anastomoses)
Chorioangioma
Villitis (TORCH)
Villitis (unknown origin)
Avascular villi
Ischemic villous necrosis
Vasculitis (decidual arteritis)
Multiple infarctions
Syncytial knots
Chronic separation (abruptio placentae)
Diffuse fibrinosis
Hydatidiform change
Abnormal insertion
Single umbilical artery
Fetal vessel thrombosis
Circumvallate placenta

Fetal Disorders

Chromosomal Disorders Associated with IUGR

Trisomies 8, 13, 18, 21
Short-arm deletion in chromosome 4
Long-arm deletion in chromosome 13
Long-arm deletion in chromosome 21
Triploidy
XO karyotype
XXY, XXXY, XXXXY karyotypes
XXXXX karyotype

Metabolic Disorders Associated with IUGR

Agenesis of pancreas
Congenital absence of islets of Langerhans
Congenital lipodystrophy
Galactosemia (?)
Generalized gangliosidosis type I
Hypophosphatasia
I cell disease
Leprechaunism
Maternal phenylketonuria
Maternal renal insufficiency
Maternal Gaucher disease
Menkes syndrome
Transient neonatal diabetes mellitus

Syndromes Associated with IUGR

Aarskog-Scott syndrome
Anencephaly
Bloom syndrome
de Lange syndrome
Dubowitz syndrome
Dwarfism (e.g., achondrogenesis, achondroplasia)
Ellis–van Creveld syndrome
Familial dysautonomia
Fanconi pancytopenia
Meckel-Gruber syndrome
Microcephaly
Möbius syndrome
Multiple congenital anomalads
Osteogenesis imperfecta
Potter disease
Prader-Willi syndrome
Progeria
Prune-belly syndrome
Radial aplasia; thrombocytopenia
Robert syndrome
Russell-Silver syndrome
Seckle syndrome
Smith-Lemli-Opitz syndrome
VATER and VACTERL
Williams syndrome

Congenital Infections Associated with IUGR

Rubella
Cytomegalovirus
Toxoplasmosis
Malaria
Syphilis
Varicella
Chagas disease

TORCH, congenital intrauterine infections: toxoplasmosis, other (syphilis), rubella, cytomegalovirus, herpes; VACTERL, syndrome of vertebral, anal, cardiac, tracheoesophageal, renal, and limb anomalies; VATER; syndrome of vertebral, anal, tracheoesophageal, and renal anomalies.

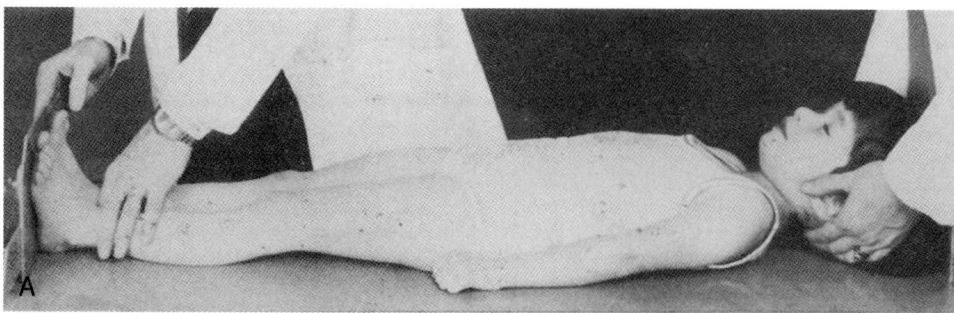

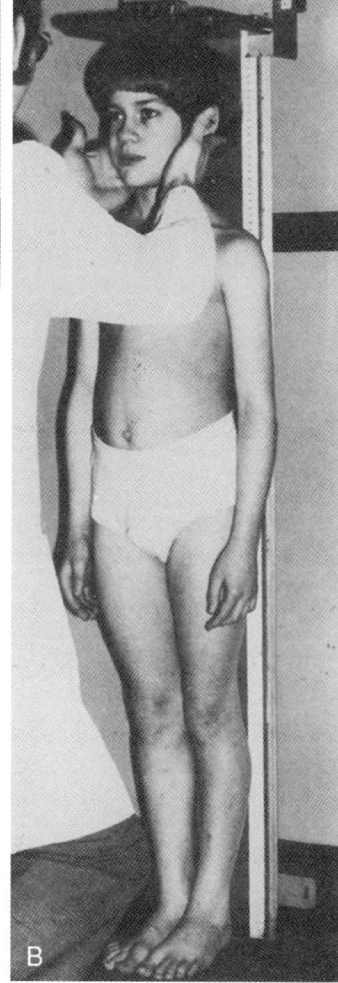

Figure 60-3. A, Technique for measuring length. B, Technique for measuring erect height. (From Wilson JD, Foster DW [eds]: Williams Textbook of Endocrinology, 8th ed. Philadelphia, WB Saunders, 1992, pp 1106-1107.)

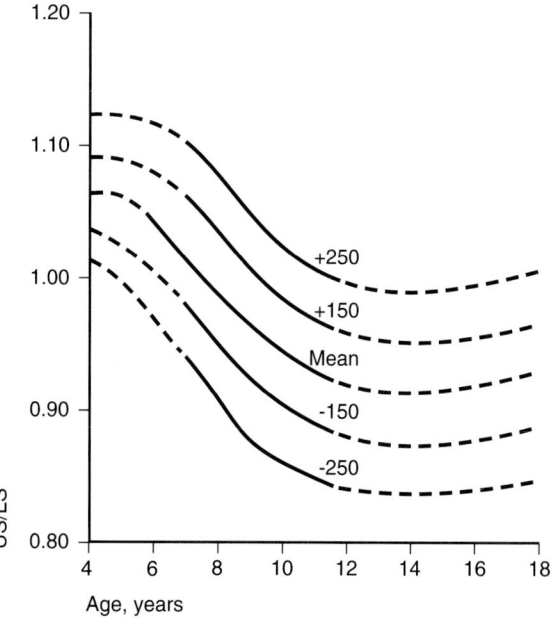

Figure 60-4. Normal upper-to-lower segment ratios (US/LS) for white children. (From McKusick V: Hereditable Disorders of Connective Tissue, 4th ed. St. Louis, CV Mosby, 1972.)

in boys) mediate the pubertal growth spurt. This probably involves direct effects of sex steroids on bone growth as well as indirect steroid-induced amplification of GH secretion. Sexual precocity (true precocious puberty, or congenital adrenal hyperplasia) tends to accelerate linear growth transiently as a result of premature or excessive production of sex steroids or both. If not successfully treated, these conditions advance osseous maturation, leading to premature epiphyseal fusion and short adult height (see Chapter 31). Absence of sex steroids (hypogonadism) in the absence of other abnormalities does not tend to limit growth.

CAUSES OF SHORT STATURE

Understanding the factors that influence childhood growth leads directly to an understanding of the causes of short stature and to the differential diagnosis of short stature for an individual child (Table 60-3; see Table 60-1). It is helpful to assess derangements of growth, in part, by the relationships among the child's chronologic age, growth rate, height age, weight age, and bone age (Table 60-4).

FAMILIAL OR GENETIC CAUSES

The two most frequent causes of short stature in children are familial and have traditionally been viewed as variants of normal. These are

Table 60-3. Differential Diagnosis of and Therapy for Common Causes of Short Stature

	GH Deficiency: May Include Gonadotropin, TRH, TSH, ACTH Deficiencies	Constitutional Delay of Growth and Development	Familial Short Stature	Deprivational Dwarfism	Turner Syndrome	Hypo-thyroidism	Chronic Disease
Family history	Rare	Frequent	Always	No	No	Variable	Variable
Phenotypic sex	Both	Male > female	Both	Both	Female	Both	Both
Facies	Immature or with midline defect (e.g., cleft palate or optic hypoplasia)	Normal	Normal	Normal	Turner facies or normal	Coarse or normal	Normal
Sexual development	Delayed if gonadotropin deficient	Delayed	Normal	Delayed	Generally prepubertal	Usually delayed, may be precocious if condition is severe	Often delayed
Bone age	Delayed	Delayed	Normal	Usually delayed; growth arrest lines	Delayed	Delayed	Often delayed
Dentition	Delayed	Slight delay	Normal	Variable	Normal	Delayed	Normal
Hypoglycemia	Variable	No	No	No	No	No	No
Karyotype	Normal	Normal	Normal	Normal	45, XO or partial deletion of X chromosome or mosaic	Normal	Normal
Free T_4	Low or normal	Normal	Normal	Normal or low	Normal: hypo-thyroidism may be acquired	Low	Normal
Stimulated growth hormone	Low	Normal	Normal	Possibly high	Usually normal	Low or normal	Variable
Insulin-like growth factor I	Low	Normal for bone age	Normal	Low or normal	Low normal	Low or normal	Low or normal (depending on nutritional status)
Therapy	Replace deficiencies	Reassurance; sex steroids to initiate secondary sexual development in selected patients	None; GH therapy controversial	Change or improve environment	Sex hormone replacement, GH	T_4	Treat primary disease

Modified from Styne DM: Endocrine disorders. In Berhman RE, Kliegman RM (eds): Nelson Essentials of Pediatrics, 2nd ed. Philadelphia, WB Saunders, 1994, p 618-619.

ACTH, adrenocorticotropic hormone; GH, growth hormone; T_4, thyroxine; TRH, thyrotropin-releasing hormone; TSH, thyroid stimulating hormone.

familial short stature and constitutional delay in growth and development. In addition, genetic disorders can cause short stature.

Familial Short Stature

The child with familial short stature comes from a short but otherwise normal family. The child's height is in keeping with the genetic endowment, and the child is otherwise healthy. Typically, one or both parents (and often other family members) are about 1.5 to 2 standard deviations below the mean in height. The child is usually noted to be small in relation to peers by early childhood. Although the growth channel is low, it should parallel the normal growth curve. Continued deviation away from the normal growth curve (indicating a subnormal growth velocity) is not typical and should raise concerns about a disorder other than familial short stature (Fig. 60-5). Stature that is out of keeping with the family pattern or that is extremely low (2.5 to 3 or more standard deviations below the mean) raises similar concerns. The review of systems is generally negative in the otherwise healthy child, as are the physical examination findings (aside from short stature). The height-to-weight ratio, body proportions, muscularity, and pubertal development are normal for age. Abnormalities found on review of systems or physical examination should prompt consideration of other diagnoses.

Laboratory study findings, including bone age, are normal. The normal bone age suggests that the short child's "room for growth" is not greater than that of other children of the same age, which indicates that the adult height is likely to be shorter than average. Actual predictions of adult height can be made, although the accuracy is variable; the predicted height is in keeping with family heights.

Table 60-4. Terms Used in the Evaluation of Short Children

Height age: the age for which the child's height would be average

Weight age: the age for which the child's weight would be average

Bone age: the age for which the child's osseous development, as assessed by radiographs of the wrist and sometimes the knee, would be average

Growth rate or *growth velocity*: the number of centimeters (or inches) the child grows in 1 year

Familial short stature is generally believed to represent one end of the normal spectrum of height. It has been suggested that some of these children may have subtle disorders of GH or its receptor, but this has not been conclusively proved. In addition, inherited pathologic conditions, such as hypochondroplasia, may manifest in a manner similar to familial short stature and should be considered in the evaluation, particularly if the short stature is marked.

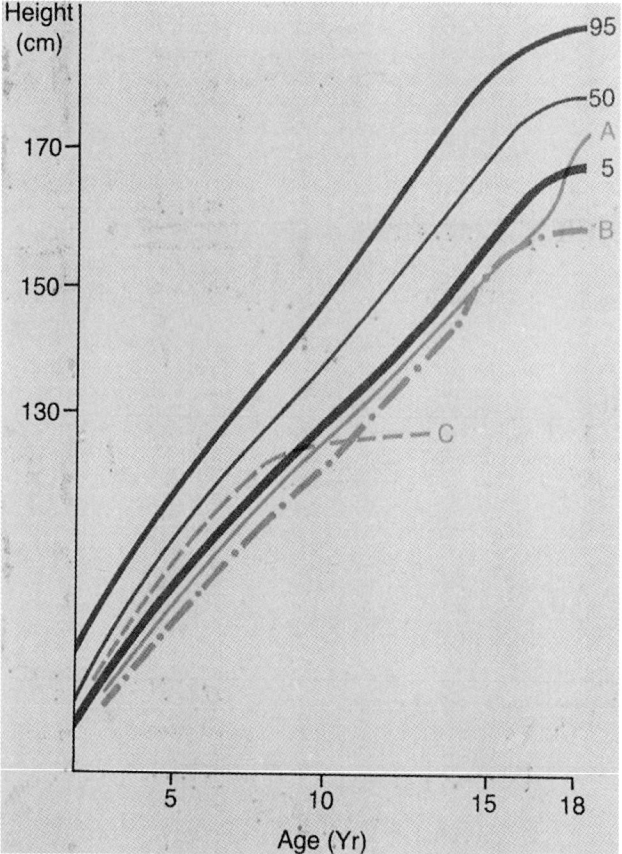

Figure 60-5. Patterns of linear growth. Normal growth percentiles (5th, 50th, 95th) are shown along with typical growth curves for constitutional delay of growth and adolescence (A), familial short stature (B), and acquired pathologic growth failure (C) (e.g., acquired primary hypothyroidism). (From Styne DM: Endocrine disorders. In Behrman RE, Kliegman RM [eds]: Nelson Essentials of Pediatrics, 2nd ed. Philadelphia, WB Saunders, 1994, p 616.)

Constitutional Delay in Growth and Development

Constitutional delay in growth and development is a growth pattern that is traditionally also considered a variant of normal (see Fig. 60-5). It is recognized predominantly in boys and accounts for a high proportion of referrals for growth evaluation. The children often begin to show moderate short stature during early to middle childhood but are otherwise healthy. They have delayed onset of puberty and therefore a delayed growth spurt. One or both parents (or other family members) usually have a history of delayed puberty, a late adolescent growth spurt, with eventual cessation of growth during late adolescence or into the third decade of life. The affected parent usually is of normal adult stature. Otherwise, the history and review of systems are generally negative. The physical examination findings are generally normal except for delayed onset of puberty in children of an appropriate age.

Laboratory test results are normal, with the important exception of a delayed bone age (bone age < chronologic age). It suggests that the child has more "room to grow" than the average age-matched child and that the child is likely to reach an adult height closer to the mean than to the current height percentile. Some children have mixed familial short stature and constitutional delay in growth and development; they tend to have both delayed puberty and a short predicted adult height.

Although constitutional delay is generally believed to represent a normal variant, it has been suggested that some children with this condition may have subtle dysregulation of GH secretion. Chronic illness may also mimic constitutional delay in growth and development and should be considered in the differential diagnosis. It is sometimes difficult to distinguish children with constitutional delay in growth and development from the more unusual condition of central (hypothalamic/pituitary) hypogonadism; a positive family history of delayed but normal puberty and growth, a normal sense of smell (to exclude Kallmann syndrome), and normal neurologic findings favor constitutional delay. Sometimes a gonadotropin-releasing hormone (GnRH) test, a GnRH analog test, or a sensitive assay of bioactive luteinizing hormone may help to distinguish the conditions.

The management of constitutional delay in growth and development involves reassurance and sometimes a short course of low-dose sex steroids. The use of GH therapy in this condition is a subject of investigation.

Genetic Abnormalities

A variety of genetic disorders—including chromosomal aberrations, specific gene defects, and syndromes of unknown origin—are associated with short stature (Table 60-5). Some of the most prominent are described as follows.

Turner Syndrome

Turner syndrome and its variants (*gonadal dysgenesis*) are common causes of short stature in girls, with an incidence of 1 per 2500 liveborn girls. It is caused by the absence or abnormality of an X chromosome, the classic form being 45,XO. A short stature homeobox gene (*SHOX*) on the pseudoautosomal region of the sex chromosome has been implicated in the short stature phenotype of Turner syndrome. This gene may also have a role in some cases of idiopathic short stature. The major clinical features of Turner syndrome include short stature and ovarian failure (Fig. 60-6). By early childhood, marked short stature is usually noted and there is progressive deviation of height away from the normal growth curve. Linear growth is further attenuated during the teenage years. The natural history includes a mean adult height of 142 cm (4 feet, 8 inches). Even in girls with Turner syndrome, adult height is influenced by the height of the parents. Breast enlargement and menses

Table 60-5. Examples of Syndromes Associated with Short Stature*

Syndrome	Genetics	Major Features
Noonan (Turner-like)	Sporadic, occasionally AD	Short stature, mental retardation, webbed neck, cryptorchidism, pulmonic stenosis
Russell-Silver (Silver)	Sporadic, occasionally AD	Small stature of prenatal onset, asymmetry, occasionally chromosomal abnormalities, small triangular face, *café au lait* spots, occasionally fasting hypoglycemia in infancy, usually normal intelligence
Bloom	AR	Short stature of prenatal onset, malar hypoplasia, facial telangiectatic eczema, chromosomal fragility, malignancies
Williams	Sporadic	Moderate short stature of prenatal onset, cardiac anomalies (especially supravalvular aortic stenosis), hypercalcemia infrequent, unusual facies
Fetal alcohol	Environmental	Prenatal growth failure, microcephaly, short palpebral fissures, intellectual or behavioral impairment, joint and cardiac anomalies
Fanconi	AR	Short stature, radial hypoplasia, pigmentation, strabismus, small phallus/cryptorchidism, mental retardation, pancytopenia with time, chromosome fragility, leukemia
Laurence-Moon-Biedl	AR	Obesity, mental deficiency, polydactyly/syndactyly, retinitis pigmentosa, hypogonadism
Prader-Willi	Deletion in chromosome 15	Obesity, hypotonia, mental retardation, hypogonadism, small hands and feet

*Excluding those with chromosomal abnormalities and excluding bone dysplasias.

AD, autosomal dominant; AR, autosomal recessive.

generally fail to occur as a result of ovarian failure. However, the presence of pubertal development should not deter consideration of the diagnosis because approximately 10% of patients have some residual ovarian tissue rather than streak gonads. In a few cases, fertility has been reported. In addition to short stature and ovarian failure, there may be a history of a slightly small birth size and dysmorphic features, including webbed neck, low posterior hairline, lymphedema beginning in the neonatal period (manifesting mainly as puffy hands and feet), increased carrying angle of the arm, pigmented nevi, short fourth metacarpals, nail abnormalities, and renal and cardiac anomalies (coarctation of the aorta). In view of the wide range of phenotypes in this condition, absence of dysmorphic features should not preclude consideration of Turner's syndrome in short girls.

A karyotype analysis is necessary to confirm or rule out the diagnosis of Turner syndrome in any girl with short stature of unknown origin. Additional laboratory features may include abnormally high levels of the gonadotropins, luteinizing hormone, and follicle-stimulating hormone (FSH), which are indicative of ovarian failure; however, levels may be normal in middle childhood because of normal central nervous system suppression of gonadotropin secretion at that time.

Although short stature in Turner syndrome is not believed to result from GH deficiency, treatment of Turner syndrome involves GH therapy (typically in higher doses than required for classical GH deficiency) from the time the child's height falls below the fifth percentile on normal growth charts. This treatment increases adult

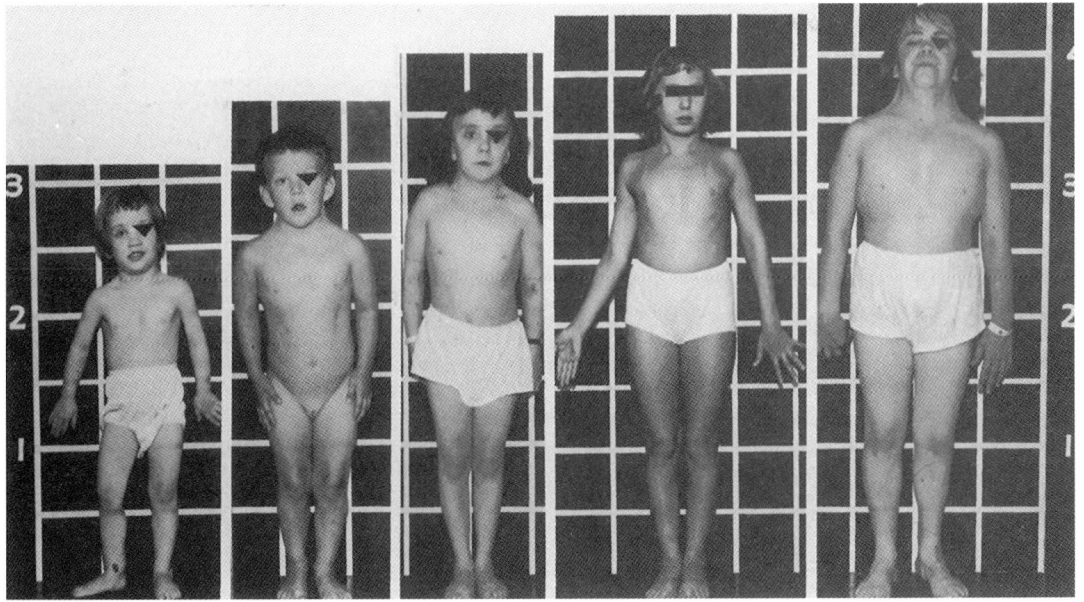

Figure 60-6. Five girls with 45,XO syndrome illustrating the variability of features such as webbed neck and broad chest. (From Lemli L, Smith D: The XO syndrome. A study of the differentiated phenotype in 25 patients. J Pediatr 1963;63:577-588.)

height in many girls with Turner syndrome. Oxandrolone may also increase the growth of girls with Turner syndrome, although its androgen activity may be troublesome. Ovarian failure in Turner syndrome is managed by sex steroid replacement therapy, beginning in adolescence.

Prader-Willi Syndrome

Prader-Willi syndrome is marked by infantile hypotonia with poor feeding, hypogonadism, mental retardation, acromicria, later onset obesity with a voracious appetite, and short stature (average adult heights, 147 cm [4 feet, 9 inches] in girls and 155 cm [5 feet, 1 inch] in boys). Prader-Willi syndrome results from the absence of a segment of paternally inherited chromosome 15. This may occur through a chromosomal deletion of the paternal chromosome or by inheritance of two complete copies of chromosome 15 from the patient's mother. Genetic testing is readily available.

Down Syndrome

A prominent feature in Down syndrome is short stature. The cause of impaired growth is not known. It is independent of the hypothyroidism that may also occur in this condition. The short stature has traditionally not been amenable to treatment.

BONE DYSPLASIAS

Bone dysplasias (*osteochondrodystrophies*) constitute a group of disorders in which there is innate failure of bone or cartilage to grow normally. Abnormal body proportions are characteristic of these conditions (disproportionate short stature), although there are some exceptions. Many bone dysplasias are inherited, often in an autosomal dominant pattern. Bone ages are not reliable indicators of osseous maturity in these conditions. Examples of bone dysplasias are described as follows and in Table 60-6.

Achondroplasia

Achondroplasia is the classic example of an osteochondrodystrophy (Fig. 60-7). The incidence is 1 per 10,000. This condition is caused by a mutation in the fibroblast growth factor receptor 3 gene. Short stature, body disproportion with short limbs, and a relatively large head are often noted at birth. Progressive deceleration of growth rate begins in infancy, and the humerus and femur are particularly shortened. In addition, there may be hydrocephalus as a result of narrowing of the foramen magnum, kyphosis, stenosis of the spinal canal, and

vertebral disk lesions. The diagnosis is clinical and is supported by characteristic radiologic features that include small cuboid vertebral bodies and anterior beaking of the first or second lumbar vertebra. The average adult height is 125 cm (4 feet, 1 inch) in girls and 131 cm (4 feet, 3 inches) in boys. There is no effective medication for short stature in this condition.

Hypochondroplasia

Hypochondroplasia, an allelic variant of achondroplasia, manifests with short stature and dysmorphic features that are often more mild than in achondroplasia. In particular, there are few craniofacial abnormalities, and body disproportion may be subtle. Newborns may be slightly small, but short stature generally becomes apparent by age 3 years. The short stature is minimally disproportionate with relatively short limbs. The hands and feet are usually stubby. Genu varum may occur. Radiologic hallmarks include metaphyseal indentation and flaring as well as hypoplasia of the ilia with small greater sciatic notches. Some reports suggest a beneficial effect of GH.

MALNUTRITION

Worldwide, malnutrition resulting from poverty is the commonest cause of short stature. In North America, malnutrition may arise from inadequate intake secondary to poverty or deprivation, poor intake secondary to overt or occult chronic illness (e.g., inflammatory bowel disease, renal failure), or inability to utilize food intake (malabsorption; see Chapter 15). Weight tends to be depressed to a greater degree than height (weight age < height age). The history should include review of the child's food intake (often best obtained by a 3-day diet record), appetite, and detailed review of systems. Specific nutritional disorders, such as rickets, may also lead to short stature.

CHRONIC ILLNESS

Chronic illnesses, such as inflammatory bowel disease, celiac disease, renal dysfunction, and chronic inflammation, lead to short stature. The mechanisms of impaired growth include poor appetite or poor intake (e.g., inflammatory bowel disease, renal dysfunction), malabsorption (e.g., celiac disease), medications (e.g., chronic glucocorticoids for severe asthma), chronic acidosis (e.g., renal tubular acidosis), and secondary endocrine dysfunction (e.g., high levels of insulin-like growth factor [IGF] binding protein in renal failure). Although the primary disorder is evident in many cases, short stature is sometimes the presenting feature of the chronic disease. This occurs notably in inflammatory bowel disease, celiac disease, and renal dysfunction.

Table 60-6. **Examples of Bone Dysplasias (Osteochondrodystrophies)**

Disorder	Genetics	Characteristics
Achondroplasia	AD	Most common osteochondrodystrophy, short limbs, macrocephaly, low nasal bridge, caudal narrowing of spinal canal, occasionally hydrocephalus
Hypochondroplasia	AD	Short stature, short limbs, relative lack of craniofacial features in comparison with achondroplasia
Acromesomelic dysplasia	AR	Short distal limbs, kyphosis, frontal prominence
Kniest syndrome	Sporadic	Flat facies, enlarged joints, platyspondyly
Kozlowski spondylometaphyseal dysplasia	AD	Short spine, pectus carinatum, irregular metaphyses
Schmid metaphyseal chondrodysplasia syndrome	AD	Metaphyseal dysostosis, tibial bowing, flared lower ribs

AD, autosomal dominant; AR, autosomal recessive.

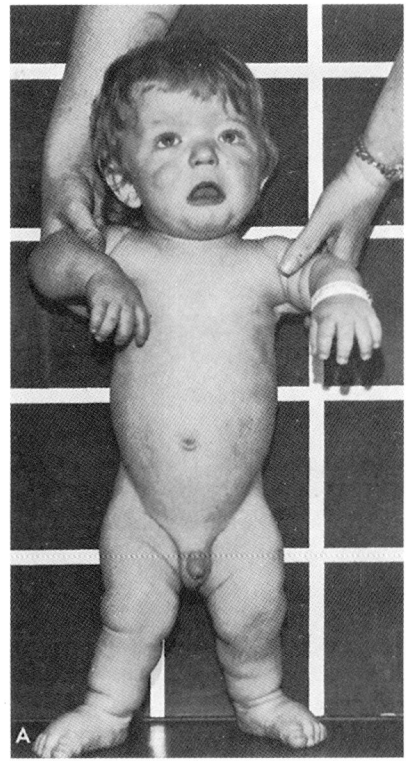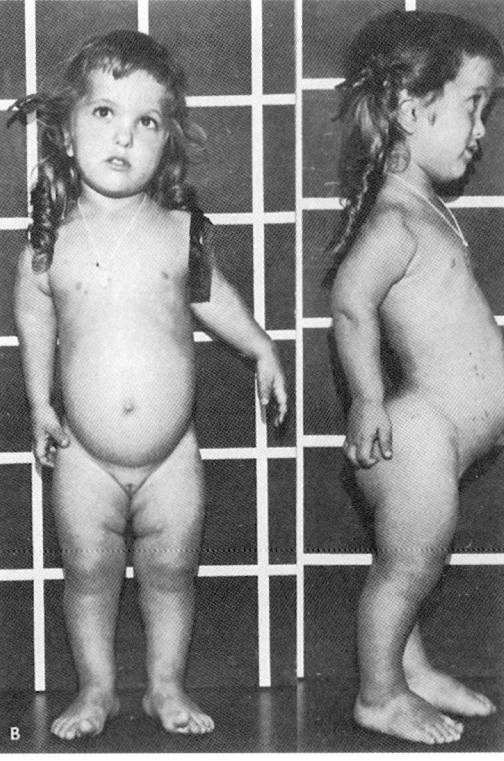

Figure 60-7. Achondroplasia. **A,** One-year-old boy with height age of 4 months. (From Smith DW: Compendium on shortness of stature. J Pediatr 1967;70:504.) **B,** Four-year-old girl with height age of 20 months. (From Jones KL [ed]: Smith's Recognizable Patterns of Human Malformation, 4th ed. Philadelphia, WB Saunders, 1988.)

The history typically reveals that the child had been growing normally until some point. Then the growth rate slowed, which is suggestive of onset of an illness. The history may reveal a clear earlier diagnosis of chronic illness or may instead include symptoms suggestive of the underlying disorder (e.g., loss of appetite, diarrhea, mouth sores, fevers as in inflammatory bowel disease). The physical examination typically shows that the weight is more depressed than the height. There may also be features indicative of the underlying disorder (e.g., pallor, buttock adipose tissue wasting, edema as in celiac disease).

Laboratory studies that screen for chronic illness (complete blood cell count, erythrocyte sedimentation rate, chemistry profile, urinalysis) may at times provide clues to the diagnosis. If indicated by the clinical features and/or screening laboratory studies, definitive diagnosis requires directed tests (e.g., endoscopy and biopsy for inflammatory bowel disease or celiac disease, sweat chloride test for cystic fibrosis).

The management of these conditions rests on specific therapy directed at the underlying condition (e.g., gluten-free diet for celiac disease). When the disease is adequately treated, the growth rate often improves. GH therapy is approved for the treatment of short stature in children with renal insufficiency.

EMOTIONAL DEPRIVATION

Deprivation can stunt growth in two ways. First, a child may be deprived of food (an example of malnutrition); in this case, the child's weight is generally depressed more than the height. Second, a child who is emotionally deprived may have profound short stature without apparent malnutrition. In this case, the height is depressed more than the weight (Fig. 60-8). The child may have the clinical features of GH deficiency and may in fact show laboratory evidence of hypopituitarism. When placed in a more nurturing environment, the child grows markedly, and the GH levels revert to normal. This disorder may be difficult to diagnose, and the social history is

critical. The diagnosis ultimately rests on significant improvement of growth once the environment improves.

ENDOCRINE DISORDERS

Growth Hormone Deficiency

GH is essential for postnatal growth, and children who lack it are extremely stunted. GH deficiency may be congenital or acquired. The congenital form may be idiopathic, associated with midline defects (absence of the septum pellucidum and optic nerve hypoplasia [septooptic dysplasia], cleft palate, holoprosencephaly, single central incisor), or related to genetic abnormalities in components of the GH regulatory axis (including defects in the genes for GH, transcription factors controlling GH [e.g., Pit-1, Prop-1], or the GH-releasing hormone receptor). In rare cases, functional GH deficiency may be caused by an abnormal GH molecule. GH deficiency may be acquired secondary to birth injury, head injury, cranial irradiation, and midline tumors or masses (craniopharyngioma). Both congenital and acquired forms may be associated with isolated GH deficiency or with multiple pituitary hormone deficiencies (panhypopituitarism).

The presenting features differ according to whether the condition is congenital or acquired and according to the origin of GH deficiency. Affected infants are often normal in birth size, although statistical analysis suggests that, as a group, they are somewhat small. Some newborns with congenital GH deficiency have hypoglycemia (see Chapter 61); they may also have jaundice with a hepatitis-type picture; affected boys may have micropenis (particularly if there is also gonadotropin deficiency). Other infants with congenital GH deficiency show no signs in the neonatal period but show slow growth later in infancy. Poor linear growth usually becomes clear by age 3 years.

In acquired forms of GH deficiency, there may be a history of a precipitating event (cranial irradiation, head trauma) or a history suggestive of an intracranial lesion (headaches, vomiting, visual

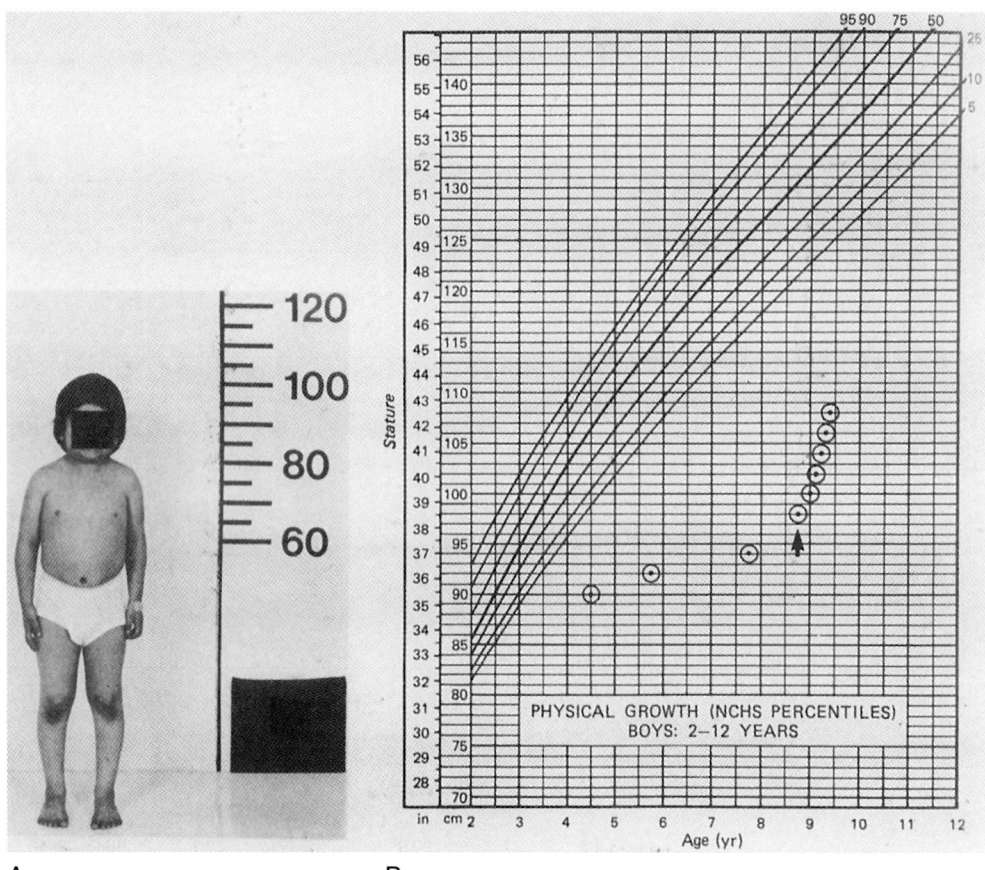

Figure 60-8. A, Photograph and growth chart of a boy with deprivation dwarfism (psychosocial dwarfism). Between ages 6 and 8 $^{7}/_{12}$ years, he had chemical evidence of growth hormone (GH) deficiency. **B,** After placement in a chronic care facility (*arrow*), his growth rate improved markedly, and his GH levels reverted to normal. NCHS, National Center for Health Statistics. (From Styne DM: Growth. In Greenspan FS, Forsham PH [eds]: Basic and Clinical Endocrinology, 3rd ed. Los Altos, Calif, Appleton & Lange, 1991.)

A   B

disturbances). Affected children often have normal growth until the onset of the disorder; thereafter, their growth is attenuated.

On physical examination, children with GH deficiency are typically short and look younger than their actual age. The children are classically described as chubby or cherubic, and their heights are depressed more than their weights (height age < weight age). They may have high-pitched voices, delayed dentition, and poor musculature. In congenital GH deficiency, there may be midline defects and, in boys, microphallus. In acquired GH deficiency, there may be evidence of the underlying disturbance (bitemporal hemianopsia, optic atrophy, or papilledema in midline tumors such as craniopharyngioma; dermatitis, scalp lesions, hepatosplenomegaly in Langerhans cell histiocytosis). Those with panhypopituitarism may show failure to enter or to progress normally through puberty.

Classically, the diagnosis of GH deficiency is based on short stature, with a slow growth rate for age, delayed bone age (bone age = height age < chronologic age), absence of another disorder to account for short stature, and subnormal GH levels (<7 or 10 ng/mL) in response to two pharmacologic stimuli (clonidine, arginine, L-dopa with or without propranolol, insulin-induced hypoglycemia). Although false-positive and false-negative results have been reported with the GH stimulation tests, no generally accepted alternative has emerged. Random GH levels are of no value in the diagnosis of GH deficiency. The GH tests must be performed in a euthyroid individual. Levels of IGF-I tend to be low in patients with GH deficiency and may be used to screen for GH deficiency; they are also affected by age and puberty. IGF binding protein 3 levels may also provide clues to GH deficiency. Once the diagnosis of GH deficiency is made, magnetic resonance imaging is performed to assess the possibility that an intracranial tumor or structural abnormality is causing the GH deficiency. Evaluation of other pituitary hormones is also needed. Children with GH deficiency respond well to GH therapy

and often more than double their rates of growth once treatment is begun. Traditionally, GH therapy for GH deficiency has stopped after adult height is reached; however, there is interest in the use of lower doses of GH for GH-deficient adults as a means of maintaining muscle mass, preventing osteoporosis, and enhancing well-being. GH has been approved by the FDA for these purposes.

There is controversy about whether the classic definition of GH deficiency is too rigid and whether there may be children with mild or subtle forms of GH deficiency who are missed by the classic criteria.

Another disorder of the GH-IGF axis is GH insensitivity from end-organ resistance to GH. This results from hereditary disorders in the GH receptor (e.g., Laron syndrome) and from cellular defects distal to the GH receptor, and is associated with high circulating levels of GH, low levels of GH binding protein, and low levels of IGF-I. Defects in IGF-I and its receptor have also been described. Studies to assess the effect of IGF-I therapy in these conditions are under way.

Hypothyroidism

Hypothyroidism impairs linear growth (see Fig. 60-5). Thyroid deficiency may be congenital or acquired (Fig. 60-9). In view of the usefulness of neonatal thyroid screening programs, it is very uncommon for congenital hypothyroidism to cause short stature.

Acquired hypothyroidism in children usually results from autoimmune thyroiditis (see Chapter 49). Children with Turner syndrome, Down syndrome, Klinefelter syndrome, or diabetes mellitus are at increased risk for autoimmune hypothyroidism, as are children with a family history of autoimmune disease. Acquired hypothyroidism tends to manifest most commonly in older children and teenagers. Often there are few complaints except for slow growth

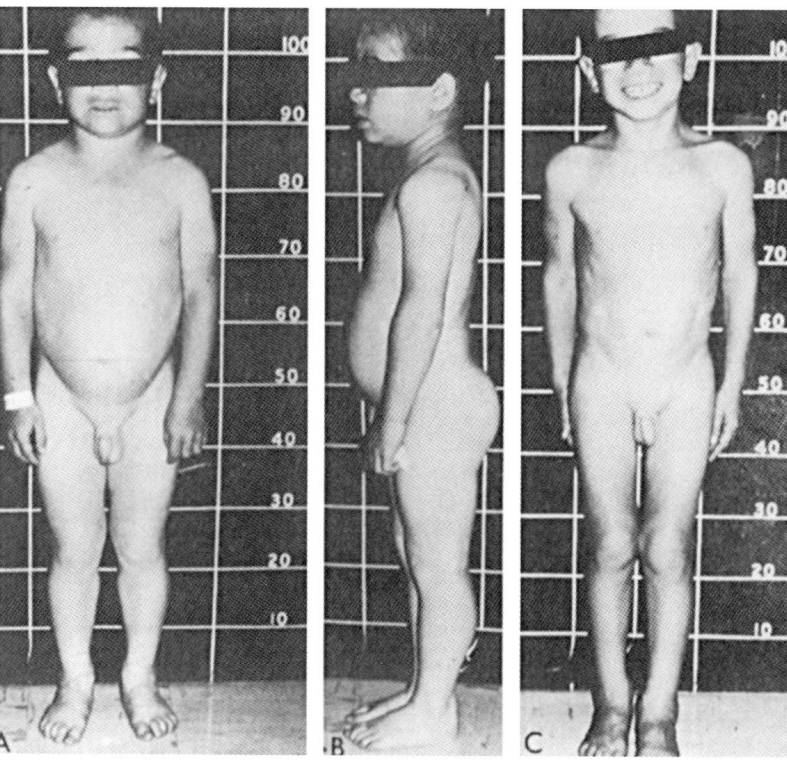

Figure 60-9. A and B, A 10-year-old boy with acquired hypothyroidism, before treatment. Note short stature, immature body proportions, sleepy expression, generalized myxedema, and protuberant abdomen. C, After 4 months of thyroid hormone therapy, the child has grown, has lost myxedema, and has a bright facial expression. (From Kaplan SA [ed]: Clinical Pediatric and Adolescent Endocrinology. Philadelphia, WB Saunders, 1982, p 93.)

(after previously normal growth), weight gain, a goiter, or a combination of these. Other symptoms (dry hair or skin, constipation, cold intolerance) are less common. Postmenarchal girls may have amenorrhea or, in rare cases, galactorrhea. School performance is generally not impaired. On physical examination, the major features are a height suggestive of deceleration from the previous growth curve, a goiter, and relative obesity (weight age > height age). The physical examination may also reveal bradycardia, dry hair or skin, and delayed reflexes.

In acquired hypothyroidism, the laboratory test results often include a high level of thyroid-stimulating hormone (TSH) and a low or low-normal free thyroxine (T_4) level or free thyroxine index (FTI). The presence of positive thyroid antibodies (antithyroglobulin, antimicrosomal antibodies) is consistent with autoimmune thyroiditis. A low or normal TSH level in the presence of low free T_4 or FTI suggests that the child does not have a primary problem of the thyroid but instead may have a hypothalamic/pituitary abnormality leading to deficiency of TSH (alternatively, the child could have euthyroid sick syndrome, a concomitant feature of serious illness). The bone age is often significantly delayed in hypothyroidism.

The treatment of hypothyroidism is thyroid replacement therapy (L-thyroxine). Monitoring of free T_4 (or FTI) and TSH is essential for optimizing the dose of medication. Unduly large doses may advance osseous maturation or lead to symptoms of thyroid excess.

Glucocorticoid Excess (Cushing Syndrome)

Cushing syndrome results from excessive levels of glucocorticoids. Whether endogenous or exogenous, glucocorticoids markedly stunt growth. In general, because such conditions are acquired, the history reveals a child previously growing well whose growth velocity slows. The child typically continues to gain weight at a rapid rate, even though linear growth is attenuated. This is in contrast to exogenous obesity, in which affected children tend to grow at normal or rapid rates. The history may indicate that the child was treated with oral, topical (especially with occlusive dressings), or intradermal

glucocorticoids at high doses or for long durations. Alternate-day oral glucocorticoids are much less likely to attenuate growth than are daily doses. In endogenous Cushing syndrome, the findings may include acne, evidence of virilization, or large appetite. Hyperpigmentation may occur when Cushing syndrome is secondary to excessive adrenocorticotropic hormone (ACTH) levels. This may be caused by ACTH from a pituitary tumor (Cushing disease) or from a nonpituitary source (ectopic ACTH syndrome).

The physical examination usually reveals short stature with relative obesity. Many affected children have the moon face and plethora characteristic of Cushing syndrome. A buffalo hump, striae, acne, and hypertension may also be present. Marked virilization is worrisome, because it may be a sign of an adrenal tumor.

The diagnosis of endogenous Cushing syndrome is based on demonstrating abnormally high glucocorticoid production (on 24-hour urine sample for free cortisol, normalized to creatinine) and failure to suppress cortisol production adequately in response to exogenous glucocorticoid. A screening test for capacity to suppress cortisol secretion in response to exogenous glucocorticoid is the overnight dexamethasone suppression test. This involves the child taking 0.3 mg/m^2 of dexamethasone at 11:00 PM (the standard dose of dexamethasone in adults is 1 mg), followed by a measurement of circulating cortisol the following morning; a normal cortisol level after dexamethasone is less than 5 μg/mL. False-positive results may occur in the setting of obesity, chronic illness, or stress. If cortisol production is excessive or is not suppressed in an overnight dexamethasone test, formal high- and low-dose dexamethasone tests are needed to define the presence and nature of hypercortisolism. If the child shows biochemical evidence of Cushing syndrome, further investigations, including computed tomography, magnetic resonance imaging, and measurement of ACTH levels, are needed to determine whether a pituitary tumor (commonest cause), an adrenal tumor, or ectopic ACTH production is present. Exogenous Cushing syndrome is usually evident from the history and physical examination results; when necessary, the diagnosis can be confirmed by failure of the child to secrete cortisol normally after administration of ACTH (ACTH stimulation test), together with clinical evidence of Cushing syndrome.

Treatment involves the removal of excess glucocorticoids either by reducing or discontinuing exogenous steroids if medically feasible or, in the case of endogenous hypercortisolism caused by a pituitary or adrenal tumor, by surgery.

Other Endocrine Disorders

Diabetes mellitus, when poorly controlled, can lead to slow linear growth. This probably results from lack of biologically available nutrients. The diagnosis should be apparent from the history. However, because of the risk of autoimmune thyroiditis, slow-growing children with diabetes should also be checked for hypothyroidism.

Diabetes insipidus, when poorly controlled or untreated, may lead to slow growth. This is presumed to reflect poor caloric intake in association with intense thirst. High fluid intake in central diabetes insipidus is dramatically decreased with vasopressin; treatment of nephrogenic diabetes insipidus is more challenging (see Chapter 62).

IATROGENIC CAUSES

Treatments for medical conditions may secondarily impair growth. The classic example is glucocorticoids. Spinal irradiation for treatment of malignancies may stunt growth by limiting further spinal growth; this is associated with a high U/L. It has also been suggested that certain treatments for hyperactivity (sympathomimetic agents suppress appetite) may interfere with growth.

EVALUATING THE CHILD WITH SHORT STATURE

HISTORY

Pregnancy and Birth History

Did the mother have illnesses or take medication during the pregnancy? Maternal illness or use of certain drugs can cause poor fetal growth.

What was the birth weight and length? Intrauterine growth retardation may lead to continuing small stature.

Did the baby have perinatal problems such as unexplained hypoglycemia, prolonged jaundice, or, in boys, a small phallus? These are suggestive of congenital GH deficiency.

Did the baby have other perinatal problems (hypoxia, puffy extremities)? These may provide clues to the underlying cause of short stature (hypoxia might lead to hypopituitarism; puffy extremities in a girl are suggestive of Turner syndrome).

Infancy and Childhood

What was the child's growth pattern? Establishing a child's growth pattern necessitates obtaining previous height measurements and plotting them on standard growth charts. The child who has been short but growing at a normal rate and paralleling the fifth percentile is more likely to have familial or constitutional short stature. The child whose height deviates progressively away from the normal curve (especially after 24 months of age) is much more likely to have an underlying medical disorder. When this progressive deviation occurs from early childhood and continues, it often represents a congenital disorder (e.g., Turner syndrome, congenital GH deficiency). However, growth attenuation that occurs after a sustained period of normal growth suggests that a disorder has been acquired (e.g., acquired GH deficiency, inflammatory bowel disease).

Two periods of life may be associated with crossing of percentiles in normal children. During the first 24 months of life, normal children may shift height percentiles while establishing their own growth channels and thereafter tend to maintain the final channel throughout childhood. It may be difficult to distinguish this normal change in growth channel from a true abnormality, and assessing the child's growth in relation to genetic endowment and general well-being may be helpful. Children with constitutional delay of growth and pubertal development may have a prolonged slowdown of growth before entering puberty.

What were the child's developmental milestones? How is the school performance? Slow development or poor school performance may indicate a central disorder or may represent part of a syndrome (e.g., Prader-Willi syndrome). Hypothyroidism acquired after age 3 years usually does not interfere with school performance, although inadequately treated congenital hypothyroidism often leads to intellectual impairment. This question may also elicit a history of emotional problems.

Has the child had any serious illnesses or been on medication? Chronic illness often impedes growth, as do certain medications (glucocorticoids). A history of nonendocrine medical problems may also provide clues to the underlying disorder (e.g., the presence of aortic coarctation may be suggestive of Turner syndrome).

What has been the impact of short stature on the child? This will help to assess the emotional ramifications of short stature and may help to clarify the particular concerns or questions of the parents.

REVIEW OF SYSTEMS

How is the child's appetite? What does the child eat in a typical 3-day period (often best described by a formal diet record)? Adequate caloric intake is needed for growth. Inadequate intake may be a symptom of underlying chronic disease.

Does the child have abdominal pain, diarrhea, unexplained fevers, mouth or anal sores, or joint pain? These symptoms suggest occult inflammatory bowel disease.

Does the child have neck swelling, lethargy, constipation, cold intolerance, or weight gain without much increase in height? These are among the symptoms of acquired hypothyroidism.

Does the child have headaches, vomiting, or visual disturbances? Symptoms of central nervous system dysfunction, raised intracranial pressure, or both, suggest the possibility of acquired hypopituitarism in association with a central lesion such as a tumor or hydrocephalus.

Has the child begun pubertal development (appropriate for a child of pubertal age)? Puberty influences growth. Children with constitutional delay in growth and development have delayed puberty and often have an exaggerated nadir of growth velocity before puberty begins. However, the more puberty is delayed, the greater the likelihood of a medical disorder such as hypogonadism. Delayed puberty may be a manifestation of hypogonadism (Turner syndrome), or it may be secondary to a growth-impeding disorder (hypothyroidism or hypopituitarism).

FAMILY HISTORY

What were the heights of parents and other family members at the child's age, and when did they undergo puberty? What are the current heights of parents and family members? The most frequent causes of short stature are familial short stature and constitutional delay in growth and development. In the former, a family history of short stature is elicited. In the latter, a family history of delayed puberty is elicited. The child's height may be assessed more formally in relation to that of the parents with the use of midparental height charts. Some familial disorders (e.g., hypochondroplasia) are associated with short stature.

Who lives at home? Who are the primary caregivers? Because deprivation can lead to stunted growth, it is important to have a sense of the family situation, although it is often extremely difficult to define this fully.

PHYSICAL EXAMINATION

Height and *weight* should each be plotted carefully on growth charts. The degree of short stature in relation to peers is ascertained. Previous height measurements provide an index of the child's pattern of growth. The height-to-weight ratio should be noted. Weight that is depressed more than height in a short child is suggestive of chronic illness or malnutrition. In contrast, a child who is short but chubby is more likely to have an endocrine disorder or syndrome (e.g., GH deficiency, hypothyroidism, Cushing syndrome, Prader-Willi syndrome).

Exogenous obesity is usually associated with relatively tall stature. Disproportionate short stature (especially short legs and arms, leading to a high U/L or short arm span or both) is characteristic of many osteochondrodystrophies. Shortness of lower limbs may also occur in hypothyroidism.

The presence of *dysmorphic features* is often suggestive of a syndrome or genetic disorder (e.g., Turner syndrome, Noonan syndrome). Midline defects are suggestive of hypopituitarism.

Goiter, delayed dentition, bradycardia, dry hair or skin, or delayed reflexes may be suggestive of hypothyroidism.

Cherubic or doll-like appearance, high-pitched voice, delayed dentition, poor musculature, or relative adiposity may be suggestive of GH deficiency.

Bitemporal hemianopsia, papilledema, optic atrophy, or accelerating head circumference in a young child is suggestive of a central nervous system abnormality (craniopharyngioma) causing hypopituitarism.

The *stage of puberty* is noted. Delayed puberty is compatible with constitutional delay in growth and development, hypogonadism, panhypopituitarism, severe hypothyroidism, or chronic illness. The degree of pubertal development also is often correlated with the bone age, thus indicating the growth potential.

CLINICAL SYNTHESIS AND LABORATORY EVALUATION

If a child is *moderately short* (1.5 to 2 standard deviations below normal for age), is growing in parallel to the normal height curve, has a family history of short stature or delayed puberty, and is otherwise healthy, it is reasonable to conduct no further investigations initially and simply to follow the growth carefully. A bone age may be helpful for indicating growth potential and distinguishing, to some degree, familial short stature from constitutional delay in growth and development.

The bone age is the age at which the observed degree of bone maturation would be typical. Bone growth is normally accompanied by a predictable sequence, rate, and structure of bone maturation. Bone age correlates more closely with overall body maturation than does height or chronologic age. The degree of bone maturation is inversely proportional to the amount of epiphyseal cartilage growth remaining and therefore can be used cautiously to predict adult height; the more delayed the bone age, the greater the growth potential is as long as no medical disorder is present. Despite their usefulness, predictions of adult height have intrinsic variability.

If on follow-up it appears that the child's growth is decelerating, further studies may be needed (Tables 60-7 and 60-8).

If a child is *more markedly short* (>2 to 2.5 standard deviations below the mean), has a decelerating growth pattern (crossing percentiles), is short for the genetic endowment, or is unwell, further investigations are needed. The specific investigations depend on the clinical findings. If there is clear evidence of a specific disorder (e.g., disproportionate short stature suggestive of osteochondrodystrophies, a goiter suggestive of hypothyroidism, dysmorphic features suggestive of Turner syndrome), the appropriate investigations (skeletal survey, thyroid function tests, or karyotype, respectively) are needed. If the specific disorder is not clear, screening tests are needed to assess growth potential (bone age), hypothyroidism (free T_4 or FTI, TSH), and the possibility of chronic illness as a cause of short stature (complete blood cell count, differential and platelet count, erythrocyte sedimentation rate, chemistry profile, urinalysis). Girls with unexplained short stature should be assessed for Turner syndrome by karyotype analysis. Levels of IGF-I and IGF binding protein 3 may provide clues to the presence or absence of GH deficiency.

If results of these tests are normal, the child's height may be monitored carefully at 3- to 4-month intervals to establish the growth velocity; a slow growth velocity for age warrants evaluation for possible GH deficiency or other disorders. Alternatively, if the child's stature or well-being is excessively impaired, GH stimulation tests may be undertaken as part of the initial evaluation once the child is established to be euthyroid.

Table 60-7. Screening Tests for Evaluating Short Stature

Test	Rationale
CBC	*Anemia:* nutritional, chronic disease, malignancy, Fanconi
	Leukocytosis: inflammation, infection
	Leukopenia: bone marrow failure syndromes
	Thrombocytopenia: malignancy, infection, Fanconi
ESR and CRP	Inflammation of infection, inflammatory diseases, malignancy
SMA 20 (electrolytes, liver enzymes, BUN)	Signs of acute or chronic hepatic, renal, adrenal dysfunction; hydration and acid-base status
Urinalysis	Signs of renal dysfunction, hydration, water and salt homeostasis; renal tubular acidosis
Karyotype	Determines Turner or other chromosomal syndromes
Cranial imaging (MRI, CT)	Assesses hypothalmic-pituitary tumors (craniopharyngioma, glioma, germinoma) or congenital midline defects
Bone age	Compare with height age and eventual height potential
IGF-1, IGF BP3	Reflect GH status
Free thyroxine, TSH	Detect hypothyroidism
Prolactin	Elevated in hypothalamic dysfunction or destruction

From Styne DM: Endocrine disorders. In Behrman RE, Kliegman RM (eds): Nelson Essentials of Pediatrics, 2nd ed. Philadelphia; WB Saunders, 1994, p 618-620.

BP3, binding protein 3; BUN, blood urea nitrogen; CBC, complete blood count; CRP, C-reactive protein; CT, computed tomography; ESR, erythrocyte sedimentation rate; GH, growth hormone; IGF, insulin-like growth factor; MRI, magnetic resonance imaging; TSH, thyroid-stimulating hormone.

Table 60-8. Approach to Laboratory Tests in the Evaluation of Short Stature

If a child has significant short stature, a slow growth rate, and/or is short for midparental height:
  a. If there is strong clinical evidence as to the cause, perform specific directed studies (e.g., in a child with short stature, goiter, and clinical evidence of hypothyroidism, check free T$_4$ and TSH)
  b. If the cause of short stature is not evident clinically, perform screening tests:
    CBC with differential and platelet count, ESR, chemistry profile, urinalysis, free T$_4$ or free thyroxine index, TSH measurement, bone age estimate (IGF-I and IGF binding protein 3 are also checked by some physicians)
If the screening test results are normal, either:
  a. Recheck growth rate in 3 to 6 mo; if growth rate is low, perform further studies (karyotype in girls, GH stimulation tests)

                                  or

  b. If the child is markedly short or there is other reason for immediate concern, may perform above tests (e.g., karyotype, GH stimulation tests) as part of the initial evaluation (note: the child should be proven euthyroid before GH stimulation tests are undertaken)

CBC, complete blood cell count; ESR, erythrocyte sedimentation rate; GH, growth hormone; IGF, insulin-like growth factor; T$_4$, thyroxine; TSH, thyroid-stimulating hormone.

THERAPEUTIC OPTIONS

SPECIFIC TREATMENT OF THE PRIMARY DISORDER

If a child is found to have a clear medical condition causing short stature and for which treatment is available (e.g., hypothyroidism, GH deficiency), the appropriate treatment (thyroid replacement therapy or GH therapy, respectively) improves growth markedly as long as the epiphyses remain open. Often, such children experience accelerated (catch-up) growth for some time after appropriate treatment is instituted. Complete compensation for growth failure is unlikely to occur if the disorder was many years in duration or occurred very close to the onset of normal puberty.

Sex Steroids

Sex steroid treatments may be administered to adolescents with constitutional delay of growth and development. Boys with delayed puberty may be treated with testosterone enanthate (50 to 100 mg/month intramuscularly for approximately 3 to 6 months) to gradually bring about secondary sexual characteristics and some linear growth. This is often gratifying for boys and is followed by gradual spontaneous pubertal development. The low dose of testosterone is designed to avoid undue advancement of bone age and loss of growth potential. Bone age should be monitored.

Counseling

Reassurance and counseling should be available for all patients. For many children with familial short stature or constitutional delay in growth and development, it is reassuring to be told that they are normal and are likely to reach a normal adult height or one in keeping with the family heights. This is particularly true for children with delayed puberty, in whom the discrepancy in height in comparison with peers (who have gone through their pubertal growth spurts) is

Table 60-9. Red Flags in the Evaluation of Short Stature

Height > 2-2.5 standard deviations below the mean for age
Subnormal growth velocity
Abnormal body proportions
Abnormal height:weight ratio
Dysmorphic features
Goiter
Abnormal central nervous system and ophthalmologic examinations

disconcerting. It is helpful if parents do not dwell on the child's height but focus on the child's strengths. Gymnastics, wrestling, soccer, and swimming are often activities at which short children are not at a disadvantage and in which they may excel.

Growth Hormone Therapy

There is consensus for the use of GH therapy in children with short stature caused by classical GH deficiency, Turner syndrome, and chronic renal failure. The U.S. Food and Drug Administration has approved GH for children with chronic renal failure, those with Prader-Willi syndrome, and some children with persistent growth failure after being born small for gestational age, and use of GH in these situations is evolving. GH therapy for short children in whom no underlying cause of impaired growth can be identified (idiopathic short stature) is controversial. The issues include whether there may be subtle forms of GH deficiency or GH insensitivity not detected by current methods, whether additional diseases associated with short stature are best treated with GH, and whether GH treatment may increase the height of short, otherwise normal children. The FDA has approved GH therapy for such children when heights are more than 2.25 standard deviations below the mean with growth rates unlikely to permit attainment of an adult height in the normal range.

Potential side effects of GH have included fluid retention and pseudotumor cerebri, slipped capital femoral epiphyses (it is not clear whether this is secondary to rapid growth or GH treatment

Table 60-10. Conditions Not to Miss

Hypoglycemia in a full-term newborn who has size appropriate for gestational age and whose mother does not have diabetes mellitus	Rule out hypopituitarism
Hypoglycemia and microphallus in a newborn boy	Rule out hypopituitarism
Obesity in a child who is short	Rule out hypothyroidism, growth hormone deficiency, Cushing syndrome, Prader-Willi syndrome, Laurence-Moon-Biedl syndrome
Shortness in a child with a goiter	Rule out hypothyroidism
Shortness in a child with headache, vomiting, or visual disturbance	Rule out hypopituitarism secondary to central nervous system lesion, including craniopharyngioma or hydrocephalus

itself), GH-neutralizing antibodies (rarely of clinical impact), growth of nevi, hyperinsulinism, and glucose intolerance. Because GH has been used for non–GH-deficient children for a relatively short time, currently unforeseen long-term side effects are possible.

Studies are under way to assess the effectiveness of combined therapy with GH and GnRH agonist (to promote growth while suppressing puberty) in children with isolated GH deficiency and those with short stature of unknown cause.

SUMMARY AND RED FLAGS

Short stature may be a variant of normal development or may indicate a serious underlying problem. When short stature is associated with a slow growth velocity, progressive deviation from the child's previous growth channel, obesity, headache, vomiting, dysmorphic features, or a goiter, or if short height is inconsistent with the family history, a search for an underlying medical disorder should be undertaken (Tables 60-9 and 60-10). Understanding how to measure a child accurately, performing simple proportion measurements, and calculating growth velocity are skills that all pediatricians must have in order to diagnose short stature and identify associated disease states and syndromes.

REFERENCES

Diagnosing Growth Disorders

American Academy of Pediatrics Section on Endocrinology and Committee on Genetics and the American Thyroid Association Committee on Public Health: Newborn screening for congenital hypothyroidism: Recommended guidelines. Pediatrics 1993;91:1203-1209.

LaFranchi S: Diagnosis and treatment of hypothyroidism in children. Compr Ther 1987;13:20-30.

Parks JS, Brown MR, Hurley DL, et al: Heritable disorders of pituitary development. J Clin Endocrinol Metab 1999;84:4362-4370.

Roche AF, Wellens R, Attie KM, et al: The timing of sexual maturation in a group of white U.S. youths. J Pediatr Endocrinol Metab 1995;8:11-18.

Saenger P, Wiklund KA, Conway GS, et al: Recommendations for the diagnosis and management of Turner syndrome. J Clin Endocrinol Metab 2001;86:3061-3069.

Savage MO, Blum WF, Ranke MB, et al: Clinical features and endocrine status in patients with growth hormone insensitivity (Laron syndrome). J Clin Endocrinol Metab 1993;77:1465-1471.

Tanner J, Davies P: Clinical longitudinal standards for height and height velocity for North American children. J Pediatr 1985;107:317-329.

Tanner J, Goldstein H, Whitehouse R: Standards for children's height at ages 2-9 years allowing for height of parents. Arch Dis Child 1970;45: 755-762.

Growth

Jones KL: Smith's Recognizable Patterns of Human Malformation, 4th ed. Philadelphia, WB Saunders, 1988.

Kliegman R: Intrauterine growth retardation: Determinants of aberrant fetal growth. In Fanaroff AA, Martin RG (eds): Neonatal-Perinatal Medicine, 5th ed. St. Louis, Mosby–Year Book, 1997, pp 203-240.

Rosenfield RL, Cuttler L: Somatic growth and maturation. In DeGroot L, Jameson L (eds): Endocrinology. Philadelphia, WB Saunders, 2001, pp 477-502.

Growth Hormone

American Academy of Pediatrics: Considerations related to use of recombinant human growth hormone in children. Pediatrics. 1997;99: 122-129.

Bercu BB: The growing conundrum. Growth hormone treatment of the non–growth hormone deficient child. JAMA 1996;276:567-568.

Blethen SL, Allen DB, Graves D, et al: Safety of recombinant deoxyribonucleic acid–derived growth hormone. The National Cooperative Growth Study experience. J Clin Endocrinol Metab 1996;81: 1704-1710.

Cuttler L, Silvers JB, Singh J, et al: Short stature and growth hormone therapy; a national survey of physician recommendation patterns. JAMA 1996;276:531-537.

FDA talk paper: FDA approves humatrope for short stature. Available at: http://www.fda.gov/bbs/topics/answers/2003/ans01242.html

Finkelstein BS, Imperiale TF, Speroff T, et al: Effect of growth hormone therapy on height in children with idiopathic short stature: A meta-analysis. Arch Pediatr Adolesc Med 2002;156:230-240.

Finkelstein BS, Silvers JB, Marrero U, et al: Insurance coverage, physician recommendations, and access to emerging treatments. Growth hormone therapy for childhood short stature. JAMA 1998;279:663-668.

Goddard A, Covello R, Luoh S, et al: Mutations of the growth hormone receptor in children with idiopathic short stature. N Engl J Med 1995;333:1093-1098.

Guyda HJ: Use of growth hormone in children with short stature and normal growth hormone secretion: A growing problem. Trends Endocrinol Metab 1994;5:334-340.

Hintz RL, Attie KM, Baptista J, Roche A: Effect of growth hormone treatment on adult height of children with idiopathic short stature. Genentech Collaborative Group. N Engl J Med 1999;340:502-507.

Lantos J, Siegler M, Cuttler L: Ethical dilemmas in growth hormone therapy. JAMA 1989;261:1148-1154.

Lippe BM, Nakamoto JM: Conventional and nonconventional uses of growth hormone. Recent Prog Horm Res 1994;48:179-225.

Oberfield SE: Growth hormone use in normal, short children—A plea for reason. N Engl J Med 1999;340:557-559.

Rosenfeld RG, Frane J, Attie KM, et al: Six-year results of a randomized, prospective trial of human growth hormone and oxandrolone in Turner syndrome. J Pediatr 1992;121:49-55.

Vance ML, Mauras N: Growth hormone therapy in adults and children. N Engl J Med 1999;341:1206-1216.

61 Hypoglycemia

Charles A. Stanley*

Hypoglycemia is an acute, life-threatening medical emergency that may result in seizures, permanent brain damage, or even sudden death. Because there are many causes of hypoglycemia, including hormonal disorders, metabolic defects, and drugs or toxins, a comprehensive strategy for diagnosis and treatment is necessary. An important approach to evaluating hypoglycemic disorders is based on the metabolic and endocrine systems involved in fasting adaptation. This "fasting systems" approach takes advantage of the fact that all of the disorders causing hypoglycemia in infants and children, with one or two exceptions, involve impaired fasting. The integrity of these various systems is reflected in the plasma concentrations of critical fuels and hormones at the point of hypoglycemia. Specimens of plasma and urine at the time of hypoglycemia are known as the *critical samples* and should be routinely obtained immediately before treatment begins.

DEFINITION OF HYPOGLYCEMIA

Devising a uniform definition, one applicable to all age groups, of low blood glucose (hypoglycemia) is difficult. This is in part related to a large number of affected patients who are otherwise well, particularly newborns, that may have a low blood glucose level without any obvious signs and symptoms (*asymptomatic hypoglycemia*).

Attempts have been made to define hypoglycemia by taking either a statistical or a clinical approach. The statistical approach relates to defining hypoglycemia when the blood glucose concentration falls outside a described limit (2 standard deviations of the mean glucose concentration measured in that population); the clinical approach defines the blood glucose concentration threshold at which clinical signs and symptoms appear (and disappear by correcting the low glucose concentration). The wide range of blood glucose concentrations at which clinically overt signs may appear has led to uncertainty in definition.

When comparing reported glucose values, the clinician must recognize some technical factors. Unless a free-flow blood sample is obtained from the infant with minimal pain, the glucose values are likely to vary greatly. Second, whole blood glucose values are slightly lower than those of plasma because of the dilution by the fluid in the red blood cells. Finally, hematocrit also influences the blood glucose concentration. This is particularly important in newborns, whose hematocrit values can vary in a wide range. A high hematocrit level results in lower blood glucose concentration; the opposite is true for low hematocrit values.

Plasma glucose concentrations are normally maintained within a very narrow range of 70 to 100 mg/dL. Glucose levels vary little with the usual schedule of overnight fasting and daytime feedings in infants and children, as in adults. A plasma glucose value below 40 mg/dL is commonly taken as the clinical definition of hypoglycemia. However, subtle signs and symptoms of neuroglycopenia can be documented at plasma glucose levels below 70 mg/dL and are more apparent at glucose levels below 60 or 50 mg/dL. For provocative tests, such as fasting studies, a glucose level of 50 mg/dL can be taken as sufficiently low for judging fuel and hormonal responsiveness. The response to a given level of plasma glucose can vary, depending on the underlying disorder. For example, patients with glucose-6-phosphatase deficiency (type 1 glycogen storage disease; see later discussion) may appear asymptomatic at glucose levels below 40 mg/dL, because they have concomitant elevations of plasma lactate, which can partially replace the glucose needed by the brain. On the other hand, children with defects in fatty acid oxidation can become very ill at plasma glucose levels as high as 60 mg/dL, because they have no alternative (e.g., ketones) to glucose as a fuel for the brain and other tissues such as heart and skeletal muscle.

In the past, it was common practice to accept lower standards for glucose levels in newborns because of the high frequency of low plasma glucose levels on the day of birth. It should be stressed, however, that these lower values represent a purely "statistical" definition of normal; there is no evidence that the neonatal brain has less need for glucose than do the brains of older children or adults. Specific maturational delays in several of the fasting systems adequately explain why infants have such a high risk of hypoglycemia during the first 12 to 24 hours after delivery. The use of different glucose standards for newborns should be discouraged, and the same treatment goals for hypoglycemia should be applied to newborns and older children: that is, to maintain plasma glucose levels above 60 mg/dL at all times.

REGULATION OF BLOOD GLUCOSE CONCENTRATION

Glucose is the primary fuel for the brain and, because the brain has no reserve stores, it must be continually supplied with glucose during periods of short- or long-term fasting. Within 2 to 3 hours after a meal, glucose absorption from the intestine ceases, and the liver becomes the major source of glucose for the brain and other tissues. As shown in Figure 61-1, the liver produces glucose through a combination of glycogenolysis and gluconeogenesis. Gluconeogenesis provides approximately 25% of hepatic glucose production in the early phases of fasting; the rate of gluconeogenesis is determined largely by rates of protein turnover and remains constant throughout fasting. Hepatic glycogenolysis provides the majority of glucose production early in a fast, but by 12 hours, liver glycogen stores become depleted. The body must then begin to depend on release of fatty acids by lipolysis from stores of fat in adipose tissue. Most tissues can oxidize free fatty acids directly and thus minimize their use of glucose. The major exception is the brain, which is unable to directly oxidize free fatty acids, because they cannot transit the blood-brain barrier. However, partial oxidation of free fatty acids in the liver produces ketones (β-hydroxybutyrate and acetoacetate), which are readily oxidized by the brain, further minimizing cerebral glucose consumption.

*This chapter is an updated and edited version of the chapter by Satish C. Kalhan and Thomas F. Riley that appeared in the first edition.

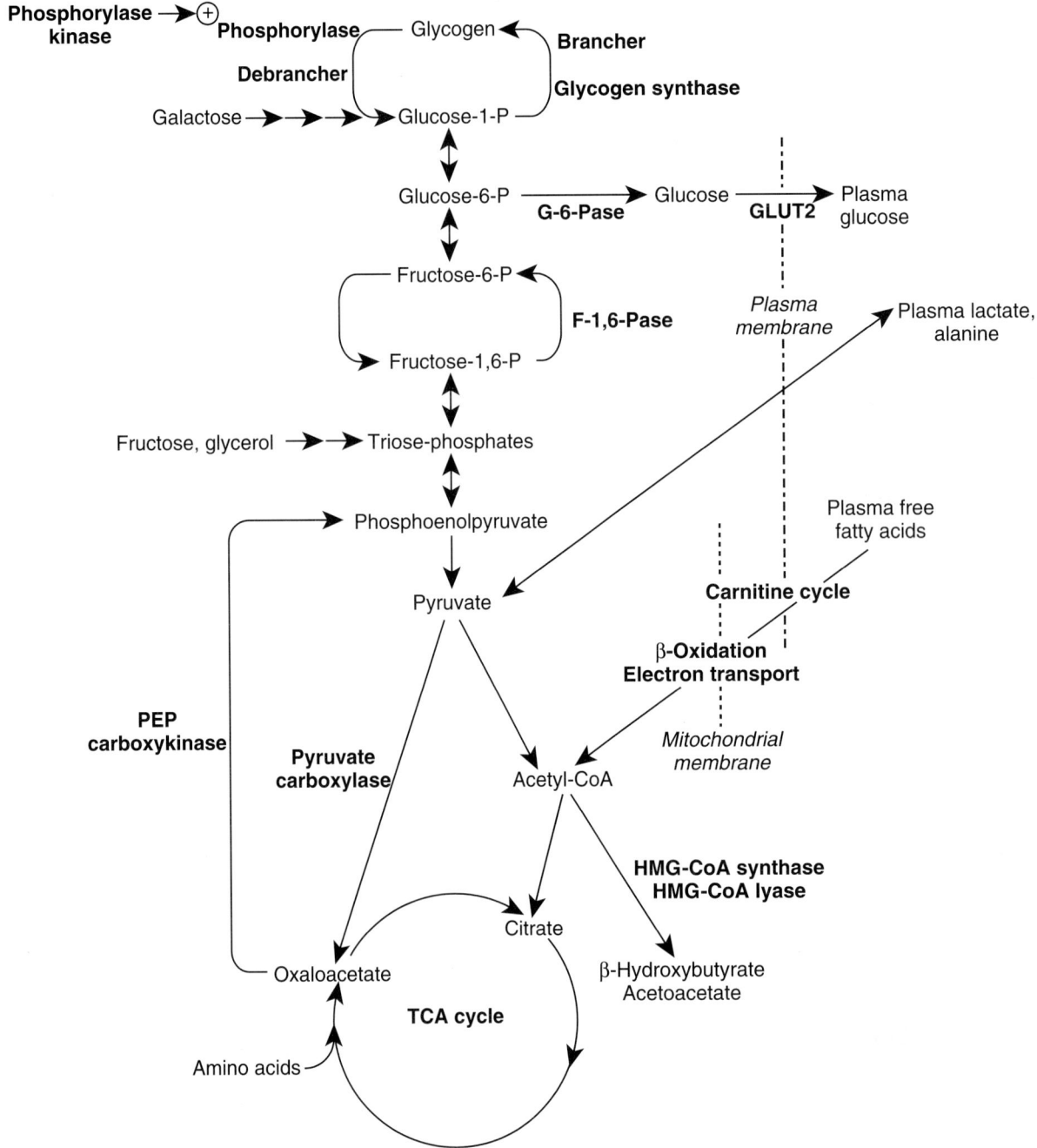

Figure 61-1. Metabolic systems of fasting adaptation. Shown are the pathways of hepatic gluconeogenesis, glycogenolysis, and ketogenesis. Key enzyme steps are in boldface. Enzyme steps in gluconeogenesis: pyruvate carboxylase, phosphoenolpyruvate (PEP) carboxykinase, fructose-1,6-bisphosphatase (F-1,6-Pase), glucose-6-phosphatase (G-6-Pase), and the plasma membrane glucose transporter 2 (GLUT-2). Enzyme steps in glycogenolysis: glycogen synthase, glycogen brancher enzyme, glycogen phosphorylase kinase, glycogen phosphorylase, and glycogen debrancher enzyme. Steps in ketogenesis include a series of enzyme steps in the carnitine cycle for transporting fatty acids across the mitochondrial membrane, enzymes of the β-oxidation cycle, enzymes of electron transport, and enzymes of ketone synthesis (3-hydroxy-3-methylglutaryl–coenzyme A [HMG-CoA] synthase and HMG-CoA lyase). P, phosphate; TCA, tricarboxylic acid.

Metabolic systems and hormones normally prevent hypoglycemia during fasting (Table 61-1). The actions of insulin and the counterregulatory hormones are summarized in Table 61-2. The integration of these systems is demonstrated by the changes in plasma concentrations of the major fuels and hormones during the course of fasting (Fig. 61-2). Plasma glucose concentrations gradually decline over the course of the fast as liver glycogen reserves are depleted. In infants and young children, with their larger ratio of brain to body mass, glucose levels fall faster than in older children and adults and may reach 50 mg/dL by 24 to 30 hours of fasting. Plasma levels of lactate, a representative gluconeogenic precursor, decline during the course of fasting as hepatic gluconeogenesis is stimulated and protein turnover slows. Plasma free fatty acid levels begin to rise quickly after 12 to 20 hours of fasting in response to the fall in insulin concentrations as glucose declines. The increased availability of fatty acids is accompanied by a 10- to 20-fold rise in plasma ketone levels as hepatic

Table 61-1. Metabolic Systems and Hormones Regulating Blood Glucose

Metabolic Systems

Hepatic gluconeogenesis
Hepatic glycogenolysis
Adipose tissue lipolysis
Fatty acid oxidation (liver and peripheral organs) and hepatic ketogenesis

Hormonal Systems

Insulin
Counter-regulatory hormones
    Glucagon
    Cortisol
    Growth hormone
    Epinephrine

oxidation of fatty acids is activated. Determining the circulating levels of these fuels and hormones at the point of hypoglycemia provides the most important information for diagnosing the cause of hypoglycemia.

CLINICAL MANIFESTATIONS

A variety of signs and symptoms may occur in patients with hypoglycemia (Table 61-3). They can be divided into two categories. Those in the first category result from activation of the autonomic nervous system and release of the counterregulatory hormone epinephrine. Those in the second category are secondary to inadequate delivery of glucose to the brain.

CAUSES OF TRANSIENT NEONATAL HYPOGLYCEMIA

Hypoglycemia is a common problem in newborns. The majority of cases are transient, although the neonatal period is also the time when inherited disorders are most likely to manifest. The differential diagnosis of hypoglycemia is extensive (Table 61-4).

NORMAL NEWBORNS

As many as 30% of normal, full-term newborns and those of size appropriate for gestational age may be unable to maintain plasma glucose levels above 50 mg/dL if they fast for the first 6 hours after delivery. By the second day of life, however, the frequency of plasma glucose concentrations below 50 mg/dL drops to less than 1%, which indicates a rapid maturation of fasting adaptation. The extremely poor fasting tolerance on the day of birth can be explained by lack of development of key enzymes in the pathways of both

hepatic gluconeogenesis and ketogenesis. Transcription of these genes is delayed until after delivery but becomes well activated by the end of the first 24 hours. Glucagon and cortisol may be important for activation of enzymes involved in gluconeogenesis. Ingestion of long-chain fats (e.g., in colostrum) may be important for triggering transcription of the two enzymes of ketogenesis. Thus, on the day of birth, all newborns can be viewed as having impaired fasting adaptation. In the absence of other risk factors, hypoglycemia in the first day may necessitate only feeding and follow-up blood glucose determination to ensure that further workup is not necessary. Breast-fed babies are at special risk for hypoglycemia when, as often occurs, there are problems initiating milk production.

NEWBORNS SMALL FOR GESTATIONAL AGE AND PREMATURE INFANTS

Hypoglycemia is significantly more common in premature infants and those small for gestational age because of decreased stores of glycogen, fat, and protein. In addition, the enzymes necessary for gluconeogenesis may be less developed than in normal full-term infants.

INFANTS OF DIABETIC MOTHERS

Infants born to mothers with any type of diabetes, including gestational diabetes, are at risk for hypoglycemia because of oversecretion of insulin during the first few days after delivery. This transient hyperinsulinemia occurs because maternal hyperglycemia stimulates fetal insulin secretion and, after delivery, affected infants have difficulty in downregulating insulin secretion to adapt to the withdrawal of the hyperglycemia. Because of the growth-stimulating effects of insulin on the fetus, infants of diabetic mothers are often large for gestational age. Hypoglycemia should be treated with intravenous glucose support, and the problem should resolve promptly, within 1 to 2 days. Prolonged hyperinsulinism (HI) in infants of diabetic mothers should raise the suspicion of either a genetic form of HI or perinatal stress-induced HI (see the following section). Other problems of infants of diabetic mothers are noted in Table 61-5.

PERINATAL STRESS-INDUCED HYPERINSULINISM

Some infants with perinatal disorders, such as birth asphyxia or intrauterine growth retardation, may have severe problems with hypoglycemia for prolonged periods, ranging from a few days to a few months after birth. This form of transient HI has not been well recognized, but it is probably not rare. The mechanism appears to be HI; oral diazoxide, which decreases insulin secretion, provides good control of hypoglycemia in these infants.

ERYTHROBLASTOSIS FETALIS

An association between hypoglycemia and erythroblastosis fetalis caused by Rh incompatibility occurs in infants who are anemic at birth (cord hemoglobin <10 g/dL). The low blood glucose levels in

Table 61-2. Hormonal Regulation of Fasting Metabolic Systems

Hormone	Hepatic Glycogenolysis	Hepatic Gluconeogenesis	Adipose Tissue Lipolysis	Hepatic Ketogenesis
Insulin	Inhibits	Inhibits	Inhibits	Inhibits
Glucagon	Stimulates	—	—	—
Cortisol	—	Stimulates	—	—
Growth hormone	—	—	Stimulates	—
Epinephrine	Stimulates	Stimulates	Stimulates	Stimulates

From Sperling, MA (ed): Pediatric Endocrinology, 2nd ed. Philadelphia, WB Saunders, 2002.

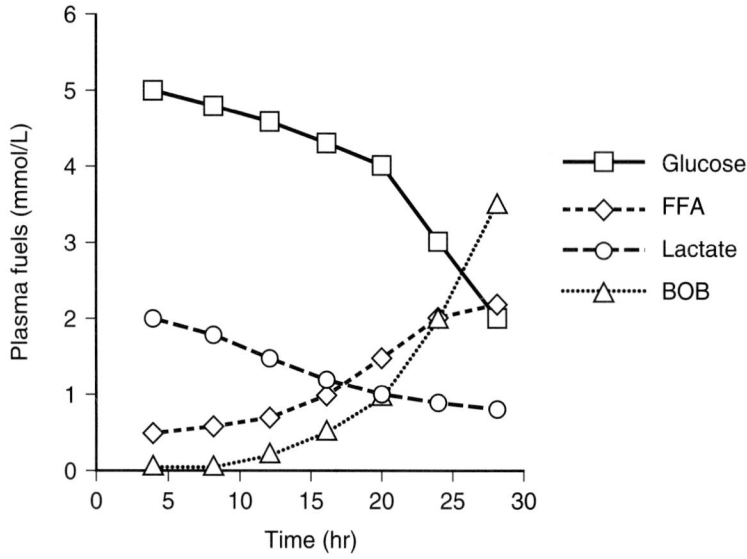

Figure 61-2. Changes in plasma levels of key fuels during fasting in a normal child. Note that plasma glucose declines toward hypoglycemic values by 24 hours as hepatic glycogen reserves become depleted. Plasma levels of lactate, a representative gluconeogenic substrate, decline gradually during the fast as hepatic gluconeogenesis is activated. Late in fasting, levels of plasma free fatty acids (FFA) increase as lipolysis is stimulated, followed by a dramatic rise in β-hydroxybutyrate that reflects the increase in the rates of hepatic fatty acid oxidation and ketone synthesis. BOB, β-hydroxybutyrate.

these infants have been attributed to high plasma insulin concentration. The cause of these high insulin levels remains undefined. The current prevention and management of Rh sensitization have markedly reduced the incidence of erythroblastosis and of fetal and neonatal anemia. Nonetheless, such infants require careful monitoring of plasma glucose concentration soon after birth.

Table 61-3. Manifestations of Hypoglycemia in Childhood

Features Associated with Activation of Autonomic Nervous System and Epinephrine Release*

Anxiety[†]
Perspiration[†]
Palpitation (tachycardia)[†]
Pallor
Tremulousness
Weakness
Hunger
Nausea
Emesis
Angina (with normal coronary arteries)

Features Associated with Cerebral Glucopenia

Headache[†]
Mental Confusion[†]
Visual disturbances (↓ acuity, diplopia)[†]
Organic personality changes[†]
Inability to concentrate[†]
Dysarthria
Staring
Seizures
Ataxia, incoordination
Somnolence, lethargy
Coma
Stroke, hemiplegia, aphasia
Paresthesias
Dizziness
Amnesia
Decerebrate or decorticate posture

From Behrman RE, Kliegman RM, Jenson HB (eds): Nelson Textbook of Pediatrics, 17th ed. WB Saunders, Philadelphia, 2003.

*Some of these features are attenuated if the patient is receiving β-adrenergic blocking agents.

[†]Common.

INTRAPARTUM MATERNAL GLUCOSE ADMINISTRATION

Administration of excessive glucose quantities to the mother during labor results in maternal as well as fetal hyperglycemia. Increased fetal glucose concentration causes increased fetal insulin secretion and fetal HI. If the glucose has been administered to the mother immediately before the infant's birth, the infant is born with high insulin levels. In addition, high fetal blood glucose and insulin levels may also cause an increase in fetal blood lactate concentration and metabolic acidosis. These effects are more pronounced if the mother has received infusions of glucose for a prolonged time. An acute administration of large amounts of glucose-containing fluids (e.g., to prevent hypotension in women receiving conduction anesthetics) leads to acute fetal hyperglycemia, HI, and metabolic acidosis. The HI of the fetus continues transiently in the neonatal period and leads to hypoglycemia.

MATERNAL DRUG THERAPY

The various pharmacologic agents administered to the mother for the treatment of medical problems that can influence blood glucose levels in the newborn can be divided into two broad categories:

1. Some drugs, including oral hypoglycemic agents, can *directly* affect blood glucose. Oral hypoglycemic agents, such as chlorpropamide and sulfonylureas, are administered by some physicians for the treatment of gestational diabetes. Because these drugs are easily transported across the placenta, the infant is born with a certain amount of drug present in the circulation. These drugs, particularly those with prolonged effects, may result in profound hypoglycemia that tends to persist until the drug is removed, either by its own clearance or by exchange transfusion.

2. Some drugs are administered to the mother with *indirect* effects (the more common contributor to neonatal hypoglycemia). β-Sympathomimetic agents commonly used for the prevention and treatment of premature labor can result in maternal hyperglycemia by increasing hepatic glucose production and decreasing glucose utilization. Maternal hyperglycemia, in turn, can initiate fetal hyperglycemia and HI, which can cause hypoglycemia in the newborn.

BECKWITH-WIEDEMANN SYNDROME

The clinical features of infants born with Beckwith-Wiedemann syndrome (BWS) consist of macroglossia, abdominal wall defects

Table 61-4. Causes of Hypoglycemia in Children

Transient Neonatal Hypoglycemia

Inadequate substrate
  Prematurity
  Small for gestational age
Excessive insulin
  Infants of diabetic mothers
  Perinatal stress-induced hyperinsulinism
  Erythroblastosis fetalis
  Intrapartum maternal glucose administration
  Maternal hypoglycemic agent
  Beckwith-Wiedemann syndrome
  Maternal prenatal hyperglycemia
Multiple mechanisms
  Normal newborn

Persistent Hypoglycemia in Neonates and Children

Hyperinsulinism
  Recessive KATP channel HI
  Focal KATP channel HI
  Dominant KATP channel HI
  Dominant glutamate dehydrogenase HI
    (hyperinsulinism/hyperammonemia syndrome)
  Dominant glucokinase HI
  Insulinoma
  Insulin reaction
  Oral hypoglycemics
  Surreptitious insulin (Munchausen syndrome by proxy)
Counterregulatory hormone deficiencies
  Hypopituitarism
  Isolated cortisol deficiency
  Epinephrine deficiency
Defects in gluconeogenesis
  Glucose-6-phosphatase deficiency (GSD types 1a and 1b)
  GLUT-2 deficiency (Fanconi-Bickel syndrome)
  Fructose-1,6-diphosphatase deficiency
  Pyruvate carboxylase deficiency
Defects in glycogenolysis
  Debrancher deficiency (GSD type 3)
  Phosphorylase deficiency (GSD type 6)
  Phosphorylase kinase deficiency (GSD type 9)
  Glycogen synthase deficiency (GSD type 0)
Fatty acid oxidation disorders
Other metabolic causes of hypoglycemia
  GLUT-1 deficiency
  Hereditary fructose intolerance
  Galactosemia
Reactive hypoglycemia
  GDH-HI, hyperinsulinism/hyperammonemia syndrome
  Post-Nissen hypoglycemia (late dumping syndrome)
  Hereditary fructose intolerance

GLUT, glucose transporter; GSD, glycogen storage disease; HI, hyperinsulinism; KATP, adenosine triphosphate–sensitive potassium.

(omphalocele, umbilical hernia), somatic gigantism, visceromegaly (liver, kidney, spleen), and hypoglycemia. Other possible features include ear anomalies, such as creases on the lobe; cardiac defects; renal abnormalities; hemihypertrophy; and neonatal polycythemia. These infants are prone to intraabdominal malignancies, including Wilms tumor, hepatoblastoma, rhabdomyosarcoma, and neuroblastoma. Most cases of BWS are sporadic, although approximately 15% are inherited through autosomal dominance. BWS appears to be caused by abnormal genomic imprinting involving multiple genes at chromosome 11p15.

Early recognition of hypoglycemia is extremely important for appropriate clinical management because there is an association in

BWS between hypoglycemia and intellectual impairment. Any infant born with an omphalocele should be monitored for potential hypoglycemia. Approximately 50% of newborns with BWS have hypoglycemia; 80% of cases are mild and transient. The remaining 20% of cases are more prolonged and difficult to control. HI is the principal mechanism of the hypoglycemia. At autopsy, hypertrophy and hyperplasia of the islet of Langerhans have been observed. Treatment depends on the severity of the hypoglycemia; it may include frequent feedings, intravenous dextrose, medications such as diazoxide or octreotide, and, in severe cases, partial pancreatectomy. If managed medically, the hypoglycemia eventually resolves over weeks to months of care.

CAUSES OF PERSISTENT HYPOGLYCEMIA IN INFANTS AND CHILDREN

HYPERINSULINISM

Congenital HI is the most common cause of recurrent hypoglycemia in infants and children. Previously, this disorder was referred to as nesidioblastosis, leucine-sensitive hypoglycemia, or idiopathic hypoglycemia of infancy. Most affected patients present during infancy, and macrosomia may be present at birth as a result of high insulin levels, which act as a growth factor in utero. Excessive insulin secretion during fasting suppresses all of the fasting systems, including hepatic glucose production, lipolysis, and ketogenesis. Thus, hypoglycemia results from both overuse and underproduction of glucose. Because lipolysis and ketosis are inhibited, levels of alternative fuels remain low, which increases the risk of seizures and permanent brain injury. There are several genetic defects of pancreatic β cell insulin secretion in children with HI (Fig. 61-3).

Recessive KATP Channel Hyperinsulinism

This is the most severe form of congenital HI. Affected infants are usually large for gestational age and present with symptoms of hypoglycemia, such as seizures, in the first days after birth. The hypoglycemia is often extremely severe, and treatment may require intravenous glucose infusions at 20 to 30 mg/kg/minute (four to six times normal) to maintain plasma glucose in the normal range of 70 to 100 mg/dL. This disorder is caused by genetic defects of the β cell plasma membrane adenosine triphosphate–dependent potassium (KATP) channel (see Fig. 61-3). The channel is encoded by two adjacent genes located on chromosome 11p: sulfonylurea receptor type 1 (*SUR1*) and *Kir6.2*. Common founder mutations of *SUR1* have been identified in Ashkenazi Jews and in Finland, but most affected patients have one of a large number of "private" (rare and unique) mutations. Medical management with diazoxide or octreotide (which acts like somatostatin) may be tried (see Fig. 61-3) but is rarely effective. Most infants require surgical near-total (98%) pancreatectomy to achieve control of hypoglycemia. As noted in the following section, about 50% of infants with severe HI who require surgery have diffuse disease caused by these recessive KATP channel mutations; the remainder have focal lesions that are potentially curable by surgical resection.

Focal KATP Channel Hyperinsulinism

Approximately half the infants with severe neonatal-onset HI have focal lesions of the pancreas that are potentially curable by surgical resection. The molecular defect in these infants involves the same KATP channel genes as in recessive KATP channel HI through a two-hit mechanism: loss of heterozygosity for the maternal chromosome 11p and expression of a paternally derived *SUR1* or *Kir6.2* mutation. Histologically, the focal lesions usually appear as adenomatosis. The clinical features are identical to those of infants with recessive KATP channel HI, including diazoxide unresponsiveness

Table 61-5. Pathophysiologic Mechanisms of Morbidity and Mortality of Infants of Diabetic Mothers

Problem	Pathophysiologic Mechanism
Fetal demise	Acute placental failure?
	Hyperglycemia–lactic acidosis–hypoxia?
Macrosomia	Hyperinsulinism
Respiratory distress syndrome	Insulin antagonism of cortisol induction of surfactant synthesis
Wet lung syndrome	Cesarean delivery
Hypoglycemia	↓ Glucose and fat mobilization–hyperinsulinemia
Polycythemia	Erythropoietic "macrosomia"?
	Mild fetal hypoxia?
	↓ O_2 delivery to fetus–HbA_{1c}?
Hypocalcemia	↓ Neonatal parathyroid hormone
	↓ Magnesium
Hyperbilirubinemia	↑ Erythropoietic mass
	↑ Bilirubin production
	Immature hepatic conjugation?
	Oxytocin induction
Congenital malformations (central nervous system, heart, skeletal)	Hyperglycemia
	Insulin as teratogen?
	Vascular accident?
Renal vein thrombosis	Polycythemia
	Dehydration
Neonatal small left colon syndrome	Immature gastrointestinal motility
Cardiomyopathy	Reversible septal hypertrophy
	↑ Glycogen
	↑ Muscle
Family psychological stress	High-risk pregnancy
	Fear of diabetes in infant
Subsequent development of insulin-dependent diabetes	Genetic HLA markers

Adapted from Kliegman RM, Fanaroff AA: Developmental metabolism and nutrition. In Gregory GA (ed): Pediatric Anesthesiology, 2nd ed. New York, Churchill Livingstone, 1989, p 236. Hb, hemoglobin; HLA, human leukocyte antigen.

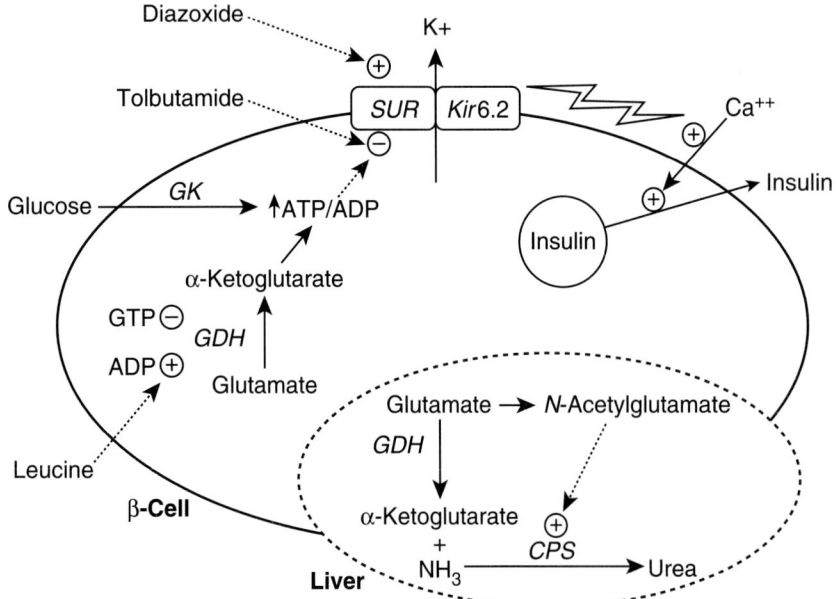

Figure 61-3. Pathways of pancreatic β cell insulin secretion. Increases in plasma concentrations of glucose lead to increased pancreatic β cell glucose oxidation rates and elevations of intracellular adenosine triphosphate (ATP). The increase in the ratio of ATP to adenosine diphosphate subsequently acts via the sulfonylurea receptor type 1 (SUR1) component of the ATP-sensitive potassium (KATP) channel to inhibit potassium efflux, resulting in membrane depolarization and activation of a voltage-gated calcium ion channel. The rise in intracellular calcium triggers release of insulin from secretory granules into the plasma. Genes involved in congenital hyperinsulinism include glucokinase; glutamate dehydrogenase (GDH); SUR1; and the ion pore component of the KATP channel, Kir6.2. Note that leucine triggers β cell insulin secretion by allosterically activating GDH to increase oxidation of glutamate, which subsequently leads to inhibition of the KATP channel. As shown in the inset of liver pathways of glutamate metabolism, in the hyperinsulinism/hyperammonemia syndrome, overactivity of GDH leads to excessive ammonia production from glutamate and also decreases the availability of glutamate for synthesis of N-acetylglutamate, a required allosteric activator of the first step in ureagenesis. Note that SUR1 mediates both tolbutamide activation of insulin release and diazoxide inhibition of insulin release. Somatostatin inhibits insulin release at a more distal site in the pathway. ADP, adenosine diphosphate; ATP, adenosine triphosphate; CPS, carbamyl phosphate synthetase; GDH, glutamate dehydrogenase; GK, glucokinase; GTP, guanosine triphosphate; SUR, sulfonylurea receptor.

and hypoglycemia that is extremely difficult to control. Methods to diagnose and localize focal pancreatic adenomatosis preoperatively include acute insulin response tests to secretagogues such as calcium and tolbutamide, selective pancreatic arterial calcium stimulation of insulin release with venous sampling, and transhepatic portal venous insulin sampling.

Dominant KATP Channel Hyperinsulinism

One family has been reported with HI caused by a dominantly expressed mutation of the SUR1 gene, rather than the usual recessive disease described previously.

Dominant Glutamate Dehydrogenase Hyperinsulinism

Dominantly expressed mutations of glutamate dehydrogenase overactivity have been identified in children with the unusual combination of HI plus hyperammonemia (HI/HA). As in many dominant diseases, the majority of cases arise from de novo mutations, and only 20% are familial. Hypoglycemic symptoms often do not manifest in the neonatal period, and the disorder may not be recognized until the affected patient is an adult. Birth weights of affected infants are normal. In addition to hypoglycemia, affected individuals have persistent but asymptomatic hyperammonemia in the range of 70 to 150 μmol/L (see Fig. 61-3). The mutations affect the pathway of leucine-stimulated insulin secretion, and patients can have protein-sensitive hypoglycemia, as well as fasting hypoglycemia. Diazoxide is effective in controlling hypoglycemia.

Dominant Glucokinase Hyperinsulinism

This extremely rare disorder causes mild fasting hypoglycemia as a result of a dominant gain-of-function mutation of islet glucokinase (see Fig. 61-3). Birth weights of affected infants are normal, and the age at onset of hypoglycemic symptoms ranges from infancy to adulthood. Diazoxide therapy has been effective in controlling plasma glucose levels.

Insulinoma

Acquired insulinomas are the most common form of HI in adults but are rare in childhood, especially in early infancy. These are usually isolated, benign tumors, but multiple adenomas may occur in association with the familial multiple endocrine neoplasia syndromes. In contrast to focal congenital HI, insulinomas may be detectable by imaging procedures such as computed tomography, magnetic resonance imaging, radioactive octreotide scans, or transduodenal ultrasonography. Surgical resection is the treatment of choice.

Insulin Reaction, Oral Hypoglycemic Agents, and Surreptitious Insulin Administration

Insulin-induced hypoglycemia is a common occurrence in insulin-treated diabetic patients and may also occur in patients with type 2 diabetes who are taking oral hypoglycemics agents, such as glyburide, that stimulate insulin secretion. Surreptitious insulin administration should always be included in the differential diagnosis of unexplained hypoglycemia and, in young children, may occur as part of Munchausen syndrome by proxy. Exogenous human or animal insulin use can be demonstrated by assays showing elevated plasma insulin values with simultaneous suppression of plasma C peptide (use of insulin lispro may not be detectable with some insulin immunoassays).

COUNTERREGULATORY HORMONE DEFICIENCIES

Hypopituitarism

Hypopituitarism with isolated deficiency of growth hormone, and particularly with deficiencies of both growth hormone and adrenocorticotropin hormone, predisposes to fasting hypoglycemia. In affected older infants, hypoglycemia may occur after 10 to 14 hours of fasting. Newborns with hypopituitarism sometimes present with much more severe hypoglycemia, which can closely mimic the KATP channel form of congenital HI, including increased glucose requirements of 10 to 20 mg/kg/minute and an inappropriate glycemic response to glucagon when patients are hypoglycemic. Liver disease resembling progressive cholestatic jaundice may occur in these newborns and does not resolve until replacement therapy is begun for the deficient hormones. Hypotonia and, in affected boys, a small phallus may also be present.

A number of syndromes, such as midline craniofacial defects, septo-optic dysplasia, and Russell-Silver dwarfism, may be associated with hypopituitarism. Infant boys characteristically have microphallus, which is a useful diagnostic sign.

Isolated Cortisol Deficiency

Fasting hypoglycemia may occur in infants and children with adrenal insufficiency of various causes, including adrenocorticotropin hormone deficiency and primary adrenal insufficiency (Addison disease), or as a consequence of adrenal suppression resulting from exogenous glucocorticoid administration. Hypoglycemia is uncommon in the presentation of newborns with congenital adrenal hyperplasia, but once glucocorticoid replacement treatment is begun, these children also acquire the risk for adrenal crises and hypoglycemia if not given supplemental doses during intercurrent illness.

Epinephrine Deficiency

Catecholamine deficiency is extremely rare and has been described as secondary to adrenal hemorrhage in infants small for gestational age. These patients may present for the first time during childhood with hypoglycemia during fasting. The diagnosis is confirmed by measurement of plasma or urinary catecholamine levels. Some affected children may show evidence, on abdominal films, of previous adrenal hemorrhage in the form of adrenal calcification.

Fasting hypoglycemia has been observed occasionally in children treated with β-blocking agents, such as propranolol. The mechanism appears to be suppression of lipolysis as a result of the interference with epinephrine stimulation of adipose tissue; this suppression impairs the third stage of fasting adaptation. Hypoglycemia may occur after 12 or more hours of fasting. Hypoglycemic attacks may be associated with acute hypertension as a result of the unopposed α-adrenergic effects of epinephrine.

METABOLIC ENZYME DEFECTS

Hepatic Gluconeogenesis

The genetic metabolic defects in hepatic gluconeogenesis lead to fasting hypoglycemia associated with increased plasma concentrations of gluconeogenic precursors, such as lactate and alanine.

Glucose-6-Phosphatase Deficiency (Glycogen Storage Disease Type 1a and Type 1b). This is the most common form of the glycogen storage disorders, although, as shown in Figure 61-1, deficiency of glucose-6-phosphatase is actually a gluconeogenic defect, inasmuch as it blocks the release of glucose from both gluconeogenesis and glycogenolysis. As a result, hypoglycemia

occurs within 2 to 3 hours after a meal, as soon as intestinal carbohydrate absorption is complete. Affected infants usually do not present with symptomatic hypoglycemia, because the associated elevations of lactate provide an alternative fuel for the brain when the glucose level is low. Instead, the manifestation is usually growth failure late in the first year. The liver is massively enlarged as a result of fat and glycogen deposition and extends into the left upper quadrant and down into the pelvis. Associated abnormalities include elevations of plasma triglyceride (up to 2000 to 4000 mg/dL) and hyperuricemia. Treatment is aimed at correcting the frequent cycling into fasting that leads to growth failure by a combination of high-carbohydrate meals together with either uncooked cornstarch or continuous intragastric dextrose infusions. Carbohydrates that cannot be converted to glucose, such as galactose in milk, fructose in fruits, and sucrose, should be limited. The type 1b variant is caused by deficiency of the microsomal glucose-6-phosphate translocase and is associated with the additional problem of neutropenia, leading to mouth ulcers and skin infections. Treatment with granulocyte colony–stimulating factor has been beneficial in these patients.

Glucose Transporter 2 Deficiency (Fanconi-Bickel Syndrome).

A small number of infants have been described with a combination of hepatomegaly, increased liver glycogen store, renal Fanconi syndrome, and galactose intolerance. This recessively inherited disorder is due to a defect in glucose transporter 2 (GLUT-2), a plasma membrane glucose transporter, which is expressed in liver, kidney, and pancreatic β cells. GLUT-2 is necessary to export free glucose from the cytosol into the plasma (see Fig. 61-1). Deficiency of GLUT-2 interferes with glucose release from the liver not only from glycogenolysis but also from gluconeogenesis and from other sugars, such as galactose and fructose.

Fructose-1,6-Diphosphatase Deficiency.

This defect blocks gluconeogenesis immediately above the triose-phosphates (see Fig. 61-1). Affected children present in the first year or the neonatal period with life-threatening attacks of hypoglycemia and lactic acidemia provoked by fasting stress. Moderate fatty hepatomegaly is commonly seen together with hyperuricemia. Fructose ingestion can precipitate hypoglycemia and lactic acidemia. During controlled fasting, plasma glucose can be maintained in the normal range until 8 to 12 hours, because glycogenolysis remains normal. Treatment with avoidance of prolonged fasting and restriction of fructose-containing foods and glycerol is effective in avoiding hypoglycemia.

Pyruvate Carboxylase Deficiency.

Pyruvate carboxylase is one of the four key gluconeogenic enzymes (see Fig. 61-1). It also plays an important role in pyruvate oxidation because it generates oxaloacetate needed to maintain tricarboxylic acid (TCA) cycle activity. The clinical features are often dominated by the defect in pyruvate oxidation and include those of Leigh syndrome and congenital lactic acidemia. However, affected infants are also susceptible to the development of symptomatic hypoglycemia after 8 to 10 hours of fasting.

Hepatic Glycogenolysis

Defects in hepatic glycogenolysis are associated with abbreviated fasting tolerance, leading to hypoglycemia and hyperketonemia. Defects can occur in either the synthesis or breakdown of hepatic glycogen (see Fig. 61-1). Debrancher enzyme deficiency is the most severe of these defects.

Debrancher Enzyme Deficiency (Type 3 Glycogen Storage Disease).

Children with this disorder usually present in the first year of life with growth delay and massive hepatomegaly. Symptomatic hypoglycemia is not common, because plasma ketone levels are usually elevated and provide the brain with alternative substrate when the glucose level is low. Hypoglycemia develops quickly, often within 3 to 6 hours after a meal. Treatment with uncooked cornstarch to prolong glucose absorption is useful in preventing hypoglycemia and improving growth. Problems caused by hypoglycemia are ameliorated later in childhood as body mass increases. However, half or more of patients with debrancher enzyme deficiency are at risk for developing progressive muscle weakness and/or cardiomyopathy by the second and third decades of life.

Phosphorylase/Phosphorylase Kinase Deficiency.

The manifestations of either of these two enzyme defects clinically resemble a very mild form of debrancher enzyme deficiency. Affected infants present with enlarged livers, often in association with impaired growth. Symptomatic hypoglycemia is unusual. Fasting tests show a pattern of accelerated starvation with early onset of hyperketonemia. Treatment to reduce fasting intervals to less than 4 to 6 hours (e.g., with uncooked cornstarch) is helpful in correcting the failure to thrive. As in debrancher enzyme deficiency, the fasting disturbance becomes less apparent as body mass increases, and the hepatomegaly and growth delay may totally resolve by the end of the first decade. Liver phosphorylase deficiency is recessively inherited; both recessive inheritance and X-linked inheritance have been reported for phosphorylase kinase deficiency.

Glycogen Synthase Deficiency.

A small number of patients with deficiency of glycogen synthase have been reported. They have presented with episodes of symptomatic, hyperketotic hypoglycemia after fasts of 10 to 12 hours. Mild hepatomegaly may be present as a result of the increased deposition of triglycerides that is common in all of the glycogenoses. Treatment with uncooked cornstarch at bedtime may be helpful in avoiding symptomatic episodes of early morning hypoglycemia.

Fatty Acid Oxidation Disorders

Genetic defects in fatty acid oxidation interfere with the ketotic phase of fasting adaptation. The most common of the disorders is medium-chain acyl–coenzyme A (CoA) dehydrogenase (MCAD) deficiency. Children with MCAD deficiency present with acute attacks of life-threatening coma and hypoketotic hypoglycemia that are usually precipitated by fasting stresses of 12 hours or longer. Attacks are triggered by intercurrent illnesses that impair feeding, especially gastroenteritis. The clinical features mimic Reye syndrome, with coma, elevated liver transaminase levels, and mild hepatomegaly with steatosis. More severe forms of fatty acid oxidation disorders also involve skeletal and cardiac muscle and may manifest with cardiomyopathy and chronic muscle weakness or acute episodes of rhabdomyolysis. More than 12 different defects in the pathway of fatty acid oxidation have been identified; all are recessively inherited. Many states have neonatal screening programs in which dual tandem mass spectrometry of blood spot acyl-carnitine profiles are used to detect MCAD deficiency and several of the other fatty acid oxidation disorders. This is important for presymptomatic detection and treatment, because the mortality rate at the first presentation may be higher than 25%.

Other Metabolic Causes of Hypoglycemia

Glucose Transporter 1 Deficiency.

Isolated hypoglycorrhachia (low cerebrospinal fluid glucose level) in association with normal concentrations of plasma glucose has been demonstrated in a number of infants with intractable seizures in early infancy caused by a deficiency of glucose transporter 1 (GLUT-1). GLUT-1 is the plasma membrane carrier protein responsible for glucose transport across the blood-brain barrier, as well as into red blood cells. Affected patients are heterozygous for a GLUT-1 mutation and have persistently low levels of spinal fluid glucose, ranging from 20 to

30 mg/dL. Seizures may begin in the neonatal period and respond poorly to treatment with antiseizure drugs. Progressive brain damage, microcephaly, and developmental delay occur in untreated patients. Several patients have been reported to respond very well to treatment with a ketogenic diet, which restricts carbohydrates and keeps plasma levels of ketones elevated to 3 to 6 mEq/L.

Hereditary Fructose Intolerance. Hereditary fructose intolerance is caused by a recessively inherited deficiency of hepatic fructose-aldolase, which transforms fructose-1-phosphate to the triose phosphates. Affected patients cannot metabolize dietary fructose or sucrose (table sugar) in the liver or intestinal mucosa for conversion to glucose. Chronic fructose intake in young infants may cause liver dysfunction, acidemia, failure to thrive, hyperuricemia, and, ultimately, liver failure. In affected older children, ingestion of fructose causes severe abdominal pain, and these children may learn by experience to avoid fructose and thus escape identification. Fasting tolerance is normal, but ingestion of large amounts of fructose may provoke postprandial hypoglycemia by tying up intracellular phosphate and thus blocking glycogenolysis. Treatment is avoidance of dietary sources of fructose.

Galactosemia (Galactose-1-Phosphate Uridyl Transferase Deficiency). This is a serious inborn error of metabolism wherein many of the long-term consequences of the metabolic defect can potentially be prevented by early intervention. For this reason, all infants born in the United States are screened for galactosemia in the neonatal period. Absence of galactose-1-phosphate uridyl transferase prevents the conversion of galactose to glucose and results in accumulation of galactose-1-phosphate in the liver and other tissues. It has been suggested that accumulation of this metabolite inhibits the enzyme involved in the conversion of glucose-1-phosphate to glucose-6-phosphate and thus decreases the production of glucose from glycogen, thereby producing hypoglycemia. Depending on the magnitude of the defect, affected infants may present in the immediate neonatal period or later in infancy. The patients do not tolerate galactose or lactose. Intolerance to lactose in milk, the major nutrient containing galactose, is evident soon after birth when feedings are initiated. The infant may present with vomiting, failure to thrive, hepatomegaly, and indirect or direct hyperbilirubinemia. In severe or untreated cases, lenticular opacities, aminoaciduria, and mental retardation may occur. In untreated patients, progressive hepatomegaly, cirrhosis, and hepatic failure may develop. Affected infants are at increased risk for *Escherichia coli* sepsis.

Any infant with persistent jaundice, hepatomegaly, and failure to thrive should be tested for galactosemia. A presumptive diagnosis can be made by the presence of reducing sugar (Clinitest positive) that is not glucose (i.e., the glucose enzyme test result is negative) in the urine. This test should be performed while the infant is being fed a galactose-containing formula. The diagnosis should be confirmed by measuring the enzyme activity in the red blood cells.

Treatment consists of elimination of galactose from the diet. In spite of treatment, which results in prevention of hepatic disease and of mental retardation, many affected older children demonstrate learning and behavior problems.

REACTIVE HYPOGLYCEMIA

Reactive or postprandial hypoglycemia is extremely rare in the pediatric age range and, even in adults, is probably vastly overdiagnosed. Only three situations in infants and children present with reactive hypoglycemia:

Glutamate Dehydrogenase–Hyperinsulinism, Hyperinsulinism/Hyperammonemia Syndrome. This form of congenital HI has been discussed previously. Affected children have fasting hypoglycemia but, because of their leucine sensitivity, may also develop symptomatic hypoglycemia within 30 to 90 minutes of eating a high-protein meal.

Post–Nissen Fundoplication Hypoglycemia (Late Dumping Syndrome). As in adults who have had gastric surgery, infants who have undergone Nissen fundoplication procedures for gastroesophageal reflux can develop recurrent attacks of postprandial hypoglycemia. The hypoglycemia may be severe enough to produce seizures and permanent brain damage. The mechanism is thought to involve rapid gastric emptying that leads to a rapid rise in plasma glucose accompanied by a delayed but excessive insulin response, which is followed by a precipitous fall in plasma glucose to hypoglycemic levels 30 to 90 minutes after a meal.

Hereditary Fructose Intolerance. As noted previously, patients with this disorder develop acute abdominal discomfort and hypoglycemia within a short period of time after an oral load of fructose (e.g., fruit, fruit juice, or sucrose).

DIAGNOSIS OF HYPOGLYCEMIA

CRITICAL SAMPLES

Tests on the specimens of blood and urine obtained at the time of hypoglycemia provide the key information for diagnosis. Ideally, these specimens are collected during hypoglycemia, immediately before treatment is begun. It is best to collect some extra tubes of plasma and urine just before giving intravenous dextrose, to set aside for later decisions about which tests to order. Tests should include plasma glucose measurement, chemistry profiles (including bicarbonate, transaminases, uric acid, triglycerides, and creatine kinase), measurement of major fuels (lactate, free fatty acids, β-hydroxybutyrate), and measurement of hormones (insulin, cortisol, growth hormone). Urine should be tested for ketones and saved for metabolic screening. Additional tests to consider are described in the following sections. Figure 61-4 shows a paradigm for diagnosis of different hypoglycemic disorders that is based on analysis of the critical samples.

FASTING STUDY

In some cases in which the diagnosis has not been established, it is necessary to reproduce the hypoglycemia by performing a formal fasting test. This should be done only in a well-controlled situation with adequate monitoring by experienced medical and nursing staff. Fasting tests are usually begun at the 8 PM bedtime snack but may be started later in order to ensure that hypoglycemia occurs during the middle of the day, when staff members are available. Specimens are obtained at frequent intervals until the blood glucose reaches 50 mg/dL and the final specimens are taken (see previous section on critical samples).

USEFUL "CASUAL SPECIMEN" TESTS

Only a few tests are informative except at times of hypoglycemia. These include plasma acyl-carnitine profiles and plasma total and free carnitine levels (for suspected fatty acid oxidation defects) and plasma ammonia (for the HI/HA syndrome).

GLUCAGON STIMULATION

If HI is suspected, a glucagon stimulation test at the onset of hypoglycemia (50 mg/dL) may be confirmatory. A glycemic response exceeding 30 mg/dL is consistent with HI, because the normal

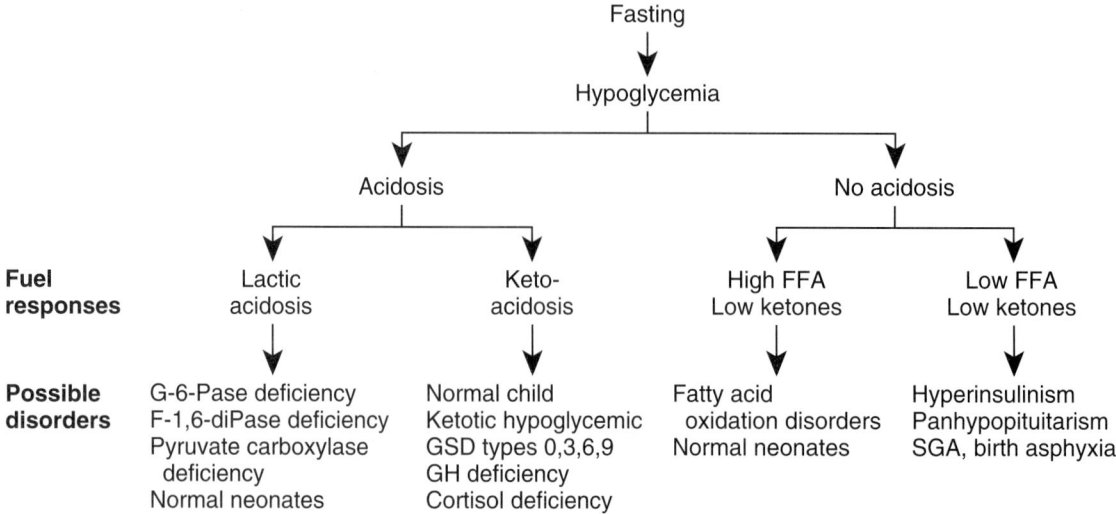

Figure 61-4. Algorithm for diagnosis of hypoglycemia, based on fasting fuel responses. F-1,6-diPase, fructose-1,6-diphosphatase; FFA, free fatty acid; G-6-Pase, glucose-6-phosphatase; GH, growth hormone; GSD, glycogen storage disease; SGA, small for gestational age.

response would be to have depleted liver glycogen reserves well before reaching hypoglycemia.

ACUTE INSULIN RESPONSE TESTS FOR HYPERINSULINISM

β cell responsiveness to different secretagogues (calcium, leucine, glucose, tolbutamide) can be used to define specific genetic forms of HI and to distinguish focal from diffuse pancreatic disease preoperatively.

PLASMA ACYL-CARNITINE PROFILE

Dual tandem mass spectrometry methods have been developed for analyzing plasma acyl-carnitine profiles and other metabolites in small samples, such as filter paper blood spots. These assays are useful for screening for most of the genetic fatty acid oxidation disorders (e.g., MCAD deficiency) and should be performed before patients suspected to have such a defect begin a formal fasting test. Many states incorporate these methods for neonatal screening of up to 30 different inborn errors of metabolism. Some fatty acid oxidation defects do not cause abnormal acyl-carnitine profiles; examples include carnitine palmityl-transferase 1 deficiency, carnitine transporter deficiency, and β-hydroxy-β-methylglutaryl-CoA dehydrogenase deficiency. These disorders must be investigated with additional in vivo and in vitro tests.

URINARY ORGANIC ACID QUANTITATION

Assays of urinary metabolites by gas chromatography–mass spectrometry are also useful in identifying specific defects in fatty acid oxidation. Abnormalities are most pronounced during activation of lipolysis, such as at the end of a diagnostic fasting test or in the "critical sample" urine collected at the time of an acute illness.

CULTURED CELLS

For in vitro diagnosis of fatty acid oxidation defects, cultured cells from patients, such as skin fibroblasts or lymphoblasts, may be useful for testing overall pathway activity, for assaying activities of candidate enzymes, or as a source of DNA for mutation analysis. Most enzymes in the pathway are expressed in cultured cells, with the exception of 3-hydroxy-3-methylglutaryl–CoA synthase, which is restricted to liver, intestine, and kidney.

MUTATION ANALYSIS

Mutation identification is useful for confirmation of diagnosis and genetic counseling. In a limited number of disorders, common mutations that can be easily screened for as a primary diagnostic test have been identified. These include MCAD deficiency, glucose-6-phosphatase deficiency, the common *SUR1* mutations present in infants with KATP channel HI who are of Ashkenazi Jewish or Finnish origins, and the HI/HA syndrome. Easy access to information about disease-associated mutations is available through the Online Mendelian Inheritance in Man (OMIM) web site (*http://www.ncbi.nlm.nih.gov/Omim/*).

TREATMENT OF HYPOGLYCEMIA

This section addresses glucose directed treatment for hypoglycemia emergencies. Specific therapies for metabolic-hormonal diseases are mentioned in the earlier sections under each of the disorders. The initial treatment of hypoglycemia is to promptly raise the plasma glucose level to normal and maintain it in the range of 80 to 100 mg/dL. For long-term management, the minimum goal of therapy is to keep the plasma glucose level above 60 mg/dL at all times.

Whenever treatment begins in a patient with new-onset hypoglycemia, every effort should be made to collect the critical samples for diagnosis. One extra tube of 5 mL of plasma or serum (green-top or red-top tube) is sufficient to measure key chemistry levels, fuels, and hormones. An extra tube of 10 mL or more of urine should also be collected for urinary organic acid quantitation.

For emergency treatment of hypoglycemia, a bolus of dextrose, 200 mg/kg, is given rapidly, and then a continuous infusion is begun to run at a rate equal to at least normal hepatic glucose output (about 4 to 6 mg/kg/minute). With 10% dextrose solutions, this means a bolus of 2 mL/kg followed by continuous infusion at maintenance rates. Infants with HI may require considerably higher rates of dextrose infusion, up to 20 to 30 mg/kg/minute. Infants with fatty acid oxidation disorders should receive sufficient dextrose to ensure that insulin secretion is stimulated enough to suppress lipolysis—that is, 10% dextrose at 8 to 10 mg/kg/minute—and to maintain all plasma glucose levels slightly above 100 mg/dL. Glucagon may be used to treat hypoglycemia on an emergency basis, but *only* if the hypoglycemia is known to be caused by HI; a dose of 1 mg should be used at all ages to avoid undertreatment.

SUMMARY AND RED FLAGS

Hypoglycemia has many manifestations and must be thought of as a cause of nonspecific signs in newborns. It is a readily treatable cause of lethargy, coma, and seizures. Other affected children have signs of catecholamine excess. Untreated symptomatic hypoglycemia is life-threatening and can produce significant, irreversible central nervous system injury.

Red flags include metabolic acidosis (inborn errors of metabolism, sepsis); a positive family history (inborn errors of metabolism, hyperinsulinism, hypoglycemic agents); hypoketonuria and high glucose infusion rates (hyperinsulinism); onset during adolescence (drugs or alcohol); hepatomegaly (glycogen storage disease, other inborn errors of metabolism); feeding intolerance (galactosemia); or recurrent or a family history of emesis, lethargy, coma, or sudden infant death syndrome (medium-chain acyl dehydrogenase deficiency).

REFERENCES

General

Cornblath M, Hawdon JM, Williams AF, et al: Controversies regarding definition of neonatal hypoglycemia: Suggested operational thresholds. Pediatrics 2000;105:1141-1145.

Online Mendelian Inheritance in Man. Available at *http://www.ncbi.nlm.nih.gov/Omim/* (accessed November 4, 2003).

Scriver CR, Sly WS, Childs B, et al (eds): The Metabolic and Molecular Basis of Inherited Disease, 8th ed. New York, McGraw-Hill, 2001.

Stanley CA, Baker L: The causes of neonatal hypoglycemia. N Engl J Med 1999;340:1200-1201.

Stanley CA, Thornton PS, Finegold DN, et al: Hypoglycemia in neonates and infants. In Sperling MA (ed): Pediatric Endocrinology. Philadelphia, WB Saunders, 2002.

Thornton PS, Finegold DN, Stanley CA, et al: Hypoglycemia in the infant and child. In Sperling MA (ed): Pediatric Endocrinology. Philadelphia, WB Saunders, 2002.

Hyperinsulinism

Aynsley-Green A, Hussain K, Hall J, et al: Practical management of hyperinsulinism in infancy. Arch Dis Child Fetal Neonatal Ed 2000;82:F98-F107.

Collins JE, Leonard JV, Teale D, et al: Hyperinsulinaemic hypoglycaemia in small for dates babies. Arch Dis Child 1990;65:1118-1120.

DeVivo DC, Trifiletti RR, Jacobson RI, et al: Defective glucose transport across the blood-brain barrier as a cause of persistent hypoglycorrhachia, seizures, and developmental delay. N Engl J Med 1991;325:703-709.

Ferry RJ Jr, Kelly A, Grimberg A, et al: Calcium-stimulated insulin secretion in diffuse and focal forms of congenital hyperinsulinism. J Pediatr 2000;137:239-246.

Glaser B, Kesavan P, Heyman M, et al: Familial hyperinsulinism caused by an activating glucokinase mutation. N Engl J Med 1998;338:226-230.

Glaser B, Thornton P, Otonkoski T, et al: Genetics of neonatal hyperinsulinism. Arch Dis Child Fetal Neonatal Ed 2000;82:F79-F86.

Grimberg A, Ferry RJ, Kelly A, et al: Dysregulation of insulin secretion in children with congenital hyperinsulinism due to sulfonylurea receptor mutations. Diabetes 2001;50:322-328.

Huopio H, Reimann F, Ashfield R, et al: Dominantly inherited hyperinsulinism caused by a mutation in the sulfonylurea receptor type 1. J Clin Invest 2000;106:897-906.

MacMullen C, Fang J, Hsu BYL, et al: Hyperinsulinism/hyperammonemia syndrome in children with regulatory mutations in the inhibitory GTP binding domain of glutamate dehydrogenase. J Clin Endocrinol Metab 2001;86:1782-1787.

Munns CFJ, Batch JA: Hyperinsulinism and Beckwith-Wiedemann syndrome. Arch Dis Child Fetal Neonatal Ed 2001;84:F67-F69.

Santer R, Schneppenheim R, Dombrowski A, et al: Mutations in GLUT2, the gene for the liver-type glucose transporter, in patients with Fanconi-Bickel syndrome. Nat Genet 1997;17:324-326.

Stanley CA: Hyperinsulinism in infants and children. Pediatr Clin North Am 1997;44:363-374.

Fatty Acid Oxidation Disorders

Stanley CA, Hale DE: Genetic disorders of mitochondrial fatty acid oxidation. Curr Opin Pediatr 1994;6:476.

Treem WR, Shoup ME, Hale DE, et al: Acute fatty liver of pregnancy, hemolysis, elevated liver enzymes, and low platelets syndrome, and long chain 3-hydroxyacyl–coenzyme A dehydrogenase deficiency. Am J Gastroenterol 1996;91:2293-2300.

Ziadeh R, Hoffman EP, Finegold DN, et al: Medium chain acyl–CoA dehydrogenase deficiency in Pennsylvania: Neonatal screening shows high incidence and unexpected mutation frequencies. Pediatr Res 1995;37:675.

62 Polyuria and Urinary Incontinence

Cynthia G. Pan

Urinary incontinence is a normal developmental stage. When present beyond a certain age defined by parental and societal expectations, it can cause concern and anxiety in the patient and family. Urinary incontinence can also be a symptom of significant pathologic processes. The challenge to the clinician is identifying the child with an organic disorder among the many who are proceeding along a normal developmental track.

VOIDING PHYSIOLOGY

Urinary continence is dependent on normal bladder function and normal urine production. Normal development of bladder function results in the storage and release of urine in a socially and physically acceptable way. During storage, the detrusor muscle is relaxed, and the capacity of the bladder allows urine to be held for several hours. Micturition is then voluntary, with coordinated detrusor contraction and sphincter relaxation, resulting in complete bladder emptying. The bladder capacity in children learning to be toilet trained is variable, being dependent on their own sensation of bladder fullness. The maximum functional bladder capacity may differ greatly among children when measured by home diaries. Cystometry, a method of measuring bladder volume, can be estimated by the following formula:

$$\text{cystometric bladder capacity (in milliliters)} = 30 \text{ mL} + (30 \times \text{age in years}).$$

Although the innervation of the bladder is predominantly autonomic, bladder function is under control of cortical function. Thus, a complex integration of visceral and somatic innervation is necessary for normal voiding, which perhaps explains the wide spectrum in the ages for urinary continence. Parasympathetic neural activity provides the primary input during micturition, leading to relaxation of the urethral smooth muscle and initiating detrusor contractions. Pelvic nerves conducting parasympathetic activity form a reflex arc with the centrally located pontine micturition center. The thoracolumbar sympathetic branch, via hypogastric and pelvic sympathetic nerves, innervates the detrusor to relax and the urinary sphincter to contract during urine storage.

Urinary continence thus relies on the abilities to (1) store urine without leakage, (2) release urine voluntarily and completely, and (3) interrupt micturition voluntarily. The third ability is indicative of fully coordinated cortical-autonomic function.

TOILET TRAINING

The age at which toilet training is achieved is influenced by cultural factors as well as the individual temperament of the child. The achievement of daytime urinary continence follows the attainment of bowel control. There is evidence that the age of daytime and nighttime continence has increased worldwide in the past century.

Data suggest a change in parental attitudes toward the toilet training process and their expectations. Temperament of the child and cognitive ability may play a less significant role. Among social factors, children of single parents are successfully toilet trained at an earlier age, whereas enrollment in day care does not have a significant influence. Consistent findings are the predictive factors of gender and race: Girls are toilet trained earlier than boys, and African American children are trained earlier than white children.

URINE VOLUME AND SOLUTE DIURESIS

Polyuria is the overproduction of urine. Polyuria is a symptom that is fixed and therefore occurs during both the daytime and the nighttime. "Nocturnal polyuria," a symptom proposed in a subset of patients with primary nocturnal enuresis, is discussed separately. Overproduction of urine indicates a defect in one of several mechanisms regulating water and solute homeostasis. Identification of children with incontinence caused by polyuria is essential for diagnosing a variety of disorders (Table 62-1).

Urine production varies, depending on the intake of fluids and solute, activity, caloric expenditure, and the environment. The volume reflects the maintenance of normal fluid and electrolyte balance (1) through regulation of plasma osmolality by vasopressin and through the thirst mechanism and (2) by regulation of extracellular volume and solute (mainly sodium) homeostasis by the kidney. The sensation of thirst occurs when plasma osmolality rises above a threshold between 280 to 290 mOsm/L. Release of vasopressin, a peptide produced by the hypothalamus, parallels the sensation of thirst and then acts on receptors in the collecting ducts of the kidney to diminish water excretion and to concentrate the urine. Hypovolemia is also a stimulant for vasopressin. Once serum osmolality is restored to normal, vasopressin release is inhibited, and renal water excretion increases. Maintenance of extracellular fluid volume depends on sodium homeostasis and directly affects urine volume. It involves the interaction of several systems, including (1) the renin-angiotensin system, (2) atrial natriuretic peptide, and (3) the sympathetic nervous system.

Among patients with primary nocturnal enuresis, there is a subset of patients with "nocturnal polyuria," in which larger volumes of more dilute urine is produced than in patients who remain dry. Responsiveness to the administration of vasopressin analogues, such as desmopressin acetate (1-deamino[8-D-arginine] vasopressin [DDAVP]), differentiates such patients into responders and nonresponders.

HISTORY

The history should begin with careful questioning to determine whether the patient has polyuria. The presence of polyuria suggests a variety of metabolic, systemic, and kidney diseases, whereas the absence of polyuria places the focus on the lower urinary tract (Table 62-2; see Table 62-1).

Table 62-1. Causes of Urinary Incontinence

With Polyuria

Osmotic diuresis (urine osmolality > plasma osmolality)
  Diabetes mellitus
Central diabetes insipidus
Nephrogenic diabetes insipidus
  Primary
    X-linked (most common)
    Autosomal recessive
    Autosomal dominant
  Secondary
    Obstructive uropathy
    Chronic renal failure
    Juvenile nephronophthisis
    Fanconi syndrome (e.g., cystinosis)
    Hypokalemia
    Hypercalcemia
    Bartter syndrome
    Gitelman syndrome
    Sickle cell disease
    Renal tubular acidosis
    Medications (e.g., lithium)
    Interstitial nephritis

Without Polyuria

Primary nocturnal enuresis*
Dysfunctional voiding syndromes
Neuropathic bladder
Anatomic defects of the urinary tract

*Some cases may be characterized by nocturnal polyuria.

POLYURIA

Polyuria, the excessive production of urine, can result from the absence of release of antidiuretic hormone (ADH), the failure of the kidney to respond to ADH, or an osmotic diuresis. Polyuria always results in polydipsia. Both symptoms are often associated in young children with urinary incontinence. It is often easier to query parents as to whether the volume of fluid intake by the child is excessive rather than to obtain an estimate of the volume of urine output.

Table 62-2. Secondary and Acquired Forms of Nephrogenic Diabetes Insipidus

Acquired

Chronic pyelonephritis
Tubulointerstitial nephritis
Chronic renal failure secondary to obstructive uropathy
Drug-induced tubulopathy

Congenital

Renal tubular acidosis
Nephrocalcinosis
Cystinosis
Sickle cell nephropathy
Juvenile nephronophthisis
Renal dysplasia
Cystic kidney disease
Bartter syndrome
Storage diseases (tyrosinemia, Fabry disease)

The first clue to polydipsia in infants is irritability and "hunger" after a successful feeding of formula or breast milk. In young children, favoring water over solids or milk, as well as seeking water in unusual places (e.g., toilets), can be a sign of polydipsia. Waking to seek fluids at night in a consistent pattern is also a sign of polydipsia. Parental stories of bed linens being soaked despite a "double diaper" or training pull-on diaper, are remarkable, especially when recounted by experienced parents who are able to compare the child to other healthy siblings.

An osmotic diuresis leading to polyuria may be an early sign of diabetes mellitus. The previously dry child may develop secondary nocturnal or even daytime enuresis. Associated symptoms include polydipsia and polyphagia with poor weight gain, and fatigue. Children with central diabetes insipidus (CDI) and the genetic forms of nephrogenic diabetes insipidus (NDI) produce very large amounts of hypotonic urine. Along with polyuria and enuresis, these children may have a history of frequent hospitalizations for dehydration, often provoked by relatively minor illnesses. The dehydration is often associated with moderate or severe hypernatremia. Failure to thrive may develop as a result of a preference of low-calorie–containing fluids over solid foods. The secondary causes of NDI may include a partial defect in the mechanism for renal concentrating, and urinary incontinence may be the only symptom (see Table 62-2). Conversely, other children may also have growth retardation as a result of associated chronic renal failure or the associated metabolic abnormalities (e.g., metabolic acidosis in renal tubular acidosis [RTA] or rickets in Fanconi syndrome).

VOIDING HISTORY

In the presence of enuresis but the absence of polyuria, a voiding history helps to determine whether additional evaluation is warranted. Is the urinary incontinence nocturnal only, or is daytime incontinence also present? Does the patient have stool incontinence? Voiding frequency is sometimes difficult to ascertain in a school-age child, and an assignment to keep a diary of voiding can be given on the first visit. This should include information on both bladder and bowel habits, specifically urine volumes and when urinary incontinence occurs. Urine-holding patterns with overflow incontinence are most easily identifiable with a diary. Incontinence can be a symptom of a urinary tract infection (UTI) (see Chapter 23). Associated symptoms may include dysuria, frequency, and urgency. Other urinary symptoms such as dysuria, urgency, dampness in the underwear, or other signs of UTI, can all be signs of dysfunctional elimination. Asking parents for specific observations—such as (1) the sudden urge to void followed by incontinence or (2) maneuvers to prevent urine leakage, such as squatting and pressing the heel of the foot into the perineum—elicits clues to a hyperactive detrusor muscle. Incontinence may occur with giggling, with physical stress while jumping, or with activities that require Valsalva maneuvers.

Secondary enuresis is defined as enuresis occurring after a dry period of at least 6 consecutive months and can be the first sign of an acquired renal or metabolic disease. Fecal soiling or constipation may be an accompanying sign of dysfunctional elimination, but it should first raise suspicion for an occult spinal lesion such as spina bifida or a tethered cord. In addition, continuous dribbling, a poor urinary stream, or recurrent infections may be a sign of anatomic or neuropathic lesions (Table 62-3).

PRIMARY NOCTURNAL ENURESIS

The patient with nocturnal enuresis (bedwetting) is typically without any major daytime symptoms. Enuresis is considered primary when the patient has not had any dry periods for greater than 6 months. Toilet training for daytime control is often achieved easily. The frequency of wet nights should be ascertained to gauge the magnitude of the problem. A family history of nocturnal enuresis increases

Table 62-3. Red Flags

Polyuria
Polydipsia
Failure to thrive
Poor urinary stream
Encopresis
Secondary enuresis
Abnormal gait
Recurrent urinary tract infections
Cutaneous lesions over lumbosacral spine
Diminished lower extremity reflexes
Abnormal genitalia
Palpable bladder
Hypertension
Headache
Visual disturbances
Obstructive sleep apneas

a patient's risk for nocturnal enuresis. If both parents have a history of enuresis, the rate of recurrence in offspring may be as high as 70% to 80%. If the father had primary nocturnal enuresis, the child has a fivefold to sevenfold increase in risk.

BEHAVIORAL ISSUES

Social stressors should be ascertained because psychological factors are important in the occurrence of secondary enuresis. Other psychiatric issues, such as attention-deficit/hyperactivity disorder, have been associated with a higher incidence of daytime and nighttime incontinence. It has been widely accepted, however, that primary nocturnal enuresis is not a psychiatric disorder and that affected children are often emotionally well adjusted. Nonetheless, care should be taken not to underestimate the sequelae of enuresis in the older school-age child, who may feel "abnormal" among peers. Evaluation of the patient should always include inquiring how the patient and other family members are reacting to the problem and how it may be interfering with social or school issues.

Finally, primary nocturnal enuresis may be a sleep disorder or a disorder of arousal. Patients with severe nocturnal enuresis may have defects in arousal to auditory stimuli. Inquiry into symptoms of sleep apnea should also be made, such as snoring or restless sleep, as it is may lead to altered arousal states leading to nocturnal enuresis in patients with sleep apnea (see Chapter 5).

PHYSICAL EXAMINATION

In all affected patients, their growth should be evaluated, because failure to thrive can be seen in many of the metabolic disorders that produce polyuria. The presence of hypertension suggests underlying renal or urologic abnormalities. Careful evaluation of the lower back may reveal cutaneous abnormalities such as hair tufts, pits, dimpling, or vascular malformations, which are possible signs of spina bifida occulta or tethered cord. A significant deviation of the gluteal cleft may also suggest the possibility of spinal dysraphism. The abdominal examination is important for detecting a distended bladder, suprapubic tenderness, or significant stool retention. A neurologic examination should include assessment of lower extremity deep tendon reflexes, observation of the gait, and evaluation of perineal sensation and anal sphincter tone, again screening for the possibility of a neuropathic bladder. Anatomic abnormalities leading to incontinence should be sought by inspection of the genitalia. In girls, the examination includes a search for fused labial folds and dribbling

urine from an ectopic ureter. In boys, the phallus should be inspected for the presence of epispadias or undescended testicles.

DIAGNOSIS

The presence or absence of polyuria helps guide the necessary laboratory and radiologic testing (Figs. 62-1 and 62-2). An immediate urinalysis is critical for differentiating the glycosuria of diabetes mellitus from the low specific gravity (osmolality) of diabetes insipidus or the proteinuria and/or hematuria of chronic renal disease.

A water deprivation test, to examine urine concentrating capacity of patients when diabetes insipidus is suspected, should be done in a hospital setting, with close observation of and attention to urine and serum osmolarity, urine output, and weight loss. In patients with significant polyuria, dehydration and hyperosmolarity are easily precipitated with several hours of water deprivation. For patients with a less suspect history of polyuria, a first morning void after an overnight fast should be sufficient for checking urine osmolarity or specific gravity.

In some patients, the problem can be better defined with a home voiding diary, which outlines how often and how much they are voiding, and when urinary incontinence, constipation, or encopresis occurs.

LABORATORY ASSESSMENT

Routine laboratory examination in patients with just enuresis is very basic and in most cases is unrevealing. When polyuria or polydipsia is present, a screening urinalysis and then appropriate blood chemistry studies are important for confirming diabetes mellitus or electrolyte disorders such as metabolic acidosis (RTA), metabolic alkalosis (Bartter syndrome), hypercalcemia, and hypokalemia. Hypernatremia can be seen in the severe forms of diabetes insipidus. UTI should be sought in most patients with incontinence by obtaining a urinalysis and urine culture. A urinalysis also helps screen for occult, chronic glomerular or tubular renal disease. Hematuria or proteinuria can be a sign of renal disease, although its absence does not exclude this possibility. Glycosuria, when associated with normal serum glucose, can indicate tubulointerstitial disease, where proximal tubular injury results in a lowered threshold for glucose reabsorption (see Table 62-2).

IMAGING AND CYSTOMETRY

Radiologic imaging is not necessary in most patients with primary nocturnal enuresis. In select patients with daytime symptoms or a suspect history or urinalysis, renal ultrasonography may provide information regarding acquired or congenital renal diseases. Images of the bladder can reveal urologic abnormalities, including poor bladder emptying or thickened bladder wall. A voiding cystourethrogram is indicated only in patients with a questionable urinary stream, continuous dribbling (aberrant ectopic ureter), or suspected spinal cord lesions with lower extremity neurologic signs. Magnetic resonance imaging of the lower spine should be reserved for patients with cutaneous signs, neurologic or orthopedic symptoms of the lumbar-sacral spine, or complex spinal bone deformities seen on plain radiographs. All patients with central diabetes insipidus must undergo cerebral magnetic resonance imaging with specific focus on the hypothalamic-pituitary region.

Cystometry examination is useful for a select group of patients with a history of dysfunctional voiding symptoms whose response to therapy is poor. Bladder instability is characterized by involuntary contractions at more than 15 cm of water pressure during filling. Small bladder capacity is almost always a functional problem, not anatomic.

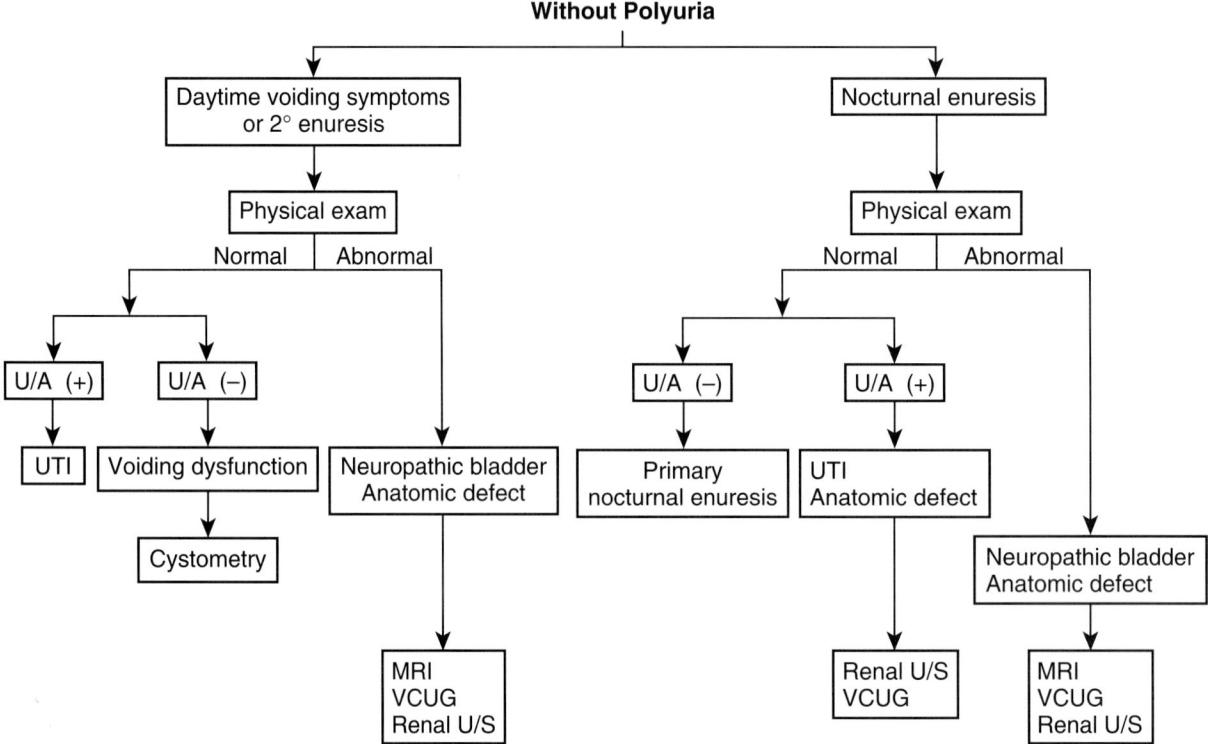

Figure 62-1. Diagnosis of enuresis without polyuria. MRI, magnetic resonance imaging; U/A, urinalysis; U/S, ultrasonography; UTI, urinary tract infection; VCUG, voiding cystourethrogram.

DIFFERENTIAL DIAGNOSIS

PRIMARY NOCTURNAL ENURESIS

Primary nocturnal enuresis (bedwetting) is considered abnormal in most social contexts after the age of 5 years. The majority of affected patients have no daytime symptoms. It is a common problem, but only a small proportion of patients actually seek medical advice.

The prevalence, when the condition is defined as a wet night more than once a month, is estimated at 10% among 6-year-olds, 5% among 10-year-olds, and 0.5% to 1.0% among teens and young adults. The spontaneous cure rate is approximately 15% per year. The incidence of pure primary nocturnal enuresis without other symptoms is twice as common among boys than among girls. The pathophysiologic mechanism is multifactorial; explanations include defects in osmoregulation, small bladder capacity, and disorders of sleep or arousal states.

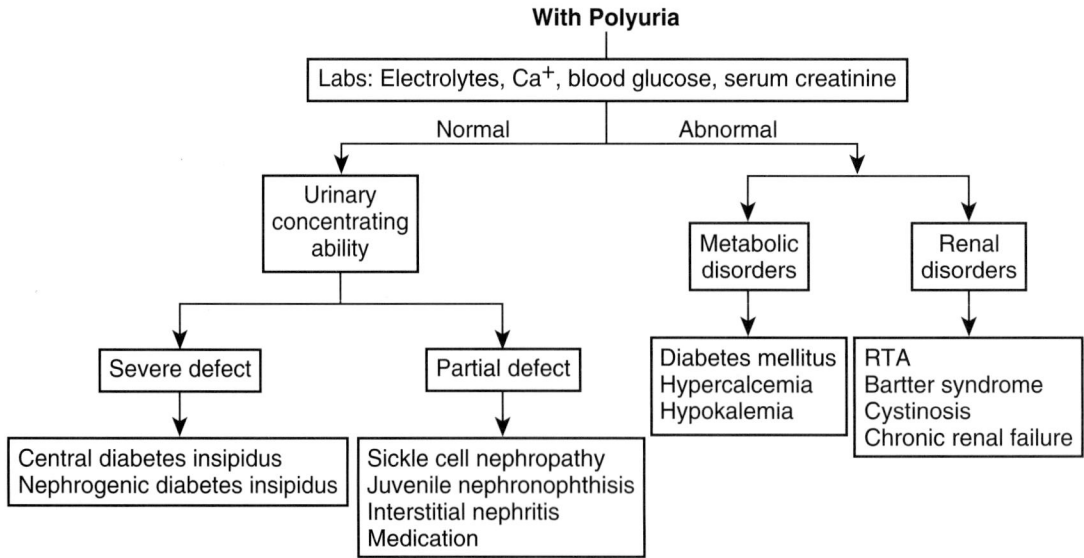

Figure 62-2. Diagnosis of enuresis with polyuria. RTA, renal tubular acidosis.

DYSFUNCTIONAL VOIDING

This occurs when there is an imbalance or lack of coordination of activity between the detrusor muscle activity (bladder contracture) and the bladder neck or external sphincter activity (bladder outlet control). This poor coordination can, over time, cause a wide spectrum of disorders, including incontinence. The severity depends on the balance of forces among the detrusor activity, bladder neck, and external sphincter. In the extreme case, high bladder pressures produce acquired urologic abnormalities, including hydronephrosis, vesicoureteral reflux (VUR), and renal damage. Dysfunctional voiding is often classified as mild, moderate, or severe. Early recognition can lead to proper management and avoidance of long-term sequelae.

Mild Voiding Dysfunction

Daytime urinary frequency is characterized by frequency and urgency every 15 to 20 minutes. This is usually associated with incontinence or mild pain and occurs in children aged 3 to 8 years. The condition is also usually self-limiting. A thorough history should be documented, a careful physical examination conducted, and urinalysis performed to rule out other pathologic processes. *Giggle incontinence* is most often seen in girls and is characterized by incontinence after laughter. It too is usually self-limiting. *Stress incontinence* follows athletic activities such as running or jumping and landing; it is common with activities such as gymnastics and cheerleading. Timely bladder emptying before exercise is effective in preventing this problem. *Postvoid dribbling* can occur in young girls who develop habits of incomplete voiding or can result from urine that is collected in the vagina during voiding. Sitting with the knees slightly apart or sitting on the toilet facing backwards eliminates this problem.

Moderate Voiding Dysfunction

There are two extremes in the spectrum of moderate dysfunctional voiding. Over time, *urine holding,* as infrequent as once every 8 to 12 hours, results in incontinence as well as recurrent UTIs. This can be a consequence of behaviors developed when the young child is learning voluntary contraction of the external sphincter muscle while toilet training. It may also develop when a child goes to school or camp and does not want to use an unfamiliar or embarrassing toilet. The child learns additional maneuvers to void infrequently, such as squatting and pressing the heel of the foot in the perineum. Dysfunctional voiding occurs over time when the child is unable to relax the external sphincter in coordination with detrusor activity during voiding. This results in incomplete and inefficient bladder emptying.

The overactive bladder, or *unstable bladder,* is the most common abnormality. Low-quantity, frequent voiding leading to incontinence is secondary to delayed resolution of uninhibited bladder contractions that normally resolve as the child matures. This asynchronous activity between detrusor muscle and sphincter contraction leads to higher intravesical pressures. Urgency and urge incontinence are the most common symptoms, but recurrent UTIs and VUR may result as well. Complications may include thickening, trabeculations, or diverticula of the bladder. High bladder pressure can also cause hydroureter and hydronephrosis.

Severe Dysfunctional Voiding

This is often referred to as the "nonneurogenic neurogenic bladder," a syndrome representing the extreme end of the spectrum of dysfunctional voiding. Inappropriate voluntary contraction of the external sphincter during voiding produces high intravesical pressure and a functional outlet obstruction, leading to abnormal bladder function, hydronephrosis, and possibly renal failure. With time, the voiding pattern becomes habitual, and the anatomic changes impede the ability to void normally. Biofeedback and clean intermittent straight catheterization may restore bladder emptying and function and prevent renal failure.

NEUROPATHIC BLADDER

The neuropathic bladder most often occurs in patients with spina bifida, an open or closed congenital spinal cord fusion defect. This results in distortion of normal neural tissues in the spinal cord or nerve roots. The range of anomalies includes meningocele, lipomeningocele, primary tethered cord, dermoid cyst, syrinx, and sacral agenesis. Closed defects can be initially asymptomatic and manifest during toilet training years with incontinence, recurrent UTIs, or orthopedic problems in later childhood. Many children who present with symptoms have a cutaneous finding over the lumbosacral spine noted since birth. The severity of the symptoms does not seem to predict the severity of the bladder dysfunction or renal damage. Despite lesser neurologic deficits in closed spina bifida, affected patients have demonstrated bladder dysfunction as severe as that observed in open spina bifida. Acute spinal injury (trauma), compression (tumor), or infection (transverse myelitis) may produce similar bladder conditions such as acute urinary retention.

ANATOMIC DEFECTS

Posterior Urethral Valves and Urethral Obstruction

This is the most common form of urinary obstruction leading to kidney failure. It is a result of persistence of fetal folds in the posterior urethra, which act as a valve to create urinary obstruction. Poor urinary stream and bladder distention are the most common urinary complaints, but dribbling and incontinence are also observed. UTI can be the presenting problem, and, when it is diagnosed in young boys, especially infants, posterior urethral valves should always be sought.

Prune-belly syndrome is another important cause of urethral obstruction. Early obstruction during embryogenesis leads to hydronephrosis, hydroureter, abdominal distention, abdominal musculature deficiency, and excessive skin folds, thus giving the wrinkly "prune" appearance of the abdomen in severe cases. A spectrum of renal dysplasia can result.

Renal Duplication

This is a result of duplication of the ureteric bud during embryogenesis, causing a double collecting system, or two ureters. Duplicated ureters can open separately inside the bladder, but in rare cases, an ectopic ureter can end in the vagina, urethra, or vestibule, leading to dribbling and incontinence.

Vesicoureteral Reflux

VUR is the backward flow of urine from the bladder into the ureters. Normal insertion of the ureter into the bladder submucosal wall forms a flap-valve mechanism that prevents urine backup during filling and contraction. Congenital VUR is secondary to shorter ureteric segments in the bladder wall. Urine flow mechanics are disrupted by the constant filling of the bladder with urine that has flowed backward and then returns to the emptied bladder. The inability to completely empty the bladder eliminates an important defense against UTIs. Secondary VUR can be associated with dysfunctional voiding. Dyssynergia between detrusor contraction and sphincter relaxation can result in VUR and recurrent UTIs. Urethral obstruction leading to high intravesical pressure also leads to VUR, poor bladder emptying, and thus UTIs and incontinence.

METABOLIC DISORDERS

Hypercalcemia

This is an uncommon electrolyte disorder in children but can be observed in primary hyperparathyroidism, vitamin D intoxication, immobilization, Williams syndrome, malignancy, and idiopathic hypercalcemia of infancy. Polyuria is a symptom of hypercalcemia and is a result of its inhibitory effect on Na^+, K^+-ATPase function in renal tubules. This leads to renal sodium and water losses and thus to polyuria and volume contraction. In chronic hypercalcemia, increased calcium excretion over time can lead to nephrocalcinosis, tubular damage, and poor urinary concentrating ability, thus enhancing polyuria.

Hypokalemia

This is another electrolyte disorder that induces polyuria. In children, it occurs clinically as a result of diuretic use, aldosterone excess states, Cushing syndrome, and intrinsic renal disorders that affect potassium handling. The latter includes disorders such as RTA, Bartter syndrome, or renal injury from nephrotoxic medications. Hypokalemia interferes with water reabsorption in the collecting duct of the kidneys.

Diabetes Mellitus

Polyuria and urinary incontinence can be the first symptoms of diabetes mellitus and are secondary to hyperglycemia and the osmotic diuresis resulting from chronic glycosuria. The renal threshold for reabsorption of glucose is exceeded when the blood glucose level is higher than approximately 180 mg/dL. If oral intake of fluid decreases, as occurs when diabetic ketoacidosis causes anorexia and emesis, significant dehydration and shock frequently develop.

CENTRAL DIABETES INSIPIDUS

In CDI, the lack of circulating ADH prevents concentration of the urine, leading to high quantities of dilute urine. The defect can be complete or partial, and thus the degree of polyuria is variable. In complete CDI, the massive polyuria can lead to severe dehydration and hypernatremia. CDI can be secondary to intracranial surgery, head trauma, or tumor involving the nuclei of the hypothalamus (where ADH is produced) or the neurohypophysial axis itself. There is also an idiopathic form and familial forms of CDI. In the idiopathic form, infiltrative diseases such as Langerhans cell histiocytosis (Letterer-Siwe syndrome) should be sought. A significant proportion of young children initially diagnosed with idiopathic CDI have been found to have histiocytosis in subsequent years. Treatment is with ADH or its analogues.

RENAL CONCENTRATING DEFECTS

Renal Tubular Acidosis

In distal (type 1) RTA, the most common form of RTA, there is a defect in the tubular secretion of hydrogen ions and decreased formation of NH_4^+ cations in the urine. In children, the presentation includes failure to thrive, polyuria, and polydipsia. Hypokalemia is a common finding and can be profound, leading to weakness. Hypercalcuria and low urine citrate excretion combine to produce nephrocalcinosis. The autosomal recessive form of the disease is frequently associated with hearing loss. There are also autosomal dominant forms of the disease. Distal RTA may be secondary to medications (e.g., amphotericin) or a variety of conditions, including interstitial nephritis, obstructive uropathy, nephrocalcinosis, renal transplantation, sickle cell disease, and systemic lupus erythematosus.

Proximal RTA is less common and is a primary defect in bicarbonate reabsorption in the proximal tubule. When associated with other proximal tubular defects, such as salt wasting, phosphate wasting, glycosuria, and aminoaciduria, it is referred to as Fanconi syndrome. Manifesting in infancy to early adulthood, cystinosis is the most common cause of proximal RTA in children. This autosomal recessive disorder results from a defect in cystine transport and results in the lysosomal accumulation of cystine throughout the body. The infantile form usually manifests in the first year of life. Without intervention, this form results in end-stage renal failure. Acidosis, rickets, polyuria, and severe failure to thrive are hallmarks of the disease. Early intervention with oral cysteamine to bind cysteine has dramatically improved the outcome in affected patients. Proximal RTA is a feature of several other genetic disorders manifesting in childhood (such as galactosemia, tyrosinemia, hereditary fructose intolerance, glycogen storage disease type I, Lowe syndrome, Wilson disease, osteopetrosis) or ingestion of toxins (heavy metals, outdated tetracyclines, carbonic anhydrase inhibitors).

Sickle Cell Disease

Hemoglobin S is a genetic defect in hemoglobin A that results in red blood cells that deform under low oxygen tension (see Chapter 48). The renal medulla is a site with high osmolality, low oxygen tension, and relative acidosis, all conditions that promote sickling. This results in occlusion of blood vessels and damage to the renal medulla, the primary site where the urine is concentrated. The resultant decreased ability to concentrate leads to a higher incidence of nocturnal enuresis in affected patients.

Nephronophthisis

Juvenile nephronophthisis is an autosomal recessive disorder that leads to end-stage renal failure between preadolescence and early adulthood. Patients have high urine output because of poor renal concentrating ability and renal salt wasting. Patients may have primary or secondary nocturnal enuresis. The salt wasting causes salt craving, and patients have a preference for salty foods or even eat salt directly from the saltshaker. A small percentage of these patients have retinitis pigmentosa, which may cause blindness at birth or later in life. Patients may present with symptoms of chronic renal failure (see Chapter 26).

Nephrogenic Diabetes Insipidus

The congenital form of NDI is often diagnosed before toilet training, but it can lead to urinary incontinence in later childhood. Infants may present with severe dehydration, seizures, and central nervous system injury or death. In families in which the diagnosis has already been made, early intervention in infants can prevent these symptoms and lead to an excellent outcome. Most patients have the X-linked form of the disease, which is caused by a mutated ADH receptor. Female carriers may be mildly affected. The autosomal recessive and autosomal dominant forms of NDI are caused by mutations in aquaporin, the water channel that allows uptake of water in the collecting duct.

TREATMENT

PRIMARY NOCTURNAL ENURESIS

Establishing whether the primary nocturnal enuresis is the only symptom or whether there are associated symptoms such as diurnal incontinence, constipation, sleep disorders, or behavioral issues, such as attention-deficit/hyperactivity disorder, is necessary before a treatment strategy is developed.

Many families simply want reassurance that there is not an organic explanation. It is also helpful to let the family and child know that almost all patients "outgrow" primary nocturnal enuresis. Positive reinforcement for dry nights, dispelling any negative attitudes, and avoiding blame enhance the child's self-esteem. If treatment is sought, the enuresis alarm has a high success rate, but patient selection is important. These devices are designed to awaken patients when micturition begins and result in the development of increased bladder capacity. Its effect may not be seen for up to 12 weeks, and therefore the family and patient must be highly motivated. Older patients who are ready to take charge of the problem and who do not have difficulty waking are the best candidates.

Pharmacologic therapy for primary nocturnal enuresis includes the use of DDAVP, an ADH analogue. There is probably a subpopulation of patients with enuresis who have "nocturnal polyuria," which led to the drug's popularity, but there is evidence that this is independent of vasopressin secretion. DDAVP is most effective in children with a positive family history of primary nocturnal enuresis, with normal bladder capacity, and who are older than 7 years. Its safety profile has been excellent, but patients should be given careful instruction on restricting fluid intake after the bedtime dose. There are occasional reports of hyponatremic seizures in children who drink excessively while taking DDAVP.

Patients with small bladder capacity and diurnal symptoms tend not to respond to DDAVP; these patients may benefit from anticholinergic therapy, such as oxybutynin. Combination therapy involving a bed alarm plus DDAVP or DDAVP plus anticholinergic therapy may be helpful in select patients.

Imipramine, a tricyclic antidepressant, has been shown to be effective, but its side effects and toxicity have limited its use for this benign condition. Patients with enuresis and other behavioral problems who take selective serotonin reuptake inhibitors have reported improvement in the enuresis. This may be an appropriate option in this population.

DYSFUNCTIONAL VOIDING

Treatment of mild voiding dysfunction should begin with nonpharmacologic management. Children should be instructed to void on a regular schedule, typically every 1 to 2 hours, even if they do not feel the urge to void. This encourages voiding when the patient is relaxed and will lead to fewer contractions of the external sphincter during micturition. Keeping a diary of the voiding schedule involves the child in management and makes him or her more aware of bladder habits. Aggressive management of constipation (see Chapter 21) improves good bladder emptying and decreases bladder instability.

When incontinence continues despite nonpharmacologic methods, anticholinergic therapy should be added in the treatment of a child with an overactive or unstable bladder. Oxybutynin should be started at a low dosage and titrated to its maximum dosage if necessary. The minimum effective dosage should be used to minimize side effects.

Patients with recurrent UTIs who develop urine-holding patterns that lead to overflow incontinence may benefit from a trial of antibiotic prophylaxis. This may keep the child free of infection and may prevent the painful urination that reinforces exaggerated external sphincter contraction and urine holding.

Biofeedback is reserved for patients with moderate to severe dysfunctional voiding. Patients can learn to increase bladder capacity and inhibit detrusor contractions through this method.

POLYURIA

The treatment of polyuria depends on the cause. In certain disorders, such as diabetes mellitus, hypokalemia, or hypercalcemia, the underlying disorder can be corrected. The high urine output in central diabetes insipidus decreases markedly with the use of DDAVP.

In contrast, there is no effective therapy for reducing urine output in patients with disorders such as juvenile nephronophthisis or obstructive uropathy.

The hereditary forms of NDI cause massive polyuria. A combination of sodium restriction and a thiazide diuretic can decrease this high urine output by producing a subtle volume depletion that results in less water being delivered to the collecting duct. The addition of a nonsteroidal antiinflammatory drug can, by reducing renal blood flow, further decrease urine output in patients with NDI. The use of indomethacin, one such drug, also reduces the high urine output in Bartter syndrome. Despite therapy, patients with Bartter syndrome and NDI continue to have high urine output, and the family should be counseled that a delay in achieving nighttime continence is expected.

NEUROPATHIC BLADDER AND ANATOMIC DISORDERS

The treatment of these disorders depends on the specific defect. In patients with neuropathic bladders resulting from spina bifida, chronic intermittent catheterization of the bladder may be the only way to achieve continence. Uninhibited bladder contractions may necessitate anticholinergic therapy as an adjunct.

Anatomic disorders such as posterior urethral valves or VUR, may still necessitate medical therapy or biofeedback after corrective surgery. Urodynamic testing can be very helpful in this population to define the problem leading to incontinence.

SUMMARY AND RED FLAGS

The majority of children with voiding problems do not have an organic problem. The workup consists of a thorough history and physical examination. Red flags that indicate the need for diagnostic tests are listed in Table 62-3.

REFERENCES

Voiding Physiology

Brazelton TB: A child-oriented approach to toilet training. Pediatrics 1962;29:21-128.

Mattsson S, Lindstrom S: Diuresis and voiding pattern in healthy school children. Br J Urol 1994;76:783-789.

Neveus T, Lackgren G, Tuvemo T, et al: Enuresis—Background and treatment. Scand J Urol Nephrol Suppl 2000;20:1-44.

Neveus T, Lackgren G, Tuvemo T, Stenberg A: Osmoregulation and desmopressin pharmacokinetics in enuretic children. Pediatrics 1999;103: 65-70.

Schum TR, McAuliffe TL, Simms MD, et al: Factors associated with toilet training in the 1990s. Ambul Pediatr 2001;1:79-86.

Taubman B: Toilet training and toileting refusal for stool only: A prospective study. Pediatrics 1997;99:54-58.

Signs and Symptoms

Fernandes E, Vernier R, Gonzalez R: The unstable bladder in children. J Pediatr 1991;118:831-837.

Fisher R, Frank D: Detrusor instability; day and night time wetting, urinary tract infections. Arch Dis Child 2000;83:135-137.

Issenman RM, Filmer RB, Gorski PA: A review of bowel and bladder control development in children: How gastrointestinal and urologic conditions relate to problems in toilet training. Pediatrics 1999;103:1346-1352.

Diagnostics

Mayo ME, Burns MW: Urodynamic studies in children who wet. Br J Urol 1990;65:641-645.

Pippi Salle JL, Capolicchio G, Houle A, et al: Magnetic resonance imaging in children with voiding dysfunction: Is it indicated? J Urol 1998;160:1080-1083.

Specific Disorders

Austin PF, Ritchey ML: Dysfunctional voiding. Pediatr Rev 2000;21: 336-340.

Barakat LP, Smith-Whitley K, Schulman S, et al: Nocturnal enuresis in pediatric sickle cell disease. J Dev Behav Pediatr 2001;22:300-305.

Bichet DG: Nephrogenic diabetes insipidus. Am J Med 1998;105:431-432.

Butler RJ, Holland P: The three systems: A conceptual way of understanding nocturnal enuresis. Scand J Urol Nephrol 2000;34:270-277.

Dinneen MD, Duffy PG, Barratt TM, Ransley PG: Persistent polyuria after posterior urethral valves. Br J Urol 1995;75:236-240.

Heninger E, Otto E, Imm A, et al: Improved strategy for molecular genetic diagnostics in juvenile nephronophthisis. Am J Kid Dis 2001;37:1131-1139.

Homsy YL: Dysfunctional voiding syndromes and vesicoureteral reflux. Pediatr Nephrol 1994;8:116-121.

Johnston LB, Borzyskowski M: Bladder dysfunction and neurological disability at presentation in closed spina bifida. Arch Dis Child 1998; 79:33-38.

Mikkelsen EJ: Enuresis and encopresis: Ten years of progress. Acad Child Adolesc Psychiat 2001;40:1146-1158.

Neveus T, Hetta J, Cnattingius S, et al: Depth of sleep and sleep habits among enuretic and incontinent children. Acta Pediatr 1999;88:748-752.

Readett DR, Morris J, Serjeant GR: Determinants of nocturnal enuresis in homozygous sickle cell disease. Arch Dis Child 1990;65:615-618.

Rodriguez-Soriano J, Vallo A: Renal tubular acidosis. Pediatr Nephrol 1990;4:268-275.

Rushton HG: Wetting and functional voiding disorders. Urol Clin North Am 1995;22:75-93.

Von Gontard A, Eiberg H, Hollman E, et al: Molecular genetics of nocturnal enuresis: Linkage to a locus on chromosome 22. Scand J Urol Nephrol Suppl 1999;202:76-80.

Yeung CK, Chiu HN, Sit FKY: Sleep disturbance and bladder dysfunction in enuretic children with treatment failure: Fact or fiction? Scand J Urol Nephrol Suppl 1999;202:20-23.

Treatment

Klauber GT: Clinical efficacy and safety of desmopressin in the treatment of nocturnal enuresis. J Pediatr 1989;114:719-722.

Oredsson AF, Jorgensen TM: Changes in nocturnal bladder capacity during treatment with the bell and pad for monosymptomatic nocturnal enuresis. J Urol 1998;160:166-169.

Schulman SL, Quinn CK, Plachter N, Kodman-Jones C: Comprehensive management of dysfunctional voiding. Pediatrics 1999;103:658.

Tullus K, Bergstrom R, Fosdal I, et al, for the Swedish Enuresis Trial Group: Efficacy and safety during long-term treatment of primary monosymptomatic nocturnal enuresis with desmopressin. Acta Pediatr 1999;88: 1274-1278.

Wiener JS, Mischca TS, Hampton J, et al: Long-term efficacy of simple behavioral therapy for daytime wetting in children. J Urol 2000;164: 786-790.

Wille S: Comparison of desmopressin and enuresis alarm for nocturnal enuresis. Arch Dis Child 1986;61:30-33.

Yamanishi T, Yasuda K, Murayama N, et al: Biofeedback training for detrusor overactivity in children. J Urol 2000;164:1686-1690.

Index

Page numbers followed by f refer to figures; page numbers followed by t refer to tables.